U0267477

ANDREWS' DISEASES OF THE SKIN: CLINICAL DERMATOLOGY

安德鲁斯临床皮肤病学

（第 13 版）

WILLIAM D. JAMES, MD
Paul R. Gross Professor of Dermatology
Department of Dermatology
University of Pennsylvania School of Medicine
Philadelphia, PA, USA

DIRK M. ELSTON, MD
Professor and Chairman
Department of Dermatology and Dermatologic Surgery
Medical University of South Carolina
Charleston, SC, USA

JAMES R. TREAT, MD
Associate Professor of Clinical Pediatrics and Dermatology
Perelman School of Medicine at the University of Pennsylvania
Fellowship and Education Directors, Pediatric Dermatology
Children's Hospital of Philadelphia
Philadelphia PA, USA

MISHA A. ROSENBACH, MD
Associate Professor of Dermatology and Internal Medicine
Perelman School of Medicine at the University of Pennsylvania
Philadelphia, PA, USA

ISAAC M. NEUHAUS, MD
Assistant Professor
Dermatologic Surgery and Laser Center
University of California
San Francisco, USA

北京大学医学出版社
Peking University Medical Press

ANDELUSI LINCHUANG PIFUBINGXUE (DI 13 BAN)

图书在版编目（CIP）数据

安德鲁斯临床皮肤病学：第13版：英文 /（美）威廉·詹姆斯 (WILLIAM D. JAMES) 等主编. – 北京：北京大学医学出版社, 2021.1

书名原文：ANDREWS' DISEASES OF THE SKIN: CLINICAL DERMATOLOGY, 13TH EDITION

ISBN 978-7-5659-2297-8

Ⅰ.①安… Ⅱ.①威… Ⅲ.①皮肤病学－医学院校－教材－英文 Ⅳ.①R751

中国版本图书馆CIP 数据核字(2020) 第 209922 号

北京市版权局著作权合同登记号：图字：01-2020-5332

Elsevier (Singapore) Pte Ltd.
3 Killiney Road, #08-01 Winsland House I, Singapore 239519
Tel: (65) 6349-0200; Fax: (65) 6733-1817

安德鲁斯临床皮肤病学（第13版）

主　　编：WILLIAM D. JAMES, DIRK M. ELSTON, JAMES R. TREAT, MISHA A. ROSENBACH, ISAAC M. NEUHAUS

出版发行：北京大学医学出版社

地　　址：（100083）北京市海淀区学院路 38 号　北京大学医学部院内

电　　话：发行部 010-82802230；图书邮购 010-82802495

网　　址：http ://www.pumpress.com.cn

E－mail：booksale@bjmu.edu.cn

印　　刷：北京金康利印刷有限公司

经　　销：新华书店

责任编辑：冯智勇　　责任校对：靳新强　　责任印制：李　啸

开　　本：889 mm×1194 mm　1/ 16　印张：61.5　字数：1930 千字

版　　次：2021 年 1 月第 1 版　2021 年 1 月第 1 次印刷

书　　号：ISBN 978-7-5659-2297-8

定　　价：350.00 元

版权所有，违者必究

（凡属质量问题请与本社发行部联系退换）

For my wife Ann, my son Dan and his family Wynn,
Declan and Driscoll and my daughter Becca. You make
my life joy-filled with your love.
—WDJ

To my wife and best friend, Kathy, and our wonderful
children, Carly and Nate.
—DME

To my incredible wife and our 2 amazing girls, thank
you for filling our lives with joy and love.
—JRT

To Jake, Lara, and Anna, my loving and supportive
family – thank you for your support and your patience
with me during all those weekends I had to work. I love
you all so very much.
—MAR

To my amazing ladies- Tammy, Leah, Josie and Anna.
—IMN

The Authors

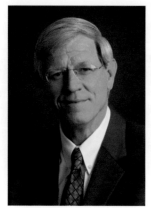

William D. James, MD

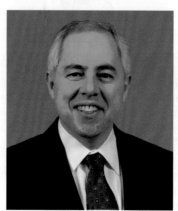

Dirk M. Elston, MD

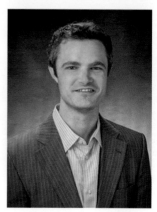

James R. Treat, MD

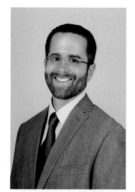

Misha A. Rosenbach, MD

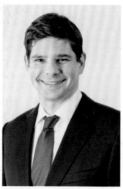

Isaac M. Neuhaus, MD

Preface and Acknowledgments to the Thirteenth Edition

Andrews' remains as it was from the beginning: an authored text whose one volume is filled with clinical signs, symptoms, diagnostic tests, and therapeutic pearls. The authors are committed to keeping *Andrews'* as an excellent tool for anyone who needs help in diagnosing a patient with a clinical conundrum or treating a patient with a therapeutically challenging disease. This edition retains Drs. James, Elston and Neuhaus but we were saddened that Dr. Berger decided the 12th edition was his last. However, we are excited that two new experts have joined the team. Dr. Jim Treat is a superb pediatric dermatologist who was recruited to update many areas of the book. He is knowledgeable in investigations which have led to reclassification of diseases, insights into etiopathogenesis, and newer treatments. He also has updated the vascular anomalies portion of the text, reflecting the continuing improvements in our understanding of these important primarily pediatric conditions. Additionally, Dr. Misha Rosenbach agreed to add his expertise to *Andrews'*. He is a dually board certified internist and dermatologist who has prominent roles in the Medical Dermatology Society and Dermatology Hospitalist group. Dr. Rosenbach was able to update and revamp the adverse drug reaction section, as so many of the new chemotherapeutic agents and small molecular/targeted inhibitors are inducing novel eruptions. New diseases such as the interferonopathies and those along the JAK/STAT pathway, and updated therapeutics in such conditions as autoimmune blistering conditions are also described in his sections of the text.

Andrews' is primarily intended for the practicing dermatologist. It is meant to be used on the desktop of his or her clinic, giving consistent, concise advice on the whole spectrum of clinical situations faced in the course of a busy workday. While we have been true to our commitment to a single-volume work, we provide our text in a convenient online format as well. Because of its relative brevity but complete coverage of our field, many find the text ideal for learning dermatology the first time. It has been a mainstay of the resident yearly curriculum for many programs. We are hopeful that trainees will learn clinical dermatology by studying the clinical descriptions, disease classifications, and treatment insights that define Andrews'. We believe that students, interns, internists or other medical specialists, family practitioners, and other health professionals who desire a comprehensive dermatology textbook will find that ours meets their needs. Long-time dermatologists will hopefully discover Andrews' to be the needed update that satisfies their lifelong learning desires. On our collective trips around the world, we have been gratified to see our international colleagues studying *Andrews'*. Thousands of books have been purchased by Chinese and Brazilian dermatologists alone.

Many major changes have been made to this edition. The new authorship team has worked closely to continue to improve the quality of our text. The surgical chapters have been updated and expanded by Isaac Neuhaus. He has added more videos to complement those already online. He has as well information on new cosmetic procedures. We thank him for his continued work to improve this portion of our textbook. We have tried to ensure that each entity is only discussed once, in a complete yet concise manner. In order to do this we have had to make decisions regarding the placement of disease processes in only one site. Clearly, netrophilic eccrine hidradenitis, for example, could be presented under drug eruptions, netrophilic reactive conditions, infection or cancer-associated disease, or with eccrine disorders. The final decisions are a team effort and made in the interest of eliminating redundancy. This allows us to present our unified philosophy in treating patients in one dense volume.

Medical science continues to progress with break-neck speed. Our understanding of the etiology of certain conditions has now led us to recategorize well-recognized disease states and dictated the addition over many newly described entities. Molecular investigative techniques, technologic breakthroughs, and designer therapeutics lead the way in providing advances in our specialty. We cover the new understanding following from such discoveries as new tools in the diagnosis and treatment of lymphoma; new staging, diagnostic modalities and treatment for melanoma and non-melanoma skin cancers; new treatment paradigms for hair disorders; and new biologics for psoriasis and JAK inhibitors for alopecia area and vitilago. We have attempted to define therapeutics in a fashion that emphasizes those interventions with the highest level of evidence, but also present less critically investigated therapeutic options. To care for our patients we need a large array of options. Not all are fully supported by formal evidence, yet are helpful to individual patients.

Extensive revisions were necessary to add this wealth of new information. We selectively discarded older concepts. By eliminating older, not currently useful information we maintain the brief but complete one-volume presentation that we and all previous authors have emphasized. Additionally, older references have been updated. The classic early works are not cited; instead we have chosen to include only new citations and let the bibliographies of the current work provide the older references as you need them. A major effort in this edition was to reillustrate the text with hundreds of new color images. Many have been added to the printed text; you will also find a number only in the online version. Enjoy! We have looked to our own collections to accomplish this. Two years ago we published an Atlas to accompany this textbook. Many newer photos in our text are included in the Atlas. The Atlas has over 3000 images covering the depth and breadth of our specialty and is a superb companion to this textbook. We are able to present these photos due to many hours of personal effort, the generosity of our patients, and a large number of residents and faculty of the programs in which we currently work or have worked in the past. Additionally, friends and colleagues from all parts of the globe have allowed us to utilize their photographs. They have given their permission for use of these wonderful educational photos to enhance your understanding of dermatology and how these diseases affect our patients. We cannot thank them enough.

All of the authors recognize the importance of our mentors, teachers, colleagues, residents, and patients in forming our collective expertise in dermatology. Dirk and Bill were trained in military programs, and our indebtedness to this fellowship of clinicians in unbounded. Jim and Misha were trained and continue to teach, see patients and publish at the University of Pennsylvania. Isaac is a product of our sister institution, The University of California, San Francisco. The other institutions we have called home, including Walter Reed, Geisinger Medical Center, Brooke in San Antonio, the Cleveland Clinic, and the Medical University of South Carolina, nurtured us and expanded our horizons. Our friendship goes well beyond the limits of our profession; it is wonderful to work with people you not only respect as colleagues, but also enjoy as closely as family. Jennifer Lu and Barbara Lang provided expert assistance throughout the revision process to Bill. He is indebted to them for their hard work. Finally, we are proud to be a part of the Elsevier team and have such professionals as Charlotta Kryhl, Louise Cook, and Andrew Riley supporting us every step of the way.

WDJ
DME
JRT
MAR
IMN
2019

Contents

1 Skin: Basic Structure and Function, 1

2 Cutaneous Signs and Diagnosis, 11

3 Dermatoses Resulting From Physical Factors, 18

4 Pruritus and Neurocutaneous Dermatoses, 46

5 Eczema, Atopic Dermatitis, and Noninfectious Immunodeficiency Disorders, 63

6 Contact Dermatitis and Drug Eruptions, 92

7 Erythema and Urticaria, 140

8 Connective Tissue Diseases, 157

9 Mucinoses, 184

10 Seborrheic Dermatitis, Psoriasis, Recalcitrant Palmoplantar Eruptions, Pustular Dermatitis, and Erythroderma, 191

11 Pityriasis Rosea, Pityriasis Rubra Pilaris, and Other Papulosquamous and Hyperkeratotic Diseases, 205

12 Lichen Planus and Related Conditions, 215

13 Acne, 231

14 Bacterial Infections, 252

15 Diseases Resulting From Fungi and Yeasts, 291

16 Mycobacterial Diseases, 324

17 Hansen Disease, 336

18 Syphilis, Yaws, Bejel, and Pinta, 347

19 Viral Diseases, 362

20 Parasitic Infestations, Stings, and Bites, 421

21 Chronic Blistering Dermatoses, 453

22 Nutritional Diseases, 475

23 Diseases of Subcutaneous Fat, 485

24 Endocrine Diseases, 496

25 Abnormalities of Dermal Fibrous and Elastic Tissue, 505

26 Errors in Metabolism, 515

27 Genodermatoses and Congenital Anomalies, 547

28 Dermal and Subcutaneous Tumors, 587

29 Epidermal Nevi, Neoplasms, and Cysts, 636

30 Melanocytic Nevi and Neoplasms, 686

31 Macrophage/Monocyte Disorders, 704

32 Cutaneous Lymphoid Hyperplasia, Cutaneous T-Cell Lymphoma, Other Malignant Lymphomas, and Allied Diseases, 731

33 Diseases of the Skin Appendages, 750

34 Disorders of the Mucous Membranes, 794

35 Cutaneous Vascular Diseases, 813

36 Disturbances of Pigmentation, 862

37 Dermatologic Surgery, 881

38 Cutaneous Laser Surgery, 909

39 Cosmetic Dermatology, 922

Index, 934

Contents

1. Skin: Basic Structure and Function. 1
2. Cutaneous Signs and Diagnosis of Disease. 7
3. Dermatoses Resulting From Physical Factors. 18
4. Pruritus and Neurocutaneous Dermatoses.
5. Atopic Dermatitis, Eczema, and Noninfectious Immunodeficiency Disorders.
6. Contact Dermatitis and Drug Eruptions.
7. Erythema and Urticaria. 140
8. Connective Tissue Diseases. 155

21. Chronic Blistering Dermatoses. 458
22. Nutritional Diseases. 470
23. Diseases of Subcutaneous Fat. 487
24. Endocrine Diseases. 490
25. Abnormalities of Dermal Fibrous and Elastic Tissue. 503
26. Errors in Metabolism. 522
27. Genodermatoses and Congenital Anomalies. 541
28. Dermal and Subcutaneous Tumors. 587
29. Epidermal Nevi, Neoplasms, and Cysts. 626

31. Lymphoma, Leukemia, and Allied Diseases. 721
32. Diseases of the Skin Appendages. 750

37. Bacterial Infections.
18. Cutaneous Candidiasis. 900
39. Cosmetic Dermatology. 942

17. Hansen Disease. 336
18. Syphilis, Yaws, Bejel, and Pinta. 347
19. Viral Diseases. 362
20. Parasitic Infestations, Stings, and Bites.

Index.

1 Skin: Basic Structure and Function

Skin is composed of three layers: the epidermis, dermis, and subcutaneous fat (panniculus) (Fig. 1.1). The outermost layer, the epidermis, is composed of viable keratinocytes covered by a layer of keratin, the stratum corneum. The principal component of the dermis is the fibrillar structural protein collagen. The dermis lies on the panniculus, which is composed of lobules of lipocytes separated by collagenous septa that contain the neurovascular bundles.

There is considerable regional variation in the relative thickness of these layers. The epidermis is thickest on the palms and soles, measuring approximately 1.5 mm. It is very thin on the eyelid, where it measures less than 0.1 mm. The dermis is thickest on the back, where it is 30–40 times as thick as the overlying epidermis. The amount of subcutaneous fat is generous on the abdomen and buttocks compared with the nose and sternum, where it is meager.

EPIDERMIS AND ADNEXA

During the first weeks of life, the fetus is covered by a layer of nonkeratinizing cuboidal cells called the periderm (Fig. 1.2). Later, the periderm is replaced by a multilayered epidermis. Adnexal structures, particularly follicles and eccrine sweat units, originate during the third month of fetal life as downgrowths from the developing epidermis. Later, apocrine sweat units develop from the upper portion of the follicular epithelium and sebaceous glands from the midregion of the follicle. Adnexal structures appear first in the cephalic portion of the fetus and later in the caudal portions.

The adult epidermis is composed of three basic cell types: keratinocytes, melanocytes, and Langerhans cells. An additional cell, the Merkel cell, can be found in the basal layer of the palms and soles, oral and genital mucosa, nail bed, and follicular infundibula. Located directly above the basement membrane zone, Merkel cells contain intracytoplasmic dense-core neurosecretory-like granules and, through their association with neurites, act as slow-adapting touch receptors. They have direct connections with adjacent keratinocytes by desmosomes and contain a paranuclear whorl of intermediate keratin filaments. Both polyclonal keratin immunostains and monoclonal immunostaining for keratin 20 stain this whorl of keratin filaments in a characteristic paranuclear dot pattern. Merkel cells also label for neuroendocrine markers such as chromogranin and synaptophysin.

Keratinocytes

Keratinocytes are of ectodermal origin and have the specialized function of producing keratin, a complex filamentous protein that not only forms the surface coat (stratum corneum) of the epidermis but also is the structural protein of hair and nails. Multiple distinct keratin genes have been identified and consist of two subfamilies, acidic and basic. The product of one basic and one acidic keratin gene combines to form the multiple keratins that occur in many tissues. Mutations in the genes for keratins 5 and 14 are associated with epidermolysis bullosa simplex. Keratin 1 and 10 mutations are associated with epidermolytic hyperkeratosis. Mild forms of this disorder may represent localized or widespread expressions of mosaicism for these gene mutations.

The epidermis can be divided into the innermost basal layer (stratum germinativum), the malpighian or prickle layer (stratum spinosum), the granular layer (stratum granulosum), and the horny layer (stratum corneum). On the palms and soles, a pale clear to pink layer, the stratum lucidum, is noted just above the granular layer (Fig. 1.3). When the skin in other sites is scratched or rubbed, the malpighian and granular layers thicken, a stratum lucidum forms, and the stratum corneum becomes thick and compact. Histones appear to regulate epidermal differentiation, and histone deacetylation suppresses expression of profilaggrin. Slow-cycling stem cells provide a reservoir for regeneration of the epidermis. Sites rich in stem cells include the deepest portions of the rete, especially on palmoplantar skin, as well as the hair bulge. Stem cells divide infrequently in normal skin, but in cell culture they form active, growing colonies. They can be identified by their high expression of β1-integrins and lack of terminal differentiation markers. Stem cells can also be identified by their low levels of desmosomal proteins, such as desmoglein 3. The basal cells divide, and as their progeny move upward, they flatten and their nucleus disappears. Abnormal keratinization can manifest as parakeratosis (retained nuclei), as corps ronds (round, clear to pink, abnormally keratinized cells), or as grains (elongated, basophilic, abnormally keratinized cells).

During keratinization, the keratinocyte first passes through a synthetic and then a degradative phase on its way to becoming a horn cell. In the synthetic phase, within its cytoplasm the keratinocyte accumulates intermediate filaments composed of a fibrous protein, keratin, arranged in an α-helical coiled pattern. These tonofilaments are fashioned into bundles, which converge on and terminate at the plasma membrane, where they end in specialized attachment plates called desmosomes. The degradative phase of keratinization is characterized by the disappearance of cell organelles and the consolidation of all contents into a mixture of filaments and amorphous cell envelopes. This programmed process of maturation resulting in death of the cell is called terminal differentiation. Terminal differentiation is also seen in the involuting stage of keratoacanthomas, where the initial phase of proliferation gives way to terminal keratinization and involution. Degradation of the mitochondrial network within keratinocytes occurs with aging. Oxidation injury to keratinocytes occurs with environmental exposure and thermal burns, and can be partially prevented by vitamin C in the form of L-ascorbic acid.

Premature programmed cell death, or apoptosis, appears in hematoxylin and eosin (H&E)–stained sections as scattered bright-red cells, some of which may contain small, black pyknotic nuclei. These cells are present at various levels of the epidermis, because this form of cell death does not represent part of the normal process of maturation. Widespread apoptosis is noted in the verrucous phase of incontinentia pigmenti. It is also a prominent finding in catagen hairs, where apoptosis results in the involution of the inferior segment of the hair follicle.

In normal skin, the plasma membranes of adjacent cells are separated by an intercellular space. Electron microscopic histochemical studies have shown that this interspace contains glycoproteins and lipids. Lamellar granules (Odland bodies or membrane-coating granules) appear in this space, primarily at the interface between the granular and cornified cell layers. Lamellar granules contribute to skin cohesion and impermeability. Conditions such as lamellar ichthyosis and Flegel hyperkeratosis demonstrate abnormal lamellar granules. Glycolipids such as ceramides

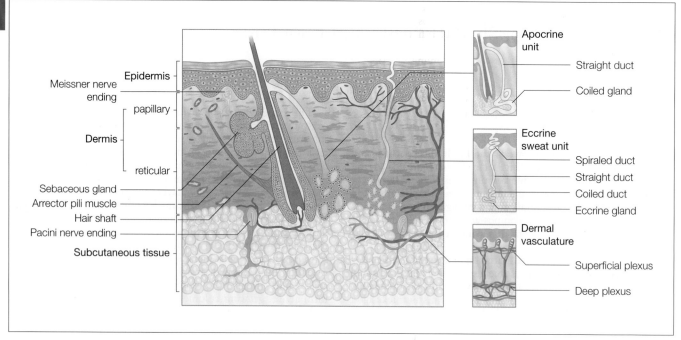

Fig. 1.1 Diagrammatic cross section of the skin and panniculus.

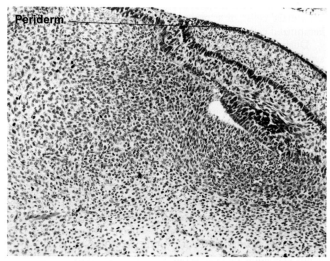

Fig. 1.2 In early fetal life, a cuboidal periderm is present, rather than an epidermis. Fetal skin, H&E × 40.

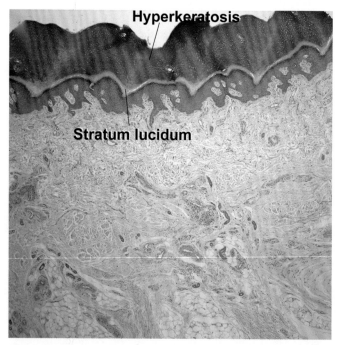

Fig. 1.3 Volar skin demonstrating a thick corneum and dermis, H&E × 100.

contribute a water-barrier function to skin and are typically found in topical products meant to restore the epidermal barrier. Lamellar bodies form abnormally in the absence of critical ceramides such as glucosylceramide, or there is disproportion of critical lipids. Desmosomal adhesion depends on cadherins, including the calcium-dependent desmogleins and desmocollins. Antibodies to these molecules result in immunobullous diseases, but desmogleins function not only in adhesion but also in differentiation. The binding of the desmoglein 1 cytoplasmic tail to the scaffolding-protein Erbin downregulates the Ras-Raf pathway to promote stratification and differentiation of keratinocytes in the epidermis.

Keratinocytes of the granular zone contain, in addition to the keratin filament system, keratohyaline granules, composed of amorphous particulate material of high sulfur-protein content. This material, profilaggrin, is a precursor to filaggrin, so named because it is thought to be responsible for keratin filament aggregation. Conversion to filaggrin takes place in the granular layer, and this forms the electron-dense interfilamentous protein matrix of mature epidermal keratin. Kallikrein-related peptidase 5, a serine protease secreted from lamellar granules, appears to function in profilaggrin cleavage.

Keratohyalin is hygroscopic, and repeated cycles of hydration and dehydration contribute to normal desquamation of the stratum corneum. Ichthyosis vulgaris is characterized by a diminished or absent granular layer, contributing to the retention hyperkeratosis noted in this disorder. Keratohyalin results in the formation of soft, flexible keratin. Keratin that forms in the absence of keratohyaline granules is typically hard and rigid. Hair fibers and nails are composed of hard keratin.

Keratinocytes play an active role in the immune function of the skin. In conditions such as allergic contact dermatitis, these cells participate in the induction of the immune response, rather than acting as passive casualties. Keratinocytes secrete a wide array of cytokines and inflammatory mediators, including tumor necrosis factor–alpha (TNF-α). They also can express molecules on their surface, such as intercellular adhesion molecule 1 (ICAM-1) and major histocompatibility complex (MHC) class II molecules, suggesting that keratinocytes actively respond to immune effector signals.

During wound healing, epithelial cell migration occurs before dermal remodeling. Tight junction proteins claudin-1 and occludin are critical for effective migration. Downregulation of claudin-1 expression results in delayed migration and reduced epithelial proliferation. For occludin, downregulation impairs wound healing when cells are also subjected to mechanical stress. Wound healing occurs best in a moist environment but can be impaired by excessive maceration.

Melanocytes

Melanocytes are derived from the neural crest and by the eighth week of development can be found within the fetal epidermis. In normal, sun-protected trunk epidermis, melanocytes reside in the basal layer at a frequency of about 1 in every 10 basal keratinocytes. Areas such as the face, shins, and genitalia have a greater density of melanocytes, and in heavily sun-damaged facial skin, Mart-1 immunostaining can demonstrate ratios of melanocytes to basal keratinocytes that approach 1 : 1. Recognition of the variation in melanocyte/keratinocyte ratio is critical in the interpretation of biopsies of suspected lentigo maligna (malignant melanoma in situ) on sun-damaged skin.

Racial differences in skin color are not caused by differences in the number of melanocytes. It is the number, size, and distribution of the melanosomes or pigment granules within keratinocytes that determine differences in skin color. Pale skin has fewer melanosomes, and these are smaller and packaged within membrane-bound complexes. Dark skin has more melanosomes, and these tend to be larger and singly dispersed. Chronic sun exposure can stimulate melanocytes to produce larger melanosomes, thereby making the distribution of melanosomes within keratinocytes resemble the pattern seen in dark-skinned individuals.

In histologic sections of skin routinely stained by H&E, the melanocyte appears as a cell with ample amphophilic cytoplasm or as a clear cell in the basal layer of the epidermis. The apparent halo is an artifact formed during fixation of the specimen. This occurs because the melanocyte, lacking tonofilaments, cannot form desmosomal attachments with keratinocytes. Keratinocytes also frequently demonstrate clear spaces but can be differentiated from melanocytes because they demonstrate cell-cell junctions and a layer of cytoplasm peripheral to the clear space.

The melanocyte is a dendritic cell. Its dendrites extend for long distances within the epidermis, and any one melanocyte is therefore in contact with a great number of keratinocytes; together they form the so-called epidermal melanin unit. Keratinocytes actively ingest the tips of the melanocytic dendrites, thus imbibing the melanosomes.

Melanosomes are synthesized in the Golgi zone of the cell and pass through a series of stages in which the enzyme tyrosinase acts on melanin precursors to produce the densely pigmented granules. Melanocytes in red-haired individuals tend to be rounder and to produce more pheomelanin. The melanocortin 1 receptor (MC1R) is important in the regulation of melanin production. Loss-of-function mutations in the *MC1R* gene bring about a change

from eumelanin to pheomelanin production, whereas activating gene mutations can enhance eumelanin synthesis. Most redheads are compound heterozygotes or homozygotes for a variety of loss-of-function mutations in this gene.

Antimicrobial peptides, including cathelicidin and β-defensins, are key components of the innate immune system. They protect against infection, are implicated in the pathogenesis of atopic dermatitis, and play a role in control of pigmentation. The β-defensins encompass a class of small, cationic proteins important to both the innate and the adaptive immune system. β-Defensin 3 also functions as a melanocortin receptor ligand.

Eumelanin production is optimal at pH 6.8, and changes in cellular pH also result in alterations of melanin production and the eumelanin/pheomelanin ratio. Within keratinocytes, melanin typically forms a cap over the nucleus, where it presumably functions principally in a photoprotective role. Evidence of keratinocyte photodamage in the form of pyrimidine dimer formation can be assessed using gas chromatography–mass spectrometry or enzyme-linked immunosorbent assays. Pigment within melanocytes also serves to protect the melanocytes themselves against photodamage, such as ultraviolet A (UVA)–induced membrane damage.

Areas of leukoderma, or whitening of skin, can be caused by very different phenomena. In vitiligo, the affected skin becomes white because of destruction of melanocytes. In albinism, the number of melanocytes is normal, but they are unable to synthesize fully pigmented melanosomes because of defects in the enzymatic formation of melanin. Local areas of increased pigmentation can result from a variety of causes. The typical freckle results from a localized increase in production of pigment by a near-normal number of melanocytes. Black "sunburn" or "ink spot" lentigines demonstrate basilar hyperpigmentation and prominent melanin within the stratum corneum. Nevi are benign proliferations of melanocytes. Melanomas are their malignant counterpart. Melanocytes and keratinocytes express neurotrophins (ectodermal nerve growth factors). Melanocytes release neurotrophin 4, but the release is downregulated by ultraviolet B (UVB) irradiation, suggesting neurotrophins as possible targets for therapy of disorders of pigmentation. Melanocytes express toll-like receptors (TLRs) and stimulation by bacterial lipopolysaccharides increases pigmentation. Melatonin and its metabolites protect melanocytes from UVB damage.

Langerhans Cells

Langerhans cells are normally found scattered among keratinocytes of the stratum spinosum. They constitute 3%–5% of the cells in this layer. As with melanocytes, Langerhans cells are not connected to adjacent keratinocytes by the desmosomes. The highest density of Langerhans cells in the oral mucosa occurs in the vestibular region, and the lowest density is in the sublingual region, suggesting the latter is a relatively immunologically "privileged" site.

At the light microscopic level, Langerhans cells are difficult to detect in routinely stained sections. However, they appear as dendritic cells in sections impregnated with gold chloride, a stain specific for Langerhans cells. They can also be stained with CD1α or S-100 immunostains. Ultrastructurally, they are characterized by a folded nucleus and distinct intracytoplasmic organelles called Birbeck granules. In their fully developed form, the organelles are rod shaped with a vacuole at one end, resembling a tennis racquet. The vacuole is an artifact of processing.

Functionally, Langerhans cells are of the monocyte-macrophage lineage and originate in bone marrow. They function primarily in the afferent limb of the immune response by providing for the recognition, uptake, processing, and presentation of antigens to sensitized T lymphocytes and are important in the induction of delayed-type sensitivity as well as humoral immunity. Once an antigen is presented, Langerhans cells migrate to the lymph nodes. Hyaluronan (hyaluronic acid) plays a critical role in Langerhans cell maturation and migration. Langerhans cells express langerin, membrane adenosine triphosphatase (ATPase, CD39), and CCR6, whereas CD1α+ dermal dendritic cells express macrophage mannose receptor, CD36, factor XIIIa, and chemokine receptor 5, suggesting different functions for these two CD1α+ populations. If skin is depleted of Langerhans cells by exposure to UV radiation, it loses the ability to be sensitized until its population of Langerhans cell is replenished. Macrophages that present antigen in Langerhans cell–depleted skin can induce immune tolerance. In contrast to Langerhans cells, which make interleukin-12 (IL-12), the macrophages found in the epidermis 72 hours after UVB irradiation produce IL-10, resulting in downregulation of the immune response. At least in mice, viral immunity appears to require priming by CD8α+ dendritic cells, rather than Langerhans cells, suggesting a complex pattern of antigen presentation in cutaneous immunity.

Vaccine studies suggest the importance of various cutaneous dendritic cells. Microneedle delivery of vaccine into skin can provoke CD8+ T-cell expansion mediated by CD11c(+) CD11b(+) langerin-negative dendritic cells. Intradermal immunization is dependent on Langerhans cells to stimulate follicular T helper cells and germinal center formation.

Chen Y, et al: Biomaterials as novel penetration enhancers for transdermal and dermal drug delivery systems. Drug Deliv 2013; 20: 199.

Homberg M, et al: Beyond expectations: novel insights into epidermal keratin function and regulation. Int Rev Cell Mol Biol 2014; 311: 265.

Janjetovic Z, et al: Melatonin and its metabolites protect human melanocytes against UVB-induced damage. Sci Rep 2017; 7: 1274.

Levin C, et al: Critical role for skin-derived migratory DCs and Langerhans cells in T(FH) and GC responses after intradermal immunization. J Invest Dermatol 2017; 137: 1905.

Mellem D, et al: Fragmentation of the mitochondrial network in skin in vivo. PLoS One 2017; 12: e0174469.

Pielesz A, et al: The role of topically applied l-ascorbic acid in ex-vivo examination of burn-injured human skin. Spectrochim Acta A Mol Biomol Spectrosc 2017; 185: 279.

Roberts N, et al: Developing stratified epithelia. Wiley Interdiscip Rev Dev Biol 2014; 3: 389.

Volksdorf T, et al: Tight junction proteins claudin-1 and occludin are important for cutaneous wound healing. Am J Pathol 2017; 187: 1301.

Whitehead F, et al: Identifying, managing and preventing skin maceration. J Wound Care 2017; 26: 159.

DERMOEPIDERMAL JUNCTION

The junction of the epidermis and dermis is formed by the basement membrane zone (BMZ). Ultrastructurally, this zone is composed of four components: the plasma membranes of the basal cells with the specialized attachment plates (hemidesmosomes); an electron-lucent zone called the lamina lucida; the lamina densa (basal lamina); and the fibrous components associated with the basal lamina, including anchoring fibrils, dermal microfibrils, and collagen fibers. At the light microscopic level, the periodic acid–Schiff (PAS)–positive basement membrane is composed of the fibrous components. The basal lamina is synthesized by the basal cells of the epidermis. Type IV collagen is the major component of the basal lamina. Type VII collagen is the major component of anchoring fibrils. The two major hemidesmosomal proteins are BP230 (bullous pemphigoid antigen 1) and BP180 (bullous pemphigoid antigen 2, type XVII collagen).

In the upper permanent portion of the anagen follicle, plectin, BP230, BP180, α6β4-integrin, laminin 5, and type VII collagen show essentially the same expression as that found in the interfollicular epidermis. Laminin 5 (laminin-332) is a component of the

lamina lucida/lamina densa interface, and collagen IV is the major component of the lamina densa. Staining in the lower, transient portion of the hair follicle, however, is different. All BMZ components diminish and may become discontinuous in the inferior segment of the follicle. Hemidesmosomes are also not apparent in the BMZ of the hair bulb. The lack of hemidesmosomes in the deep portions of the follicle may relate to the transient nature of the inferior segment, whereas abundant hemidesmosomes stabilize the upper portion of the follicle.

The BMZ is considered to be a porous semipermeable filter, which permits exchange of cells and fluid between the epidermis and dermis. It further serves as a structural support for the epidermis and holds the epidermis and dermis together. The BMZ also helps regulate growth, adhesion, and movement of keratinocytes and fibroblasts, as well as apoptosis. Much of this regulation takes place through activation of integrins and syndecans. Extracellular matrix protein 1 demonstrates loss-of-function mutations in lipoid proteinosis, resulting in reduplication of the basement membrane.

Breitkreutz D, et al: Skin basement membrane. Biomed Res Int 2013; 2013: 179784.

El Domyati M, et al: Immunohistochemical localization of basement membrane laminin 5 and collagen IV in adult linear IgA disease. Int J Dermatol 2015; 54: 922.

Hashmi S, et al: Molecular organization of the basement membrane zone. Clin Dermatol 2011; 29: 398.

EPIDERMAL APPENDAGES (ADNEXA)

Eccrine and apocrine glands, ducts, and pilosebaceous units constitute the skin adnexa. Embryologically, they originate as downgrowths from the epidermis and are therefore ectodermal in origin. Hedgehog signaling by the transducer known as *smoothened* appears critical for hair development. Abnormalities in this pathway contribute to the formation of pilar tumors and basal cell carcinoma. In the absence of hedgehog signaling, embryonic hair germs may develop instead into modified sweat gland or mammary epithelium.

Although the various adnexal structures serve specific functions, all can function as reserve epidermis, in that reepithelialization occurs after injury to the surface epidermis, principally because of the migration of keratinocytes from the adnexal epithelium to the skin surface. It is not surprising, therefore, that skin sites such as the face or scalp, which contain pilosebaceous units in abundance, reepithelialize more rapidly than skin sites such as the back, where adnexa of all types are comparatively scarce. Once a wound has reepithelialized, granulation tissue is no longer produced. Deep, saucerized biopsies in an area with few adnexa will slowly fill with granulation tissue until they are flush with the surrounding skin. In contrast, areas rich in adnexa will quickly be covered with epithelium. No more granulation tissue will form, and the contour defect created by the saucerization will persist.

The pseudoepitheliomatous hyperplasia noted in infections and inflammatory conditions consists almost exclusively of adnexal epithelium. Areas of thin intervening epidermis are generally evident between areas of massively hypertrophic adnexal epithelium.

Eccrine Sweat Units

The intraepidermal spiral duct, which opens directly onto the skin surface, is called the *acrosyringium*. It is derived from dermal duct cells through mitosis and upward migration. The acrosyringium is composed of small polygonal cells with a central round nucleus surrounded by ample pink cytoplasm. In the stratum corneum overlying an actinic keratosis, the lamellar spiral acrosyringeal keratin often stands out prominently against the compact red parakeratotic keratin produced by the actinic keratosis.

The straight dermal portion of the duct is composed of a double layer of cuboidal epithelial cells and is lined by an eosinophilic cuticle on its luminal side. The coiled secretory acinar portion of the eccrine sweat gland may be found within the superficial panniculus. In areas of skin such as the back that possess a thick dermis, the eccrine coil is found in the deep dermis, surrounded by an extension of fat from the underlying panniculus. An inner layer of epithelial cells, the secretory portion of the gland, is surrounded by a layer of flattened myoepithelial cells. The secretory cells are of two types: large, pale, glycogen-rich cells and smaller, darker-staining cells. The pale glycogen-rich cells are thought to initiate the formation of sweat. The darker cells may function similar to cells of the dermal duct, which actively reabsorb sodium, thereby modifying sweat from a basically isotonic to a hypotonic solution by the time it reaches the skin surface. Sweat is similar in composition to plasma, containing the same electrolytes, but in a more dilute concentration. Physical conditioning in a hot environment results in production of larger amounts of extremely hypotonic sweat in response to a thermal stimulus. This adaptive response allows greater cooling with conservation of sodium.

In humans, eccrine sweat units are found at virtually all skin sites. In most other mammals, the apocrine gland is the major sweat gland.

Physiologic secretion of sweat occurs as a result of many factors and is mediated by cholinergic innervation. Heat is a prime stimulus to increased sweating, but other physiologic stimuli, including emotional stress, are important as well. During early development, there is a switch between adrenergic and cholinergic innervation of sweat glands. Some responsiveness to both cholinergic and adrenergic stimuli persists. Cholinergic sweating involves a biphasic response, with initial hyperpolarization and secondary depolarization mediated by the activation of calcium and chloride ion conductance. Adrenergic secretion involves monophasic depolarization and is dependent on cystic fibrosis transmembrane conductance regulator GCl. Cells from patients with cystic fibrosis demonstrate no adrenergic secretion. Vasoactive intestinal polypeptide may also play a role in stimulating eccrine secretion.

Apocrine Units

Apocrine units develop as outgrowths not of the surface epidermis, but of the infundibular or upper portion of the hair follicle. Although immature apocrine units are found covering the entire skin surface of the human fetus, these regress and are absent by the time the fetus reaches term. The straight excretory portion of the duct, which opens into the infundibular portion of the hair follicle, is composed of a double layer of cuboidal epithelial cells.

The coiled secretory gland is located at the junction of the dermis and subcutaneous fat (Fig. 1.4). It is lined by a single layer of cells, which vary in appearance from columnar to cuboidal. This layer of cells is surrounded by a layer of myoepithelial cells. Apocrine coils appear more widely dilated than eccrine coils, and apocrine sweat stains more deeply red in H&E sections, contrasting with the pale pink of eccrine sweat.

The apices of the columnar cells project into the lumen of the gland and in histologic cross section appear as if they are being extruded (decapitation secretion). Controversy surrounds the mode of secretion in apocrine secretory cells, whether merocrine, apocrine, holocrine, or all three. The composition of the product of secretion is only partially understood. Protein, carbohydrate, ammonia, lipid, and iron are all found in apocrine secretion. It appears milky white, although lipofuscin pigment may rarely produce dark shades of brown and gray-blue (apocrine chromhidrosis). Apocrine sweat is odorless until it reaches the skin surface, where it is altered by bacteria, which makes it odoriferous. Apocrine secretion is mediated by adrenergic innervation and by circulating catecholamines of adrenomedullary origin. Vasoactive intestinal polypeptide may also play a role in stimulating apocrine secretion.

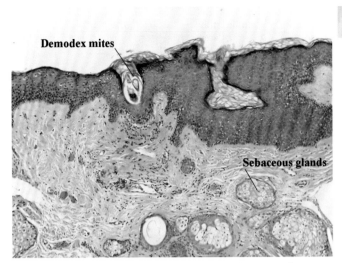

Fig. 1.4 Axillary skin is rugose and demonstrates large apocrine glands. Axillary skin, H&E × 40.

Apocrine excretion is episodic, although the actual secretion of the gland is continuous. Apocrine gland secretion in humans serves no known function. In other species, it has a protective as well as a sexual function, and in some species, it is important in thermoregulation as well.

Although occasionally found in an ectopic location, apocrine units of the human body are generally confined to the following sites: axillae, areolae, anogenital region, external auditory canal (ceruminous glands), and eyelids (glands of Moll). They are also generally prominent in stroma of the sebaceous nevus of Jadassohn. Apocrine glands do not begin to function until puberty.

Hair Follicles

During embryogenesis, mesenchymal cells in the fetal dermis collect immediately below the basal layer of the epidermis. Epidermal buds grow down into the dermis at these sites. The developing follicle forms at an angle to the skin surface and continues its downward growth. At this base, the column of cells widens, forming the bulb, and surrounds small collections of mesenchymal cells. These papillary mesenchymal bodies contain mesenchymal stem cells with broad functionality. At least in mice, they demonstrate extramedullary hematopoietic stem cell activity, representing a potential therapeutic source of hematopoietic stem cells and a possible source of extramedullary hematopoiesis in vivo.

Along one side of the fetal follicle, two buds are formed; an upper bud develops into the sebaceous gland, and a lower bud becomes the attachment for the arrector pili muscle. A third epithelial bud develops from the opposite side of the follicle above the level of the sebaceous gland anlage and gives rise to the apocrine gland. The uppermost portion of the follicle, which extends from its surface opening to the entrance of the sebaceous duct, is called the infundibular segment. It resembles the surface epidermis, and its keratinocytes may be of epidermal origin. The portion of the follicle between the sebaceous duct and the insertion of the arrector pili muscle is the isthmus. The inner root sheath fully keratinizes and sheds within this isthmic portion. The inferior portion includes the lowermost part of the follicle and the hair bulb. Throughout life, the inferior portion undergoes cycles of involution and regeneration.

Hair follicles develop sequentially in rows of three. Primary follicles are surrounded by the appearance of two secondary follicles; other secondary follicles subsequently develop around the principal

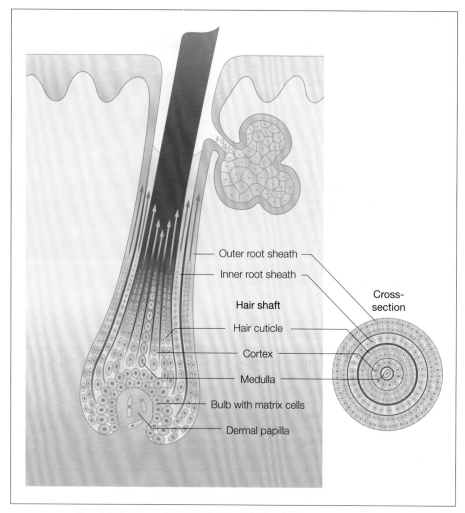

Fig. 1.5 Anatomy of the hair follicle. Additional eFigures are available.

units. The density of pilosebaceous units decreases throughout life, possibly because of dropout of the secondary follicles. In mouse models, signaling by molecules designated as ectodysplasin A and noggin is essential for the development of primary hair follicles and induction of secondary follicles. Arrector pili muscles contained within the follicular unit interconnect at the level of the isthmus.

The actual hair shaft, as well as an inner and an outer root sheath, is produced by the matrix portion of the hair bulb (Fig. 1.5). The sheaths and contained hair form concentric cylindrical layers. The hair shaft and inner root sheath move together as the hair grows upward until the fully keratinized, inner root sheath sheds at the level of the isthmus. The epidermis of the upper part of the follicular canal is contiguous with the outer root sheath. The upper two portions of the follicle (infundibulum and isthmus) are permanent; the inferior segment is completely replaced with each new cycle of hair growth. On the scalp, anagen, the active growth phase, lasts about 3–5 years. Normally, about 85%–90% of all scalp hairs are in the anagen phase, a figure that decreases with age and decreases faster in individuals with male-pattern baldness (as length of anagen decreases dramatically). Scalp anagen hairs grow at a rate of about 0.37 mm/day. Catagen, or involution, lasts about 2 weeks. Telogen, the resting phase, lasts about 3–5 months. Most sites on the body have a much shorter anagen and much longer telogen, resulting in short hairs that stay in place for long periods without growing longer. Prolongation of the anagen phase results in long eyelashes in patients with acquired immunodeficiency syndrome (AIDS).

Human hair growth is cyclic, but each follicle functions as an independent unit and regulatory T cells play a role in control of follicular stem cells and hair regeneration (Fig. 1.6). Humans do not shed hair synchronously, as most animals do. Each hair follicle undergoes intermittent stages of activity and quiescence. Synchronous termination of anagen or telogen results in telogen effluvium. Most commonly, telogen effluvium is the result of early release from anagen, such as that induced by a febrile illness, surgery, or weight loss.

Pregnancy is typically accompanied by retention of an increased number of scalp hairs in anagen, as well as a prolongation of telogen. Soon after delivery, telogen loss can be detected as abnormally prolonged telogen hairs are released. At the same time, abnormally prolonged anagen hairs are converted synchronously to telogen. Between 3 and 5 months later, a more profound effluvium is noted. Patients receiving chemotherapy often have hair loss because the drugs interfere with the mitotic activity of the hair matrix, leading to the formation of a tapered fracture. Only anagen hairs are affected, leaving a sparse coat of telogen hairs on the scalp. As the matrix recovers, anagen hairs resume growth without having to cycle through catagen and telogen.

The growing anagen hair is characterized by a pigmented bulb and an inner root sheath. Histologically, catagen hairs are best identified by the presence of many apoptotic cells in the outer root sheath. Telogen club hairs have a nonpigmented bulb with a shaggy lower border. The presence of bright-red trichilemmal keratin bordering the club hair results in a flamethrower-like

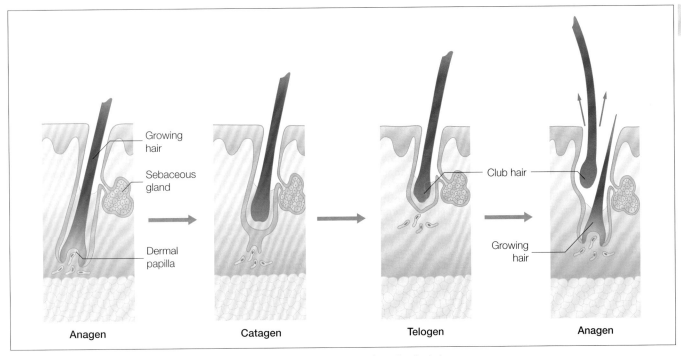

Fig. 1.6 Phases of the growth cycle of a hair.

appearance in vertical H&E sections. As the new anagen hair grows, the old telogen hair is shed.

The scalp hair of white people is round; pubic hair, beard hair, and eyelashes are oval. The scalp hair of black people is also oval, and this, along with curvature of the follicle just above the bulb, causes black hair to be curly. Uncombable hair is triangular with a central canal. Hair shape is at least partially controlled by the trichohyalin gene.

Hair color depends on the degree of melanization and distribution of melanosomes within the hair shaft. Melanocytes of the hair bulb synthesize melanosomes and transfer them to the keratinocytes of the bulb matrix. Larger melanosomes are found in the hair of black persons; smaller melanosomes, which are aggregated within membrane-bound complexes, are found in the hair of white persons. Red hair is characterized by spherical melanosomes. Graying of hair results from a decreased number of melanocytes, which produces fewer melanosomes. Repetitive oxidative stress causes apoptosis of hair follicle melanocytes, resulting in normal hair graying. Premature graying is related to exhaustion of the melanocyte stem cell pool.

Although the genetics of balding is complex, it is known that polymorphisms in the androgen receptor gene are carried on the X chromosome, inherited from the mother. The genetics of female pattern hair loss is less clear, because polymorphisms in the androgen receptor do not appear to be associated with female-pattern hair loss, and adrenal androgens may play a larger role.

Sebaceous Glands

Sebaceous glands are formed embryologically as an outgrowth from the upper portion of the hair follicle. They are composed of lobules of pale-staining cells with abundant lipid droplets in their cytoplasm. At the periphery of the lobules, basaloid germinative cells are noted. These cells give rise to the lipid-filled pale cells, which are continuously being extruded through the short sebaceous duct into the infundibular portion of the hair follicle. The sebaceous duct is lined by a red cuticle that undulates sharply

in a pattern resembling a shark's teeth. This same undulating cuticle is seen in steatocystoma and some dermoid cysts.

Sebaceous glands are found in greatest abundance on the face and scalp, although they are distributed throughout all skin sites except the palms and soles. They are always associated with hair follicles, except at the following sites: tarsal plate of the eyelids (meibomian glands), buccal mucosa and vermilion border of the lip (Fordyce spots), prepuce and mucosa lateral to the penile frenulum (Tyson glands), labia minora, and female areola (Montgomery tubercles).

Most lipids produced by the sebaceous gland are also produced elsewhere in the body. Wax esters and squalene are unique secretory products of sebaceous glands. Sebocytes express histamine receptors, and antihistamines can reduce squalene levels, suggesting that antihistamines could play a role in modulating sebum production. Skin lipids contribute to the barrier function, and some have antimicrobial properties. Antimicrobial lipids include free sphingoid bases derived from epidermal ceramides and fatty acids (e.g., sapienic acid) derived from sebaceous triglycerides.

Ali N, et al: Regulatory T cells in skin facilitate epithelial stem cell differentiation. Cell 2017; 169: 1119.

Horsley V, et al: T(regs) expand the skin stem cell niche. Dev Cell 2017; 41: 455.

Maryanovich M, et al: T-regulating hair follicle stem cells. Immunity 2017; 46: 979.

Patzelt A, et al: Drug delivery to hair follicles. Expert Opin Drug Deliv 2013; 10: 787.

Nails

Nails act to assist in grasping small objects and in protecting the fingertip from trauma and serve a sensory function. Pacinian corpuscle-like structures are present in the nail bed of human fetuses, but are difficult to identify in adults. Fingernails grow an average of 0.1 mm/day, requiring about 4–6 months to replace a complete nail plate. The growth rate is much slower for toenails, with 12–18 months required to replace the great toenail.

The keratin types found in the nail are a mixture of epidermal and hair types, with the hair types predominating. Nail isthmus keratinization differs from that of the nail bed in that keratin 10 is only present in nail isthmus. Brittle nails demonstrate widening of the intercellular space between nail keratinocytes on electron microscopy.

Whereas most of the skin is characterized by rete pegs that resemble an egg crate, the nail bed has true parallel rete ridges. These ridges result in the formation of splinter hemorrhages when small quantities of extravasated red blood cells mark their path. The nail cuticle is formed by keratinocytes of the proximal nailfold, whereas the nail plate is formed by matrix keratinocytes. Endogenous pigments tend to follow the contour of the lunula (distal portion of matrix), whereas exogenous pigments tend to follow the contour of the cuticle. The dorsal nail plate is formed by the proximal matrix, and the ventral nail plate is formed by the distal matrix with some contribution from the nail bed. The location of a melanocytic lesion within the matrix can be assessed by the presence of pigment within the dorsal or ventral nail plate.

Baswan S, et al: Understanding the formidable nail barrier. Mycoses 2017; 60: 284.

Kim JH, et al: Pacinian corpuscle-like structure in the digital tendon sheath and nail bed. Anat Cell Biol 2017; 50: 33.

DERMIS

The constituents of the dermis are mesodermal in origin except for nerves, which, as with melanocytes, derive from the neural crest. Until the sixth week of fetal life, the dermis is merely a pool of scattered dendritic-shaped cells containing acid mucopolysaccharide, which are the precursors of fibroblasts. By the 12th week, fibroblasts are actively synthesizing reticulum fibers, elastic fibers, and collagen. A vascular network develops, and by the 24th week, fat cells have appeared beneath the dermis. During fetal development, Wnt/β-catenin signaling is critical for differentiation of ventral versus dorsal dermis, and the dermis then serves as a scaffold for the adnexal structures identified with ventral or dorsal sites.

Infant dermis is composed of small collagen bundles that stain deeply red. Many fibroblasts are present. In adult dermis, few fibroblasts persist; collagen bundles are thick and stain pale red. Two populations of dermal dendritic cells are noted in the adult dermis. Factor XIIIa–positive dermal dendrocytes appear to give rise to dermatofibromas, angiofibromas, acquired digital fibrokeratomas, pleomorphic fibromas, and fibrous papules. CD34+ dermal dendrocytes are accentuated around hair follicles but exist throughout the dermis. They disappear from the dermis early in the course of morphea. Their loss can be diagnostic in subtle cases. CD34+ dermal dendrocytes reappear in the dermis when morphea responds to UVA1 light treatment.

The principal component of the dermis is collagen, a family of fibrous proteins comprising at least 15 genetically distinct types in human skin. Collagen serves as the major structural protein for the entire body; it is found in tendons, ligaments, and the lining of bones, as well as in the dermis. Collagen represents 70% of the dry weight of skin. The fibroblast synthesizes the procollagen molecule, a helical arrangement of specific polypeptide chains that are subsequently secreted by the cell and assembled into collagen fibrils. Collagen is rich in the amino acids hydroxyproline, hydroxylysine, and glycine. The fibrillar collagens are the major group found in the skin.

Type I collagen is the major component of the dermis. The structure of type I collagen is uniform in width, and each fiber displays characteristic cross-striations with a periodicity of 68 nm. Collagen fibers are loosely arranged in the papillary and adventitial (periadnexal) dermis. Large collagen bundles are noted in the reticular dermis (dermis below level of postcapillary venule). Collagen I messenger ribonucleic acid (mRNA) and collagen III mRNA are both expressed in the reticular and papillary dermis and are downregulated by UV light, as is the collagen regulatory proteoglycan decorin. This downregulation may play a role in photoaging.

Type IV collagen is found in the BMZ. Type VII collagen is the major structural component of anchoring fibrils and is produced predominantly by keratinocytes. Abnormalities in type VII collagen are seen in dystrophic epidermolysis bullosa, and autoantibodies to this collagen type characterize acquired epidermolysis bullosa. Collagen fibers are continuously being degraded by proteolytic enzymes called "spare collagenases" and replaced by newly synthesized fibers. Additional information on collagen types and diseases can be found in Chapter 25.

The fibroblast also synthesizes elastic fibers and the ground substance of the dermis, which is composed of acid mucopolysaccharides and fibronectin. They can be stimulated to produce fibronectin by agents such as phytosphingosine-1-phosphate and epidermal growth factor.

Elastic fibers differ both structurally and chemically from collagen. They consist of aggregates of two components: protein filaments and elastin, an amorphous protein. The amino acids desmosine and isodesmosine are unique to elastic fibers. Elastic fibers in the papillary dermis are fine, whereas those in the reticular dermis are coarse. The extracellular matrix or ground substance of the dermis is composed of sulfated acid mucopolysaccharide, principally chondroitin sulfate and dermatan sulfate, neutral mucopolysaccharides, and electrolytes. Sulfated acid mucopolysaccharides stain with colloidal iron and with alcian blue at both pH 2.5 and pH 0.5. They stain metachromatically with toluidine blue at both pH 3.0 and pH 1.5. Hyaluronan (hyaluronic acid) is a minor component of normal dermis but is the major mucopolysaccharide that accumulates in pathologic states. It stains with colloidal iron, and with both alcian blue and toluidine blue (metachromatically), but only at the higher pH for each stain.

Collagen is the major stress-resistant material of the skin. Elastic fibers contribute little to resisting deformation and tearing of skin but have a role in maintaining elasticity. *Connective tissue disease* is a term generally used to refer to a clinically heterogeneous group of autoimmune diseases, including lupus erythematosus, scleroderma, and dermatomyositis. Scleroderma involves the most visible collagen abnormalities, as collagen bundles become hyalinized and the space between collagen bundles diminishes. Both lupus and dermatomyositis produce increased dermal mucin, mostly hyaluronic acid. Bullous lupus has autoantibodies directed against type VII collagen.

Defects in collagen synthesis have been described in a number of inheritable diseases, including Ehlers-Danlos syndrome, X-linked cutis laxa, and osteogenesis imperfecta. Defects in elastic tissue are seen in Marfan syndrome and pseudoxanthoma elasticum.

Vasculature

The dermal vasculature consists principally of two intercommunicating plexuses. The subpapillary plexus, or upper horizontal network, contains the postcapillary venules and courses at the junction of the papillary and reticular dermis (Fig. 1.7). This plexus furnishes a rich supply of capillaries, end arterioles, and venules to the dermal papillae. The deeper, lower horizontal plexus is found at the dermal-subcutaneous interface and is composed of larger blood vessels than those of the superficial plexus. Nodular lymphoid infiltrates surrounding this lower plexus are typical of early inflammatory morphea. The vasculature of the dermis is particularly well developed at sites of adnexal structures. Associated with the vascular plexus are dermal lymphatics and nerves.

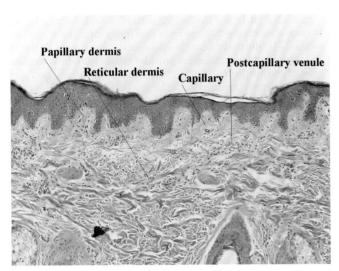

Fig. 1.7 Below the epidermis, the papillary dermis is composed of fine, nonbundled collagen. Capillaries are present within the papillary dermis, and the postcapillary venule sits at the junction of the papillary and reticular dermis. H&E × 40.

Muscles

Smooth muscle occurs in the skin as arrectores pilorum (erectors of the hairs), as the tunica dartos (or dartos) of the scrotum, and in the areolas around the nipples. The arrectores pilorum are attached to the hair follicles below the sebaceous glands and, in contracting, pull the hair follicle upward, producing gooseflesh. The presence of scattered smooth muscle throughout the dermis is typical of anogenital skin.

Smooth muscle also comprises the muscularis of dermal and subcutaneous blood vessels. The muscularis of veins is composed of small bundles of smooth muscle that crisscross at right angles. Arterial smooth muscle forms a concentric, wreathlike ring. Specialized aggregates of smooth muscle cells (glomus bodies) are found between arterioles and venules and are especially prominent on the digits and at the lateral margins of the palms and soles. Glomus bodies serve to shunt blood and regulate temperature. Most smooth muscle expresses desmin intermediate filaments, but vascular smooth muscle instead expresses vimentin. Smooth muscle actin is consistently expressed by all types of smooth muscle.

Striated (voluntary) muscle occurs in the skin of the neck as the platysma muscle and in the skin of the face as the muscles of expression. This complex network of striated muscle, fascia, and aponeuroses is known as the superficial muscular aponeurotic system (SMAS).

Nerves

In the dermis, nerve bundles are found together with arterioles and venules as part of the neurovascular bundle. In the deep dermis, nerves travel parallel to the surface, and the presence of long, sausage-like granulomas following this path is an important clue to the diagnosis of Hansen disease.

Touch and pressure are mediated by Meissner corpuscles found in the dermal papillae, particularly on the digits, palms, and soles, and by Vater-Pacini corpuscles located in the deeper portion of the dermis of weight-bearing surfaces and genitalia. Mucocutaneous end organs are found in the papillary dermis of modified hairless skin at the mucocutaneous junctions: the glans, prepuce, clitoris, labia minora, perianal region, and vermilion border of the lips. Temperature, pain, and itch sensation are transmitted by

unmyelinated nerve fibers that terminate in the papillary dermis and around hair follicles. Impulses pass to the central nervous system by way of the dorsal root ganglia. Histamine-evoked itch is transmitted by slow-conducting unmyelinated C-polymodal neurons. Signal transduction differs for sensations of heat and cold and in peripheral nerve axons.

Postganglionic adrenergic fibers of the autonomic nervous system regulate vasoconstriction, apocrine gland secretions, and contraction of arrector pili muscles of hair follicles. Cholinergic fibers mediate eccrine sweat secretion.

Mast Cells

Mast cells play an important role in the normal immune response, as well as immediate-type sensitivity, contact allergy, and fibrosis. Measuring 6–12 microns in diameter, with ample amphophilic cytoplasm and a small round central nucleus, normal mast cells resemble fried eggs in histologic sections. In telangiectasia macularis eruptiva perstans (TMEP mastocytosis), they are spindle shaped and hyperchromatic, resembling large, dark fibroblasts. Mast cells are distinguished by containing up to 1000 granules, each measuring 0.6–0.7 micron in diameter. Coarse particulate granules, crystalline granules, and granules containing scrolls may be seen. On the cell's surface are 100,000–500,000 glycoprotein receptor sites for immunoglobulin E (IgE). There is heterogeneity to mast cells with type I, or connective tissue mast cells found in the dermis and submucosa, and type II, or mucosal mast cells found in the bowel and respiratory tract mucosa.

Mast cell granules stain metachromatically with toluidine blue and methylene blue (in Giemsa stain) because of their high content of heparin. They also contain histamine, neutrophil chemotactic factor, eosinophil chemotactic factor of anaphylaxis, tryptase, kininogenase, and β-glucosaminidase. Slow-reacting substance of anaphylaxis (leukotrienes C4 and D4), leukotriene B4, platelet-activating factor, and prostaglandin D2 are formed only after IgE-mediated release of granules. Mast cells stain reliably with the Leder ASD–chloracetase esterase stain. Because this stain does not rely on the presence of mast cell granules, it is particularly useful in situations when mast cells have degranulated. In forensic medicine, fluorescent labeling of mast cells with antibodies to the mast cell enzymes chymase and tryptase is useful in determining the timing of skin lesions in regard to death. Lesions sustained while living show an initial increase and then a decline in mast cells. Lesions sustained postmortem demonstrate few mast cells.

Cutaneous mast cells respond to environmental changes. Dry environments result in an increase in mast cell number and cutaneous histamine content. In mastocytosis, mast cells accumulate in skin because of abnormal proliferation, migration, and failure of apoptosis. The terminal deoxynucleotidyl transferase–mediated deoxyuridine triphosphate–biotin nick end labeling (TUNEL) method is used to assess apoptosis and demonstrates decreased staining in mastocytomas. Proliferation usually is only moderately enhanced.

SUBCUTANEOUS TISSUE (FAT)

Beneath the dermis lies the panniculus, with lobules of fat cells or lipocytes separated by fibrous septa composed of collagen and large blood vessels (Fig. 1.8). The collagen in the septa is continuous with the collagen in the dermis. Just as the epidermis and dermis vary in thickness according to skin site, so does the subcutaneous tissue. The panniculus provides buoyancy and functions as a repository of energy and an endocrine organ. It is an important site of hormone conversion, such as that of androstenedione into estrone by aromatase. Leptin, a hormone produced in lipocytes, regulates body weight through the hypothalamus and influences how we react to flavors in food. Various substances can affect lipid accumulation within lipocytes. Obestatin is a polypeptide that

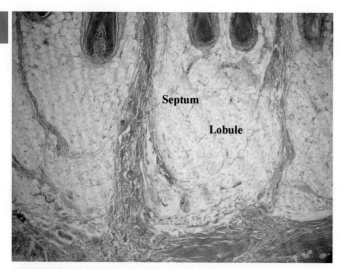

Fig. 1.8 The lobules of the subcutaneous fat are separated by fibrous septae. H&E × 40.

reduces feed intake and weight gain in rodents. (–)Ternatin, a highly *N*-methylated cyclic heptapeptide that inhibits fat accumulation, produced by the mushroom *Coriolus versicolor*, has similar effects in mice. Study of these molecules provides insight into the molecular basis of weight gain and obesity. Abnormal fat distribution and insulin resistance are seen in Cushing syndrome and as a result of antiretroviral therapy. In obese children and adolescents developing diabetes, severe peripheral insulin resistance is associated with intramyocellular and intraabdominal lipocyte lipid accumulation.

Certain inflammatory dermatoses, known as the panniculitides, principally affect this level of the skin, producing subcutaneous nodules. The pattern of the inflammation, specifically whether it primarily affects the septa or the fat lobules, serves to distinguish various conditions that may be clinically similar.

Abraham SN, et al: Mast cell-orchestrated immunity to pathogens. Nat Rev Immunol 2010; 10: 440.

Kwon SB, et al: Phytosphingosine-1-phosphate and epidermal growth factor synergistically restore extracellular matrix in human dermal fibroblasts in vitro and in vivo. Int J Mol Med 2017; 39: 741.

Mikesh LM, et al: Proteomic anatomy of human skin. J Proteomics 2013; 84: 190.

Purohit T, et al: Smad3-dependent CCN2 mediates fibronectin expression in human skin dermal fibroblasts. PLoS One 2017; 12: e0173191.

2 Cutaneous Signs and Diagnosis

In some patients, the appearance of skin lesions may be so distinctive that the diagnosis is clear at a glance. In others, subjective symptoms and clinical signs alone are inadequate, and a complete history and laboratory examination, including a biopsy, are essential to arrive at a diagnosis.

The same disease may show variations under different conditions and in different individuals. The appearance of the lesions may have been modified by previous treatment or obscured by extraneous influences, such as scratching or secondary infection. Subjective symptoms may be the only evidence of a disease, as in pruritus, and the skin appearance may be generally unremarkable. Although history is important, the diagnosis in dermatology is most frequently made based on the objective physical characteristics and location or distribution of one or more lesions that can be seen or felt. Therefore careful physical examination of the skin is paramount in dermatologic diagnosis.

CUTANEOUS SIGNS

Typically, most skin diseases present with lesions that have distinct characteristics. They may be uniform or diverse in size, shape, and color or may be in different stages of evolution or involution. The original lesions are known as the primary lesions, and identification of such lesions is the most important aspect of the dermatologic physical examination. They may continue to full development or be modified by regression, trauma, or other extraneous factors, producing secondary lesions.

Primary Lesions

Primary lesions are of the following forms: macules (or patches), papules (or plaques), nodules, tumors, wheals, vesicles, bullae, and pustules.

Macules (Maculae, Spots)

Macules are variously sized, circumscribed changes in skin color, without elevation or depression (nonpalpable) (Fig. 2.1). They may be circular, oval, or irregular and may be distinct in outline or may fade into the surrounding skin. Macules may constitute the whole lesion or part of the eruption or may be merely an early phase. If the lesions become slightly raised, they are then designated papules or, in some cases, morbilliform eruptions.

Patches

A patch is a large macule, 1 cm or greater in diameter, as may be seen in nevus flammeus or vitiligo.

Papules

Papules are circumscribed, solid elevations with no visible fluid, varying in size from a pinhead to 1 cm (Fig. 2.2). They may be acuminate, rounded, conical, flat topped, or umbilicated and may appear white (as in milium), red (eczema), yellowish (xanthoma), or black (melanoma).

Papules are generally centered in the dermis and may be concentrated at the orifices of the sweat ducts or at the hair follicles. They may be of soft or firm consistency. The surface may be smooth or rough. If capped by scales, they are known as squamous papules, and the eruption is called papulosquamous.

Some papules are discrete and irregularly distributed, as in papular urticaria, whereas others are grouped, as in lichen nitidus. Some persist as papules, whereas those of the inflammatory type may progress to vesicles or to pustules, or they may erode before regression takes place.

The term "maculopapular" should not be used. There is no such thing as a "maculopapule," although there may be both macules and papules in an eruption. Typically, such eruptions are morbilliform.

Plaques

A plaque is a broad papule (or confluence of papules), 1 cm or more in diameter (Fig. 2.3). It is generally flat but may be centrally depressed.

Nodules

Nodules are morphologically similar to papules but are larger than 1 cm in diameter. Nodules most frequently are centered in the dermis or subcutaneous fat.

Tumors

Tumors are soft or firm, freely movable or fixed masses of various sizes and shapes, but usually are greater than 2 cm in diameter. General usage dictates that the word "tumor" means a neoplasm. They may be elevated or deep seated and in some cases are pedunculated (neurofibromas). Tumors have a tendency to be rounded. Their consistency depends on the constituents of the lesion. Some tumors remain stationary indefinitely, whereas others increase in size or break down.

Wheals (Hives)

Wheals are evanescent, edematous, plateaulike elevations of various sizes (Fig. 2.4). They are usually oval or of arcuate contours, pink to red, and surrounded by a "flare" of macular erythema. Wheals may be discrete or may coalesce. These lesions often develop quickly (minutes to hours). Because the wheal is the prototypic lesion of urticaria, diseases in which wheals are prominent are frequently described as "urticarial" (e.g., urticarial vasculitis). Dermatographism, or pressure-induced whealing, may be evident.

Vesicles (Blisters)

Vesicles are circumscribed, fluid-containing elevations 1–0 mm in size (Fig. 2.5). They may be clear from serous exudate or red from serum mixed with blood. The apex may be rounded, acuminate, or umbilicated, as in eczema herpeticum. Vesicles may be discrete, irregularly scattered, grouped (e.g., herpes zoster), or linear, as in allergic contact dermatitis from urushiol (poison ivy/oak). Vesicles may arise directly or from a macule or papule and generally lose their identity in a short time. They may break spontaneously or develop into bullae through coalescence or enlargement. The

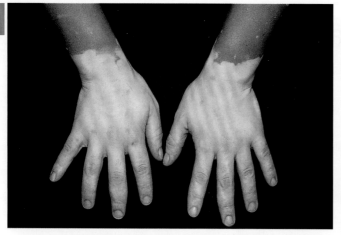

Fig. 2.1 Macular depigmentation, vitiligo.

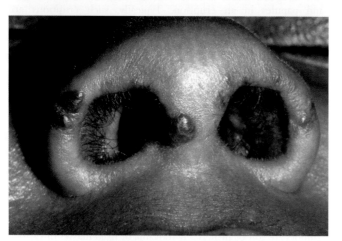

Fig. 2.2 Sarcoidosis (papules).

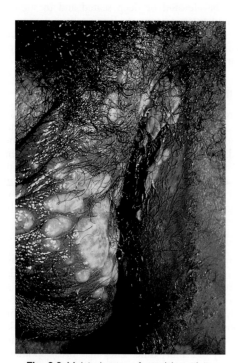

Fig. 2.3 Moist plaques of condyloma lata.

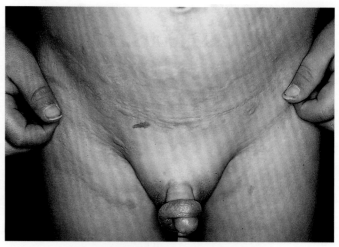

Fig. 2.4 Acute urticaria.

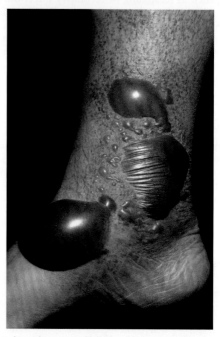

Fig. 2.5 Piroxicam hypersensitivity (vesicles and bullae, some with hemorrhage).

inflammatory process may lead to pustule formation. When the contents are of a seropurulent character, the lesions are known as vesicopustules. Vesicles have either a single cavity (unilocular) or several compartments (multilocular).

Bullae

Bullae are rounded or irregularly shaped blisters containing serous or serosanguineous fluid. They differ from vesicles only in size, being larger than 1 cm (see Fig. 2.5). They are usually unilocular but may be multilocular. Bullae may be located superficially in the epidermis, so their walls are flaccid and thin and subject to rupture spontaneously or from slight injury. After rupture, remnants of the thin walls may persist and, together with the exudate, may dry to form a thin crust. Alternatively the broken bleb may leave a raw and moist base, which may be covered with seropurulent or purulent exudate. Less frequently, irregular vegetations may appear on the base (as in pemphigus vegetans). When subepidermal, the bullae are tense, do not rupture easily, and are often present when the patient is examined.

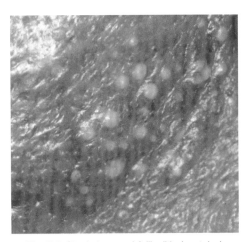

Fig. 2.6 Staphylococcal folliculitis (pustules).

Nikolsky sign refers to the diagnostic maneuver of putting lateral pressure on unblistered skin in a patient with a bullous eruption; a positive result occurs when the epithelium shears off. Asboe-Hansen sign refers to the extension of a blister to adjacent, unblistered skin when pressure is put on the top of the blister. Both these signs demonstrate the principle that in some diseases, the extent of microscopic vesiculation is more than what is evident by simple inspection. These findings are useful in evaluating the severity of pemphigus vulgaris and severe bullous drug reactions. Hemorrhagic bullae are common in pemphigus, herpes zoster, severe bullous drug reactions, and lichen sclerosus. The cellular contents of bullae may be useful in cytologically confirming the diagnosis of pemphigus, herpes zoster, and herpes simplex.

Pustules

Pustules are small elevations of the skin containing purulent material, usually necrotic inflammatory cells (Fig. 2.6). They are similar to vesicles in shape and usually have an inflammatory areola. Pustules are usually white or yellow centrally but have a red tinge if they also contain blood. They may originate as pustules or may develop from papules or vesicles, passing through transitory early stages, during which they are known as papulopustules or vesicopustules.

Secondary Lesions

Secondary lesions are of many types; the most important are scales, crusts, erosions, ulcers, fissures, and scars.

Scales (Exfoliation)

Scales are dry or greasy, laminated masses of keratin. The body ordinarily is constantly shedding imperceptible tiny, thin fragments of stratum corneum. When the formation of epidermal cells is rapid or the process of normal keratinization is disturbed, pathologic exfoliation results, producing scales. These scales vary in size; some are fine, delicate, and branny, as in tinea versicolor, whereas others are coarser, as in eczema and ichthyosis, and still others are stratified, as in psoriasis. Scales vary in color from white-gray to yellow or brown from the admixture of dirt or melanin. Occasionally, they have a silvery sheen from trapping of air between their layers; these are micaceous scales, characteristic of psoriasis. When scaling occurs, it usually suggests a pathologic process in the epidermis, and parakeratosis is often present histologically.

Crusts (Scabs)

Crusts are dried serum, pus, or blood, usually mixed with epithelial and sometimes bacterial debris. When crusts become detached, the base may be dry or red and moist.

Excoriations and Abrasions (Scratch Marks)

An excoriation is a punctate or linear abrasion produced by mechanical means, usually involving only the epidermis but sometimes reaching the papillary layer of the dermis. Excoriations are caused by scratching with the fingernails in an effort to relieve itching. If the skin damage is the result of mechanical trauma or constant friction, the term "abrasion" may be used. Frequently, there is an inflammatory areola around the excoriation or a covering of yellowish dried serum or red dried blood. Excoriations may provide access for pyogenic microorganisms and the formation of crusts, pustules, or cellulitis, occasionally associated with enlargement of the neighboring lymphatic glands. In general, the longer and deeper the excoriations, the more severe is the pruritus that provoked them. Lichen planus is an exception, however, in which pruritus is severe, but excoriations are rare.

Fissures (Cracks, Clefts)

A fissure is a linear cleft through the epidermis or into the dermis. These lesions may be single or multiple and vary from microscopic to several centimeters in length with sharply defined margins. Fissures may be dry or moist, red, straight, curved, irregular, or branching. They occur most often when the skin is thickened and inelastic from inflammation and dryness, especially in regions subjected to frequent movement. Such areas are the tips and flexural creases of the thumbs, fingers, and palms; the edges of the heels; the clefts between the fingers and toes; at the angles of the mouth; the lips; and around the nares, auricles, and anus. When the skin is dry, exposure to cold, wind, water, and cleaning products (soap, detergents) may produce a stinging, burning sensation, indicating microscopic fissuring is present. This may be referred to as chapping, as in "chapped lips." When fissuring is present, pain is often produced by movement of the parts, which opens or deepens the fissures or forms new ones.

Erosions

Loss of all or portions of the epidermis alone, as in impetigo, produces an erosion. It may or may not become crusted, but it heals without a scar.

Ulcers

Ulcers are rounded or irregularly shaped excavations that result from complete loss of the epidermis plus some portion of the dermis. They vary in diameter from a few millimeters to several centimeters (Fig. 2.7). Ulcers may be shallow, involving little beyond the epidermis, as in dystrophic epidermolysis bullosa, the base being formed by the papillary layer, or they may extend deeply into the dermis, subcutaneous tissues, or deeper, as with leg ulcers. Ulcers heal with scarring.

Scars

Scars are composed of new connective tissue that has replaced lost substance in the dermis or deeper parts resulting from injury or disease, as part of the normal reparative process. Their size and shape are determined by the form of the previous destruction. Scarring is characteristic of certain inflammatory processes and is therefore of diagnostic value. The pattern of scarring may be characteristic of a particular disease. Lichen planus and discoid

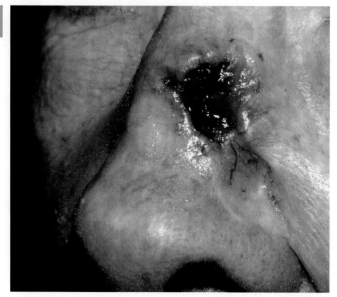

Fig. 2.7 Basal cell carcinoma (ulcer). (Courtesy Steven Binnick, MD.)

lupus erythematosus, for example, have inflammation that is in relatively the same area anatomically, yet discoid lupus characteristically causes scarring as it resolves, whereas lichen planus rarely results in scarring of the skin. Both processes, however, cause scarring of the hair follicles when occurring on the scalp. Scars may be thin and atrophic, or the fibrous elements may develop into neoplastic overgrowths, as in hypertrophic scars or keloids. Some individuals and some areas of the body, especially the anterior chest and upper back, are especially prone to hypertrophic scarring. Scars first tend to be pink or violaceous, later becoming white, glistening, and, rarely, hyperpigmented. Scars are persistent but usually become softer, less elevated, and less noticeable over years.

GENERAL DIAGNOSIS

Interpretation of the clinical picture may be difficult because identical clinical lesions may have many different causes. Moreover, the same skin disease may give rise to diverse eruptions. Thus for each specific type of primary morphologic lesion, there is a differential diagnosis of the conditions that could produce that lesion. Also, there is a parallel list of all the variations that a single skin disease can cause; for example, lichen planus may have hyperpigmented patches, violaceous plaques, hypertrophic papules, and, rarely, minute papules.

Being superficial, skin lesions can be easily observed and palpated. Magnification may be easily applied, enhancing visualization of the fine details of the lesions. Smears and cultures may be readily obtained for bacteria and fungi. Biopsy and histologic examination of skin lesions are usually minor procedures, making histopathology an important component of many dermatologic evaluations. The threshold for biopsy should be low. This is especially true of inflammatory dermatoses, potentially infectious conditions, and skin disorders in immunosuppressed and hospitalized patients in whom clinical morphology may be atypical. Once therapy is begun empirically, histologic features may be altered by the treatment, making pathologic diagnosis more difficult.

History

Knowledge of the patient's age, health, occupation, hobbies, diet, and living conditions is important, as well as the onset, duration, and course of the disease and the response to previous treatment.

The family history of similar disorders and other related diseases may be useful.

A complete drug history is one of the most important aspects of a thorough history. This includes prescription and over-the-counter medications, supplements, herbal products, eyedrops, and suppositories. Drug reactions are frequent and may simulate many different skin diseases clinically and histologically. It is equally important to inquire about topical agents that have been applied to the skin and mucous membranes for medicinal or cosmetic purposes, because these agents may cause cutaneous or systemic reactions.

A complete medical history that includes other medical diagnoses of the patient is essential. Certain skin diseases are specific to or associated with other conditions, such as cutaneous Crohn disease and pyoderma gangrenosum in Crohn disease. Travel abroad, the patient's environment at home and at work, seasonal occurrences and recurrences of the disease, and the temperature, humidity, and weather exposure of the patient are all important factors in a dermatologic history. Habitation in certain parts of the world predisposes to distinctive diseases for that particular geographic locale, including San Joaquin Valley fever (coccidioidomycosis), Hansen disease, leishmaniasis, and histoplasmosis. Sexual orientation and practices may be relevant, as in genital ulcer diseases and human immunodeficiency virus (HIV) infection.

Examination

Examination should be conducted in a well-lit room. Natural sunlight is the ideal illumination. Abnormalities of melanin pigmentation (e.g., vitiligo, melasma) are more clearly visible under ultraviolet (UV) light. A Wood's light (365 nm) is most often used and is also valuable for the diagnosis of some types of tinea capitis, tinea versicolor, and erythrasma.

A magnifying lens is of inestimable value in examining small lesions. It may be necessary to palpate the lesion for firmness and fluctuation; rubbing will elucidate the nature of scales, and scraping will reveal the nature of the lesion's base. Pigmented lesions, especially in infants, should be rubbed in an attempt to elicit Darier sign (whealing), as seen in urticaria pigmentosa. Dermoscopy is an important part of the examination of neoplasms.

The entire eruption must be seen to evaluate distribution and configuration. This is optimally done by having the patient completely undress and viewing from a distance to take in the whole eruption at once. "Peek-a-boo" examination, by having the patient expose one anatomic area after another while remaining clothed, is not optimal because the examination of the skin will be incomplete, and the overall distribution is difficult to determine. After the patient is viewed at a distance, individual lesions are examined to identify primary lesions and to determine the evolution of the eruption and the presence of secondary lesions.

Diagnostic Details of Lesions

Distribution

Lesions may be few or numerous, and in arrangement they may be discrete or may coalesce to form patches of peculiar configuration. Lesions may appear over the entire body or may follow the lines of cleavage (pityriasis rosea), dermatomes (herpes zoster), or lines of Blaschko (epidermal nevi) (Fig. 2.8). Lesions may form groups, rings, crescents, or unusual linear patterns. A remarkable degree of bilateral symmetry is characteristic of certain diseases, such as dermatitis herpetiformis, vitiligo, and psoriasis.

Evolution

Some lesions appear fully evolved. Others develop from smaller lesions, then remain the same during their entire existence (e.g.,

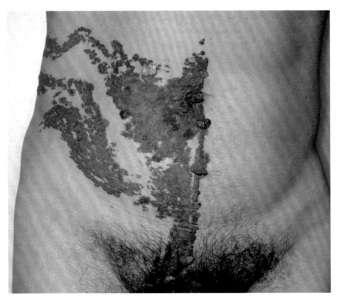

Fig. 2.8 Linear epidermal nevus (blaschkoid).

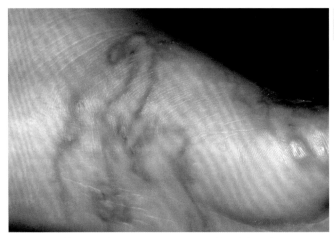

Fig. 2.9 Cutaneous larva migrans (serpiginous).

warts). When lesions succeed one another in a series of crops, as in varicella and dermatitis herpetiformis, a polymorphous eruption results, with lesions in various stages of development or involution all present at the same time.

Involution

Certain lesions disappear completely, whereas others leave characteristic residual pigmentation or scarring. Residual dyspigmentation, although a significant cosmetic issue, is not considered a scar. The pattern in which lesions involute may be useful in diagnosis, as with the typical keratotic papule of pityriasis lichenoides varioliformis acuta.

Grouping

Grouping is a characteristic of dermatitis herpetiformis, herpes simplex, and herpes zoster. Small lesions arranged around a large one are said to be in a corymbose (corymbiform) arrangement. Concentric annular lesions are typical of borderline Hansen disease and erythema multiforme. These are sometimes said to be in a "cockade" pattern, referring to the tricolor cockade hats worn by French revolutionists. Flea and other arthropod bites are usually grouped and linear (breakfast-lunch-and-dinner sign). Grouped lesions of various sizes may be called agminated.

Configuration

Certain terms are used to describe the configuration that an eruption assumes either primarily or by enlargement or coalescence. Lesions in a line are called linear, and they may be confluent or discrete. Lesions may form a complete circle with normal-appearing skin centrally (annular) or a portion of a circle (arcuate or gyrate), or may be composed of several intersecting portions of circles (polycyclic). If the eruption is not straight but does not form parts of circles, it may be serpiginous (Fig. 2.9). Round lesions may be small, like drops, called guttate; or larger, like a coin, called nummular. Unusual configurations that do not correspond to these patterns or to normal anatomic or embryonic patterns should raise the possibility of an exogenous dermatosis or factitia.

Color

The color of the skin is determined by melanin, oxyhemoglobin, reduced hemoglobin, lipid, and carotene. Not only do the proportions of these components affect the color, but also their depth within the skin, the thickness of the epidermis, and hydration play a role. The Tyndall effect modifies the color of skin and of lesions by the selective scattering of light waves of different wavelengths. The blue nevus and mongolian spots are examples of this light dispersion effect, in which brown melanin in the dermis appears blue-gray.

The color of lesions may be valuable as a diagnostic factor. Dermatologists should be aware that there are many shades of pink, red, and purple, each of which tends to suggest a diagnosis or disease group. Interface reactions such as lichen planus or lupus erythematosus are described as violaceous. Lipid-containing lesions are yellow, as in xanthomas (Fig. 2.10) or steatocystoma multiplex. The orange-red (salmon) color of pityriasis rubra pilaris is characteristic. The constitutive color of the skin determines the quality of the color one observes with a specific disorder. In dark-skinned persons, erythema is difficult to perceive. Pruritic lesions in African Americans may evolve to be small, shiny, flat-topped papules with a violaceous hue, from the combination of erythema and pigment incontinence. These lichenified lesions would be suspected of being lichenoid by the untrained eye, but may be in fact eczematous.

Patches lighter in color than the normal skin may be completely depigmented or may have lost only part of their pigment (hypopigmented). This is an important distinction because certain conditions are or may be hypopigmented, such as tinea versicolor, Hansen disease, ash-leaf macules of tuberous sclerosis, hypomelanosis of Ito, seborrheic dermatitis, and idiopathic guttate hypomelanosis. True depigmentation should be distinguished from this; it suggests vitiligo, nevus depigmentosus, halo nevus, scleroderma, morphea, or lichen sclerosus.

Hyperpigmentation may result from epidermal or dermal causes. It may be related to either increased melanin or deposition of other substances. Epidermal hyperpigmentation occurs in nevi, melanoma, café au lait spots, melasma, and lentigines. These lesions are accentuated when examined with a Wood's light. Dermal pigmentation occurs subsequent to many inflammatory conditions (postinflammatory hyperpigmentation) or from deposition of metals, medications, medication-melanin complexes, or degenerated dermal material (ochronosis). These conditions are not enhanced when examined by a Wood's light. The hyperpigmentation following inflammation is most frequently the result of dermal melanin deposition, but in some conditions, such as lichen aureus, is caused

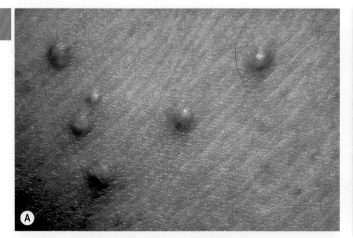

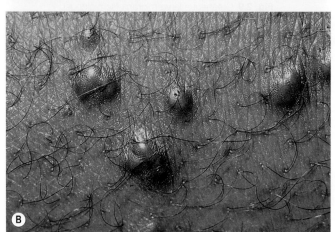

Fig. 2.10 Eruptive xanthoma. (A) Yellow color easily discerned on white skin. (B) Yellow color subtler in brown or black skin.

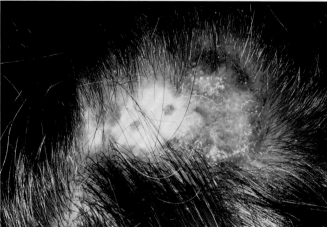

Fig. 2.11 Scalp plaque with scarring alopecia hyperpigmentation and depigmentation, discoid lupus erythematosus.

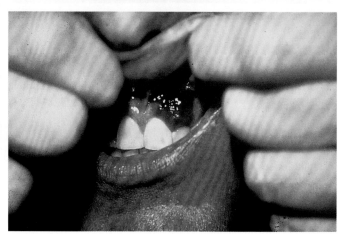

Fig. 2.12 Oral Kaposi sarcoma.

by iron. Dermal iron deposition appears more yellow-brown or golden than dermal melanin.

Texture/Consistency

Palpation is an essential part of the physical examination of lesions. Does the lesion blanch on pressure? If not, it may be purpuric. Is it fluctuant? If so, it may have free fluid in it. If there is a nodule or tumor, does it sink through a ring into the panniculus, like a neurofibroma? Is it hard enough for calcification to be suspected, or merely very firm, like a keloid or dermatofibroma?

Hyperesthesia/Anesthesia

Certain conditions may be associated with increased or decreased sensation. For example, the skin lesions of borderline and tuberculoid Hansen disease typically are anesthetic in their centers. In complex regional pain syndrome spontaneous pain and tenderness on palpation are characteristic. In other neuropathic conditions such as notalgia paresthetica, the patient may perceive both pruritus and hyperesthesia. Neurally mediated itch may be accompanied by other neural sensations, such as heat or burning. The combination of pruritus with other neural symptoms suggests the involvement of nerves in the pathologic process.

Hair, Nails, and Oral Mucosa

Involvement of hair-bearing areas by certain skin disorders causes characteristic lesions. Discoid lupus, for example, causes scarring alopecia with characteristic dyspigmentation (Fig. 2.11). On the skin, the lesions may be much less characteristic. Diffuse hair loss may be seen in certain conditions, such as acrodermatitis enteropathica, and may be a clue to the diagnosis. In addition, loss of hair within a skin lesion may suggest the diagnosis, such as the alopecia seen in the tumid plaques of follicular mucinosis.

Some skin disorders cause characteristic changes of the nails, even when the periungual tissue is not involved. The pitting seen in psoriasis and alopecia areata may be useful in confirming these diagnoses when other findings are not characteristic. In addition, the nails and adjacent structures may be the sole site of pathology, as in candidal paronychia.

The complete skin examination includes examination of the oral mucosa. Oral lesions are characteristically found in viral syndromes (exanthems), lichen planus, HIV-associated Kaposi sarcoma (Fig. 2.12), and autoimmune bullous diseases (pemphigus vulgaris).

Self-Examination

Patients at risk for the development of skin cancer should be taught the correct method of skin self-examination, specifically, the ABCDEs of melanoma detection and the types of lesions that might represent basal cell carcinoma or squamous cell carcinoma.

3 Dermatoses Resulting From Physical Factors

The body requires a certain amount of heat, but beyond definite limits, insufficient or excessive amounts are injurious. The local action of excessive heat causes burns or scalds; undue cold causes chilblains, frostbite, and congelation. Thresholds of tolerance exist in all body structures sensitive to electromagnetic wave radiation of varying frequencies, such as x-rays and ultraviolet (UV) rays. The skin, which is exposed to so many external physical forces, is more subject to injuries caused by this radiation than any other organ.

HEAT INJURIES

Thermal Burns

Injury of varying intensity may be caused by the action of excessive heat on the skin (Fig. 3.1). If this heat is extreme, the skin and underlying tissue may be destroyed. The changes in the skin resulting from dry heat or scalding are classified in four degrees, as follows:

- *First-degree burns* of the skin result merely in an active congestion of the superficial blood vessels, causing erythema that may be followed by epidermal desquamation (peeling). Ordinary sunburn is the most common example of a first-degree burn. The pain and increased surface heat may be severe, and some constitutional reaction can occur if the involved area is large.
- *Second-degree burns* are subdivided into superficial and deep forms.
  - In the superficial second-degree burn, there is a transudation of serum from the capillaries, which causes edema of the superficial tissues. Vesicles and bullae are formed by the serum gathering beneath the outer layers of the epidermis. Complete recovery without scarring is usual in patients with superficial burns.
  - The deep second-degree burn is pale and anesthetic. Injury to the reticular dermis compromises blood flow and destroys appendages, so healing takes more than 1 month and results in scarring.
- *Third-degree burns* involve loss of the full thickness of the dermis and often some of the subcutaneous tissues. Because the skin appendages are destroyed, there is no epithelium available for regeneration of the skin. An ulcerating wound is produced, which on healing leaves a scar.
- *Fourth-degree burns* involve the destruction of the entire skin, including the subcutaneous fat, and any underlying tendons.

Both third-degree and fourth-degree burns require grafting for closure. All third- and fourth-degree burns are followed by constitutional symptoms of varying severity, depending on the size of the involved surface, the depth of the burn, and particularly the location of the burned surface. The more vascular the involved area, the more severe are the symptoms.

The prognosis is poor for any patient in whom a large area of skin surface is involved, particularly if more than two thirds of the body surface has been burned. Women, infants, and toddlers all have a greater risk of death from burns than men. Excessive scarring, with either keloid-like scars or flat scars with contractures, may produce deformities and dysfunction of the joints, as well as chronic ulcerations from impairment of local circulation. Delayed postburn blistering may occur in partial-thickness wounds and skin graft donor sites. It is most common on the lower extremities and is self-limited. Although burn scars may be the site of development of carcinoma, evidence supports only the possibility of a modest excess of squamous cell carcinomas in burn scars. With modern reconstructive surgery, this unfortunate end result can be minimized.

Treatment

Immediate first aid for minor thermal burns consists of prompt cold applications (ice water, or cold tap water if no ice is available), which are continued until pain does not return on stopping them.

The vesicles and bullae of second-degree burns should not be opened but should be protected from injury because they form a natural barrier against contamination by microorganisms. If they become tense and unduly painful, the fluid may be evacuated under strictly aseptic conditions by puncturing it with a sterile needle, allowing collapse onto the underlying wound. Excision of full-thickness and deep dermal wounds that will not reepithelialize within 3 weeks (as soon as hemodynamic stability is achieved, normally 2–3 days) reduces wound infections, shortens hospital stays, and improves survival. Additionally, contractures and functional impairment may be mitigated by such intervention. Skin grafting, or coverage with biologic dressings such as allograft or xenograft skin, cultured epidermal autografts, or skin substitutes also assist in healing. The role of early ablative laser treatments to prevent disabling scars and its use in improving fully formed scars is an area of active investigation. The most superficial wounds may be dressed with greasy gauze, whereas silver-containing dressings are used for their antibiotic properties in intermediate wounds.

Fluid resuscitation, treatment of inhalation injury and hypercatabolism, monitoring and early intervention of sepsis, pain control, environmental control, and nutritional support are key components of the critical care of burns. Intensive care management in a burn center is recommended for patients with partial-thickness wounds covering more than 10% of the body surface, if involving the face, hands, feet, genitalia, perineum, or joints; if secondary to electrical, chemical, or inhalation injury; in patients with special needs; and for any full-thickness burn.

Electrical Burns

Electrical burns may occur from contact or as a flash exposure. A contact burn is small but deep, causing some necrosis of the underlying tissues. Low-voltage injuries usually occur in the home, are treated conservatively, and generally heal well. Oral commissure burns may require reconstructive procedures (Fig. 3.2). High-voltage burns are often occupational; internal damage may be masked by minimal surface skin change and may be complicated by subtle and slowly developing sequelae. Early surgical intervention to improve circulation and repair vital tissues is helpful in limiting loss of the extremity.

Flash burns usually cover a large area and, being similar to any surface burn, are treated as such. Lightning may cause burns after a direct strike, where an entrance and an exit wound are visible. This is the most lethal type of strike, and cardiac arrest

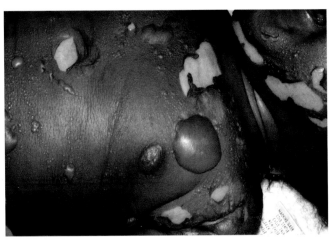

Fig. 3.1 Hot water burn. (Courtesy Steven Binnick, MD.)

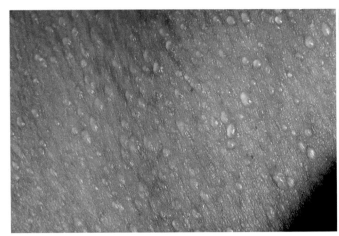

Fig. 3.3 Miliaria crystallina.

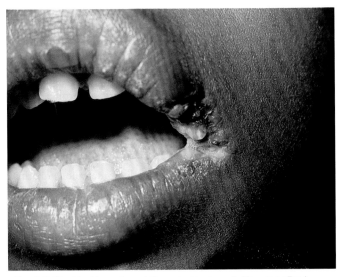

Fig. 3.2 Electrical burn from biting electrical cord. (Courtesy Paul Hong, MD.)

or other internal injuries may occur. Other types of lightning strike are indirect and result in the following burns:

- Linear burns in areas on which sweat was present
- Burns in a feathery or arborescent pattern, which is believed to be pathognomonic
- Punctate burns with multiple, deep, circular lesions
- Thermal burns from ignited clothing or heated metal, which may occur if the patient was speaking on a cell phone or listening to an iPod or similar device when struck

Hot Tar Burns

Polyoxyethylene sorbitan in bacitracin zinc–neomycin–polymyxin B (e.g., Neosporin) ointment, vitamin E ointment, and sunflower oil are excellent dispersing agents that facilitate the removal of hot tar from burns.

Alemayehu H, et al: Management of electrical and chemical burns in children. J Surg Res 2014; 190: 210.
Carta T, et al: Use of mineral oil Fleet enema for the removal of a large tar burn. Burns 2015; 41: e11.

Compton CC: The delayed postburn blister. Arch Dermatol 1992; 128: 24.
El-Zawahry BM, et al: Ablative CO2 fractional resurfacing in treatment of thermal burn scars. J Cosmet Dermatol 2015; 14: 324.
Esteban-Vives R, et al: Second-degree burns with six etiologies treated with autologous noncultured cell-spray grafting. Burns 2016; 42: e99.
Heffernan EJ, et al: Thunderstorms and iPods. N Engl J Med 2007; 357: 198.
Kalantar Motamedi MH, et al: Prevalence and pattern of facial burns. J Oral Maxillofac Surg 2015; 73: 676.
Russell KW, et al: Lightning burns. J Burn Care Res 2014; 35: e436.
Saracoglu A, et al: Prognostic factors in electrical burns. Burns 2014; 40: 702.
Sheridan RL, Greenhalgh D: Special problems in burns. Surg Clin North Am 2014; 94: 781.
Sokhal AK, et al: Clinical spectrum of electrical burns. Burns 2017; 43: 182.
Wallingford SC, et al: Skin cancer arising in scars: a systematic review. Dermatol Surg 2011; 37: 1239.
Wang KA, et al: Epidemiology and outcome analysis of hand burns. Burns 2015; 41: 1550.

Miliaria

Miliaria, the retention of sweat as a result of occlusion of eccrine sweat ducts, produces an eruption that is common in hot, humid climates, such as in the tropics and during the hot summer months in temperate climates. *Staphylococcus epidermidis*, which produces an extracellular polysaccharide substance, induces miliaria in an experimental setting. This polysaccharide substance may obstruct the delivery of sweat to the skin surface. The occlusion prevents normal secretion from the sweat glands, and eventually pressure causes rupture of the sweat gland or duct at different levels. The escape of sweat into the adjacent tissue produces miliaria. Depending on the level of the injury to the sweat gland or duct, several different forms are recognized.

Miliaria Crystallina

Miliaria crystallina is characterized by small, clear, superficial vesicles with no inflammatory reaction (Fig. 3.3). It appears in bedridden patients whose fever produces increased perspiration or when clothing prevents dissipation of heat and moisture, as in bundled children. Hypernatremia without fever may induce it.

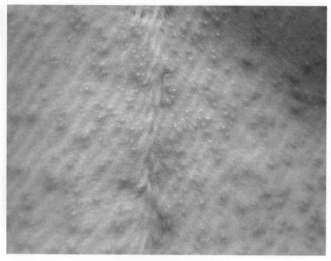

Fig. 3.4 Miliaria rubra.

The lesions are generally asymptomatic, and their duration is short-lived because they tend to rupture at the slightest trauma. Drugs such as isotretinoin, adrenergic/cholinergic drugs, and doxorubicin may induce it. The lesions are self-limited; no treatment is required.

Miliaria Rubra (Prickly Heat)

The lesions of miliaria rubra appear as discrete, extremely pruritic, erythematous papulovesicles (Fig. 3.4) accompanied by a sensation of prickling, burning, or tingling. They later may become confluent on a bed of erythema. The sites most frequently affected are the antecubital and popliteal fossae, trunk, inframammary areas (especially under pendulous breasts), abdomen (especially at the waistline), and inguinal regions; these sites frequently become macerated because evaporation of moisture has been impeded. Exercise-induced itching or that of atopic dermatitis may also be caused by miliaria rubra. The site of injury and sweat escape is in the prickle cell layer, where spongiosis is produced.

Miliaria Pustulosa

Miliaria pustulosa is preceded by another dermatitis that has produced injury, destruction, or blocking of the sweat duct. The pustules are distinct, superficial, and independent of the hair follicle. The pruritic pustules occur most frequently on the intertriginous areas, flexural surfaces of the extremities, scrotum, and back of bedridden patients. Contact dermatitis, lichen simplex chronicus, and intertrigo are some of the associated diseases, although pustular miliaria may occur several weeks after these diseases have subsided. Recurrent episodes may be a sign of type I pseudohypoaldosteronism, because salt-losing crises may precipitate miliaria pustulosa or rubra, with resolution after stabilization.

Miliaria Profunda

Nonpruritic, flesh-colored, deep-seated, whitish papules characterize miliaria profunda. It is asymptomatic, usually lasts only 1 hour after overheating has ended, and is concentrated on the trunk and extremities. Except for the face, axillae, hands, and feet, where there may be compensatory hyperhidrosis, all the sweat glands are nonfunctional. The occlusion is in the upper dermis. Miliaria profunda is observed only in the tropics and usually follows a severe bout of miliaria rubra.

Postmiliarial Hypohidrosis

Postmiliarial hypohidrosis results from occlusion of sweat ducts and pores, and it may be severe enough to impair an individual's ability to perform sustained work in a hot environment. Affected persons may show decreasing efficiency, irritability, anorexia, drowsiness, vertigo, and headache; they may wander in a daze.

It has been shown that hypohidrosis invariably follows miliaria, and that the duration and severity of the hypohidrosis are related to the severity of the miliaria. Sweating may be depressed to half the normal amount for as long as 3 weeks.

Tropical Anhidrotic Asthenia

Tropical anhidrotic asthenia is a rare form of miliaria with long-lasting poral occlusion, which produces anhidrosis and heat retention.

Treatment

The most effective treatment for miliaria is to place the patient in a cool environment. Even a single night in an air-conditioned room helps to alleviate the discomfort. Circulating air fans can also be used to cool the skin. Anhydrous lanolin resolves the occlusion of pores and may help to restore normal sweat secretions. Hydrophilic ointment also helps to dissolve keratinous plugs and facilitates the normal flow of sweat. Soothing, cooling baths containing colloidal oatmeal or cornstarch are beneficial if used in moderation. Patients with mild cases may respond to dusting powders, such as cornstarch or baby talcum powder.

Chao CT: Hypernatremia-related miliaria crystallina. Clin Esp Nephrol 2014; 18: 831.

Haque MS, et al: The oldest new finding in atopic dermatitis. JAMA Dermatol 2013; 149: 436.

Mowad CM, et al: The role of extracellular polysaccharide substance produced by *Staphylococcus epidermidis* in miliaria. J Am Acad Dermatol 1995; 20: 713.

Onal H, et al: Miliaria rubra and thrombocytosis in pseudohypoaldosteronism. Platelets 2012; 23: 645.

Erythema Ab Igne

Erythema ab igne is a persistent erythema—or the coarsely reticulated residual pigmentation resulting from it—that is usually produced by long exposure to excessive heat without the production of a burn (Fig. 3.5). It begins as a mottling caused by local hemostasis and becomes a reticulated erythema, leaving pigmentation. Multiple colors are simultaneously present in an active patch, varying from pale pink to old rose or dark purplish brown. After the cause is removed, the affection tends to disappear gradually, but sometimes the pigmentation is permanent.

Histologically, an increased amount of elastic tissue in the dermis is noted. The changes in erythema ab igne are similar to those of actinic elastosis. Interface dermatitis and epithelial atypia may be noted.

Erythema ab igne on the legs results from habitually warming them in front of open fireplaces, space heaters, or car heaters. Similar changes may be produced on the lower back or at other sites of an electric heating pad application, on the upper thighs with laptop computers, or on the posterior thighs from heated car seats. The reason for chronically exposing the skin to heat may be pain from an underlying cancer, or from a condition which predisposes to a feeling of cold, such as anorexia nervosa. The condition occurs also in cooks, silversmiths, and others exposed over long periods to direct moderate heat.

Epithelial atypia, which may lead to Bowen disease and squamous cell carcinoma, has rarely been reported to occur overlying erythema

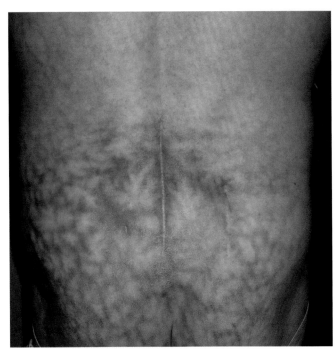

Fig. 3.5 Erythema ab igne.

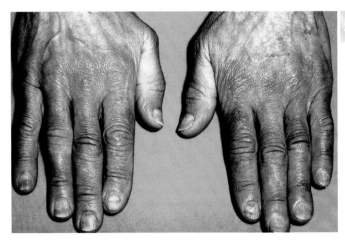

Fig. 3.6 Acrocyanosis.

ab igne. In remote areas of Kashmir, Kangri fire pots can induce erythema ab igne and cancer within the affected area. Treatment with 5-fluorouracil (5-FU), imiquimod, or photodynamic therapy may be effective in reversing this epidermal alteration.

The use of emollients containing α-hydroxy acids or a cream containing fluocinolone acetonide 0.01%, hydroquinone 4%, and tretinoin 0.05% may help reduce the unsightly pigmentation, as may treatment with the Q-switched neodymium-doped yttrium-aluminum-garnet (Nd:YAG) laser.

Brodell D, et al: Automobile seat heater-induced erythema ab igne. Arch Dermatol 2012; 148: 264.

Dessinoti C, et al: Erythema ab igne in three girls with anorexia nervosa. Pediatr Dermatol 2016; 333: e149.

Kim HW, et al: Erythema ab igne successfully treated with low fluenced 1,064-nm Q-switched neodymium-doped yttrium aluminum garnet laser. J Cosmet Laser Ther 2014; 16: 147.

Riahi RR, et al: Practical solutions to prevent laptop-induced erythema ab igne. Int J Dermatol 2014; 53: e395.

Wani I: Kangri cancer. Surgery 2010; 147: 586.

Wharton JB, et al: Squamous cell carcinoma in situ arising in the setting of erythema ab igne. J Drugs Dermatol 2008; 7: 488.

COLD INJURIES

Exposure to cold damages the skin by at least three mechanisms:

- Reduced temperature directly damages the tissue, as in frostbite and cold immersion foot.
- Vasospasm of vessels perfusing the skin prevents adequate perfusion of the tissue and causes vascular injury and consequent tissue injury (pernio, acrocyanosis, and frostbite).
- In unusual circumstances, adipose tissue is predisposed to damage by cold temperatures because of fat composition or location (cold panniculitis; see Chapter 23).

Outdoor workers and recreationalists, military service members, alcoholic persons, and homeless people are particularly likely to sustain cold injuries. Maneuvers to treat orthopedic injuries or heatstroke and cooling devices for other therapeutic use may result in cold injuries ranging from acrocyanosis to frostbite. Holding ice coated with salt (salt and ice challenge) will induce cold-induced blistering.

Heil K, et al: Freezing and non-freezing cold weather injuries. Br Med Bull 2016; 117: 79.

Roussel LO, et al: Tweens feel the burn. Int J Adolesc Med Health 2016; 28: 217.

Acrocyanosis

Acrocyanosis is a persistent blue discoloration of the entire hand or foot worsened by cold exposure. The hands and feet may be hyperhidrotic (Fig. 3.6). It occurs chiefly in young women. Cyanosis increases as the temperature decreases and changes to erythema with elevation of the dependent part. The cause is unknown. Smoking should be avoided. Acrocyanosis is distinguished from Raynaud syndrome by its persistent (rather than episodic) nature and lack of tissue damage (ulceration, distal fingertip resorption).

Acrocyanosis with swelling of the nose, ears, and dorsal hands may occur after inhalation of butyl nitrite. Interferon alpha-2a and beta may induce it. Repeated injection of the dorsal hand with narcotic drugs may produce lymphedema and an appearance similar to the edematous phase of scleroderma. This so-called puffy hand syndrome may include erythema or a bluish discoloration of the digits. Patients with anorexia nervosa frequently manifest acrocyanosis as well as perniosis, livedo reticularis, and acral coldness. It may improve with weight gain. Approximately one third of patients with skin findings of POEMS syndrome (polyneuropathy, organomegaly, endocrinopathy, M component, skin changes) have acrocyanosis. Also, in patients with a homozygous mutation in *SAMDH1* and cerebrovascular occlusive disease, acrocyanosis was frequent.

Acral vascular syndromes, such as gangrene, Raynaud phenomenon, and acrocyanosis, may be a sign of malignancy. In 47% of 68 reported cases, the diagnosis of cancer coincided with the onset of the acral disease. If such changes appear or worsen in an elderly patient, especially a man, without exposure to vasoconstrictive drugs or prior autoimmune or vascular disorders, a paraneoplastic origin should be suspected.

Del Giudice P, et al: Hand edema and acrocyanosis. Arch Dermatol 2006; 142: 1084.

Dessinoti C, et al: Erythema ab igne in three girls with anorexia nervosa. Pediatr Dermatol 2016; 333: e149.

Kurklinsky AK, et al: Acrocyanosis. Vasc Med 2011; 16: 288.

Masuda H, et al: Bilateral foot acrocyanosis in an interferon-β-treated MS patient. Intern Med 2016; 55: 319.

Miest RY, et al: Cutaneous manifestations in patients with POEMS syndrome. Int J Dermatol 2013; 52: 1349.

Poszepczynska-Guigné E, et al: Paraneoplastic acral vascular syndrome. J Am Acad Dermatol 2002; 47: 47.

Xin B, et al: Homozygous mutation in *SAMHD1* gene causes cerebral vasculopathy and early onset stroke. Proc Natl Acad Sci USA 2011; 108: 5372.

Pernio (Chilblains, Perniosis)

Pernio constitutes a localized erythema and swelling caused by exposure to cold. Blistering and ulcerations may develop in severe cases. In people predisposed by poor peripheral circulation, even moderate exposure to cold may produce chilblains. Cryoglobulins, cryofibrinogens, antiphospholipid antibodies, or cold agglutinins may be present and pathogenic. Chilblain-like lesions may occur in discoid and systemic lupus erythematosus (SLE; chilblain lupus), particularly the TREX1-associated familial type, as a presenting sign of leukemia cutis, or if occurring in infancy may herald the Nakajo-Nishimura syndrome or the Aicardi-Goutières and Singleton-Merten syndrome. The chronic use of crack cocaine and its attendant peripheral vasoconstriction will lead to perniosis with cold, numb hands and atrophy of the digital fat pads, especially of the thumbs and index fingers, as well as nail curvature.

Pernio occur chiefly on the feet, hands, ears, and face, chiefly in women; onset is enhanced by dampness (Fig. 3.7). In surgery technicians, the hands are affected if an orthopedic cold therapy system is used; the skin under the device develops the lesions. The lateral thighs are involved in women equestrians who ride on cold, damp days and the hips in those wearing tight-fitting jeans with a low waistband. Wading across cold streams may produce similar lesions. Nondigital lesions of cold injury can be nodular.

Patients with chilblains are often unaware of the cold injury when it is occurring, but later burning, itching, and redness call it to their attention. The affected areas are bluish red, with the color partially or totally disappearing on pressure, and are cool to the touch. Sometimes the extremities are clammy because of excessive sweating. As long as the dampness and cold exposure continues, new lesions will continue to appear. Investigation into an underlying cause should be undertaken in patients with pernio that is recurrent, chronic, extending into warm seasons, or poorly responsive to treatment.

Pernio histologically demonstrates a lymphocytic vasculitis. There is dermal edema, and a superficial and deep perivascular, tightly cuffed, lymphocytic infiltrate. The infiltrate involves the vessel walls and is accompanied by characteristic "fluffy" edema of the vessel walls.

Treatment

The affected parts should be protected against further exposure to cold or dampness. If the feet are involved, woolen socks should be worn at all times during the cold months. Because patients are often not conscious of the cold exposure that triggers the lesions, appropriate dress must be stressed, even if patients say they do not sense being cold. Because central cooling triggers peripheral vasoconstriction, keeping the whole body (not just the affected extremity) warm is critical. Heating pads may be used judiciously to warm the parts. Smoking is strongly discouraged.

Nifedipine, 20 mg three times a day, has been effective. Vasodilators such as nicotinamide, 500 mg three times a day, or dipyridamole, 25 mg three times a day, or the phosphodiesterase inhibitor sildenafil, 50 mg twice daily, may be used to improve circulation. Pentoxifylline and hydroxychloroquine may be effective. Spontaneous resolution occurs without treatment in 1–3 weeks. Systemic corticoid therapy is useful in chilblain lupus.

Al-Sudany NK: Treatment of primary perniosis with oral pentoxifylline (a double-blind placebo-controlled randomized therapeutic trial). Dermatol Ther 2016; 29: 263.

Baker JS, Miranpuri S: Perniosis a case report with literature review. J Am Podiatr Med Assoc 2016; 106: 138.

Ferrara G, Cerroni L: Cold-associated perniosis of the thighs ("equestrian-type" chilblain). Am J Dermatopathol 2016; 38: 726.

Günther C, et al: Familial chilblain lupus due to a novel mutation in the exonuclease III domain of 3′ repair exonuclease 1 (TREX1). JAMA Dermatol 2015; 151: 426.

Kanazawa N: Nakajo-Nishimura syndrome. Allergol Int 2012; 61: 197.

King JM, et al: Perniosis induced by a cold-therapy system. Arch Dermatol 2012; 148: 1101.

Mireku KA, et al: Tender macules and papules on the toes. JAMA Dermatol 2014; 150: 329.

Payne-James JJ, et al: Pseudosclerodermatous triad of perniosis, pulp atrophy and parrot-beaked clawing of the nails. J Forensic Leg Med 2007; 14: 65.

Tran C, et al: Chilblain-like leukaemia cutis. BMJ Case Rep 2016 Apr 19; 2016.

Weismann K, et al: Pernio of the hips in young girls wearing tight-fitting jeans with a low waistband. Acta Derm Venereol 2006; 86: 558.

Frostbite

When soft tissue is frozen and locally deprived of blood supply, the damage is called frostbite. The ears, nose, cheeks, fingers, and

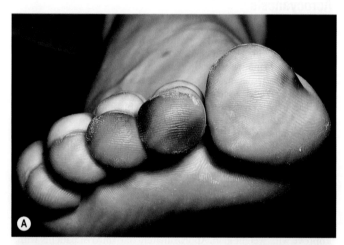

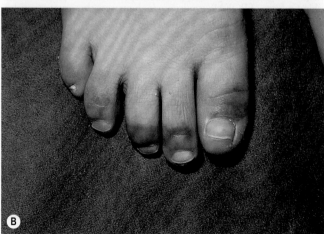

Fig. 3.7 Chilblains (pernio) in adult (A) and child (B).

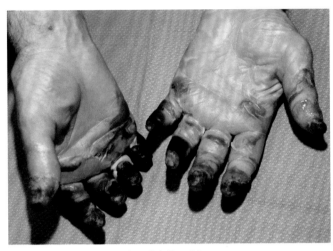

Fig. 3.8 Frostbite.

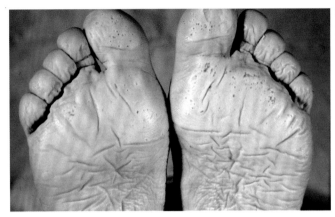

Fig. 3.9 Tropical immersion foot. (Courtesy Steven Binnick, MD.)

toes are most often affected. The frozen part painlessly becomes pale and waxy. Various degrees of tissue destruction similar to that caused by burns are encountered. These are erythema and edema, vesicles and bullae, superficial gangrene, deep gangrene, and injury to muscles, tendons, periosteum, and nerves (Fig. 3.8). The degree of injury is directly related to the temperature and duration of freezing. African Americans are at increased risk of frostbite. Arthritis of the small joints of the hands and feet may appear months to years later.

Treatment

Early treatment of frostbite before swelling develops should consist of covering the part with clothing or with a warm hand or other body surface to maintain a slightly warm temperature so that adequate blood circulation can be maintained. Rapid rewarming in a water bath between 37°C and 43°C (100°F and 110°F) is the treatment of choice for all forms of frostbite. Rewarming should be delayed until the patient has been removed to an area where there is no risk of refreezing. Slow thawing results in more extensive tissue damage. Analgesics should be administered because of the considerable pain experienced with rapid thawing. When the skin flushes and is pliable, thawing is complete. The use of tissue plasminogen activator to lyse thrombi decreases the need for amputation if given within 24 hours of injury. Infusion of the vasodilator iloprost may be used if available. Supportive measures such as bed rest, a high-protein/high-calorie diet, wound care, and avoidance of trauma are imperative. Any rubbing of the affected part should be avoided, but gentle massage of proximal portions of the extremity that are not numb may be helpful.

The use of anticoagulants to prevent thrombosis and gangrene during the recovery period has been advocated. Pentoxifylline, ibuprofen, and aspirin may be useful adjuncts. Antibiotics should be given as a prophylactic measure against infection, and tetanus immunization should be updated. Recovery may take many months. Injuries that affect the proximal phalanx or the carpal or tarsal area, especially when accompanied by a lack of radiotracer uptake on bone scan, have a high likelihood of requiring amputation. Whereas prior cold injury is a major risk factor for recurrent disease, sympathectomy may be preventive against repeated episodes. Arthritis may be a late complication.

Heil K, et al: Freezing and non-freezing cold weather injuries. Br Med Bull 2016; 117: 79.
Johnson-Arbor K: Digital frostbite. N Engl J Med 2014; 370: e3.

McIntosh SE, et al: Wilderness Medical Society practice guidelines for the prevention and treatment of frostbite. Wilderness Environ Med 2014; 25: S43.
Wang Y, et al: Frostbite arthritis. Am J Phys Med Rehabil 2016; 95: e28.

Immersion Foot Syndromes

Trench Foot

Trench foot results from prolonged exposure to cold, wet conditions without immersion or actual freezing. The term is derived from trench warfare in World War I, when soldiers stood, sometimes for hours, in trenches with a few inches of cold water in them. Fishermen, sailors, and shipwreck survivors may be seen with this condition. The lack of circulation produces edema, paresthesias, and damage to the blood vessels. Similar findings may complicate the overuse of ice, cold water, and fans by patients trying to relieve the pain associated with erythromelalgia. Gangrene may occur in severe cases. Treatment consists of removal from the causal environment, bed rest, and restoration of the circulation. Other measures, such as those used in the treatment of frostbite, should be employed.

Warm Water Immersion Foot

Exposure of the feet to warm, wet conditions for 48 hours or more may produce a syndrome characterized by maceration, blanching, and wrinkling of the soles and sides of the feet (Fig. 3.9). Itching and burning with swelling may persist for a few days after removal of the cause, but disability is temporary. This condition was often seen in military service members in Vietnam but has also been seen in persons wearing insulated boots.

Warm water immersion foot should be differentiated from tropical immersion foot, seen after continuous immersion of the feet in water or mud at temperatures above 22°C (71.6°F) for 2–10 days. This was known as "paddy foot" in Vietnam. It involves erythema, edema, and pain of the dorsal feet, as well as fever and adenopathy (Fig. 3.10). Resolution occurs 3–7 days after the feet have been dried.

Warm water immersion foot can be prevented by allowing the feet to dry for a few hours in every 24 or by greasing the soles with a silicone grease once a day. Recovery is usually rapid if the feet are thoroughly dry for a few hours.

Adnot J, et al: Immersion foot syndromes. In: James WD (ed): Military Dermatology. Washington, DC: Office of the Surgeon General, 1994.

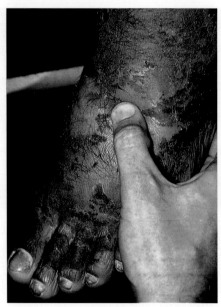

Fig. 3.10 Tropical immersion foot. (Courtesy James WD [ed]: Textbook of Military Medicine, Office of the Surgeon General, United States Army, 1994.)

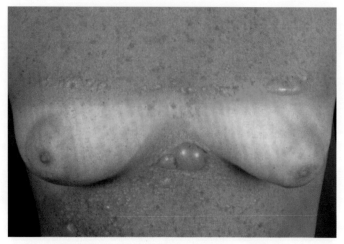

Fig. 3.11 Acute sunburn. (Courtesy Dr. L. Lieblich.)

Davis MD: Immersion foot associated with the overuse of ice, cold water, and fans. J Am Acad Dermatol 2013; 69: 169.
Olson Z, Kman N: Immersion foot. J Emerg Med 2015; 49: e45.

ACTINIC INJURY

Sunburn and Solar Erythema

The solar spectrum has been divided into different regions by wavelength. The parts of the solar spectrum important in photomedicine include UV radiation (below 400 nm), visible light (400–760 nm), and infrared radiation (beyond 760 nm). Visible light has limited biologic activity, except for stimulating the retina. Infrared radiation is experienced as radiant heat. Below 400 nm is the UV spectrum, divided into three bands: UVA, 320–400 nm; UVB, 280–320 nm; and UVC, 200–280 nm. UVA is divided into two subcategories: UVA I (340–400 nm) and UVA II (320–340 nm). Virtually no UVC reaches the Earth's surface because it is absorbed by the ozone layer above the Earth.

The minimal amount of a particular wavelength of light capable of inducing erythema on an individual's skin is called the minimal erythema dose (MED). Although the amount of UVA radiation is 100 times greater than UVB radiation during midday hours, UVB is up to 1000 times more erythemogenic than UVA, and so essentially all solar erythema is caused by UVB. The most biologically effective wavelength of radiation from the sun for sunburn is 308 nm. Although it does not play a significant role in solar erythema, UVA is of major importance in patients with drug-induced photosensitivity and also play a role in photoaging and cutaneous immunosuppression.

The amount of UV exposure increases at higher altitudes, is substantially larger in temperate climates in the summer months, and is greater in tropical regions. UVA may be reflected somewhat more than UVB from sand, snow, and ice. Whereas sand and snow reflect as much as 85% of the UVB, water allows 80% of the UV to penetrate up to 3 feet. Cloud cover, although blocking substantial amounts of visible light, is a poor UV absorber. During the middle 4–6 hours of the day, the intensity of UVB is 2–4 times greater than in the early morning and late afternoon.

Clinical Signs and Symptoms

Sunburn is the normal cutaneous reaction to sunlight in excess of an erythema dose. UVB erythema becomes evident at around 6 hours after exposure and peaks at 12–24 hours, but the onset is sooner and the severity greater with increased exposure. The erythema is followed by tenderness and in severe cases, blistering, which may become confluent (Fig. 3.11). Discomfort may be severe; edema typically occurs in the extremities and face; chills, fever, nausea, tachycardia, and hypotension may be present. In severe cases, such symptoms may last for as long as a week. Desquamation is common about 1 week after sunburn, even in areas that have not blistered.

After UV exposure, skin pigment undergoes two changes: immediate pigment darkening (IPD, Meirowsky phenomenon) and delayed melanogenesis. IPD is maximal within hours after sun exposure and results from metabolic changes and redistribution of the melanin already in the skin. It occurs after exposure to long-wave UVB, UVA, and visible light. With large doses of UVA, the initial darkening is prolonged and may blend into the delayed melanogenesis. IPD is not photoprotective. Delayed tanning is induced by the same wavelengths of UVB that induce erythema, begins 2–3 days after exposure, and lasts 10–14 days. Delayed melanogenesis by UVB is mediated through the production of DNA damage and the formation of cyclobutane pyrimidine dimers (CPD). Therefore, although UVB-induced delayed tanning does provide some protection from further solar injury, it is at the expense of damage to the epidermis and dermis. Tanning is not recommended for sun protection. Commercial tanning bed–induced tanning, while increasing skin pigment, does not increase UVB MED and is therefore not protective for UVB damage. Such tanning devices have been shown to cause melanoma, and their use for tanning purposes should be banned. An individual's inherent baseline pigmentation, ability to tan, and susceptibility to burns are described as the person's "skin type." Skin type is used to determine starting doses of phototherapy and sunscreen recommendations and reflects the risk of development of skin cancer and photoaging (Table 3.1).

Exposure to UVB and UVA causes an increase in the thickness of the epidermis, especially the stratum corneum. This increased epidermal thickness leads to increased tolerance to further solar radiation. Patients with vitiligo may increase their UV exposure without burning by this mechanism.

Treatment

Once redness and other symptoms are present, treatment of sunburn has limited efficacy. The damage is done, and the inflammatory

TABLE 3.1 Skin Types (Phototypes)

Skin Type	Baseline Skin Color	Sunburn and Tanning History
I	White	Always burns, never tans
II	White	Always burns, tans minimally
III	White	Burns moderately, tans gradually
IV	Olive	Minimal burning, tans well
V	Brown	Rarely burns, tans darkly
VI	Dark brown	Never burns, tans darkly black

cascades are triggered. Prostaglandins, especially of the E series, are important mediators. Aspirin (acetylsalicylic acid [ASA]) and nonsteroidal antiinflammatory drugs (NSAIDs), including indomethacin, have been studied, as well as topical and systemic steroids. Medium-potency (class II) topical steroids applied 6 hours after the exposure (when erythema first appears) provide a small reduction in signs and symptoms. Oral NSAIDs and systemic steroids have been tested primarily before or immediately after sun exposure, so there is insufficient evidence to recommend their routine use, except immediately after solar overexposure. Therefore treatment of sunburn should be supportive, with pain management (using acetaminophen, ASA, or NSAIDs), plus soothing topical emollients or corticosteroid lotions. In general, a sunburn victim experiences at least 1 or 2 days of discomfort and even pain before much relief occurs.

Prophylaxis

Sunburn is best prevented. Use of the UV index facilitates taking adequate precautions to prevent solar injury. Numerous educational programs have been developed to make the public aware of the hazards of sun exposure. Despite this, sunburn and excessive sun exposure continue to occur in the United States and Western Europe, especially in white persons under age 30, more than 50% of whom report at least one sunburn per year. Sun protection programs have the following four main messages:

- Avoid midday sun.
- Seek shade.
- Wear sun-protective clothing.
- Apply a sunscreen.

The period of highest UVB intensity, between 9 AM and 3–4 PM, accounts for the vast majority of potentially hazardous UV exposure. This is the time when the angle of the sun is less than 45 degrees, or when a person's shadow is shorter than his or her height. In temperate latitudes, it is almost impossible to burn if these hours of sun exposure are avoided. Trees and artificial shade provide substantial protection from UVB. Foliage in trees provides the equivalent of sun protection factor (SPF) 4–50, depending on the density of the greenery. Clothing can be rated by its ability to block UVB radiation. The scale of measure is the UV protection factor (UPF), analogous to SPF in sunscreens. Although it is an in vitro measurement, UPF correlates well with the actual protection the product provides in vivo. In general, denser weaves, washed older clothing, and loose-fitting clothes screen UVB more effectively. Wetting a fabric may substantially reduce its UPF. Laundering a fabric in a Tinosorb-containing material (SunGuard) will add substantially to the UPF of the fabric. Hats with at least a 4-inch brim all around are recommended.

A sunscreen's efficacy in blocking the UVB (sunburn-inducing) radiation is expressed as an SPF. This is the ratio of the number of MEDs of radiation required to induce erythema through a film of sunscreen (2 mg/cm²) compared with unprotected skin. Most persons apply sunscreens in too thin a film, so the actual

"applied SPF" is about half that on the label. Sunscreen agents include UV-absorbing chemicals (chemical sunscreens) and UV-scattering or blocking agents (physical sunscreens). Available sunscreens, especially those of high SPFs (>30), usually contain both chemical sunscreens (e.g., *p*-aminobenzoic acid [PABA], PABA esters, cinnamates, salicylates, anthranilates, benzophenones, benzylidene camphors such as ecamsule [Mexoryl], dibenzoylmethanes [Parsol 1789, in some products present as multicompound technology Helioplex], and Tinosorb [S/M]) and physical agents (zinc oxide or titanium dioxide). Sunscreens are available in numerous formulations, including sprays, gels, emollient creams, and wax sticks. Sunscreens may be water resistant, with some maintaining their SPF after 40 minutes of water immersion and others maintaining their SPF after 80 minutes of water immersion.

For skin types I to III (see Table 3.1), daily application of a broad-spectrum sunscreen with an SPF of 30 in a facial moisturizer, foundation, or aftershave is recommended. For outdoor exposure, a sunscreen of SPF 30 or higher is recommended for regular use. In persons with severe photosensitivity and at times of high sun exposure, high-intensity sunscreens of SPF 30+ with inorganic blocking agents may be required. Application of the sunscreen at least 20 minutes before and 30 minutes after sun exposure has begun is recommended. This dual-application approach will reduce the amount of skin exposure by twofold to threefold over a single application. Sunscreen should be reapplied after swimming or vigorous activity or toweling. Sunscreen failure occurs mostly in men, from failure to apply it to all the sun-exposed skin or failure to reapply sunscreen after swimming. Sunscreens may be applied to babies (under 6 months) on limited areas. Vitamin D supplementation is recommended with the most stringent sun protection practices. The dose is 600 IU daily for those 70 and younger and 800 IU for older patients.

Photoaging and cutaneous immunosuppression are mediated by UVA as well as UVB. For this reason, sunscreens with improved UVA coverage have been developed. Those containing excellent protection for both UVB and UVA are identified on the label by the words "broad spectrum," and these sunscreens should be sought by patients.

Aguilera J, et al: New advances in protection against solar ultraviolet radiation in textiles for summer clothing. Photochem Photobiol 2014; 90: 1199.

Almutawa F, Buabbas H: Photoprotection. Dermatol Clin 2014; 32: 439.

Cohen LE, Grant RT: Sun protection. Clin Plast Surg 2016; 43: 605.

Faurschou A, et al: Topical corticosteroids in the treatment of acute sunburn. Arch Dermatol 2008; 144: 620.

Fisher DE, et al: Indoor tanning. N Engl J Med 2010; 363: 901.

Lim HW, et al: Adverse effects of ultraviolet radiation from the use of indoor tanning equipment. J Am Acad Dermatol 2011; 64: 893.

Mallett KA, et al: Rates of sunburn among dermatology patients. JAMA Dermatol 2015; 151: 231.

Polefka PG, et al: Effects of solar radiation on the skin. J Cosmet Dermatol 2012; 11: 134.

Thompson AE: Suntan and sunburn. JAMA 2015; 314: 638.

Ephelis (Freckle) and Lentigo

Freckles are small (<0.5 cm) brown macules that occur in profusion on the sun-exposed skin of the face, neck, shoulders, and backs of the hands. They become prominent during the summer when exposed to sunlight and subside, sometimes completely, during the winter when there is no exposure. Blonds and redheads with blue eyes and of Celtic origin (skin types I or II) are especially susceptible. Ephelides may be genetically determined and may

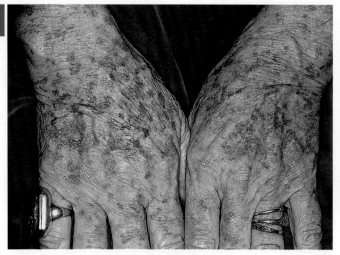

Fig. 3.12 Solar lentigines.

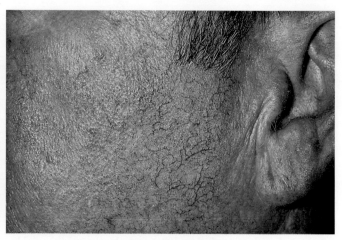

Fig. 3.13 Dermatoheliosis.

recur in successive generations in similar locations and patterns. They usually appear at about age 5 years.

Ephelis must be differentiated from lentigo simplex. The lentigo is a benign, discrete hyperpigmented macule appearing at any age and on any part of the body, including the mucosa. The intensity of the color is not dependent on sun exposure. The solar lentigo appears at a later age, mostly in persons with long-term sun exposure. The backs of the hands and face (especially the forehead) are favored sites (Fig. 3.12).

Histologically, the ephelis shows increased production of melanin pigment by a normal number of melanocytes. Otherwise, the epidermis is normal, whereas the lentigo has elongated rete ridges that appear to be club shaped.

Freckles and solar lentigines are best prevented by appropriate sun protection. Cryotherapy, topical retinoids, hydroquinone, intense pulse light, undecylenoyl phenylalanine, and lasers are effective in the treatment of solar lentigines.

Hafner C, et al: The absence of *BRAF, FGFR3,* and *PIK3CA* mutations differentiates lentigo simplex from melanocytic nevus and solar lentigo. J Invest Dermatol 2009; 129: 2730

Imhof L, et al: A prospective trial comparing Q-switched ruby laser and a triple combination skin-lightening cream in the treatment of solar lentigines. Dermatol Surg 2016; 42: 853.

Praetorius C, et al: Sun-induced freckling. Pigment Cell Melanoma Res 2014; 27: 339.

Photoaging (Dermatoheliosis)

The characteristic changes induced by chronic sun exposure are called photoaging or dermatoheliosis. An individual's risk for developing these changes correlates with the person's skin type (see Table 3.1). Risk for melanoma and nonmelanoma skin cancer is also related to skin type. The persons most susceptible to the deleterious effects of sunlight are those of skin type I: blue-eyed, fair-complexioned persons who do not tan. They are frequently of Irish or other Celtic or Anglo-Saxon descent. Individuals who develop photoaging have the genetic susceptibility and have had sufficient actinic damage to develop skin cancer, and they therefore require more frequent and careful cutaneous examinations.

Chronic sun exposure and chronologic aging are additive. Cigarette smoking is also important in the development of wrinkles, resulting in the inability of observers to distinguish solar-induced from smoking-induced skin aging accurately. The areas primarily affected by photoaging are those regularly exposed to the sun: the V area of the neck and chest, back and sides of the neck, face,

backs of the hands and extensor arms, and in women the skin between the knees and ankles. The skin becomes atrophic, scaly, wrinkled, inelastic, or leathery with a yellow hue (milian citrine skin). In some persons of Celtic ancestry, dermatoheliosis produces profound epidermal atrophy without wrinkling, resulting in an almost translucent appearance of the skin through which hyperplastic sebaceous glands and prominent telangiectasias are seen (Fig. 3.13). These persons are at high risk for nonmelanoma skin cancer. Pigmentation is uneven, with a mixture of poorly demarcated, hyperpigmented and white atrophic macules observed. The photodamaged skin appears generally darker because of these irregularities of pigmentation; in addition, dermal hemosiderosis occurs from actinic purpura. Solar lentigines occur on the face and dorsa of the hands.

Many of the textural and tinctorial changes in sun-damaged skin are caused by alterations in the upper dermal elastic tissue and collagen. This process is called solar (actinic) elastosis, which imparts a yellow color to the skin. Many clinical variants of solar elastosis have been described, and an affected individual may simultaneously have many of these changes. Small yellowish papules and plaques may develop along the sides of the neck. They have been variably named "striated beaded lines" (the result of sebaceous hyperplasia) or "fibroelastolytic papulosis" of the neck, which is caused by solar elastosis. At times, usually on the face or chest, this elastosis may form a macroscopic, translucent papule with a pearly color that may closely resemble a basal cell carcinoma (actinic elastotic plaque). Similar plaques may occur on the helix or antihelix of the ear (elastotic nodules of the ear). Poikiloderma of Civatte refers to reticulate hyperpigmentation with telangiectasia, and slight atrophy of the sides of the neck, lower anterior neck, and V of the chest. The submental area, shaded by the chin, is spared (Fig. 3.14). Poikiloderma of Civatte frequently presents in fair-skinned men and women in their mid to late thirties or early forties. Cutis rhomboidalis nuchae (sailor's or farmer's neck) is characteristic of long-term, chronic sun exposure (Fig. 3.15). The skin on the back of the neck becomes thickened, tough, and leathery, and the normal skin markings are exaggerated. Nodular elastoidosis with cysts and comedones occurs on the inferior periorbital and malar skin (Favre-Racouchot syndrome) (Fig. 3.16) on the forearms (actinic comedonal plaque) or helix of the ear. These lesions appear as thickened yellow plaques studded with comedones and keratinous cysts. The ears may exhibit one or more firm nodules on the helix, known as weathering nodules. Biopsy reveals fibrosis and cartilage metaplasia.

Telangiectasias over the cheeks, ears, and sides of the neck may develop. Because of the damage to the connective tissue of the dermis, skin fragility is prominent, and patients note skin tearing from trivial injuries. This is known as dermatoporosis. Most

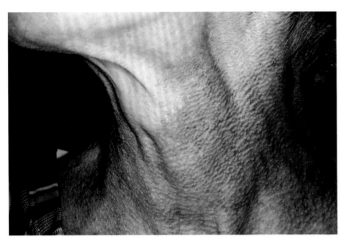

Fig. 3.14 Poikiloderma of Civatte.

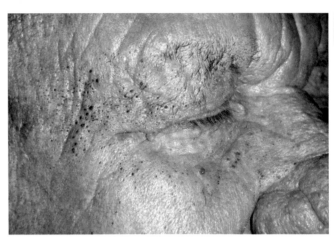

Fig. 3.16 Favre-Racouchot.

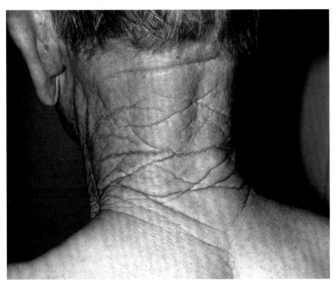

Fig. 3.15 Cutis rhomboidalis nuchae.

frequently, patients complain that even minimal trauma to their extensor arms leads to an ecchymosis, a phenomenon called actinic purpura. As the ecchymoses resolve, dusky brown macules remain for months, increasing the mottled appearance of the skin. Deep dissecting hematomas may result as well, causing large areas of necrosis. Again, minor trauma may lead to a painful deep bruise or simply erythema, without fever. This severe complication of dermatoporosis occurs primarily on the legs of elderly women, many of whom are taking anticoagulants or systemic steroids. Slowly growing erythematous plaques called acquired elastotic hemangiomas, which show horizontal proliferation of capillary blood vessels in the upper dermis, may also appear on the sun-damaged skin of the arms and neck. White stellate pseudoscars on the forearms are a frequent complication of this enhanced skin fragility. In some patients, soft, flesh-colored to yellow papules and nodules coalesce on the forearms to form a cordlike band extending from the dorsal to the flexural surfaces (solar elastotic bands).

Both UVB and UVA radiation induce reactive oxygen species (ROS) and hydrogen peroxide. Acting through activator protein 1 (AP-1), transcription of various matrix-degrading enzymes is upregulated, specifically matrix metalloproteinase 1 (MMP-1;

collagenase), MMP-3 (stromelysin 1), and MMP-9 (gelatinase). In darkly pigmented persons, UV exposure does not activate MMP-1, in part explaining the protective effect of skin pigmentation against photoaging. In chronologically aged skin, MMP-1 levels are also increased through AP-1. Thus chronologic aging and photoaging may be mediated through an identical biochemical mechanism.

Histologically, chronically sun-exposed skin demonstrates homogenization and a faint blue color of the connective tissue of the upper reticular dermis, so-called solar elastosis. This "elastotic" material is derived largely from elastic fibers, stains with histochemical stains for elastic fibers, and demonstrates marked increased deposition of fibulin 2 and its breakdown products. Types I and III collagen are decreased. Characteristically, there is a zone of normal connective tissue immediately below the epidermis and above the elastotic material.

Colloid Milium

There are two forms of colloid milium: adult and juvenile. In both the adult and the juvenile form of colloid milium, the primary skin lesion is a translucent, flesh colored or slightly yellow, 1–5 mm papule. Minimal trauma may lead to purpura from vascular fragility. Histologically, the colloid consists of intradermal, amorphous fissured eosinophilic material. In adult colloid milium, lesions appear in the sun-exposed areas of the hands, face, neck, forearms, and ears in middle-age and older adults, usually men. Lesions often coalesce into plaques and may rarely be verrucous. Petrochemical exposures have been associated with adult colloid milium. Pigmented forms of colloid milium are associated with hydroquinone use. Lesions have been induced by tanning bed exposure, and they can be unilateral, usually in commercial drivers. Adult colloid milium may be considered a papular variant of solar elastosis. The colloid material is derived from elastic fibers, and solar elastosis is found adjacent to the areas of colloid degeneration histologically.

Juvenile colloid milium is much rarer. It develops before puberty, and there may be a family history. The lesions are similar to the adult form but appear initially on the face, later extending to the neck and hands. Sun exposure also appears to be important in inducing lesions of juvenile colloid milium. Juvenile colloid milium, ligneous conjunctivitis, and ligneous periodontitis may appear in the same patient and are probably of similar pathogenesis. Histologically, juvenile colloid milium can be distinguished from adult colloid milium by the finding of keratinocyte apoptosis in the overlying epidermis. The colloid material in juvenile colloid milium is derived from the apoptotic keratinocytes and stains for cytokeratin.

Treatment with fractional photothermolysis or MAL-photodynamic therapy may be effective for colloid milium.

Prevention and Treatment

Because both UVB and UVA are capable of inducing the tissue-destructive biochemical pathways implicated in photoaging, sun protection against both portions of the UV spectrum is the primary prevention required against photoaging. Because photoaging, as with other forms of radiation damage, appears to be cumulative, reducing the total lifetime UV exposure is the goal. The guidelines previously outlined for sunburn prophylaxis should be followed.

The regular use of emollients or moisturizing creams on the areas of sun damage will reduce scaling and may improve fragility by making the skin more pliable. α-Hydroxy acids may improve skin texture when used in lower, nonirritating concentrations. Topical tretinoin, adapalene, and tazarotene can improve the changes of photoaging. Changes are slow and irritation may occur. Chemical peels, resurfacing techniques, laser and other light technologies (for vascular alterations, pigmented lesions, and dermal alterations), botulinum toxins, and soft tissue augmentation are all used to treat the consequences of photoaging. The surgical and laser treatments of photoaging are discussed in Chapter 38.

Balus L, et al: Fibroelastolytic papulosis of the neck. Br J Dermatol 1997; 137: 461.

Bilaç C, et al: Chronic actinic damage of facial skin. Clin Dermatol 2014; 32: 752.

Calderone DC, Fenske NA: The clinical spectrum of actinic elastosis. J Am Acad Dermatol 1995; 32: 1016.

Carniol PJ, et al: Current status of fractional laser resurfacing. JAMA Facial Plast Surg 2015; 17: 360.

Chung HT, et al: Firm papules on the auricular helix. JAMA Dermatol 2013; 149: 475.

Desai C, et al: Colloid milium. Arch Dermatol 2006; 142: 784.

Han A, et al: Photoaging. Dermatol Clin 2014; 32: 291.

Kaya G, et al: Deep dissecting hematoma. Arch Dermatol 2008; 144: 1303.

Li YL, et al: Infrared-induced adult colloid milium treated with fractionated CO_2 laser. Dermatol Ther 2014; 27: 68.

Mancebo SE, et al: Sunscreens. Dermatol Clin 2014; 32: 427.

Martorell-Calatayud A, et al: Definition of the features of acquired elastotic hemangioma reporting the clinical and histopathological characteristics of 14 patients. J Cutan Pathol 2010; 37: 460.

Martorell-Calatayud A, et al: Familial juvenile colloid milium. J Am Acad Dermatol 2011; 64: 203.

Mehregan D, et al: Adult colloid milium. Int J Dermatol 2011; 50: 1531.

Pittayapruek P, et al: Role of matrix metalloproteinases in photoaging and photocarcinogenesis. Int J Mol Sci 2016; 17: 868.

Poon F, et al: Mechanisms and treatments of photoaging. Photodermatol Photoimmunol Photomed 2015; 31: 65.

Riahi RR, et al: Topical retinoids. Am J Clin Dermatol 2016; 17: 265.

Sanches Silveira JE, Myaki Pedroso DM: UV light and skin aging. Rev Environ Health 2014; 29: 243.

Skotarczak K, et al: Photoprotection. Eur Rev Med Pharmacol Sci 2015; 19: 98.

Tierney E, et al: Photodynamic therapy for the treatment of cutaneous neoplasia, inflammatory disorders, and photoaging. Dermatol Surg 2009; 35: 725.

Tierney E, et al: Treatment of poikiloderma of Civatte with ablative fractional laser resurfacing. J Drugs Dermatol 2009; 8: 527.

Wang B: Photoaging. J Cutan Med Surg 2012; 15: 374.

Zeng YP, et al: A split-face treatment of adult colloid milium using a non-ablative, 1550-nm, erbium-glass fractional laser. J Eur Acad Dermatol Venereol 2016; 30: 490.

PHOTOSENSITIVITY

Photosensitivity disorders include cutaneous reactions that are chemically induced (from an exogenous source), metabolic (inborn errors such as the porphyrias, resulting in production of endogenous photosensitizers), idiopathic, and light exacerbated (genetic and acquired). Phototoxicity and the idiopathic disorders are discussed here; the other conditions are covered in later chapters.

Chemically Induced Photosensitivity

A number of substances known as photosensitizers may induce an abnormal reaction in skin exposed to sunlight or its equivalent. The result may be a greatly increased sunburn response without allergic sensitization called phototoxicity. Phototoxicity may occur from both externally applied (phytophotodermatitis and berloque dermatitis) and internally administered chemicals (phototoxic drug reaction). In contrast, photoallergic reactions are true allergic sensitizations triggered by sunlight, produced either by internal administration (photoallergic drug reaction) or by external contact (photoallergic contact dermatitis). Chemicals capable of inducing phototoxic reactions may also produce photoallergic reactions.

In the case of external contactants, the distinction between phototoxicity and photoallergy is usually straightforward. Phototoxicity occurs on initial exposure, has an onset of less than 48 hours, occurs in the vast majority of persons exposed to the phototoxic substance and sunlight, and shows a histologic pattern similar to sunburn. By contrast, photoallergy occurs only in sensitized persons, may have a delayed onset (up to 14 days, the period of initial sensitization), and shows histologic features of allergic contact dermatitis.

Action Spectrum

Chemicals known to cause photosensitivity (photosensitizers) are usually resonating compounds with a molecular weight of less than 500 daltons. Absorption of radiant energy (sunlight) by the photosensitizer produces an excited state; returning to a lower-energy state gives off energy through fluorescence, phosphorescence, charge transfer, heat, or formation of free radicals. Each photosensitizing substance absorbs only specific wavelengths of light, called its absorption spectrum. The specific wavelengths of light that evoke a photosensitive reaction are called the action spectrum. The action spectrum is included in the absorption spectrum of the photosensitizing chemical. The action spectrum that produces phototoxicity is mostly in the long ultraviolet (UVA) region and may extend into the visible light region (320–425 nm).

Photosensitivity reactions occur only when there is sufficient concentration of the photosensitizer in the skin, and when the skin is exposed to a sufficient intensity and duration of light in the action spectrum of that photosensitizer. The intensity of the photosensitivity reaction is generally dose dependent and is worse with a greater dose of photosensitizer and greater light exposure.

Phototoxic Reactions

A phototoxic reaction is a nonimmunologic reaction that develops after exposure to a specific wavelength and intensity of light in the presence of a photosensitizing substance. It is a sunburn-type reaction, with erythema, tenderness, and even blistering occurring only on the sun-exposed parts. This type of reaction can be elicited in many persons who have no previous history of exposure or sensitivity to that particular substance, but individual susceptibility

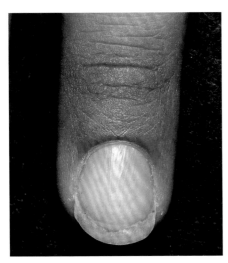

Fig. 3.17 Photo-onycholysis from minocycline.

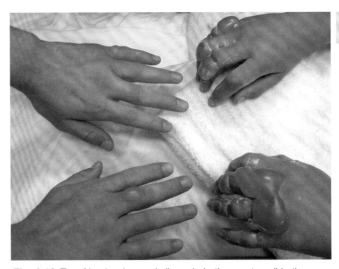

Fig. 3.18 Two friends who made limeade in the sun to sell in the summer.

varies widely. In general, to elicit a phototoxic reaction, a considerably greater amount of the photosensitizing substance is necessary than that needed to induce a photoallergic reaction. The erythema begins, as with any sunburn, within 2–6 hours but worsens for 48–96 hours before beginning to subside. Exposure of the nail bed may lead to onycholysis, called photo-onycholysis (Fig. 3.17). Phototoxic reactions, especially from topically applied photosensitizers, may cause marked hyperpigmentation, even without significant preceding erythema.

Phototoxic Tar Dermatitis. Coal tar, creosote, crude coal tar, or pitch, in conjunction with sunlight exposure, may induce a sunburn reaction associated with a severe burning sensation. These volatile hydrocarbons may be airborne, so the patient may give no history of touching tar products. The burning and erythema may continue for 1–3 days. Although up to 70% of white persons exposed to such a combination develop this reaction, persons with type V or VI skin are protected by their constitutive skin pigmentation. After the acute reaction, hyperpigmentation occurs, which may persist for years. Coal tar or its derivatives may be found in cosmetics, drugs, dyes, insecticides, and disinfectants.

Phytophotodermatitis. Furocoumarins in many plants may cause a phototoxic reaction when they come in contact with skin that is exposed to UVA light. This is called phytophotodermatitis. Several hours after exposure, a burning erythema occurs, followed by edema and the development of vesicles or bullae. An intense residual hyperpigmentation results that may persist for weeks or months. The intensity of the initial phototoxic reaction may be mild and may not be recalled by the patient despite significant hyperpigmentation. Fragrance products containing bergapten, a component of oil of bergamot, will produce this reaction. If a fragrance containing this 5-methoxypsoralen or other furocoumarin is applied to the skin before exposure to the sun or tanning lights, berloque dermatitis may result. This hyperpigmentation, which may be preceded by redness and edema, occurs primarily on the neck and face. Artificial bergapten-free bergamot oil and laws limiting the use of furocoumarins in Europe and the United States have made this a rare condition. However, "Florida Water" and "Kananga Water" colognes, formerly popular in the Hispanic, African American, and Caribbean communities, contain this potent photosensitizer and can still be ordered online, as can other aromatherapy products containing furocoumarins.

Most phototoxic plants are in the Umbelliferae, Rutaceae (rue), Compositae, and Moraceae families. Incriminated plants include

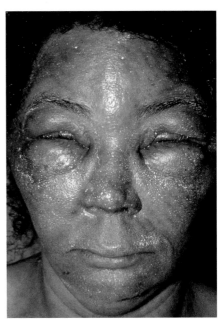

Fig. 3.19 Severe phytophototoxicity.

agrimony, angelica, atrillal, bavachi, buttercup, common rice, cowslip, dill, fennel, fig, garden and wild carrot, garden and wild parsnip, gas plant, goose foot, zabon, lime and Persian lime (Fig. 3.18), lime bergamot, masterwort, mustard, parsley, St. John's wort, and yarrow. In Hawaii, the anise-scented mokihana berry *(Pelea anisata)* was known to natives for its phototoxic properties (mokihana burn). It is a member of the rue family. Exposure through limes used to flavor gin and tonics and Mexican beer may result in phototoxic reactions in outdoor bartenders and their customers. Home tanning solutions containing fig leaves can produce phytophotodermatitis. These conditions may be widespread and severe enough to require burn unit management (Fig. 3.19).

Occupational disability from exposure to the pink rot fungus *(Sclerotinia sclerotiorum),* present on celery roots, occurs in celery farmers. In addition, disease-resistant celery contains furocoumarins and may produce phytophotodermatitis in grocery workers. Usually, insufficient sensitizing furocoumarin is absorbed from dietary exposure; however, ingested herbal remedies may cause systemic phototoxicity.

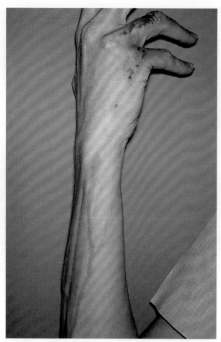

Fig. 3.20 Phytophotodermatitis; the patient had rinsed her hair with lime juice on the beach in Mexico.

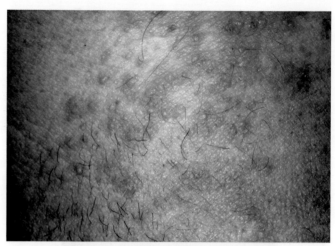

Fig. 3.21 Polymorphous light eruption, papular type.

Dermatitis bullosa striata pratensis (grass or meadow dermatitis) is a phytophotodermatitis caused by contact not with grass, but with yellow-flowered meadow parsnip or a wild, yellow-flowered herb of the rose family. The eruption consists of streaks and bizarre configurations with vesicles and bullae that heal with residual hyperpigmentation. The usual cause is sunbathing in fields containing the phototoxic plants. Similarly, tourists in the tropics may rinse their hair with lime juice outdoors, and streaky hyperpigmentation of the arms and back will result where the lime juice runs down (Fig. 3.20).

Blistering phytophotodermatitis must be differentiated from rhus dermatitis. The vesicles and bullae of rhus are not necessarily limited to the sun-exposed areas, and itching is the most prominent symptom. Lesions continue to occur in rhus dermatitis for a week or more. In phytophotodermatitis, the reaction is limited to sun-exposed sites, a burning pain appears within 48 hours, and marked hyperpigmentation results. The asymmetry, atypical shapes, and streaking of the lesions are helpful in establishing the diagnosis. These features may lead to a misdiagnosis of child abuse.

Treatment of a severe, acute reaction is similar to the management of a sunburn, with cool compresses, mild analgesics if required, and topical emollients. Use of topical steroids and strict sun avoidance immediately after the injury may protect against the hyperpigmentation. The hyperpigmentation is best managed by "tincture of time."

Carlsen K, et al: Phytophotodermatitis in 19 children admitted to hospital and their differential diagnosis. J Am Acad Dermatol 2007; 57: S88.

Krakowski AC, et al: Severe photo-oxidative injury from over-the-counter skin moisturizer. J Emerg Med 2015; 49: e105.

Machado M, et al: Phytophotodermatitis. BMJ Case Rep 2015 Dec 23; 2015.

Maloney FJ, et al: Iatrogenic phytophotodermatitis resulting from herbal treatment of an allergic contact dermatitis. Clin Exp Dermatol 2006; 31: 39.

Moustafa GA, et al: Skin disease after occupational dermal exposure to coal tar. Int J Dermatol 2015; 54: 868.

Pfurtscheller K, Trop M: Phototoxic plant burns. Pediatr Dermatol 2014; 31: e156.

Raam R, et al: Phytophotodermatitis. Ann Emerg Med 2016; 67: 554.

Sasseville D: Clinical patterns of phytodermatitis. Dermatol Clin 2009; 27: 299.

Zaias N, et al: Finger and toenail onycholysis. J Eur Acad Dermatol Venereol 2015; 29: 848.

Idiopathic Photosensitivity Disorders

This idiopathic group includes the photosensitivity diseases for which no cause is known. These disorders are not associated with external photosensitizers (except for some cases of chronic actinic dermatitis) or inborn errors of metabolism.

Polymorphous Light Eruption

Polymorphous light eruption (PLE, PMLE) is the most common form of photosensitivity. In various studies of Northern European white persons, a history of PLE can be elicited in between 5% and 20% of the adult population. It represents about one quarter of all photosensitive patients in referral centers. All races and skin types can be affected. The onset is typically in the first four decades of life, and females outnumber males by 2 : 1 or 3 : 1. The pathogenesis is unknown, but a family history may be elicited in 10%–50% of patients. Some investigators report that 10%– 20% of patients with PLE may have positive antinuclear antigens (ANAs) and a family history of lupus erythematosus. Photosensitive SLE patients may give a history of PLE-like eruptions for years before the diagnosis of SLE is made. PLE patients should be followed for the development of symptoms of SLE.

Clinically, the eruption may have several different morphologies, although in the individual patient, the morphology is usually constant. The papular (or erythematopapular) variant is the most common, but papulovesicular, eczematous, erythematous, and plaquelike lesions also occur (Fig. 3.21). Plaquelike lesions are more common in elderly patients and may closely simulate lupus erythematosus, with indurated, erythematous, fixed lesions. In African Americans, a pinpoint papular variant has been observed, closely simulating lichen nitidus but showing spongiotic dermatitis histologically (Fig. 3.22). Scarring and atrophy do not occur; in darkly pigmented races, however, marked postinflammatory hyperpigmentation or hypopigmentation may be present. In some patients, pruritus only, without an eruption, may be reported (PLE sine eruptione). Some of these patients will develop typical PLE later in life.

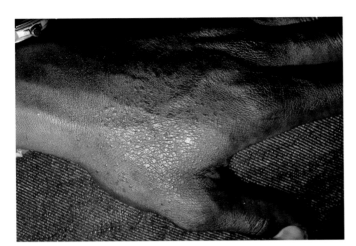

Fig. 3.22 Polymorphous light eruption, micropapular variant resembling lichen nitidus.

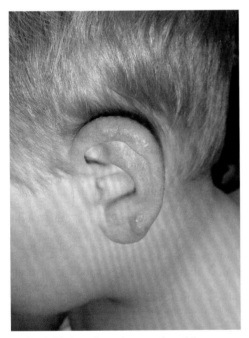

Fig. 3.23 Juvenile spring eruption of the ears.

The lesions of PLE appear most often 1–4 days after exposure to sunlight, although patients may report itching and erythema during sun exposure and development of lesions within the first 24 hours. A change in the amount of sun exposure appears to be more critical than the absolute amount of radiation. Patients living in tropical climates may be free of eruption, only to develop disease when they move to temperate zones, where there is more marked seasonal variation in UV intensity. Areas of involvement include the face, the V area of the chest, neck, and arms. In general, for each individual, certain areas are predisposed. Typically, however, areas protected during the winter, such as the extensor forearms, are particularly affected, whereas areas exposed all year (face and dorsa of hands) may be relatively spared. The eruption appears most frequently in the spring. The eruption often improves with continued sun exposure (hardening), so patients may be clear of the condition in the summer or autumn.

An unusual variant of PLE is juvenile spring eruption of the ears (Fig. 3.23). This occurs most frequently in boys age 5–12 years but may also be found in young adult males. It presents in the spring, often after sun exposure on cold but sunny days. The typical lesions are grouped small papules or papulovesicles on the helices. Lesions may form visible vesicles and crusting. Juvenile spring eruption of the ears is self-limited and does not scar. UVA is the inducing spectrum, and some patients also have lesions of PLE elsewhere. The histologic picture is identical to that of PLE. Another localized variant of PLE is spring and summer eruption of the elbows, but this occurs in adults, equally in men and women.

Histologically, a perivascular, predominantly T-cell infiltrate is present in the upper and middle dermis. There is often edema and endothelial swelling, with occasional neutrophils. Epidermal changes are variable, with spongiosis and exocytosis most often observed. Occasionally, a virtual absence of findings microscopically may paradoxically be reported and has been referred to as pauci-inflammatory photodermatitis.

The reported action spectrum of PLE varies, possibly depending on the different ethnic backgrounds of reported populations. UVA is most often responsible; however, UVB and both wavelengths in combination are also frequently necessary. Patients often report eruptions following sun exposure through window glass. Although rare, visible light sensitivity can also occur. Typically, women are more sensitive than men to UVA only, and men are more sensitive to visible light. Men, although the minority of PLE patients, tend to have more severe PLE and broader wavelengths of sensitivity. Most patients react more in affected sites, and in some, lesions can only be induced in affected areas. Phototesting produces variable results. One protocol produced positive results in 83% of tested patients using four exposures of UVB, UVA, or a combination in previously affected sites. However, the light sources are not readily available, and reported protocols vary widely. In clinical practice, the diagnosis is usually made clinically.

The differential diagnosis of PLE includes lupus erythematosus, photosensitive drug eruption, prurigo nodularis, and photoallergic contact dermatitis. Histopathologic examination, ANA testing, and direct immunofluorescence (DIF) are helpful in distinguishing these diseases. Serologic testing alone may not distinguish PLE from SLE because of the possibility of positive ANA tests in PLE patients. Lupus erythematosus may present initially with photosensitivity before other features of lupus occur. Sebaceous neutrophilic adenitis, is characterized by erythematous circinate plaques on the head, neck, and upper chest and has been reported in the first to second month of spring. Histologically, neutrophilic infiltration of the sebaceous glands occurs, sometimes forming microabscesses. Although it may be photoinduced, it may also be idiopathic as in the cases reported in the genital area. Acute pustular folliculitis is a recurrent eruption of the head and neck that may be photoinduced, viral associated, or idiopathic. It resolves in most cases spontaneously in several days. The presence of follicular pustules distinguishes the photoinduced cases from PLE.

Therapeutically, most patients with mild PLE can be managed by avoiding the sun and using barrier protection and high-SPF, broad-spectrum sunscreens. It is critical that the sunblocks contain specific absorbers or blockers (ecamsule, avobenzone, titanium dioxide, zinc oxide) of long-wave UVA because this is the most common triggering wavelength. Sunblocks containing more than one of these agents are more effective. DermaGard film can be applied to windows at home and in the car to block the transmission of almost all UVB and UVA rays while allowing visible light to be transmitted. Degradation does occur, so the film should be replaced every 5 years. These measures of photoprotection are critical for all patients, because they are free of toxicity and reduce the amount and duration of other therapies required. Patient education is important in the management of PLE. Phototesting may be required to convince patients that they are UV sensitive and will also determine the action spectrum.

The use of topical tacrolimus ointment at night or twice daily, combined with the previous measures for sun avoidance and the use of sunscreens, controls PLE in many patients. At times, topical steroids, frequently of super or high potency and in several daily to weekly pulses, are necessary to control the pruritus and clear the eruption. Antihistamines may be used for pruritus. Systemic corticosteroids in short courses may be necessary, especially in the spring. In patients whose condition is not controlled by these measures, hardening in the spring with UVB, narrow-band (NB) UVB, or psoralen plus UVA (PUVA) can dramatically decrease the sun sensitivity of patients with PLE, and up to 80% can be controlled with phototherapy. In the most sensitive patients, systemic steroids may be needed at the inception of the phototherapy. Systemic hydroxychloroquine sulfate, 200–400 mg/day, may be used. It has a delayed onset and is best instituted in the late winter to prevent spring outbreaks. Chloroquine or quinacrine may be effective if hydroxychloroquine is not, but in general, antimalarials are inferior to phototherapy. In the most severe cases, management with azathioprine, cyclosporine, thalidomide, or mycophenolate mofetil may be considered. If these agents are used in a patient considered to have PLE, an evaluation for chronic actinic dermatitis should be performed because patients with PLE rarely require these agents.

Actinic Prurigo

Actinic prurigo probably represents a variant of PLE; it is most often seen in Native Americans of North and Central America and Colombia. The incidence in Mexico has been reported at between 1.5% and 3.5%. It has been reported in Europe, Australia, and Japan as well. The female/male ratio is between 2 : 1 and 6 : 1. Actinic prurigo in Native Americans in the United States begins before age 10 in 45% of cases and before age 20 in 72%. Up to 75% of patients have a positive family history (hereditary PLE of Native Americans). In Europe, 80% of cases occur before age 10. In the Inuit Canadian population, onset is later and frequently in adulthood.

In childhood, lesions begin as small papules or papulovesicles that crust and become impetiginized. They are intensely pruritic and frequently excoriated. In children, the cheeks, distal nose, ears, and lower lip are typically involved. Cheilitis may be the initial and only feature for years. Conjunctivitis is seen in 10%–20% of patients (limbal-type vernal catarrh). Lesions of the arms and legs are also common and usually exhibit a prurigo nodule–like configuration (Fig. 3.24). The eruption may extend to involve

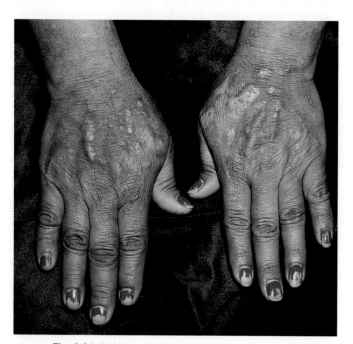

Fig. 3.24 Actinic prurigo, prurigo nodularis–like lesions.

sun-protected areas, especially the buttocks, but lesions in these areas are always less severe. In adults, chronic, dry papules and plaques are most typical, and cheilitis and crusting occur less frequently. Skin lesions tend to persist throughout the year in the tropics but are clearly worse during periods of increased sun exposure. In temperate and high-latitude regions, lesions occur from March through the summer and substantially remit in the winter. Hardening, as seen with PLE, does not occur. In up to 60% of patients with actinic prurigo that present before age 20, the condition improves or resolves within 5 years, whereas adults usually have the disease throughout life.

Initial therapy is identical to that for PLE. Thalidomide has been used effectively and safely over many years for this condition. In patients refractory to or intolerant of thalidomide, cyclosporine can be effective. Topical cyclosporine 2% may be effective in controlling limbal lesions of actinic prurigo–associated conjunctivitis.

Boonstra HE, et al: Polymorphous light eruption. J Am Acad Dermatol 2000; 42: 199.

Chantorn R, et al: Photosensitivity disorders in children. J Am Acad Dermatol 2012; 67: 1093.e1.

Gruber-Wackernagel A, et al: Polymorphous light eruption. Dermatol Clin 2014; 32: 315.

Honigsmann H: Polymorphous light eruption. Photodermatol Photoimmunol Photomed 2008; 24: 155.

Kerr AC: Actinic prurigo deterioration due to degradation of DermaGard window film. Br J Dermatol 2007; 157: 609.

LaBerge L, et al: Actinic superficial folliculitis in a 29-year-old man. J Cutan Med Surg 2012; 16: 191.

Millard TP, et al: Familial clustering of PLE in relatives of patients with lupus erythematosus. Br J Dermatol 2001; 144: 334.

Molina-Riuz AM, et al: Spring and summer eruption of the elbows. J Am Acad Dermatol 2013; 68: 306.

Patel DC, et al: Efficacy of short-course oral prednisolone in PLE: a randomized controlled trial. Br J Dermatol 2000; 143: 828.

Plaza JA, et al: Actinic prurigo cheilitis. Am J Dermatopathol 2016; 38: 418.

Schornagel IJ, et al: Diagnostic phototesting in PLE. Br J Dermatol 2005; 153: 1220.

Stratigos AJ, et al: Juvenile spring eruption. J Am Acad Dermatol 2004; 50: 57.

Su W, et al: Photodermatitis with minimal inflammatory infiltrate. Am J Dermatopathol 2006; 28: 482.

Tohyama M, et al: Two cases of genital neutrophilic sebaceous adenitis. J Dermatol 2016; 43: 1221.

Trelles AS, et al: A new case of sebaceous neutrophilic adenitis. J Am Acad Dermatol 2009; 60: 887.

Valbuena, MC et al: Actinic prurigo. Dermatol Clin 2014; 32: 335

Van de Pas CB, et al: An optimal method of photoprovocation of PLE. Arch Dermatol 2004; 140: 286.

Yong Gee SA, et al: Long-term thalidomide for actinic prurigo. Australas J Dermatol 2001; 42: 281.

Brachioradial Pruritus

PLE may present initially and only on the brachioradial area. This type of brachioradial eruption was the initial pattern of brachioradial pruritus described and was termed solar pruritus (Fig. 3.25). The majority of cases of brachioradial pruritus, especially those characterized by severe, refractory, intractable pruritus and secondary severe lichenification, are now thought to represent a form of neuropathic pruritus, sometimes related to cervical spine disease (see Chapter 4). Sunlight may be an eliciting factor and cervical spine disease a predisposing factor in patients with brachioradial pruritus. To identify those patients in whom photosensitivity plays a prominent role, a high-SPF (UVA/UVB)

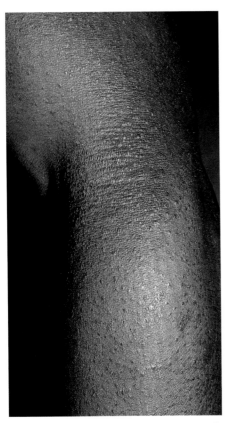

Fig. 3.25 Polymorphous light eruption, brachioradial distribution.

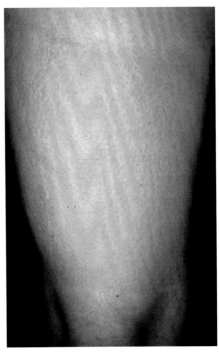

Fig. 3.26 Solar urticaria.

sunscreen should be applied to one arm only for several weeks. In patients with PLE, this usually leads to improvement of that one arm compared with the contralateral unprotected arm. In patients with primarily neuropathic disease, sunscreen application leads to minimal improvement. The capsaicin patch provides both itch relief and a physical barrier but is expensive.

Solar Urticaria

Solar urticaria is most common in women age 20–40. Within seconds to minutes after light exposure, typical urticarial lesions appear and resolve in 1–2 hours, rarely lasting more than 24 hours (Fig. 3.26). Delayed reactions rarely occur. Chronically exposed sites may have some reduced sensitivity. In severe attacks, syncope, bronchospasm, and anaphylaxis may occur.

Patients with solar urticaria may be sensitive to wavelengths over a broad spectrum. The wavelengths of sensitivity and the minimal urticarial doses (MUDs) may vary with anatomical site and over time within the same patient. UVA sensitivity is the most common, but visible light sensitivity is also frequently reported. The photosensitivity can be passively transferred, and irradiation of the patient's serum with the activating wavelength followed by reinjection will create a wheal in the patient, but not in an unaffected patient. This suggests the presence of a circulating photoinducible allergen to which the individual patient with solar urticaria is sensitive. In some patients, an inhibition spectrum may be identified that inhibits the binding of the endogenous photoallergen to mast cells.

Solar urticaria is virtually always idiopathic. Rarely, medications such as tetracycline (but not minocycline), chlorpromazine, progestational agents, and repirinast have been reported to induce solar urticaria. Erythropoietic protoporphyria and more rarely porphyria cutanea tarda may present with lesions simulating solar urticaria. There are rare reports of solar urticaria in patients with lupus erythematosus.

The diagnosis of solar urticaria is usually straightforward from the history. Phototesting is useful to determine the wavelengths of sensitivity and to ascertain the MUD if UVA desensitization is being considered.

Because many patients have sensitivity in the UVA or even visible range, broad-spectrum sunscreens should be instituted. Antihistamines, especially the nonsedating H1 agents loratadine, cetirizine HCl, and fexofenadine, may increase the MUD 10-fold or more. Higher doses, twice or more the standard recommendation, may be required. These drugs, plus sun avoidance and broad-spectrum sunscreens, are the first-line therapy. The leukotriene receptor antagonist motelukast may provide additive efficacy when used in combination with the above regimen. PUVA or increasing UVA exposures are effective in more difficult cases, with PUVA having greater efficacy. Rush hardening may induce UVA tolerance, allowing patients to begin PUVA therapy. PUVA is effective, even if the patient is not sensitive to UVA. Cyclosporine (4.5 mg/kg/day) and intravenous immune globulin at various doses and time frames have been anecdotally reported as effective. For the most difficult cases, plasmapheresis may be used to remove the circulating photoallergen, allowing PUVA to be given and leading to remission. Multiple reports attest to positive responses in some patients with the use of omalizumab.

Aubin F, et al: Severe and refractory solar urticaria treated with intravenous immunoglobulins. J Am Acad Dermatol 2014; 71: 948.

Beattie PE, et al: Characteristics and prognosis of idiopathic solar urticaria. Arch Dermatol 2003; 139: 1149.

Botto NC, et al: Solar urticaria. J Am Acad Dermatol 2008; 59: 909.

de Dios-Velázquez Á, et al: Effectiveness of omalizumab in severe solar urticaria. Ann Allergy Asthma Immunol 2016; 116: 260.

Goetze S, Elsner P: Solar urticaria. J Dtsch Dermatol Ges 2015; 13: 1250.

Levi A, Enk CD: Treatment of solar urticaria using antihistamine and leukotriene receptor antagonist combinations tailored to disease severity. Photodermatol Photoimmunol Photomed 2015; 31: 302.

Metz M, et al: Retreatment with omalizumab results in rapid remission in chronic spontaneous and inducible urticaria. JAMA Dermatol 2014; 150: 288.

Mori N, et al: Successful treatment with UVA rush hardening in a case of solar urticaria. Eur J Dermatol 2014; 24: 117.

Steinke S, et al: Cost-effectiveness of an 8% capsaicin patch in the treatment of brachioradial pruritus and notalgia paresthetica, two forms of neuropathic pruritus. Acta Derm Venereol 2017; 97: 71.

Veien NK, et al: Brachioradial pruritus. Acta Derm Venereol 2011; 91: 183

Yap LM, et al: Drug-induced solar urticaria due to tetracycline. Australas J Dermatol 2000; 41: 181.

Hydroa Vacciniforme

Hydroa vacciniforme is a rare, chronic photodermatosis with onset in childhood. Boys and girls are equally represented, but boys present earlier and on average have longer-lasting disease. There is a bimodal onset, between ages 1 and 7 and between 12 and 16. The natural history of the typical disorder is spontaneous remission before age 20, but rare cases in young adults do occur. Within 6 hours of exposure, stinging begins. At 24 hours or sooner, erythema and edema appear, followed by the characteristic 2–4 mm vesicles. Over the next few days, these lesions rupture, become centrally necrotic, and heal with a smallpox-like scar. Lesions tend to appear in crops with disease-free intervals. The ears, nose, cheeks, and extensor arms and hands are affected. Subungual hemorrhage, ocular involvement, or oral ulcerations may occur.

Histologically, early lesions show intraepidermal vesiculation and dermal edema that evolve into a subepidermal blister. Necrotic lesions show reticular degeneration of keratinocytes, with epidermal necrosis flanked by spongiosis with a dense perivascular infiltrate of neutrophils and lymphocytes. Dermal vessels may be thrombosed, simulating vasculitis. Lesions may be reproduced by repetitive UVA, with the action spectrum in the 330–360 nm range.

The differential diagnosis includes PLE, actinic prurigo, and erythropoietic protoporphyria. Porphyrin levels are normal in hydroa vacciniforme. In erythropoietic protoporphyria, the burning typically begins within minutes of sun exposure, and over time patients develop diffuse, thickened, waxlike scarring, rather than the smallpox-like scars of hydroa vacciniforme. Histologic evaluation, DIF and porphyrin studies are useful in distinguishing these two conditions. Treatment is principally to avoid sunlight exposure and to use broad-spectrum sunscreens that block in the UVA range. Prophylactic NB UVB phototherapy in the early spring may be effective. Choloroquine and systemic corticosteroids have provided relief in some cases.

A subset of children and less often adults with photosensitive hydroa vacciniforme–like skin lesions manifest facial swelling, indurated nodules or progressive ulcers, fever, and liver damage. Oral, esophageal, or colonic ulcerations may occur. Hypersensitivity to mosquito bites may also be seen. These patients may develop Epstein-Barr virus (EBV)–associated natural killer (NK) cell/T-cell lymphomas and die of this or a hemophagocytic syndrome. The hydroa vacciniforme–like skin lesions may precede the diagnosis of the lymphoma by up to a decade. Initially the patient may appear to have typical hydroa vacciniforme of the self-limited type; older age is more concerning for a complex course. This is therefore a disease spectrum, with both typical and severe hydroa vacciniforme being EBV associated. Treatment of the lymphoma may lead to clearing of these lesions.

Chantorn R, et al: Photosensitivity disorders in children. J Am Acad Dermatol 2012; 67: 1093.e1.

Eminger LA, et al: Epstein-Barr virus: dermatologic associations and implications: part II. J Am Acad Dermatol 2015; 72: 21.

Gupta G, et al: Hydroa vacciniforme. J Am Acad Dermatol 2000; 42: 208.

Hall LD, et al: Epstein-Barr virus: dermatologic associations and implications: part I. J Am Acad Dermatol 2015; 72: 1.

Magaña M, et al: Clinicopathologic features of hydroa vacciniforme-like lymphoma. Am J Dermatopathol 2016; 38: 20.

Miyake T, et al: Survival rates and prognostic factors of Epstein-Barr virus-associated hydroa vacciniforme and hypersensitivity to mosquito bites. Br J Dermatol 2015; 172: 56.

Nitiyarom R, Wongpraparut C: Hydroa vacciniforme and solar urticaria. Dermatol Clin 2014; 32: 345.

Poligone B: Risk of mortality in hydroa vacciniforme and hypersensitivity to mosquito bites. Br J Dermatol 2015; 172: 5.

Chronic Actinic Dermatitis

Chronic actinic dermatitis represents the end stage of progressive photosensitivity in some patients. It has replaced the terms persistent light reactivity, actinic reticuloid, photosensitive eczema, and chronic photosensitivity dermatitis. The basic components of this disease are as follows:

- Persistent, chronic, eczematous eruption in the absence of exposure to known photosensitizers
- Usually, broad-spectrum photosensitivity with decreased MED to UVA and/or UVB and at times visible light
- Histology consistent with a chronic dermatitis, with or without features of lymphoma

Clinically, chronic actinic dermatitis predominantly affects middle-age or elderly men. In the United States patients with skin types V and VI may be disproportionately affected (Fig. 3.27). Skin lesions consist of edematous, scaling, thickened patches and plaques that tend to be confluent. Lesions occur primarily or most severely on the exposed skin and may spare the upper eyelids, behind the ears, and the bottom of wrinkles. Involvement of unexposed sites often occurs, progressing to erythroderma in the most severe cases. Marked depigmentation resembling vitiligo

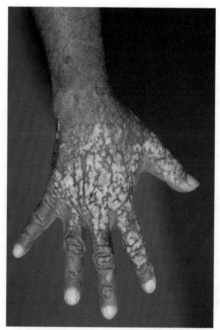

Fig. 3.27 Chronic actinic dermatitis.

may result. Patients may not realize their condition is exacerbated by exposure to light. It may persist in all seasons.

The pathogenesis of this syndrome is unknown. In some patients, a preceding topical or oral photosensitizer may be implicated, but chronic actinic dermatitis fails to improve with discontinuation of the inciting agent. In about one third of patients, photopatch testing yields a positive response to previously applied agents, especially musk ambrette, sunscreen ingredients, *p*-phenylenediamine, and hexachlorophene. Patch testing to standard agents may have a positive result in about 30% of patients, but no particular relevance is found. However, in approximately 65% of European patients, sesquiterpene lactone contact sensitivity from Compositae has been identified. In addition, more than 75% of men over age 60 with sesquiterpene lactone sensitivity have abnormal phototesting results. CD8 (suppressor/cytotoxic) T cells are disproportionately represented in the cutaneous infiltrates in the majority of patients and less frequently in the peripheral blood. IgE levels may be elevated.

In this clinical setting, diagnosis of chronic actinic dermatitis is established by histologic evaluation and phototesting. Phototesting often reproduces the lesions. About 65% of patients are sensitive to UVA, UVB, and visible light; 22% to UVA and UVB; and 5% to UVB or UVA only. The finding of photosensitivity to UVA and UVB helps to differentiate chronic actinic dermatitis from drug-induced photosensitivity, in which patients usually exhibit only UVA photosensitivity. PLE, photoallergic contact dermatitis, airborne contact dermatitis, and mycosis fungoides or Sézary syndrome must be excluded. PLE is excluded by the broad-spectrum–reduced MED in chronic actinic dermatitis, although some patients may begin with a PLE-like disease that later meets the criteria for chronic actinic dermatitis. Contact dermatitis is excluded by patch and photopatch testing. Mycosis fungoides may be difficult to differentiate from chronic actinic dermatitis in cases with atypical histology. Phototesting is critical in these patients. Mycosis fungoides will manifest a T-cell receptor rearrangement in lesional skin or peripheral blood and usually shows a CD4 (helper) T-cell predominance.

Therapy for chronic actinic dermatitis includes identifying possible topical photosensitizers by photopatch testing and scrupulously avoiding them. Maximum sun avoidance and broad-spectrum sunscreens are essential. Topical tacrolimus is useful in many patients. Topical and systemic steroids are effective in some patients, but chronic toxicity of systemic steroids limits chronic use. Azathioprine, 50–200 mg/day, is the most reproducibly effective treatment and may be required annually during periods of increased sun intensity. Low-dose PUVA or NB UVB can be effective when used with topical and systemic steroids, but patients may also be intolerant of this approach. Hydroxyurea, 500 mg twice daily, cyclosporine, thalidomide, and mycophenolate mofetil may also be used. Immunosuppressive agents may allow patients to tolerate PUVA therapy. With careful management, about 2 in 10 patients will lose their photosensitivity within 5 years, 1 in 4 by 10 years, and 1 in 3 of patients by 15 years. Most of the remaining will improve over this time with only one of 20 worsening in a study by Wolverton et al.

Beach RA, et al: Chronic actinic dermatitis. J Cutan Med Surg 2009; 13: 121.

Chew AL, et al: Contact and photocontact sensitization in chronic actinic dermatitis. Contact Dermatitis 2010; 62: 42.

Choi D, et al: Evaluation of patients with photodermatoses. Dermatol Clin 2014; 32: 267.

Dawe RS, et al: The natural history of chronic actinic dermatitis. Arch Dermatol 2000; 136: 1215.

Ibbotson S: How should we diagnose and manage photosensitivity? J R Coll Physicians Edinb 2014; 44: 308.

Ma Y, et al: Treatment with topical tacrolimus favors chronic actinic dermatitis. J Dermatol Treat 2010; 21: 171.

Paek SY, Lim HW: Chronic actinic dermatitis. Dermatol Clin 2014; 32: 355.

Wolverton JE, et al: The natural history of chronic actinic dermatitis. Dermatitis 2014; 25: 27.

Photosensitivity and HIV Infection

Photosensitivity resembling PLE, actinic prurigo, or chronic actinic dermatitis is seen in about 5% of patients with human immunodeficiency virus (HIV) infection. In general, photosensitivity is seen when the CD4 count is below 200 (often <50), except in persons with a genetic predisposition (Native Americans). Photosensitivity may be the initial manifestation of HIV disease. African American patients are disproportionately represented among patients with HIV photosensitivity. Photosensitivity may be associated with ingestion of a photosensitizing medication, especially NSAIDs, efavirenz (an antiretroviral) or trimethoprim-sulfamethoxazole, but the skin eruption often does not improve even when the medication is discontinued. Histologically, the lesions may show subacute or chronic dermatitis, often with a dense dermal infiltrate with many eosinophils. Histology identical to PLE, lichen planus, or lichen nitidus may also occur. When the CD4 count is below 50, especially in black patients, chronic actinic dermatitis with features of actinic prurigo is typical. Widespread vitiliginous lesions may develop. Therapy is difficult, but thalidomide may be beneficial.

Bilu D, et al: Clinical and epidemiological characterization of photosensitivity in HIV-positive individuals. Photodermatol Photoimmunol Photomed 2004; 20: 175.

Isaacs T, et al: Annular erythema and photosensitivity as manifestations of efavirenz-induced cutaneous reactions. J Antimicrob Chemother 2013; 68: 2871.

Maurer TA, et al: Thalidomide treatment for prurigo nodularis in HIV-infected subjects. Arch Dermatol 2004; 140: 845.

Mercer JJ, et al: Photodermatitis with subsequent vitiligo-like leukoderma in HIV infection. Int J Dermatol 2016; 55: e306.

RADIODERMATITIS

The major target within the cell by which radiation damage occurs is the DNA. The effects of ionizing radiation on the cells depend on the amount of radiation, its intensity (exposure rate), and the characteristics of the individual cell. Rapidly dividing cells and anaplastic cells in general have increased radiosensitivity compared with normal tissue. When radiation therapy is delivered, it is frequently fractionated (i.e., divided into small doses). This allows the normal cells to recover between doses.

When the dose is large, cell death results. In small amounts, the effect is insidious and cumulative. Mitosis is arrested temporarily, with consequent retardation of growth. The exposure rate affects the number of chromosome breaks. The more rapid the delivery of a certain amount of radiation, the greater is the number of chromosome breaks.

Acute Radiodermatitis

When an "erythema dose" of ionizing radiation is given to the skin, there is a latent period of up to 24 hours before visible erythema appears. This initial erythema lasts 2–3 days but may be followed by a second phase beginning up to 1 week after the exposure and lasting up to 1 month. When the skin is exposed to a large amount of ionizing radiation, an acute reaction develops, the extent of which will depend on the amount, quality, genetic susceptibility, and duration of exposure. Such radiation reaction occurs in the treatment of malignancy and in accidental overexposure. The reaction is manifested by initial erythema, followed by a second phase of erythema at 3–6 days (Fig. 3.28). Vesication, edema, and

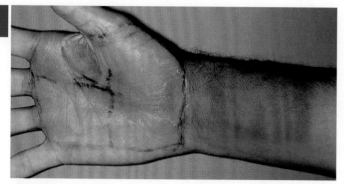

Fig. 3.28 Acute radiation burn during treatment of epithelioid sarcoma.

erosion or ulceration may occur, accompanied by pain. The skin develops a dark color that may be mistaken for hyperpigmentation but that desquamates. This type of radiation injury may subside in several weeks to several months, again depending on the amount of radiation exposure. Skin that receives a large amount of radiation will never return to normal. It will lack adnexal structures, will be dry, atrophic, and smooth, and will be hypopigmented or depigmented. Cutaneous necrosis may complicate yttrium-90 synovectomy, a treatment given for chronic synovitis.

Eosinophilic, Polymorphic, and Pruritic Eruption Associated With Radiotherapy

The polymorphic, pruritic eruption arising several days to several months after radiotherapy for cancer tends to favor the extremities. Acral excoriations, erythematous papules, vesicles, and bullae occur. It is not necessarily limited to the areas of radiation treatment. Histologically, a superficial and deep perivascular lymphohistiocytic infiltrate with eosinophils is present. Topical steroids, antihistamines, and UVB are all effective, and spontaneous resolution also occurs.

Chronic Radiodermatitis

Chronic exposure to "suberythema" doses of ionizing radiation over a prolonged period will produce varying degrees of damage to the skin and its underlying parts after a variable latent period ranging from several months to several decades. Radiodermatitis may also occur on the back or flank after fluoroscopy and roentgenography for diagnostic or therapeutic purposes (Fig. 3.29).

Telangiectasia, atrophy, and hypopigmentation with residual focal increased pigment (freckling) may appear (Fig. 3.30). The skin becomes dry, thin, smooth, and shiny. The nails may become striated, brittle, and fragmented. The capacity to repair injury is substantially reduced, resulting in ulceration from minor trauma. The hair becomes brittle and sparse. In more severe cases, these chronic changes may be followed by radiation keratoses and carcinoma. Additionally, subcutaneous fibrosis, thickening, and binding of the surface layers to deep tissues may present as tender, erythematous plaques 6–12 months after radiation therapy (Fig. 3.31). It may resemble erysipelas or inflammatory metastases.

Radiation Cancer

After a latent period averaging 20–40 years, various malignancies may develop, most frequently basal cell carcinoma (BCC), followed by squamous cell carcinoma (SCC). These may appear in sites of prior radiation, even if there is no evidence of chronic radiation damage. Sun damage may be additive to radiation therapy, increasing the appearance of nonmelanoma skin cancers. SCCs arising in sites of radiation therapy metastasize more frequently than

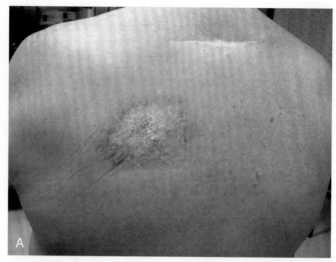

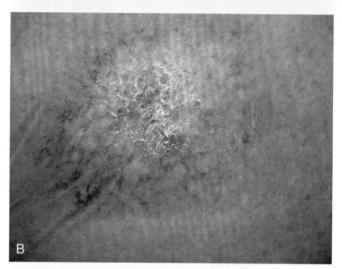

Fig. 3.29 (A) Fluoroscopy-induced radiodermatitis. (B) Close-up of Fig. 3.29A.

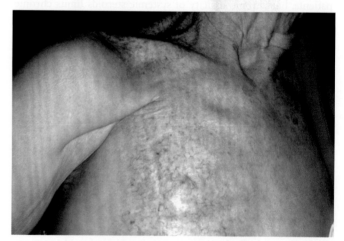

Fig. 3.30 Chronic radiodermatitis.

purely sun-induced SCCs. In some patients, either type of tumor may predominate. Location plays some role; SCCs are more common on the arms and hands, whereas BCCs are seen on the head and neck and lumbosacral area (Fig. 3.32). Other radiation-induced cancers include angiosarcoma, Kaposi sarcoma, malignant

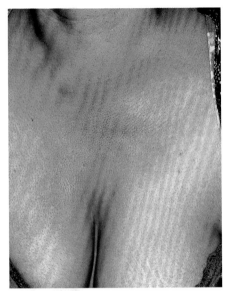

Fig. 3.31 Delayed radiation reaction 8 months after therapy.

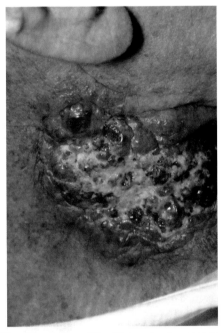

Fig. 3.32 Chronic radiodermatitis with basal cell cancer as a complication. (Courtesy Steven Binnick, MD.)

fibrous histiocytoma, sarcomas, and thyroid carcinoma. The incidence of malignant neoplasms increases with the passage of time.

Treatment

Acute radiodermatitis may be reduced with a topical corticosteroid ointment combined with an emollient cream applied twice a day and instituted at the onset of therapeutic radiotherapy. However the skin should be gently cleansed and dried shortly before radiation treatment. Chronic radiodermatitis without carcinoma requires little or no attention except protection from sunlight and the extremes of heat and cold. Careful cleansing with mild soap and water, the use of emollients, and occasionally hydrocortisone ointment are the only requirements for good care.

The early removal of precancerous keratoses and ulcerations is helpful in preventing the development of cancers. For radiation keratoses treatment with cryosurgery, 5-FU, imiquimod cream, ingenol, or topical 5-aminolevulinic acid (ALA)–photodynamic therapy may be sufficient. If the keratosis feels infiltrated, a biopsy is indicated. Radiation ulcerations should be studied by excisional or incisional biopsy if they have been present for 3 months or longer. Complete removal by excision is frequently required to obtain healing and exclude focal carcinoma in the ulceration. Radiation-induced nonmelanoma skin cancers are managed by standard methods. The higher risk of metastasis from radiation-induced SCCs mandates careful follow-up and regular regional lymph node evaluation.

Balter S, et al: Patient skin reactions from interventional fluoroscopy procedures. Am J Roentgenol 2014; 202: 335.
Cota C, et al: Localized post-radiation Kaposi sarcoma in a renal transplant immunosuppressed patient. Am J Dermatopathol 2014; 36: 270.
Davis MM, et al: Skin cancer in patients with chronic radiation dermatitis. J Am Acad Dermatol 1989; 20: 608.
Huang A, Glick SA: Genetic susceptibility to cutaneous radiation injury. Arch Dermatol Res 2017; 309: 1.
James WD, et al: Late subcutaneous fibrosis following megavoltage radiotherapy. J Am Acad Dermatol 1980; 3: 616.
Oztürk H, et al: Treatment of skin necrosis after radiation synovectomy with yttrium-90. Rheumatol Int 2008; 28: 1067.
Singh M, et al: Radiodermatitis. Am J Clin Dermatol 2016; 17: 277.
van Kester MS, Quint KD: Eosinophilic, polymorphic, and pruritic eruption associated with radiotherapy on the skin of the right breast. JAMA Oncol 2016; 2: 677.
Watt TC, et al: Radiation-related risk of basal cell carcinoma. J Natl Cancer Inst 2012; 104: 1240.
Wei KC, et al: STROBE—radiation ulcer. Medicine (Baltimore) 2015; 94: e2178.

MECHANICAL INJURIES

Mechanical factors may induce distinctive skin changes. Pressure, friction, and the introduction of foreign substances (as by injection) are some of the means by which skin injuries may occur.

Callus

Callus is a nonpenetrating, circumscribed hyperkeratosis produced by pressure. It occurs on parts of the body subject to intermittent pressure, particularly the palms and soles, and especially the bony prominences of the joints. Those engaged in various sports, certain occupations, or other repetitive activity develop callosities of distinctive size and location as stigmata. Examples are surfer's nodules, boxer's knuckle pads, jogger's toe, rower's rump, playstation thumb, milker's callus, tennis toe (Fig. 3.33), jogger's nipple, prayer callus, the yoga sign, neck callosities of violinists, pillar knocker's knuckles, bowler's hand, and Russell sign. The latter are calluses, small lacerations, or abrasions on the dorsum of the hand overlying the metacarpophalangeal and interphalangeal joints and are seen as a clue to the diagnosis of bulimia nervosa.

The callus differs from the clavus in that it has no penetrating central core and is a more diffuse thickening. Callus tends to disappear spontaneously when the pressure is removed. Most problems are encountered with calluses on the soles. Poorly fitting shoes, orthopedic problems of the foot caused by aging or a deformity of the foot exerting abnormal pressure, and high activity level are some of the etiologic factors to be considered in painful callosities of the feet.

Padding to relieve the pressure, paring of the thickened callus, and use of keratolytics such as 40% salicylic acid plasters are

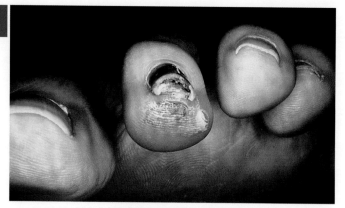

Fig. 3.33 Tennis toe.

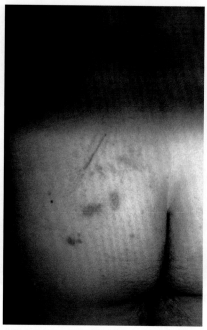

Fig. 3.34 Fire coral cuts. (Courtesy Steven Binnick, MD.)

effective means of relieving painful callosities. Use of 12% ammonium lactate lotion or a urea-containing cream is often helpful.

Clavus (Corns)

Corns are circumscribed, horny, conical thickenings with the base on the surface and the apex pointing inward and pressing on subjacent structures. There are two varieties: the hard corns, which occur on the dorsa of the toes, or subungually on the soles, and the soft corns, which occur between the toes and are softened by the macerating action of sweat. In a hard corn, the surface is shiny and polished, and when the upper layers are shaved off, a core is noted in the densest part of the lesion. It is this core that causes a dull/boring or sharp/lancinating pain by pressing on the underlying sensory nerves. Corns arise at sites of friction or pressure, and when these causative factors are removed, they spontaneously disappear. Frequently, a bony spur or exostosis is present beneath both hard and soft corns of long duration, and unless this exostosis is removed, cure is unlikely. The soft interdigital corn usually occurs in the fourth interdigital space of the foot. Frequently, there is an exostosis at the metatarsophalangeal joint that causes pressure on the adjacent toe. These are soft, soggy, and macerated so that they appear white. Treatment by simple excision may be effective.

Plantar corns must be differentiated from plantar warts. Squeezing the lesion laterally will induce pain in a wart, while pressing perpendicularly will produce pain in a corn. Paring off the surface keratin until either the pathognomonic elongated dermal papillae of the wart with its blood vessels or the clear horny core of the corn can be clearly seen is another option. Porokeratosis plantaris discreta is a sharply marginated, cone-shaped, rubbery lesion that commonly occurs beneath the metatarsal heads. Multiple lesions may occur. It has a 3:1 female predominance, is painful, and is frequently confused with a plantar wart or corn. Keratosis punctata of the creases may be seen in the creases of the toes, where it may be mistaken for a corn.

The relief of pressure or friction by corrective footwear or the application of a ring of soft felt wadding around the region of the corn will often bring a good result. Soaking the feet in hot water and paring the surface by means of a scalpel blade or pumice stone leads to symptomatic improvement. Salicylic acid is successful when carefully and diligently used. After careful paring of the corn with emphasis on removing the center core, 40% salicylic acid plaster is applied. Soaking the foot for ½ hour before reapplying the medication enhances the effect. After 48 hours, the plaster is removed, the white macerated skin is rubbed off, and a new plaster is reapplied. This is continued until the corn is gone. Punch excisions of small lesions and the Er:YAG laser ablation are other options. It should be stressed that removal of any underlying bony abnormality, if present, is often necessary to effect a cure.

Pseudoverrucous Papules and Nodules

These striking 2–8 mm, shiny, smooth, red, moist, flat-topped round lesions in the perianal area of children are considered to be a result of encopresis or urinary incontinence. There is a similarity to lesions affecting urostomy or elderly incontinent patients. Protection of the skin will help eliminate them. Similar lesions have been described in women who repeatedly apply an antifungal (Vagisil) to the groin area.

Coral Cuts

A severe type of skin injury may occur from the cuts of coral skeletons (Fig. 3.34). The abrasions and cuts are painful, and local therapy may provide little or no relief. Healing may take months. As a rule, if secondary infection is guarded against, such cuts heal as well as any others. The possibility of *Mycobacterium marinum* infection must be considered in persistent lesions.

Pressure Ulcers (Decubitus)

The bedsore, or decubitus, is a pressure ulcer produced anywhere on the body by prolonged pressure. The pressure sore is caused by ischemia of the underlying structures of the skin, fat, and muscles as a result of sustained and constant pressure. Usually, it occurs in chronically debilitated persons who are unable to change position in bed. The bony prominences of the body are the most frequently affected sites. About 95% of all pressure ulcers develop on the lower body, with 65% in the pelvic area and 30% on the legs. The ulcer usually begins with erythema at the pressure point; in a short time a "punched-out" ulcer develops. Necrosis with a grayish pseudomembrane is seen, especially in the untreated ulcer. Potential complications of pressure ulcers include sepsis, local infection, osteomyelitis, fistulas, and SCC.

More than 100 risk factors have been identified, with diabetes mellitus, peripheral vascular disease, cerebrovascular disease, sepsis, and hypotension being prominent. Pressure ulcers are graded according to a four-stage system, with the earliest being recognized by changes in skin temperature, tissue consistency, and sensation. The lesion first appears as an area of persistent redness. Stage II is a superficial ulcer involving the epidermis and/or dermis. The deeper stage III ulcers damage the subcutaneous fat and stage IV, the muscle, bone, tendon, or joint capsule.

Prevention relies on redistributing pressure at a minimum interval of 2 hours. Treatment consists of relief of the pressure on the affected parts by frequent change of position, meticulous nursing care, and use of air-filled products, liquid-filled flotation devices, or foam products. Other measures include ulcer care, management of bacterial colonization and infection, surgical repair if necessary, continual education, adequate nutrition, management of pain, and provision of psychosocial support.

Ulcer care is critical. Debridement may be accomplished by sharp, mechanical, enzymatic, and autolytic measures, at least once weekly. In some patients, operative care will be required. Stable heel ulcers are an exception; debridement is unnecessary if only a dry eschar is present. Wounds should be cleaned initially and each dressing changed by a nontraumatic technique. Normal saline rather than peroxide or povidone-iodine is best. Selection of a dressing should ensure that the ulcer tissue remains moist and the surrounding skin dry.

Occlusive dressings include more than 300 products, generally classified as films, alginates, foams, hydrogels, hydrofibers, and hydrocolloid dressings. Transparent films are used only for stage II ulcers because they provide light drainage, whereas hydrofibers are used only for full-thickness stage III and IV ulcers. Surgical debridement and closure with flaps and reconstructive procedures may be necessary. Adjuvant therapies such as ultrasound, laser, UV radiation, hyperbaric oxygen, electrical stimulation, radiant heat, application of growth factors, cultured keratinocyte grafts, skin substitutes, and miscellaneous topical and oral agents are being investigated to determine their place in the treatment of these ulcers.

At times, anaerobic organisms colonize these ulcers and cause a putrid odor. The topical application of metronidazole eliminates this odor within 36 hours.

Friction Blisters

The formation of vesicles or bullae may occur at sites of combined pressure and friction and may be enhanced by heat and moisture. The feet of military recruits in training, the palms of oarsmen who have not yet developed protective calluses, and the fingers of drummers (drummer's digits) are examples of those at risk. The size of the bulla depends on the site of the trauma. If the skin is tense and uncomfortable, the blister should be drained, but the roof should not be completely removed because it may act as its own dressing.

In studies focusing on the prevention of friction blisters of the feet in long-distance runners and soldiers, acrylic fiber socks with drying action have been found to be effective. Additionally, pretreatment with a 20% solution of aluminum chloride hexahydrate for at least 3 days has been shown to reduce foot blisters significantly after prolonged hiking, but at the expense of skin irritation. Emollients decrease the irritation but reduce the overall effectiveness of the treatment.

Fracture Blisters

Fracture blisters overlie sites of closed fractures, especially the ankle and lower leg. The blisters appear a few days to 3 weeks after the injury and are thought to be caused by vascular compromise. Fracture blisters may create complications such as infection and scarring, especially if blood filled or in diabetic patients. The blisters generally heal spontaneously in 5–14 days but may cause delay of surgical reduction of the fracture.

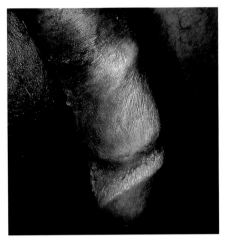

Fig. 3.35 Sclerosing lymphangitis of penis.

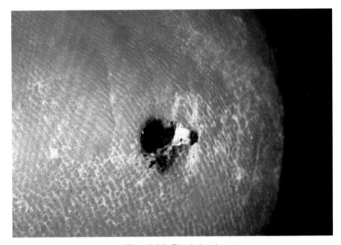

Fig. 3.36 Black heel.

Sclerosing Lymphangiitis

This lesion is a cordlike structure encircling the coronal sulcus of the penis or running the length of the shaft and has been attributed to trauma during vigorous sexual play (Fig. 3.35). Most if not all cases result from a superficial thrombophlebitis and thus has been renamed Mondor disease of the penis. Some early reports favor a lymphatic origin of some cases; CD31 and D240 stains will allow differentiation of future cases. Treatment is not necessary; sclerosing lymphangiitis follows a benign, self-limiting course.

Black Heel

Synonyms for black heel include talon noir and calcaneal petechiae. A sudden shower of minute, black, punctate macules occurs most often on the posterior edge of the plantar surface of one or both heels (Fig. 3.36), but sometimes distally on one or more toes. Black heel is often seen in basketball, volleyball, tennis, or lacrosse players. Seeming confluence may lead to mimicry of melanoma. The bleeding is caused by shearing stress of sports activities. Paring with a No. 15 blade and performing a guaiac test will confirm the diagnosis. Treatment is unnecessary.

Subcutaneous Emphysema

Free air occurring in the subcutaneous tissues is detected by the presence of cutaneous crepitations. Gas-producing organisms, especially *Clostridia*, and leakage of free air from the lungs or

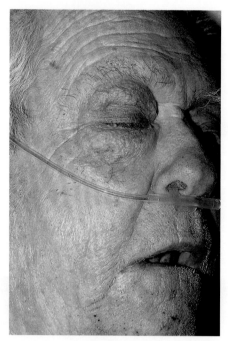

Fig. 3.37 Subcutaneous emphysema. (Courtesy Curt Samlaska, MD.)

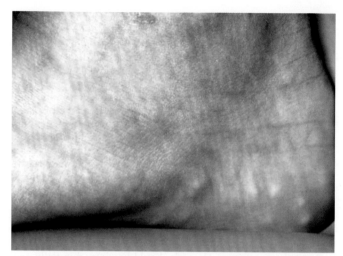

Fig. 3.38 Piezogenic papules. (Courtesy Paul Hong, MD.)

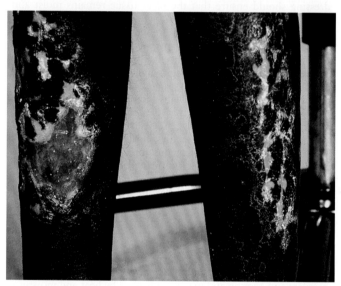

Fig. 3.39 Ulceration secondary to "skin popping."

gastrointestinal tract are the most common causes (Fig. 3.37). Samlaska et al. reviewed the wide variety of causes of subcutaneous emphysema, including penetrating and nonpenetrating injuries, iatrogenic causes occurring during various procedures in hospitalized patients, spontaneous pneumomediastinum such as may occur with a violent cough, childbirth, asthma, Boerhaave syndrome (esophageal rupture after vomiting or the Heimlich maneuver), intraabdominal causes such as inflammatory bowel disease, cancer, perirectal abscess, pancreatitis or cystitis, dental procedures when using air pressure instruments and high-speed drills, and factitial disease.

Traumatic Asphyxia

Cervicofacial cyanosis and edema; multiple petechiae of the face, neck, and upper chest; and bilateral subconjunctival hemorrhage may occur after prolonged crushing injuries of the thorax or upper abdomen. Such trauma reverses blood flow in the superior vena cava or its tributaries.

Painful Fat Herniation

Also called painful piezogenic pedal papules, this rare cause of painful feet represents fat herniations through thin fascial layers of the weight-bearing parts of the heel (Fig. 3.38). These dermatoceles become apparent when weight is placed on the heel and disappear as soon as the pressure is removed. These fat herniations are present in many people, but the majority experience no symptoms. However, extrusion of the fat tissue together with its blood vessels and nerves may initiate pain on prolonged standing. Avoidance of prolonged standing will relieve this pain. Other options include taping of the foot, use of compression stockings, or use of plastic heel cups or padded orthotic devices to restrict the herniations. Laing et al. found that 76% of 29 patients had pedal papules, and interestingly, by placing pressure on the wrists, found 86% to have piezogenic wrist papules.

Narcotic Dermopathy

Heroin (diacetylmorphine) is a narcotic prepared for injection by dissolving the heroin powder in boiling water and then injecting it. The favored route of administration is intravenous. This results in thrombosed, cordlike, thickened veins at the sites of injection. Subcutaneous injection ("skin popping") can result in multiple, scattered ulcerations, which heal with discrete atrophic scars (Fig. 3.39). In addition, amphetamines, cocaine, and other drugs may be injected. Subcutaneous injection may result in infections, complications of bacterial abscess and cellulitis, or sterile nodules, apparently acute foreign body reactions to the injected drug or the adulterants mixed with it. These lesions may ulcerate. Chronic persistent firm nodules, a combination of scar and foreign body reaction, may result. If cocaine is being injected, it may cause ulcers because of its direct vasospastic effect. Addicts will continue to inject heroin and cocaine into the chronic ulcer bed. Cocaine-associated vasculitis caused by levamisole is discussed in Chapter 35.

The cutaneous manifestations of injection of heroin and other drugs also include camptodactylia, edema of the eyelids, persistent nonpitting edema of the hands, urticaria, abscesses, atrophic scars, and hyperpigmentation. Pentazocine abuse leads to a typical clinical picture of tense woody fibrosis, irregular punched-out ulcerations, and a rim of hyperpigmentation at injection sites. Extensive calcification may occur within the thickened sites.

Arosi I, et al: Pathogenesis and treatment of callus in the diabetic foot. Curr Diabetes Rev 2016; 12: 179.

Babu AK, et al: Sclerosing lymphangitis of penis—literature review and report of 2 cases. Dermatol Online J 2014; 20: 13030/qt7gq9h1v9.

Bae JM, et al: Differential diagnosis of plantar wart from corn, callus and healed wart with the aid of dermoscopy. Br J Dermatol 2009; 160: 220.

Balevi A, et al: How I do it: treatment of plantar calluses and corns with an erbium-doped yttrium aluminum garnet laser. Dermatol Surg 2016; 42: 1304.

Del Giudice P: Cutaneous complications of intravenous drug abuse. Br J Dermatol 2004; 150: 1.

Diamond S, et al: National outcomes after pressure ulcer closure. Am Surg 2016; 82: 903.

Fleming JD, et al: Pentazocine-induced cutaneous scarring. Clin Exp Dermatol 2013; 39: 115.

Garrido-Ruiz MC, et al: Vulvar pseudoverrucous papules and nodules secondary to a urethral-vaginal fistula. Am J Dermatopathol 2011; 33: 410.

Googe AB, et al: Talon noir. Postgrad Med J 2014; 90: 730.

Haitz KA, et al: Periorbital subcutaneous emphysema mistaken by unilateral angioedema during dental crown preparation. JAMA Dermatol 2014; 150: 907.

Halawi MJ: Fracture blisters after primary total knee arthroplasty. Am J Orthop (Belle Mead NJ) 2015; 44: E291.

Hennings C, et al: Illicit drugs. J Am Acad Dermatol 2013; 69: 135.

Jensen P, et al: Cryotherapy caused widespread subcutaneous emphysema mimicking angioedema. Acta Derm Venereol 2014; 94: 241.

Knapik JJ: Prevention of foot blisters. J Spec Oper Med 2014 Summer; 14: 95.

Laing VB, et al: Piezogenic wrist papules. J Am Acad Dermatol 1991; 24: 415.

Levine SM, et al: An evidence-based approach to the surgical management of pressure ulcers. Ann Plast Surg 2012; 69: 482.

Mailler-Savage EA, et al: Skin manifestations of running. J Am Acad Dermatol 2006; 55: 290.

Niederhauser A, et al: Comprehensive programs for preventing pressure ulcers. Adv Skin Wound Care 2012; 25: 167.

Patruno C, et al: Instrument-related skin disorders in musicians. Dermatitis 2016; 27: 26.

Reddy M, et al: Treatment of pressure ulcers: a systematic review. JAMA 2008; 300: 2647.

Rocha Bde O, et al: Piezogenic pedal papules. An Bras Dermatol 2015; 90: 928.

Rudolph RI: Skin manifestations of cocaine use. J Am Acad Dermatol 2009; 60: 346.

Samlaska CP, et al: Subcutaneous emphysema. Adv Dermatol 1996; 11: 117.

Strumia R: Skin signs of anorexia nervosa. Dermatoendocrinology 2009; 1: 268.

Tayyib N, Coyer F: Effectiveness of pressure ulcer prevention strategies for adult patients in intensive care units. Worldviews Evid Based Nurs 2016; 13: 432.

Wilcox JR, et al: Frequency of debridements and time to heal. JAMA Dermatol 2013; 149: 1050.

Wolf R, Wolf D: Playstation thumb. Int J Dermatol 2014; 53: 617.

Zaiac MN, et al: Clinical pearl: the squeeze maneuver. Cutis 2016; 97: 202.

FOREIGN BODY REACTIONS

Tattoo

Tattoos result from the introduction of insoluble pigments into the skin. They may be traumatic, cosmetic, or medicinal in nature

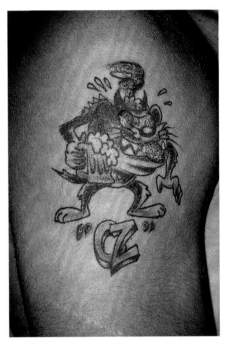

Fig. 3.40 Red tattoo reaction. (Courtesy Curt Samlaska, MD.)

and may be applied by a professional or an amateur. Pigment is applied to the skin, and needles pierce the skin to force the material into the dermis. Pigments used include carmine, indigo, vermilion, India ink, chrome green, magnesium (lilac color), Venetian red, aluminum, gold, titanium (white color) or zinc oxide, lead carbonate, copper, iron, logwood, azo and naptha-derived pigments, quinacridones, cobalt blue, cinnabar (mercuric sulfide), and cadmium sulfide. Cadmium, cobalt, mercury, and lead are not often used; however, occasional photosensitive reactions to cadmium, which was used for yellow color or to brighten the cinnabar red, are still seen. "Invisible tattoos," seen only under UV light, have ingredients such as polymethylmethacrylate and melamine that may cause granulomatous reactions.

Tattoo-associated dermopathies may be reactive (allergic, lichenoid, granulomatous, or photosensitive) (Fig. 3.40) or infective (inoculation of syphilis, infectious hepatitis, tuberculosis, HIV, warts, molluscum, Hansen disease) or may induce a Koebner response in patients with active lichen planus or psoriasis. Discoid lupus erythematosus has been reported to occur in the red-pigmented portion of tattoos. Tattoos over nevi may delay the diagnosis of melanoma. Occasionally, the tattoo marks may become keloidal. Severe allergic reactions to "temporary tattoos" (painting of pigments such as henna on surface of skin) occur when the allergen *p*-phenylenediamine is added to make the color more dramatic.

Red tattoos are the most common cause of delayed reactions, with the histologic findings typically showing a lichenoid process. Occasionally, a pseudolymphomatous reaction may occur in red tattoos. Dermatitis in areas of red (mercury), green (chromium), or blue (cobalt) have been described in patients who are patch test positive to these metals. Sarcoidal, foreign body, and allergic granulomatous reactions may also occur within tattoos; aluminum may induce such reactions.

Treatment of such reactions is with topical or intralesional steroids. Excision is also satisfactory when the lesions are small enough and situated so that ellipsoid excisions are feasible. Reactions may also be successfully treated with Q-switched lasers, at times combined with ablative fractional resurfacing Generalized allergic reactions occasionally occur; prevention by treatment with oral steroids and antihistamines has been suggested. Tattoo darkening can occur, as well as no response to laser treatment. Caution must be used when treating flesh-colored and pink-red tattoos because they may darken after treatment, likely caused by the reduction of ferric oxide to ferrous oxide. White ink, composed mostly of titanium dioxide, is often used to brighten green, blue, yellow, and purple tattoos. Laser irradiation reduces titanium to a blue-colored pigment. Test areas are recommended when treating light-colored facial tattoos. CO_2 resurfacing lasers used conservatively are an alternative to the Q-switched lasers in such patients (see Chapter 38).

Paraffinoma (Sclerosing Lipogranuloma)

Injection of oils into the skin for cosmetic purposes, such as the smoothing of wrinkles and the augmentation of breasts, was popular in the past. Paraffin, camphorated oil, cottonseed or sesame oil, mineral oil, and beeswax may produce plaquelike indurations with ulcerations within months and up to 40 years. Several reports document penile paraffinomas caused by self-injection. When petroleum jelly (Vaseline) gauze or a topical ointment is used to dress unsutured wounds, lipogranulomas or inflammatory mild erysipelas-like lesions with marked tenderness may occur. A radiofrequency device successfully treated a facial paraffinoma. Surgical removal must be wide and complete.

Granulomas

Silicone Granuloma

Liquid silicones, composed of long chains of dimethyl siloxy groups, are biologically inert. Silicones have been used for correcting wrinkles, reducing scars, and building up atrophic depressed areas of the skin. Many case reports detail granulomatous reactions to silicone, some with migration and reactive nodules at points distant from the injection site (Figs. 3.41 and 3.42). Acupuncture needles are coated with silicone, and granulomas may occur at the entry points. The incidence of the nodular swellings, which may be quite destructive and treatment resistant, remains unknown. It is clear that, if used off label, medical-grade silicone injected in small volume should be the rule, and it should not be injected into the penis or the glandular tissue of the breast.

For breast augmentation, silicone may be used as Silastic implants. If trauma causes rupture of the bag, subcutaneous fibrotic nodules often develop. Bioplastique consists of polymerized silicone particles dispersed in a gel carrier. When used for lip augmentation, nodules may develop. Histologically, these are foreign body granulomas.

Treatment of silicone granulomas is often not successful. Surgical removal may lead to fistulas, abscesses, and marked deformity. Both minocycline, 100 mg twice daily for several months, and imiquimod cream have been anecdotally useful.

Mercury Granuloma

Mercury may cause foreign body giant cell or sarcoidal-type granulomas (Fig. 3.43), pseudolymphoma, or membranous fat necrosis. It is usually identifiable as egg-shaped, extracellular, dark-gray to black, irregular globules. The gold lysis test is positive in tissues. Energy-dispersive radiographic spectroscopy may be done and will identify mercury by the characteristic emission spike. Such testing may be helpful in identifying any foreign substance suspected to have been implanted accidentally or intentionally by the patient. Systemic toxicity or embolus may develop from mercury and may result in death. Therefore excision is necessary and can be accomplished under x-ray guidance.

Beryllium Granuloma

Beryllium granuloma is seen as a chronic, persistent, granulomatous inflammation of the skin with ulceration that may follow accidental laceration, usually in an occupational setting.

Zirconium Granuloma

A papular eruption involving the axillae is sometimes seen as an allergic reaction in those shaving their armpits and using a

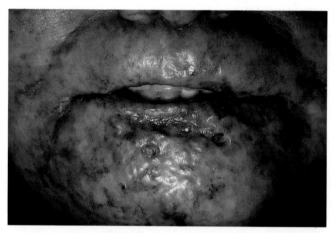

Fig. 3.42 Silicone granuloma.

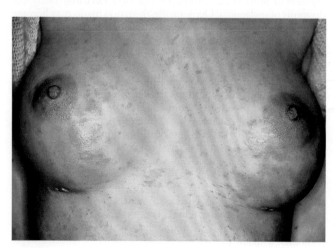

Fig. 3.41 Silicone reaction.

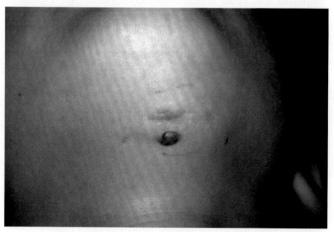

Fig. 3.43 Mercury granuloma from thermometer.

deodorant containing zirconium (Fig. 3.44). Although zirconium was eliminated from aerosol-type deodorants in 1978, aluminum-zirconium complex is present in some antiperspirants. Additionally, various poison ivy lotions contain zirconium compounds. The lesions are brownish red, dome-shaped, shiny papules. This is an acquired, delayed-type, allergic reaction resulting in a granuloma of the sarcoidal type. After many months, the lesions involute spontaneously.

Silica Granuloma

Automobile crashes and other types of trauma may produce tattooing of dirt (silicon dioxide) into the skin, which induces silica granulomas (Fig. 3.45). These typically present as black or blue papules or macules arranged in a linear fashion. At times, the granulomatous reaction to silica may be delayed for many years, with the ensuing reaction being both chronic and disfiguring. The granulomas may be caused by amorphous or crystalline silicon dioxide (quartz), magnesium silicate (talcum), or complex polysilicates (asbestos). Talc granulomas of the skin and peritoneum may develop after surgery from the talcum powder used on surgical gloves. Silica granulomas have a statistical association with systemic sarcoidosis, and silica may act as a stimulus for granuloma formation in patients with latent sarcoidosis.

Removal of these granulomas is fraught with difficulties. The best method of care is immediate and complete removal to prevent these reactions. Excision and systemic steroids have been used, but recurrences are common. Some reactions may subside spontaneously after 1–12 months. Dermabrasion or simple abrasion with a hard-bristled toothbrush is a satisfactory method for the removal of dirt accidentally embedded into the skin of the face or scalp.

Carbon Stain

Discoloration of the skin from embedded carbon usually occurs in children from improper use of firearms (Fig. 3.46) or fireworks or from a puncture wound by a pencil, which may leave a permanent black mark of embedded graphite, easily mistaken for a metastatic melanoma. Narcotic addicts who attempt to clean needles by flaming them with a lighted match may tattoo the carbon formed on the needle as it is inserted into the skin.

Carbon particles may be removed immediately after their deposition using a toothbrush and forceps. This expeditious and meticulous early care results in the best possible cosmetic result. If the particles are left in place long enough, they are best removed using the Q-switched Nd:YAG laser at 1064 nm. In one series

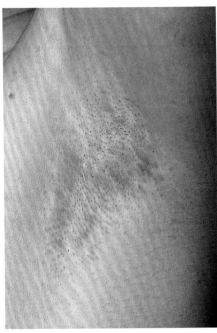

Fig. 3.44 Aluminum-zirconium granuloma secondary to antiperspirant use.

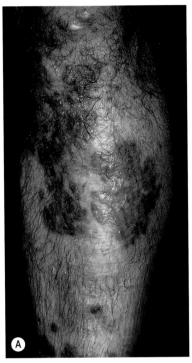
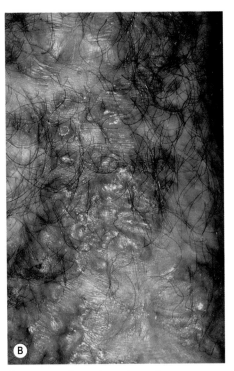

Fig. 3.45 (A and B) Silica granuloma years after motorcycle crash.

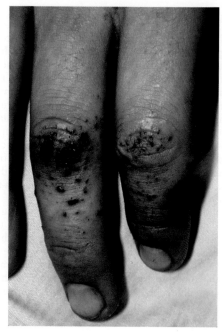

Fig. 3.46 Carbon stain, gunshot wound.

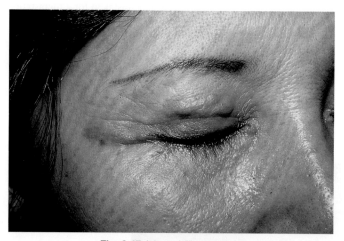

Fig. 3.47 Injected filler reaction.

success was reported in 50 of 51 treated tattoos with an average of 1.7 treatments. However, microexplosions producing poxlike scars have occurred with each laser pulse. Alternatively, dermabrasion may be used.

Injected Filler Substances

Injected or implanted filler substances used for facial rejuvenation may produce foreign body or sarcoidal granulomas. Palpable thickening and nodules (Fig. 3.47), which are occasionally painful, have been reported with collagen, hyaluronic acid and acrylic hydrogels, and polylactic acid, polyalkylimide, and polymethylmethacrylate microspheres. The reaction may be delayed for years; at times, patients are reluctant to admit to these prior cosmetic interventions and frequently cannot name the filler used. Topical, intralesional, or systemic steroids, sometimes augmented by tacrolimus, and minocycline or doxycycline have been reported to be helpful medical interventions.

Alani RM, et al: Acupuncture granulomas. J Am Acad Dermatol 2001; 45: S225.

Altemyer MD, et al: Cutaneous mercury granuloma. Cutis 2011; 88: 189.

Antonovitch DD, et al: Development of sarcoidosis in cosmetic tattoos. Arch Dermatol 2005; 141: 869.

Bachmeyer C, et al: Penile paraffinoma developing during treatment with pegylated interferon alfa-2a for chronic hepatitis C virus infection. Arch Dermatol 2011; 147: 1232.

Bassi A, et al: Tattoo-associated skin reaction. Biomed Res Int 2014; 2014: 1.

Bernstein S, et al: A gunpowder tattoo in a 6-year-old girl. Pediatr Dermatol 2016; 33: e210.

Boztepe G, et al: Cutaneous silica granuloma. Eur J Dermatol 2005; 15: 194.

Choudhary S, et al: Lasers for tattoo removal. Lasers Med Sci 2010; 25: 619.

El-Khalawany M, et al: Dermal filler complications. Ann Diagn Pathol 2015; 19: 10.

England RW, et al: Immediate cutaneous hypersensitivity after treatment of tattoo with Nd:YAG laser. Ann Allergy Asthma Immunol 2002; 89: 215.

Fusade T, et al: Treatment of gunpowder traumatic tattoo by Q-switched Nd:YAG laser. Dermatol Surg 2000; 26: 1057.

Garcovich S, et al: Lichenoid red tattoo reaction. Eur J Dermatol 2010; 22: 93.

Gaudron S, et al: Azo pigments and quinacridones induce delayed hypersensitivity in red tattoos. Contact Dermatitis 2015; 72: 97.

Gormley RH, et al: Role for trauma in introducing pencil "lead" granuloma in the skin. J Am Acad Dermatol 2010; 62: 1074.

Hexsel D, de Morais MR: Management of complications of injectable silicone. Facial Plast Surg 2014; 30: 623.

Hou M, et al: Cutaneous silica granuloma with generalized involvement of lymph nodes. J Dermatol 2011; 38: 697.

Islam PS, et al: Medical complications of tattoos. Clin Rev Allergy Immunol 2016; 50: 273.

Kazandjieva J, et al: Tattoos: dermatological complications. Clin Dermatol 2007; 25: 375.

Kim HK, et al: Facial paraffinoma treated with a bipolar radio-frequency device. Int J Dermatol 2015; 54: 89.

Kim JH, et al: Treatment algorithm of complications after filler injection. J Korean Med Sci 2014; 29: S176.

Klontz KL, et al: Adverse effects of cosmetic tattooing. Arch Dermatol 2005; 141: 918.

Montemarano AD, et al: Cutaneous granulomas caused by an aluminum-zirconium complex. J Am Acad Dermatol 1997; 37: 496.

Mortimer NJ, et al: Red tattoo reactions. Clin Exp Dermatol 2003; 28: 508.

Paul S, et al: Granulomatous reaction to liquid injectable silicone for gluteal enhancement. Dermatol Ther 2015; 28: 98.

Ross EV, et al: Tattoo darkening and nonresponse after laser treatment. Arch Dermatol 2001; 137: 33.

Rossman MD: Chronic beryllium disease. Appl Occup Environ Hyg 2001; 16: 615.

Senet P, et al: Minocycline for the treatment of cutaneous silicone granulomas. Br J Dermatol 1999; 140: 963.

Seok J, et al: Delayed immunologic complications due to injectable fillers by unlicensed practitioners. Dermatol Ther 2016; 29: 41.

Shimizu I, et al: Metal-induced granule deposition with pseudoochronosis. J Am Acad Dermatol 2010; 63: 357.

Suvanasuthi S, et al: *Mycobacterium fortuitum* cutaneous infection from amateur tattoo. J Med Assoc Thai 2012; 95: 834.

Tammaro A, et al: Contact allergic dermatitis to gold in a tattoo. Int J Immunopathol Pharmacol 2011; 24: 1111.

Timko AL, et al: In vitro quantitative chemical analysis of tattoo pigments. Arch Dermatol 2001; 137: 143.

Tsang M, et al: A visible response to an invisible tattoo. J Cutan Pathol 2012; 39: 877.

Vagefi MR, et al: Adverse reactions to eyeliner tattoo. Ophthal Plast Reconstr Surg 2006; 22: 48.

Wilken R, et al: Intraoperative localized urticarial reaction during Q-switched Nd:YAG laser tattoo removal. J Drugs Dermatol 2015; 14: 303.

Woodward J, et al: Facial filler complications. Facial Plast Surg Clin North Am 2015; 23: 447.

4 Pruritus and Neurocutaneous Dermatoses

PRURITUS

Pruritus, commonly known as itching, is a sensation exclusive to the skin. It may be defined as the sensation that produces the desire to scratch. Pruritogenic stimuli are first responded to by keratinocytes, which release a variety of mediators, and fine intraepidermal C-neuron filaments. Approximately 5% of the afferent unmyelinated C neurons respond to pruritogenic stimuli. Itch sensations in these nerve fibers are transmitted via the lateral spinothalamic tract to the brain, where a variety of foci generate both stimulatory and inhibitory responses. The sum of this complicated set of interactions appears to determine the quality and intensity of itch.

Itching may be elicited by many normally occurring stimuli, such as light touch, temperature change, and emotional stress. Chemical, mechanical, and electrical stimuli may also elicit itching. The brain may reinterpret such sensations as being painful or causative of burning or stinging sensations. A large group of neuromediators and their receptors have been identified. Some of the most important mediators are histamine and the H4 receptor, tryptase and its proteinase-activated receptor type 2, opioid peptides and the mu (μ) and kappa (κ) opioid receptors, leukotriene B4, prostaglandins such as PGE, thymic stromal lymphopoietin, acetylcholine, cytokines such as interleukin-31 (IL-31), and a variety of neuropeptides and vasoactive peptides (e.g., nerve growth factor, substance P) and their receptors (e.g., TRPV1). Investigation is ongoing to discover the relative importance of each of these mediators and to determine the clinical circumstances under which therapeutic targeting of these molecules will lead to relief of symptoms.

Itch has been classified into four primary categories, as follows:

- Pruritoceptive itch, initiated by skin disorders
- Neurogenic itch, generated in the central nervous system and caused by systemic disorders
- Neuropathic itch, caused by anatomic lesions of the central or peripheral nervous system
- Psychogenic itch, the type observed in parasitophobia

An overlap or mixture of these types may be causative in any individual patient.

Patterns of Itching

There are wide variations in itching from person to person, and a person may have a variation in reactions to the same stimulus. Heat will usually aggravate preexisting pruritus. Stress, absence of distractions, anxiety, and fear may all enhance itching. Itching tends to be most severe during undressing for bed.

Severe pruritus, with or without prior skin lesions, may be paroxysmal in character with a sudden onset, often severe enough to awaken the patient. It may stop instantly and completely as soon as pain is induced by scratching. However, the pleasure of scratching is so intense that the patient, despite the realization of damaging the skin, is often unable to stop short of inflicting such damage (Fig. 4.1). Itching of this distinctive type is characteristic of a select group of dermatoses: lichen simplex chronicus, atopic dermatitis, nummular eczema, dermatitis herpetiformis, neurotic excoriations, eosinophilic folliculitis, uremic pruritus, prurigo simplex, paraneoplastic itch (usually secondary to lymphoma), and prurigo nodularis. In general, only these disorders produce such intense pruritus and scratching as to induce bleeding. In individual cases, other diseases may manifest such severe symptoms.

Treatment

General guidelines for therapy of the itchy patient include keeping cool and avoiding hot baths or showers and wool clothing, which is a nonspecific irritant, as is xerosis. Many patients note itching increases after showers, when they wash with soap and then dry roughly. Using soap only in the axilla and inguinal area, patting dry, and applying a moisturizer can often help prevent such exacerbations. If itching is severe, a trial of "soaking and smearing" may provide significant relief (see winter itch later in this chapter). Patients often use an ice bag or hot water to ease pruritus; however, hot water can irritate the skin, is effective only for short periods, and over time exacerbates the condition.

Relief of pruritus with topical remedies may be achieved with topical anesthetic preparations. Many contain benzocaine, which may produce contact sensitization. Pramoxine in a variety of vehicles, lidocaine 5% ointment, eutectic mixture of lidocaine and prilocaine (EMLA) ointment, and lidocaine gel are preferred anesthetics that may be beneficial in localized conditions. EMLA and lidocaine may be toxic if applied to large areas. Topical antihistamines are generally not recommended, although doxepin cream may be effective for mild pruritus when used alone. Doxepin cream may cause contact allergy or a burning sensation, and somnolence may occur when doxepin is used over large areas. Topical lotions that contain menthol or camphor feel cool and improve pruritus. They may be kept in the refrigerator to enhance this soothing effect. Other lotions have specific ceramide content designed to mimic that of the normal epidermal barrier. Capsaicin, by depleting substance P, can be effective, but the burning sensation present during initial use frequently causes patients to discontinue its use. Topical steroids and calcineurin inhibitors effect a decrease in itching through their antiinflammatory action and therefore are of limited efficacy in neurogenic, psychogenic, or systemic disease–related pruritus.

Phototherapy with ultraviolet B (UVB), UVA, and psoralen plus UVA (PUVA) may be useful in a variety of dermatoses and pruritic disorders. Many oral agents are available to treat pruritus. Those most frequently used by nondermatologists are the antihistamines. First-generation H1 antihistamines, such as hydroxyzine and diphenhydramine, may be helpful in nocturnal itching, but their efficacy as antipruritics is disappointing in many disorders, except for urticaria and mastocytosis. Doxepin is an exception in that it can reduce anxiety and depression and is useful in several pruritic disorders. Sedating antihistamines should be prescribed cautiously, especially in elderly patients because of their impaired cognitive ability. The nonsedating antihistamines and H2 blockers are only effective in urticaria and mast cell disease. Opioids are involved in itch induction. In general, activation of μ-opioid receptors stimulates itch, whereas κ-opioid receptor stimulation inhibits itch perception; however, the interaction is complex. Additionally, opioid-altering agents such as naltrexone, naloxone, nalfurafine, and butorphanol have significant side effects and varying modes of delivery (intravenous, intranasal, oral). Initial reports of benefit in one condition are often followed by conflicting reports on further study. Specific recommendations in select pruritic

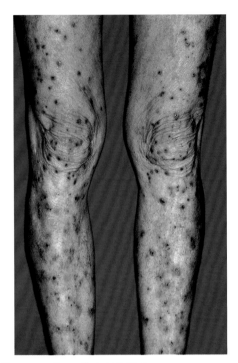

Fig. 4.1 Severe pruritus with excoriations.

conditions are detailed in those sections. These agents appear most useful for cholestatic pruritus. Central reduction of itch perception may be effected by anticonvulsants, such as gabapentin and pregabalin, and antidepressants, such as mirtazapine and the selective serotonin reuptake inhibitors (SSRIs). These take 8–12 weeks to attain full onset of action. Thalidomide, through a variety of direct neural effects, immunomodulatory actions, and hypnosedative effects, is also useful in select patients.

Chan IH, Murrell DF: Itch management. Curr Probl Dermatol 2016; 50: 54.

Elmariah SB, et al: Topical therapies for pruritus. Semin Cutan Med Surg 2011; 30: 118.

Matsuda KM, et al: Gabapentin and pregabalin for the treatment of chronic pruritus. J Am Acad Dermatol 2016; 75: 619.

Matterne U, et al: Prevalence, correlates and characteristics of chronic pruritus. Acta Derm Venereol 2011; 91: 674.

Misery L, et al: Neuropathic pruritus. Nat Rev Neurol 2014; 10: 408.

Pereira MP, et al: Chronic pruritus in the absence of skin disease. Am J Clin Dermatol 2016; 17: 337.

Sharma D, Kwatra SG: Thalidomide for the treatment of chronic refractory pruritus. J Am Acad Dermatol 2016; 74: 363.

Ständer S, et al: Emerging drugs for the treatment of pruritus. Expert Opin Emerg Drugs 2015; 20: 515.

Stull C, et al: Advances in the therapeutic strategies for the treatment of pruritus. Expert Opin Pharmacother 2016; 17: 671.

Valdes-Rodriguez R, et al: Chronic pruritus in the elderly. Drugs Aging 2015; 32: 201.

Weisshaar I, et al: European guideline on chronic pruritus. Acta Derm Vernereol 2012; 92: 563.

Yosipovitch G, et al: Chronic pruritus. N Engl J Med 2013; 368: 1625.

Internal Causes of Pruritus

Itching may be present as a symptom in a number of internal disorders. The intensity and duration of itching vary from one disease to another. The most important internal causes of itching include liver disease, especially obstructive and hepatitis C (with or without evidence of jaundice or liver failure), renal failure, diabetes mellitus, hypothyroidism and hyperthyroidism, hematopoietic diseases (e.g., iron deficiency anemia, polycythemia vera), neoplastic diseases (e.g., lymphoma [especially Hodgkin disease and cutaneous T-cell lymphoma], leukemia, myeloma), internal solid-tissue malignancies, intestinal parasites, carcinoid, multiple sclerosis, acquired immunodeficiency syndrome (AIDS), connective tissue disease (particularly dermatomyositis) and neuropsychiatric diseases, especially anorexia nervosa.

The pruritus of Hodgkin disease is usually continuous and at times is accompanied by severe burning. The incidence of pruritus is 10%–30% and is the first symptom of this disease in 7% of patients. Its cause is unknown. The pruritus of leukemia, except for chronic lymphocytic leukemia, has a tendency to be less severe than in Hodgkin disease.

Internal organ cancer may be found in patients with generalized pruritus that is unexplained by skin lesions. However, no significant overall increase of malignant neoplasms can be found in patients with idiopathic pruritus. A suggested workup for chronic, generalized pruritus includes a complete history, thorough physical examination, and laboratory tests, including complete blood count (CBC) and differential; thyroid, liver, and renal panels; fasting blood glucose; hepatitis C serology; human immunodeficiency virus (HIV) antibody (if risk factors are present); urinalysis; stool for occult blood; serum protein electrophoresis; and chest x-ray evaluation. Presence of eosinophilia on the CBC is a good screen for parasitic diseases, but if the patient has been receiving systemic corticosteroids, blood eosinophilia may not be a reliable screen for parasitic diseases, and stool samples for ova and parasites should be submitted. Additional radiologic studies or specialized tests are performed as indicated by the patient's age, history, and physical findings. A biopsy for direct immunofluorescence is occasionally helpful to detect dermatitis herpetiformis or pemphigoid.

Treatment of the itch associated with some of these internal conditions is discussed later in this chapter or under those specific diseases in other chapters; however, in other conditions listed previously treatment of the underlying disease state (e.g., treating the cancer, replacing thyroid hormone in hypothyroidism) causes relief of the pruritus. Be aware that disease specific therapies can exacerbate itching during treatment, for instance in cancer patients treated with biologic agents such as the anti EGFR monocolonal antibiodies.

Cassano N, et al: Chronic pruritus in the absence of specific skin disease. Am J Clin Dermatol 2010; 11: 399.

Rowe B, Yosipovitch G: Malignancy-associated pruritus. Eur J Pain 2016; 20: 19.

Santoni M, et al: Risk of pruritus in cancer patients treated with biological therapies. Crit Rev Oncol Hematol 2015; 96: 206.

Tarikci N, et al: Pruritus in systemic diseases. Scientific World Journal 2015; 2015: 803752.

Weisshaar I, et al: European guideline on chronic pruritus. Acta Derm Vernereol 2012; 92: 563.

Chronic Kidney Disease

Chronic kidney disease (CKD) is the most common systemic cause of pruritus; 20%–80% of patients with chronic renal failure have itching. The pruritus is often generalized, intractable, and severe; however, dialysis-associated pruritus may be episodic, mild, or localized to the dialysis catheter site, face, or legs.

The mechanism of pruritus associated with CKD is multifactorial. Xerosis, secondary hyperparathyroidism, increased serum histamine levels, hypervitaminosis A, iron deficiency anemia, and

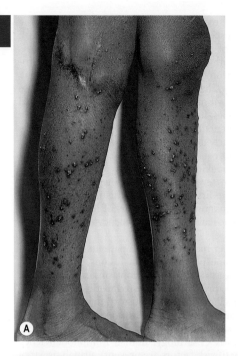

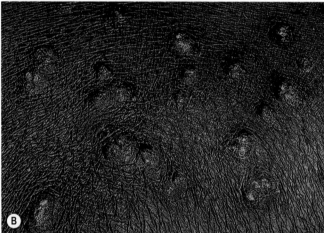

Fig. 4.2 (A) Acquired perforating dermatosis of uremia. (B) Close-up view of A.

neuropathy have been implicated. Complications such as acquired perforating disease, lichen simplex chronicus, and prurigo nodularis may develop and contribute to the degree and severity of pruritus (Fig. 4.2).

Many patients have concomitant xerosis, and aggressive use of emollients, including "soaking and smearing" (see winter itch later in this chapter), may help. A trial of γ-linolenic acid cream twice daily was effective, as was one using baby oil. Gabapentin given three times weekly at the end of hemodialysis sessions can be effective, but its renal excretion is decreased in CKD, so a low initial dose of 100 mg after each session with slow upward titration is recommended. A mainstay of CKD-associated pruritus has been narrow-band (NB) UVB phototherapy, but a randomized controlled trial (RCT) failed to confirm its efficacy. Broad-band UVB may be best in the CKD patient. Naltrexone, topical tacrolimus, and ondansetron also were reported to be useful in initial trials, but subsequent studies indicated these agents are ineffective. Nalfurafine, 5 μg once daily after supper, has demonstrated improvement

and was relatively well tolerated over a 1-year study. Thalidomide, intranasal butorphanol, and intravenous lidocaine are less practical options. Patients on peritoneal dialysis have a lower severity of pruritus than those on hemodialysis. Renal transplantation will eliminate pruritus.

Berger TG, et al: Pruritus and renal failure. Semin Cutan Med Surg 2011; 30: 99.
Combs SA, et al: Pruritus in kidney disease. Semin Nephrol 2015; 35: 383.
Ko MJ, et al: Narrowband ultraviolet B phototherapy for patients with refractory uraemic pruritus. Br J Dermatol 2011; 165: 633.
Mettang T: Uremic itch management. Curr Probl Dermatol 2016; 50: 133.
Mettang T, Kremer AE: Uremic pruritus. Kidney Int 2015; 87: 685.
Wu HY, et al: A comparison of uremic pruritus in patients receiving peritoneal dialysis and hemodialysis. Medicine (Baltimore) 2016; 95: e2935.

Biliary Pruritus

Chronic liver disease with obstructive jaundice may cause severe generalized pruritus, and 20%–50% of patients with jaundice have pruritus. Intrahepatic cholestasis of pregnancy, primary sclerosing cholangitis, and hereditary cholestatic diseases such as Alagille syndrome all have pruritus in common. Another disease, primary biliary cirrhosis, is discussed separately next because of its many other cutaneous manifestations. Hepatitis C may be associated with pruritus as well.

Itching of biliary disease is probably caused by central mechanisms. The pathophysiology is not well understood, but it appears that lysophosphatidic acid, formed by the action of the enzyme autotaxin on lysophosphatidylcholine, is central. The serum conjugated bile acid levels do not correlate with the severity of pruritus, and the theory invoking endogenous opioids as the main cause has not been upheld.

Pruritus of chronic cholestatic liver disease is improved with cholestyramine, 4 to 16 g daily. Rifampin, 150 to 300 mg/day, may be effective but should be used with caution because it may cause hepatitis. Naltrexone, up to 50 mg/day, is useful but has significant side effects. If used, naltrexone should be started at $\frac{1}{4}$ tablet (12.5 mg) and increased by $\frac{1}{4}$ tablet every 3 to 7 days until pruritus improves. Sertraline, 75 to 100 mg/day, is another option. UVB phototherapy was effective in a small case series. Ursodeoxycholic acid is effective for the pruritus in intrahepatic cholestasis of pregnancy, but not for the itching from other causes. Liver transplantation is the definitive treatment for end-stage disease and provides dramatic relief from the severe pruritus.

Primary Biliary Cirrhosis. Primary biliary cirrhosis occurs almost exclusively in women older than 30. Itching may begin insidiously and may be the presenting symptom in a quarter to half of patients. With time, extreme pruritus develops in almost 80% of patients. This almost intolerable itching is accompanied by jaundice and a striking melanotic hyperpigmentation of the entire skin; the patient may turn almost black, except for a hypopigmented "butterfly" area in the upper back. Eruptive xanthomas, planar xanthomas of the palms (Fig. 4.3), xanthelasma, and tuberous xanthomas over the joints may be seen.

Dark urine, steatorrhea, and osteoporosis occur frequently. Serum bilirubin, alkaline phosphatase, serum ceruloplasmin, serum hyaluronate, and cholesterol values are increased. The antimitochondrial antibody test is positive. The disease is usually relentlessly progressive with the development of hepatic failure. Several cases have been accompanied by scleroderma.

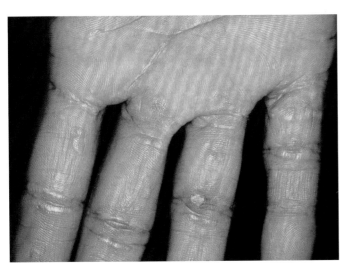

Fig. 4.3 Primary biliary cirrhosis with plane xanthomas.

Bunchornatavakul C, et al: Pruritus in chronic cholestatic lever disease. Clin Liver Dis 2012; 16: 331.

Carey EJ, et al: Primary biliary cirrhosis. Lancet 2015; 386: 1565.

Decock S, et al: Cholestasis-induced pruritus treated with ultraviolet B phototherapy. J Hepatol 2012; 57: 637.

Hegade VS, et al: Drug treatment of pruritus in liver diseases. Clin Med (London) 2015; 15: 354.

Kremer AE, et al: Pathogenesis and management of pruritus in PBC and PSC. Dig Dis 2015; 33 Suppl 2: 164.

Polycythemia Vera. More than one third of patients with polycythemia vera report pruritus; it is usually induced by temperature changes or several minutes after bathing. The cause is unknown.

Aspirin has been shown to provide immediate relief from itching; however, there is a risk of hemorrhagic complications. PUVA and NB UVB are also effective. A marked improvement is noted after an average of six treatments, with complete remission often occurring in 2–10 weeks. Paroxetine, 20 mg/day, produced clearing or near-complete clearing in a series of nine patients. Interferon (IFN) alpha-2 has been shown to be effective for treating the underlying disease and associated pruritus.

Saini KS, et al: Polycythemia vera–associated pruritus and its management. Eur J Clin Invest 2010; 40: 828.

PRURITIC DERMATOSES

Winter Itch

Asteatotic eczema, eczema craquelé, and xerotic eczema are other names for this pruritic condition. Winter itch is characterized by pruritus that usually first manifests and is most severe on the legs and arms. Extension to the body is common; however, the face, scalp, groin, axillae, palms, and soles are spared. The skin is dry with fine flakes (Fig. 4.4). The pretibial regions are particularly susceptible and may develop eczema craquelé, exhibiting fine cracks in the eczematous area that resemble the cracks in old porcelain dishes.

Frequent and lengthy bathing with plenty of soap during the winter is the most frequent cause. This is especially prevalent in elderly persons, whose skin has a decreased rate of repair of the epidermal water barrier and whose sebaceous glands are less productive. Low humidity in overheated rooms during cold weather contributes to this condition. In a study of 584 elderly individuals,

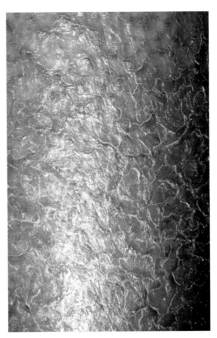

Fig. 4.4 Winter itch.

the prevalence of asteatosis (28.9%) was second only to seborrheic dermatitis as the most common finding.

Treatment consists of educating the patient on using soap only in the axillae and inguinal area and lubricating the skin with emollients immediately after showering. Preparations containing lactic acid or urea applied after bathing are helpful in some patients but may cause irritation and may worsen itching in patients with erythema and eczema.

For those with more severe symptoms, long-standing disease, or a significant inflammatory component, a regimen referred to as "soaking and smearing" is dramatically effective. The patient soaks in a tub of plain water at a comfortable temperature for 20 minutes before bedtime. Immediately on exiting the tub, without drying, triamcinolone, 0.025%–0.1% ointment, is applied to the wet skin. This will trap the moisture, lubricate the skin, and allow for excellent penetration of the steroid component. An old pair of pajamas is then donned, and the patient will note relief even on the first night. The nighttime soaks are repeated for several nights, after which the ointment alone suffices, with the maintenance therapy of limiting soap use to the axillae and groin, and moisturization after showering. Plain petrolatum may be used as the lubricant after the soaking if simple dryness without inflammation is present. Folliculitis may complicate this therapy.

Gutman A, et al: Soak and smear therapy. Arch Dermatol 2005; 141: 1556.

Kimura N, et al: Prevalence of asteatosis and asteatotic eczema among elderly residents in facilities covered by long-term care insurance. J Dermatol 2013; 40: 770.

Pruritus Ani

Pruritus is often centered on the anal or genital area (less frequently in both), with minimal or no pruritus elsewhere. Anal neurodermatitis is characterized by paroxysms of violent itching, when the patient may tear at the affected area until bleeding is induced. Manifestations are identical to lichen simplex chronicus elsewhere on the body. Specific etiologic factors should always be sought and generally can be classified as dermatologic disease, local irritants (which may coexist with colorectal and anal causes), and infectious agents.

Allergic contact dermatitis is a common dermatologic cause or secondary complication of pruritus ani. It occurs from various medicaments, fragrance in toilet tissue, or preservatives in moist toilet tissue, with one study reporting 18 of 40 consecutive patients being patch test positive. Seborrheic dermatitis, psoriasis, lichen planus, lichen sclerosis, and atopic dermatitis all may cause perianal itching, and an examination of other classic sites of involvement with these conditions should be carefully undertaken. Extramammary Paget disease and Bowen disease, although not often itchy, may be present and will not improve with therapy. Biopsy of resistant dermatitic-appearing skin should be done in nonresponsive pruritus ani.

Irritant contact dermatitis from gastrointestinal contents, such as hot spices or cathartics, or failure to cleanse the area adequately after bowel movements may be causal. Anatomic factors may lead to leakage of rectal mucus on to perianal skin and thus promote irritation. Physical changes such as hemorrhoids, anal tags, fissures, and fistulas may aggravate or produce pruritus.

Mycotic pruritus ani is characterized by fissures and a white, sodden epidermis. Scrapings are examined directly with potassium hydroxide mounts, and cultures will usually reveal *Candida albicans*, *Epidermophyton floccosum*, or *Trichophyton rubrum*. Other sites of fungal infection, such as the groin, toes, and nails, should also be investigated. Erythrasma in the groin and perianal regions may also occasionally produce pruritus. The diagnosis is established by coral red fluorescence under the Wood's light. β-Hemolytic streptococcal infections have also been implicated, especially in young children. The use of tetracyclines may cause pruritus ani, most often in women, by inducing candidiasis. Diabetic patients are susceptible to perianal candidiasis.

Pinworm infestations may cause pruritus ani, especially in children and sometimes in their parents. Nocturnal pruritus is most prevalent. Other intestinal parasites, such as *Taenia solium*, *T. saginata*, amebiasis, and *Strongyloides stercoralis*, may produce pruritus. Pediculosis pubis may cause anal itching; however, attention is focused by the patient on the pubic area, where itching is most severe. Scabies may be causative but often will also involve the finger webs, wrists, axillae, areolae, and genitalia.

Lumbosacral radiculopathy also may be present with pruritus ani, as assessed by radiographs and nerve conduction studies; paravertebral blockade may help these patients.

Treatment

Meticulous toilet care should be followed, no matter what the cause of the itching. After defecation, the anal area should be cleansed whenever possible, washed with mild soap and water. Cleansing with wet toilet tissue is advisable in all cases. Medicated cleansing pads (Tucks) should be used regularly. A variety of moist toilet tissue products are now available. Contact allergy to preservatives in these products is occasionally a problem. An emollient lotion (Balneol) is helpful for cleansing without producing irritation.

Once the etiologic agent has been identified, a rational and effective treatment regimen may be started. Topical corticosteroids are effective for most noninfectious types of pruritus ani; however, use of topical tacrolimus ointment will frequently suffice and is safer. Pramoxine, a nonsteroidal topical anesthetic, is also often effective, especially in a lotion form combined with hydrocortisone. In pruritus ani, as well as in pruritus scroti and vulvae, it is sometimes best to discontinue all topical medications and treat with plain water sitz baths at night, followed immediately by plain petrolatum applied over wet skin. This soothes the area, provides a barrier, and eliminates contact with potential allergens and irritants.

Abu-Asi MJ, et al: Patch testing is clinically important for patients with peri-anal dermatoses and pruritus ani. Contact Dermatitis 2016; 74: 298.

Nasseri YY, et al: Pruritus ani: diagnosis and treatment. Gastroenterol Clin North Am 2013; 42: 801.
Sahnan K, et al: Anal itching. BMJ 2016; 355: i4931.
Silvestri DL, et al: Pruritus ani as a manifestation of systemic contact dermatitis. Dermatitis 2011; 22: 50.
Suys E, et al: Randomized study of topical tacrolimus ointment as possible treatment for resistant idiopathic pruritus ani. J Am Acad Dermatol 2012; 66: 327.

Pruritus Scroti

The scrotum of an adult is a susceptible site for circumscribed neurodermatitis (lichen simplex chronicus) (Fig. 4.5). Psychogenic pruritus is probably the most frequent type of itching seen. Why it preferentially affects the scrotum, or in women the vulva (see pruritus vulvae), is unclear. Lichenification may result, can be extreme, and may persist for many years despite intensive therapy.

Infectious conditions may complicate or cause pruritus on the scrotum but are less common than idiopathic scrotal pruritus. Fungal infections, except candidiasis, usually spare the scrotum. When candidal infection affects the scrotum, burning rather than pruritus is frequently the primary symptom. The scrotum is eroded, weepy, or crusted. The scrotum may be affected to a lesser degree in cases of pruritus ani, but this pruritus usually affects the midline, extending from the anus along the midline to the base of the scrotum, rather than the dependent surfaces of the scrotum, where pruritus scroti usually occurs. Scrotal pruritus may be associated with allergic contact dermatitis from topical medications, including steroidal agents.

Topical corticosteroids are the mainstay of treatment, but caution should be exercised. The "addicted scrotum syndrome" may be caused by the use of high-potency topical steroidal agents. As with facial skin, after attempts to wean patients off the steroid, severe burning and redness may occur. Although usually seen after chronic use, this may occur even with short-term high-potency steroids. The scrotum is frequently in contact with inner thigh skin, producing areas of occlusion, which increases the penetration of topical steroid agents. Topical tacrolimus ointment is useful in overcoming the effects of overuse of potent topical steroids. Another alternative is gradual tapering to less potent corticosteroids. Other useful nonsteroidal alternatives include topical pramoxine, doxepin, and simple petrolatum, which is applied after a sitz bath as described for pruritus ani.

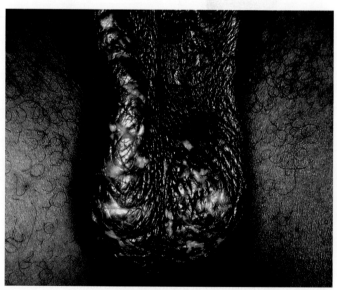

Fig. 4.5 Pruritus scroti.

Krishnan A, et al: Scrotal dermatitis. Oman Med J 2013; 28: 302.

Tan ES, et al: Effective treatment of scrotal lichen simplex chronicus with 0.1% tacrolimus ointment. J Eur Acad Dermatol Venereol 2015; 29: 1448.

Pruritus Vulvae

The vulva is a common site for pruritus of different causes. Pruritus vulvae (Fig. 4.6) is the counterpart of pruritus scroti. In a prospective series of 141 women with chronic vulvar symptoms, the most common causes were unspecified dermatitis (54%), lichen sclerosus (13%), chronic vulvovaginal candidiasis (10%), dysesthetic vulvodynia (9%), and psoriasis (5%). In prepubertal children, such itching is most frequently irritant in nature, and girls generally benefit from education about improved hygienic measures.

Vaginal candidiasis is a frequent cause of pruritus vulvae. This is true especially during pregnancy and when oral antibiotics are taken. The inguinal, perineal, and perianal areas may be affected. Microscopic examination for *Candida albicans* and cultures for fungus should be performed. *Trichomonas vaginalis* infection may cause vulvar pruritus. For the detection of *T. vaginalis*, examination of vaginal secretions is often diagnostic. The organism is recognized by its motility, size (somewhat larger than a leukocyte), and piriform shape.

Contact dermatitis from sanitary pads, contraceptives, douche solutions, fragrance, preservatives especially in moist towelettes, colophony, benzocaine, corticosteroids, and a partner's condoms may account for vulvar pruritus. Urinary incontinence should also be considered. Lichen sclerosus is another frequent cause of pruritus in the genital area in middle-age and elderly women. Lichen planus may involve the vulva, resulting in pruritus and mucosal changes, including erosions and ulcerations, resorption of the labia minora, and atrophy.

When burning rather than itching predominates, the patient should be evaluated for signs of sensory neuropathy.

Treatment

Candidiasis and *Trichomonas* treatments are discussed in Chapters 15 and 20, respectively. Lichen sclerosus responds best to pulsed dosing of high-potency topical steroids or to topical tacrolimus or pimecrolimus. Topical steroidal agents and topical tacrolimus may be used to treat psychogenic pruritus or irritant or allergic reactions. The use of silk fabric underwear may limit irritation. Patch testing will assist in identifying the inciting allergen. High-potency topical steroids are effective in treating lichen planus, but other options are also available (see Chapter 12). Topical lidocaine, topical pramoxine, or an oral tricyclic antidepressant (TCA) may be helpful in select cases. Phototherapy using a comb light device may be effective. Any chronic skin disease that does not respond to therapy should prompt a biopsy.

Caro-Bruce E, et al: Vulvar pruritus in a postmenopausal woman. CMAJ 2014; 186: 688.

Haverhock E, et al: Prospective study of patch testing in patients with vulvar pruritus. Australas J Dermatol 2008; 49: 80.

Ozalp SS, et al: Vulval pruritus. J Obstet Gynaecol 2015; 35: 53.

Utas S, et al: Patients with vulvar pruritus. Contact Dermatitis 2008; 58: 296.

Virgili A, et al: Phototherapy for vulvar lichen simplex chronicus. Photodermatol Photoimmunol Photomed 2014; 30: 332.

Puncta Pruritica (Itchy Points)

"Itchy points" consists of one or two intensely itchy spots in clinically normal skin, sometimes followed by the appearance of seborrheic keratoses at exactly the same site. Curettage, cryosurgery, punch biopsy, or botulinum toxin A injection of the itchy points may cure the condition.

Boyd AS, et al: Puncta pruritica. Int J Dermatol 1992; 31: 370.

Salardini A, et al: Relief of intractable pruritus after administration of botulinum toxin A. Clin Neuropharmacol 2008; 31: 303.

Aquagenic Pruritus and Aquadynia

Aquagenic pruritus is itching evoked by contact with water of any temperature. Most patients experience severe, prickling discomfort within minutes of exposure to water or on cessation of exposure to water. There are two groups of patients: about one third consist of an older, primarily male population who have polycythemia vera, hypereosinophilic syndrome, or myelodysplastic syndrome, and two thirds are younger women who develop aquagenic pruritus as young adults and who have no known underlying disease and may have a family history of similar symptoms.

Aquagenic pruritus must be distinguished from xerosis as water may be perceived as an irritant in severely dry skin, and in these cases an initial trial of "soaking and smearing," as previously described for winter itch, is recommended. Treatment options for aquagenic pruritus include the use of antihistamines, sodium bicarbonate dissolved in bath water, propranolol, atenolol, SSRIs, acetylsalicylic acid (ASA, aspirin), pregabalin, montelukast, and NB UVB or PUVA phototherapy. One patient found tight-fitting clothing settled the symptoms after only 5 minutes.

Shelley et al. reported two patients with widespread burning pain that lasted 15–45 minutes after water exposure, calling this reaction "aquadynia" and considering the disorder a variant of aquagenic pruritus. Clonidine and propranolol seemed to provide some relief.

Cao T, et al: Idiopathic aquagenic pruritus. Dermatol Ther 2015; 28: 118.

Heitkemper T, et al: Aquagenic pruritus. J Dtsch Dermatol Ges 2010; 8: 797–804.

Herman-Kideckel SM, et al: Successful treatment of aquagenic pruritus with montelukast. J Cut Med Surg 2012; 16: 151–152.

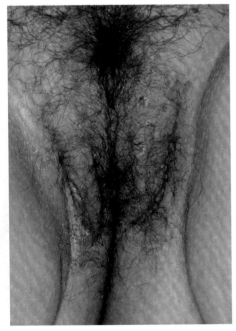

Fig. 4.6 Lichen simplex chronicus of the vulva.

Koh MJA, et al: Aquagenic pruritus responding to combine ultraviolet A/narrowband ultraviolet B therapy. Photodermatol Photoimmunol Photomed 2009; 25: 169–170.

Shelley WB, et al: Aquadynia. J Am Acad Dermatol 1998; 38: 357.

Scalp Pruritus

Pruritus of the scalp, especially in elderly persons, is rather common. Lack of excoriations, scaling, or erythema excludes inflammatory causes of scalp pruritus such as seborrheic dermatitis, psoriasis, dermatomyositis, or lichen simplex chronicus. Most such cases remain are neuropathic or idiopathic, but some represent chronic folliculitis. Treatment with topical tar shampoos, salicylic acid shampoos, corticosteroid topical gels, mousse, shampoos, and liquids can be helpful. In patients who have severe scalp pruritus with localized itch, an intralesional injection of corticosteroid suspension may provide relief. Minocycline or oral antihistamines may be helpful. In other patients, low doses of antidepressants, such as doxepin, are useful.

Cohen AD, et al: Similarities between neuropathic pruritus sites and lichen simplex chronicus sites. Isr Med Assoc J 2014; 16: 88.

Shumway NK, et al: Neurocutaneous disease: Neurocutaneous dysesthesias. J Am Acad Dermatol 2016; 74: 215.

Drug-Induced Pruritus

Medications should be considered a possible cause of pruritus with or without a skin eruption. For example, pruritus is frequently present after opioid use. Also, chloroquine and to a lesser degree other antimalarials produce pruritus in many patients, especially African Americans, treated for malaria. SSRIs and drugs causing cholestatic liver disease are other frequent causes.

Hydroxyethyl starch (HES) is used as a volume expander, a substitute for human plasma. One third of all patients treated will develop severe pruritus with long latency of onset (3–15 weeks) and persistence. Up to 30% of patients have localized symptoms. Antihistamines are ineffective.

Ebata T: Drug-induced itch management. Curr Probl Dermatol 2016; 50: 155.

Ständer S, et al: Hydroxyethyl starch-induced pruritus. Acta Derm Venereol 2014; 94: 282.

Chronic Pruritic Dermatoses of Unknown Cause

Prurigo simplex is the preferred term for the chronic itchy idiopathic dermatosis described here. Papular dermatitis, subacute prurigo, "itchy red bump" disease, urticarial dermatitis, the eruption of senescence of Berger, and Rosen papular eruption in black men most likely represent variations of prurigo simplex. The term prurigo continues to lack nosologic precision.

Prurigo simplex is characterized by the lesion known as the prurigo papule, which is dome shaped and topped with a small vesicle. The vesicle is usually present only transiently because of its immediate removal by scratching, so that a crusted papule is more frequently seen. Prurigo papules are present in various stages of development and are seen mostly in middle-age or elderly persons of both genders. The trunk and extensor surfaces of the extremities are common sites, symmetrically distributed. Other areas include the face, neck, lower trunk, and buttocks. The lesions usually appear in crops, so that papulovesicles and the late stages of scarring may be seen at the same time. At times eczematous morphology may be intermixed.

The histopathology of prurigo simplex is nonspecific but often suggests an arthropod reaction. Spongiosis accompanied by a perivascular mononuclear infiltrate with some eosinophils is often found.

Many conditions may cause pruritic erythematous papules. Scabies, atopic dermatitis, insect bite reactions, papular urticaria, dermatitis herpetiformis, contact dermatitis, pityriasis lichenoides et varioliformis acuta (PLEVA), transient acantholytic dermatosis (TAD), papuloerythroderma of Ofuji, dermatographism, and physical urticarias should be considered. Biopsy may be helpful in differentiating dermatitis herpetiformis, PLEVA, TAD, and on occasion, unsuspected scabies.

Treatment

The medications for initial treatment of prurigo simplex and its variants should be topical corticosteroids and oral antihistamines. Early in the disease process, moderate-strength steroids should be used; if the condition is found to be unresponsive, a change to high-potency forms is indicated. "Soaking and smearing" may be necessary. Intralesional injection of triamcinolone will eradicate individual lesions. For more recalcitrant disease, UVB or PUVA therapy may be beneficial. If such interventions do not provide relief, low-dose azathioprine, mycophenolate, or methotrexate may be needed.

Berger TG, et al: Pruritus in elderly patients—eruptions of senescence. Semin Cutan Med Surg 2011; 30: 113.

Clark AR, et al: Papular dermatitis (subacute prurigo, "itchy red bump" disease). J Am Acad Dermatol 1998; 38: 929.

Hannon GR, et al: Urticarial dermatitis. J Am Acad Dermatol 2014; 70: 264.

Prurigo Pigmentosa

Prurigo pigmentosa is a rare dermatosis of unknown cause characterized by the sudden onset of erythematous papules or vesicles that leave reticulated hyperpigmentation when they heal (Fig. 4.7). The condition mainly affects Japanese, although numerous cases

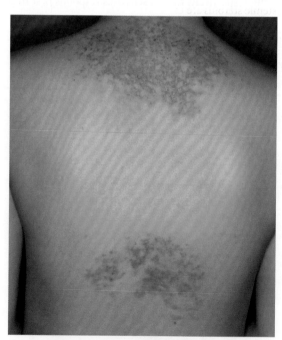

Fig. 4.7 Prurigo pigmentosa. (Courtesy Department of Dermatology, Keio University School of Medicine, Tokyo, Japan.)

have been reported in Caucasians. Women outnumber men 2:1. The mean age of onset is 25. It is associated with weight loss, dieting, anorexia, post bariatric surgery, pregnancy, diabetes, and ketonuria. It is exacerbated by heat, sweating, and friction and thus occurs most often in the winter and spring. The areas most frequently involved are the upper back, nape, clavicular region, and chest. Mucous membranes are spared. Histology of early lesions shows neutrophils in the dermal papillae and epidermis. Following this, a lichenoid dermatitis with variable psoriasiform hyperplasia occurs. Direct immunofluorescence yields negative findings. The cause is unknown. Minocycline, 100–200 mg/day, is the treatment of choice. Dapsone and alteration of the diet are also effective; topical steroids are not effective. Recurrence and exacerbations are common.

Beutler BD, et al: Prurigo pigmentosa. Am J Clin Dermatol 2015; 16: 533.

Hijazi M, et al: Prurigo pigmentosa. Am J Dermatopathol 2014; 36: 800–806.

Zeng X, et al: Prurigo pigmentosa. J Eur Acad Dermatol Venereol 2016; 30: 1794.

Papuloerythroderma of Ofuji

A rare disorder most often found in Japan, papuloerythroderma of Ofuji (PEO) is characterized by flat-topped, red-to-brown pruritic papules that spare the skinfolds, producing bands of uninvolved cutis, the so-called deck-chair sign. Almost all patients are over age 55, with clear male predominance. Frequently, there is associated blood eosinophilia. Skin biopsies reveal a dense lymphohistiocytic infiltrate, eosinophils in the papillary dermis, and increased Langerhans cells. Malignancies have occurred in 21% of reported cases, but the timing and course do not always often correlate with PEO. Reported malignancies include T-cell lymphomas, B-cell lymphomas, Sézary syndrome, and visceral carcinomas. Drugs (e.g., aspirin, ranitidine, furosemide) and infections (e.g., HIV, hepatitis C) may induce the condition. Severe atopic dermatitis and cutaneous T-cell lymphoma may present with identical morphologic finding of PEO. History will assist in making the diagnosis of atropic dermatitis, whereas biopsy may reveal findings diagnostic of eruptions.

Systemic steroids are the treatment of choice and may result in long-term remission. Topical or systemic steroids, tar derivatives, emollients, systemic retinoids, cyclosporine, UVB, and PUVA may also be therapeutic. UV therapy, with or without steroids, is favored.

Teraki Y, et al: High incidence of internal malignancy in papuloerythroderma of Ofuji. Dermatology 2013; 224: 5.

Torchia D, et al: Papuloerythroderma 2009. Dermatology 2010; 220: 311.

Lichen Simplex Chronicus

Also known as circumscribed neurodermatitis, lichen simplex chronicus results from long-term chronic rubbing and scratching, more vigorously than a normal pain threshold would permit, with the skin becoming thickened and leathery. The normal markings of the skin become exaggerated (Fig. 4.8), so that the striae form a crisscross pattern, producing a mosaic in between composed of flat-topped, shiny, smooth quadrilateral facets. This change, known as lichenification, may originate on seemingly normal skin or may develop on skin that is the site of another disease, such as atopic or allergic contact dermatitis or ringworm. Such underlying etiologies should be sought and, if found, treated specifically. Paroxysmal pruritus is the main symptom.

Circumscribed, lichenified pruritic patches may develop on any part of the body; however, lichen simplex chronicus has a

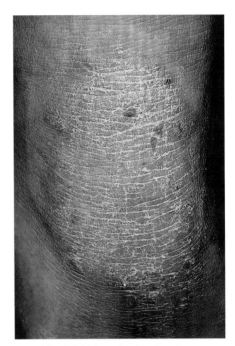

Fig. 4.8 Lichen simplex chronicus.

predilection for the back and sides of the neck, the scalp, the upper eyelid, the orifice of one or both ears, the palm, soles, or often the wrist and ankle flexures. The vulva, scrotum, and anal areas are common sites, although the genital and anal areas are seldom involved at the same time. The eruption may be papular, resembling lichen planus; and in other cases the patches are excoriated, slightly scaly or moist, and rarely, nodular. Persistent rubbing of the shins or upper back may result in dermal deposits of amyloid and the subsequent development of lichen or macular amyloidosis, respectively.

The onset of this dermatosis is usually gradual and insidious. Chronic scratching of a localized area may be a response to an inciting dermatitis; however, scratching of the localized site continues long after the original insult and becomes a habit. It may be associated with anxiety disorders and in depressed patients, with erectile dysfunction.

Treatment. Cessation of pruritus is the goal with lichen simplex chronicus. It is important to stress the need for the patient to avoid scratching the areas involved if the sensation of itch is ameliorated. Recurrences are frequent, even after the most thorough treatment, and in some cases the clearance of one lesion will see the onset of another elsewhere.

A high-potency steroid cream or ointment should be used initially but not indefinitely because of the potential for steroid-induced atrophy. Occlusion of medium-potency steroids may be beneficial. Use of a steroid-containing tape to provide both occlusion and antiinflammatory effects may have benefit. Treatment can be shifted to the use of medium- to lower-strength topical steroid creams as the lesions resolve. Topical doxepin, capsaicin, or pimecrolimus cream or tacrolimus ointment provides significant antipruritic effects and is a good adjunctive therapy.

Intralesional injections of triamcinolone suspension, using a concentration of 2.5–5 mg/mL, may be required. Too superficial an injection invites the twin risks of epidermal and dermal atrophy and depigmentation, which may last for many months. The suspension should not be injected into infected lesions because it may cause abscess. Botulinum toxin A injection may be curative. In the most severe cases, complete occlusion with an Unna boot may break the cycle.

Aschoff R, et al: Topical tacrolimus for the treatment of lichen simplex chronicus. J Dermatol Treat 2007; 18: 15.

Cohen AD, et al: Similarities between neuropathic pruritus sites and lichen simplex chronicus sites. Isr Med Assoc J 2014; 16: 88.

Juan CK, et al: Lichen simplex chronicus associated with erectile dysfunction. PLoS One 2015; 10: e0128869.

Liao YH, et al: Increased risk of lichen simplex chronicus in people with anxiety disorder. Br J Dermatol 2014; 170: 890.

Prurigo Nodularis

Prurigo nodularis is a disease with multiple itchy nodules mainly on the extremities (Fig. 4.9), especially on the anterior surfaces of the thighs and legs. A linear arrangement is common. The individual lesions are pea sized or larger, firm, and erythematous or brownish. When fully developed, they become verrucous or fissured. The course of the disease is chronic, and the lesions evolve slowly. Itching is severe but usually confined to the lesions themselves. Bouts of extreme pruritus often occur when these patients are under stress. Prurigo nodularis is one of the disorders in which the pruritus is characteristically paroxysmal: intermittent, unbearably severe, and relieved only by scratching to the point of damaging the skin, usually inducing bleeding and often scarring.

The cause of prurigo nodularis is unknown; multiple factors may contribute, including atopic dermatitis, hepatic diseases (including hepatitis C), HIV disease, pregnancy, renal failure, lymphoproliferative disease, stress, and insect bites. Pemphigoid nodularis may be confused with prurigo nodularis clinically.

The histologic findings are those of compact hyperkeratosis, irregular acanthosis, multinucleated keratinocytes, and a perivascular mononuclear cell infiltrate in the dermis. Dermal collagen may be increased, especially in the dermal papillae, and subepidermal fibrin may be seen, both evidence of excoriation. In cases associated with renal failure, transepidermal elimination of degenerated collagen may be found.

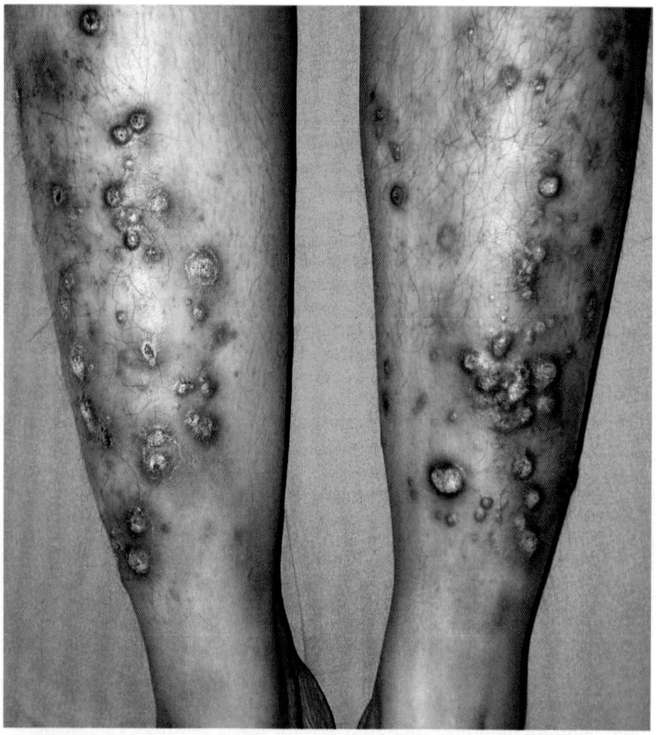

Treatment. The initial treatment of choice for prurigo nodularis is intralesional or topical administration of steroids. Usually, superpotent topical products are required, but at times, lower-strength preparations used with occlusion may be beneficial, as when administered as the "soak and smear" regimen. The use of steroids in tape (Cordran) and prolonged occlusion with semipermeable dressings, such as used for treating nonhealing wounds, can be useful in limited areas. Intralesional steroids will usually eradicate individual lesions, but unfortunately, many patients have too extensive disease for these local measures. PUVA, NB UVB, and UVA alone have been shown to be effective in some patients. The combination product containing calcipotriene and betamethasone dipropionate ointment, calcitriol ointment, or tacrolimus ointment applied topically twice daily may be therapeutic and steroid sparing. Isotretinoin, 1 mg/kg/day for 2–5 months, may benefit some patients. Managing dry skin with emollients and avoidance of soap, with administration of antihistamines, antidepressants, or anxiolytics, is of moderate benefit in allaying symptoms.

Good results have been obtained with thalidomide, lenalidomide, pregabalin, and cyclosporine. With thalidomide, onset may be rapid or slow, and sedation may occur; initial dose is 100 mg/day, titered to the lowest dose required. Patients treated with thalidomide are at risk for developing a dose-dependent neuropathy at cumulative doses of 40–50 g. Lenalidomide, an analog of thalidomide, has less problems with neuropathy but may cause myelosuppression, venous thrombosis, and Stevens-Johnson syndrome. Methotrexate, 7.5–20 mg weekly produced improvement in 10 of 13 treated patients. Pregabalin, 75 mg/day for 3 months, improved 23 of 30 patients in one study. Cyclosporine at doses of 3–4.5 mg/kg/day has also been shown to be effective in treating recalcitrant disease. Cryotherapy may be used adjunctively. Multimodal therapy, combining topical and systemic therapies, can improve results.

Andersen TP, et al: Thalidomide in 42 patients with prurigo nodularis Hyde. Dermatology 2011; 223: 107–112.

Kanavy H, et al: Treatment of refractory prurigo nodularis with lenalidomide. Arch Dermatol 2012; 148: 794–796.

Mazza M, et al: Treatment of prurigo nodularis with pregabalin. J Clin Pharm Ther 2013; 38: 16–18.

Nakamura M, Koo JY: Phototherapy for the treatment of prurigo nodularis. Dermatol Online J 2016; 22: 13030/qt4b077778z.

Sorenson E, et al: Successful use of a modified Goeckerman regimen in the treatment of generalized prurigo nodularis. J Am Acad Dermatol 2015; 72: e40.

Spring P, et al: Prurigo nodularis. Clin Exp Dermatol 2014; 39: 468.

Sweeney SA, et al: Grape cells (multinucleated keratinocytes) in noninfectious dermatoses. Am J Dermatopathol 2015; 37: e143.

Tsianakas A, et al: Prurigo nodularis management. Curr Probl Dermatol 2016; 50: 94.

Psychodermatology

Some purely cutaneous disorders are psychiatric in nature, their cause being directly related to psychopathologic causes in the absence of primary dermatologic or other organic causes. Delusions of parasitosis, psychogenic (neurotic) excoriations, factitial dermatitis, and trichotillomania compose the major categories of psychodermatology. The differential diagnosis for these four disorders is twofold, requiring the exclusion of organic causes and the definition of a potential underlying psychological disorder.

Fig. 4.9 Prurigo nodularis. (Courtesy Debabrata Bandyopadhyay, MD.)

Bromidrosiphobia is another delusional disorder. Body dysmorphic disorder is a spectrum of disease; some severely affected patients are delusional, whereas others have more insight and are less functionally impaired.

Psychosis is characterized by the presence of delusional ideation, which is defined as a fixed misbelief that is not shared by the patient's subculture. Monosymptomatic hypochondriacal disorder is a form of psychosis characterized by delusions regarding a particular hypochondriacal concern. In contrast to schizophrenia, there are no other mental deficits, such as auditory hallucination, loss of interpersonal skills, or presence of other inappropriate actions. Patients with monosymptomatic hypochondriacal psychosis often function appropriately in social settings, except for a single fixated belief that there is a serious problem with their skin or with other parts of their body.

Butler DC, et al: Psychotropic medications in dermatology. Semin Cutan Med Surg 2013; 32: 126.
Fried RG: Nonpharmacologic treatments of psychodermatologic conditions. Semin Cutan Med Surg 2013; 32: 119.
Kuhn H, et al: Psychocutaneous disease. J Am Acad Dermatol 2017; 76: 779.
Leon A, et al: Psychodermatology. Semin Cutan Med Surg 2013; 32: 64.

Skin Signs of Psychiatric Illness

The skin is a frequent target for the release of emotional tension. Some of the signs described here may become repetitive compulsions that impair normal life functions and may be manifestations of an obsessive-compulsive disorder. Self-injury by prolonged, compulsive repetitious acts may produce various mutilations, depending on the act and site of injury.

Self-biting may be manifested by biting the nails (onychophagia) or recurrent manipulation of components of the nail unit (onychotillomania) (Fig. 4.10), skin (most frequently the forearms, hands, and fingers), and lip. Dermatophagia is a habit or compulsion, conscious or subconscious. Bumping of the head produces lacerations and contusions, which may be so severe as to produce cranial defects and life-threatening complications. Compulsive repetitive handwashing may produce an irritant dermatitis of the hands (Fig. 4.11).

Bulimia, with its self-induced vomiting, results in Russell sign—crusted papules on the dorsum of the dominant hand from cuts by the teeth. Clenching of the hand produces swelling and ecchymosis of the fingertips and subungual hemorrhage.

Self-inflicted lacerations may be of suicidal intent. Lip licking produces increased salivation and thickening of the lips. Eventually, the perioral area becomes red and produces a distinctive picture resembling the exaggerated mouth makeup of a clown. Pressure produced by binding the waistline tightly with a cord will eventually lead to atrophy of the subcutaneous tissue.

Psychopharmacologic agents, especially the newer atypical antipsychotic agents, and behavioral therapy alone or in combination with these agents are the treatments of choice.

Kestenbaum T: Obsessive-compulsive disorder in dermatology. Semin Cutan Med Surg 2013; 32: 83.
Kuhn H, et al: Psychocutaneous disease. J Am Acad Dermatol 2017; 76: 779.
Rieder EA, et al: Onychotillomania. J Am Acad Dermatol 2016; 75: 1245.
Singal A, Daulatabad D: Nail tic disorders. Indian J Dermatol Venereol Leprol 2017; 83: 19.
Strumia R: Eating disorders and the skin. Clin Dermatol 2013; 31: 80.

Delusional Infestation (Delusions of Parasitosis)

Delusional infestation (Ekbom syndrome) is a firm fixation in a person's mind that he or she suffers from a parasitic infestation of the skin. At times, close contacts may share the delusion (folie a deux or trios). The belief is so fixed that the patient often pick small pieces of epithelial debris from the skin and bring them to be examined, insisting that the offending parasite is contained in such material. Samples of alleged parasites enclosed in assorted containers, paper tissue, or sandwiched between adhesive tape are so characteristic that it is referred to as the "matchbox" or "ziplock" sign. Usually, the only symptom is pruritus or a stinging, biting, or crawling sensation. Intranasal formication, or a crawling sensation of the nasal mucosa, is common in this condition. Cutaneous findings may range from none to excoriations, prurigo nodularis, and frank ulcerations.

Frequently, these patients have paranoid tendencies. Women are affected 2 : 1 over men, often during middle or old age, although there is a bimodal peak, with some patients presenting in their 20s or 30s. The condition has been reported to be associated with schizophrenia, bipolar disorders, depression, anxiety disorders, and

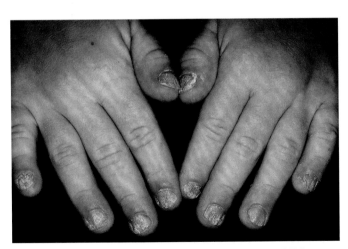
Fig. 4.10 Onychophagia. (Courtesy Curt Samlaska, MD.)

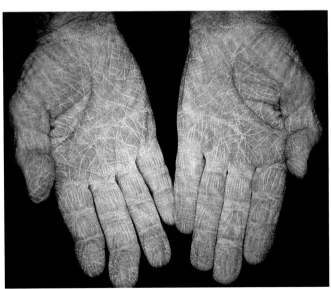
Fig. 4.11 Irritant dermatitis from chronic handwashing.

obsessional states but is usually a monosymptomatic hypochondriacal disorder. A variety of organic conditions may be causative and should be considered. They include cocaine, alcohol, and amphetamine abuse; dementia and other neurologic conditions (e.g., multiple sclerosis, central nervous system tumors, epilepsy, Parkinson disease); malignancies, particularly lymphoma and leukemia; cerebrovascular disease; endocrine disorders; infectious diseases; pellagra; and vitamin B_{12} deficiency. A variety of medications, including gabapentin, antiparkinsonian and antihistaminic drugs, and corticosteroids, may also produce this condition. Some of these agents may produce cutaneous symptoms, particularly pruritus, which may contribute to the delusion.

The differential diagnosis is influenced by the cutaneous findings and history. Initial steps should be directed at excluding a true infestation, such as scabies, or an organic cause. A thorough history, particularly in reference to therapeutic and recreational drug use (e.g., amphetamines, alcohol, cocaine), review of systems, and physical examination should be performed. Many consider Morgellons disease simply to be another name for delusions of parasitosis. Patients complain of crawling, biting, burning, or other sensations that cause them to be intensely anxious. Often, granules or fibers are provided by the patient for analysis. Many patients have associated psychiatric conditions.

A skin biopsy is frequently performed, more to reassure the patient than to uncover occult skin disease. Screening laboratory tests to exclude systemic disorders should be obtained: CBC; urinalysis; liver, renal, and thyroid function tests; iron studies; serum glucose and serum B_{12}; folate; and electrolyte levels. Once organic causes have been eliminated, the patient should be evaluated to determine the cause of the delusions. Schizophrenia, monosymptomatic hypochondriacal psychosis, psychotic depression, dementia, and depression with somatization are considerations in the differential diagnosis.

Management of this difficult problem varies. Although referral to a psychiatrist may seem best, most frequently the patient will reject suggestions to seek psychiatric help. The dermatologist is cautioned against confronting the patient with the psychogenic nature of the disease. It is preferable to develop trust, which will usually require several visits. If pharmacologic treatment is undertaken, the patient may accept it if the medication is presented as one that will alter the perception of this bothersome sensation. Pimozide was the long-standing treatment of choice given at relatively low dosages, in the 1–4 mg range. Although this strategy has limited side effects, newer, atypical antipsychotic agents, such as risperidone (0.5–6 mg/day), olanzapine (2.5–20 mg/day), quetiapine (25–600 mg/day), and aripiprazole (2–30 mg/day), are safer and considered the appropriate first-line agents, although the experience with them is more limited. With appropriate pharmacologic intervention, at least 50% of patients will likely remit.

Elliott A, et al: Cocaine bugs. Am J Addict 2012; 21: 180.

Hylwa SA, et al: Delusional infestation, including delusions of parasitosis. Arch Dermatol 2011; 147: 1041.

Lewis EC et al: Delusions of parasitosis. Semin Cutan Med Surg 2013; 32: 73.

Martins AC, et al: Delusional infestation. Int J Dermatol 2016; 55: 864.

Mohandas P, et al: Morgellons disease. 2017 Jul 14: 1.

Reichenberg JS, et al: Patients labeled with delusions of parasitosis compose a heterogenous group. J Am Acad Dermatol 2013; 68: 41.

Rodríguez-Cerdeira C, et al: Delusional infestation. Am J Emerg Med 2017; 35: 357.

Schairer D, et al: Psychology and psychiatry in the dermatologist's office. J Drug Dermatol 2012; 11: 543.

Vulink NC: Delusional infestation. Acta Derm Venereol 2016; 96: 58.

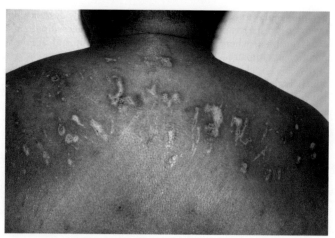
Fig. 4.12 Psychogenic excoriations. (Courtesy Steven Binnick, MD.)

Excoriation Disorder

This condition is also called psychogenic excoriations, neurotic excoriations or skin picking disorder. Many persons have unconscious compulsive habits of picking at themselves, and at times the tendency is so persistent and pronounced that excoriations of the skin result. The lesions are caused by picking, digging, or scraping and usually occur on parts readily accessible to the hands. These patients admit their actions induce the lesions but cannot control their behavior.

The excavations may be superficial or deep and are often linear. The bases of the ulcers are clean or covered with a scab. Right-handed persons tend to produce lesions on their left side and left-handed persons on their right side. There is evidence of past healed lesions, usually with linear scars, or rounded hyperpigmented or hypopigmented lesions, in the area of the active excoriations. The face, upper arms, and upper back are common sites for these excoriations (Fig. 4.12). Sometimes the focus is on acne lesions, producing acne excoriée.

Most of these patients are otherwise healthy adults leading normal lives. The organic differential diagnosis is vast and includes any condition that may manifest with excoriations. The most common psychopathologies associated with neurotic excoriations are depression, obsessive-compulsive disorder, and anxiety.

The treatment of choice is doxepin because of its antidepressant and antipruritic effects; doses are slowly increased to 100 mg or higher, if tolerated. Many alternatives to doxepin may be indicated, especially in those affected by an obsessive-compulsive component. N-acetylcysteine 1200 to 3000 mg/day is safe and tolerable option, which is now being studied in many psychodermatologic conditions. It has been shown to be effective in this excoriation disorder. Treatment is difficult, often requiring a combined psychiatric and pharmacologic intervention. It is important to establish a constructive patient-therapist alliance. Training in diversion strategies during "scratching episodes" may be helpful. An attempt should be made to identify specific conflicts or stressors preceding onset. The therapist should concentrate on systematic training directed at the behavioral reaction pattern. There should be support and advice given with regard to the patient's social situation and interpersonal relations.

Grant JE, et al: N-Acetylcysteine in the treatment of excoriation disorder. JAMA Psychiatry 2016; 73: 490.

Koblenzer CS, et al: Neurotic excoriations and dermatitis artefacta. Semin Cutan Med Surg 2013; 32: 95.

Kuhn H, et al: Psychocutaneous disease. J Am Acad Dermatol 2017; 76: 779.

Misery L, et al: Psychogenic skin excoriations. Acta Derm Venereol 2012, 92: 416.

Torales J, et al: Alternative therapies for excoriation (skin picking) disorder. Adv Mind Body Med 2017 Winter; 31: 10.

Factitious Dermatitis and Dermatitis Artefacta

Factitious dermatitis is the term applied to self-inflicted skin lesions with the intent to elicit sympathy, escape responsibility, or collect disability insurance. Malingering applies to the latter two cases, where material gain is the objective. This contrasts with the usual dermatitis artefacta patient, who has an unconscious goal of gaining attention and assuming the sick patient role. Most patients are adults in midlife, with women affected three times more often than men. The vast majority have multiple lesions and are unemployed or on sick leave. These skin lesions are provoked by mechanical means or by the application or injection of chemical irritants and caustics. These patients often have a "hollow" history, unable to detail how the lesions appeared or evolved. The lesions may simulate other dermatoses but usually have a distinctive, geometric, bizarre appearance (Fig. 4.13), often with a shape and arrangement not encountered in other disorders. The lesions are generally distributed on parts easily reached by the hands, tend to be linear and arranged regularly and symmetrically, and are rarely seen on the dominant hand.

When chemicals are used, red streaks or guttate marks are often seen beneath the principal patch, where drops of the chemical have accidentally run or fallen on the skin. According to the manner of production, the lesions may be erythematous, vesicular, bullous, ulcerative, or gangrenous. The more common agents of destruction used are the fingernails, pointed instruments, hot metal, chemicals (e.g., carbolic, nitric, or acetic acid), caustic potash or soda, turpentine, table salt, urine, and feces. The lesions are likely to appear in crops. At times the only sign may be the indefinitely delayed healing of an operative wound, which is purposely kept open by the patient. Tight cords or clothing tied around an arm or leg may produce factitious lymphedema, which may be mistaken for postphlebitic syndrome or nerve injury, as well as other forms of chronic lymphedema.

Subcutaneous emphysema, manifesting as cutaneous crepitations, may be factitial in origin. Recurrent migratory subcutaneous emphysema involving the extremities, neck, chest, or face can be induced through injections of air into tissue with a needle and syringe. Circular pockets and bilateral involvement without physical findings, indicating contiguous spread from a single source, suggest a factitial origin. Puncturing the buccal mucosa through to facial skin with a needle and puffing out the cheeks can produce alarming

results. Neck and shoulder crepitation is also a complication in manic patients that results from hyperventilation and breath holding.

The organic differential diagnosis depends on the cutaneous signs manifested, such as gas gangrene for patients with factitious subcutaneous emphysema and the various forms of lymphedema for factitious lymphedema. A subset of these patients have Munchausen syndrome. They tend to cause lesions that closely simulate known conditions, and they create an intricate, often fantastic story surrounding the problem. Admissions to the hospital with extensive workup often result. Parents may induce lesions on their child to gain attention, so-called Munchausen by proxy, which is really child abuse. Considerations for psychopathology in dermatitis artefacta include borderline personality disorders and psychosis.

Proof of diagnosis is sometimes difficult. Occlusive dressings may be necessary to protect the lesions from ready access by the patient. It is usually best not to reveal any suspicion of the cause to the patient and to establish the diagnosis definitively without the patient's knowledge. If the patient is hospitalized, a resourceful, cooperative nurse may be useful in helping to establish the diagnosis. When injection of foreign material is suspected, examination of biopsy material by spectroscopy may reveal talc or other foreign material. Additionally epidermal multinucleated keratinocytes may be present as a clue.

Treatment should ideally involve psychotherapy, but typically the patient promptly rejects the suggestion and goes to another physician to seek a new round of treatment. It is best for the dermatologist to maintain a close relationship with the patient and provide symptomatic therapy and nonjudgmental support. SSRIs may address associated depression and anxiety. Very-low-dose atypical antipsychotics may also be added, if needed. Consultation with an experienced psychiatrist is prudent.

Alcántara Luna S, et al: Dermatitis artefacta in childhood. Pediatr Dermatol 2015; 32: 604.

Gutierrez D, et al: Epidermal multinucleated keratinocytes. J Cutan Pathol 2016; 43: 880.

Koblenzer CS, et al: Neurotic excoriations and dermatitis artefacta. Semin Cutan Med Surg 2013; 32: 95.

Ucmak D, et al: Dermatitis artefacta. Cutan Ocul Toxicol 2014; 33: 22.

Trichotillomania

Trichotillomania (trichotillosis or hair pulling disorder) is characterized by an abnormal urge to pull out the hair. The sites involved are generally the frontal region of the scalp, eyebrows, eyelashes, and the beard. The classic presentation is the "Friar Tuck" form of vertex and crown alopecia. There are irregular areas of hair loss, which may be linear or bizarrely shaped. Infrequently, adults may pull out pubic hair. Hairs are broken and show differences in length (Fig. 4.14). The pulled hair may be ingested, and occasionally the trichobezoar will cause obstruction. When the tail extends from the main mass in the stomach to the small or large intestine, Rapunzel syndrome is the diagnosis. The nails may show evidence of onychophagy (nail biting), but no pits are present. The disease is seven times more common in children than in adults, and girls are affected 2.5 times more often than boys.

Trichotillomania often develops in the setting of psychosocial stress in the family, which may involve school problems, sibling rivalry, moving to a new house, hospitalization of a parent, or a disturbed parent-child relationship.

Differentiation from alopecia areata is possible because of the varying lengths of broken hairs present, the absence of nail pitting, and the microscopic appearance of the twisted or broken hairs in contrast to the tapered fractures of alopecia areata. Other organic disorders to consider are androgenic alopecia, tinea capitis,

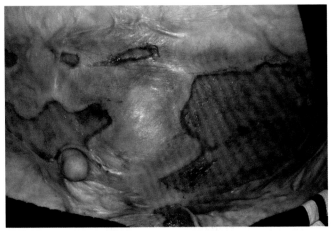

Fig. 4.13 Factitial ulcers and scarring.

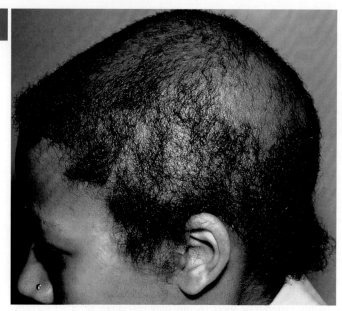

Fig. 4.14 Trichotillomania.

monilethrix, pili torti, pseudopelade of Brocq, traction alopecia, syphilis, nutritional deficiencies, and systemic disorders such as lupus and lymphoma. Trichoscopy reveals broken hairs of varying lengths; some may be frayed, longitudinally split, or coiled. If necessary, a biopsy can be performed and is usually quite helpful. It reveals traumatized hair follicles with perifollicular hemorrhage, fragmented hair in the dermis, empty follicles, pigmented casts, and deformed hair shafts (trichomalacia). Multiple catagen hairs are typically seen. An alternative technique to biopsy, particularly for children, is to shave a part of the involved area and observe for regrowth of normal hairs. The differential diagnosis for this impulse control disorder should include underlying comorbid psychopathology, such as an obsessive-compulsive disorder (most common), depression, or anxiety.

In children, the diagnosis should be addressed openly, and referral to a child psychiatrist for cognitive-behavioral therapy (CBT) should be encouraged. Habit-reversal training is often part of the treatment. In adults with the problem, psychiatric impairment may be severe. Pharmacotherapy with clomipramine or olanzapine is the most effective of the studied medications, but SSRIs are most often prescribed and may help any associated depression or anxiety. N-acetylcysteine also shows promise especially in adults; it is available in health food stores and is relatively inexpensive and well tolerated. Trichobezoars require surgical removal.

Harrison JP, et al: Pediatric trichotillomania. Curr Psychiatry Rep 2012; 14: 188.

Huynh M, et al: Trichotillomania. Semin Cutan Med Surg 2013; 32: 88.

Keuthen NJ, et al: Getting the word out: cognitive-behavioral therapy for trichotillomania (hair-pulling disorder) and excoriation (skin-picking) disorder. Ann Clin Psychiatry 2015; 27: 10.

Kim SC, et al: Large trichobezoar causing Rapunzel syndrome. Medicine (Baltimore) 2016; 95: e3745.

Miteva M, et al: Pigmented casts. Am J Dermatopathol 2014; 36: 58.

Taylor M, Bhagwandas K: N-acetylcysteine in trichotillomania. Br J Dermatol 2014; 171: 1253.

Woods DW, et al: Diagnosis, evaluation, and management of trichotillomania. Psychiatr Clin North Am 2014; 37: 301.

Dermatothlasia

Dermatothlasia is a cutaneous neurosis characterized by a patient's uncontrollable desire to rub or pinch himself or herself to form bruised areas on the skin, sometimes as a defense against pain elsewhere.

Olfactory Reference Syndrome

Also called bromidrosiphobia or delusions of bromhidrosis, this is a monosymptomatic delusional state in which a person is convinced that his or her sweat has a repugnant odor that keeps other people away. The patient is unable to accept any evidence to the contrary. Three quarters of patients with bromidrosiphobia are male, with an average age of 25. Atypical antipsychotic agents or pimozide may be beneficial. It may be an early symptom of schizophrenia.

Body Dysmorphic Disorder (Dysmorphic Syndrome, Dysmorphophobia)

Body dysmorphic disorder is the excessive preoccupation of having an ugly body part. It is most common in young adults of either gender. The concern is frequently centered about the nose, mouth, genitalia, breasts, or hair. Objective evaluation will reveal a normal appearance or slight defect. These patients are usually seen in dermatologic practice, especially among those presenting for cosmetic surgery evaluation. Patients may manifest obsessional features, spending long periods inspecting the area. Associated depression and social isolation along with other comorbidities present a high risk of suicide. The SSRIs accompanied by CBT give the best results for those with this somatoform disorder. More severely affected patients have delusions that may lead to requests for repeated surgeries of the site and require antipsychotic medications.

Buhlmann U, et al: Perceived ugliness. Curr Psychiatry Rep 2011; 13: 283.

Conrado LA, et al: Body dysmorphic disorder among dermatologic patients. J Am Acad Dermatol 2010; 63: 235.

Ipser JC, et al: Pharmacotherapy and psychotherapy for body dysmorphic disorder. Cochrane Database Syst Rev 2009; (1): CD005332.

Rieder E: Approaches to the cosmetic patient with potential body dysmorphia. J Am Acad Dermatol 2015; 73: 304.

Sarwer DB, et al: Body image dysmorphic disorder in persons who undergo aesthetic medical treatments. Aesthet Surg J 2012; 32: 9999.

Vashi NA: Obsession with perfection. Clin Dermatol 2016; 34: 788.

CUTANEOUS DYSESTHESIA SYNDROMES

Cutaneous dysesthesia syndromes are characterized by pain and burning sensations without objective findings. Many patients report coexisting pruritus or transient pruritus associated with the dysesthesia.

Shumway NK, et al: Neurocutaneous disease: neurocutaneous dysesthesias. J Am Acad Dermatol 2016; 74: 215.

Scalp Dysesthesia

Scalp dysesthesia occurs primarily in middle-age to elderly women. Cervical spine degenerative disk disease is frequently present. The hypothesis is that chronic tension is placed on the occipitofrontalis muscle and scalp aponeurosis. In one series, gabapentin helped four of the seven patients seen in follow-up. A psychiatric overlay is frequently associated, and treatment with low-dose antidepressants may also be helpful. If a history of a prior brow or face lift is elicited, surgical trauma to the face or scalp nerves may account for the symptoms.

Thornsberry LA, et al: Scalp dysesthesia related to cervical spine disease. JAMA Dermatol 2013; 149: 200.

Burning Mouth Syndrome (Glossodynia, Burning Tongue)

Burning mouth syndrome (BMS) is divided into two forms: a primary type characterized by a burning sensation of the oral mucosa, with no dental or medical cause, and secondary BMS, caused by a number of conditions, including lichen planus, candidiasis, vitamin or nutritional deficiencies (e.g., low B_{12}, iron, or folate), hypoestrogenism, parafunctional habits, diabetes, hypothyroidism, HIV, herpes simplex viral shedding, dry mouth, contact allergies, cranial nerve injuries, and medication side effects. Identification of the underlying condition and its treatment will result in relief of secondary BMS.

Primary BMS occurs most frequently in postmenopausal women. They are particularly prone to a feeling of burning of the tongue, mouth, and lips, with no objective findings. Symptoms vary in severity but are more or less constant. Patients with BMS often complain that multiple oral sites are involved. Management with topical applications of clonazepam, capsaicin, doxepin, or lidocaine can help. Oral administration of α-lipoic acid, SSRIs or TCAs, gabapentin, pregabalin, and benzodiazepines has been reported to be effective. The most common, best studied, and most successful therapy is provided by the antidepressant medications, because many patients are depressed as well.

Burning lips syndrome may be a separate entity; it appears to affect both men and women equally and occurs in individuals between ages 50 and 70. The labial mucosa may be smooth and pale, and the minor salivary glands of the lips are frequently dysfunctional. Treatment with α-lipoic acid showed improvement in 2 months in a double-blind controlled study.

Crow HC, et al: Burning mouth syndrome. Oral Maxillofac Surg Clin North Am 2013; 25: 67.
Lewis AK, et al: An overview of burning mouth syndrome for the dermatologist. Clin Exp Dermatol 2016; 41: 119.
Lynde CB, et al: Burning mouth syndrome. J Cutan Med Surg 2014; 18: 174.
McMillan R, et al: Interventions for treating burning mouth syndrome. Cochrane Database Syst Rev 2016; 11: CD002779.
Nagel MA, et al: Burning mouth syndrome due to herpes simplex virus type 1. BMJ Case Rep 2015; 2015: bcr2015209488.
Steele JC: The practical evaluation and management of patients with symptoms of a sore burning mouth. Clin Dermatol 2016; 34: 449.

Vulvodynia

Vulvodynia is defined as vulvar discomfort, usually described as burning pain, occurring without medical findings. It is chronic, defined as lasting 3 months or longer. Two subtypes are seen, the localized and generalized subsets. Both may occur only when provoked by physical contact, as a spontaneous pain, or mixed in type. Vulvar pain may be secondary to many specific underlying disorders, but when caused by infections (most often candidal or herpetic), inflammatory conditions (e.g., lichen planus, autoimmune blistering disease), neoplastic disorders (e.g., extramammary Paget disease, squamous cell carcinoma), neurologic etiologies (e.g., spinal nerve compression, herpetic neuralgia), or previous radiotherapy, these conditions are treated appropriately, and the patient's condition is not categorized as vulvodynia. Thus the diagnosis of vulvodynia is a diagnosis of exclusion.

The pain experienced may be debilitating. It may be accompanied by pelvic floor abnormalities, headaches, fibromyalgia, irritable bowel syndrome, and interstitial cystitis. Psychosocial problems result and may be exacerbated by stress, depression, or anxiety or may lead to such conditions over time. A male counterpart may be seen and has been called burning genital skin syndrome and dysesthetic penodynia or scrotodynia.

Treatment should always include patient and partner education and psychological support, including sex therapy and counseling, as appropriate. Spontaneous remission occurs in 90% of patients, but half recur within 6–30 months. Topical anesthetics and lubricants, such as petrolatum, applied before intercourse may be tried initially. Elimination of irritants, treatment of atopy with topical tacrolimus (allowing for the discontinuance of topical steroids, which have usually been tried without success), and the use of antihistamines for dermatographism may be helpful. Pelvic floor physical therapy and at times cognitive behavioral therapy may be useful. Vulvodynia is considered among the chronic pain syndromes that can have a psychological impact. Treatment then centers on the use of TCAs, SSRIs, and neuroleptics, chiefly gabapentin or pregabalin. Other interventions, such as botulinum toxin A and surgery, may be considered in individual patients, but the evidence for any of these therapies is limited.

De Andres J, et al: Vulvodynia—an evidence-based literature review and proposed treatment algorithm. Pain Pract 2016; 16: 204.
Edwards L: Vulvodynia. Clin Obstet Gynecol 2015; 58: 143.
Goldstein AT, et al: Vulvodynia. J Sex Med 2016; 13: 572.
Havemann LM, et al: Vulvodynia. J Low Genit Tract Dis 2017; 21: 150.
Reed BD, et al: Remission, relapse, and persistence of vulvodynia. J Womens Health (Larchmt) 2016; 25: 276.

Notalgia Paresthetica

Notalgia paresthetica is a unilateral sensory neuropathy characterized by infrascapular pruritus, burning pain, hyperalgesia, and tenderness, often in the distribution of the second to sixth thoracic spinal nerves. A pigmented patch localized to the area of pruritus is often found, caused by postinflammatory change. Macular amyloidosis may be produced by chronic scratching. In most patients, degenerative changes in the corresponding vertebrae are seen, leading to spinal nerve impingement. When this is present, physical therapy, nonsteroidal antiinflammatory drugs (NSAIDs), gabapentin, oxycarbazepine, and muscle relaxants may be helpful, as may paravertebral blocks.

Topical capsaicin, corticosteroids, tacrolimus, or lidocaine patch has been effective, but relapse occurs in most patients after discontinuing use. Botulinum toxin A injections were reported to be successful, although an RCT failed to show efficacy. When it was effective excellent long-term results may occur, and injections may be repeated as necessary. NB UVB is also an option.

Chiriac A, et al: Notalgia paresthetica, a clinical series and review. Pain Pract 2016; 16: E90.
Maari C, et al: Treatment of nostalgia paresthetica with botulinum toxin A. J Am Acad Dermatol 2014; 70: 1139.
Maciel AA, et al: Efficacy of gabapentin in the improvement of pruritus and quality of life of patients with notalgia paresthetica. An Bras Dermatol 2014; 89: 570.
Ochi H, et al: Notalgia paresthetica. J Eur Acad Dermatol Venereol 2016; 30: 452.
Perez-Perez L, et al: Notalgia paresthesica successfully treated with narrow-band UVB. J Eur Acad Dermatol Venereol 2010; 24: 730.

Brachioradial Pruritus

This condition is characterized by itching localized to the brachioradial area of the arm. To relieve the burning, stinging, or even painful quality of the itch, patients will frequently use ice packs. The majority will have the sun-induced variety, a variant of polymorphous light syndrome that usually responds well to broad-spectrum sunscreens (see Chapter 3). In the remaining patients, cervical spine pathology is frequently found on radiographic evaluation. Searching for causes of the abnormality should include discussion of spinal injury, such as trauma, arthritis, or chronic repetitive microtrauma, whiplash injury, or assessment for a tumor in the cervical spinal column.

Gabapentin, botulinum A toxin, topical amitriptyline-ketamine or capsaicin 8% patch, aprepitant, carbamazepine, cervical spine manipulation, neck traction, antiinflammatory medications, physical therapy, and surgical resection of a cervical rib have all been successful in individual patients with brachioradial pruritus.

Ally MS, et al: The use of aprepitant in brachioradial pruritus. JAMA Dermatol 2013; 149: 627.
Kavanagh GM, et al: Botulinum A toxin and brachioradial pruritus. Br J Dermatol 2012; 166: 1147.
Marziniak M, et al: Brachioradial pruritus as a result of cervical spine pathology. J Am Acad Dermatol 2011; 65: 756.
Poterucha TJ, et al: Topical amitriptyline-ketamine for the treatment of brachioradial pruritus. JAMA Dermatol 2013; 149: 148.
Steinke S, et al: Cost-effectiveness of an 8% capsaicin patch in the treatment of brachioradial pruritus and notalgia paraesthetica, two forms of neuropathic pruritus. Acta Derm Venereol 2017; 97: 71.

Meralgia Paresthetica (Roth-Bernhardt Disease)

Persistent numbness and periodic transient episodes of burning or lancinating pain on the anterolateral surface of the thigh characterize Roth-Bernhardt disease. The lateral femoral cutaneous nerve innervates this area and is subject to entrapment and compression along its course. Sensory mononeuropathies besides notalgia paresthetica and meralgia paresthetica include mental and intercostal neuropathy and cheiralgia, gonyalgia, and digitalgia paresthetica.

Meralgia paresthetica occurs most frequently in middle-age adults. Although some series show an association with obesity, others do not. Additionally, diabetes mellitus is twice as common in these patients than in the general population. Among diabetics, meralgia paresthetica is seven times more common than seen in patients without diabetes. Alopecia localized to the area innervated by the lateral femoral nerve may be a skin sign of this disease. The pelvic compression test and the Tinel test are two physical findings based on relieving pressure on the nerve, or percussing it which can help verify the diagnosis at the bedside. External compression may occur from tight-fitting clothing, cell phones, or other heavy objects in the pockets or worn on belts, or seat belt injuries from automobile crashes. Internal compression from arthritis of the lumbar vertebrae, a herniated disk, pregnancy, intraabdominal disease that increases intrapelvic pressure, iliac crest bone graft harvesting, diabetes, neuroma, and rarely a lumbar spine or pelvic tumor have been reported causes in individual patients.

The diagnostic test of choice is somatosensory-evoked potentials of the lateral femoral cutaneous nerve. Local anesthetics (e.g., lidocaine patch), NSAIDs, rest, avoidance of aggravating factors, and weight reduction may lead to improvement; indeed, 70% of patients have spontaneous improvement, aided by conservative measures. Gabapentin is useful in various neuropathic pain disorders. Pulsed frequency neuomodulation and acupuncture are other nonsurgical methods that may be helpful. If such interventions

fail and a nerve block rapidly relieves symptoms, local infiltration with corticosteroids is indicated. Surgical decompression of the lateral femoral cutaneous nerve can produce good to excellent outcomes but should be reserved for patients with intractable symptoms who responded to nerve blocks but not corticosteroids. If the nerve block does not result in symptom relief, computed tomography (CT) scan of the lumbar spine as well as pelvic and lower abdominal ultrasound examinations to assess for tumors are indicated.

Karwa KA, et al: Smart device neuropathy. J Neurol Sci 2016; 370: 132.
Khalil N, et al: Treatment for meralgia paresthetica. Cochrane Database Syst Rev 2012; 12: CD004159.
Lee JJ, et al: Clinical efficacy of pulsed radiofrequency neuromodulation for intractable meralgia paresthetica. Pain Physician 2016; 19: 173.
Shumway NK, et al: Neurocutaneous disease: neurocutaneous dysesthesias. J Am Acad Dermatol. 2016; 74: 215.

Complex Regional Pain Syndrome

Encompassing the descriptors reflex sympathetic dystrophy, causalgia, neuropathic pain, and Sudek syndrome, complex regional pain syndrome (CRPS) is characterized by burning pain, hyperesthesia, and trophic disturbances resulting from injury to a peripheral nerve. The continuing pain is disproportionate to the injury, which may have been a crush injury, laceration, fracture, hypothermia, sprain, burn, or surgery. It usually occurs in one of the upper extremities, although leg involvement is also common. The characteristic symptom is burning pain aggravated by movement or friction. The skin of the involved extremity becomes shiny, cold, and atrophic and may perspire profusely. Additional cutaneous manifestations include bullae, erosions, edema, telangiectases, hyperpigmentation, ulcerations, and brownish red patches with linear fissures (Fig. 4.15).

The intensity of the pain in CRPS patients varies from trivial burning to a state of torture accompanied by extreme hyperesthesia and frequently hyperhidrosis. Not only is the part subject to an intense burning sensation, but also a touch of the finger also causes exquisite pain. Exposure to the air is avoided with scrupulous care, and the patient walks carefully, carrying the limb tenderly with the sound hand. Patients are tremulous and apprehensive, and they keep the hand constantly wet, finding relief in the moisture rather than in the temperature of the application. A condition resembling permanent chilblains or even trophic ulcers may be present.

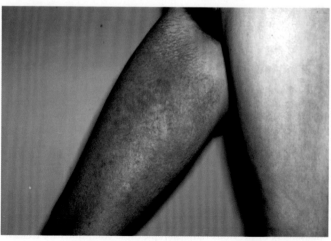

Fig. 4.15 Complex regional pain syndrome.

The syndrome usually begins with severe, localized, burning pain. focal edema, muscle spasm, stiffness or restricted mobility, and vasospasm affecting skin color and temperature. These may be followed by a diffusion of the pain and edema, diminished hair growth, brittle nails, joint thickening, and onset of muscle atrophy. Finally, irreversible trophic changes, intractable pain involving the entire limb, flexor contractures, marked atrophy of the muscles, severe limitation in joint and limb mobility, and severe osteoporosis result.

Not all patients will have all the features of CRPS, and an early diagnosis improves the chance of cure. The four major components are categorized as sensory, vasomotor, sudomotor/edema, and motor/trophic. Signs pertaining to at least two of these categories and symptoms relating to three are necessary to meet the Budapest diagnostic criteria. A three-phase technetium bone scan is helpful in confirming the diagnosis of CRPS.

Consultation with a neurologist or an anesthesiologist specializing in pain is advisable. Osteoporosis is a frequent complication, and studies using pamidronate, a powerful inhibitor of bone absorption, have been shown to improve symptoms of pain, tenderness, and swelling significantly. Pain relief which allows for physical mobilization and massage is helpful. Additionally psychological intervention with patients, their families, and caregivers is important as they often require ongoing support, education, and counseling.

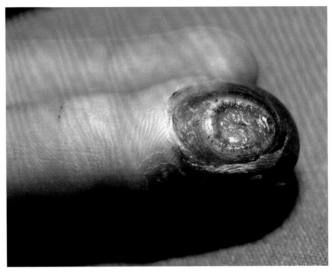

Fig. 4.16 Neuropathic ulcer of the hand in a diabetic patient.

Dietz FR, Compton SP: Outcomes of a simple treatment for complex regional pain syndrome type I in children. Iowa Orthop J 2015; 35: 175.

Fisher E, et al: Psychological therapies (remotely delivered) for the management of chronic and recurrent pain in children and adolescents. Cochrane Database Syst Rev 2015; 3: 1.

Goebel A: Complex regional pain syndrome in adults. Rheumatology 2011; 50: 1739.

Kabani R, Brassard A: Dermatological findings in early detection of complex regional pain syndrome. JAMA Dermatol 2014; 150: 640.

Marinus J, et al: Clinical features and pathophysiology of complex regional pain syndrome. Lancet Neurol 2011; 10: 637.

Slobodin G, et al: Pamidronate treatment in rheumatology practice. Clin Rheumatol 2009, 28: 1359.

Weissmann S, Uziel Y: Pediatric complex regional pain syndrome. Pediatr Rheumatol Online J 2016; 14: 29.

Wertli M, et al: Prognostic factors in complex regional pain syndrome. J Rehabil Med 2013; 45: 225.

Trigeminal Trophic Syndrome

Interruption of the peripheral or central sensory pathways of the trigeminal nerve may result in a slowly enlarging, unilateral, uninflamed ulcer on ala nasi or adjacent cheek skin. The nasal tip is spared. It may infrequently occur elsewhere on the face, scalp, ear, or palate. The neck has been reported to be affected in the so-called cervical trophic syndrome, secondary to herpes zoster–associated nerve injury. Onset of ulceration varies from weeks to several years after nerve injury from trauma, herpes zoster, or stroke. Biopsy to exclude tumor or a variety of granulomatous or infectious etiologies is usually indicated. The cause is self-inflicted trauma to the anesthetic skin; the appropriate treatment is to prevent this by occlusion or with psychotropic medication, which is often successful. Scarring may be severe.

Brewer JD, et al: The treatment of trigeminal trophic syndrome with a thermoplastic dressing. Dermatol Surg 2016; 42: 438.

Fischer AA, et al: Cervical trophic syndrome. Cutis 2014; 93: E6.

Sawada T, et al: Trigeminal trophic syndrome. J Dermatol 2014; 41: 525.

Mal Perforans Pedis

Also known as neuropathic ulceration or perforating ulcer mal perforans is a chronic ulcerative disease seen on the sole or hand in conditions that result in loss of pain sensation at a site of constant trauma (Fig. 4.16). The primary cause lies in the posterolateral tracts of the cord (in arteriosclerosis and tabes dorsalis), lateral tracts (in syringomyelia), or peripheral nerves (in diabetes or Hansen disease).

In most patients, mal perforans begins as a circumscribed hyperkeratosis, usually on the ball of the foot. This lesion becomes soft, moist, and malodorous and later exudes a thin, purulent discharge. A slough slowly develops, and an indolent necrotic ulcer is left that lasts indefinitely. Whereas the neuropathy renders the ulceration painless and walking continues, plantar ulcers in this condition have a surrounding thick callus. Deeper perforation and secondary infection often lead to osteomyelitis of the metatarsal or tarsal bones.

Treatment consists of relief of pressure on the ulcer through use of a total-contact cast and debridement of the surrounding callosity. Removable off-loading devices were found to be significantly less effective in a systematic review and meta-analysis. Administration of local and systemic antibiotics is sometimes helpful.

Bus SA: The role of pressure offloading on diabetic foot ulcer healing and prevention of recurrence. Plast Reconstr Surg 2016; 138: 179S.

Morona JK, et al: Comparison of the clinical effectiveness of different off-loading devices for the treatment of neuropathic foot ulcers in patients with diabetes. Diabetes Metab Res Rev 2013; 29: 183.

Sciatic Nerve Injury

Serious sciatic nerve injury can result from improperly performed injections into the buttocks. Older patients are more susceptible to injection-induced sciatic nerve injury because of their decreased muscle mass or the presence of debilitating disease. The most common scenario for nerve damage is improper needle placement. Other common causes of sciatic neuropathy are hip surgery complications, hip fracture and dislocation, and compression by benign and malignant tumors. A paralytic footdrop is the most common finding. There is sensory loss and absence of sweating over the distribution of the sciatic nerve branches. The skin of the affected extremity becomes thin, shiny, and often edematous.

Surgical exploration, guided by nerve action potentials, with repair of the sciatic nerve is worthwhile and is most successful if done soon after injury.

Topuz K, et al: Early surgical treatment protocol for sciatic nerve injury due to injection. Br J Neurosurg 2011; 25: 509.

Syringomyelia

Syringomyelia results from cystic cavities inside the cervical spinal cord caused by alterations of cerebrospinal fluid flow. Compression of the lateral spinal tracts produces sensory and trophic changes on the upper extremities, particularly in the fingers. The disease begins insidiously and gradually causes muscular weakness, hyperhidrosis, and sensory disturbances, especially in the thumb and index and middle fingers. The skin changes are characterized by dissociated anesthesia with loss of pain and temperature sense but retention of tactile sense. Burns are the most frequent lesions noted. Bullae, warts, and trophic ulcerations occur on the fingers and hands, and eventually contractures and gangrene occur. Other unusual features include hypertrophy of the limbs, hands, or feet

and asymmetric scalp hair growth with a sharp midline demarcation. The disease must be differentiated chiefly from Hansen disease. Unlike Hansen disease, syringomyelia does not interfere with sweating or block the flare around a histamine wheal.

Early surgical treatment allows for improvement of symptoms and prevents progression of neurologic deficits.

Blegvad C, et al: Syringomyelia. Acta Neurochir (Wien) 2014; 156: 2127.

Hereditary Sensory and Autonomic Neuropathies

A number of inherited conditions are characterized by variable degrees of motor and sensory dysfunctions combined with autonomic alterations. From a dermatologic standpoint, altered pain and temperature sensation, trophic changes, sweating abnormalities, ulcers of the hands and feet, and, in some patients, self-mutilating behavior may be present. These five syndromes and their variants are now known to be secondary to disease-producing mutations in 12 genes.

Rotthier A, et al: Mechanisms of disease in hereditary sensory and autonomic neuropathies. Nat Rev Neurol 2012; 8: 73.

5 Eczema, Atopic Dermatitis, and Noninfectious Immunodeficiency Disorders

ECZEMA

The word *eczema* seems to have originated in 543 AD and is derived from the Greek word *ekzein*, meaning to "to boil forth" or "to effervesce." The term encompasses such disorders as dyshidrotic eczema and nummular eczema (NE), but at times is used synonymously for atopic dermatitis (atopic eczema). The acute stage generally presents as a red edematous plaque that may have grossly visible, small, grouped vesicles. Subacute lesions present as erythematous plaques with scale or crusting. Later, lesions may be covered by a drier scale or may become lichenified. In most eczematous reactions, severe pruritus is a prominent symptom. The degree of irritation at which itching begins (the itch threshold) is lowered by stress. Itching is often prominent at bedtime and usually results in insomnia. Heat and sweating may also provoke episodes of itching.

Histologically, the hallmark of all eczematous eruptions is a serous exudate between cells of the epidermis (spongiosis), with an underlying dermal perivascular lymphoid infiltrate and exocytosis (lymphocytes present in overlying epidermis singly or in groups). Spongiosis is generally out of proportion to the lymphoid cells in the epidermis. This is in contrast to mycosis fungoides, which demonstrates minimal spongiosis confined to the area immediately surrounding the lymphocytes.

In most eczematous processes, spongiosis is very prominent in the acute stage, where it is accompanied by minimal acanthosis or hyperkeratosis. Subacute spongiotic dermatitis demonstrates epidermal spongiosis with acanthosis and hyperkeratosis. Chronic lesions may have minimal accompanying spongiosis, but acute and chronic stages may overlap because episodes of eczematous dermatitis follow one another. Scale corresponds to foci of parakeratosis produced by the inflamed epidermis. A crust is composed of serous exudate, acute inflammatory cells, and keratin. Eczema, regardless of cause, will manifest similar histologic changes if allowed to persist chronically. These features are related to chronic rubbing or scratching and correspond clinically to lichen simplex chronicus or prurigo nodularis. Histologic features at this stage include compact hyperkeratosis, irregular acanthosis, and thickening of the collagen bundles in the papillary portion of the dermis. The dermal infiltrate at all stages is predominantly lymphoid, but an admixture of eosinophils may be noted. Neutrophils generally appear in secondarily infected lesions. Spongiosis with many intraepidermal eosinophils may be seen in the early spongiotic phase of pemphigoid, pemphigus, and incontinentia pigmenti, as well as some cases of allergic contact dermatitis.

ATOPIC DERMATITIS (ATOPIC ECZEMA)

Atopic dermatitis (AD) is a chronic, inflammatory skin disease characterized by pruritus and a chronic course of exacerbations and remissions. It is associated with other atopic conditions, including food allergies, asthma, allergic rhinoconjunctivitis, eosinophilic esophagitis, and eosinophilic gastroenteritis. Because AD usually precedes the appearance of these other atopic conditions, it has been proposed that AD is the first step in an "atopic march" whereby sensitization to allergens through the skin may lead to allergic responses in the airways or digestive tract. Although this sequence of atopic conditions does occur in many children, whether the AD is causal in the development of the other manifestations of atopy is unproved but plausible. For this reason, early and effective treatment of AD is encouraged in an effort to prevent other atopic conditions. The genetic defect(s) predisposing at-risk individuals to the development of AD is the same for asthma and allergic rhinoconjunctivitis, and thus it has been difficult to prove that AD is causal in the development of other atopic conditions.

Epidemiology

The prevalence of AD, asthma, and allergic rhinoconjunctivitis increased dramatically in the last half of the 20th century, becoming a major health problem in many countries. The increase began first in the most developed nations, and as the standard of living has increased worldwide, so has the prevalence of AD. Rates of AD are about 30% in the most developed nations and exceed 10% in many countries, resulting in a worldwide cumulative prevalence of 20%. In the most developed nations, the rates of AD plateaued in the 1990s, whereas developing nations have rates that continue to increase. Factors associated with high rates of AD are high latitude (perhaps associated with low levels of annual sun exposure) and lower mean annual temperature. A role for exposure to allergens thought to "trigger" AD is not supported by epidemiologic studies. Iceland has a very high rate of AD (27%) yet has no dust mites, few trees, and low pet ownership. However, children in Iceland often have positive skin prick tests to environmental allergens (24%). This questions the value of such tests in predicting causal environmental allergens in AD. Girls are slightly more likely to develop AD. In the United States an increased risk of AD during the first 6 months of life is noted in infants with African and Asian race/ethnicity, male gender, greater gestational age at birth, and a family history of atopy, particularly a maternal history of eczema. Other factors that increase the risk for the development of AD early in childhood include consumption of a Western diet, birth order (first children at greater risk), and delivery by cesarean section, all of which alter the intestinal microbiome. Exposure to antibiotics prenatally during the first or second and third trimesters also increases risk of AD. Therefore biodiversity in the gut microbiome seems to be protective. Gut colonization with *Clostridium* cluster I is associated with development of AD. Dog ownership before age 1 year decreases the risk of developing AD by age 4, but cat ownership has no effect. The hygiene hypothesis suggests that being raised on a farm lowers the risk of AD whereas living in modernized, cleaner indoor environments leads to a higher risk of AD.

About 50% of cases of AD appear in the first year of life, the vast majority within the first 5 years of life, and the remaining cases of "adult" AD usually before age 30. Atopy is now so common in the population that most individuals have a family history of atopy. Elevated immunoglobulin E (IgE) levels are not diagnostic of atopic disease in the adult. Therefore elevated IgE and a family history of "atopy" in an adult with new-onset dermatitis should not be used to confirm the diagnosis of adult AD. Adult AD should only be considered when the dermatitis has a characteristic distribution and when other significant diagnoses, such as allergic contact dermatitis, photodermatitis, and cutaneous T-cell lymphoma, have been excluded. Rather, a dermatologist should infrequently make the diagnosis of adult "atopic dermatitis" for a dermatitis appearing for the first time after age 30.

Genetic Basis and Pathogenesis

Eighty percent of identical twins show concordance for AD. A child is at increased risk of developing AD if either parent is affected. More than one quarter of offspring of atopic mothers develop AD in the first 3 months of life. If one parent is atopic, more than half the children will develop allergic symptoms by age 2. This rate rises to 79% if both parents are atopic. All of these findings strongly suggested a genetic cause for AD. Filaggrin is a protein encoded by the gene *FLG*, that resides in the epidermal differentiation complex (EDC) on chromosome 1q21. Filaggrin is processed by caspase 14 during terminal keratinocyte differentiation into highly hydroscopic pyrrolidone carboxylic acid and urocanic acid, collectively known as the "natural moisturizing factor" (NMF). Null mutations in *FLG* lead to reduction in NMF, which probably contributes to the xerosis that is almost universal in AD. Transepidermal water loss (TEWL) is increased. This may be caused by subclinical dermatitis, but also by abnormal delivery of lamellar body epidermal lipids (especially ceramide) to the interstices of the terminally differentiated keratinocytes. The resulting defective lipid bilayers retain water poorly, leading to increased TEWL and clinical xerosis. Ichthyosis vulgaris is caused by mutations in the *FLG* gene and is frequently associated with AD. Four *FLG* mutations have an estimated combined allelic frequency of 7%–10% in individuals of European descent. Different *FLG* gene mutations are associated with AD in other ethnicities although the rates do not necessarily match AD prevalence, demonstrating that the disease is multifactorial. Filaggrin 2 (*FLG2*), also in the EDC and with similar function to *FLG*, is associated with persistent AD in African Americans. Inheriting one null *FLG* mutation slightly increases one's risk of developing AD, and inheriting two mutations, either as a homozygote or a compound heterozygote, dramatically increases one's risk. Between 42% and 79% of persons with one or more *FLG* null mutations will develop AD. However, 40% of carriers with *FLG* null mutations never have AD. *FLG* mutations are associated with AD that presents early in life, tends to persist into childhood and adulthood, and is associated with wheezing in infancy and with asthma. *FLG* mutations are also associated with allergic rhinitis and keratosis pilaris, independent of AD. Hyperlinear palms are strongly associated with *FLG* mutations, with a 71% positive predictive value (PPV) for marked palmar hyperlinearity. *LAMA3* gene mutations, encoding the alpha chain of laminin 5, may also predispose to AD. In murine models, decreased Claudin 3 expression can lead to leakage of sweat in the superficial dermis contributing to impaired sweating in atopic dermatitis.

Not all cases of AD are associated with *FLG* mutations. AD patients often demonstrate immunologic features consistent with a T-helper 2 (Th2) phenotype, with elevated IgE, eosinophils on skin biopsy, and positive skin tests and radioallergosorbent test (RAST). The cytokines, especially interleukin-4 (IL-4) and interleukin-13 (IL-13), that are released due to the Th2 immune response play an important role in AD by increasing inflammatory cell infiltration and stimulating the inflammatory feedback loop. Basophils and innate type 2 lymphoid cells can also secrete IL-4 and IL-13. Thymic stromal lymphopoietin (TSLP) is an important interleukin-7 (IL-7)–like cytokine that, through its interaction with Th2 cells, basophils, mast cells, and dendritic cells, promotes the secretion and production of Th2 cytokines and the development of inflammatory Th2 CD4+ T cells (through production of OL40L). TSLP is produced by keratinocytes and is found in high levels in AD skin lesions. In addition, interleukin-31 (IL-31) is produced by Th2 and Th22 cells. IL-31 binds directly to nerves leading to itching and also downregulates expression of filaggrin. The JAK-STAT pathway is also critical in causing overactivation of the

TH2 response and itch. Interleukin-17 (IL-17) and interleukin-22 (IL-22), which are released by Th17 cells, are also elevated in AD. Thus AD appears to represent a disorder characterized by a barrier defect that activates a specific Th2 response leading to a cycle of inflammation mediated by various inflammatory signals. The cytokines produced then worsen the already defective barrier. This leads to a vicious cycle of barrier failure and progressive inflammation, producing a chronic, relapsing, pruritic disorder, and explains why moisturization alone is not enough once the inflammatory cascade has started.

Cotter DG, et al: Emerging therapies for atopic dermatitis: JAK inhibitors. Journal of the American Academy of Dermatology 2018; 78(3): S53-62.

Yamaga K, et al: Claudin-3 Loss Causes Leakage of Sweat from the Sweat Gland to Contribute to the Pathogenesis of Atopic Dermatitis. Journal of Investigative Dermatology 2018; 138(6): 1279-87.

Prevention in High-Risk Children

Extensive studies have been undertaken to determine whether it is possible to prevent the development of AD in children at high risk—those with parents or siblings with atopy. The most promising studies now repeated multiple times show that early moisturization, starting before 3 weeks of life, with thick emollient, may prevent AD in children at high risk of developing AD. Twice daily moisturization with various emollients such as petrolatum, sunflower seed oil, and others leads to an approximately 50% reduction in the expected rate of AD development in the first 6 months of life. This supports the idea that breaks in the skin barrier are an essential step in developing AD.

Switching to soy formula does not appear to reduce the risk of developing AD. Prolonged exclusive breastfeeding beyond 3–4 months of age is not protective for the development of AD. Extensively hydrolyzed casein formulas may be used as a supplement or substitute for breast milk during the first 4 months of life. Maternal allergen avoidance during pregnancy does not reduce the risk of AD in the offspring. Probiotic administration during and after pregnancy has been shown to decrease AD incidence by 14% based on data from a meta-analysis. However, the type of probiotic to use, exactly when to start, and the safety during pregnancy are not fully elucidated. House dust mite (HDM) avoidance does not reduce AD, even in sensitized individuals, and high levels of HDMs in the environment in early life reduce AD risk.

Food Allergy

The role of food allergy in AD is complicated, and the purported role of foods in AD has changed in recent years. Approximately 35% of children with moderate to severe AD have food allergies. However, 85% of children with AD will have elevated IgE to food or inhalant allergens, making a diagnosis of food allergy with serum or prick tests alone challenging due to the high false-positive rate of testing. Before food allergy testing is undertaken, treatment of the AD should be optimized. Parents are often seeking a "cause" for the child's AD, when in fact it could be controlled with appropriate topical measures. Food restriction diets can be difficult and could put the child at risk for malnourishment and possibly development of allergy and should never be pursued without the oversight of an allergist and nutritionist to ensure proper nutrition. Food allergy should be pursued only in younger children with moderate to severe AD in whom standard treatments have failed. These children should also have a history of possible triggering of AD by specific food exposures. Testing, if performed, should be targeted foods to which the child is likely to be exposed, but generally wheat, egg, soy, cow's milk, and peanut testing has been the most relevant to the AD. Double-blind placebo-controlled food challenges are the "gold standard" for diagnosing food allergy. Skin prick tests have a high negative predictive value (>95%) but a PPV of only 30%–65%. For example, more than 8% of the U.S. population has a positive prick test to peanut, but only 0.4% are actually clinically allergic. Possible food allergy detected by testing should be confirmed by clinical history. A positive RAST or skin prick test for a food that the child rarely or never ingests is probably not causally relevant to the child's AD. Higher serum IgE levels and larger wheal sizes (>8–10 mm) are associated with greater likelihood of reacting to these foods when challenged. About 90% of food allergy is caused by a limited number of foods, as follows:

- Infants: cow's milk, egg, soybean, wheat
- Children (2–10 years): cow's milk, egg, peanut, tree nuts, fish, crustacean shellfish, sesame, kiwi fruit
- Older children: peanut, tree nuts, fish, shellfish, sesame, pollen-associated foods

Breastfeeding mothers must avoid the incriminated foods if their infant has been diagnosed with a food allergy.

There has been a rapid rise in peanut allergy in the United States. Recommendations to limit peanut exposure in childhood has been revised. A large randomized placebo control trial showed that early exposure in children at high risk for peanut allergy (due to strong family history of atopy) decreased the rate of development of peanut allergy by 86%. Therefore the revised guidelines that were developed in conjunction with dermatologists and allergists for peanut exposure are based on AD in the child. Of course a whole peanut should never be given to an infant due to choking hazard; therefore this was done with smooth peanut butter or the peanut snack Bamba (trademark).

1. Children with severe AD or egg allergy should be considered for peanut testing before exposure to peanuts around 4–6 months of age.
2. Mild to moderate AD: Introduce peanuts around 6 months.
3. No AD or food allergy: Introduce peanuts in accordance with family and cultural preferences.

Aeroallergens

It is debated how much of a role aeroallergens play in the pathophysiology of AD. Although early exposure to allergens may lessen the incidence of AD, exposure to dust mites, animal allergens, mold, pollen, tree allergens, and other airborne allergens in those who are allergic may exacerbate AD. Testing for IgE responses to aeroallergens may not be predictive of their effect on patients with AD. In patients who note worsening around specific allergens, they should avoid these. Common allergens to avoid if possible include tobacco smoke, pollen, house dust mites, cats, and dogs (if allergic) although early exposure to dogs may prevent AD. Reduction of dust mite exposure can be achieved through vacuuming with a filtered vacuum, using dust mite covers on mattresses, avoidance of stuffed animals, and wall-to-wall carpeting if feasible.

Clinical Manifestations

AD can be divided into three stages: infantile AD, occurring from 2 months to 2 years of age; childhood AD, from 2–10 years; and adolescent/adult AD. In all stages, pruritus is the hallmark. Itching often precedes the appearance of lesions, thus the concept that AD is "the itch that rashes." Useful diagnostic criteria include those of Hannifin and Rajka, the UK Working Party, and the American Academy of Dermatology's Consensus Conference on Pediatric Atopic Dermatitis (Boxes 5.1 and 5.2). These criteria have specificity at or above 90% but have much lower sensitivities (40%–100%). Therefore these criteria are useful for enrolling patients in studies and ensuring that they have AD, but less practical in diagnosing a specific patient with AD.

BOX 5.1 Criteria for Atopic Dermatitis

MAJOR CRITERIA

Must have three of the following:
1. Pruritus
2. Typical morphology and distribution
   - Flexural lichenification in adults
   - Facial and extensor involvement in infancy
3. Chronic or chronically relapsing dermatitis
4. Personal or family history of atopic disease (e.g., asthma, allergic rhinitis, atopic dermatitis)

MINOR CRITERIA

Must also have three of the following:
1. Xerosis
2. Ichthyosis/hyperlinear palms/keratosis pilaris
3. IgE reactivity (immediate skin test reactivity, RAST test positive)
4. Elevated serum IgE
5. Early age of onset
6. Tendency for cutaneous infections (especially *Staphylococcus aureus* and HSV)
7. Tendency to nonspecific hand/foot dermatitis
8. Nipple eczema
9. Cheilitis
10. Recurrent conjunctivitis
11. Dennie-Morgan infraorbital fold
12. Keratoconus
13. Anterior subcapsular cataracts
14. Orbital darkening
15. Facial pallor/facial erythema
16. Pityriasis alba
17. Itch when sweating
18. Intolerance to wool and lipid solvents
19. Perifollicular accentuation
20. Food hypersensitivity
21. Course influenced by environmental and/or emotional factors
22. White dermatographism or delayed blanch to cholinergic agents

HSV, Herpes simplex virus; *IgE,* immunoglobulin E; *RAST,* radioallergosorbent assay.

BOX 5.2 Modified Criteria for Children With Atopic Dermatitis

ESSENTIAL FEATURES
1. Pruritus
2. Eczema
   - Typical morphology and age-specific pattern
   - Chronic or relapsing history

IMPORTANT FEATURES
1. Early age at onset
2. Atopy
3. Personal and/or family history
4. IgE reactivity
5. Xerosis

ASSOCIATED FEATURES
1. Atypical vascular responses (e.g., facial pallor, white dermatographism)
2. Keratosis pilaris/ichthyosis/hyperlinear palms
3. Orbital/periorbital changes
4. Other regional findings (e.g., perioral changes/periauricular lesions)
5. Perifollicular accentuation/lichenification/prurigo lesions

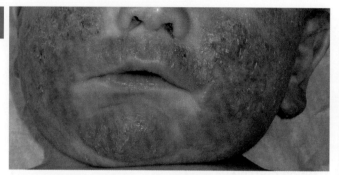

Fig. 5.1 Atopic dermatitis.

Eichenfield LF, et al: Consensus conference on pediatric atopic dermatitis. J Am Acad Dermatol 2003; 49: 1088-95
Hanifin JM, et al: Diagnostic features of atopic dermatitis. Acta Derm Venereol (Stockh) 1980; (Suppl. 92): 44-7

Infantile Atopic Dermatitis

Fifty percent or more of AD cases present in the first year of life, but usually not until after 2 months. Widespread dermatitis in children under 2 months may be from an irritant, ichthyosis, or a hallmark of severe immunodeficiency. AD in infancy usually begins as erythema and scaling of the cheeks (Fig. 5.1). The eruption may extend to the scalp, neck, forehead, wrists, extensor extremities, and buttocks. There can be overlap with seborrheic dermatitis on the scalp and in the folds, but papular or nodular involvement in the axillae and inguinal folds is more typical of scabies infestation. Children with AD who have *FLG* gene mutations specifically have more cheek and extensor arm/hand involvement. There may be significant exudate; secondary effects from scratching, rubbing, and infection include crusts, infiltration, and pustules, respectively. Occlusion of saliva due to teething, extensive breastfeeding, and drooling may cause the cheeks and upper chest to flare and thick emollients can help prevent this. Breastfeeding should not be curtailed. The infiltrated plaques eventually take on a characteristic lichenified appearance. The infantile pattern of AD usually disappears by the end of the second year of life.

Worsening of AD is often observed in infants after immunizations and viral infections likely due to activation of the immune system. Partial remission may occur during the summer, with relapse in winter. This may relate to the therapeutic effects of ultraviolet (UV) B light and humidity in many atopic patients, as well as the aggravation by wool and dry air in the winter. Extensive airborne environmental allergies may lead to worsening in the warmer months.

Childhood Atopic Dermatitis

During childhood, lesions tend to be less exudative. The classic locations are the antecubital and popliteal fossae (Fig. 5.2), flexor wrists, ankles, eyelids, face, and around the neck. Lesions are often lichenified, indurated plaques. These are intermingled with isolated, excoriated, 2–4 mm papules that are scattered more widely over the uncovered parts. Nummular morphology and involvement of the feet are more common in childhood AD.

Pruritus is a constant feature, and most of the cutaneous changes are secondary to it. Itching is paroxysmal. Scratching induces lichenification and may lead to secondary infection. A vicious cycle may be established, the itch-scratch cycle, as pruritus leads to scratching, and scratching causes secondary changes that in them cause itching. Instead of scratching causing pain, in the atopic patient the "pain" induced by scratching is perceived as itch and induces more scratching. The scratching impulse is beyond the control of the patient. Severe bouts of scratching occur during

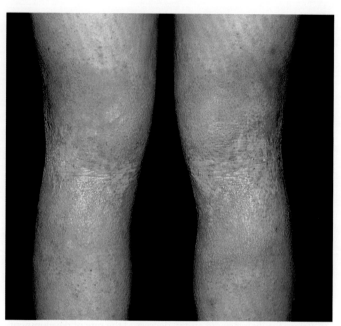

Fig. 5.2 Flexural involvement in childhood atopic dermatitis.

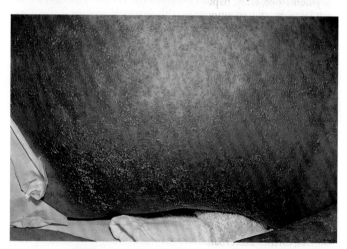

Fig. 5.3 Severe, widespread atopic dermatitis.

sleep, leading to poor rest and chronic tiredness in atopic children. This can affect school performance. Parents often scold children who are scratching, and this leads to more anxiety and thus more scratching.

Severe AD involving a large percentage of the body surface area (BSA) can be associated with growth retardation (Fig. 5.3). Restriction diets and steroid use may exacerbate growth impairment. Aggressive management of such children with phototherapy or systemic immunosuppressive agents may allow for rebound growth. Children with severe AD may also have substantial psychological disturbances. Parents should be questioned with regard to school performance and socialization. Although using light therapy and systemic immunosuppressive or immunomodulatory therapy in children can be daunting for patients and practitioners, the benefits to quality of life can dramatically outweigh the risks.

Atopic Dermatitis in Adolescents and Adults

Most adolescents and adults with AD will give a history of childhood disease. AD will begin after age 18 years in only 6%–14% of patients diagnosed with AD. One exception is the patient who moves from a humid, tropical region to a more temperate area of higher latitude. This climatic change is often associated with the appearance of AD. In older patients, AD may occur as localized

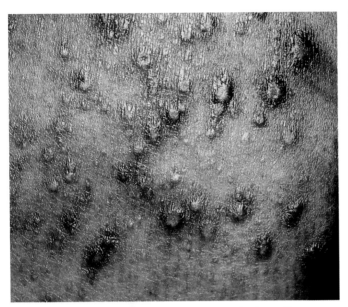

Fig. 5.4 Prurigo-like papules in adult atopic dermatitis.

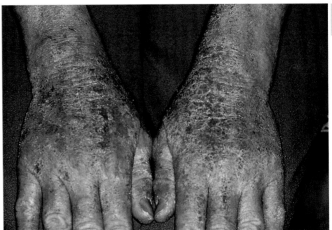

Fig. 5.5 Atopic hand dermatitis.

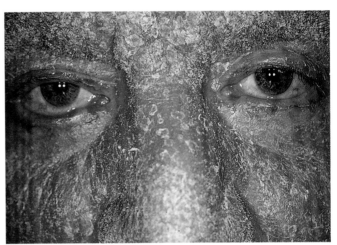

Fig. 5.6 Periocular atopic dermatitis.

erythematous, scaly, papular, exudative, or lichenified plaques. In adolescents, the eruption often involves the classic antecubital and popliteal fossae, front and sides of the neck, forehead, and area around the eyes. In older adults, the distribution is generally less characteristic, and localized dermatitis may be the predominant feature, especially hand, nipple, or eyelid eczema. At times, the eruption may generalize, with accentuation in the flexures. The skin generally is dry and somewhat erythematous. Lichenification and prurigo-like papules are common (Fig. 5.4). Papular lesions tend to be dry, slightly elevated, and flat topped. They are almost always excoriated and often coalesce to form plaques. Staphylococcal colonization is common. In darker-skinned patients, the lesions are often hyperpigmented, frequently with focal hypopigmented areas related to healed excoriations.

Itching usually occurs in crises or paroxysms. Adults frequently complain that flares of AD are triggered by acute emotional upsets. Stress, anxiety, and depression reduce the threshold at which itch is perceived and result in damage to the epidermal permeability barrier, further exacerbating AD. Atopic persons may sweat poorly and may complain of severe pruritus related to heat or exercise. Physical conditioning and liberal use of emollients improve this component, and atopic patients can participate in competitive sports.

Even in patients with AD in adolescence or early adulthood, improvement usually occurs over time, and dermatitis is uncommon after middle life. In general, these patients retain mild stigmata of the disease, such as dry skin, easy skin irritation, and itching in response to heat and perspiration. They remain susceptible to a flare of their disease when exposed to a specific allergen or environmental situation. Photosensitivity develops in approximately 3% of AD patients and may manifest as either a polymorphous light eruption–type reaction or simply exacerbation of the AD by UV exposure. The average age for photosensitive AD is the middle to late thirties. Human immunodeficiency virus (HIV) infection can also serve as a trigger, and new-onset AD in an at-risk adult should lead to counseling and testing for HIV if warranted.

The hands, including the wrists, are frequently involved in adults, and hand dermatitis is a common problem for adults with a history of AD. It is common for irritant or atopic hand dermatitis to appear in young women after the birth of a child, when increased exposure to soaps and water triggers their disease. There is a new trend in children who can buy kits or mix their own various household liquids such as glue, borax, contact solution, baking soda and others to make "slime". This can lead to irritant dermatitis or worsening of hand atopic dermatitis. Wet work is a major factor in hand eczema in general, including those patients with AD.

Atopic hand dermatitis can affect both the dorsal and the palmar surface (Fig. 5.5). Keratosis punctata of the creases, a disorder seen almost exclusively in black persons, is also more common in atopic patients. Patients with AD have frequent exposure to preservatives and other potential allergens in the creams and lotions that are continually applied to their skin. Contact allergy may manifest as chronic hand eczema. Patch testing can help differentiate an allergic contact dermatitis.

Eyelids are often involved (Fig. 5.6). In general, the involvement is bilateral and the condition flares with cold weather. As in hand dermatitis, irritants and allergic contact allergens must be excluded by a careful history and patch testing.

Gittler JK, et al: "Slime" May Not be so Benign: A Cause of Hand Dermatitis. The Journal of pediatrics. 2018.

Associated Features and Complications

Cutaneous Stigmata

A linear transverse fold just below the edge of the lower eyelids, known as the Dennie-Morgan fold, is indicative of the atopic diathesis, although it may be seen with any chronic dermatitis of the lower lids. In atopic patients with eyelid dermatitis, increased folds and darkening under the eyes is common. When there is extensive facial involvement, the nose is still typically spared. This is called the "headlight sign." The axillary vault and inguinal folds are also typically spared likely due to high humidity in these areas.

A prominent nasal crease may also be noted due to chronic upward wiping of the nose when there is rhinitis secondary to seasonal allergies. This is called the "nasal salute." When taken together with other clinical findings, these remain helpful clinical signs.

The less involved skin of atopic patients is frequently dry and slightly erythematous and may be scaly. Histologically, the apparently normal skin of atopic patients is frequently inflamed subclinically. The dry, scaling skin of AD may represent low-grade dermatitis. Pityriasis alba is a form of subclinical dermatitis, frequently atopic in origin. It presents as poorly marginated, hypopigmented, slightly scaly patches on the cheeks, upper arms, and trunk, typically in children and young adults with types III to V skin. It usually responds to emollients and mild topical steroids, preferably in an ointment base.

Keratosis pilaris (KP) consists of horny follicular lesions of the outer aspects of the upper arms, legs, cheeks, and buttocks and is often associated with AD, AD and occurs in patients with filagrin mutations. The keratotic papules on the face may be on a red background, a variant of KP called keratosis pilaris rubra faceii. KP is often refractory to treatment. Moisturizers alone are only partially beneficial. Some patients will respond to topical lactic acid, urea, or retinoids but they can easily irritate the skin of atopic patients and should be avoided in young children. If older patients desire, treatment should begin with applications only once or twice a week. KP must be differentiated from follicular eczema which tends to affect the trunk and is often more prominent in patients with skin types III-VI.

Thinning of the lateral eyebrows (Hertoghe sign) is sometimes present. This apparently occurs from chronic rubbing caused by pruritus and subclinical dermatitis. Hyperkeratosis and hyperpigmentation, which produce a "dirty neck" appearance, are also common in AD patients.

Vascular Stigmata

White dermatographism is blanching of the skin at the site of stroking or scratching. Chronic exposure to the vasoconstrictive effects of topical and oral steroids may lead to erythroderma due to vasodilation when steroids are tapered. This can lead to dysesthesias and belies the importance of using maintenance therapies that limit steroid exposure or lessen strength.

Atopic patients are at increased risk of developing various forms of urticaria, including contact urticaria. Episodes of contact urticaria may be followed by typical eczematous lesions at the affected site because skin that is scratched may flare with AD.

Ophthalmologic Abnormalities

Up to 10% of patients with AD develop cataracts, either anterior or posterior subcapsular. Posterior subcapsular cataracts in atopic individuals are indistinguishable from corticosteroid-induced cataracts. Development of cataracts is more common in patients with severe dermatitis. Keratoconus is an uncommon finding, occurring in approximately 1% of atopic patients. Contact lenses, keratoplasty, and intraocular lenses may be required to treat this condition. Environmental allergies may also lead to allergic rhinoconjunctivitis.

Susceptibility to Infection

Chronic eczematous lesions are often colonized with *Staphylococcus aureus*. *Staphylococcus epidermitis* may actually be protective as it is predominates in patients with fewer flares. In addition, the apparently normal nonlesional skin of atopic patients may also be colonized by *S. aureus*. The finding of increasing numbers of pathogenic staphylococci on the skin of a patient with AD is frequently associated with weeping and crusting of skin lesions, retroauricular and infraauricular and perinasal fissures, folliculitis, and adenopathy. In a flaring atopic patient, the possibility of

secondary infection must be considered. IgE antibodies directed against *Staphylococcus* and its toxins have been documented in some atopic individuals. Staphylococcal production of superantigens is another possible mechanism for staphylococcal flares of disease. Treatment of lesions of AD with topical steroids is associated with reduced numbers of pathogenic bacteria on the surface, even if antibiotics are not used. Despite the frequent observation that the presence of staphylococcal infection of lesions of AD is associated with worsening of disease, it has not been proven that oral antibiotics make a long term difference in the course of AD. Nonetheless, treatment of the "infected" AD patient with oral antibiotics is a community standard of dermatologists worldwide.

With the widespread presence of antibiotic-resistant *S. aureus*, dermatologists have shifted from the chronic use of oral antibiotics in managing patients with frequent flares of AD associated with staphylococcal infection. Rather, dilute sodium hypochlorite (bleach) baths and reduction of nasal carriage have become the basis for preventing infection-triggered AD. The typical formula is one quarter of a US cup (approximately 60 milliliters) of plain, unscented, NOT concentrated, NOT splashproof bleach per 20 gallon bathtub of water. In patients with AD and frequent infections, chronic suppressive oral antibiotic therapy may stabilize the disease. Options include cephalosporins, trimethoprim-sulfamethoxazole (TMP-SMX), clindamycin, and (in older patients) doxycycline. Identifying and treating *S. aureus* carriers in the family and pets may also be of benefit. An unusual complication of *S. aureus* infection in patients with AD is subungual infection, with osteomyelitis of the distal phalanx. In atopic patients with fever who appear very toxic, the possibility of streptococcal infection must be considered. These children may require hospital admission and intravenous antibiotics. Group A streptococcal superinfection of AD typically presents with a more vesiculopustular look that may mimic herpes simplex virus (HSV). Culture of the skin can differentiate and guide therapy typically with a penicillin- or cephalosporin-based antibiotic.

Patients with AD have increased susceptibility to viral super-infection, especially from HSV, varicella-zoster virus (VZV), enteroviruses (Coxsackie), vaccinia, and molluscum. *Kaposi varicelliform infection* is a term used to describe an acute vesicular eruption on top of AD and is usually caused by HSV, VZV, or enterovirus superinfection. Eczema herpeticum is seen most frequently in young children and is usually associated with HSV type 1 transmitted from a caretaker or sibling. Once infected, there can be frequent flares of eczema herpeticum. Eczema herpeticum presents as the sudden appearance of vesicular, pustular, crusted, or eroded lesions concentrated in the areas of dermatitis (Fig. 5.7). The patients may have a fever and appear toxic. The lesions may continue to spread, and most of the skin surface may become involved. Secondary staphylococcal or streptococcal infection is common, and local edema and regional adenopathy frequently occur. If lesions of eczema herpeticum occur on or around the eyelids, ophthalmologic evaluation is recommended. The severity of eczema herpeticum is quite variable, but most cases require systemic antiviral therapy and an antistaphylococcal antibiotic. Delayed administration of acyclovir in hospitalized patients is associated with prolonged hospital stay. Genetic variants in TSLP and interferon regulatory factor 2 (IFR-2) in addition to DOCK 8 mutations are associated with AD and eczema herpeticum.

Recently a more virulent form of "hand foot and mouth" caused by enterovirus A6 instead of the typical A16 (also termed *Coxsackie A16*) has been recognized and labeled "eczema coxsackium." Superinfection with the A6 strain often leads to very widespread papules and vesicles with low-grade fever. There will typically be at least a few lesions on the palms and soles and in the mouth but there is not the typical predominance in these areas compared with areas of AD. Therapy is supportive.

Vaccination against smallpox is contraindicated in persons with AD, even when the dermatitis is in remission. Widespread and even fatal vaccinia can occur in patients with an atopic diathesis.

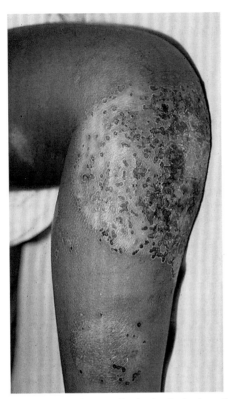

Fig. 5.7 Recurrent herpes simplex in atopic dermatitis.

Atopic individuals may also develop extensive flat warts or molluscum contagiosum (MC). If the infection is extremely exuberant, an immunodeficiency such as DOCK-8 mutation should be ruled out. A common presentation of MC in children is a new patch of AD in an unusual area such as an axilla due to MC causing an immune response leading to a flare of AD. Chemical therapies such as salicylic acid and cantharidin may cause severe irritation within lesions of AD. Destruction with curettage (for molluscum), cryosurgery, or electrosurgery may be required to clear the lesions.

Differential Diagnosis

Typical AD in infancy and childhood is straightforward because of its characteristic morphology; predilection for symmetric involvement of the face, neck, and antecubital and popliteal fossae; and association with food allergy, asthma, and allergic rhinoconjunctivitis. Dermatoses that may resemble AD include seborrheic dermatitis (especially in infants), irritant or allergic contact dermatitis, nummular dermatitis, photodermatitis, scabies, and cases of psoriasis with an eczematous morphology. Certain immunodeficiency syndromes (see later discussion) may exhibit a dermatitis remarkably similar or identical to AD. In older patients with new onset dermatitis, cutaneous T cell lymphoma and allergic contact dermatitis should be considered.

Histopathology

The histology of AD varies with the stage of the lesion, with many of the changes induced by scratching. Hyperkeratosis, acanthosis, and excoriation are common. Staphylococcal colonization may be noted histologically. Although eosinophils may not be seen in the dermal infiltrate, staining for eosinophil major basic protein (MBP) reveals deposition in many cases.

General Management

Education and Support

Parental and patient education is of critical importance in the management of AD. In the busy clinic setting, dermatologists frequently have insufficient time to educate patients adequately regarding the multiple factors that are important in managing AD. Educational formats that have proved effective have been immediate nursing education on the correct use of medications, weekly evening educational sessions, and multidisciplinary day treatment venues. There are also now multiple online resources from major academic centers, professional societies, and associations that can be helpful. In all cases, "written action plans" outlining a "stepwise approach" have been important for parent/patient education. In addition, patients with chronic disease often become disenchanted with medical therapies or simply "burn out" from having to spend significant amounts of time managing their skin disease. The psychological support that can be incorporated into educational sessions can help motivate parents/patients and keep them engaged in the treatment plan. Having a child with AD is extremely stressful and generates significant stress within the family. Sleep is lost by both the patient and the parents. Supportive educational techniques and sometimes professional behavioral health consultation can help the family cope with this burden. In addition, the dermatologist must consider the complexity and time commitment of any prescribed regimen and ensure that the parents/patient understand and are committed to undertaking the treatments proposed.

Barrier Repair

AD patients have an impaired epidermal barrier. The cornerstone of treatment and prevention of AD lies in addressing this problem. Patients should moisturize daily, especially immediately after bathing, ideally while the skin is still damp within a few minutes of getting out of the water. This may be with petrolatum or a petrolatum-based product, an oil-based product, a dimethicone-based product, vegetable shortening, or a "barrier repair" moisturizer that contains the essential lipids of the epidermal barrier. These special barrier repair moisturizers have similar benefits in AD to low-potency topical steroids. They are easier to apply and, if available to the patient, may enhance compliance. Petrolatum and petrolatum-based moisturizers are most often recommended and are often the least expensive. However, men with significant body hair, AD patients triggered by heat, and the very rare patient with true allergic contact dermatitis to petrolatum may be unable to tolerate petrolatum-based agents. Moisturizers should ideally be fragrance and formaldehyde free because these are two of the most common allergens in patients with AD. The ratio and content of ceramides in the epidermis of patients with AD is abnormal. Moisturizers with ceramides added have been shown to provide some benefit beyond the actual emollient. Patients should be instructed on the barrier-damaging properties of soaps, hot water, and scrubbing. The pH of the skin that promotes normal epidermal function is slightly acidic (the acid mantle) so synthetic detergents that have a more acidic pH are preferred to more basic soaps that have a high concentration of surfactant. Detergent use should be restricted to the axilla, groin, face, soles, and scalp. Oil-based cleansers can be used to "wash" the skin without water. For flares of AD, the soak and smear technique (soak in tub, then seal in water with a heavy moisturizer or medicated ointments) or wet dressings (wet wraps) with topical steroids can be very effective. In dry climates, AD patients may note some benefit with humidifiers. α-Hydroxy acid–containing products (lactic acid, glycolic acid) can be irritating and can exacerbate inflamed AD. These products should only be used for the xerosis of AD when there is absolutely no inflammation or pruritus.

Antimicrobial Therapy

When the AD patient has evidence of infection, treatment with topical or systemic antibiotics may be appropriate. Rather than treating once an infection occurs, it appears that the key in AD is to reduce nasal staphylococcal carriage preemptively and to keep the skin decolonized from *Staphylococcus*. Dilute sodium hypochlorite (bleach) baths have rapidly become a mainstay in AD patients. Twice-weekly bathing in a tepid bath with one quarter of a US cup (approximately 60 ml) of standard household bleach (5–6%) diluted in 20 gallons of water dramatically improves AD on the trunk and extremities, but less so on the face. For a smaller baby bathtub this is typically 2.5 mL = ½ teaspoon per gallon of water. Many bleach manufacturers make splashless or double-concentrated bleach, which should be avoided. This treatment combines decolonization of the skin with hydration, addressing two of the major factors in worsening of AD. Dilute bleach baths have been shown to decrease Nuclear Factor (NF) kappa-beta and thus may serve a role as a primary antiinflammatory therapy as well. Adequate moisturizing after bathing is critical. Intranasal application of mupirocin is beneficial in reducing nasal carriage although resistance is emerging. In 80% of families, at least one parent is carrying the same staphylococcal strain as a colonized AD child. If the AD patient has recurrent infections, other carriers in the family and their pets are sought and treated aggressively. Recurrent infections, especially furunculosis, are a cardinal feature of children and adults with AD who have systemic immunologic abnormalities, especially hyper-IgE syndrome.

Environmental Factors

Stress, heat, sweating, and external irritants may precipitate an attack of itching and flare in the AD patient. Wool garments should be avoided. Addressing these triggers may improve the AD. Itch nerves are more active at higher temperatures, so overheating should be avoided. Irritants and allergens in the numerous products that AD patients may use can lead to flares of AD. Patients should avoid products that contain common allergens and should be evaluated for allergic contact dermatitis if a topical agent is associated with worsening of their AD.

Antipruritics

The primary treatment for the pruritus of AD is to reduce the severity of the AD. Antihistamines are frequently used for the pruritus of AD but are mainly beneficial for their sedative properties. If the patient has environmental allergies that lead to itch, the scratched skin can flare with AD, so in these patients long-acting histamine-2 blockers such as cetirizine, loratadine, and fexofenadine may help by decreasing the symptoms of the environmental allergies. Sedating antihistamines can lose some of their sedative effect if used consistently, so ideally they are only used when needed. Diphenhydramine, hydroxyzine, and doxepin can all be efficacious. Nonsedating antihistamines do not appear to benefit the pruritus of AD in standard doses. In some patients, gabapentin, selective serotonin reuptake inhibitors (SSRIs), mirtazapine, and even opiate antagonists may reduce pruritus. Applying ice during intense bouts of itch may help to "break" an itch paroxysm. Moisturizing lotions containing menthol, phenol, or pramoxine can be used between steroid applications to moisturize and reduce local areas of severe itch. More widespread use of topical doxepin (Sinequan) is limited by systemic absorption and sedation.

Specific Treatment Modalities

Topical Corticosteroid Therapy

Topical corticosteroids are the most common class of medications, along with moisturizers, used for the treatment of AD. They are effective and economical. Ointments are preferred because they can serve a double purpose as an emollient, they do not burn when applied, and they typically have fewer ingredients leading to lower of a chance of allergic contact dermatitis.

In infants, low-potency steroid ointments, are preferred. Regular application of emollients must be emphasized. Once corticosteroid receptors are saturated, additional applications of a steroid preparation contribute nothing more than an emollient effect. In most body sites, once-daily application of a corticosteroid is almost as effective as more frequent applications, at lower cost and with less systemic absorption and likely increased compliance. In some areas, twice-daily applications may be beneficial, but more frequent applications are almost never of benefit. Steroid phobia is common in parents and patients with AD. Less frequent applications of lower-concentration agents or intermittent use of steroids 2–5 times weekly, with emphasis on moisturizing, address these concerns. It can also be useful to point out that the human body must produce endogenous steroids daily to function. Application of topical corticosteroids under wet wraps or vinyl suit occlusion especially after soaking in a tub of water (soak and smear) can increase efficiency. For refractory areas, a stronger corticosteroid may be used. A more potent molecule is more appropriate than escalating concentrations of a weaker molecule because the effect of the latter plateaus rapidly as receptors become saturated, and the potent medication should be stopped when the flare subsides. Because AD is an inflammatory cascade that must be halted, it is important not to undertreat. Undertreatment leads to loss of faith on the part of the patient/parents and prolongs the suffering of the patient. For severe disease, using more potent topical steroids in short bursts of a few days to a week can help gain control of the disease. In refractory and relapsing AD, twice-weekly steroid application to the areas that commonly flare may reduce flares. Another maintenance method is to mix 1 part of hydrocortisone 2.5% ointment in with 1 to 4 parts of the patient's preferred emollient 2–5 days per week, lessening the amount this is used as tolerated.

In older children and adults, medium-potency steroids are often used, except on the face, where milder steroids or calcineurin inhibitors are preferred. For thick plaques and lichen simplex chronicus–like lesions, extremely potent steroids may be necessary. Ointments are more effective because of their moisturizing properties and require no preservatives, reducing the likelihood of allergic contact dermatitis. If an atopic patient worsens or fails to improve after the use of topical steroids and moisturizers, the possibility of allergic contact dermatitis to a preservative or the corticosteroids must be considered. Contact allergy to the corticosteroid itself can occur. Corticosteroid allergy seldom manifests as acute worsening of the eczema. Instead, it manifests as a flare of eczema whenever the corticosteroid is discontinued, even for a day. This may be difficult to differentiate from stubborn AD.

Although the potential for local and even systemic toxicity from corticosteroids is real, the steroid must be strong enough to control the pruritus and remove the inflammation. Even in small children, strong topical steroids may be necessary in weekly pulses to control severe flares. Monitoring of growth parameters should be carried out in infants and young children.

Ideally prevention of AD flares is with just emollients, but patients with more severe disease often need some consistent antiinflammatory medicines (similar to the paradigm used for asthma). Maintenance therapy with topical steroids as discussed earlier can be with twice-weekly application, mixing a low-potency steroid in with an emollient or with nonsteroidal antiinflammatory medications.

Topical Calcineurin Inhibitors

Topical calcineurin inhibitors (TCIs) such as tacrolimus or pimecrolimus offer an alternative to topical steroids. Systemic absorption is generally not significant with either of these agents.

Although a 0.03% tacrolimus ointment is marketed for use in children, it is unclear whether it really offers any safety advantage over the 0.1% formulation. Patients may experience a warm or stinging feeling in the skin when the medicines are first started. This tends to resolve and tolerability is improved if the ointment is applied to "bone-dry" skin. Patients experience less burning if eczematous patches are treated initially with a corticosteroid, with transition to a TCI after partial clearing. Improvement tends to be steady, with progressively smaller areas requiring treatment. TCIs are particularly useful on the eyelids and face, in areas prone to steroid atrophy, when steroid allergy is a consideration, or when systemic steroid absorption is a concern. Tacrolimus is more effective than pimecrolimus, with tacrolimus 0.1% ointment equivalent to triamcinolone acetonide 0.1%, and pimecrolimus equivalent to a class V or VI topical corticosteroid. There is a black box warning on calcineurin inhibitors in the United States, but a recent study that followed patients after marketing found no increase in malignancy in over 26,000 patient-years studied.

Topical Phosphodiesterase Inhibitors

Crisaborole is an antiinflammatory topical PDE4 inhibitor introduced in 2017 for AD in children over 2 years. It can be used on the face and skinfolds without concern for striae but may sting when applied. It may be most useful as a maintenance medication or for mild to moderate disease.

Tar

Crude coal tar 1%–5% in white petrolatum or hydrophilic ointment USP, or liquor carbonis detergens (LCDs) 5%–20% in hydrophilic ointment USP, is sometimes helpful for an area of refractory AD. Tar preparations are especially beneficial when used for intensive treatment for adults in an inpatient or day care setting, especially in combination with UV phototherapy. Goeckerman therapy with tar and UVB in a day treatment setting will lead to improvement in more than 90% of patients with refractory AD, and prolonged remission can be induced.

Phototherapy

If topical modalities fail to control AD, phototherapy is another step on the therapeutic ladder. Narrow-band (NB) UVB is highly effective and has replaced broadband UV for treating AD. When acutely inflamed, AD patients may tolerate UV poorly. Initial treatment with soak and smear topical steroids or a systemic immunosuppressive may cool off the skin enough to institute UV treatments. Patients with significant erythema must be introduced to UV at very low doses to avoid nonspecific irritancy and flaring of the AD. Often, the initial dose is much lower and the dose escalation much slower than in patients with psoriasis. In acute flares of AD, UVA I can be used. For patients unresponsive to NB UVB, photochemotherapy with psoralen plus UVA (PUVA) can be effective but the benefits must outweigh the risks. It requires less frequent treatments, and can be given either topically (soak/bath PUVA) or systemically (oral PUVA).

Systemic Therapy

Dupilumab is an IL-4 receptor inhibitor that thus blocks the function of IL-4 and IL-13. It is an injection given every 2 weeks after a loading dose and decreases pruritus and Eczema Area and Severity Index (EASI) scores. It is the first targeted systemic therapy for AD. The most common significant side effect is keratoconjunctivitis.

Systemic Corticosteroids. In general, systemic corticosteroids should be avoided due to concerns for reexacerbation when the steroids are stopped. Some will use systemic steroids to control acute exacerbations. In patients requiring systemic steroid therapy, short courses (≤3 weeks) are preferred. If repeated or prolonged courses of systemic corticosteroids are required to control the AD, phototherapy or a steroid-sparing systemic therapy should be considered. Chronic corticosteroid therapy for AD frequently results in significant steroid-induced side effects such as striae, infection, bony changes, and growth delay. Osteoporosis in women requires special consideration and should be addressed with a bisphosphonate early in the course of therapy when bone loss is greatest. Preventive strategies, such as calcium supplements, vitamin D supplementation, bisphosphonates, regular exercise, and smoking cessation, should be strongly encouraged. Dual-energy x-ray absorptiometry (DEXA) scans are recommended.

Cyclosporine

Cyclosporine (cyclosporin A) is highly effective in the treatment of severe AD, but the response is rarely sustained after the drug is discontinued. It is very useful to gain rapid control of severe AD. Cyclosporine has been shown to be safe and effective in both children and adults, although probably tolerated better in children. Potential long-term side effects, especially renal disease and hypertension, require careful monitoring, with attempts to transition the patient to a potentially less toxic agent if possible. The dose range is 3–5 mg/kg in children and 150–300 mg in adults, with a better and more rapid response at the higher end of the dose range. Cyclosporin should not be used long term due to risks of renal and other toxicity. Rebound flaring of AD is possible and can be significant after stopping cyclosporin A, and a plan should be in place for this eventuality.

Methotrexate

Methotrexate has a long history of safe use in children for other diseases. Recently studies have been published demonstrating that its efficacy is similar to cyclosporine, although the onset to action is significantly slower and it is not FDA approved for this indication. Doses are similar to what is used in psoriasis (0.3–0.6 mg/kg given once weekly (up to 25 mg) in children and 10–25 mg weekly in adults. Patients on methotrexate should take folic acid as well. The time to relapse with methotrexate may be longer than with cyclosporine. Switching from oral to subcutaneous administration may increase the benefit.

Other Immunosuppressive Agents

Several other immunosuppressive agents have demonstrated efficacy in patients with AD. They include axathioprine and mycophenolate mofetil. These agents do not appear to be as quick to work as cyclosporine. Patients with FLG mutations respond to azathioprine and methotrexate, but the response is slower than in those without FLG mutations. However, over time they may have a better safety profile, so patients requiring long-term immunosuppression may benefit from one of these agents. The dosing of azathioprine is guided by the serum thiopurine methyltransferase level. Mycophenolate mofetil (MMF) is generally well tolerated and, as with azathioprine, takes about 6 weeks to begin to reduce the AD. Unfortunately, the response of AD patients to MMF is variable, with 20%–40% not responding. If cyclosporin A is not to be used, the choice of steroid-sparing agent is personalized to the patient's risk factors and tolerance of the medication. Hydroxyurea, as used for psoriasis in the past, can be effective in AD if other steroid-sparing agents fail, as well as in the patient with liver disease.

Intravenous immune globulin (IVIG) has had some limited success in managing AD, but its high cost precludes it use, except when other reasonable therapeutic options have been exhausted. There are also reports of a dyshidrotic flare of dermatitis on the hands in patients on IVIG. Interferon-γ (IFN-γ) given by daily injection has demonstrated efficacy in both children and adults with severe AD but is very rarely used. IFN-γ is well tolerated but can cause flulike symptoms. Omalizumab can be considered in refractory cases, but only 20% of patients achieve a 50% or greater reduction of their AD. Infliximab has not been beneficial in AD. Ustekinumab has been effective in a few reports, because the inflammatory cascade triggering and maintaining AD does involve Th17 cells.

Traditional Chinese herb mixtures have shown efficacy in children and in animal models for AD. The active herbs appear to be ophiopogon tuber and Schisandra fruit. Chinese herbs are usually delivered as a brewed tea to be drunk daily. Their bitter taste makes them difficult to palate, and there is a risk of allergy from herbal products.

Management of Acute Flare

Initially, the precipitating cause of the flare should be sought. Recent stressful events may be associated with flares. Secondary infection with *S. aureus* is one of the most common causes for flares and will manifest with pustules and honey-colored erosions. Less frequently, HSV or coxsackievirus may be involved. Pityriasis rosea may also cause AD to flare. The development of contact sensitivity to an applied medication or photosensitivity must be considered.

In the patient with an acute flare, treating triggers may lead to improvement (see earlier discussion). Soaking and smearing (wet wrapping) is recommended as first-line treatment. Often, 3–4 days of such intensive home therapy will break a severe flare. A short course of systemic corticosteroids may be of benefit as a last resort.

Agusti-Mejias AM, et al: Severe refractory atopic dermatitis in an adolescent patient successfully treated with ustekinumab. Ann Dermatol 2013; 25: 3.

Andreae DA, Wang J: Immunologic effects of omalizumab in children with severe refractory atopic dermatitis. Pediatrics 2014; 134: S160.

Annesi-Maesano I, et al: Time trends in prevalence and severity of childhood asthma and allergies from 1995 to 2002 in France. Allergy 2009; 64: 798.

Benninger MS, et al: Prevalence of atopic disease in patients with eosinophilic esophagitis. Int Forum Allergy Rhinol 2017; 7: 757.

Byrd AL, et al: *Staphylococcus aureus* and *Staphylococcus epidermidis* strain diversity underlying pediatric atopic dermatitis. Sci Transl Med 2017; 9.

Cao L, et al: Long-term effect of early-life supplementation with probiotics on preventing atopic dermatitis. J Dermatolog Treat 2015; 26: 537.

Damm JA, et al: The influence of probiotics for preterm neonates on the incidence of atopic dermatitis. Arch Dermatol Res 2017; 309: 259.

Du Toit G, et al: Randomized trial of peanut consumption in infants at risk for peanut allergy. N Engl J Med 2015; 372: 803.

Dvorakova V, et al: Methotrexate for severe childhood atopic dermatitis. Pediatr Dermatol 2017; 34: 528.

Eichenfeld LF, et al: Guidelines of care for the management of atopic dermatitis. Section 1. J Am Acad Dermatol 2014; 70: 2.

Eichenfeld LF, et al: Guidelines of care for the management of atopic dermatitis. Section 2. J Am Acad Dermatol 2014; 71:116.

Epstein TG, et al: Opposing effects of cat and dog ownership and allergic sensitization on eczema in an atopic birth cohort. J Pediatr 2011; 158: 2.

Fleischer DM, et al: Primary prevention of allergic disease through nutritional interventions. J Allergy Clin Immunol 2013; 1: 29.

Flohr C, Mann J: New approaches to the prevention of childhood atopic dermatitis. Allergy 2014; 69: 56.

Flohr C, Mann J: New insights into the epidemiology of childhood atopic dermatitis. Allergy 2014; 69: 3.

Gao PS, et al: Genetic variants in interferon regulatory factor 2 (IRF2) are associated with atopic dermatitis and eczema herpeticum. J Invest Dermatol 2012; 132: 650.

Gao PS, et al: Genetic variants in thymic stromal lymphopoietin are associated with atopic dermatitis and eczema herpeticum. J Allergy Clin Immunol 2010; 125: 6.

Gittlem JK, et al: Progressive activation Th2/Th22 cytokines and selective epidermal proteins characterizes acute and chronic atopic dermatitis. J Allergy Clin Immunol 2012; 130: 6.

Goujon C, et al: Methotrexate versus cyclosporine in adults with moderate-to-severe atopic dermatitis. J Allergy Clin Immunol Pract 2017 Sep 26. Epub ahead of print.

Haeck IM, et al: Enteric-coated mycophenolate sodium versus cyclosporine as a long-term treatment in adult patients with severe atopic dermatitis. J Am Acad Dermatol 2011; 64: 6.

Hotze M, et al: Increased efficacy of omalizumab in atopic dermatitis patients with wild-type filaggrin status and higher serum levels of phosphatidylcholines. Allergy 2014; 69: 132.

Huang JT, et al: Treatment of *Staphylococcus aureus* colonization in atopic dermatitis decreases disease severity. Pediatrics 2009; 123: e808.

Luca NJ, et al: Eczema herpeticum in children: clinical features and factors predictive of hospitalization. J Pediatr 2012; 161: 4.

Margolis DJ, et al: Filaggrin-2 variation is associated with more persistent atopic dermatitis in African American subjects. J Allergy Clin Immunol 2014; 133: 784.

Margolis DJ, et al: Thymic stromal lymphopoietin variation, filaggrin loss of function, and the persistence of atopic dermatitis. JAMA Dermatol 2014; 150: 254.

Otsuka A, et al: The interplay between genetic and environmental factors in the pathogenesis of atopic dermatitis. Immunol Rev 2017; 278: 246.

Ozkaya E: Adult-onset atopic dermatitis. J Am Acad Dermatol 2005; 52: 579.

Penders J, et al: Establishment of the intestinal microbiota and its role for atopic dermatitis in early childhood. J Allergy Clin Immunol 2013; 132: 601.

Polcari I, et al: Filaggrin gene mutations in African Americans with both ichthyosis vulgaris and atopic dermatitis. Pediatr Dermatol 2014; 31: 489.

Rahman SI, et al: The methotrexate polyglutamate assay supports the efficacy of methotrexate for severe inflammatory skin disease in children. J Am Acad Dermatol 2013; 70: 252.

Ricci G, et al: Three years of Italian experience of an educational program for parents of young children affected by atopic dermatitis. Pediatr Dermatol 2009; 26: 1.

Ring J, et al: Guidelines for treatment of atopic eczema (atopic dermatitis). J Eur Acad Dermatol Venereol 2012; 26: 1176.

Rupnik H, et al: Filaggrin loss-of-function mutations are not associated with atopic dermatitis that develops in late childhood or adulthood. Br J Dermatol 2015; 172: 455.

Salimi M, et al: A role for IL-25 and IL-33-driven type-2 innate lymphoid cells in atopic dermatitis. J Exp Med 2013; 210: 13.

Sidbury R, et al: Guidelines of care for the management of atopic dermatitis: section 3. J Am Acad Dermatol 2014; 71: 327.

Sidbury R, et al: Guidelines of care for the management of atopic dermatitis: section 4. J Am Acad Dermatol 2014; 71: 1218.

Simpson EL, et al: Emollient enhancement of the skin barrier from birth offers effective atopic dermatitis prevention. J Allergy Clin Immunol 2014; 134: 818.

Stemmler S, et al: Association of variation in the *LAMA3* gene, encoding the alpha-chain of laminin 5, with atopic dermatitis in a German case-control cohort. BMC Dermatol 2014; 14: 17.

Stott B, et al: Human IL-31 is induced by IL-4 and promotes Th2-driven inflammation. J Allergy Clin Immunol 2013; 132: 2.

Thomsen SF, et al: Outcome of treatment with azathioprine in severe atopic dermatitis. Br J Dermatol 2015; 172: 1122.

Van Drongelen V, et al: Reduced filaggrin expression is accompanied by increased *Staphylococcus aureus* colonization of epidermal skin models. Clin Exp Allergy 2014; 44: 1515.

Wang WL, et al: Thymic stromal lymphopoietin. Int Arch Allergy Immunol 2013; 160: 18.

Regional Eczemas

Some eczema is different clinically based on location. Localized eczema can be from AD, contact dermatitis (both allergic and irritant), sebopsoriasis, and others as reviewed here.

Ear Eczema

Eczema of the ears or otitis externa may involve the helix, postauricular fold, and external auditory canal. By far the most frequently affected site is the external canal, where eczema is often a manifestation of seborrheic dermatitis or allergic contact dermatitis caused by topical medications, especially neomycin (Fig. 5.8), benzocaine, and preservatives or earphones. Secretions of the ear canal derive from the specialized apocrine and sebaceous glands, which form cerumen. Rubbing, wiping, scratching, and picking exacerbate the condition. Secondary bacterial colonization or infection is common. Infection is usually caused by staphylococci, streptococci, or *Pseudomonas. Pseudomonas aeruginosa* can result in malignant external otitis with ulceration and sepsis. Earlobe dermatitis in people with pierced ears is virtually pathognomonic for metal contact dermatitis (especially nickel).

Treatment should be directed at removal of causative agents, such as topically applied allergens. First, examine the ear with an otoscope and be sure there is not a perforated tympanic membrane. If there is drainage from a perforated tympanic membrane, management should be in consultation with an otolaryngologist. This purulent fluid can be the cause of an ear eczema—infectious eczematoid dermatitis. If the tympanic membrane is intact, scales and cerumen should be removed by gentle lavage with an ear syringe. A topical steroid otic solution can be used for noninfectious causes. For very weepy lesions, aluminum acetate optic solution (e.g., Domeboro) may be drying and beneficial.

Eyelid Dermatitis

Eyelid dermatitis is most often related to AD or allergic contact dermatitis, or both (see Chapter 6). Allergic conjunctivitis in an atopic patient may lead to rubbing and scratching of the eyelid and result in secondary eyelid dermatitis. Seborrheic dermatitis, psoriasis, and airborne dermatitis are other possible causes. Most patients with eyelid dermatitis are female. When an ocular medication contains an allergen, the allergen passes through the nasolacrimal duct, and dermatitis may also be noted below the nares in addition to the eyelids. Some cases of eyelid contact dermatitis are caused by substances transferred by the hands to the eyelids. If eyelid dermatitis occurs without associated AD, an allergen is detected in more than 50% of cases. More than 25% of patients with AD and eyelid dermatitis will also have allergic contact dermatitis contributing to the condition. Fragrances and balsam of Peru, metals (nickel and gold), paraphenylenediamine, quaternium 15, oleamidopropyl dimethylamine, thiuram (in rubber pads used to apply eyelid cosmetics), and tosylamide formaldehyde (in nail polish) are common allergens causing eyelid dermatitis. In medications, preservatives such as cocamidopropyl betaine and active agents such as phenylephrine hydrochloride, sodium cromoglycate, papain, and idoxuridine have all been implicated.

Eyelid dermatitis requires careful management, often in collaboration with an ophthalmologist. The most important aspect is to identify and eliminate any possible triggering allergens as noted previously. Patch testing for standard allergens, as well as the patient's ocular medications, is highly recommended. Preservative-free eye medications should be used. The ophthalmologist should monitor the patient for conjunctival complications, measure the intraocular pressure, and monitor for the development of cataracts, especially in patients with AD who have an increased risk for cataracts. Initially, topical corticosteroids and petrolatum-based emollients are recommended. If the dermatitis is persistent, the patient may be transitioned to TCIs or crisaborole to reduce the long-term risk of ocular steroid complications. The TCIs are often not initially tolerated on inflamed eyelids due to the burning. If there is an associated allergic conjunctivitis, or in patients who fail treatment with topical medications applied to the eyelid, ocular instillation of cyclosporine ophthalmic emulsion (Restasis) can be beneficial. Cromolyn sodium ophthalmic drops may be used to stabilize mast cells in the eyelid and reduce pruritus. In balsam of Peru–allergic patients, a balsam elimination diet may benefit.

Breast Eczema (Nipple Eczema)

Eczema of the breasts usually affects the areolae and may extend onto the surrounding skin (Fig. 5.9). The area around the base of the nipple is usually spared, and the nipple itself is less frequently affected. The condition is more common in women but can be seen in infants as well. Usually, eczema of the nipples is of the moist type with oozing and crusting. Painful fissuring is frequently seen, especially in nursing mothers. AD is a frequent cause, and nipple eczema may be the sole manifestation of AD in adult women. It frequently presents during breastfeeding. The role of secondary infection with bacteria and *Candida* should be considered in breastfeeding women. Other causes of nipple eczema are allergic contact dermatitis and irritant dermatitis. Irritant dermatitis occurs from friction (jogger's nipples), or from poorly fitting brassieres with seams in women with asymmetric and large breasts. In patients in whom eczema of the nipple or areola has persisted for more than 3 months, especially if it is unilateral, a biopsy is mandatory to rule out the possibility of Paget disease of the breast. Topical corticosteroids or TCIs are often effective in the treatment of non-Paget eczema of the breast. Nevoid hyperkeratosis of the nipples is a chronic condition that may mimic nipple eczema, but it is not responsive to corticosteroids.

Nipple eczema in the breastfeeding woman is a therapeutic challenge and can be from AD, ACD, irritant dermatitis, infection or food allergy. A lactation consultant or nurse may be helpful in managing these patients, because poor positioning during breastfeeding is a common cofactor in the development of nipple eczema. The dermatitis may appear in an atopic woman when her child begins to ingest solid foods rarely due to contact dermatitis to a

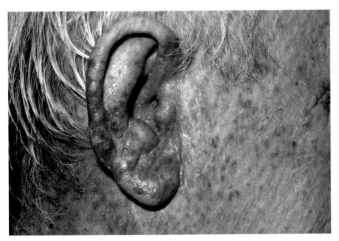

Fig. 5.8 Ear eczema.

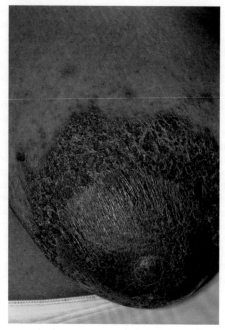

Fig. 5.9 Nummular eczema of the breast.

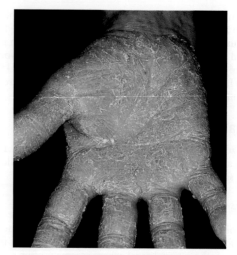

Fig. 5.10 Hand eczema.

food. Allergic contact dermatitis may develop to topical protective creams (containing vitamin A and E, aloe, lanolin, chamomile, or preservatives). Staphylococcal superinfection may develop and can be identified by culture. Oral antibiotics are the preferred treatment for bacterial secondary infection.

Candidal infection of the areola may present as normal skin, erythema, or an acute or chronic eczema. The area of the areola immediately adjacent to the nipple tends to be involved, sometimes with fine hairline cracks. Associated conditions include oral thrush in the infant, antibiotic use, and a personal history of vaginal candidiasis in mother. Cultures are typically positive from the affected areola/nipple. Oral thrush in the infant in the setting of nipple eczema in the mother would warrant treatment of the mother and infant. Patients frequently complain of severe pain, especially with nursing. Analgesia may be required, and breastfeeding may need to be suspended for a period. Pumping and the use of a silicone nipple shield may be helpful. Therapy with topical or systemic antifungal agents may be required. Topical gentian violet 0.5%, applied once daily to the nipple for up to 1 week, may be helpful but should not be ingested by the infant. Guaiazulene (Azulon) is a dark-blue hydrocarbon used in Europe for nipple "cracks" with breastfeeding.

Hand Eczema

Hand eczema is a common and important skin condition. The genetic risk factors for the development of hand dermatitis are unknown but patients with AD are more susceptible. The risk for persistence of the hand eczema is doubled if there is associated eczema at other sites at presentation, if there is a childhood history of AD, and if the onset of the hand eczema was before age 20. Atopic patients with the *FLG* null mutation may have a specific form of hand dermatitis characterized by dorsal hand and finger dermatitis, volar wrist involvement, and hyperlinear palms, but limited palmar dermatitis. Hand eczema is the most common occupational skin condition, accounting for more than 80% of all occupational dermatitides. About 1 per 1000 workers are affected annually. Women are at increased risk, most of which is accounted for by a "spike" in the rate of hand eczema in the 20–29 age-group, when increased environmental exposures increase women's risk (e.g., child care). As noted above, children with new hand dermatitis

should be asked about making or handling "slime" which is an often home-made play substance that can cause irritant or allergic contact dermatitis.

Chronic hand eczema, especially if severe, significantly reduces the patient's quality of life and can be associated with symptoms of depression. Persons at high risk for hand eczema can be identified and counseled to avoid high-risk occupations such as those that involve consistent exposure to water or sensitizing chemicals such as hairdressers. If occupational hand eczema develops, some occupation-specific strategies can lead to improvement and prevent recurrence.

The evaluation and management of hand eczema has been hampered by the lack of a uniform classification system and a dearth of controlled therapeutic trials. The diagnostic dilemma in hand dermatitis is in part related to two factors. The clinical appearance of the skin eruption on the palms and soles may be very similar, independent of the etiology. In addition, virtually all chronic hand dermatitis demonstrates a chronic dermatitis histologically, again independent of pathogenic cause. For instance, psoriasis on the palms and soles may show the same spongiosis as a dermatitis (Fig. 5.10). As a result, the proposed classification schemes rely on a combination of morphologic features, history of coexistent illnesses, occupational exposure, and results of patch testing. The different types of hand eczema are as follows:

1. Allergic contact dermatitis (with or without an additional irritant component)
2. Irritant hand dermatitis
3. Atopic hand eczema (with or without an additional irritant component)
4. Recurrent vesicular (or vesiculobullous) hand eczema
5. Hyperkeratotic hand eczema
6. Pulpitis (chronic fingertip dermatitis)
7. Nummular dermatitis

A complete history, careful examination of the rest of the body surface, and frequently patch testing are essential in establishing a diagnosis. Patch testing is recommended in all patients with chronic hand eczema. Allergens in the environment, especially shower gels and shampoos, in the workplace, and in topical medications may be important in any patient. Patch testing must include broad screens of common allergens or allergic contact dermatitis may be missed.

The role of ingested nickel in the development of hand eczema in nickel-allergic patients is controversial. Some practitioners treat such patients with low-nickel diets and even disulfiram chelation with reported benefit. However, the risk of development of hand eczema in adulthood is independent of nickel allergy. Similarly, the role of low-balsam diets in the management of balsam of Peru–allergic patients with hand eczema is unclear.

Wet work, defined as skin in liquids or gloves for more than 2 hours per day, or handwashing more than 20 times per day, is a strong risk factor for hand eczema. High-risk occupations include those that entail wet work and those with exposure to potential allergens. "high-risk" occupations include bakers, hairdressers, dental surgery assistants, kitchen workers/cooks, butchers, health care workers, cleaners, physicians/dentists/veterinarians, and laboratory technicians. In about 5% of patients with hand eczema, especially if severe, it is associated with prolonged missed work, job change, and job loss. In health care workers, the impaired barrier poses a risk for infection by blood-borne pathogens.

Almost one third of baker's apprentices develop hand dermatitis within 12 months of entering the profession. Among hairdressers, the incidence approaches 50% after several years. Both irritant dermatitis and allergic contact dermatitis are important factors, with glyceryl monothioglycolate and ammonium persulfate being the most common allergens among hairdressers. Cement workers have a high rate of hand dermatitis related to contact allergy, alkalinity, and hygroscopic effects of cement. Dorsal hand dermatitis in a cement worker suggests contact allergy to chromate or cobalt. The addition of ferrous sulfate to cement has no effect on irritant dermatitis, but reduces the incidence of allergic chromate dermatitis by two thirds.

Among patients with occupational hand dermatitis, atopic patients are disproportionately represented. Hand dermatitis is frequently the initial or only adult manifestation of an atopic diathesis. The likelihood of developing hand eczema is greatest in patients with AD, more common if the AD was severe, but is still increased in incidence in patients with only respiratory atopy. One third to one half of patients with hand eczema have atopy. Atopic patients should receive career counseling in adolescence to consider avoidance of occupations that are likely to induce hand dermatitis.

Contact urticaria syndrome may present as immediate burning, itching, or swelling of the hands, but a chronic eczematous phase may also occur. Latex is an important cause of the syndrome, but raw meat, lettuce, garlic, onion, carrot, tomato, spinach, grapefruit, orange, radish, fig, parsnip, cheese, or any number of other foods may be implicated.

Vesiculobullous Hand Eczema (Pompholyx, Dyshidrosis). Primary lesions of dyshidrosis are deep-seated multilocular vesicles resembling tapioca on the sides of the fingers (Fig. 5.11), palms, and soles. The eruption is symmetric and pruritic, with pruritus often preceding the eruption. Coalescence of smaller lesions may lead to bulla formation severe enough to prevent ambulation. Individual outbreaks resolve spontaneously over several weeks. Acute pompholyx, also known as cheiropompholyx if it affects the hands, presents with severe, sudden outbreaks of intensely pruritic vesicles. Idiopathic acute vesicular hand dermatitis is not related to blockage of sweat ducts, although palmoplantar hyperhidrosis is common in these patients, and control of hyperhidrosis improves the eczema. Bullous tinea or an id reaction from a dermatophyte should be excluded, and patch testing should be considered to rule out allergic contact dermatitis.

Chronic Vesiculobullous Hand Eczema. In chronic cases, the lesions may be hyperkeratotic, scaling, and fissured, and the "dyshidrosiform" pattern may be recognized only during exacerbations. The pruritic 1–2 mm vesicles tend to be most pronounced at the sides of the fingers. In long-standing cases, the nails may become dystrophic. The distribution of the lesions is, as a rule, bilateral and roughly symmetric.

Hyperkeratotic Hand Dermatitis. The eruption presents as hyperkeratotic, fissure-prone, erythematous areas of the middle or proximal palm. Vesicles are not seen. The volar surfaces of the fingers may also be involved (Fig. 5.12). Plantar lesions occur in about 10% of patients. Males outnumber females by 2 : 1, and the patients are usually older adults. Histologically, the lesions show chronic spongiotic dermatitis. The most important differential diagnosis is psoriasis, and some of the patients with chronic hyperkeratotic hand dermatitis will ultimately prove to be psoriatic. The presence of sharply demarcated plaques, nail pitting, or occasional crops of pustules is an important clue to psoriatic hand involvement.

Pulpitis (Fingertip Hand Dermatitis). This hyperkeratotic and fissuring eczema affects primarily the fingertips and may extend to merge with eczema of the palm. Vesicles can occur. Involvement of the three fingers of the dominant hand suggests a contact dermatitis (irritant or allergic), whereas similar involvement of the nondominant hand suggests vegetables and other items related to food preparation that are held in this hand for cutting (e.g., garlic).

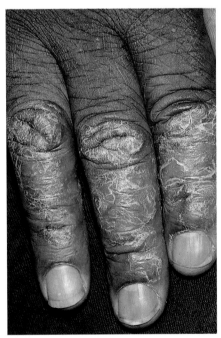

Fig. 5.12 Hyperkeratotic hand dermatitis.

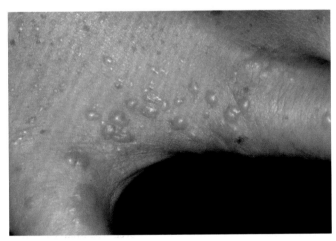

Fig. 5.11 Pompholyx.

Treatment. The hands are essential for work both in and out of the home. Treatment regimens must be practical and must allow patients to function as normally as possible. The efficacy of some of the treatments depends on the morphology of the eruption and the diagnostic classification (see previous discussion).

Protection. Vinyl gloves may be worn during wet work, especially when detergents are used. Although vinyl gloves protect against chemicals, they do not prevent exposure to heat through the glove or the macerating effect of sweat, which accumulates under the gloves. Wearing white cotton gloves under the vinyl gloves can prevent this. Vinyl gloves are also much less durable than rubber gloves. Rubber gloves may be used at home if patients do not exhibit allergy to rubber chemicals or latex. For rough work, such as gardening, wearing protective cloth or leather gloves is essential.

Barrier Repair. Moisturizing is a critical component of the management of hand dermatitis. Application of a protective moisturizing cream or ointment after each handwashing or water exposure is recommended. Creams require a preservative and have a higher risk of contact sensitivity and often burn when applied. Ointments tend to have few ingredients and do not generally require a preservative. At night, even during periods of remission, a heavy moisturizing ointment should be applied to the hands after soaking in water. If palmar dryness is present, occlusion of the moisturizer with a plastic bag or vinyl gloves is recommended. White petrolatum is inexpensive and nonsensitizing and remains a valuable agent in the treatment of hand dermatitis. Jars of moisturizers can be contaminated with *S. aureus.*

Topical Agents. Potent and ultrapotent topical corticosteroids are first-line pharmacologic therapy. Their efficacy is enhanced by presoaking and occlusion (soak and smear technique or wet dressings). A single application with occlusion at night is often more effective than multiple daytime applications. The treatment is continued until the hands are clear, and then either emollients are substituted or maintenance treatment with the topical steroid two or three times weekly is continued to prevent recurrence. In refractory cases, ultrapotent corticosteroids may be used for 2–3 weeks, then on weekends, with a milder corticosteroid applied during the week.

The TCIs may be of benefit in some mildly affected patients. Soaks with a tar bath oil or applications of 20% LCD or 2% crude coal tar in an ointment base may be of benefit, especially in patients with hyperkeratotic hand eczema. Bexarotene gel can be beneficial in up to 50% of patients with refractory hand eczema.

Phototherapy. Phototherapy in the form of high-dose UVA I, soak or cream PUVA, and oral PUVA can be effective but the risks of chronic photo damage and skin cancer must be discussed with patients.. Given the thickness of the palms, UVA irradiation should be delivered 30 minutes after soaking, as opposed to bath PUVA, which can be done immediately after bathing.

Grenz ray radiotherapy is rarely used due to long-term risk of malignancy.

Botulinum Toxin A. In patients with palmoplantar hyperhidrosis and associated hand eczema, treatment of the hyperhidrosis with intradermal injections of botulinum toxin A leads to both dramatic resolution of the sweating and clearing of the hand eczema. The hand eczema returns when the sweating returns.

Iontophoresis, which also reduces sweating, can similarly improve hand dermatitis. This illustrates the importance of wetness in the exacerbation of hand eczema.

Systemic Agents. The systemic agents used to treat severe chronic hand dermatitis are identical to those used for AD. Systemic steroids are recommended only to control acute exacerbations. For example, patients with infrequent but severe outbreaks of pompholyx may benefit from a few weeks of systemic steroids, starting at about 1 mg/kg/day. Patients with persistent, severe hand dermatitis should be considered for alternative, steroid-sparing therapy. Oral retinoids may have a place in the management of hand dermatitis. Alitretinoin (not available in the United States), may lead to complete or near-complete clearance of chronic refractory hand eczema in about 50% of patients, especially those with hyperkeratotic hand eczema. The onset of response is delayed, with some patients achieving optimal benefit only after more than 6 months of treatment. Acitretin, may have similar benefit and of course should not be used in women of childbearing potential.

Workplace Modifications. The incidence of hand dermatitis in the workplace can be reduced by identifying major irritants and allergens, preventing exposure through engineering controls, substituting less irritating chemicals when possible, enforcing personal protection and glove use, and instituting organized worker education. Hand eczema classes have been documented to reduce the burden of occupational dermatitis. It is important to note that prevention of exposure to a weak but frequent irritant can have more profound effects than removal of a strong but infrequently contacted irritant.

Proper gloves are essential in industrial settings. Nitrile gloves are generally less permeable than latex gloves. Gloves of ethylene vinyl alcohol copolymer sandwiched with polyethylene are effective against epoxy resin, methyl methacrylate, and many other organic compounds. Latex and vinyl gloves offer little protection against acrylates. The 4H (4 hour) glove and nitrile are best in this setting. As hospitals transition to nonlatex gloves, it is important to note that even low-protein, powder-free latex gloves reduce self-reported skin problems among health workers.

Clin Cosmet Investig Dermatol. 2010; 3: 59–65
Ann Dermatol. 2017 Jun; 29(3): 385–387

Diaper (Napkin) Dermatitis

Diaper dermatitis has dramatically decreased as a result of highly absorbable disposable diapers. Nonetheless, dermatitis of the diaper area in infants remains a common cutaneous disorder. The highest prevalence occurs between 6 and 12 months of age. Diaper dermatitis is also seen in adults with urinary or fecal incontinence who wear diapers.

Irritant diaper dermatitis is the most common type of dermatitis and is an erythematous dermatitis due to skin contact with urine and feces that is usually limited to the convex exposed surfaces. The folds remain unaffected, in contrast to intertrigo, inverse psoriasis, and candidiasis, where the folds are frequently involved. In severe cases of irritant dermatitis, there may be superficial erosion or even ulceration (Jacquet erosive diaper dermatitis), violaceous plaques and nodules (granuloma gluteal infantum), or pseudoverrucous papules and nodules; these three entities are part of a disease spectrum and can simulate herpetic infections or genital warts. The tip of the penis may become irritated and crusted, with the baby urinating frequently and spots of blood appearing on the diaper.

Excessive hydration with maceration of the skin is the primary causal factor in diaper dermatitis. The absence of diaper dermatitis in societies where children do not wear diapers clearly implicates the diaper environment as the cause of the eruption. Many parents will incorrectly switch to cloth diapers when diaper dermatitis occurs even though the superabsorbent modern diapers are much more effective at preventing diaper dermatitis by wicking urine and stool to some extent away from the skin. Moist skin is more easily abraded by friction of the diaper as the child moves. Wet skin is more permeable to irritants. Skin wetness also allows the growth of bacteria and yeast. Bacteria raise the local pH, increasing the activity of fecal lipases and proteases, which leads to more skin breakdown. *Candida albicans* is frequently a secondary invader and, when present, produces typical satellite erythematous lesions or pustules at the periphery as the dermatitis spreads. *S. aureus* and group A β-hemolytic streptococci can infect diaper dermatitis. Breastfeeding is associated with less frequent diaper dermatitis, and diarrhea is a risk factor.

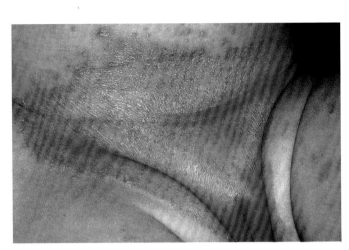

Fig. 5.13 Napkin psoriasis.

The differential diagnosis of diaper dermatitis should include napkin psoriasis (Fig. 5.13), seborrheic dermatitis, AD, langerhans cell histiocytosis, tinea cruris, acrodermatitis enteropathica, aminoacidurias, biotin deficiency, and congenital syphilis. Allergic contact dermatitis is becoming more frequently recognized as a cause of dermatitis in the diaper area. Allergens include sorbitan sesequioleate, fragrances, disperse dye, cyclohexylthiopthalimide, and mercaptobenzothiazole (in rubber diaper covers). Given the skill of most pediatricians in the management of diaper dermatitis, dermatologists should think about these conditions in infants who have failed the standard interventions used by pediatricians. Refractory diaper dermatitis may require a biopsy to exclude some of these conditions.

Prevention is the best treatment. Diapers that contain superabsorbent gel have been proved effective in preventing diaper dermatitis in both neonates and infants. They work by absorbing the wetness away from the skin and by buffering the pH. Cloth diapers and regular disposable diapers are equal in their propensity to cause diaper dermatitis and are inferior to the superabsorbent gel diapers. The frequent changing of diapers is also critical: every 2 hours for newborns and every 3–4 hours for older infants. The renewed popularity of cloth and bamboo diapers as more natural and ecologic has led to a reemergence of severe diaper dermatitis in some European countries.

Protecting the skin of the diaper area is vital. Zinc oxide paste and petrolatum are both effective barriers, preventing the urine and stool from contacting the dermatitis. If simple improved hygiene and barrier therapy are not effective, the application of anticandidal agents in addition to a very-low-potency topical steroid for a few days can aid in healing.

Circumostomy Eczema

Eczematization of the surrounding skin frequently occurs after an ileostomy or colostomy. It is estimated that 75% of ileostomy patients have some postoperative sensitivity as a result of the leakage of intestinal fluid onto unprotected skin. As the consistency of the intestinal secretion becomes viscous, the sensitization subsides. Proprietary medications containing karaya powder have been helpful; 20% cholestyramine (an ion-exchange resin) in a petrolatum-based moisturizer and topical sucralfate as a powder or emollient are effective treatments. Absorbent silicone protective layers can be placed around the ostomy to provide protection against the tube rubbing and absorption of any leaking intestinal contents. Psoriasis may also appear at ostomy sites, especially in patients with inflammatory bowel disease (IBD) being treated with tumor necrosis factor (TNF) inhibitors who develop psoriasis as a complication. Topical treatment may be difficult because the appliance adheres poorly after the topical agents are applied. A topical corticosteroid spray may be used and will not interfere with appliance adherence. Contact dermatitis to the ostomy bag adhesive can be problematic, and even supposedly hypoallergenic ostomy bags may still trigger dermatitis in these patients.

Autosensitization (Id Reactions) and Conditioned Irritability

The presence of a localized, chronic, and usually severe focus of dermatitis may affect distant skin in two ways. Patients with a chronic localized dermatitis may develop dermatitis at distant sites from scratching or irritating the skin. This is called "conditioned irritability." The most common scenario is distant dermatitis in a patient with a chronic eczematous leg ulcer.

Autoeczematization (id reaction) refers to the spontaneous development of widespread dermatitis or dermatitis distant from a local inflammatory focus. The agent causing the local inflammatory focus is not the direct cause of the dermatitis at the distant sites. Autoeczematization most frequently presents as a generalized acute vesicular eruption with a prominent dyshidrosiform component on the hands. The most common associated condition is a chronic eczema of the legs, with or without ulceration. The "angry back" or "excited skin" syndrome observed with strongly positive patch tests, and the local dermatitis seen around infectious foci (infectious eczematoid dermatitis), may represent a limited form of this reaction.

Patients with a variety of infectious disorders may also present with an id reaction. The most classic pattern is characterized by symmetrically distributed minute papules that have a predilection for the face, upper ears, and trunk. The most common causes are tinea capitis or an allergic contact dermatitis. Therapy of tinea capitis with griseofulvin can lead to an id reaction soon after therapy that can be mistaken for an allergic reaction to griseofulvin. Proper management is to continue the griseofulvin and treat symptomatically with topical steroids or antihistamines if necessary. Id reactions can also be vesicular on the hands in response to an inflammatory tinea of the feet. Nummular eczematous lesions or pityriasis rosea–like lesions may occur in patients with head or pubic louse infestation. Id reactions clear when the focus of infection or infestation is treated, but topical or systemic antiinflammatory agents may be required until the triggering infection is eradicated.

Juvenile Plantar Dermatosis

Juvenile plantar dermatosis is an eczematous disorder of children from age 3 years to puberty although rarely it persists into adulthood. It usually begins as a patchy, symmetric, smooth, red glazed patch on the base or medial surface of the great toes, sometimes with fissuring and desquamation. Unlike tinea, it spares the interdigital spaces. Lesions evolve into red scaling patches involving the weight-bearing and frictional areas of the feet, usually symmetrically. The skin ends up appearing like parchment paper and it fissures easily. The forefoot is usually much more involved than the heel. The eruption is disproportionately more common in atopic children. In some patients, a similar eruption occurs on the fingers. Histologically, there is psoriasiform acanthosis and a sparse, largely lymphocytic infiltrate in the upper dermis, most dense around sweat ducts at their point of entry into the epidermis. Spongiosis is often present, and the stratum corneum is thin but compact.

The disease is caused by the repeated maceration of the feet due to occlusive shoes often worn without socks, especially athletic shoes, sandals, or rubber shoes, or by the abrasive effects of pool surfaces or diving boards. Thin, nonabsorbent, synthetic socks may contribute to the problem, but socks that soak up excess water must be changed when soaked.

The diagnosis of plantar dermatosis is clinical, especially if there is a family or personal history of atopy and the toe webs are spared. Treatment involves avoidance of maceration. Foot powders, thick absorbent socks, absorbent insoles, and having alternate pairs of shoes to wear to allow the shoes to dry out are all beneficial. Topical corticosteroid medications are of limited value and often are no more effective than occlusive barrier protection. Petrolatum or urea preparations can sometimes be of benefit. Most cases clear within 4 years of diagnosis.

Allergic contact dermatitis may play a significant role in plantar dermatoses in childhood. In one study from Scotland, 50% of children with "inflammatory dermatitis" of the soles had relevant positive patch tests, and 4 of 14 children with typical juvenile plantar dermatitis also had a relevant contact allergen. Refractory plantar dermatitis in childhood should suggest allergic contact dermatitis.

Xerotic Eczema

Xerotic eczema is also known as winter itch, eczema craquelé, and asteatotic eczema. These vividly descriptive terms are all applied to dehydrated skin showing redness, dry scaling, and fine crackling that may resemble crackled porcelain or the fissures in the bed of a dried lake. The primary lesion is an erythematous patch covered with an adherent scale. As the lesion enlarges, fine cracks in the epidermis occur (Fig. 5.14). Nummular lesions may occur. Xerotic "nummular" eczema is less weepy than classic nummular dermatitis. Favored sites are the anterior shins, extensor arms, and flank. Elderly persons are particularly predisposed, and xerosis is the most common cause of pruritus in older individuals. Xerotic eczema is seen most frequently during the winter, when there is low relative humidity. Bathing with hot water and harsh soaps contributes. The epidermal water barrier is impaired, and TEWL is increased. Epidermal barrier repair begins to decrease after age 55, correlated with an increase in epidermal pH (see later discussion). The loss of barrier repair ability is improved by acidifying the epidermis, showing the benefit of mild acids in treating xerosis. Heterozygous null mutation of the *FLG* gene is associated with xerosis.

Taking short tepid showers, limiting use of soap to soiled and apocrine-bearing areas, using acid pH synthetic detergents, and promptly applying an emollient after bathing are usually effective.

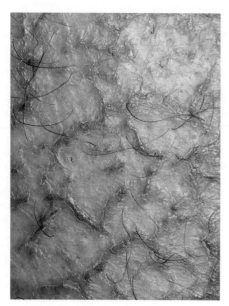

Fig. 5.14 Eczema craquelé.

White petrolatum and emollients containing 10% urea or 5% lactic acid are effective. Topical corticosteroids in ointment vehicles are useful for inflamed areas.

Pruritic Dermatitis in Elderly Persons

Pruritic skin conditions are common in elderly patients, appearing around age 55 and increasing in severity with age. Males are more often affected, and Asians and Caucasians more frequently have pruritus as seniors than African Americans or Hispanics.

The dermatoses seen in this age-group are typically eczematous or papular. The eczematous plaques may resemble nummular dermatitis, a feature recognized by Marion Sulzberger when he coined the phrase "exudative discoid and lichenoid chronic dermatitis," or "oid-oid disease." The pathogenic basis of this component of dermatitis in elderly persons may be related to barrier failure due to loss of acidification of the epidermis. In addition, patients often have urticarial papules on the trunk and proximal extremities that resemble insect bites. These lesions are termed *subacute prurigo* and histologically demonstrate features of an arthropod assault, with superficial and deep perivascular lymphohistiocytic infiltrates, dermal edema, and at times interstitial eosinophils. Lesions of transient acantholytic dermatitis or eosinophilic folliculitis may also occur. This component of the eruption may be related to the tendency of elderly individuals to have an immune system that skews toward Th2 because of loss of Th1 function parallel to what occurs in the setting of AD. For this reason, some practitioners consider this "adult atopic dermatitis." However, it is unknown whether these conditions have a genetic basis, or more likely, given the time of onset, are caused by acquired barrier and immune system abnormalities. In these patients, allergic contact dermatitis and photodermatitis may be present or develop. Patch testing may identify important allergens, avoidance of which leads to improvement.

Certain medication may also cause a similar eruption. Calcium channel blockers may be associated with pruritic dermatitis, but stopping them will clear only about one quarter of patients taking that class of medication. If there is widespread pruritic dermatitis, a biopsy should be performed to rule out cutaneous T-cell lymphoma. Treatment for these patients is similar to that of AD patients, with oral antipruritics, emollients, and topical corticosteroids (soak and smear) as first-line therapy. In refractory cases, phototherapy (UVB or PUVA), Goeckerman therapy (UVB plus crude coal tar) in a day treatment setting, and immunosuppressive agents can be effective. Inadvertent use of phototherapy in the patient with coexistent photosensitivity will lead to an exacerbation of pruritic dermatitis.

Nummular Eczema (Discoid Eczema)

NE usually begins on the lower legs, dorsa of the hands, or extensor surfaces of the arms. In younger adults, females predominate, but most patients older than 40 are male. Alcohol consumption has been associated with NE in adult males. A single lesion often precedes the eruption and may be present for some time before other lesions appear. The primary lesions are discrete, coin-shaped, erythematous, edematous, vesicular, and crusted patches (Fig. 5.15). Most lesions are 2–4 cm in diameter. Lesions may form after trauma (conditioned hyperirritability). As new lesions appear, the old lesions expand as tiny papulovesicular satellite lesions appear at the periphery and fuse with the main plaque. In severe cases, the condition may spread into palm-sized or larger patches. Pruritus is usually severe and of the same paroxysmal, compulsive quality and nocturnal timing seen in AD and prurigo nodularis.

AD frequently has nummular morphology in adolescents, but in atopy the lesions tend to be more chronic and lichenified. Histologically, NE is characterized by acute or subacute spongiotic dermatitis. The skin lesions of nummular dermatitis are frequently

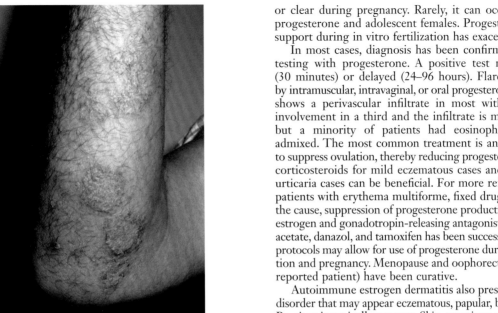

Fig. 5.15 Nummular eczema. (Courtesy Steven Binnick, MD.)

colonized with *S. aureus*, in frequency similar to that seen in AD. Relevant positive patch tests are found in one quarter to one third of patients with NE. This may represent the primary cause of the dermatitis or a secondary allergy that developed from products used to treat the NE.

Initial treatment consists of simple soaking and greasing with an occlusive ointment, and once-daily or twice-daily application of a potent or superpotent topical corticosteroid cream or ointment then switched to a nonsteroidal topical medication such as a calcineurin inhibitor or crisaborole. Ointments are more effective, and occlusion may be necessary as nummular dermatitis can be very recalcitrant. If secondary staphylococcal infection is present, an antibiotic with appropriate coverage can be used. Stopping alcohol consumption may improve response. A sedating antihistamine, doxepin, or gabapentin at bedtime can help with sleep and reduce nighttime scratching. In some cases refractory to topical agents, intralesional or systemic corticosteroid therapy may be required. In patients unresponsive to topical steroids, phototherapy with NB UVB, bath (soak), or oral PUVA can be effective. For refractory plaques, the addition of topical tar as 2% crude coal tar or 20% LCD may be beneficial.

HORMONE-INDUCED DERMATOSES

Autoimmune progesterone dermatitis (APD) may appear as urticarial papules, deep gyrate lesions, papulovesicular lesions, an eczematous eruption, targetoid lesions, or a fixed drug reaction. Urticarial and erythema multiforme–like lesions are most characteristic. Lesions typically appear 5–7 days before menses, and improve or resolve a few days following menses. Pruritus is common. Onset is typically in the third and fourth decades of life. Familial cases have been reported. When urticaria is the predominant skin lesion, there is a generalized distribution, and it may be accompanied by laryngospasm and anaphylactoid reactions. Oral erosions may be present and cyclical, and a case of erythema multiforme associated with APD in an HIV patient has been reported. Many of the reported patients had received artificial progestational agents before the onset of the eruption. In some, it appeared during a normal pregnancy. The eruption may worsen or clear during pregnancy. Rarely, it can occur in males given progesterone and adolescent females. Progesterone luteal-phase support during in vitro fertilization has exacerbated the disease.

In most cases, diagnosis has been confirmed by intradermal testing with progesterone. A positive test may be immediate (30 minutes) or delayed (24–96 hours). Flares may be induced by intramuscular, intravaginal, or oral progesterone. Histopathology shows a perivascular infiltrate in most with some interstitial involvement in a third and the infiltrate is mostly lymphocytes, but a minority of patients had eosinophils or neutrophils admixed. The most common treatment is an oral contraceptive to suppress ovulation, thereby reducing progesterone levels. Topical corticosteroids for mild eczematous cases and antihistamines in urticaria cases can be beneficial. For more refractory cases or in patients with erythema multiforme, fixed drug, or anaphylaxis as the cause, suppression of progesterone production with conjugated estrogen and gonadotropin-releasing antagonists such as leuprolide acetate, danazol, and tamoxifen has been successful. Desensitization protocols may allow for use of progesterone during in vitro fertilization and pregnancy. Menopause and oophorectomy (except in one reported patient) have been curative.

Autoimmune estrogen dermatitis also presents as a cyclic skin disorder that may appear eczematous, papular, bullous, or urticarial. Pruritus is typically present. Skin eruptions may be chronic but are exacerbated premenstrually or occur only immediately before the menses. Characteristically, the dermatosis clears during pregnancy and at menopause. Intracutaneous skin testing with estrone produces a papule lasting longer than 24 hours or an immediate urticarial wheal (in patients with urticaria). Injections of progesterone yield negative results, ruling out autoimmune progesterone dermatitis. Tamoxifen is effective in some cases.

Agner T, et al: Hand eczema severity and quality of life. Contact Dermatitis 2008; 59: 43.

Asai J, et al: Case of autoimmune progesterone dermatitis presenting as fixed drug eruption. J Dermatol 2009; 36: 643.

Bonamonte D, et al: Nummular eczema and contact allergy. Dermatitis 2012; 23: 153.

Cvetkovski RS, et al: Prognosis of occupational hand eczema. Arch Dermatol 2006; 142: 305.

Darling MI, et al: Sole dermatitis in children. Pediatr Dermatol 2012; 29: 254.

Delle Sedie A, et al: Psoriasis, erythema nodosum, and nummular eczema onset in an ankylosing spondylitis patient treated with infliximab. Scand J Rhematol 2007; 36: 403.

Detrixhe A et al: Autoimmune progesterone dermatitis. Arch Gynecol Obstet 2017; 296: 1013.

Drayer SM, et al: Autoimmune progesterone dermatitis presenting as Stevens-Johnson syndrome. Obstet Gynecol 2017; 130: 881.

Grunnet KM, et al: Autoimmune progesterone dermatitis manifesting as mucosal erythema multiforme in the setting of HIV infection. JAAD Case Rep 2016; 3: 22.

Guillet MH, et al: A 3-year causative study of pompholyx in 120 patients. Arch Dermatol 2007; 143: 1504.

Gunes T, et al: Guaiazulene. J Matern Fetal Neonatal Med 2013; 26: 197.

Heimall LM, et al: Beginning at the bottom: evidence-based care of diaper dermatitis. MCN Am J Matern Child Nurs 2012; 37: 10.

Honda T, et al: Autoimmune progesterone dermatitis that changed its clinical manifestation from anaphylaxis to fixed drug eruption-like erythema. J Dermatol 2014; 41: 447.

Isaksson M, et al: Children with atopic dermatitis should always be patch-tested if they have hand or foot dermatitis. Acta Derm Venereol 2015; 95: 583.

Jacob SE: Ciclosporin ophthalmic emulsion: a novel therapy for benzyl alcohol–associated eyelid dermatitis. Contact Dermatitis 2008; 58: 169.

James T, et al: The histopathologic features of autoimmune progesterone dermatitis. J Cutan Pathol 2017; 44: 70.

Kim WJ, et al: Features of *Staphylococcus aureus* colonization in patients with nummular eczema. Br J Dermatol 2013; 168: 656.

Kontochristopoulos G, et al: Letter: regression of relapsing dyshidrotic eczema after treatment of concomitant hyperhidrosis with botulinum toxin-A. Dermatol Surg 2007; 33: 1289.

Krupa Shankar DS, Shrestha S: Relevance of patch testing in patients with nummular dermatitis. Indian J Dermatol Venereol Leprol 2005; 71: 406.

Lakshmi C, Srinivas CR: Hand eczema. Indian J Dermatol Venereol Leprol 2013; 78: 569.

Le K, Wood G: A case of autoimmune progesterone dermatitis diagnosed by progesterone pessary. Australas J Dermatol 2011; 52: 139.

Lee M, et al: A case of autoimmune progesterone dermatitis misdiagnosed as allergic contact dermatitis. Allergy Asthma Immunol Res 2011; 3: 141.

Lerbaek A, et al: Incidence of hand eczema in a population-based twin cohort. Br J Dermatol 2007; 157: 552.

Li CH, et al: Diaper dermatitis. J Int Med Res 2012; 40: 1752.

Lundov MD, et al: Creams used by hand eczema patients are often contaminated with *Staphylococcus aureus*. Acta Derm Venereol 2012; 92: 441.

Lynde C, et al: Extended treatment with oral alitretinoin for patients with chronic hand eczema not fully responding to initial treatment. Clin Exp Dermatol 2012; 37: 712.

Mauruani A, et al: Re-emergence of papulonodular napkin dermatitis with use of reusable diapers. Eur J Dermatol 2013; 23: 246.

Mutasim DF, et al: Bullous autoimmune estrogen dermatitis. J Am Acad Dermatol 2003; 49: 130.

Petering H, et al: Comparison of localized high-dose UVA1 irradiation versus topical cream psoralen-UVA for treatment of chronic vesicular dyshidrotic eczema. J Am Acad Dermatol 2004; 50: 68.

Poffet F, et al: Autoimmune progesterone dermatitis. Dermatol 2011; 223: 32.

Prieto-Garcoa A, et al: Autoimmune progesterone dermatitis. Fertil Steril 2011; 95: 1121.e9.

Stamatas GN, Tierney NK: Diaper dermatitis. Pediatr Dermatol 2014; 31: 1.

Thyssen JP, et al: Filaggrin null-mutations may be associated with a distinct subtype of atopic hand eczema. Acta Derm Venereol 2010; 90: 528.

Thyssen JP, et al: Xerosis is associated with atopic dermatitis, hand eczema and contact sensitization independent of filaggrin gene mutations. Acta Derm Venereol 2013; 93: 406.

Wollina U: Pompholyx. Am J Clin Dermatol 2010; 11: 305.

Yu J, et al: Patch test series for allergic perineal dermatitis in the diapered infant. Dermatitis 2017; 28: 70.

IMMUNODEFICIENCY SYNDROMES

Primary immunodeficiency diseases (PIDs) are important to the dermatologist. PIDs may present with skin manifestations, and the dermatologist may be instrumental in referring appropriate patients for immunodeficiency evaluation. These conditions have also given us tremendous insight into the genetic makeup and functioning of the immune system. The PIDs can be classified as those with predominantly antibody deficiency, impaired cell-mediated immunity (cellular immunodeficiencies, T cells, natural killer [NK] cells), combined B-cell and T-cell deficiencies, defects of phagocytic function, complement deficiencies, and well-characterized syndromes with immunodeficiency. More than 150 PIDs have been identified, as of the 2005 classification. Many of the original paradigms of PIDs have been refuted. PIDs are not rare, can be sporadic (not familial), can have adult onset, can be autosomal dominant, have incomplete penetrance, and may even spontaneously improve over time.

The dermatologist should suspect a PID in patients with chronic, severe, atypical or recalcitrant infections, and the type of immunodeficiency can at times be suggested by the clinical situation. Skin infections, especially chronic and recurrent bacterial skin infections, can be the initial manifestation of a PID with neutropenia, elevated IgE, or T-helper cell immunodeficiency. Fungal (especially *Candida*) and viral infections (warts, molluscum) suggest a PID of helper T cells or a specific monogenetic defect (STAT1 gain of function, IL-17, DOCK-8). Not all immunodeficiencies present with infections, but rather an inflammatory phenotype. Eczematous dermatitis and erythroderma, at times closely resembling severe atopic or seborrheic dermatitis, may affect the skin of PID patients due to maternal engraftment graft-versus-host disease (GVHD). They may be refractory to standard therapies. Granuloma formation, autoimmune disorders, and vasculitis are other cutaneous manifestations seen in some forms of primary immunodeficiency. The PIDs in which a specific infection or finding is the more common presentation are discussed in other chapters, including chronic mucocutaneous candidiasis (Chapter 15); Hermansky-Pudlak, Chédiak-Higashi, and Griscelli syndromes with pigmentary anomalies (Chapter 36); and cartilage-hair hypoplasia syndrome with disorders of hair (Chapter 27). The conditions described next are the most important PID conditions with which dermatologists should be familiar.

Al-Herz W, et al: Primary immunodeficiency diseases. Front Immunol 2011; 2: 54.

Mohiuddin MS, et al: Diagnosis and evaluation of primary panhypogammaglobulinemia. J Allergy Clin Immunol 2013; 131: 1717.

Ozcan E, et al: Primary immune deficiencies with aberrant IgE production. J Allergy Clin Immunol 2008; 122: 1054.

Rezaei N, et al: Primary immunodeficiency diseases associated with increased susceptibility to viral infections and malignancies. J Allergy Clin Immunol 2011; 127: 1329.

Schwartzfarb EM, et al: Pyoderma gangrenosum in a patient with Bruton's X-linked agammaglobulinemia. J Clin Aesthet Dermatol 2008; 1: 26.

Disorders of Antibody Deficiency

X-Linked Agammaglobulinemia

Also known as Bruton syndrome, X-linked agammaglobulinemia (XLA) is caused by mutations in the *BTK* gene (Bruton tyrosine kinase), which is essential for the development of B lymphocytes. XLA typically presents between 4 and 12 months of life, when maternal immunoglobulins wane. The affected boys present with infections of the upper and lower respiratory tracts, gastrointestinal (GI) tract, skin, joints, and central nervous system (CNS). The infections are usually caused by *Streptococcus pneumoniae*, *S. aureus*, *Haemophilus influenzae*, *Helicobacter*, and *Pseudomonas*. Recurrent skin staphylococcal infection may be a prominent component of this condition. Atopic-like dermatitis and pyoderma gangrenosum have been described. Hepatitis B, enterovirus, and rotavirus infections are common in XLA patients, and one third develop a rheumatoid-like arthritis. Enterovirus infection may result in a dermatomyositis-meningoencephalitis syndrome. Pyoderma gangrenosum has been reported in a patient, although this would absolutely be a diagnosis of exclusion because these patients can have such unusual skin infections. Kawasaki disease and polyarteritis nodosa have been reported in affected patients. An absence of palpable lymph nodes is characteristic.

Immunoglobulin A (IgA), IgM, IgD, and IgE are virtually absent from the serum, although IgG may be present in small amounts. The spleen and lymph nodes lack germinal centers, and plasma cells are absent from the lymph nodes, spleen, bone marrow, and connective tissues. In XLA, B cells usually only make up 0.1% of circulating peripheral blood lymphocytes (normal 5%–20%). More than 500 different mutations have been identified in the *BTK* gene in XLA patients. Some of these mutations only partially compromise the gene, so some patients may have milder phenotype and up to 7% circulating B cells, making differentiation from common variable immunodeficiency difficult. In addition to mutations in the *BTK* gene, mutations in other genes required for immunoglobulin production, such as *IGHM*, *CD79A*, *CD79B*, *IGLLa*, *BLNK*, and *LRRC8A*, can be responsible for panhypogammaglobulinemia.

Treatment with gamma globulin has enabled many patients to live into adulthood. The maintenance dose required can vary considerably from patient to patient. High-dose IVIG may also lead to improvement of pyoderma gangrenosum–like lower extremity ulcerations. Chronic sinusitis and pulmonary infection remain problematic because of the lack of IgA, and chronic sinopulmonary infections require repeated pulmonary function monitoring.

Chen XF, et al: Clinical characteristics and genetic profiles of 174 patients with X-linked agammaglobulinemia. Medicine (Baltimore) 2016; 95: e4544.

Dua J, et al: *Pyoderma gangrenosum*–like ulcer caused by *Helicobacter cinaedi* in a patient with X-linked agammaglobulinaemia. Clin Exp Dermatol 2012; 37: 642.

Hunter HL, et al: Eczema and X-linked agammaglobulinaemia. Clin Exp Dermatol 2008; 33: 148.

Sharma D, et al: A child with X-linked agammaglobulinemia and Kawasaki disease. Rheumatol Int 2017; 37: 1401.

Tan Q, et al: Pyoderma gangrenosum in a patient with X-linked agammaglobulinemia. Ann Dermatol 2017; 29: 476.

Isolated IgA Deficiency (OMIM 137100)

An absence or marked reduction of serum IgA (<7 mg/dL) is the most common immunodeficiency state. Patients with RAG-1 mutations can also present selective IgA deficiency. The incidence varies greatly based on ethnic background: about 1 : 150 in the Arab Peninsula and Spain, 1 : 225–1 : 300 in the United States, and 1 : 14,000–18,000 in Japan. Certain medications appear to induce selective IgA deficiency, including phenytoin, sulfasalazine, cyclosporine, nonsteroidal antiinflammatory drugs (NSAIDs), and hydroxychloroquine. The genetic cause in most cases is unknown.

From 10%–15% of all symptomatic immunodeficiency patients have IgA deficiency. Most IgA-deficient patients, however, are completely well. Of those with symptoms, half have repeated infections of the GI and respiratory tracts, and one quarter have autoimmune disease. Allergies such as anaphylactic reactions to transfusion or IVIG, asthma, and AD are common in the symptomatic group. There is an increased association of celiac disease, dermatitis herpetiformis, and IBD. Vitiligo, alopecia areata, and other autoimmune diseases (e.g., systemic lupus erythematosus [SLE], dermatomyositis, scleroderma, thyroiditis, rheumatoid arthritis, polyarteritis-like vasculitis, Sjögren syndrome) and ulcerative gingivitis have all been reported to occur in these patients. Malignancy is increased in adults with IgA deficiency.

Azzi L, et al: Oral manifestations of selective IgA-deficiency. J Biol Regul Homeost Agents 2017; 31: 113.

Kato T, et al: RAG1 deficiency may present clinically as selective IgA deficiency. J Clin Immunol 2015; 35: 280.

Paradela S, et al: Necrotizing vasculitis with a polyarteritis nodosa–like pattern and selective immunoglobulin A deficiency. J Cutan Pathol 2008; 35: 871.

Yel L: Selective IgA deficiency. J Clin Immunol 2010; 30: 10.

Common Variable Immunodeficiency

Common variable immunodeficiency (CVID) is a heterogeneous disorder and is the most common immunodeficiency syndrome after IgA deficiency. Patients have low levels of IgG and IgA, and 50% also have low levels of IgM. Lymphocyte counts may be normal or low. Multiple genetic defects have been found in CVID, including mutations in *ICOS* (CVID type 1), *TNFRSF13B* (type 2), *CD19* (type 3), *TNFRSF13C* (type 4), *MS4A1* (type 5), *CD81* (type 6), *CR2* (type 7), *LRBA* (type 8), *PRKCD* (type 9), and *NFKB2* (CVID 10). These patients do not form antibodies to bacterial antigens, and have recurrent sinopulmonary infections. They have a predisposition to autoimmune disorders, such as vitiligo and alopecia areata, GI abnormalities, lymphoreticular malignancy (10-fold increase of lymphoma), and gastric carcinoma. Noninfectious granulomas have been reported in as many as 22% of CVID (Fig. 5.16). In some patients with CVID and multiple other immunodeficiencies, vaccine strain rubella has been found within the granulomas. Therefore it is hypothesized that the granulomas form due to difficulty processing the live rubella vaccination that is often given before diagnosis of CVID. Seven percent of CVID patients with granulomas have cutaneous granulomas, and virtually all patients with cutaneous granulomas also have visceral granulomas. These patients are more often female and have higher risk for lymphoma than other CVID patients. The granulomas can show multiple histologic patterns: granuloma annulare-like, sarcoidal, and even caseating. They show a CD4/CD8 ratio of less than 1, distinguishing these granulomas from sarcoidosis. CVID patients who develop granulomas have more severe depletion of isotype-switched memory B cells and naïve T cells, an immunologic profile also seen in ataxia telangiectasia patients with cutaneous granulomas.

Replacement of the reduced immunoglobulins with IVIG may help reduce infections. Topical, systemic, and intralesional corticosteroids may be used for the granulomas, depending on their extent. Infliximab and etanercept have been effective in steroid-refractory cases.

Lin JH, et al: Etanercept treatment of cutaneous granulomas in common variable immunodeficiency. J Allergy Clin Immunol 2006; 117: 878.

Neven B, et al: Cutaneous and visceral chronic granulomatous disease triggered by a rubella virus vaccine strain in children with primary immunodeficiencies. Clin Infect Dis 2017; 64: 83.

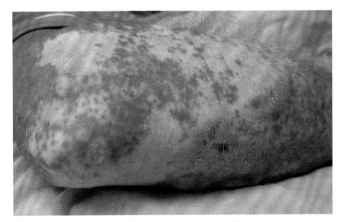

Fig. 5.16 Common variable immunodeficiency with granulomas in vitiligo.

Class-Switch Recombination Defects (Formerly Immunodeficiency With Hyper-IgM)

This group of diseases includes defects that are combined T-cell and B-cell abnormalities, such as CD40 deficiency (*CD40*) and CD40 ligand deficiency (*CD40LG*), and disorders of primary B cells, such as cytidine deaminase (*AICDA*) and uracil-DNA glycosylase (*UNG*) deficiencies. Class-switch recombination defects are rare, and the different genetic diseases included in this group appear to have different clinical manifestations. These patients experience recurrent sinopulmonary infections, diarrhea, and oral and anogenital ulcers. Neutropenia may be associated with the ulcers. Recalcitrant human papillomavirus (HPV) infections (typically flat warts) may occur.

Hypomorphic mutations in *NEMO* or *IKBKG* are associated with hypogammaglobulinemia and elevated IgM and may be associated with anhidrotic ectodermal dysplasia with immunodeficiency. *NEMO* mutations cause X-linked recessive disorders with lymphocytosis and elevated CD3 and CD4 cells and low levels of NK cells. The mother may have mild stigmata of incontinentia pigmenti. These male infants present within the first few months of life with hypohidrosis, delayed tooth eruption, and immunodeficiency. Hair may be absent. Frequent infections of the skin and respiratory tract are common. The eruption has been characterized as an "atopic dermatitis–like eruption," although some patients may have prominent intertriginous lesions resembling seborrheic dermatitis. Treatment is bone marrow transplantation.

Mancini AJ, et al: X-linked ectodermal dysplasia with immunodeficiency caused by *NEMO* mutation. Arch Dermatol 2008; 144: 342.

Qamar N, et al: The hyper IgM syndromes. Clin Rev Allergy Immunol 2014; 46: 120.

Thymoma With Immunodeficiency

Thymoma with immunodeficiency, also known as Good syndrome, occurs in adults in whom profound hypogammaglobulinemia and benign thymoma appear almost simultaneously. It is now classified predominantly as an antibody deficiency disorder. There is a striking deficiency of B and pre-B cells. One patient who developed vulvovaginal gingival lichen planus and severe oral herpes simplex has also been reported. Myelodysplasia and pure red blood cell aplasia may occur. Patients are at risk for fatal opportunistic pulmonary infections with fungi and *Pneumocystis*. Thymectomy does not prevent the development of the infectious or lymphoreticular complications. Supportive therapy with IVIG, granulocyte-macrophage colony-stimulating factor (GM-CSF), and transfusions may be required.

Aydintug YS, et al: Thymoma with immunodeficiency with multiple recurrent oral herpetic infections. Journal of Dental Sciences 2016; 11: 103.

Moutasim KA, et al: A case of vulvovaginal gingival lichen planus in association with Good's syndrome. Oral Surg Oral Med Oral Pathol Oral Radiol Endod 2008; 105: e57.

Disorders With T-Cell Deficiency

T-cell deficiency states can result from lack of thymic tissue, enzyme defects toxic to T lymphocytes (purine nucleoside phosphorylase deficiency), failure to express surface molecules required for immune interactions (CD3, major histocompatibility complex [MHC] class I and II), or defects in signaling molecules.

Digeorge Syndrome

DiGeorge syndrome is an autosomal dominant disorder that in 50% of cases is caused by hemizygous deletion of 22q11-pter and rarely by deletions in 10p. Many cases are sporadic. Most DiGeorge syndrome patients have the congenital anomalies and only minor thymic anomalies. They present with hypocalcemia or congenital heart disease. The syndrome includes congenital absence of the parathyroids and an abnormal aorta. Aortic and cardiac defects are the most common cause of death. DiGeorge syndrome is characterized by a distinctive facies: notched, low-set ears, micrognathia, shortened philtrum, and hypertelorism. Patients with these DiGeorge congenital malformations and complete lack of thymus are deemed to have "complete DiGeorge syndrome." Cell-mediated immunity is absent or depressed, and few T cells with the phenotype of recent thymus emigrants are found in the peripheral blood or tissues. Opportunistic infections are common despite normal immunoglobulin levels. Maternally derived GVHD may occur in these patients. A small subset of patients with complete DiGeorge syndrome develop an eczematous dermatitis, lymphadenopathy, and an oligoclonal T-cell proliferation. The condition may present as an atopic-like dermatitis, severe and extensive seborrheic dermatitis, or an erythroderma. This is called "atypical complete DiGeorge syndrome." Biopsies show features of a spongiotic dermatitis with eosinophils, necrotic keratinocytes with satellite necrosis, and characteristically perieccrine and intraeccrine inflammation. This resembles the histology of grade 1 or 2 GVHD, lichen striatus, and some cases of mycosis fungoides. One African American patient with DiGeorge syndrome developed a granulomatous dermatitis. The treatment for complete DiGeorge syndrome is thymic transplantation.

Davies EG: Immunodeficiency in DiGeorge syndrome and options for treating cases with complete athymia. Front Immunol 2013; 4: 322.

Gaudinski MR, Milner JD: Atopic dermatitis and allergic urticaria. Immunol Allergy Clin North Am 2017; 37: 1.

Jyonouchi H, et al: SAPHO osteomyelitis and sarcoid dermatitis in a patient with DiGeorge syndrome. Eur J Pediatr 2006; 165: 370.

Seminario-Vidal L, et al: Dermatological clues to the diagnosis of atypical complete DiGeorge syndrome. Dermatol Online J 2016 Nov 15; 22.

Miscellaneous T-Cell Deficiencies and Severe Combined Immunodeficiency

IPEX Syndrome

The immune dysregulation, polyendocrinopathy, enteropathy, X-linked recessive (IPEX) syndrome is a rare disorder presenting neonatally with the classic triad of autoimmune enteropathy, endocrinopathy (diabetes, thyroiditis), and eczematous dermatitis affecting males. Elevated IgE levels, eosinophilia, and food allergies, plus the eczematous dermatitis, all are manifestations of Th2 skewing of the immune system. Patients present with diffuse and severe erythematous exudative plaques resembling AD. Secondary infection is common, and staphylococcal septicemia can occur. The skin eruption may be follicularly based or may lead to prurigo nodularis. The scalp develops hyperkeratotic psoriasiform plaques. Cheilitis and onychodystrophy can occur. Alopecia areata, chronic urticaria, and bullous pemphigoid are cutaneous autoimmune manifestations of IPEX syndrome.

The IPEX syndrome is caused by mutations in *FOXP3* (forkhead box P3 protein), the master control gene for regulatory T-cell (Treg) development. IPEX like disease may also be caused by loss-of-function mutations in *CD25*, *STAT5b*, and *ITCH* and gain-of-function mutations in *STAT1* (signal transducer and activator of transcription 1). *FOXP3* is necessary for the development of Tregs, which are required to maintain immune homeostasis and mediate peripheral tolerance to "self" and nonself antigens. The enteropathy may be driven by autoantibodies to villin, and these autoantibodies can be used diagnostically. Treatment is immunomodulator therapy or bone marrow transplantation.

Severe Combined Immunodeficiency

Severe combined immunodeficiency (SCID) is a heterogeneous group of genetic disorders characterized by severely impaired cellular and humoral immunity. Severe T-cell deficiency and low lymphocyte count are found in virtually all SCID patients. Candidiasis (moniliasis) of the oropharynx and skin, intractable diarrhea, and pneumonia are the triad of findings that usually lead to the diagnosis of SCID. In addition, severe recurrent infections may occur, caused by *Pseudomonas, Staphylococcus,* Enterobacteriaceae, or *Candida.* Overwhelming viral infections are the usual cause of death. Engraftment of maternally transmitted or transfusion-derived lymphocytes can lead to GVHD. The initial seborrheic dermatitis–like eruption may represent maternal engraftment GVHD. This cutaneous eruption may be asymptomatic but tends to generalize. Infants with a widespread dermatitis but who lack any palpable lymph nodes should raise suspicion for SCID. More severe eczematous dermatitis and erythroderma may develop with alopecia. Cutaneous granulomas have been reported. In addition a higher rate of dermatofibroma sarcoma protuberans (DFSP) had been reported in SCID due to adenosine deaminase.

Deficiency or total absence of circulating T lymphocytes characterizes SCID. Immunoglobulin levels are consistently very low, but B-cell numbers may be reduced, normal, or increased. The thymus is very small; its malformed architecture at autopsy is pathognomonic.

The inheritance is either autosomal recessive or X-linked. Forty percent of SCID cases are X-linked and caused by deficiency of a common γ-chain that is an essential component of the IL-2 receptor. Twenty percent are caused by adenosine deaminase (ADA) deficiency and 6% from *Jak3* mutations.

Prenatal diagnosis and carrier detection are possible for many forms of SCID. The definitive treatment is hematopoietic stem cell transplantation (HSCT, bone marrow transplantation). This should ideally be carried out before age 3½ months for optimal outcome. The success rate approaches 90%. In utero HSCT has been successful in X-linked SCID. SCID patients rarely live longer than 2 years without transplantation. On average, 8 years after successful HSCT, SCID patients may develop severe HPV infection with common warts, flat warts, or even epidermodysplasia verruciformis. The development of HPV infections in SCID patients after HSCT is only seen in patients with either *Jak3* or γ-chain (gamma c) deficiency, but more than 50% of these patients may develop this complication.

Miscellaneous Genetic Disorders of Cellular Immunity

The *TAP1* and *TAP2* gene deficiencies are extremely rare autosomal recessive disorders that result in severe reduction of MHC class I expression on the surface of cells. CD8 cells are decreased, but CD4 cells are normal, as are B-cell numbers and serum immunoglobulins. Three forms of disease occur. The patient with the first phenotype develops severe bacterial, fungal, and parasitic infection and dies by age 3. The patient with the second phenotype is completely asymptomatic. The third group is the most common. Group 3 patients present in childhood with recurrent and chronic bacterial respiratory infections. These lead to bronchiectasis and eventually fatal respiratory failure in adulthood. The skin abnormalities appear in late childhood or more frequently in young adulthood (after age 15). Necrotizing granulomatous lesions appear as plaques or ulcerations on the lower legs and on the midface around the nose. The perinasal lesions are quite destructive and resemble "lethal midline granuloma" or Wegener granulomatosis. Nasal polyps with necrotizing granulomatous

histology also occur. One patient also developed leukocytoclastic vasculitis.

The ZAP-70 (ζ-chain [TCR]–associated protein kinase of 70 kD) deficiency is an autosomal recessive disorder of considerable heterogeneity. This enzyme is required for T-cell receptor (TCR) intracellular signaling. Patients present before age 2 years with recurrent bacterial, viral, and opportunistic infections, diarrhea, and failure to thrive. They have a lymphocytosis with normal CD4, NK, and B cells and decreased CD8 cells. Some patients develop an exfoliative erythroderma, eosinophilia, and elevated IgE levels.

Omenn syndrome (OMIM 603554; histiocytic medullary reticulosis) is a rare disorder that presents at birth or in the neonatal period. Classic Omenn was caused by defects in molecules involved in the variable diversity and joining V(D)J process. It is also caused by hypomorphic mutations in some of the genes that cause SCID. Both antibody production and cell-mediated immune function are impaired. Genetic mutations causing Omenn syndrome occur in *RAG1* and *RAG2* (90% of cases, classic Omenn), *DCLRE1C* (encoding ARTEMIS), *DNA-ligIV, IL7Rα, IL2Rγ, CHD7, ADA,* and *RNRP.* These mutations all result in defective T-cell development and oligoclonal, abnormally activated T cells. Clinical features include severe exfoliative erythroderma, eosinophilia, alopecia, *Pneumocystis jiroveci* and viral pneumonias, colitis, hepatosplenomegaly, lymphadenopathy, hypogammaglobulinemia, and elevated IgE.

De la Morena MT, Nelson RP Jr: Recent advances in transplantation for primary immune deficiency diseases. Clin Rev Allergy Immunol 2014; 46: 131.

Dvorak CC, et al: The natural history of children with severe combined immunodeficiency. J Clin Immunol 2013; 33: 1156.

Gadola SD, et al: TAP deficiency syndrome. Clin Exp Immunol 2000; 121: 173.

Halabi-Tawil M, et al: Cutaneous manifestations of immune dysregulation, polyendocrinopathy, enteropathy, X-linked (IPEX) syndrome. Br J Dermatol 2009; 160: 645.

Horino S, et al: Selective expansion of donor-derived regulatory T cells after allogeneic bone marrow transplantation in a patient with IPEX syndrome. Pediatr Transplant 2014; 18: e25.

Kelly BT, et al: Screening for severe combined immunodeficiency in neonates. Clin Epidemiol 2013; 5: 363.

Lampasona V, et al: Autoantibodies to harmonin and villin are diagnostic markers in children with IPEX syndrome. PLoS One 2013; 8: e78664.

Lee PP, et al: The many faces of *ARTEMIS*-deficient combined immunodeficiency. Clin Immunol 2013; 149: 464.

Marrella V, et al: Omenn syndrome does not live by V(D)J recombination alone. Curr Opin Allergy Clin Immunol 2011; 11: 525.

Moins-Teisserenc HT, et al: Association of a syndrome resembling Wegener's granulomatosis with low surface expression of HLA class-I molecules. Lancet 1999; 354: 1598.

Reichert SL, et al: Identification of a novel nonsense mutation in the FOXP3 gene in a fetus with hydrops. Am J Med Genet A 2016; 170A: 226.

Shearer WT, et al: Establishing diagnostic criteria for severe combined immunodeficiency disease (SCID), leaky SCID, and Omenn syndrome. J Allergy Clin Immunol 2013; 133: 1092.

Uzel G, et al: Dominant gain-of-function *STAT1* mutations in *FOXP3* wild-type immune dysregulation–polyendocrinopathy–enteropathy–X-linked–like syndrome. J Allergy Clin Immunol 2013; 131: 161.

Verbsky JW, Chatila TA: Immune dysregulation, polyendocrinopathy, enteropathy, X-linked (IPEX) and IPEX-related disorders. Curr Opin Pediatr 2013; 25: 708.

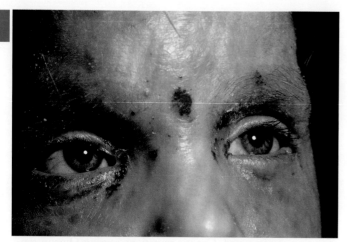

Fig. 5.17 Eczematous eruption with purpura in Wiskott-Aldrich syndrome.

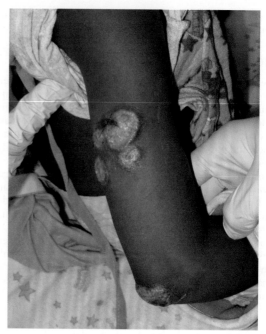

Fig. 5.18 Granulomatous lesions in ataxia teleangiectasia.

Wiskott-Aldrich Syndrome

Wiskott-Aldrich syndrome, an X-linked recessive syndrome, consists of a triad of chronic eczematous dermatitis resembling AD (Fig. 5.17); increased susceptibility to bacterial infections, such as pyoderma or otitis media; and thrombocytopenic purpura with small platelets. Levels of IgM are variable, IgA is normal to high, and IgE is elevated, as is IgG. On a complete blood cell count the mean platelet volume (MPV) is decreased. T cells (especially naïve T cells) are low in infancy and progressively decline in number and activity over time. Untreated survival is about 15 years, with death from infection, bleeding, or lymphoma (25% of patients).

The genetic cause of Wiskott-Aldrich syndrome is a mutation in the *WASP* gene. This gene codes for a protein called WASP, which is universally expressed in hematopoietic cells and is critical in the reorganization of the actin cytoskeleton in hematopoietic cells in response to external stimuli. The hematopoietic cells of affected patients cannot polarize or migrate in response to physiologic stimuli, accounting for the protean clinical features of the syndrome. Wiskott-Aldrich syndrome occurs when mutations in *WASP* lead to absence or truncation of the WASP protein (WASP – mutations). Mutations that result in normal length but some loss of function in the WASP protein (WASP + mutations) result in two different syndromes: X-linked thrombocytopenia (XLT) and intermittent X-linked thrombocytopenia. Gain-of-function mutations in WASP cause X-linked neutropenia. Patients with XLT may also have an atopic-like dermatitis, but this is usually milder than the severe and difficult to control eczema affecting patients with the full Wiskott-Aldrich syndrome. WASP/XLT patients may also develop autoimmune disease, especially autoimmune hemolytic anemia, vasculitis, Henoch-Schönlein–like purpura, and IBD. High IgM is associated with the development of autoimmune disease.

Treatment is with platelet transfusions, antibiotics, and IVIG, if required. Low dose IL2 is in trials and targeted gene therapy has been attempted. Often, splenectomy is performed to help control bleeding, but this leads to increased risk of sepsis and is not routinely recommended. Immunosuppressive therapy or rituximab may be used to control autoimmune complications. Bone marrow transplantation from a human leukocyte antigen (HLA)–identical sibling as early as possible in the disease course provides complete reversal of the platelet and immune dysfunction, as well as improvement or clearing of the eczematous dermatitis. Survival at 7 years with a matched sibling donor transplant approaches 90%.

Jyonouchi S, et al: Phase I trial of low-dose interleukin 2 therapy in patients with Wiskott-Aldrich syndrome. Clin Immunol 2017; 179: 47.
Massaad MJ, et al: Wiskott-Aldrich syndrome. Ann NY Acad Sci 2013; 1285: 26.

Ataxia Telangiectasia

Ataxia telangiectasia is an autosomal recessive condition caused by mutations in a single gene on chromosome 11 (*ATM*), which encodes a protein called ATM. When ATM is absent, the cell cycle does not stop to repair DNA damage, particularly double-stranded breaks, or for B(D)J recombination of immunoglobulin and TCR genes. This results in immunodeficiency and an increased risk for malignancy. The initial prominent skin feature is progressive ocular and cutaneous telangiectasias starting at age 3–6 years. These begin on the bulbar conjunctiva but later develop on the eyelids, ears, and flexors of the arms and legs. The ATM protein seems to be important in maintaining mitochondrial homeostasis, and this defect may be responsible for the premature aging (with loss of subcutaneous fat and graying of hair) and neurodegeneration.

Cutaneous noninfectious granulomas may occur and can be ulcerative and painful (Fig. 5.18). Rubella virus has been recovered by PCR from active ulcerations. Live vaccinations such the measles mumps and rubella vaccination should not be given to immunodeficient children, but because AT presents typically after age 1, children are often already vaccinated. Therefore the likely mechanism of granuloma formation is the ineffective processing of the rubella (or other infectious antigens) in live vaccinations. The granulomas tend to worsen with biopsy and manipulation. Other cutaneous features include large, irregular segmental café au lait spots, vitiligo, seborrheic dermatitis, AD, recurrent impetigo, and acanthosis nigricans. Late tightening of the skin can occur and resembles acral sclerosis. Sinopulmonary infections are common, especially otitis media, sinusitis, bronchitis, and pneumonia. Varicella (at times severe), herpes simplex, molluscum contagiosum, and herpes zoster can occur. Refractory warts occur in more than 5% of patients. Aside from candidal esophagitis, unusual opportunistic infections are rare.

Lymphopenia is common, with reduction of both B and T cells occurring in the majority of patients. Th-cell counts can be less than 200. IgA, IgG4, IgG2, and IgE deficiencies can all be present. Paradoxically, IgM, IgA, and IgG can be elevated in some patients, including the presence of monoclonal gammopathy in more than 10%. The immunologic abnormalities are not progressive. Lymphoma risk is increased more than 200-fold (especially B-cell lymphoma), and leukemia (especially T-cell chronic lymphocytic leukemia) is increased 70-fold. Treatment includes high vigilance for infection and malignancy. In patients with low CD4 counts, prophylaxis to prevent *Pneumocystis* pneumonia can be considered. When IgG deficiency is present and infections are frequent, IVIG may be beneficial. IVIG and intralesional corticosteroids may be used for the cutaneous granulomas. Carriers of ataxia telangiectasia have an increased risk for breast cancer. Because of the accumulation of chromosomal breaks after radiation exposure, both the ataxia telangiectasia patients and the carriers should minimize radiation exposure.

Ambrose M, Gatti RA: Pathogenesis of ataxia-telangiectasia. Blood 2013; 121: 4036.
Neven B, et al: Cutaneous and visceral chronic granulomatous disease triggered by a rubella virus vaccine strain in children with primary immunodeficiencies. Clin Infect Dis 2016; 64: 83.

Primary Immunodeficiency Diseases Associated With Warts

Depressed T-cell function, either iatrogenic or genetic, is associated with an increased risk of HPV infection. However, a few PIDs are associated with a particular burden of HPV infection, and HPV infection may be an initial or prominent component of the syndrome. HPV vaccine may activate the immune system to help clear recalcitrant verrucae in some patients. Epidermodysplasia verruciformis is discussed in Chapter 19.

WHIM Syndrome

The warts, hypogammaglobulinemia, infections, and myelokathexis (WHIM) syndrome is an autosomal dominant disorder with hypogammaglobulinemia, reduced B-cell numbers, and neutropenia. The most common genetic cause is a gain of function mutation of the *CXCR4* gene. Additional mutations that are not in the *CXCR4* gene can also cause WHIM, but all of them lead to functional hyperactivity of *CXCR4*. *CXCR4* causes retention of neutrophils in the bone marrow and is the basis of the neutropenia and myelokathexis (increased apoptotic neutrophils in bone marrow). There is profound loss of circulating CD27+ memory B cells, resulting in hypogammaglobulinemia, with the observation that WHIM patients have normal antibody response to certain antigens but fail to maintain this antibody production. However, normal immunoglobulin levels do not exclude the diagnosis of WHIM. Almost 80% of WHIM patients have warts at the time of their diagnosis (Fig. 5.19). These include common and genital wart types. A significant number of female WHIM patients have cervical and vulval dysplasia, which can progress to carcinoma. WHIM patients have disproportionately more HPV infections than SCID patients but have little problem resolving other viral infections. However, they may develop Epstein-Barr virus (EBV)–induced lymphomas. The vast majority of patients in early childhood have recurrent sinopulmonary infections, skin infections, osteomyelitis, and urinary tract infections. Recurrent pneumonias lead to bronchiectasis. There is a CXCR4 antagonist in trials but standard treatment is G-CSF, IVIG, prophylactic antibiotics, and aggressive treatment of infections. There is one report recently of a cure of WHIM by chromothripsis in a hematopoietic stem cell. Chromothripsis is a catastrophic disruption of chromosomes

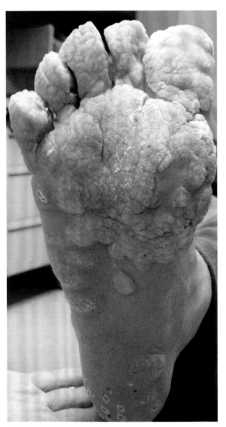

Fig. 5.19 Warts in WHIM syndrome.

in a cell in this case the new stem cell had a selective advantage due to the lack of the WHIM mutation. Untreated, the HPV infections can progress to fatal carcinomas, and therefore male patients must be regularly examined by dermatologists and female patients by gynecologists; a low threshold for biopsy of genital lesions is required.

DOCK8 Deficiency

Deficiency in DOCK8 (dedicator of cytokinesis 8) are associated with hyper-IgE syndrome (see later discussion). However, unlike other genetic causes of hyper-IgE, DOCK8 deficiency is uniquely associated with a susceptibility to cutaneous viral infections, including HSV, molluscum contagiosum, and HPV (Fig. 5.20). Warts can be flat or verrucous and affect about two thirds of patients.

GATA2 Deficiency (WILD Syndrome)

GATA2 is an important transcription factor involved in hematopoiesis maintenance of the stem cell compartment. GATA2 deficiency leads to a constellation of syndromes characterized by myelodysplasia, opportunistic infections, and leukemia. Patients have profound monocytopenia, often neutropenia, and NK, B, and dendritic cell lymphocytopenia. T-cell counts are variable. More than 75% of patients have severe or disseminated HPV infection, usually verruca plana or verruca vulgaris, and the HPV infection is first manifestation in the majority of patients, usually in adolescence or early adulthood. Severe cervical HPV infection can also occur and may lead to cancer. Thirty percent of patients develop a corticosteroid-responsive panniculitis. GATA2 has a role in lymphatic development and when the constellation includes lymphedema, it has been named WILD syndrome (warts,

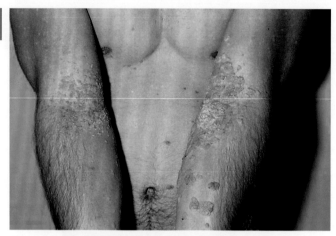

Fig. 5.20 Warts in DOCK8 immunodeficiency. (Courtesy Edward W. Cowen, MD.)

immunodeficiency, lymphedema, and dysplasia). The genetic defect in WILD patients can be missed on typical sanger sequencing because the mutation can be large and extend into exons. The WILD syndrome is rare and presents at age 6 months with lower extremity lymphedema that is progressive and later may involve the upper extremities and groin. Venous thrombosis occurs in 25% and lymphedema in 11% of patients of all patients with GATA2 mutations. Allogeneic HSCT seems to be curative.

Badolato R, et al: How I treat warts, hypogammaglobulinemia, infections, and myelokathexis syndrome. Blood 2017; 130: 2491.

Dorn JM, et al: WILD syndrome is GATA2 deficiency. J Allergy Clin Immunol Pract 2017; 5: 1149.

Leiding JW, et al: Warts and all: HPV in primary immunodeficiencies. J Allergy Clin Immunol 2012; 130: 1030.

McDermott DH, et al: Chromothriptic cure of WHIM syndrome. Rare Dis 2015; 3: e1073430.

Minegishi Y, Saito M: Cutaneous manifestations of hyper-IgE syndrome. Allergol Int 2012; 61: 191.

Sanal O, et al: Additional diverse findings expand the clinical presentation of DOCK8 deficiency. J Clin Immunol 2012; 32: 698.

Smith SP, et al: Clearance of recalcitrant warts in a patient with idiopathic immune deficiency following administration of the quadrivalent human papillomavirus vaccine. Clin Exp Dermatol 2017; 42: 306.

Spinner MA, et al: GATA2 deficiency. Blood 2014; 123: 809.

Defects of Phagocyte Number, Function, or Both

Chronic Granulomatous Disease

Chronic granulomatous disease (CGD) is a rare disorder caused by mutations in one of the genes that encode the subunits of the superoxide-generating phagocyte NADPH oxidase system responsible for the respiratory burst involved in organism killing. CGD is characterized by repeated and recurrent bacterial and fungal infections of the lungs, skin, lymph nodes, and bones. Gingivostomatitis (aphthous-like ulcerations) and a seborrheic dermatitis of the periauricular, perinasal, and perianal area are characteristic. The dermatitis is frequently infected with *S. aureus*, and regional adenopathy and abscesses may complicate the infections. The term *suppurative dermatitis* is used in the immunology literature to describe this seborrheic-like dermatitis with secondary infection, analogous to the "infective dermatitis" seen in human T-cell lymphotropic virus (HTLV)–1 infection. In addition to *S. aureus*,

Serratia species are often isolated from skin abscesses and osteomyelitis. *Aspergillus* is the most common agent causing pneumonia in CGD patients. In tuberculosis-endemic areas, CGD patients frequently develop active tuberculosis or prolonged scarring, abscesses, or disseminated infection following bacille Calmette-Guérin (BCG) immunization.

There are four types of CGD, one X-linked and three autosomal recessive. The X-linked form is the most common (65%–75% of CGD patients) and is caused by a mutation in the *CYBB* gene, which leads to a total absence of NADPH oxidase activity. In autosomal recessive forms, mutations in the genes encoding for the remaining three oxidase components have been described: p22-phox (*CYBA*), p47-phox (*NCF1*), and p67-phox (*NCF2*). One patient with a mutation in p40-phox (*NCF4*) has been described. The X-linked variant has the most severe phenotype. Compared with the autosomal recessive CGD patients, the X-linked patients present at an earlier age (14 vs. 30 months) and are diagnosed at an earlier age (3–5 vs. 6–13 years). The lack of superoxide generation apparently causes disease, not because the bacteria are not being killed by the superoxide, but because the superoxide is required to activate proteases in phagocytic vacuoles that are needed to kill infectious organisms.

Granuloma formation is characteristic of CGD and can occur in the GI tract, liver, bladder, bone, and lymph nodes. Up to 40% of biopsies from these organs will demonstrate granulomas, at times with identifiable fungal or mycobacterial organisms. These patients are often receiving prophylactic antibiotics, however, so organisms are frequently not found. Subcorneal pustular eruptions can also be seen in CGD patients. In the intestinal tract, the GI symptoms and granuloma formation can present in a similar fashion to inflammatory bowel disease.

The diagnosis of CGD is made by demonstrating low reduction of yellow nitroblue tetrazolium (NBT) to blue formazan in the "NBT test." Dihydrorhodamine 123 flow cytometry (DHR), chemiluminescence production, and the ferricytochrome *c* reduction assay are also confirmatory. Western blot analysis for NADPH oxidase expression and DNA sequencing can pinpoint the genetic mutation.

Female carriers of the X-linked form of CGD have a mixed population of normal and abnormal phagocytes and therefore show intermediate NBT reduction and two discrete populations with DHR testing. The majority of carriers have skin complaints including a malar rash, discoid lupus erythematosus (DLE)–like lesions, adult acne and skin abscesses. The lesions are clinically DLE-like, but histologically, the interface component is often absent, and the lesions resemble tumid lupus. Direct immunofluorescence examination is usually negative, as is common in tumid lupus erythematosus (LE). Less frequently, CGD patients themselves have been described as having similar LE-like lesions, or "arcuate dermal erythema." Despite these findings, the vast majority of patients with LE-like skin lesions, both carriers and CGD patients, are antinuclear antibody (ANA) negative. Raynaud phenomenon can occur. More than half will report a photosensitive dermatitis, 40% have oral ulcerations, and one third have joint complaints.

Treatment of infections should be early and aggressive. There should be a low threshold to biopsy skin lesions, as they may reveal important and potentially life-threatening infections. Patients usually receive chronic TMP-SMX prophylaxis, chronic oral anti-*Aspergillus* agent (such as itraconazole, posaconazole or voriconazole), and IFN-γ injections. Voriconazole can lead to severe photodamage and skin malignancy, so chronic therapy in CGD patients should be used with extreme caution. Thalidomide has been used for the colitis. Bone marrow or stem cell transplantation has been successful in restoring enzyme function, reducing infections, and improving the associated bowel disease. However, survival is *not* increased with bone marrow transplantation, so this is not routinely undertaken. Recently IL-1 blockade was found to be effective at decreasing the inflammation of CGD.

Battersby AC, et al: Inflammatory and autoimmune manifestations in X-linked carriers of chronic granulomatous disease in the United Kingdom. J Allergy Clin Immunol 2017; 140: 628.

de Luca A, et al: IL-1 receptor blockade restores autophagy and reduces inflammation in chronic granulomatous disease in mice and in humans. Proc Natl Acad Sci U S A 2014; 111: 3526.

Grimm MJ et al: Chronic granulomatous disease and aspergillosis. In *Immunogenetics of Fungal Diseases*, 2017 (pp. 105–120). Springer International Publishing.

Ho H, et al: P203 thalidomide as an alternative therapy for steroid-refractory colitis in chronic granulomatous disease. Ann Allergy Asthma Immunol 2016; 117: S82.

Lee PP, et al: Susceptibility to mycobacterial infections in children with X-linked chronic granulomatous disease. Pediatr Infect Dis J 2008; 27: 224.

Leiding JW, Holland SM: Chronic granulomatous disease. GeneReviews [Internet].

Raptaki M, et al: Chronic granulomatous disease. J Clin Immunol 2013; 33: 1302.

Leukocyte Adhesion Deficiency

This rare autosomal recessive disorder has three types. Leukocyte adhesion deficiency (LAD) type I is caused by a mutation in the common chain (CD18) of the β2-integrin family (*ITGB2*). It is characterized by recurrent bacterial infections of the skin and mucosal surfaces, especially gingivitis and periodontitis. The remnant umbilical cord is often delayed in separation during infancy. Skin ulcerations from infection may continue to expand. Cellulitis and necrotic abscesses, especially in the perirectal area, can occur. Minor injuries may lead to pyoderma gangrenosum–like ulcerations that heal slowly. Infections begin at birth, and omphalitis with delayed separation of the cord is characteristic. Neutrophilia is marked, usually 5–20 times normal, and the count may reach up to 100,000 during infections. Despite this, there is an absence of neutrophils at the sites of infection, demonstrating the defective migration of neutrophils out of the blood vessels in these patients. LAD type I patients are affected either severely (<1% of normal CD18 expression) or moderately (2.5%–10% of normal expression.) Patients with moderate disease have less severe infections and survive into adulthood, whereas patients with severe disease often die in infancy.

LAD type II is caused by a mutation in *SLC35C1*, which results in a general defect in fucose metabolism which results in decreased fucosylation of selectin ligands on leukocytes. This leads to impaired tethering and rolling on activated endothelial cells. Severe mental retardation, short stature, a distinctive facies, and the rare hh blood phenotype are the features. Initially, these patients have recurrent cellulitis with marked neutrophilia, but the infections are not life threatening. After age 3 years, infections become less of a problem and patients develop chronic periodontitis.

LAD type III is caused by a mutation in the gene *FERMT3* and is characterized by severe recurrent infections, bleeding tendency (from impaired platelet function), and marked neutrophilia.

LAD1 patients can have abnormal IL12 and 23 activity and thus ustekinumab was recently tried with excellent success. Bone marrow transplantation is an option for patients with severe LAD type I and LAD type III.

Hajishengallis G, et al: Role of bacteria in leukocyte adhesion deficiency-associated periodontitis. Microb Pathog 2016; 94: 21.

Harris ES et al: Lessons from rare maladies. Curr Opin Hematol 2013; 20: 16.

Mellouli F, et al: Successful treatment of *Fusarium solani* ecthyma gangrenosum in a patient affected by leukocyte adhesion deficiency type 1 with granulocytes transfusions. BMC Dermatology 2010; 10: 10.

Moutsopoulos NM, et al: Interleukin-12 and interleukin-23 blockade in leukocyte adhesion deficiency type 1. N Engl J Med 2017; 376: 1141.

Simpson BN, et al: A new leukocyte hyperadhesion syndrome of delayed cord separation, skin infection, and nephrosis. Pediatrics 2014; 133: e257.

Stepensky PY, et al: Leukocyte adhesion deficiency type III. J Pediatr Hematol Oncol 2015; 37: 264.

Hyperimmunoglobulinemia E Syndrome

There are at least multiple defined mutations that cause hyperimmunoglobulinemia E syndrome (HIES; also called hyper-IgE syndrome). The autosomal dominant form is caused by a mutation in *STAT3*, and the autosomal recessive form by mutations in *DOCK8* and rarely in tyrosine kinase 2 (TYK2) or phosphoglucomutase 3 (PGM3). The autosomal recessive forms of HIES are clinically somewhat different and are described separately.

Autosomal dominant HIES was first called Job syndrome or Buckley syndrome. The classic triad is an AD-like eczematous dermatitis, recurrent skin and lung infections, and high serum IgE, although IgE is elevated in atopy generally. The skin disease is the first manifestation of STAT3 deficiency and begins at birth in 19% of cases, within the first week of life in more than 50%, and in the first month in 80%. This is very helpful clinically because AD does not usually start until the second or third month of age. The initial eruption is noted first on the face or scalp, but quickly generalizes to affect the face, scalp, and body. The rash favors the shoulder, arms, chest, and buttocks. The newborn rash begins as pink papules and pustules that coalesce into crusted plaques that may initially be diagnosed as "neonatal acne." Histologically, these papules are intraepidermal eosinophilic pustules. The dermatitis evolves to bear a close resemblance to AD, often very severe, and occurs in 100% of autosomal dominant HIES patients. Staphylococcal infection of the dermatitis is common. There can be "cold" abscesses due to the lack of inflammation typically present to fight infection. IgE levels are above 2000 in 95% of patients with autosomal dominant HIES, but since only a small percentage of children with IgE levels above 2000 actually have HIES, other features must be used to confirm the diagnosis. Recurrent pyogenic pneumonia is the rule, starting in childhood. Because of the lack of neutrophilic inflammation in abscesses and pneumonia, symptoms may be lacking and lead to a delay in diagnosis. Although antibiotic treatment clears the pneumonia, healing is abnormal, with the formation of bronchiectasis and pneumatoceles, a characteristic feature of HIES. Mucocutaneous candidiasis is common, typically thrush, vaginal candidiasis, and candidal onychomycosis. Musculoskeletal abnormalities are common, including scoliosis, osteopenia, minimal trauma fractures (55%), and hyperextensibility, leading to premature degenerative joint disease. Retention of some or all of the primary teeth is a characteristic feature. Other oral manifestations include median rhomboid glossitis, high-arch palate, and abnormally prominent wrinkles on the oral mucosa. Arterial aneurysms are common, including Chiari 1 malformation (40%) and coronary vascular abnormalities (60%). The latter can cause myocardial infarction. Autosomal dominant HIES patients have a characteristic facies, developing during childhood and adolescence. Features include facial asymmetry, broad nose, deep-set eyes, and a prominent forehead. The facial skin is rough, with large pores. There is an increased risk of malignancy, predominantly B-cell non-Hodgkin lymphoma, but cutaneous squamous cell carcinoma has also been reported. Laboratory abnormalities are limited to eosinophilia and an elevated IgE. In adults, IgE levels may become normal. Functional Th17 studies can help in diagnosis. A scoring system developed at the National Institutes of Health (NIH) can accurately identify patients with HIES, selecting those in whom genetic testing could be considered.

Autosomal recessive HIES is caused by *DOCK8*, TYK2, or PGM3 mutations and is less common. Patients with *DOCK8* mutations also have severe eczema and recurrent skin and lung infections, although the lung infections resolve without pneumatoceles (except in PGM3). TYK2 has only been described in a small number of patients who had high IgE and atopy. Food allergies are often present in autosomal recessive HIES caused by *DOCK8* mutation, as is decreased IgM. The main cutaneous difference is patients with *DOCK8* mutations are predisposed to exuberant cutaneous viral infections, especially warts, molluscum contagiosum, herpes simplex, and varicella-zoster, as well as systemic viral infections, including EBV and cytomegalovirus (CMV). They also develop mucocutaneous candidiasis. Neurologic disease is much more common in autosomal recessive HIES, ranging from facial paralysis to hemiplegia. Autosomal recessive HIES patients have normal facies, no fractures, and normal shedding of primary dentition, but a dramatic increase in malignancy, especially leukemia.

Treatment for HIES is aimed at decreasing infection and maintaining skin barrier. Infections are suppressed with bleach baths and chronic antibiotic prophylaxis (usually with TMP-SMX); antifungal agents may be used for candidal infections of the skin and nails. Topical antiinflammatories are used to manage the eczema, and in severe cases, systemic therapy can be considered but should be used with caution. Bisphosphonates are used for osteopenia. The role of IVIG, antihistamines, dupilumab, and omalizumab (antibody against IgE) is unknown. In patients with autosomal recessive HIES, hematopoietic cell transplantation (HCT) is recommended because of the high risk of malignancy and CNS infarction. Autosomal dominant HIES patients with malignancy should be considered for HCT because it can reverse the HIES, reducing the infectious complications following HCT.

Mogensen TH: STAT3 and the hyper-IgE syndrome. JAKSTAT 2013; 2: e23435.

Rael EL, et al: The hyper-IgE syndromes. World Allergy Organ J 2012; 5: 79.

Sasihuseyinoglu AS, et al: Squamous cell carcinoma with hyper-IgE syndrome. J Pediatr Hematol Oncol 2017 Sep 8. Epub ahead of print.

Woellner C, et al: Mutations in *STAT3* and diagnostic guidelines for hyper-IgE syndrome. J Allergy Clin Immunol 2010;125: 424.

Yang L, et al: Hyper-IgE syndromes. Curr Opin Pediatr 2014; 26: 697.

Zhang Q, et al: Recent advances in *DOCK8* immunodeficiency syndrome. J Clin Immunol 2016; 36: 441.

Complement Deficiency

The complement system is an effector pathway of proteins that results in membrane damage and chemotactic activity. Four major functions result from complement activation: cell lysis, opsonization/phagocytosis, inflammation, and immune complex removal. In the "classical" complement pathway, complement is activated by an antigen-antibody reaction involving IgG or IgM. Some complement components are directly activated by binding to the surface of infectious organisms; this is called the "alternate" pathway. The central component common to both pathways is C3. In the classical pathway, antigen-antibody complexes sequentially bind and activate three complement proteins, C1, C4, and C2, leading to the formation of C3 convertase, an activator of C3. The alternate pathway starts with direct activation of C3. From activated C3, C5–C9 are sequentially activated. Cytolysis is induced mainly through the membrane attack complex (MAC), which is made up of the terminal components of complement. Opsonization is mainly mediated by a subunit of C3b, and inflammation by subunits of C3, C4, and C5.

Inherited deficiencies of complement are usually autosomal recessive traits. Deficiencies of all 11 components of the classical pathway, as well as inhibitors of this pathway, have been described. Genetic deficiency of the C1 inhibitor is the only autosomal dominant form of complement deficiency and results in hereditary angioedema (see Chapter 7). In general, deficiencies of the early components of the classical pathway result in autoimmune connective tissue diseases, whereas deficiencies of the late components of complement lead to recurrent neisserial sepsis or meningitis. Overlap exists, and patients with late-component deficiencies may exhibit connective tissue diseases, and patients with deficiencies of early components, such as C1q, may manifest infections. Deficiency of C3 results in recurrent infections with encapsulated bacteria such as *Pneumococcus, H. influenzae*, and *Streptococcus pyogenes*. C3 inactivator deficiency, as with C3 deficiency, results in recurrent pyogenic infections. Properdin (component of alternate pathway) dysfunction is inherited as an X-linked trait and predisposes to fulminant meningococcemia. Deficiency of C9 is the most common complement deficiency in Japan but is uncommon in other countries. Most patients appear healthy. MASP2 deficiency, resulting in absent hemolytic activity by the lectin pathway, is considered a complement deficiency and results in a syndrome resembling SLE and increased pyogenic infection. Factor I deficiency results in recurrent infections, including *Neisseria meningitides.* Partially deficient family members may also have increased infections.

C2 deficiency is the most common complement deficiency in the United States and Europe. Most patients are healthy, but SLE-like syndromes develop in 10%. C1q-, C3-, and C4-deficient patients have SLE at rates of 90%, 31%, and 75%, respectively, and C1r deficiency was recently reported in early-onset SLE. Complement deficiency–associated SLE typically has early onset, photosensitivity, less renal disease, and Ro/La autoantibodies in two thirds of patients. C2- and C4-deficient patients with LE typically have subacute annular morphology (Fig. 5.21), Sjögren syndrome, arthralgias, and oral ulcerations. CH50 is a functional assay of the complement system and is typically low in active systemic lupus. Cell-bound complement activity products such as C4d and C3d, which are the byproducts of complement activation, are deposited on other cells such as erythrocytes and can be detected to monitor systemic lupus disease activity. Frequent infections, anaphylactoid purpura, dermatomyositis, vasculitis, and cold urticaria may be seen. A patient with C1q deficiency presented with macrophage activating syndrome. Renal disease, anti-dsDNA antibodies, and anticardiolipin antibodies are uncommon. Patients with C4 deficiency may have lupus and involvement of the palms and soles.

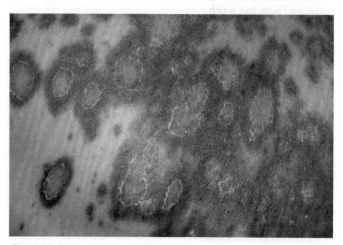

Fig. 5.21 Subacute lupus erythematosus as can be seen in complement deficiency disorders.

Many of the complement component deficiencies can be acquired as an autoimmune phenomenon or a paraneoplastic finding. Examples include acquired angioedema, as when C1 inhibitor is the target, or lipodystrophy and nephritis, when C3 convertase is the target.

When complement deficiency is suspected, a useful screening test is a CH50 (total hemolytic complement) determination, because deficiency of any of the complement components will usually result in CH50 levels that are dramatically reduced or zero.

Demirkaya E, et al: Brief report: deficiency of complement 1r subcomponent in early-onset systemic lupus erythematosus. Arthritis Rheumatol 2017; 69: 1832.

Kosaka S, et al: Cutaneous vasculitic and glomerulonephritis associated with C4 deficiency. Clin Exp Dermatol 2013; 38: 492.

Lintner KE, et al: Early components of the complement classical activation pathway in human systemic autoimmune diseases. Front Immunol 2016; 7: 36.

Lipsker D, Hauptmann G: Cutaneous manifestations of complement deficiencies. Lupus 2010; 19: 1096.

Sozeri B, et al: Complement-4 deficiency in a child with systemic lupus erythematosus presenting with standard treatment-resistant severe skin lesion. ISRN Rhematol 2011; 10.

Tichaczek-Goska D: Deficiencies and excessive human complement system activation in disorders of multifarious etiology. Adv Clin Exp Med 2012; 21: 105.

Wisner E, et al: P197 Macrophage activation syndrome as the initial presentation of C1q deficiency. Ann Allergy Asthma Immunol 2016; 117: S80.

Graft-Versus-Host Disease

GVHD occurs most frequently in the setting of HSCT but may also occur following organ transplantation or in the rare situation of transfusion of active lymphoid cells into an immunodeficient child postpartum or even in utero. Blood transfusions with active lymphocytes (nonradiated whole blood) from family members or in populations with minimal genetic variability, given to an immunodeficient patient, can result in GVHD. HSCT from a monozygotic twin (syngeneic) or even from the patient's own stem cells (autologous) can rarely induce a mild form of GVHD.

Development of GVHD requires three elements. First, the transplanted cells must be immunologically competent. Second, the recipient must express tissue antigens that are not present in the donor and therefore are recognized as foreign. Third, the recipient must be unable to reject the transplanted cells. Immunologic competence of the transplanted cells is important, because ablating them too much may lead to failure of engraftment, or, more often, incomplete eradication of the recipient's malignancy (graft-vs.-tumor effect). Therefore some degree of immunologic competence of the transplanted cells is desired. For this reason, the prevalence of GVHD still remains about 50% after HSCT. Another important factor in determining the development and severity of the GVHD is the preconditioning regimen. Chemotherapy and radiation cause activation of dendritic cells (antigen-presenting cells [APCs]) in tissues with high cell turnover—the skin, gut, and liver. These APCs increase their expression of HLA and other minor cell surface antigens, priming them to interact with transplanted lymphoid cells. Host APCs are important in presenting these antigens to the active lymphoid donor cells. Cytokines, especially IL-2, TNF-α, and IFN-γ, are important in enhancing this host-donor immunologic interaction. Reducing this early inflammatory component in GVHD can delay the onset of the GVHD but may not reduce the prevalence. The indications for HSCT, age limits, and allowable degree of HLA incompatibility have resulted in greater use of HSCT, increasing the number of persons at risk for GVHD.

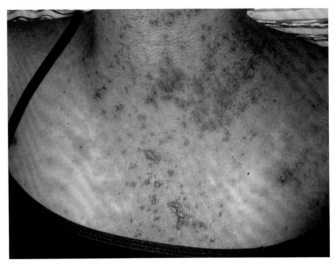

Fig. 5.22 Acute graft-versus-host disease. (Courtesy Jennifer Huang, MD.)

Initially, only reactions that occurred within the first 100 days after transplantation were considered acute GVHD, but it is now recognized that classic acute GVHD can occur up to 1 year or more after HSCT, especially with tapering of anti-GVHD immunosuppressives. Acute GVHD is based on the clinical presentation, *not* the time of onset after transplantation. In acute GVHD, the cutaneous eruption typically begins between the 14th and 42nd days after transplantation, with a peak at day 30 (Fig. 5.22). Acute GVHD is characterized by an erythematous morbilliform eruption of the face and trunk, which may become confluent and result in exfoliative erythroderma. Ear involvement is common. It often begins with punctate lesions corresponding to hair follicles and eccrine ducts, resembling keratosis pilaris. In many cases, a fine scale can be appreciated on the skin lesions. GVH is often described as more monomorphous than similar-appearing morbilliform drug eruptions, and tends to involve the upper back, rather than the lower back and dependent areas. GVHD is staged clinically, with stage 1 as less than 25% BSA, stage 2 as 25%–50% BSA, stage 3 as greater than 50% BSA, and stage 4 as erythroderma with bullae. In children, the diaper area is often involved. The eruption may appear papular and eczematous, involving web spaces, periumbilical skin, and ears, and bears some resemblance to scabies.

The differential diagnosis for the eruption of acute GVHD includes the eruption of lymphocyte recovery, engraftment syndrome, viral exanthem, and drug eruption. The cutaneous histology in the early phases of acute GVHD may not be able to completely distinguish these entities. Grade IV GVHD is characterized by full-thickness slough and may resemble toxic epidermal necrolysis, and it may be impossible to distinguish the two entities clinically or histologically. The mucous membranes and the conjunctivae can be involved as well, which can be difficult to distinguish from chemotherapy-induced and infectious mucositis. Often, about the same time, the patient develops the other characteristic features of acute GVHD: cholestatic hepatitis with elevated bilirubin and high-volume diarrhea. Autologous GVHD usually involves only the skin and is self-limited, and it is thought to occur from preconditioning regimen–induced loss of "self-tolerance."

The "eruption of lymphocyte recovery" is a mild, self-limited morbilliform eruption that may be associated with a brief fever, occurring when lymphocyte counts first return following chemotherapy. This can closely resemble GVHD, though without liver or gut involvement; patients may progress to overt aGVHD. Engraftment syndrome is a combination of symptoms that occur about the time of engraftment and neutrophil recovery. Patients develop fever (without infectious source), diarrhea, pulmonary infiltrates with hypoxia, and capillary leak syndrome with edema and weight gain. It occurs as soon as 7 days after autologous HSCT and 11–16 days after allogeneic transplants. The associated skin eruption is clinically and histologically identical to acute GVHD. Ocular involvement with keratitis can occur. This syndrome occurs in 7%–59% of post-HSCT patients and is a significant cause of morbidity and mortality in autologous peripheral blood progenitor cell transplant patients. It is mediated by cytokine production and neutrophil infiltration of the organs damaged by the conditioning chemotherapy, especially the lungs. Administration of G-CSF and autologous transplantation are risk factors for its development. Treatment is high-dose systemic corticosteroids.

With improved support for GVHD patients after HSCT, more are surviving, and 60%–70% develop chronic GVHD (cGVHD). It is the second most common cause of death in HSCT patients. It is unclear whether cGVHD is mediated by the same pathologic mechanisms as acute GVHD. Certain conditioning regimens may increase risk of cGVHD, particularly total body irradiation and the risk of scleroderma-like cGVHD. Chronic disease has features more typical of an autoimmune disease. Diagnostic criteria have been adopted, with "diagnostic" and "distinctive" cutaneous manifestations. The most common diagnostic feature, occurring in 80% of patients who develop cGVHD, is a lichen planus–like eruption. It typically occurs 3–5 months after grafting, usually beginning on the hands and feet but becoming generalized. It may present with a malar rash resembling LE. The chronic interface dermatitis can leave the skin with a poikilodermatous appearance. Similar lichen planus–like lesions may occur on the oral mucosa and can result in pain and poor nutrition. Lichen sclerosus–like lesions can also occur. Involvement of the vaginal or esophageal mucosa can result in severe scarring and strictures. About 20% of men with cGVHD have genital skin changes, and 13% have cGVHD of the penis. cGVHD of the skin and oral mucosa is associated with genital involvement. Lichen sclerosus–like lesions, phimosis, and inflammatory balanitis are most common; 80% of men with penile cGVHD report erectile dysfunction. Patients may underreport their genital cGVH, and a thorough physical and history is important.

Sclerosis is the other "diagnostic" family of skin lesions. This can include lesions resembling superficial morphea, which can have overlying lichen sclerosus–like changes. The morphea-like lesions demonstrate an isomorphic response, favoring areas of pressure, especially the waistband and brassiere-band areas. Deeper sclerotic lesions resembling eosinophilic fasciitis (resulting in joint contractures, Fig. 5.23) and restriction of the oral commissure due to sclerosis can occur. These sclerotic plaques may ulcerate.

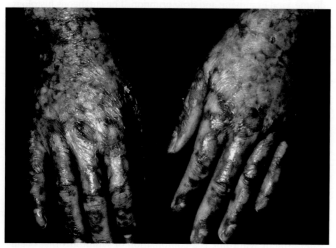

Fig. 5.23 Chronic graft-versus-host disease.

The extent of involvement of the deep tissues, such as muscle and fascia, cannot be easily defined by clinical examination and may be aided by magnetic resonance imaging. Rarely, the myositis of cGVHD may be accompanied by a skin eruption similar to dermatomyositis. Other features of GVHD may include depigmentation resembling vitiligo; scarring or nonscarring alopecia; nail dystrophy (e.g., longitudinal ridging, brittle thin nails, pterygium, nail loss); and xerostomia and other, Sjögren-like mucosal symptoms. Atypical forms of GVHD resembling Pityriasis Rubra Pilaris (PRP), psoriasis, eczematous eruptions, isolated follicular hyperkeratosis, and Pityriasis Rosea (PR)-like eruptions have been reported. GVHD associated angiomatosis, with vascular lesions within sclerotic-type cGVHD, is a newly described and challenging subtype of cGVHD.

Biopsy may not be necessary to diagnose GVHD, particularly aGVHD. Punch biopsy is generally adequate, unless evaluating scleroderma-like disease, where incisional biopsy is preferred. Histologically, aGVHD demonstrates vacuolar interface dermatitis. Individual keratinocyte necrosis with adjacent lymphocytes (satellite necrosis) is typically present, suggesting cell-mediated cytotoxicity. The height and extent of keratinocyte necrosis, bulla formation, and slough are used in grading schemes (grade 0 is normal, grade 1 is basal vacuolization, grade 2 includes necrotic epidermal cells, grade 3 has clefting, and grade 4 has bulla formation). Eosinophils may be more common in drug reactions, but can be seen in GVH and cannot be used to distinguish the two. GVHD inflammation histologically often involves follicles, corresponding to the characteristic clinical perifollicular inflammation. Elafin has been proposed as a possible marker for GVHD but cannot reliably distinguish GVHD from drug reactions, though high levels of elafin may correspond to a poorer prognosis. The histologic findings in early disease may be nonspecific, and many treatment protocols do not depend on histologic features to initiate therapy. A background of epidermal disorder and atypia may be present in later lesions of acute GVHD, but similar epidermal changes may be seen after chemotherapy and may be unreliable in distinguishing GVHD from drug reactions. Chronic GVHD demonstrates lichenoid dermatitis or dermal sclerosis with hyalinization of collagen bundles and narrowing of the space between bundles.

Acute GVHD is managed on the skin with topical corticosteroids, TCIs, and rarely UV phototherapy. Most patients have associated systemic symptoms, in which case systemic corticosteroids, tacrolimus, and occasionally other suppressive agents are instituted. When aGVH is not responsive to steroids, multidisciplinary discussions and individual regimens based on comorbidities, infectious history, and status of underlying disease are often necessary. Mesenchymal stem cells, antithymocyte globulin, and extracorporeal photopheresis (ECP) are novel options being evaluated. TNF inhibitors, rituximab, and targeted small molecule inhibitors are also being studied. Ruxolitinib and other JAK inhibitors have shown promise in early studies and are being actively evaluated for both acute and chronic GVHD. For cGVHD, ECP can be considered as a nonsuppressive, disease-stabilizing, steroid-sparing agent for patients unresponsive to these first-line therapies. Phototherapy, particularly UVA-based regimens (PUVA with or without retinoids, UVA1), may improve sclerotic cGVHD. Rituximab has shown some benefit in steroid-refractory cGVHD. Sirolimus and everolimus appear to have activity against fibrosis and may be useful in fibrotic cGVHD. Imatinib may also be useful in cGVHD with fibrosis. Hydroxychloroquine has also been reported. In cGVHD, topical steroids may help lichen planus–like disease but are unlikely to affect scleroderma-like disease. Physical therapy is essential in patients with sclerosis, especially if it involves joints.

Graft-Versus-Host Disease in Solid-Organ Transplantation

Transplantation of a solid organ into a partially immunosuppressed host may result in GVHD, because the organ may contain immune cells. The prevalence of GVHD after solid-organ transplantation is extremely low, about 1% at one center over 15 years with more than 2000 transplants. The risk for developing GVHD after solid-organ transplantation is related to the type of organ transplanted and depends on the amount of lymphoid tissue that the organ contains. The risk profile is small intestine > liver/pancreas > kidney > heart. In liver and small intestine transplants the risk is 1%–2%, but when it occurs the mortality rate is 85%. Close matching increases the risk of GVHD in organ transplantation, because the immunocompetent recipient cells are less likely to recognize the donor lymphocytes as nonself and destroy them. Also, African American race and CMV infection increase the risk. The onset is usually 1–8 weeks following transplantation but can be delayed for years. Fever, rash, and pancytopenia are the cardinal features, with pancytopenia a frequent cause of mortality. The skin is the first site of involvement, and only cutaneous disease occurs in 15% of cases. Both acute and chronic GVHD skin findings can occur. Skin biopsies tend to show more inflammation than in HSCT-associated GVHD. In GVHD accompanying liver transplantation, the liver is unaffected because it is syngeneic with the donor lymphocytes. The diagnosis of GVHD in patients receiving organ transplantation can be aided by documenting macrochimerism in the peripheral blood and skin after the first month of transplantation.

Abu-Dalle I, et al: ECP in steroid-refractory GVHD. Biol BloodMarrow Transplant 2014; 20: 1677.

Bruggen MC, et al: Epidermal elafin expression in cGVHD. J Invest Dermatol 2015; 135: 999.

Cornejo CM, et al: Atypical manifestations of GVHD. J Am Acad Dermatol 2015; 72: 690.

Hillen U, et al: Consensus on performing skin biopsies, lab workup, evaluation of tissue samples in patients with suspected cGVHD. J Eur Acad Dermatol Venereol 2015; 29: 948.

Inamoto Y, et al: Incidence, risk factors, and outcomes of sclerosis in cGVHD. Blood 2013; 121: 5098.

Kaffenberger BH, et al: GVHD-associated angiomatosis. J Am Acad Dermatol 2014; 71: 745.

Kekre N, et al: Emerging drugs for GVHD. Expert Opin Emerg Drugs 2016; 21: 209.

Zeiser R, et al: Ruxolitinib in corticosteroid-refractory GVHD. Leukemia 2015; 29: 2062.

6 Contact Dermatitis and Drug Eruptions

CONTACT DERMATITIS

There are two types of dermatitis caused by substances coming in contact with the skin: irritant dermatitis and allergic contact dermatitis. Irritant dermatitis is an inflammatory reaction in the skin resulting from exposure to a substance that causes an eruption in most people who come in contact with it. Allergic contact dermatitis is an acquired sensitivity to various substances that produce inflammatory reactions only in those persons who have been previously sensitized to the allergen.

Irritant Contact Dermatitis

Many substances act as irritants that produce a nonspecific inflammatory reaction of the skin. This type of dermatitis may be induced in any person if there is contact with a sufficiently high concentration. No previous exposure is necessary, and the effect is evident within minutes, or a few hours at most. The concentration and type of toxic agent, duration of exposure, and condition of the skin at the time of exposure produce the variation in severity of the dermatitis from person to person, or from time to time in the same person. The skin may be more vulnerable because of maceration from excessive humidity or exposure to water, heat, cold, pressure, or friction. Dry skin, as opposed to wet skin, is less likely to react to contactants, although in chronic xerosis, as seen in elderly patients, increased sensitivity to irritants results. Thick skin is less reactive than thin skin. Atopic patients are predisposed to irritant hand dermatitis. Repeated exposure to some of the milder irritants may produce a hardening effect over time. This process makes the skin more resistant to the irritant effects of a given substance. Symptomatically, pain and burning are more common in irritant dermatitis, contrasting with the usual itch of allergic reactions. Avoidance, substitution of nonirritating agents when possible, and protection, most often by wearing gloves or using barrier creams, are the mainstays of treatment.

Alkalis

Irritant dermatitis is often produced by alkalis such as soaps, cement, detergents, bleaches, ammonia preparations, lye, drain pipe cleaners, and toilet bowl and oven cleansers (Fig. 6.1). Alkalis penetrate and destroy deeply because they dissolve keratin. Strong solutions are corrosive, and immediate application of a weak acid such as vinegar, lemon juice, or 0.5% hydrochloric acid solution will lessen their effects.

The principal compounds are sodium, potassium, ammonium, and calcium hydroxides. Occupational exposure is frequent among workers in soap manufacturing. Sodium silicate (water glass) is a caustic used in soap manufacture and paper sizing and for the preservation of eggs. Alkalis in the form of soaps, bleaching agents, detergents, and most household cleansing agents figure prominently in the causes of hand eczema. Alkaline sulfides are used as depilatories. Calcium oxide (quicklime) forms slaked lime when water is added. Severe burns may be caused in plasterers.

Acids

The powerful acids are corrosive, whereas the weaker acids are astringent. Hydrochloric acid produces burns that are less deep and more liable to form blisters than injuries from sulfuric and nitric acids (Fig. 6.2). Hydrochloric acid burns are encountered in those who handle or transport the product and in plumbers and those who work in galvanizing or tin-plate factories. Sulfuric acid produces a brownish charring of the skin, beneath which is an ulceration that heals slowly. Sulfuric acid is used more widely than any other acid in industry; it is handled principally by brass and iron workers and by those who work with copper or bronze. Nitric acid is a powerful oxidizing substance that causes deep burns; the tissue is stained yellow. Such injuries are observed in those who manufacture or handle the acid or use it in the making of explosives in laboratories. At times, nitric acid or formic acid is used in assaults secondary to interpersonal conflicts, resulting in scarring most prominently of the face, with the complication of renal failure present in a small number of cases.

Hydrofluoric acid is used widely in rust remover, in the semiconductor industry, and in germicides, dyes, plastics, and glass etching. It may act insidiously at first, starting with erythema and ending with vesiculation, ulceration, and finally necrosis of the tissue. Hydrofluoric acid is one of the strongest inorganic acids, capable of dissolving glass. Hypocalcemia, hypomagnesemia, hyperkalemia, and cardiac dysrhythmias may complicate hydrofluoric acid burns. Fluorine is best neutralized with hexafluorine solution, followed by 10% calcium gluconate solution or magnesium oxide.

Oxalic acid may produce paresthesia of the fingertips, with cyanosis and gangrene. The nails become discolored yellow. Oxalic acid is best neutralized with limewater or milk of magnesia to produce precipitation. Titanium hydrochloride is used in the manufacture of pigments. Application of water to the exposed part will produce severe burns. Therefore treatment consists only of wiping away the noxious substance.

Phenol (carbolic acid) is a protoplasmic poison that produces a white eschar on the surface of the skin. It can penetrate deep into the tissue. If a large surface of the skin is treated with phenol for cosmetic peeling effects, the absorbed phenol may produce glomerulonephritis and arrhythmias. Locally, temporary anesthesia may also occur. Phenol is readily neutralized with 65% ethyl or isopropyl alcohol.

Chromic acid burns, which may be seen in electroplating and dye production occupations, may result in extensive tissue necrosis and acute renal damage. Excision of affected skin down to the fascia should be accomplished rapidly, and hemodialysis to remove circulating chromium should start in the first 24 hours. Other strong acids that are irritants include acetic, trichloracetic, arsenious, chlorosulfonic, fluoroboric, hydriodic, hydrobromic, iodic, perchloric, phosphoric, salicylic, silicofluoric, sulfonic, sulfurous, tannic, and tungstic acids.

Treatment of acid burns consists of immediate rinsing with copious amounts of water and alkalization with sodium bicarbonate, calcium hydroxide (limewater), or soap solutions. Phosphorus burns should be rinsed off with water, followed by application of copper sulfate to produce a precipitate.

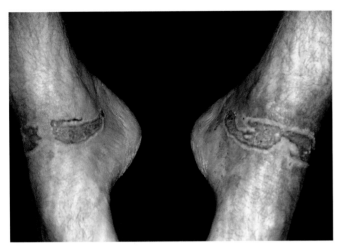

Fig. 6.1 Cement burns. (Courtesy Steven Binnick, MD.)

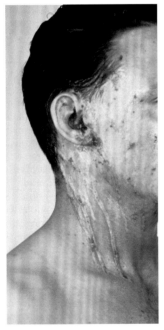

Fig. 6.2 Drip burn from acid solution.

Airbag Dermatitis

Airbags are deployed as a safety feature on cars when rapid deceleration occurs. Activation of a sodium azide and cupric oxide propellant cartridge releases nitrogen gas, which expands the bag at speeds exceeding 160 km/hour (96 miles/hour). Talcum powder, sodium hydroxide, and sodium carbonate are released into the bag. Abrasions, thermal, friction, and chemical burns and an irritant contact dermatitis may result. Superficial erythema may respond well to topical steroids, but full-thickness burns may occur and require debridement and grafting.

Other Irritants

Metal salts that act as irritants include the cyanides of calcium, copper, mercury, nickel, silver, and zinc and the chlorides of calcium and zinc. Bromine, chlorine, fluorine, and iodine are also irritants. Occupational exposure to methyl bromide may produce erythema and vesicles in the axillary and inguinal areas. Insecticides, including

2,2-dichlorovinyl dimethyl phosphate used in roach powder and fly repellents and killers, can act as irritants.

Fiberglass Dermatitis

Fiberglass dermatitis is seen after occupational or inadvertent exposure. The small spicules of glass penetrate the skin and cause severe irritation with tiny erythematous papules, scratch marks, and intense pruritus. Usually, there is no delayed hypersensitivity reaction. Wearing clothes that have been washed together with fiberglass curtains, handling air conditioner filters, or working in the manufacture of fiberglass material may produce severe folliculitis, pruritus, and eruptions that may simulate scabies or insect bites. Fiberglass is also used in thermal and acoustic installation, the wind industry, padding, vibration isolation, curtains, draperies, insulation for automobile bodies, furniture, gasoline tanks, and spacecraft. Talcum powder dusted on the flexure surfaces of the arms before exposure makes the fibers slide off the skin. A thorough washing of the skin after handling fiberglass is helpful. Patch testing to epoxy resins should be done when evaluating workers in fiberglass and reinforced-plastics operations, because an allergic contact dermatitis may be difficult to discern from fiberglass dermatitis.

Dusts

Some dusts and gases may irritate the skin in the presence of heat and moisture, such as perspiration. The dusts of lime, zinc, and arsenic may produce folliculitis. Dusts from various woods, such as teak, may incite itching and dermatitis. Dusts from cinchona bark, quinine, and pyrethrum produce widespread dermatitis. Tobacco dust in cigar factories, powdered orris root, lycopodium, and dusts of various nutshells may cause swelling of the eyelids and dermatitis of the face, neck, and upper extremities, the distribution of an airborne contact dermatitis. Dusts formed during the manufacture of high explosives may cause erythematous, vesicular, and eczematous dermatitis that may lead to generalized exfoliative dermatitis.

Capsaicin

Hand irritation produced by capsaicin in hot peppers used in Korean and North Chinese cuisine (Hunan hand) may be severe and prolonged, sometimes necessitating stellate ganglion blockade and gabapentin. Pepper spray, used by police in high concentrations and by civilians in less concentrated formulas, contains capsaicin and may produce severe burns. Cold water is not much help; capsaicin is insoluble in water. Acetic acid 5% (white vinegar) or antacids (Maalox) may completely relieve the burning, even if applied an hour or more after the contact. Application should be continued until the area can be dried without return of the discomfort.

Tear Gas Dermatitis

Lacrimators such as chloroacetophenone in concentrated form may cause dermatitis, with a delayed appearance about 24–72 hours after exposure. Irritation or sensitization, with erythema and severe vesiculation, may result. Treatment consists of lavage of the affected skin with sodium bicarbonate solution and instillation of boric acid solution into the eyes. Contaminated clothing should be removed.

Sulfur mustard gas, also known as yperite (dichlorodiethyl sulfide), has been used in chemical warfare. Erythema, vesicles, and bullae result from mild to moderate exposure (Fig. 6.3). Toxic epidermal necrolysis (TEN)–like appearance may follow more concentrated contact. The earliest and most frequently affected sites are areas covered by clothing and humidified by sweat, such as the groin, axillae, and genitalia.

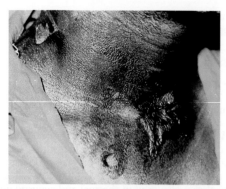

Fig. 6.3 Mustard gas burn. (Courtesy James WD: Textbook of Military Medicine. Office of the Surgeon General, United States Army, 1994.)

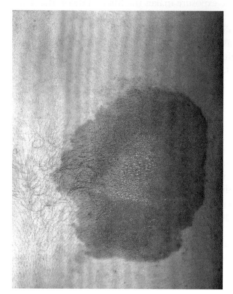

Fig. 6.4 Mace-induced reaction.

Mace is a mixture of tear gas (chloroacetophenone) in trichloroethane and various hydrocarbons resembling kerosene. It is available in a variety of self-defense sprays. Mace is a potent irritant and may cause allergic sensitization (Fig. 6.4). Treatment consists of changing clothes, then washing with oil or milk, followed by washing with copious amounts of water.

Chloracne

Workers in the manufacture of chlorinated compounds may develop chloracne, with small, straw-colored follicular plugs and papules, chiefly on the malar crescent, retroauricular areas, earlobes, neck, shoulders, and scrotum. Histologically, there is a loss of sebaceous glands and the formation of cystic structures. The synthetic waxes chloronaphthalene and chlorodiphenyl, used in the manufacture of electric insulators and in paints, varnishes, and lacquers, predispose workers engaged in the manufacture of these synthetic waxes to chloracne. Exposure to 2,6-dichlorobenzonitrile during the manufacture of a herbicide, and to 3,4,3′,4′-tetrachloroazoxybenzene, which is an unwanted intermediate byproduct in the manufacture of a pesticide, may also produce chloracne.

A contaminant in the synthesis of herbicides and hexachlorophene, 2,3,7,8-tetracholorodibenzo-*p*-dioxin, produces a chemical burn in the acute stage, but chloracne, hyperpigmentation, hirsutism, and skin fragility (with or without criteria for porphyria cutanea

tarda) are manifestations of chronic toxicity. Gastrointestinal tract cancer and malignancies of the lymphatic and hematopoietic systems are suspected to result. Although direct contact is the usual method of exposure, inhalation, ingestion, or contact with contaminated clothing may also result in chloracne. Chloracne may persist for long periods because dioxin is stored in the liver and released slowly into the circulation. Treatment is with medications used in acne vulgaris, including isotretinoin.

Hydrocarbons

Many hydrocarbons produce skin eruptions. Crude petroleum causes generalized itching, folliculitis, or acneiform eruptions. The irritant properties of petroleum derivatives are directly proportional to their fat-solvent properties and inversely proportional to their viscosity. Oils of the naphthalene series are more irritating than those of the paraffin series. Refined fractions from petroleum are less irritating than the unrefined products, although benzene, naphtha, and carbon disulfide may cause a mild dermatitis.

Lubricating and cutting oils are causes of similar cutaneous lesions. They represent a frequent cause of occupational dermatoses in machine tool operators, machinists, layout men, instrument makers, and setup men. Insoluble (neat) cutting oils are responsible for a follicular acneiform eruption on the dorsa of the hands, the forearms, face, thighs, and back of the neck. Hyperpigmentation, keratoses, and scrotal cancer have been found in those exposed to insoluble cutting oils. Soluble oils and synthetic fluids used in metalworking do not result in acne, but rather an eczematous dermatitis, usually of the dorsal forearms and hands. Approximately 50% of the time it is irritant and in the remainder it is allergic. Allergic contact dermatitis arises from various additives, such as biocides, coloring agents, and deodorizers.

Coal briquette makers develop dermatitis as a result of a tarry residue from petroleum used in their trade. Paraffin exposure leads to pustules, keratoses, and ulcerations. Shale oil workers develop an erythematous, follicular eruption that eventually leads to keratoses, which may become the sites of carcinoma. It is estimated that 50% of shale oil workers have skin problems.

Impure and low-grade paraffins and mineral oils cause similar skin eruptions. Initially, the skin changes are similar to those in chloracne. Over time, a diffuse erythema with dappled pigmentation develops. Gradually, keratoses appear, and after many years, some of these are the sites of carcinoma. Melanoderma may occur from exposure to mineral oils and lower-grade petroleum from creosote, asphalt, and other tar products. Photosensitization may play a role. Creosote is a contact irritant, sensitizer, and photosensitizer. Allergy is demonstrated by patch testing with 10% creosote in oil.

Petrolatum dermatitis may appear as a verrucous thickening of the skin caused by prolonged contact with impure petroleum jelly or, occasionally, lubricating oil. A follicular-centered process may occur in which erythematous horny nodules are present, usually on the anterior and inner aspects of the thighs. There are no comedones, and the lesions are separated by apparently normal skin.

Acne corne consists of follicular keratosis and pigmentation resulting from crude petroleum, tar oils, and paraffin. The dorsal aspects of the fingers and hands, the arms, legs, face, and thorax are the areas usually involved. The lesions are follicular horny papules, often black, and are associated at first with a follicular erythema and later with a dirty brownish or purplish spotty pigmentation, which in severe cases becomes widespread and is especially marked around the genitals. This syndrome may simulate pityriasis rubra pilaris or lichen spinulosus.

Coal tar and pitch and many of their derivatives produce photosensitization and an acneiform folliculitis of the forearms, legs, face, and scrotum. Follicular keratoses (pitch warts) may develop and later turn into carcinoma. Soot, lamp black, and the ash from peat fires produce dermatitis of a dry, scaly character, which over time forms warty outgrowths and cancer. Chimney sweep's cancer occurs under a soot wart and is usually located on the scrotum, where soot, sebum, and dirt collect in the folds of the skin. This form of cancer has virtually disappeared.

Acquired perforating disease may occur in oil field workers who use drilling fluid containing calcium chloride. Patients develop tender, umbilicated papules of the forearms that microscopically show transepidermal elimination of calcium.

Solvents

The solvents cause approximately 10% of occupational dermatitis. When solvents are applied to the hands to cleanse them, the surface oil is dissolved, and a chronic fissured dermatitis results. Additionally, peripheral neuropathy and chemical lymphangitis may occur after the solvents are absorbed through the fissured skin. Solvent sniffers may develop an eczematous eruption around the mouth and nose; erythema and edema occur. This is a direct irritant dermatitis caused by the inhalation of the solvent placed on a handkerchief.

Trichloroethylene is a chlorinated hydrocarbon solvent and degreasing agent also used in the dry-cleaning and refrigeration industry. Inhalation may produce exfoliative erythroderma, mucous membrane erosions, eosinophilia, and hepatitis.

Allergic contact dermatitis caused by alcohol is rarely encountered with lower-aliphatic alcohols. A severe case of bullous and hemorrhagic dermatitis on the fingertips and deltoid region was caused by isopropyl alcohol. Although rare, ethyl alcohol dermatitis may also be encountered. Cetyl and stearyl alcohols may provoke contact urticaria.

Ale IS, et al: Irritant contact dermatitis. Rev Environ Health 2014; 29: 195.

Angelova-Fischer I: Irritants and skin barrier function. Curr Probl Dermatol 2016; 49: 80.

Bordel-Gomez MT, et al: Fiberglass dermatitis. Contact Dermatitis 2008; 59: 120.

Das KK, et al: Management of acid burns. Burns 2015; 41: 484.

Fartasch M: Wet work and barrier function. Curr Probl Dermatol 2016; 49: 144.

Flammiger A, et al: Sulfuric acid burns. Cutan Ocul Toxicol 2006; 25: 55.

Goon AT, et al: A case of trichloroethylene hypersensitivity syndrome. Arch Dermatol 2001; 137: 274.

Greenwood JE, et al: Alkalis and skin. J Burn Care Res 2016; 37: 135.

Herzemans-Boer M, et al: Skin lesions due to methyl bromide. Arch Dermatol 1988; 124: 917.

Jia X, et al: Adverse effects of gasoline on the skin of gasoline workers. Contact Dermatitis 2002; 46: 44.

Mostosi C, Simonart T: Effectiveness of barrier creams against irritant contact dermatitis. Dermatology 2016; 232: 353.

Patterson AT, et al: Skin diseases associated with Agent Orange and other organochlorine exposures. J Am Acad Dermatol 2016; 74: 143.

Saxena AK, et al: Multimodal approach for the management of Hunan hand syndrome. Pain Prac 2013; 13: 227.

Schep LJ, et al: Riot control agents. J R Army Med Corps 2015; 161: 94.

Steinritz D, et al: Medical documentation, bioanalytical evidence of an accidental human exposure to sulfur mustard and general therapy recommendations. Toxicol Lett 2016; 244: 112.

Tan CH, et al: Contact dermatitis. Clin Dermatol 2014; 32: 116.

Wang X, et al: A review of treatment strategies for hydrofluoric acid burns. Burns 2014; 40: 1447.

Wu JJ, et al: A case of air bag dermatitis. Arch Dermatol 2002; 138: 1383.

Yin S: Chemical and common burns in children. Clin Pediatr (Phila) 2017; 56: 8S.

Allergic Contact Dermatitis

Allergic contact dermatitis results when an allergen comes into contact with previously sensitized skin. It is caused by a specific acquired hypersensitivity of the delayed type, also known as cell-mediated (type IV) hypersensitivity. These sensitizers do not cause demonstrable skin changes on initial contact. Persons may be exposed to allergens for years before finally developing hypersensitivity. Genetic variability in the immunologic processes leading to sensitization and other factors, such as concentration of the allergen applied, its vehicle, timing and site of the exposure, presence of occlusion, age, gender, and race of the patient, and presence of other skin or systemic disorders, likely determine whether any given exposure will result in sensitization. Once sensitized, however, subsequent outbreaks may result from extremely slight exposure.

Childhood exposures do result in allergy, and the frequency of allergy in this age group is increasing. The most common relevant allergens in young children are nickel, cobalt, fragrance, lanolin, and neomycin. In adolescents potassium dichromate and Myroxylon pereirae become significant. Sensitivity is rarely lost over the years; older patients have similar rates of allergy as adults.

Occasionally, dermatitis may be induced when the allergen is taken internally by a patient first sensitized by topical application, as with substances such as cinnamon oil or various medications. The anamnestic response is termed systemic contact dermatitis. It may appear first at the site of the prior sensitization or past positive patch test, but may spread to a generalized morbilliform or eczematous eruption. Additional morphologic patterns include vesicular hand eczema, urticaria, erythema multiforme, vasculitis, or symmetric drug-related intertriginous and flexural exanthema (SDRIFE). Formerly called baboon syndrome, SDRIFE is a deep-red-violet eruption on the buttocks, genital area, inner thighs, and sometimes the axillae.

The most common causes of contact dermatitis in the United States are toxicodendrons (poison ivy, oak, or sumac), nickel, balsam of Peru (*Myroxylon pereirae*), neomycin, fragrance, formaldehyde and the formaldehyde-releasing preservatives, bacitracin, and rubber compounds. Frequent positive reactions to gold and thimerosal do not often correlate with the clinical exposure history. Gold reactions, which may be prolonged, can be correlated in some cases with oral gold exposure or occupational dermatitis, but in most cases, the relevance is questionable. Thimerosal reactions are probably related to its use as a preservative in common vaccines and skin-testing material. It also serves as a marker for piroxicam photosensitivity.

Eczematous delayed-type hypersensitivity reaction, as exemplified by allergic contact dermatitis and the patch test, must be distinguished from immediate-type hypersensitivity reaction. The latter presents within minutes of exposure with urticaria and is proved with a scratch test. It should be kept in mind, however, that persons who develop contact urticaria to a substance may concomitantly have a type IV delayed-type sensitization and eczema from the same allergen.

In some patients, impetigo, pustular folliculitis, and irritation or allergic reactions from applied medications are superimposed on the original dermatitis. A particularly vexing situation is when allergy to topical corticosteroids complicates an eczema, in which case the preexisting dermatitis usually does not flare, but simply does not heal as expected. The cutaneous reaction may also provoke a hypersusceptibility to various other, previously innocuous substances, which continues the eczematous inflammatory response indefinitely.

These eruptions resolve when the cause is identified and avoided. For acute generalized allergic contact dermatitis, treatment with systemic steroidal agents is effective, beginning with 40–60 mg/day of prednisone in a single oral dose, and tapering slowly to topical steroids. When the eruption is limited in extent and severity, local application of topical corticosteroid creams, lotions, or aerosol sprays is preferred.

Testing for Sensitivity

Patch Test. The patch test is used to detect hypersensitivity to a substance that is in contact with the skin so that the allergen may be determined and corrective measures taken. So many allergens can cause allergic contact dermatitis that it is impossible to test a person for all of them. In addition, a good history and observation of the pattern of the dermatitis, its localization on the body, and its state of activity are helpful in determining the cause. The patch test is confirmatory and diagnostic, but only within the framework of the history and physical findings; it is rarely helpful if it must stand alone. Interpretation of the relevance of positive tests and the subsequent education of patients are challenging in some cases. The Contact Allergen Management Program (CAMP) provides names of alternative products that may be used by patients when an allergen is identified. This is available through the American Contact Dermatitis Society.

The patch test consists of application of substances suspected to be the cause of the dermatitis to intact uninflamed skin. Patch testing may be administered by the thin-layer rapid-use epicutaneous (TRUE) test or by individually prepared patches. The TRUE test has resulted in more screening for allergic contact dermatitis than in the past, but if it does not reveal the allergen for a highly suspect dermatitis, testing with an expanded series will on average yield relevant allergens in more than half of these patients. Dermatitis originating in the workplace will almost always require individualized testing.

Test substances are applied usually to the upper back, although if only one or two are applied, the upper outer arm may be used. Each patch should be numbered to avoid confusion. The patches are removed after 48 hours (or sooner if severe itching or burning occurs at the site) and read. The patch sites need to be evaluated again at day 4 or 5 because positive reactions may not appear earlier. Some allergens may take up to day 7 to show a reaction, and the patient should be advised to return if such a delayed reaction occurs. Erythematous papules and vesicles with edema are indicative of allergy (Fig. 6.5). Occasionally, patch tests for potassium iodide, nickel, or mercury will produce pustules at the site of the test application. Usually no erythema is produced; therefore the reaction has no clinical significance.

Strong patch test reactions may induce a state of hyperirritability ("excited skin syndrome") in which adjacent tests that would otherwise be negative appear as weakly positive. Weakly positive tests in the presence of strong tests do not prove sensitivity. The skin and mucous membranes vary widely in the ability to react to antigens. The oral mucosa is more resistant to primary irritants and is less liable to be involved in allergic reactions. This may be because the keratin layer of the skin more readily combines with haptens to form allergens. Also, the oral mucosa is bathed in saliva, which cleanses and buffers the area and dilutes irritants. However, patch testing for various types of oral signs and symptoms, such as swelling, tingling and burning, perioral dermatitis, and the appearance of oral lichen planus, is useful in determining a cause in many cases.

Potent topical corticosteroids, ultraviolet (UV) light, prednisone, and the acquired immunodeficiency syndrome (AIDS) have been reported to interfere with the reliability of patch testing. Expert opinion regarding patch testing while on other immunosuppressants (e.g., methotrexate, azathioprine, biologics) is that these are less likely to produce unreliable testing. However, with all of these, false-negative reactions may result; the value of testing in such circumstances is that if a positive reaction occurs, a diagnosis may be made. Vitiliginous skin is less reactive than normally pigmented adjacent skin.

Provocative Use Test. The provocative use test may be used to screen products used by the patient. Products that are made to stay on the skin once applied (as opposed to shampoos or soaps) are rubbed on normal skin of the inner aspect of the forearm several times daily for 5 days. A pink itchy patch will indicate the need to avoid the product. Further testing to its individual ingredients will help identify replacement products. This test may also confirm a positive closed patch test reaction to ingredients of the personal care product.

Photopatch Test. The photopatch test is used to evaluate for contact photoallergy to such substances as sulfonamides, phenothiazines, p-aminobenzoic acid, oxybenzone, 6-methyl coumarin, musk ambrette, and tetrachlorosalicylanilide. A standard patch test is applied for 48 hours; this is then exposed to 5 to 15 J/m² of UVA and read after another 48 hours. To test for 6-methyl coumarin sensitivity, the patch is applied in the same manner but for only 30 minutes before light exposure, rather than for 48 hours. A duplicate set of nonirradiated patches is used in testing for the presence of routine delayed hypersensitivity reactions. Also, a site of normal skin is given an identical dose of UVA to test for increased sensitivity to light without prior exposure to chemicals. There is a steady increase in incidence of photoallergy to sunscreening agents and a decreasing incidence of such reactions to fragrance.

Regional Predilection

Familiarity with certain contactants and the typical dermatitis they elicit on specific parts of the body will assist in diagnosis of the etiologic agent.

Head and Neck. The scalp is relatively resistant to the development of contact allergies; however, involvement may be caused by hair dye, hair spray, shampoo, or permanent wave solutions. The surrounding glabrous skin, including the ear rims and backs of the ears, may be much more inflamed and suggestive of the cause. Persistent otitis of the ear canal may be caused by sensitivity to neomycin, an ingredient of most aural medications. The eyelids are the most frequent site for nail polish dermatitis. Volatile gases, false-eyelash adhesive, fragrances, eye medications, preservatives,

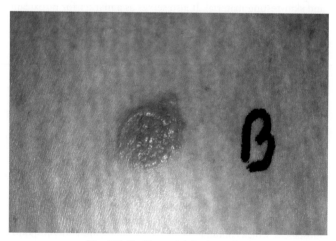
Fig. 6.5 Positive patch test reaction.

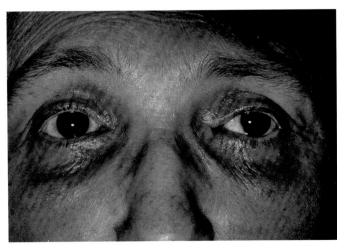

Fig. 6.6 Eyelid dermatitis.

fragrances in cleansing materials. Almost half of women with pruritus vulvae have one or more relevant allergens; often these are medicaments, fragrances, or preservatives.

Lower Extremities. The shins may be the site of rubber dermatitis from elastic stockings. Feet are sites for shoe dermatitis, most often attributable to rubber sensitivity, chrome-tanned leather, dyes, or adhesives. Application of topical antibiotics to stasis ulcers frequently leads to sensitivity and allergic contact dermatitis.

Bangash HK, Petronic-Rosic V: Acral manifestations of contact dermatitis. Clin Dermatol 2017; 35: 9.

Bourke I, et al: Guidelines for the management of contact dermatitis. Br J Dermatol 2009; 160: 946.

Bryden AM, et al: Photopatch testing of 1155 patients. Br J Dermatol 2006; 155: 737.

Diepgen TL, et al: Guidelines for diagnosis, prevention and treatment of hand eczema—short version. J Dtsch Dermatol Ges 2015; 13: 77.

Feser A, et al: Periorbital dermatitis. Br J Dermatol 2008; 159: 858.

Jean SE, et al: Contact dermatitis in leg ulcer patients. J Cutan Med Surg 2009; 13: S38.

Kockentiet B, et al: Contact dermatitis in athletes. J Am Acad Dermatol 2007; 56: 1048.

Mahler V: Hand dermatitis—differential diagnoses, diagnostics, and treatment options. J Dtsch Dermatol Ges 2016; 14: 7.

Martin SF: Immunological mechanisms in allergic contact dermatitis. Curr Opin Allergy Clin Immunol 2015; 15: 124.

Mowad CM: Contact dermatitis. Dermatol Clin 2016; 34: 263.

Mowad CM, et al: Allergic contact dermatitis. J Am Acad Dermatol 2016; 74: 1029 and 1043.

Pelletier JL, et al: Contact dermatitis in pediatric. Pediatr Ann 2016; 45: e287.

Rashid RS, Shim TN: Contact dermatitis. BMJ 2016; 353: i3299.

Rodrigues DF, Goulart EM: Patch-test results in children and adolescents. An Bras Dermatol 2016; 91: 64.

Schalock PC, et al: American Contact Dermatitis Society Core Allergen Series. Dermatitis 2017; 28: 141.

Scheman A, et al: Contact allergy cross-reactions. Dermatitis 2017; 28: 128.

Schlosser BJ: Contact dermatitis of the vulva. Dermatol Clin 2010; 28: 697.

Thyssen JP, et al: The epidemiology of contact allergy in the general population. Contact Dermatitis 2007; 57: 287.

Torgerson RR, et al: Contact allergy in oral disease. J Am Acad Dermatol 2007; 57: 315.

Veien NK: Systemic contact dermatitis. Int J Dermatol 2011; 50: 1445.

Warshaw EM, et al: Positive patch test reactions in older individuals. J Am Acad Dermatol 2012; 66: 229.

Wentworth AB, Davis MD: Patch testing with the standard series when receiving immunosuppressive medications. Dermatitis 2014; 25: 195.

Winnicki M, et al: A systematic approach to systemic contact dermatitis and symmetric drug-related intertriginous and flexural exanthema (SDRIFE). Am J Clin Dermatol 2011; 12: 171.

Dermatitis Resulting From Plants

A large number of plants, including trees, grasses, flowers, vegetables, fruits, and weeds, are potential causes of dermatitis. Eruptions from them vary considerably in appearance but are usually vesicular and accompanied by marked edema. After previous exposure and sensitization to the active substance in the plant, the typical dermatitis results from reexposure. The onset is usually a few hours or days after contact. The characteristic linearly grouped

mascara, rubber in sponges used to apply cosmetics, and eye shadow are also frequently implicated (Fig. 6.6). Perioral dermatitis and cheilitis may be caused by flavoring agents in dentifrices and gum, as well as fragrances, shellac, medicaments, and sunscreens in lipstick and lip balms. Perfume dermatitis may cause redness just under the ears or on the neck. Earlobe dermatitis is indicative of nickel sensitivity. Photocontact dermatitis may involve the entire face and may be sharply cut off at the collar line or extend down on to the sternum in a V shape. There is a typical clear area under the chin where there is little or no exposure to sunlight. The left cheek and left side of the neck (from sun exposure while driving) may be the first areas involved.

Trunk. The trunk is an infrequent site; however, the dye or finish of clothing may cause dermatitis. The axilla may be the site of deodorant dermatitis and clothing-dye dermatitis; involvement of the axillary vault suggests the former; of the axillary folds, the latter. In women, brassieres cause dermatitis from the material itself, the elastic, or the metal snaps or underwires.

Arms. The wrists may be involved because of jewelry or the backs of watches and clasps, all of which may contain nickel. Wristbands made of leather are a source of chrome dermatitis.

Hands. Innumerable substances may cause allergic contact dermatitis of the hands, which typically occurs on the backs of the hands and spares the palms. Florists will often develop fingertip or palmar lesions. A hand dermatitis that changes from web spaces to fingertips or from palms to dorsal hands should trigger patch testing. Poison ivy and other plant dermatitides frequently occur on the hands and arms. Rubber glove sensitivity must be kept constantly in mind. Usually, irritancy is superimposed on allergic contact dermatitis of the hands, altering both the morphologic and histologic clues to the diagnosis.

Abdomen. The abdomen, especially the waistline, may be the site of rubber dermatitis from the elastic in pants and undergarments. The metallic rivets in blue jeans may lead to periumbilical dermatitis in nickel-sensitive patients, as may piercings of the umbilicus.

Groin. The groin is usually spared, but the buttocks and upper thighs may be sites of dermatitis caused by dyes. The penis is frequently involved in poison ivy dermatitis. Condom dermatitis may also occur. The perianal region may be involved from the "caine" medications in suppositories, as well as preservatives and

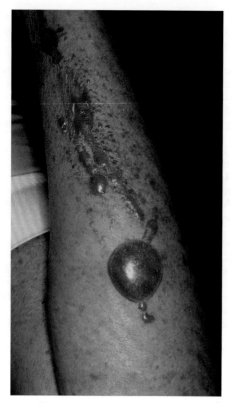

Fig. 6.7 Acute poison ivy reaction.

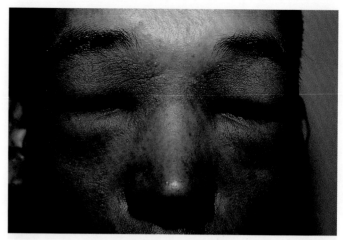

Fig. 6.8 Acute poison ivy reaction.

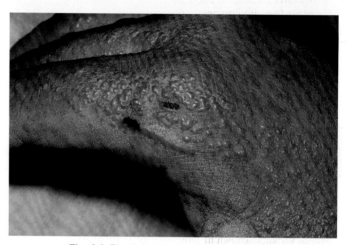

Fig. 6.9 Black dot sign in poison ivy reaction.

lesions are probably produced by brushing the skin with a leaf edge or a broken twig or by carriage of the allergen under the nails. Contrary to popular belief, the contents of vesicles are not capable of producing new lesions.

***Toxicodendron* (Poison Ivy).** *Toxicodendron* dermatitis includes dermatitis from members of the Anacardiaceae family of plants: poison ivy (*T. radicans*, or *Rhus radicans*), poison oak *(T. diversilobum, R. diversaloba)*, poison sumac *(T. vernix, R. vernix)*, Japanese lacquer tree, cashew nut tree (allergen in nutshell), mango (allergen in rind, leaves, or sap), Rengas tree, and Indian marking nut tree. The ginkgo (allergen in fruit pulp), spider flower or silver oak, *Gluta* species of trees and shrubs in Southeast Asia, Brazilian pepper tree, also known as Florida holly, and poisonwood tree contain almost identical antigens.

Toxicodendron dermatitis appears within 48 hours of exposure of a person previously sensitized to the plant. It usually begins on the backs of the fingers, interdigital spaces, wrists, and eyelids, although it may begin on the ankles or other parts that have been exposed. Marked pruritus is the first symptom; inflammation, vesicles, and bullae may then appear. The vesicles are usually grouped and often linear (Fig. 6.7). Large bullae may be present, especially on the forearms and hands. The eyelids are puffy and worse in the morning, improving as the day progresses (Fig. 6.8). Pruritus ani and involvement of the genital areas occur frequently. A black lacquer deposit may occur in which the sap of the plant has been oxidized after being bound to the stratum corneum (Fig. 6.9). Untreated *Toxicodendron* dermatitis usually lasts 2–3 weeks.

The fingers transfer the allergen to other parts, especially the forearms and the male prepuce, which become greatly swollen. However, once the causative oil has been washed off, there is no spreading of the allergen. Some persons are so susceptible that direct contact is not necessary, the allergen apparently being carried by objects with prior exposure to the catechol. Occasionally, eating the allergen, as occurred in a patient who ingested raw cashew

nuts in an imported pesto sauce, may result in SDRIFE (see earlier) or a systematized allergic contact dermatitis with the morphology of a generalized erythematous papular eruption.

The cause is an oleoresin known as urushiol, of which the active agent is a mixture of catechols. This and related resorcinol allergens are present in many plants and also in *Philodendron* species, wood from *Persoonia elliptica*, wheat bran, and marine brown algae.

The most striking diagnostic feature is the linearity of the lesions. It is rare to see vesicles arranged linearly except in plant-induced dermatitis. A history of exposure in the country or park to plants that have shiny leaves in groups of three, followed by the appearance of vesicular lesions within 2 days, usually establishes the diagnosis.

Eradication of plants having grouped "leaves of three" growing in frequented places is one easy preventive measure, as is recognition of the plants to avoid. An excellent resource is a pamphlet available from the American Academy of Dermatology. If the individual is exposed, washing with soap and water within 5 minutes may prevent an eruption. Protective barrier creams are available that are somewhat beneficial. Quaternium-18 bentonite has been shown to prevent or diminish experimentally produced poison ivy dermatitis.

Innumerable attempts have been made to immunize against poison ivy dermatitis by oral administration of the allergen or subcutaneous injections of oily extracts. To date, no accepted method of immunization is available. Repeated attacks do not confer immunity, although a single severe attack may achieve this by what has been called massive-dose desensitization.

When the diagnosis is clear and the eruption severe or extensive, systemic steroidal agents are effective, beginning with 40–60 mg of prednisone in a single oral dose daily, tapered off over a 3-week period. When the eruption is limited in extent and severity, local application of topical corticosteroid creams, lotions, or aerosol sprays is preferred. Time-honored calamine lotion without phenol is helpful and does no harm. Antihistaminic ointments should be avoided because of their sensitization potential. This also applies to the local application of the "caine" topical anesthetics.

Other *Toxicodendron*-Related Dermatitides. Lacquer dermatitis is caused by a furniture lacquer made from the Japanese lacquer tree, used on furniture, jewelry, or bric-a-brac. Antique lacquer is harmless, but lacquer less than 1 or 2 years old is highly antigenic. Cashew oil is extracted from the nutshells of the cashew tree (*Anacardium occidentale).* This vesicant oil contains cardol, a phenol similar to urushiol in poison ivy. The liquid has many commercial applications, such as the manufacture of brake linings, varnish, synthetic glue, paint, and sealer for concrete.

Mango dermatitis is uncommon in natives of mango-growing countries (e.g., Philippines, Guam, Hawaii, Cuba) who have never been exposed to contact with *Toxicodendron* species. Many persons who have been so exposed, however, whether or not they had dermatitis from it, are sensitized by one or a few episodes of contact with the peel of the mango fruit. The palms carry the allergen, so the eyelids and the male prepuce are often early sites of involvement.

Ginkgo tree dermatitis simulates *Toxicodendron* dermatitis with its severe vesiculation, erythematous papules, and edema. The causative substances are ginkgolic acids from the fruit pulp of the ginkgo tree. Ingestion of the ginkgo fruit may result in perianal dermatitis. Ginkgo biloba given orally for cerebral disturbances is made from a leaf extract so it does not elicit a systemic contact allergy when ingested.

Flowers and Houseplants. Among the more common houseplants, the velvety-leafed philodendron, *Philodendron crystallinum* (and its several variants), known in India as the "money plant," is a frequent cause of contact dermatitis. The eruption is often seen on the face, especially the eyelids, carried there by hands that have watered or cared for the plant. English ivy follows philodendron in frequency of cases of occult contact dermatitis. Primrose dermatitis affects the fingers, eyelids, and neck with a punctate or diffuse erythema and edema. Formerly found most frequently in Europe, the primrose is now a common U.S. houseplant. Primin, a quinone, is the causative oleoresin abounding in the glandular hairs of the plant *Primula obconica.*

The popular cut flower, the Peruvian lily, is the most common cause of allergic contact dermatitis in florists. When handling flowers of the genus *Alstroemeria,* the florist uses the thumb and second and third digits of the dominant hand. Because it is chronic, fissured hyperkeratotic dermatitis results, identical to the "tulip fingers" seen among sensitized tulip workers (see Fig. 6.10). Testing is done with the allergen tuliposide A. It does not penetrate nitrile gloves. The geranium, scorpion flower (*Phacelia crenulata* or *P. campanularia*), hydrangea, creosote bush (*Larvia tridentata), Heracula,* daffodil, foxglove, pooja, lisianthus, lilac, lady slipper, magnolia, and tulip and narcissus bulbs are other flowers that commonly cause allergic reactions among florists. The poinsettia and oleander almost never cause dermatitis, despite their reputation for it, although they are toxic if ingested.

Chrysanthemums frequently cause dermatitis, with the hands and eyelids of florists most often affected. The α-methylene portion of the sesquiterpene lactone molecule is the antigenic site, as it is in the other genera of the Compositae family.

A severe inflammatory reaction with bulla formation may be caused by the prairie crocus (*Anemone patens* L.), the floral emblem of the province of Manitoba. Several species of ornamental "bottle

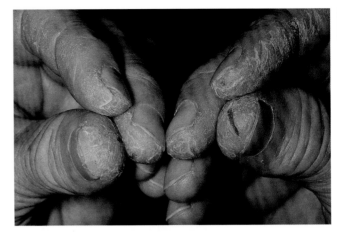

Fig. 6.10 Chronic fissured fingertip dermatitis in a florist.

brush" from Queensland (*Grevillea banksii, G. Robyn Gordon, G. robusta),* may cause allergic contact dermatitis. It is exported to the United States and other Western countries. The allergen is a long-chain alkyl resorcinol. Cross-sensitivity to *Toxicodendron* has been demonstrated. Treatment of all these plant dermatitides is the same as that recommended for toxicodendron dermatitis.

Contact dermatitis may be caused by handling many other flowers, such as the geranium, scorpion flower (*Phacelia crenulata* or *P. campanularia*), hydrangea, creosote bush (*Larvia tridentata), Heracula,* daffodil, foxglove, lilac, lady slipper, magnolia, and tulip and narcissus bulbs. The poinsettia and oleander almost never cause dermatitis, despite their reputation for it, although they are toxic if ingested.

Parthenium hysterophorus is a photosensitizing weed. The well-deserved reputation for harmfulness of dieffenbachia, a common, glossy-leafed house plant, rests on the high content of calcium oxalate crystals in its sap, which burn the mouth and throat severely if any part of the plant is chewed or swallowed. Severe edema of the oral tissues may result in complete loss of voice, thus its common nickname, "dumb cane." It does not appear to sensitize. The castor bean, the seed of *Ricinus communis,* contains ricin, a poisonous substance (phytotoxin). Its sap contains an antigen that may cause anaphylactic hypersensitivity and also dermatitis.

Fruit and Vegetables. Many vegetables may cause contact dermatitis, including asparagus, carrot, celery, cow-parsnip, cucumber, garlic, Indian bean, mushroom, onion, parsley, tomato, and turnip. Onion and celery, among other vegetables, have been incriminated in the production of contact urticaria and even anaphylaxis. Several plants, including celery, fig, lime, and parsley, can cause a phototoxic dermatitis because of the presence of psoralens. Phototoxic contact dermatitis from plants is discussed more fully in Chapter 3.

Trees. Trees with timber and sawdust that may produce contact dermatitis include ash, birch, cedar, cocobolo, elm, Kentucky coffee tree, koa, mahogany, mango, maple, mesquite, milo, myrtle, pine, and teak. The latex of fig and rubber trees may also cause dermatitis, usually of the phototoxic type. Melaleuca oil (tea tree oil), which may be applied to the skin to treat a variety of maladies, can cause allergic contact dermatitis, primarily through the allergen D-limonene (Fig. 6.11). The exotic woods, especially cocobolo and rosewood are prominent among allergens that may produce erythema multiforme (EM) after cutaneous exposure. *Toxicodendron,* tea tree oil, various medicaments, and a variety of other allergens may induce this reaction.

Tree-Associated Plants. Foresters and lumber workers can be exposed to allergenic plants other than trees. Lichens are a group

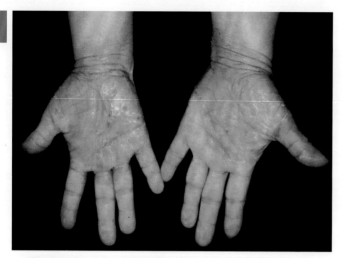

Fig. 6.11 Tea tree oil dermatitis. (Courtesy Glen Crawford, MD.)

of plants composed of symbiotic algae and fungi. Foresters and wood choppers exposed to these lichens growing on trees may develop severe allergic contact dermatitis. Exposure to the lichens may also occur from firewood, funeral wreaths, and also fragrances added to aftershave lotions (oak moss and tree moss). Sensitization is produced by D-usnic acid and other lichen acids contained in lichens. The leafy liverwort (*Frullania nisquallensis*), a forest epiphyte growing on tree trunks, has produced allergic dermatitis in forest workers. The eruption is commonly called "cedar poisoning." It resembles *Toxicodendron* dermatitis; its attacks are more severe during wet weather. The allergen is sesquiterpene lactone.

Pollens and Seeds. The pollens in ragweed are composed of two antigens. The protein fraction causes the respiratory symptoms of asthma and hay fever, and the oil-soluble portion causes contact dermatitis. Ragweed oil dermatitis is a seasonal disturbance seen mainly during the ragweed growing season from spring to fall. Contact with the plant or with wind-blown fragments of the dried plant produces the typical dermatitis. The oil causes swelling and redness of the lids and entire face, and a red blotchy eruption on the forearms that, after several attacks, may become generalized, with lichenification. It closely resembles chronic atopic dermatitis, with lichenification of the face, neck, and major flexures, and severe pruritus. The distribution also mimics that of photodermatitis, with ragweed dermatitis differentiated by its involvement of the upper eyelids and the retroauricular and submental areas. Chronic cases may continue into the winter, although signs and symptoms are most severe at the height of the season. Sesquiterpene lactones are the cause. Coexistent sensitization to pyrethrum may account for prolongation of ragweed dermatitis. Men outnumber women in hypersensitivity reactions; farmers outnumber patients of all other occupations.

Marine Plants. Numerous aquatic plants are toxic or produce contact dermatitis. Algae are the worst offenders. Freshwater plants are rarely of concern. Seaweed dermatitis is a type of swimmer's eruption produced by contact with a marine blue-green alga, *Lyngbya majuscula Gomont*. The onset is within a few minutes of leaving the ocean, with severe itching and burning, followed by dermatitis, blisters, and deep, painful desquamation that affects the areas covered by the bathing suit, especially the scrotum, perineum, and perianal areas and occasionally the breasts in women). Patch tests with the alga are neither necessary nor helpful because it is a potent irritant. Bathing in fresh water within 10 or 15 minutes of leaving the ocean may prevent the dermatitis. The

Bermuda fire sponge may produce contact erythema multiforme. Trawler fishermen in the Dogger Bank area of the North Sea develop allergic dermatitis after contact with *Alcyonidium hirsutum*. This seaweed-like animal colony becomes caught in nets and produces erythema, edema, and lichenification on the fishermen's hands and wrists.

Plant-Associated Dermatitis. The residua of various insecticides on plants may also produce dermatitis. This is especially true of sprays containing arsenic and malathion. Randox (2-chloro-*N*,*N*-diallyl-acetamide) has been reported as the cause of hemorrhagic bullae on the feet of farmers. Lawn care companies spray herbicides and fungicides throughout the spring, summer, and fall. Dryene, thiuram, carbamates, and chlorothalonil are potential sensitizers in these workers, whose clothing frequently becomes wetted while spraying.

Barbs, bristles, spines, thorns, spicules, and cactus needles are some of the mechanical accessories of plants that may produce dermatitis. Sabra dermatitis is an occupational dermatitis resembling scabies. It is seen among pickers of the prickly pear cactus plant. It also occurs in persons handling Indian figs in Israel, where the condition is seen from July to November. The penetration of minute, invisible thorns into the skin is the cause. *Agave americana* is a low-growing plant used for ornamental purposes in many southwestern U.S. communities. Trimming during landscaping can induce an irritant dermatitis caused by calcium oxalate crystals. The stinging nettle is a common weed that bears tiny spines with biologically active substances such as histamine that produce itching and urticaria within minutes of contact.

Plant Derivatives. Sensitizing substances derived from plants are found in the oleoresin fractions that contain camphors, essential oils, phenols, resins, and terpenes. The chief sensitizers are the essential oils. These may be localized in certain parts of the plant, such as in the peel of citrus fruits, leaves of the eucalyptus tree, and bark of the cinnamon tree. Aromatherapy, an increasingly popular treatment for relief of stress, involves either inhaling or massaging with essential oils; this may cause allergic contact dermatitis in therapists or clients. Exposure to botanical extracts through many cosmetics and homeopathic remedies has resulted in an increasing number of reports of allergic contact sensitivity to individual ingredients, especially tea tree oil.

Cinnamon oil (*Cassia* oil) is a common flavoring agent, especially in pastries. Hand dermatitis in pastry bakers is often caused by cinnamon. It is also used as a flavor for lipstick, bitters, alcoholic and nonalcoholic beverages, toothpaste, and chewing gum. Perioral dermatitis may be caused by cinnamon in chewing gum. A 5% cinnamon solution in olive oil is used for patch testing. Eugenol, clove oil, and eucalyptus oil are used by dentists, who may acquire contact dermatitis from them. Anise, peppermint, and spearmint oils may cause sensitization.

Nutmeg, paprika, and cloves are causes of spice allergy. Fragrance mix is a useful indicator allergen. Lemon oil from lemon peel or lemon wood may cause sensitization in the various handlers of these substances. Citric acid may cause dermatitis in bakers. Lime oil in lime-scented shaving cream or lotion may cause photoallergy. *Myroxylon pereirae* contains numerous substances, including essential oils similar to the oil of lemon peel. It is known to cross-react with vanilla, cinnamon, and many other substances. Vanillin is derived from the vanilla plant and frequently produces contact dermatitis, vanillism, in those connected with its production and use.

Turpentine frequently acts as an irritant and as an allergic sensitizer (carene). It is contained in paints, paint thinners, varnishes, and waxes.

Arberer W: Contact allergy and medicinal plants. J Dtsch Dermatol Ges 2008; 6: 15.

Crawford GH, et al: Use of aromatherapy products and increased risk of hand dermatitis in massage therapists. Arch Dermatol 2004; 140: 991.

de Groot AC, Schmidt E: Tea tree oil. Contact Dermatitis 2016; 75: 129.

Ferreira O, et al: Erythema multiforme–like lesions revealing allergic contact dermatitis to exotic woods. Cutan Ocul Toxicol 2012; 31: 61.

Foti C, et al: Occupational contact dermatitis caused by *Eustoma exaltatum russellianum* (lisianthus). Contact Dermatitis 2014; 71: 59.

Ghorpade A: Contact dermatitis caused by Indian marking nut juice used to relieve ankle pain. Int J Dermatol 2014; 53: 117.

Gladman AC: *Toxicodendron* dermatitis. Wilderness Environ Med 2006; 17: 120.

Hershko K, et al: Exploring the mango–poison ivy connection. Contact Dermatitis 2005; 52: 3.

Higgins C, et al: Eucalyptus oil. Contact Dermatitis 2015; 72: 344.

Jack AR, et al: Allergic contact dermatitis to plant extracts in cosmetics. Semin Cutan Med Surg 2013; 32: 140.

Lakshmi C: Fingertip eczema to pooja flowers. Indian J Dermatol Venereol Leprol 2015; 81: 514.

Linares T, et al: Phytodermatitis caused by *Agave americana.* Allergol Immunopathol (Madr) 2011; 39: 184.

McClanahan C, et al: Black spot poison ivy. Int J Dermatol 2014; 53: 752.

Sharma VK, et al: *Parthenium* dermatitis. Photochem Photobiol Sci 2013; 12: 85.

Swinnen I, et al: An update on airborne contact dermatitis: 2007–2011. Contact Dermatitis 2013; 68: 232.

Veien NK: Systemic contact dermatitis. Int J Dermatol 2011; 50: 1445.

Verma P, et al: Severe marking-nut dermatitis. Dermatitis 2012; 23: 293.

Dermatitis From Clothing

A predisposition to contact dermatitis from clothing occurs in persons who perspire freely or who are obese and wear clothing that tends to be tight. Depending on the offending substance, various regions of the body will be affected. Regional location is helpful in identifying the sensitizing substance. The axillary folds are often involved; the vaults of the axillae are usually spared. Sites of increased perspiration and sites where evaporation is impeded, such as the intertriginous areas, will tend to leach dyes from fabrics to produce dermatitis. Areas where the material is tight against the skin, such as the waistband or neck, are frequently involved (Fig. 6.12). The thighs are affected when pants contain the offending allergen. The hands, face, and undergarment sites are usually spared, but otherwise these reactions may be scattered and generalized. Secondary changes of lichenification and infection occur frequently because of the chronicity of exposure.

Cotton, wool, linen, and silk fabrics were used exclusively before the advent of synthetic fabrics. Most materials are now blended in definite proportions with synthetics to produce superior lasting and esthetic properties. Dermatitis from cotton is virtually non-existent. In most cases, there is no true sensitization to wool. Wool acts as an irritant because of the barbs on its fibers. These barbs may produce severe pruritus at points of contact with the skin, especially in the intertriginous areas. In persons with sensitive skin, such as those with atopic dermatitis, the wearing of wool is not advisable because of its mechanical irritative properties. Silk is a sensitizer, but rarely; the nature of the allergen is not known. Many patients believe their detergent is the source of a dermatitis, but this is rarely the case.

Numerous synthetic fibers are available for clothing and accessory manufacture, all of which again are remarkably free of

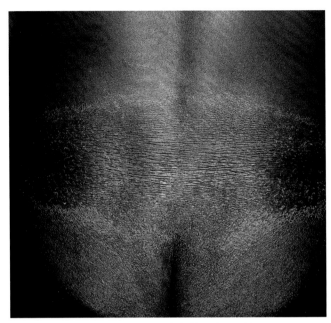

Fig. 6.12 Waistband clothing dermatitis.

sensitizing properties. Polyvinyl resins are the plastics used in such apparel as raincoats, rainhoods, wristbands, suspenders, plastic mittens, and gloves. These also are only infrequently found to be causes of contact dermatitis.

The most common causes of clothing dermatitis are the fabric finishers, dyes, and rubber additives. Fabric finishers are used to improve the durability, appearance, and feel of a material. Anti-wrinkling and crease-holding chemicals are mostly resins, which are incorporated into the fibers as they are being manufactured or applied to the finished fabric. Fabrics are treated to make them less vulnerable to the effects of perspiration and ironing. Clothing may be treated with these substances to make it dry rapidly after washing. They are used to make clothing fabrics shrink resistant and water and stain repellent. When all these uses are taken into consideration, the low incidence of dermatitis from these form-aldehyde resin materials is remarkable.

Ethylene urea melamine formaldehyde resin and dimethylol dihydroxyethylene urea formaldehyde resin are the best screening agents. Many persons also react to formaldehyde and the formaldehyde-releasing preservatives such as quaternium 15. Avoidance of exposure of the skin to formaldehyde resin is most difficult. New clothes should be thoroughly washed twice before wearing the first time. Even with this precaution, however, allergens may still be present in sufficient quantities to continue the dermatitis. T-shirts, sweat-shirts and pants, white underclothes suitable for bleaching, and garments of mixed synthetic fibers with cotton fibers added to make them drip-dry are most likely to cause problems in these patients.

Synthetic fabrics such as polyester and acetate liners in women's clothing are also prime causes, and women are more affected than men. Even infants may be affected, however, with dyes in diapers accounting for some cases. Many patients do not react to para-phenylene diamine, but only to the disperse dye allergens. The best screening agents are disperse blue 106 and 124. Lymphomatoid contact allergy may result from clothing dye reactivity.

Suspected fabrics may be soaked in water for 15 minutes and applied under a patch for 72–96 hours. Jeans, Spandex, silk, 100% linen, 100% nylon, and 100% cotton that is not wrinkle resistant or colorfast are best tolerated. Spandex is a nonrubber (but elastic) polyurethane fiber. It is widely used for garments such as girdles, brassieres, and socks, but is generally safe in the United States because it is free of rubber additives.

Carlson RM, et al: Diagnosis and treatment of dermatitis due to formaldehyde resin in clothing. Dermatitis 2004; 15: 169.

Coman G, et al: Textile allergic contact dermatitis. Rev Environ Health 2014; 29: 163.

Donovan J, et al: Allergic contact dermatitis from formaldehyde textile resins in surgical uniforms and nonwoven textile masks. Dermatitis 2007; 18: 40.

Malinauskiene L, et al: Contact allergy from disperse dyes in textiles. Contact Dermatitis 2013; 68: 65.

Mobolaji-Lawal M, Nedorost S: The role of textiles in dermatitis. Curr Allergy Asthma Rep 2015; 15: 17.

Narganes LM, et al: Lymphomatoid dermatitis caused by contact with textile dyes. Contact Dermatitis 2013; 68: 62.

Reich HC, et al: Allergic contact dermatitis from formaldehyde textile resins. Dermatitis 2010; 21: 65.

Zug KA, et al: The value of patch testing patients with a scattered generalized distribution of dermatitis. J Am Acad Dermatol 2008; 59: 426.

Shoe Dermatitis

Footwear dermatitis may begin on the dorsal surfaces of the toes and may remain localized to that area indefinitely (Fig. 6.13). There is erythema, lichenification, and, in severe cases, weeping and crusting. Secondary infection is frequent. In severe cases, an id reaction may be produced on the hands, similar to the reaction from fungal infection of the feet. A diagnostic point is the normal appearance of the skin between the toes, which has no contact with the offending substance. In fungal infections, the toe webs are usually involved. Another pattern seen is involvement of the sole with sparing of the instep and flexural creases of the toes. Also, purpuric reactions may occur to components of black rubber mix. Hyperhidrosis and atopy predispose to development of shoe allergy.

Shoe dermatitis is most frequently caused by the rubber accelerators mercaptobenzothiazole, carbamates, and tetramethylthiuram disulfide. Potassium dichromate in leather and the adhesives used in synthetic materials (especially *p*-tert-butylphenol formaldehyde resin) are also common shoe allergens. Diisocyanates are used in making foam rubber padding for athletic shoes and may cause allergy. Dimethyl fumarate is a preservative used in

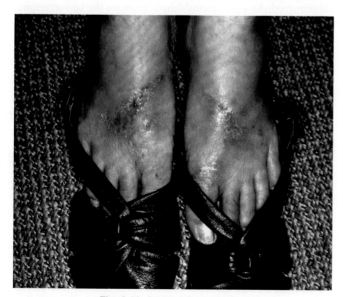

Fig. 6.13 Acute shoe dermatitis.

antihumidity sachets. It is a volatile substance and may deposit on shoes during its transport. Dimethyl fumarate is highly allergenic, and several outbreaks of shoe dermatitis in Europe have occurred secondary to this allergen. Other causative agents are felt, cork liners, formaldehyde, dyes, asphalt, and tar. Shoe refresher sprays may also induce allergy. Patch testing with pieces of various shoe parts may be done by soaking them for 15 minutes in water and applying them to the back for 72–96 hours. Once the allergen has been identified, selection of shoes without the offending substance will lead to resolution. Unfortunately, this is a difficult process, because most shoes are made in areas without mandatory labeling requirements, and plastic, wooden, or fabric shoes that contain fewer allergens are often impractical.

Castando-Tardan MP, et al: Allergic contact dermatitis to Crocs. Contact Dermatitis 2008; 58: 248.

Matthys E, et al: Shoe allergic contact dermatitis. Dermatitis 2014; 25: 163.

Mowitz M, Pontén A: Foot dermatitis caused by didecyldimethylammonium chloride in a shoe refresher spray. Contact Dermatitis 2015; 73: 374.

Švecová D, et al: Footwear contact dermatitis from dimethyl fumarate. Int J Dermatol 2013; 52: 803.

Washaw EM, et al: Shoe allergens. Dermatitis 2007; 18: 191.

Dermatitis From Metals and Metal Salts

Metal dermatitis is most frequently caused by nickel and chromates. Usually, with the exception of nickel, the pure metals generally do not cause hypersensitivity; only when they are incorporated into salts do they cause reactions. Most objects containing metal or metal salts are combinations of several metals, some of which may have been used to plate the surface, thereby enhancing its attractiveness, durability, or tensile strength. For this reason, suspected metal-caused dermatitis should be investigated by doing patch tests to several of the metal salts.

Patients have developed a variety of dermatoses, most often eczematous in type, after placement of an orthopedic, gynecologic, or dental implant or a pacemaker/defibrillator or endovascular device. When patients are symptomatic with an eczematous process after implantation, patch testing will allow evaluation of allergy by testing with an extended tray, metals, and bone cement. A positive diagnosis of allergy at a minimum requires the appearance of a chronic dermatitis after placement, no other cause, a positive patch test for the suspected metal (or with drug-eluting stents, the drug), and healing after removal. This scenario is exceedingly uncommon; the removal of the foreign material needs to be judged as necessary, reasonable, and safe, and no objective criteria exist to determine the necessity. Dental and gynecologic implants are more frequently replaced; some patients do improve. Patch testing before placement does not seem to predict complications and is therefore not recommended.

Black Dermatographism. Black or greenish staining under rings, metal wristbands, bracelets, and clasps is caused by the abrasive effect of cosmetics or other powders containing zinc or titanium oxide on gold jewelry. This skin discoloration is black because of the deposit of metal particles on skin that has been powdered and that has metal, such as gold, silver, or platinum, rubbing on it. Abrasion of the metal results because some powders are hard (zinc oxide) and can abrade the metal.

Nickel. Because we are all constantly exposed to nickel, nickel dermatitis is a frequent occurrence. Although still most common among women, sensitization is increasing among men. A direct relationship between prevalence of nickel allergy and number of pierced sites has been documented. Nickel produces more cases of allergic contact dermatitis than all other metals combined.

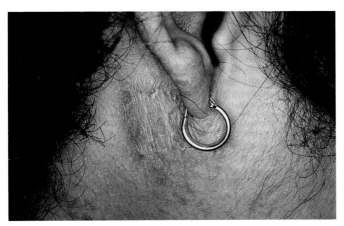

Fig. 6.14 Nickel dermatitis caused by earring.

Erythematous and eczematous eruptions, sometimes with licheni-fication, appear beneath earrings (Fig. 6.14), bracelets, rings, wrist watches, clasps, and jeans buttons. The snaps on clothing have been implicated in producing allergy in children; nickel is the most common cause of allergic contact dermatitis in children as well as adults. Laptop computers, cell phones, electronic cigarettes, and microneedling devices are newer products capable of causing nickel dermatitis. Metals, including nickel, are increasingly being recognized as a cause of cosmetic allergies. Nickel ranks highly on lists of occupationally induced allergic contact dermatitis.

Nickel dermatitis is seen most frequently on the earlobes. Piercing the earlobes with nickel-plated instruments or wearing nickel-plated jewelry readily induces nickel sensitivity. Earlobes should be pierced only with stainless steel instruments, and only stainless steel earrings should be worn until the ears have healed. Exposure to the metal may not be readily apparent most of the time. Even with gold jewelry, the clasps and solder may contain nickel. Nickel objects may be plated with chrome but may still cause nickel dermatitis through the leaching of some of the nickel through the small pores of the chromium plating.

Nickel oxides in green paints may produce nickel dermatitis. Homeopathic and complementary medicaments may also contain enough nickel to produce a contact allergy. Sweat containing sodium chloride may combine with nickel to form nickel chloride. This affects the degree of nickel dermatitis, being more severe in persons who perspire profusely.

The diagnosis is established by a positive patch test reaction to nickel sulfate. Nickel may be detected by applying dimethyl-glyoxime solution to the test object. In the presence of nickel, the cotton swab used to apply the solution will turn orange-pink. A positive test always means that nickel is present, but a negative test does not rule out its presence. Sweat, blood, or saline may leach nickel from stainless steel.

Prophylactic measures should include the reduction of perspira-tion in those sensitive to nickel. Topical corticosteroids applied before exposure to nickel, such as before putting on a wristband, may be successful. Clasps and other objects are available in plastic material so that some of the exposure to nickel may be decreased. Polyurethane varathane 91 applied in three coats will give protection for several months. Treatment of nickel dermatitis consists of the application of topical corticosteroids. In Europe, laws regulating the maximum content of nickel in jewelry have led to a marked decrease in sensitization. Dr. Sharon Jacob is leading an effort to have a similar law passed in the United States.

Hand eczema and pompholyx in nickel-sensitive or cobalt-sensitive patients have rarely been aggravated by ingested metals in the diet. In severe, treatment-resistant dermatitis, a specific diet low in nickel and cobalt may be tried.

Chromium. The chromates are strongly corrosive and irritating to the skin and may act as primary irritants or as sensitizers to produce allergic contact dermatitis. Besides affecting employees in chromate works, chrome dermatitis is encountered among tanners, painters, dyers, photographers, polishers, welders, aircraft workers, diesel engine workers, and those involved with the bleaching of crude oils, tallows, and fats. Traces of dichromates in shoe leather and gloves may cause eczema of the feet and hands. Many zippers are chromium plated, and the nickel underneath may be the causative agent. Chromium metal and stainless steel do not produce contact dermatitis.

Zinc chromate paint is a source of dermatitis. Matches, hide glues, chrome alloys, cigarette lighters, and leather hatbands, sandals, or camera cases may cause chrome dermatitis. Anticorrosion solutions used for refrigeration and other recirculation systems often contain chromates that produce dermatitis. Most workers in the cement industry who have cement eczema show positive patch tests to dichromates. Cement eczema is often a primary irritant dermatitis complicated by allergic contact dermatitis to the hexavalent chromates. The incidence of cement dermatitis has decreased significantly over the years, believed to be the result of the addition of ferrous sulfate, delivery of premixed cement to the job site, and improved education.

The skin changes are multiform, ranging from a mild follicular dermatitis to widespread nodular and crusted eruptions, all being worse on exposed parts. Often the eruptions are slow to clear up, lasting from a few weeks to 6 months after contact has ceased. Heavy exposure of industrial workers to chromates may produce chrome ulcers on the backs of the hands and forearms, usually beginning around a hair follicle, or in the creases of the knuckles or finger webs. The hole begins as a small abrasion that deepens and widens as its edges grow thick, eventually forming a conical, indolent ulceration. Chrome ulcers may also arise on—and perforate—the nasal septum. Arsenic exposure may result in similar ulcers.

Diagnosis of chrome sensitivity is made by a positive patch test to potassium dichromate in petrolatum. The hexavalent chrome compounds are the most frequent cause of chrome dermatitis because these penetrate the skin more easily than the trivalent form. Both forms are sensitizers. Even with avoidance of chromate-containing materials, chromate-induced dermatitis is often persistent.

Mercury. The mercurials may act not only as irritants but also as sensitizers. Thimerosal is a mercuric-containing preservative; it is an allergen that is rarely relevant. Allergy to this compound is likely to have been caused by exposure during childhood vac-cinations and to tincture of merthiolate antiseptic. In general, these patients tolerate repeated vaccinations well. Most individuals are sensitized to the ethyl mercuric component of thimerosal; however, those who react to the thiosalicylic acid portion develop photodermatitis to piroxicam. Mercury in amalgam dental fillings has been shown in multiple large studies to cause oral lichenoid eruptions. The relationship is especially strong when the oral lesion, often with a painful erosion present, is apposed to a gold or amalgam filling. In many cases, when sensitivity is proved by patch testing and fillings are replaced, involution of the oral findings occurs.

Cobalt. Cobalt is frequently combined with nickel as a contami-nant, and patients allergic to cobalt typically are also allergic to nickel. The metals have similar properties but do not produce cross-reactions. Cobalt dermatitis may occur in those involved in the manufacture of polyester resins and paints, hard metals used for cutting and drilling tools, and cement. Cobalt dermatitis may also occur in producers of pottery, ceramics, metal alloys, glass, carbides, and pigments. Individuals may be exposed to cobalt in hair dye, flypaper, and vitamin B_{12}. Blue tattoo pigment contains

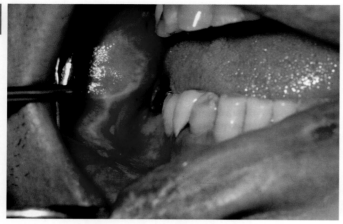

Fig. 6.15 Oral lichenoid dermatitis due to gold.

cobalt oxide. Rarely, cobalt chloride may cause nonimmunologic local release of vasoreactive materials, with a local urticarial response.

Gold. Gold dermatitis may rarely occur from the wearing of gold jewelry. A predisposing factor in such patients is the presence of dental gold. Oral lichenoid eruptions have also been reported with gold, similar to the situation with mercury-containing amalgams (Fig. 6.15). It is not uncommon to see positive reactions to gold when patch-testing patients with facial, eyelid, or widespread dermatitis of unknown cause. Although it is difficult to make a direct clinical correlation with any one piece of jewelry, occasionally patients will clear if they stop wearing all gold jewelry. One possible explanation is that titanium dioxide in sunscreen products may liberate gold particles from jewelry. In most patients, however, there is a lack of relevance. Gold reactions on patch testing may be delayed in onset and remain inflamed for months.

Other Metals. Most other common metals are not important in causing contact dermatitis. Platinum dermatitis may occur from exposure to platinum salts and sprays in industry. Platinum rings, earrings, white gold spectacles, clasps, and other jewelry cause eruptions resembling those caused by nickel. Zinc, aluminum, copper sulfate, titanium, and antimony dermatitis rarely occur, although these metals may act as irritants.

Atanaskova Mesinkovska N, et al: The effect of patch testing on surgical practices and outcomes in orthopedic patients with metal implants. Arch Dermatol 2012; 148: 687.

Borowska S, Brzóska MM: Metals in cosmetics. J Appl Toxicol 2015; 35: 551.

Bregnbak D, et al: Chromium allergy and dermatitis. Contact Dermatitis 2015; 73: 261.

Chen JK, Lampel HP: Gold contact allergy. Dermatitis 2015; 26: 69.

Crépy MN: Skin diseases in musicians. Eur J Dermatol 2015; 25: 375.

Fage SW, et al: Copper hypersensitivity. Contact Dermatitis 2014; 71: 191.

Fage SW, et al: Titanium. Contact Dermatitis 2016; 74: 323.

Fowler JF Jr: Cobalt. Dermatitis 2016; 27: 3.

Goldenberg A, et al: Nickel allergy in adults in the U.S. Dermatitis 2015; 26: 216.

Gölz L, et al: Nickel hypersensitivity and orthodontic treatment. Contact Dermatitis 2015; 73: 1.

Honari G, et al: Hypersensitivity reactions associated with endovascular devices. Contact Dermatitis 2008; 59: 7.

Jacob SE, et al: Nickel allergy and our children's health. Pediatr Dermatol 2015; 32: 779.

Maridet C, et al: The electronic cigarette. Contact Dermatitis 2015; 73: 49.

Mislankar M, et al: Low nickel diet scoring system for systemic nickel allergy. Dermatitis 2013; 24: 190.

Pacheco KA: Allergy to surgical implants. J Allergy Clin Immunol Pract 2015; 3: 683.

Stuckert J, et al: Low cobalt diet for dyshidrotic eczema. Contact Dermatitis 2008; 59: 361.

Teo Wendy ZW, Schalock PC: Hypersensitivity reactions to implanted metal devices. J Investig Allergol Clin Immunol 2016; 26: 279.

Thomas P, et al: DKG statement on the use of metal alloy discs for patch testing in suspected intolerance to metal implants. J Dtsch Dermatol Ges 2015; 13: 1001.

Thyssen JP, et al: Patch test reactivity to metal allergens following regulatory intervention. Contact Dermatitis 2010; 63: 102.

Warshaw EM, et al: Body piercing and metal allergic contact sensitivity. Dermatitis 2014; 25: 255.

Contact Stomatitis

The role of contact allergy in oral symptomatology is significant. Approximately 30% of patients with oral symptoms will have relevant allergens, most frequently metals used in dental fillings, food additives (flavorings and antioxidants), and dental products (acrylic monomers, epoxy resins, hardeners used in prosthodontics and dental impression materials). Chewing gums and dentifrices may also produce contact stomatitis. Ingredients responsible for this are hexylresorcinol, thymol, dichlorophen, oil of cinnamon, and mint.

Clinical signs may be bright erythema of the tongue and buccal mucosa with scattered erosions. Angular cheilitis may also develop. Oral lichenoid lesions may be caused by sensitization to metals in dental fillings and gold caps or crowns.

Batchelor JM, et al: Allergic contact stomatitis caused by a polyether dental impression material. Contact Dermatitis 2010; 63: 296.

de Groot A: Contact allergy to (ingredients of) toothpastes. Dermatitis 2017; 28: 95.

Isaac-Renton M, et al: Cinnamon spice and everything not nice: many features of intraoral allergy to cinnamic aldehyde. Dermatitis 2015; 26: 116.

Johns DA, et al: Allergic contact stomatitis from bisphenol-a-glycidyl dimethacrylate during application of composite restorations. Indian J Dent Res 2014; 25: 266.

Krishen C, et al: Dental allergic contact dermatitis. Dermatitis 2012; 23: 222.

O'Gorman SM, Torgerson RR: Contact allergy in cheilitis. Int J Dermatol 2016; 55: e386.

Sharma R, et al: Role of dental restoration materials in oral mucosal lichenoid lesions. Indian J Dermatol Venereol Leprol 2015; 81: 478.

Torgerson RR, et al: Contact allergy in oral disease. J Am Acad Dermatol 2007; 57: 315.

Zug KA, et al: Patch-testing North American lip dermatitis patients. Dermatitis 2008; 19: 202.

Rubber Dermatitis

Rubber dermatitis generally occurs on the hands from wearing rubber gloves, as by surgeons, nurses, and homemakers. The eruption is usually sharply limited to the gloved area but may spread up the forearms. Rubber dermatitis also develops from exposure to condoms, diaphragms, swim goggles (Fig. 6.16), caps and scuba masks, wet suits, bandages for chronic leg ulcers, respirators, gas

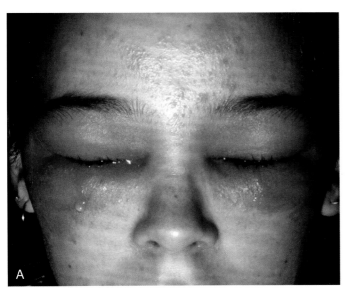

Fig. 6.16 Rubber dermatitis from swim goggles.

masks, rubber sheets, and cosmetic sponges. Shoe dermatitis may be caused by rubber allergy to insoles or sneakers.

Natural and synthetic rubbers are used separately or in combination to make the final rubber product. The chemicals added in the rubber manufacturing process, most importantly the accelerators and antioxidants, are the common causes of allergic contact dermatitis. A similar list of additives is present in neoprene, a synthetic rubber, but also includes the dialkyl thioureas. These are not in the standard patch trays and thus may escape detection unless applied as a supplemental allergen. Elastic in underwear is chemically transformed by laundry bleach into a potent sensitizing substance. The allergen is permanent and cannot be removed by washing. The offending garments must be thrown out and the use of bleaches interdicted.

Accelerators. During the manufacturing process, chemicals are used to hasten the vulcanization of rubber. Among the numerous chemicals available, tetramethylthiuram disulfide, mercaptobenzothiazole, and diphenylguanidine are frequently used. Tetramethylthiuram disulfide and its analogs, known as disulfiram and thiuram, may produce contact dermatitis when moist skin is exposed to the finished rubber product. In a 10-year study of 636 cases of allergy to rubber additives, thiuram mix was by far the most common sensitizer. Mercaptobenzothiazole is most often the cause in shoe allergy and thiuram in glove allergy.

Antioxidants. Antioxidants are used to preserve rubber. Amine antioxidants, such as phenyl-α-naphthylamine, are most effective. Hydroquinone antioxidants may cause depigmentation of the skin, as well as allergic contact dermatitis. A frequent antioxidant sensitizer, propyl *p*-phenylenediamine, is used in tires, heavy-duty rubber goods, boots, and elastic underwear.

Bendewald MJ, et al: An 8-year retrospective review of patch testing with rubber allergens. Dermatitis 2010; 21:33.
Cao LY, et al: Allergic contact dermatitis to synthetic rubber gloves. Arch Dermatol 2010; 146: 1001.
Higgins CL, et al: Occupational skin disease among Australian healthcare workers. Contact Dermatitis 2016; 75: 213.
Ibler KS, et al: Prevalence of delayed-type and immediate-type hypersensitivity in healthcare workers with hand eczema. Contact Dermatitis 2016; 75: 223.

Schwensen JF, et al: Contact allergy to rubber accelerators remains prevalent. J Eur Acad Dermatol Venereol 2016; 30: 1768.
Warshaw EM, et al: Positive patch-test reactions to mixed dialkyl thioureas. Dermatitis 2008; 19: 190.

Adhesive Dermatitis

Cements, glues, and gums may cause adhesive dermatitis. Formaldehyde resin adhesives contain free formaldehyde, naphtha, glue, and disinfectants. Synthetic resin adhesives contain plasticizers; hide glues may contain chromates from the tanned leather, and other glues incorporate preservatives such as formaldehyde. Dental bonding adhesives may contain acrylic monomers and epoxy resins and hardeners. Pressure-sensitive adhesives contain rubber and acrylates, and anaerobic adhesives have primarily acrylates.

Vegetable gums, such as gum tragacanth, gum arabic, and karaya, may be used in denture adhesives, hair wave lotions, topical medications, toothpastes, and depilatories, and many cause contact dermatitis. Resins are used in adhesive tapes and in various adhesives such as tincture of benzoin. Turpentine is frequently found in rosin; abietic acid in the rosin is the causative sensitizer.

Adhesive tape reactions are frequently irritant in nature. Allergic reactions to adhesive tape itself are caused by the rubber components, accelerators, antioxidants, and various resins or turpentine. Some adhesive tapes contain acrylate polymers rather than rubber adhesives. These acrylates may cause allergic contact dermatitis. Pressure-sensitive adhesives are increasingly used. Allergens present in these adhesives include rosin, rubber accelerators, antioxidants, acrylates, hydroquinones, lanolin, thiourea compounds, and *N*-dodecylmaleamic compounds.

Bennike, NH, et al: Please, label the label; a case report of occupational allergic contact dermatitis caused by methylisothiazolinone in adhesive labels. Contact Dermatitis 2016; 75: 314.
Bhargava K, et al: Eyelid allergic contact dermatitis caused by ethyl cyanoacrylate–containing eyelash adhesive. Contact Dermatitis 2012; 67: 306.
Corazza M, et al: Allergic contact dermatitis in a volleyball player due to protective adhesive taping. Eur J Dermatol 2011; 21: 430.
Davis MD, Stuart MJ: Severe allergic contact dermatitis to Dermabond Prineo, a topical skin adhesive of 2-octyl cyanoacrylate increasingly used in surgeries to close wounds. Dermatitis 2016; 27: 75.
Jacobs M, et al: Peristomal allergic contact dermatitis caused by stoma adhesive paste containing N-butyl monoester of polymethyl vinyl ether maleic acid. Contact Dermatitis 2015; 73: 314.
Lau YN, et al: Use of skin adhesive in dermatological surgery. Clin Exp Dermatol 2014; 39: 773.
Özkaya E, Kavlak Bozkurt P: Allergic contact dermatitis caused by self-adhesive electrocardiography electrodes. Contact Dermatitis 2014; 70: 121.
Schwensen JF, et al: Sensitization to cyanoacrylates caused by prolonged exposure to a glucose sensor set in a diabetic child. Contact Dermatitis 2016; 74: 124.

Synthetic Resin Dermatitis

The many varieties of synthetic resins preclude adequate discussion of each. The reactions during the manufacture of these substances are more common than those in their finished state.

Epoxy Resins. The epoxy resins in their liquid (noncured, monomer) form may produce severe dermatitis, especially during the manufacturing process. The fully polymerized or cured product is nonsensitizing. Nonindustrial exposure is usually to epoxy resin glues, nail lacquers, and artificial nails. Epoxy resins are used in the home as glues and paints (bathtub and refrigerator). Artists and sculptors frequently use epoxy resins.

Epoxy resins consist of two or more components, the resin and the curing agent. Approximately 90% of allergic reactions are to the resin and 10% to the hardener. The numerous curing agents include the amines, phenolic compounds, peroxides, and polyamides. These may be irritants and/or allergens. The resin, based on an acetone and phenol compound known as bisphenol A, in its raw state may cause allergic contact dermatitis. BIS-GMA, a combination of bisphenol A and glycidyl methacrylate, is the main allergen in dental bonding agents. Epoxy resins are used also as stabilizers and plasticizers. Their use in the manufacture of polyvinyl chloride (plastic) film has caused dermatitis from plastic handbags, beads, gloves, and panties.

Polyester Resins. Ordinarily, completely cured or polymerized resins are not sensitizers. The unsaturated polyester resins are dissolved and later copolymerized with vinyl monomers. Such polyester resins are used for polyester plasticizers, polyester fibers (Dacron), and polyester film (Mylar). The unsaturated polyester resins, on the other hand, will produce primary irritation in their fabrication or among sculptors. The dermatitis occurs typically as an eczematous eruption on the back of the hands, wrists, and forearms. Polyester resins are incorporated into other plastic material as laminates to give them strength; applications include boat hulls, automobile body putty, safety helmets, fuel tanks, lampshades, and skylights.

Acrylic Monomers. Cyanoacrylates are used widely as adhesives in a variety of home and commercial products. They are generally a rare cause of contact dermatitis. Multifunctional acrylic monomers may produce allergic or irritant contact dermatitis. Pentaerythritol triacrylate, trimethylolpropane triacrylate, and hexanediol diacrylate are widely used acrylic monomers. Printers handling multifunctional acrylic monomers in printing inks and acrylic printing plates may present with an erythematous, pruritic eruption, mainly of the hands and arms, swelling of the face, and involvement of the eyelids.

Orthopedic surgeons experience contact dermatitis from the use of acrylic bone cement (methyl methacrylate monomer) used in mending hip joints. Dentists and dental technicians are exposed when applying this to teeth. The sensitizer passes through rubber and polyvinyl gloves and may additionally cause paresthesias. In patients who are allergic to their acrylate dental prosthesis, coating this with UV light–cured acrylate lacquer may allow it to be worn without adverse effects.

Benzoyl peroxide is a popular acne remedy. It is also used for bleaching flour and edible oils and for curing plastics, such as acrylic dentures. Infrequently, an allergic contact dermatitis may result.

Aalto-Korte K, et al: Contact allergy to epoxy hardeners. Contact Dermatitis 2014; 71: 145.

Aalto-Korte K, et al: Occupational allergic contact dermatitis caused by epoxy chemicals. Contact Dermatitis 2015; 73: 336.

Bowen C, et al: Allergic contact dermatitis to 2-octyl cyanoacrylate. Cutis 2014; 94: 183.

Kocak O, Gul U: Patch test results of the dental personnel with contact dermatitis. Cutan Ocul Toxicol 2014; 33: 299.

Shmidt E, et al: Patch-testing with plastics and glues series allergens. Dermatitis 2010; 21: 269.

Strazzula L, et al: Fingertip purpura in a dental student. JAMA Dermatol 2014; 150: 784.

Cosmetic Dermatitis

Cutaneous reactions to cosmetics may be divided into irritant, allergic, and photosensitivity reactions. More than half the reactions

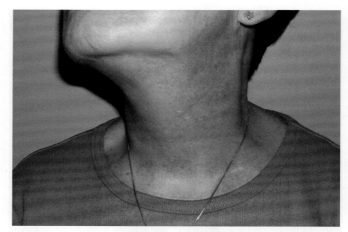

Fig. 6.17 Fragrance allergy, lyral.

occur on the face and are caused primarily by skin care products, nail cosmetics, shaving preparations, and deodorants. The leading cause of allergic contact dermatitis associated with cosmetics is from fragrance. A close second is preservatives, such as methylchloroisothiazolinone/methyllisothiazolinone, 2-bromo-2-nitropropane-1,3-diol, quaternium 15, methyldibromo glutaronitrile, and imidazolidinyl urea. The third leading cause is *p*-phenylenediamine in hair dye. It is recommended that patch testing with the patient's own product, as long as it is applied to the skin as a leave-on product, be part of the evaluation.

Fragrances. Almost all cosmetic preparations, skin care products, and many medications contain fragrance; even those labeled "nonscented" often contain a masking fragrance that may be a sensitizer. Even "fragrance-free" products have been documented to contain the raw fragrance ingredients, such as rose oil in "all-natural" products. Fragrances are the most common cosmetic ingredient causing allergic contact dermatitis. Photodermatitis, irritation, contact urticaria, and dyspigmentation are other types of reactions that fragrances may produce.

The most common individual allergens identified are cinnamic alcohol, oak moss, cinnamic aldehyde, hydroxy citronellal, musk ambrette, isoeugenol, geraniol, coumarin, lyral (Fig. 6.17), and eugenol. Hyperperoxides of linalool and oxidized limonene are newer important fragrance allergens. Frequently, unspecified allergens are the cause, because they are not listed on labels, and fragrances are combinations of many different ingredients. *Myroxylon pereirae* (balsam of Peru) will identify approximately half of those often unsuspected cases of allergic dermatitis, and additional testing with the fragrance mixes will identify over 90%. Additionally, a natural fragrance mixture of jasmine absolute, ylang-ylang oil, narcissus absolute, spearmint oil, and sandalwood oil is recommended. Other essential oils may be missed if not individually tested. Fragrance mixes should be prepared the day of application as evaporation may compromise their reliability. New products should be tested for tolerance in patients with a history of fragrance sensitivity.

At least 1% of the population have fragrance sensitivity. Women still outnumber men, but as the frequency of fragrance contact reactions has increased over the years, men have shown a steeper increase in sensitivity. Fragrance is one allergen that may be transferred by skin-to-skin contact to a sensitive person, causing connubial contact dermatitis. Ingestion of balsam-related foods, such as tomatoes, citrus fruits, and spices, may cause a flare in some sensitive patients. In particularly difficult-to-treat patients, balsam-restricted diets may be beneficial but are not easy to follow.

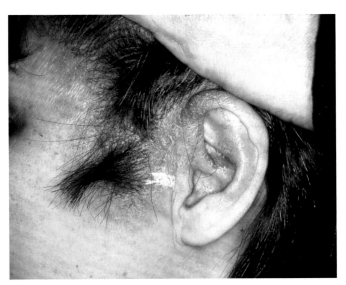

Fig. 6.18 Hair dye allergy.

Hair Dyes. Permanent hair dyes incorporate *p*-phenylenediamine (PPDA), a popular but potent sensitizer that may cross-react with many chemicals. In rinses and tints, the azo dyes, acid violet 6B, water-soluble nigrosine, and ammonium carbonate may sensitize and cross-react with PPDA. Workers in the manufacture of PPDA, furriers, hairdressers, and those in the photographic and rubber vulcanization industries develop eruptions first on the back of the hands, wrists, forearms, eyelids, and nose, consisting of an eczematous, erythematous, oozing dermatitis. It will penetrate most protective gloves, but not nitrile gloves. Lichenification and scaling are seen in the chronic type. In those with dyed hair, sensitivity is manifested by itching, redness, and puffiness of the upper eyelids, tops of the ears, temples, and back of the neck (Fig. 6.18). Beard/mustache dermatitis may be caused by coloring of the facial hair and eyelid dermatitis by dying eyelashes. PPDA added to temporary henna tattoos to make them darker has resulted in acute vesicular allergic reactions, some with scarring and hyperpigmentation. Kumkum is a common cosmetic in India, primarily smeared on the forehead of women to denote their marital status; one of many reported allergens in the product is PPDA.

For those sensitive to this type of hair dye, use of semipermanent or temporary dyes might be the solution. In the case of sensitivity to these alternatives, vegetable dyes such as henna may be tried. Metallic dyes are usually not favored by women but are frequently used by men as "hair color restorers." The metallic hair dyes may contain nickel, cobalt, chromium, or lead. Hair dyes containing FD&C and D&C dyes often do not cross-react with PPDA and 70% of PPDA-sensitive patients exposed to a dye containing the less allergenic PPDA derivative 2-methoxymehtyl-PPD tolerated it.

Other Hair Products. Hair bleach products incorporate peroxides, persulfates, and ammonia, which may act as primary irritants. Hair bleaches that contain ammonium persulfate, a primary irritant, may produce a local urticarial and a generalized histamine reaction.

Several types of permanent wave preparations exist. The alkaline permanent wave preparations, which use ammonium thioglycolate, are rarely if ever sensitizers and usually cause only hair breakage and irritant reactions. The hot type, or acid perm, is a common sensitizer, the allergen being glyceryl monothioglycolate. Cosmetologists are at risk for development of hand dermatitis. The glyceryl monothioglycolate persists in the hair for at least 3 months after application and may cause a long-lasting dermatitis.

It readily penetrates rubber and vinyl gloves. A more neutral pH permanent wave solution is less allergenic than the acid perms; however, allergy to cysteamine hydrochloride found in neutral permanent wave products may occur. This allergen does not penetrate household-weight latex gloves, and hair waved with it does not produce allergic reactions in sensitized individuals. Also, it is an amine salt, not a thioglycolate, so cross-reactivity is unlikely.

Hair straighteners using greases and gums are not sensitizers; however, the perfume incorporated in these preparations can be sensitizing. Thioglycolates are also used, and hair breakage may occur with these products.

Hair sprays may contain shellac, gum arabic, sunscreens, and synthetic resins as sensitizers, and allergic reactions occur infrequently. Lanolin is frequently incorporated into aerosol sprays.

Chemical depilatories containing calcium thioglycolate and the sulfides and sulfhydrates may cause primary irritant dermatitis. Mechanical hair removers include the mercaptans, waxes, and resins; resins may produce allergic dermatitis.

Hair tonics and lotions with tincture of cinchona produce allergic sensitization; tincture of cantharidin and salicylic acid cause primary irritation. Resorcin, quinine sulfate, and perfumes such as bay rum are also sensitizers.

Nail Products. Nail lacquers may contain tosylamide/formaldehyde resin and are a frequent cause of eyelid and neck dermatitis. Polishes free of this resin are available. Nail polish removers are solvents such as acetone, which can cause nail brittleness. The acrylic monomers in artificial nails, as well as the ethyl cyanoacrylate glue required to attach the prosthetic nail, may produce allergic sensitivity. Photoinitiating agents, such as benzophenone, used in photo-bonded acrylic sculptured nails are other potential allergens.

Lipsticks. Various R and C dyes, sunscreens, shellac, flavoring agents, preservative, and lipstick perfumes may cause sensitization reactions. Lipsticks are tested as is. Lip plumpers may cause contact urticaria in those being kissed. Propolis is found in many so-called natural products, including lip balms, toothpastes, lotions, shampoos, and other cosmetics. Its main allergens are two types of caffeates.

Eye Makeup. In mascara, eye shadow, and eyeliners, preservatives, shellac, metals, base wax, and perfumes are the components that may produce sensitization, but this occurs rarely. False-positive reactions to some mascaras occur when a closed patch test is used. This is caused by the irritative qualities of the solvents. An open or nonocclusive patch test is recommended. A provocative use test in the antecubital fossae may ultimately be necessary. The rubber sponges used to apply eye makeup, nickel in the tools used, or cocamidopropylbetaine in eye makeup remover also cause eyelid dermatitis.

Sunscreens. *p*-Aminobenzoic acid (PABA) and its derivatives (e.g., padimate O, padimate A, glycerol PABA), dibenzoylmethanes, salicylates, cinnamates, and benzophenones are photosensitizers as well as sensitizers. The benzophenones (most often benzophenone-3) and dibenzoylmethanes are the most common sunscreen allergens and photoallergens. These agents frequently are found in various other cosmetic products. The physical blockers titanium dioxide and zinc oxide do not cause allergy. If allergy to PABA exists, its derivatives should be avoided, and the patient should be aware that thiazides, sulfonylurea antidiabetic medication, azo dyes, *p*-aminosalicylic acid, benzocaine, and PPDA all may cause dermatitis from cross-reactions.

Bleaching Creams. Hydroquinones are occasional sensitizers. Ammoniated mercury is a sensitizing agent formerly used in bleaching creams.

Lanolin. The fatty alcohol lanolin is rarely a sensitizer on normal skin, so it usually does not produce dermatitis when exposure is with cosmetic and skin care products. It provokes allergic reactions more frequently in therapeutic agents used by atopic patients and in emollient products that may be used postsurgically.

Dentifrices and Mouthwashes. Dentifrices and mouthwashes contain sensitizers, such as the essential oils used as flavoring agents, preservatives, formalin, antibiotics, and antiseptics. Circumoral dermatitis and cheilitis may be caused by tartar-control types of dentifrice.

Axillary Antiperspirants. Aluminum salts, such as aluminum chloride and chlorhydroxide, and zinc salts, such as zinc chloride, act as primary irritants and may rarely produce a folliculitis. Aluminum chlorhydrate is considered to be the least irritating antiperspirant. Zirconium salt preparations, now removed from all antiperspirants, produced a granulomatous reaction. Zirconium-aluminum complexes, however, are often used as the active ingredient in topical antiperspirants and may produce granulomas. Quaternary ammonium compounds in some roll-on deodorants may produce allergic contact dermatitis.

Axillary Deodorants and Feminine Hygiene Sprays. Fragrances, bacteriostats, and propellants cause the majority of the reactions seen with these products. Deodorants that contain cinnamic aldehyde can induce irritation on axillary skin even when tolerated on healthy skin in other sites.

Cosmetic Intolerance Syndrome. Occasionally, a patient will complain of intense burning or stinging after applying any cosmetic. The patient usually has only subjective symptoms, but objective inflammation may also be present. The underlying cause may be difficult to document, even after thorough patch, photopatch, and contact urticaria testing. Endogenous disease, such as seborrheic dermatitis, rosacea, or atopic dermatitis, may complicate the assessment. Avoidance of all cosmetics, with only glycerin being allowed, for 6–12 months is often necessary to calm the reactive state. Adding back cosmetics one at a time, no more frequently than one a week, may then be tolerated.

Antelmi A, et al: Are gloves sufficiently protective when hairdressers are exposed to permanent hair dyes? An in vivo study. Contact Dermatitis 2015; 72: 229.

Beleznay K, et al: Analysis of the prevalent of allergic contact dermatitis to sunscreen. J Cutan Med Surg 2014; 18: 15.

Bourgeois P, Goossens A: Allergic contact cheilitis caused by menthol in toothpaste and throat medication. Contact Dermatitis 2016; 75: 113.

Bråred Christensson J, et al: Positive patch test reactions to oxidized limonene. Contact Dermatitis 2014; 71: 264.

Cheng J, Zug KA: Fragrance allergic contact dermatitis. Dermatitis 2014; 25: 232.

Das S, et al: Shellac. Dermatitis 2011; 22: 220.

de Groot AC: Propolis. Dermatitis 2013; 24: 263.

de Groot AC, Roberts DW: Contact and photocontact allergy to octocrylene. Contact Dermatitis 2014; 70: 193.

Diepgen TL, et al: Prevalence of fragrance contact allergy in the general population of five European countries. Br J Dermatol 2015; 173: 1411.

Elliott JF, et al: Severe intractable eyelid dermatitis probably caused by exposure to hydroperoxides of linalool in a heavily fragranced shampoo. Contact Dermatitis 2017; 76: 114.

Ghazavi MK, et al: Photo-allergic contact dermatitis caused by isoamyl P-methoxycinnamate in an "organic" sunscreen. Contact Dermatitis 2011; 64: 115.

González-Muñoz P, et al: Allergic contact dermatitis caused by cosmetic products. Actas Dermosifiliogr 2014; 105: 822.

Haylett AK, et al: Sunscreen photopatch testing. Br J Dermatol 2014; 171: 370.

Heurung AR, et al: Adverse reactions to sunscreen agents. Dermatitis 2014; 25: 289.

Jacob SE, et al: Nickel ferrule applicators. Pediatr Dermatol 2015; 32: e62.

Jefferson J, et al: Update on nail cosmetics. Dermatol Ther 2012; 25: 481.

Kock M, et al: Continuous usage of a hair dye product containing 2-methoxymethyl-para-phenylenediamine by hair-dye-allergic individuals. Br J Dermatol 2016; 174: 1042.

Landers MC, et al: Permanent wave dermatitis. Am J Contact Dermat 2003; 14: 157.

Le Q, et al: The rising trend in allergic contact dermatitis to acrylic nail products. Australas J Dermatol 2015; 56: 221.

Leventhal JS, et al: Crystal deodorant-induced axillary granulomatous dermatitis. Int J Dermatol 2014; 53: e59.

Lev-Tov H, et al: The sensitive skin syndrome. Indian J Dermatol 2012; 57: 419.

Lopez IE, et al: Clues to diagnosis of connubial contact dermatitis to paraphenylenediamine. Dermatitis 2014; 25: 32.

Miest RY, et al: Diagnosis and prevalence of lanolin allergy. Dermatitis 2013; 24: 119.

Montgomery R, et al: Contact allergy resulting from the use of acrylate nails is increasing in both users and those who are occupationally exposed. Contact Dermatitis 2016; 74: 120.

Mowitz M, et al: Fragrance patch tests prepared in advance may give false-negative reactions. Contact Dermatitis 2014; 71: 289.

Nardelli A, et al: Results of patch testing with fragrance mix 1, fragrance mix 2, and their ingredients, and *Myroxylon pereirae* and *colophonium*, over a 21-year period. Contact Dermatitis 2013; 68: 307.

Panasoff J: Cheilitis caused by to mint-containing toothpastes. Contact Dermatitis 2016; 75: 260.

Panfili E, et al: Temporary black henna tattoos and sensitization to para-phenylenediamine (PPD). Int J Environ Res Public Health 2017; 14: E421.

Park ME, Zippin JH: Allergic contact dermatitis to cosmetics. Dermatol Clin 2014; 32: 1.

Sabroe RA, et al: Contact allergy to essential oils cannot always be predicted from allergy to fragrance markers in the baseline series. Contact Dermatitis 2016; 74: 236.

Scheman A, et al: Balsam of Peru. Dermatitis 2013; 24: 153.

Uter W, et al: Coupled exposure to ingredients of cosmetic products. Contact Dermatitis 2014; 70: 219.

Preservatives

Preservatives are added to any preparation that contains water to kill microorganisms and prevent spoilage. Such products include moist materials such as baby wipes, which when used in either infants or adults can produce reactions caused by preservatives. The most important class is formaldehyde and the formaldehyde-releasing compounds, including quaternium 15 (the leading preservative sensitizer in the United States), imidazolidinyl urea, diazolidinyl urea, DMDM hydantoin, and 2-bromo-2-nitropropane-1,3-diol.

Kathon CG, or methylchloroisothiazolinone/methylisothiazolinone (MCI/MI), and Euxyl K 400 (methyldibromoglutaronitrile and phenoxyethanol in 1 : 4 ratio) are other important preservative allergens. MCI/MI is widely used in cosmetics and personal care products such as baby wipes and moist towelettes, but may be found in medical devices, and in industrial products such as cutting oils, household detergents, paints, and glues. MCI is a stronger allergen, however use of MI alone in high concentrations has led to a increase in primary sensitization to it. Testing should be to each chemical separately. In Euxyl K 400, the methyldibromoglutaronitrile component produces the allergic response. This preservative may produce false-negative results on testing, so repeat open testing is indicated if a specific leave-on product is suspected of causing allergy. European regulations limit exposure to methyldibromoglutaronitrile. As with similar laws regulating nickel in Europe, allergy to this preservative is also lowering in incidence over time.

Tea tree oil is an additive to some natural products that may serve as an antimicrobial. It is a frequent sensitizer as many products include this oil as a "natural" antimicrobial agent. Sorbic acid is a rare sensitizer among the preservatives; however, it is a cause of facial flushing and stinging through its action as an inducer of nonimmunologic contact urticaria. Benzalkonium chloride is widely used but a rare sensitizer. Triclosan and benzyl alcohol are weak sensitizers. Thimerosal is discussed earlier.

Formaldehyde and Formaldehyde-Releasing Agents. Formaldehyde is used rarely, primarily in shampoos. Because it is quickly diluted and washed away, sensitization through this exposure is rare. Formaldehyde releasers are polymers of formaldehyde that may release small amounts of formaldehyde under certain conditions. Allergy may be to the formaldehyde-releasing preservatives (which act as antibacterial and antifungal agents in their own right) or to the released formaldehyde. Cross-reactivity among them is common, so when allergy is proved to one compound and avoidance does not clear the eruption, screening for clinically relevant reactions to the others is indicated. This may be done by repetitive open application testing to the leave-on product or by extended patch testing.

Parabens. Allergic contact dermatitis may develop from parabens, which are used in cosmetics, foods, drugs, dentifrices, and suppositories. The paraben esters (methyl, ethyl, propyl, and butyl p-hydroxybenzoates) are used in low concentrations in cosmetics and rarely cause dermatitis. They are found in higher concentration in topical medicaments and may be the cause of allergic reactions. Parabens, which are frequently used as bacteriostatic agents, are capable of producing immunologically mediated, immediate systemic hypersensitivity reactions. Cross-reactivity to p-phenylenediamine and benzocaine occurs in some individuals.

Other Important Preservatives. Iodopropynyl butylcarbamate is a wood and paint preservative that is being used more commonly in cosmetics and personal care products. This accounts for its reported higher importance among preservative allergens. The hands are the most frequent area sensitized. Gallates are antioxidant preservatives that are also emerging as important allergens; propyl gallate is the most commonly reported gallate allergen. It usually produces hand and facial eruptions as it is most commonly encountered by patients in cosmetics and personal care products. p-Chloro-metaxylenol (PCMX), a chlorinated phenol antiseptic is used in many over-the-counter products with the disinfectant properties of p-chloro-metacresol to which it is cross-reactive.

Aerts O, et al: Contact allergy caused by methylisothiazolinone. Eur J Dermatol 2015; 25: 228.
Cheng S, et al: Contact sensitivity to preservatives in Singapore. Dermatitis 2014; 25: 77.
Chow ET, et al: Frequency of positive patch test reactions to preservatives. Australas J Dermatol 2013; 54: 31.
Curry EJ, et al: Benzyl alcohol allergy. Dermatitis 2005; 16: 203.
Hauksson I, et al: Formaldehyde in cosmetics in patch tested dermatitis patients with and without contact allergy to formaldehyde. Contact Dermatitis 2016; 74: 145.
Holcomb ZE, et al: Gallate contact dermatitis. Dermatitis 2017; 28: 115.
Murad A, Marren P: Prevalence of methylchloroisothiazolinone and methylisothiazolinone contact allergy in facial dermatitis. J Eur Acad Dermatol Venereol 2016; 30: 60.
Pontén A, Bruze M: Formaldehyde. Dermatitis 2015; 26: 3.
Warshaw EM, et al: North American contact dermatitis group patch test results. Dermatitis 2015; 26: 49.
Wilson M, et al: Chloroxylenol. Dermatitis 2007; 18: 120.
Yim E, et al: Contact dermatitis caused by preservatives. Dermatitis 2014; 25: 215.
Yu SH, et al: Patch testing for methylisothiazolinone and methylchloroisothiazolinone-methylisothiazolinone contact allergy. JAMA Dermatol 2016; 152: 67.

Vehicles

Formulation of topically applied products is complex, and additives are blended to make a pleasant base for carriage of the active ingredient to the skin. Various emulsifiers, humectants, stabilizers, surfactants, and surface active agents are used to make esthetically pleasing preparations. These may cause irritation, erythema, and allergy. The surfactant cocamidopropyl betaine produces dermatitis of the head and neck in consumers and the hands in hairdressers, often from its presence in shampoos. Sorbitan sesquioleate is an emulsifier in the fragrance I mix. It may produce false-positive results to fragrance in the few patients sensitive to it. Propolis and lanolin are discussed previously under "Cosmetic Dermatitis."

Propylene Glycol. Propylene glycol is widely used as a vehicle for topical medications, cosmetics (especially antiperspirants), and various emollient lotions. It is used in the manufacture of automobile brake fluid and alkyd resins, as a lubricant for food machinery, and as an additive for food colors and flavoring agents. Propylene glycol must be considered as a sensitizer able to produce contact dermatitis, and it can cause a flare of the contact dermatitis when ingested. It is tested as a 4% aqueous solution, but irritant reactions or false-negative results are common. A use test of the implicated propylene glycol–containing products may be required.

Ethylenediamine. Ethylenediamine is used as a stabilizer in medicated creams. It may cause contact dermatitis and cross-react with internally taken aminophylline, which consists of theophylline and ethylenediamine. Hydroxyzine is a piperazine derivative that is structurally based on a dimer of ethylenediamine, to which patients sensitive to the stabilizer may develop a generalized itchy, red eruption that recurs each time hydroxyzine is taken orally.

Bennike NH, Johansen JD: Sorbitan sesquioleate; a rare cause of contact allergy in consecutively patch tested dermatitis patients. Contact Dermatitis 2016; 74: 242.
Goossens RA: Allergic contact dermatitis from the vehicle components of topical pharmaceutical products. Immunol Allergy Clin North Am 2014; 34: 663.
Jacob SE, et al: Cocamidopropyl betaine. Dermatitis 2008; 19: 157.
Reid N, et al: Worsening of contact dermatitis by oral hydroxyzine: a case report. Dermatol Online J 2013; 19: 4.
Warshaw EM, et al: Positive patch-test reactions to propylene glycol. Dermatitis 2009; 20: 14.
Welling JD, et al: Chronic eyelid dermatitis secondary to cocamidopropyl betaine allergy in a patient using baby shampoo eyelid scrubs. JAMA Ophthalmol 2014; 132: 357.

Topical Drug Contact Dermatitis

Drugs, in addition to their pharmacologic and possible toxic action, also possess sensitizing properties. Sensitization may occur not only from topical application (Fig. 6.19) but also from ingestion, injection, or inhalation. Some drugs, such as the antihistamines, including topical doxepin, sensitize much more frequently when applied topically than when taken orally. With the advent of transdermal patches for delivery of medications (e.g., nitroglycerin, hormones, nicotine, clonidine, fentanyl, lidocaine, and scopolamine)

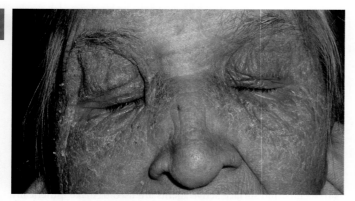

Fig. 6.19 Contact dermatitis to eyedrops. (Courtesy Shyam Verma, MBBS, DVD.)

reports of sensitization have been increasing. Clonidine induces the highest rate of allergic reactions. At times, EM-like reactions may occur with transdermally applied drugs.

Some drugs may produce sensitization of the skin when applied topically; if the medication is taken later internally, an acute flare at the site of the contact dermatitis may result. This anamnestic (recalled) eruption or systemic contact dermatitis can occur with antihistamines, sulfonamides, and penicillin. The same is true of the local anesthetic ointments containing "caine" medications, but not as a rule with lidocaine allergy. Usually, if sensitization occurs when using transdermal patches, the drugs do not cause systemic contact dermatitis when taken orally. The important topical medications that cause irritation or allergic contact dermatitis are discussed next.

Local Anesthetics. Physicians and dentists may develop allergic contact dermatitis from local anesthetics. In addition, the continued use of these local anesthetics as antipruritic ointments and lotions causes sensitization of the skin. Benzocaine is a frequently used topical antipruritic and is the most common topical sensitizer of this group. Itchy dermatitis of the anogenital area may be caused by a topical anesthetic.

Local anesthetics may be divided into two groups. The first group includes the *p*-aminobenzoic acid esters, such as benzocaine, butethamine, chloroprocaine, procaine (Novacaine), and tetracaine. The second group, which sensitizes much less frequently, includes the amides, such as dibucaine (Nupercainal), lidocaine (Lido-Mantle, EMLA, Lidoderm patch, LMX, Xylocaine), mepivacaine (Carbocaine), and prilocaine. In addition, the preservative methylparaben, frequently found in these prepared solutions, may cause hypersensitivity reactions that can easily be misattributed to the local anesthetics. It should be kept in mind that numerous cross-reactions are seen in benzocaine-sensitive individuals. These are discussed earlier in the sections on sunscreens and preservatives. Lidocaine can induce contact urticaria as well. Finally pramoxine has a distinctive structure and is not an amide nor an ester anesthetic. It may rarely induce contact allergy of both the immediate and delayed types.

Antimicrobials. Physicians, dentists, nurses, and other medical personnel, as well as patients, especially those with chronic leg ulcers, may develop contact dermatitis from various antibiotics. Neomycin and bacitracin are the most common sensitizers in the United States. Neomycin sulfate has been incorporated into innumerable ointments, creams, and lotions, including underarm deodorants, otic and ophthalmologic preparations, and antibiotic creams and ointments available without prescription. The signs of neomycin sensitivity may be those of a typical contact dermatitis but are often signs of a recalcitrant skin eruption that has become lichenified and even hyperkeratotic. This may result because many topical agents contain several types of antibiotic but also often have corticosteroids present. This picture may be seen in persistent external otitis, lichen simplex chronicus of the nuchal area, or dermatophytosis between the toes. A late-appearing reaction on patch testing can occur, so an assessment at day 7 is recommended.

Allergy to bacitracin increased dramatically because of its use after minor surgical procedures. After clean surgical procedures, white petrolatum is as effective in wound healing as antibiotic ointment and does not carry the allergenic potential. Petrolatum should be used after clean cutaneous surgery; antibiotic ointments are not necessary. There is a high rate of co-reaction (not cross-reaction) with neomycin because of simultaneous exposures. Contact urticaria and anaphylaxis are reported more often with bacitracin than with other antibiotics.

Mafenide acetate, the topical antimicrobial found in Sulfamylon, a burn remedy, may cause allergic contact dermatitis, as can metronidazole. Polymyxin B is an uncommon sensitizer.

Antifungal Agents. Allergic contact dermatitis to imidazole and other antifungal agents may occur. There is a high cross-reactivity rate among miconazole, isoconazole, clotrimazole, and oxiconazole because of their common chemical structure.

Corticosteroids. Numerous reports of large series of patients who have developed allergy to common corticosteroid preparations emphasize the need for a high index of suspicion when treating patients with chronic dermatitis who fail to improve, or who worsen, when topical steroidal agents are used. Once sensitized to one type of corticosteroid, cross-sensitization may occur. The corticosteroids have been separated into the following four structural classes:

- Class A is the hydrocortisone, tixocortol pivalate group.
- Class B is the triamcinolone acetonide, budesonide group.
- Class C is the betamethasone group.
- Class D is the hydrocortisone-17-butyrate group.

There are frequent cross-reactions between classes B and D. Tixocortol pivalate and budesonide have been found to be the best screening agents, finding 93% of steroid allergies. Patch testing to the implicated leave-on product may be useful. An empiric trial of desoximetasone (Topicort) or mometasone (Elocon) in the absence of patch testing will give the best chance of selecting a topical steroid with an extremely low risk of sensitization.

Alfalah M, et al: Contact allergy to polymyxin B among patients referred to patch testing. Dermatitis 2016; 27: 119.

Corbo MD, et al: Lidocaine allergy. Dermatitis 2016; 27: 68.

Cronin H, et al: Anaphylactic reaction to bacitracin ointment. Cutis 2009; 83: 127.

Fathi R, et al: Identifying and managing local anesthetic allergy in dermatologic surgery. Dermatol Surg 2016; 42: 147.

Foti C, et al: Contact dermatitis to topical acne drugs. Dermatol Ther 2015; 28: 323.

Gilissen L, Goossens A: Frequency and trends of contact allergy to and iatrogenic contact dermatitis caused by topical drugs over a 25-year period. Contact Dermatitis 2016; 75: 290.

Hylwa SA, Warshaw E: Contact allergy to pramoxine (pramocaine). Dermatitis 2014; 25: 147.

Jean SE, et al: Contact dermatitis in leg ulcer patients. J Cutan Med Surg 2009; 13: S38.

Kim SJ, Goldberg BJ: Anaphylaxis due to topical pramoxine. Ann Allergy Asthma Immunol 2015; 114: 72.

Kot M, et al: Contact allergy in the population of patients with chronic inflammatory dermatoses and contact hypersensitivity to corticosteroids. Postepy Dermatol Alergol 2017; 34: 253.

Musel AL, et al: Cutaneous reactions to transdermal therapeutic systems. Dermatitis 2006; 17: 109.

Nihawan RI, et al: Systemic contact dermatitis. Dermatol Clin 2009; 27: 355.

Otani IM, Banerji A: Immediate and delayed hypersensitivity reactions to corticosteroids. Curr Allergy Asthma Rep 2016; 16: 18.

Sasseville K: Contact dermatitis from topical antibiotics. Eur J Dermatol 2011; 3: 311.

Tang MM, et al: Severe cutaneous allergic reactions following topical antifungal therapy. Contact Dermatitis 2013; 68: 56.

Timmermans MW, et al: Allergic contact dermatitis from EMLA cream. J Dtsch Dermatol Ges 2009; 7: 237.

To D, et al: Lidocaine contact allergy is becoming more prevalent. Dermatol Surg 2014; 40: 1367.

Vatti RR, et al: Hypersensitivity reactions to corticosteroids. Clin Rev Allergy Immunol 2014; 47: 26.

Occupational Contact Dermatitis

Workers in various occupations are prone to contact dermatitis from primary irritants and allergic contactants. In certain occupations, it is a common occurrence. Irritant contact dermatitis occurs more frequently in the workplace, but it tends to be less severe and less chronic than allergic contact dermatitis. Occupational skin disease has declined over the past 30 years but still constitutes approximately 10% of all occupational disease cases. Agriculture, forestry, and fishing have the highest incidence of occupational skin disease, with the manufacturing and health care sectors contributing many cases as well.

Irritant contact dermatitis is often present in wet-work jobs, and allergy occurs in hairdressers, machinists, and many others with unique exposures to multiple sensitizing chemicals. The hands are the parts most affected and are involved in 60% of allergic reactions and 80% of irritant dermatitis. Epoxy resin is an allergen overrepresented when evaluating occupational patients. The allergens most frequently encountered in occupational cases are carba mix, thiuram mix, epoxy resin, formaldehyde, and nickel.

Management

Occupational contact dermatitis is managed by eliminating contact of the skin with irritating and sensitizing substances. The work environment should be carefully controlled, with use of all available protective devices to prevent accidental and even planned exposures. Personal protective measures, such as frequent clothing changes, cleansing showers, protective clothing, and protective barrier creams, should be used as appropriate. Hand-cleansing procedures should be thoroughly surveyed, with particular attention to the soaps available and the solvents used.

Treatment of the dermatitis follows closely that recommended for *Toxicodendron* dermatitis. Topical corticosteroid preparations are especially helpful in the acute phase. For dry, fissured hands, soaking them in water for 20 minutes at night followed immediately on removing (without drying them) with triamcinolone 0.1% ointment will help hydrate and heal. Topical tacrolimus ointment and pimecrolimus cream may assist in maintenance therapy, along with high-lipid content moisturizing creams. When rubber and polyvinyl gloves cannot be used against irritant and allergenic substances, protective skin creams may offer a solution but are often impractical. A wide variety is available, but two main types are used: for "wet work," to protect against acids, alkalis, water-based paints, coolants, and cutting oils with water; and for "dry work," to protect against oils, greases, cutting oils, adhesive, resins, glues, and wood preservatives.

Unfortunately, despite the best efforts at treatment and prevention, the prognosis for occupational skin disease is guarded. One third to one quarter heal, and another one third to one half improve, with the remainder the same or worse. A change or discontinuance of the job does not guarantee relief; many individuals continue to have persistent postoccupational dermatitis. The importance of thorough patient education cannot be overemphasized. Atopic patients, males with chromate allergy, females with nickel allergy, those with a delay in diagnosis before institution of treatment, and construction industry workers fare the worst, whereas irritation from metalworking fluids, reactions to urushiols in foresters, and allergic contact dermatitis to acrylic monomers or amine curing agents is usually short-lived.

Bauer A, et al: Intervention for preventing occupational irritant hand dermatitis. Cochrane Database Syst Rev 2010; 6: CD004414.

de Groot AC: New contact allergens. Dermatitis 2015; 26: 199.

Friis UF, et al: Occupational irritant contact dermatitis diagnosed by analysis of contact irritants and allergens in the work environment. Contact Dermatitis 2014; 71: 364.

Higgins CL, et al: Occupational skin disease among Australian healthcare workers. Contact Dermatitis 2016; 75: 213.

Holness DL: Occupational skin allergies. Curr Allergy Asthma Rep 2014; 14: 410.

Kasemsarn P, et al: The role of the skin barrier in occupational skin diseases. Curr Probl Dermatol 2016; 49: 135.

Lugović-Mihić L, et al: Occupational contact dermatitis amongst dentists and dental technicians. Acta Clin Croat 2016; 55: 293.

Lukács J, et al: Occupational contact urticaria caused by food—a systematic clinical review. Contact Dermatitis 2016; 75: 195.

Mälkönen T, et al: Long-term follow-up study of occupational hand eczema. Br J Dermatol 2010; 163: 999.

Nicholson PJ, et al: Evidence-based guidelines for the prevention, identification and management of occupational contact dermatitis and urticaria. Contact Dermatitis 2010; 63: 177.

Oreskov KW, et al: Glove use among hairdressers. Contact Dermatitis 2015; 72: 362.

Otani IM, Banerji A: Immediate and delayed hypersensitivity reactions to proton pump inhibitors. Curr Allergy Asthma Rep 2016; 16: 17.

Slodownik D, et al: Occupational factors in skin diseases. Curr Probl Dermatol 2007; 35: 173.

Sohrabian S, et al: Contact dermatitis in agriculture. J Agromed 2007; 12: 3.

Whitaker P: Occupational allergy to pharmaceutical products. Curr Opin Allergy Clin Immunol 2016; 16: 101.

Wiszniewska M, Walusiak-Skorupa J: Recent trends in occupational contact dermatitis. Curr Allergy Asthma Rep 2015; 15: 43.

Contact Urticaria

Contact urticaria may be defined as a wheal and flare reaction occurring when a substance is applied to the intact skin. Urticaria is only one of a broad spectrum of immediate reactions, including pruritus, dermatitis, local or general urticaria, bronchial asthma, orolaryngeal edema, rhinoconjunctivitis, gastrointestinal distress, headache, or anaphylactic reaction. Any combination of these is subsumed under the expression "syndrome of immediate reactions."

Contact urticaria may be nonimmunologic (no prior sensitization), immunologic, or of unknown mechanism. The nonimmunologic type is the most common and may be caused by direct release of vasoactive substances from mast cells. The allergic type tends to be the most severe, because anaphylaxis is possible. The third type has features of both other types.

Nonimmunologic Mechanism. The nonimmunologic type of reaction induces contact urticaria in almost all exposed individuals. Examples of this type of reaction are seen with nettle rash (plants), dimethyl sulfoxide (DMSO), sorbic acid, benzoic acid, cinnamic aldehyde, cobalt chloride, and Trafuril.

Immunologic Mechanism. The immunologic reaction is of the immediate (immunoglobulin E [IgE]–mediated) type of hypersensitivity. Latex, potatoes, phenylmercuric propionate, and many other allergens have been reported to cause this type.

Uncertain Mechanism. The uncertain type of reaction occurs with agents that produce contact urticaria and a generalized histamine type of reaction but lack a direct or immunologic basis for the reaction.

Substances Causing Contact Urticaria. Many different substances can elicit such a reaction. Universal precautions not only led to a marked increase in delayed-type hypersensitivity reaction to rubber additives, but also to many reports of contact urticaria and anaphylaxis to latex. Most of these reactions occur in health professionals. Reactions are characterized by itching and swelling of the hands within a few minutes of donning the gloves, usually resolving within an hour after removing them. In patients with continued exposure, the eruption may eventually appear as chronic eczema. Glove powder may aerosolize the allergen and produce more generalized reactions. Although these reactions may occur on the job, many cases present as death or near-death events when sensitized individuals undergo surgery or other procedures, especially when there is mucosal exposure (e.g., dental care, rectal examination, childbirth).

In addition to health care workers, who have a reported incidence of 3%–10%, atopic persons and spina bifida patients are other risk groups for the development of type I allergy to latex protein. The sensitized individual should also be aware that up to 50% of patients have a concomitant fruit allergy to foods such as banana, avocado, kiwi, chestnut, and passion fruit.

Contact urticaria is seen in homemakers and food workers who handle raw vegetables, raw meats and fish, shellfish, and other foods. Raw potatoes have been shown to cause not only contact urticaria but also asthma at the same time. It has been seen in hairdressers who handle bleaches and hair dyes containing ammonium persulfate, in whom the contact urticaria is accompanied by swelling and erythema of the face, followed by unconsciousness. Caterpillars, moths, and hedgehogs may cause contact urticaria just by touching the skin.

Additional substances inducing this reaction are oatmeal, flour, meat, turkey skin, calf liver, banana, lemon, monoamylamine, benzophenone, nail polish, tetanus antitoxin, streptomycin, cetyl alcohol, stearyl alcohol, estrogenic cream, cinnamic aldehyde, sorbic acid, benzoic acid, castor bean, lindane, carrots, spices, wool, silk, dog and cat saliva, dog hairs, horse serum, ammonia, sulfur dioxide, formaldehyde, acrylic monomers, exotic woods, wheat, cod liver oil, and aspirin.

Bacitracin ointment may cause anaphylactic reactions when applied topically, especially to chronic leg ulcers; however, it may rarely occur after application to acute wounds (Fig. 6.20).

Testing. The usual closed patch tests do not show sensitivity reactions. Instead, open patch tests are performed for eliciting immediate-type hypersensitivity. The substance is applied to a 1-cm² area on the forearm and observed for 20–30 minutes for erythema that evolves into a wheal and flare response. When foods are tested, a small piece of the actual food is placed on the skin. Rubber glove testing can be done by applying one finger of a latex glove to a moistened hand for 15 minutes. If no reaction is observed, the entire glove is worn for another 15–20 minutes. The radioallergosorbent test (RAST) detects 75% of latex-allergic individuals. Prick, scratch, or intradermal testing is undertaken only when there are problems of interpretation of the open patch tests. These tests have produced anaphylactic reactions and should only be attempted when support for this complication is available.

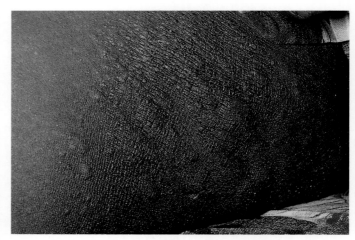

Fig. 6.20 Contact urticaria caused by bacitracin applied to punch biopsy site.

Management. Avoidance of the offending substance is best, but if this is not possible, antihistamines are of benefit. If generalized urticaria or asthmatic reactions occur, systemic glucocorticoids are best. For anaphylaxis, epinephrine and supportive measures are needed.

Barbaud A, et al: Occupational protein contact dermatitis. Eur J Dermatol 2015; 25: 527.

Bensefa-Colas L, et al: Occupational contact urticarial. Br J Dermatol 2015; 173: 1453.

Cronin H, et al: Anaphylactic reaction to bacitracin ointment. Cutis 2009; 83: 127.

Firoz EF, et al: Lip plumper contact urticaria. J Am Acad Dermatol 2009; 60: 861.

Gimenez-Arnau A, et al: Immediate contact skin reactions, an update of contact urticaria, contact urticarial syndrome and protein contact dermatitis. Eur J Dermatol 2010; 20: 552.

Ibler KS, et al: Prevalence of delayed-type and immediate-type hypersensitivity in healthcare workers with hand eczema. Contact Dermatitis 2016; 75: 223.

Lukács J, et al: Occupational contact urticaria caused by food—a systematic clinical review. Contact Dermatitis 2016; 75: 195.

Miceli Sopo S, et al: Contact urticaria on eczematous skin by kiwifruit allergy. Allergol Immunopathol (Madr) 2015; 43: 474.

Orb Q, et al: Prevalence and interest in the practice of scratch testing for contact urticaria. Dermatitis 2014; 25: 366.

Williams JD, et al: Occupational contact urticaria. Br J Dermatol 2008; 159: 125.

DRUG REACTIONS

Epidemiology

Adverse drug reactions (ADRs) are a common cause of dermatologic consultation. In a large French study, about 1 in 200 inpatients on medical services developed a drug eruption, compared with 1 in 10,000 on surgical services. In the United States, similar studies have shown a reaction rate of 2%–3% for medical inpatients. In only about 55% of patients who were carefully evaluated was it possible to attribute a specific medication definitely as the cause of the eruption. Simple exanthems (75%–95%) and urticaria (5%–6%) account for the vast majority of drug eruptions. Females are 1.3–1.5 times more likely to develop drug eruptions, except in children under age 3 years, with boys more likely to be affected than girls. Aminopenicillins cause drug eruptions in 1.2%–8% of exposures and trimethoprim-sulfamethoxazole (TMP-SMX) in 2.8%–3.7%. About 20% of emergency department visits for adverse events caused by medications are related to antibiotics, mainly penicillins and cephalosporins. Nonsteroidal antiinflammatory drugs (NSAIDs) have a reaction rate of about 1 in 200. In contrast, reaction rates for digoxin, lidocaine, prednisone, codeine, and acetaminophen are less than 1 in 1000.

Patients with immune dysregulation (lupus, HIV, bone marrow transplant) and multiple drug exposures have higher rates of reactions. Patients with human immunodeficiency virus (HIV) or Epstein-Barr virus (EBV) infection have dramatically increased rates of exanthematous reactions to certain antibiotics. Hypersensitivity syndromes from multiple drug classes have been associated with reactivation of latent viral infections, primarily human herpesvirus (HHV) 6 and HHV-7, but also EBV and cytomegalovirus (CMV). Certain human leukocyte antigen (HLA) types in specific populations, may increase risk for drug reactions for specific medications, with personalized pharmacogenomics emerging as a strategy to prevent ADRs

Evaluation

All patients with a suspected drug reaction should be evaluated for primary lesion morphology and distribution of the rash, checked for concerning, atypical, or high-risk features, and examined for any extracutaneous manifestations. Four basic rules should always be applied in evaluating the patient with a suspected ADR, as follows:

1. The patient is probably on unnecessary medications, and all of these should be stopped. Pare down the medication list to the bare essentials.
2. The patient must be asked about nonprescription medications and pharmaceuticals delivered by other means (e.g., eyedrops, suppositories, implants, injections, patches, dialysates, radiocontrast agents, recreational drugs, herbal supplements, vitamins, minerals, and more).
3. Regardless of how atypical the patient's cutaneous reaction, always consider medication as a possible cause. In patients with unusual reactions, searching the medical literature and calling the manufacturer for prior reports may be useful.
4. The timing of drug administration must correlate with the appearance of the eruption. A drug chart lists all the drugs given to the patient in the left column, with the dates along the lower axis, and the course of the drug eruption at the top. Lines extend from left to right for the dates of administration of each medication. These are directly below the course of the eruption. This graphic representation of the timing of medication administration and eruption is a very handy tool in assigning plausibility to a certain medication causing an eruption. It is important to consider dose changes, concomitant medications that may affect drug levels, comorbid illnesses that may affect metabolism (i.e., kidney injury), and whether patients have changed from brand name to generic drug types.

An important step in evaluating a patient with a potential ADR is to diagnose the cutaneous eruption by clinical pattern (e.g., exanthema, urticaria, vasculitis, pustular, hypersensitivity syndrome). Regularly updated manuals (e.g., Litt) or similar Internet databases are strongly recommended as reference sources for this information. Attribution scoring systems exist, but are generally used in clinical research settings (Naranjo scale, Kramer criteria). The following questions provide a framework for evaluation:

- Has the suspected medication been reported to cause the reaction the patient is experiencing? How frequently? Has the patient had a previous reaction to any medications?
- What are other possible causes of the patient's eruption? For example, an exanthem could be related to an associated viral illness, not the medication.

- When did the eruption appear relative to the administration of the suspected medication?
- Certain reactions are known to be related to rate of administration (vancomycin red man syndrome) or cumulative dose (lichenoid reactions to gold). Could the rate or dose be causing this patient's reaction?
- Does the eruption clear when the suspected medication is stopped? Because certain eruptions may clear with continuation of the drug, however, this is a useful, but not irrefutable, criterion to ascribe a specific reaction to a medication.
- Does the reaction recur with rechallenge?

Skin testing may be useful in evaluating type I (immediate) hypersensitivity reactions. It is most frequently used in evaluating adverse reactions to penicillin, local anesthetics, insulin, and vaccines. RAST has demonstrated a 20% false-negative rate in penicillin type I allergy; thus, in their current form, RASTs cannot replace skin testing. Intradermal, skin prick, and patch testing are also reported to be beneficial in some patients with morbilliform reactions, acute generalized exanthematous pustulosis, drug reaction with eosinophilia and systemic symptoms (DRESS), or, if done within the site of the eruption, fixed-drug reaction. Lymphocyte transformation tests reveal T-cell sensitization to drugs by measuring the response of peripheral blood mononuclear cells, although false-positive (and negative) results are possible, depending on the type of eruption and timing of testing. The enzyme-linked immunospot (ELISpot) assay, cytokine profiling, and ELISA testing for cytotxic mediators are also utilized in research settings. These are typically utilized for severe cutaneous adverse reactions (SCARs), such as anticonvulsant or sulfonamide hypersensitivity reaction or Stevens-Johnson syndrome (SJS). Serum measurement of drug-specific IgEs may also be used in some cases.

The patient should be given concrete advice about the reaction. The primary concern is whether the patient can continue on or retake the medication in question. This requires carefully weighing the severity of the eruption, likelihood of true reaction, risks and benefits of reexposure, and alternate treatment options (and risk of cross-reactivity) for the condition for which the drug was prescribed. Unusual reactions should be reported to regulatory agencies and the manufacturer for pharmacovigiliance and postmarketing identification of potentially important reaction patterns.

Pathogenesis

The pathogenesis of the various ADRs varies by subtype. Most common cutaneous ADRs are type I (urticarial reactions, IgE mediated) or type IV (delayed). Type IV, delayed-type reactions, can be subdivided into type IVa (T-helper 1 [Th1] cells, interferon [IFN]-γ/tumor necrosis factor–α [TNF-α] mediated), type IVb (T-helper 2 [Th2], interleukin [IL]-4/IL-5/IL-13), type IVc (cytotoxic T cells, granzyme), and type IVd (neutrophils, CXCL-8, granulocyte-macrophage colony-stimulating factor [GM-CSF]), which correlates with the clinical morphologic pattern of the ADR. T cells in the dermis in acute generalized exanthematous pustulosis (AGEP, an example of a type IVd reaction) secrete IL-8, a neutrophil-attracting chemokine. In drug rash (reaction) with eosinophilia and systemic symptoms (DRESS, a type IVb reaction), they secrete IL-5 and eotaxin, recruiting eosinophils. As a consequence of T-helper cell activation, memory T cells are produced, resulting in recurrence of many eruptions on rechallenge.

Large molecules, such as rat- or mouse-derived antibodies, can be immunogenic. Most medications, however, are too small to be recognized as antigens by immunologically active cells. The medication is the hapten, and the immunologically active molecule is a medication-protein complex or hapten-carrier complex. Some medications, such as penicillin, are active enough to bind directly to proteins. Most, however, need to be metabolized to more active or more immunogenic forms to bind to proteins and cause an

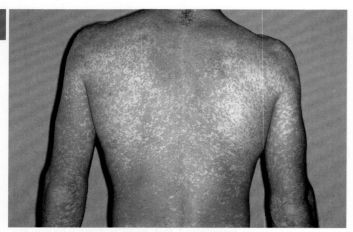

Fig. 6.21 Morbilliform (exanthematous) drug eruption caused by exposure to an antibiotic.

immunologic reaction. The drug metabolites can also be toxic to cells, causing direct cell damage. Drug metabolism varies by drug class, but frequently occurs in the cytochrome P450 system in the liver.

There has also been a proposed model for ADRs in which the drug or a metabolite binds directly to T cells or Langerhans cells in close opposition to sentinel T cells in the skin. This direct binding could activate the T cell–Langerhans cell interactive unit, resulting in the production of biologically active molecules. This would explain how some drug eruptions occur soon after exposure or with the first exposure to a medication. It could also explain a dose-dependent effect in drug eruptions. Also, a systemic viral infection may have already activated the immune cells in the skin, reducing their threshold for activation by drug binding. Once the T cell is activated, it may produce a variety of reactions, as follows:

1. T cells stimulate IFN-γ production and a Th1 response. This type of reaction could be "bullous" but without extensive epidermal necrosis (contact dermatitis).
2. T cells could be activated to function in a Th2 manner and stimulate eosinophil ingress through Th2 cytokines (DRESS).
3. T cells could activate cytotoxic (CD8+) T cells, which would secrete perforin/granzyme B and Fas ligand, resulting in keratinocyte apoptosis (SJS/ toxic epidermal necrolysis [TEN]).
4. T cells, through chemokine (CXCL8) and cytokine (IL-8, GM-CSF) production, recruit neutrophils, resulting in pustular exanthems (AGEP).

Th17 cells are implicated in many drug eruptions, and sulfamethoxazole induces a T-cell switch mechanism based on the TCRVβ20-1 domain altering peptide–HLA recognition. Dermal CD4+/CD25+/Foxp3 regulatory T cells (Tregs) are reduced in severe bullous drug eruptions such as TEN. Circulating Tregs expressing skin-homing molecules are increased in early drug-induced hypersensitivity syndrome (DIHS, DHS). The cells are immunologically active early in the course of the eruption, enter the skin, and can effectively suppress the immune response. However, they become functionally deficient later, perhaps explaining the occasional development of autoimmune phenomena months after DIHS, as well as the tendency of DIHS reactions to relapse, recur, or fail to resolve. In severe drug reactions, micro-RNA-18a-5p downregulates the expression of the antiapoptotic B-cell lymphoma/leukemia-2–like protein 10 (BCL2L10), promoting apoptosis.

Clinical Morphology

Cutaneous drug reactions are initially discussed here by morphologic pattern. In addition to the cutaneous eruption, some reactions

may be associated with other systemic symptoms or findings. The modifier "simple" is used to describe reactions without systemic symptoms or internal organ involvement. "Complex" reactions are those with systemic findings. This includes drug induced hypersensitivity syndrome (DIHS, DHS), which is synonymous with drug reaction with eosinophilia and systemic symptoms (DRESS), and drug induced delayed multiorgan hypersensitivity syndrome.

Drug reactions may cause cutaneous lesions and findings identical to a known disease or disorder. These may be of similar or disparate pathogenesis. For example, true serum sickness caused by the injection of foreign proteins, such as antithymocyte globulin, is associated with circulating immune complexes. Medications, notably cefaclor, induce a serum sickness–like reaction not associated with circulating immune complexes. Vancomycin-induced linear IgA bullous disease is nearly identical to the de novo disease. Calcium channel blockers (CCBs) and IFN are associated with eczematous eruptions.

Exanthems (Morbilliform or Maculopapular Reactions)

Exanthems are the most common form of adverse cutaneous drug eruption. They are characterized by erythema, often with small papules throughout. Exanthems tend to occur within the first 2 weeks of treatment but may appear later, or even up to 10 days after the medication has been stopped. Lesions tend to appear first proximally, especially in the groin and axilla, generalizing within 1 or 2 days. The face is typically spared; facial involvement should prompt consideration for DRESS. Pruritus is usually prominent, helping to distinguish a drug eruption from a viral exanthema or graft-versus-host disease. Antibiotics, especially semisynthetic penicillins and TMP-SMX, are the most common causes of this reaction pattern (Fig. 6.21). Ampicillin-amoxicillin given during EBV infection causes an exanthem in 29%–69% of adults and 100% of children. TMP-SMX given to AIDS patients causes exanthems in about 40%. Antimalarials given to patients with dermatomyositis cause exanthems in 25%. Certain quinolones cause exanthems at a high rate: 4% overall and 30% in young women.

Morbilliform eruptions may rarely be restricted to a previously sunburned site, the so-called "UV recall–like" phenomenon. The sunburn may have occurred 1–7 months before the drug eruption. This pattern of eruption must be distinguished from a true UV recall caused by antimetabolites (see later section, "Adverse Reactions to Chemotherapeutic Agents").

In the case of simple exanthems, treatment is supportive. The eruption will clear within 2 weeks of stopping the offending medication, and it may clear even if the drug is continued. Topical corticosteroids and antipruritics may be of benefit and allow the course of therapy to be completed. Rechallenge usually results in the reappearance of the eruption, except in the setting of HIV. In many HIV-infected patients with simple reactions to TMP-SMX, reexposure by slow introduction or full-dose reexposure may be tolerated. Infrequently in HIV patients, however, and rarely in persons with normal immune function, rechallenge may result in a more severe blistering reaction. The use of patch and intradermal testing for the confirmation of the incriminated drug in morbilliform exanthems is not standardized. Only 2%–10% of patients who experience the eruption on rechallenge will have a positive patch or intradermal test.

Cutaneous findings identical to simple exanthems may occur as part of DRESS. Most patients with DRESS will have facial involvement, facial edema, ear involvement, and many will have hand edema, all of which are uncommon in simple exanthems. In contrast to simple exanthems, in complex exanthems the inciting agent must be stopped immediately, and rechallenge should rarely be undertaken. Even outside the setting of DRESS, higher eosinophil counts correlate with more severe ADRs.

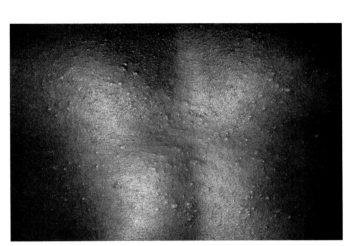

Fig. 6.22 Phenytoin-induced drug reaction with eosinophilia and systemic symptoms.

Barbaud A: Skin testing and patch testing in non-IgE-mediated drug allergy. Curr Allergy Asthma Rep 2014; 14: 442.

Garon SL, et al: Pharmacogenomics of off-target adverse drug reactions. Br J Clin Pharmacol 2017; 83: 1896.

Harp JL, et al: Severe cutaneous adverse reactions: impact of immunology, genetics, and pharmacology. Semin Cutan Med Surg 2014; 33: 17.

Hoetzenecker W, et al: Adverse cutaneous drug eruptions. Semin Immunopathol 2016; 38: 75.

Naldi L, Crotti S: Epidemiology of cutaneous drug-induced reactions. G Ital Dermatol Venereol 2014; 149: 207.

Porebski G, et al: *In vitro* drug causality assessment in Stevens-Johnson syndrome—alternatives for lymphocyte transformation test. Clin Exp All 2013; 43: 1027.

Scripcaru G, et al: Adverse drug events. PLoS One 2017; 12: ePub ahead of print.

Teo Y, et al: Cutaneous adverse drug reaction referrals to a liaison dermatology service. Br J Dermatol 2017; 177: 141.

Young JWS, Shear NH: Cutaneous drug reactions in the elderly. Drugs Aging 2017; 11: ePub ahead of print.

Drug-Induced Hypersensitivity Syndrome or Drug Reaction With Eosinophilia and Systemic Symptoms

DIHS/DRESS is a severe cutaneous eruption with associated systemic involvement, where host genetic factors, medication exposure, plus frequent viral reactivation, lead to activated T cells and create a multiorgan inflammatory reaction. The overall incidence of DRESS is between 1/1000 and 1/10,000 individuals. Genetic factors appear to play an important role in DRESS. Polymorphisms in drug metabolizing enzymes (CYP450, N-acetyltransferase) can lead to reduced activity and increased active drug metabolites. Specific HLA-alleles are associated with the development of DRESS in certain populations.

All patients with DRESS share the characteristic features of fever, rash, and internal organ involvement. Characteristic features include the following:

- Rash developing late (>2, often 4–8 weeks) after the inciting medication is started
- Long-lasting symptoms after discontinuation of the causative drug
- Fever (>38°C)
- Multiorgan involvement

- CBC abnormalities (usually an eosinophilia, but may have activated lymphocytosis instead):
  - Eosinophilia (>1500 absolute eosinophilia; criteria vary, with some groups citing counts greater than 1500/µL and others more than 700/µL or above 10% if the leukocyte count is lower than 4000/µL)
  - Lymphocyte activation (lymphocytosis, atypical lymphocytosis, lymphadenopathy)
- Frequent reactivation of HHV-6, HHV-7, EBV, and CMV (60%–80% of cases demonstrate HHV family reactivation)

Seven major medications/classes of medication are commonly implicated, though DRESS may occur with drugs from almost any category: (1) anticonvulsants—phenytoin, carbamazepine, phenobarbital, and lamotrigine primarily (can occur with the other antiepileptic agents as well); (2) long-acting sulfonamides—sulfamethoxazole, sulfadiazine, and sulfasalazine (but *not* all sulfa-containing medications—sulfonylureas, thiazine diuretics, furosemide, and acetazolamide); (3) allopurinol; (4) nevirapine; (5) abacavir; (6) dapsone; and (7) minocycline. DRESS has been reported with multiple other agents as well, including, but not limited to, antimicrobial agents (vancomycin, cephalosporins, fluoroquinolones, antituberculosis agents, other antibiotics), biologic agents (tocilizumab, IL-1 inhibitors, and more), targeted chemotherapeutics (vismodegib, imatinib, and more), other antiviral agents (telaprevir for hepatitis C before its removal from the market, raltegravir, and others), antipyretic agents (acetaminophen, ibuprofen, diclofenac, celecoxib), and more. Diagnosis of DRESS should be made based on clinical and laboratory features, and drug exposure history, with consideration given to any potential inciting agent, regardless of drug class.

The skin eruption accompanying DRESS/DIHS is typically morbilliform (with variable follicular accentuation [Fig. 6.22] and occasional 2-zone targetoid lesions), and can vary from faint and mild to severe with exfoliative erythroderma. Facial erythema and edema with periorbital sparing often accompanies the skin eruption, and there may be impetigo-like crusting on the chin and/or superficial fine pustules, especially on the face. Mucositis is uncommon but may occur, typically in the mouth and milder than that of SJS. Patients with DRESS, AGEP, and SJS/TEN may share overlapping features and these SCARs may coexist; patients should be managed based on which features predominate and are most severe. In DRESS, adverse prognostic indicators include tachycardia, leukocytosis, tachypnea, coagulopathy, thrombocytopenia, and gastrointestinal bleeding. The internal organ involvement described in DRESS can be divided into two types: (1) organ dysfunction occurring during or immediately associated with the acute episode and (2) delayed involvement/late sequelae, possibly with an autoimmune basis. The first category includes hepatitis, interstitial nephritis, interstitial pneumonitis, and myocarditis, with rare other organ involvement (colitis/intestinal bleeding, encephalitis/aseptic meningitis, sialadenitis). Late sequelae include delayed myocarditis, autoimmune diseases from 4.8% up to 10% of patients (thyroiditis/Graves, type 1 diabetes, vitiligo), syndrome of inappropriate secretion of antidiuretic hormone (SIADH), or rarely Systemic lupus erythematosus (SLE). Mortality rates from DRESS are cited as 5% to up to 10% of patients, usually from complications of fulminant hepatic involvement, myocarditis, or renal/lung disease. It is important to note that the manifestations of the syndrome may vary by drug (and possibly ethnicity, as patients of certain backgrounds are more likely to develop DRESS from certain agents); dapsone hypersensitivity has a weaker association with eosinophilia, and allopurinol hypersensitivity has more renal involvement, whereas minocycline-associated DRESS may have more pulmonary involvement.

Skin biopsy is not required to confirm a diagnosis of DRESS. The histopathologic features may vary, with epidermal spongiosis, interface dermatitis, superficial epidermal pustules (resembling

AGEP), and apoptotic keratinocytes (resembling EM) reported. Atypical lymphocytes can be seen; eosinophils may be observed but are not required. Small studies suggest a more severe histopathologic phenotype (with EM-like features) may be more associated with a severe illness.

First-line treatment for DRESS involves identifying and stopping the causative agent, and initiation of antiinflammatory therapy, generally with high dose systemic corticosteroids (1–2 mg/kg/day, sometimes administered in divided doses). Pulse intravenous (IV) steroids, intravenous immune globulin (IVIG), cyclosporine, and other agents have been employed in severe or recalcitrant cases. Patients often require a long, slow steroid taper over weeks to months after initial onset.

Anticonvulsant Hypersensitivity Syndrome

The terms anticonvulsant hypersensitivity syndrome is now thought of as a subset of DRESS, and can be seen with phenytoin, phenobarbital, carbamazepine, lamotrigine, zonisamide, levetiracetam and other anticonvulsants. The estimated incidence of this condition is 1:1000 to 1:10,000 patients treated with these medications. Carbamazepine is currently the most common anticonvulsant causing DRESS, because it is also used to treat neuropathic pain, bipolar disorder, and schizophrenia, though lamotrigine has a higher rate on an individual basis (and patients with DRESS from lamotrigine may be less likely to develop an eosinophilia). Anticonvulsant hypersensitivity syndrome may occur at any dose, though slow upward titration of these agents may be associated with lower rates of severe reactions. Coadministration of valproate may increase the risk of DRESS with other agents. Certain HLA-haplotypes confer increased risk of DRESS (carbamazepine HLA A*31:01), and there are evolving recommendations existing for pretreatment genetic testing in some populations (such as exists in testing for HLA B*1502 in patients before carbamazepine therapy to prevent SJS).

Because many of the anticonvulsants are metabolized through the same pathway, cross-reactions are frequent, making selection of an alternative agent quite difficult. The rate of cross-reactivity among phenytoin, phenobarbital, and carbamazepine is 70%. In vitro tests are commercially available and may aid in selecting an agent to which the patient will not cross-react. Valproate, levetiracetam, and newer antiepileptics are generally considered safer alternatives for patients sensitive to aromatic anticonvulsants.

Allopurinol Hypersensitivity Syndrome

Allopurinol hypersensitivity syndrome typically occurs in patients with preexisting renal failure, or in those who develop acute kidney injury and whose dosing of allopurinol is not adjusted. Often, affected patients are treated unnecessarily for asymptomatic hyperuricemia, with clear indications for therapy present in only about one third of these patients. They are often given a dose not adjusted for their coexisting renal disease and are frequently taking a thiazide diuretic. Weeks to many months (average 7 weeks) after the allopurinol is begun, the patient develops a morbilliform eruption (50% of cases) that often evolves to an exfoliative erythroderma (20%) (Fig. 6.23). Bullae may occur, especially on the palms and soles, and oral ulcers may be present. Associated with the dermatitis are fever, eosinophilia, sometimes hepatitis (70% of cases), and typically worsening of renal function (40%–80%, the higher percentage in those with preexisting renal disease). Lung involvement and adenopathy occur infrequently. About 25% of patients die as a result of this syndrome, often from cardiovascular complications. Dialysis does not appear to accelerate the resolution of the eruption, suggesting that if a drug metabolite is responsible, it is not dialyzable. There is a strong association between HLA-B-5801 and the development of allopurinol hypersensitivity syndrome in the Han Chinese, but not in other races. HHV reactivation

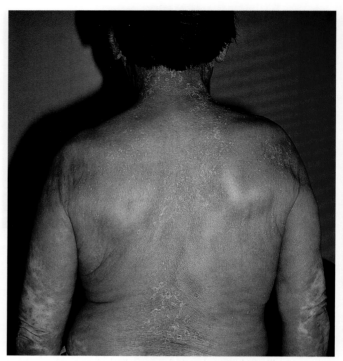
Fig. 6.23 Allopurinol hypersensitivity syndrome.

may be associated. This syndrome may be steroid responsive but is extremely slow to resolve, frequently lasting for months after allopurinol has been stopped. Very gradual tapering of systemic corticosteroids with monitoring of eosinophil count and renal function is essential. Too rapid tapering may lead to relapse of the syndrome.

Sulfonamide Hypersensitivity Syndrome

Fewer than 0.1% of treatment courses with sulfonamides are complicated by a hypersensitivity syndrome. It typically begins 3 weeks after starting the medication but may occur as soon as 1 week, faster than most other DRESS reactions. The skin eruption is similar to others, though patients may be erythrodermic. Patients are often slow acetylators, unable to detoxify the toxic and immunogenic metabolites generated during the metabolism of the sulfonamides. Patients with sulfonamide hypersensitivity syndrome may develop antibodies that recognize microsomal proteins to which the reactive metabolite of the sulfonamides binds. Hepatitis, nephritis/nephropathy, pneumonitis, myocarditis or pericarditis, and pancreatitis can all occur as a part of the syndrome. The hepatitis may be fulminant and life threatening. Patients who are allergic to antimicrobial sulfonamides are usually tolerant of other types of sulfa moieties, and should not all be labeled allergic to "sulfa." Zonisamide, a sulfonamide anticonvulsant, cross-reacts with sulfonamides but not other anticonvulsants.

Minocycline Hypersensitivity Syndrome

Minocycline hypersensitivity syndrome occurs in young adults, sometimes in the context of acne therapy. Deficiency of glutathione S-transferases is common in affected individuals and is more common in persons of African Caribbean descent. Females are more often affected. Minocycline may be detected in the blood of these patients up to 17 months after its discontinuation, suggesting that slow metabolism and persistent levels of medication may play a role. Minocycline hypersensitivity syndrome usually begins 2–4 weeks after starting the minocycline, and demonstrates typical skin findings of DRESS. Headache and cough are common complaints. Liver involvement occurs in 75% of patients and renal disease in 17%. Minocycline hypersensitivity is particularly associated with pneumonitis. This may progress to respiratory distress syndrome. It can be life threatening, but most patients survive. Myocarditis has also been reported. Patients with minocycline-induced DRESS may be at higher risk of developing long-term/delayed autoimmune sequelae.

Dapsone Hypersensitivity Syndrome

Dapsone hypersensitivity syndrome occurs in less than 1% of patients given this medication. It usually begins 4 weeks or more after starting dapsone. Hemolytic anemia and methemoglobinemia may be present. A morbilliform eruption that heals with desquamation is most characteristic. Icterus and lymphadenopathy occur in 80% of patients. Eosinophilia is typically *not* present. Liver involvement is a mixture of hepatocellular and cholestatic. The bilirubin is elevated in 85%, partly attributable to the hemolysis, and hypoalbuminemia is characteristic. Liver involvement is often severe and may be fatal. As with the hypersensitivity syndromes previously discussed, corticosteroids are the mainstay of treatment.

Cho YT, et al: Drug reaction with eosinophilia and systemic symptoms (DRESS). Int J Mol Sci 2017; 18: 1243.

Dar WR, et al: Levetiracetam induced drug reaction with eosinophilia and systemic symptom syndrome. Indian J Dermatol 2016; 61: 235.

Dibek Misirlioglu E, et al: Severe cutaneous adverse drug reactions in pediatric patients. J Allergy Clin Immunol Pract 2017; 5: 757.

Ghattaoraya GS, et al: Human leucocyte antigen-adverse drug reaction associations. Int J Immunogenetics 2017; 44: 7.

Husain Z, et al: DRESS syndrome. J Am Acad Dermatol 2013; 68: 693.e1.

Kirchhof MG, et al: Cyclosporine treatment of drug-induced hypersensitivity syndrome. JAMA Dermatol 2016; 152: 1254.

Lonowski S, et al: Vitiligo. Br J Dermatol 2016; 175: 642.

Ortonne N, et al: Histopathology of drug rash with eosinophilia and systemic symptoms syndrome. Br J Dermatol 2015; 173: 50.

Pavlos R, et al: Severe delayed drug reactions. Immunol Allergy Clin N Am 2017; 37: 785.

Shiohara T, et al: Prediction and management of drug reaction with eosinophilia and systemic symptoms (DRESS). Expert Opin Drug Metab Toxicol 2017; 13: 701.

Su SC, et al: Severe cutaneous adverse reactions. Int J Mol Sci 2016; 17: e1890.

Wang L, Mei XL: Drug reaction with eosinophilia and systemic symptoms. Chin Med J 2017; 130: 943.

Stevens-Johnson Syndrome and Toxic Epidermal Necrolysis

SJS and TEN (Lyell syndrome, nonstaphylococcal scaled skin syndrome) exist on a continuum, representing different levels of severity of an acute blistering drug eruption. The term *erythema multiforme* is a source of some confusion. Historically, EM minor refers to the syndrome of true 3-zone target lesions, often symmetrically on acral surfaces, with mild mucositis of one site; this is now generally seen in association with HSV (see Chapter 7), termed *herpes-associated EM* (HAEM). Most historical cases of EM major/majus are now simply referred to as SJS. An SJS-like illness with severe mucositis can be seen due to mycoplasma, particularly in children, which some have referred to as mycoplasma-induced rash and mucositis (suggesting it is a distinct entity from SJS or EM; Fuchs syndrome may also refer to this entity). EM and SJS/

TEN appear to be distinct entities with largely unrelated pathophysiology and demographics, and many are moving away from use of the term EM minor, EM major/majus, and EM-like drug eruption.

SJS, SJS/TEN overlap, and TEN are related, severe, potentially fatal SCARs. Fortunately, these are uncommon reactions, with an incidence of 0.4–1.2 per million person-years for TEN and 1.2–6.0 per million person-years for SJS. SJS is defined as <10% epidermal detachment, TEN as >30% epidermal detachment, and SJS/TEN overlap as 10%–30% detachment, measured at the worst extent of the disease.

- Both SJS and TEN are most frequently induced by the same medications.
- Patients initially presenting with SJS may progress to extensive skin loss resembling TEN.
- The histologic findings of TEN and SJS are indistinguishable.
- Both are increased by the same magnitude in HIV infection.

There are specific HLA-haplotypes that confer an increased risk in some ethnic populations for the development of these SCARs. In Han Chinese, the HLA haplotype HLA-B*1502 is present in the vast majority of carbamazepine-induced SJS/TEN patients and is present in about 10% of the Han Chinese population in general; this haplotype has also been shown to confer risk in other Asian populations. HLA typing should be performed in all Asians before starting carbamazepine, because the prevalence of HLA-B*1502 is 5%–10% in Asians in the United States and Asia, and testing before drug administration may markedly decrease or eliminate the risk of SJS in this setting.

More than 100 medications have been reported to cause SJS and TEN. In adults, common inciting medications are TMP-SMX (1–3 : 100,000), sulfadoxine plus pyrimethamine (Fansidar-R) (10 : 100,000), nevirapine, lamotrigine (1 : 1000 adults and 3 : 1000 children), and carbamazepine (14 : 100,000). Antibiotics (especially long-acting sulfa drugs and penicillins), other anticonvulsants, antiinflammatories (NSAIDs), and allopurinol are also frequent causes. Currently, in Europe, allopurinol is the most common cause of SJS and TEN. In children SJS/TEN is most often caused by sulfonamides and other antibiotics, antiepileptics, and acetaminophen. SJS/TEN from TMP-SMX is significantly more common in the spring. Establishing causality of a drug can sometimes be difficult; the ALDEN score has been proposed as a tool to help establish causality. Rechallenge can be dangerous and is discouraged, so in vitro methods have been developed. Lymphocyte granulysin expression, Granzyme B-ELISpot, and IFN-γ production assays together provided a sensitivity of 80% and specificity of 95% but are still used primarily in a research setting. It is important to identify the causative agent; if the culprit is stopped within 24 hours of blister development, mortality is reduced from 26% to 5%. As many patients are on multiple agents, similar principles apply as outlined in the introduction section. It is important to note classes of medications with relatively low rates of SCAR: β-blockers, angiotensin-converting enzyme (ACE) inhibitors, CCBs, diuretics, and most antidiabetic agents.

The clinical presentation may start with fever and influenza-like symptoms preceeding the eruption by a few days. Skin lesions appear on the face and trunk and rapidly spread, usually within 4 days, to their maximum extent. Initial lesions are often deep-red/dusky macules, sometimes with a central nonblanching zone (2-zone lesions, targetoid lesions, atypical targets, "SJS with spots"); these may centrally desquamate or may form atypical targets with purpuric centers that coalesce, form bullae (Fig. 6.24), then slough. In SJS virtually always, two or more mucosal surfaces are inflamed, with peeling, erosions, and hemorrhagic crust forming. The oral mucosa and conjunctiva are most frequently affected (Fig. 6.25), but physical examination should include thorough inspection of

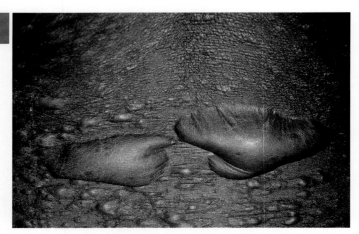

Fig. 6.24 Bullous drug reaction.

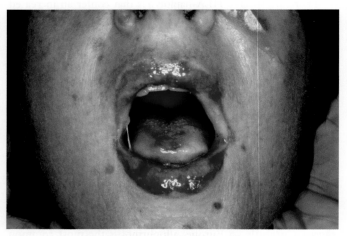

Fig. 6.25 Stevens-Johnson syndrome.

T cells, NK cells, and Th17 cells appear to play a role in mediating the disease. In addition, keratinocyte necrosis can be induced by the binding of soluble Fas ligand (sFasL) to Fas (also known as the death receptor or CD95). Soluble Fas ligand is elevated in the blood of patients with TEN, and its level correlates with body surface area (BSA) involvement. In addition, the peripheral blood mononuclear cells of patients with TEN secrete Fas ligand on exposure to the incriminated drug. The sera of patients with TEN induce necrosis of cultured keratinocytes, and a monoclonal antibody to Fas ligand in a dose-dependent manner inhibits keratinocyte necrosis exposed to TEN patient sera.

A skin biopsy is usually performed. Frozen-section analysis may lead to a rapid diagnosis, either by submitting the roof of a blister or portion of sloughed skin, or performing a biopsy of an area of impending necrosis. The histology of TEN and SJS is similar. There is a lymphocytic infiltrate at the dermoepidermal junction (DEJ) with necrosis of keratinocytes that at times may be full thickness. There is typically cellular necrosis out of proportion to the infiltrate. Paraneoplastic pemphigus may be excluded with direct immunofluorescence (DIF). Patients with graft-versus-host disease (GVHD) may also demonstrate a TEN-like picture with identical histology, although prominent follicular involvement may occasionally be a clue favoring GVHD.

Management of SJS/TEN patients is complex and requires multidisciplinary, coordinated care, often in an experienced intensive care unit or burn unit. There exists some controversy over optimal supportive care and therapeutic interventions, with little high quality evidence to guide decision making. Patients with SJS/TEN have fluid and electrolyte imbalances, hypercatabolism, and sometimes acute respiratory distress syndrome (ARDS), may be hypercoaguable, and are at risk for bacteremia from loss of the protective skin barrier. Their metabolic and fluid requirements are less than in burn victims (generally fluid resuscitation is approximately two thirds that of a burn victim's requirements based on the Parkland formula for skin loss), but nutritional support and monitoring for sepsis are critical. In addition to extent of skin loss, age, known malignancy, tachycardia, renal failure (particularly patients requiring dialysis), hyperglycemia, and low bicarbonate are all risk factors for having a higher mortality risk with SJS/TEN. SCORTEN, the most common model used to predict mortality, gives 1 point for each of these findings, with a 3.2% mortality rate for 0–1 points, and a 90% mortality rate for 5 or more points. However, respiratory tract involvement, not included in the SCORTEN, is also a poor prognostic sign. About one quarter of TEN patients have bronchial involvement. In TEN, epithelial detachment of the respiratory mucosae and associated ARDS are associated with a mortality rate of 70%. Supportive care is essential. Appropriate consultation with specialists to manage any affected mucosa is advised (ophthalmology for eyes and often amniotic membranes, gynecology for vaginal, urology consideration for severe urethral inflammation). When mucosal surfaces are eroded, they can adhere and scar; this is particularly common in the eyes or vaginal area, and care should be taken to separate eroded sites with nonstick dressings. General principles of skin care include limiting trauma and avoiding tape-to-skin, placing IV lines at uninvolved sites, keeping the skin moist to assist in healing, and using nonstick dressings. Silver-impregnated dressings may be used, and skin substitutes have been explored as well. Generally it is advised to leave involved epidermis in place to serve as a natural biologic dressing.

In the past corticosteroids were used, but more recently there exists controversy. Many European experts use cyclosporine (3-6mg/kg/day divided dosing), whereas in the United States many use IVIG (1 g/kg/day for 4 days) with or without corticosteroids. Early, high-dose steroids for a short period may be helpful in some cases. Etanercept has recently been reported as beneficial in a moderate sized study in Asia. There exists no consensus for the optimal systemic intervention for SJS/TEN.

all mucosal surfaces (oral, ocular, urethral, vaginal, anal). The patient may have photophobia, difficulty with swallowing, rectal erosions, dysuria, and/or cough, indicative of ocular, alimentary, urinary, and respiratory tract involvement, respectively. In other patients, dusky macular erythema is present in a local or widespread distribution over the trunk. Mucosal involvement may not be found. The epidermis in the areas of macular erythema rapidly becomes detached from the dermis, leading to extensive skin loss, often much more rapidly than occurs in the patients with atypical targets and extensive mucosal involvement. "Pure TEN" is a conceptual way of thinking of such patients. Rarely, SJS/TEN patients may present with lesions predominantly in sun-exposed areas, with a clear history of a recent significant sun exposure. This suggests that, in rare cases, SJS/TEN may be photo induced or photo exacerbated. Patients with SJS/TEN may have internal involvement similar to patients with DRESS/DIHS. These most frequently include eosinophilia, hepatitis, and worsening renal function.

Keratinocyte death in SJS and TEN is proposed to occur through more than one potential mechanism, and the relative importance of each of these mechanisms in SJS and TEN is not known. There is likely an immune response triggered to a drug-tissue complex. Activated cytotoxic T cells and natural killer (NK) cells produce granulysin, TNF-α, TRAIL, and perforin-granzyme B, all of which can induce keratinocyte necrosis. T-cell, NK-cell, and NKT-cell–derived granullysin is a key mediator of tissue damage, and serum (and blister) granulysin levels may correlate with disease severity. Effector memory CD8+ T cells, regulatory

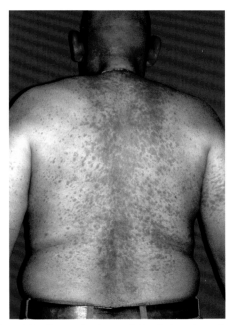

Fig. 6.26 Phenytoin plus radiation-induced reaction.

The proposed mechanism of action of IVIG in TEN is by IVIG blocking the binding of sFasL to Fas, stopping keratinocyte apoptosis. The presence of cytotoxic T lymphocytes and NK cells within the dermis subjacent to the necrotic epidermis suggests that immunosuppressive agents that block immune function could also be effective in SJS or TEN. Cyclosporine is the most promising agent. If considered, immunosuppressive treatment should be used as soon as possible, given as a short trial to see if the process may be arrested, and then tapered rapidly to avoid the risk of continued immunosuppression in a patient with substantial loss of skin. A prospective trial of thalidomide was discontinued because of excessive mortality rates in the active treatment arm. Data are mixed regarding systemic corticosteroid therapy for skin disease, and there is a clear risk of sepsis and potential for steroids to impair wound healing. Systemic and topical steroid therapy for ocular involvement may improve outcomes, as may topical cyclosporine. In patients with SJS/TEN who also have systemic involvement, as seen in DIHS (considered by some as SJS/TEN representing the cutaneous eruption of DIHS), systemic corticosteroids should be given early and tapered as rapidly as possible.

For patients who survive, the average time for epidermal regrowth is 3 weeks. The most common sequelae are ocular scarring and vision loss. The only predictor of eventual visual complications is the severity of ocular involvement during the acute phase. A sicca-like syndrome with dry eyes may also result, even in patients who never had clinical ocular involvement during the acute episode. Other complications include cutaneous scarring, altered taste, eruptive melanocytic lesions, hair, sweating, and nail abnormalities. Transient, widespread verrucous hyperplasia resembling confluent seborrheic keratoses has also been reported.

Canavan TN, et al: Mycoplasma pneumonia-induced rash and mucositis as a syndrome distinct from Stevens-Johnson syndrome and erythema multiforme. J Am Acad Dermatol 2015; 72: 239.

Carr DF, Pirmohamed M: Biomarkers of adverse drug reactions. Exp Biol Med (Maywood) 2017; ePub ahead of print.

Chung WH, et al: Granulysin is a key mediator for disseminated keratinocyte death in Stevens-Johnson syndrome and toxic epidermal necrolysis. Nat Med 2008; 14: 1343.

Chung WH, et al: Severe cutaneous adverse drug reactions. J Dermatol 2016; 43: 758.

Creamer D, et al: UK guidelines for the management of Stevens-Johnson syndrome/toxic epidermal necrolysis in adults 2016. J Plast Reconstr Aesthet Surg 2016;69: e119.

Harris V, et al: Review of toxic epidermal necrolysis. Int J Mol Sci 2016; 17: e2135.

Maverakis E, et al: Stevens-Johnson syndrome and toxic epidermal necrolysis standard reporting and evaluation guidelines. JAMA Dermatol 2017; 153: 587.

McCullough M, et al: Steven Johnson syndrome and toxic epidermal necrolysis in a burn unit. Burns 2017; 43: 200.

Micheletti RG, et al: SJS/TEN: A multicenter retrospective study from the US. J Invest Dermatol 2018; 138(11): 2315-2321.

Mockenhaupt M, et al: Stevens-Johnson syndrome and toxic epidermal necrolysis. J Invest Dermatol 2008; 128: 35.

Roujeau JC: Re-evaluation of 'drug-induced' erythema multiforme in the medical literature. Br J Dermatol 2016; 175: 642.

Roujeau JC, Bastuji-Garin S: Systematic review of treatments for Stevens-Johnson syndrome and toxic epidermal necrolysis using the SCORTEN score as a tool for evaluating mortality. Ther Adv Drug Saf 2011; 2: 87.

Roujeau JC, et al: New evidence supporting cyclosporine efficacy in epidermal necrolysis. J Invest Dermatol 2017; 137: 2047.

Schwartz RA, et al: Toxic epidermal necrolysis. J Am Acad Dermatol 2013; 69: 173. e1.

Wang CW, et al: Randomized, controlled trial of TNF-a antagonist in severe cutaneous adverse reactions. J Clin Invest 2018; 128(3): 985-996.

Zimmermann S, et al: Systemic immunomodulating therapies for Stevens-Johnson syndrome and toxic epidermal necrolysis. JAMA Dermatol 2017; 153: 514.

Radiation-Induced Epidermal Necrolysis

This rare reaction may occur if phenytoin is given prophylactically in neurosurgical patients who are receiving whole-brain radiation therapy and systemic steroids. As the dose of steroids is being reduced, erythema and edema initially appear on the head in the radiation ports. This evolves over 1 or 2 days to lesions with the clinical appearance and histology of SJS or even TEN. The eruption spreads caudad, and mucosal involvement may occur (Fig. 6.26). A similar syndrome has been reported with the use of amifostine, phenobarbital, or levetiracetam during radiation for head and neck cancers. This EM syndrome can rarely be seen with radiation therapy alone. If amifostine is used to reduce acute and chronic, radiation-associated head and neck xerostomia, there is a significant risk of SJS/TEN.

Barbosa LA, Teixeira CB: Erythema multiforme associated with prophylactic use of phenytoin during cranial radiation therapy. Am J Health-Syst Pharm 2008; 65: 1048.

Chodkiewicz HM, et al: Radiation port erythema multiforme. Skinmed 2012; 10: 390.

Elazzazy S, et al: Toxic epidermal necrolysis associated with antiepileptic drugs and cranial radiation therapy. Case Rep Oncol Med 2013; 2013: 415031.

Vern-Gross TZ, Kowal-Vern A: Erythema multiforme, Stevens Johnson syndrome, and toxic epidermal necrolysis syndrome in patients undergoing radiation therapy. Am J Clin Oncol 2014; 37: 506.

Human Immunodeficiency Virus Disease and Drug Reactions

Patients infected with HIV, especially those with Th-cell counts between 25 and 200, are at increased risk for the development of adverse reactions to medications, which may adversely affect treatment adherence. Morbilliform reactions to TMP-SMX occur in 45% or more of AIDS patients being treated for *Pneumocystis jiroveci* (formerly *P. carinii*) pneumonia. In two thirds of patients without life-threatening reactions, TMP-SMX treatment can be continued with simple conservative support, and the eruption may resolve. Associated hepatitis or neutropenia may require discontinuation of the drug. A similar increased rate of reaction to amoxicillin-clavulanate is also seen, and patients have been described with sensitivity to multiple antituberculosis agents, especially streptomycin and ofloxacin. If the dermatitis is treatment limiting but the eruption is not life threatening, low-dose rechallenge/desensitization may be attempted. It is successful in 65%–85% of patients in the short term and in more than 50% in the long term. In fact, initial introduction of TMP-SMX for prophylaxis by dose escalation reduces the rate of adverse reactions as well. However, rechallenge at full dose may have the same rate of recurrent eruptions as does introduction by dose escalation. Low-dose rechallenge is usually safe, but severe acute reactions may occur, including marked hypotension. Although most ADRs occur in the first few days of rechallenge, reactions may appear months after restarting TMP-SMX and may be atypical in appearance. The mechanism of this increased adverse reaction to TMP-SMX is unknown.

Severe bullous reactions, SJS, and TEN are 100–1000 times more common per drug exposure in patients with AIDS. These reactions are usually caused by sulfa drugs, especially long-acting ones, but may be caused by many agents. Nevirapine, a nonnucleoside reverse transcriptase inhibitor, has been associated with a high rate of severe drug eruptions, including SJS/TEN. Most of these ADRs are cutaneous and occur in the first 6 weeks of treatment. This high rate of reaction can be reduced by starting with a lower lead-in dose and by concomitant treatment with prednisone during the induction period. Nevirapine hypersensitivity syndrome presents with fever, hepatitis, or rash. More than 1% of patients will develop SJS/TEN. Multiple HLA-alleles in different populations have been reported as conferring elevated risk for nevirapine-associated SCARs (C*04:01 in Malawi, DRB1*01:01 in Europeans, and B*35 in Asian groups). Hepatitis, but not cutaneous reactions, is seen more often in patients with CD4 counts above 200 to 250. Fixed drug eruptions (FDEs) are also frequently seen in patients with HIV infection. Abacavir is associated with a potentially life-threatening hypersensitivity syndrome (DRESS-like, with fever, rash, and gastrointestinal or pulmonary symptoms) in 8% of patients. It usually occurs in the first 6 weeks of treatment but can occur within hours of the first dose. Rechallenge in these patients may lead to life-threatening hypotension and death. Abacavir hypersensitivity usually occurs in patients who are HLA-B*5701 positive, and screening of patients for this HLA type and not exposing patients with this HLA type to abacavir has decreased the number of cases of abacavir hypersensitivity syndrome. Patch testing is very sensitive and can be used to confirm abacavir hypersensitivity.

Aciclovir, nucleoside and nonnucleoside reverse transcriptase inhibitors (except nevirapine), and protease inhibitors are uncommon causes of ADRs. Many reactions attributed to these agents may actually be coexistent HIV-associated skin disorders, especially folliculitis, which are common in patients with AIDS. Regarding HAART-specific cutaneous adverse reactions, older antiretroviral agents were more likely to cause lipodystrophy (Stavudine, protease inhibitors) than newer regimens. HAART agents have been reported to cause hyperpigmentation (Emtricitabine), including of the nails (Zidovudine), and injection site reactions (ISRs; Enfuvirtide).

Introcaso CE, et al: Cutaneous toxicities of antiretroviral therapy for HIV. J Am Acad Dermatol 2010; 63: 549, 563.

Stewart A, et al: Severe antiretroviral-associated skin reactions in South African patients. Pharmacoepidemiol Drug Saf 2016; 25: 1313.

Tseng J, et al: HIV-associated toxic epidermal necrolysis at San Francisco General Hospital. J Int Assoc Provid AIDS Care 2017; 16: 37.

Weldegebreal F, et al: Magnitude of adverse drug reaction and associated factors among HIV-infected adults on antiretroviral therapy in Hiwot Fana specialized hospital, eastern Ethiopia. Pan Afr Med J 2016; 24: 255.

Fixed Drug Reactions (Eruptions)

Fixed drug reactions are common. FDEs are so named because they recur at the same site with each exposure to the medication. The time from ingestion of the offending agent to the appearance of symptoms is between 30 minutes and 8 hours, averaging 2 hours. In most patients, six or fewer lesions occur, and often only one. Infrequently, FDEs may be multifocal with numerous lesions (generalized) and can blisters, termed *generalized bullous fixed drug eruption* (GBDFE), which can mimic SJS/TEN (Fig. 6.27). They may present anywhere on the body, but half occur on the oral and genital mucosa. FDEs represent 2% of all genital ulcers evaluated at clinics for sexually transmitted diseases and can occur in young boys. In males, lesions are usually unifocal and can affect the glans or shaft of the penis. FDE of the vulva is often symmetric, presenting as an erosive vulvitis, with lesions on the labia minora and majora and extending to the perineum. Other unusual variants of FDE include eczematous, urticarial, papular, purpuric, linear, giant, and psoriasiform. At times, some lesions of FDE will not reactivate with exposure because of a presumed "refractory period" that may last from weeks to months.

Clinically, an FDE begins as a red round/oval patch that can develop a dusky, intensely inflamed central portion and resemble an iris or target lesion similar to erythema multiforme, which may blister and erode. Lesions of the genital and oral mucosae usually present as erosions. Most lesions are 1 to several cm in diameter, but larger plaques may occur, mimicking cellulitis. Characteristically, prolonged or permanent postinflammatory hyperpigmentation results, although a nonpigmenting variant of an FDE is recognized. With repeated or continued ingestion of the offending medication, new lesions may be added, sometimes eventuating in a clinical picture similar to SJS with similar morbidity and mortality. Histologically, an interface dermatitis occurs with subepidermal vesicle formation, necrosis of keratinocytes, and a mixed superficial and deep infiltrate of neutrophils, eosinophils, and mononuclear cells. Pigment incontinence is usually marked, correlating with the pigmentation resulting from repeated FDEs at the same site. Because biopsies are generally performed during the acute stage of a recurrence, the stratum corneum is normal. Papillary dermal fibrosis and deep perivascular pigment incontinence are often present from prior episodes.

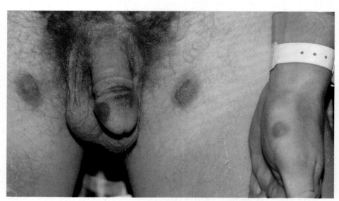

Fig. 6.27 Fixed drug reactions caused by aspirin.

Medications inducing FDEs are usually those taken intermittently. Many of the NSAIDs, especially pyrazolone derivatives, paracetamol, naproxen, oxicams, and mefenamic acid, cause FDE, with a special predilection for the lips. Sulfonamides, trimethoprim, and TMP-SMX are now responsible for the majority of genital FDEs. Barbiturates, tetracyclines, fluconazole, fluoroquinolones, phenolphthalein, acetaminophen, cetirizine, celecoxib, dextromethorphan, hydroxyzine/cetirizine/levocetirizine, quinine, lamotrigine, phenylpropanolamine, erythromycin, metformin, sildenafil, mycophenolate, chemotherapeutic agents, and Chinese and Japanese herbs are also among the long list of possible causes. The risk of developing a FDE has been linked to HLA-B22. Patch tests with various concentrations of the offending medication can reproduce the lesion when placed on affected, but not on unaffected, skin. Tape-stripping the skin before applying the suspected medication in various vehicles may increase the likelihood of a positive patch test.

Occasionally, FDEs do not result in long-lasting hyperpigmentation. The so-called nonpigmenting FDE is distinctive and has two variants. The pseudocellulitis or scarlatiniform type is characterized by large, tender, erythematous plaques that resolve completely within weeks, only to recur on reingestion of the offending drug. Pseudoephedrine hydrochloride is by far the most common culprit. The second variant is SDRIFE (formerly baboon syndrome; see "Allergic Contact Dermatitis" earlier). SDRIFE preferentially affects the buttocks, groin, and axillae with erythematous, fixed plaques, and is most commonly due to antibiotic agents, particularly aminopenicillins. Histologically, a giant cell lichenoid dermatitis can be seen in this setting. Fixed sunlight eruption has been reported as multiple FDE-like lesions occurring in response to sunlight.

The diagnosis of FDE is often straightforward and is elucidated by the history. Antibiotics manufactured overseas are readily available in many ethnic markets, including reports of such agents as trimethoprim/sulfamethoxazole in over-the-counter cold medications, and the formulations may not be carefully regulated. In some patients, the reaction may be to a dye in a medication rather than the active ingredient. Fixed drug reaction may rarely be related to foods, including residual antibiotics in meat products and quinine contained in tonic water. Confirmation with provocation tests can be performed. Because of the "refractory period," provocation tests need to be delayed at least 2 weeks from the last eruption. If an oral provocation test is considered, the initial challenge should be 10% of the standard dose, and patients with widespread lesions (SJS/TEN–like) should not be challenged. Patch testing using a drug concentration of 10%–20% in petrolatum or water applied to a previously reacted site is the recommended approach. In most patients, the treatment is simply to stop the medication. Desensitization can be successful.

Lesions of an FDE contain intraepidermal CD8+ T cells with the phenotypic markers of resident memory T cells. Tissue resident memory T cells are thought to remain in the skin to provide immunity to infection (e.g., herpes simplex virus). In FDE, once the medication is stopped, the abundant CD4+/FoxP3 T cells (Tregs) are believed to downregulate the eruption. In SJS/TEN patients, such Tregs are found in much fewer numbers than in FDE, which may explain the progression of SJS/TEN even after stopping the trigger. Resident mast cells in lesions of FDE may be the cells initially activated with drug exposure, explaining the rapid onset of the lesion.

Bhari N, et al: Fixed drug eruption due to three antihistamines of a same chemical family. Dermatol Ther 2017; 30: ePub 2016 Sep 9.

Flowers H, et al: Fixed drug eruptions: presentation, diagnosis, and management. South Med J 2014; 107: 724.

Game D, et al: Fixed sunlight eruption. Photodermatol photoimmunol photomed 2017; 33: 222.

Georgesen C, et al: A generalized fixed drug eruption associated with mycophenolate. JAAD Case Rep 2017; 3: 98.

Hoetzenecker W, et al: Adverse cutaneous drug eruptions: current understanding. Semin Immunopathol 2016; 38: 75.

Hughey LC: Approach to the hospitalized patient with targetoid lesions. Dermatol Ther 2011; 24: 196.

Acute Generalized Exanthematous Pustulosis

Also known as toxic pustuloderma and pustular drug eruption, AGEP is an uncommon reaction with an incidence of 1–5 cases per million per year. The average age in Europe is in the fifties and about one decade younger in Israel. Children can be affected. Women have been affected slightly more than men until recently, when a strong female predominance was suggested. There may be a genetic predisposition, with HLA*B51, DR11, and DQ3 more association with AGEP. Drugs are the most common cause of this reaction pattern, although AGEP has also been reported after mercury exposure. AGEP following infections and insect bites, such as from the *Loxosceles* spider (e.g., brown recluse), has been reported, but some of these patients have also received antibiotics. A localized variant, "acute localized exanthematous pustulosis" (ALEP), has been rarely reported, usually acutely after antibiotic exposure.

The eruption is of sudden onset, within 1 day in many cases associated with antibiotics, and averaging 11 days in other cases. The rash is accompanied by fever in most patients. Initially, there is a scarlatiniform erythema. The eruption evolves and disseminates rapidly, consisting usually of more than 100 nonfollicular pinpoint pustules less than 5 mm in diameter; dermoscopy may aid in identifying pustules in some early cases (Fig. 6.28). The face and flexural folds are commonly affected first, with extension to the trunk and limbs. Nikolsky sign may be positive. Facial edema may be seen, and mucous membrane involvement is uncommon, and if present usually affects only one surface and is nonerosive. Laboratory abnormalities typically include a leukocytosis with neutrophilia (90%) and at times an eosinophilia (30%). Typically, the entire self-limited episode lasts up to 15 days. Characteristically, widespread superficial desquamation occurs as the eruption clears. AGEP can recur with seconder-exposure to the medication.

In more than 90% of patients, drugs are the cause of AGEP. Frequently implicated medications include antibiotics (penicillin and macrolide classes in particular, plus clindamycin, minocycline, sulfonamides, antimycotic agents, vancomycin, and quinolones), antiepileptic agents, and antihypertensives, particularly CCBs

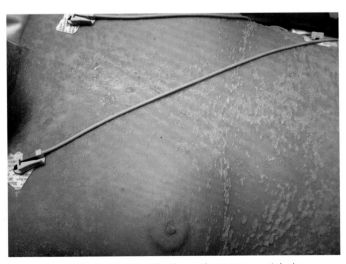

Fig. 6.28 Acute generalized exanthematous pustulosis.

(especially diltiazem, though cross-reactivity between CCBs has been described). Hydroxychloroquine is frequently implicated, including in atypical, prolonged courses, but may also induce psoriasis, and it is important to distinguish the two. Corticosteroids, allopurinol, oxicam NSAIDs, pseudoephedrine, terazosin, omeprazole, and sennoside have also caused AGEP. Chemotherapeutic agents, including small molecule/multikinase inhibitors and other targeted agents, are being reported as inciting agents with increasing frequency. Radiocontrast material and some forms of dialysates have been shown to cause AGEP. Infectious agents implicated include viruses (enteroviruses, CMV, EBV, hepatitis), rarely vaccinations, and other infections (mycoplasma, and other bacterial infections), though concomitant antibiotics were occasionally employed and may have been the inciting agent.

In the classic case, the diagnosis is straightforward, with the characteristic sudden and rapid onset, widespread pustulation, and self-limited course. Due to the severity of the eruption and potential for widespread erythroderma, patients with certain comorbidities may be at risk for complications such as high output heart failure. The facial edema and pustulation can simulate DRESS/DIHS from anticonvulsants. Cases of overlap between SJS/TEN, DRESS, an dAGEP exist, and patients with mixed features should be evaluated for each and treated based on the most severe features. Pustular psoriasis, especially pustular psoriasis of pregnancy, can be difficult to differentiate from AGEP. If there are no characteristic lesions of psoriasis elsewhere and no prior personal or family history of psoriasis, distinguishing these two entities may be impossible, and the patient may need to be followed for a final diagnosis to be made. A microbial pustulosis in the setting of a connective tissue disease can also resemble AGEP, but lesions are usually localized to the flexors, and the course is more chronic.

Histologically, early lesions show marked papillary edema, neutrophil clusters in the dermal papillae, and perivascular eosinophils. There may be an associated leukocytoclastic vasculitis. Well-developed lesions show intraepidermal or subcorneal spongiform pustules. Severe cases may demonstrate an interface dermatitis similar to EM. The presence of eosinophils and the marked papillary edema help to distinguish this eruption from pustular psoriasis, though pustular psoriasis of pregnancy is often associated with tissue eosinophilia.

Patch testing with the suspected agent may reproduce a pustular eruption on an erythematous base at 48 hours in about 50% of patients. Patch testing rarely will result in a recrudescence of AGEP. AGEP is mediated by T cells, and shares overlapping features and inflammatory pathways with pustular psoriasis, with dermal IL-17 and IL-23 and epidermal IL-8. IFN-γ, IL-4/IL-5, and GM-CSF are also increased. *IL36RN* gene mutations have been demonstrated in both AGEP and pustular psoriasis patients.

Most patients with AGEP can be managed with topical corticosteroids and antihistamines. In over one third of cases, systemic corticosteroids may be required. In severe cases, cyclosporine, infliximab, or etanercept have rapidly stopped the pustulation and appeared to have hastened the resolution of the eruption.

Alegre-Sanchez A, et al: Sorafenib-induced acute generalized exanthematous pustulosis. Actas Dermosifiliogr 2017; 108: 599.

Alniemi DT, et al: Acute generalized exanthematous pustulosis. Int J Dermatol 2017; 56: 405.

Errichetti E, et al: Dermoscopy as an auxiliary tool in the early differential diagnosis of acute generalized exanthematous pustulosis (AGEP) and exanthematous (morbilliform) drug eruption. J Am Acad Dermatol 2016; 74: e29.

Hwang SJ, et al: Ipilimumab-induced acute generalized exanthematous pustulosis in a patient with metastatic melanoma. Melanoma Res 2016; 26: 417.

Kostopoulos TC, et al: Acute generalized exanthematous pustulosis. J Eur Acad Dermatol Venereol 2015; 29: 209.

Pearson KC, et al: Prolonged pustular eruption from hydroxychloroquine. Cutis 2016; 97: 212.

Saénz de Santa Maria García M, et al: Acute generalized exanthematous pustulosis due to diltiazem. J Allergy Clin Immunol Pract 2016; 4: 765.

Szatkowski J, Schwartz RA: Acute generalized exanthematous pustulosis (AGEP). J Am Acad Dermatol 2015; 73: 843.

Thienvibul C, et al: Five-year retrospective review of acute generalized exanthematous pustulosis. Dermatol Res Pract 2015; ePub 2015 Dec 10.

Drug-Induced Pseudolymphoma

At times, exposure to medication may result in cutaneous inflammatory patterns that resemble lymphoma. These pseudolymphomatous drug eruptions may resemble either T-cell or B-cell lymphomas. The most common drug-induced pseudolymphoma is one resembling cutaneous T-cell lymphoma (CTCL) clinically and histologically. The most common setting in which these pseudolymphomas occur is a drug-induced hypersensitivity syndrome (DRESS/DIHS), in which infrequently the histology may resemble CTCL. More rarely, medications may induce plaques or nodules, usually in elderly white men after many months of treatment. Lymphadenopathy and circulating Sézary cells may also be present. CD30+ cells may be present in the infiltrate. Usually, other features (e.g., keratinocyte necrosis, dermal edema) help to distinguish these reactions from true lymphoma. Importantly, T-cell receptor gene rearrangements in the skin and blood may be positive (or show pseudoclones) in these drug-induced cases, representing a potential pitfall for the unwary physician. Importantly, patients with angioimmunoblastic T-cell lymphoma can very closely resemble patients with DRESS, leading to delays in diagnosis. Pseudolymphoma resolves with discontinuation of the medication. The medication groups primarily responsible are anticonvulsants, antimicrobial agents (sulfa drugs, vancomycin, rifampin, others), antihypertensives (ACE inhibitors, β-blockers, CCBs, thiazides), and antidepressants or anxiolytics. Vaccinations and herbal supplements can also induce pseudolymphoma.

Mangana J, et al: Angioimmunoblastic T-cell lymphoma mimicking drug reaction with eosinophilia and systemic symptoms (DRESS Syndrome). Case Rep Dermatol 2017; 9: 74–79.

Urticaria/Angioedema

Urticarial drug eruptions are the second most common type of cutaneous adverse drug eruption, and can be induced by immunologic and nonimmunologic mechanisms. In either case, clinically the lesions are pruritic wheals or angioedema (Fig. 6.29). Urticaria, especially extensive disease, around the face or mouth, may be part of a more severe anaphylactic reaction with bronchospasm, laryngospasm, or hypotension. Immediate hypersensitivity skin testing and sometimes RAST is useful in evaluating risk for these patterns of reaction. Most patients are acutely managed with antihistamine therapy, with severe cases requiring systemic corticosteroids.

Aspirin and NSAIDs are the most common causes of nonimmunologic urticarial reactions. They alter prostaglandin metabolism, enhancing degranulation of mast cells. They may therefore also exacerbate chronic urticaria of other causes. The nonacetylated salicylates (trilisate and salsalate) do not cross-react with aspirin in patients experiencing bronchospasm and may be safe alternatives. Some patients have urticaria to only one medication in this family, without cross-reaction with other NSAIDs, suggesting that specific IgE-mediated mechanisms may also be possible in NSAID-induced urticaria. Other agents causing nonimmunologic urticaria include radiocontrast material, opiates, tubocurarine, and polymyxin B. Pretesting does not exclude the possibility of anaphylactoid reaction

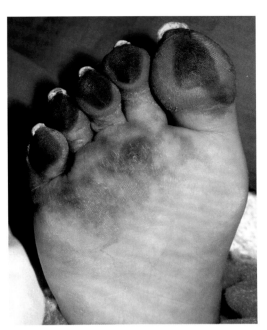

Fig. 6.29 Angioedema. (Courtesy Steven Binnick, MD.)

to radiocontrast material. The use of low-osmolarity radiocontrast material and pretreatment with antihistamines, systemic steroids, and in those with a history of asthma, theophylline, may reduce the likelihood of reaction to radiocontrast material.

Immunologic urticaria is most often associated with penicillin and related β-lactam antibiotics and relates to the minor determinants rather than the β-lactam ring. It is associated with IgE antibodies to penicillin or its metabolites. Skin testing with major and minor determinants is useful in evaluating patients with a history of urticaria associated with penicillin exposure. Patients with penicillin allergy have an increased rate of reaction to cephalosporins. In the case of cefaclor, half of anaphylactic reactions occur in patients with a history of penicillin allergy. Third-generation cephalosporins, especially cefdinir, are much less likely to induce a reaction in a penicillin-allergic patient than are first- or second-generation agents.

Bupropion is often used for depression and smoking cessation. It can induce urticaria, which may be severe and associated with hepatitis and a serum sickness like syndrome. Two antihistamines, cetirizine and hydroxyzine, may induce urticaria, an apparent paradox that may lead to confusion in the clinical setting.

Angioedema is a known complication of the use of ACE inhibitors and angiotensin II antagonists. Blacks are at almost 5 times greater risk than whites. Lisinopril and enalapril produce angioedema more frequently than captopril. Angioedema typically occurs within a week of starting therapy but may begin after months of treatment. The episodes may be severe, requiring hospitalization in up to 45% of patients, intensive care in up to 27%, and intubation in up to 18%. One quarter of patients affected give a history of previous angioedema. The angioedema appears to be dose dependent, because it may resolve with decreased dose. All these factors suggest that the angioedema may represent a consequence of a normal pharmacologic effect of the ACE inhibitors. The blocking of kininase II by ACE inhibitors may increase tissue kinin levels, enhancing urticarial reactions and angioedema. Although this is dose dependent, ACE inhibitor users with one episode of angioedema have a 10-fold risk of a second episode, and the recurrent episodes may be more severe. The treatment of urticaria is discussed in Chapter 7.

Red Man Syndrome

The IV infusion of vancomycin may be complicated by a characteristic reaction called "red man syndrome." With rapid infusions, due to a direct toxic effect of vancomycin on mastocytes, rapid degranulation may occur. A macular eruption appears initially on the back of the neck, sometimes spreading to the upper trunk, face, and arms. Angioedema has been described. There is associated pruritus and "heat," as well as hypotension that may be severe enough to cause cardiac arrest. Oral vancomycin has caused a similar reaction in a child. Children with systemic juvenile idiopathic arthritis (JIA) may have potentially fatal macrophage activation syndrome during or after a "red man reaction" from vancomycin, and thromboses have occurred in patients with sickle cell disease. The red man reaction is caused by elevated blood histamine. Red man syndrome can be prevented in most patients by reducing the rate of infusion of the antibiotic, or by pretreatment with H1 and H2 antihistamines. Although typically reported with vancomycin, similar "anaphylactoid" reactions have been seen with ciprofloxacin, cefepime, amphotericin B, rifampin, infliximab, and teicoplanin.

Asero R, et al: Clinical management of patients with a history of urticaria/angioedema induced by multiple NSAIDs. Int Arch Allergy Immunol 2013; 160: 126.
Bruniera FR, et al: The use of vancomycin with its therapeutic and adverse effects. Eur Rev Med Pharmacol Sci 2015; 19: 694.
Kowalski ML, et al: Approaches to the diagnosis and management of patients with a history of nonsteroidal anti-inflammatory drug-related urticaria and angioedema. J Allergy Clin Immunol 2015; 136: 245.

Photosensitivity Reactions (Photosensitive Drug Reactions)

Medications may cause phototoxic, photoallergic, and lichenoid reactions, accelerated photoaging, and photodistributed telangiectasias, as well as pseudoporphyria. The mechanisms of photosensitivity are discussed in Chapter 3. In many cases, the mechanism for drug-induced photosensitivity is unknown, though some have speculated damage occurs through the generation of reactive oxygen species. Most medication-related photosensitivity is triggered by radiation in the UVA range, partly because (1) most photosensitizing drugs have absorption spectra in the UVA and short-visible range (315–430 nm), and (2) UVA penetrates into the dermis where the photosensitizing drug is present. The most common causes of photosensitivity are NSAIDs, TMP-SMX, thiazide diuretics and related sulfonylureas, quinine and quinidine, phenothiazines, and certain tetracyclines; some less commonly prescribed medications have very high per-patient rates of photosensitivity and toxicity, such as voriconazole and vemurafenib. Numerous other medications in many classes induce photosensitivity less frequently.

Phototoxic reactions are related to the dose of both the medication and the UV irradiation. Reactions can occur in anyone if sufficient thresholds are reached and do not require prior exposure or participation by the immune system. Persons of higher skin types are at lower risk of developing phototoxic eruptions in some studies. There is individual variation in the amount of photosensitivity created by a standard dose of medication, independent of serum concentration. This remains unexplained but reflects the clinical setting, where interindividual variability in development of phototoxic eruptions is seen. Reactions can appear from hours to days after exposure. Tetracyclines, amiodarone, and NSAIDs are common culprits. The reaction may present as immediate burning with sun exposure (amiodarone, chlorpromazine) or exaggerated sunburn (fluoroquinolone antibiotics, chlorpromazine, amiodarone, thiazide diuretics, quinine, tetracyclines). Hyperpigmentation may complicate phototoxic reactions and may last for many months.

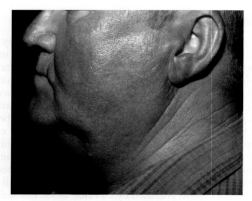

Fig. 6.30 Amiodarone hyperpigmentation.

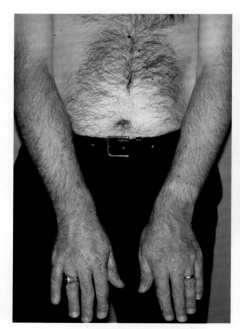

Fig. 6.31 Piroxicam photosensitivity.

Treatment may include dose reduction and photoprotection by a sunblock with strong coverage through the whole UVA spectrum.

Photoallergic reactions are typically eczematous and pruritic, may first appear weeks to months after drug exposure, and involve the immune system. Unfortunately, in the patient with photoallergy to systemic medications, photopatch testing is infrequently positive and of limited clinical value. In general, photoallergic reactions are not as dependent on drug dose as phototoxic reactions. Photosensitivity of both the phototoxic and the photoallergic type may persist for months to years after the medication has been stopped. Photosensitivity reactions to various drugs are discussed individually next, emphasizing the characteristic patterns seen with each medication group.

Amiodarone photosensitivity develops in up to 75% of treated patients and occurs after a cumulative dose of 40 g and at least 4 months on therapy. A reduced minimal erythema dose (MED) to UVA, but not UVB, occurs, and gradually returns to normal between 12 and 24 months after stopping the medication. Stinging and burning may occur as soon as 30 minutes after sun exposure. Less frequently, a dusky, blue-red erythema of the face and dorsa of the hands occurs (Fig. 6.30). At times, papular reactions are also seen. This reaction may be dose dependent, and acute burning may be relieved by dose reduction; amiodarone has a long half-life and can persist for weeks to months after stopping. Narrow-band UVB may desensitize patients with persistent phototoxicity after stopping amiodarone.

The NSAIDs, especially piroxicam, are frequently associated with photosensitivity (Fig. 6.31). The characteristic reaction is a vesicular eruption of the dorsa of the hands, sometimes associated with a dyshidrosiform pattern on the lateral aspects of the hands and fingers. In severe cases, even the palms may be involved. Histologically, this reaction pattern shows intraepidermal spongiosis, exocytosis, and perivascular inflammatory cells—a pattern typical of photoallergy. However, this reaction may occur on the initial exposure to the medication, but phototoxicity tests in animals and humans have been negative. Patients with photosensitivity to piroxicam may also react to thiosalicylic acid, a common sensitizer in thimerosal. Half of patients having a positive patch test to thimerosal with no prior exposure to piroxicam test positive to piroxicam. This suggests that piroxicam reactions seen on initial exposure to the medication may be related to sensitization during prior thimerosal exposure.

Sulfonamide antibiotics, related hypoglycemic agents, and the sulfonylurea diuretics may all be associated with photosensitivity reactions. Notably, patients may tolerate one of the medications from this group, but when additional members of the group are added, clinical photosensitivity occurs. The typical pattern is erythema, scale, and, in chronic cases, lichenification and hyperpigmentation.

Fluoroquinolone antibiotics are frequently associated with photosensitivity reactions. Sparfloxacin is highly photosensitizing; enoxacin, ciprofloxacin, and sitafloxacin are mildly photosensitizing; and levofloxacin rarely, if ever, causes photosensitivity.

Photodistributed lichenoid reactions have been reported most often from thiazide diuretics, quinidine, and NSAIDs, but also occur from diltiazem and clopidogrel bisulfate. They present as erythematous patches and plaques. Sometimes, typical Wickham striae are observed in the lesions. Histologically, photodistributed lichenoid reactions are often indistinguishable from idiopathic lichen planus. Marked hyperpigmentation may occur, especially in persons of higher skin types (IV–VI) and diltiazem-induced cases. The lichenoid nature of the eruption may not be clinically obvious, and histology is required to confirm the diagnosis. This hyperpigmentation may persist for months. UVA-associated phototoxicity is also common with vemurafenib, with reduced UVA MED in 94% of those tested.

Azathioprine can cause photosensitivity to UVA, and there are scattered reports of antimalarial agents inducing photosensitivity. These reactions rare reactions are important to keep in mind as the diseases for which these agents may be prescribed, such as connective tissue disorders, can also exhibit photosensitivity.

Some newer medications have generated multiple reports of photosensitivity, including combination antivirals for hepatitis C, particularly simeprevir; newer chemotherapeutic agents (discussed at length later in the chapter), including vemurafenib, which is strikingly photosensitizing; and emerging reports with other agents (imatinib, ibrutinib, vandetanib, EGF-receptor inhibitors, and more). Flutamide has been reported to induce photoleukomelanoderma, a mosaic mix of hypopigmentation and hyperpigmentation after erythema in sun-exposed areas.

Voriconazole, a second-generation triazole, has been associated with an unusual combination of photosensitive phenomena. Photosensitivity occurs in 8%–10% of patients taking voriconazole for more than 12 weeks. It appears to be UVA induced, and is not dose dependent. Usually, the photosensitivity is mild, with facial erythema and chelitis, and may resemble a sunburn. In these cases, with the use of sun protection and topical treatment, voriconazole can be continued. Occasionally, more severe reactions occur. Pseudoporphyria, eruptive lentigines, atypical nevi, premature aging, and even the development of melanoma and highly aggressive and potentially fatal squamous cell carcinomas (SCCs) have been reported. Multiple studies, including a large 20-year retrospective study of lung cancer patients, have shown that voriconazole is an independent risk factor for SCC development, and 17% can be unusually aggressive. Any exposure to voriconazole is associated with a 2.6-fold increased risk of SCC, and the risk increases with cumulative exposure. Affected patients can closely resemble patients with xeroderma pigmentosa. Photodistributed granuloma annulare has also been seen. This severe form of photosensitivity rapidly resolves on stopping voriconazole. Patients with aggressive SCC or melanoma are advised to stop voriconazole and transition to an alternate agent if possible; posaconazole can be an effective alternative. Emerging studies suggest hydrochlorothiazide may be associated with an increased risk of skin cancer.

Photodistributed telangiectasia is a rare complication of CCBs (nifedipine, felodipine, amlodipine). UVA appears to be the action spectrum. Cefotaxime has also been reported to produce this reaction. Corticosteroids, oral contraceptives, isotretinoin, IFNs, lithium, thiothixene, methotrexate, and other medications may induce telangiectasia, but not through photosensitivity.

Pseudoporphyria is a photodistributed bullous reaction clinically and histologically resembling porphyria cutanea tarda (Fig. 6.32). Patients present with blistering on sun-exposed skin of the face and hands and skin fragility. Varioliform scarring occurs in 70% of patients. Facial scarring is especially common in children with pseudoporphyria. Hypertrichosis is rarely found; dyspigmentation and sclerodermoid changes are not reported. Porphyrin studies are normal. The blistering usually resolves gradually once the offending medication is stopped. However, skin fragility may persist for years. Naproxen is the most frequently reported cause. Up to 12% of children with JIA treated with NSAIDs may develop pseudoporphyria. Pseudoporphyria has also been reported to other NSAIDs (oxaprozin, nabumetone, ketoprofen, mefenamic acid; but not piroxicam), tetracycline, furosemide, nalidixic acid, isotretinoin, acitretin, 5-fluorouracil, bumetanide, dapsone, oral contraceptives, rofecoxib, celecoxib, cyclosporine, imatinib, vemurafenib, voriconazole, and pyridoxine. Tanning booth (sunbed) exposure and even excessive sun exposure can produce pseudoporphyria. Cases in women outnumber men by 24:1. Some women with sunbed-induced pseudoporphyria are taking oral contraceptives. Patients on dialysis may develop pseudoporphyria, and *N*-acetylcysteine in doses up to 600 mg twice daily may lead to improvement in these cases. Histologically, a pauciinflammatory

subepidermal vesicle is seen. DIF may show immunoglobulin and complement deposition at the DEJ and perivascularly, as seen in porphyria cutanea tarda.

Banerjee D, et al: Safety and tolerability of direct-acting anti-viral agents in the new era of hepatitis C therapy. Aliment Pharmacol Ther 2016; 43: 674.

Batrani M, et al: Imatinib mesylate-induced pseudoporphyria in a patient with chronic myeloid leukemia. Indian J Dermatol Venereol Leprol 2016; 82: 727.

Drago F, et al: Porphyrin elevation in a patient on treatment with simeprevir. Am J Gastroenterol 2016; 111: 1368.

Higashiyama A, et al: Flutamide-induced photoleukomelanoderma. J Dermatol 2016; 43: 1105.

Jaworski K, et al: Cutaneous adverse reactions of amiodarone. Med Sci Monit 2014; 20: 2369.

Khandpur S, et al: Drug-induced photosensitivity. Br J Dermatol 2017; 176: 902.

O'Gorman SM, Murphy GM: Photosensitizing medications and photocarcinogenesis. Photodermatol Photoimmunol Photomed 2014; 30: 8.

Pedersen SA, et al: Hydrochlorothiazide use and risk of non-melanoma skin cancer. J Am Acad Dermatol 2018; 78: 673-681.

Williams K, et al: Voriconazole-associated cutaneous malignancy. Clin Infect Dis 2014; 58: 997.

Anticoagulant-Induced Skin Necrosis

Both warfarin and heparin induce lesions of cutaneous necrosis, although by different mechanisms. Obese, postmenopausal women are predisposed, and lesions tend to occur in areas with abundant subcutaneous fat, such as the breast, abdomen, thigh, or buttocks. The clinical appearance overlaps with calciphylaxis, and patients with warfarin-induced calciphylaxis have been described.

Warfarin-induced skin necrosis (WISN) usually occurs 3–5 days after therapy is begun, and a high initial dose increases the risk. Patients with a much more delayed onset (up to 15 years) are ascribed to noncompliance, drug-drug interactions, or liver dysfunction. WISN occurs in 1:1000 to 1:10,000 patients treated with warfarin. Hereditary or acquired deficiency of protein C, and less often protein S, is associated with warfarin necrosis. Other hypercoaguable states, such as antithrombin III or factor V Leiden mutations, or lupus anticoagulant syndrome may be associated as well. Lesions begin as red, painful plaques that develop petechiae, then form a large bulla (Fig. 6.33). Necrosis follows. Priapism can complicate warfarin necrosis. A less common variant seen in patients

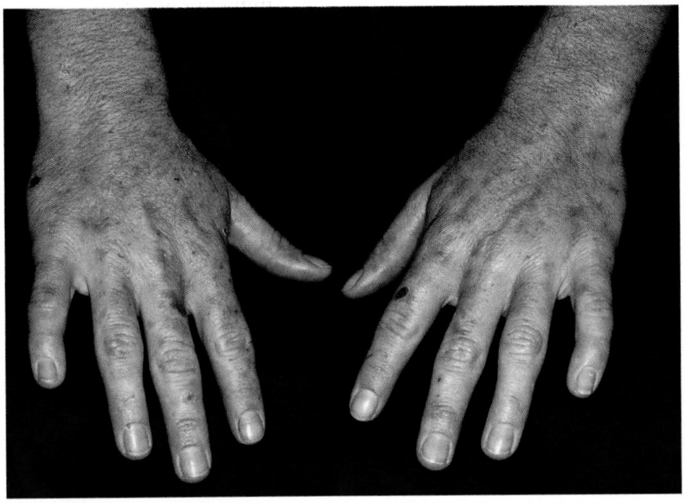

Fig. 6.32 Sixteen-year-old with scarring from pseudo–porphyria cutanea tarda reaction to tetracycline.

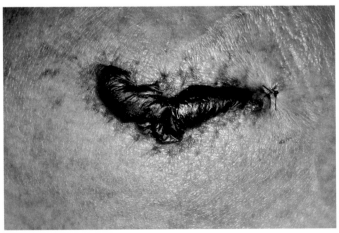

Fig. 6.33 Warfarin-induced necrosis. (Courtesy Steven Binnick, MD.)

with a deep venous thrombosis (DVT) of an extremity is necrosis of a distal extremity, usually the one with the DVT. Warfarin-induced venous limb necrosis is most often seen in cancer patients, but also in the setting of heparin-induced thrombocytopenia (HIT) and antiphospholipid syndrome.

Early in warfarin treatment, the serum levels of the vitamin K–dependent antithrombotic protein C fall. Because the half-life of antithrombotic protein C is shorter than that of the vitamin K–dependent prothrombotic factors II, X, and IX, an acquired state of reduced protein C level occurs before the clotting factors are reduced. This creates a temporary prothrombotic state. This is more likely to occur if the levels of protein C are already low, if other antithrombotic proteins are deficient, or if the patient has an associated hypercoagulable state. This explains why the syndrome does not always recur with gradual reinstitution of warfarin, and why it has been reported to resolve with continued warfarin treatment. Histologically, noninflammatory thrombosis with fibrin in the vessels is seen. Treatment is to stop the warfarin, administer vitamin K to reverse the warfarin, and begin heparin or low-molecular-weight (LMW) heparin. Administration of purified protein C can rapidly reverse the syndrome, as well as associated priapism. Other vitamin K antagonists, such as fluindione, may cause a similar reaction. Rivaroxaban, a direct inhibitor of activated factor X that does not inhibit other vitamin K–dependent proteins, may be considered an alternative anticoagulant. Dabigatran etexilate has been suggested for prevention of WISN in the patient with protein C deficiency.

Heparin induces necrosis both at the sites of local injections and in a widespread pattern when infused intravenously or given by local injection. Local reactions are the most common. Heparin can also induce local allergic reactions at injection sites, which are distinct from the necrosis syndrome. Independent of its method of delivery, heparin-induced skin necrosis lesions present as tender red plaques that undergo necrosis, usually 6–12 days after the heparin treatments are started. Intraepidermal hemorrhagic bullae have also been described. Unfractionated heparin is more likely to cause this complication than fractionated LMW heparin, and postsurgical patients are at greater risk than medical patients. Even the heparin used for dialysis or to flush arterial catheters may be associated with cutaneous necrosis.

Some necrotic reactions to local injections, and most disseminated reactions occurring with IV heparin, are associated with HIT. Patients with underlying prothrombotic conditions, such as factor V Leiden and prothrombin mutations or elevated levels of factor VIII, may develop severe skin lesions if they develop HIT and heparin necrosis. A heparin-dependent antiplatelet antibody is the pathogenic basis of HIT and apparently of heparin-induced skin necrosis. This antibody causes both the thrombocytopenia and the aggregation of platelets in vessels, leading to thrombosis (white clot syndrome). The antibody may appear up to 3 weeks after the heparin has been discontinued, so the onset of the syndrome may be delayed. Histologically, fibrin thrombi are less reproducibly found in affected tissues, because the vascular thrombosis is the result of platelet aggregation, not protein deposition. The process may not only produce infarcts in the skin, but also cause arterial thrombosis of the limbs, heart, lung, and brain, resulting in significant morbidity or mortality. Bilateral adrenal necrosis caused by hemorrhagic infarction can occur and, if not detected early, may lead to death from acute addisonian crisis. The syndrome must be recognized immediately in any patient receiving heparin with late-developing thrombocytopenia. The treatment is to stop the heparin and give a direct thrombin inhibitor and vitamin K. After the platelet count has returned to normal, warfarin therapy is typically given for 3–6 months. Patients with HIT cannot be treated with warfarin immediately, as the warfarin would be ineffective in stopping the thrombosis (it is *not* anti-thrombotic) and may worsen the thrombosis by enhancing coagulation. The diagnosis of HIT can be delayed because the antiplatelet antibody may not be present while the platelet count is falling. Adding warfarin at this time can lead to disastrous widespread acral thrombosis resembling disseminated intravascular coagulation (DIC).

Skin necrosis has also been associated with other anticoagulants, such as fluindione enoxaparin. Patients with cancer, an acquired prothrombotic state, are at increased risk for DVT. If they are treated with heparin and develop HIT, patients are at extreme risk for development of a prothrombotic state if treated with warfarin. In this setting, digital and limb gangrene has occurred in the face of normal peripheral pulses and supertherapeutic anticoagulation by standard measures (international normalized ratio). The consumptive coagulopathy induced by the cancer is the underlying trigger.

Adya KA, et al: Anticoagulants in dermatology. Indian J Dermatol Venereol Leprol 2016; 82: 626.

Bakoyiannis C, et al: Dabigatran in the treatment of warfarin-induced skin necrosis. Case Rep Dermatol Med 2016; ePub 2016 Mar 27.

Beggal K, et al: Skin necrosis due to fluindione treatment. J Wound Care 2014; 23: s16.

Vitamin K Reactions

Several days to 2 weeks after injection of vitamin K, an allergic reaction at the injection site may occur (Fig. 6.34). Most affected patients have liver disease and are being treated for elevated prothrombin time. The lesions are pruritic red patches or plaques that can be deep seated, involving the dermis and subcutaneous tissue. There may be superficial vesiculation. Lesions occur most often on the posterior arm and over the hip or buttocks. Plaques on the hip tend to progress around the waist and down the thigh, forming a "cowboy gunbelt and holster" pattern. Small, generalized eczematous papules may occur on other skin sites in severe reactions. These reactions usually persist for 1–3 weeks, but may persist much longer, or resolve only to recur spontaneously. On testing, patients with this pattern of reaction are positive on intradermal testing to the pure vitamin K_1.

In Europe a second pattern of vitamin K reaction has been reported. Subcutaneous sclerosis with or without fasciitis appears at the injection site many months after vitamin K treatment. There may have been a preceding acute reaction as previously described. Peripheral eosinophilia may be found. These pseudosclerodermatous reactions have been termed *Texier disease* and last several years.

The addition of vitamin K_1 to cosmetics has led to allergic contact dermatitis from the vitamin K, confirmed by patch testing.

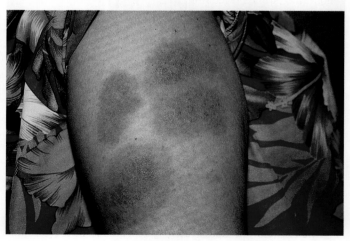

Fig. 6.34 Vitamin K allergy.

Injection Site Reactions

In addition to allergic reactions, as described with vitamin K, cutaneous necrosis may occur at sites of medication injections. These are of two typical forms: those associated with IV infusions and those related to intramuscular (IM) injections. Pharmacologic agents that extravasate into tissue during IV infusion may cause local tissue necrosis, resulting from inherent tissue-toxic properties. These include chemotherapeutic agents (fluorouracil in particular, but multiple agents), calcium salts, radiocontrast material, and nafcillin. IM injections may produce a syndrome called embolia cutis medicamentosa, livedoid dermatitis, or Nicolau syndrome. Immediately after injection, local intense pain occurs and the overlying skin blanches (ischemic pallor). Within minutes to hours, the site develops an erythematous macule that evolves into a livedoid violaceous patch with dendrites. This becomes hemorrhagic, then ulcerates, often forming a deep ulcer many centimeters in diameter. Eventually, over weeks to months, the ulcer heals with an atrophic scar. Muscle and liver enzymes may be elevated, and neurologic symptoms and sequelae occur in one third of patients. The circulation of the limb may be affected, rarely leading to amputation. Nicolau syndrome has been seen with injection of many unrelated agents, including NSAIDs, local anesthetics, corticosteroids, antibiotics, IFN-α, sedatives, vaccines, and medroxyprogesterone acetate (Depo-Provera). There may be a particular risk with refrigerated medications that may contain crystals, which are meant to be warmed before injection. It appears to be caused by periarterial injection leading to arterial thrombosis. IFN-β injections into subcutaneous tissue of the abdomen, buttocks, or thighs of patients with multiple sclerosis has resulted in similar lesions. Patient education and autoinjectors can prevent this complication. Biopsy of the IFN ISRs resembles lupus panniculitis. Vitamin B₁₂ also produces localized sclerodermoid reactions. Treatment of Nicolau syndrome is conservative: dressing changes, debridement, bed rest, and pain control. Surgical intervention is rarely required.

IFN injections, as well as subcutaneous injections of pain medication, allergy shots, and Depo-Provera, have also been reported to cause subcutaneous sarcoid-like granulomatous lesions. Fusion inhibitors, such as enfuvirtide, have very high rates of local ISRs. TNF inhibitors and other biologic agents, particularly anakinra, may frequently induce localized injection-site reactions, which in some cases can be severe enough to be treatment limiting. Calcinosis cutis may develop at injection sites, including from antithrombotic agents. Injection-site dermatitis has been reported with agents such as diclofenac, docetaxel, ketoprofen, piroxicam and others. Insulin pumps and injections have led to localized panniculitis-like nodules. One case of injection-site pseudolymphoma has been reported from a GM-CSF–producing tumor cell vaccine.

Abbott J, et al: Isolated subcutaneous sarcoid-like granulomatous inflammation occurring at injection sites. JAAD Case Rep 2017; 3: 74.

Al-Benna S, et al: Extravasation injuries in adults. ISRN Dermatol 2013; 2013: 856541.

Ball RA, et al: Injection site reactions with the HIV-1 fusion inhibitor enfuvirtide. J Am Acad Dermatol 2003; 49: 826.

Kaiser C, et al: Injection-site reactions upon anakinra administration. Rhematol Int 2012; 32: 295.

Kim DH, et al: Nicolau syndrome involving whole ipsilateral limb induced by intramuscular administration of gentamycin. Indian J Dermatol Venereol Leprol 2014; 80: 96.

Oh YJ, et al: A study about the cause and clinicopathologic findings of injection-induced dermatitis. Ann Dermatol 2015; 27: 721.

Staser K, et al: Injection-site cutaneous pseudolymphoma induced by a GM-CSF-producing tumor cell vaccine. JAMA Dermatol 2017; 153: 332.

Drug-Induced Pigmentation

Pigmentation of the skin may result from drug administration. The mechanism may be postinflammatory hyperpigmentation in some patients but frequently is related to actual deposition of the drug in the skin.

Minocycline induces many types of hyperpigmentation, which may occur in various combinations. Classically, three types of pigmentation are described. Type I is a blue-black discoloration appearing in areas of prior inflammation, often acne, sarcoidal plaques, or surgical scars (Fig. 6.35). This may be the most common type seen by dermatologists. It does not appear to be related to the total or daily dose of exposure. In all other types of pigmentation resulting from minocycline, the incidence increases with total dose, with up to 40% of treated patients experiencing hyperpigmentation with more than 1 year of therapy. The second type (type II) is the appearance of a similar-colored pigmentation on the normal skin of the anterior shins. In most cases, types I and II minocycline pigmentation occur after 3 months to several years of treatment. Generalized black hyperpigmentation has occurred after several days or a few weeks of treatment in Japanese patients. In type I and type II minocycline hyperpigmentation, histologic evaluation reveals pigment granules within macrophages in the dermis and at times in the fat, resembling a tattoo. These granules usually stain positively for both iron and melanin. At times, the macrophages containing minocycline are found only in the subcutaneous fat. Stains for iron may be negative in some cases. Calcium stains may also be positive because minocycline binds calcium. The least common type (type III) is generalized, muddy-brown hyperpigmentation, accentuated in sun-exposed areas. Tigecycline may produce similar hyperpigmentation. Histologic examination reveals only increased epidermal and dermal melanin. This may represent the consequence of a low-grade photosensitivity reaction.

In addition to the skin, minocycline types I and II pigmentation may also involve the sclera, conjunctiva, bone, thyroid, ear cartilage (simulating alkaptonuria), nail bed, oral mucosa, and permanent teeth (Fig. 6.36). Black veins have been reported following sclerotherapy in a patient on minocycline. Tetracycline staining of the teeth is usually related to childhood or fetal exposure, is brown, and is accentuated on the gingival third of the teeth. Dental hyperpigmentation caused by minocycline, in contrast, occurs in adults, is gray or gray-green, and is most marked in the midportion of the tooth. Some patients with affected teeth do not have hyperpigmentation elsewhere. The blue-gray pigmentation of the skin may be improved with the Q-switched ruby laser and pulsed dye laser, or fractional photothermolysis.

Chloroquine, hydroxychloroquine, and quinacrine all may cause a blue-black pigmentation of the face, extremities, ear cartilage,

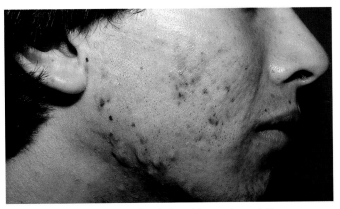

Fig. 6.35 Minocycline-induced hyperpigmentation.

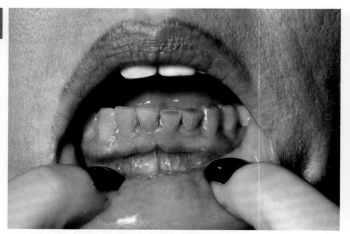

Fig. 6.36 Minocycline hyperpigmentation.

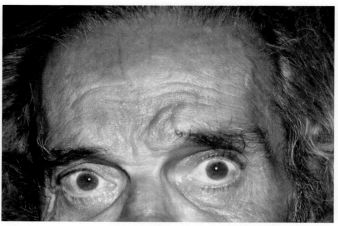

Fig. 6.37 Chlorpromazine hyperpigmentation.

oral mucosa, and nails, in up to 29% of patients. Generally this occurs after long duration or higher cumulative dose (over 300 g). Pretibial hyperpigmentation is the most common pattern and is similar to that induced by minocycline. The gingiva or hard palate may also be discolored. Quinidine may also rarely cause such a pattern of hyperpigmentation. Quinacrine is yellow and concentrated in the epidermis. Generalized yellow discoloration of the skin and sclera (mimicking jaundice) occurs reproducibly in patients but fades within 4 months of stopping the drug. In dark-skinned patients, this color is masked and less significant cosmetically. Histologically pigment granules are present within macrophages in the dermis.

Amiodarone causes photosensitivity in 30%–57% of treated patients after 3–6 months. In 1%–10% of patients, a slate-gray hyperpigmentation develops in the areas of photosensitivity. The pigmentation gradually fades after the medication is discontinued. Histologically, periodic acid–Schiff (PAS)–positive, yellow-brown granules are seen within the cytoplasm of macrophages in the dermis. Electron microscopy reveals membrane-bound structures resembling lipid-containing lysosomes. It responds to treatment with the Q-switched ruby laser.

Clofazimine treatment is reproducibly complicated by the appearance of a pink discoloration that gradually becomes reddish blue or brown and is concentrated in the lesions of patients with Hansen disease. This pigmentation may be disfiguring and is a major cause of noncompliance with this drug in the treatment of Hansen disease. Histologically, a PAS-positive, brown, granular pigment is variably seen within foamy macrophages in the dermis. This has been called "drug-induced lipofuscinosis."

Zidovudine causes a blue or brown hyperpigmentation that is most frequently observed in the nails. The lunula may be blue, or the whole nail plate may become dark brown. Diffuse hyperpigmentation of the skin, pigmentation of the lateral tongue, and increased tanning are less common. It occurs in darkly pigmented persons, is dose dependent, and clears after zidovudine is discontinued. Hydroxyurea causes a similar pattern of hyperpigmentation, including the melanonychia.

Chlorpromazine, thioridazine, imipramine, and clomipramine may cause a slate-gray hyperpigmentation in sun-exposed areas after long periods of ingestion (Fig. 6.37). Frequently, corneal and lens opacities are also present, so all patients with hyperpigmentation from these medications should have an ophthalmologic evaluation. The pigmentation from the phenothiazines fades gradually over years, even if the patient is treated with another phenothiazine. The corneal, but not the lenticular, changes also resolve. Imipramine hyperpigmentation has been reported to disappear within 1 year. Histologically, in sun-exposed but not sun-protected skin, numerous refractile golden-brown granules

are present within macrophages in the dermis, along with increased dermal melanin. The slate-gray color comes from a mixture of the golden-brown pigment of the drug and the black color of the melanin viewed in the dermis.

The heavy metals gold, silver, and bismuth produce blue to slate-gray hyperpigmentation. Pigmentation occurs after years of exposure, predominantly in sun-exposed areas, and is permanent. Silver is by far the most common form of heavy metal–induced pigmentation seen by dermatologists. It occurs in two forms, local or systemic. Local argyria typically follows the topical use of silver sulfadiazine or silver-containing dressings (Acticoat). Blue-gray pigmentation occurs at the site of application. Implantation into the skin by needles or pierced jewelry may lead to focal areas of argyria. Systemic argyria can also arise from topical application to the skin (in burn and epidermolysis bullosa patients), by inhalation, by mucosal application (nose drops or eyedrops), or by ingestion. Patients may purchase or build devices that allow them to make colloidal silver solutions, which they then ingest in the belief that it will improve their health. After several months of such exposure, the skin becomes slate-gray or blue-gray, primarily in areas of sun exposure. Histologically, granules of silver are found in basement membranes around adnexal (especially eccrine) and vascular structures. Sun exposure leads to the silver binding to either sulfur or selenium in the skin, increasing deposition. The deposited silver activates tyrosinase, increasing pigmentation. Most patients with argyria have no systemic symptoms or consequences of the increased silver in their body. Q-switched 1064-nm neodymium-doped yttrium-aluminum-garnet (Nd:YAG) laser may be used. Gold deposition was more common when gold was used as a treatment for rheumatoid arthritis. Cutaneous chrysiasis also presents as blue-gray pigmentation, usually after a cumulative dose of 8 g. Chrysiasis is also more prominent in sun-exposed sites. Dermatologists should remain aware of this condition, because patients treated with gold, even decades earlier, may develop disfiguring hyperpigmentation after Q-switched laser therapy for hair removal or lentigines lightening. Chrysiasis has been treated effectively in one patient using repeated 595-nm pulsed dye laser therapy. Bismuth also pigments the gingival margin. Histologically, granules of the metals are seen in the dermis and around blood vessels. Arsenical melanosis is characterized by black, generalized pigmentation or by a pronounced truncal hyperpigmentation that spares the face, with scattered depigmented macules that resemble raindrops.

The CCB diltiazem can cause a severe photodistributed hyperpigmentation. This is most common in African American or Hispanic women and occurs about 1 year after starting therapy. The lesions are slate-gray or gray-blue macules and patches on the face, neck, and forearms. Perifollicular accentuation is noted.

Histology shows a sparse lichenoid dermatitis with prominent dermal melanophages. The action spectrum of the drug appears to be in the UVB range, but hyperpigmentation is induced by UVA irradiation. The mechanism appears to be postinflammatory hyperpigmentation from a photosensitive lichenoid eruption rather than drug or drug metabolite deposition. Treatment is broad-spectrum sunscreens, stopping the diltiazem, and bleaching creams if needed. Other CCBs can be substituted without the reappearance of the hyperpigmentation.

Some chemotherapeutic agents have been reported to result in pigmentary changes of the skin, hair, and nails (see later discussion). Imatinib in particular has multiple reports of melasma-like hyperpigmentation particularly in darker skin types, and may also cause darkening in other sites, such as the palate. Multiple other agents can cause darkening of the hair, including antiviral drugs, valproate, retinoids, and CCBs; propofol has been reported to cause the hair to appear green in one case.

Periocular hyperpigmentation occurs in patients treated with prostaglandin analogs for glaucoma. These agents also cause pigmentation of the iris. Eyelash length increases. The periocular hyperpigmentation may gradually resolve when the medications are discontinued.

Bahloul E, et al: Hydroxychloroquine-induced hyperpigmentation in systemic diseases. Lupus 2017; 26: 1304.
Ghunawat S, et al: Imatinib induced melisma-like pigmentation. Indian J Dermatol Venereol Leprol 2016; 82: 409.
Nguyen AL, et al: Longitudinal melanonychia on multiple nails induced by hydroxyurea. BMJ Case Rep 2017; 2017: bcr2016218644.
Ricci F, et al: Drug-induced hair colour changes. Eur J Dermatol 2016; 26: 531.
Riemenschneider K, et al: Successful treatment of minocycline-induced pigmentation with combined use of Q-switched and pulsed dye lasers. Photodermatol Photoimmunol Photomed 2017; 33: 117.
Star P, et al: Black veins. J Cutan Pathol 2017; 44: 83.

Vasculitis and Serum Sickness–Like Reactions

Leukocytoclastic vasculitis (LCV) is a rare reaction but can be induced by many medications. Propylthiouracil and hydralazine are frequent culprits (and can induce antineutrophil cytoplasmic antibody). Biologic agents (TNF inhibitors, rituximab, ustekinumab), cocaine (with or without levamisole), and even montelukast and statins have been reported as inciting agents for drug-induced vasculitis. Antibiotics (minocycline, nafcillin, ciprofloxacin, vancomycin, and others) are common culprits in the inpatient setting. Targeted chemotherapeutic agents, particularly immunotherapy/checkpoint inhibitors, have demonstrated multiple autoimmune-pattern eruptions, including vasculitis (see later discussion).

True serum sickness is caused by foreign proteins such as antithymocyte globulin, with resulting circulating immune complexes. In the patient with true serum sickness, purpuric lesions tend to be accentuated along the junction between palmoplantar and glabrous skin (Wallace line).

Serum sickness–like reactions refer to adverse reactions that have similar symptoms to serum sickness, but in which immune complexes are not found. This reaction was particularly common with cefaclor, occurring in 1%–2% of patients. Patients present with fever, an urticarial rash, and arthralgias 1–3 weeks after starting the medication, without the vasculitis, hypocomplementemia, or nephropathy of true serum sickness. Antibiotics are the most frequent culprits (especially β-lactams and minocycline), but other agents such as bupropion, influenza vaccination, NSAIDs, and rituximab have been reported to cause serum sickness–like reactions.

Lichenoid Reactions

Lichenoid reactions can be seen with many medications, including gold, hydrochlorothiazide, furosemide, NSAIDs, aspirin, antihypertensives (ACE inhibitors, β-blockers, CCBs), terazosin, quinidine, proton pump inhibitors, pravastatin, phenothiazines, anticonvulsants, antituberculous drugs, ketoconazole, sildenafil, imatinib, antivirals for hepatitis C, and antimalarials. Hepatitis B immunization may trigger a lichenoid eruption. Checkpoint inhibitors for cancer therapy are an emerging class of agents with high rates of lichenoid reactions (see later discussion). Lichenoid reactions may be photodistributed (lichenoid photoeruption) or generalized, and drugs causing lichenoid photoeruptions may also induce more generalized ones. In either case, the lesions may be plaques (occasionally with Wickham striae), small papules, or exfoliative erythema. Photolichenoid reactions favor the extensor extremities, including the dorsa of the hands. Oral involvement is less common in lichenoid drug reactions than in idiopathic lichen planus but can occur (and with imatinib may be severe). It appears as either plaques or erosions. The lower lip is frequently involved in photolichenoid reactions. The nails may also be affected and can be the only site of involvement. Lichenoid drug eruptions can occur within months to years of starting the offending medication and may take months to years to resolve once the medication has been stopped. Histologically, inflammation occurs along the DEJ, with necrosis of keratinocytes and a dermal infiltrate composed primarily of lymphocytes. Eosinophils are useful, if present, but are not common in photolichenoid reactions. The histology is often similar to idiopathic lichen planus, though eosinophils may be more prominent, and a clinical correlation is required to determine whether the lichenoid eruption is drug induced. If the drug is essential, the course of treatment may be tolerated with corticosteroid therapy.

Lichenoid reactions may be restricted to the oral mucosa, especially if induced by dental amalgam. In these patients, the lesions are topographically related to the dental fillings or to metal prostheses. Patients may be patch test positive to mercury, or less often gold, cobalt, or nickel, in up to two thirds of cases. Amalgam replacement will result in resolution of the oral lesions in these cases. Patients with cutaneous lesions of lichen planus and oral lesions do not improve with amalgam removal. An unusual form of eruption is the "drug-induced ulceration of the lower lip." Patients present with a persistent erosion of the lower lip that is tender but not indurated. It is induced by diuretics and resolves slowly once they are discontinued.

Grau RG: Drug-induced vasculitis. Curr Rheumatol Rep 2015; 17: 71.
MacArthur KM, et al: Severe small-vessel vasculitis temporally associated with administration of ustekinumab. J Drugs Dermatol 2016; 15: 359.
Mirouse A, et al: Systemic vasculitis associated with vemurafenib treatment. Medicine (Baltimore) 2016; 95: e4988.
Morgado B, et al: Leukocytoclastic vasculitis with systemic involvement associated with ciprofloxacin therapy. Cureus 2016; 8: e900.
Pingili CS, et al: Vancomycin-induced leukocytoclastic vasculitis and acute renal failure due to tubulointerstitial nephritis. Am J Case Rep 2017; 18: 1024.
Yorulmaz A, et al: Demographic and clinical characteristics of patients with serum sickness-like reaction. Clin Rheumatol 2017; ePub ahead of print.

Adverse Reactions to Chemotherapeutic Agents

Patients undergoing treatment for cancer can develop skin manifestations due to their disease, paraneoplastic conditions, chemotherapeutic agents, immunosuppression-related conditions and infections, and supportive medications. Patients who undergo bone marrow transplants can develop reactions due to engraftment syndrome, the eruption of lymphocyte recovery (nonspecific erythematous macules as lymphocyte count recovers), or GVHD (see Chapter 5) as well.

Chemotherapeutic agents can cause adverse reactions by multiple potential mechanisms. Adverse reactions may be related to toxicity either directly to the mucocutaneous surfaces (stomatitis, alopecia), or reflected in the skin, such as purpura resulting from thrombocytopenia. The use of localizing cooling devices to limit blood flow, and reduce chemotherapy delivery to sites of toxicity may help prevent or alleviate some side effects, such as nail damage or hair loss. Chemotherapeutic agents can also act as antigens inducing classic immunologic reactions, or as immunotherapy may stimulate autoimmune reactions through their intended mechanism of anticancer action. Chemotherapy reactions can be grouped by skin reaction pattern, or by drug class. Most reactions are assessed using the common terminology criteria for adverse events (CTCAE) grading scale to determine whether dose reduction, interval prolongation, or alternate agents are necessary. Xerosis (17%–20%), pruritus (17%–20%), and nonspecific erythematous papular eruptions are fairly common and managed with supportive care.

Dermatologists are rarely confronted with the acute hypersensitivity reactions seen during infusion of chemotherapeutic agents. These reactions resemble type I allergic reactions, with urticaria and hypotension, and can be prevented by premedication with systemic corticosteroids and antihistamines in most cases.

Toxic Erythema of Chemotherapy (Chemotherapy-Induced Acral Erythema, Palmoplantar Erythrodysesthesia Syndrome, Hand-Foot Syndrome, Intertriginous Eruptions)

The unifying term *toxic erythema of chemotherapy* was proposed by Bolognia in 2008. Many traditional chemotherapeutic agents can induce this relatively common reaction (taxanes, especially docetaxel, cytarabine, anthracyclines, 5-fluorouracil [5-FU] capecitabine, methotrexate, and others less commonly). In the case of pegylated liposomal doxorubicin, localization of the chemotherapeutic agent to the sweat glands has been demonstrated, and one report demonstrated a strikingly intertriginous/flexural erythema and peeling that spared only one axilla, which had been previously radiated and lacked adnexal structures. Cases of neutrophilic eccrine hidradenitis and syringometaplasia, all induced by the same agents, suggest that the eccrine glands are unique targets for adverse reactions to antineoplastic agents.

The initial manifestation is often dysesthesia or tingling of the palms and soles, usually 2–3 weeks after administration of chemotherapy. This is followed in a few days by painful, symmetric erythema and edema most pronounced over the distal pads of the digits. Painful erythema and skin peeling can occur and the skin becomes dusky, deep red-brown, and may blister and desquamate either superficially or involving most of the epidermis (Fig. 6.38). The desquamation is often the most prominent part of the syndrome. The eruption generally involves sites of contact, friction, rubbing, or high concentrations of eccrine ducts/sweat, presumably due to accumulation of toxic metabolites plus occlusion or mild trauma. A localized plaque of fixed erythrodysesthesia has been described proximal to the infusion site of docetaxel, and cytarabine can cause striking localized ear erythema.

The histopathology is nonspecific, with necrotic keratinocytes and vacuolar changes along the basal cell layer. Acute GVHD is in the differential diagnosis. Histologic evaluation may not be useful in the acute setting to distinguish these syndromes. The clinical distribution, timing, and presence or absence of extracutaneous involvement (gastrointestinal or liver findings of GVHD) are more helpful.

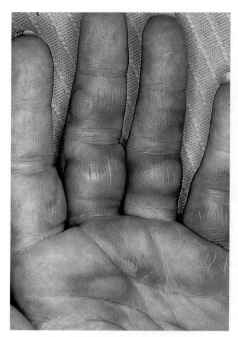

Fig. 6.38 Hand-foot syndrome.

Most patients require only local supportive care. Cold compresses and elevation are helpful, and cooling the hands during treatment may reduce the severity of the reaction. Modification of the dose schedule can be beneficial. Pyridoxine, 100–150 mg daily, decreased the pain of 5-FU–induced acral erythema in one study, but benefits are not proven. Cox-2 inhibitors have also been suggested. Local or systemic corticosteroids may be considered, depending on the severity. Lidocaine patches may help with pain. IVIG has been reported to be beneficial in a methotrexate-induced case of acral erythema. Cyclosporine has been reported to result in worsening of the condition.

Sorafenib and sunitinib are small, multikinase-inhibiting molecules with blocking activity for numerous tyrosine kinases, including vascular endothelial growth factor (VEGF), platelet-derived growth factor (PDGFRβ), and c-kit ligand (stem cell factor). Both agents induce a condition similar to acral erythema, also referred to as hand-foot skin reaction (HFSR). Patients also present with acral pain and dysesthesia, but usually less severe than with classic chemotherapeutic agents. In contrast to classic acral erythema, multikinase inhibitor–induced HFSR causes lesions over areas of friction, either blisters or patchy hyperkeratotic plaques. The HFSR is dose dependent, high grade in 9% of cases (with blisters, ulceration, and functional loss) and results in the sorafenib being stopped in about 1% of patients. The addition of another VEGF inhibitor, bevacizumab, leads to worse HFSR. Olmutinib was reported to induce a palmoplantar keratoderma in 3 patients. The development of hand-foot syndrome in patients receiving sorafenib for metastatic renal cell carcinoma is associated with better tumor response and improved progression-free survival.

Histologically, there are horizontal layers of necrotic keratinocytes within the epidermis (if biopsy is taken in first 30 days) or in the stratum corneum (later biopsies). Topical tazarotene, 40% urea, heparin ointment, and fluorouracil cream have been used to treat HFSR from multikinase inhibitors.

Neutrophilic eccrine hidradenitis is discussed in Chapter 33.

Chemotherapy-Induced Dyspigmentation

Many traditional chemotherapeutic agents (especially the antibiotics bleomycin, doxorubicin, and daunorubicin) and the alkylating

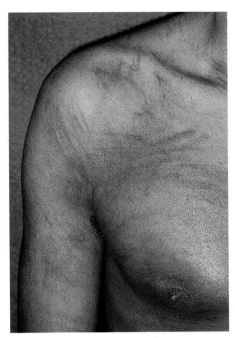

Fig. 6.39 Bleomycin-induced flagellate hyperpigmentation.

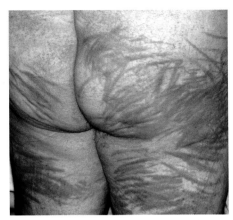

Fig. 6.40 Shiitake mushroom–induced dermatitis. (Courtesy Don Adler, DO.)

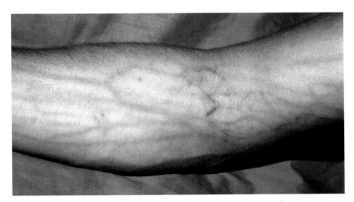

Fig. 6.41 Methotrexate-induced vascular hyperpigmentation. (Courtesy Steven Binnick, MD.)

agents (cyclophosphamide and busulfan) cause various patterns of cutaneous hyperpigmentation; the risk of pigmentary changes with targeted chemotherapeutic agents is gaining recognition. Adriamycin (doxorubicin) causes marked hyperpigmentation of the nails, skin, and tongue. This is most common in black patients and appears in locations where constitutional hyperpigmentation is sometimes seen. Hydroxyurea can also cause this pattern of hyperpigmentation. Cyclophosphamide causes transverse banding of the nails or diffuse nail hyperpigmentation beginning proximally. Bleomycin and 5-FU cause similar transverse bands. Busulfan and 5-FU induce diffuse hyperpigmentation that may be photoaccentuated.

Bleomycin induces characteristic flagellate erythematous urticarial wheals associated with pruritus within hours or days of infusion (Fig. 6.39). Lesions continue to appear for days to weeks. Although investigators have not always been able to induce lesions, the pattern strongly suggests scratching is the cause. Bleomycin hyperpigmentation may be accentuated at areas of pressure, strongly supporting trauma as the cause of the peculiar pattern. Patients may present with linear erythematous wheals 1–2 days after eating raw or cooked shiitake mushrooms (Fig. 6.40). This so-called toxicodermia, or shiitake flagellate dermatitis, is thought to be caused by a toxic reaction to lentinan, a polysaccharide component of the mushrooms. It is self-limited and resolves within days to weeks of its appearance, but can be treated with topical corticosteroids to relieve the associated pruritus some patients experience. Other associations with flagellate eruptions include adult-onset Still disease, dermatomyositis, and docetaxel therapy.

5-FU, and less frequently other chemotherapeutic agents such as methotrexate, may produce a serpentine hyperpigmentation overlying the veins proximal to an infusion site (Fig. 6.41). This represents hyperpigmentation from a direct cytotoxic effect of the chemotherapeutic agent.

Targeted chemotherapeutic agents may also induce a variety of patterns of pigmentary changes, with one review showing 17% of patients with skin and 21% of patients with hair pigmentation sequelae. Most established is imatinib, which leads to dose-related generalized or localized hypopigmentation in 40% or more of pigmented persons (possibly due to inhibiting tyrosinase activity). Paradoxic hyperpigmentation of the skin, nails, and hair caused by imatinib has been reported. It starts an average of 4 weeks

after treatment and progresses over time if treatment with imatinib is continued. Patients also complain of an inability to tan and "photosensitivity." Imatinib-induced pseudoporphyria has been reported. One patient with vitiligo had significant progression with imatinib therapy. Multikinase inhibitors (such as cabozantinib, pazopanib, sorafenib, and sunitinib) may inhibit *C-kit*, which is a regulator of melanogenesis, and may induce skin pigmentary changes through this mechanism, such as sunitinib-related depigmentation of the hair after 5–6 weeks of treatment. Sunitinib may lead to yellow pigmentation of the skin from the drug or its metabolites being deposited, though some mTOR inhibitors have also been reported to cause yellowing (temsirolimus). Eruptive melanocytic nevi and lentigines with an acral predisposition have been seen with sorafenib therapy. Ipilimumab, pembrolizumab, and nivolumab are immune-stimulating agents that likely induce vitiligo through autoimmune-activited CD8+ T cells targeting the melanocytes. EGF-receptor inhibitors, VEGF-receptor inhibitors, and other targeted agents have also been reported to cause both skin and hair hypopigmentation as well. Although in general targeted agents induce less alopecia (14% overall) than cytoxic chemotherapy, some (particularly vismodegib, at over 50%) have high rates.

Palifermin-Associated Papular Eruption

Palifermin is a recombinant human keratinocyte growth factor sometimes used to reduce the severity and duration of mucositis in patients undergoing hematopoietic stem cell transplantation. An intertriginous erythema accompanied by oral white confluent plaques and small lichenoid papules developed in one patient receiving palifermin therapy. A direct hyperproliferative effect of the keratinocyte growth factor is the proposed mechanism.

Chemotherapy-Induced Pseudocellulitis

Gemcitabine has been reported to cause a bilateral bright red leg syndrome, which can mimic cellulitis. It has also been described as causing a lipodermatosclerosis-like eruption, possibly after the pseudocellulitis. Pemetrexed has also been noted to cause a similar eruption. Both of these reactions have been reported in sites of lymphedema or swelling, possibly through impaired lymphatic drainage leading to drug accumulation in the tissues. The bilaterality and symmetry may help distinguish from infection. Biopsy may demonstrate eosinophils within a mixed infiltrate.

Scleroderma-Like Reactions

Patients treated with the taxanes (docetaxel, paclitaxel) or pemetrexed have been reported to develop an acute, diffuse, infiltrated edema of the extremities and/or head. This occurs after one to several courses. The affected areas, specifically the lower extremities, evolve over months to become sclerotic and at times painful. Flexion contractures of the palm, digits, and large joints may occur. Biopsies of the initial lesion show lymphangiectasia and a diffuse infiltration with mononuclear cells in the superficial dermis. Late fibrotic lesions demonstrate marked dermal fibrosis. Discontinuation of the therapy leads to resolution in most cases.

Exudative Hyponychial Dermatitis

Repeated chemotherapeutic cycles can lead to patterned nail changes due to recurrent growth interruption (Beau lines). More severe nail toxicity is common (20%–44% in most studies, though some report as high as 89%) during chemotherapy for breast cancer, especially with taxanes (particularly docetaxel). Subungual hemorrhage, subungual abscesses, paronychia, subungual hyperkeratosis, and onychomadesis all occur, though onycholysis is most common, and can be severe. All these reactions probably represent various degrees of toxicity to the nail bed. Protective clear polish, clipping the nails back, using cotton gloves, and avoiding trauma are helpful; frozen gloves during chemotherapy may help prevent the reaction.

Cutaneous Side Effects of Epidermal Growth Factor Receptor Inhibitors

Epidermal growth factor receptor (EGFR) inhibitors are used for a variety of tumors, and include both monoclonal antibodies (cetuximab and panitumumab) and tyrosine kinase inhibitors. EGFR is expressed by basal keratinocytes, sebocytes, and the outer root sheath, explaining why up to 90% of patients treated with EGFR inhibitors may develop cutaneous side effects, including xerosis (19%), pruritus (24%), trichomegaly, hair curling, and signs of skin aging, and painful periungual or finger pulp fissures and paronychia (with or without periungual pyogenic granulomas) may develop in 15%–25% (Fig. 6.42).

The most common side effect is an acneiform rash, which is severe in up to 18% of cases. The severity of the reaction may indicate more drug metabolism and possibly better tumor response rates. When severe, however, the eruption can be dose limiting. The eruption begins 7–10 days after initiation of therapy, attaining maximum severity in the second week. The seborrheic areas of the scalp, central face, upper back, and retroauricular regions are mainly affected. The primary lesion is a follicular papule or pustule with few or no comedones. Crusting and confluence can occur. Cultures should be performed to rule out secondary infection in patients with severe disease. Radiation therapy during EGFR

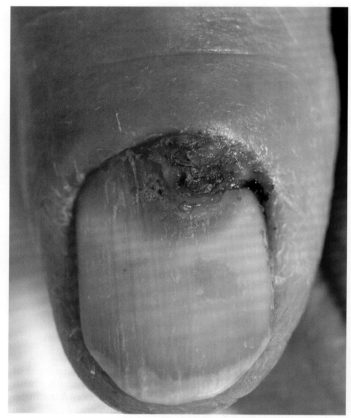

Fig. 6.42 Epidermal growth factor receptor (EGFR) inhibitor–induced paronychia.

inhibitor therapy will enhance the skin toxicity, but previously radiated skin is often spared from inhibitor toxicity. Treatment is oral tetracycline antibiotics and corticosteroids. It is recommended that prophylactic sun protection and oral doxycycline be used in many cases. Effective topical therapies have included metronidazole, clindamycin, hydrocortisone, pimecrolimus, tretinoin, and possibly dapsone. In the most severe cases, isotretinoin or acitretin can be used. TNF-α and IL-1 are involved in the pathogenesis of EGFR inhibitor toxicity. Etanercept and anakinra, therefore, may also be therapeutically useful.

Other Cutaneous Side Effects of Multikinase Inhibitors

In addition to the reactions previously listed, multikinase inhibitors may cause other skin reactions. Psoriasis exacerbation, acral psoriasiform hyperkeratosis, and pityriasis rosea-like eruptions have been described with imatinib. Both imatinib and sunitinib cause facial edema, with a periocular predilection. Increased vascular permeability caused by PDGFR inhibition has been the proposed mechanism. Dasatinib has caused a lobular panniculitis. Bevacizumab, a VEGF inhibitor, causes bleeding, painful distal subungual splinter hemorrhages, and wound healing complications. Extensive cutaneous surgery should probably be delayed for 60 days after bevacizumab therapy, and 28 days should elapse after surgery before initiation of bevacizumab therapy. Bevacizumab has also been associated with ulceration of striae distensae (Fig. 6.43). VEGF inhibitors in general can lead to mucosal bleeding (epistaxis).

BRAF-Inhibitor Reactions

BRAF mutations are common in melanoma and other malignancies. Targeted BRAF inhibitors (vemurafenib, dabrafenib) have been

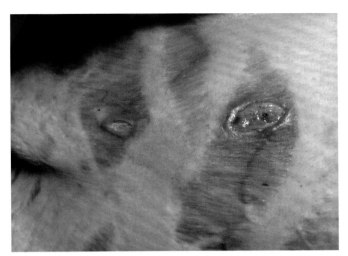

Fig. 6.43 Bevacizumab-induced ulceration of striae. (Courtesy Farber SA, Samimi S, Rosenbach M. Ulcerations within striae distensae associated with bevacizumab therapy. J Am Acad Dermatol 2015;72;1:e33-35.)

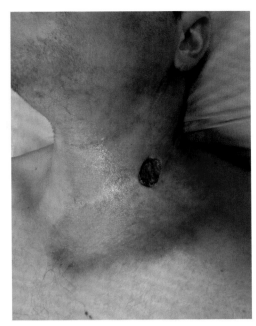

Fig. 6.44 Radiation recall induced by vemurafenib.

successfully used to treat metastatic melanoma, but may have a number of cutaneous adverse effects. Many patients exhibit pruritus and can develop a nonspecific eruption, and these agents are very photosensitizing. Verrucous keratoses resembling warts occur in more than 50% of patients. Patients may develop palmoplantar hyperkeratosis and curly hair. From 20%–30% of patients develop SCCs, including keratoacanthoma (KA)-type lesions, which may be eruptive early in treatment. BRAF-inhibitors can induce changes in existing nevi, and eruptive nevi. Radiation recall may be seen. A panniculitis has been reported in some patients. MEK inhibitors typically cause a papulopustular eruption, but have also been reported to cause a dusky erythema. When used in combination, patients on combined BRAF/MEK inhibitions have fewer of the BRAF-inhibitor–related side effects. Sorafenib is a multikinase inhibitor with BRAF-inhibitory activity, and has also been associated with the rapid development of multiple keratoacanthomas or SCCs, as well as eruptive melanocytic lesions. Bexarotene was reported as therapeutic in a patient with sorafenib-induced squamoproliferative lesions. Multiple monomorphous, follicular, keratotic skin-colored papules resembling keratosis pilaris can develop during sorafenib treatment. Histologically, these papules show hyperplasia of the follicular isthmus or follicular hyperkeratosis with plugging. Facial and scalp erythema and dysesthesia occur in about 60% of sorafenib-treated patients.

Checkpoint Inhibitors and Immunotherapy

Immunotherapy for cancer is a rapidly emerging area, with an explosion of indications for the novel class of anticancer agents, immune-checkpoint inhibitors. Ipilimumab is an anti CTLA-4 antibody used for metastatic melanoma, and can cause a maculopapular rash, alopecia, and fairly commonly vitiligo. Currently pembrolizumab and nivolimuab are approved PD-1 receptor inhibitors, with agents targeting the PD-1 ligand PD-L1 and other agents being rapidly developed. These drugs have many immune-mediated side effects, including cutaneous reactions. Nonspecific rash is common (15%–29%), as is pruritus (12%); vitiligo occurs in 7%–9% of patients (especially when the drugs are used to treat melanoma). Lichenoid reactions, both clinically and histologically, are also fairly common, including oral lichenoid mucositis. Patients who had skin reactions have been reported to have longer progression-free survival in small studies. Reports

of rare reactions, such as vasculitis, granulomatous eruptions (sarcoidosis, granuloma annulare), panniculitis, lupus-like reactions, and SJS/TEN also exist. Alopecia may develop in these patients as well, an unlike traditional cytotoxic chemotherapy, may be alopecia areata or universalis pattern. Eruptive keratoacanthomas were reported in three patients. Interestingly, there are multiple reports of PD-1-inhibitor–induced autoimmune bullous eruptions resembling bullous pemphigoid with anti BP-180 antibodies. Most immune-mediated reactions are managed with topical or systemic corticosteroids.

Radiation Enhancement and Recall Reactions

Radiation dermatitis, in the form of intense erythema and vesiculation of the skin, may be observed in radiation ports. Administration of many chemotherapeutic agents, during or about the time of radiation therapy, may induce an enhanced radiation reaction. In some patients, however, months to years after radiation treatment, the administration of a chemotherapeutic agent may induce a reaction within the prior radiation port, with features of radiation dermatitis (Fig. 6.44). This phenomenon has been termed "radiation recall," reported with numerous chemotherapeutic agents (gemcitabine, small molecule inhibitors, tamoxifen, methotrexate, taxanes, and multiple other agents), high-dose IFN-α, and simvastatin. Besides the skin, internal structures such as the gut may also be affected. A similar reaction of reactivation of a sunburn after methotrexate therapy also occurs. Exanthems restricted to prior areas of sunburn are not true radiation recall, but may represent "locus minoris resistentiae," or a nonspecific eruption showing up at a site of prior damage.

Belum VR, et al: Characterisation and management of dermatologic adverse events to agents targeting the PD-1 receptor. Eur J Cancer 2016; 60: 12.

Bolognia JL, et al: Toxic erythema of chemotherapy. J Am Acad Dermatol 2008; 59: 524.

Capriotti K, et al: The risk of nail changes with taxane chemotherapy. Br J Dermatol 2015; 173: 842.

Chen KL, et al: Olmutinib-induced palmoplantar keratoderma. Br J Dermatol 2017; ePub ahead of print.

Dai J, et al: Pigmentary changes in patients treated with targeted anticancer agents. J Am Acad Dermatol 2017; 77: 902.

Freites-Martinez A, et al: Eruptive keratoacanthomas associated with pembrolizumab therapy. JAMA Dermatol 2017; 153: 694.

Gaughan EM: Sarcoidosis, malignancy, and immune checkpoint blockade. Immunotherapy 2017; 9: 1051.

Gorcsey L, et al: Papular eruption associated with palifermin. J Am Acad Dermatol 2014; 71: 101.

Hofheinz RD, et al: Recommendations for the prophylactic management of skin reactions induced by epidermal growth factor receptor inhibitors in patients with solid tumors. Oncologist 2016; 21: 1483.

Ishikawa K, et al: Pemetrexed-induced scleroderma-like conditions in the lower legs of a patient with non-small cell lung carcinoma. J Dermatol 2016; 43: 1071.

Kaunitz GJ, et al: Cutaneous eruptions in patients receiving immune checkpoint blockade. Am J Surg Pathol 2017; 41: 1381.

Lacouture ME, et al: Ipilimumab in patient with cancer and the management of dermatologic adverse events. J Am Acad Dermatol 2014; 71: 161.

Macdonald JB, et al: Cutaneous adverse effects of targeted therapies. J Am Acad Dermatol 2015; 72: 203.

Mittal A, et al: Gemcitabine-associated acute lipodermatosclerosis-like eruption. JAAD Case Rep 2017; 3: 190.

Naidoo J, et al: Autoimmune bullous skin disorders with immune checkpoint inhibitors targeting PD-1 and PD-L1. Cancer Immunol Res 2016; 4: 383.

Patel U, et al: MEK inhibitor-induced dusky erythema. JAMA Dermatol 2015; 151: 78.

Sanlorenzo M, et al: Pembrolizumab cutaneous adverse events and their association with disease progression. JAMA Dermatol 2015; 151: 1206.

Shah VV, et al: Scalp hypothermia as a preventative measure for chemotherapy-induced alopecia. J Eur Acad Dermatol Venereol 2017; ePub ahead of print.

Shao K, et al: Lupus-like cutaneous reaction following pembrolizumab. J Cutan Pathol 2017; ePub ahead of print.

Sibaud V, et al: Dermatological adverse events with taxane chemotherapy. Eur J Dermatol 2016; 26: 427.

Sibaud V, et al: Oral lichenoid reactions associated with anti-PD-1/PD-L1 therapies. J Eur Acad Dermatol Venereol 2017; e464.

Tracey EH, et al: Pemetrexed-induced pseudocellulitis reaction with eosinophilic infiltrate on ski biopsy. Am J Dermatopathol 2017; 39: e1.

Valentine J, et al: Incidence and risk of xerosis with targeted anticancer therapies. J Am Acad Dermatol 2015; 72: 656.

Wu J, et al: Granuloma annulare associated with immune checkpoint inhibitors. J Eur Acad Dermatol Venereol 2017; ePub ahead of print.

Zarbo A, et al: Immune-related alopecia (areata and universalis) in cancer patients receiving immune checkpoint inhibitors. Br J Dermatol 2017; 176: 1649.

Cutaneous Adverse Reactions to Traditional Immunosuppressants Used in Dermatology

Azathioprine is used as a steroid-sparing agent for dermatologic conditions and can cause a hypersensitivity syndrome. In addition, neutrophilic dermatoses resembling Sweet syndrome appear with azathioprine therapy and resolve with its discontinuation. Photosensitivity can also occur with azathioprine, despite its frequent use in severe photodermatoses.

Methotrexate can cause erosive skin lesions in two patterns. Ulceration or erosion of psoriatic plaques may be a sign that the patient is taking a midweek dose of methotrexate. This can be associated with severe methotrexate marrow toxicity. If renal failure is present or occurs during low-dose methotrexate therapy, a severe bullous eruption resembling TEN can occur. This apparently represents severe cutaneous toxicity from the prolonged blood and skin levels of methotrexate that result from reduced excretion because of coexistent renal disease and drug-drug interactions, and is more common in older patients, patients with renal disease, and higher dose without folic acid supplementation. If this scenario is recognized, leucovorin rescue should be prescribed.

Adverse Reactions to Cytokines

Cytokines, which are normal mediators of inflammation or cell growth, are increasingly used in the management of malignancies and to ameliorate the hematologic complications of disease or its treatment. Skin toxicity is a common complication of the use of these agents. Many cause local inflammation and ulceration at the injection site in a large number of the patients treated. More widespread papular eruptions are also frequently reported.

Granulocyte colony-stimulating factor (G-CSF) has been associated with the induction of several neutrophil-mediated disorders, most often Sweet syndrome or bullous pyoderma gangrenosum. These occur about 1 week after cytokine therapy is initiated and are present despite persistent neutropenia in peripheral blood. A rare complication of G-CSF is a thrombotic and necrotizing panniculitis. Both G-CSF and GM-CSF may exacerbate leukocytoclastic vasculitis. IFN-α, IFN-γ, and G-CSF have been associated with the exacerbation of psoriasis. Rarely, linear IgA disease can be induced by IFN-α. G-CSF can also cause granulomatous dermatitides. IFN therapy can induce granulomatous lesions, both systemic granulomatous processes and localized granulomatous reactions at injection sites. Anakinra and rarely erythropoietin can cause similar granulomatous skin reactions.

IL-2 frequently causes diffuse erythema, followed by desquamation, pruritus, mucositis (resembling aphthosis), glossitis, and flushing. Erythroderma with blistering or TEN-like reactions can occur and may be dose limiting. Administration of iodinated contrast material within 2 weeks of IL-2 therapy is associated with a hypersensitivity reaction in 30% of patients. Fever, chills, angioedema, urticaria, and hypotension may occur. Subcutaneous injections of IL-2 can lead to injection site nodules or necrosis. Histologically, a diffuse panniculitis with noninflammatory necrosis of the involved tissue is present.

Aleissa M, et al: Azathioprine hypersensitivity syndrome. Case Rep Dermatol 2017; 19: 6.

Chen TJ, et al: Methotrexate-induced epidermal necrosis. J Am Acad Dermatol 2017; 77: 247.

Colafrancesco S, et al: Response to interleukin-1 inhibitors in 140 Italian patients with adult-onset Still's disease. Front Pharmacol 2017; 8: 369.

Ilyas M, et al: Cutaneous toxicities from transplantation-related medications. Am J Transplant 2017; 17: 2782.

Ozaki S, et al: Granulocyte colony-stimulating factor-induced granulomatous dermatitis with enlarged histiocytes clinically manifesting as painful edematous nodules with high fever similar to Sweet's syndrome. J Dermatol 2015; 42: 414.

Adverse Reactions to Biologic Agents

Tumor Necrosis Factor Inhibitors

The TNF inhibitors are associated with palmoplantar pustulosis, pustular folliculitis, new or worsening of psoriasis, interface dermatitis, neutrophilic eccrine hidradenitis, Sweet syndrome, lupus (systemic and subacute cutaneous), granulomatous reactions (sarcoidosis, granuloma annulare), and vasculitis. ISRs are common with etanercept therapy for rheumatologic disease, with 20%–40% of patients developing ISR. ISRs present as erythematous, mildly

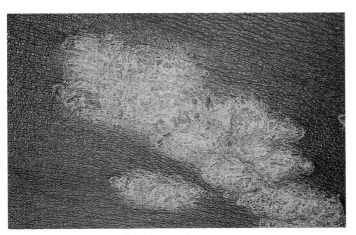

Fig. 6.45 Plaque-type psoriasis.

swollen plaques, appearing 1–2 days after the injection. Pruritus occurs in 20% of patients. ISR is most common early in the treatment course (median number of injections, four) and stops appearing with continued treatment. Individual lesions resolve over 2–3 days. Recall ISR (reappearance of eruption at previous ISR site) occurs in 40% of patients. This adverse reaction appears to be mediated by CD8+ T cells. IL-1 (anakinra) therapy is associated with high rates of local ISRs (>50% in one study of 140 patients) and diffuse rash (25% of patients), which may be urticarial.

The paradoxic appearance of psoriasis or a psoriasiform dermatitis is now a well-recognized complication of TNF inhibitor therapy. It occurs with all of the TNF inhibitors. The psoriasis can appear from days to years after anti-TNF therapy. There is no age or gender predisposition. Several clinical patterns have been described. Palmoplantar pustulosis represents about 40% of cases. Generalized pustular disease may accompany the palmoplantar lesions. Plaque-type psoriasis occurs in about one third of TNF inhibitor–induced psoriasis (Fig. 6.45). New-onset guttate psoriasis occurs in 10% of cases. Stopping the TNF inhibitor led to improvement or resolution in the vast majority of patients. In some cases, therapy was continued and the eruption resolved. Experts disagree as to whether switching to a different anti-TNF agent may be tolerated in these patients. Many patients have been rechallenged with other TNF inhibitors. In severe cases, this is probably not prudent, but in milder or localized cases, this could be considered. The psoriasis caused by anti-TNF agents can be treated with topical corticosteroids, UV phototherapy, topical vitamin D analogs, methotrexate, acitretin, cyclosporine, or other antipsoriatic biologics. The proposed mechanism for the appearance with psoriasis with anti-TNF therapy is either overactivity of Th1 cells or increased IFN-α production by skin-resident plasmacytoid dendritic cells. Systemic IFN-α and topical imiquimod (an IFN inducer) have been reported to exacerbate psoriasis, supporting this hypothesis. Sarcoidosis induced by anti-TNF agents could also be related to increased IFN production.

Many patients on biologic therapy may develop new antinuclear antibodies (ANAs; 11% of etanercept patients for RA, similar rates with infliximab), though most of those do not have overt lupus. True drug-induced lupus (DIL) with features of SLE may occur. It begins on average after 41 weeks of treatment. Compared with DIL from other medications, the TNF inhibitors cause more skin disease with malar rash, discoid lesions, and photosensitivity. Many of the patients fulfill the American Rheumatology Association (ARA) criteria for SLE, and significant internal organ involvement can occur, including renal and central nervous system (CNS) involvement. Etanercept seems to cause skin lesions more frequently. Etanercept patients also developed vasculitis more often. The vast

majority of patients improve about 10 months after therapy has been discontinued. Switching from one TNF inhibitor to another has been reported to be successful. Subacute cutaneous lupus erythematosus (SCLE) may also occur. This is important to keep in mind as the appearance may be psoriasiform, rather than the classic annular morphology, and can be mistaken for TNF-induced psoriasis. Dermatomyositis has also been caused by TNF inhibitor treatment.

Vasculitis is also a well-recognized complication of treatment with TNF inhibitors. Etanercept is the most common agent reported to induce vasculitis. The lesions of vasculitis may begin around the injection sites in some etanercept-induced vasculitis cases. More than 85% of patients present with skin lesions, usually a leukocytoclastic vasculitis. Ulcerations, nodules, digital lesions, chilblains, livedo, and other morphologies have also been described. Visceral vasculitis occurs in about one quarter of patients. They may be ANA positive or antineutrophil cytoplasmic antibody (ANCA) positive (usually p-ANCA) or may have cryoglobulins. Drug-induced antiphospholipid syndrome with TNF inhibitors can be associated with DIL or vasculitis and presents with thrombosis as well as cutaneous lesions. Some patients with TNF inhibitor–induced vasculitis have died. Stopping the TNF inhibitor leads to resolution of the vasculitis in more than 90% of cases. Rechallenge leads to new vasculitic lesions in 75% of cases. Other neutrophilic disorders induced by TNF inhibitors include Sweet syndrome–like reactions and neutrophilic eccrine hidradenitis. New onset vitiligo has also been reported with a variety of biologics, primarily the TNF inhibitors.

Lichenoid drug eruptions have been reported from anti-TNF agents. They are typically pruritic and affect areas typically involved by lichen planus: the flexor wrists. However, gluteal cleft lesions are also common. In some cases, the lichenoid eruption superimposes itself on psoriatic lesions, presenting as an exacerbation of the "psoriasis." Biopsies show features of both lichen planus and psoriasis, and stopping the anti-TNF therapy leads to improvement of the "psoriasis." Despite these agents' immunosuppressive properties, patients can still develop allergic contact dermatitis while taking them, and patch testing during anti-TNF treatment may identify relevant allergens. It appears that patients receiving anti-TNF agents are at slightly increased risk for development of nonmelanoma skin cancers, especially if they also have used methotrexate.

Other Biologic Agents

Recent years have seen the introduction of numerous other classes of biologic agents with specific targets, many of which can induce nonspecific rashes (eczematous, urticarial) and ISRs. Ustekinumab (IL-12/IL-23 inhibitor) has also been reported to induce psoriasis, sarcoidosis, small vessel vasculitis, bullous pemphigoid, and tumid lupus in scattered reports. The IL-17 inhibitors and new IL-23–specific inhibitors appear to be overall well tolerated, with no specific signal for cutaneous adverse events. Omalizumab (mAb against IgE receptor) is well tolerated, with rare anaphylactic reactions. Dupilumab (IL-4/IL-13 inhibitor), recently approved for atopic dermatitis, appears to be well tolerated, with trials demonstrating ISRs as the primary skin issue. Rituximab (anti-CD20 mAb) is generally well tolerated, but as a chimeric antibody patients can develop hypersensitivity reactions and serum sickness.

JAK Inhibitors

The janus-kinase signal transducer and activation of transcription (JAK-STAT) is involved in a broad set of interleukin and IFN signaling, and many inflammatory conditions involve this pathway. JAK inhibitors are being used for a growing list of skin conditions, including vitiligo, alopecia areata, atopic dermatitis, psoriasis, and small case reports of benefit in GVHD and dermatomyositis. JAK inhibitors are generally well tolerated, with the notable exception being high rates of varicella-zoster virus reactivation.

Beck LA, et al: Dupilumab treatment in adults with moderate-to-severe atopic dermatitis. N Engl J Med 2014; 371: 130.

Damsky W, et al: JAK inhibitors in dermatology. J Am Acad Dermatol 2017; 76: 736.

Guarneri C, et al: Ustekinumab-induced drug eruption resembling lymphocytic infiltration (of Jessner-Kanof) and lupus erythematosus tumidus. Br J Clin Pharmacol 2016; 81: 792.

Karmacharya P, et al: Rituximab-induced serum sickness. Semin Arthritis Rheum 2015; 45: 334.

MacArthur KM, et al: Severe small-vessel vasculitis temporally associated with administration of ustekinumab. J Drugs Dermatol 2016; 15: 359.

Mery-Bossard L, et al: New-onset vitiligo and progression of pre-existing vitiligo during treatment with biological agents in chronic inflammatory diseases. J Eur Acad Dermatol Venereol 2017; 31: 181.

Onsun N, et al: Bullous pemphigoid during ustekinumab therapy in a psoriatic patient. Eur J Dermatol 2017; 27: 81.

Powell JB, et al: Acute systemic sarcoidosis complicating ustekinumab therapy for chronic plaque psoriasis. Br J Dermatol 2015; 172: 834.

Suh HY, et al: Exacerbation of infliximab-induced paradoxical psoriasis after ustekinumab therapy. J Dermatol 2017; ePub ahead of print.

Mercury

Mercury may induce multiple cutaneous syndromes. The classic syndrome is acrodynia, usually in infancy, also known as calomel disease, pink disease, and erythrodermic polyneuropathy. The skin changes are characteristic and almost pathognomonic: painful swelling of the hands and feet, sometimes associated with considerable itching of these parts. The hands and feet are also cold, clammy, and pink or dusky red. The erythema is usually blotchy but may be diffuse. Hemorrhagic puncta are frequently evident. Over the trunk, a blotchy macular or papular erythema is usually present. Stomatitis and loss of teeth may occur. Constitutional symptoms consist of moderate fever, irritability, marked photophobia, increased perspiration, and a tendency to cry most of the time. There is always moderate upper respiratory inflammation with throat soreness. The infant may have hypertension, hypotonia, muscle weakness, anorexia, and insomnia. Albuminuria and hematuria are usually present. The diagnosis is made by finding mercury in the urine.

An exanthem may occur from inhalation of mercury vapors or absorption by direct contact. A diffuse, symmetric, erythematous morbilliform eruption in the flexors and proximal extremities begins within a few days of exposure. Accentuation in the groin and medial thighs produces a "baboon syndrome" appearance. The eruption burns or itches, and small follicular pustules appear. Extensive desquamation occurs with resolution. Old broken thermometers or the application of mercury-containing skin-lightening creams and herbal medications are potential sources. In Haiti, elemental mercury is applied to surfaces for religious purposes and may result in contamination of those coming in contact.

Mercury is also a possible cause of foreign body granulomas and hyperpigmentation at sites of application. An eruption of 1–2 mm, minimally pruritic papules and papulovesicles on the palms (all patients) and soles, arms, and trunk has also been ascribed to levels of mercury in the blood at near the upper limits considered to be safe. Treatment with a seafood-free diet and chelation with succimer led to resolution of the eruption in some patients. Nummular dermatitis improved in two mercury patch test–positive patients when their dental amalgam was removed.

Halogenoderma

Bromoderma and Fluoroderma

Bromides and fluorides produce distinctive follicular eruptions: acneiform, papular, or pustular. Vegetative, exudative plaques studded with pustules may develop, resembling Sweet syndrome, pyoderma gangrenosum, or an orthopoxvirus infection. Any area of skin may be affected, but bromoderma and especially fluoroderma tend to affect the lower extremities more than iododerma. Histologically, the lesions show epidermal hyperplasia with intraepidermal and dermal neutrophilic abscesses. There is rapid involution of the lesions on cessation of bromide ingestion. Excessive cola or soft-drink consumption or ingestion of bromine-containing medications (ipratropium bromide, dextromethorphan hydrobromide, potassium bromide, pipobroman, Medecitral, sedatives) may be the cause of a bromoderma. Serum bromide level is elevated and confirms the diagnosis. Fluoroderma has been associated with intensive use of dental fluoride treatments.

Iododerma

Iodides may cause a wide variety of skin eruptions. The most common sources of exposure are oral and IV contrast materials and when iodides are used to treat thyroid disease. Application of povidone-iodine to the skin, mucosa, or as a tub soak has produced iododerma. The most common type is the acneiform eruption with numerous acutely inflamed follicular pustules, each surrounded by a ring of hyperemia (Fig. 6.46). Dermal bullous lesions are also common and may become ulcerated and crusted, resembling pyoderma gangrenosum or Sweet syndrome. The eruption may involve the face, upper extremities, trunk, and even the buccal mucosa. Acne vulgaris and rosacea are unfavorably affected by iodides. Acute iododerma may follow IV radiocontrast studies in patients with renal failure. The lesions may be associated with severe leukocytoclastic vasculitis, intraepidermal spongiform pustules, and suppurative folliculitis. The lesions respond to prednisone.

Chalela JG, Aguilar L: Iododerma from contrast material. N Engl J Med 2016; 374: 2477.

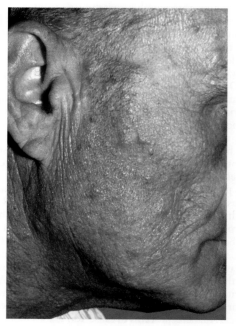

Fig. 6.46 Follicular iododerma.

Oda F, et al: Bromoderma mimicking pyoderma gangrenosum caused by commercial sedatives. J Dermatol 2016; 43: 564.

Park JD, et al: Human exposure and health effects of inorganic and elemental mercury. J Prev Med Public Health 2012; 45: 344–352.

Drug-Induced Autoimmune Diseases

Lupus Erythematosus

Drug-induced SLE is rarely associated with skin lesions. It occurs in older patients and affects men as frequently as women. The symptoms are generally mild and include fever, myalgias/arthralgias, and serositis. This form of DIL is associated with a positive ANA, homogeneous pattern, and antihistone antibodies, but a negative anti-dsDNA antibody and normal complement levels. Procainamide, hydralazine, quinidine, captopril, isoniazid, minocycline, carbamazepine, propylthiouracil, sulfasalazine, and the statins are among the reported agents triggering this form of DIL. The TNF inhibitors, especially etanercept, may also cause an SLE-like syndrome but with prominent skin lesions. Women are favored, and nephropathy and CNS involvement can occur. Again, the affected patients are ANA positive, but also anti-dsDNA antibody positive, and more than half are hypocomplementemic. Methimazole has been implicated in bullous SLE.

Numerous medications have been reported to produce cutaneous lesions characteristic of SCLE. The eruption begins days to years after starting the medications. Hydrochlorothiazide, diltiazem (and other calcium channel blockers), and terbinafine have been traditionally the most common causative agents, but proton pump inhibitors (due to being widely available) and TNF inhibitors are rapidly rising toward the top of the list of causative agents. Other causes include ACE inhibitors, statins, anticonvulsants, NSAIDs, paclitaxel, doxycycline, and even agents used to treat lupus (e.g., hydroxychloroquine, leflunomide) can induce SCLE. Patients with SCLE may also be ANA positive, but in addition have positive anti-SSA antibodies; antihistone antibodies are less common than in DIL. Cutaneous lesions are photod, but not photodistributed, annular or papulosquamous thin plaques. Treatment is as for SCLE, with sun avoidance, and topical and systemic corticosteroids as required. Drug withdrawal results in resolution over weeks to months. The positive serologies may decrease as the eruption improves. The pathogenesis of drug-induced SCLE is unknown, but most causative agents also cause both photosensitive and lichenoid drug eruptions. Patients with SCLE are more likely to be HLA-B8 or DR3 haplotype.

Hydroxyurea Dermopathy

Chronic use of hydroxyurea for chronic myelogenous leukemia, thrombocythemia, or psoriasis may be associated with the development of cutaneous lesions characteristic of dermatomyositis. Scaly, linear erythema of the dorsal hands, accentuated over the knuckles, is noted. There may be marked acral atrophy and telangiectasia. Elbow and eyelid involvement characteristic of dermatomyositis may also be seen. Biopsy shows vacuolar degeneration of the basal cells and an interface lymphocytic infiltrate. The skin lesions tend to improve over months, although the atrophy may not improve. Muscle disease is less common. Patients with hydroxyurea can also develop ulcerations on the lateral ankles, occasionally with withdrawal of therapy.

Bullous Dermatoses

Linear IgA disease is frequently associated with medication exposure, especially vancomycin (but also other antibiotics, NSAIDs, lithium, infliximab, and other agents). Men and women are equally affected, and the eruption usually begins within 2 weeks of vancomycin therapy. Clinical morphology is variable and can include flaccid or tense bullae, vesicles, erythematous papules or plaques, exanthematous morbilliform eruptions typical of a drug exanthem, and targetoid papules. TEN or severe SJS may be simulated, but mucosal involvement is only 30%–45% and conjunctival involvement, 10%. Histology will show subepidermal blistering with neutrophils and eosinophils in biopsies taken from bullous lesions with linear IgA on DIF. In cases with morbilliform and TEN/SJS–like lesions, the DIF is essential to make the diagnosis, as histology may show only a vacuolar/lichenoid dermatitis with eosinophils. Treatment is to stop the offending drug, use systemic corticosteroids in severe cases, or dapsone at 100–200 mg daily.

Drug-induced pemphigoid and other blistering disorders are discussed in Chapter 21.

Leukotriene Receptor Antagonist–Associated Churg-Strauss Syndrome

Asthma patients being treated with leukotriene receptor antagonists may develop a syndrome resembling Churg-Strauss vasculitis. It occurs 2 days to 10 months after the leukotriene receptor antagonist has been started. Inhaled fluticasone has also been reported to produce this syndrome. Involvement may be limited to the skin. Features of the syndrome include peripheral eosinophilia, pulmonary infiltrates, and, less often, neuropathy, sinusitis, pericardial effusion, and cardiomyopathy. Skin lesions occur in about half the patients and are usually purpuric and favor the lower legs. Histologically, the skin lesions show LCV with significant tissue eosinophilia. Perinuclear ANCA (p-ANCA) may be positive. Withdrawal of leukotriene receptor antagonist therapy may lead to improvement, but systemic therapy may be required. The neuropathy may be permanent. The pathogenesis of this drug-induced syndrome is unknown. Unopposed leukotriene B4 activity, a potent chemoattractant for eosinophils and neutrophils, may explain the clinical findings.

Adler NR, et al: Piperacillin-tazobactam induced linear IgA bullous dermatosis presenting clinically as Stevens-Johnson syndrome/toxic epidermal necrolysis overlap. Clin Exp Dermatol 2017; 42: 299.

Alniemi DT, et al: Subacute cutaneous lupus erythematosus. Mayo Clin Proc 2017; 92: 406.

Bryant KD, et al: Linear IgA dermatosis after infliximab infusion for ulcerative colitis. JAAD Case Rep 2016; 2: 448.

Calapai G, et al: Montelukast-induced adverse drug reactions. Pharmacology 2014; 94: 60.

Grönhagen CM, et al: Subacute cutaneous lupus erythematosus and its association with drugs. Br J Dermatol 2012; 167: 296.

Lomicova I, et al: A case of lupus-like syndrome in a patient receiving adalimumab and a brief review of the literature on drug-induced lupus erythematosus. J Clin Pharm Ther 2017; 42: 363.

Michaelis TC, et al: An update in drug-induced subacute cutaneous lupus erythematosus. Dermatol Online J 2017; 23.

Adverse Reactions to Corticosteroids

Cutaneous reactions may result from topical, intralesional, subcutaneous, or systemic delivery of corticosteroids.

Topical Application

The prolonged topical use of corticosteroid preparations may produce distinctive changes in the skin. The appearance of these side effects depends on four factors: strength of the steroid, area to which it is applied, amount of coexistent sun damage at the site of application, and patient's predisposition to certain side

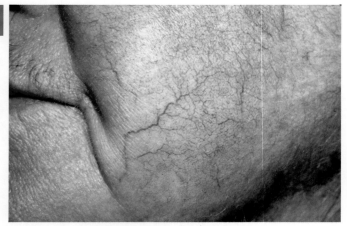

Fig. 6.47 Topical steroid-induced atrophy. (Courtesy Steven Binnick, MD.)

effects. Atrophy, striae, telangiectasia, skin fragility, and purpura are the changes most frequently seen. The most striking changes of telangiectasia are seen in fair-skinned individuals who use fluorinated corticosteroids on the face (Fig. 6.47). The changes in the skin are enhanced by occlusion. When these side effects occur, the strength of the steroid should be reduced or substituted with pimecrolimus or tacrolimus. Weekly pulse dosing of a potent topical corticosteroid can also reduce the incidence of side effects. Adjunctive measures to reduce steroid requirement could include addition of topical doxepin, pramoxine, or menthol and camphor to the regimen. Usually, the telangiectases disappear a few months after corticosteroid applications are stopped.

When corticosteroid preparations are applied to the face over weeks or months, persistent erythema with telangiectases, and often small pustules, may occur. Perioral dermatitis and rosacea may be caused by topical corticosteroids. Steroid rosacea has been reported from long-term use of 1% hydrocortisone cream. For this reason, the authors do not recommend chronic topical corticosteroid preparations of any strength in the adjunctive treatment of rosacea. A topical calcineurin inhibitor may be used instead as an antiinflammatory, although it can also induce a rosacea-like eruption. When a rosacea-like eruption appears in the setting of a topical antiinflammatory, a pustule should be opened and the contents examined for overgrowth of *Demodex* mites.

Repeated application of corticosteroids to the face, scrotum, or vulva may lead to marked atrophy of these tissues, including the red scrotum syndrome. The tissues become "addicted" to the topical steroid, so that withdrawing treatment results in severe itching or burning and intense erythema. Topical application of corticosteroids can produce epidermal atrophy with hypopigmentation. If used over large areas, sufficient topical steroids may be absorbed to suppress the hypothalamic-pituitary axis. This may affect the growth of children with atopic dermatitis and has led to addisonian steroid dependency and also Cushing syndrome. Atopic children with more than 50% BSA involvement have short stature. This may be related to their increased use of potent topical corticosteroids. In addition, bone mineral density is reduced in adults with chronic atopic dermatitis severe enough to require corticosteroid preparations stronger than hydrocortisone.

Injected Corticosteroids

Intralesional injection of corticosteroids is valuable in the management of many dermatoses. The injection of corticosteroids may produce subcutaneous atrophy at the site of injection. The injected corticosteroid may also migrate along lymphatic channels, causing not only local side effects but also linear, atrophic, hypopigmented hairless streaks. These may take years to resolve. These complications are best avoided by injecting directly into the lesion, not into the fat, and using only the minimal concentration and volume required. Triamcinolone acetonide, not hexacetonide, should be used for injecting cutaneous lesions.

Intramuscular steroid injections should always be given into the buttocks with a long needle (at least 1½ inches in adults). Injection of corticosteroids into the deltoid muscle sometimes causes subcutaneous atrophy. The patient becomes aware of the reaction by noticing depression and depigmentation at the site of injection. There is no pain, but it is bothersome cosmetically. The patient may be assured that this will fill in eventually but may take several years.

Systemic Corticosteroids

Prolonged use of corticosteroids may produce numerous changes of the skin. In addition, steroids have a profound effect on the metabolism of many tissues, leading to predictable, and sometimes preventable, complications. IM injections are not a safer delivery method than oral administration.

The skin may become thin and fragile. Spontaneous tearing may occur from trivial trauma. Purpura and ecchymoses are especially seen over the dorsal forearms in many patients over age 50, caused by aggravation of actinic purpura.

Cushingoid changes may occur, most commonly the alteration in fat distribution. Buffalo hump, facial and neck fullness, increased supraclavicular and suprasternal fat, gynecomastia, protuberant or pendulous abdomen, and flattening of the buttocks may occur. Aggressive dietary management with reduction in carbohydrate and caloric intake may ameliorate these changes.

Steroid-induced acne may develop as small, firm monomorphic follicular papules on the forehead, cheeks, and chest. Even inhaled corticosteroids for pulmonary disease can cause acne. Steroid acne can persist as long as the corticosteroids are continued. The management is similar to acne vulgaris with topical preparations and oral antibiotics.

Striae may be widely distributed, especially over the abdomen, buttocks, and thighs.

There may be generalized skin dryness (xerosis). The skin may become thin and fragile; keratosis pilaris may develop; persistent erythema of the skin in sun-exposed areas may occur, and erythromelanosis may rarely occur.

Hair loss occurs in about half of patients receiving long-term corticosteroids in large doses. There may be thinning and brittle fracturing along the hair shaft. Hair growth may be increased on the bearded area and on the arms and back with fine, vellus hairs.

Systemic complications may occur during prolonged systemic steroid therapy, including hypertension, peptic ulcer disease, diabetes, mood changes, cataracts, aseptic necrosis of the hip, and osteoporosis. Bone loss can occur early in the course of corticosteroid therapy, so it should be managed preemptively. Effective management can reduce steroid-induced osteoporosis. All patients with anticipated treatment courses longer than 1 month should be supplemented with calcium and vitamin D (1.0–1.5 g calcium and 400–800 U cholecalciferol daily). Smoking should be stopped and alcohol consumption minimized. Bone mineral density can be accurately measured at baseline with dual-energy x-ray absorptiometry (DEXA) scan and followed during corticosteroid therapy. Fracture risk assessment is essential, and most patients warrant up-front treatment with bisphosphonates (premenopausal women and younger men are a possible exception, depending on individual risks). Hypogonadism, which contributes to osteoporosis, can be treated in men and women with testosterone or estrogen, respectively. Implementation of bone loss prevention strategies by dermatologists is unacceptably low. Patients on concurrent aspirin or NSAIDs should consider proton pump inhibitor prophylaxis.

Patients are at risk for infection and should receive appropriate vaccination. Pneumocystis pneumonia (PCP) prophylaxis remains controversial and is not widely used.

Caplan A, et al: Prevention and management of glucocorticoid-induced side effects. J Am Acad Dermatol 2017; 76: 1.

6

FLUSHING

Flushing presents with transient erythema, usually localized to the face, neck, and upper trunk, and a sensation of warmth. Flushing may be physiologic or pathologic; though normally benign, causes range from emotions to hormones to medications and malignancy.

Menopausal flushing may be associated with perspiration, as is flushing induced by high ambient temperature, fever, or consumption of alcohol or hot or spicy foods and beverages. Flushing associated with medications, histamine, or serotonin is generally dry. Menopausal flushing may be age related, may be induced by oophorectomy or medication (tamoxifen, leuprolide acetate, treptorelin, clomiphene citrate, danazol), and may begin long before menses cease. Paraxetine, other antidepressants, or gabapentin may help. Men may also experience climacteric flushing after orchiectomy or antiandrogen therapy (flutamide).

Flushing may occur through thermoregulation. Blushing, or emotional flushing, may be either emotionally or physiologically induced. Simple facial redness may occur in individuals with translucent skin and is called anatomically predisposed blushing. Intense flushing may be associated with rosacea. In patients with rosacea, exercise, ambient heat or cold, spicy foods, alcohol, and hot beverages are common triggers for flushing. Topical cinnamic aldehyde can induce flushing. Drugs associated with flushing include niacin, hormonal agents, serotonin agonists, calcium channel blockers, cyclosporine, chemotherapeutic agents, antimicrobials (vancomycin, metronidazole, rifampin), disulfiram, bromocriptine, intravenous contrast material, vasodilators (nicotinic acid, nitroglycerine, sildenafil and related drugs), and glucocorticoids. Severe serotonin toxicity with flushing can be precipitated by the combination of a monoamine oxidase inhibitor and a selective serotonin reuptake inhibitor (SSRI). Reduced or absent methylnicotinate-induced flushing has been noted in patients with schizophrenia. This lack of flushing in response to methylnicotinate has been used for diagnostic psychiatric testing. Flushing after induction of general anesthesia with agents such as thiopental and muscle relaxants is more common in patients prone to blushing. It appears to be neuronally mediated rather than related to histamine release. Endogenous vasoactive substances are associated with flushing in carcinoid syndrome, mastocytosis, medullary thyroid carcinoma, and pheochromocytoma.

Some food additives, such as nitrites, sulfites, and spicy foods with capsaicin, can induce flushing; monosodium glutamate (MSG) has been reported to as well, but remains controversial. Nitrites are found in deli meats and cured meats, and sulfites are found in wine, dried fruit, prepared foods, and fresh grapes and potatoes. Scombroid fish poisoning from improperly refrigerated fish presents with flushing and systemic symptoms within 10–30 minutes of eating. Alcohol may produce flushing in patients using topical calcineurin inhibitors. Individuals who flush without an identifiable cause should be investigated for dietary triggers and subtle manifestations of rosacea.

Many cases of flushing remain idiopathic. Atypical causes or mimics include superior vena cava syndrome, thyroid disease, and malignancies (mastocytosis, pheochromocytoma, carcinoid syndrome, and others). Urinary catecholamines and serotonin and histamine metabolites should be measured if an endogenous cause is suspected.

The Women's Health Initiative studies concerning hormone replacement therapy (HRT) suggested that breast cancer risk is increased by combinations of estrogen and progestogen taken for longer than 5 years. Unopposed estrogen can increase the risk of endometrial carcinoma in premenopausal women. HRT does not appear to lower the risk of cardiac events, and the risks of long-term therapy often outweigh the benefits. Short-term HRT may still be very helpful in the management of perimenopausal flushing, because alternatives have generally been disappointing. Menopausal flushing may also respond to low-dose oral or transdermal estrogen. Flushing can be reduced by avoidance of alcohol, caffeine, and spicy foods. Niacin-induced flushing is mediated by prostaglandin D2 (PGD2). PGD2 shows some response to aspirin, as well as the PGD2 receptor-1 antagonist laropiprant.

Sadeghian A, et al: Etiologies and management of cutaneous flushing: malignant causes. J Am Acad Dermatol 2017; 77: 405.
Sadeghian A, et al: Etiologies and management of cutaneous flushing: nonmalignant causes. J Am Acad Dermatol 2017; 77: 391.

ERYTHEMAS

The term *erythema* means blanchable redness (hyperemia) of the skin. A number of reactive skin conditions are referred to as erythema. These include toxic erythemas related to viral and bacterial infections, erythema multiforme, erythema nodosum, and the gyrate (figurate) erythemas.

Erythema Palmare

Erythema palmare, or persistent palmar erythema, is usually most marked on the hypothenar areas and is associated with an elevated level of circulating estrogen. Cirrhosis, hepatic metastases, and pregnancy are common causes. Hereditary palmar erythema (Lane disease) has been rarely reported.

Generalized Erythema

Generalized erythema may be caused by medications, bacterial toxins, or viral infection. It is often uneven in distribution, being most noticeable on the chest, proximal extremities, and face. In general, these reactions are self-limited and resolve when the offending medication is stopped or the associated infection is treated or resolves. Specific exanthems associated with bacterial or viral infections are discussed in Chapters 14 and 19.

Erythema Toxicum Neonatorum

Erythema toxicum neonatorum occurs in a quarter to under half of healthy full-term newborns, usually on the second or third day of life. Because it is so common, dermatologists are usually consulted only for the most florid or atypical cases. Characteristically, the broad erythematous flare is much more prominent than the small follicular papule or pustule it surrounds (Fig. 7.1). Lesions involve the face, trunk, and proximal extremities and appear rarely on the soles or palms. There may be confluent erythema on the face. Fever is absent, and the eruption generally disappears by the

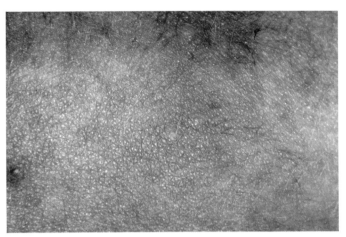

Fig. 7.1 Erythema toxicum neonatorum.

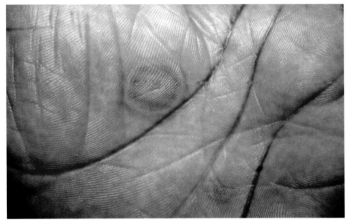

Fig. 7.2 Erythema multiforme, target lesions.

10th day. Erythema toxicum must be distinguished from miliaria, bacterial folliculitis, neonatal herpes, and scabies. When the rash is atypical, smears of the pustules demonstrating eosinophils are adequate to confirm the diagnosis. Rarely, a biopsy is required and demonstrates folliculitis containing eosinophils and neutrophils.

Durieux-Verde M, et al: Erythema palmare hereditarium (Lane's disease). Ann Dermatol Venereol 2016; 143: 32.
Reginatto FP, et al: Prevalence and characterization of neonatal skin disorders in the first 72h of life. J Pediatr 2017; 93: 238.

Erythema Multiforme

In 1860 von Hebra first described erythema exudativum multiforme. The original disease described by von Hebra is now called erythema multiforme minor (minus) or herpes simplex–associated erythema multiforme. It is strongly associated with a preceding herpetic infection. When multiple mucous membranes are involved, the lesions are more intense, and fever or arthralgias accompany the eruption, erythema multiforme major (majus) is diagnosed. This is most often caused by *Mycoplasma* infection. In contrast, Stevens-Johnson syndrome (SJS) and toxic epidermal necrolysis (TEN) usually represent adverse reactions to medications (see Chapter 6). As treatment and prognosis are related in part to the inciting agent, it is useful to classify erythema multiforme (EM) as follows:

- Herpes simplex–associated EM (HAEM)
- Erythema multiforme major (most often caused by *Mycoplasma*; some suggest the term *mycoplasma pneumonia-induced rash and mucositis*)
- Chronic oral EM
- Contact dermatitis–induced EM (see Chapter 6)
- Radiation-induced EM (see Chapter 6)
- Idiopathic

Clinical Features

HAEM (erythema multiforme minor) is a recurrent self-limited disease, usually of young adults, occurring seasonally in the spring and fall, with each episode lasting 1–4 weeks. The individual clinical lesions begin as sharply marginated, erythematous macules, which become raised, edematous papules over 24–48 hours. The lesions may reach several centimeters in diameter. Typically, a ring of erythema forms around the periphery, and centrally the lesions become flatter, more purpuric, and dusky. This lesion is the classic "target" or "iris" lesion with three zones: central dusky purpura; an elevated, edematous, pale ring; and surrounding macular erythema (Figs. 7.2 and 7.3). The central area may be bullous.

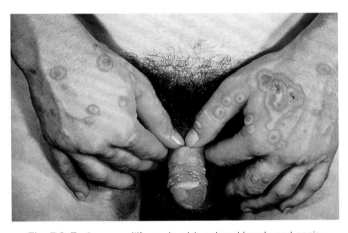

Fig. 7.3 Erythema multiforme involving dorsal hands and penis.

Typical targets are best observed on the palms and soles. Lesions generally appear symmetrically and acrally, with initial involvement most frequently on the dorsal hands. The dorsal feet, extensor limbs, elbows, knees, palms, and soles typically become involved. In about 10% of patients, more widespread lesions occur on the trunk. The Koebner phenomenon or photoaccentuation may be observed. Mucosal involvement occurs in 25% of cases and is usually limited to the oral mucosa. Oral lesions may appear as indurated plaques, target lesions, or erosions (Fig. 7.4).

An atypical variant of HAEM has been described in women. It consists of outbreaks of unilateral or segmental papules and plaques that may be few in number or solitary. Lesions may be up to 20 cm in diameter. The plaques are erythematous and evolve to have a dusky center, which desquamates. Subcutaneous nodules resembling erythema nodosum may be simultaneously present. Histologic examination shows features of EM, and herpes simplex virus (HSV) DNA may be identified in the lesions by polymerase chain reaction (PCR). Acyclovir suppression prevents the lesions.

Erythema multiforme major is frequently accompanied by a febrile prodrome and sometimes arthralgias. It occurs in all ages, is centered on the extremities and face, but more often than EM minor may include truncal lesions, which are papular and erythematous to dusky in color. Mucous membrane disease is prominent and often severely involves the oral mucosa and lips with hemorrhagic sloughing; less commonly the genital and ocular mucosa may be involved as well (Fig. 7.5). SJS is distinguished morphologically by the presence of purpura or bullae in macular lesions of the trunk (Fig. 7.6). In children, polycyclic urticarial

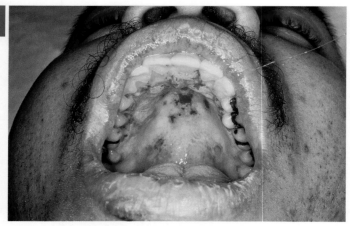

Fig. 7.4 Mucosal lesions of erythema multiforme.

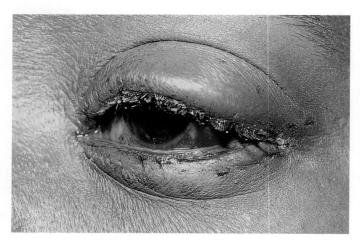

Fig. 7.5 Ocular erythema multiforme.

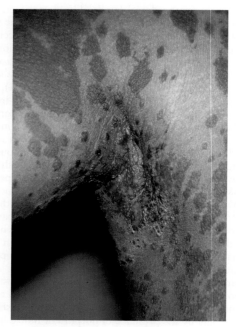

Fig. 7.6 Stevens-Johnson syndrome.

lesions often become dusky centrally and are frequently misdiagnosed as EM. This presentation of urticaria has been dubbed "urticaria multiforme." It represents urticaria, and histologic changes of EM are never present.

Etiologic Factors

Typical EM minor is usually associated with a preceding orolabial HSV infection. HAEM lesions appear 1–3 weeks (average 10 days) after the herpes outbreak. Episodes of EM minor may not follow every episode of herpes, and some EM outbreaks will not be preceded by a clinically recognizable herpetic lesion. Using PCR and in situ hybridization techniques, HSV DNA and antigens have been found in the lesions of EM minor. The majority of "idiopathic" cases of EM minor are associated with recurrent HSV infection, and patients may be successfully treated with suppressive antiviral regimens. Autoantibodies have been reported to a number of desmosomal adherence molecules, but whether these are pathogenic or incidental (due to epitope spreading from repeated exposure) is unclear. EM major is associated with *Mycoplasma* infections, although a minority may result from herpes simplex and a reaction to medications.

Histopathology

The histologic features are similar in HAEM and EM major and are not predictive of etiology. The extent of epidermal involvement depends on the duration of the lesion and where in the lesion the biopsy is taken. All lesions are characterized by cellular necrosis. Biopsies of EM demonstrate a normal basket-weave stratum corneum and a vacuolar interface reaction. Vacuoles and foci of individual cell necrosis are present and out of proportion to the number of lymphocytes. The dermal infiltrate is largely mononuclear and tends to be primarily around the upper dermal vessels and along the dermoepidermal junction. Activated T lymphocytes are present in lesions of EM, with cytotoxic or suppressor cells more prominent in the epidermis and helper T cells in the dermis. Leukocytoclastic vasculitis is not observed. Eosinophils may be present but are rarely prominent. The presence of eosinophils is not predictive of the etiology. Histologically, EM must be distinguished from the following:

- Fixed drug eruption, which often has a deeper infiltrate, eosinophils and neutrophils, papillary dermal fibrosis, and melanophages
- Graft-versus-host disease (GVHD), which typically has a more compact stratum corneum and involves the follicles
- Pityriasis lichenoides, which characteristically has a lymphocyte in every vacuole, erythrocyte extravasation, and neutrophil margination within dermal vessels
- Lupus erythematosus, which has compact hyperkeratosis, a deeper periadnexal infiltrate, dermal mucin, and basement membrane zone thickening

Differential Diagnosis

When characteristic target lesions are present, the diagnosis of EM is established clinically. When bullae are present, EM major must be distinguished from bullous arthropod reactions and autoimmune bullous diseases: pemphigus if mucous membrane involvement is prominent, and bullous pemphigoid if lesions are small and erythema is prominent at the periphery of the bulla. Paraneoplastic pemphigus may produce atypical target lesions, mucosal involvement, and a vacuolar interface dermatitis and may appear similar to *Mycoplasma*-induced EM major. Use of direct immunofluorescence may be necessary to exclude this possibility.

Treatment

Treatment of EM is determined by its cause and extent. EM minor is generally related to HSV, and prevention of herpetic outbreaks is central to control of the subsequent episodes of EM. A sunscreen lotion and sunscreen-containing lip balm should be used daily on the face and lips to prevent ultraviolet B (UVB)–induced outbreaks of HSV. If this does not prevent recurrence or if genital HSV is the cause, chronic suppressive doses of an oral antiviral drug (valacyclovir, 500 mg to 1 g/day, or famciclovir) may be used. If this dose is ineffective, it may be increased. This will prevent recurrences in up to 90% of HSV-related cases. Intermittent treatment with systemic antivirals or the use of topical antivirals is of minimal benefit in preventing HAEM. It should be noted that most cases of EM minor (HAEM) are self-limited, and symptomatic treatment may be all that is required. Symptoms related to oral lesions often respond to topical "swish and spit" mixtures containing lidocaine, diphenhydramine (Benadryl), and kaolin. In extensive cases of EM minor, intermittent steroids, or chronic dapsone, cyclosporine, azathioprine, or thalidomide may occasionally be helpful. Apremilast and rituximab have recently been reported for recalcitrant cases. If HSV infection is present, concurrent antivirals should be used. For patients with widespread EM unresponsive to the previous therapies, management is as for severe drug-induced SJS (see Chapter 6).

Oral Erythema Multiforme

A unique subset of EM is limited to or most prominent in the oral cavity. Clinically, patients are otherwise well; 60% are female, with a mean age of 43 years. The minority, about 25%, have recurrent, self-limited, cyclic disease. The oral cavity is the only site of involvement in 45%, in 30% there is oral and lip involvement, and in 25% the skin is also involved. All portions of the oral cavity may be involved, but the tongue, gingiva, and buccal mucosa are usually most severely affected. Lesions are almost universally eroded, with or without a pseudomembrane. There are no well-designed trials of treatment for oral EM, but the treatments previously listed for EM minor are typically used; topical corticosteroids may be helpful (fluocinonide gel 0.05%). "Swish and spit" mixtures containing lidocaine, diphenhydramine, and kaolin are helpful for symptomatic relief; patients should be warned the anesthetic effect may dampen their gag reflex.

Canavan TN, et al: Mycoplasma pneumonia-induced rash and mucositis as a syndrome distinct from Stevens-Johnson syndrome and erythema multiforme. J Am Acad Dermatol 2015; 72: 239.

Chen T, et al: Apremilast for treatment of recurrent erythema multiforme. Dermatol Online J 2017 Jan 15; 23.

Ellis E, et al: Circulating plakin autoantibodies in a patient with erythema multiforme major. Australas J Dermatol 2014; 55: 266.

Hirsch G, et al: Rituximab, a new treatment for difficult-to-treat chronic erythema multiforme major? J Eur Acad Dermatol Venereol 2016; 30: 1140.

Oak AS, et al: Treatment of antiviral-resistant recurrent erythema multiforme with dapsone. Dermatol Ther 2017; 30.

Roujeau JC, et al: Re-evaluation of 'drug-induced' erythema multiforme in the medical literature. Br J Dermatol 2016; 175: 650.

Siedner-Weintraub Y, et al: Paediatric erythema multiforme. Acta Derm Venereol 2017; 97: 489.

Gyrate Erythemas (Figurate Erythemas)

The gyrate erythemas are characterized by clinical lesions that are round (circinate), ringlike (annular), polycyclic (figurate), or

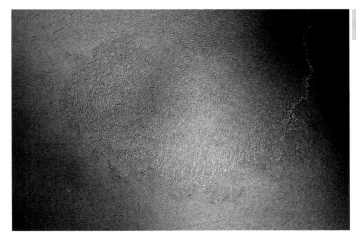

Fig. 7.7 Erythema annulare centrifugum.

arcuate. The primary lesions are erythematous and slightly elevated. There may be a trailing scale, as in erythema annulare centrifugum. In some of these diseases, the lesions are transient and migratory, and in some they are fixed. Gyrate erythemas often represent the cutaneous manifestations of an infection, malignancy, or drug reaction. Certain diseases in this group have specific causes (erythema marginatum of rheumatic fever, carrier state of chronic granulomatous disease, erythema migrans of Lyme borreliosis) and are discussed in the relevant chapters.

Erythema Annulare Centrifugum

Erythema annulare centrifugum (EAC) is the most common gyrate erythema. It is characterized by asymptomatic annular or polycyclic lesions that grow slowly (2–3 mm/day), rarely reaching more than 10 cm in diameter. Characteristically, there is a trailing scale at the inner border of the annular erythema (Fig. 7.7). The surface is typically devoid of crusts or vesicles, although atypical cases with telangiectasia and purpura have been described. Lesions usually occur on the trunk and proximal extremities. Mucosal lesions are absent.

Histologically, the epidermis will show mild focal spongiosis and parakeratosis. Within the superficial dermis and at times the deep dermis, lymphocytes are organized tightly around the blood vessels in a pattern described as a "coat sleeve" arrangement. The gyrate erythemas are divided into the superficial and deep types, but these histologic types do not correlate with etiology.

Waxing and waning in severity, EAC tends to be recurrent over months to years. Most cases eventually subside spontaneously. While active, the eruption is often responsive to topical steroids. Topical calcipotriol has also been reported to be successful.

The majority of EAC cases are idiopathic. Some cases are clearly associated with dermatophytosis or the ingestion of molds, such as those in blue cheese. Other foods, such as tomatoes, are sometimes implicated, and a dietary journal may be helpful. Medications are implicated in some cases, and internal cancer has been found (solid organ and hematologic). Annually recurrent EAC has been reported. Laboratory tests should be dictated by the physical examination and associated signs and symptoms. In one study of 66 patients, 48% had an associated cutaneous fungal infection such as tinea pedis, and 13% had internal malignancies.

The differential diagnosis of EAC includes conditions that can have annular configuration, including granuloma annulare, secondary syphilis, tinea, subacute cutaneous lupus erythematosus, sarcoidosis, Hansen disease, erythema marginatum, erythema migrans, annular urticaria, and mycosis fungoides. Histologic examination,

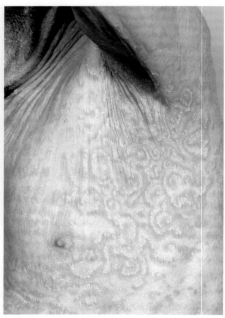

Fig. 7.8 Erythema gyratum repens. (Courtesy Donald Lookingbill, MD.)

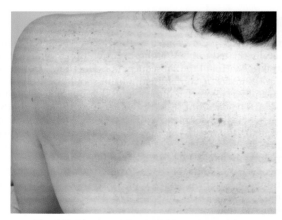

Fig. 7.9 Wells syndrome (eosinophilic cellulitis).

clinical features, and basic laboratory examinations will usually allow these diseases to be excluded.

Erythema Gyratum Repens

Erythema gyratum repens (EGR) is a rare disease that is striking and unique in appearance. Lesions consist of undulating wavy bands of slightly elevated erythema with trailing scale over the entire body. Lesions migrate rapidly (up to 1 cm/day) and are characteristically concentric, giving the skin a "wood grain" appearance (Fig. 7.8).

Pruritus may be severe, and blood eosinophilia is often found. In more than 70% of patients, an underlying malignancy is found. Lung cancer is the most common associated malignancy, although a wide range of neoplasms has been described. The skin eruption precedes the detection of the malignancy by an average of 9 months. Given the high frequency of malignant disease, patients with EGR should have extensive evaluations to exclude internal malignancy. If the carcinoma is removed, the lesions clear. Otherwise, the eruption is generally resistant to treatment, although cetirizine and topical corticosteroids have been reported to improve individual cases. EGR may rarely occur due to other causes, including medications, infections (pulmonary tuberculosis, cryptogenic organizing pneumonia), or other systemic diseases (rheumatoid arthritis). These patients respond to discontinuation of the implicated medication or to treatment of the underlying condition.

Eosinophilic Annular Erythema

Adults or children may develop bilateral annular erythema, usually presenting on the trunk and often symmetric. Females are the favored sex. Histologically a dense perivascular and interstitial lymphocytic infiltrate with many eosinophils is seen but without flame figures. Spontaneous resolution may occur. Hydroxychloroquine and/or prednisone are favored treatments when needed, though phototherapy, nicotinamide, and other treatments have been used. Normally an isolated occurrence, there are reports in the setting of thymoma, prostate cancer, and autoimmune pancreatitis.

Neutrophilic figurate erythema of infancy is a variant with a dermal neutrophilic infiltrate and karyorrhexis on biopsy.

Abarzua A, et al: Eosinophilic annular erythema in childhood. An Bras Dermatol 2016; 91: 503.
Endo Y, et al: Erythema gyratum repens preceding the onset of rheumatoid arthritis. Eur J Dermatol 2013; 23: 399.
Mandel VD, et al: Annually recurring erythema annulare centrifugum. J Med Case Rep 2015; 9: 236.
Mu EW, et al: Paraneoplastic erythema annulare centrifugum eruption (PEACE). Dermatol Online J 2015 Dec 16; 21.
Ogawa K, et al: Eosinophilic annular erythema in a patient with autoimmune pancreatitis. J Dermatol 2016; 43: 1380.
Samotij D, et al: Erythema gyratum repens associated with cryptogenic organizing pneumonia. Indian J Dermatol Venereol Leprol 2016; 82: 212.

EOSINOPHILIC CELLULITIS (WELLS SYNDROME)

In 1971 Wells described four patients with acute onset of plaques resembling cellulitis that persisted for many weeks (Fig. 7.9). Wells syndrome occurs at all ages, and pruritus is common. The condition is typically recurrent, and individual episodes may be prolonged. Degranulation of dermal eosinophils produces the flame figures seen in histologic sections. These consist of dermal collagen with adherent eosinophil granules. Eosinophilic panniculitis may also be present.

It is unclear whether Wells syndrome is a distinct disorder sui generis or a reaction pattern to many possible allergic stimuli. Many (perhaps most) cases represent arthropod reactions. It has also been associated with onchocerciasis, intestinal parasites, varicella, mumps, immunization, drug reactions that include interferon (IFN) and the anti–tumor necrosis factor (TNF)–α biologic agents, hypereosinophilic syndrome, myeloproliferative diseases, angioimmunoblastic lymphadenopathy, solid organ malignancies, atopic diathesis, inflammatory bowel disease (IBD), eosinophilic granulomatosis with polyangiitis (EGPA, Churg-Strauss syndrome), and fungal infection. Reports of Wells in association with chronic lymphocytic leukemia may represent another form of exuberant arthropod response in that disease. Most cases resolve without therapy; treatment may include topical and intralesional corticosteroids, oral antihistamines, or tacrolimus ointment. Systemic therapy for severe cases may include doxycycline, minocycline, phototherapy, antimalarials, dapsone, colchicine, sulfasalazine, low-dose prednisone, azathioprine, cyclosporine. Despite that some cases may be caused by exposure to TNF inhibitors, adalimumab has been used as well. Any underlying disease or triggering factor, including arthropod bites, should be eliminated.

Kambayashi Y, et al: Eosinophilic cellulitis induced by subcutaneous administration of interferon-β. Acta Derm Venereol 2013; 93: 755.

Qiao J, et al: Flame figures associated with eosinophilic dermatosis of hematologic malignancy. Int J Clin Exp Pathol 2013; 6: 1683.

Rabler F, et al: Treatment of eosinophilic cellulitis (Wells syndrome). J Eur Acad Dermatol Venereol 2016; 30: 1465.

Rajpara A, et al: Recurrent paraneoplastic Wells syndrome in a patient with metastatic renal cancer. Dermatol Online J 2014 Jun 15; 20.

Simpson JK, et al: Influenza vaccination as a novel trigger of Wells syndrome in a child. Pediatr Dermatol 2015; 32: e171.

Stuhr PM, et al: Wells syndrome associated with chronic lymphocytic leukemia. An Bras Dermatol 2015; 90: 571.

REACTIVE NEUTROPHILIC DERMATOSES

As with the gyrate erythemas, the reactive neutrophilic dermatoses tend to follow certain stimuli, such as acute upper respiratory tract infections (URIs) or medications, or are associated with underlying diseases, such as IBD and hematologic malignancy. Some of the neutrophilic dermatoses share common triggers, and clinical features may overlap. Patients may exhibit the simultaneous or sequential appearance of two or more of the conditions. Most often is the combination of typical lesions of Sweet syndrome on the upper body and erythema nodosum (EN)–like lesions on the legs. In these patients, histology often enables the diagnosis of subcutaneous Sweet syndrome for the EN-type lesions, allowing one diagnosis to be made. In occasional cases, however, it may be difficult to establish the diagnosis firmly as one of the neutrophilic reactive dermatoses. For these reasons, it is clinically useful to think of these diseases as forming a spectrum of conditions expressed in certain individuals by a group of stimuli with various overlapping morphologies.

Erythema Nodosum

Erythema nodosum is discussed in Chapter 23.

Sweet Syndrome (Acute Febrile Neutrophilic Dermatosis)

Since its first description in 1964 by Dr. Robert Sweet, as a recurrent febrile dermatosis in women, the spectrum of this syndrome has expanded. Sweet syndrome primarily affects adults, and females outnumber males (reports vary with ranges from 3:1 up to 8:1 predominance, though some recent reports demonstrate near equivalent sex distribution). In younger adults, female predominance is marked, but in persons older than 50, the gender ratio is more equal, and cases associated with malignancy have a 1:1 ratio. In children, boys and girls are equally affected. In Europe, cases are more common in the spring and fall. Four main subtypes of Sweet syndrome have been described, based on their pathogenesis: the classic type (majority of cases), cases associated with neoplasia (3%–35% of cases), cases associated with inflammatory disease (3%–16%), and cases associated with pregnancy (1%–4%); drug-induced cases exist as well (1%–26%).

The clinical features of all four subtypes are similar, although dusky bullous lesions that overlap with pyoderma gangrenosum (PG) are more common in patients with associated leukemia. The primary skin lesion is a sharply marginated, rapidly extending, tender, erythematous or violaceous, painful, elevated plaque, 2–10 cm in diameter. Lesions may appear intensely edematous ("juicy"), or merely indurated (Fig. 7.10). They typically involve the face (Fig. 7.11), neck, upper trunk, and extremities. Lesions may burn but do not itch. The surface of the plaques may develop pseudovesiculation or pustulation as a result of an intense dermal

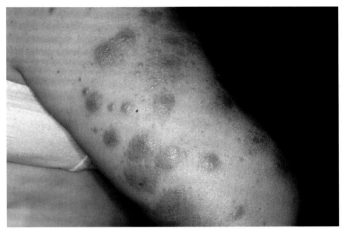

Fig. 7.10 Sweet syndrome with acute myelogenous leukemia.

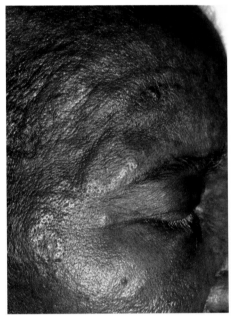

Fig. 7.11 Sweet syndrome.

inflammatory infiltrate and accompanying dermal edema. Pathergy or koebnerization may occur in 25%–30% of patients, from trauma, biopsies, peripheral IV lines, and rarely from phototherapy or radiation. Clinical morphologic variants more recently described include immunocompromised patients with deep necrosis simulating necrotizing fasciitis and patients whose lesions were extremely large and described as giant cellulitis–like in appearance.

More than three quarters of Sweet syndrome patients have systemic findings. The most common is fever, present in 50%–80% of patients. Arthritis, arthralgias, or myalgias occur in one third to two thirds of cases. About 30% of patients have conjunctivitis or episcleritis. Other ocular manifestations include periorbital inflammation, dacryoadenitis, limbal nodules, peripheral ulcerative keratitis, glaucoma, iritis, and choroiditis. Oral lesions resembling aphthae occur in 2% or 3% of classic cases, but in 10% or more of those associated with hematologic malignancy. Cough, dyspnea, and pleuritis may represent pulmonary involvement. Pulmonary infiltrates and effusions are often seen on chest radiographs of such patients. Rarely, there may be cardiac, renal, hepatic, intestinal, and neurologic involvement. Multifocal sterile osteomyelitis may occur.

Laboratory findings include an elevated sedimentation rate (90%), neutrophilia (70%), leukocytosis (60%), and a left shift (increased bands; 50%). Patients with complete blood count (CBC) abnormalities may be more likely to have an underlying malignancy. Antineutrophilic cytoplasmic antibodies (ANCAs) have been rarely reported. In most cases, an attack lasts 3–6 weeks and then resolves. Recurrences may be seen with the same precipitating cause, such as URI. Persistent cases, with new lesions erupting before the old lesions resolve, may continue for many years.

The histologic hallmark of Sweet syndrome is a nodular and diffuse dermal infiltrate of neutrophils with karyorrhexis and massive papillary dermal edema. Leukocytoclastic vasculitis may be present focally, and this does not exclude a diagnosis of Sweet syndrome. Upper dermal edema may be so intense as to form subepidermal bullae. Leukemic cells may be present in the infiltrate, and clonal restriction of neutrophils has even been seen in Sweet syndrome not associated with malignancy.

Histologic variants described as histiocytic or lymphocytic Sweet syndrome have been reported. These entities are somewhat controversial, as Sweet syndrome is by definition a neutrophilic dermatosis. Occasionally, the main infiltrating cell resembles histiocytes, but in some studies with immunohistochemical stains, they are found to be immature myeloid cells, with positive myeloperoxidase stains. These can be mistaken for, and must be distinguished from, leukemia cutis. Patients with histiocytoid Sweets are more likely to have an underlying hematologic disorder or malignancy concurrent or shortly after the diagnosis is made.

The majority of cases of Sweet syndrome follow a URI or viral gastroenteritis and are therefore acute and self-limited. Other associated conditions include infections with *Yersinia*, toxoplasmosis, histoplasmosis, salmonellosis, tuberculosis, tonsillitis, vaccination, and vulvovaginal infections. Sweet syndrome has been reported in association with IBD and Behçet syndrome, and can develop in sites of lymphedema.

Hematologic malignancies or solid tumors are present in about 10% (3%–35% range) of reported cases. Sweet syndrome often presents early in the course of the cancer, but may present months to years before a diagnosis of malignancy is made. Sweet syndrome may occur with myelodysplastic syndromes or with hemoproliferative malignancies including leukemias (usually acute myelogenous) and lymphomas. One study reported an increased frequency of FLT3 mutations or del(5q) karyotype in AML patients with Sweets. Solid tumors are of any type but are most often genitourinary, breast (in women), or gastrointestinal (in men). Anemia is found in 93% of men and 71% of women with malignancy-associated Sweet syndrome. Thrombocytopenia is seen in half. Solitary, bullous, or ulcerative lesions are more frequently associated with malignancy, as is the histiocytoid histopathologic pattern.

Pregnancy-associated Sweet syndrome typically presents in the first or second trimester with lesions on the head, neck, trunk, and less often on the upper extremities. Lower-extremity lesions resembling EN may occur. The condition may resolve spontaneously or clear with topical or systemic corticosteroids. It may recur with subsequent pregnancies, but there seems to be no risk to the fetus.

Many drug therapies have been associated with Sweet-like reactions in the skin. The strongest association exists for granulocyte colony-stimulating factor (G-CSF). All-*trans*-retinoic acid (ATRA) and the new class of FLT3-inhibitors, which also have been reported to cause sweets, are, like G-CSF, often used in the treatment of diseases (such as leukemia) that themselves can be associated with Sweets, making causality assessments a challenge. Oral contraceptives, radiation therapy fields, radiocontrast dye, IFNs, interleukin-2 (IL-2), abatacept, TNF inhibitors, allopurinol, vaccines, multiple antineoplastic agents (bortezomib, gemcitabine, BRAF inhibitors, multikinase inhibitors,

---

BOX 7.1 Revised Diagnostic Criteria for Diagnosis of Sweet Syndrome[a]

MAJOR CRITERIA

1. Abrupt onset of erythematous plaques or nodules, occasionally with vesicles, pustules, or bullae
2. Nodular and diffuse neutrophilic infiltration in the dermis with karyorrhexis and massive papillary dermal edema

MINOR CRITERIA

1. Preceded by a respiratory infection, gastrointestinal tract infection, or vaccination, or associated with the following:
   - Inflammatory disease or infection
   - Myeloproliferative disorders or other malignancy
   - Pregnancy
2. Malaise and fever (>38°C [100.4°F])
3. Abnormal laboratory findings ≥3 of the following:
   - Erythrocyte sedimentation rate >20 mm/hr
   - C-reactive protein elevated
   - Leukocytosis >8000/mm^3
   - Left shift with >70% neutrophils
4. Excellent response to treatment with systemic corticosteroids

[a]Both major criteria and two minor criteria are needed for diagnosis.

---

immunotherapy), anticonvulsants, antimicrobials (trimethoprim-sulfamethoxazole, minocycline, and many others), and azathioprine have been implicated. ATRA and FLT3 inhibitors cause terminal differentiation of some leukemic clones and are used to treat promyelocytic leukemia. After about 2 weeks of treatment, Sweet-like lesions may appear. Induction of the skin lesions appears to be related to the desired pharmacologic effect of the medication. ATRA has been reported to cause scrotal ulcers with neutrophils on histopathology; this is likely a site-specific manifestation of Sweet syndrome.

The two major criteria for the diagnosis of Sweet syndrome are the presence of red edematous plaques and a biopsy demonstrating neutrophils, karyorrhexis, and marked papillary dermal edema. Minor criteria include associated symptoms or conditions, laboratory findings, and response to therapy. Patients should have both major criteria and two of the four minor criteria for diagnosis (Box 7.1). Sweet syndrome is a diagnosis of exclusion, and often tissue culture is necessary to exclude infection. Bowel bypass syndrome has skin lesions that, on histologic examination, are identical to those of Sweet syndrome; fever and arthritis also accompany bowel bypass syndrome. Although it is easy to distinguish classic EN from Sweet syndrome, these two conditions share many features. Both occur most often in young adult women and frequently follow URIs. Both may be associated with pregnancy, underlying malignancy, and IBD. In both, fever and arthritis may occur, along with leukocytosis with neutrophilia. There are many reports of simultaneous or sequential EN and Sweet syndrome in the same patient. Leukemia-associated Sweet syndrome may overlap with pyoderma gangrenosum. A search for an underlying cause should be undertaken, especially in persons over age 50 and those with anemia, thrombocytopenia, histiocytoid pathology, or lesions that are bullous or necrotic. The standard treatment is systemic corticosteroids, with approximately 1–2 mg/kg/day of oral prednisone. This will result in resolution of fever and skin lesions within days. Topical or intralesional steroids may be tried for mild disease but are often ineffective. Dapsone, colchicine, potassium iodide (which may rarely cause paradoxic worsening similar to iododerma), sulfapyridine, doxycycline, clofazimine, and nonsteroidal antiinflammatory drugs (NSAIDs) may be helpful in chronic or refractory disease. Granulocyte adsorption apheresis,

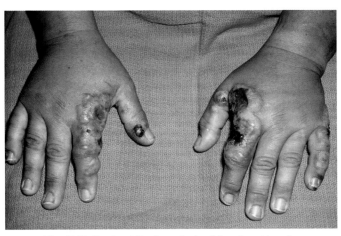

Fig. 7.12 Neutrophilic dermatosis of the dorsal hands.

cyclosporine, intravenous immune globulin (IVIG), thalidomide/lenalidomide, methotrexate, rituximab, TNF inhibitors, and anakinra have been used for severe cases. Medication should be continued for several weeks to prevent relapse.

Neutrophilic Dermatosis of the Dorsal Hands

Neutrophilic dermatosis of the dorsal hands (NDDH) is a rare disease, which many consider a localized variant of Sweet syndrome, with similar age and sex distribution, presentation, and disease associations. Lesions of NDDHs present as edematous, pustular, or ulcerative nodules or plaques localized to the dorsal hands (Fig. 7.12); as palmar involvement has been described, some argue that the term NDDH is unnecessarily restrictive. Histologically, papillary dermal edema and a nodular and diffuse neutrophilic infiltrate with karyorrhexis are noted. Leukocytoclastic vasculitis may be present focally. Individual flares respond to prednisone and dapsone, but recurrences are common.

Neutrophilic Eccrine Hidradenitis

Neutrophilic eccrine hidradenitis is discussed in Chapter 33.

Marshall Syndrome

The rare Marshall syndrome is characterized by skin lesions resembling Sweet syndrome, which are followed by acquired cutis laxa. Cases occur primarily in children. Small red papules expand to urticarial, targetoid plaques with hypopigmented centers. Histologic evaluation of the skin lesions usually shows a neutrophilic dermatosis virtually identical to Sweet syndrome. Occasionally, an eosinophilic infiltrate will be found. The lesions resolve with destruction of the elastic tissue at the site, producing soft, wrinkled, skin-colored protuberant plaques that can be pushed into the dermis. Elastic tissue in other organs may also be affected, especially the heart and lungs. Some cases may be associated with α_1-antitrypsin deficiency.

Baquerizo Nole KL, et al: Ketoconazole-induced Sweet syndrome. Am J Dermatopathol 2015; 37: 419.

Cheraghi N, et al: Azathioprine hypersensitivity presenting as neutrophilic dermatosis and erythema nodosum. Cutis 2016; 98: e7.

Chu CH, et al: Lymphedema-associated neutrophilic dermatosis. J Dermatol 2016; 43: 1062.

Costa-Silva M, et al: Neutrophilic dermatosis of the dorsal hands: a restrictive designation for an acral entity. Acta Dermatovenereol Alp Pannonica Adriat 2016; 25: 85.

Ghoufi L, et al: Histiocytoid Sweet syndrome is more frequently associated with myelodysplastic syndromes than the classical neutrophilic variant. Medicine (Baltimore) 2016; 95: e3033.

Gormley R, et al: Ipilimumab-associated Sweet syndrome in a melanoma patient. J Am Acad Dermatol 2014; 71: e211.

Kaminska EC, et al: Giant cellulitis-like Sweet syndrome in the setting of autoimmune disease. J Am Acad Dermatol 2014; 71: e94.

Kazmi SM, et al: Characteristics of Sweet syndrome in patients with acute myeloid leukemia. Clin Lymphoma Myeloma Leuk 2015; 15: 358.

Kroshinsky D, et al: Necrotizing Sweet syndrome. J Am Acad Dermatol 2012; 67: 945.

Larson AR, et al: Systemic lupus erythematosus-associated neutrophilic dermatosis. Adv Anat Pathol 2014; 21: 248.

Nelson CA, et al: Neutrophilic dermatoses. J Am Acad Dermatol 2018; accepted/in press.

Nelson CA, et al: Sweet syndrome in patients with and without malignancy. J Am Acad Dermatol 2018; 78: 303-9.

Nofal A, et al: Neutrophilic dermatosis of the dorsal hands. Int J Dermatol 2015; 54: e66.

Peroni A, et al: Histiocytoid Sweet syndrome is infiltrated predominantly by M2-like macrophages. J Am Acad Dermatol 2015; 72: 131.

Wolf R, et al: Acral manifestations of Sweet syndrome. Clin Dermatol 2017; 35: 81.

Pyoderma Gangrenosum

Brunsting is credited with the initial clinical description of PG in 1930. PG is a rare disease that affects people of all ages, most commonly in the 40s to 60s, with a female predominance. Childhood cases are rare. Approximately 50% of patients with PG have an associated underlying medical condition or trigger, particularly inflammatory bowel disease, but also inflammatory arthritides and hematologic disorders (myelodysplastic syndrome, leukemia, immunoglobulin A [IgA] paraproteinemia, others); drug-induced cases exist but are rare. There are five clinical subtypes, with ulcerative the most common; others include bullous, vegetative, pustular, and peristomal.

Classic PG begins as an inflammatory pustule with a surrounding halo that enlarges and begins to ulcerate. A primary lesion may not always be seen as it can rapidly expand. Approximately 20%–30% of patients may exhibit pathergy, development of lesions from mild trauma. Satellite violaceous papules may appear just peripheral to the border of the ulcer and break down to fuse with the central ulcer, or multiple small erosions may develop concurrently and run together, resembling "cheese cloth" initially. Fully developed lesions are painful ulcers with undermined, purple to gray borders (Fig. 7.13). Lesions tend to be on the lower extremities and trunk. Lesions heal with characteristic thin, atrophic, crosslike "cribriform" scars.

Bullous PG is more superficial and less destructive than the ulcerative type. These red plaques become dusky and develop superficial erosions. These lesions have considerable overlap with "bullous Sweet syndrome" and are usually seen in patients with hematologic disorders (leukemia or myelodysplasia), and some argue whether these patients should not simply be diagnosed with Sweet syndrome.

Pustular PG consists of pustules that generally do not progress to ulcerative lesions. This forme fruste of PG is most often seen in IBD patients but can occur in other settings. Pyostomatitis vegetans and subcorneal pustular dermatosis are two other pustular neutrophilic diseases reported in association with PG, sometimes in patients with IgA gammopathy.

Vegetative PG is the least aggressive form of PG. Lesions present as chronic, superficial, cribriform ulcerations, usually of the trunk, that enlarge slowly and have elevated borders and clean

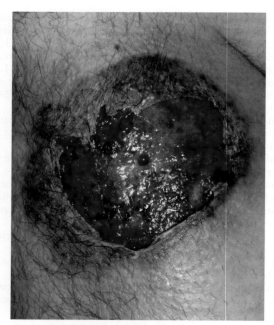

Fig. 7.13 Pyoderma gangrenosum.

bases. The lesions are rarely painful, generally respond to relatively conservative treatments, and are usually not associated with underlying systemic disease.

PG is rare in children. More than 40% of these patients have underlying IBD, and another 18% have leukemia. An association of childhood acquired immunodeficiency syndrome (AIDS) and PG has been documented. About one quarter of children with PG have no underlying disease. Genital and head/neck lesions can occur in children.

Overall, approximately 50% of patients with PG have an associated disease, most often IBD—both Crohn disease and ulcerative colitis. Between 1.5% and 5% of patients with IBD develop PG. The two diseases may flare together or run an independent course. Surgical removal of the diseased intestine may lead to complete remission of PG, or lesions may persist or first appear after removal of the affected bowel. If an ostomy is created, PG may present with peristomal erosions and ulcers, clinically similar to classic PG, but isolated to the abdomen near the stoma. Postoperative PG has also been reported following breast reconstructive surgery, and misdiagnoses of PG as necrotizing fasciitis leading to extensive debridement can be another dramatic presentation of postsurgical PG.

Many other associated conditions have been reported. Leukemia (chiefly acute or chronic myelogenous leukemia), myeloma, monoclonal gammopathy (chiefly IgA), polycythemia vera, myeloid metaplasia, chronic active hepatitis, hepatitis C, human immuno-deficiency virus (HIV) infection, systemic lupus erythematosus, pregnancy, PAPA syndrome (see Autoinflammatory Syndromes next), and Takayasu arteritis are among the many diseases seen in conjunction with PG. Monoclonal gammopathy, usually IgA, is found in up to 10% of PG patients. Granulomatosis with poly-angiitis (GPA; formerly Wegener) can present with "malignant pyoderma," cutaneous ulcerations that resemble PG but may in fact be cutaneous vasculitis. More than one third of PG patients have arthritis, usually an asymmetric, seronegative, monoarticular arthritis of the large joints. Children with congenital deficiency of leukocyte adhesion glycoproteins (LAD) develop PG-like lesions. There are increasing reports of PG occurring in hidradenitis suppurativa patients. Patients with PG may rarely develop

extracutaneous organ inflammation, particularly sterile neutrophilic pulmonary infiltrates; the eyes, spleen, and musculoskeletal system may also be involved.

Early biopsies of PG show a suppurative folliculitis. The affected follicle is often ruptured. As the lesions evolve, they demonstrate suppurative inflammation in the dermis and subcutaneous fat. Massive dermal edema and epidermal neutrophilic abscesses are present at the violaceous, undermined border. These features are not diagnostic, and infectious causes must be excluded.

The clinical picture of PG, in the classic ulcerative form, is characteristic. Because no diagnostic serologic or histologic features exist, however, PG remains a diagnosis of exclusion. Clinical and pathologic correlation, coupled with extensive testing to exclude alternative etiologies, is essential. Many cases exist of PG being incorrectly diagnosed and patients treated with inappropriate immunosuppression. The initial workup of the patient includes studies necessary to ensure that the proper diagnosis is made, as well as to investigate possible associated diseases. Biopsy, tissue culture, evaluation for potential associated diseases such as IBD, hematologic disorders, inflammatory arthritis, and other entities is recommended. One large study of 356 cases of PG demonstrated that IBD is more common in patients younger than age 65 years, and malignancies and hematologic disorders are more common in patients over 65. Multiple infections, including mycobacteria, deep fungi, gummatous syphilis, synergistic gangrene, and amebiasis, must be excluded with cultures and special studies. Other disorders frequently misdiagnosed as PG include vascular occlusive or chronic venous disease, vasculitis, cancer, and exogenous tissue injury, including factitial disease. PG has been reported in association with levamisole-tainted cocaine.

The most difficult diagnosis to exclude is factitial disease. The clinical lesions may be strikingly similar, evolving from small papulopustules to form ulcerations that do not heal. Histologic evaluation will often simply show suppurative dermatitis, because the injected or applied caustic substance may not be identifiable (urine, disinfectants, drain cleaner). Even the most experienced clinician may misdiagnose factitial disease as PG.

Pyoderma gangrenosum may be misdiagnosed as a spider bite if there is only a solitary lesion on an extremity. Spider bites tend to evolve more rapidly and may be associated with other systemic symptoms or findings, such as disseminated intravascular coagulation.

Management of PG is challenging. Successful treatment requires both halting the inflammatory process and healing a large wound. Appropriate response to therapy is one of the minor diagnostic criteria, and if patients fail to respond, the diagnosis of PG should be questioned. If there is an underlying disease present, that should be identified and treated. The treatment is determined by the severity of disease and rate of progression. In rapidly progressive cases, aggressive early management may reduce morbidity.

Local treatment includes both proper wound care and medica-tion to reduce inflammation; compresses or whirlpool baths are followed by the use of ointment or hydrophilic occlusive dressings. In solitary lesions or slowly progressive cases, application of potent topical corticosteroids, intralesional steroid injections, topical dapsone, or topical tacrolimus may be beneficial, although pathergy may be seen at sites of injection. The absorption of tacrolimus in large or multiple wounds may lead to systemic blood levels. Topical timolol has recently been described as beneficial in isolated reports. In general, the vegetative type will respond to topical or local measures.

For most cases, systemic treatment is indicated, with TNF inhibitors (infliximab in particular), systemic corticosteroids, and cyclosporine representing first-line treatments. Systemic corticosteroids can be extremely effective, with initial doses in the range of 1–2 mg/kg. If control is achieved, the dose may be rapidly tapered. If corticosteroid reduction is not possible, a steroid-sparing agent may be added. Severe patients may require pulse methylprednisolone for 3–5 days, followed by prednisone tapering as the lesions heal. Initial doses of cyclosporine of approximately 4–5 mg/kg/day are effective in most cases, with the STOP GAP trial supporting efficacy at the 4-mg dose. The response is independent of any underlying cause. Infliximab has been shown to be effective in randomized trials, and is given in doses of about 5 mg/kg at weeks 0, 2, and 6 and then every 6–8 weeks.

Alternative treatment options or steroid-sparing agents for patients unable to taper include etanercept, adalimumab, alefacept, ustekinumab, mycophenolate mofetil (MMF), granulocyte apheresis IVIG, alkylating agents, and thalidomide. Anti–IL-1β agents such as canakinumab have been used in small studies with promising results. Systemic tacrolimus has been reported to help severe, recalcitrant cases. Sulfapyridine, sulfasalazine, salicylazosulfapyridine, dapsone, methotrexate, azathioprine, and minocycline generally are somewhat less effective but may be useful adjuncts or tried for patients with either mild disease, or contraindications/comorbidities that preclude more potent agents.

Patients typically show response within 1–2 weeks of initiation of therapy, with reduced pain, decreased exudate, and less erythema and edema. Systemic therapy should be tapered as the inflammation recedes. Often patients have a large wound, but the inflammation is under control—ongoing high-dose immunosuppression may not be necessary in these cases. Optimal wound care is essential, including compression if edema is present, though caution should be used to avoid compression-induced pathergy. Most wound care consists of keeping the wound clean and avoiding colonization, biofilm, or infection; Vaseline and impregnated nonstick gauze may help avoid trauma with dressing changes. Alginates or other absorptive dressings may be required for very exudative wounds. Epidermal allografts or autografts may be applied soon after PG is controlled. Pathergy is rarely noted at the donor site when patients are receiving adequate immunosuppressive therapy.

Ashchyan HJ, et al: Neutrophilic dermatoses. J Am Acad Dermatol 2018; ePub ahead of print.

Ashchyan HJ, et al: The association of age with clinical presentation and comorbidities of pyoderma gangrenosum. JAMA Dermatol 2018; 154: 409-13.

Barbosa NS, et al: Clinical features, causes, treatments, and outcomes of peristomal pyoderma gangrenosum in 44 patients. J Am Acad Dermatol 2016; 75: 931.

Binus AM, et al: Pyoderma gangrenosum. Br J Dermatol 2011; 165: 1244.

Braswell SF, et al: Pathophysiology of pyoderma gangrenosum. J Am Acad Dermatol 2015; 73: 691.

Herberger K, et al: Treatment of pyoderma gangrenosum. Br J Dermatol 2016; 175: 1070.

Jeong HS, et al: Pyoderma gangrenosum associated with levamisole-adulterated cocaine. J Am Acad Dermatol 2016; 74: 892.

Kolios AG et al: Canakinumab in adults with steroid-refractory pyoderma gangrenosum. Br J Dermatol 2015; 173: 1216.

Moreira C, et al: Topical timolol for the treatment of pyoderma gangrenosum. BMJ Case Rep 2017 Jan 27; 2017.

Ormerod AD, et al: Comparison of the two most commonly used treatments for pyoderma gangrenosum. BMJ 2015; 350: h2958.

Patel DK, et al: Pyoderma gangrenosum with pathergy. J Plast Reconstr Aesthet Surg 2017; 70: 884.

Patel F, et al: Effective strategies for the management of pyoderma gangrenosum. Acta Derm Venereol 2015; 95: 525.

Sadati MS, et al: Recalcitrant cases of pyoderma gangrenosum responding dramatically to systemic tacrolimus. G Ital Dermatol Venereol 2017; 152: 308.

Schoch JJ, et al: Pediatric pyoderma gangrenosum. Pediatr Dermatol 2017; 34: 39.

Thomas KS, et al: Clinical outcomes and response of patients applying topical therapy for pyoderma gangrenosum. J Am Acad Dermatol 2016; 75: 940.

Tolkachjov SN, et al: Postoperative pyoderma gangrenosum. Mayo Clin Proc 2016; 91: 1267.

Vacas AS, et al: Pyoderma gangrensoum. Int J Dermatol 2017; 56: 386.

AUTOINFLAMMATORY SYNDROMES

The autoinflammatory syndromes are a group of disorders characterized by bouts of systemic inflammation related to dysregulation of the innate immune system. There are over 30 monogenic diseases described, many of which are related to excessive IFN and/or IL-1 signaling, sometimes referred to as inflammasomopathies or interferonopathies. These generally cause hereditary periodic fevers along with clinical and laboratory evidence of inflammation. These conditions present most often in children with episodes that often include fever and symptoms related to the skin, gastrointestinal (GI) tract, eyes, chest, musculoskeletal system, and central nervous system. Inflammatory skin lesions are often prominent manifestations, especially acne, PG, and erysipelas-like and urticaria-like lesions. Nonspecific elevations of erythrocyte sedimentation rate (ESR) and C-reactive protein (CRP) are often seen.

Familial Mediterranean fever (FMF) is the most common monogenic inherited autoinflammatory syndrome and was the first recognized. FMF is an autosomal recessive disease caused by mutation in the *MEFV* gene, which produces pyrin, and affects IL-1b production downstream, but approximately 30% of patients with a similar phenotype lack a detectable gene defect. Clinically it is characterized by recurrent attacks of 12–72 hours of fever and a monoarthritis with overlying erysipelas-like erythema. Multiple diagnostic criteria have been proposed. Peritonitis, pleuritis, arthritis, and vasculitis, including Henoch-Schönlein purpura, may also occur in these patients, who usually present before the teenage years. Colchicine is the mainstay of treatment for FMF patients and can reduce the risk of associated amyloidosis. Anti–IL-1 treatment can be used in patients who fail to improve on colchicine.

The PAPA syndrome is an autosomal dominant disorder characterized by pyogenic sterile arthritis, PG, and acne and is caused by proline-serine-threonine-phosphatase–interacting protein 1 *(PSTPIP1)* or CD2-binding protein 1 *(CD2BP1)* gene mutations. PSTPIP1/CD2BP1, a tyrosine-phosphorylated protein involved in cytoskeletal organization, interacts with pyrin, the gene product important in the pathogenesis of FMF. Pyogenic arthritis, PG, acne, and suppurative hidradenitis (PA-PASH) syndrome has also been described, and PG, acne, and suppurative hidradenitis (PASH) syndrome has been reported with PSTPIP1 mutations as well.

The TNF-receptor–associated periodic syndrome (TRAPS) is similar to FMF but shows autosomal dominant inheritance, longer attacks, and a lack of response to colchicine. TRAPS is associated with mutations in the *TNFRSF1A* gene, resulting in decreased serum-soluble TNF receptor and excessive IL-1b secretion. TRAPS and deficiency of the IL-36 receptor antagonist (DITRA) are the most common autoinflammatory syndromes with onset in adulthood. Febrile episodes of 1–3 weeks are accompanied by periorbital edema, abdominal pain, myalgia, and a painful, distally migrating erythematous or urticarial-like plaques often overlying areas of myalgia. NSAIDs or prednisone can treat the acute episodes; anti–TNF-receptor antagonists or anakinra and other anti–IL-1 agents may prevent bouts.

An autosomal recessive DITRA is due to mutations in *IL36RN* leading to episodes of generalized pustular psoriasis, nail dystrophy, and geographic tongue. Treatment is as for pustular psoriasis. Deficiency of the IL-1 receptor antagonist (DIRA) also manifests as a pustular eruption, although onset is in the neonatal period.

Bone lesions, oral ulcers, and other findings are all reversed dramatically by anakinra, though steroids and traditional psoriasis treatments, including retinoids, have been used.

Deficiency of IL-1 receptor antagonist (DIRA) is a very rare autosomal recessive disease due to mutations in *IL1RN* that can present with neonatal sterile osteomyelitis, periostitis, and pustulosis. Deficiency of ADA2 (DADA2 syndrome) due to *CECR1* mutations has been described as early-onset stroke, intermittent fevers, and systemic vasculopathy, which can present with livedo racemosa, polyarteritis nodosa, or Raynaud phenomenon. TNF inhibitors are often used.

The recessively inherited hyper-IgD syndrome (HIDS), associated with mutations in the mevalonate kinase *(MVK)* gene, leading to MVK deficiency, also increases IL-1 and presents with hereditary periodic fever. Patients have fevers, lymphadenopathy, GI, musculoskeletal, and neurologic issues, in addition to mucocutaneous findings. Two thirds of patients manifest various morbilliform or urticarial eruptions and may develop aphthous stomatitis or genital ulcerations. NSAIDs, TNF inhibitors, or anti–IL-1 agents are generally used, though statins and colchicine have also been tried with limited success.

There are three autosomal dominant cryopyrin-associated periodic syndromes associated with mutations of *NLRP3*, which encodes cryopyrin and is involved in the IL-1 pathway. Familial cold autoinflammatory syndrome is characterized by fever, cold urticaria, conjunctivitis, and arthralgia elicited by generalized exposure to cold. Patients with Muckle-Wells syndrome manifest most often in adolescence with acute febrile inflammatory episodes comprising abdominal pain, arthritis, urticaria, hearing loss, and multiorgan amyloidosis. Neonatal-onset multisystem inflammatory disease is characterized by fever, chronic meningitis, uveitis, sensorineural hearing loss, urticarial rash, and a deforming arthritis. Patients may also have dysmorphic facial appearance, clubbing of the fingers, mild mental retardation, and papilledema. A second familial cold autoinflammatory syndrome is similar in its clinical findings but is related to mutations in the *NALP12* gene. Given the characteristic overproduction of IL-1, the mainstay of treatment is anti–IL-1 therapy with anakinra or canakinumab.

Blau syndrome is an autosomal dominant disease with arthritis, uveitis, granulomatous inflammation, and camptodactyly. It is associated with mutations in the *NOD2* gene, which also predisposes to Crohn disease and early-onset sarcoidosis. Another acquired syndrome, consisting of dermatitis, fever, arthritis, and serositis, without autoantibody formation and with the occurrence of a *NOD2* mutation, has been described in 22 patients. The dermatitis was polymorphic, but many patients had papules and plaques on the face, trunk, and extremities. Biopsies were also variable. The authors named it NOD2-associated autoinflammatory disease; the only effective therapy was prednisone or topical corticosteroids. Last, two patients with urticarial lesions that burned rather than itched had accompanying fever, or arthralgias, and/or laboratory markers of systemic inflammation, such as a high ESR or CRP. They did not respond to antihistamines but did respond to anakinra, suggesting their urticarial lesions were mediated by IL-1 and fit into this acquired autoinflammatory disease spectrum. This disease was dubbed "neutrophilic urticaria with systemic inflammation," which is differentiated from prior reports of neutrophilic urticaria.

Interferon-mediated diseases can cause autoinflammatory syndromes due to upregulated IFN signaling. These are very rare, but the list of identified gene mutations and syndromes is growing. Given signaling through the Janus kinases (JAKs), signal transducer and activator of transcription (STAT) pathway, experimental treatments with JAK inhibitors or IFN-targeting therapies are often employed. Aicardi-Goutières syndrome involves mutations in *TREX1* and involves neurologic disease, developmental delay, and a variety of skin rashes, including chilblain lesions. Stimulator of interferon genes-associated vasculopathy with onset in infancy (SAVI) patients present with erythematous or purpuric patches and plaques on cold-sensitive areas such as the cheeks, nose, ears, and acral sites. These may ulcerate and cause tissue loss. Chronic atypical neutrophilic dermatosis with lipodystrophy and elevated temperature (CANDLE) involves mutations in proteasome components, which leads to increased cell stress and proinflammatory cytokines. Patients present in the newborn period with fever; swollen purplish red eyelids; red and purplish papules and plaques of the trunk, neck, and extremities; and lipodystrophy of the face, along with other systemic findings. The skin biopsy reveals atypical cells of the myelocytic lineage in the dermis. It is caused by a mutation in the *PSMB8* gene.

Calderon-Castrat X, et al: PSTPIP1 gene mutation in PASH syndrome. Br J Dermatol 2016; 175: 194.

Chia J, et al: Failure to thrive, interstitial lung diseases, and progressive digital necrosis with onset in infancy. J Am Acad Dermatol 2016; 74: 186.

Jain A, et al: Vasculitis and vasculitis-like manifestations in monogenic autoinflammatory syndromes. Rheumatol Int 2017; ePub.

Manthiram K, et al: The monogenic autoinflammatory diseases define new pathways in human innate immunity and inflammation. Nat Immunol 2017; 18: 832.

Oda H, et al: Genomics, biology, and human illness. Rheum Dis Clin North Am 2017; 43: 327.

Pichard DC, et al: Early-onset stroke, PAN, and livedo racemosa. J Am Acad Dermatol 2016; 75: 449.

Sag E, et al: Autoinflammatory diseases with periodic fevers. Curr Rheumatol Rep 2017; 19: 41.

Torrelo A: CANDLE syndrome as a paradigm of proteasome-related autoinflammation. Front Immunol 2017; 8: 927.

URTICARIA (HIVES)

Urticaria is a vascular reaction of the skin characterized by the appearance of wheals (Fig. 7.14), generally surrounded by a red halo or flare and associated with severe itching, stinging, or pricking sensations. These wheals are caused by localized edema. Clearing of the central region may occur, and lesions may coalesce, producing an annular or polycyclic pattern. Subcutaneous swellings (angioedema) may or may not accompany the wheals. When angioedema is not present, and fever, malaise, and joint/bone pain coexist, an autoinflammatory or autoimmune condition should be considered.

Schnitzler syndrome is another diagnosis to consider. This rare acquired disorder is a combination of chronic nonpruritic urticaria, fever of unknown origin, disabling bone pain, hyperostosis, increased ESR, and monoclonal immunoglobulin M (IgM)

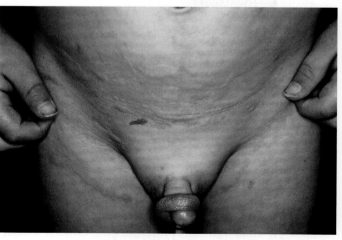

Fig. 7.14 Acute urticaria.

gammopathy. Pruritus is not generally a feature. The age of onset ranges from 29–77 years, without gender predilection. The skin biopsy most often reveals a predominant neutrophilic perivascular and interstitial infiltrate, although about one third of cases are mononuclear. In some patients, the IgM gammopathy progresses to neoplasia, especially Waldenström macroglobulinemia. Effective therapy for patients with Schnitzler syndrome has included anakinra, rituximab, tocilizumab, rilonacept, and canakinumab.

Classification

Acute urticaria evolves over days to weeks, producing evanescent wheals that, individually, rarely last more than 12 hours, with complete resolution of the urticaria within 6 weeks of onset. Daily episodes of urticaria and/or angioedema lasting more than 6 weeks are designated chronic urticaria. Chronic urticaria predominantly affects adults and is twice as common in women as in men.

More than 50% of cases of chronic urticaria are of unknown causation and are called chronic spontaneous urticaria. Physical stimuli may produce urticarial reactions and represent up to 35% of cases of chronic urticaria. The physical urticarias include dermatographic, cold, heat, cholinergic, aquagenic, solar, vibratory, galvanic, and exercise-induced cases. Physical urticaria usually coexists with chronic spontaneous urticaria.

Etiologic Factors

In general, infections, ingestants, inhalants, and injections should be considered as possible underlying causes of urticaria. In acute spontaneous cases, URIs and viral infections are the most common etiologies in children. Drugs (e.g., NSAIDs, antibiotics) and foods are other common causes in both adults and children. Clues suggesting physical urticaria as both a primary cause and as a coexistent second etiology should be sought historically.

In addition to streptococcal and viral URIs, the possibility of localized infection in the tonsils, a tooth, sinuses, gallbladder, prostate, bladder, or kidney should be considered. Treatment with antibiotics for *Helicobacter pylori* has led to resolution of the urticaria. Chronic viral infections, such as hepatitis B and C, may cause urticaria (Fig. 7.15). Acute infectious mononucleosis and psittacosis

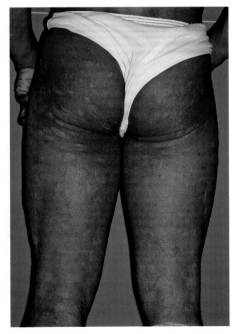

Fig. 7.15 Urticaria secondary to hepatitis B.

may also be triggering conditions. Helminths may cause urticaria and include *Ascaris, Ankylostoma, Strongyloides, Filaria, Echinococcus, Schistosoma, Trichinella, Toxocara,* and liver fluke.

The most allergenic foods are chocolate, shellfish, nuts, peanuts, tomatoes, strawberries, melons, pork, cheese, garlic, onions, eggs, milk, and spices. Food allergens that may cross-react with latex include chestnuts, bananas, passion fruit, avocado, and kiwi. Food additives and preservatives are also implicated in some cases. Natural food additives that may be implicated in urticaria include yeasts, salicylates, citric acid, egg, and fish albumin. Synthetic additives include azo dyes, benzoic acid derivatives, sulfite, and penicillin.

Inhalants that have caused urticaria include grass pollens, house dust mites, feathers, formaldehyde, acrolein (produced when frying with lard or by smoking cigarettes containing glycerin), castor bean or soybean dust, cooked lentils, cottonseed, animal dander, cosmetics, aerosols, pyrethrum, and molds.

Injections of both prescribed and recreational drugs, as well as vaccinations, should be considered in the historical data obtained.

Nonimmunologic mechanisms can produce mast cell degranulation. Common triggers include opiates, polymyxin B, tubocurarine, radiocontrast dye, aspirin, other NSAIDs, vancomycin, tartrazine, and benzoate.

Physical (Inducible) Urticarias

Specific physical stimuli cause up to 35% of all urticarias and occur most frequently in persons age 17–40. The most common form is dermatographism, followed by cholinergic urticaria and cold urticaria. Several forms of physical urticaria may occur in the same patient. Physical urticarias, particularly dermatographic, delayed pressure, cholinergic, and cold urticarias, are frequently found in patients with chronic idiopathic urticaria. Provocative testing off of all treatment at sites not recently affected by urticaria is a useful diagnostic maneuver, and repeated testing with treatment may help gauge therapeutic response. Treatment may be avoidance of the provocative stimulus and often antihistamines, as discussed later for chronic urticaria.

Dermatographism. Dermatographism is a sharply localized edema or wheal, with a surrounding erythematous flare occurring in seconds to minutes after the skin has been stroked (Fig. 7.16). It affects 2%–5% of the population. Dermatographism may arise spontaneously after drug-induced urticaria and persist for months. It has also been reported to be associated with the use of the H2 blocker famotidine. It may occur in hypothyroidism and hyperthyroidism, infectious diseases, diabetes mellitus, and during onset of menopause. It may be a cause of localized or generalized pruritus. Antihistamines suppress this reaction. The addition of an H2 antihistamine may be of benefit. Phototherapy has been used for severe cases.

Cholinergic Urticaria. Cholinergic urticaria, produced by the action of acetylcholine on the mast cell, is characterized by minute, highly pruritic, punctate wheals or papules 1–3 mm in diameter and surrounded by a distinct erythematous flare (Fig. 7.17). These lesions occur primarily on the trunk and face. The condition spares the palms and soles. Lesions persist for 30–90 minutes and are followed by a refractory period of up to 24 hours. Bronchospasm may occur. Familial cases have been reported.

The lesions may be induced in the susceptible patient by increasing the core body temperature with either exercise or a warm bath to raise core temperature by 0.7–1.0°C (1.2–1.8°F). In some cases, an attack may be aborted by rapid cooling of the body, as by taking a cold shower. Cholinergic dermatographism is noted in some patients.

Antihistamines suppress this reaction. The addition of an H2 antihistamine may be of benefit. Antihistamines have been combined with other agents, such as montelukast and propranolol. Attenuated

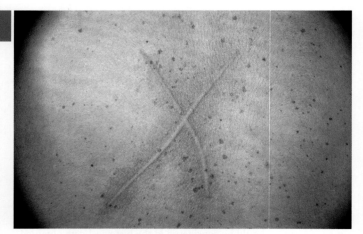

Fig. 7.16 Dermatographism.

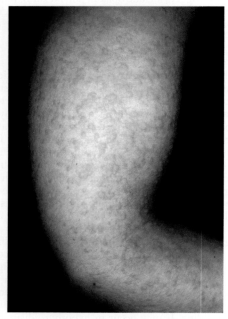

Fig. 7.17 Cholinergic urticaria.

androgens, such as danazol, may be of benefit in patients with refractory cholinergic urticaria. Omalizumab has been used in a refractory case.

Adrenergic Urticaria. Adrenergic urticaria may occur alone or may coexist with cholinergic urticaria. Bouts of urticaria are mediated by norepinephrine. The eruption consists of small (1–5 mm) red macules and papules with a pale halo, appearing within 10–15 minutes of emotional upset, coffee, or chocolate. Serum catecholamines, norepinephrine, dopamine, and epinephrine may rise greatly during attacks, whereas histamine and serotonin levels remain normal. Propranolol, 10 mg four times daily, is effective; atenolol has been ineffective. Anxiolytic benzodiazepines have been used in a refractory case. A provocative test consists of intradermal administration of 3–10 ng of norepinephrine.

Cold Urticaria. Exposure to cold may result in edema and whealing on the exposed areas, usually the face and hands. The urticaria does not develop during chilling, but on rewarming. This heterogeneous group of disorders is classified into primary (essential), secondary, and familial cold urticaria.

Primary (essential) cold urticaria is not associated with underlying systemic diseases or cold-reactive proteins. Symptoms are usually localized to the areas of cold exposure, although respiratory and cardiovascular compromise may develop. Fatal shock may occur when these persons go swimming in cold water or take cold showers. This type of cold urticaria usually begins in adulthood. It usually yields a positive ice cube test result. Antihistamines suppress this reaction. The addition of an H2 antihistamine may be of benefit. Desensitization by repeated, increased exposures to cold has been effective in some cases. Anti–IL-5 therapy with reslizumab or omalizumab has been reported to help severe cases, with one randomized trial of 31 patients stopped early due to benefit from omalizumab at 150 mg or 300 mg doses. In many patients, cold urticaria will resolve after months, although about 50% of patients have symptomatic disease for years. As a provocative test, a plastic-wrapped ice cube is applied to the skin for 5–20 minutes. If no wheal develops, the area should be fanned for an additional 10 minutes. The use of a combination of cold and moving air is, in some cases, more effective in reproducing lesions than cold alone. The provocative test is not performed if secondary cold urticaria is being considered.

Secondary cold urticaria is associated with an underlying systemic disease, such as cryoglobulinemia. Other associations include cryofibrinogenemia, multiple myeloma, secondary syphilis, hepatitis, and infectious mononucleosis. Patients may have headache, hypotension, laryngeal edema, and syncope. An ice cube test is not recommended because it can precipitate vascular occlusion and tissue ischemia.

Familial cold autoinflammatory syndrome is grouped with the other autoinflammatory syndromes discussed earlier. The lesions produce a burning sensation rather than itching. They may have cyanotic centers and surrounding white halos and last for 24–48 hours. They may be accompanied by fever, chills, headache, arthralgia, myalgia, and abdominal pain. A prominent feature is leukocytosis, which is the first observable response to cold. Familial cold urticaria will yield a negative ice cube test result.

Heat Urticaria. Within 5 minutes of the skin being exposed to heat above 43°C (109.4°F), the exposed area begins to burn and sting, then becomes red, swollen, and indurated. This rare type of urticaria may also be generalized and is accompanied by cramps, weakness, flushing, salivation, and collapse. Heat desensitization may be effective. As a provocative test, apply a heated cylinder, 45°C (113°F), to a small area of skin on the upper body for 5 minutes.

Solar Urticaria. Solar urticaria appears soon after unshielded skin is exposed to sunlight. It is classified by the wavelengths of light that precipitate the reaction. Visible light can trigger solar urticaria, and sunscreens may not prevent it. Angioedema may occasionally occur. Solar urticaria may be a manifestation of porphyria, leukocytoclastic vasculitis, and EGPA (Churg-Strauss syndrome). Treatment is sun avoidance, sunscreens, antihistamines, or repetitive phototherapy; omalizumab has been recently used with success. (Solar urticaria is reviewed more extensively in Chapter 3.)

Pressure Urticaria (Delayed Pressure Urticaria). Pressure urticaria is characterized by the development of swelling with pain that usually occurs 3–12 hours after local pressure has been applied. It occurs most frequently on the feet after walking and on the buttocks after sitting. It is unique in that there may be a latent period of as long as 24 hours before lesions develop. Arthralgias, fever, chills, and leukocytosis can occur. The pain and swelling last for 8–24 hours. Pressure urticaria may be seen in combination with other physical urticarias. As a provocative test, a 15-lb weight is suspended from the shoulder by a 3-cm strap for 20 minutes and the area inspected after 4–8 hours (Fig. 7.18).

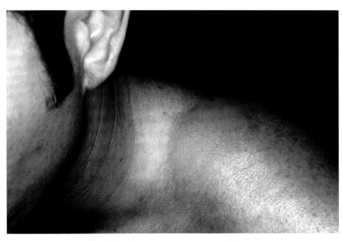

Fig. 7.18 Delated pressure urticaria.

Antihistamines may suppress this reaction. The addition of an H2 antihistamine or montelukast may be of benefit. Systemic corticosteroids are often therapeutic but are generally unsuitable for long-term use. Tranexamic acid, high-dose IVIG, TNF inhibitors, IL-1 inhibitors, and omalizumab have been used in refractory cases.

Exercise-Induced Urticaria. Although both cholinergic urticaria and exercise urticaria are precipitated by exercise, they are distinct entities. Raising the body temperature passively will not induce exercise urticaria, and the lesions of exercise urticaria are larger than the tiny wheals of cholinergic urticaria. Urticarial lesions appear 5–30 minutes after the start of exercise. Anaphylaxis may be associated. Atopy is common in these patients, and some have documented food allergy. Some patients only have such a reaction after eating celery before exercise. Avoiding these allergens may improve symptoms.

Antihistamines suppress the exercise-induced reaction. The addition of an H2 antihistamine may be of benefit. Self-injectable epinephrine kits are recommended for rare patients with episodes of anaphylaxis manifesting with respiratory symptoms. Exercise is a provocative test but may require priming with the identified food allergens.

Vibratory Angioedema. Vibratory angioedema, a form of physical urticaria, may be an inherited autosomal dominant trait or may be acquired after prolonged occupational vibration exposure. Dermatographism, pressure urticaria, and cholinergic urticaria may occur in affected patients. Plasma histamine levels are elevated during attacks. The appearance of the angioedema is usually not delayed. The treatment is antihistamines. As a provocative test, laboratory vortex vibration is applied to the forearm for 5 minutes.

Aquagenic Urticaria. The rare aquagenic urticaria is elicited by water or seawater at any temperature. Pruritic wheals develop immediately or within minutes at the sites of contact of the skin with water, irrespective of temperature or source, and clear within 30–60 minutes. Sweat, saliva, and even tears can precipitate a reaction. Aquagenic urticaria may be familial in some cases or associated with atopy or cholinergic urticaria. Systemic symptoms have been reported, including wheezing, dysphagia, and respiratory distress. The pathogenesis is unknown but may be associated with water-soluble antigens that diffuse into the dermis and cause histamine release from sensitized mast cells.

Whealing may be prevented by pretreatment of the skin with petrolatum. Antihistamines suppress this reaction. The addition

of an H2 antihistamine may be of benefit. PUVA appears to prevent skin lesions but may not prevent the symptoms of pruritus. The provocative test is to apply water compresses, 35°C (95°F), to the skin of the upper body for 30 minutes.

Galvanic Urticaria. Galvanic urticaria has been described after exposure to a galvanic device for iontophoresis used to treat hyperhidrosis. The relationship of this condition to other forms of physical urticaria remains to be established.

Pathogenesis/Histopathology

Capillary permeability results from the increased release of histamine from the mast cells situated around the capillaries. The mast cell is the primary effector cell in urticarial reactions. Other mediators include IL-1 in the autoinflammatory conditions discussed earlier and bradykinin in angioedema associated with angiotensin-converting enzyme (ACE) inhibitors and in the hereditary and acquired angioedema syndromes discussed shortly.

About one third of patients with chronic idiopathic urticaria have circulating functional histamine-releasing IgG autoantibodies that bind to the high-affinity IgE receptor. Some patients have IgG that does not bind the IgE receptor, but rather causes mast cell degranulation. Thyroid autoantibodies are often present in women with chronic idiopathic urticaria, but clinically relevant thyroid disease is seldom present. Even in those with thyroid disease, treatment of the thyroid disorder generally does not affect the course of the urticaria.

The histopathologic changes in acute urticaria include mild dermal edema and margination of neutrophils within postcapillary venules. Later, neutrophils migrate through the vessel wall into the interstitium, and eosinophils and lymphocytes are also noted in the infiltrate. Karyorrhexis and fibrin deposition within vessel walls are absent, helping to differentiate urticaria from vasculitis.

A subset of patients have urticarial lesions with biopsies that show a preponderance of neutrophils; this has been called neutrophilic urticaria. Patients with such histology may present with acute urticaria, chronic urticaria, or physical urticaria. Because neutrophils are typically present in urticaria in general, it is likely that cases of neutrophilic urticaria simply represent urticaria with upregulation of some mast cell–derived cytokines. Some of these may be cases of urticarial vasculitis where the damaged vessels are not visualized. Dapsone may be an alternate therapy for neutrophil-predominant urticaria as well.

Diagnosis

Diagnosis of urticaria and angioedema is usually made on clinical grounds. Burning lesions in a fixed location for more than 24 hours or resolving with bruising suggest urticarial vasculitis, the urticarial phase of an immunobullous eruption, EM, granuloma annulare, sarcoidosis, or cutaneous T-cell lymphoma. If individual wheals last for longer than 24 hours, a skin biopsy should be performed.

Clinical Evaluation

Laboratory evaluation should be driven by associated signs and symptoms. Random tests in the absence of a suggestive history or physical findings are rarely cost-effective and are not recommended. A practical evaluation is limited to a detailed history and a thorough physical examination. Questions to ask include a history of the timing, duration, and frequency of wheals and any associated angioedema; possible association with foods, drugs, febrile illness, occupation, travel, or hobbies; and a family or personal history of atopy, or potential physical causes. A history of aspirin or NSAID ingestion should trigger their avoidance because these drugs may not only cause urticaria, but also aggravate preexisting disease.

If the urticaria is acute and recurrent, food allergy may be suggested by a food diary. Serum radioallergosorbent tests (RASTs) can be used to detect specific IgE, and elimination diets can occasionally be beneficial in some patients. If urticaria does not occur, suspected foods are added one by one and reactions observed.

Angioedema in the absence of urticaria may be related to hereditary angioedema (HAE) or an ACE inhibitor. C1 esterase deficiency does not cause hives, only angioedema, and measurement of C4 is indicated. If C4 is low, an evaluation of C1 esterase inhibitor is appropriate.

In patients with chronic spontaneous urticaria, a directed history and physical examination should elicit signs or symptoms of thyroid disease, connective tissue disease, changes in bowel or bladder habits, vaginal or urethral discharge, other localized infection, jaundice, or risk factors for hepatitis or Lyme disease. Positive findings should prompt appropriate screening tests. Although sinus x-ray films, a panoramic dental film, streptococcal throat culture, abdominal ultrasonography, and urinalysis with urine culture (with prostate massage in men) may reveal the most common occult infections triggering urticaria, positive cases are almost always associated with some signs or symptoms suggestive of the diagnosis. For example, if the patient has a history of sinus difficulties, particularly if there is palpable tenderness over the maxillary or ethmoid sinuses, radiologic sinus evaluation is recommended. Last, a routine CBC with differential, liver function testing, and ESR or CRP level may be done to help decide if infection may be a causal factor. In areas where parasitic disease is common, eosinophilia is an inexpensive screening test with a fair yield.

If the history suggests a physical urticaria, the appropriate challenge test should be used to confirm the diagnosis. Lesions that burn rather than itch, resolve with purpura, or last longer than 24 hours should prompt a biopsy to exclude urticarial vasculitis. If lesions burn rather than itch, and if patients have associated fever, arthralgias, or other evidence of systemic inflammation and antihistamines are not effective, an acquired autoinflammatory syndrome should be considered, and a trial of anakinra may be useful.

Treatment

Acute Urticaria

The mainstay of treatment of acute urticaria is administration of antihistamines. In adults, nonsedating antihistamines pose a lower risk of psychomotor impairment. If the cause of the acute episode can be identified, avoiding that trigger should be stressed. In patients with acute urticaria that does not respond to antihistamines, systemic corticosteroids are generally effective, but histamine-nonresponsive urticaria should prompt consideration for whether there is an underlying disease or continuing trigger present.

For severe reactions, including anaphylaxis, respiratory and cardiovascular support is essential. Patients should be monitored in the hospital. A 0.3-mL dose of a 1:1000 dilution of epinephrine is administered every 10–20 minutes as needed. In young children, a half-strength dilution is used. In rapidly progressive cases, intubation or tracheotomy may be required. Adjunctive therapy includes intramuscular antihistamines (25–50 mg hydroxyzine or diphenhydramine every 6 hours as needed) and systemic corticosteroids (250 mg hydrocortisone or 50 mg methylprednisolone intravenously every 6 hours for 2–4 doses).

Chronic Urticaria

In chronic spontaneous urticaria, the goal of therapy is to alleviate symptoms. The mainstay of treatment is administration of antihistamines. These should be taken on a daily basis; antihistamines should *not* be prescribed to be taken only as needed. Second-generation H1 antihistamines (cetirizine, desloratadine, fexofenadine, acrivastine,

ebastine, mizolastine) are large, lipophilic molecules with charged side chains that bind extensively to proteins, preventing the drugs from crossing the blood-brain barrier; thus they produce less sedation in most patients than the third-generation antihistamine levocetirizine. Long-acting forms are available, and the long half-life of these antihistamines and reduced sedation result in improved compliance and efficacy. First-line treatment is the use of a second- or third-generation nonsedating antihistamine such as cetirizine, in standard dosage. If after 2 weeks the symptoms persist, the dosage should be increased up to 4 times the standard dosage, usually adding a second pill in the evening, then a third in the AM and a fourth in the AM to a maximum of 4 pills per day, two in the morning and two in the evening. If this is ineffective, another nonsedating antihistamine may be tried. Some experience indicates that fexofenadine is less likely to work at higher-than-standard dosages, so this is not escalated if there is no response at standard dosage. Cetirizine and some of the other second-generation antihistamines can cause drowsiness in some individuals, particularly in higher doses or when combined with other antihistamines.

Although some add an H2 blocker such as ranitidine as well, evidence is conflicting on whether this is an effective strategy. Ranitidine should not be used alone for treatment of urticaria because it may interfere with feedback inhibition of histamine release. Also, doxepin, a tricyclic antidepressant with potent H1 antihistaminic activity, may be useful, but evidence is weak. Doxepin is frequently dosed at bedtime, so much of the drowsiness and dry mouth are gone by morning. The same is true for first-generation antihistamines; if any is added to the previous second-generation strategy, it should only be used at night.

If it is necessary to consider other therapies, the following guidance is offered. Mycophenolate, cyclosporine, and prednisone are often effective, but the potential for side effects limits their clinical utility. At least 20% of patients, and up to 50% in some studies, will continue to have chronic spontaneous urticaria after 5 years, and chronic suppressive agents should be avoided if possible. Dapsone, colchicine, and sulfasalazine may be most useful if the biopsy shows a preponderance of neutrophils, and they may be added to antihistamine treatment if some response to the latter has been obtained. Hydroxychloroquine, leukotriene receptor antagonists such as montelukast, and even phototherapy may have some benefit in individual patients. Also, their more satisfactory safety profile makes these therapies worth considering as alternatives to medications such as MMF, omalizumab, and methotrexate, which show more evidence of efficacy. Omalizumab, a recombinant humanized monoclonal antibody that binds to free IgE, is effective in many patients with chronic spontaneous urticaria in doses of 150–300 mg every 4 weeks, with a good safety profile.

Topical corticosteroids, topical antihistamines, and topical anesthetics have no role in the management of chronic urticaria. For local treatment, tepid or cold tub baths or showers may be freely advocated if cold is not a trigger. Topical camphor and menthol can provide symptomatic relief. Sarna lotion contains menthol, phenol, and camphor.

In about one third of patients with chronic idiopathic urticaria, autoantibodies bind to high-affinity IgE receptors. Unfortunately, testing for this condition is not well standardized, has false-positive results, and is impractical. If chronic spontaneous urticaria is nonresponsive to the previous approach, patients may require more aggressive management, including chronic immunosuppressive therapy, plasmapheresis, or IVIG.

Angioedema

Angioedema is an acute, evanescent, circumscribed edema that usually affects the most distensible tissues, such as the eyelids, lips (Fig. 7.19), earlobes, and external genitalia, or the mucous membranes of the mouth, tongue, or larynx. The swelling occurs in

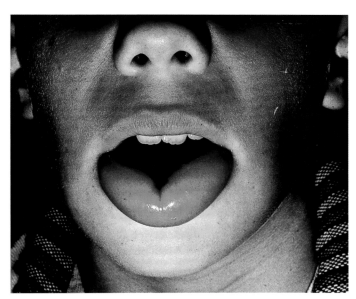

Fig. 7.19 Angioedema of the lips.

the deep dermis or in the subcutaneous tissues and as a rule is only slightly tender, with the overlying skin unaltered, edematous, or rarely ecchymotic. There may be a diffuse swelling on the hands, forearms, feet, and ankles. Frequently, the condition begins during the night and is found on awakening. Angioedema may target the GI and respiratory tracts, resulting in abdominal pain, coryza, asthma, and respiratory problems. Respiratory tract involvement can produce airway obstruction. Anaphylaxis and hypotension may also occur.

There are two distinct subsets of angioedema. The first is considered a deep form of urticaria and may be observed as solitary or multiple sites of angioedema alone or in combination with urticaria. The action of histamine creates vasomotor lability, and pruritus may be a significant feature. The second subgroup, angioedema associated with C1 esterase inhibitor deficiency, or that related to ACE inhibitors, is not associated with hives, or pruritus. Symptoms of pain predominate, and this deficiency is mediated by bradykinin.

Hereditary Angioedema

Also known as Quincke edema, HAE was originally described and named by Osler in 1888. HAE characteristically appears before age 20. Sudden attacks of angioedema occur as frequently as every 2 weeks throughout the patient's life, lasting for 2–5 days. Swelling is typically asymmetric, and urticaria or itching does not occur. The presentation may overlap with that of the autoinflammatory syndromes.

Patients may experience local swelling in subcutaneous tissues (face, hands, arms, legs, genitals, buttocks); abdominal organs (stomach, intestines, bladder), mimicking surgical emergencies; and the upper airway (larynx), which can be life threatening. There is minimal response to antihistamines, epinephrine, or corticosteroids. Mortality rate is high, often caused by laryngeal edema. GI edema is manifested by nausea, vomiting, and severe colic, and it may simulate appendicitis so closely that appendectomy is mistakenly performed. The factors that trigger attacks are minor trauma, surgery, sudden changes of temperature, or sudden emotional stress.

Inherited in an autosomal dominant fashion, HAE is estimated to occur in 1 in 50,000–150,000 persons. There are three phenotypic forms of the disease. Type I is characterized by low antigenic and

functional plasma levels of a normal C1 esterase inhibitor protein (C1-EI). Type II is characterized by the presence of normal or elevated antigenic levels of a dysfunctional protein. Type III demonstrates normal C1-EI function and normal complement. The majority of patients are women. Criteria for type III include a long history of recurrent attacks of skin swelling, abdominal pain, or upper airway obstruction; absence of urticaria; familial occurrence; normal C1-EI and C4 concentrations; and failure of treatment with antihistamines, corticosteroids, and C1-EI concentrate.

The screening test of choice for types I and II is a C4 level. C4 will be low (<40% of normal) as a result of continuous activation and consumption. In addition to depressed C4 levels, patients with types I and II also have low C1, C1q, and C2 levels. If the clinical picture and screening tests are positive, a titer of C1-EI should be ordered. C1-EI is a labile protein, and sample decay is common. A low C1-EI in the presence of normal C4 levels should raise the suspicion of sample decay, rather than true HAE.

The treatment of choice for acute HAE types I and II is plasma-derived or recombinant C1 inhibitor or contact system modulators such as ecallantide or icatibant. Short-term prophylaxis (e.g., for patients undergoing dental care, endoscopy, or intubation for surgery) can be obtained from C1 inhibitor replacement therapy or danazol, an attenuated androgen. Lanadelumab, a monoclonal antibody inhibitor of plasma kallikrein, has been studied for prophylactic therapy. Estrogens in oral contraceptives, in contrast, may precipitate attacks. Attenuated androgens, C1 inhibitors, and in some cases antifibrinolytics are useful for long-term prophylaxis. Patients with type III do not respond to C1-EI replacement but may respond to danazol. Multiple agents are being evaluated to aid in the treatment of HAE, including C1 esterase inhibitor concentrates, recombinant C1INH, monoclonal antibodies against kallikrein, oral kallikrein inhibitors, and factor XIIa–blocking monoclonal antibodies.

Acquired C1 Esterase Inhibitor Deficiency

Some patients present with symptoms indistinguishable from HAE, but with onset after the fourth decade of life and lacking a family history. As in HAE, there is no associated pruritus or urticaria. This condition is subdivided into acquired angioedema I and II and an idiopathic form. Acquired angioedema I is a rare disorder associated with lymphoproliferative disease. These associations include lymphomas (usually B cell), chronic lymphocytic leukemia, monoclonal gammopathy, myeloma, myelofibrosis, Waldenström macroglobulinemia, and breast carcinoma. Some patients have detectable autoantibodies to C1-EI. Worsening of stable HAE has been the presenting sign of lymphoma. Part of the management of this condition is to treat the causative associated condition.

Acquired angioedema II is an extremely rare disease defined by the presence of autoantibodies to C1-EI. It is important to realize that autoantibodies directed against C1-EI may also be found in acquired angioedema I, particularly in patients with B-cell lymphomas, so the diagnosis of acquired angioedema II is made only when no such underlying condition exists.

The pathophysiology of acquired angioedema I is unknown but may be related to increased catabolism of C1-EI; many patients with the disorder have been shown to produce normal amounts of C1-EI. In acquired angioedema II, hepatocytes and monocytes are able to synthesize normal C1-EI; however, a subpopulation of B cells secretes autoantibodies to the functional region of the C1-EI molecule.

Management of acute attacks in acquired angioedema I is directed toward replacement of C1-EI with plasma-derived or recombinant C1 inhibitor. Some patients develop progressive resistance to the infusions. Antifibrinolytic agents, such as aminocaproic acid or tranexamic acid, may be beneficial and are more effective than antiandrogen therapy. Synthetic androgens, such as danazol, may be helpful in angioedema I. However, androgens are ineffective in treating patients with acquired angioedema II, stressing the importance of identifying these patients. Immunosuppressive therapy has been shown to be effective in the treatment of acquired angioedema II by decreasing autoantibody production. Systemic corticosteroids may be temporarily effective.

Episodic Angioedema With Eosinophilia

Episodic angioedema or isolated facial edema may occur with fever, weight gain, eosinophilia, and elevated eosinophil major basic protein (Gleich syndrome). The disorder is not uncommon, and there is no underlying disease. Increased levels of IL-5 have been documented during periods of attack. Treatment options include administration of systemic steroidal medications, imatinib, antihistamines, and IVIG.

Anaphylaxis

Anaphylaxis is an acute and often life-threatening immunologic reaction, frequently heralded by scalp pruritus, diffuse erythema, urticaria, or angioedema. Bronchospasm, laryngeal edema, hyperperistalsis, hypotension, and cardiac arrhythmia may occur. Antibiotics (especially penicillins), other drugs, and radiographic contrast agents are the most common causes of serious anaphylactic reactions. Hymenoptera stings are the next most frequent cause, followed by ingestion of crustaceans and other food allergens. Atopic dermatitis is frequently associated with anaphylaxis, regardless of origin. Causative agents can be identified in up to two thirds of cases, and recurrent attacks are the rule. Exercise-induced anaphylaxis often depends on priming by prior ingestion of a specific food, or food in general, and aspirin may be an additional exacerbating factor.

Chen M, et al: Emerging therapies in hereditary angioedema. Immunol Allergy Clin North Am 2017; 37: 585.

Heelan K, et al: Symptomatic dermatographism treated with NB-UVB. J Dermatolog Treat 2015; 26: 365.

Hogan SR, et al: Adrenergic urticaria. J Am Acad Dermatol 2014; 70: 763.

Kawakami Y, et al: Refractory case of adrenergic urticaria successfully treated with clotiazepam. J Dermatol 2015; 42: 635.

Koumaki D, et al: Successful treatment of refractory cholinergic urticaria with omalizumab. Int J Dermatol 2017; ePub ahead of print.

Gusdorf L, et al: Schnitzler syndrome. Curr Rheumatol Rep 2017; 19: 46.

Holm JG, et al: Diagnostic properties of provocation tests for cold, heat, and delayed-pressure urticaria. Eur J Dermatol 2017; 27: 406.

Joshi S, et al: Biologics in the management of chronic urticaria. J Allergy Clin Immunol Pract 2017; 5: 1489.

Maurer M, et al: Benefit from reslizumab treatment in chronic spontaneous urticaria and cold urticaria. J Eur Acad Dermatol Venereol 2017; ePub ahead of print.

Maurer M, et al: Omalizumab treatment in patients with chronic inducible urticaria. J Allergy Clin Immunol 2017; ePub ahead of print.

Metz M, et al: Omalizumab is effective in cold urticaria—a randomized placebo-controlled trial. J Allergy Clin Immunol 2017;140: 864.

Perez-Ferriols A, et al: Solar urticaria. Actas Dermosifiliogr 2017; 108: 132.

Pezzolo E, et al: Heat urticaria. Br J Dermatol 2016; 175: 473.

Quintero OP, et al: Rapid response to omalizumab in 3 cases of delayed pressure urticaria. J Allergy Clin Immunol Pract 2017; 5: 179.

Radonjic-Hoesli S, et al: Urticaria and angioedema. Clin Rev Allergy Immunol 2017; ePub ahead of print.

Riedl MA, et al: An open-label study of lanadelumab for prevention of attacks in hereditary angioedema. Clin Transl Allergy 2017; 7: 36.

Rodriguez-Jimenez P, et al: Response to omalizumab in solar urticaria. Actas Dermosifiliogr 2017; 108: 53.

8 Connective Tissue Diseases

Lupus erythematosus (LE), dermatomyositis (DM), scleroderma, rheumatoid arthritis, Sjögren syndrome, eosinophilic fasciitis, relapsing polychondritis, and related disorders are classified as connective tissue diseases. Basic to all these is a complex array of autoimmune responses that target or affect collagen or ground substance.

LUPUS ERYTHEMATOSUS

Lupus may manifest as a systemic disease or in purely cutaneous forms. Cutaneous manifestations of LE are classified as in Box 8.1.

Chronic Cutaneous Lupus Erythematosus

Discoid Lupus Erythematosus

Discoid lupus erythematosus (DLE) generally occurs in young adults, with women outnumbering men 2:1. Lesions begin as dull-red macules or indurated plaques that develop an adherent scale, then evolve with atrophy, scarring, and pigment changes (Fig. 8.1). In darker-skinned individuals, lesions typically demonstrate areas of both hyperpigmentation and depigmentation. In lighter-skinned patients, the plaques may appear gray or have minimal pigment alteration. The hyperkeratosis characteristically extends into patulous follicles, producing carpet tacklike spines on the undersurface of the scale.

Localized Discoid Lupus Erythematosus. Discoid lesions are usually localized above the neck, particularly on sun-exposed sites such as the scalp, bridge of the nose, malar areas, lower lip, and ears (Fig. 8.2). The concha of the ear and external canal are frequently involved. Typical lesions are disk-shaped areas of erythema, with follicular plugging, which progress to develop atrophy, scarring, and pigment alteration. Some patients present with periorbital edema and erythema. On the scalp, most lesions begin as erythematous patches or plaques that evolve into white, often depressed, hairless patches. Perifollicular erythema and the presence of easily extractable anagen hairs are signs of active disease. Scarred areas may appear completely smooth or may demonstrate dilated follicular openings in the few remaining follicles. Itching and tenderness are common but rarely severe. On the lips, lesions may be gray or red and hyperkeratotic. They may be eroded and are usually surrounded by a narrow, red inflammatory zone (Fig. 8.3). In one study, 24% of DLE patients had mucosal involvement of the mouth, nose, eye, or vulva. Rarely, aggressive squamous cell carcinoma (SCC) may arise in long-standing lesions of DLE.

Patients with cutaneous lupus erythematosus (CLE) may develop systemic disease over time, sometimes with a lengthy delay (8–10 years), though overall only a small percentage (5%–23% reported, though more often the number is less than 15%) of patients with localized DLE will go on to meet criteria for systemic lupus erythematosus (SLE), usually due to cutaneous and mucosal criteria. Although progression from purely cutaneous DLE to SLE occurs infrequently, patients with SLE frequently have discoid lesions. These patients generally have systemic involvement early in the course of their disease, rather than evolving from chronic cutaneous

LE to SLE. Fever and arthralgia are common in patients with SLE and discoid lesions. In patients with systemic symptoms, abnormal laboratory tests, such as elevation of antinuclear antibodies (ANAs), antibodies to double-stranded (ds) DNA and C1q, leukopenia, hematuria, and proteinuria, help to identify patients with SLE and suggest a prognosis.

Generalized Discoid Lupus Erythematosus. Generalized DLE is less common than localized DLE. All degrees of severity are encountered. Most often, the thorax and upper extremities are affected, as well as the head and neck (Fig. 8.4). The scalp may become quite bald with striking patterns of hyperpigmentation and depigmentation. Diffuse scarring may involve the face and upper extremities. Laboratory abnormalities, such as an elevated erythrocyte sedimentation rate (ESR), elevated ANAs, single-stranded (ss) DNA antibodies, and leukopenia, are more common with this form of LE than with localized DLE, and as such patients with generalized DLE are more likely to meet criteria for systemic lupus.

Childhood Discoid Lupus Erythematosus. Among children with DLE, a low frequency of photosensitivity and a higher rate of association with SLE have been noted, with one recent study showing 15% of patients with DLE had concurrent SLE, and 26% of the remaining patients eventually met SLE criteria. In most other respects, the clinical presentation and course are similar to those in adults.

Histology. The epidermis may demonstrate effacement of the rete ridge pattern or irregular acanthosis. Compact hyperkeratosis without parakeratosis is characteristic, and follicular plugging is typically prominent. Hydropic degeneration of the basal layer of the epidermis and follicular epithelium results in pigmentary incontinence. A patchy perivascular and periadnexal lymphoid inflammatory infiltrate occurs in the superficial and deep dermis. The infiltrate characteristically surrounds vessels, follicles, and the eccrine coil. Increased mucin is often present, though is not a reliable mechanism to distinguish lupus from mimickers. Thickening of the basement membrane zone (BMZ) may be prominent.

The histology varies with the stage of the lesion. Acute lesions show only patchy lymphoid inflammation and vacuolar interface dermatitis. Lesions established for several months begin to show hyperkeratosis, BMZ thickening, and dermal mucin. Chronic, inactive lesions show atrophy, with postinflammatory pigmentation and scarring throughout the dermis. At this stage, the inflammatory infiltrate is sparse to absent. Pilosebaceous units, except for "orphaned" arrector muscles, are destroyed. At this stage, the dermis appears fibrotic, but an elastic tissue stain can still distinguish the diffuse dermal scar of lupus from the focal, wedge-shaped, superficial scars of lichen planopilaris (LPP) or folliculitis decalvans. Direct immunofluorescence (DIF) testing of lesional skin is positive in more than 75% of cases, provided the lesions have been active for at least several months and usually demonstrate strong, continuous granular deposition of immunoglobulin and complement located at the dermoepidermal junction (DEJ).

Differential Diagnosis. Discoid LE must often be differentiated from seborrheic dermatitis, rosacea, lupus vulgaris, sarcoidosis, drug eruptions, actinic keratosis, Bowen disease, lichen planus (LP), tertiary syphilis, and polymorphous light eruption (PMLE).

BOX 8.1 Classification of Cutaneous Manifestations of Lupus Erythematosus

I. CHRONIC CUTANEOUS LE

A. Discoid LE
   1. Localized
   2. Disseminated
B. Verrucous (hypertrophic) LE (Behçet): usually acral and often lichenoid
C. Lupus erythematosus–lichen planus overlap
D. Chilblain LE
E. Tumid lupus
F. Lupus panniculitis (LE profundus)
   1. With no other involvement
   2. With overlying discoid LE
   3. With systemic LE

II. SUBACUTE CUTANEOUS LE

A. Papulosquamous
B. Annular
C. Syndromes commonly exhibiting similar morphology
   1. Neonatal LE
   2. Complement deficiency syndromes
   3. Drug induced

III. ACUTE CUTANEOUS LE: LOCALIZED OR GENERALIZED ERYTHEMA OR BULLAE, GENERALLY ASSOCIATED WITH SLE

LE, Lupus erythematosus; *SLE,* systemic lupus erythematosus.

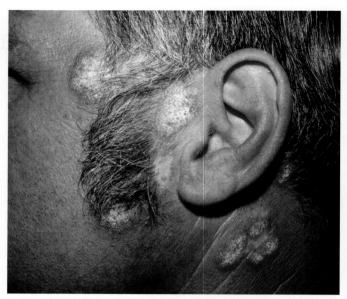

Fig. 8.2 Discoid lupus erythematosus. (Courtesy Steven Binnick, MD.)

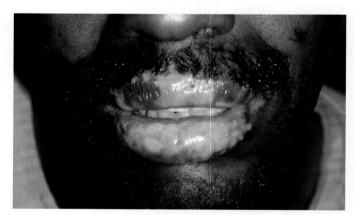

Fig. 8.3 Discoid lupus erythematosus.

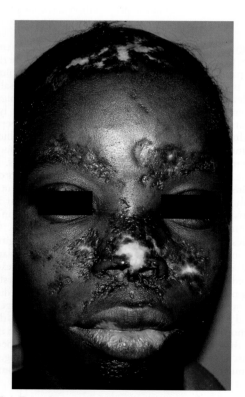

Fig. 8.1 Extensive scarring from discoid lupus erythematosus.

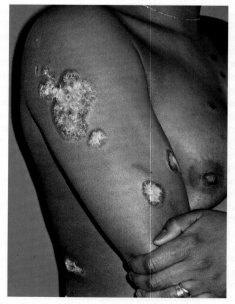

Fig. 8.4 Generalized discoid lupus erythematosus.

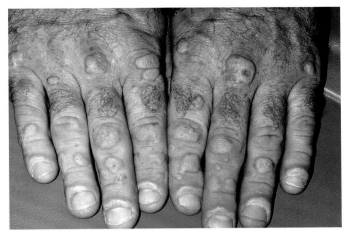

Fig. 8.5 Hypertrophic lupus erythematosus. (Courtesy Steven Binnick, MD.)

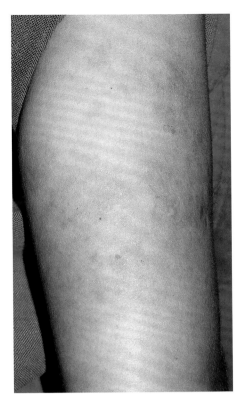

Fig. 8.6 Tumid lupus.

Seborrheic dermatitis does not show atrophy, alopecia, or dilated follicles and has greasy, yellowish scale without follicular plugs. Acral, lip, and scalp lesions of chronic cutaneous LE may demonstrate lichenoid dermatitis histologically. In these cases, the presence of continuous granular immunoglobulin in addition to cytoid bodies is a helpful distinguishing feature.

In rosacea, atrophy does not occur, and pustules are almost always found. Apple-jelly nodules (granulomas) are seen with diascopy in lupus vulgaris. Sunlight-sensitizing agents, such as sulfonamides, may produce lesions similar to LE, because phototoxic reactions demonstrate vacuolar interface dermatitis. It may be necessary to differentiate syphilis and sarcoid by biopsy and serologic testing. PMLE is distinguished by the absence of scarring and the presence of intensely edematous plaques and papules. DIF is generally negative or nonspecific in PMLE.

Hypertrophic Lupus Erythematosus

Nonpruritic papulonodular lesions may occur on the arms and hands, resembling keratoacanthoma or hypertrophic LP (Fig. 8.5). The lips and scalp may also demonstrate lesions that resemble LP or LPP. Dermoscopy may help distinguish hypertrophic LE from SCC, but biopsy is often needed. Histologic sections of these lesions typically demonstrate lichenoid dermatitis, and a careful examination for other characteristic skin lesions of LE or LP, as well as DIF testing, may be critical in establishing a diagnosis. BMZ thickening, dermal mucin, eccrine coil involvement, and subcutaneous nodular lymphoid infiltrates are features of LE that are not found in LP. Recent reports suggesting the pattern and number of plasmacytoid dendritic cells may be helpful in distinguishing SCC from hypertrophic LE.

Lupus Erythematosus–Lichen Planus Overlap Syndrome

In addition to the cases of hypertrophic LE with lichenoid histology previously discussed, there are patients with a true overlap syndrome with features of both LE and LP. The lesions are usually large, atrophic, hypopigmented, red or pink patches and plaques. Pigment abnormalities become prominent over time, and fine telangiectasia and scaling are usually present. The extensor aspects of the extremities and midline back are typically affected. Prominent palmoplantar involvement is characteristic and tends to be the most troublesome feature for these patients. Nail dystrophy and anonychia may occur. Scarring alopecia and oral involvement have been noted in some patients. The histology of individual lesions has features of LP and/or LE. One study suggested that higher

CD3 and CD34 may favor LP over DLE, but this has not been widely examined. DIF may help differentiate the two, but they may share overlapping features. Response to treatment is poor, although potent topical corticosteroids, dapsone, thalidomide, or isotretinoin may be effective. Some patients require immunosuppressive therapy with agents such as mycophenolate mofetil (MMF) or azathioprine. It should also be noted that antimalarials can occasionally produce a lichenoid drug eruption. A rare variant of chronic CLE termed the *pigmented macular variant* has been described, with lichenoid to gray pigmentation in sun exposed areas; although these patients display interface reaction on biopsy and may have seropositivity, systemic disease is rare, and it is unclear if this represents a rare subtype of lupus or another lichenoid entity. Patients respond to topical steroids, sun protection, and hydroquinone.

Chilblain Lupus Erythematosus

Chilblain LE (Hutchinson) is a chronic, unremitting form of LE affecting the fingertips, rims of ears, calves, and heels, especially in women. It is usually preceded by DLE on the face. Systemic involvement is sometimes seen. Mimicry of sarcoidosis may be striking. Cryoglobulins and antiphospholipid antibody (APLA) should also be sought. Familial chilblain lupus has been linked to mutations in a number of genes, particularly *TREX-1*, and is considered part of the group of genetic diseases termed *interferonopathies*.

Tumid Lupus Erythematosus

Tumid LE is a rare but distinctive entity. Patients present with edematous erythematous plaques, usually on the trunk (Fig. 8.6). Histologically, the lesions demonstrate a patchy superficial and deep perivascular and periadnexal lymphoid infiltrate that frequently affects the eccrine coil. Dermal mucin deposition is typical and

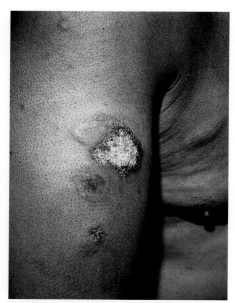

Fig. 8.7 Lupus panniculitis with overlying discoid lupus erythematosus.

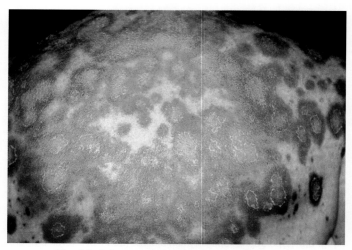

Fig. 8.8 Subacute cutaneous lupus erythematosus.

may be striking. The lesions generally respond readily to antimalarials. Tumid LE shares many features with reticular erythematous mucinosis, and some authorities consider them to be closely related entities.

Lupus Erythematosus Panniculitis (Lupus Erythematosus Profundus)

Patients with the panniculitis type of LE develop subcutaneous nodules that are usually firm, sharply defined, and nontender. The proximal extremities are typically involved. Usually, the overlying skin is normal, but overlying discoid or tumid lesions may occur (Fig. 8.7). Some cases are discovered incidentally when an unrelated lesion is biopsied. The lesions may progress to deep depressions, or "dells," from loss of the panniculus. LE panniculitis is characteristically chronic and occurs most often in women between ages 20 and 45. Many patients have DLE at other sites or less typically, in the overlying skin.

Histologic sections demonstrate lymphoid nodules in the subcutaneous septa, necrosis of the fat lobule, and fibrinoid or hyaline degeneration of the remaining lipocytes. Lipomembranous change, resembling frost on a windowpane, is more typical of stasis panniculitis (lipodermatosclerosis), but it may be noted focally in LE panniculitis. The overlying epidermis may show basal liquefaction and follicular plugging or may be normal. Dermal lymphoid nodules or vertical columns of lymphoid cells may be seen in fibrous tract remnants. Dermal mucin may be prominent, and dermal collagen hyalinization (resembling that seen in morphea) may be present. Continuous granular deposition of immunoglobulin and C3 may be seen at the DEJ. In active cases, abundant fibrin is usually noted in the panniculus.

The most important entity to consider in the differential diagnosis is subcutaneous panniculitis–like T-cell lymphoma (SPTCL). Important clues include the presence of lipocytes, rimmed by atypical lymphocytes with nuclear molding, and the presence of constitutional symptoms. Erythrophagocytosis may be present focally, and T-cell clonality can usually be demonstrated. The infiltrate may be CD8 dominant or may label strongly for CD56, as in natural killer cell lymphoma, or CD30, as in anaplastic lymphoma. CD5 and CD7 expression may be reduced (aberrant

loss of pan-T markers). Unfortunately, T-cell clonality, erythrophagocytosis, CD8 predominance, and loss of CD5 or CD7 may also be seen in patients with LE panniculitis who respond to antimalarials or corticosteroids and do not progress to clinical lymphoma. Taken together, these data suggest that some cases of lymphoma may be virtually indistinguishable from LE panniculitis, or that some cases of LE panniculitis represent an abortive lymphoid dyscrasia. Patients diagnosed with lupus panniculitis should be monitored for progression.

Subacute Cutaneous Lupus Erythematosus

In 1979 Sontheimer, Thomas, and Gilliam described a clinically distinct subset of cases of LE to which they gave the name subacute cutaneous lupus erythematosus (SCLE). Patients are most often white women age 15–40. SCLE patients make up approximately 10%–15% of the LE population. Lesions are scaly and evolve as polycyclic annular lesions (Fig. 8.8) or psoriasiform plaques, although rare widespread cases of erythrodermic SCLE or patients resembling SJS/TEN have been described. The lesions vary from red to pink with faint violet tones. The scale is thin and easily detached, and telangiectasia or dyspigmentation may be present. Follicles are not involved, the lesions tend to be transient or migratory, and there is no scarring. Lesions tend to occur on sun-exposed surfaces of the face and neck, the V portion of the chest and back, and the sun-exposed areas of the arms. Photosensitivity is prominent in about half of patients. Concomitant DLE is present in 20% of cases.

About three quarters of patients have arthralgia or arthritis, 20% have leukopenia, and 80% have a positive ANA test (usually in a particulate pattern). Between 20% and 50% of patients meet the American Rheumatology Association (ARA) criteria for a diagnosis of SLE. The majority of cases have antibodies to Ro/SSA antigen, and most are positive for human leukocyte antigen (HLA) DR3. La/SSB may also be present, and many patients have overlap features with Sjögren syndrome. The disease generally runs a mild course, and renal, central nervous system (CNS), or vascular complications are unusual. An association with autoimmune thyroid disease has been noted. Most patients respond to sun protection and antimalarial agents. From 12%–30% of cases may be drug induced. Medication-induced SCLE is traditionally most often related to hydrochlorothiazide due to its wide use, but proton pump inhibitors are increasingly recognized, perhaps due to over-the-counter availability. Drug-induced SCLE may also be seen with angiotensin-converting enzyme (ACE) inhibitors, calcium channel blockers (CCBs), interferons (IFNs), anticonvulsants, griseofulvin, glyburide, piroxicam, penicillamine, spironolactone, terbinafine, statins, voriconazole, and chemotherapeutic agents. Chemotherapeutic agents implicated include fluorouracil, capecitabine, cemcitabine, docetaxel, paclitaxel, and doxorubicin, with emerging reports of nivolumab, other checkpoint inhibitors, and small molecule kinase inhibitors such as masitinib. TNF inhibitors are increasingly recognized as the triggering drug and are important to keep in mind due to the potential for psoriasiform SCLE to resemble psoriasis, which can lead to a misdiagnosis of TNF-induced psoriasis—photosensitivity is a clue to SCLE in these cases. Case reports describe both topical terbinafine and imiquimod inducing SCLE-like eruptions as well.

Histopathology

Vacuolar interface dermatitis is a universal finding in active SCLE lesions. Mild hyperkeratosis and parakeratosis may be present. Chronic changes of DLE, such as follicular plugging, BMZ thickening, and heavy lymphoid aggregates, are usually lacking. Dermal mucin is variable. DIF is positive in lesional skin in only about one third of cases. A dustlike particulate deposition of immunoglobulin G (IgG) in epidermal nuclei of Ro-positive patients may be present and is a helpful diagnostic finding.

Neonatal Lupus Erythematosus

Most infants with neonatal lupus are girls, born to mothers who carry the Ro/SSA antibody. These infants have no skin lesions at birth, but develop them during the first few weeks of life. Annular erythematous macules and plaques may appear on the head and extremities (Fig. 8.9). Periocular involvement (raccoon eyes) may be prominent. With time, the lesions fade and become atrophic. Telangiectasia or dermal mucinosis in an acral papular pattern may be the predominant findings in some cases. Telangiectatic macules or angiomatous papules may be found in sun-protected sites such as the diaper area, may occur independently of active lupus skin lesions, and may be persistent. The skin lesions usually resolve spontaneously by 6 months of age, and usually heal without significant scarring, although atrophy and telangiectatic mats may persist. Dyspigmentation and persistent telangiectasias may remain for months to years. Half the mothers are asymptomatic at delivery, although many will subsequently develop arthralgia, Sjögren syndrome, or other mild systemic findings.

Although the skin lesions are transient, half the patients have an associated isolated congenital heart block, usually third degree, which is permanent. Some infants have only this manifestation of LE, and for cardiac lesions alone, there is no female predominance. In children with cutaneous involvement, thrombocytopenia and hepatic disease may occur as frequently as cardiac disease. Close monitoring is recommended for at least the first 3 months

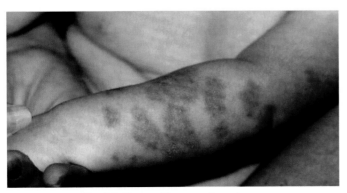

Fig. 8.9 Neonatal lupus erythematosus.

of life, and by 9 months of life most cases resolve, with only 10% of infants with persistent antibodies at that time.

There is a strong association with Ro/SSA autoantibody. Almost all mothers, and thus almost all infants, are positive for this antibody, although some mothers are also positive for La/SSB, and some with only U1RNP antibodies have been described. Infants with only U1RNP antibodies have not developed heart block. There is linkage to HLA-DR3 in the mother. The risk that a second child will have neonatal LE is approximately 25%. Japanese infants apparently differ in that they may express anti-dsDNA antibodies, and 8% progress to SLE. In unselected women with anti-Ro antibodies, only 1%–2% will have an infant with neonatal LE.

Complement Deficiency Syndromes

Although deficiency of many complement components may be associated with LE-like conditions, deficiencies of the early components, especially C2 and C4, are most characteristic. Many such cases are found to have photosensitive annular SCLE lesions and Ro/SSA antibody formation. Patients with C4 deficiency often have hyperkeratosis of the palms and soles. Heterozygous deficiency of either complement component C4A or C4B has a frequency of approximately 20% in white populations. Homozygous deficiency of both is rare, and affected patients may present with SLE with mesangial glomerulonephritis, membranous nephropathy, and severe skin lesions. Although frequently asymptomatic, homozygous C2 deficiency can cause severe infections, SLE, and atherosclerosis.

Systemic Lupus Erythematosus

Young to middle-aged women are predominantly affected by SLE, manifesting a wide range of symptoms and signs. Skin involvement occurs in 80% of cases and is often helpful in arriving at a diagnosis. Its importance is suggested by the fact that 4 of the 11 American College of Rheumatology (ACR) criteria for the diagnosis of SLE are mucocutaneous findings. The diagnostic criteria are as follows:

1. Malar rash
2. Discoid rash
3. Photosensitivity
4. Oral ulcers (21%)
5. Arthritis
6. Proteinuria >0.5 g/day or casts
7. Neurologic disorders (seizures or psychosis in the absence of other known causes)
8. Pleuritis/pericarditis
9. Blood abnormalities (e.g., hemolytic anemia, leukopenia, thrombocytopenia)
10. Immunologic disorders, including anti-dsDNA antibody, anti-Sm, APLAs (based on IgG or IgM anticardiolipin antibodies, lupus anticoagulant [LA], or false-positive serologic test for syphilis known for at least 6 months)
11. Positive ANA blood test

For identification of patients in clinical studies, a patient may be said to have SLE if four or more of these criteria are satisfied, serially or simultaneously. It is important to note that many patients present with autoantibodies, arthralgia, and constitutional signs, but do not meet ACR criteria for SLE. With time, patients may evolve to meet all criteria. The Systemic Lupus International Collaborating Clinics (SLICC) group revision of the ACR criteria results in greater sensitivity with equal specificity. According to the SLICC rule, the patient must manifest at least four criteria (including at least one clinical criterion and one immunologic criterion) *or* must have biopsy-proven lupus nephritis in the presence of either ANAs or anti-dsDNA antibodies. Many patients with DLE or SCLE meet criteria for SLE due to mucocutaneous criteria.

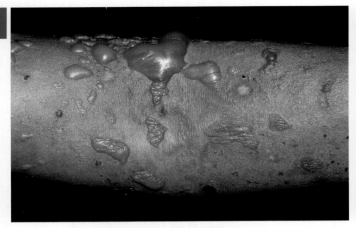

Fig. 8.10 Bullous lupus erythematosus.

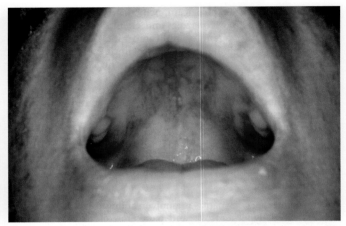

Fig. 8.11 Oral lupus erythematosus.

Cutaneous Manifestations

The characteristic butterfly facial erythema seen in patients with SLE is a common manifestation of acute cutaneous LE. The eruption usually begins on the malar area and the bridge of the nose. There may be associated edema. The nasolabial crease if often strikingly spared, unlike in DM. The ears and chest may also be the sites of early lesions. Biopsies at all sites show interface dermatitis and a scant perivascular lymphoid infiltrate. The eruption may last a day to several weeks and resolves without scarring. There may be more widespread erythema in some cases.

Bullous lesions of lupus erythematosus (BLE) occur as single or grouped vesicles or bullae, often widespread, with a predilection for sun-exposed areas (Fig. 8.10). Rarely, the lesions may itch. Most sets of published criteria require that patients with BLE meet ACR criteria for SLE, but some patients have identical bullous lesions and less than four ACR criteria. Histologically, neutrophils accumulate at the DEJ and within dermal papillae. In bullous lesions, there is a subepidermal bulla or superficial dermal edema containing neutrophils. Fluorescence with IgG, IgM, IgA, or C3 is typically present in a continuous, granular pattern at the BMZ on DIF testing. Neutrophils are found in or below the lamina densa on immunofluorescent electron microscopy. Most of these patients are HLA-DR2 positive. The recognition of this subset as distinct is made clear by its often dramatic therapeutic response to dapsone. Epidermolysis bullosa acquisita is histopathologically and immunopathologically identical, because both diseases are mediated by circulating antibodies against type VII collagen. Dapsone is usually ineffective in epidermolysis bullosa acquisita.

A variety of vascular lesions occur in 50% of SLE patients. Often, fingertips or toes show edema, erythema, or telangiectasia. Nailfold capillary loops in LE are more likely to show wandering glomeruloid loops, whereas DM and scleroderma capillary loops demonstrate symmetric dilation and dropout of vessels. Capillary loops in the Osler-Weber-Rendu syndrome demonstrate ectasia of half the capillary loop. Erythema multiforme (EM)–like lesions may predominate, termed Rowell syndrome. Rarely, lupus may present with TEN-like lesions due to intense interface inflammation leading to blistering.

In addition to periungual telangiectasia, red or spotted lunulae may be present in patients with SLE, as in RA. The palms, soles, elbows, knees, or buttocks may become persistently erythematous or purplish, sometimes with overlying scale. Diffuse, nonscarring hair loss is common. Short hairs in the frontal region are called "lupus hairs." These hairs result from a combination of chronic telogen effluvium and increased hair fragility.

Mucous membrane lesions are seen in 20%–30% of SLE patients. Conjunctivitis, episcleritis, and nasal and vaginal ulcerations

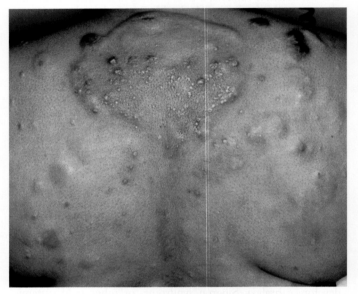

Fig. 8.12 Papulonodular mucinosis.

may occur. Oral mucosal hemorrhages, erosions, shallow angular ulcerations with surrounding erythema, and gingivitis are common (Fig. 8.11). Erythema, petechiae, and ulcerations may occur on the hard palate.

Multiple eruptive dermatofibromas have been described in SLE. Leg ulcers, typically deeply punched out and with very little inflammation, may be seen on the pretibial or malleolar areas. Many of these patients present with a livedoid pattern, and many have an antiphospholipid antibody. Sneddon syndrome is composed of livedo reticularis and strokes related to a hyalinizing vasculopathy.

Calcinosis cutis is uncommon but may be dramatic. Also seen infrequently are plaquelike or papulonodular depositions of mucin. These reddish purple to skin-colored lesions are often present on the trunk and arms or head and neck (Fig. 8.12). Last, a symmetric papular eruption of the extremities may occur. These skin-colored to erythematous lesions with a smooth, ulcerated or umbilicated surface may show vasculitis or, in older lesions, a palisaded granulomatous inflammation. These occur in patients with SLE, RA, or other immune complex–mediated disease. This eruption has been referred to as palisaded neutrophilic and granulomatous dermatitis of immune complex disease (Fig. 8.13).

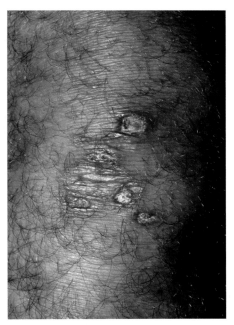

Fig. 8.13 Palisaded neutrophilic granulomatous dermatitis.

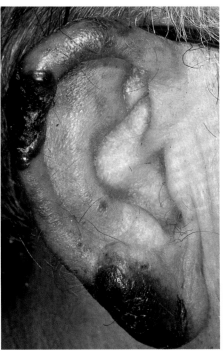

Fig. 8.14 Cutaneous thrombosis in antiphospholipid antibody syndrome.

Systemic Manifestations

Most organs can be involved in SLE; the symptoms and findings are often caused by immune complex disease, especially vasculitis. The earliest changes noted may be transitory or migratory arthralgia, often with periarticular inflammation. Fever, weight loss, pleuritis, adenopathy, or acute abdominal pain may occur. Arthralgia is often the earliest abnormality and may remain the sole symptom for some time. About 95% of SLE patients will manifest this symptom. Arthralgia, deforming arthropathy, and acute migratory polyarthritis resembling RA may all occur as manifestations of SLE. Avascular necrosis of the femoral head has been observed. Although this is a known complication of systemic corticosteroid therapy, it has also occurred in patients with SLE who have never taken corticosteroids.

Patients with SLE have a higher rate of peripheral arterial disease compared with controls. Thrombosis in vessels of various sizes and thromboembolism may be a recurring event (Fig. 8.14). It may be attributed to a plasma constituent, paradoxically called "lupus anticoagulant" (LA) because it causes prolonged coagulation studies in vitro but thrombosis in vivo. The finding of an LA is usually associated with APLAs. These may be anticardiolipin antibodies, but other APLA types—antiphosphatidylserine, antiphosphatidylinositol, and antiphosphatidylethanolamine—may occur. APLAs and elevated homocysteine may each increase the risk of thrombosis. APLAs are associated with early-onset organ damage. SLE patients with APLAs have higher mortality. Many, but not all, patients have a false-positive blood test for syphilis. In one study, inflammatory lesions of SLE and infections were the most common causes of death during the initial 5 years of disease, whereas thromboses were the most common cause of death after the first 5 years.

Renal involvement is a predictor of poor prognosis. It may be of either nephritic or nephrotic type, leading in either case to chronic renal insufficiency with proteinuria and azotemia. Patients with lupus who are ANCA positive have higher rates of damage. Active nephritis is unlikely in the absence of anti-dsDNA. Both anti-dsDNA antibody and anti-C1q antibody are of relatively high specificity for active nephritis. Hypercholesterolemia and hypo-albuminemia may occur. Immunoglobulin and complement components have been found localized to the BMZ of glomeruli, where vasculitis produces the characteristic "wire-loop" lesion.

Myocarditis is indicated by cardiomegaly and gallop rhythm, but the electrocardiographic (ECG) changes are usually not specific. Pericarditis, the most frequent cardiac manifestation, and endo-carditis also occur. Patients with SLE have accelerated athero-sclerosis and elevated risk for cardiovascular morbidity and mortality. Raynaud phenomenon (RP) occurs in about 15% of patients, who have less renal disease and consequently lower mortality rates.

The CNS may be involved with vasculitis, manifested by hemiparesis, convulsions, epilepsy, diplopia, retinitis, and choroiditis. Livedo reticularis is a marker for patients at risk for CNS lesions (Sneddon syndrome; see earlier). Depression and anxiety are common in patients with SLE, and other psychiatric and personality have been reported as well.

Idiopathic thrombocytopenic purpura is occasionally the forerunner of SLE. Coombs-positive hemolytic anemia, neutro-penia, and lymphopenia are other hematologic findings. The severity of thrombocytopenia may be a prognostic marker, but can also be followed as a biomarker for response to treatment. Gastro-intestinal (GI) involvement may produce symptoms of nausea, vomiting, and diarrhea, and patients may develop intestinal pseudo obstruction. Frequently, the intestinal wall and the mesenteric vessels show vasculitis. Pulmonary involvement with pleural effu-sions, interstitial lung disease, pulmonary artery hypertension (PAH), and acute lupus pneumonitis may be present. Patients with SLE, pericardial effusions, and anti-RNP antibodies have higher rates of PAH. Sjögren syndrome (keratoconjunctivitis sicca) and Hashimoto thyroiditis are associated with SLE. Overlap with any of the connective tissue diseases may be seen, occurring in approximately 25% of patients. Muscular atrophy may accompany extreme weakness so that DM may be suspected. Myopathy of the vacuolar type may produce muscular weakness, myocardial disease, dysphagia, and achalasia of the esophagus. Steroid myopathy may also occur, and antimalarials may rarely induce myopathy.

The serum aldolase level may be elevated with a normal creatine phosphokinase.

A history of exposure to excessive sunlight before the onset of the disease or before an exacerbation is sometimes obtained. Some patients may have only mild constitutional symptoms for weeks or months, but immediately after exposure to strong sunlight, they may develop the facial eruption and severe disease complications.

Hydralazine, procainamide, sulfonamides, penicillin, anticonvulsants, minocycline, and isoniazid have been implicated as causes of drug-induced LE. Penicillamine induces (or unmasks) true SLE. HLA-DR4 individuals, who are slow acetylators, are predisposed to develop hydralazine-induced LE. Antibody to the histone complex H2A-H2B is closely associated with disease. Most drug-induced SLE is associated with a positive ANA, and antibodies directed against histones. Exceptions include penicillamine and etanercept, which may induce or unmask native disease with anti-dsDNA antibodies. L-Canavanine, an amino acid found in alfalfa sprouts and tablets, can also induce or worsen SLE. TNF-inhibitors can induce a variety of types of lupus, with infliximab surpassing etanercept as the most commonly reported culprit. Patients with anti–chimeric antibodies may be ANA positive, and patients with TNF-induced lupus frequently display a malar rash, photosensitivity, and meet ACR criteria for lupus.

Childhood Systemic Lupus Erythematosus

The onset of childhood SLE occurs between ages 3 and 15, with girls outnumbering boys 4 : 1. The skin manifestations may be the typical butterfly eruption on the face and photosensitivity. In addition, there may be morbilliform, bullous, purpuric, ulcerating, or nodose lesions. The oral mucosa is frequently involved. Skin eruptions may be associated with joint, renal, neurologic, and GI disease. Weight loss, fatigue, hepatosplenomegaly, lymphadenopathy, and fever are other manifestations. Pediatric patients with SLE and APLAs, specifically lupus anticoagulants, are at high risk of developing thromboembolic events.

Pregnancy and Female Hormones

Women with LE may have successful pregnancies, but they might have difficulty conceiving, and miscarriages occur with greater frequency, especially among those with APLAs. The course of pregnancy may be entirely normal, with remission of the LE, or the symptoms of LE may become worse. Risk of fetal death is increased in women with a previous history of fetal loss and anticardiolipin or anti-Ro antibodies. For the patient with these antibodies but without a history of previous fetal loss, the risk of fetal loss or neonatal lupus is low. In most cases, the pregnancy itself is well tolerated, although a flare of SLE may occur during the postpartum period. Although several studies failed to demonstrate a clinically significant association between oral contraceptive (OC) use and flares of SLE, recently a UK epidemiologic study found an increased risk of SLE with current use of OC, and the U.S. Nurses' Health Study suggested that OC and HRT were associated with SLE. There is a high incidence of thromboses in women with APLAs, and OCs containing second- or third-generation progestogens may induce a higher risk. One female-to-male transgender patient experienced significant improvement after testosterone therapy.

Etiology

Genetics plays an important role in LE, with over 100 loci identified in association with sLE. Many of these gene targets are involved in recognition of nucleic acid, type 1 IFN production, and immune signaling. Taken together, these data suggest polygenetic susceptibility to LE. A family history of connective tissue disease is a strong risk factor for all forms of LE. Monozygotic twins, however, display a low concordance rate, with lupus in approximately one fourth of cases. Some skin lesions of LE follow lines of Blaschko, suggesting postzygotic mutation or loss of heterozygosity for a genetic locus. Understanding of lupus genetics is rapidly evolving.

The C-reactive protein (CRP) response is defective in patients with flares of SLE, and the gene locus for CRP maps to 1q23.2 within an interval linked with SLE. Gene polymorphisms in *APRIL*, a member of the TNF family, have also been linked with SLE. Increased expression of TNF-α and IFN-inducible proteins are noted in cutaneous LE. Polymorphisms of the *C1qA* gene are associated with both systemic and cutaneous LE. HLA-DR3 confers risk for SLE, and C4 null alleles in Europeans is a specific genetic risk factor for SLE. Linkage varies in different ethnic groups and different clinical subsets of lupus.

Whole exome sequencing has helped identify rare monogenic variants of SLE and SLE-like diseases. *CYBB* mutations have an X-linked inheritance, and carriers have a higher risk of DLE and SLE. Mutations in *DNASE1L3* are associated with SLE with early onset and anti-dsDNA abs. *TREX1* mutations are associated with familial chilblain lupus.

Several aspects of the altered immune response are worth particular attention. T-suppressor cell function is reduced in patients with LE. Overproduction of γ-globulins by B cells and reduced clearance of immune complexes by the reticuloendothelial system may contribute to complement-mediated damage. Externalization of cellular antigens, such as Ro/SSA in response to sunlight, may lead to cell injury by way of antibody-dependent cellular cytotoxicity. Abnormal apoptosis or reduced clearance of apoptotic cells may lead to increased exposure of nucleosome antigens and antinucleosome antibodies.

Both ultraviolet (UV) B and UVA can upregulate antigen expression and cytokines, including IL-1, TNF-α, and LFA-1, causing release of sequestered antigens and free radical damage, with UV B felt to be the most pathologically relevant. All these mechanisms may contribute to photosensitivity and UV-induced flares of systemic disease. Air pollutants have been considered a potential trigger, due to increased concentrations of SLE in urban areas and a small Canadian study suggesting a possible link. Tobacco smoke is highly associated with cutaneous LE, but not with systemic LE, and may interfere with the efficacy of antimalarial therapy. Minimal credible data exist regarding other possible aggravating dietary factors, but some reports have implicated excess calories, excess protein, high fat (especially saturated and ω-6 polyunsaturated fatty acids), excess zinc, and excess iron.

Laboratory Findings

There may be hemolytic anemia, thrombocytopenia, lymphopenia, or leukopenia; ESR usually is greatly elevated during active disease but nonspecific. Coombs test may be positive, there is a biologic false-positive test for syphilis, and a rheumatoid factor (RF) may be present. IgG levels may be high, the albumin/globulin ratio is reversed, and serum globulin is increased, especially the γ-globulin or α2 fraction. Albumin, red blood cells, and casts are the most frequent findings in the urine.

Immunologic Findings

1. *ANA test.* This is positive in 95% of cases of SLE. Human substrates, such as Hep-2 or KB tumor cell lines, are far more sensitive than mouse substrates, and the historical entity "ANA-negative lupus" is quite rare now. ANA pattern has some correlation with clinical subsets, such as a shrunken peripheral pattern in SLE with renal disease, a fine particulate pattern in subacute cutaneous LE, and a homogeneous pattern with antihistone antibodies.
2. *Double-stranded DNA. Anti-dsDNA, anti–native DNA.* This is specific, but not very sensitive. It indicates a high risk of renal

disease, and correlates with a shrunken peripheral ANA pattern and positive DIF in sun-protected skin.

3. *Anti-Sm antibody.* Sensitivity is less than 10%, but specificity is very high.

4. *Antinuclear ribonucleic acid protein (anti-nRNP).* Very high titers are present in mixed connective tissue disease (MCTD). Lower titers may be seen in SLE.

5. *Anti-La antibodies.* These are common in SCLE and Sjögren syndrome, and occasionally found in SLE.

6. *Anti-Ro antibodies.* These are found in about 25% of SLE and 40% of Sjögren patients. They are more common in patients with SCLE (70%), neonatal LE (95%), C2- and C4-deficient LE (50%–75%), late-onset LE (75%), and Asian patients with LE (50%–60%). Photosensitivity may be striking, and externalization of the antigen is seen after UV exposure.

7. *Serum complement.* Low levels indicate active disease, often with renal involvement.

8. *Lupus band test. Direct cutaneous immunofluorescence.* Continuous granular deposits of immunoglobulins and complement along the DEJ occur in more than 75% of well-established lesions of DLE. In SLE, it usually is positive in sun-exposed skin. A positive test in normal, protected skin correlates with the presence of anti-dsDNA antibodies and renal disease. The lupus band test is seldom performed, because the same population of patients can be detected with anti-dsDNA antibodies.

9. *Anti-ssDNA antibody.* This test is sensitive but not specific. Many patients are photosensitive. An IgM isotope seen in DLE may identify a subset of patients at risk for developing systemic symptoms.

10. *Antiphospholipid antibodies.* Both the anticardiolipin antibody and the LA are subtypes of APLAs. These are associated with a syndrome that includes venous thrombosis, arterial thrombosis, spontaneous abortions, and thrombocytopenia. Livedo reticularis is a frequent skin finding, and nonfading acral microlivedo, with small, pink cyanotic lesions on the hands and feet, is a subtle clue to the presence of APLAs. These antibodies may occur in association with lupus and other connective tissue disease, or as a solitary event. In the latter case, it is referred to as the primary antiphospholipid syndrome.

Differential Diagnosis

Diagnostically, SLE must be differentiated from DM, EM, polyarteritis nodosa, acute rheumatic fever, RA, pellagra, pemphigus erythematosus (Senear-Usher syndrome), drug eruptions, hyperglobulinemic purpura, Sjögren syndrome, and myasthenia gravis. The SLE patient may have fever, arthralgia, weakness, lassitude, diagnostic skin lesions, increased ESR, cytopenias, proteinuria, immunoglobulin deposition at DEJ, and positive ANA test. Biopsies of skin lesions and involved kidney may also be diagnostic.

Treatment

Some general measures are important for all patients with LE. Exposure to sunlight must be avoided, and broad spectrum, high sun protection factor (SPF) sunscreen should be used daily. Photosensitivity is frequently present even if the patient denies it, and all patients must be educated about sun avoidance and sunscreen use. Smokers should be encouraged and assisted in quitting. The patient should also avoid exposure to excessive cold, to heat, and to localized trauma. Biopsies and scar revision will often provoke a flare of the disease. Women with SLE have an increased risk of osteoporosis, independent of corticosteroid use. Bone density should be monitored and calcium and vitamin D supplementation considered, especially with strict photoprotection. Vitamin D repletion was shown to improve response to some medications. Some women will benefit from bisphosphonate

therapy, especially if corticosteroids are used. The most rapid bone loss with corticosteroid therapy occurs at the onset of treatment, so bisphosphonate therapy should not be delayed. Patients who will be treated with immunosuppressive agents should receive a tuberculin skin test, appropriate vaccinations, and thorough physical examination. Aggressive treatment is often necessary for discoid lesions and scarring alopecia. The slowly progressive nature of these lesions, and the lack of systemic involvement, may lead to inappropriate therapeutic complacency. The result is slow, progressive disfigurement.

Local Treatment. The application of potent or superpotent topical corticosteroids is beneficial in LE patients. Occlusion may be necessary and may be enhanced by customized vinyl appliances (especially for oral lesions) or surgical dressings. Tape containing corticosteroid (Cordran) is sometimes helpful. The single most effective local treatment is the injection of corticosteroids into the lesions. Triamcinolone acetonide, 2.5–10 mg/mL, is injected at intervals of 4–6 weeks. No more than 40 mg of triamcinolone should be used at one time. Steroid atrophy is a valid concern, but so are the atrophy and scar produced by the disease. The minimal intralesional dose needed to control the disease should be used; when the response is poor, however, it is generally better to err on the slightly more aggressive side of treatment than to undertreat. Topical calcineurin inhibitors may also be useful as second-line topical therapy. Topical retinoids have scattered reports of benefits, particularly for hypertrophic lesions. Cryosurgery has been used but may induce scarring, dyspigmentation, and flared. Although lupus is a photosensitive disorder, UVA-I therapy appears to be a useful adjuvant treatment modality in some patients; all light should be used with caution. Photodynamic therapy has been reported as effective. Lasers such as the PDL 585–595 nm laser have been used to treat individual lesions with improvement, but patients should be treated cautiously at low fluence if attempted.

Systemic Treatment. The safest class of systemic agent for LE is the antimalarials. Retinoids may be particularly helpful in treating hypertrophic LE. Systemic immunosuppressive agents are often required to manage recalcitrant cases or patients with systemic manifestations. Thalidomide can be effective, but its use is limited by the risk of teratogenicity and neuropathy. Methotrexate is often the next traditional systemic agent selected. Dapsone is the drug of choice for bullous systemic LE and may be effective in some cases of SCLE and DLE. Oral prednisone is generally reserved for acute flares of disease. Biologic agents and new targeted therapies are now used for refractory disease. One study of 73 antimalarial-refractory CLE patients showed that thalidomide was effective in 10 of 11, methotrexate in 10 of 19, dapsone in 8 of 18, belimumab in 6 of 16, MMF in 9 of 25, and azathioprine in 3 of 12.

Antimalarials. Hydroxychloroquine (Plaquenil), at a dose of 5 mg/kg/day or less, has an excellent safety profile and is generally used as first-line systemic therapy in most forms of cutaneous LE, with two thirds of patients responding. If no response occurs after 3 months, another agent should be considered. Chloroquine (Aralen) is effective at 250 mg/day for an average adult but is difficult to procure and has higher rates of ocular toxicity. Quinacrine (Atabrine), 100 mg/day, may be added to hydroxychloroquine because it adds no increased risk of retinal toxicity. Quinacrine is also difficult to procure and carries a higher risk of yellowish pigmentation than the other antimalarials. Systemic treatment can sometimes be reduced or stopped during the winter months. A Cochrane group review of randomized controlled trials (RCTs) concluded that hydroxychloroquine and acitretin appear to be of similar efficacy, although adverse effects are more severe and occur more often with acitretin.

Ocular toxicity is rare with doses of hydroxychloroquine of 5 mg/kg/day or less, and tends to occur in older patients, patients with liver or kidney disease, or after 5 years of therapy.

Ophthalmologic consultation should be obtained before, and approximately annually (depending on risk factors, this may not be necessary in the first few years of treatment). The finding of any visual field defect or pigmentary abnormality is an indication to stop antimalarial therapy.

Other reported side effects with antimalarials include hair loss, lichenoid eruptions, erythroderma, EM, purpura, urticaria, nervousness, tinnitus, abducens nerve paralysis, toxic psychoses, leukopenia, and thrombocytopenia. Antimalarials, except in very small doses, will exacerbate skin disease or cause hepatic necrosis in patients with porphyria cutanea tarda. They may also worsen or induce psoriasis. Quinacrine produces a yellow discoloration of the skin and conjunctivae. Antimalarials have also been known to produce blue-black pigmentation of the hard palate, nail beds, cartilage of the ears, alae nasi, and sclerae. Nausea, vomiting, anorexia, and diarrhea may develop. Aplastic anemia has rarely been noted in long-term therapy. A patient's brown or red hair may rarely turn light blond. Morbilliform eruptions are rare in patients with lupus, but occur in a quarter of patients with DM.

Corticosteroids. Systemic corticosteroids are highly effective for widespread or disfiguring lesions, but disease activity often rebounds quickly when the drug is discontinued. Because of long-term side effects, corticosteroid treatment should be limited to short courses to treat flares of disease or to obtain initial control while antimalarial therapy is being initiated. In patients with renal or neurologic involvement, corticosteroids should be administered in doses adequate to control the disease while treatment with a steroid-sparing regimen is initiated. Treatment with 1000 mg/day intravenous methylprednisolone for 3 days, followed by oral prednisone, 0.5–1 mg/kg/day, is effective in quickly reversing most clinical and serologic signs of activity of lupus nephritis. In general, the corticosteroid dose should be optimized to the lowest possible that controls symptoms and laboratory abnormalities.

Traditional Immunosuppressive Therapy. Aggressive treatment protocols with agents such as pulse cyclophosphamide (with hydration and mesna to prevent bladder toxicity) have greatly improved the outcome of renal LE. Other immunosuppressive agents (e.g., azathioprine, methotrexate, MMF), are often employed as steroid-sparing agents for refractory cutaneous disease. Methotrexate is often effective; patients with concomitant renal disease may be at higher risk of severe methotrexate toxicity, and all patients should receive folic acid concurrently. Some authorities have suggested that azathioprine is inferior to MMF in the treatment of cutaneous lesions.

Other Therapy. Isotretinoin therapy, 0.2–1 mg/kg/day, may be effective, especially in patients with hypertrophic or lichenoid lesions of LE. Rapid relapse may be noted when the drug is discontinued. Dapsone, clofazimine, acitretin, IFN alpha-2a, auranofin (oral gold), high-dose intravenous immune globulin (IVIG), and efalizumab have all been reported as effective in anecdotal use or limited trials. Thalidomide may be effective in antimalarial-refractory CLE, but is often limited by side effects including peripheral neuropathy. Lenalidomide may be more effective with lower rates of neurotoxicity and fewer side effects, and has increasingly been used to treat recalcitrant cases of CLE and SCLE, with response rates nearing 90%. Apremilast reduced disease activity in a pilot study of eight patients. Belimumab, a monoclonal antibody against B lymphocyte stimulator, was approved for SLE, but effects on cutaneous disease remain unclear. Anti-CD20 monoclonal antibody (rituximab) has been used successfully to treat life-threatening refractory SLE with renal and CNS involvement, as well as for hypocomplementemic urticarial vasculitis and refractory cutaneous lesions, though an RCT for SLE did not demonstrate success. Rituximab is also used for dapsone-resistant cases of BLE. Interleukin-6 (IL-6)–receptor inhibition with tocilizumab appears promising but may cause neutropenia. Sirukumab, another IL-6 antibody, was used in a study of 31 patients, with 91% experiencing adverse events and a nonsignificant decrease in disease activity.

Janus kinase (JAK) inhibitors are being explored for multiple interferonopathies and may have a role in treating lupus, and targeted anti-IFN antibodies are being evaluated as well. Ustekinumab has been reported as beneficial in a few cases of recalcitrant DLE.

Aggarwal N: Drug-induced subacute cutaneous lupus erythematosus associated with proton pump inhibitors. Drugs Real World Outcomes 2016; 3: 145.

Arkin LM, et al: The natural history of pediatric-onset discoid lupus erythematosus. J Am Acad Dermatol 2015; 72: 628.

Böckle BC, Sepp NT: Smoking is highly associated with discoid lupus erythematosus and lupus tumidus. Lupus 2015; 24: 669.

Chasset F, Arnaud L: Targeting interferons and their pathways in systemic lupus erythematosus. Autoimmun Rev 2018; 17: 44.

Costa-Reis P, et al: Monogenic lupus. Curr Opin Immunol 2017; 49: 87.

Deng Y, et al: Updates in lupus genetics. Curr Rheumatol Rep 2017; 19: 68.

Elman SA, et al: Development of classification criteria for discoid lupus. J Am Acad Dermatol 2017; 77: 261.

Ezra N, et al: Voriconazole-induced subacute cutaneous lupus erythematosus. Skinmed 2016; 14: 461.

Fennira F, et al: Lenalidomide for refractory chronic and subacute cutaneous lupus. J Am Acad Dermatol 2016; 74: 1248.

Fiehn C: Familial chilblain lupus. Curr Rheumatol Rep 2017; 19: 61.

Fruchter R, et al: Characteristics and alternative treatment outcomes of antimalarial-refractory cutaneous lupus erythematosus. JAMA Dermatol 2017; 153: 937.

Garza-Mayers AC, et al: Review of treatment for discoid lupus erythematosus. Dermatol Ther 2016; 29: 274.

Giacomel J, et al: Dermoscopy of hypertrophic lupus. J Am Acad Dermatol 2015; 72: s33.

Gulati G, Brunner HI: Environmental triggers in systemic lupus erythematosus. Semin Arthritis Rheum 2017 Oct 5; ePub ahead of print.

Jessop S, et al: Drugs for discoid lupus erythematosus. Cochrane Database Syst Rev 2017; 5: CD002954.

Khullar G, et al: Pigmented macular variant of chronic cutaneous lupus erythematosus. Clin Exp Dermatol 2017; 42: 793.

La Paglia GMC, et al: One year in review 2017: systemic lupus. Clin Exp Rheumatol 2017; 35: 551.

Liu RC, et al: Subacute cutaneous lupus erythematosus induced by nivolumab. Australas J Dermatol 2017 Jul 20; ePub ahead of print.

Maguiness SM, et al: Imiquimod-induced subacute cutaneous lupus erythematosus-like changes. Cutis 2015; 95: 349.

Mayor-Ibarguren A, et al: Subacute cutaneous lupus erythematosus induced by mitotane. JAMA Dermatol 2016; 152: 109.

Momen SE, et al: Tumour necrosis factor antagonist-induced lupus. Br J Dermatol 2017 Aug 3; ePub ahead of print.

Nieto-Rodriguez D, et al: Subacute cutaneous lupus erythematosus induced by masitinib. Int J Dermatol 2017; 56: 1180.

Nutan F, et al: Cutaneous lupus. J Investig Dermatol Symp Proc 2017; 18: s64.

Ramachandran SM, et al: Topical drug-induced subacute cutaneous lupus erythematosus isolated to the hands. Lupus Sci Med 2017; 4: e000207.

Ramezani M, et al: Diagnostic value of immunohistochemistry staining of Bcl-2, CD34, CD20 and CD3 for distinction between discoid lupus erythematosus and lichen planus. Indian J Pathol Microbiol 2017; 60: 172.

Rees F, et al: The worldwide incidence and prevalence of systemic lupus erythematosus. Rheumatology (Oxford) 2017; 56: 1945.

Romero-Mate A, et al: Successful treatment of recalcitrant discoid lupus erythematosus with ustekinumab. Dermatol Online J 2017; 23.

Shovman O, et al: Diverse patterns of anti-TNF-α-induced lupus. Clin Rheumatol 2017 Oct 23; ePub ahead of print.

Tiao J, et al: Using the American College of Rheumatology (ACR) and Systemic Lupus International Collaborating Clinics (SLICC) criteria to determine the diagnosis of systemic lupus erythematosus (SLE) in patients with subacute cutaneous lupus erythematosus (SCLE). J Am Acad Dermatol 2016; 74: 862.

Vincent JG, et al: Specificity of dermal mucin in the diagnosis of lupus erythematosus. J Cutan Pathol 2015; 42: 722.

Walsh NM, et al: Plasmacytoid dendritic cells in hypertrophic discoid lupus. J Cutan Pathol 2015; 42: 32.

Wieczorek IT, et al: Systemic symptoms in the progression of cutaneous to systemic lupus. JAMA Dermatol 2014; 150: 291.

Zuppa AA, et al: Neonatal lupus. Autoimmun Rev 2017; 16: 427.

DERMATOMYOSITIS

DM is typically characterized by inflammatory myositis and skin disease, although the hypomyopathic type (DM with subclinical) or amyopathic (with absent muscle disease) also occur. Muscle involvement without skin changes is called polymyositis (PM). With or without skin lesions, weakness of proximal muscle groups is characteristic.

Skin Findings

Usually the disease begins with erythema and edema of the face and eyelids. Eyelid involvement may be characterized by pruritic and scaly pink patches, edema, and pinkish violet (heliotrope) discoloration or bullae (Fig. 8.15). Edema and pinkish violet discoloration are often signs of inflammation in the underlying striated orbicularis oculi muscle, rather than the skin itself; the patient's eyelids may be tender to the touch.

Other skin changes include erythema, scaling, and swelling of the upper face, often with involvement of the eyebrows and scalp; scalp erythema alone may be the initial sign. Pruritus may be striking. Over time, some lesions may develop a reticulated pattern of white scarring. Extensor surfaces of the extremities are often pink, red, or violaceous with an atrophic appearance or overlying scale. The similarity to psoriasis can be striking, and patients may suffer severe flares of DM if they are inappropriately treated with phototherapy for presumed psoriasis. Photosensitivity to natural sunlight is common as well. Firm, slightly pitting edema may be seen over the shoulder girdle, arms, and neck (Fig. 8.16). Associated erythema and scale (with or without poikiloderma) over the shoulder regions is known as the "shawl sign." Similar changes on the hip are called the "holster sign." Pruritus may be severe, especially on the scalp, and is much more common in DM than in psoriasis or LE.

On the hands, telangiectatic vessels often become prominent in the proximal nailfolds. Enlarged capillaries of the nailfold appear as dilated, sausage-shaped loops with adjacent avascular regions, similar to those changes observed in scleroderma but without the associated sclerodactyly. There may be cuticular overgrowth with an irregular, frayed appearance (Fig. 8.17). A pink to reddish purple atrophic or scaling eruption often occurs over the knuckles, knees, and elbows (Gottron sign). Flat-topped, polygonal, violaceous papules over the knuckles (Gottron papules) are less common but highly characteristic of DM (Fig. 8.18). Hyperkeratosis, scaling, fissuring, and hyperpigmentation over the fingertips, sides of the thumb, and fingers, with occasional involvement of the palms, is referred to as "mechanic's hands" and has been reported in 70% of patients with antisynthetase antibodies (Fig. 8.19). Intermittent fever, malaise, anorexia, arthralgia, and marked weight loss are typically present at this stage.

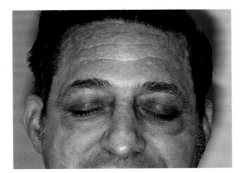

Fig. 8.15 Heliotrope rash in patient with dermatomyositis.

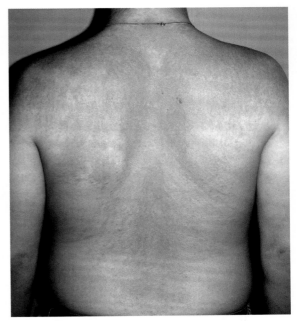

Fig. 8.16 Dermatomyositis, shawl sign. (Courtesy Steven Binnick, MD.)

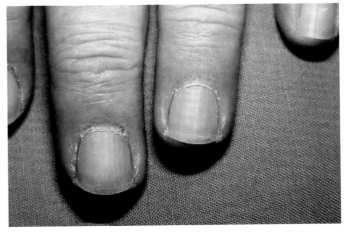

Fig. 8.17 Dermatomyositis, frayed cuticles (Samitz sign).

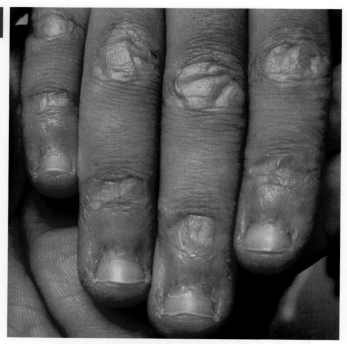

Fig. 8.18 Dermatomyositis, Gottron papules.

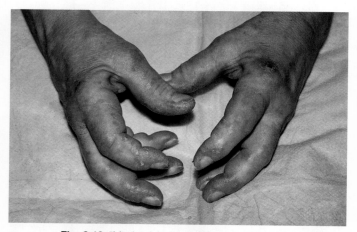

Fig. 8.19 "Mechanic's hands" in dermatomyositis.

Rarely, large, persistent ulcerations in flexural areas or over pressure points may develop. Ulceration in the early stages of DM has been reported to be associated with a higher incidence of cancer and a poor prognosis, but the authors have seen many patients with ulcerative DM without associated cancer. In later stages, ulceration may merely be a manifestation of pressure or trauma to atrophic areas. Rare manifestations of DM include clinical findings of pityriasis rubra pilaris (Wong variant of DM) or generalized subcutaneous edema. Rarely, bullous DM may develop, which portends a poor prognosis, with associated severe inflammatory myopathy or lung disease. In approximately 5% of patients, a flagellate pattern mimicking bleomycin-induced linear edematous streaks or erythroderma may be seen.

Although the classic cutaneous manifestations of DM can be seen with patients with anti-Mi2 antibodies, recently other specific patterns of cutaneous findings that may correlate with certain disease-specific antibodies have been described. Dave Fiorentino has championed many of these subphenotyping efforts. Hypopigmented and telangiectatic ("red on white") patches, palmar hyperkeratotic papules, and psoriasis-like lesions may be associated with autoantibodies to TIF-1γ. Ovoid palatal violaceous erythema has also been reported. These patients have lower rates of ILD and arthritis, but this autoantibody appears to be associated with higher rates of malignancy (see later discussion). Patients with anti-MDA5 antibodies usually have clinically amyopathic DM, but display high rates of cutaneous ulcerations, digital tip ulcerations, swollen and puffy fingers, "inverse Gottron" lesions with papules on the flexural creases of the digits, which may ulcerate, and have high rates of vasculopathy and severe, rapidly progressive, often fatal interstitial lung disease. Patients with this phenotype may also have an elevated serum ferritin.

Calcium deposits in the skin and muscles occur in more than half of children with DM and are found infrequently in adults, although recently anti-NXP2 antibodies have been shown to be more associated with calcinosis cutis; in adults it is also a marker of an increased rate of malignancy. Calcification is related to duration of disease activity and its severity. Calcinosis of the dermis, subcutaneous tissue, and muscle occurs mostly on the upper half of the body around the shoulder girdle, elbows, and hands. Ulcerations and cellulitis are frequently associated with this debilitating and disabling complication of DM.

Muscle Changes

In patients with severe DM, early and extensive muscular weakness occurs, with acute swelling and pain. The muscle weakness is seen symmetrically, most frequently involving the shoulder girdle and sometimes the pelvic region, as well as the hands. The patients may notice difficulty in lifting even the lightest objects. They may be unable to raise their arms to comb their hair, and rising from a chair may be impossible without "pushing off" with the arms. Patients often complain of pain in the legs when standing barefoot or of being unable to climb stairs. Difficulty in swallowing, talking, and breathing, caused by weakness of the involved muscles, may be noted early in the disease, and as with cutaneous phenotypes, may turn out to be more common with certain disease-specific antibodies, as over 75% of patients with anti-SAE antibodies develop dysphagia. Some patients with severe diaphragmatic disease require mechanical ventilation. Cardiac failure may be present in the terminal phase of the disease.

Skin involvement frequently precedes muscle involvement, but some patients have typical skin findings of DM but never develop clinically apparent muscle involvement. These cases have been termed *amyopathic DM* or *DM sine myositis*. However, muscle inflammation often is present but not symptomatic, identified only via laboratory or radiographic testing, and the term *hypomyopathic* is preferred. Muscle enzymes (creatine kinase [CK] and aldolase), electromyography (EMG), and magnetic resonance imaging (MRI) may be required to detect subtle involvement.

Diagnostic Criteria

The following criteria are used to define DM/PM:

- Skin lesions
- Heliotrope rash (red-purple edematous erythema on upper palpebra)
- Gottron papules or sign (red-purple flat-topped papules, atrophy, or erythema on extensor surfaces and finger joints)
- Proximal muscle weakness (upper or lower extremity and trunk)
- Elevated serum CK or aldolase level
- Muscle pain on grasping or spontaneous pain
- Myogenic changes on EMG (short-duration, polyphasic motor unit potentials with spontaneous fibrillation potentials)
- Positive anti–Jo-1 (histadyl tRNA synthetase) antibody
- Nondestructive arthritis or arthralgias

- Systemic inflammatory signs (fever >37°C at axilla, elevated serum CRP level or accelerated ESR of >20 mm/hr by Westergren method)
- Pathologic findings compatible with inflammatory myositis

Patients with the first criterion, skin lesions, and four of the remaining criteria have DM. Patients lacking the first criterion but with at least four of the remaining criteria have PM. Some patients with DM have little evidence of myopathy, and drug eruptions may mimic the characteristic rash. In particular, hydroxyurea has been associated with a DM-like eruption. Antisynthetase antibody syndrome presents with variable systemic manifestations, mainly PM, interstitial lung disease, cutaneous lesions, and Raynaud phenomenon. These criteria may evolve as our understanding of the specific phenotypes correlating to subsets of DM-specific antibodies expands.

Associated Diseases

DM may overlap with other connective tissue diseases. Sclerodermatous changes are the most frequently observed; this is called sclerodermatomyositis. Antibodies such as anti-Ku and anti-PM/scl may be present in this subgroup. Mixed connective tissue disease associated with high anti-ribonucleoprotein (RNP), RA, LE, and Sjögren syndrome may occur concomitantly. DM may be associated with interstitial lung disease (ILD), which is frequently the cause of death, particularly in patients with anti-MDA5 DM who present with rapidly progressive ILD. The presence of anti–Jo-1 antibody, as well as other antisynthetase antibodies, such as anti–PL-7, anti–PL-12, anti-DJ, and anti-EJ, correlates well with the development of pulmonary disease. All patients with DM should routinely be screened for ILD.

Neoplasia With Dermatomyositis

In adults, malignancy is frequently associated with DM, with an overall relative risk 4–5 times the general population. The malignancy is discovered before, simultaneously, or after the DM at near-equal rates. The highest probability of finding an associated tumor occurs within 2 years of the diagnosis. Factors associated with malignancy include age, constitutional symptoms, rapid onset of DM, lack of Raynaud phenomenon, and a grossly elevated ESR or CK level. Anti–TIF1-γ and anti-NXP2 antibodies in adults may a marker for an even higher rate of malignancy. Malignancy is most frequently seen in patients in the fifth and sixth decades of life. Routine "age-appropriate screening" may be inadequate to uncover a significant number of malignancies, as some cancers, such as ovarian cancer and nasopharyngeal cancer, are strongly overrepresented in DM patients, and not captured on routine surveillance. In addition to history and physical examination, a stool guaiac test for occult blood (Hemoccult) or colonoscopy, mammography, pelvic examination and pap smear, chest radiography, and computed tomography (CT) scans of the abdominal, pelvic, and thoracic areas may be indicated. Transvaginal ultrasound or abdominal MRI may be necessary to evaluate the endometrium and ovaries. Tumor markers such as CA19-9 and CEA-125 should be considered. Some clinicians advocate for positron emission tomography imaging, as it may take patients a long time to obtain all of the individual screening tests; cost-benefit analyses are ongoing. Periodic rescreening may be of value, but the appropriate interval for screening has not been established, with most experts suggesting intense screening initially, within the first 3 years, followed by symptom-based and age-appropriate surveillance.

Childhood Dermatomyositis (Fig. 8.20)

Several features of childhood DM differ from the adult form. Two childhood variants exist. The more common Brunsting type has

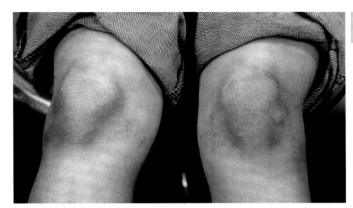

Fig. 8.20 Dermatomyositis, Gottron sign.

a slow course, progressive weakness, calcinosis, and steroid responsiveness. Calcinosis may involve intermuscular fascial planes or may be subcutaneous. The second type, the Banker type, is characterized by a vasculitis of the muscles and GI tract, rapid onset of severe weakness, steroid unresponsiveness, and high mortality rate. Internal malignancy is seldom seen in children with either type (even in children with the malignancy-associated antibodies), but insulin resistance may be present. Calcinosis cutis is more common in children with severe disease.

Etiology

Evidence indicates that muscle findings in DM are related to humoral immunity, a vasculopathy mediated by complement deposition, lysis of endomysial capillaries, and resulting muscle ischemia. In contrast, PM and inclusion-body myositis are related to clonally expanded CD8+ cytotoxic T cells invading muscle fibers and causing necrosis through the perforin pathway. The initial immune response in DM includes a type I IFN signature with an IFN-α/β–induced cascade with secondary stimulation of IFN-γ. Many autoantibodies may be present in DM, some of which are disease specific and can identify specific subgroups, indicating a possible role for B cells in the disease.

Both healthy individuals and children with juvenile DM may demonstrate persistence of maternal microchimerism, but the incidence is higher in children with juvenile DM. This has also been demonstrated in patients with other connective tissue diseases, such as scleroderma. The finding may be an epiphenomenon or may be part of a pathogenic alloimmune response. An inherited predisposition has been demonstrated, and studies of juvenile DM gene expression have shown DQA1*0501 in 85% of patients.

Viral or bacterial infections may produce an abnormal immune response, and human herpesvirus 6 reactivation has been reported. Fulminant disease may be related to an endotheliotropic viral infection. Epitopes of group A β-hemolytic streptococcal M protein have sequence homology with myosin and can elicit both cell-mediated cytotoxicity and TNF-α production when incubated with mononuclear cells from children with active juvenile DM. The TNF-α-308A allele is associated with increased TNF-α synthesis in juvenile DM patients and with increased thrombospondin 1 and small-vessel occlusion. Interestingly, as with LE, DM can be induced by anti-TNF biologic agents. In adults with PM and DM, endothelial damage occurs early. Pathogenic factors in adults include IL-1α, transforming growth factor–β (TGF-β), and myoblast production of IL-15. Cases associated with terbinafine may be related to apoptosis induced by the drug. DM is relatively rarely induced by medications, but atorvastatin has been reported, and the emerging reports of autoimmune diseases in the setting of checkpoint inhibitor therapy include cases of DM.

Incidence

The disease is twice as prevalent in women as in men and 4 times as common in black as in white patients. There is a bimodal peak, the smaller one seen in children and the larger peak in adults age 40–65.

Histopathology

The histologic changes in DM are similar to those of LE. The two may be indistinguishable, although lesions of DM tend to become atrophic more often. Lesions typically demonstrate thinning of the epidermis, hydropic degeneration of the basal layer, BMZ thickening, papillary dermal edema, and a perivascular and periadnexal lymphocytic infiltrate in the superficial and deep dermis with increased dermal mucin. Scattered melanophages are present in the superficial dermis. Compared with LE, DM shows less eccrine coil involvement and fewer vertical columns of lymphocytes in fibrous tract remnants. Subcutaneous lymphoid nodules and panniculitis are rarely seen in DM. Certain subtypes and different lesion morphologies demonstrate different histopathologic findings, such as the dusky or ulcerated lesions in anti-MDA5 DM patients, which histologically often show vascular plugging and dermal necrosis. Characteristic changes are found in the muscles. The deltoid, trapezius, and quadriceps muscles seem to be almost always involved and are good biopsy sites. Muscle bundles demonstrate lymphoid inflammation and atrophy, which preferentially affects the periphery of the muscle bundle. Muscle biopsy is directed to those areas found to be most tender or in which EMG demonstrates myopathy. MRI is a useful aid in identifying active sites for muscle biopsy and may obviate the need for biopsy in some cases. The short T1 inversion recovery (STIR) magnetic resonance images are best and can be used to localize disease and longitudinally assess results of treatment.

Laboratory Findings

The serum CK levels are elevated in most patients. Aldolase, lactic dehydrogenase (LDH), and transaminases (AST in particularly, but also ALT) are other indicators of active muscle disease. There may be leukocytosis, anemia with low serum iron, and an increased ESR. Ferritin may be elevated. Positive ANA tests are seen in 60%–80% of patients; with the expanded profile of DM-specific antibodies being discovered, more than two thirds of DM patients may have identifiable myositis-specific antibodies.

Cutaneous DIF is positive in at least one third of cases, with a higher yield in well-established lesion (at least 3–6 months old). Cytoid bodies are often seen, although continuous granular staining with IgG, IgM, and IgA may be seen.

X-ray studies with barium swallow may show weak pharyngeal muscles. MRI of the muscles is an excellent way to assess activity of disease noninvasively.

The EMG studies for diagnosis show spontaneous fibrillation, polyphasic potential with voluntary contraction, short duration potential with decreased amplitude, and salvos of muscle stimulation.

Chest imaging and pulmonary function testing should be performed to evaluate for signs of interstitial lung disease.

Differential Diagnosis

DM must be differentiated from erysipelas, SLE, angioedema, drug eruptions, trichinosis, and EM. Aldosteronism, with adenoma of adrenal glands and hypokalemia, may also cause puffy heliotrope eyelids and face. Hydroxyurea may produce an eruption resembling DM.

Treatment

Prednisone is the mainstay of acute treatment for DM patients, at doses beginning with 1 mg/kg/day, until severity decreases and muscle enzymes are almost normal. The dosage is reduced with clinical response. The aspartate transaminase (AST, SGOT)/alanine transaminase (ALA/SGOT) and CK return to normal levels as remission occurs. Methotrexate and MMF are used as steroid-sparing agents and should be started early in the course of treatment to reduce steroid side effects. Because of the increased risk of ILD with methotrexate, some avoid this agent in patients with pulmonary disease or anti–Jo-1 antibodies, and many clinicians use MMF as the steroid-sparing drug of choice. This may be particularly helpful in patients with interstitial lung disease, due to possible antifibrotic effects. Azathioprine is less expensive than MMF, but skin disease may not respond as well. If patients do not respond adequately to methotrexate, MMF, or azathioprine, are often used. Rituximab may help muscle disease, but is less effective for skin disease. In severe cases tacrolimus in particular, but also cyclosporine or cyclophosphamide may be beneficial. Anti–TNF-α treatment with infliximab has proved a rapidly effective therapy for some patients with myositis. Etanercept has also been used, but some studies have found little improvement or flares of muscle disease. Because anti-TNF therapy has been shown to induce DM, patients should be monitored carefully. Leflunomide, an immunomodulatory drug used to treat RA, has been effective as adjuvant therapy.

In severe juvenile DM, pulse IV methylprednisone or oral prednisone are effective for acute management, but some data suggest that corticosteroids may not be necessary in many children treated with methotrexate or IVIG. Rituximab appears promising in the treatment of refractory disease. Onset of calcinosis is associated with delays in diagnosis and treatment, as well as longer disease duration. Calcinosis related to DM has been treated with aluminum hydroxide, alendronate, diphosphonates, diltiazem, probenecid, colchicine, low doses of warfarin, sodium thiosulfate, and surgery with variable, but usually poor, results. Autologous stem cell transplantation has been reported as successful.

The skin lesions may respond to systemic therapy; however, response is unpredictable, and skin disease may persist despite involution of the myositis. Because DM is photosensitive, sunscreens with high SPF (>30) should be used daily, and patients should be counseled about sun avoidance. Topical corticosteroids may be helpful in some patients. Antimalarials such as hydroxychloroquine at 200–400 mg/day (2–5 mg/kg/day in children) have been shown to be useful in abating the eruption of DM, although adverse cutaneous reactions occur in one fourth of patients, and up to one half of those who react to hydroxychloroquine will also react to chloroquine. Beyond the traditional immunosuppressant agents discussed previously, IVIG (0.5–1g/kg/d for 2 days each month) may be beneficial, particularly for skin disease. IVIG has been associated with thromboembolic events, including deep venous thrombosis, pulmonary embolism, myocardial infarction, and cerebrovascular accident (stroke), and this risk must be weighed against the benefits of the drug; some utilize concomitant aspirin. IVIG has been successfully used even in recalcitrant cases of severe anti-MDA5 pattern disease with rapidly progressive-ILD and vasculopathy. Case reports and series suggest dapsone can help cutaneous DM. Biologic agents have been utilized with increasing frequency in small reports, including anakinra, TNF inhibitors, tocilizumab, and abatacept. Recently the JAK inhibitor ruxolitinib has been reported to be dramatically beneficial for refractory cases of DM. Cannabinoids appear to reduce DM-associated inflammatory cytokines and are being actively studied. Other agents under investigation include sifalimumab and belimumab.

In pregnant patients who require treatment, evidence supports the use of topical corticosteroids and topical calcineurin inhibitors. Published evidence also suggests that systemic corticosteroids, hydroxychloroquine, and azathioprine may be used in pregnancy when necessary.

Prognosis

Major causes of death in DM patients are cancer, ischemic heart disease, and lung disease. Independent risk factors include failure to induce clinical remission, white blood cell count above 10,000/mm³, temperature greater than 38°C (100.4°F) at diagnosis, older age, shorter disease history, and dysphagia. Early aggressive therapy in juvenile cases is associated with a lower incidence of disabling calcinosis cutis.

Bernet L, et al: Ovoid palatal patch in dermatomyositis. JAMA Dermatol 2016; 152: 1049.

Eichenfield DZ, et al: Zebra stripes in dermatomyositis. J Eur Acad Dermatol Venereol 2017; 31: e7.

Fang YF, et al: Malignancy in dermatomyositis and polymyositis. Clin Rheumatol 2016; 35: 1977.

Femia AN, et al: IVIG for refractory cutaneous dermatomyositis. J Am Acad Dermatol 2013; 69: 654.

Fiorentino DF, et al: Distinctive cutaneous and systemic features associated with anti-TIF-1γ antibodies in dermatomyositis. J Am Acad Dermatol 2015; 72: 449.

Fiorentino DF, et al: Most patients with cancer-associated dermatomyositis have antibodies to NXP-2 or TIF-1γ. Arthritis Rheum 2013; 65: 2954.

Fujimoto M, et al: Recent advances in dermatomyositis-specific autoantibodies. Curr Opin Rheumatol 2016; 28: 636.

Ge Y, et al: The efficacy of tacrolimus in patients with refractory dermatomyositis/polymyositis. Clin Rheumatol 2015; 34: 2097.

Hayashi M, et al: Mycophenolate mofetil for patients with interstitial lung diseases in amyopathic dermatomyositis with anti-MDA-5 antibodies. Clin Rheumatol 2017; 36: 239.

Hornung T, et al: Remission of recalcitrant dermatomyositis treated with ruxolitinib. N Engl J Med 2014; 371: 2537.

Ishibuchi H, et al: Successful treatment with dapsone for skin lesions of amyopathic dermatomyositis. J Dermatol 2015; 42: 1019.

Jordan M, Ghoreschi K: Anti-melanoma differentiation-associated protein 5 autoantibodies as a marker for dermatomyositis-associated interstitial lung disease. Br J Dermatol 2017; 176: 294.

Koguchi-Yoshioka H, et al: Intravenous immunoglobulin contributes to the control of antimelanoma differentiation-associated protein 5 antibody-associated dermatomyositis with palmar violaceous macules/papules. Br J Dermatol 2017; 177: 1442.

Komai E, et al: Atorvastatin-induced dermatomyositis. Acta Cardiol 2015; 70: 373.

Li L, et al: Assessment of anti-MDA5 antibody as a diagnostic biomarker in patients with dermatomyositis-associated interstitial lung disease or rapidly progressive interstitial lung disease. Oncotarget 2017; 8: 76129.

Merlo G, et al: Specific autoantibodies in dermatomyositis. Arch Dermatol Res 2017; 309: 87.

Moghadam-Kia S, et al: Antimelanoma differentiation-associated gene 5 antibody. J Rheumatol 2017; 44: 319.

Muro Y, et al: Cutaneous manifestations in dermatomyositis. Clin Rev Allergy Immunol 2016; 51: 293.

Olazagasti JM, et al: Cancer risk in dermatomyositis. Am J Clin Dermatol 2015; 16: 89.

Qiang JK, et al: Risk of malignancy in dermatomyositis and polymyositis. J Cutan Med Surg 2017; 21: 131.

Robinson ES, et al: Cannabinoid reduces inflammatory cytokines, TNF-α, and type I interferons in dermatomyositis in vitro. J Invest Dermatol 2017; 137: 2445.

Saini I, et al: Calcinosis in juvenile dermatomyositis. Rheumatol Int 2016; 36: 961.

Sheik Ali S, et al: Drug-associated dermatomyositis following ipilimumab therapy. JAMA Dermatol 2015; 151: 195.

Wright NA, et al: Cutaneous dermatomyositis in the era of biologicals. Semin Immunopathol 2016; 38: 113.

SCLERODERMA

Scleroderma disorders comprise a group of diseases characterized by thickening and sclerosis of the skin. This includes both localized, skin-only diseases, and systemic diseases. Localized scleroderma generally refers to morphea-spectrum disorders, including morphea (localized, generalized, profunda, atrophic, and pansclerotic types) or linear scleroderma (with or without melorheostosis or hemiatrophy). Systemic sclerosis includes limited systemic sclerosis (also known as CREST syndrome) and diffuse systemic sclerosis (at higher risk of significant internal organ disease). These disorders are characterized by the appearance of circumscribed or diffuse, hard, smooth, ivory-colored areas that are immobile and give the appearance of hidebound skin.

Cutaneous Types

Localized Morphea

The morphea form of scleroderma is twice as common in women as men and occurs in childhood as well as adult life. It presents most often as macules or plaques a few centimeters in diameter, but also may occur as bands or in guttate lesions or nodules. Rose or violaceous macules may appear first, followed by smooth, hard, somewhat depressed, yellowish white or ivory lesions. The lesions are most common on the trunk (Fig. 8.21) but also occur on the extremities.

The margins of the areas are generally surrounded by a lilac border or by telangiectases. Within the patch, skin elasticity is lost, and when it is picked up between the thumb and index finger,

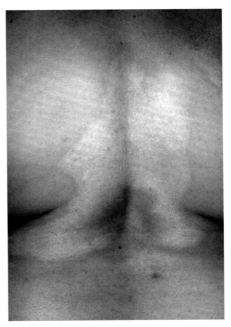

Fig. 8.21 Morphea.

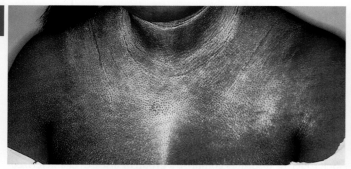

Fig. 8.22 Generalized morphea.

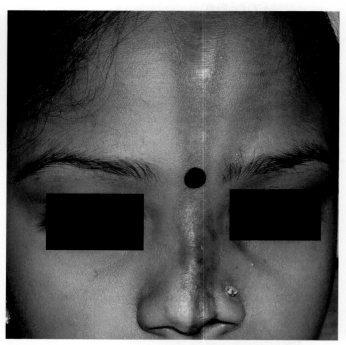

Fig. 8.23 Linear morphea. (Courtesy Debabrata Bandyopadhyay, MD.)

it feels rigid. The follicular orifices may be unusually prominent, leading to a condition that resembles pigskin.

In guttate morphea, multiple small, chalk-white, flat or slightly depressed macules occur over the chest, neck, shoulders, or upper back. The lesions are not very firm and may be difficult to separate clinically from guttate lichen sclerosus et atrophicus (LSA).

Morphea–Lichen Sclerosus Et Atrophicus Overlap

Some patients present with lesions of both morphea and LSA, typically women with widespread morphea who have LSA lesions separated from morphea or overlying morphea. When the changes are seen above dermal changes of morphea, the characteristic inflammatory lymphoid band of LSA is lacking, suggesting that the superficial homogenization is actually a manifestation of morphea rather than a separate disease process.

Generalized Morphea

Widespread involvement by indurated plaques with pigmentary change characterizes generalized morphea. Muscle atrophy may be present, but no visceral involvement (Fig. 8.22). These patients may have autoantibodies to topoisomerase, though antibody testing is not generally necessary, and diagnosis is made clinically. Patients may lose their wrinkles as a result of the firmness and contraction of skin. Spontaneous involution is less common with generalized morphea than with localized lesions. If very widespread, these patients can be mistaken as having systemic sclerosis; importantly, this type of morphea generally spares the hands and face and is not associated with Raynaud phenomenon.

Pansclerotic Morphea

Pansclerotic morphea manifests as sclerosis of the dermis, panniculus, fascia, muscle, and at times the bone. The patient has disabling limitation of joint motion. This devastating disorder can also be mistaken for systemic sclerosis, though again patients lack some of the internal involvement and vascular components of that disorder.

Morphea Profunda

Most types of morphea involve the dermis and little to none of the panniculus. Morphea profunda involves deep subcutaneous tissue, including fascia. There is clinical overlap with eosinophilic fasciitis, eosinophilia myalgia syndrome, and the Spanish toxic oil syndrome. The latter two conditions were related to contaminants found in batches of tryptophan or cooking oil. Unlike eosinophilic fasciitis, morphea profunda shows little response to corticosteroids and tends to run a more chronic debilitating course.

Linear Scleroderma/Linear Morphea

These linear lesions may extend the length of the arm or leg and may follow lines of Blaschko. Two thirds of cases are diagnosed in patients under 18, but adult cases do occur, and women are the majority of patients. Lesions may also occur parasagittally on the frontal scalp and extend partly down the forehead (en coup de sabre; Fig. 8.23). The Parry-Romberg syndrome, which manifests as progressive hemifacial atrophy, epilepsy, exophthalmos, and alopecia, may be a form of linear scleroderma. When the lower extremity is involved, there may be associated spina bifida, faulty limb development, hemiatrophy, or flexion contractures. Melorheostosis, seen on radiographs as a dense, linear cortical hyperostosis, may occur. At times, linear lesions of the trunk merge into more generalized involvement. Physical therapy of the involved limb is of paramount importance to prevent contractures and frozen joints. Patients may have additional associated autoimmune diseases.

Atrophoderma of Pasini and Pierini

In 1923 Pasini described a peculiar form of atrophoderma which some have considered within the spectrum of morphea. The disease consists of brownish gray, oval, round or irregular, smooth atrophic lesions depressed below the level of the skin, with a well-demarcated, sharply sloping "cliff-drop" border. Some of the appearance of depression is an optical illusion related to the color change. Atrophoderma occurs mainly on the trunk of young, predominantly female, patients (Fig. 8.24). The lesions are usually asymptomatic and may measure 20 cm or more in diameter. Linear atrophoderma of Moulin is a related condition that follows lines of Blaschko. Rarely congenital cases have been described.

Biopsies of atrophoderma demonstrate a reduction in the thickness of the dermal connective tissue, including alteration in elastic fibers (more so than collagen fiber changes characteristic of classic variants of morphea). Because the changes may be subtle, a biopsy should include normal-appearing skin so that a comparison may be made.

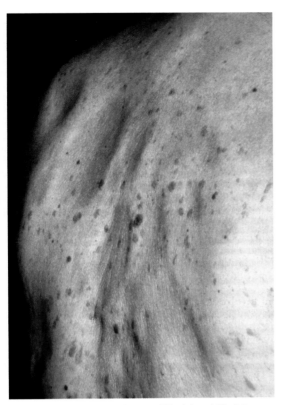

Fig. 8.24 Atrophoderma of Pasini and Pierini.

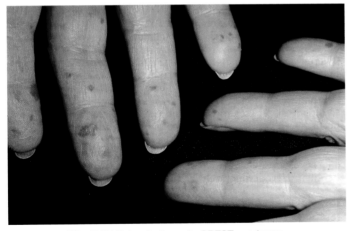

Fig. 8.25 Telangiectases in CREST syndrome.

Systemic Types

CREST Syndrome

This variant of systemic scleroderma has the most favorable prognosis because of the usually limited systemic involvement (limited systemic sclerosis [LcSSc]). Patients with CREST syndrome develop *c*alcinosis cutis, *R*aynaud phenomenon, *e*sophageal dysmotility, *s*clerodactyly, and *t*elangiectasia (Fig. 8.25). Patients may present with sclerodactyly, severe heartburn, or telangiectatic mats. The mats tend to have a smooth outline, in contrast to the mats of the Osler-Weber-Rendu syndrome, which tend to exhibit an irregular outline with more radiating vessels. This

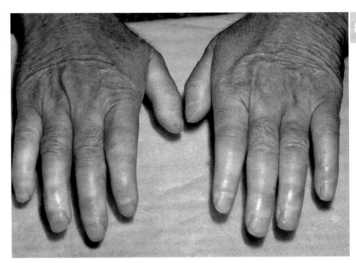

Fig. 8.26 Sclerodactyly.

form of scleroderma generally lacks serious renal or pulmonary involvement, though a subset may develop ILD or pulmonary hypertension. Patients typically have skin involvement limited to the hands, feet, face, and forearms. Anticentromere antibodies are highly specific for the CREST syndrome, being positive in 50%–90% of cases and only 2%–10% of patients with progressive sclerosis.

Progressive Systemic Sclerosis

Progressive systemic sclerosis (SSc) is a generalized disorder of connective tissue in which there is thickening of dermal collagen bundles, as well as fibrosis and vascular abnormalities in internal organs. RP is the first manifestation of SSc in more than half the cases. Other patients present with "woody edema" of the hands, which can precede the classic skin thickening. This form of scleroderma tends to involve the truncal skin as well. The heart, lungs, GI tract, kidney, and other organs are frequently involved. Women are affected 3 times more often than men, with peak age of onset between the third and fifth decades. Patients may have anti–Scl-70 antibodies (45%) and/or anti-RNA polymerase antibodies.

Classic criteria include either proximal sclerosis or two or all of the following:

1. Sclerodactyly (Fig. 8.26)
2. Digital pitting scars of the fingertips or loss of substance of the distal finger pad
3. Bilateral basilar pulmonary fibrosis

Localized forms of scleroderma must be excluded. These criteria have been shown to be 97% sensitive and 98% specific for the diagnosis. The ACR has proposed an expanded list of criteria for SSc, as follows:

1. *Skin changes:* tightness, thickening, and nonpitting induration, sclerodactyly, proximal scleroderma; changes proximal to the metacarpophalangeal or metatarsophalangeal joints and affecting other parts of the extremities, face, neck, or trunk (thorax or abdomen), digital pitting, loss of substance from the finger pad, bilateral firm but pitting finger or hand edema, abnormal skin pigmentation (often "pepper and salt"). The changes are usually bilateral and symmetric and almost always include sclerodactyly. The modified Rodnan skin score is typically used to measure skin involvement and estimate skin thickness using palpation.

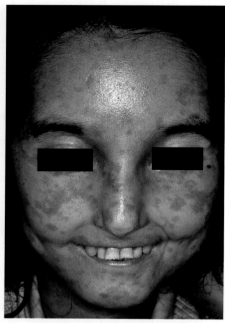

Fig. 8.27 Facial involvement in scleroderma.

2. *Raynaud phenomenon:* at least two-phase color change in fingers and often toes consisting of pallor, cyanosis, and reactive hyperemia.
3. *Visceral manifestations:* bibasilar pulmonary fibrosis not attributable to primary lung disease, lower (distal) esophageal dysphagia, lower (distal) esophageal dysmotility, colonic sacculations.

There exists a rare variant of scleroderma termed *systemic sclerosis sine scleroderma* in which patients only have internal organ involvement.

Skin Findings. In the earlier phases of scleroderma, affected areas are erythematous and swollen. Patients are frequently misdiagnosed as having carpal tunnel syndrome and may even have positive EMG results. RP is often present and suggests the correct diagnosis. Over time, sclerosis supervenes. The skin becomes smooth, yellowish, and firm and shrinks so that the underlying structures are bound down. The earliest changes often occur insidiously on the face and hands, and in more advanced stages these parts become "hidebound," so the face is expressionless, the mouth is constricted (Fig. 8.27), and the hands are clawlike. The facial skin appears drawn, stretched, and taut, with loss of lines of expression. The lips are thin, contracted, and radially furrowed; the nose appears sharp and pinched; and the chin may be puckered. The "neck sign" is described as a ridging and tightening of the neck on extension, occurring in 90% of patients with scleroderma.

The disease may remain localized to the hands and feet for long periods (acrosclerosis). The fingers become semiflexed, immobile, and useless, the overlying skin hard, inelastic, incompressible, and pallid. The terminal phalanges are boardlike and indurated. In the "round finger-pad sign," the fingers lose their normal peaked contour and appear as rounded hemispheres when viewed from the side. This process may lead to loss of pulp on the distal digit. Trophic ulcerations and gangrene may occur on the tips of the fingers and knuckles, which may be painful or insensitive. In pterygium inversum unguis, the distal part of the nail bed remains adherent to the ventral surface of the nail plate; it may be seen in scleroderma and LE or may be idiopathic. Dilated nailfold capillary loops are present in 75% of systemic sclerosis patients. Symmetrically dilated capillaries are seen adjacent to avascular areas. Nailfold capillary hemorrhage in two or more fingers is highly specific for scleroderma and correlates with the anticentromere antibody.

Keloid-like nodules may develop on the extremities or the chest, either as an extremely rare isolated skin phenomenon (nodular scleroderma), or within other areas of sclerosis. There may be a widespread diffuse calcification of the skin, as shown by radiographs. A diffuse involvement of the chest may lead to a cuirass-like restraint of respiration. Late in the course of the disorder, hyperpigmented or depigmented spots or a diffuse bronzing may be present. The most characteristic pigmentary change is a loss of pigment in a large patch with perifollicular pigment retention within it. Perifollicular pigmentation may appear in response to UV light exposure. Pigment may also be retained over superficial blood vessels. The affected areas become hairless, and atrophy is often associated with telangiectasia. Bullae and ulcerations may develop, especially on the distal parts of the extremities.

Rarely patients may have true overlap of morphea and systemic sclerosis. In one review of 370 patients with SSc, 12 (3.2%) of patients had coexistent morphea, generally in patients with limited cutaneous SSc.

Internal Involvement. Sclerosis may involve most of the internal organs. Esophageal involvement is seen in more than 90% of SSc patients; the distal two thirds of the esophagus is affected, leading to dysphagia and reflux esophagitis. Small intestinal atonia may lead to constipation, malabsorption, or diarrhea. Pulmonary fibrosis with arterial hypoxia, dyspnea, and productive cough may be present. Progressive nonspecific interstitial fibrosis, with bronchiectasis and cyst formation, is the most frequent pathologic change. Pulmonary hypertension and right-sided heart failure are ominous signs, occurring in 5%–10% of patients. The cardiac involvement produces dyspnea and other symptoms of congestive heart failure. Sclerosis of the myocardium also produces conduction changes and may result in arrhythmia. Pericarditis, hypertension, and retinopathy may be present.

The skeletal manifestations include articular pain, swelling, and inflammation. Polyarthritis may be the first symptom in SSc. There is limitation of motion as a result of skin tautness, followed by ankylosis and severe contractual deformities. The hand joints are involved most frequently. There may be resorption and shortening of the phalanges and narrowing of the joint spaces. Osteoporosis and sclerosis of the bones of the hands and feet may occur, as well as decalcification of the vault of the skull.

Childhood SSc has identical cutaneous manifestations. RP occurs less often, whereas cardiac wall involvement is more common and is responsible for half of deaths. Renal disease is unusual. Familial scleroderma rarely occurs.

Prognosis. The course of SSc is variable. Renal disease accounts for some early mortality, but pulmonary disease remains the major cause of death. The patient's age at disease onset is a significant risk factor for pulmonary arterial hypertension. Cardiac disease also correlates with a poor prognosis, whereas GI involvement contributes mainly to morbidity. ANA patterns predict different subsets of disease with varying prognosis. Anticentromere antibodies correlate with CREST syndrome and a good prognosis, whereas Scl-70 and ANA correlate with a poorer prognosis. Malignancy may be associated with SSc in up to 10% of patients, with lung and breast cancer the most frequent associated malignancies. The presence of many telangiectases is strongly associated with the presence of pulmonary vascular disease.

Laboratory Findings. In SSc, ANA testing is positive in more than 90% of patients. As noted, several of these antibodies identify specific clinical subsets of patients. The antinucleolar pattern is considered most specific for systemic sclerosis and when present as the only pattern, it is highly specific for systemic sclerosis.

When antibodies to such nucleolar antigens as RNA polymerase t and fibrillarin are present, diffuse sclerosis, generalized telangiectasia, and internal organ involvement are often seen. The homogeneous ANA pattern is seen in patients with PM-Scl antibodies, the marker for PM-SSc overlap. The true speckled or anticentromere pattern is sensitive and specific for the CREST variant. Patients with antibodies to Scl-70 tend to have diffuse truncal involvement, pulmonary fibrosis, and digital pitted scars, but a lower incidence of renal disease. Antibodies to nuclear RNP are found in patients with Raynaud phenomenon, polyarthralgia, arthritis, and swollen hands. Very high RNP titers define MCTD. These patients are fairly homogeneous and the term is not synonymous with connective tissue overlap. Anti-ssDNA antibodies are common in linear scleroderma. Anti-Rpp25 chemiluminescence and anti-Th/To by immunoprecipitation correlate with limited cutaneous and internal involvement. Anti-U11 RNP, Scl-70, Th/To, and TRIM/Ro52 have been related to ILD and poor survival. RNA pol III is associated with diffuse disease, but low risk of ILD. Cryoglobulins are only found in about 3% of patients with SSc, but the presence of cryoglobulinemic vasculitis is associated with a poor prognosis. Monoclonal gammopathy has rarely been reported in association with morphea, particularly morphea profunda.

Radiographic Findings. The GI tract is almost always involved. Esophagography, esophageal manometry, and a 24-hour pH study may be helpful. In early esophageal involvement, a barium swallow in the usual upright position may be reported as normal, but if the patient is supine, barium will often be pool in the flaccid esophagus. The stomach may atonic resulting in delayed emptying time, and involvement of the intestine may cause producing a characteristic radiographic picture of persistently dilated intestinal loops long after the barium has passed through. CT scan of the chest may reveal interstitial lung disease. Echocardiography may detect both direct cardiac involvement and pulmonary hypertension. Cardiac MRI may be preferred to identify heart fibrosis. Cutaneous calcinosis may be visualized on plain radiography, though that is rarely required.

Histology

Systemic and localized forms of scleroderma show similar histologic changes, although lymphoid infiltrates tend to be heavier in the acute phase of morphea. In the acute phase, there is a perivascular lymphocytic infiltrate with plasma cells that is heaviest at the junction of the dermis and subcutaneous fat. Collagen bundles become hyalinized, and the space between adjacent bundles is lost. Loss of CD34+ dermal dendritic cells is an early finding.

Dermal sclerosis typically results in a rectangular punch biopsy specimen. As the dermis replaces the subcutaneous tissue, eccrine glands appear to be in the midportion of the thickened dermis. The subcutaneous fat is quantitatively reduced, and adventitial fat (fat that normally surrounds adnexal structures on trunk) is lost. Collagen abuts directly on the adnexal structures. Elastic fibers in the reticular dermis may be prominent and stain bright red, and the papillary dermis may appear pale and edematous. In advanced lesions, the inflammatory infiltrate may be minimal. Pilosebaceous units are absent, and eccrine glands and ducts are compressed by surrounding collagen.

On DIF testing of skin, the nucleolus may be stained in the keratinocytes if antinucleolar circulating antibodies are present. A "pepper-dot" epidermal nuclear reaction pattern may be seen in CREST patients who have anticentromere antibodies in their serum.

Differential Diagnosis

Myxedema is softer and associated with other signs of hypothyroidism. Diabetic scleredema tends to be erythematous and affects the central back in a pebbly pattern. Scleromyxedema begins with discrete papules but may assume an appearance similar to SSc. A paraprotein is typically present. Sclerodactyly may be confused with digital changes of Hansen disease and syringomyelia. Eosinophilic fasciitis (EF) lacks RP and is more treatment responsive. The skin is thickened, edematous, and erythematous and has a coarse, peau d'orange appearance, unlike its sclerotic, taut appearance in scleroderma. The hands and face are usually spared in EF, and when the arms are involved, the blood vessels draw inward when the arms are raised, producing a "dry riverbed" appearance. EF of the forearms may cause finger contraction and can be mistaken for SSc.

In vitiligo, the depigmentation is the sole change in the skin, and sclerosis is absent. Scleroderma in the atrophic stage may closely resemble acrodermatitis chronica atrophicans (ACA), but ACA shows more attenuation of collagen fibers and a diffuse lymphohistiocytic infiltrate. Lyme titers may be positive.

Dermal fibrosis is a major feature of chronic, sclerodermoid graft-versus-host disease (GVHD), porphyria cutanea tarda, phenylketonuria, carcinoid syndrome, juvenile-onset diabetes, progeria, and the Werner, Huriez, and Crow-Fukase (POEMS) syndromes. Occupational exposure to silica, epoxy resins, polyvinyl chloride (PVC), and vibratory stimuli (jackhammer or chainsaw) may produce sclerodermoid conditions. Chemicals (e.g., PVC), bleomycin, isoniazid, pentazocine, valproate sodium, epoxy resin vapor, vitamin K (after injection), contaminated Spanish rapeseed oil (toxic oil syndrome), contaminated tryptophan (eosinophilia-myalgia syndrome), nitrofurantoin, and hydantoin may also induce various patterns of fibrosis. Gadolinium-containing contrast agents may rarely induce nephrogenic systemic fibrosis (NSF) in patients with kidney dysfunction, which can closely resemble SSc. The "stiff skin syndrome," also known as congenital fascial dystrophy, is characterized by stony-hard induration of the skin and deeper tissues of the buttocks, thighs, and legs, with joint limitation and limb contractures. The disease begins in infancy. Scleroderma-like symptoms may be the presenting features of multiple myeloma and amyloidosis. IgG4-related disease presents with soft tissue sclerosis, elevated serum IgG4, and increased IgG4-positive plasma cells in a variety of tissues.

Pathogenesis

The pathogenesis of systemic sclerosis and morphea involves vasculopathy, fibrosis, and inflammation, and may result from a combination of environmental exposures and genetic risk factors resulting in epigenetic changes, including DNA methylation and histone modification, leading to the observed phenotype. It has been suggested that the autoimmune mechanisms may be due to microchimerism resulting in alloimmune graft-versus-host reactions. Both anticardiolipin and anti–β2-glycoprotein I antibodies appear to play roles in pathogenesis. The plasma D-dimer concentration correlates with macrovascular complications. *Borrelia afzelii* and *Borrelia garinii* are related to the development of morphea-like lesions in some cases. Other environmental agents may be involved. Epidemiologic studies support the role of organic solvents and certain chemicals. In women, there is an association with teaching and working in the textile industry. Genetically *HLA DRB1, DQB1, DQA1, DPB1* genes, and variants in *STAT4, IRF5,* and *CD247* have been reported in association with SSc, with one study also suggesting GSDMA and PRDM1 gene loci as conferring risk. *HLA-DRB1* and B37 may be risk alleles for morphea. One case control study identified occupational exposure to heavy metals including antimony, cadmium, lead, mercury, molybdenum, palladium, and zinc as potential risk factors for SSc. Morphea has been reported following trauma, subcutaneous medication injections, and there are multiple radiation-induced cases.

The immune mechanisms involved are complex. Certain chemokines and cytokines that have been identified as potentially involved include NFKB, STAT4, IFN-γ, and interleukins. CXCL9 appears to be an important chemokine and has been proposed as a possible biomarker of disease activity in morphea. Upregulated proteins and messenger RNAs include monocyte chemoattractant protein 1 (MCP-1), pulmonary and activation-regulated chemokine, macrophage inflammatory protein 1 (MIP-1), IL-4, IL-6, IL-8, CRP, platelet-derived growth factor receptor–β (PDGFR-β), and possibly TGF-β. These factors may stimulate extracellular matrix production, TGF-β production and activation, and chemoattraction of T cells. Various target antigens have been proposed, including a protein termed *protein highly expressed in testis* (PHET), which is ectopically overexpressed in scleroderma dermal fibroblasts. Serum antibodies to a recombinant PHET fragment have been detected in 9 (8.4%) of 107 scleroderma patients, but in none of 50 SLE patients or 77 healthy controls.

The macrophage receptor protein CD163 is upregulated in scleroderma, and increased levels of soluble CD163 correlate with disease progression. Expression of CD40 is increased on fibroblasts in lesional skin, and ligation of CD40 by recombinant human CD154 results in increased production of IL-6, IL-8, and MCP-1 in a dose-dependent manner. These phenomena are not shown in normal fibroblasts with the addition of CD154. Lesion skin of early-stage scleroderma contains T cells preferentially producing high levels of IL-4. CD4+ T-helper 2 (Th2)–like cells can inhibit collagen production by normal fibroblasts and the inhibition is mediated by TNF-α. The inhibition is dominant over the enhancement induced by IL-4 and TGF-β. To be inhibitory, Th2 cells require activation by CD3 ligation. Th2 cells are less potent than T-helper 1 (Th1) cells in inhibiting collagen production by normal fibroblasts, and fibroblasts from involved skin are resistant to inhibition. Because Th2 cells reduce type I collagen synthesis through the effect of TNF-α, TNF-α blockade by new biologics should be approached with caution. Drug-induced morphea has been related to the cathepsin K inhibitor balicatib, used for osteoporosis. Capecitabine, an oral prodrug of 5-fluorouracil used in the treatment of metastatic colon and breast carcinoma, has been associated with a hand-foot syndrome with sclerodactyly. Onset of systemic sclerosis with digital ulcers has been reported during IFN-β therapy for multiple sclerosis.

Treatment

Although effective treatment is available for many of the visceral complications of SSc, treatment for the skin disease remains unsatisfactory. Spontaneous improvement may be seen in some children and in some cases of localized scleroderma. Physical therapy emphasizing range of motion for all joints as well as the mouth is important. Exposure to cold is to be avoided, and smoking is forbidden. Among patients with scleroderma, smokers are 3 to 4 times more likely than never-smokers to incur digital vascular complications. Although early treatment may be beneficial, end-stage fibrosis or inactive morphea may not respond to even high-dose suppression. The future lies with early aggressive intervention before the development of fibrosis and organ damage. Monitoring treatment response is important. The Rodnan score can be used to measure skin disease. Objective measures of improvement of skin sclerosis can be obtained by means of durometer measurements and high-resolution ultrasound. The course of microangiopathic changes can be evaluated with serial nailfold videocapillaroscopy.

RP is managed with vasodilating drugs—CCBs, angiotensin II receptor antagonists, topical nitrates, and prostanoids—as the mainstay of medical therapy. CCBs such as nifedipine (Procardia XL), 30–60 mg/day, are often used as first-line therapy. Some patients who experience worsening of esophageal reflux with nifedipine do better with diltiazem (Cardizem CD), 120–180 mg/day. Phosphodiesterase-5 (PDE-5) inhibitors can reduce the frequency and severity of RP attacks. Antioxidants such as vitamin C have been used, but data are mixed. Both sildenafil (Viagra) and IV or inhaled iloprost are useful in the treatment of both pulmonary hypertension and RP. Ginkgo biloba has been shown to have some efficacy in a double-blind trial. Oral L-arginine has reversed digital necrosis in some patients with RP and improved symptoms in others. Fluoxetine has been reported to improve RP in one small study. Botulinum toxin, topical nitroglycerin, and warming—both maintaining a warm core, and direct hand warming—on a regular basis may also be effective. Bosentan, an oral, dual endothelin receptor antagonist, has been effective in preventing and treating scleroderma-related ulcers, and oral treprostinil diethanolamine has been shown to improve skin perfusion in an open label trial. Digital ulcers may benefit from IV iloprost, bosentan, and/or PDE-5 inhibitors.

Systemic sclerosis should be managed in conjunction with an experienced rheumatologist and other organ-specific experts, and managed based on their disease subset, pattern of organ involvement, and comorbidities. Diffuse SSc should be treated with immunosuppression, generally methotrexate, mycophenolate mofetil, or cyclophosphamide as first-line treatment. Azathioprine or mycofenolate are often used after cyclophosphamide for maintenance. Systemic corticosteroids have been used, but evidence of benefit is limited and patients must be monitored closely for scleroderma renal crisis. TNF blockade has shown some benefit in reducing fibrosis, but has also triggered onset of disease. Rituximab has resulted in resolution of limited disease associated with anti-TNF therapy. Extracorporeal phototherapy has been used in the past. IVIG was helpful for internal involvement in one retrospective study in France. Abatacept has been reported as beneficial in a small randomized trial. Tyrosine kinase inhibitors are being actively studied due to their activity on pathways involved in fibrosis, including imatinib and nilotinib. Similarly, anti-IFN therapy, agents that target TGF-β1 signaling, and inhibitors of histone deacetylase are being actively explored. Although there is strong evidence that the ACE inhibitors are disease modifying for scleroderma renal crisis, better RCTs are still needed. Epo-prostenol is used to treat pulmonary hypertension in scleroderma, based largely on evidence that it can be lifesaving in the treatment of primary pulmonary hypertension. Other promising drugs for visceral involvement include bosentan (for pulmonary hypertension and ischemic ulcers), cyclophosphamide (for alveolitis), IFN-γ (for interstitial pulmonary fibrosis), IV prostaglandins (for vascular disease), and sildenafil (for pulmonary hypertension and Raynaud phenomenon). Bone marrow and nonmyeloablative allogeneic hematopoietic stem cell transplantation has shown dramatic and sustained benefits in some patients.

For localized scleroderma/morphea, management depends on the type of disease. If there is no inflammation, and simply bound down tissue, it is doubtful whether active antiinflammatory or suppressive therapy is helpful. If there is active inflammation, topical therapy with corticosteroids tacrolimus, or calcipotriene may be helpful for plaque disease. Topical imiquimod 5% was helpful in one small study. Deeper disease or recalcitrant plaque disease can be treated with phototherapy with NB-UVB and photochemotherapy, especially with UVA I. Generalized morphea or linear morphea may be treated with methotrexate, with or without corticosteroids, generally as first-line treatment. Myco-phenolate is second line after methotrexate. Severe or recalcitrant cases may be treated with agents similar to SSc. Cyclosporine has been shown to be effective in a retrospective study of 12 patients with morphea. Widespread morphea has been treated with hydroxychloroquine, TNF inhibitors, oral calcitriol, retinoic acid, penicillamine, colchicine, and oral tacrolimus as well. Halofuginone, an inhibitor of collagen type I synthesis, can decrease collagen synthesis in the tight-skin mouse and murine GVHD, and application of halofuginone caused a reduction in skin scores in a pilot study with scleroderma patients.

Calcinosis tends to be challenging to treat. Surgical removal, CCBs, bisphosphonates, colchicine, minocycline, and other agents have been employed with limited success. Carbon dioxide (CO_2) laser vaporization has produced remission of symptoms in cutaneous calcinosis of CREST syndrome. Emerging reports of sodium thiosulfate, both systemically and locally, show mixed results.

Bali G, et al: Cyclosporine reduces sclerosis in morphea. Dermatology 2016; 232: 503.

Barsotti S, et al: One year in review 2016: systemic sclerosis. Clin Exp Rheumatol 2016; 34: 3.

Careta MF, et al: Localized scleroderma. An Bras Dermatol 2015; 90: 62.

Charita P, et al: Genomic and genetic studies of systemic sclerosis. Hum Immunol 2017; 78: 153.

Chen JK, et al: Characterization of patient with clinical overlap of morphea and systemic sclerosis. J Am Acad Dermatol 2016; 74: 1272.

Desbois AC, et al: Systemic sclerosis. Autoimmun Rev 2016; 15: 417.

Dytoc M, et al: Topical imiquimod 5% for plaque-type morphea. J Cutan Med Surg 2015; 19: 132.

Endo J, et al: The association between morphea profunda and monoclonal gammopathy. Dermatol Online J 2016; 22.

Fruchter R, et al: Characteristics and treatment of postirradiation morphea. J Am Acad Dermatol 2017; 76: 19.

Jacobe H, et al: Major histocompatibility complex class I and class II alleles may confer susceptibility to or protection against morphea. Arthritis Rheumatol 2014; 66: 3170.

Kowal-Bielecka O, et al: Update of EULAR recommendations for the treatment of systemic sclerosis. Ann Rheum Dis 2017; 76: 1327.

Kumanovics G, et al: Assessment of skin involvement in systemic sclerosis. Rheumatology (Oxford) 2017; 56: v53.

Marie I, et al: systemic sclerosis and exposure to heavy metals. Autoimmun Rev 2017; 16: 223.

Mazori DR, et al: Characteristics and treatment of adult-onset linear morphea. J Am Acad Dermatol 2016; 74: 577.

O'Brien JC, et al: Transcriptional and cytokine profiles identify CXCL9 as a biomarker of disease activity in morphea. J Invest Dermatol 2017; 137: 1663.

Sanges S, et al: Intravenous immunoglobulins in systemic sclerosis. Autoimmun Rev 2017; 16: 377.

Spierings J, et al: Nodular scleroderma. Arthritis Rheumatol 2015; 67: 3157.

Terao C, et al: Transethnic meta-analysis identifies GSDMA and PRDM1 as susceptibility genes to systemic sclerosis. Ann Rheum Dis 2017; 76: 1150.

Thomas RM, et al: Retinoic acid for treatment of systemic sclerosis and morphea. Dermatol Ther 2017; 30.

Viera-Damiani G, et al: Idiopathic atrophoderma of Pasini and Pierini. J Am Acad Dermatol 2017; 77: 930.

Wolf R, et al: The role of skin trauma in the distribution of morphea. J Am Acad Dermatol 2015; 72: 560.

EOSINOPHILIC FASCIITIS

In 1974 Lawrence Shulman described a disorder that he called diffuse eosinophilic fasciitis. Classically, patients had engaged in strenuous muscular activity for a few days or weeks before the acute onset of weakness, fatigability, and pain and swelling of the extremities. The prodrome was followed by severe induration of the skin and subcutaneous tissues of the forearms and legs. A favorable response to corticosteroids was noted. Since the initial description, environmental exposures have been rarely reported as possible triggers for the syndrome, including L-tryptophan contaminated with 1,1′-ethylidenebis, *Borrelia*, and exposure to trichloroethylene. Some consider this disease to be a variant of

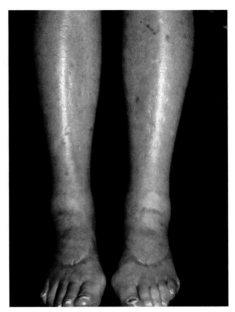

Fig. 8.28 Eosinophilic fasciitis.

scleroderma, though it lacks the vascular and internal manifestations. Polycythemia vera, metastatic colorectal carcinoma, and multiple myeloma have been associated in a limited number of patients, suggesting that some cases may represent a paraneoplastic phenomenon.

The skin is usually edematous and erythematous, with a coarse peau d'orange appearance, and a "pseudocellulite" appearance most noticeable inside the upper arms, thighs, or flanks. The hands and face are usually spared. When the patient holds the arms laterally or vertically, linear depressions occur within the thickened skin. This "groove sign" or "dry riverbed sign" follows the course of underlying vessels (Fig. 8.28). This contrasts with scleroderma, in which the skin remains smooth and taut. Limitation of flexion and extension of the limbs and contracture may develop in 50% of patients, and patients may be unable to stand fully erect. Physical therapy is important. In contrast to scleroderma, RP is absent. Tightening of the forearm may retract the fingers, and it is important to distinguish EF from SSc. Associated systemic abnormalities have included carpal tunnel syndrome, peripheral neuropathy, seizures, posterior ischemic optic neuropathy, pleuropericardial effusion, pancytopenia, anemia, antibody-mediated hemolytic anemia, thrombocytopenia, Sjögren syndrome, lymphadenopathy, pernicious anemia, and IgA nephropathy. Patients with EF are frequently misdiagnosed initially. Detected cytokine abnormalities are similar to those in atopic patients, but with a striking elevation of TGF-β1. Th17-mediated inflammation may be involved. ESR is generally increased, and hypergammaglobulinemia is common. Many patients (10%–40%) exhibit a peripheral eosinophilia. Increased production of IL-5 and clonal populations of circulating T cells have been reported.

Biopsy shows a patchy lymphohistiocytic and plasma cell infiltrate in the fascia and subfascial muscle, with massive thickening of the fascia and deep subcutaneous septa. Eosinophils may or may not be present in the affected fascia. The inflammatory infiltrate is mainly composed of macrophages and lymphocytes, often with a CD8+ T lymphocyte predominance. CT and MRI have both been used to demonstrate fascial thickening and may obviate the need for biopsy in some cases.

Early treatment is ideal, but sometimes delayed due to failure to recognize EF. Patients are often treated with initially high-dose steroids, and then weekly methotrexate, and may do better with combination therapy than corticosteroids alone. The response to systemic corticosteroids is generally excellent. In responders, complete recovery is usual within 1–3 years. Some patients have also demonstrated a response to histamine blockers, including hydroxyzine and cimetidine. Patients with a prolonged course unresponsive to systemic corticosteroids are sometimes diagnosed as overlap cases with morphea profunda. In refractory cases, hydroxychloroquine, cyclosporine azathioprine, psoralen plus UVA (PUVA), bath PUVA, extracorporeal photochemotherapy, IVIG, rituximab, mycophenolate, sirolimus, and other immunosuppressive regimens have been used with variable success. Recently high-dose IV pulse methotrexate was reported as helpful. Both infliximab and IV cyclophosphamide used with moderate- to high-dose prednisolone have been reported as effective in refractory cases.

Mertens JS, et al: High-dose IV pulse methotrexate in patients with eosinophilic fasciitis. JAMA Dermatol 2016; 152: 1262.
Mertens JS, et al: Long-term outcome of eosinophilic fasciitis. J Am Acad Dermatol 2017; 77: 512.
Oza VS, et al: Treatment of eosinophilic fasciitis with sirolimus. JAMA Dermatol 2016; 152: 488.
Wright NA, et al: Epidemiology and treatment of eosinophilic fasciitis. JAMA Dermatol 2016; 152: 97.

MIXED CONNECTIVE TISSUE DISEASE

Patients with a constellation of overlapping clinical and serologic features of other connective tissue diseases, including SSc, myositis, rheumatoid arthritis, and lupus, may be diagnosed with MCTD. It is unclear whether MCTD is a final diagnosis or whether it represents an overlap syndrome and that overtime patients with MCTD may end up better characterized as a specific autoimmune disease, often SSc or SLE. MCTD is defined by the presence of Raynaud phenomenon, arthralgias, swollen joints, esophageal dysfunction, muscle weakness, and sausage-like appearance of the fingers (Fig. 8.29), together with the presence of high titer anti-RNP antibodies in the absence of anti-Sm antibodies. The term is not synonymous with "overlap syndrome," a combination of diseases in which each disease complies with the diagnostic criteria for that disorder. MCTD is not synonymous with undifferentiated connective tissue disease (UCTD)—patients with connective tissue disease who have not yet developed a defined disease. Only about 4% of patients with UCTD go on to develop MCTD.

The ANA test typically demonstrates a particulate pattern in MCTD, reflecting the high titers of nuclear RNP antibodies (anti-RNP antibodies). In addition, particulate epidermal nuclear

IgG deposition on DIF study of skin is a distinctive finding in MCTD. Anti–TS1-RNA antibodies appear to define a subpopulation with predominance of lupus-like clinical features. Patients with a younger age of onset and those with pulmonary hypertension, Raynaud phenomenon, and livedo reticularis have a higher risk of mortality. Causes of death include pulmonary fibrosis and pulmonary arterial hypertension, cardiovascular events, renal disease, CNS disease, thrombotic thrombocytopenic purpura, and infection.

For acute treatment, corticosteroids such as prednisone (1 mg/kg/day) are effective for inflammatory features such as arthritis and myositis. As with LE, MCTD may be associated with an independent risk of osteoporosis, and the long-term morbidity associated with corticosteroid treatment can be significant. Bisphosphonate therapy and therapy with a steroid-sparing agent should be considered early. In general, the LE features of MCTD are the most likely to improve with therapy, and the scleroderma features are the least likely to improve. Generally, the prognosis is better than that of scleroderma, largely related to the lower incidence of renal disease. Life-threatening complications refractory to other treatment often respond to rituximab. In the setting of thrombocytopenia, the response rate is 80%.

Gunnarsson R, et al: Mixed connective tissue disease. Best Pract Res Clin Rheumatol 2016; 30: 95.
Pepmueller PH: Undifferentiated connective tissue disease, mixed connective tissue disease, and overlap syndromes in rheumatology. Mo Med 2016; 113: 136.
Ungprasert P, et al: Epidemiology of mixed connective tissue disease, 1985-2014. Arthritis Care Res 2016; 68: 1843.

NEPHROGENIC SYSTEMIC FIBROSIS

NSF is a fibrosing skin condition that resembles scleromyxedema histologically. It usually develops in patients with renal insufficiency on hemodialysis, although it has been noted in patients with acute renal failure who had never undergone dialysis. Gadolinium-containing MRI contrast agents are considered the trigger, and incidence of NSF has decreased since their use has been limited in patients with renal failure. Cases typically develop weeks to months after gadolinium, but may develop many years (3–10) after exposure. Concurrent infection, increased serum phosphate and calcium concentrations, iron, and acidosis may play important roles in pathogenesis. Clinical findings of NSF include thickened sclerotic or edematous papules and plaques involving the extremities and trunk. Yellow scleral plaques and scleral telangiectasia resembling conjunctivitis have been described. Gadolinium within cutaneous sclerotic bodies, termed *gadolinium-associated plaques*, has been reported. Soft tissue calcification is rare but may be extensive when it occurs. Clinically, NSF differs from scleromyxedema by the lack of involvement of the face, absence of plasma cells, and lack of paraproteinemia. Deep tissue or systemic involvement is generally absent but may occur.

Histologic sections demonstrate plump bipolar CD34+ spindle cells with dendrites extending along both sides of elastic fibers (tram track sign), many new collagen bundles, and increased mucin. With time, thickened collagen bundles become prominent in the reticular dermis. Ossification with trapped elastic fibers appears to be fairly specific for gadolinium exposure. Myofibroblasts have been noted in lesional skin. Immunohistochemical staining for CD34 and procollagen I in the spindle cells of NFD suggests that many of the dermal cells of NFD may represent circulating fibrocytes recruited to the dermis. The CD34 positivity in NFD contrasts with the loss of CD34+ cells in morphea.

Effective therapy remains elusive. Improved renal function appears to improve NSF, including renal transplantation, which may be significantly helpful. Topical retinoids, steroids, and vitamin D analogs are not effective. Immunosuppressive therapy appears

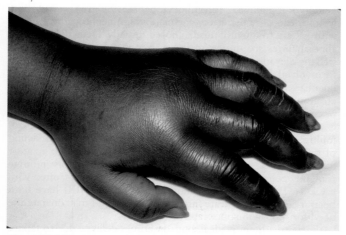

Fig. 8.29 Mixed connective tissue disease. (Courtesy Steven Binnick, MD.)

to be of little benefit. In three cases evolving after liver transplantation, treatment with basiliximab, MMF, calcineurin inhibitor, and prednisone did not stop the development of "woody" skin induration of the distal extremities, erythematous papules, and contractures. Some data support a beneficial effect from phototherapy, extracorporeal photopheresis, or IV sodium thiosulfate, tyrosine kinase inhibitors, and rapamycin. All patients should be referred for physical therapy.

Bandino JP, et al: Gadolinium presence within cutaneous sclerotic bodies confirmed by laser ablation inductively coupled plasma mass spectrometry. JAMA Dermatol 2017 Nov 8; ePub ahead of print.

Gathings RM, et al: Gadolinium-associated plaques. JAMA Dermatol 2015; 151: 316.

Larson KN, et al: Nephrogenic systemic fibrosis manifesting a decade after exposure to gadolinium. JAMA Dermatol 2015; 151: 1117.

Thomsen HS: Nephrogenic systemic fibrosis. Acta Radiol 2016; 57: 643.

Wilson J, et al: Nephrogenic systemic fibrosis. J Am Acad Dermatol 2017; 77: 235.

SJÖGREN SYNDROME (SICCA SYNDROME)

Sjögren syndrome is a chronic autoimmune disorder characterized by lymphocytic infiltration of the exocrine glands, particularly the salivary and lacrimal glands. One third of patients present with extraglandular manifestations, such as vasculitis. Most patients are age 50 or older, and more than 90% are women. Genes associated with Sjögren syndrome generally fall in the NF-kB, IFN signaling, lymphocyte signaling, and antigen presentation pathways. *IRF5*, a gene in IFN signaling and B-cell differentiation, may confer risk. Secondary Sjögren syndrome is defined as xerostomia and keratoconjunctivitis sicca in patients with other connective tissue diseases. The presence of arthritis, leukopenia, proteinuria, or low complement levels suggests secondary Sjögren syndrome. These patients have lower incidences of xerostomia and ILD compared with patients who have primary Sjögren syndrome.

Xerostomia may produce difficulty in speech and eating, increased tooth decay, thrush, and decreased taste (hypogeusia). Patients frequently suck on sour candies to stimulate what little salivary secretions remain, and those unfamiliar with the condition may blame the habit of sucking lemon drops for the ensuing tooth decay. Sjögren syndrome alters the composition of saliva, producing a decrease in salivary amylase and carbonic anhydrase, along with an increase in lactoferrin, β2-microglobulin, cystatin C, sodium, and lysozyme C.

Rhinitis sicca (dryness of nasal mucous membranes) may induce nasal crusting and decreased olfactory acuity (hyposmia). Vaginal dryness and dyspareunia may develop. Dry eyes are painful, feel gritty or scratchy, and produce discharge and blurry vision. Fatigue is a prominent symptom. In addition, there may be laryngitis, gastric achlorhydria, thyroid enlargement resembling Hashimoto thyroiditis, malignant lymphoma, thrombotic thrombocytopenic purpura, painful distal sensory axonal neuropathy, and splenomegaly.

Skin manifestations of Sjögren syndrome include vasculitis, xerosis, pruritus, and annular erythema. Decreased sweating occurs. Asian patients have been described who develop erythematous, indurated, annular dermal plaques, primarily on the face. This is different from the annular lesions of SCLE, which show epidermal change and histologic changes of lupus. Patients may also present with an overlap of Sjögren syndrome and LE. A common finding in these patients is Ro/SSA antibody positivity. These patients are also at risk of neonatal lupus. SCLE patients with Sjögren syndrome have a worse prognosis than patients with SCLE not associated with Sjögren syndrome. Patients may have low levels of vitamin

D, and some data suggest that it may play a role in disease pathogenesis.

Patients with Sjögren syndrome and cutaneous vasculitis also have a significant incidence of peripheral, renal, or CNS vasculitis. Cutaneous vasculitis may present as purpura of the legs, which may be palpable or nonpalpable. Sjögren vasculitis accounts for most patients with Waldenström benign hypergammaglobulinemic purpura; about 30% of these patients will have or will develop Sjögren syndrome, and a high percentage have SSA and SSB antibodies. Other cutaneous vascular manifestations are urticarial vasculitis, digital ulcers, and petechiae. Histologically, a leukocytoclastic vasculitis is found at the level of the postcapillary venule, with expansion of the vascular wall, fibrin deposition, and karyorrhexis, but no necrosis of the endothelium.

Labial salivary gland biopsy from inside the lower lip is usually regarded as the most definitive test for Sjögren syndrome. Typically, there is a dense lymphocytic infiltrate with many plasma cells and fewer histiocytes in aggregates within minor salivary glands. More than one focus of 50 or more lymphocytes is typically present per 4 mm^2 of the tissue biopsy. Lymphoepithelial islands predominate early, whereas glandular atrophy predominates in the late stages. At this stage, few lymphoid aggregates are present. Xerostomia is diagnosed by the Schirmer test and reflects diminished glandular secretion from the lacrimal glands. Imaging studies are also helpful.

Classically, the diagnosis is made when there is objective evidence for two of three major criteria: (1) xerophthalmia, (2) xerostomia, and (3) an associated autoimmune, rheumatic, or lymphoproliferative disorder. These criteria may be too restrictive, however, because patients are increasingly being identified with predominantly extraglandular disease. The lack of sicca symptoms or anti-SSA or anti-SSB antibodies does not exclude Sjögren syndrome. Numerous serologic abnormalities are associated with Sjögren syndrome or its associated conditions. Antibodies to fodrin, a major component of the membrane cytoskeleton of most eukaryotic cells, are present in some populations with primary and secondary Sjögren syndrome. IgA and IgG antibodies against α-fodrin are detected in 88% and 64%, respectively, in some studies. In other populations, fodrin antibodies are less helpful. About 80% of patients have anti-Ro/SSA antibodies; half as many have anti-La/SSB antibodies. The RF is usually positive, and elevated ESR, serum globulin, and CRP and high titers of IgG, IgA, and IgM are common. Cryoglobulins may be demonstrated. Dendritic cells are increased in tissue during the early phases of the disease.

The aquaporin family of water channels (proteins freely permeated by water but not protons) appears to be an important target in the pathogenesis of Sjögren syndrome. Both duct and secretory cells are targets for the activation of CD4+ T cells. IL-12 and IFN-γ are upregulated. It appears that Th1 cytokines mediate the functional interactions between antigen-presenting cells (APCs) and CD4+ T cells in early lesions.

Patients with Sjögren syndrome are predisposed to the development of lymphoreticular malignancies, especially non-Hodgkin B-cell lymphoma. Both malignant and nonmalignant extraglandular lymphoproliferative processes occur. Cases of pseudolymphoma have the potential for regression or for progression to overt B-cell lymphoma. Patients with palpable purpura, low C4, and mixed monoclonal cryoglobulinemia are at higher risk for lymphoma.

The differential diagnosis of Sjögren syndrome includes sarcoidosis, lymphoma, amyloidosis, and human immunodeficiency virus (HIV) disease. HIV produces diffuse infiltrative lymphocytosis syndrome (DILS), which is characterized by massive parotid enlargement; prominent renal, lung, and GI manifestations; and a low frequency of autoantibodies.

Treatment for Sjögren syndrome has largely been symptomatic, but disease-modifying therapy is also becoming a reality. Artificial lubricants are helpful for eye symptoms as well as oral, nasal, and vaginal dryness. Topical lubricants are useful for xerosis. In hot climates, patients with impaired sweating must be counseled to avoid heatstroke. Secretagogs such as pilocarpine and cevimeline, along with topical fluoride, are used for dry mouth. In all trials, mechanical stimulation by the lozenge may play a significant role in improvement of symptoms, as reflected in a high placebo response. Acid maltose lozenges are less expensive and remain useful for symptomatic relief. Secretagogs may also have a role in the treatment of dry eyes. Topical cyclosporine is often employed as well. Pilocarpine has been shown to have a beneficial effect on subjective eye symptoms, as well as improvement of rose bengal staining. For patients with systemic disease, there is a lack of high-quality evidence to guide therapy. Hydroxychloroquine is often used, and depending on severity and type of symptoms, immunosuppressive agents are frequently used. Severe disease may require high-dose steroids, and cryoglobulinemia may require plasma exchange or rituximab. TNF inhibitors show some promise.

Garcia-Carrasco M, et al: Vitamin D and Sjögren syndrome. Autoimmune Rev 2017; 16: 587.

Gupta S, Gupta N: Sjögren syndrome and pregnancy. Perm J 2017; 21.

Reksten TR, et al: Genetics in Sjögren syndrome. Rheum Dis Clin North Am 2016; 42: 435.

Saraux A, et al: Treatment of primary Sjögren syndrome. Nat Rev Rheumatol 2016; 12: 456.

Reactive Palisading Granulomatous Dermatitis

Rheumatoid arthritis (RA) is a fairly common inflammatory arthritis that can occur at any age, and occurs in women 2–3 times more than in men. HLA-DRB1 contributes to disease risk, and more specific alleles have been identified in different populations and with varying clinical significance. Polymorphisms in STAT-4 and IL-10 genes confer risk. Beyond genetic factors, environmental exposures and epigenetics appears to play a role, particularly cigarette smoke. The most common skin finding is the development of rheumatoid nodules (RNs), which occur in 20% of patients, particularly those with high titers of RF. There may be annular erythemas, purpura, bullae, shallow ulcers, and gangrene of the extremities. Many diseases have been reported to occur in association with RA, such as erythema elevatum diutinum, pyoderma gangrenosum, Felty syndrome, IgA vasculitis, linear IgA disease, Sjögren syndrome, bullous pemphigoid, and yellow nail syndrome. Treatment of RA with disease-modifying drugs has reduced the burden of destructive disease for patients, and treatment paradigms are rapidly evolving.

Methotrexate remains a mainstay of treatment, with corticosteroids serving as temporary bridging agents primarily. Other disease-modifying antirheumatic drugs (DMARDs) include sulfasalazine and hydroxychloroquine. Biologic agents are being used with increasing frequency, including TNF inhibitors, IL-6 antagonists, abatacept, and rituximab, along with the JAK inhibitors. Methotrexate-treated RA patients have an increased incidence of melanoma. Of interest to dermatologists, extracts from the *Rhus* family of plants have shown some benefit in limited studies.

Rheumatoid Nodules

Subcutaneous nodules are seen in 20%–30% of patients (Fig. 8.30). They may arise anywhere on the body but most frequently are found over the bony prominences, especially on the extensor surface of the forearm just below the elbow and the dorsal hands. The lesions are nontender, firm, skin-colored, round nodules, which may or may not be attached to the underlying tissue. Frequently, they are attached to the fibrous portions of the periarticular capsule, or they may be free in the subcutaneous tissue. RNs can easily be mistaken for xanthomas because of a yellow color (pseudoxanthomatous variant). They are seen most commonly when there is a high RF. RNs may also occur in 5%–7%

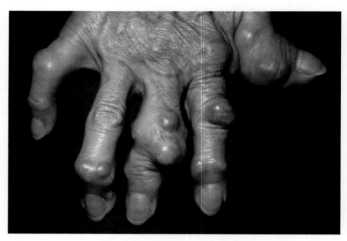

Fig. 8.30 Rheumatoid nodules.

of patients with SLE, especially around small joints of the hands, with variable RF positivity. Accelerated RN may occur with the appearance of multiple RNs, typically following initiation of a treatment for RA, most commonly methotrexate (but may also occur in the setting of TNF or hydroxychloroquine therapy). Histologic examination of the RN shows intensely staining eosinophilic necrobiosis surrounded by histiocytes in palisade arrangement. There is scant to absent mucin staining, distinguishing from subcutaneous granuloma annulare.

RNs are differentiated from Heberden nodes, which are tender, hard, bony exostoses on the dorsolateral aspects of the distal interphalangeal joints of patients with degenerative joint disease. Nodules or tophi of gout are characterized by masses of feathery urate crystals surrounded by a chronic inflammatory infiltrate often containing foreign body giant cells.

Rarely, RA patients present with multiple ulcerated nodules and high RF, but no active joint disease. This variant of rheumatoid disease without destructive joint disease is designated "rheumatoid nodulosis." These patients may instead have subcutaneous granuloma annulare (GA) rather than RA.

Rheumatoid Vasculitis

This is a rare complication with declining incidence, typically seen in late-stage, severe RA. Peripheral vascular lesions appear as localized purpura, nailfold infarcts, cutaneous ulceration, and digital ischemia and gangrene of the distal parts of the extremities. Additionally, papular lesions located primarily on the hands have been described as rheumatoid papules. These show a combination of vasculitis and palisading granuloma formation. An RF is typically present. Peripheral neuropathy is frequently associated with the vasculitis. The presence of RNs may help to distinguish these lesions of vasculitis from SLE, polyarteritis nodosa, eosinophilic granulomatosis with polyangiitis (Churg-Strauss), Buerger disease (thromboangiitis obliterans), and the dysproteinemias. Prednisone and cytotoxic agents are frequently used, as in other forms of vasculitis. Hydroxychloroquine and aspirin may be protective. Rituximab has also been used successfully.

Rheumatoid Neutrophilic Dermatosis

Chronic urticaria–like plaques characterized histologically by a dense neutrophilic infiltrate have been described in patients with debilitating RA (Fig. 8.31). The differential diagnosis includes erythema elevatum diutinum and Sweet syndrome. Patients have been treated with steroids, dapsone, or other RA-targeting therapies.

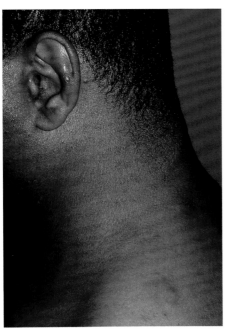

Fig. 8.31 Rheumatoid neutrophilic dermatosis presents with urticarial plaques.

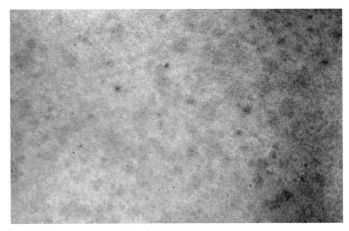

Fig. 8.32 Still disease.

Reactive Palisading Granulomatous Dermatitis

Reactive granulomatous dermatitis may be seen in patients with RA, such as interstitial granulomatous dermatitis (IGD) with arthritis, which shares significant overlap with palisaded neutrophilic and granulomatous dermatitis. IGD can present with round to oval erythematous or violaceous plaques on the flanks, axillae, inner thighs, and lower abdomen. Linear, slightly red or skin-colored cords extending from the upper back to the axilla called the "rope sign" have been described. When the lesions resolve, they may leave behind hyperpigmentation and a slightly wrinkled appearance. Arthritis may occur before, during, or after the eruption and tends to affect multiple joints of the upper extremities. IGD and related disorders can also occur with other autoimmune diseases, including SLE, and with hematologic disorders. Medication-induced cases have been rarely described, particularly with CCBs.

Histologically, a moderate to dense inflammatory infiltrate is seen through the reticular dermis, composed mostly of histiocytes distributed interstitially around discrete bundles of sclerotic collagen, which may demonstrate a "floating sign" as the inflammatory collection peels away from the normal collagen. Variable numbers of neutrophils and eosinophils are seen. Mucin, necrobiosis, vasculitis, and vacuolar change are usually absent or mild. The eruption is typically asymptomatic and may spontaneously involute after many months or years. If therapy is required, intralesional corticosteroids, methotrexate, hydroxychloroquine, dapsone, etanercept, ustekinumab, tocilizumab, and cyclosporine have been used, though most treatment is directed at the underlying disease.

Palisaded neutrophilic and granulomatous dermatitis represents another reactive granulomatous disorder and usually associated with a well-defined connective tissue disease, most commonly SLE, or RA. It often presents with eroded or ulcerated, symmetrically distributed umbilicated papules or nodules on the elbows, knuckles, and knees. The biopsy may reveal interstitial neutrophils and leukocytoclastic debris, with leukocytoclastic vasculitis in 30% of cases, accompanied by varying degrees of collagen degeneration. Palisaded granulomatous infiltrates with dermatofibrosis and scant neutrophilic debris are seen in older lesions. Mucin is absent, helping differentiate from interstitial GA.

Angelotti F, et al: Pathogenesis of rheumatoid arthritis. Clin Exp Rheumatol 2017; 35: 368.

Canete JD, et al: Safety profile of biological therapies for treating rheumatoid arthritis. Expert Opin Biol Ther 2017; 17: 1089.

Ferro F, et al: Novelties in the treatment of rheumatoid arthritis. Clin Exp Rheumatol 2017; 35: 721.

Fujio Y, et al: Rheumatoid neutrophilic dermatosis with blister formation. Australas J Dermatol 2014; 55: e12.

Makol A, et al: Vasculitis associated with rheumatoid arthritis. Rheumatology (Oxford) 2014; 53: 890.

Makol A, et al: Rheumatoid vasculitis. Curr Opin Rheumatol 2015; 27: 63.

Rosenbach M, et al: Reactive granulomatous dermatitis. Dermatol Clin 2015; 33: 373.

Singh JA, et al: Biologics or tofacitinib for people with rheumatoid arthritis naïve to methotrexate. Cochrane Database Syst Rev 2017; CD012657.

Tilstra JS, et al: Rheumatoid nodules. Dermatol Clin 2015; 33: 361.

Xue Y, et al: Skin signs of rheumatoid arthritis and its therapy-induced cutaneous side effects. Am J Clin Dermatol 2016; 17: 147.

Juvenile Rheumatoid Arthritis (Juvenile Idiopathic Arthritis)

Juvenile rheumatoid arthritis (JRA) is not a single disease but a group of disorders characterized by arthritis and young age of onset. The subset called Still disease accounts for only 20% of the patients. It shows skin manifestations in about 40% of young patients age 7–25 years. An eruption consisting of evanescent, nonpruritic, salmon-pink, macular, or papular lesions on the trunk and extremities may precede the onset of joint manifestations by many months (Fig. 8.32). Patients generally have extremely high serum ferritin levels. Neutrophilic panniculitis has been described. The systemic symptoms of fever and serositis usually recur over weeks each afternoon. Most patients remit permanently by adulthood. TNF-α IL-1, IL-6, IL-18, and IFN-γ are implicated in the pathogenesis of JRA, as are phagocyte-specific S100-proteins, such as S100A8, S100A9, and S100A12. Steroid-sparing agents are useful to decrease steroid-associated toxicity. The dose-response curve for methotrexate plateaus with parenteral administration of 15 mg/m²/week. Refractory disease has been treated with biologic agents as described, pulse methylprednisolone, and cyclophosphamide.

Anakinra and canakinumab have been employed and may be helpful.

Castaneda S, et al: Adult-onset Still's disease. Best Pract Res Clin Rheum 2016; 30: 222.
Colafrancesco S, et al: Presentation and diagnosis of adult-onset Still's disease. Expert Rev Clin Immunol 2015; 11: 749.

Fibroblastic Rheumatism

Fibroblastic rheumatism is a rare condition characterized by bilateral distal polyarthritis, flexion contractures, cutaneous nodules, sclerodactylitis, thickened palmar fascia, and Raynaud phenomenon. Biopsy demonstrates a fibroblastic proliferation with a collagenous stroma varying from smooth muscle actin–positive cellular fascicles to paucicellular areas with randomly arranged spindle or stellate cells. Elastic fibers are typically absent. Standard therapy includes immunosuppressive agents, typically methotrexate and oral corticosteroids, although some patients have responded to physical therapy without immunosuppressive treatment. Interferon has also been used. One patient has been reported with elevated lead levels, of unclear significance.

Zou XW, et al: Fibroblastic rheumatism. Clin Exp Dermatol 2015; 40: 309.

Paraneoplastic Rheumatism

Paraneoplastic syndromes resembling adult Still disease have been associated with a variety of neoplasms, including gastric carcinoma, lung carcinoma, and lymphoma. Patients with new onset of rheumatologic disease should be screened for signs and symptoms suggesting neoplasm.

Symmetric Synovitis

Symmetric seronegative synovitis is an idiopathic form of arthritis sometimes associated with idiopathic edema. Symmetric synovitis may also be a manifestation of Blau syndrome, an early-onset granulomatous disease with symmetric arthritis and recurrent uveitis, related to the caspase recruitment domain gene *CARD15/NOD2* and considered by some to be a form of early-onset sarcoidosis.

RELAPSING POLYCHONDRITIS

Relapsing polychondritis is characterized by intermittent episodes of inflammation of the articular and nonarticular cartilage resulting in chondrolysis and collapse of the involved cartilage. The course of the disease is chronic and variable, with episodic flares. Both genders are equally affected, with age between the third to sixth decade, most commonly around age 50, though pediatric and elderly cases may occur. Dissolution of the cartilage involves the ears, nose, and respiratory tract. The eye, joints, inner ear, and heart may rarely be involved. During bouts of inflammation, the bright-red involvement of the ears is confined to the cartilaginous portion while the earlobes remain conspicuously normal (Fig. 8.33). The affected areas are swollen and tender. There may be conductive deafness as a result of the obstruction produced by the swollen cartilage. The nasal septal cartilage is similarly involved to produce rhinitis, with crusting and bleeding and eventually saddle nose. Involvement of the bronchi, larynx, and epiglottis produces hoarseness, coughing, and dyspnea. Endobronchial ultrasonography has been used to facilitate the diagnosis of relapsing polychondritis. Migratory arthralgia and atypical chest pain are often present. Patients evaluated for chest pain are often released without treatment and with a diagnosis of costochondritis. Ocular disease most often presents as conjunctivitis, scleritis, or iritis. Perforation of the globe may occur. Complete heart block has been reported as a presenting sign. Michet criteria include auricular,

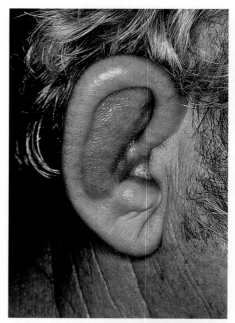

Fig. 8.33 Relapsing polychondritis characteristically involves cartilaginous portions of the ear but spares the lobe.

nasal, or laryngotracheal chondritis as major criteria, and ocular inflammation, hearing loss/vestibular dysfunction, or seronegative arthritis as minor criteria, requiring two major or one major and two minor criteria. The MAGIC syndrome is a combination of Behçet disease and relapsing polychondritis (mouth and genital ulcers with inflamed cartilage).

Cell-mediated immunity and antibodies against cartilage and collagen (primarily IgG anti–type II collagen antibodies, though reports of other types exist), in titers corresponding with disease activity. Elevations in ESR, CRP levels, and urinary type II collagen neoepitope levels correlate with disease activity. A second connective tissue disease or other autoimmune disease is present in about one third of patients with relapsing polychondritis, and some cases appear to be paraneoplastic, occurring in association with hematopoietic malignancies. Limited data suggest that serum levels of Th1 cytokines (IFN-γ, IL-12, IL-2) may correlate better with disease activity than those of Th2 cytokines (IL-4, IL-5, IL-6, IL-10). Monocyte chemoattractant protein 1 levels, macrophage inflammatory protein, and IL-8 are increased during disease flares.

Histologically, a predominantly neutrophilic infiltrate is noted in the perichondrium. Varying degrees of chondrolysis may be present. DIF often demonstrates a lupus-like, continuous granular band of immunoglobulin and complement in the perichondrium.

NSAIDs, corticosteroids, or traditional immunosuppressants have been used. Biologics are increasingly being evaluated for this disorder. Dapsone, colchicine, hydroxychloroquine, leflunomide, and IVIG may be varyingly effective. Dapsone may reduce frequency of flares but is usually inadequate for the disease. Systemic corticosteroids should be used to treat acute flares, but most patients require a steroid-sparing immunosuppressive drug. Methotrexate, azathioprine, MMF, cyclosporine, TNF-α inhibitors, abatacept, anakinra, tocilizumab, and rituximab have been used, but only about half of the patients experienced a good response. Sustained response to etanercept has been reported, even after failure to respond to infliximab. Cyclophosphamide may be used for extremely severe disease.

Mathian A, et al: Relapsing polychondritis. Best Pract Res Clin Rheumatol 2016; 30: 316.

Salles M, et al: Sustained response to tocilizumab in a patient with relapsing polychondritis complicated by aortitis. Clin Exp Rheumatol 2017; 103: 223.

Smylie A, et al: Relapsing polychondritis. Am J Clin Dermatol 2017; 18: 77.

9 Mucinoses

Within the dermis is a fibrillar matrix, termed *ground substance*, composed of proteoglycans and glycosaminoglycans. These acid mucopolysaccharides, produced by fibroblasts, are highly hygroscopic, binding about 1000 times their own volume in water. They are critical in holding water in the dermis and are responsible for dermal volume and texture. Normally, the sulfated acid mucopolysaccharide chondroitin sulfate and heparin are the primary dermal mucins. In certain diseases, fibroblasts produce abnormally large amounts of acid mucopolysaccharides, usually hyaluronic acid. These acid mucopolysaccharides (mucin) accumulate in large amounts in the dermis and may be visible histopathologically as pale-blue, granular or amorphous material between collagen bundles. They are often not visualized with hematoxylin and eosin stains because the water they bind is removed in processing, so the presence of increased mucin is suspected by the presence of large, empty spaces between the collagen bundles. Acid mucopolysaccharides can be detected by special stains, such as colloidal iron, alcian blue, and toluidine blue. Incubation of the tissue with hyaluronidase eliminates the staining, confirming the presence of hyaluronic acid.

Increased dermal mucin may result from many diseases and is a normal component of wound healing. The mucinoses are diseases in which production of increased amounts of mucin is the primary process. Mucin may also accumulate in the skin as a secondary phenomenon in lupus erythematosus, dermatomyositis, Degos disease, granuloma annulare, and cutaneous tumors, or after therapies such as psoralen plus ultraviolet A (PUVA) or retinoids. The genetic diseases in which mucin accumulates as a result of inherited metabolic abnormalities are termed the *mucopolysaccharidoses* (see Chapter 26). Myxedema and pretibial myxedema are reviewed in Chapter 24.

LICHEN MYXEDEMATOSUS

The terminology used to describe disorders in the lichen myxedematosus group has varied widely over the years; the 2001 classification of Rongioletti and Rebora is used here. A generalized form, scleromyxedema, is usually accompanied by a monoclonal gammopathy (lambda more commonly than kappa) and may have systemic organ involvement. Five localized forms are recognized, characterized by a lack of a monoclonal antibody and systemic disease. Also, patients may have disease that does not fit into these subsets, and their condition is termed atypical or intermediate in type. Mucin deposition secondary to thyroid disease is excluded from the classification.

Generalized Lichen Myxedematosus

Scleromyxedema affects both men and women and generally appears between ages 30 and 80. It is chronic and progressive. The primary lesions are multiple, waxy, 2–4 mm, dome-shaped or flat-topped papules (Fig. 9.1). They may coalesce into plaques (Fig. 9.2) or may be arranged in linear arrays. Less often, urticarial, nodular, or even annular lesions are seen. The dorsal hands, face, elbows, and extensor extremities are most frequently affected (Fig. 9.3). Mucosal lesions are absent.

A diffuse infiltration develops, leading to "woody" sclerosis of the skin. A reduced range of motion of the mouth, hands, and extremities may follow (Fig. 9.4). On the glabella and forehead, coalescence of lesions leads to the prominent furrowing of a "leonine facies." At the proximal interphalangeal joint, induration surrounding a centrally depressed area has been called the "doughnut sign." Pruritus may occur.

Scleromyxedema is often associated with visceral disease. Gastrointestinal findings are most common. Dysphagia from esophageal involvement often occurs, and the stomach or intestine may also be affected. Pulmonary complications with dyspnea caused by restrictive or obstructive disease are also common. Proximal muscle weakness with an inflammatory myopathy or a nonspecific vacuolar change may occur. Carpal tunnel syndrome occurs in 10% of patients. Arthralgia or inflammatory arthritis frequently develop. Disease-specific adenopathy and renal impairment may be present.

The most serious systemic findings are cardiac, hematologic, and neurologic manifestations. Peripheral neuropathies and central nervous system disturbances can occur, including confusion, dizziness, dysarthria, ascending paralysis, seizures, syncope, and coma. The latter conditions have been called "dermato-neuro syndrome" and may be due to disruption in perfusion by the excessive immunoglobulins leading to an encephalopathy. Middle-aged men are most frequently affected, and one third of these patients demonstrate recurrent symptoms. Plasmapheresis and intravenous immune globulin (IVIG) may result in dramatic recovery from this life-threatening emergency. Visceral disease can be fatal.

Criteria for inclusion in the scleromyxedema category include mucin deposition, fibroblast proliferation and fibrosis, normal thyroid function tests, and presence of a monoclonal gammopathy. Approximately 10% of patients do not have a gammopathy on initial evaluation. Association with hepatitis C, diabetes mellitus, and multiple sclerosis has also been reported. The gammopathy is usually an immunoglobulin G–λ (IgG-λ) type, suggesting an underlying plasma cell dyscrasia. Bone marrow examination may be normal or may reveal increased numbers of plasma cells or frank multiple myeloma.

Clinical and histologic features are usually diagnostic. Skin biopsies of early papular lesions demonstrate a proliferation of fibroblasts with mucin and many small collagen fibers. The papules generally appear more fibrotic than mucinous. Over time, fibroblast nuclei become less numerous, and collagen fibers become thickened.

Many clinical findings in scleromyxedema are also found in systemic scleroderma, including cutaneous sclerosis, Raynaud phenomenon, dysphagia, and carpal tunnel syndrome. This distinction in some cases may be difficult without a biopsy. Other infiltrative disorders, such as amyloidosis, must be excluded. Nephrogenic systemic fibrosis presents with skin thickening in the setting of renal failure and gadolinium exposure (see Chapter 8). In its earliest form, it includes mucin along with collagen deposition with a proliferation of CD34+ cells in the dermis. The histologic findings are identical to those of scleromyxedema, and a first report referred to a scleromyxedema-like disease associated with renal failure. The clinical findings are dominated by fibrosis (see Chapter 8).

Treatment of scleromyxedema is difficult and usually undertaken in concert with an oncologist. Therapy is targeted to treat the gammopathy (if present). Typical therapies may include immunosuppressive agents, especially melphalan, bortezomib, or cyclophosphamide, with or without plasma exchange and high-dose prednisone. IVIG has also been used with success. Thalidomide and the newer thalidomide analog lenalinomide have shown benefit

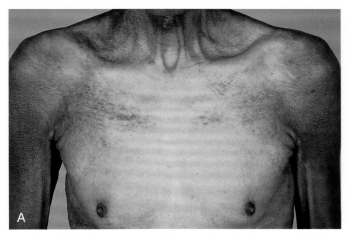

Fig. 9.1 Scleromyxedema. (Courtesy Douglas Pugliese, MD.)

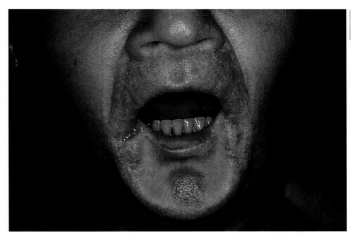

Fig. 9.4 Scleromyxedema. (Courtesy Rui Tavares Bello, MD.)

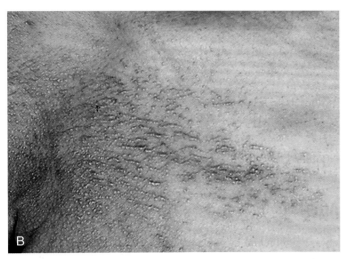

Fig. 9.2 Scleromyxedema. (Courtesy Douglas Pugliese, MD.)

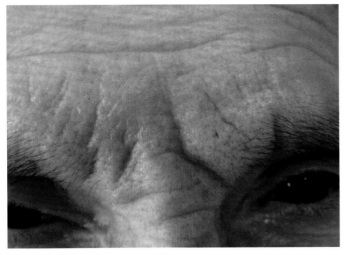

Fig. 9.3 Scleromyxedema. (Courtesy Rui Tavares Bello, MD.)

in patients with or without a paraproteinemia and may provide a long-term maintenance option. Temporary remission of progressive visceral disease may occur. These short-term benefits must be weighed against the increase in malignancies and sepsis complicating such therapy. Chances of remission are enhanced by the use of autologous stem cell transplantation with high-dose melphalan.

Skin-directed therapy may also be used. Physical therapy is indicated. Retinoids, plasmapheresis, extracorporeal photochemo-therapy, grenz ray and electron beam therapy, PUVA, thalidomide, interferon-α (IFN-α), cyclosporine, topical dimethyl sulfoxide, and topical and intralesional hyaluronidase and corticosteroids have all produced improvement in the skin of select patients. Many others, however, have not benefited, and visceral disease is usually not affected. Ultraviolet B (UVB) light and IFN-α have exacerbated scleromyxedema.

Occasional patients are reported who spontaneously remit even after many years of disease; however, scleromyxedema remains a therapeutic challenge, and the overall prognosis is poor.

Localized Lichen Myxedematosus

The localized variants of lichen myxedematosus lack visceral involvement or an associated gammopathy. As a group, they are benign but often persistent. No therapy is reliably effective in any of the localized forms of lichen myxedematosus. Because there is no gammopathy, visceral involvement, or associated thyroid disease in any of the variants, often no treatment is needed. Shave excision or carbon dioxide (CO$_2$) ablation are other options for individual lesions. Spontaneous resolution may occur in all varieties.

Discrete Papular Lichen Myxedematosus

Discrete papular lichen myxedematosus is characterized by the occurrence of waxy, 2–5 mm, firm, flesh-colored papules, usually confined to the limbs or trunk. The papules may have an erythematous or yellowish hue, may coalesce into nodules or plaques, and may number into the hundreds. Nodules may occasionally be the predominant lesion present, with few or absent papules. The underlying skin is not indurated, and there is no associated gammopathy or internal involvement. Biopsy reveals the presence of mucin in the upper and middle dermis. Fibroblast proliferation is variable, but collagen deposition is minimal. The slow accumulation of papules is the usual course, without the development of a gammopathy or internal manifestations. Occasional cases may spontaneously involute.

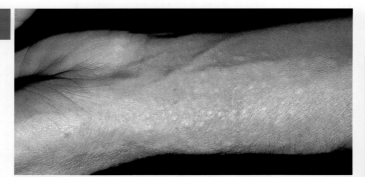

Fig. 9.5 Acral persistent papular mucinosis.

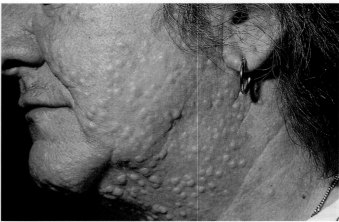

Fig. 9.6 Self-healing papular mucinosis.

Patients with advanced human immunodeficiency virus (HIV) disease have been reported to develop mucinous papules, usually widespread, unassociated with a paraprotein. It is usually seen in patients diagnosed with acquired immunodeficiency syndrome (AIDS), in patients with multiple infectious complications. These lesions may occur in association with an eczematous dermatitis or on normal skin. If associated with an eczematous dermatitis, the lesions often clear if the eczema is controlled. Lesions on normal skin may respond to systemic retinoid therapy. Intralesional hyaluronidase has been used for lesions of papular mucinosis. At times, spontaneous remission occurs. The authors have also seen a patient with AIDS and true scleromyxedema with visceral involvement, and two patients have been reported with acral persistent papular mucinosis.

Acral Persistent Papular Mucinosis

Patients with acral persistent papular mucinosis have a few to more than 100 bilaterally symmetric, 2–5 mm, flesh-colored papules localized to the hands and wrists (Fig. 9.5). The knees, calves, or elbows may also be involved in a minority of patients. The face and trunk are spared. Women outnumber men by 5 : 1. The course is one of persistence and slow progression. Two involved sisters have been reported. Histologically, there is a collection of upper dermal mucin with minimal or no increase in fibroblasts. Electrocoagulation of these lesions was reported to result in no recurrence in 6 months and topical tacrolimus was also reported to have some benefit.

Self-Healing Papular Mucinosis

Self-healing papular mucinosis occurs in a juvenile and an adult form. The juvenile variant, also called self-healing juvenile cutaneous mucinosis, is a rare but distinct disorder characterized by the sudden onset of skin lesions and polyarthritis. Children, usually between ages 5 and 15, are affected. Familial cases are reported. Skin lesions are ivory-white papules of the head, neck, trunk, and typically the periarticular regions; deep nodules on the face and periarticular sites; and hard edema of the periorbital area and face. An acute arthritis affects the knees, elbows, and hand joints. In the adult form, papular lesions occur, usually without the associated joint symptoms (Fig. 9.6). Histology of the skin lesions reveals dermal mucin with minimal fibroblastic proliferation or collagen deposition. Although the initial presentation is worrisome, the prognosis is excellent. Spontaneous resolution without sequelae occurs over several months.

Papular Mucinosis of Infancy

Also referred to as cutaneous mucinosis of infancy, this rare syndrome occurs at birth or within the first few months of life. Skin-colored,

yellow, pink or translucent, grouped or discrete, 2–8 mm papules develop on the trunk or upper extremities, especially the back of the hands. A case of familial cutaneous mucinosis of infancy has been reported. Patients with Carney complex can also have widespread myxomas, which can look similar. Biopsies of papular mucinosis show very superficial upper dermal mucin without proliferation of fibroblasts. Existing lesions remain static; new lesions continue to accumulate gradually. Similar lesions may sometimes be noted in association with neonatal lupus erythematosus.

Nodular Lichen Myxedematosus

Patients may have multiple nodules on the trunk or extremities.

Atypical or Intermediate Lichen Myxedematosus

The cutaneous mucinoses are all relatively uncommon. In a literature dominated by case reports, individual patients have been found who do not fit well into the previously described scheme. For example, some patients with acral persistent papular mucinosis have a paraprotein, with localized papular mucinosis and immunoglobulin A (IgA) nephropathy, whereas others with apparently classic scleromyxedema with visceral lesions may not have a detectable circulating paraprotein.

Abbot RA, et al: Widespread papules in a patient with HIV. Clin Exp Dermatol 2010; 35: 801.

Andre Jorge F, et al: Treatment of acral persistent popular mucinosis with electrocoagulation. J Cutan Med Surg 2011; 15: 227.

Blum M, et al: Scleromyxedema. Medicine (Baltimore) 2008; 87: 10.

Brunet-Possenti F, et al: Combination of intravenous immunoglobulins and lenalidomide in the treatment of scleromyxedema. J Am Acad Dermatol 2013; 69: 319.

Canueto J, et al: The combination of bortezomib and dexamethasone is an efficient therapy for relapsed/refractory scleromyxedema. Eur J Haematol 2012; 88: 450.

Concheiro J, et al: Discrete papular lichen myxedematosus. Clin Exp Dermatol 2009; 34: e608.

Dinneen A et al: Scleromyxedema. J Am Acad Dermatol 1995; 33: 37.

Donato ML, et al: Scleromyxedema. Blood 2006; 107: 463.

Feliciani C, et al: Adult self-healing popular mucinosis on genital skin. Clin Exp Dermatol 2009; 34: e760.

Fleming KE, et al: Scleromyxedema and the dermato-neuro syndrome. J Cutan Pathol 2012; 39: 508.

Hummers LK: Scleromyxedema. Curr Opin Rheumatol 2014; 26: 658.

Jun JY, et al: Acral persistent papular mucinosis with partial response to tacrolimus ointment. Ann Dermatol 2016; 28: 517.

Lee WS, et al: Cutaneous focal mucinosis arising from the chin. J Craniofac Surg 2010; 21: 1639.

Luo DQ, et al: Acral persistent papular mucinosis. J Dtsch Dermatol Ges 2011; 9: 354.

Ramamurthi A, et al: Hyaluronidase in the treatment of papular dermal mucinosis. J Surg Dermatol 2016; 1: 61.

Rampino M, et al: Scleromyxedema. Int J Dermatol 2007; 46: 864.

Rongioletti F, et al: Scleromyxedema. J Am Acad Dermatol 2013; 69: 66.

Rongioletti F, et al: Treatment of localized lichen myxedematosus of discrete type with tacrolimus ointment. J Am Acad Dermatol 2008; 58: 530.

Savran Y, et al: Dermato-neuro syndrome in a case of scleromyxedema. Eur J Rheumatol 2015; 2: 160.

Wang P, et al: Localized papular mucinosis with IgA nephropathy. Arch Dermatol 2011; 147: 599.

Wilson J, et al: Nephrogenic systemic fibrosis. J Am Acad Dermatol 2017; 77: 235.

Yamamoto M, et al: Plaque-type focal mucinosis. Int J Dermatol 2011; 50: 893.

Zeng R, et al: Nodular lichen myxedematosus during childhood. Pediatr Dermatol 2014; 31: e160.

SCLEREDEMA

Scleredema is a skin disease characterized by a stiffening and hardening of the subcutaneous tissues, as if infiltrated with paraffin. It occurs in two forms: with and without diabetes mellitus. In the more generalized, nondiabetic condition, a sudden onset after an infection, typically streptococcal, may occur. This reactive variant may also present as a drug eruption. In other cases, onset is insidious and chronic and has no preceding infection. In the more common diabetes-associated disease, a long-lasting induration of the upper back is characteristic.

In cases not associated with diabetes, females outnumber males by 2:1. The onset can be from childhood through adulthood. Skin tightness and induration begin on the neck and/or face, spreading symmetrically to involve the arms, shoulders, back, and chest. The distal extremities are spared. The patient may have difficulty opening the mouth or eyes and a masklike expression as a result of the infiltration. The involved skin, which is waxy and of woodlike consistency, gradually transitions into normal skin with no clear demarcation. Associated findings occur in variable numbers of patients and can include dysphagia caused by tongue and upper esophageal involvement, cardiac arrhythmias, and an associated paraproteinemia, usually an IgG type. Myeloma may be present. There may be pleural, pericardial, or peritoneal effusion.

In about half the patients in whom scleredema follows an infection, spontaneous resolution will occur in months to a few years. In one patient whose disease had a sudden onset after beginning infliximab treatment for rheumatoid arthritis, the condition resolved quickly after discontinuation of the medicine and did not recur after etanercept was initiated. The remaining patients with nondiabetic scleredema have a prolonged course. Therapy is generally of no benefit, but patients may live with the disease for many years. Cyclosporine, UVA I, pulsed dexamethasone, tamoxifen, IVIG, and extracorporeal photopheresis have reportedly been effective in individual patients. Bortezomib induced remission in one patient with myeloma-associated scleredema.

In the second group, which in most dermatologists' experience is the more common type, there is an association with late-onset, insulin-dependent diabetes. Men outnumber women by 10:1.

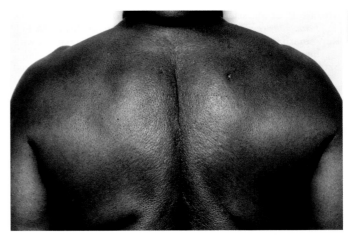

Fig. 9.7 Scleredema.

Affected men tend to be obese. The lesions are of insidious onset and long duration, presenting as woody induration and thickening of the skin of the middle-upper back, neck, and shoulders (Fig. 9.7). There is a sharp step-off from the involved to the normal skin. Persistent erythema and folliculitis may involve the affected areas. The associated diabetes is of long duration and is difficult to control. Further, patients often have complications of their diabetes, such as nephropathy, atherosclerotic disease, retinopathy, and neuropathy. Control of the diabetes does not affect the course of the scleredema. No paraprotein is detected, and no visceral involvement is seen. Lesions are persistent and usually unresponsive to treatment. Intravenous penicillin, electron beam alone or in combination with photon irradiation, narrow-band UVB, and both bath and systemic PUVA, in one case combined with colchicine, and frequency-modulated electromagnetic neural stimulation have each been effective in individual patients. Although low-dose methotrexate was successful in one patient, it was ineffective in a case series of seven patients.

The histology of both forms is identical. The skin is dramatically thickened, with the dermis often expanded twofold to threefold. There is no hyalinization, such as that seen in scleroderma, but rather the thick, dermal collagen bundles are separated by clear spaces that may contain visible mucin (hyaluronic acid). The amount of mucin is variable and usually only prominent in early lesions. In late lesions, slightly widened spaces between thick collagen bundles are the sole finding, because the amount of mucin is scant.

Aichelburg MC, et al: Successful treatment of poststreptococcal scleredema adultorum Buschke with intravenous immunoglobulins. Arch Dermatol 2012; 148: 1126.

Alsaeedi SH, et al: Treatment of scleredema diabeticorum with tamoxifen. J Rheumatol 2010; 37: 2636.

Beers WH, et al: Scleredema adultorum of Buschke. Semin Arthritis Rheum 2006; 35: 355.

Gandolfi A, et al: Improvement in clinical symptoms of scleredema diabeticorum by frequency-modulated electromagnetic neural stimulation. Diabetes Care 2014; 37: e233.

Ioannidou DI, et al: Scleredema adultorum of Buschke presenting as periorbital edema. J Am Acad Dermatol 2005; 52: 41.

Kokpol C, et al: Successful treatment of scleredema diabeticorum by combining local PUVA and colchicine. Case Rep Dermatol 2012; 4: 265.

Kroft EB et al: Ultraviolet A phototherapy for sclerotic skin diseases. J Am Acad Dermatol 2008; 59: 1017.

Kurihara Y, et al: Case of diabetic scleredema. J Dermatol 2011; 38: 693.

Morais P, et al: Scleredema of Buschke following *Mycoplasma pneumoniae* respiratory infection. Int J Dermatol 2011; 50: 454.

Ranganathan P: Infliximab-induced scleredema in a patient with rheumatoid arthritis. J Clin Rheumatol 2005; 11: 319.

Szturz P, et al: Complete remission of multiple myeloma associated scleredema after bortezomib-based treatment. Leuk Lymphoma 2013; 54: 1324.

Yachoui R, et al: Scleredema in a patient with AIDS-related lipodystrophy syndrome. Case Rep Endocrinol 2013; 2013: 943798.

RETICULAR ERYTHEMATOUS MUCINOSIS (REM SYNDROME, PLAQUELIKE CUTANEOUS MUCINOSIS)

Reticular erythematous mucinosis (REM) favors women in the third and fourth decades of life. The eruption frequently appears after intense sun exposure. Clinical lesions are erythematous plaques or reticulated patches that are several centimeters in diameter and usually in the midline of the chest and back (Fig. 9.8). Evolution is gradual, photosensitivity may be present, and lesions may be induced with UVB. Onset or exacerbation with oral contraceptives, menses, and pregnancy is another feature. Serologic tests for lupus erythematosus (LE) are negative.

Histologically, there are varying degrees of lymphocytic infiltration around dermal vessels, with deposits of mucin in the dermis. Direct immunofluorescence is negative, but focal vacuolar interface dermatitis is sometimes seen. Treatment with antimalarials is successful in most cases. The pulsed dye laser has led to resolution in two patients.

Lesions of REM have also been reported to occur on the face, arms, abdomen, and groin. When evaluating patients with mucinous smooth-surfaced erythematous lesions it is important to consider the possibility of connective tissue disease. Plaquelike or papulo-nodular lesions in sites away from the central chest and back may infrequently herald the development of systemic LE, discoid LE, dermatomyositis, or scleroderma.

Tumid LE is a subset of chronic cutaneous lupus character-ized by erythematous papules, nodules, and plaques that most often involve the face, extensor aspects of the arms, shoulders, V of the neck, and upper back. Histology more often has a deep perivascular and panfollicular location and commonly reveals direct immunofluorescence activity than REM. REM also tends to have more superficial mucin and lymphocytes with fewer plasmocytoid dendritic cells. Tumid LE is photoinducible and responsive to antimalarials. Although serologic abnormalities occur in a small percentage of patients, this is usually a skin-limited condition.

Cinotti E, et al: Reticular erythematous mucinosis. J Eur Acad Dermatol Venereol 2015; 29: 689.

Clarke JT: Recognizing and managing reticular erythematous mucinosis. Arch Dermatol 2011; 147: 715.

Kreuter A, et al: Clinical features and efficacy of antimalarial treatment for reticulated erythematous mucinosis. Arch Dermatol 2011; 147: 710.

Susok L, et al: Complete clearance of reticular erythematous mucinosis with quinacrine monotherapy. Arch Dermatol 2012; 148: 768.

Thareja S, et al: Reticulated erythematous mucinosis. Int J Dermatol 2012; 51: 903.

Wristen CC, et al: Plaque-like cutaneous mucinosis. Am J Dermatopathol 2012; 34: e50.

FOLLICULAR MUCINOSIS (ALOPECIA MUCINOSA)

Alopecia mucinosa is characterized by inflammatory plaques with alopecia that demonstrate mucinous deposits in the outer root sheath of the hair follicle on histopathology. The plaques may be simply hypopigmented or erythematous and scaly, eczematous, or composed of flesh-colored, follicular papules (Fig. 9.9). There may be only one lesion, especially on the head and neck, or multiple sites may be present. The plaques are firm and coarsely rough to the palpating finger. They are distributed mostly on the face, neck, and scalp but may appear on any part of the body. Itching may or may not be present. Alopecia occurs regularly in lesions on the scalp and frequently in lesions located elsewhere. Some papules show a comedo-like black central dot that corresponds to a broken hair or the mucin itself and in children can simulate a nevus comedonicus. The follicular involvement may cause the surface of a patch to resemble keratosis pilaris. Sensory dissociation, with hot-cold perception alterations or anesthesia to light touch, has been reported in some lesions, with a resultant misdiagnosis of leprosy.

The term *alopecia mucinosa* may be used to describe the disease process, and *follicular mucinosis* to describe the histologic features. The disease may be limited to skin and benign (primary follicular mucinosis) or may be associated with follicular mycosis fungoides (Fig. 9.10). When lesions are solitary or few in number and cluster on the head and neck of individuals younger than 40, the condition usually follows a benign, chronic course, even when the infiltrate is found to be clonal in nature. Widespread lesions in an older patient, however, will usually be found to be cutaneous T-cell lymphoma (CTCL) at initial presentation or will progress to lymphoma within 5 years. These two subsets are not exclusive,

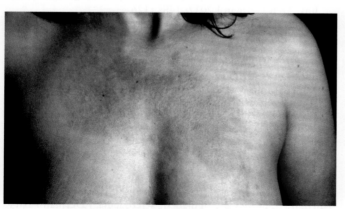

Fig. 9.8 Reticulated erythematous mucinosis.

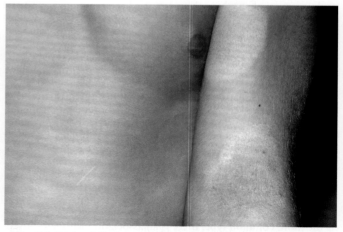

Fig. 9.9 Benign follicular mucinosis. (Courtesy Steven Binnick, MD.)

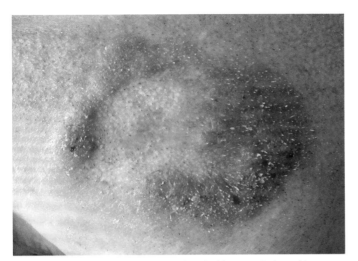

Fig. 9.10 Follicular mucinosis associated with mycosis fungoides. (Courtesy Ellen Kim, MD.)

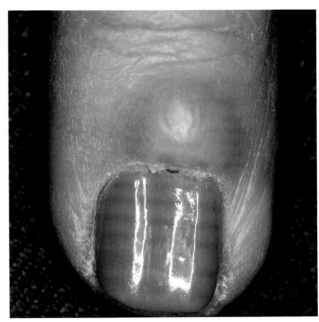

Fig. 9.11 Myxoid cyst. Note nail deformity. (Courtesy Steven Binnick, MD.)

however, and no clinical or histologic criteria absolutely distinguish them in the absence of diagnostic findings of CTCL.

Histologically, follicular mucinosis demonstrates large collections of mucin within the sebaceous gland and outer root sheath. The mucin typically stains as hyaluronic acid. A mixed dermal infiltrate is present. When the condition occurs in association with CTCL, the perifollicular infiltrate is atypical but not generally epidermotropic, and considerable admixture of eosinophils and plasma cells is present. The additional finding of the presence of syringolymphoid hyperplasia should raise concern that lymphoma is or will become evident. T-cell receptor gene rearrangement studies that indicate clonality are also supportive but do not alone predict an aggressive course.

Spontaneous involution of primary follicular mucinosis may occur, especially in young children. Topical corticosteroids produce improvement and are favored for localized disease, especially in children. Hydroxychloroquine is an excellent first-line systemic therapy. Dapsone, PUVA, radiation therapy, IFN alpha-2b, minocycline, isotretinoin, photodynamic therapy, imiquimod, and indomethacin have been effective in individual cases. Follicular mycosis fungoides, with or without associated mucin, is more refractory to treatment and has a worse prognosis than classic CTCL. All patients should be followed for progression of disease.

Alikhan A, et al: Pediatric follicular mucinosis. Pediatr Dermatol 2013; 30: 192.

Alonso de Celada RM, et al: Treatment of primary follicular mucinosis with imiquimod 5% cream. Pediatr Dermatol 2014; 31: 406.

Lehman JS, et al: Folliculotropic mycosis fungoides. Arch Dermatol 2010; 146: 662.

Schneider SW, et al: Treatment of so-called idiopathic follicular mucinosis with hydroxychloroquine. Br J Dermatol 2010; 163: 420.

White FN, et al: Acneiform follicular mucinosis responding to hydroxychloroquine. Arch Dermatol 2011; 147: 130.

Zvulunov A, et al: Clinical and histopathologic spectrum of alopecia mucinosa/follicular mucinosis and its natural history in children. J Am Acad Dermatol 2012; 67: 1174.

CUTANEOUS FOCAL MUCINOSIS

Focal mucinosis is characterized by a solitary nodule or papule. Lesions are asymptomatic and usually occur on the face, neck, trunk, or extremities. They appear in adulthood. Histologically, the lesion is characterized by a loose dermal stroma containing large quantities of mucin together with numerous dendritic-shaped fibroblasts. The clinical appearance is not distinctive and at times may suggest a cyst, basal cell carcinoma, or neurofibroma. Treatment is surgical excision.

Lee WS, et al: Cutaneous focal mucinosis arising from the chin. J Craniofac Surg 2010; 21: 1639.

Takemura N, et al: Cutaneous focal mucinosis. J Dermatol 2005; 32: 1051.

MYXOID CYSTS

Myxoid cysts, also called synovial and digital mucous cysts, occur most frequently on the dorsal or lateral terminal digits of the hands but may also occur on the toes. These lesions present as solitary, 5–7 mm, opalescent or skin-colored cysts. They may occur as asymptomatic swellings of the proximal nailfold, as subungual growths, or over the distal interphalangeal joint. Women are more frequently affected, and osteoarthritis is often present in the adjacent distal interphalangeal joint. Myxoid cysts that can be reduced with pressure communicate directly with the joint space.

Multiple myxoid cysts are associated with connective tissue disease. Young children, even infants, may present with multiple digital mucous cysts as the initial manifestation of juvenile rheumatoid arthritis.

When a synovial cyst is present beneath the proximal nailfold, a characteristic groove may be formed in the nail plate by pressure of the lesion on the nail matrix (Fig. 9.11). Those located beneath the nail cause a transverse nail curvature and a red or blue discoloration of the lunula. Nail integrity typically is compromised, leading to distal or longitudinal splitting or onycholysis. The diagnosis can be confirmed by magnetic resonance imaging or surgical exploration. Myxoid cysts contain a clear, viscous, sticky fluid that may spontaneously drain. These cysts do not have an epithelial lining, but rather a compacted fibrous wall.

Treatment depends on the site of the myxoid cyst. The repeated puncture technique for cysts located beneath the proximal nailfold may achieve a cure rate of up to 70%, but multiple punctures

(>40) may be required. This technique may be complicated by local tissue or joint infection. Steroids may be injected into the tissue after draining the cyst. Intralesional injection of sodium tetradecyl sulfate has an 80% response rate. Destruction by cryotherapy, CO_2 laser ablation, curettage, and fulguration are alternatives with similar cure rates, but these therapies result in scarring.

Surgical approaches that reflect the skin overlying the cyst and either excise or tie off the communication to the joint, which may be visualized by injecting the myxoid cyst with methylene blue, have a cure rate greater than 90%.

Li K, et al: Digital mucous cysts. Cutan Med Surg 2010; 14: 199.
Park SE, et al: Treatment of digital mucous cysts with intralesional sodium tetradecyl sulfate injection. Dermatol Surg 2014; 40: 1249.

CHAPTER REFERENCES

Rongioletti F, et al: Cutaneous mucinoses. Am J Dermatopathol 2001; 23: 257.
Yaqub A, et al: Localized cutaneous fibrosing disorders. Rheum Dis Clin North Am 2013; 39: 347.

10

Seborrheic Dermatitis, Psoriasis, Recalcitrant Palmoplantar Eruptions, Pustular Dermatitis, and Erythroderma

SEBORRHEIC DERMATITIS

Clinical Features

Seborrheic dermatitis is common, occurring in 2%–5% of the population. It is a chronic, superficial, inflammatory disease with a predilection for the scalp, eyebrows, eyelids, nasolabial creases, lips, ears (Fig. 10.1), sternal area, axillae, submammary folds, umbilicus, groins, and gluteal crease. The disease is characterized by scaling on an erythematous base. The scale often has a yellow, greasy appearance. Itching may be severe. Dandruff (pityriasis sicca) represents a mild form of seborrheic dermatitis. An oily type, pityriasis steatoides, is accompanied by erythema and an accumulation of thick crusts.

Other types of seborrheic dermatitis on the scalp include arcuate, polycyclic, or petaloid patches and psoriasiform, exudative, or crusted plaques. The disease frequently spreads beyond the hairy scalp to the forehead, ears, postauricular regions, and neck. On these areas, the patches have convex borders and are reddish yellow or yellowish. In dark-skinned individuals, arcuate and petaloid lesions typically involve the hairline. In extreme cases, the entire scalp is covered by a greasy, dirty crust with an offensive odor. In infants, yellow or brown scaling lesions on the scalp, with accumulated adherent epithelial debris, are called "cradle cap."

Erythema and scaling are often seen in the eyebrows. The lids may show fine, yellowish white scales and faint erythema. The edges of the lids may be erythematous and granular (marginal blepharitis), and the conjunctivae may be injected. If the glabella is involved, fissures in the wrinkles at the inner end of the eyebrow may accompany the fine scaling. In the nasolabial creases and on the alae nasi, there may be yellowish or reddish yellow scaling macules, sometimes with fissures. In men, folliculitis of the beard area is common.

In the ears, seborrheic dermatitis may be mistaken for an infectious otitis externa. There is scaling in the aural canals, around the auditory meatus, usually with marked pruritus. The postauricular region and skin under the lobe may be involved. In these areas, the skin often becomes red, fissured, and swollen. In the axillae, the eruption begins in the apices, bilaterally, and later progresses to neighboring skin. This pattern resembles that of allergic contact dermatitis to deodorant, but differs from that of clothing dermatitis (which involves periphery of axillae but spares the vault). The involvement may vary from simple erythema and scaling to more pronounced petaloid patches with fissures. The inframammary folds and the umbilicus may be involved. The presternal area is a favored site on the trunk.

Seborrheic dermatitis is common in the groin and gluteal crease, where its appearance may closely simulate tinea cruris or candidiasis. In these areas, the appearance often overlaps with that of inverse psoriasis. In fact, many of these patients have an overlap of the two conditions (sebopsoriasis or seborrhiasis) in the groin, as well as the scalp. The lesions may also become generalized and progress to an exfoliative erythroderma (erythroderma desquamativum),

especially in infants. A minority of these infants will have evidence of immunosuppression. In adults, generalized eruptions may be accompanied by adenopathy and may simulate mycosis fungoides or psoriatic erythroderma.

Seborrheic dermatitis may be associated with several internal diseases. Parkinson disease is often accompanied by severe refractory seborrheic dermatitis involving the scalp and face, with waxy, profuse scaling. A unilateral injury to the innervation of the face, or a stroke, may lead to unilateral localized seborrheic dermatitis. Patients with acquired immunodeficiency syndrome (AIDS) have an increased incidence of seborrheic dermatitis. An increased incidence has also been noted in patients who are seropositive for human immunodeficiency virus (HIV) but have not developed other signs of clinical disease. Diabetes mellitus (especially in obese persons), sprue, malabsorption disorders, epilepsy, neuroleptic drugs (e.g., haloperidol), and reactions to arsenic and gold have all produced seborrheic dermatitis–like eruptions.

Etiology and Pathogenesis

The etiology of this common disorder is complex but may be related to the presence of the lipophilic yeast *Malassezia ovalis (Pityrosporum ovale)*, which produces bioactive indoles, oleic acid, malssezin, and indole-3-carbaldehyde. The density of yeast has been correlated with the severity of the disease, and reduction of the yeast occurs with response to therapy. *M. ovalis* may also be abundant on the scalps of patients who have no clinical signs of the disease, and the yeast may only be pathogenic in predisposed individuals. Heavy colonization with *Staphylococcus epidermidis* has also been noted.

Patients with seborrheic dermatitis may show upregulation of interferon (IFN)–γ, expressed interleukin-6 (IL-6), expressed IL-1β, and IL-4. Expression of cytotoxicity-activating ligands and recruitment of natural killer (NK) cells have also been noted.

Histology

The epidermis demonstrates regular acanthosis with some thinning of the suprapapillary plates. Varying degrees of spongiosis and lymphocyte exocytosis are noted. A characteristic finding is the presence of a focal scale crust adjacent to the follicular ostia.

Differential Diagnosis

Some cases of seborrheic dermatitis bear a close clinical resemblance to psoriasis, and the two conditions may overlap. Patients with psoriasis tend to have more pronounced erythema and heavier silvery scales that peel in layers. Removal of scales in psoriasis may disclose bleeding points (Auspitz sign). This sign is common but lacks great specificity. Severe itching favors seborrheic dermatitis. Characteristic psoriasis elsewhere (nail pitting, balanitis) may resolve the question. Impetigo of the scalp, especially when associated with pediculosis, may cause difficulty in differentiation. Scalp impetigo can be an indolent crusted dermatosis associated with failure to thrive. Langerhans cell histiocytosis may also resemble seborrheic dermatitis, but typically demonstrates

191

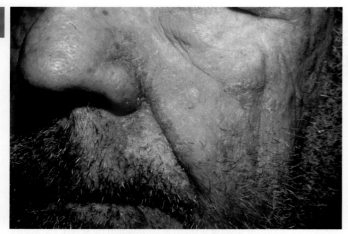

Fig. 10.1 Seborrheic dermatitis.

yellow-brown perifollicular papules and groin fissuring. Crusted scabies of the scalp can also be confused with seborrheic dermatitis, and *Trichophyton tonsurans* often produces a subtle seborrheic scale. In subtle cases of tinea, a moist gauze pad rubbed vigorously on the scalp will typically dislodge short, broken potassium hydroxide (KOH)–positive hairs. This can be the fastest way to make the diagnosis.

Treatment

Agents suitable for use on glabrous skin include corticosteroid creams, gels, sprays, and foams. Corticosteroids tend to produce a rapid effect with high clearance rates, but on the face, even medium-potency corticosteroids can produce steroid rosacea. For this reason, antifungal agents and topical calcineurin inhibitors (CNIs) are often used. Ketoconazole, ciclopirox, sertaconazole, tacrolimus, pimecrolimus, zinc pyrithione, and *Quassia amara* extract preparations are all effective alone and in combination. The antifungals are now available in a wide range of vehicles, including foams, gels, and liquids. Surfactant-based pronosomal formulations can improve drug delivery. Proniosomes are particles coated with a nonionic surfactant. Bifonazole shampoo has been effective in treating infants and small children. Topical CNIs may be associated with a burning sensation, especially on moist skin, and may produce flushing if patients consume alcohol. Patients generally tolerate these agents better after initial treatment with a corticosteroid. An open, randomized, prospective, comparative study of topical pimecrolimus 1% cream versus topical ketoconazole 2% cream found the two to be equally effective, but side effects were somewhat more common with pimecrolimus. Preliminary studies suggest oral itraconazole and oral terbinafine may show some efficacy. Oral fluconazole showed marginal benefit. Study results with topical metronidazole have been mixed.

When secondary bacterial infection is present, a topical or oral antibiotic may be required. In patients infected with HIV, lithium succinate ointment has been used for facial disease. Lithium gluconate 8% ointment has compared favorably with ketoconazole 2% emulsion in healthy adults and was more effective in terms of control of scaling and symptoms. Sodium sulfacetamide products, with or without sulfur, are effective in some refractory patients.

For scalp disease, selenium sulfide, ketoconazole, tar, zinc pyrithione, fluocinolone, and resorcin shampoos are effective. In many patients, these agents may be used two to three times a week, with a regular shampoo used in between as required. White patients often prefer antifungal foams and gels, as well as corticosteroid solutions, foams, gels, and sprays, whereas some black patients prefer ointment or oil preparations.

Itching of the external ear canal usually responds to a topical corticosteroid, CNIs, or antifungals (e.g., ketoconazole, ciclopirox). Some patients require the use of a class 1 corticosteroid on weekends to control refractory pruritus. Cortisporin otic suspension (neomycin, polymyxin B, hydrocortisone) can bring about prompt clearing, but contact dermatitis to neomycin may complicate the use of some Cortisporin products. Desonide otic lotion (0.05% desonide, 2% acetic acid) is also effective and may be better tolerated than Domeboro otic solution (aluminum acetate).

Sodium sulfacetamide drops or ointment may be effective for seborrheic blepharitis. Oral tetracyclines can also be effective and have been shown to decrease the density of microorganisms in the affected follicles. Steroid preparations are suitable for short-term use but may induce glaucoma and cataracts. Daily gentle cleansing with a cotton-tipped applicator and baby shampoo in water can reduce symptoms. In severe cases, oral antibiotics or oral antifungals may be combined with topical agents. Low-dose isotretinoin has also been shown to be effective in refractory disease.

An Q, et al: High *Staphylococcus epidermidis* colonization and impaired permeability barrier in facial seborrheic dermatitis. Chin Med J (Engl) 2017; 130: 1662.

Balighi K, et al: Hydrocortisone 1% cream and sertaconazole 2% cream to treat facial seborrheic dermatitis. Int J Womens Dermatol 2016; 3: 107.

de Souza Leão Kamamoto C, et al: Low-dose oral isotretinoin for moderate to severe seborrhea and seborrheic dermatitis. Int J Dermatol 2017; 56: 80.

Gupta AK, et al: Topical treatment of facial seborrheic dermatitis. Am J Clin Dermatol 2017; 18: 193.

Kastarinen H, et al: Topical anti-inflammatory agents for seborrhoeic dermatitis of the face or scalp. Cochrane Database Syst Rev 2014; 5: CD009446.

PSORIASIS

Clinical Features

Psoriasis is a common, chronic, and recurrent inflammatory disease of the skin characterized by circumscribed, erythematous, dry, scaling plaques of various sizes, usually covered by silvery white lamellar scales. The lesions are usually symmetrically distributed and have a predilection for the scalp, nails, extensor surfaces of the limbs, umbilical region, and sacrum. It usually develops slowly but may be exanthematous, with the sudden onset of numerous guttate (droplike) lesions (Fig. 10.2). Subjective symptoms, such as itching or burning, may be present and may cause extreme discomfort.

The early lesions are small, erythematous macules covered with dry, silvery scales from the onset. The lesions increase in size by peripheral extension and coalescence. The scales are micaceous, meaning they peel in layers, and are looser toward the periphery and adherent centrally. When removed, bleeding points appear (Auspitz sign). Although plaques typically predominate, lesions may be annular or polycyclic. Old patches may be thick and covered with tough lamellar scales like the outside of an oyster shell (psoriasis ostracea). Descriptive terms applied to the diverse appearance of the lesions include psoriasis *guttata*, in which the lesions are the size of water drops; psoriasis *follicularis*, in which tiny, scaly lesions are located at the orifices of hair follicles; psoriasis *figurata*, *annulata*, or *gyrata*, in which curved linear patterns are produced by central involution; psoriasis *discoidea*, in which central involution does not occur and solid patches persist; and psoriasis *rupioides*, in which crusted lesions occur, resembling syphilitic rupia. The term *chronic plaque psoriasis* is often applied to stable lesions of the trunk and extremities. Inverse psoriasis predominates in intertriginous areas (Fig. 10.3). Pustular variants of psoriasis may be chronic on the palms and soles (Fig. 10.4),

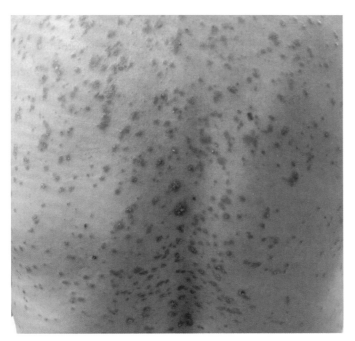

Fig. 10.2 Guttate psoriasis.

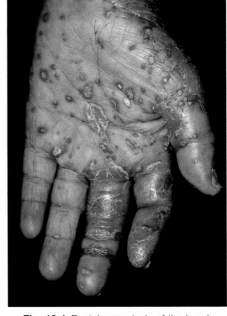

Fig. 10.4 Pustular psoriasis of the hand.

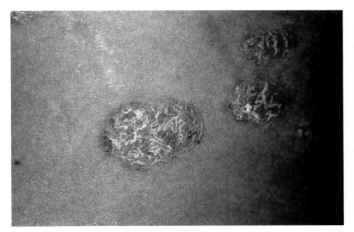

Fig. 10.3 Psoriasis.

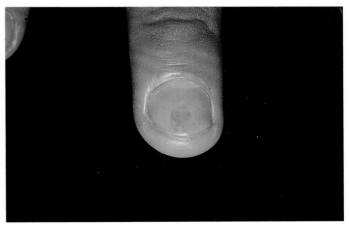

Fig. 10.5 Nail with oil spot of psoriasis.

or these may be eruptive and accompanied by severe toxicity and hypocalcemia.

Involved nails can demonstrate distal onycholysis, random pitting caused by parakeratosis from the proximal matrix (Fig. 10.5), oil spots (yellow areas of subungual parakeratosis from the distal matrix; Fig. 10.6), or salmon patches (nail bed psoriasis). Thick, subungual hyperkeratosis may resemble onychomycosis.

Types

Seborrheic-Like Psoriasis

Some cases of psoriasis overlap with seborrheic dermatitis. Seborrheic lesions may predominate on the face, under the breasts, and in the scalp, flexures, and axillae. Lesions in these areas are moist and erythematous, with yellow, greasy, soft scales, rather than dry and micaceous scales. Terms such as sebopsoriasis and seborrhiasis may be used to describe the condition of such patients.

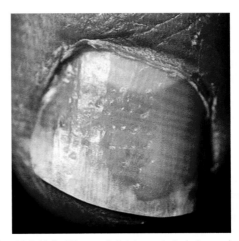

Fig. 10.6 Nail pitting and distal onycholysis in psoriasis.

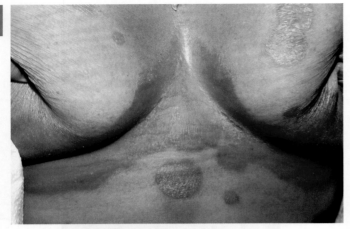

Fig. 10.7 Inverse psoriasis. (Courtesy Steven Binnick, MD.)

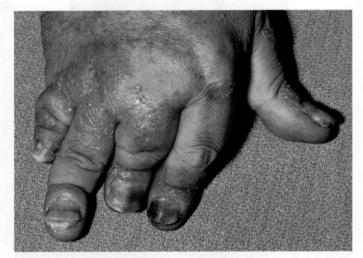

Fig. 10.8 Psoriatic arthritis.

Inverse Psoriasis

Inverse psoriasis selectively and often exclusively involves folds, recesses, and flexor surfaces, such as the ears, axillae, groin, inframammary folds (Fig. 10.7), navel, intergluteal crease, penis, lips, and web spaces. Other areas, such as the scalp and nails, may be involved.

"Napkin" Psoriasis

Napkin psoriasis, or psoriasis in the diaper area, is characteristically seen in infants between 2 and 8 months of age. Lesions appear as brightly erythematous, sharply demarcated patches of skin involving much of the diaper area. The lesions typically clear with topical therapy, but psoriasis may reappear in adulthood.

Psoriatic Arthritis

Five clinical patterns of psoriatic arthritis occur, as follows:

1. Asymmetric distal interphalangeal joint involvement with nail damage (16%)
2. Arthritis mutilans with osteolysis of phalanges and metacarpals (5%) (Fig. 10.8)
3. Symmetric polyarthritis-like rheumatoid arthritis (RA), with clawhand (15%)
4. Oligoarthritis with swelling and tenosynovitis of one or a few hand joints (70%)
5. Ankylosing spondylitis alone or with peripheral arthritis (5%)

Most radiographic findings resemble those in RA, but certain findings are highly suggestive of psoriasis. These include erosion of terminal phalangeal tufts (acrosteolysis), tapering or "whittling" of phalanges or metacarpals with "cupping" of proximal ends of phalanges ("pencil in a cup deformity"), bony ankylosis, osteolysis of metatarsals, predilection for distal interphalangeal and proximal interphalangeal joints, relative sparing of metacarpophalangeal and metatarsophalangeal joints, paravertebral ossification, asymmetric sacroiliitis, and rarity of "bamboo spine" when the spine is involved. Almost half the patients with psoriatic arthritis have type human leukocyte antigen (HLA)–B27.

Rest, splinting, passive motion, and nonsteroidal antiinflammatory drugs (NSAIDs) may provide symptomatic relief but do not prevent deformity. Methotrexate, cyclosporine, tacrolimus, anti-TNF, anti-IL-17 and anti-IL-12/23 agents are disease-modifying drugs that prevent deformity.

Guttate Psoriasis

In the distinctive guttate form of psoriasis, typical lesions are the size of water drops, 2–5 mm in diameter. Lesions typically occur as an abrupt eruption after acute infection, such as a streptococcal pharyngitis. Guttate psoriasis occurs mostly in patients under age 30. This type of psoriasis usually responds rapidly to broad-band ultraviolet B (UVB) at erythemogenic doses. Suberythemogenic doses often have little impact on the lesions. This is one of the few forms of psoriasis where broad-band UVB may have an advantage over narrow-band (NB) UVB. Minimal erythemogenic (erythema) dose (MED) testing is recommended to allow for appropriately aggressive treatment. Recurrent episodes may be related to pharyngeal carriage of the responsible streptococcus by the patient or a close contact. A course of a semisynthetic penicillin (e.g., dicloxacillin, 250 mg four times daily for 10 days) with rifampin (600 mg/day for adults) may be required to clear chronic streptococcal carriage.

Generalized Pustular Psoriasis (von Zumbusch Psoriasis)

Typical patients with generalized pustular psoriasis have plaque psoriasis and often psoriatic arthritis. The onset is sudden, with formation of lakes of pus periungually, on the palms, and at the edge of psoriatic plaques. Erythema occurs in the flexures before the generalized eruption appears. This is followed by a generalized erythema and more pustules (Fig. 10.9). Pruritus and intense burning are often present. Mucous membrane lesions are common. The lips may be red and scaly, and superficial ulcerations of the tongue and mouth occur. Geographic or fissured tongue frequently occurs (Fig. 10.10).

The patient is frequently ill with fever, erythroderma, hypocalcemia, and cachexia. A number of cases of acute respiratory distress syndrome associated with pustular and erythrodermic psoriasis have been reported. Other systemic complications include pneumonia, congestive heart failure, and hepatitis.

Episodes are often provoked by withdrawal of systemic corticosteroids. The authors have also observed generalized pustular psoriasis as the presenting sign of Cushing disease. Other implicated drugs include iodides, coal tar, terbinafine, minocycline, hydroxychloroquine, acetazolamide, and salicylates. There is usually a strong familial history of psoriasis. Generalized pustular psoriasis may occur in infants and children with no implicated drug. It may also occur as an episodic event punctuating the course of localized acral pustular psoriasis.

Acitretin is the drug of choice in this severe disease. The response is generally rapid. Isotretinoin is also effective. Cyclosporine,

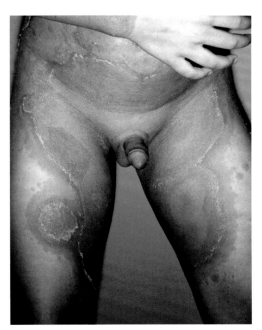

Fig. 10.9 Pustular psoriasis.

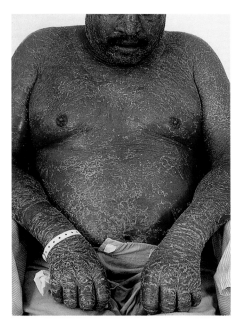

Fig. 10.11 Erythrodermic psoriasis.

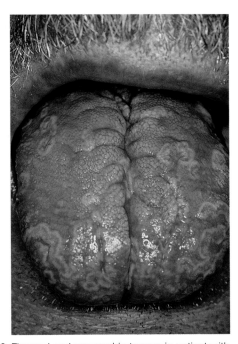

Fig. 10.10 Fissured and geographic tongue in patient with generalized pustular psoriasis.

methotrexate, and biologic agents are alternatives. In some cases, dapsone is effective in doses of 50–100 mg/day.

Acrodermatitis Continua (of Hallopeau)

Typical patients develop acral erythematous plaques studded with pustules. The nail beds are heavily involved, and the fingernails float away on lakes of pus, resulting in anonychia. Hyperkeratosis often ensues, and the fingertips become increasingly painful, tapering to long, keratotic points. Occasionally, patients may develop generalized pustular flares. Acrodermatitis continua is discussed

in more detail later (see Dermatitis Repens under Recalcitrant Palmoplantar Eruptions, later in this chapter).

Impetigo Herpetiformis

The term *impetigo herpetiformis* has been applied to pustular psoriasis of pregnancy. Flexural erythema, studded with pustules, often occurs initially, followed by a generalized pustular flare and increasing toxicity. These patients are pregnant, so systemic retinoids are not appropriate. Many patients only respond to delivery, and early delivery should be strongly considered as soon as it is safe for the infant. Alternatively, patients may respond to prednisone, 1 mg/kg/day. The corticosteroid can also contribute to neonatal lung maturity.

Keratoderma Blennorrhagicum (Reiter Syndrome)

Keratoderma blennorrhagicum resembles psoriasis both histologically and clinically, except for its tendency for thicker keratotic lesions. Patients are often positive for HLA-B27 and develop reactive arthritis and skin disease after a bout of urethritis or enteritis.

Erythrodermic Psoriasis

Patients with psoriasis may develop a generalized erythroderma (Fig. 10.11). Erythrodermic psoriasis is covered in greater detail in Chapter 11 under Exfoliative Dermatitis.

Course

The course of psoriasis is unpredictable. It usually begins on the scalp or elbows and may remain localized in the original region for years. Chronic disease may also be almost entirely limited to the fingernails. Involvement over the sacrum may easily be confused with candidiasis or tinea. Onset may also be sudden and widespread.

Two of the chief features of psoriasis are its tendency to recur and its persistence. The isomorphic response (Koebner phenomenon) is the appearance of typical lesions of psoriasis at sites of even trivial injury (Fig. 10.12). Lesions may occur at sites of

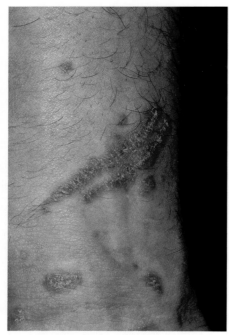

Fig. 10.12 Koebner phenomenon in psoriasis.

scratches, incisions, and burns. Lesions may first appear after viral exanthema or pityriasis rosea. The isomorphic response may occur if psoriatic lesions are severely burned during phototherapy. With a reduction in light dosage, the erythema and burning resolve, and the plaques begin to clear. Woronoff ring is concentric blanching of the erythematous skin at or near the periphery of a healing psoriatic plaque. It is often the first sign that the patient's psoriasis is responding to phototherapy.

The palms and soles are sometimes exclusively affected, showing discrete, dry, erythematous scaling patches, circumscribed verrucous thickenings, or pustules on an erythematous base. The patches usually begin in the midportion of the palms or on the soles and gradually expand. Psoriasis of the palms and soles is typically chronic and extremely resistant to treatment.

Many studies report an association between hepatitis C and psoriasis, and hepatitis C virus (HCV) has also been implicated in psoriatic arthritis. If treatment of psoriasis is to include a potentially hepatotoxic drug, such as methotrexate, a full hepatitis panel should be obtained. Also, IFN treatment of the hepatitis can further exacerbate or induce psoriasis. Anti–tumor necrosis factor (TNF)–α therapy shows promise in the treatment of psoriasis, even in the setting of chronic HCV infection.

Inheritance

In a large study of psoriasis in monozygotic twins, heritability was high and environmental influence low. Patients with psoriasis often have relatives with the disease, and the incidence typically increases in successive generations. Multifactorial inheritance is likely. Analysis of population-specific HLA haplotypes has provided evidence that susceptibility to psoriasis is linked to major histocompatibility complex (MHC) classes I and II on human chromosome 6. A number of genetic loci are linked to psoriasis, including *PSORS1* on chromosome 6 and within the MHC, and *PSORS2* on chromosome 17q. Also, there are two subsets that differ in age of onset and frequency of HLA associations. Early onset is type I psoriasis and is associated mostly with Cw6, B57, and DR7. Late onset is type II and predominantly features Cw2. *PSORS9* has also been confirmed as a susceptibility locus for psoriasis.

A variety of other HLA associations have been reported. It is believed that any individual who has B13 or B17 carries a fivefold risk of developing psoriasis. In pustular psoriasis, HLA-B27 may be seen, whereas B13 and B17 are increased in guttate and erythrodermic psoriasis. In palmoplantar pustulosis, there is an association with HLA-B8, Bw35, Cw7, and DR3. HLA typing is a research tool for population-based studies, but of limited value in assessing an individual patient.

Epidemiology

Psoriasis occurs with equal frequency in men and women. Between 1% and 2% of the U.S. population has psoriasis. It occurs less frequently in the tropics. It is less common in North American and West African black persons. Native (Indian) Americans and native Fijians rarely have psoriasis. The onset of psoriasis is at a mean age of 27 years, but the range is wide, from the neonatal period to the seventies. Severe emotional stress tends to aggravate psoriasis in almost half of those studied.

In pregnancy, there is a distinct tendency for improvement or even temporary disappearance of lesions in the majority of women studied. After childbirth, there is a tendency for exacerbation of lesions. Paradoxically, pregnancy is also the milieu for impetigo herpetiformis, and psoriasis may behave differently from one pregnancy to another in the same patient.

A high prevalence of celiac disease has been noted in patients with psoriasis. Lymphoma also has an increased incidence in these patients, and psoriasis has been linked to the metabolic syndrome and a higher risk of cardiovascular disease, although early age of onset does not appear to correlate with greater risk. Patients should be screened for comorbidities.

Pathogenesis

Psoriasis is a hyperproliferative disorder, but the proliferation is driven by a complex cascade of inflammatory mediators. Psoriasis appears to represent a mixed T-helper 1 (Th1) and Th17 inflammatory disease. Th17 cells appear to be more proximal in the inflammatory cascade. T cells and cytokines play pivotal roles in the pathophysiology of psoriasis. Overexpression of type 1 cytokines, such as IL-2, IL-6, IL-8, IL-12, IFN-γ, and TNF-α, has been demonstrated, and overexpression of IL-8 leads to the accumulation of neutrophils. The main signal for Th1 development is IL-12, which promotes intracellular IFN-γ production. In animal models, shifting from Th1 to Th2 responses improves psoriasis. IL-4 is capable of inducing Th2 responses and improving psoriasis. Reduced expression of the antiinflammatory cytokines IL-1RA and IL-10 has been found, and polymorphisms for IL-10 genes correlate with psoriasis. IL-10 is a type 2 cytokine with major influence on immunoregulation, inhibiting type 1 proinflammatory cytokine production. Patients receiving established traditional therapies show rising levels of IL-10 messenger RNA expression, suggesting that IL-10 may have antipsoriatic capacity.

IL-15 triggers inflammatory cell recruitment, angiogenesis, and production of inflammatory cytokines, including IFN-γ, TNF-α, and IL-17, all of which are upregulated in psoriatic lesions. The interplay is complex, but IL-17 appears to be proinflammatory, and IL-22 may serve to retard keratinocyte differentiation. IL-23 stimulates survival, as well as proliferation of Th17 cells. Circulating NK cells are reduced in psoriasis.

Streptococci

Streptococci play a role in some patients. Patients with psoriasis report sore throat more often than controls. β-Hemolytic streptococci of Lancefield groups A, C, and G can cause exacerbation of chronic plaque psoriasis. Th1 cells recognize cell wall extract

CHAPTER 10 Seborrheic Dermatitis, Psoriasis, Recalcitrant Palmoplantar Eruptions, Pustular Dermatitis, and Erythroderma **197**

10

isolated from group A streptococci. HLA variation has a significant effect on the immune response to group A streptococci.

Stress

Various studies have shown a positive correlation between stress and severity of disease. In almost half of patients studied, stress appears to play a significant role.

Drug-Induced Psoriasis

Psoriasis may be induced by β-blockers, lithium, antimalarials, terbinafine, calcium channel blockers, captopril, glyburide, granulocyte colony-stimulating factor, interleukins, interferons, and lipid-lowering drugs. Systemic steroids may cause rebound or pustular flares. Antimalarials are associated with erythrodermic flares, but patients traveling to malaria-endemic regions should take appropriate prophylaxis. Often, drugs such as doxycycline or mefloquine are appropriate for the geographic area, but when a quinine derivative offers the best protection, it is generally better to take the prophylactic doses of a quinine derivative than to risk disease and full-dose treatment.

Pathology

Histologically, all psoriasis is pustular. The microscopic pustules include spongiform intraepidermal pustules, and Munro microabscesses within the stratum corneum. In early guttate lesions, focal parakeratosis is noted within the stratum corneum. The parakeratotic focus typically has an outline resembling a seagull. Neutrophils are generally noted immediately above the focus of parakeratosis, but in some sections the neutrophils will not be visible as a result of sampling error. In plaque psoriasis, neutrophilic foci are so numerous that they are rarely missed. Neutrophilic microabscesses are generally present at multiple levels in the stratum corneum, usually on top of small foci of parakeratosis. These foci generally alternate with areas of orthokeratotic stratum corneum, suggesting that the underlying spongiform pustules arise in a rhythmic fashion. The granular layer is absent focally, corresponding to areas producing foci of parakeratosis. In well-developed plaques, there is regular epidermal acanthosis with long, bulbous rete ridges, thinning over the dermal papillae, and dilated capillaries within the dermal papillae. The last two findings correlate with the Auspitz sign. The stratum corneum may be entirely parakeratotic but still shows multiple small, neutrophilic microabscesses at varying levels. Spongiosis is typically scant, except in the area immediately surrounding collections of neutrophils.

In pustular psoriasis, geographic tongue, and Reiter syndrome, intraepidermal spongiform pustules tend to be much larger. Grossly pustular lesions often have little associated acanthosis. In Reiter syndrome, the stratum corneum is often massively thickened, with prominent foci of neutrophils above parakeratosis, alternating with orthokeratosis.

Acral lesions often demonstrate nondiagnostic features histologically. Spongiosis is typically prominent in these lesions and often leads to a differential diagnosis of psoriasis or chronic psoriasiform spongiotic dermatitis. Foci of neutrophils often contain serum and may be interpreted as impetiginized crusting.

On direct immunofluorescence testing, the stratum corneum demonstrates intense fluorescence with all antibodies, complement, and fibrin. This fluorescence is independent of the fluorescent label, as it has been noted in hematoxylin and eosin–stained sections and frozen unstained sections. The same phenomenon of stratum corneum autofluorescence has been noted in some cases of candidiasis that demonstrate a psoriasiform histology.

Psoriasis can generally be distinguished from dermatitis by the paucity of edema, relative absence of spongiosis, tortuosity of the capillary loops, and presence of neutrophils above foci of parakeratosis. Neutrophils in the stratum corneum are often seen in tinea, impetigo, candidiasis, and syphilis, but they rarely are found atop parakeratosis alternating with orthokeratosis rhythmically. In psoriasiform syphilis, the rete ridges are typically long and slender; a vacuolar interface dermatitis is usually present; dermal blood vessels appear to have no lumen because of endothelial swelling; and plasma cells are present in the dermal infiltrate. About one third of biopsies of syphilis lack plasma cells, but the remaining characteristics still suggest the correct diagnosis. Psoriasiform lesions of mycosis fungoides exhibit epidermotropism of large lymphocytes with little spongiosis. The lymphocytes are typically larger, darker, and more angulated than the lymphocytes in the dermis. There is associated papillary dermal fibrosis, and the superficial perivascular infiltrate is asymmetrically distributed around the postcapillary venules, favoring the epidermal side ("bare underbelly sign").

Clinical Differential Diagnosis

Psoriasis must be differentiated from dermatomyositis (DM), lupus erythematosus (LE), seborrheic dermatitis, pityriasis rosea, lichen planus, eczema, and psoriasiform syphilid. The distribution in psoriasis is on the extensor surfaces, especially of the elbows and knees, and on the scalp; DM shares this distribution, whereas LE generally lacks involvement of the extensor surfaces. Patients with DM may exhibit a heliotrope sign, atrophy, poikiloderma, and nailfold changes. Advanced lesions of discoid LE often demonstrate follicular hyperkeratosis (carpet tack sign). Seborrheic dermatitis has a predilection for the eyebrows, nasolabial angle, ears, sternal region, and flexures. The scales in psoriasis are dry, white, and shiny, whereas those in seborrheic dermatitis are greasy and yellowish. On removal of the scales in psoriasis, blood oozes from the capillaries (Auspitz sign), whereas this does not occur in seborrheic dermatitis.

In pityriasis rosea, the eruption is located on the upper arms, trunk, and thighs, and the duration is over weeks. Lesions are typically oval and follow skin tension lines. Individual lesions show a crinkling of the epidermis and collarette scaling. A herald patch is frequently noted. Lichen planus chiefly affects the flexor surfaces of the wrists and ankles. Often the violaceous color is pronounced. In darker-skinned individuals, the lesions have a tendency to pronounced hyperpigmentation. The nails are not pitted as in psoriasis, but longitudinally ridged, rough, and thickened. Pterygium formation is characteristic of lichen planus.

Hand eczema may resemble psoriasis. In general, psoriatic lesions tend to be more sharply marginated, but at times the lesions are indistinguishable. Psoriasiform syphilid has infiltrated copper-colored papules, often arranged in a figurate pattern. Serologic tests for syphilis are generally positive, but prozone reactions may occur, and the serum may have to be diluted to obtain a positive test. Generalized lymphadenopathy and mucous patches may be present.

Treatment

Topical therapy, intralesional triamcinolone, excimer laser, light emitting diode (LED), and other forms of focused light may be suitable for limited plaques. Phototherapy remains highly cost-effective for widespread psoriasis. Cyclosporine has a rapid onset of action but is generally not suitable for sustained therapy. Methotrexate remains the systemic agent against which others are compared. Biologic agents can produce dramatic responses at dramatic expense.

Topical Treatment

Corticosteroids. Topical application of corticosteroids in creams, ointments, lotions, foams, and sprays is the most frequently prescribed therapy for localized psoriasis. Class I steroids are suitable for 2-week courses of therapy on most body areas. Therapy can be continued with pulse applications on weekends to reduce the incidence of local adverse effects. On the scalp, corticosteroids in propylene glycol, gel, foam, and spray bases are preferred by most white patients. Black patients may find them drying and may prefer oil and ointment preparations. Low- to medium-strength creams are preferred in the intertriginous areas and on the face. To augment effectiveness of topical corticosteroids in areas with thick keratotic scale, the area should be hydrated before application and covered with an occlusive dressing of polyethylene film (plastic wrap) or a sauna suit. Side effects include epidermal atrophy, steroid acne, miliaria, and pyoderma.

Intralesional injections of triamcinolone are helpful for refractory plaques. Triamcinolone acetonide (Kenalog) suspension, 10 mg/mL, may be diluted with sterile saline to make a concentration of 2.5–5 mg/mL. Good results are also obtained in the treatment of psoriatic nails by injecting triamcinolone into the region of the matrix and the lateral nailfold. A digital block can be performed before injection to provide anesthesia. Injections are given once a month until the desired effect is achieved.

Tars. Crude coal tar and tar extracts such as liquor carbonis detergens (LCD) can be compounded into agents for topical use. Tar bath oils and shampoos are readily available. Oil of cade (pine tar) or birch tar in concentrations of 5%–10% may also be incorporated into ointments. The odor of all tars may be offensive, and relapse is more rapid than with topical agents such as calcipotriene.

Anthralin. Anthralin is effective but is irritating and stains skin, clothing, and bedding. To avoid these drawbacks, short-contact anthralin treatment (SCAT) can be helpful, with anthralin washed off after 15–30 minutes. Anthralin exerts a direct effect on keratinocytes and leukocytes by suppressing neutrophil superoxide generation and inhibiting monocyte-derived IL-6, IL-8, and TNF-α.

Tazarotene. Tazarotene is a nonisomerizable retinoic acid receptor–specific retinoid. It appears to treat psoriasis by modulating keratinocyte differentiation and hyperproliferation, as well as by suppressing inflammation. Combining its use with a topical corticosteroid and weekend pulse therapy can decrease irritation.

Calcipotriene. Vitamin D_3 affects keratinocyte differentiation partly through its regulation of epidermal responsiveness to calcium. Treatment with the vitamin D analog calcipotriene (Dovonex) in ointment, cream, or solution form has been effective in the treatment of plaque-type and scalp psoriasis. Combination therapy with calcipotriene and high-potency steroids may provide greater response rates, fewer side effects, and steroid sparing. Calcipotriene is unstable in the presence of many other topical agents and degrades in the presence of UV light. Monitoring of serum calcium levels in adults is not required. Calcipotriene plus betamethasone dipropionate is more effective than either agent alone.

Macrolactams (Calcineurin Inhibitors). Topical macrolactams such as tacrolimus and pimecrolimus are especially helpful for thin lesions in areas prone to atrophy or steroid acne. The burning associated with these agents can be problematic but may be avoided by prior corticosteroid treatment and application to dry skin rather than after bathing.

Salicylic Acid. Salicylic acid is used as a keratolytic agent in shampoos, creams, and gels. It can promote the absorption of other topical agents. Widespread application may lead to salicylate toxicity, manifesting with tinnitus, acute confusion, and refractory hypoglycemia, especially in patients with diabetes and those with compromised renal function.

Ultraviolet Light. Phototherapy is a cost-effective and underused modality for psoriasis. In most cases, sunlight improves psoriasis. However, severe burning of the skin may cause the Koebner phenomenon and an exacerbation. Artificial UVB light is produced by fluorescent bulbs in broad-band or NB spectrum. Maximal effect is usually achieved at MEDs. Although suberythemogenic doses can be effective, the response is slower than with erythemogenic regimens. With treatment, a tanning response occurs, and the dose must be increased to maintain efficacy. Maintenance UVB phototherapy after clearing contributes to the duration of remission and is justified for many patients.

Using a monochromator, it has been shown that wavelengths of 254, 280, and 290 nm are ineffective; at 296, 300, 304, and 313 nm, however, there is clearing. NB UVB (peak emission about 311 nm) is now widely available.

Goeckerman Technique. Goeckerman therapy remains an effective and cost-effective method of treatment even in patients with poor responses to biologic agents. In its modern form, a 2%–5% tar preparation is applied to the skin, and a tar bath is taken at least once a day. The excess tar is removed with mineral or vegetable oil, and UV light is given. In psoriasis day care centers, patients clear in an average of 18 days, and 75% remain free of disease for extended periods. The addition of a topical corticosteroid to the Goeckerman regimen shortens the time required for remission. Phototoxic reactions (tar smarts) may result from UVA generated by the predominantly UVB bulbs.

Ingram Technique. Ingram therapy consists of a daily coal tar bath in a solution such as 120 mL LCD to 80 L of warm water. This is followed by daily exposure to UV light for increasing periods. An anthralin paste is then applied to each psoriatic plaque. Talcum powder is sprinkled over the lesions, and stockinette dressings are applied. Modern versions of the technique employ SCAT.

PUVA Therapy. High-intensity longwave UV radiation (UVA) given 2 hours after ingestion of 8-methoxypsoralen (Oxsoralen-Ultra), twice a week, is highly effective, even in severe psoriasis. Most patients clear in 20–25 treatments, but maintenance treatment is needed.

Although PUVA therapy is highly effective, in patients with less than 50% of the skin surface affected, UVB may be as effective. Polyethylene sheet bath PUVA is another therapeutic alternative to oral psoralen–UVA. The patient is immersed in a psoralen solution contained in plastic sheeting that conforms to the patient's body.

Oral psoralen can produce cataracts, and protective eyewear must be used. PUVA therapy is a risk factor for skin cancer, including squamous cell carcinoma (SCC) and melanoma. Arsenic exposure is a more significant cofactor than prior exposure to methotrexate, UVB, or concomitant use of topical tar. Men treated without genital protection are at an increased risk of developing SCC of the penis and scrotum. Although the risk of cancer is dose related, there is no definitive threshold dose of cumulative PUVA exposure above which carcinogenicity can be predicted.

Surgical Treatment

In patients with pharyngeal colonization by streptococci, an excellent response has been reported after tonsillectomy. More effective antibiotic regimens, such as a 10-day course of dicloxacillin combined with rifampin (600 mg/day for adult), have largely replaced tonsillectomy.

Hyperthermia

Local hyperthermia can clear psoriatic plaques, but relapse is usually rapid. Microwave hyperthermia may produce significant complications, such as pain over bony prominences and tissue destruction.

Occlusive Treatment

Occlusion with surgical tape or dressings can be effective as monotherapy or when combined with topical drugs.

Systemic Treatment

Corticosteroids. The hazards of the injudicious use of systemic corticosteroids must be emphasized. There is great risk of "rebound" or induction of pustular psoriasis when therapy is stopped. Corticosteroid use is generally restricted to unique circumstances, such as impetigo herpetiformis when expeditious delivery is not possible.

Methotrexate. This folic acid antagonist remains the standard against which other systemic treatments are measured. Methotrexate has a greater affinity for dihydrofolic acid reductase than does folic acid. The indications for methotrexate include psoriatic erythroderma, psoriatic arthritis, acute pustular psoriasis (von Zumbusch type), or widespread body surface area (BSA) involvement. Localized pustular psoriasis or palmoplantar psoriasis that impairs normal function and employment may also require systemic treatment.

It is important to ensure the patient has no history of liver or kidney disease. Methotrexate can be toxic to the liver, and decreased renal clearance can enhance toxicity. Other important factors to consider are alcohol abuse, cryptogenic cirrhosis, severe illness, debility, pregnancy, leukopenia, thrombocytopenia, active infectious disease, immunodeficiency, anemia, colitis, and ability to comply with directions. Hepatic enzymes, bilirubin, serum albumin, creatinine, alkaline phosphatase, complete blood count, platelet count, hepatitis serology (B and C), HIV antibody, a test for tuberculosis, and urinalysis should all be evaluated before starting treatment. Patients with hypoalbuminemia have a higher risk of developing pulmonary complications.

The need for liver biopsy remains controversial. Biopsy is not without risks and is not usually performed in the setting of methotrexate therapy for rheumatic disease. However, patients with psoriasis have a greater risk of liver disease than other patient populations. Weekly blood counts and monthly liver enzyme assessment are recommended at the onset of therapy or when the dosage is changed, but hepatitis fibrosis can occur without elevations in liver enzymes. Monitoring of aminoterminal procollagen III peptide may reduce or eliminate the need for liver biopsy.

Numerous treatment schedules have evolved, and the liquid for injection may be dosed orally in orange juice as a less expensive alternative to pills. The authors recommend either three divided oral doses (12 hours apart) weekly, weekly single doses orally, or single weekly subcutaneous injections. The weekly dose varies from 5 mg to more than 50 mg, with most patients requiring 15–30 mg a week. Once a single dose exceeds 25 mg, oral absorption is unpredictable, and subcutaneous injections are recommended. Midweek doses can result in severe toxicity and must be avoided. Oral or cutaneous ulceration may be a sign that the patient has taken a midweek dose. Oral folic acid has been reported to decrease side effects, especially nausea, and doses of 1–4 mg/day are used. Oral folic acid is not adequate for the treatment of overdosage, and leukovorin must be used in such cases.

Cyclosporine. The therapeutic benefit of cyclosporine in psoriatic disease may be related to downmodulation of proinflammatory epidermal cytokines. The microemulsion formulation Neoral has greater bioavailability and is now standard. Doses of 2–5 mg/kg/day generally produce rapid clearing of psoriasis, with both efficacy

and risk being dose related. Unfortunately, the lesions recur rapidly as well, and transition to another form of therapy is required. Treatment durations of up to 6 months are associated with a low incidence of renal complications, but blood pressure and serum creatinine must be monitored and doses adjusted accordingly. Usually, the dose is reduced if the baseline creatinine increases by one third. Some data support the feasibility of pulse dosing for a few days each week for both the induction and the maintenance of response in psoriasis patients.

Diet. The antiinflammatory effects of fish oils rich in n-3 polyunsaturated fatty acids (PUFAs) have been demonstrated in RA, inflammatory bowel disease, psoriasis, and asthma. The n-3 and n-6 PUFAs affect a variety of cytokines, including IL-1, IL-6, and TNF. Herbal remedies have also been used with variable effects. Many of these products are unpalatable, and their efficacy does not compare favorably to pharmacologic agents.

Oral Antimicrobial Therapy. The association of streptococcal pharyngitis with guttate psoriasis is well established. *Staphylococcus aureus* and streptococci secrete exotoxins that act as superantigens, producing massive T-cell activation, and pharyngeal colonization should be addressed as previously noted. Oral bile acid supplementation has been shown to improve psoriasis, presumably by affecting the microflora and endotoxins in the gut. Oral ketoconazole, itraconazole, and other antibiotics have shown efficacy in a limited number of patients with psoriasis.

Retinoids. Oral treatment with the aromatic retinoid ethylester etretinate has been effective in many patients with psoriasis, especially in pustular disease. Because of its long half-life, etretinate has been replaced by acitretin. Alcohol ingestion can convert acitretin to etretinate and is discouraged. 13-*Cis*-retinoic acid can also produce good results in some patients with pustular psoriasis. All these drugs are potent teratogens, and elevated triglyceride levels may complicate therapy. Combinations of retinoic acids with photochemotherapy can be effective in chronic plaque psoriasis, resulting in lowered cumulative doses of light.

Dapsone. Dapsone use is limited largely to palmoplantar pustulosis or other variants of pustular psoriasis. Even in this setting, it is a second- or third-line agent with limited efficacy.

Biologic Agents

A number of biologic agents are available that can produce dramatic responses in some patients with psoriasis; all are expensive. Retrospective analysis using BSA multiplied by physician's global assessment as an endpoint suggests that outcomes with biologic agents are superior to those with other systemic agents, despite the patients taking biologics having a higher baseline severity and a greater number of previous treatments.

Several agents block TNF-α. Infliximab is a chimeric monoclonal antibody (mAb) to TNF-α and requires intravenous infusion; etanercept is a fusion protein of human TNF type II receptor and the Fc region of immunoglobulin (Ig)G1; and adalimumab is a recombinant, fully human IgG1 mAb to TNF-α. Alefacept is a fusion protein of the external domain of LFA-3 and the Fc region of IgG1; it blocks T-cell activation and triggers apoptosis of pathogenic T cells, but was withdrawn from the market in the United States. Golimumab is an anti-TNF agent with less frequent dosing used in patients with psoriatic arthritis, and certolizumab has also demonstrated efficacy. Ustekinumab, a human mAb against IL-12 and IL-23, blocks the inflammatory pathway at a more proximal point than anti-TNF agents. Guselkumab is an IL-23 receptor monoclonal antibody. Ixekizumab and secukinumab are IL-17A antagonists. Brodalumab is a human, anti–IL-17RA monoclonal antibody.

Percentage of Patients Clearing With Each Drug. Published data allow for some comparisons of biologic agents, but the endpoints of some trials differ. Newer anti–IL-17 and anti-IL-23 agents can achieve PASI 100 in some patients, a dramatic improvement over previous biologic agents. The anti–IL-17 agents include secukinumab, ixekizumab, and brodalumab. A meta-analysis of published trials of the older biologics suggested that of the agents studied at the end of the induction phase (week 24), ustekinumab had the greatest probability of achieving at least 75% improvement from baseline in the psoriasis area and severity index (PASI 75), followed by infliximab, adalimumab, and etanercept. The percentage of patients reaching PASI 75 at week 10 is about 70% with infliximab at 3 mg/kg and 90% at 5 mg/kg, compared with 6% for placebo. About 35% of patients receiving etanercept, 25 mg subcutaneously twice weekly, achieve PASI 75 at 12 weeks and 45% at 24 weeks. With the 50-mg induction dose administered twice a week, about 46% of patients achieve PASI 75 at 12 weeks and 50% at 24 weeks. The data available suggest that about 53% of patients taking 40 mg of adalimumab every other week achieve PASI 75 by week 12, and about 80% of those taking 40 mg a week achieve PASI 75.

Risks. Anti-TNF agents are contraindicated with demyelinating disease and anti-IL-17 agents are contraindicated with inflammatory bowel disease. The anti-TNF agents may induce flares of psoriasis through upregulation of plasmacytoid dendritic cells. This may be a class effect. The biologic agents all suppress the normal immune response. Infliximab has been associated with reactivation of tuberculosis, demyelinating disease, and serious systemic opportunistic infection. Infliximab may also lose its effect because of neutralizing antibodies. Methotrexate or azathioprine may be needed as concomitant therapy to reduce the incidence of neutralizing antibodies and infusion reactions. Even though adalimumab is a fully human antibody, it may also induce an antibody response. Serious infections have been reported in RA patients treated with this agent. Etanercept has been associated with infection, onset, or exacerbation of multiple sclerosis, vasculitis, and LE-like manifestations. All these effects are rare and may not be statistically increased from the general population. Many of the reported complications, such as lymphoma, demyelinating disease, progressive multifocal leukoencephalopathy and infection, are not unique to any one immunosuppressive agent.

The National Psoriasis Foundation has endorsed a recommendation that all patients be screened for latent tuberculosis infection before any immunologic therapy. The Foundation recommends delaying immunologic therapy until prophylaxis for latent tuberculosis infection is completed, although noting that patients with severe disease may be treated after 1–2 months of prophylaxis. IFN-γ assays have greater specificity than tuberculin skin tests and are being used along with imaging studies to confirm tuberculosis in patients with positive skin tests.

Phosphodiesterase Inhibitors

Apremilast, a small molecule specific inhibitor of phosphodiesterase 4, has demonstrated efficacy in recalcitrant plaque psoriasis. It is also indicated for psoriatic arthritis. Diarrhea is the most common adverse effect. Other adverse reactions include nausea, depression, upper respiratory tract infection, and headache.

Janus Kinase Inhibitors

Janus kinase (JAK) inhibitors such as tofacitinib have demonstrated efficacy in the treatment of psoriasis, including nail psoriasis. The side-effect profile of tofacitinib includes dose-dependent decreases in red blood cell counts, along with transient or reversible dose-dependent decreases in neutrophil counts. Tofacitinib has also demonstrated transient increases in lymphocyte counts, primarily attributable to increases in B-cell counts.

Combination Therapy

In more severe forms of psoriasis, a combination of treatment modalities may be employed. In treating patients with methotrexate, for example, concomitant topical agents may be used to minimize the dose. Methotrexate has been combined with infliximab to reduce the incidence of neutralizing antibodies, and also has been used with acitretin in managing patients with severe, generalized pustular psoriasis. Recent evidence suggests that neutralizing antibodies correlated with loss of response to biologics other than infliximab, suggesting a broader role for combination therapy. The use of PUVA and retinoids is called Re-PUVA and has been studied extensively. Acitretin has been combined with biologic agents to treat refractory psoriasis. Combination systemic therapy has the potential to reduce overall toxicity if the toxicities of each agent are different. However, new regimens should be used with caution because of the potential for cumulative toxicity or drug interaction.

Evolving Therapies

Alternative therapies for psoriasis include mycophenolate mofetil, sulfasalazine, paclitaxel, azathioprine, fumaric acid esters, climatotherapy, and grenz ray therapy. A3 adenosine receptor agonists are also being developed. Nail disease can respond to systemic agents, topical retinoids, local triamcinolone injections, and topical 5-fluorouracil. The latter agent can cause onycholysis if applied to the free edge of the nail.

Colombo MD, et al: Cyclosporine regimens in plaque psoriasis. Scientific World Journal 2013; 2013: 805705.

Elman SA, Weinblatt M, Merola JF. Targeted therapies for psoriatic arthritis: an update for the dermatologist. Semin Cutan Med Surg. 2018 Sep;37(3):173-181. doi: 10.12788/j.sder.2018.045. PubMed PMID: 30215635.

Fitzmaurice S, et al: Goeckerman regimen for management of psoriasis refractory to biologic therapy. J Am Acad Dermatol 2013; 69: 648.

Gladman DD, et al: Treating psoriasis and psoriatic arthritis. J Rheumatol 2017; 44: 519.

Hawkes JE, Yan BY, Chan TC, Krueger JG. Discovery of the IL-23/IL-17 Signaling Pathway and the Treatment of Psoriasis. J Immunol. 2018 Sep 15;201(6):1605-1613. doi: 10.4049/jimmunol.1800013. Review. PubMed PMID: 30181299; PubMed Central PMCID: PMC6129988.

Ho D, et al: A systematic review of light emitting diode (LED) phototherapy for treatment of psoriasis. J Drugs Dermatol 2017; 16: 482.

Kim BR, et al: Methotrexate in a real-world psoriasis treatment. Ann Dermatol 2017; 29: 346.

Langley RG, et al: Efficacy and safety of guselkumab in patients with psoriasis who have an inadequate response to ustekinumab. Br J Dermatol 2018; 178: 114.

Merola JF, et al: Efficacy of tofacitinib for the treatment of nail psoriasis. J Am Acad Dermatol 2017; 77: 79.

Millsop JW, et al: Diet and psoriasis, part III. J Am Acad Dermatol 2014; 71: 561.

Mota F, et al: Importance of immunogenicity testing for cost-effective management of psoriasis patients treated with adalimumab. Acta Dermatovenerol Alp Pannonica Adriat 2017; 26: 33.

Murage MJ, Tongbram V, Feldman SR, Malatestinic WN, Larmore CJ, Muram TM, Burge RT, Bay C, Johnson N, Clifford S, Araujo AB. Medication adherence and persistence in patients with rheumatoid arthritis, psoriasis, and psoriatic arthritis: a systematic literature review. Patient Prefer Adherence. 2018 Aug 21;12:1483-1503. doi: 10.2147/PPA.S167508.

eCollection 2018. Review. PubMed PMID: 30174415; PubMed Central PMCID: PMC6110273.

Pereira R, et al: Infection and malignancy risk in patients treated with TNF inhibitors for immune-mediated inflammatory diseases. Curr Drug Saf 2017; 12: 162.

Prasad V, et al: Performance evaluation of non-ionic surfactant based tazarotene encapsulated proniosomal gel for the treatment of psoriasis. Mater Sci Eng C Mater Biol Appl 2017; 79: 168.

Saleem MD, et al: Comorbidities in patients with psoriasis. J Am Acad Dermatol 2017; 77: 191.

Spadaccini M, et al: PDE4 Inhibition and inflammatory bowel disease. Int J Mol Sci 2017; 18: E1276.

van de Kerkhof PC: Biologics for psoriasis. J Dermatolog Treat 2017; 28: 281.

Yiu ZZ, Warren RB. Ustekinumab for the treatment of psoriasis: an evidence update. Semin Cutan Med Surg. 2018 Sep;37(3):143-147. doi: 10.12788/j.sder.2018.040. PubMed PMID: 30215630.

REACTIVE ARTHRITIS WITH CONJUNCTIVITIS/ URETHRITIS/DIARRHEA (REITER SYNDROME)

The syndrome includes a characteristic clinical triad of urethritis, conjunctivitis, and arthritis. The disease occurs chiefly in young men of HLA-B27 genotype, generally following a bout of urethritis or diarrheal illness. Systemic involvement can include the gastrointestinal tract, kidneys, central nervous system, and cardiovascular system. Because few patients present with the classic triad, the American College of Rheumatology recognizes criteria for limited manifestations of the syndrome, including peripheral arthritis of more than 1-month duration in association with urethritis, cervicitis, or bilateral conjunctivitis.

Hans Reiter was a Nazi war criminal, involved with or having knowledge of involuntary sterilization as well as a study of an experimental typhus vaccine that resulted in hundreds of deaths of concentration camp internees. Some believe that he should no longer be afforded the name recognition to designate the syndrome.

Clinical Features

Any part of the triad may occur first, often accompanied by fever, weakness, and weight loss. Although the inciting urethritis may be bacterial, later manifestations include a nonbacterial urethritis with painful urination and pyuria. Cystitis, prostatitis, and seminal vesiculitis may be accompaniments. Vulvar ulceration has been reported. About one third of patients develop conjunctivitis, which may be bulbar, tarsal, or angular. Keratitis is usually superficial and extremely painful. Iritis is common, especially in recurrent cases. Infrequently, optic neuritis may occur. Uveitis correlates with axial joint disease and HLA-B27 positivity. An asymmetric arthritis may affect peripheral joints, especially weight-bearing joints. Its onset is usually sudden. Pain in one or both heels is a frequent symptom. Sacroiliitis may develop in up to two thirds of patients, most of whom are of HLA-B27 type.

The skin involvement usually begins with small, guttate, hyperkeratotic, crusted or pustular lesions of the genitals (Fig. 10.13), palms, or soles. Involvement of the glans penis (balanitis circinata) occurs in 25% of patients. Lesions on the soles and trunk often become thickly crusted or hyperkeratotic. The eruption on the soles is known as keratoderma blennorrhagicum and occurs in 10% of patients (Fig. 10.14). The buccal, palatal, and lingual mucosa may show painless, shallow, red erosions. The nails become thick and brittle, with heavy subungual keratosis. Children are much more likely to have the postdysenteric form, often with conjunctivitis and arthritis as the most prominent complaints.

The syndrome generally follows an infectious urethritis or diarrheal illness. Implicated organisms include *Chlamydia*, *Shigella*, *Salmonella*, *Yersinia*, *Campylobacter*, *Ureaplasma*, *Borrelia*,

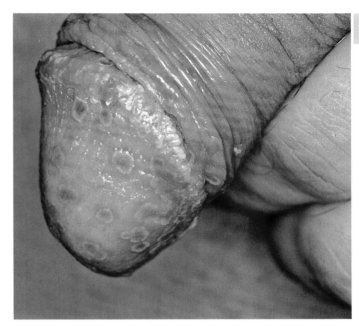

Fig. 10.13 Genital involvement in reactive arthritis.

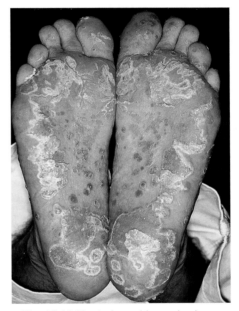

Fig. 10.14 Keratoderma blennorrhagicum.

Cryptosporidium, gonococci, and bacille Calmette-Guérin (BCG). *Chlamydia trachomatis* and *Ureaplasma urealyticum* have been isolated from the synovial fluid of affected joints, and some patients respond to antibiotic therapy. Chlamydial antigens demonstrate high homology with human sequences containing the binding motif of HLA-B27. Reiter syndrome has also been observed in HIV disease but may not be directly related to the virus, because it frequently occurs during treatment as the immune response improves. The disease has also been triggered by adalimumab and leflunomide in the setting of ankylosing spondyloarthropathy and Crohn disease.

Peripheral leukocytosis of 10,000–20,000/mm^3 and elevated erythrocyte sedimentation rate are the most consistent findings.

There is no specific test for Reiter syndrome. The differential diagnosis includes RA, ankylosing spondylitis, gout, psoriatic arthritis, gonococcal arthritis, acute rheumatic fever, chronic mucocutaneous candidiasis, and serum sickness. The presence of associated mucocutaneous lesions establishes the diagnosis. Some cases of Lyme disease overlap with Reiter syndrome. Individual skin lesions may be indistinguishable from those in psoriasis. Hyperkeratotic lesions generally have a thicker scale crust than most psoriatic plaques, but are otherwise identical.

Mucocutaneous lesions are generally self-limited and clear with topical corticosteroids. Joint disease is managed with rest and NSAIDs.

Antibiotic therapy has been effective in *Chlamydia*-triggered arthritis, but the role of antibiotics in arthritis triggered by enteric pathogens is less clear, with some studies suggesting a higher incidence in patients treated with antibiotics. Immunosuppressive agents, such as methotrexate, are used for refractory joint disease. TNF-α biologics, acitretin, and cyclosporine have been used in severe disease.

Esan OB, et al: Factors associated with sequelae of campylobacter and non-typhoidal salmonella infections. EBioMedicine 2017; 15: 100.
Schmitt SK: Reactive arthritis. Infect Dis Clin North Am 2017; 31: 265.

SUBCORNEAL PUSTULAR DERMATOSIS (SNEDDON-WILKINSON DISEASE)

In 1956 Sneddon and Wilkinson described a chronic pustular disease that occurred chiefly in middle-aged women. The pustules are superficial and arranged in annular and serpiginous patterns, especially on the abdomen, axillae, and groins. Cultures from the pustules are sterile. Oral lesions are rare. The condition is chronic, with remissions of variable duration. Some cases have followed administration of drugs including sorafenib.

Histologically, the pustules form below the stratum corneum, as in impetigo. Acantholysis is absent, but spongiform pustules may be noted in the upper epidermis. The histologic differential diagnosis includes pustular psoriasis and superficial fungal and bacterial infections.

IgA pemphigus shows significant overlap with subcorneal pustular dermatosis. Presentations of IgA pemphigus include subcorneal pustular dermatosis and intraepidermal neutrophilic IgA dermatosis types. Immunoblotting techniques have shown that human desmocollin 1 is an autoantigen for the subcorneal pustular dermatosis type of IgA pemphigus.

Localized cases may respond well to topical corticosteroids. Dapsone, 50–200 mg/day (adult), is effective for most of the remaining cases. Some patients have responded better to sulfapyridine therapy. Acitretin, NB UVB phototherapy, colchicine, azithromycin, biologic agents, and tetracycline with niacinamide may also be effective in subcorneal pustular dermatosis. Paraprotein-associated disease has resolved after treatment of the associated myeloma.

Watts PJ, et al: Subcorneal pustular dermatosis. Am J Clin Dermatol 2016; 17: 653.
Wick MR: Bullous, pseudobullous, and pustular dermatoses. Semin Diagn Pathol 2017; 34: 250.

EOSINOPHILIC PUSTULAR FOLLICULITIS

Eosinophilic pustular folliculitis (EPF) was first described in 1970 by Ofuji, although it is also referred to as sterile eosinophilic pustulosis. It occurs more often in males and is mostly reported in Asia. The mean age of onset is 35. It is characterized by pruritic, follicular papulopustules that measure 1–2 mm. The lesions tend to be grouped, and plaques usually form. New lesions may form at the edges of the plaques, leading to peripheral extension, while central clearing takes place. The most frequent site is the face, particularly over the cheeks. The trunk and upper extremities frequently are affected, and 20% have palmoplantar pustules. The distribution is usually asymmetric, and the typical course is one of spontaneous remissions and exacerbations lasting several years. The condition must be distinguished from eosinophilic folliculitis in infancy, HIV infection, and posttransplantation. A similar condition has occurred in association with HCV infection, with allopurinol, and during pregnancy.

Histologically, there is spongiosis and vesiculation of the follicular infundibulum and heavy infiltration with eosinophils. Follicular mucinosis may be present. There is a peripheral eosinophilia in half the cases, and pulmonary eosinophilia has been described. The cause is unknown; but numerous studies have implicated chemotactic substances, intercellular adhesion molecule 1 (ICAM-1), and cyclooxygenase-generated metabolites. Tryptase-positive and chymase-negative mast cells have also been implicated.

Indomethacin is effective in the vast majority of patients with eosinophilic pustular folliculitis. Topical and intralesional corticosteroids, clofazimine, minocycline, isotretinoin, UVB therapy, dapsone, colchicine, cyclosporine, topical tacrolimus, nicotine patches, infliximab, and cetirizine have also been reported as effective.

Childhood cases have been described. This subset differs from the typical cases in Asian males. Pediatric patients develop sterile pustules and papules preferentially over the scalp, although scattered clusters of pustules may occur over the trunk and extremities. Leukocytosis and eosinophilia are often present. Recurrent exacerbations and remissions usually occur, with eventual spontaneous resolution. High-potency topical steroids are the treatment of choice in pediatric patients.

Nomura T, et al: Eosinophilic pustular folliculitis. J Dermatol 2016; 43(8): 919.
Nomura T, et al: Eosinophilic pustular folliculitis. J Dermatol 2016; 43(11): 1301.

RECALCITRANT PALMOPLANTAR ERUPTIONS

Dermatitis Repens

Dermatitis repens, also known as acrodermatitis continua (see earlier) and acrodermatitis perstans, is a chronic inflammatory disease of the hands and feet. It usually remains stable on the extremities, but in rare cases, generalized pustular flares may occur. The disease usually begins distally on a digit, either as a pustule in the nail bed or as a paronychia. Extension takes place by eruption of fresh pustules with subsequent hyperkeratosis and crusting. The disease is usually unilateral at first and asymmetric throughout its entire course. As the disease progresses, one or more of the nails may become dystrophic or float away on pus. Anonychia is common in chronic cases. Some have used the term *dermatitis repens* to refer to more indolent involvement of the distal fingers.

Involvement of the mucous membranes may occur, even when the eruption of the skin is localized. Painful, circular, white plaques surrounded by inflammatory areolae are found on the tongue and may form a fibrinous membrane. Fissured or geographic tongue may occur.

Histologically, intraepithelial spongiform pustules identical to those of psoriasis are seen in the acute stage. Later stages show hyperkeratosis with parakeratosis or atrophy.

Numerous treatment options have been used, including topical corticosteroids, calcipotriene, dapsone, sulfapyridine, methotrexate, PUVA, acitretin, cyclosporine, topical mechlorethamine, anti-TNF agents, and anakinra. The choice of agent to use should consider the severity of disease and the patient's age and functional impairment. It should be noted that anti-TNF agents have triggered similar eruptions.

Palmoplantar Pustulosis (Pustular Psoriasis of Extremities)

Chronic palmoplantar pustulosis is essentially a bilateral and symmetric dermatosis (Fig. 10.15). The favorite locations are the thenar or hypothenar eminences or the central portion of the palms and soles. The patches begin as erythematous areas in which minute intraepidermal pustules form. At the beginning, these are pinhead sized; then they may enlarge and coalesce to form small lakes of pus. As the lesions resolve, denuded areas, crusts, or hyperkeratosis may persist. Palmoplantar pustulosis is strongly associated with thyroid disorders and cigarette smoking. Medications such as lithium, which aggravate psoriasis, have also been reported to induce palmoplantar pustular psoriasis.

In 1968 Kato described the first case of bilateral clavicular osteomyelitis with palmar and plantar pustulosis. In 1974 Sonozaki described persistent palmoplantar pustulosis and sternoclavicular hyperostosis. These conditions belong to the spectrum of skin and joint involvement designated by Kahn as the SAPHO syndrome (synovitis, acne, pustulosis, hyperostosis, and osteitis). Common features include palmoplantar pustulosis, acneiform eruption, and pain and swelling of a sternoclavicular joint or at sternomanubrial or costochondral junctions. There is shoulder, neck, and back pain, and limitation of motion of the shoulders and neck is common. Brachial plexus neuropathy and subclavian vein occlusion may occur. The lumbar spine and sacroiliac joints are usually spared. Chronic multifocal osteomyelitis in children may be a pediatric variant. Others have described an association between palmoplantar pustulosis and arthritis or osteitis. SAPHO syndrome may coexist with features of Behçet disease. The knees, spine, and ankles may be involved. Ivory vertebrae have been described.

The disease typically is resistant to treatment. Topical corticosteroids, retinoids, calcipotriene, and macrolactams are of some benefit. Acitretin is generally extremely effective at 1 mg/kg/day, although rebound occurs more quickly than with etretinate. Apremilast, dapsone, colchicine, tofacitanib, cyclosporine, allitretinoin, cefcapene pivoxil hydrochloride (a third-generation cephalosporin), leflunomide, and mycophenolate mofetil may be effective. Oral 8-methoxypsoralen and high-intensity UVA irradiation or soak PUVA can both be helpful, and grenz ray therapy can induce prolonged remissions in some patients. Chronic osteomyelitis in SAPHO syndrome has been reported to respond to bisphosphonates.

Pustular Bacterid

Pustular bacterid was first described by George Andrews. It is characterized by a symmetric, grouped, vesicular, or pustular eruption on the palms and soles, marked by exacerbations and remissions over long periods. Andrews regarded the discovery of a remote focus of infection, and cure on its elimination, as crucial to the diagnosis.

The primary lesions are pustules. Tiny hemorrhagic puncta intermingled with the pustules are frequently seen. When lesions are so numerous as to coalesce, they form a honeycomb-like structure in the epidermis. The disease usually begins on the midportions of the palms or soles, from which it spreads outwardly until it may eventually cover the entire flexor aspects of the hands and feet. There is no involvement of the webs of the fingers or toes, as in tinea pedis.

When the eruption is fully developed, both palms and soles are completely covered, and the symmetry is pronounced. During fresh outbreaks, the white blood count may show a leukocytosis that ranges from 12,000 to 19,000 cells/mm³ with 65%–80% neutrophils. As a rule, scaling is present in fully evolved lesions, and the scales are adherent, tough, and dry. During exacerbations, crops of pustules or vesicles make their appearance, and there is often severe itching of the areas. Tenderness may be present. Many regard this condition as a variant of psoriasis, triggered by infection.

Infantile Acropustulosis

Infantile acropustulosis is an intensely itchy vesicopustular eruption of the hands and feet (Fig. 10.16). Most cases are postscabetic, and active scabies can produce similar lesions. Lesions often predominate at the edges of the palms and soles. Individual crops of lesions clear in a few weeks, but recurrences may continue for months or years.

Histologically, a subcorneal pustule with neutrophils is noted. Eosinophils may be numerous. The lesions are easily punctured to produce smears of the inflammatory cells, so biopsies are seldom employed.

Lesions often respond to topical corticosteroids. Refractory lesions may respond to dapsone at doses of 1–2 mg/kg/day.

Koga T, et al: Successful treatment of palmoplantar pustulosis with rheumatoid arthritis, with tofacitinib. Clin Immunol 2016; 173: 147.

Kouno M, et al: Retrospective analysis of the clinical response of palmoplantar pustulosis after dental infection control and dental metal removal. J Dermatol 2017; 44: 695.

Lutz V, et al: Acitretin- and tumor necrosis factor inhibitor–resistant acrodermatitis continua of Hallopeau responsive to the interleukin 1 receptor antagonist anakinra. Arch Dermatol 2012; 148: 297.

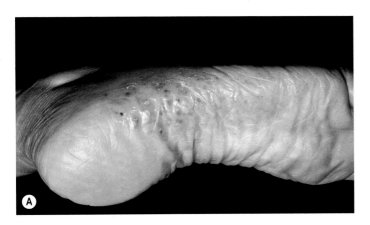

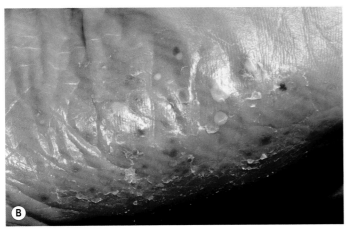

Fig. 10.15 (A) Plantar pustulosis. (B) Pustules and hyperkeratosis are typical.

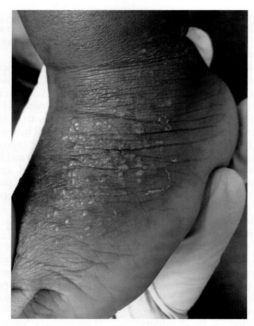

Fig. 10.16 Acropustulosis of infancy.

11 Pityriasis Rosea, Pityriasis Rubra Pilaris, and Other Papulosquamous and Hyperkeratotic Diseases

PITYRIASIS ROSEA

Clinical Features

Pityriasis rosea is a mild inflammatory exanthem characterized by salmon-colored thin papules and plaques that are at first discrete but may become confluent (Fig. 11.1). The individual patches are oval or circinate and covered with finely crinkled, dry epidermis, which often desquamates, leaving a collarette of scaling in the center. When stretched across the long axis, the scales tend to fold across the lines of stretch, the so-called hanging curtain sign or Christmas tree sign. The disease most frequently begins with a single herald or mother patch (Fig. 11.2), usually larger than succeeding lesions, which may persist 1 week or longer before others appear. This is often confused for tinea corporis because it is an isolated patch with central colarette of scale mistaken for being annular. By the time involution of the herald patch has begun, new lesions arise rapidly (Fig. 11.3). The total course is typically 3–8 weeks, and then the lesions spontaneously resolve. Relapses and recurrences are observed infrequently. The incidence is highest between ages 15 and 40, and the disease is most prevalent in the spring and autumn. Women are more frequently affected than men.

The fully developed eruption has a striking appearance because of the distribution and definite characteristics of the individual lesions. These are arranged so that the long axis of the macules runs parallel to the lines of cleavage. The eruption is usually generalized, affecting chiefly the trunk and sparing sun-exposed surfaces. Less common presentations are localized (involving neck, thighs, groins, or axillae), distribution (sparing covered areas), unilateral, papular, and segmental pattern. Children with darker skin pigmentation are particularly predisposed to the papular variant and are also more prone to facial and scalp involvement. In darker-skinned patients, the lesions often resolve with hypopigmentation. A vesicular variant has also been described, and erythema multiforme–like lesions may occur. Purpuric pityriasis rosea may manifest with petechiae and ecchymoses along Langer lines of the neck, trunk, and proximal extremities, and may rarely be a sign of an underlying leukemia. Pityriasis rosea occurring during pregnancy may be associated with premature delivery, neonatal hypotonia, and fetal loss, especially if the eruption occurs within the first 15 weeks of gestation.

When the eruption localized, it can be difficult to distinguish from unilateral laterothoracic exanthema (asymmetric periflexural exanthema of childhood). Confluent circinate patches with gyrate borders may form and may resemble tinea corporis. Rarely, the eyelids, palms and soles, scalp, or penis may be involved, and syphilis should be ruled out, especially with palm and sole involvement. Oral lesions are relatively uncommon; they are asymptomatic, erythematous macules with raised borders and clearing centers or aphthous ulcer–like lesions. They involute simultaneously with the skin lesions. Moderate pruritus may be present, particularly during the outbreak, and mild constitutional symptoms may occur before the onset.

Etiology

Pityriasis rosea is most likely a response to a virus. The most commonly implicated viruses are herpes viridae such as human herpesvirus (HHV)–6 and HHV-7. Watanabe et al. (2002) demonstrated active replication of HHV-6 or HHV-7 in mononuclear cells of lesional skin, as well as identifying the viruses in serum samples of patients including women who experienced miscarriage in association with pityriasis rosea. Although these viruses are almost universally acquired in early childhood and remain in a latent phase as mononuclear cells, the eruption is likely secondary to reactivation leading to viremia. HHV-2 and hepatitis C virus (HCV) have also been implicated in individual cases.

A pityriasis rosea–like eruption may occur as a reaction to medications such as captopril, imatinib mesylate, interferon, ketotifen, arsenicals, gold, bismuth, clonidine, methoxypromazine, tripelennamine hydrochloride, ergotamine, lisinopril, acyclovir, lithium, adalimumab, nortriptyline, lamotrigine, rituximab, imatinib, asenapine, barbiturates, or bacille Calmette-Guérin (BCG) vaccine.

Histology

The histologic features of pityriasis rosea include mild acanthosis, focal parakeratosis, and extravasation of erythrocytes into the epidermis. Spongiosis may be present in acute cases. A mild perivascular infiltrate of lymphocytes is found in the dermis. Histologic evaluation is especially helpful in excluding the conditions with which pityriasis rosea may be confused.

Differential Diagnosis

Pityriasis rosea may closely mimic seborrheic dermatitis, tinea corporis, secondary syphilis (macular syphilid), drug eruption, other viral exanthems, and psoriasis. In seborrheic dermatitis, the scalp and eyebrows are usually scaly; there is a predilection for the sternal and interscapular regions, as well as the flexor surfaces of the articulations, where the patches are covered with greasy scales. Tinea corporis is rarely so widespread. Tinea versicolor may also closely simulate pityriasis rosea but the individual lesions tend to be flatter and smaller. A positive potassium hydroxide (KOH) examination serves well to differentiate these last two. In macular syphilid, the lesions are of a uniform size and assume a brownish tint. Scaling and itching are absent or slight, and there is typically generalized adenopathy with mucous membrane lesions, palmoplantar lesions, positive nontreponemal and treponemal tests, and often the remains of a chancre. Because syphilis can so closely mimic pityriasis rosea and syphilis incidence is rising again, strong consideration for syphilis testing should be considered in patients with pityriasis rosea. Scabies and lichen planus may be confused with the papular type.

Treatment

Most patients with pityriasis rosea require no therapy because they are asymptomatic; however, the duration of the eruption may be notably reduced by several interventions. A Cochrane review cited inadequate evidence for efficacy for most published treatments;

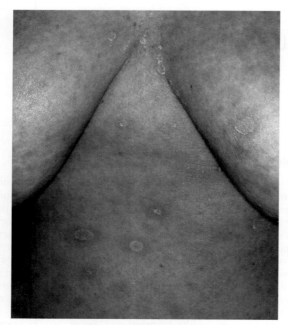

Fig. 11.1 Pityriasis rosea.

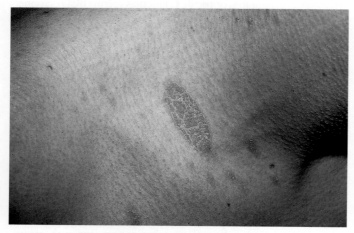

Fig. 11.2 Herald patch of pityriasis rosea.

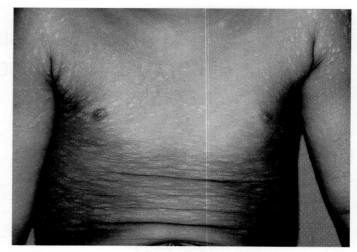

Fig. 11.3 Pityriasis rosea.

Bangash HK, et al: Pityriasis rosea–like drug eruption due to nortriptyline in a patient with vulvodynia. J Low Genit Tract Dis 2013; 17: 226.

Chuh A, et al: A position statement on the management of patients with pityriasis rosea. J Eur Acad Dermatol Venereol 2016; 30: 1670.

Drago F, et al: Evidence of human herpesvirus-6 and -7 reactivation in miscarrying women with pityriasis rosea. J Am Acad Dermatol 2014; 71: 198.

Drago F, et al: Pityriasis rosea. Dermatology 2016; 232: 431.

Ganguly S: A randomized, double-blind, placebo-controlled study of efficacy of oral acyclovir in the treatment of pityriasis rosea. J Clin Diagn Res 2014; 8: YC01.

Oh CW, et al: Pityriasis rosea–like rash secondary to intravesical bacillus Calmette-Guérin immunotherapy. Ann Dermatol 2012; 24: 360.

Relhan V, et al: Pityriasis rosea with erythema multiforme–like lesions. Indian J Dermatol 2013; 58: 242.

Sezer E, et al: Pityriasis rosea–like drug eruption related to rituximab treatment. J Dermatol 2013; 40: 495.

Sharma PK, Yadav TP, Gautam RK, Taneja N, Satyanarayana L. Erythromycin in pityriasis rosea: A double-blind, placebo-controlled clinical trial. Journal of the American Academy of Dermatology. 2000 Feb 1;42(2):241-4.

PITYRIASIS RUBRA PILARIS

Clinical Features

Pityriasis rubra pilaris (PRP) is a chronic skin disease characterized by small follicular papules that coalesce into salmon colored pink scaling patches, and often, solid confluent yellow-orange palmo-plantar hyperkeratosis. The papules are the most important diagnostic feature, being more or less acuminate (pointy), salmon colored to reddish brown, about pinhead sized, and topped by a central horny plug (Fig. 11.4). A hair, or part of one, may be embedded in the horny center. There are two peaks of during the first 5 years of life or in the fifties. Some cases of PRP are caused by genetic mutations, thus explaining their chronic recalcitrant nature.

PRP is generally symmetric and diffuse, with characteristic small islands of normal skin within the affected areas (Fig. 11.5). There is a hyperkeratosis of the palms and soles (Fig. 11.6), with a tendency to fissures. The classic disease generally manifests first by scaliness and erythema of the scalp. The eruption is limited in the beginning, having a predilection for the sides of the neck and

however, lack of evidence does not equate to lack of efficacy. The most data exists for the use of acyclovir with multiple trials showing decrease the eruption and itching. In pregnant patients, given the small risk of harm to the fetus early in pregnancy, acyclovir could be considered along with input from an obstetrician to help weigh the risks and benefits. Erythromycin has demonstrated benefit in small studies. The gastrointestinal side effects of erythromycin may limit its use. Use of ultraviolet B (UVB) light in erythema exposures may expedite the involution of the lesions after the acute inflammatory stage has passed. The erythema produced by ultraviolet (UV) treatment is followed by superficial exfoliation. Narrow Band UVB therapy may help improve individual lesions but may not shorten the course or alleviate pruritis. Corticosteroid lotions or creams provide some relief from itching. For dryness and irritation, simple emollients are recommended.

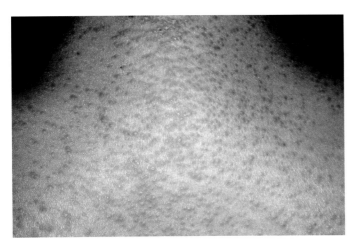

Fig. 11.4 Pityriasis rubra pilaris.

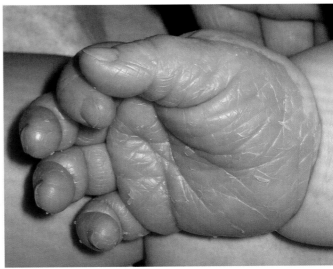

Fig. 11.6 Childhood pityriasis rubra pilaris.

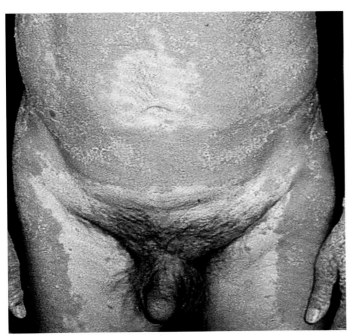

Fig. 11.5 Islands of sparing in pityriasis rubra pilaris.

trunk and the extensor surfaces of the extremities, especially the backs of the first and second phalanges. Then, as new lesions occur, extensive areas are converted into sharply marginated patches of various sizes, which look like exaggerated gooseflesh and feel like a nutmeg grater. Any part or the entire skin surface may be affected. On the soles especially, the hyperkeratosis typically extends up the sides, in the distribution of a sandal. The nails may be dull, rough, thickened, brittle, and striated, and are apt to crack and break. They are rarely, if ever, pitted. The exfoliation may become generalized and the follicular lesions less noticeable, finally disappearing and leaving a widespread dry, scaly erythroderma. The skin becomes dull red, glazed, atrophic, sensitive to slight changes in temperature, and over the bony prominences, subject to ulcerations. In the classic juvenile type, limited plaques occur on extensor surfaces, with adjacent "nutmeg-grater" papules.

The skin may be itchy or asymptomatic. The Koebner phenomenon may be present. The general health of most patients is not affected. Occasionally arthritis may accompany the eruption and rarely a protein-losing enteropathy may occur if there is very widespread involvement. A number of cases of associated malignancy

have recently been reported. It remains to be established whether these are true associations or chance findings. Both hypothyroidism and hypoparathyroidism have been reported, as has the combination of sacroiliitis and autoimmune thyroiditis.

PRP may be classified according to familial (typically autosomal dominant) or acquired types and to the onset of disease in childhood or adulthood. Griffith's classification is useful in this regard. Type I, the classic adult type, is seen most often and carries a good prognosis, with 80% involuting over a 3-year period. Most patients with the classic juvenile type (type III) have clearing of the disease in 1 year, although it may recur, even into adulthood. The atypical adult (type II) and circumscribed juvenile (type IV) form account for a minority of cases and carry a poorer prognosis for spontaneous recovery. Type V appears in infancy or early childhood and has a more chronic course that has been associated with a CARD14 mutation, likely explaining the chronic nature. CARD14 mutations have also been demonstrated in pustular psoriasis. A type VI has been proposed that is seen in patients infected with human immunodeficiency virus (HIV) and is associated with acne conglobata, hidradenitis suppurativa, or lichen spinulosus.

Etiology

Although CARD14 has been found in chronic early-onset forms, the etiology of spontaneous PRP is unknown. Either gender may be affected, with equal frequency. Both clinically and histologically, the disease has many features that suggest it is a vitamin deficiency disorder, particularly of vitamin A. Some reports of patients with low serum levels of retinol-binding protein have appeared, but this is not a reproducible finding. Streptococcal infections have rarely been implicated in children. A similar eruption has been described secondary to imatinib, sorafenib, and telaprevir.

Histology

There is hyperkeratosis, follicular plugging, and focal parakeratosis at the follicular orifice. Parakeratosis may alternate both vertically and horizontally, producing a checkerboard pattern. Acantholysis may be present, especially within adnexal structures. The inflammatory infiltrate in the dermis is composed of mononuclear cells and is generally mild. Although making an unequivocal histologic diagnosis of PRP may be difficult, the findings of psoriasis, which is the most common clinical entity in the differential diagnosis, are not present.

Diagnosis

Once fully manifested, the diagnosis of fully developed PRP is rarely difficult because of its distinctive features, such as the peculiar orange or salmon-yellow color of the follicular papules, containing a horny center, on the backs of the fingers, sides of the neck, and extensor surfaces of the limbs; the thickened, rough, and slightly or moderately scaly, harsh skin; the sandal-like palmoplantar hyperkeratosis; and the islands of normal skin in the midst of the eruption. It is distinguished from psoriasis by the scales, which in the latter are silvery and light, and overlap like shingles, and by the papules, which extend peripherally to form patches. Phrynoderma (follicular hyperkeratosis) caused by vitamin A deficiency gives a somewhat similar appearance to the skin, as may eczematous eruptions caused by vitamin B deficiency. Rheumatologic disorders, such as subacute cutaneous lupus erythematosus and dermatomyositis, may present with similar cutaneous findings.

Treatment

The management of PRP is generally with systemic retinoids, although topical tazarotene has also been reported to be of benefit. Isotretinoin, may induce prolonged remissions or cures. It may take 6–9 months for full involution to occur, and tapering of the drug may prevent recurrence. Acitretin and methotrexate have also been shown to improve PRP. Ustekinumab has shown efficacy including in patients with familial PRP from CARD14 mutations. Resolution by way of an erythema gyratum repens–like pattern has been described during methotrexate therapy. UV light may flare some patients, but in others, psoralen plus ultraviolet A (PUVA), UVA I, or narrow-band (NB) UVB, alone or in combination with retinoids, may be effective. Phototesting before initiating light therapy is recommended. Extracorporeal photochemotherapy, cyclosporine, anti–tumor necrosis factor (TNF) agents, and azathioprine have also been reported to be effective in resistant and severe cases.

Topical applications of calcineurin inhibitors, lactic acid, or urea-containing preparations may be helpful. Responses to topical corticosteroids are not very effective as a rule. Systemic corticosteroids are beneficial only for acute, short-term management, but are not recommended for chronic use. In HIV-related disease, multiagent antiviral therapy may be useful alone or in combination with retinoids.

Adnot-Desanlis L, et al: Effectiveness of infliximab in pityriasis rubra pilaris is associated with pro-inflammatory cytokine inhibition. Dermatology 2013; 226: 41.

Eastham AB, et al: Treatment options for pityriasis rubra pilaris including biologic agents. JAMA Dermatol 2014; 150: 92.

Griffiths WA. Pityriasis rubra pilaris. Clinical and experimental dermatology. 1980 Mar;5(1):105-12.

Ko CJ, et al: Pityriasis rubra pilaris. Int J Dermatol 2011; 50: 1480.

Marchetti MA, et al: Pityriasis rubra pilaris treated with methotrexate evolving with an erythema gyratum repens–like appearance. J Am Acad Dermatol 2013; 69: e32.

Mercer JM, et al: Familial pityriasis rubra pilaris. J Cutan Med Surg 2013; 17: 226.

Möhrenschlager, M. and Abeck, D., 2002. Further clinical evidence for involvement of bacterial superantigens in juvenile pityriasis rubra pilaris (PRP): report of two new cases. Pediatric dermatology, 19(6), pp.569-569.

Napolitano M, et al: Ustekinumab treatment of pityriasis rubra pilaris. J Dermatol 2017 Oct 28; ePub ahead of print.

Pampín A, et al: Successful treatment of atypical adult pityriasis rubra pilaris with oral alitretinoin. J Am Acad Dermatol 2013; 69: e105.

Paz C, et al: Sorafenib-induced eruption resembling pityriasis rubra pilaris. J Am Acad Dermatol 2011; 65: 452.

Petrof G, et al: A systematic review of the literature on the treatment of pityriasis rubra pilaris type 1 with TNF-antagonists. J Eur Acad Dermatol Venereol 2013; 27: e131.

Plana A, et al: Pityriasis rubra pilaris–like reaction induced by imatinib. Clin Exp Dermatol 2013; 38: 520.

Takeichi T, et al: Pityriasis rubra pilaris type V as an autoinflammatory disease by CARD14 mutations. JAMA Dermatol 2017; 153: 66.

SMALL PLAQUE PARAPSORIASIS

Small plaque parapsoriasis (SPP) is characterized by hyperpigmented or yellowish red scaling patches, round to oval in configuration, with sharply defined, regular borders. Most lesions occur on the trunk, and all are 1–5 cm in diameter. In the digitate variant, yellowish tan, elongated, fingerprint-like lesions are oriented along the cleavage lines, predominantly on the flank (Fig. 11.7). These lesions may at times be longer than 5 cm. There is an absence of the induration, the large, erythematous to purplish red lesions, and poikiloderma that characterize small patches of cutaneous T-cell lymphoma in its early stages. Histology can help differentiate from pityriasis lichenoides. The eruption may be mildly itchy or asymptomatic and has a male preponderance. Typical SPP rarely progresses to mycosis fungoides, although the histologic changes can overlap, and clonality may be demonstrated in SPP. Debate continues on this issue. A hypopigmented variant may have a somewhat higher rate of progression to hypopigmented mycosis fungoides. SPP has been reported in the setting of liposarcoma, with resolution of the eruption after resection of the tumor.

The histologic findings of SPP are characterized by an infiltrate in the superficial dermis composed predominantly of lymphocytes. The overlying epidermis demonstrates mild acanthosis, spongiosis, and focal overlying parakeratosis. SPP is considered to be a type of chronic spongiotic dermatitis. Lesional skin also demonstrates an increase in CD1a(+), Langerhans cells, CD1a-positive dermal dendritic cells, and CD68(+) macrophages.

Although SPP may be refractory to topical steroids alone, patients usually respond to phototherapy. Treatment with UVB, NB UVB, or natural sunlight, alone or in combination with a low-strength topical corticosteroid or simple lubricant, will usually

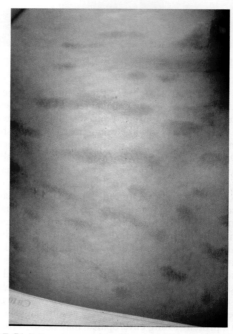

Fig. 11.7 Digitate parapsoriasis. (Courtesy Thomas Nicotori, MD.)

clear SPP. Without treatment, the patches of SPP may persist for years to decades but rarely progress to lymphoma.

Arai R, et al: Retrospective study of 24 patients with large or small plaque parapsoriasis treated with ultraviolet B therapy. J Dermatol 2012; 39: 674.

Duarte IA, et al: An evaluation of the treatment of parapsoriasis with phototherapy. An Bras Dermatol 2013; 88: 306.

El-Darouti MA, et al: Hypopigmented parapsoriasis en plaque, a new, overlooked member of the parapsoriasis family. J Am Acad Dermatol 2012; 67: 1182.

Lewin J, et al: Digitate dermatosis (small-plaque parapsoriasis). Dermatol Online J 2012; 18: 3.

Sibbald C, et al: Systematic review of cases of cutaneous T-cell lymphoma transformation in pityriasis lichenoides and small plaque parapsoriasis. Br J Dermatol 2016; 175: 807.

Takahashi H, et al: Digitate dermatosis successfully treated by narrowband ultraviolet B irradiation. J Dermatol 2011; 38: 923.

CONFLUENT AND RETICULATED PAPILLOMATOSIS (GOUGEROT AND CARTEAUD)

The eruption of confluent and reticulated papillomatosis (CARP) typically begins on the inframammary and upper lateral trunk as slightly scaly macules that may slowly spread to involve the remainder of the trunk (Fig. 11.8). There is a nummular version that simulates tinea versicolor or erythema dychromicum perstans. In light-skinned people, the lesions vary from skin colored or faintly erythematous to hyperpigmented; in more darkly pigmented people, lesions usually show hyperpigmentation, although a nonpigmenting form with fine, white scale has been described. There may be severe itching, or the lesions may be entirely asymptomatic. Familial cases have been reported. The pathophysiology is unknown, but the consistent response to minocycline and doxycycline suggests an infectious or inflammatory etiology. An actinomycete, dubbed *Dietzia papillomatosis*, has been isolated from lesional skin, although it is unknown if this is causative. Isolated cases have been associated with hypothyroidism and 15q tetrasomy syndrome.

Histologically, hyperkeratosis, acanthosis, and papillomatosis are generally seen and *Pityrosporum (Malassezia)* yeast are frequently present. The histologic changes resemble those seen in acanthosis nigricans, and the two conditions may occur together.

A variety of antibiotics have been successful in treating this papillomatosis. Minocycline or doxycycline, for 4–8 weeks, is used most often. Successful treatment has also been reported with oral fusidic acid, clarithromycin, amoxicillin, erythromycin, azithromycin, and topical mupirocin. Topical and oral retinoids have also been used successfully, either alone or in combination with topical lactic acid, urea, or alcohol. CARP associated with polycystic ovarian syndrome has responded to contraceptive therapy. One case of CARP resolved with delivery of a baby.

Pseudo–atrophoderma colli may be a related condition that occurs on the neck. It manifests as papillomatosis, pigmented, and atrophic glossy lesions with delicate wrinkling, which tend to have a vertical orientation and may respond to minocycline.

Hudacek KD, et al: An unusual variant of confluent and reticulated papillomatosis masquerading as tinea versicolor. Arch Dermatol 2012; 148: 505.

Kim H, et al: A case of confluent and reticulated papillomatosis treated with oral isotretinoin. Korean J Dermatol 2016; 54: 397.

Koguchi H, et al: Confluent and reticulated papillomatosis associated with 15q tetrasomy syndrome. Acta Derm Venereol 2013; 93: 202.

Tamraz H, et al: Confluent and reticulated papillomatosis. J Eur Acad Dermatol Venereol 2013; 27: e119.

Usta JA, et al: Confluent and reticulated papillomatosis subsiding spontaneously after delivery. Rev Med Chil 2016; 144: 1494.

PALMOPLANTAR KERATODERMA

The term *keratoderma* is frequently used synonymously with the terms *keratosis palmaris et plantaris* (KPP), *palmoplantar keratoderma* (PPK), and *tylosis*. This group of conditions is characterized by excessive formation of keratin on the palms and soles. There are hereditary and acquired PPKs. PPK nomenclature has improved over time as genetic testing has improved and the etiology of many of the PPKs has been elucidated, but there are still many historical names used. Hereditary PPK can be divided into diffuse and focal PPK, as well as PPK with and without associated features. The diffuse forms can be subdivided based on presence or absence of transgrediens (involvement onto the dorsal aspect sides of the hand/foot), and the focal forms can be further divided into punctate and striate forms. Those PPKs that are part of a syndrome such as pachyonychia congenita, Huriez syndrome, tyrosinemia II (Richner-Hanhart), Darier disease, Clouston (hidrotic ectodermal dysplasia), Naxos syndrome (keratoderma, wooly hair, and cardiomyopathy), various ichthyoses, and dyskeratosis congenita are discussed in other chapters.

Acquired types include keratoderma climactericum, arsenical keratoses, corns, calluses, porokeratosis plantaris discreta, glucan-induced keratoderma in acquired immunodeficiency syndrome (AIDS), and many skin disorders associated with palmoplantar keratoderma, such as psoriasis, paraneoplastic syndromes, PRP, lichen planus, and syphilis. Palmoplantar keratoderma has been described with multikinase inhibitors such as sorafenib. Treatment of these PPKs is aimed toward treating the primary disease or withdrawing the offending agent. Arsenical keratoses can occur from tainted water supplies, intentional poisoning, and medications containing arsenic. Arsenical keratoses have been treated with a combination of keratolytics and low-dose acitretin.

FOCAL PALMOPLANTAR KERATODERMAS

Keratosis Punctata of the Palmar Creases

Keratosis punctata of the palmar creases has also been referred to as keratotic pits of the palmar creases, punctate keratosis of the palmar creases, keratosis punctata, keratodermia punctata, hyperkeratosis penetrans, lenticular atrophia of the palmar creases, and hyperkeratosis punctata of the palmar creases. This common disorder occurs most often in patients of African descent. The

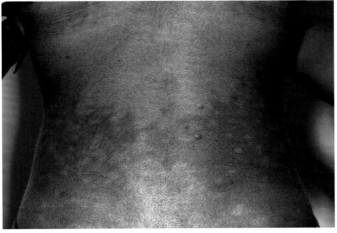

Fig. 11.8 Confluent and reticulated papillomatosis.

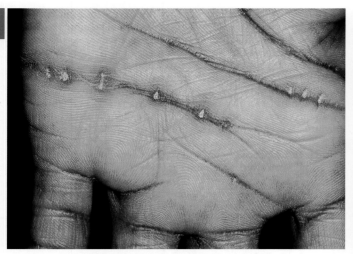

Fig. 11.9 Keratosis punctata of the palmar creases.

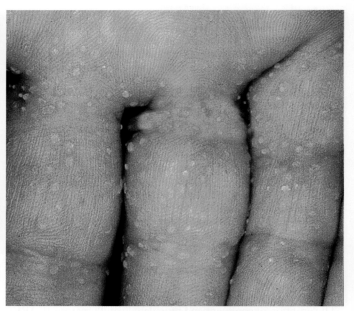

Fig. 11.11 "Music box" spiny keratoderma.

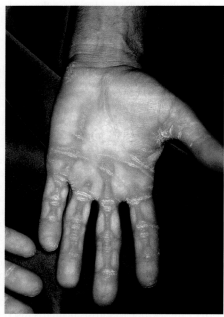

Fig. 11.10 Striate keratoderma.

primary lesion is a 1–5 mm depression filled with a comedo-like keratinous plug. The lesions localize to the creases of the palms or fingers (Fig. 11.9). The soles may be involved.

Keratosis punctata of the palmar creases has been associated with atopic dermatitis, Dupuytren contractures, pterygium inversum unguis, dermatitis herpetiformis, knuckle pads, striate keratoderma, and psoriasis, although some of these may just be disorders with a similar clinical phenotype and not truly associated. Keratolytic agents and topical retinoids have provided temporary relief. Extremely painful lesions respond to punch excision.

Striate Keratodermas

The striate keratodermas are a group of autosomal dominant palmoplantar keratodermas with streaking hyperkeratosis involving the fingers and extending onto the palm (Fig. 11.10). In some patients, mutation in desmoglein 1 (DSG-1) or desmoplakin and keratin 1 (KRT-1) have been described. In other patients,

desmosome numbers are normal, but their inner plaques are attenuated. Brunauer-Fohs-Siemens syndrome is one form with diminished desmosomes, clumping of keratin filaments, and enlarged keratohyalin granules. Striate keratoderma has also been reported in association with Rubinstein-Taybi syndrome.

Punctate Palmoplantar Keratoderma

Punctate keratoses of the palms and soles has also been referred to as punctate keratoderma, keratodermia punctata, keratosis punctata palmaris et plantaris, keratoma hereditarium dissipatum palmare et plantare, keratoderma disseminatum palmaris et plantaris, palmar keratoses, and palmar and plantar seed dermatoses. *AAGAB* as well as *COL14A1* mutations have been implicated. Spiny keratoderma of the palms and soles, known as "music box spines," is a distinct variant (Fig. 11.11).

There may be from 1 to over 40 papules, with an average in one series of 8.3. The main symptom is pruritus. The onset is between ages 15 and 68. Individuals of African descent predominate, and it more frequently affects men. The histology may show pyknotic, vacuolated epithelium, basal layer spongiosis, and dilated, occluded sweat ducts, blood vessels, and lymph vessels. Mechanical debridement may help.

Circumscribed palmar hypokeratosis is a delayed manifestation of friction and repetitive-use trauma that presents as a sharply circumscribed, erythematous patch on the palm. Histologically, thickness of the stratum corneum decreases abruptly.

Acrokeratoelastoidosis

Acrokeratoelastoidosis presents with translucent to erythematous papules at the margins of the palms. Both sporadic and autosomal dominant forms have been reported. Small, round, firm papules occur over the dorsal hands, knuckles, and lateral margins of the palms and soles. The lesions appear in early childhood or adolescence in the inherited form and progress slowly. They are most often asymptomatic. The characteristic histologic feature is dermal elastorrhexis.

The differential diagnosis includes focal acral hyperkeratosis, which occurs as a familial trait in African American patients. The lesions are marginal hyperkeratotic papules, often with a central dell and usually on both the hands and the fingers. No alteration of the collagen or elastin is present on biopsy.

Porokeratosis Plantaris Discreta

Porokeratosis plantaris discreta occurs in adults, with a 4:1 female preponderance. It is characterized by a sharply marginated, rubbery, wide-based papule that on blunt dissection reveals an opaque plug without bleeding on removal. Lesions are multiple, painful, and usually 7–10 mm in diameter. They are usually confined to the weight-bearing area of the sole, beneath the metatarsal heads. Treatment may begin with fitted foot pads to redistribute the weight. Surgical excision, blunt dissection, and cryotherapy have been successful.

Focal Acral Hyperkeratosis

Focal acral hyperkeratosis occurs in autosomal dominant and sporadic forms. Clinically, it is characterized by crateriform keratotic papules and plaques along the borders of the hands and feet. It differs from acrokeratoelastoidosis and collagenous and elastotic marginal bands by the lack of underlying dermal changes.

DIFFUSE PALMOPLANTAR KERATODERMAS

Most diffuse palmoplantar keratoderms are genetic, but they can be acquired. The most helpful clinical differentiator is the presence or absence of transgrediens. Diffuse palmoplantar keratodermas are poorly responsive to therapy; 5% salicylic acid, 12% ammonium lactate, and 40% urea have been used. Fifty percent propylene glycol in water under occlusion may help soak off the hyperkeratosis. Systemic retinoid therapy is impractical because of bone toxicity with long-term use, and topical retinoids are generally not effective.

Diffuse Palmoplantar Keratodermas without Transgrediens

Vorner and Unna-Thost PPK are caused by KRT1 and KRT9 mutations. Vorner is epidermolytic and Unna-Thost is nonepidermolytic, although there is significant overlap. Variants without epidermolytic hyperkeratosis (EHK) may have more waxy appearance. They are dominantly inherited, have marked congenital thickening of the epidermal horny layer of the palms and soles, are usually symmetric, and affect all parts equally (Fig. 11.12). There is thick yellow keratin and the arches of the feet are generally spared. The uniform thickening forms a rigid plate, which ends with characteristic abruptness at the periphery of the palm. Diffuse PPK can also be caused by DSG-1 mutations. Patients with this variant can have thickened yellow nails, and on histopathology there is acantholysis especially in the superficial epidermal layers. Bothnian type PPK is a nonepidermolytic palmoplantar keratoderma due to the aquaporin 5 (AQP5), water-channel protein.

Diffuse Palmoplantar Keratodermas with Transgrediens

Mal de Meleda type PPK is a rare, autosomal recessive form of palmoplantar keratoderma seen in individuals from the island of Meleda. The hyperkeratosis does not remain confined to the palms, and the extensor surfaces of the arms are frequently affected. Mutations in the gene encoding secreted lymphocyte antigen-6/urokinase-type plasminogen activator receptor–related protein 1 (SLURP-1) are causative.

Nagashima-type PPK is a nonprogressive, autosomal recessive form caused by mutations in SERPINB7 that resembles a mild form of mal de Meleda and is more common in Japan. There is a higher rate of melanoma in these patients possibly due to a lack of circulating Langerhans cells. PPK of Sybert shows autosomal dominant inheritance and a lack of associated systemic features and can also involve the groin, elbows, knees, and forearms.

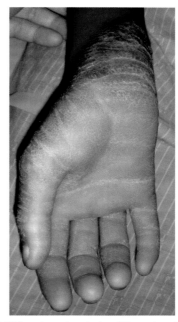

Fig. 11.12 Diffuse hyperkeratosis of the palms, Unna-Thost.

OTHER PALMOPLANTAR KERATODERMAS

Palmoplantar Keratodermas and Malignancy

Howell-Evans reported a diffuse, waxy keratoderma of the palms and soles occurring as an autosomal dominant trait associated with esophageal carcinoma. Other related features are oral leukoplakia, esophageal strictures, squamous cell carcinoma of tylotic skin, and carcinoma of the larynx and stomach. The tylosis esophageal cancer gene has been localized to chromosome 17q25. Acquired forms of palmoplantar keratoderma have also been associated with cancers of the esophagus, lung, breast, urinary bladder, and stomach.

Buschke-Fisher-Brauer is a focal PPK caused by mutations in the *AAGAB* gene. It is characterized by painful hyperkeratosis on the palms and soles that can begins most commonly in childhood and is associated with colon, breast, prostate, and lung cancer in addition to psoriasis and neurologic abnormalities.

Mutilating Keratoderma of Vohwinkel

Vohwinkel described honeycomb palmoplantar hyperkeratosis associated with starfish-like or honeycomb keratoses on the backs of the hands and feet, linear keratoses of the elbows and knees, and annular constriction (pseudo-ainhum) of the digits (Fig. 11.13), which may progress to autoamputation. Inheritance is mostly autosomal dominant, although a recessive type exists. The disease is more common in women and in Caucasians, with onset in infancy or early childhood. Reported associations include deafness, deaf-mutism, high-tone acoustic impairment, congenital alopecia universalis, pseudopelade-type alopecia, acanthosis nigricans, ichthyosiform dermatoses, spastic paraplegia, myopathy, nail changes, mental retardation, and bullous lesions on the soles. Vohwinkel keratoderma without deafness is due to a mutation loricrin and Vohwinkel with deafness is due to mutation in GJB2 (connexin 26). Other disorders caused by mutations in connexin 26 include keratisis ichthyosis deafness syndrome (KID) and is hystrix-like ichthyosis-deafnesss (HID) syndromes, as well as Bart-Pumphrey syndrome, which may also lead to deafness. There have been some reports of a response to acitretin (or etretinate) therapy helping patients with Vohwinkel.

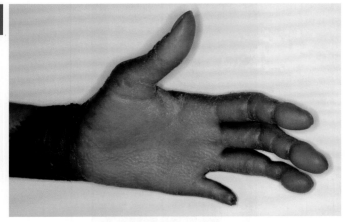

Fig. 11.13 Mutilating keratoderma of Vohwinkel.

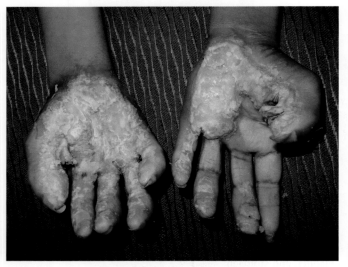

Fig. 11.14 Olmsted syndrome.

Other forms of mutilating keratoderma also occur. They lack the constricting bands, honeycomb palmoplantar hyperkeratosis, and starfish-like keratoses of Vohwinkel syndrome. The affected digits are often shortened, narrow, rigid, and tapered.

Olmsted Syndrome

Olmsted syndrome is characterized by mutilating palmoplantar keratoderma and periorificial keratotic plaques caused by mutations in TRPV3. The distinctive features of this syndrome include a congenital, sharply marginated, palmoplantar keratoderma (Fig. 11.14); constriction of the digits; linear keratotic streaks on the flexural aspects of the wrists; onychodystrophy; and periorificial keratoses. Constriction of digits may result in spontaneous amputations. Extensive grafting has sometimes been necessary. Most cases of Olmsted syndrome are sporadic. Associated abnormalities have included hyperhidrosis of the palms and soles and congenital deafness. Histologically, there is acanthosis, papillomatosis, and orthokeratotic hyperkeratosis. The finding of Ki-67 staining of suprabasal keratinocytes suggests that Olmsted syndrome is a hyperproliferative disorder of the epidermis.

Papillon-Lefèvre Syndrome

The Papillon-Lefèvre syndrome is inherited in an autosomal recessive fashion and presents with palmoplantar keratoderma and destructive periodontitis, usually beginning in young childhood. Well-demarcated, erythematous, hyperkeratotic lesions on the palms and soles may extend to the dorsal hands and feet. Hyperkeratosis may also be present on the elbows, knees, and Achilles tendon areas. Transverse grooves of the fingernails may occur. Severe gingival inflammation with loss of alveolar bone is typical. Histology reveals a psoriasiform pattern. Mutations in the gene for cathepsin C are causative in most cases. The condition usually has an early age of onset, although a late-onset variant has been reported. Some patients with late-onset disease have not shown mutations in the cathepsin C gene.

The early onset of periodontal disease has been attributed to alterations in polymorphonuclear leukocyte function caused by *Actinomyces actinomycetemcomitans*, although a variety of other bacteria have also been implicated. Acro-osteolysis and pyogenic liver abscesses may occur. There are asymptomatic ectopic calcifications in the choroid plexus and tentorium. Some patients have responded to acitretin, etretinate, or isotretinoin.

The stocking-glove distribution of the hyperkeratosis is similar to that seen in mal de Meleda. Haim-Munk syndrome is autosomal recessive with periodontal disease, keratoderma, and onychogryphosis, linked to cathepsin C gene mutations.

Keratoderma Climactericum

Keratoderma climactericum is characterized by hyperkeratosis of the palms and soles (especially the heels) beginning at about the time of menopause. The discrete, thickened, hyperkeratotic patches are most pronounced at sites of pressure such as around the rim of the sole. Fissuring of the thickened patches may be present. There is a striking resemblance to plantar psoriasis, and indeed, keratoderma climactericum may represent a form of psoriasis. Therapy consists of keratolytics such as 10% salicylic acid ointment, lactic acid creams, or 20%–30% urea mixtures. The response to topical corticosteroids is often disappointing. Acitretin is more effective than isotretinoin.

OTHER PALMOPLANTAR DERMATOSES

Collagenous and Elastotic Marginal Plaques of the Hands

Collagenous and elastotic marginal plaques of the hands are slowly progressive lesions at the margins of the palms that demonstrate thickened collagen bundles admixed with elastic fibers and amorphous basophilic elastotic material.

Keratolysis Exfoliativa (Lamellar Dyshidrosis, Recurrent Palmar Peeling)

Keratolysis exfoliativa is a superficial exfoliative dermatosis of the palms and sometimes soles. Clinically inflammation is minimal to absent, and the areas of cleaved epidermis appear as asymptomatic white spots that expand and then peel leaving a colarette of scale (Fig. 11.15). The eruption is often exacerbated by environmental factors. Many patients have an atopic background, and some have lesions of dyshidrotic eczema. Although some suggest it is a cohesion disorder of the stratum corneum, keratolysis exfoliativa more likely represents subclinical eczema. The differential diagnosis includes mild epidermolysis bullosa simplex and acral peeling skin syndrome, both of which should manifest earlier in life. The condition must also be differentiated from dermatophytosis, and a KOH examination or culture is recommended.

Because keratolysis exfoliativa is generally asymptomatic, no treatment may be necessary. In some patients, spontaneous involution occurs in a few weeks. For patients who require treatment, avoidance of wetness and friction when possible and emollients, corticosteroid preparations, tar, urea, and lactic acid or ammonium lactate may be effective.

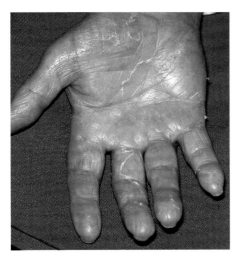

Fig. 11.15 Keratolysis exfoliativa.

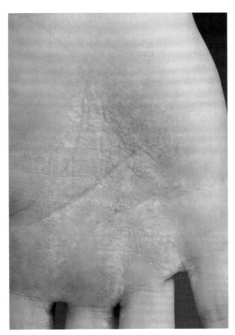

Fig. 11.16 Transient reactive papulotranslucent acrokeratoderma.

Acquired Aquagenic Syringeal Acrokeratoderma (Aquagenic Wrinkling of the Palms)

Patients with papulotranslucent acrokeratoderma, sometimes referred to as aquagenic wrinkling, develop white papules on the palms after water exposure. The skin quickly takes on a waterlogged appearance similar to what normally happens after long exposures to water in normal hosts. The lesions are sharply demarcated from the surrounding skin and appear white. There may be a central prominent pore within each white lesion (Fig. 11.16). In affected individuals the lesions appear 3–5 minutes after exposure to water and resolve within a short time of drying. Sometimes the white skin can be peeled off. The majority of patients with cystic fibrosis and approximately 10% of carriers will have aquagenic wrinkling of the palms, although there is no genotype phenotype correlation. Excess salinity of the sweat creates an osmotic gradient pulling water into the skin. It has also been reported in patients taking

aspirin or rofecoxib. Autosomal dominant inheritance has been suggested in some cases, and abnormally active AQP5 has been described in sweat glands.

Baquerizo K, et al: Atypical form of transient reactive papulotranslucent acrokeratoderma in a cystic fibrosis carrier. J Cutan Pathol 2013; 40: 413.
Biswal SG, et al: Vörner syndrome. Eur J Pediatr Dermatol 2015; 25: 138.
Bonnecaze AK, et al: Keratosis punctata of the palmar creases in a 68-year-old African-American man. BMJ Case Rep 2016 Jul 12; 2016.
Chang YY, et al: Keratolysis exfoliativa (dyshidrosis lamellosa sicca). Br J Dermatol 2012; 167: 1076.
Eytan O, et al: Olmsted syndrome caused by a homozygous recessive mutation in TRPV3. J Invest Dermatol 2014; 134: 1752.
Fuchs-Telem D, et al: Epidermolytic palmoplantar keratoderma caused by activation of a cryptic splice site in *KRT9*. Clin Exp Dermatol 2013; 38: 189.
Kosem R, et al: Cathepsin C gene 5'-untranslated region mutation in Papillon-Lefèvre syndrome. Dermatology 2012; 225: 193.
Kubo A: Nagashima-type palmoplantar keratosis. J Invest Dermatol 2014; 134: 2076e9.
Pohler E, et al: Haploinsufficiency for *AAGAB* causes clinically heterogeneous forms of punctate palmoplantar keratoderma. Nat Genet 2012; 44: 1272.
Sakiyama T, Kubo A: Hereditary palmoplantar keratoderma "clinical and genetic differential diagnosis." J Dermatol 2016; 43: 264.
Tieu KD, et al: Thickened plaques on the hands. Arch Dermatol 2011; 147: 499.
Tsutsumi R, et al: Nagashima-type palmoplantar keratosis with melanoma. Eur J Dermatol 2017; 27: 210.

EXFOLIATIVE DERMATITIS (ERYTHRODERMA)

Exfoliative dermatitis is also known as dermatitis exfoliativa, pityriasis rubra (Hebra), and erythroderma (Wilson-Brocq). Exfoliative erythroderma is not a diagnosis but a clinical phenotype that can result from various diseases including atopic dermatitis, psoriasis, PRP, medication reactions, and cutaneous T-cell lymphoma (CTCL). Patients present with extensive erythema and scaling (Fig. 11.17). Ultimately, the entire body surface is dull scarlet and covered by small, laminated scales that exfoliate profusely. An extensive telogen effluvium may be noted. In both PRP and mycosis fungoides, distinctly spared islands of skin are frequently noted. Patients with PRP also have thickened, orange palms and "nutmeg grater" follicular papules on the dorsa of the fingers (see earlier), although a palmoplantar keratoderma can be seen in CTCL as well.

Itching of the erythrodermic skin may be severe, and the onset is often accompanied by symptoms of general toxicity, including fever and chills. Transepidermal water loss is high, and secondary infections by *Staphylococcus aureus* and streptococcal infections often complicate the disease course in the absence of treatment. Severe complications include sepsis, high-output cardiac failure, acute respiratory distress syndrome, and capillary leak syndrome. The mortality rate attributable to the erythroderma approaches 7% in some series.

Etiology

Erythroderma is usually caused by exacerbation of a pre-existing dermatosis such as atopic dermatitis or psoriasis. Erythroderma can also be from severe drug reactions, idiopathic and less commonly CTCL. In children, especially infants, immunodeficiency, netherton syndrome, ichthyosis, metabolic syndrome, and infection

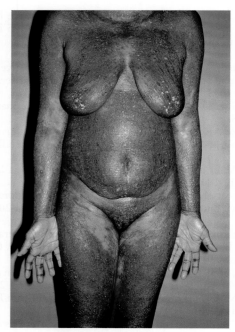

Fig. 11.17 Erythroderma.

should be considered. Atopic dermatitis presenting as erythroderma is usually observed later, after the neonatal period.

In a comparison of patients with and without HIV infection, erythroderma in the HIV-positive group was most often related to drug reactions. HIV-positive patients did not have an overall increase in the number of episodes of erythroderma.

Mycosis fungoides can be erythrodermic without meeting the criteria for the Sézary syndrome. Sézary syndrome consists of generalized exfoliative dermatitis with intense pruritus, leonine facies, alopecia, palmoplantar hyperkeratosis, and onychodystrophy. The criteria for a diagnosis of Sézary syndrome include an absolute Sézary cell count of at least 1000 cells/mm^3; a CD4/CD8 ratio of 10 or higher by flow cytometry, caused by an increase in circulating T cells or loss of expression of pan–T-cell markers; increased lymphocyte counts with evidence of a T-cell clone by Southern blot or polymerase chain reaction; or a chromosomally abnormal T-cell clone. Prognosis is poor and similar to that of patients with nodal involvement.

Hodgkin disease may show generalized exfoliative dermatitis. Fever, lymphadenopathy, splenomegaly, and hepatomegaly are frequently present. The erythrocyte sedimentation rate is elevated in most of these patients.

Histopathology

Exfoliative dermatitis may retain the histologic features of the original disease process. This is particularly true in patients with psoriasis and mycosis fungoides. Often, however, the histology is nonspecific, with hyperkeratosis, mild acanthosis, and focal parakeratosis.

Treatment

Treatment of the erythroderma should target the primary cause the treatments are covered in greater depth in the individual sectiosn that discuss those diseases. Application of a medium-strength corticosteroid after soaking and occlusion under a sauna suit are often helpful, regardless of the cause of the erythroderma. Moist pajamas can be added under the sauna suit. Acitretin, cyclosporine, and methotrexate are useful in psoriatic erythroderma. Isotretinoin, acitretin, and methotrexate are useful in erythroderma caused by PRP. TNF-α agents should be avoided if the diagnosis is in question as they can lead to significant worsening of CTCL.

Carter JB, et al: Case records of the Massachusetts General Hospital: Case 24-2013—a 53-year-old woman with erythroderma, pruritus, and lymphadenopathy. N Engl J Med 2013; 369: 559.

Chinazzo C, et al: Aquagenic wrinkling of the palms and cystic fibrosis. Dermatology 2014; 228: 60.

Dhar S, et al: Neonatal erythroderma. Indian J Dermatol 2012; 57: 475.

Dunst-Huemer KM, et al: Generalized erythroderma and palmoplantar hyperkeratosis in a patient receiving TNF-α antagonist therapy. J Cutan Pathol 2013; 40: 855.

Hulmani M, et al: Clinico-etiological study of 30 erythroderma cases from tertiary center in South India. Indian Dermatol Online J 2014; 5: 25.

Mohd Noor N, et al: Transepidermal water loss in erythrodermic patients of various aetiologies. Skin Res Technol 2013; 19: 320.

Rice SA, et al: Erythroderma in the emergency department. BMJ 2013; 346: f3613.

Yang JH, et al: Paraneoplastic erythroderma. Int J Dermatol 2013; 52: 1149.

Watanabe T, et al: Pityriasis Rosea is Associated with Systemic Active Infection with Both Human Herpesvirus-7 and Human Herpesvirus-6. J Invest Dermatol 2002; 119: 793.

LICHEN PLANUS

Lichen planus (LP) is a common, pruritic, inflammatory disease of the skin, mucous membranes, and hair follicles. It occurs throughout the world, in all races. Cutaneous LP affects 0.3% of men and 0.1% of women. Oral LP affects 1.5% of men and 2.3% of women. It may be familial in rare cases. The pattern of LP detected and the age distribution vary among various genetic and geographic groups; certain human leukocyte antigen (HLA) alleles (HLA-DR/DQ, HLA-A3), gene mutations (MTHFR), and single-nucleotide polymorphisms (tumor necrosis factor–α [TNF-α], NRP2, IGFBP4) have been reported to confer risk in select populations and subgroups. In persons of European descent, LP appears primarily after age 20 and peaks between 40 and 70. Very few cases appear after age 80. Childhood LP typically accounts for 5% or less of LP cases, although in some regions, including the Indian subcontinent, Arab countries, and Mexico, it represents 10%–20%. Race appears to be the critical factor; in the United States, LP occurs more commonly in African American children, and in the United Kingdom, for example, Indians account for 80% of childhood LP. Pathophysiologically LP is a T-cell disorder with increased Th1 cytokine expression and T-cell activity at the basement membrane zone.

The primary lesions of LP are characteristic, almost pathognomonic: small, flat-topped, polygonal papules (Fig. 12.1). The color of the lesions initially is erythematous. Well-developed lesions are violaceous, and resolving lesions are often hyperpigmented, especially in patients with darker skin. The surface is glistening and dry, with scant, adherent scales. On the surface, gray or white puncta or streaks (Wickham striae) cross the lesions—a feature seen more easily with dermoscopy. Lesions begin as pinpoint papules and expand to 0.5–1.5 cm plaques. Infrequently, larger lesions are seen. There is a predilection for the flexor wrists, trunk, medial thighs, shins, dorsal hands, and glans penis (Fig. 12.2). The face is only rarely involved, with lesions usually confined to the eyelids and lips. The palms and soles may be affected with small papules or hyperkeratotic plaques (Fig. 12.3). Certain morphologic patterns favor certain locations (e.g., annular lesions favoring penis; keratotic lesions favoring anterior shins). Lesions are often bilateral and relatively symmetric. The Koebner phenomenon occurs in LP (Fig. 12.4). Oral mucosal involvement is common.

Pruritus is often prominent in LP. The pruritus may precede the appearance of the skin lesions, and the intensity of the itch may seem out of proportion to the amount of skin disease. Most patients react to the itching of LP by rubbing rather than scratching, and thus scratch marks are usually not present, though linear papules of LP can indicate prior scratching and koebnerization.

The natural history of LP is highly variable and dependent on the site of involvement and the clinical pattern. Two thirds of patients with skin lesions will have LP for less than 1 year, and many patients spontaneously clear in the second year. Hypertrophic and mucosal disease tends to be more chronic. Recurrences are common. In older patients, and those with comorbidities such as hyperlipidemia and diabetes, LP may persist for longer duration.

Nail changes are present in approximately 5%–10% of patients (Fig. 12.5), with fingernails more often affected than toenails.

Involvement of the nail can occur as an initial manifestation, especially in children. Longitudinal ridging and splitting are most common, seen in 90% of patients with nail involvement. Onycholysis and subungual debris may be present, indicating involvement of the nail bed. The lunulae are red in 30% of patients with nail LP. Involvement of the entire matrix may lead to obliteration of the whole nail plate (anonychia). Pterygium formation is characteristic of LP of the nails, but seen in only about 20% of patients. The nail matrix is destroyed by the inflammation and replaced by fibrosis. The proximal nailfold fuses with the proximal portion of the nail bed. Dermoscopy can show pitting of the nail matrix, tachyonychia, chromonychia, onycholysis, or splinter hemorrhages. LP may be a cause of some cases of 20-nail dystrophy of childhood. In the absence of periungual lesions or pterygium formation, 20-nail dystrophy usually resolves spontaneously, and frequently in these children, no other stigmata of cutaneous or mucosal LP are found.

Involvement of the genitalia, with or without lesions at other sites, is common. On the glans or shaft of the penis, the lesions may consist of flat, polygonal papules, or these may be annular. Erosive LP can occur on the glans. Simultaneous involvement of the gingival and penile mucosa may occur. On the labia and anus, similar lesions are observed, which may be whitish because of maceration. Half of women with oral LP also have vulvovaginal LP, but in only half of these patients is the genital LP symptomatic. Vulval LP occurs in three main forms. The *classic* type presents with polygonal papules resembling cutaneous LP and affects the clitoral hood and labia minora. Pruritus is the usual symptom. Although only about 20% of women with vulval LP have *erosive* or *ulcerative* LP, this type represents the vast majority of patients seen for vulval LP, because it is usually very symptomatic. Soreness, pain, and dyspareunia are frequent complaints. Vaginal involvement with a bloody discharge can occur. Involvement is symmetric from the fourchette to the anterior vestibule. The erosions have a lacy white periphery, a good area to biopsy to confirm the diagnosis of vulval LP. Vulvovaginal-gingival syndrome is characterized by involvement at these three sites, with significant long-term sequelae due to scaring; patients may also have scarring at other mucosal sites, including the esophagus and eye. The third, and least common, form of vulval LP is the *hypertrophic* type. It involves the perineum and perianal skin (but not the vagina) with warty plaques with a violaceous edge. Pruritus is severe. Vulval splitting, vaginal stenosis, and sealing of the clitoral hood may be caused by LP. It is important to distinguish vulvovaginal LP from lichen sclerosus et atrophicus.

Conjunctival involvement is a rarely recognized complication of LP but was seen in 0.5% of patients with vulval LP in one series. It most frequently occurs in patients with involvement of other mucosal surfaces. Cicatrization, lacrimal canalicular duct scarring, and keratitis can occur. It may closely simulate mucous membrane pemphigoid. Routine histology and direct immunofluorescence (DIF) may be required to confirm the diagnosis.

Otic involvement by LP is rarely reported. It affects primarily females (80% of patients) and is associated with oral and vulval LP in more than 50% of cases, and cutaneous LP in 5 of 19 (26%). Hearing loss and external auditory canal stenosis are the most common otic complaints and complications. Four of 19 (21%) patients with otic LP also had esophageal involvement.

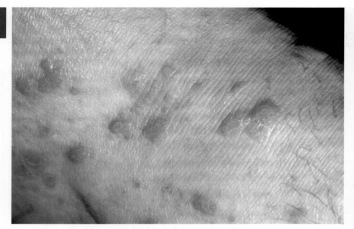
Fig. 12.1 Lichen planus. (Courtesy Steven Binnick, MD.)

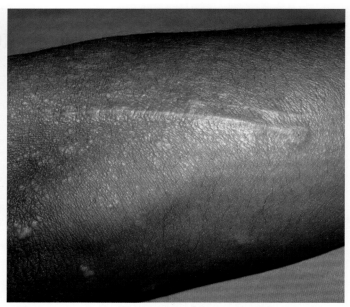
Fig. 12.4 Koebnerized lichen planus. (Courtesy Debabrata Bandyopadhyay, MD.)

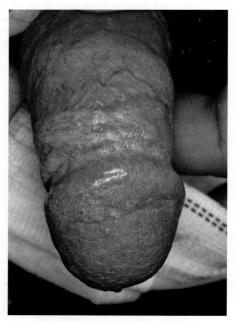
Fig. 12.2 Lichen planus of the penis.

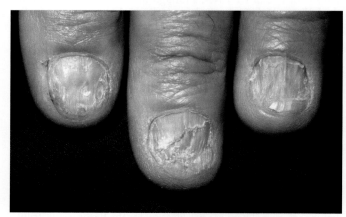
Fig. 12.5 Lichen planus of the nail.

LP of the esophagus is uncommon but increasingly being recognized, and the diagnosis is frequently delayed. One study involving endoscopy in 32 consecutive patients with LP identified 10 with probable and 10 with definitive esophageal disease. Dysphagia, odynophagia, and weight loss are typical manifestations. The proximal esophagus is more frequently affected. Most patients have coexistent oral disease. Esophageal involvement is much more common in women. One paper in the gastrointestinal literature noted that stricture formation occurs in 80% of esophageal LP and may require frequent dilations; the observed rate in dermatologic practice is much lower. Esophageal squamous cell carcinoma (SCC) may complicate esophageal LP, suggesting that, once this diagnosis is made, routine gastrointestinal evaluation is required.

Whether the many clinical variants of LP represent separate diseases or part of the LP spectrum is unknown. They all demonstrate typical LP histologically. The variants are described separately because their clinical features are distinct from classic LP. Some patients with these clinical variants may have typical cutaneous, follicular, or mucosal LP. The more common or well-known variants are described here.

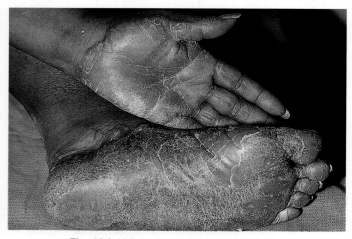
Fig. 12.3 Lichen planus of the palm and sole.

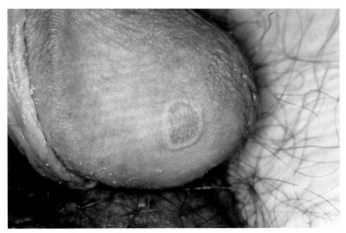

Fig. 12.6 Annular lichen planus. (Courtesy Steven Binnick, MD.)

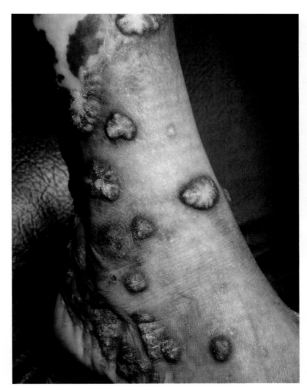

Fig. 12.7 Hypertrophic lichen planus. (Courtesy Debabrata Bandyopadhyay, MD.)

Linear Lichen Planus

Small, linear lesions caused by the Koebner phenomenon often occur in classic LP. Limitation of LP to one band or streak has also been described in fewer than 1% of patients of European descent. In Japan, however, up to 10% of cases are linear, and in India, 7% of childhood cases of LP are linear. Although originally described as following dermatomes (zosteriform), the lesions actually follow lines of Blaschko. It is more common in children but also occurs in adults. Papules with varying degrees of overlying hyperkeratosis or simple hyperpigmentation may be the presenting manifestations. There are often "skip areas" of normal skin between the individual lesions. Ipsilateral mucosal disease may be seen.

Annular and Annular Atrophic Lichen Planus

Annular LP occurs in 3%–7% of patients with LP, and is more common in men (90% of cases). Lesions with this configuration favor the axilla, penis/scrotum (Fig. 12.6), and groin. LP lesions of the mucosa, scalp, and nails are rare in patients with annular LP. Patients usually have fewer than 10 lesions. Most patients with annular LP are asymptomatic. The ringed lesions are composed of small papules and measure about 1 cm in diameter. Central hyperpigmentation may be the dominant feature. They may coalesce to form polycyclic figures. Annular lesions may also result from central involution of flat papules or plaques, forming lesions with violaceous, elevated borders and central hyperpigmented macules. A rare type of annular lichenoid dermatitis which may resemble morphea, inflammatory vitiligo, or mycosis fungoides has been described in pediatric patients termed annular lichenoid dermatitis of youth; one report from a region with endemic borrelia suggested a possible etiologic link, which has not been proven.

Hypertrophic Lichen Planus

Hypertrophic LP usually occurs on the shins but may occur anywhere. The anterior lower leg below the knee is the sole area of involvement in most patients. The typical lesions are verrucous plaques with variable amounts of scale (Fig. 12.7). At the edges of the plaques, small, flat-topped, polygonal papules may at times be discovered. Superficial inspection of the lesion often suggests psoriasis or a keratinocytic neoplasm rather than LP, but the typical appearance resembling rapidly cooled igneous rock (igneous rock sign) may be useful in suggesting LP over keratinocytic neoplasms. The lesions are of variable size but are frequently several centimeters in diameter and larger than the lesions of classic LP. Dermoscopy of hypertrophic LP may demonstrate pearly white

areas and peripheral striations, which can help distinguish it from mimickers in some cases; however, clinical diagnosis may be difficult, and biopsy is often required. Histologically, the pseudoepitheliomatous keratinocyte hyperplasia may be marked, leading to the erroneous diagnosis of SCC. Eosinophils are much more often present in the dermal infiltrate of hypertrophic LP than classic LP. True SCC may also evolve from long-standing hypertrophic LP, over long as 11–12 years. In addition, keratoacanthoma-like proliferations may occur in lesions of hypertrophic LP. This has also been called "hypertrophic lichen planus–like reactions combined with infundibulocystic hyperplasia." Hypertrophic LP is chronic and often refractory to topical therapy. Hypertrophic lupus erythematosus (LE) resembles hypertrophic LP both clinically and histologically. Hypertrophic LE tends to affect the distal extremities, face, and scalp. The finding of continuous granular immunoglobulin on DIF strongly suggests a diagnosis of hypertrophic LE rather than LP.

Erosive/Ulcerative/Mucosal Lichen Planus

Erosive LP has significant impact on quality of life, and patients with erosive LP have high levels of depression, anxiety, and stress. Ulcerative LP is rare on the skin but common on the mucous membranes. A rare ulcerative variant of cutaneous LP, or LE/LP overlap syndrome, affects the feet and toes, causing bullae, ulcerations, and permanent loss of the toenails. These chronic ulcerations on the feet are painful and disabling. Cicatricial alopecia may be present on the scalp, and the buccal mucosa may also be affected. These cases are a therapeutic challenge, and aggressive oral retinoid or immunomodulatory treatment is indicated if there is a poor response to standard topical and systemic agents. Skin grafting of the soles has produced successful results.

Oral mucosal LP is the most common form of mucosal LP, and it is usually chronic. Between 10% and 15% of patients with oral LP will also have skin lesions. Women represent 50%–75%

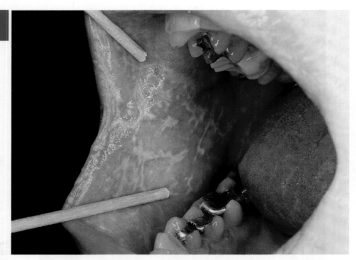

Fig. 12.8 Lichen planus, reticulate white lesions of the buccal mucosa.

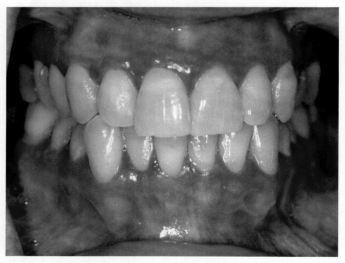

Fig. 12.9 Desquamative gingivitis in the vulvovaginal syndrome.

of patients with oral LP. Oral LP in women begins 10 years later than in men (age 57 vs. 47). Oral lesions may be reticulate (reticular), the oral version of Wickham striae (Fig. 12.8), erythematous (atrophic), or ulcerative (erosive) (Fig. 12.9); lesions are often bilateral and symmetric. The most common pattern in oral LP is the ulcerative form (40% of patients). Usually, reticulate and erythematous lesions are found adjacent to the ulcerative areas. The erythematous pattern is the predominant pattern in 37% of patients, but almost always, reticulate lesions are also seen in these patients. In oral LP, the "classic" reticulate lesions are most prominent in 23% of patients. Rarely patients may have a white plaque mimicking leukoplakia, bullous, or papular lesions. Symptoms are least common in patients with reticulate lesions; 23% are symptomatic, and then only when the tongue is involved. All patients with erosive lesions are symptomatic, usually with burning or pain. Patients may simultaneously have several patterns, so patients are characterized by the primary form they exhibit. Lesions appear on any portion of the mouth, and multisite involvement is common. The buccal mucosa is involved in 90%, the gingiva in more than 50%, and the tongue in about 40%.

On the gingiva, LP may produce desquamative gingivitis (see Fig. 12.9). Gingival involvement is particularly difficult to diagnose and often requires biopsy for both histology and DIF to confirm the diagnosis and exclude other autoimmune causes of desquamative gingivitis. Gingival involvement is associated with accelerated gingival recession. Mechanical injury from dental procedures and poorly fitting appliances may trigger or exacerbate gingival LP. On the tongue and palate, lesions are often mistaken for leukoplakia. The lower lip is involved in 15% of oral LP patients, but the upper lip in only 2%. Lower lip LP is frequently mistaken for actinic cheilitis. Imiquimod treatment can lead to exacerbation of the labial LP, with extensive erosion and crusting. Oral LP is stable but chronic, with fewer than 3% of patients having a spontaneous remission in an average 5-year follow-up. Periodontitis appears to exacerbate oral LP, especially gingival disease. Plaque control either by the patient after training or by a dental professional improves the clinical appearance and pain.

Oral lichenoid lesion (OLL), or oral lichenoid reaction (OLR), refers to an oral lesion histologically identical to oral LP (OLP) but from a different cause, such as graft-versus-host disease (GVHD), medications (antihypertensives, dapsone, nonsteroidal antiinflammatory drugs [NSAIDs], penicillamine, phenothiazines, antimalarials, oral hypoglycemics, and more), and local or systemic exposures. Gold, cobalt, indium, manganese, chrome, nickel, palladium, cinnamate, and spearmint sensitivity may induce OLLs. The most common causes, however, are the metals in dental amalgams, including mercury, copper, zinc, and tin. If the lesions in the oral mucosa are physically close to the amalgam, removal of the amalgam will lead to resolution of the OLL in 36%. In patients patch test positive to a metal in the amalgam, 44% and 47% of OLLs healed with removal of the amalgam in two studies. In patients with the OLL in strict contact with the amalgam, and there is a relevant positive patch test to a component of the amalgam, 80% to 90% or more of OLLs will heal. Patch testing, however, may not identify all patients whose OLLs improve with removal of the oral metal. Rarely, patients with metal sensitivity will also have skin and nail lesions that improve with removal of the oral metal. In one study, 6 of 10 patients with nail LP who were patch test positive to a metal in their amalgam improved with removal of the dental material or with oral disodium chromoglycate treatment.

Involvement of the vulva and vagina with LP, along with the gingiva, has been called the vulvovaginal-gingival (VVG) syndrome. Although all three of these mucous membranes may be involved, only one or two sites may be involved at any one time. The prevalence of erosive vulvar LP had been underappreciated simply because many women with oral LP did not volunteer their vulvovaginal complaints and were not asked about them. The vaginal lesions of VVG are erythematous, friable erosions that are very painful. Untreated scarring is severe and can lead to adhesions, vestibular bands, and even vaginal stenosis. In one third of patients, typical reticulate buccal LP is seen, and in up to 80% the oral mucosa is also involved. Cutaneous lesions occur in 20%–40% of VVG patients. The course of the VVG syndrome is protracted, and patients frequently have sequelae, including chronic pain, dyspareunia, and even scarring of the conjunctiva, urethra, and oral, laryngeal, pharyngeal, and esophageal mucosae. Nails are involved in about 15% of patients with VVG, compared with only 2% of patients with oral LP. The VVG syndrome is now considered to be a separate subgroup of mucosal LP that is particularly disabling, scarring, and refractory to therapy.

Bullous Lichen Planus

Two forms of LP may be accompanied by bullae. In bullous LP (BLP), individual lesions, usually on the lower extremities, will vesiculate centrally, with bullae confined to preexisting LP lesions. Histology reveals the bullae are due to a large Max-Joseph space within the extensive lichenoid inflammatory infiltrate. These lesions often spontaneously resolve. There are familiar forms of bullous lichen planus, with earlier onset and more chronic course. Recently checkpoint inhibitors such as PD-1 inhibitors (pembrolizumab) have been shown to cause bullous LP-like reactions, LP pemphigoides, and bullous pemphigoid.

LP pemphigoides describes a rare subset of patients who usually have typical LP, then, an average of 8 months later, develop blistering on their LP lesions and on normal skin. Less often, the blister and the LP lesions occur simultaneously. Clinically, these patients appear to be a combination of LP and bullous pemphigoid. Oral disease may occur and resemble either LP or mucous membrane pemphigoid. LP pemphigoides can be triggered by medications, especially angiotensin-converting enzyme (ACE) inhibitors, as well as interferon (IFN), hepatitis B virus (HBV), and psoralen plus ultraviolet A (PUVA). Pruritus may be severe, and lesions may evolve to resemble pemphigoid nodularis. Bullous pemphigoid affects an older age-group than LP pemphigoides; typical onset for LP pemphigoides is 30–50. Histologically, the LP lesions show LP, and the bullous lesions show the features of bullous pemphigoid. DIF is positive in a linear pattern, with immunoglobulin G (IgG) and C3 along the basement membrane zone (BMZ), at the roof of saline split skin. The antigen targeted by the autoantibody in LP pemphigoides is located in the same region as the bullous pemphigoid antigen, at the basal hemidesmosome. Antibodies from patients with LP pemphigoides typically bind the 180-kD bullous pemphigoid antigen, but in a different region from bullous pemphigoid sera. One case of clinical and histologic bullous LP was reported with autoantibodies to BP180, with authors suggesting chronic inflammation and damage to the BMZ may expose antigens and lead to development of overt LPP over time. LP pemphigoides tends to follow a benign and chronic course, even compared with bullous pemphigoid. Treatment of LP pemphigoides is similar to bullous pemphigoid, with potent topical steroids, systemic steroids, tetracycline, nicotinamide, intravenous immune globulin (IVIG), and immunosuppressives all being variably effective.

Hepatitis-Associated Lichen Planus

Three liver conditions have been associated with LP: hepatitis C virus (HCV), hepatitis B immunization, and primary biliary cirrhosis. HCV infection has been found in proportionately more patients with LP than in controls in numerous studies. The prevalence of HCV infection in patients with LP varies from 1.6% to 20%. There is an association with the HLA-DR6 allele. A systematic review and meta-analysis of 1807 cases of oral LP and 2519 controls revealed an odds ratio was 6.07, with OLP patients having a sixfold higher risk for HCV infection than controls. Despite multiple systematic reviews suggesting a connection, the association of HCV infection and LP has been questioned, perhaps due to geographic differences in disease prevalences. In a large series of patients with oral LP from the United States, none of the 195 patients was infected with HCV, whereas 29% of patients with oral LP from Italy had HCV. In Scotland, 20% of patients infected with HCV had oral LP, compared with 1% of seronegative patients. Although the data are conflicting, screening for HCV appears appropriate in persons from a geographic region where or a population in whom HCV infection is frequently associated with LP. The clinical features of LP in patients with hepatitis C are identical to classic LP, but LP patients with HCV infection are reported as being more likely to have erosive mucous membrane disease, and higher rates of malignancy. The HCV genome is not found in lesions of LP associated with HCV infection. The existence of underlying hepatitis cannot be predicted by clinical pattern or the results of liver function tests. Treatment of hepatitis C with IFN-α may be associated with the initial appearance of LP or exacerbation of preexisting LP. LP may occur at IFN injection sites, and skin testing may reproduce LP-like lesions. LP may improve or may not change with IFN and ribavirin treatment for hepatitis C. Improvement is usually seen toward the end of the treatment course. Most patients do not completely clear their LP. Treatment with newer antivirals for HCV, including ledipasvir-sofosbuvir, have shown conflicting results, with some responders clearing their coexistent LP, and one case of LP developing after HCV clearance.

Although less robust data support an association, HBV immunization may be associated with the appearance of LP in both children and adults. Lesions are typical of LP, and the oral mucosa may be affected. Typically, the first lesions of LP appear about 1 month after the second dose of vaccine. Lesions usually resolve after some time.

Primary biliary cirrhosis and LP may coexist. Patients with this liver abnormality also have a marked propensity to develop a lichenoid eruption while receiving D-penicillamine therapy. Xanthomas in patients with primary biliary cirrhosis may appear initially in lesions of LP, and the infiltrate, although lichenoid, may contain xanthomatous cells. Primary sclerosing cholangitis has been associated with oral LP.

Cancer Risk and Lichen Planus

The risk of malignant transformation in LP varies by morphologic type, with mucosal disease having higher rates. Rare cases of SCC of the skin occurring on the lower leg in lesions of hypertrophic LP have been reported. Cutaneous LP alone is not considered to be a condition with increased cancer risk. Oral LP and vulvovaginal LP, however, do appear to increase the risk of developing SCC. In a study of 13,100 women in Finland, LP was associated with an increased risk of cancers of the lip, tongue, oral cavity, esophagus, larynx, and vulva. About 1% of patients with oral LP will develop oral SCC. A higher risk is seen in smokers, alcoholics, and patients with HCV infection. SCC occurs in patients with erythematous or ulcerative LP, not in those with only the reticulate pattern. Of the oral LP patients who develop oral SCC, only about 45% have one cancer. The majority develop multiple cancers, and close vigilance is recommended in these patients. LP patients with erosive penile and vaginal disease also have developed SCC. The number of penile cases is too low to determine the frequency, but in patients with vulvar LP, development of SCC may be as high as 3%. Clinicians should have a low threshold to biopsy fixed erosive or leukokeratotic lesions in patients with mucosal LP. The use of oral and topical calcineurin inhibitors (CNIs) for LP has been associated with the appearance of SCC on the genitalia. There is no evidence that the medications caused the neoplasia, but if these agents are used, regular follow-up and careful examination are required.

Pathogenesis and Histology

LP is characterized by a Th1 immunologic reaction mediated by CD8+ T cells. These cells induce keratinocytes to undergo apoptosis. Although this inflammatory reaction is thought to be autoimmune, the antigen targeted by these effector T lymphocytes is unknown. The prevalence of autoimmune phenomena is not increased in patients with classic cutaneous LP, however, patient with erosive LP of the vulva (and lichen sclerosus) may have an autoimmune basis. A personal and family history of autoimmune disorders (usually thyroid disease) is present in up to 30% of patients with vulvar LP, and up to 40% have circulating autoantibodies. Patients with oral LP may also have elevated rates of thyroid disease. Patients with LP and OLP have a high rate of dyslipidemia, with elevated triglycerides, elevated low-density lipoprotein (LDL) cholesterol and reduced high-density lipoprotein (HDL) cholesterol. Inflammatory markers also are elevated in the blood of LP patients, potentially contributing to this dyslipidemia. In addition, both insulin resistance and frank type 2 diabetes mellitus are increased in patients with LP compared with controls. Both insulin resistance and dyslipidemia are cardiovascular risk factors. Adult LP patients should be evaluated appropriately. Drug induced lichenoid eruptions are common with a long list of potential triggering agents (including but not limited to checkpoint inhibitors, NSAIDs, allopurinol, oral hypoglycemic agents, anticonvulsants, cardiovascular/blood pressure medications, biologics, antimicrobials, antimalarials, antipsychotic drugs, and more, with some causing specifically photo-accentuated lichenoid eruptions, including antiviral agents such as lepidasvir/sofosbuvir).

LP pemphigoides is hypothesized to result from exposure to the immune system of epitopes in the BP180 antigen as keratinocytes are destroyed by the lichenoid inflammation. Epitope spreading can occur, and LP pemphigoides patients may also develop autoantibodies to the same epitopes as bullous pemphigoid patients.

The histologic features of LP are distinctive and vary with the stage of the lesion. In early lesions, there is an interface dermatitis along the dermoepidermal junction. As the lesion evolves, the epidermis takes on a characteristic appearance. There is destruction of the basal layer with a "sawtooth" pattern of epidermal hyperplasia, orthokeratosis, and beaded hypergranulosis. The basal cells are lost, so the basal layer is described as "squamatized." In the superficial dermis, there is a dense, bandlike infiltrate composed of lymphocytes and melanophages. "Civatte bodies" (cytoid bodies, colloid bodies) represent necrotic keratinocytes in the superficial dermis. Hypertrophic LP shows marked epidermal hyperplasia (pseudoepitheliomatous hyperplasia). Old lesions of LP show effacement of the rete ridge pattern, melanophages in the upper dermis, and occasional Civatte bodies. LP rarely demonstrates parakeratosis or eosinophils (except in hypertrophic LP, where these are characteristic). The presence of either of these suggests a different cause of lichenoid tissue reaction, such as lichenoid drug eruption. Lichen planopilaris, frontal fibrosing alopecia (FFA), and Graham-Little-Piccardi-Lasseur syndrome show the findings of LP, centered on the superficial follicular epithelium.

Lesions of LP of the skin or mucosae can demonstrate clumps of IgM on DIF, and less frequently IgA, IgG, and C3, subepidermally, corresponding to the colloid bodies. Dense, shaggy staining for fibrinogen along the BMZ is characteristic of LP. A lichenoid drug eruption may be difficult to differentiate from LP. The presence of eosinophils or parakeratosis supports the diagnosis of lichenoid drug eruption. GVHD tends to have a sparser infiltrate than LP, and the infiltrate may involve hair follicles if present. Hypertrophic LE may be histologically identical to LP, and the diagnosis is best made by clinical correlation, serologies, and DIF. In most other forms of LE, there is a greater tendency for epidermal atrophy with parakeratosis, dermal mucin is found, and follicular plugging is more prominent. The infiltrate in lupus tends to surround and involve deep portions of the appendageal structures, such as the follicular isthmus and eccrine coil. Deep, nodular, perivascular lymphoplasmacytic infiltrates and necrosis of the fat lobule with fibrin or hyalin rings are also findings characteristic of LE.

Differential Diagnosis

Classic LP (Fig. 12.10) displays lesions that are so characteristic that clinical examination is often adequate to lead to suspicion of the diagnosis. Lichenoid drug eruptions may be difficult to distinguish. A lichenoid drug reaction should be suspected if the eruption is photodistributed, scaly but not hypertrophic, and confluent or widespread—clinical features that are unusual for idiopathic LP. The presence of oral mucosa involvement may prompt suspicion of LP, but oral lesions may occasionally occur in lichenoid drug eruptions as well. Pityriasis rosea, guttate psoriasis, the small papular or lichenoid syphilid, and pityriasis lichenoides et varioliformis acuta are dermatoses that may resemble generalized LP. Mucous membrane lesions may be confused with leukoplakia, LE, mucous patches of syphilis, candidiasis, cancer, and oral lesions of autoimmune bullous diseases, such as pemphigus or cicatricial

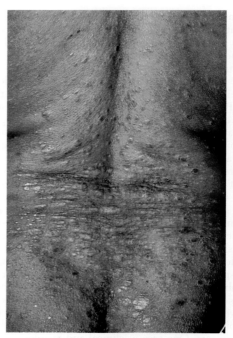

Fig. 12.10 Generalized lichen planus.

pemphigoid. On the scalp, the atrophic lesions may be mistaken for other cicatricial alopecias, such as LE, folliculitis decalvans, and pseudopelade of Brocq. Hypertrophic LP type may simulate psoriasis, LE, SCC, and keratoacanthomas. Isolated patches of LP may resemble lichen simplex chronicus.

Treatment

There is virtually no high-quality evidence for treatment of LP of the skin, scalp, or mucosae. Limited lesions may be treated with superpotent topical corticosteroids or intralesional steroid injections. Topical tacrolimus or pimecrolimus can be effective, particularly for erosive disease. Topical vitamin D derivatives have also been reported to help in small studies. In patients with widespread disease, these treatments are usually unsatisfactory. Widespread lesions respond well to systemic corticosteroids but tend to relapse as the dose is reduced. Monthly pulse dosing has been championed by dermatologists in India. Phototherapy may be effective for cutaneous LP, including narrow-band (NB) ultraviolet B (UVB), UVA I, and PUVA (topical or oral). NB UVB was superior to systemic corticosteroids in one study. A variety of lasers have been reported as helpful in isolated case reports for different morphologic and anatomic forms of LP. Photodynamic therapy with topical 5-aminolevulinic acid can be effective in genital LP. The oral retinoids—isotretinoin, alitretinoin, and acitretin, in doses similar to or slightly lower than those used for other skin conditions—may also be useful and avoid the long-term complications of systemic steroids. They are especially beneficial in patients with hypertrophic LP and palmoplantar LP. Retinoid therapy may be combined with phototherapy in refractory cases. Hydroxychloroquine in standard doses can be effective for cutaneous, oral, genital and follicular LP. Adding quinacrine, 100 mg daily, may be considered in patients with only a partial response to hydroxychloroquine. Thalidomide, 50–150 mg daily, can improve refractory oral and cutaneous LP. Griseofulvin can improve cutaneous LP. Sulfasalazine led to a partial response in 11 of 26 patients. Low-molecular-weight heparin (enoxaparin), injected subcutaneously once a week, led to remission of cutaneous and reticulate oral LP in 61% of patients and improvement in 11%. Enoxaparin is less effective than systemic steroids. Dapsone and metronidazole in small studies failed to outperform topical or phototherapy, though one small series did show 40% of patients responding to metronidazole 250 mg every 8 hours. Apremilast, a phosphodiesterase type IV inhibitor, at a dose of 20 mg twice daily, showed modest efficacy in pooled data, but pruritus was dramatically decreased.

In the most severe cases, immunosuppressive agents may be indicated. Cyclosporine, methotrexate, and mycophenolate mofetil are all options and can induce remission in severe cases of cutaneous and oral LP. The TNF inhibitors have been effective in anecdotal cases. Similarly, extracorporeal photophoresis (ECP), anakinra, rituximab, systemic tacrolimus, and IVIG have been successful in extremely refractory cases.

For oral lesions, superpotent steroids in Orabase or gel form are useful. Vinyl dental trays may be used to apply steroid ointments to the gingiva. Begin with 30-minute applications three times a day and reduce to maintenance of 20 minutes every evening. Addition of nystatin to clobetasol in Orabase may be especially effective. Overall, more than 70% of patients with vulvar LP have relief of symptoms with topical clobetasol. Intralesional injections may be used for focal unresponsive lesions. Topical tacrolimus 0.1% ointment has become standard treatment in erosive LP of the oral and genital mucosa. Burning may occur initially but can be reduced by concomitant use of topical steroids or initial use of a lower strength of tacrolimus ointment. Higher concentrations, up to 0.3%, also may be used. Most patients have a partial but significant response, with increased ability to eat with much less pain. Blood levels can be detected, independent of area of involvement, but tend to decrease over time as the oral erosions heal. Pimecrolimus can be used successfully in patients intolerant of topical tacrolimus. Sustained remissions are rare, and chronic use is usually required to maintain remission. Topical cyclosporine is comparable to topical steroids and should not be used first-line, but may be tried in recalcitrant cases. Topical retinoids may be used but are generally less desirable than topical steroids. Aloe vera gel has been used and in one study was equivalent to steroids. PUVA, photodynamic therapy, and 308-nm excimer laser have been effective in oral LP. The systemic agents recommended earlier to treat cutaneous LP may also improve mucosal disease. For VVG syndrome, corticosteroids topically and systemically are beneficial. Topical therapy with corticosteroids may be enhanced by mixing the steroid in vaginal bioadhesive moisturizer (Replens). Iontophoresis may improve delivery.

Aghbari SMH, et al: Malignant transformation of oral lichen planus and oral lichenoid lesions. Oral Oncol 2017; 68: 92.

Ahlgren C, et al: Contact allergy to gold in patients with oral lichen lesions. Acta Derm Venereol 2012; 92: 138.

Alaizari NA, et al: Hepatitis C virus infections in oral lichen planus. Aust Dent J 2016; 61: 282.

Alomari A, McNiff JM: The significance of eosinophils in hypertrophic lichen planus. J Cutan Pathol 2014; 41: 347.

Alrashdan MS, et al: Oral lichen planus. Arch Dermatol Res 2016; 308: 539.

Atzmony L, et al: Treatments for cutaneous lichen planus. Am J Clin Dermatol 2016; 17: 11.

Brauns B, et al: Intralesional steroid injection alleviates nail lichen planus. Int J Dermatol 2011; 50: 626.

Cesinaro AM: Annular lichenoid dermatitis (of youth). Am J Dermatopathol 2017; ePub ahead of print.

Cohen PR, Kurzrock R: Anakinra-responsive lichen planus in a woman with Erdheim-Chester disease. Dermatol Online J 2014; 20: 21241.

Domingues E, et al: Imiquimod reactivation of lichen planus. Cutis 2012; 89: 276.

Dreijer J, et al: Lichen planus and dyslipidaemia. Br J Dermatol 2009; 11: 626.

Friedman P, et al: Dermoscopic findings in different clinical variants of lichen planus. Dermatol Pract Concept 2015; 5: 51.

Fox LP, et al: Lichen planus of the esophagus. J Am Acad Dermatol 2011; 65: 175.

Fujii M, et al: Bullous lichen planus accompanied by elevation of serum anti-BP180 autoantibody. J Dermatol 2017; 44: e124.

Garcia-Pola MJ, et al: Thyroid disease and oral lichen planus as comorbidity. Dermatology 2016; 232: 214.

Garcia-Pola MJ, et al: Treatment of oral lichen planus. Med Clin (Barc) 2017; 149: 351.

Goettmann S, et al: Nail lichen planus. J Eur Acad Dermatol Venereol 2012; 26: 1304.

Goñi Esarte S, et al: Rituximab as rescue therapy in refractory esophageal lichen planus. Gastroenterol Hepatol 2013; 36: 264.

Gorouhi F, et al: Cutaneous and mucosal lichen planus: a comprehensive review of clinical subtypes, risk factors, diagnosis, and prognosis. ScientificWorldJournal 2014; 742826.

Gupta S, et al: Interventions for the management of oral lichen planus. Oral Dis 2017; 23: 1029.

Halonen P, et al: Cancer risk of lichen planus. Int J Cancer 2018; 142: 18.

Holló P, et al: Successful treatment of lichen planus with adalimumab. Acta Derm Venereol 2012; 92: 339.

Iraji F, et al: Comparison of the narrow band UVB versus systemic corticosteroids in the treatment of lichen planus. J Res Med Sci 2011; 16: 1578.

Ito Y, et al: Disseminated lichen planus due to a zinc allergy. J Dermatol 2012; 39: 948.

Jin X, et al: Association between -308 G/A polymorphism in TNF-α gene and lichen planus. J Dermatol Sci 2012; 68: 127.

Kanwar AJ, De D: Methotrexate for treatment of lichen planus. J Eur Acad Dermatol Venereol 2013; 27: e410.

Kern JS, et al: Esophageal involvement is frequent in lichen planus. Eur J Gastroenterol Hepatol 2016; 28: 1374.

Kurago ZB: Etiology and pathogenesis of oral lichen planus: an overview. Oral Surg Oral Med Oral Pathol Oral Radiol 2016; 122: 72.

Lade NR, et al: Blaschkoid lichen planus. Dermatol Online J 2013; 19: 17.

Le Cleach L, Chosidow O: Lichen planus. N Engl J Med 2012; 366: 723.

Lewis FM, Bogliatto F: Erosive vulval lichen planus. Eur J Obstet Gynecol Reprod Biol 2013; 171: 214.

Liakopoulou A, et al: Bullous lichen planus—a review. J Dermatol Case Rep 2017; 11: 1.

Limas C, Limas CJ: Lichen planus in children. Pediatr Dermatol 2002; 19: 204.

Lodi G, et al: Hepatitis C virus infection and lichen planus. Oral Dis 2010; 16: 601.

Lospinoso DJ, et al: Lupus erythematosus/lichen planus overlap syndrome. Lupus 2013; 22: 851.

Lucchese A, et al: Vulvovaginal gingival lichen planus. Oral Implantol (Rome) 2016; 9: 54.

Montebugnoli L, et al: Clinical and histologic healing of lichenoid oral lesions following amalgam removal. Oral Surg Oral Med Oral Pathol Oral Radiol 2012; 113: 766.

Morales-Callaghan A Jr, et al: Annular atrophic lichen planus. J Am Acad Dermatol 2005; 52: 906.

Muñoz ER, et al: Isolated conjunctival lichen planus. Arch Dermatol 2011; 147: 465.

Nagao Y, et al: Genome-wide association study identifies risk variants for lichen planus in patients with hepatitis C virus infection. Clin Gastroenterol Hepatol 2017; 15: 937.

Nakashima C, et al: Treatment of intractable oral lichen planus with intravenous immunoglobulin therapy. Eur J Dermatol 2012; 22: 693.

Nishizawa A, et al: Close association between metal allergy and nail lichen planus. J Eur Acad Dermatol 2013; 27: e231.

Pandhi D et al: Lichen planus in childhood. Pediatr Dermatol 2014, 31: 59.

Parodi A, et al: Prevalence of stratified epithelium-specific antinuclear antibodies in 138 patients with lichen planus. J Am Acad Dermatol 2007; 56: 974.

Passeron T, et al: Treatment of oral erosive lichen planus with 1% pimecrolimus cream. Arch Dermatol 2007; 143: 472.

Paul J, et al: An open-label pilot study of apremilast for the treatment of moderate to severe lichen planus. J Am Acad Dermatol 2013; 68: 255.

Payette MJ, et al: Lichen planus and other lichenoid dermatoses. Clin Dermatol 2015; 33: 631.

Quispel R, et al: High prevalence of esophageal involvement in lichen planus. Endoscopy 2009; 41: 187.

Radfar L, et al: A comparative treatment study of topical tacrolimus and clobetasol in oral lichen planus. Oral Surg Oral Med Oral Pathol Oral Radiol Endod 2008; 105: 187.

Rashed L, et al: Studying the association between methylene-tetrahydrofolate reductase (MTHFR) 677 gene polymorphism, cardiovascular risk and lichen planus. J Oral Pathol Med 2017; 46: 1023.

Rasi A, et al: Efficacy of oral metronidazole in treatment of cutaneous and mucosal lichen planus. J Drugs Dermatol 2010; 9: 1186.

Rogers RS, Bruce AJ: Lichenoid contact stomatitis. Arch Dermatol 2004; 140: 1524.

Salgado DS, et al: Plaque control improves the painful symptoms of oral lichen planus gingival lesions. J Oral Pathol Med 2013; 42: 728.

Sartori-Valinotti JC, et al: A 10-year review of otic lichen planus. JAMA Dermatol 2013; 149: 1082.

Schmidgen MI, et al: Pembrolizumab-induced lichen planus pemphigoides in a patient with metastatic melanoma. J Dtsch Dermatol Ges 2017; 15: 742.

Scott GD, et al: New-onset cutaneous lichen planus following therapy for hepatitis C with ledipasvir-sofosbuvir. J Cutan Pathol 2016; 43: 408.

Shah KM, et al: Oral lichenoid reaction due to nickel alloy contact hypersensitivity. BMJ Case Rep 2013; 2013.

Simpson RC, et al: Real-life experience of managing vulval erosive lichen planus. Br J Dermatol 2012; 167: 85.

Singal A: Familial mucosal lichen planus in three successive generations. Int J Dermatol 2005; 44: 81.

Singh S, et al: Lichen planus causing severe vulval stenosis. Int J Dermatol 2013; 52: 1398.

Suresh SS, et al: Medical management of oral lichen planus. J Clin Diagn Res 2016; 10: ZE10-5.

Thorne JE, et al: Lichen planus and cicatrizing conjunctivitis. Am J Ophthalmol 2003; 136: 239.

Thornhill M, et al: The role of histopathological characteristic in distinguishing amalgam-associated oral lichenoid reactions and oral lichen planus. J Oral Pathol Med 2006; 35: 233.

Tiwari SM, et al: Dental patch testing in patients with undifferentiated oral lichen planus. Australas J Dermatol 2017; ePub ahead of print.

Wakade DV, et al: PD-1 inhibitors induced bullous lichen planus-like reactions. Melanoma Res 2016; 26: 421.

Walton KE, et al: Childhood lichen planus. Pediatr Dermatol 2010; 27: 34.

Webber NK, et al: Lacrimal canalicular duct scarring in patients with lichen planus. Arch Dermatol 2012; 148: 224.

Wee JS, et al: Efficacy of mycophenolate mofetil in severe mucocutaneous lichen planus. Br J Dermatol 2012; 167: 36.

Weston G, et al: Update on lichen planus and its clinical variants. Int J Womens Dermatol 2015; 1: 140.

Wilk M, et al: Annular lichenoid dermatitis (of youth). Am J Dermatopathol 2017; 39: 177.

Xia J, et al: Short-term clinical evaluation of intralesional triamcinolone acetonide injection for ulcerative oral lichen planus. J Oral Pathol Med 2006; 35: 327.

Yew YW, et al: A retrospective cohort study of epidemiology and clinical outcome in lichen planus. Ann Acad Med Singapore 2016; 45: 516.

Zaraa I, et al: Lichen planus pemphigoides. Int J Dermatol 2013; 52: 406.

Zendell K: Genital lichen planus. Semin Cutan Med Surg 2015; 34: 182.

Adnexal Lichen Planus: Follicular Lichen Planus (Lichen Planopilaris) and Acrosyringeal Lichen Planus

Lichen planopilaris (LPP) is lichen planus involving the follicular apparatus. Most cases involve the scalp, and LPP is an important cause of cicatricial alopecia (Fig. 12.11; see Chapter 33). From 70%–90% or more of affected patients are women, usually about age 50. The oral mucosa may be involved in 7%–27% of patients, and 20%–40% of patients have cutaneous involvement. Patients often demonstrate perifollicular erythema and scale with progressive scarring; dermoscopy may reveal subtle signs of the folliculocentric inflammation. As with classic LP, there are reports of trauma inducing LPP. Patients may have lesions scattered throughout the scalp, clustered centrally, or on the margins; one study of 80 patients showed the FFA variant in 31% of patients with LPP. FFA is considered a variant of LPP markedly more common in postmenopausal women, with rare skin-colored papules on the upper face often lateral to the eyes, frequent loss of eyebrows, and occasionally loss of axillary and/or pubic hair. One study demonstrated an androgen excess in LPP and an androgen deficiency in patients with FFA. Graham-Little-Piccardi-Lasseur syndrome is a rare variant of LPP of the scalp with coexistent keratosis pilaris–like LPP lesions on the skin. Patients may rarely present with localized linear LPP. The rarest variant of LPP is lichen planus follicularis tumidus, formerly called agminate lichen follicularis with cysts and comedones. This presents in the retroauricular area and on the cheeks of middle-age women, where the lesions appear as tumid, red-violet plaques covered with numerous small, white-yellow cysts and comedones. The lesions resemble the plaques seen in Favre-Racouchot syndrome and phymatous cystic rosacea. The ears, chin, and scalp can be similarly involved. Other areas of LP of the skin and nails can occur in the same patient, and these may appear at about the same time. Histologically, a dense lichenoid

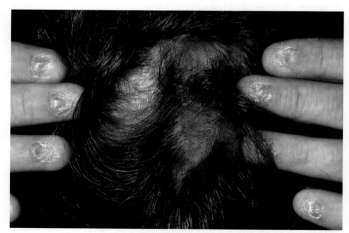

Fig. 12.11 Lichen planopilaris.

infiltrate surrounds the follicles and cysts of the affected skin. The cysts are considered secondary to the lichenoid inflammation. Favre-Racouchot syndrome, follicular mucinosis, and LE must be distinguished histologically from LPP. LPP treatment often involves potent topical corticosteroids and/or intralesional injections, with systemic options including hydroxychloroquine, tetracycline-class antibiotics, retinoids, pioglitazones, and sometimes suppressive agents such as cyclosporine, mycophenolate, methotrexate, or systemic steroids. FFA has been treated with 5-α reductase inhibitors as well. Hair transplantation may be an option once the inflammation is controlled.

LP can involve the soles and at times the palms. Lesions are typically scaly plaques that look very hyperkeratotic or psoriasiform and are usually only diagnosed by the coexistence of typical LP elsewhere or by biopsy. Less often, the lesions of LP of the palms and soles may present as petechial-like lesions, or diffuse keratoderma. When palmoplantar LP affects primarily the acrosyringium, the lesions appear as umbilicated papules or punctate keratoses. A biopsy is usually required to confirm the diagnosis, unless typical LP is present elsewhere. Palmoplantar LP can respond well to oral retinoids.

Esteban-Lucia L, et al: Update on frontal fibrosing alopecia. Actas Dermosifiliogr 2017; 108: 293.

Jiménez-Gallo D, et al: Facial follicular cysts. J Cutan Pathol 2013; 40: 818.

Lyakhovitsky A, et al: A case series of 46 patients with lichen planopilaris. J Dermatolog Treat 2015; 26: 275.

Mesinkovska NA, et al: The use of oral pioglitazone in the treatment of lichen planopilaris. J Am Acad Dermatol 2015; 72: 355.

Ranasinghe GC, et al: Prevalence of hormonal and endocrine dysfunction in patients with lichen planopilaris (LPP). J Am Acad Dermatol 2017; 76: 314.

Soares VC, et al: Lichen planopilaris epidemiology. An Bras Dermatol 2015; 90: 666.

Zeng YP, et al: Lichen planus with palmoplantar involvement. Eur J Dermatol 2011; 21: 632.

Lichen Planus Pigmentosus/Actinicus

LP pigmentosus is seen primarily in Central America, the Indian subcontinent, the Middle East, and Japan. It appears to be a form of LP restricted to certain racial groups. The persons from these genetic groups can develop the condition when they move to North America and Europe, but Caucasians from Europe and North America do not develop LP pigmentosus when they move to tropical areas where the disease is common. LP pigmentosus patients are young, usually 20–45, and men and women are equally affected. Men present a decade earlier (mean age 26 vs. 34). One study suggested a possible association with thyroid disease, usually hypothyroidism. The face and neck are primarily involved (Fig. 12.12), but the axilla, inframammary region, and groin may also be affected; ocular involvement has been reported but is extremely rare. Lesions may be unilateral. The condition is usually mild (<10% body surface area), and although patients may have associated pruritus, it is usually much milder than in patients with classic LP. Sometimes, other types of LP may coexist or classic LP papules may occur at the periphery of the lesions. In the United States persons of color may demonstrate this pattern of LP. Individual lesions are typically several millimeters to several centimeters in size, are oval in shape, and may follow lines of Blaschko.

Some patients with LP pigmentosus may have lesions predominantly in sun-exposed areas, and the diagnosis LP actinicus can be used in these cases. LP actinicus is reported most frequently in Africa, the Middle East, and the Indian subcontinent and represents a substantial proportion of LP diagnosed in these geographic areas (36% of all LP patients in an Egyptian series).

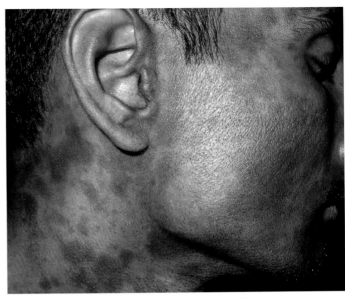

Fig. 12.12 Lichen planus pigmentosa. (Courtesy Debabrata Bandyopadhyay, MD.)

Most cases reported as LP actinicus occur in childhood through young adulthood, with 20–30 the primary decade of presentation. The disease presents in the spring or summer and is frequently quiescent in winter. Lesions favor the sun-exposed parts of the body, especially the face, which is almost always the most severely affected site. Most lesions occur on the forehead, cheeks, eyelids, and lips. Outside the face, the V area of the chest, the neck, the backs of the hands, and the lower extensor forearms are involved. Associated pruritus, the hallmark of LP, is usually described as mild or absent. Lesions are usually annular but may be reticulate or diffuse. Individual lesions are often macular but may be plaques with peripheral violaceous papules. Characteristically, lesions are hyperpigmented, sometimes with the blue-gray tinge of dermal melanin. They may resemble melasma. It is important to exclude alternate explanations for photo-distributed lichenoid eruptions, such as connective tissue diseases or chronic HIV photodermatitis, when rendering this diagnosis.

Because cases of LP pigmentosus and LP actinicus overlap, it is best to think of these conditions as a single disorder that may or may not be photoexacerbated. It is important to recognize the LP actinicus variant of LP pigmentosus because the actinicus patients do respond to sun protection, with gradual fading of their hyperpigmentation. Mucous membrane disease is significantly less common in patients with LP pigmentosus/actinicus. Histologically, any papular element will usually show features of LP. Even macular areas may show subtle evidence of an interface dermatitis, with prominent dermal melanophages.

LP pigmentosus-inversus is a unique, separate, and uncommon disorder. Lesions can be seen in patients with classic LP pigmentosus; however, this inverse pattern has a different racial distribution and has been reported in Caucasian patients as well as Asians and Hispanics. The axillae are the primary region of involvement in most patients (90%), although other skin folds such as the groin, inframammary, neck, retroauricular, and flexural areas can also be involved. As with other types of LP pigmentosus, pruritus is uncommon in the inversus type, and oral, nail, and hair involvement usually does not occur. The etiology is unknown, although a temporal association to occupational exposure to heavy metals was reported in one case, and others have suggested koebnerization from tight-fitting clothing.

The treatment of LP pigmentosus of all types is similar to other forms of LP. Topical corticosteroids and CNIs, antimalarials, retinoids, and even immunomodulators can be used. The lesions may fade slowly because they are primarily caused by melanin incontinence, and even if the active agent has stopped the interface reaction, the pigment will persist. Chemical peels and retinoids have been reported to improve the discoloration.

Erythema Dyschromicum Perstans

Erythema dyschromicum perstans is also known as "ashy dermatosis" or dermatosis cenicienta. The age of onset is virtually always before 40, but it is a chronic disease, so patients of all ages have been described, with a slight female predominance. Prepubertal children have been reported. Lesions are typically several centimeters in size and affect primarily the trunk, along with the neck and upper extremities. A characteristic very fine (several millimeters), erythematous, palpable, nonscaling border is seen at the periphery of the lesions. This is described as feeling like a small cord. Unfortunately, this leading edge (and diagnostic feature) of the disorder is only present early in the disease course (a few months). Pruritus is not reported, and typical lichenoid papules are said not to occur. Nail and mucosal involvement is not found. An association with HLA-DR4 has been suggested for Mexican patients, and rare drug-induced cases have been reported (recently with fluoxetine, omeprazole, and other agents). Unfortunately, erythema dyschromicum perstans became a catchall term for the panoply of dermatologic disorders that heal with prominent postinflammatory change in pigmented persons. It is now believed that most cases previously called erythema dyschromicum perstans are actually cases of LP pigmentosus. Childhood cases may represent idiopathic eruptive macular pigmentation. True erythema dyschromicum perstans, if it exists, is quite rare and largely restricted to certain geographic regions.

At the active border, the characteristic histologic features of erythema dyschromicum perstans are those of a lichenoid dermatitis. In the centers of the lesions, the histologic changes are those of postinflammatory pigmentation. Therapeutic agents used for LP may benefit the acute inflammatory stage but have limited effect on the pigmented lesions. Isolated reports mention some improvement of dyspigmentation in patients with NB-UVB phototherapy, retinoids, and topical tacrolimus. Some lasers have been reported to improve the appearance, occasionally in conjunction with topical tacrolimus. Spontaneous improvement has occurred, leading some to suggest that no treatment is reasonable.

Idiopathic Eruptive Macular Pigmentation

Although rarely reported, idiopathic eruptive macular pigmentation (IEMP) is not rare. Young persons (mean age 11 years in one study) presented with asymptomatic widespread brown to gray macules of up to several centimeters in diameter on the neck, trunk, and proximal extremities. Lesions are not confluent, and there is no history of preceding inflammation. At times, there is slight papillomatosis histologically, identical to that seen in confluent and reticulate papillomatosis (CARP). Unlike CARP, however, IEMP does not respond to oral minocycline. Lesions may spontaneously involute. Some cases reported as erythema dyschromicum perstans in childhood may actually represent IEMP.

Bilu D, et al: Clinical and epidemiologic characterization of photosensitivity in HIV-positive individuals. Photodermatol Photoimmunol Photomed 2004; 20: 175.

Chang SE, et al: Clinical and histological aspect of erythema dyschromicum perstans in Korea. J Dermatol 2015; 42: 1053.

Chen S, et al: Lichen planus pigmentosus-inversus. J Dermatol 2015; 42: 77.

Chiu MW, et al: Multiple brown patches on the trunk: idiopathic eruptive macular pigmentation with papillomatosis (IEMP). Arch Dermatol 2010, 146: 1301.

Chua S, et al: Ashy dermatosis (erythema dyschromicum perstans) induced by omeprazole. Int J Dermatol 2015; 54: 435.

Hsu CY, et al: Lichen planus pigmentosus inversus caused by occupational systemic sensitization to metals in a semiconductor factory worker. Dermatitis 2017; 28: 324.

Karn D, et al: Lichen planus pigmentosus. Kathmandu Univ Med J 2016; 14: 36.

Mahajan VK, et al: Erythema dyschromicum perstans. Indian J Dermatol 2015; 60: 525.

Majima Y, et al: Two cases of lichen planus-inversus. Eur J Dermatol 2013; 23: 904.

Muthu SK, et al: Low-dose oral isotretinoin therapy in lichen planus pigmentosus. Int J Dermatol 2016; 55: 1048.

Ohshima N, et al: Lichen planus pigmentosus-inversus occurring extensively in multiple intertriginous areas. J Dermatol 2012; 39: 412.

Ramírez P, et al: Childhood actinic lichen planus. Australas J Dermatol 2012; 53: e10.

Soleimani M, et al: Corneal involvement by lichen planus pigmentosus. Ocul Immunol Inflamm 2017; ePub ahead of print.

Wolff M, et al: A case of lichen planus pigmentosus with facial dyspigmentation responsive to combination therapy with chemical peels and topical retinoids. J Clin Aesthet Dermatol 2016; 9: 44.

Wolfsohl JA, et al: Improvement of erythema dyschromicum perstans using a combination of the 1,550-nm erbium-doped fractionated laser and topical tacrolimus ointment. Lasers Surg Med 2017; 49: 60.

KERATOSIS LICHENOIDES CHRONICA

Keratosis lichenoides chronica is a rare dermatosis characterized by its chronicity. In adults, the disease begins in the late twenties. Abnormal keratinization leads to typical lesions of papulonodular and hyperkeratotic and covered with gray scales. These lesions favor the extremities and buttocks, with the face involved in two thirds of patients. Although initially discrete, the lesions frequently coalesce to form linear and reticulate arrays of warty lichenoid lesions (Fig. 12.13). Lesions are infundibulocentric and acrosyringocentric. Keratotic plugs and prominent telangiectasia may be present. The palms and soles have discrete hyperkeratotic

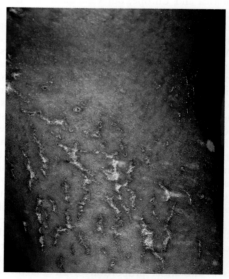

Fig. 12.13 Keratosis lichenoides chronica.

papules. There is an associated sharply marginated erythema, scaling, and telangiectasia of the face, superficially resembling seborrheic dermatitis or rosacea. Nail changes described include thickening of the nail plate, yellowing, longitudinal ridging, onycholysis, hyperkeratosis of the nail bed, paronychia, and warty lesions of the periungual areas. In addition, painful oral ulcerations occur in 25% of cases, and oral or genital involvement occurs in 50% of adult patients. Other findings include hoarseness from vocal cord edema and involvement of the eyelids (one third of patients), conjunctiva, iris, or anterior chamber. Cases have been reported in association with hepatitis, lymphoma, thyroid disease, and other systemic illnesses, but no specific links to true comorbid conditions exist.

Childhood cases are rare and differ from adult cases. Infants are affected in the first year of life and have prominent facial purpura and erythema, especially on the cheeks, and children develop alopecia more often than adults. More than half of childhood cases are familial, suggesting autosomal recessive inheritance.

Histologically, there is irregular acanthosis or epidermal atrophy with hyperkeratosis and zones of parakeratosis. A lichenoid infiltrate, consisting primarily of lymphocytes, and vacuolar alteration at the basal cell layer, but concentrated around the infundibula or acrosyringia. Marked follicular plugging and plugging of the acrosyringia are characteristic.

Topical calcipotriol, phototherapy (NB-UVB or PUVA), oral retinoids, photodynamic therapy, and sometimes systemic immunosuppressive agents, or combination therapy may all prove beneficial, though most reports highlight phototherapy and/or systemic retinoids. Keratosis lichenoides chronica rarely responds to topical or systemic steroids.

Barisani A, et al: Keratosis lichenoides chronica with an atypical clinical presentation and variable histopathological features. J Dtsch Dermatol Ges 2016; 14: 1136.
Boer A: Keratosis lichenoides chronica. Am J Dermatopathol 2006; 28: 260.
Pistoni F, et al: Keratosis lichenoides chronica. J Dermatolog Treat 2016; 27: 383.
Singh BE, et al: Pediatric onset keratosis lichenoides chronica. Pediatr Dermatol 2012; 29: 511.

LICHEN NITIDUS

Clinical Features

Lichen nitidus (LN) is a chronic inflammatory disease characterized by minute, shiny, flat-topped, pale, exquisitely discrete, uniform papules, rarely larger than 1–2 mm. Children and young adults are primarily affected. Pruritus is usually minimal or absent but may be more prominent in more generalized cases. Linear arrays of papules (Koebner phenomenon) are common, especially on the penis, forearms, and dorsal hands (Fig. 12.14). Initially, lesions are localized and often remain limited to a few areas, chiefly the penis (Fig. 12.15) and lower abdomen, the inner surface of the thighs, and the flexor aspects of the wrists and dorsal hands/forearms. In other cases, the disease assumes a more widespread distribution, and the papules fuse into erythematous, finely scaly plaques. The reddish color varies with tints of yellow, brown, or violet. Unusual variants of LN include vesicular, hemorrhagic, linear, purpuric (resembling a pigmented purpuric dermatosis), perforating, and spinous follicular (resembling lichen spinulosus).

Palm and sole involvement may occur in LN, and the disease may be restricted to these areas. It presents with multiple tiny, hyperkeratotic papules. The papules may coalesce to form diffuse hyperkeratotic plaques that fissure. The differentiation of LN from hyperkeratotic hand eczema and LP of the palms is aided by the presence of a keratotic plug in the center of lesions of

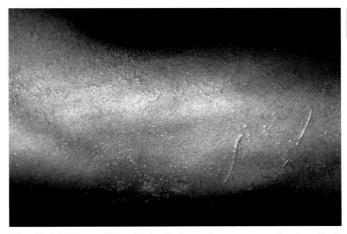

Fig. 12.14 Lichen nitidus. Note Koebner phenomenon. (Courtesy Curt Samlaska, MD.)

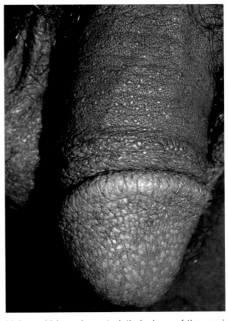

Fig. 12.15 Lichen nitidus, characteristic lesions of the penis. (Courtesy Curt Samlaska, MD.)

palmoplantar LN. Nail involvement with pitting, beaded, longitudinal ridging, and nailfold inflammation has been reported. Isolated LN on the eyelid has been reported. Oral involvement, with gray-yellow papules or petechiae of the hard palate or papules on the tongue, is rare.

A variant of LN, termed *actinic lichen nitidus*, has been reported in dark-skinned patients from the Middle East and Indian subcontinent. Cases seen in African Americans have also been termed *pinpoint, papular polymorphous light eruption* (PMLE), or known by the older term *summer actinic lichenoid eruption*. These cases all have lesions clinically and histologically identical to LN, which are limited to the sun-exposed areas of the dorsal hands, brachioradial area, and posterior neck. The LN histology may represent subacute or chronic lesions of pinpoint PMLE. Actinic LN/pinpoint papular PMLE usually responds to sun protection, with or without topical corticosteroids. Hydroxychloroquine has been used successfully in one Moroccan case.

The cause of LN is unknown. Rare familial cases do occur. LN is clinically and histologically distinct from lichen planus, and immunohistochemical studies also suggest they are distinct disorders, however, patients have had overlap of both disorders (and other lichenoid eruptions, including LN and lichen striatus), suggesting some common pathogenic basis. LN (with larger-than normal inflammatory aggregates) has been described in the setting of Crohn disease as well. LN has occurred after tattoo placement, either as an immunologic reaction to the material or due to koebnerization. One case reported LN developing within sites of vitiligo in a patient with alopecia universalis and Sjögren syndrome. Both LP and LN have been reported secondary to hepatitis B immunization and during treatment of hepatitis with IFN-α. Lichenoid eruptions have been described with increasing frequency in the setting of cancer treatment with checkpoint inhibitors, including reports of generalized LN with tremeliumumab.

LN has a characteristic histologic appearance. Dermal papillae are widened and contain a dense infiltrate composed of lymphocytes, histiocytes, and melanophages. There is an accumulation of both CD68+ histiocytes and S-100+, CD1a+ Langerhans cells in the dermal collections. Multinucleate giant cells are often present, imparting a granulomatous appearance to the infiltrate. The epidermal rete ridges on either side of the papilla form a claw-like collarette. The overlying epidermis is attenuated, and there is usually vacuolar alteration of its basal layer. Transepidermal inflammation and debris can occur in the rare subtype of perforating LN. At times, the infiltrate may extend down adjacent hair follicles and eccrine ducts, making distinction of LN from lichen scrofulosorum and lichen striatus difficult. One case series describes patients with mild cutaneous PRP displaying LN-like histopathology.

The course of LN is slowly progressive, with a tendency for remission. The lesions may remain stationary for years but often eventually disappear spontaneously and entirely. Treatment is not required because it is usually asymptomatic and self-healing. However, topical corticosteroids or CNIs can be used for localized disease. NB UVB and PUVA can be effective in generalized cases, but care must be taken to be sure that the LN in not of the actinic variety. Anecdotal reports suggest therapeutic benefit from oral retinoids (acitretin). As in LP, refractory LN cases requiring aggressive therapy may respond to cyclosporin A.

Albayrak H, et al: Lichen nitidus presenting with trachyonychia. Indian J Dermatol Venereol Leprol 2017; 83: 516.
Bilgili SG, et al: A case of generalized lichen nitidus successfully treated with narrow-band ultraviolet B treatment. Photodermatol Photoimmunol Photomed 2013; 29: 215.
Bouras M, et al: Facial actinic lichen nitidus successfully treated with hydroxychloroquine. Dermatol Online J 2013; 19: 20406.
Cho EB, et al: Three cases of lichen nitidus associated with various cutaneous diseases. Ann Dermatol 2014; 26: 505.
Fetil E, et al: Lichen nitidus after hepatitis B vaccine. Int Soc Dermatol 2004; 43: 956.
Leung AK, Ng J: Generalized lichen nitidus in identical twins. Case Rep Dermatol Med 2012; 2012: 982084.
Li AW, et al: Generalized lichen nitidus-like eruption in the setting of mogamulizumab and tremelimumab. Eur J Dermatol 2017; 27: 325.
Liu ET, et al: Lichen nitidus of the eyelids. Ophthal Plast Reconstr Surg 2017; 33: e85.
Nakamizo S, et al: Accumulation of S-100+ CD1a+ Langerhans cells as a characteristic of lichen nitidus. Clin Exp Dermatol 2011; 36: 811.
Oscoz-Jaime S, et al: Lichen nitidus arising on vitiligo. Actas Dermosifiliogr 2016; 107: 860.
Park J, et al: Persistent generalized lichen nitidus successfully treated with 0.03% tacrolimus ointment. Eur J Dermatol 2013; 23: 918.
Park JS: Lichen nitidus and lichen spinulosus or spinous follicular lichen nitidus? Clin Exp Dermatol 2011; 36: 557.
Rashidghamat E, et al: Pityriasis rubra pilaris with histologic features of lichen nitidus. J Am Acad Dermatol 2015; 73: 336.
Schelar M, et al: Generalized lichen nitidus with involvement of the palms following interferon alpha treatment. Dermatol 2007; 215: 236.
Summe HS, et al: Generalized spinous follicular lichen nitidus with perifollicular granulomas. Pediatr Dermatol 2013; 30: e20.
Synakiewicz J, et al: Generalized lichen nitidus. Postepy Dermatol Alergol 2016; 33: 488.
Tay EY, et al: Lichen nitidus presenting with nail changes. Pediatr Dermatol 2015; 32: 386.
Wanat KA, et al: Extensive lichen nitidus as a clue to underlying Crohn's disease. J Am Acad Dermatol 2012; 67: 5.
Zussman J, Smart CN: Perforating lichen nitidus. Am J Dermatopathol 2015; 37: 406.

LICHEN STRIATUS

Lichen striatus is a fairly common, self-limited eruption seen primarily in young children (mean age 3 years). Girls are affected two to three times more frequently than boys. Lesions begin as small papules that are erythematous and slightly scaly (Fig. 12.16). In more darkly pigmented persons, hypopigmentation is prominent and may be purely macular. The 1–3 mm papules coalesce to form a band 1–3 cm wide, either continuous or interrupted, which over a few weeks progresses down the extremity or around the trunk, following lines of Blaschko. An extremity is more often involved, but trunk lesions or lesions extending from the trunk onto an extremity can also occur. About 10% of cases occur on the head and face. Multiple bands infrequently occur, including bilateral cases. Lesions are usually asymptomatic, but pruritus may occur, especially in patients who are also atopic.

Nail involvement can occur if the process extends down the digit to the nail. Typically, the lichen striatus appears first on the skin, but the skin and nail abnormality may appear simultaneously. Infrequently, only the nail may be involved for months, with later appearance of the band on the skin, or the nail may remain the sole area of involvement throughout the course of the disease. Unilateral lichen striatus may be associated with bilateral nail involvement. Nail plate thinning, longitudinal ridging, splitting, and nail bed hyperkeratosis may be seen. Often, only a part of the nail is involved. The histology of involved nails is identical to that of the skin lesions.

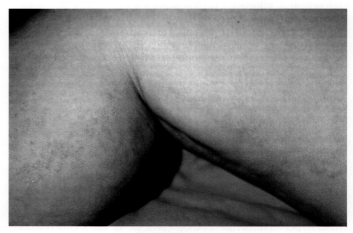

Fig. 12.16 Lichen striatus.

The active lesions of lichen striatus last for an average of 1 year but may persist for up to 4 years. Eventually, all the lesions, including dystrophic nails, spontaneously resolve without scarring. Hypopigmentation may persist for several years. Hyperpigmentation is uncommon (<5%) and should suggest a diagnosis of linear LP instead. Relapses can occur in up to 5% of cases, either in the same distribution or in a different anatomic region.

The histologic features of lichen striatus vary, partly reflecting the stage of evolution of the lesion. There may be a spongiotic dermatitis, but most frequently a lichenoid component is present. There is a bandlike infiltrate with necrotic keratinocytes at the dermoepidermal junction. Granulomatous inflammation is occasionally present. Typically, there is a dense lymphoid infiltrate around the eccrine sweat glands and ducts. This helps distinguish lichen striatus from lichen planus. One study showed Ki-67 cells increased in linear LP but not in LS. It is important to exclude mycosis fungoides as occasionally histology of LS may resemble the adnexal inflammation of folliculotropic MF.

The blaschkolinear nature of the eruption has prompted some to suggest LS represents a somatic mutation in a group of cells, which then develops the characteristic eruption in response to some environmental trigger. Multiple reports exist of simultaneous cases in siblings and families. There is also a seasonal variation, with most cases occurring in the spring and summer. Epidemic outbreaks have been reported, suggesting a viral etiology or trigger. Cases have occurred following vaccinations and viral infections such as varicella, influenza, and human herpes virus infections, and following IFN therapy. LS has been reported in children with atopic dermatitis, and in conjunction with vitiligo, though it is important to distinguish LS from segmental vitiligo in those patients. Trauma has also been reported to precipitate an outbreak of lichen striatus. Medication-induced causes are rare beyond those previously mentioned, though one report described LS developing with etanercept treatment of rheumatoid arthritis.

Adult cases of lichen striatus differ from those in childhood and are rarer and more papulovesicular, affecting multiple regions, resolving more rapidly (<2 months), and relapsing more frequently (up to one third of patients). Histologically, the lesions show more spongiotic and less lichenoid features, leading some authors to call these cases "adult blaschkitis" or "Grosshans-Marot disease." This splitting of terms probably has no clinical utility.

Usually, the diagnosis of lichen striatus is straightforward, in a young child with sudden onset of an eruption following the lines of Blaschko. The differential diagnosis could include linear LP, linear psoriasis, inflammatory linear verrucous epidermal nevus, epidermal nevus, linear cutaneous LE, and verruca plana. Histologic evaluation will usually distinguish these entities, but is rarely required.

Treatment is usually not necessary. Parents may be reassured of the uniformly excellent prognosis. Topical corticosteroids and topical CNIs may accelerate the resolution of lesions. The combination of tazarotene and topical steroid treatment has led to rapid resolution in one series. Laser treatment has been reported to clear residual discoloration. In children with an acquired nail dystrophy of one or two digits, lichen striatus must be considered, and watchful waiting might be considered before biopsying the nail.

Bae JM, et al: Effectiveness of the 308-nm excimer laser on hypopigmentation after lichen striatus: a retrospective study of 12 patients. J Am Acad Dermatol 2016; 75: 637.

Chong JH, et al: Vitiligo co-existing with lichen striatus. J Eur Acad Dermatol Venereol 2017; 31: e200.

Feely MA, Silverberg NB: Two cases of lichen striatus with prolonged active phase. Pediatr Dermatol 2014; 31: e67.

Garcia-Briz MI, et al: Lichen striatus in childhood. Actas Dermosifiliogr 2017; 108: 882.

Gupta A, et al: Bilateral lichen striatus. Indian Dermatol Online J 2017; 8: 264.

Karempelis PS, et al: Lichen striatus in a mother and son. Int J Dermatol 2014; 53: e366.

Karouni M, et al: Lichen striatus following yellow fever vaccination in an adult woman. Clin Exp Dermatol 2017; 42: 823.

Lee DY, et al: Lichen striatus in an adult treated by a short course of low-dose systemic corticosteroid. J Dermatol 2010; 38: 298.

Lora V, et al: Lichen striatus associated with etanercept treatment of rheumatoid arthritis. J Am Acad Dermatol 2014; 70: e90.

Mascolo M, et al: Lichen striatus histopathologically mimicking mycosis fungoides. J Dtsch Dermatol Ges 2014; 12: 1048.

Mask-Bull L, et al: Lichen striatus after interferon therapy. JAAD Case Rep 2015; 1: 254.

Müller CS, et al: Lichen striatus and blaschkitis. Br J Dermatol 2011; 164: 257.

Park JY, Kim YC: Lichen striatus successfully treated with photodynamic therapy. Clin Exp Dermatol 2012; 37: 562.

Patrizi A, et al: Lichen striatus: clinical and laboratory features of 115 children. Pediatr Dermatol 2004; 21: 197.

Zhou Y, et al: Lichen striatus versus linear lichen planus. Int J Dermatol 2016; 55: e204.

LICHEN SCLEROSUS (LICHEN SCLEROSUS ET ATROPHICUS)

Lichen sclerosus is a chronic disease of the skin and mucosa. The terms *lichen sclerosus et atrophicus*, *kraurosis vulvae*, and *balanitis xerotica obliterans* are synonymous but have been replaced by the single term *lichen sclerosus* (LS). LS can present from childhood to old age. Although it occurs in all races, whites and Hispanics are more frequently affected, and it is rare in African Americans. Both genders develop LS both before and after puberty, with females predominating at all ages. The prevalence is about 1.7% in the general adult female population, and about one-tenth as frequent in premenarchal girls. Transgender patients require careful evaluation as disease may occur at both surgical sites of transformed genitalia and at sites particular to the patients' gender identity, such as perianal involvement in a male-to-female patient. Patients may develop LS after bone marrow transplantation, though it is challenging to distinguish from chronic graft-versus-host.

The pathogenesis of LS is poorly understood. Autoimmune diseases (thyroid disease, vitiligo, morphea, alopecia areata, pernicious anemia) occur in one fifth to one third of women with LS but are much less common in men, with rates similar to the general population. Psoriasis is increased in women with LS, reported to occur in 7.5%–17% of patients. Autoantibodies to extracellular matrix protein 1 (ECM-1) are found in 80% of LS patients, compared with 4% of controls and 7%–10% of patients with other autoimmune diseases. The titer of the ECM-1 autoantibody correlates with the disease severity.

In females, there is a bimodal age distribution—prepubertal and postmenopausal. The initial lesions of LS are white, polygonal, flat-topped papules, plaques, or atrophic patches (Fig. 12.17). Lesions may be surrounded by an erythematous to violaceous halo. In atrophic lesions, the skin is smooth, slightly wrinkled, soft, and white. Bullae, often hemorrhagic, telangiectasias, and fixed areas of purpura may occur on the patches. About 40% of patients with LS are asymptomatic. However, when women referred to specialists are questioned, virtually 100% are symptomatic. Itching is frequently severe, especially in the anogenital area. In the genital area, fissuring and erosion may occur. This may result in dysuria, urethral and vaginal discharge, dyspareunia, and burning pain. Normal anatomic structures may be obliterated, with loss of the labia minora, clitoral hood, and urethral meatus. In women, this perineal involvement typically affects the vulvar and perianal areas, giving a figure-8 or hourglass appearance. Introital stenosis or fusion may occur. The vaginal and cervical mucosae are not

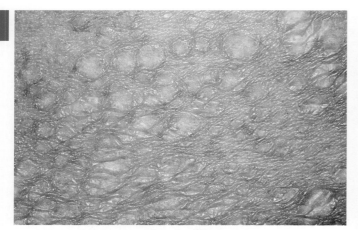

Fig. 12.17 Lichen sclerosus et atrophicus.

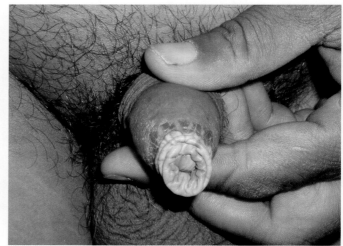

Fig. 12.19 Lichen sclerosus et atrophicus. (Courtesy Shyam Verma, MBBS, DVD.)

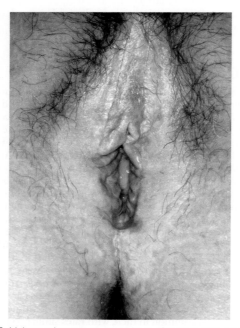

Fig. 12.18 Lichen sclerosus et atrophicus. (Courtesy Steven Binnick, MD.)

involved by LS, in contrast to LP. Prepubertal girls may also be affected and usually have vulvar and perianal lesions (Fig. 12.18). Even a relatively brief delay in diagnosis may be associated with atrophy and/or scarring.

Vulvar disease is associated with similar skin changes to those in adult women, and pruritus may be a prominent symptom. Perianal involvement may produce significant symptomatology of constipation, stool holding, and rectorrhagia caused by rectal fissures. Infantile perineal protrusion refers to a pyramidal soft tissue swelling covered by red or rose-colored skin along the median perineal raphe (skin between posterior fourchette and anus). This occurs only in girls and appears to be a manifestation of LS in some prepubertal girls. Two thirds of girls with LS have been evaluated for sexual abuse, largely because of the purpura and ecchymoses that accompany the lesions. If risk of sexual abuse is suspected, appropriate investigations must be performed.

There is clearly a relationship between the hormonal milieu and LS. Postmenopausal women are preferentially affected. Pregnancy leads to improvement and often complete resolution.

Oral contraceptive (OC) use is common in premenopausal women with LS. These OCs are often antiandrogenic. Stopping OCs and treating with standard topical agents lead to significant improvement, suggesting that the antiandrogen OCs may have accelerated the appearance of the LS. However, treatment of postmenopausal women with estrogen supplementation does not alter the incidence or course of their LS.

In males, lesions are atrophic and may be greatly hypopigmented or depigmented, resembling vitiligo, although melanosis mimicking melanoma has been reported. Lesions usually involve only the glans penis and the inner foreskin of the uncircumcised male. Infrequently, LS may extend on to the penile shaft and scrotum. If the glans is involved, hemorrhage is common, and shallow erosions may occur. LS of the glans does not usually lead to nonhealing erosions of the glans, but rather simply skin fragility. Patients often have itching and pain, but may be asymptomatic while ongoing inflammation is occurring. Phimosis and paraphimosis are common complications of LS in men (Fig. 12.19). Between 15% and 100% of circumcision specimens from prepubertal boys show features of LS. Sixty percent of acquired phimosis in boys and at least 10% in adult men are associated with LS. Most men with LS are uncircumcised, and exposure to urine appears to be an important trigger for LS in males, including in obese patients with urinary microincontinence. Circumcision is effective treatment for penile LS, with cure rates of 75%–100%. Urethral meatal stenosis may occur and requires surgical correction. One study of 301 male patients with LS revealed penile intraepithelial neoplasia in 13%, which often required biopsy diagnosis and surgical intervention. Perianal involvement by LS is rare in men and boys with penile LS, but may occur in transgender male-to-female patients.

Extragenital lesions are uncommon, but may develop in 6%–20% of patients, and are most frequent on the upper back, chest, and breasts and are usually asymptomatic. The tongue and oral mucosa may also be involved, either alone or with lesions elsewhere. Extragenital bulloue LS may rarely occur as well, with a blistering or hemorrhagic appearance. Oral LS is a rare diagnosis and appears to occur without associated skin or genital involvement. Peristomal LS around colostomy sites may occur. LS has been reported following radiation, including on the breast after radiotherapy for breast cancer, and given the histologic similarities may be hard to distinguish from radiation dermatitis. Patients having only extragenital lesions with histologic features of both LS and morphea have been reported. About one quarter of these patients have LS-like changes overlying the morphea lesions (a recognized histopathologic variant of morphea), and in three quarters the extragenital LS lesions are distinct from the morphea lesions. Genital LS is much more common in patients (usually women) with localized plaque or generalized morphea. In one study, up to 40% of patients with morphea also had genital LS. The genital area of patients with morphea should be examined for the presence of LS. Rarely, in Europe, *Borrelia* has been reported to cause extragenital LS, and treatment with antibiotics has arrested the progression of the lesions.

Lichen Sclerosus and Cancer

Although the risk is not as high as was proposed early in this century, LS of the genitalia is a condition with increased risk for genital SCC in both women and men. The lifetime risk for women who are carefully followed appears to be 5% or less but is clearly higher than for the general population. A large Finnish study of 7616 patients demonstrated a markedly elevated risk of vulvar cancer and slightly increased risk of vaginal cancer in patients with LS. About one third of cases of vulvar SCCs are associated with LS. HPV is more prevalent in male patients with LS than in female patients, with HPV16 most prevalent but multiple genotypes present; HPV alone is not the cause of LS. Human papillomavirus (HPV) appears to be associated with only about 15% of SCCs arising in women with LS. Hypertrophic vulvar lesions and age beyond 60 are risk factors for the development of SCC in women with LS. Such lesions and patients should be evaluated carefully. In men with LS, the risk for genital SCC is less than in women with LS. However, about 25% of cases of penile SCC are associated with LS. Oncogenic HPV types do not appear to be associated with LS-related penile cancer. Successful treatment and control of LS-related inflammation appears to reduce the risk of malignancy, but patients require long-term surveillance.

Histopathology

Early lesions of LS are characterized by an interface dermatitis with vacuolar alteration of keratinocytes. With evolution, the epidermis is thinned and the rete ridges are effaced. Compact orthokeratosis and follicular and eccrine plugging are present. The upper dermis is edematous, with the upper dermal collagen homogenized. Immediately beneath the altered papillary dermis, there is a sparse, bandlike and perivascular lymphoid infiltrate. In pruritic lesions, coexistent changes of lichen simplex chronicus may be seen, with epidermal acanthosis rather than atrophy.

Differential Diagnosis

Extragenital LS must be differentiated from guttate morphea and LP, especially of the atrophic type. Anogenital LS must be distinguished from genital LP, lichen simplex chronicus, vulvar intraepithelial neoplasia (SCC in situ), and extramammary Paget disease. The white color and atrophic surface are characteristic, and such areas are most fruitful if biopsied.

Treatment

The use of superpotent topical corticosteroids has dramatically changed the management of anogenital LS. These are universally accepted as the treatment of choice for all forms of genital LS. Most patients will respond to once-daily application of these agents and can subsequently be tapered to less frequent applications (once or twice a week) or to lower-strength corticosteroids. Ointment formulations are generally better tolerated, but vehicle preference and side-effect profile may vary by patient and affect adherence. Most patients can be controlled but not cured, and require ongoing maintenance therapy. Most women can achieve a symptom-free state with 30 g of clobetasol ointment used over 3 months, and patients who continued with intermittent maintenance therapy remained symptom free and developed less scaring than noncompliant patients. Patients occasionally are reluctant to use high-potency steroids due to the risk of atrophy—it is important to educate patients about the benefits of disease control outweighing those risks. Patients should be educated how to correctly apply the medication to cover the affected area, which may require a mirror and can be challenging for older patients. During treatment, coexistent candidiasis may be present or develop, and can be managed with topical or oral agents. Penile, vulvar, and prepubertal LS in girls have all been documented to respond to this form of treatment. Phimosis in young boys should be treated initially with potent topical steroids. The degree of symptomatic improvement far exceeds the objective improvement. The majority of patients have dramatic reduction in their itching and burning with topical clobetasol. However, the visible white, atrophic, scarred vulvar skin is often only minimally improved. In one study, 95% of compliant patients achieved complete symptom control; none had disease progression. In partially compliant patients, only 75% achieved complete symptom control, and 35% experienced progression. None of the fully compliant women developed vulvar SCC, but 5 of 45 (11%) of the partially compliant women did. This adds limited evidence to the impression that good control of LS is associated with better outcomes—symptomatically, functionally, and with respect to cancer development. Vulvar pain associated with LS may have a neuropathic component (as in vulvodynia), and treatment with tricyclic antidepressants (e.g., amitriptyline), gabapentin, and duloxetine hydrochloride may be tried.

Topical tacrolimus 0.1% and 0.03% ointments and pimecrolimus 1% cream have also been demonstrated to be effective in genital LS. However, since superpotent corticosteroids have proven so effective in genital LS, topical CNIs should be reserved for patients in whom topical corticosteroids are ineffective or not tolerated. Close clinical follow-up is recommended because the long-term risk of applying topical CNIs to skin predisposed to malignant degeneration is not known. Topical calcipotriol may also be of benefit. Topical testosterone was no more effective than emollient and in one trial was worse than emollients as maintenance therapy. It is no longer recommended. Hydroxychloroquine, calcitriol, topical 8% progesterone cream, topical calcipotriol, topical tretinoin, cyclosporine, and hydroxyurea can be considered in refractory cases. In one patient, intralesional adalimumab cleared LS of the glans penis. UVA-I phototherapy led to moderate improvement in some patients unresponsive to topical steroids. Patients who initially failed topical steroid treatment may respond to topical corticosteroids following the UV treatment. Intralesional steroid/anesthetic injections can be helpful for persistently symptomatic areas. Emerging reports exist of improvement with intradermal injections of autologous platelet-rich plasma. Surgical treatment can be effective, starting with cryotherapy, which has been reported as helpful in three quarters of patients with severe vulvar itch. Photodynamic therapy has brought significant improvement in multiple reports and can be considered in refractory cases. Extragenital LS is very difficult to treat. If superpotent topical steroids are ineffective, PUVA, UVA I, NB UVB, calcipotriol, or antimalarials may be tried. Given the appearance of LS-like lesions in chronic GVHD and the success of ECP in chronic GVHD, ECP has been tried in a few severe cases of extragenital LS with success.

Arnold N, et al: Extragenital bullous lichen sclerosus on the anterior lower extremities. Dermatol Online J 2017; 23.

Becker K, et al: Lichen sclerosus and atopy in boys. Br J Dermatol 2013; 168: 362.

Borghi A, et al: Clearance in vulvar lichen sclerosus. J Eur Acad Dermatol Venereol 2017; ePub ahead of print.

Brouillard C, et al: A case of cutaneous lichen sclerosus et atrophicus effectively treated by extracorporeal photochemotherapy. Photodermatol Photoimmunol Photomed 2013; 29: 160.

Celis S, et al: Balanitis xerotica obliterans in children and adolescents. J Pediatr Urol 2014; 10: 34.

Chi CC, et al: Systematic review and meta-analysis of randomized controlled trials on topical interventions of genital lichen sclerosus. J Am Acad Dermatol 2012; 67: 305.

Corazza M, et al: Mometasone furoate in the treatment of vulvar lichen sclerosus. J Dermatolog Treat 2017; ePub ahead of print.

Cusini M: Lichen sclerosus et atrophicus in males. Acta Derm Venereol 2014; 94: 499.

Davick JJ, et al: The prevalence of lichen sclerosus in patients with vulvar squamous cell carcinoma. Int J Gynecol Pathol 2017; 36: 305.

Doiron PR, Bunker CB: Obesity-related male genital lichen sclerosus. J Eur Acad Dermatol Venereol 2017; 31: 876.

Edmonds EV, et al: Extracellular matrix protein 1 autoantibodies in male genital lichen sclerosus. Br J Dermatol 2011; 165: 218.

Edmonds EV, et al: Clinical parameters in male genital lichen sclerosus. J Eur Acad Dermatol Venereol 2012; 26: 730.

Gambichler T, et al: Differential expression of connective tissue growth factor and extracellular matrix proteins in lichen sclerosus. J Eur Acad Dermatol Venereol 2012; 26: 207.

Goldstein AT, et al: A double-blind, randomized controlled trial of clobetasol versus pimecrolimus in patients with vulvar lichen sclerosus. J Am Acad Dermatol 2011; 64: e99.

Goldstein AT, et al: Intradermal injection of autologous platelet-rich plasma for the treatment of vulvar lichen sclerosus. J Am Acad Dermatol 2017; 76: 158.

Gunthert A, et al: Early onset vulvar lichen sclerosus in premenopausal women and oral contraceptives. Euro J Obstet Gynecol 2008; 137: 56.

Hald AK, Blaakaer J: The possible role of human papillomavirus infection in the development of lichen sclerosus. Int J Dermatol 2018; 57: 139.

Halonen P, et al: Lichen sclerosus and risk of cancer. Int J Cancer 2017; 140: 1998.

Kantere D, et al: Clinical features, complications, and autoimmunity in male lichen sclerosus. Acta Derm Venereol 2017; 97: 365.

Kim GW, et al: Topical tacrolimus ointment for the treatment of lichen sclerosus. J Dermatol 2012; 39: 145.

Kirtschig G: Lichen sclerosus. Dtsch Arztebl Int 2016; 113: 337.

Kravvas G, et al: The diagnosis and management of male genital lichen sclerosus. J Eur Acad Dermatol Venereol 2018; 32: 91.

Kreuter A, et al: Coexistence of lichen sclerosus and morphea. J Am Acad Dermatol 2012; 67: 1157.

Kreuter A, et al: Association of autoimmune diseases with lichen sclerosus in 532 male and female patients. Acta Derm Venereol 2013; 93: 238.

Lee A, et al: Long-term management of adult vulvar lichen sclerosus. JAMA Dermatol 2015; 151: 1061.

Lowenstein EB, Zeichner JA: Intralesional adalimumab for the treatment of refractory balanitis xerotica obliterans. JAMA Dermatol 2013; 149: 23.

Lutz V, et al: High frequency of genital lichen sclerosus in a prospective series of 76 patients with morphea. Arch Dermatol 2012; 148: 24.

Marchs-Braun N, et al: Acute urinary retention in an adolescent as the presenting symptom of lichen sclerosus et atrophicus. J Pediatr Adolesc Gynecol 2013; 26: e117.

Maronn M, et al: Constipation as a feature of anogenital lichen sclerosus in children. Pediatr 2005; 115: e230.

Mashayekhi S, et al: The treatment of vulval lichen sclerosus in prepubertal girls. Br J Dermatol 2017; 176: 307.

McMurray SL, et al: A transgender woman with anogenital lichen sclerosus. JAMA Dermatol 2017; 153: 1334.

Micheleti L, et al: Vulvar lichen sclerosus and neoplastic transformation. Low Genit Tract Dis 2016; 20: 180.

Nemer KM, Anadkat MJ: Postirradiation lichen sclerosus et atrophicus. JAMA Dermatol 2017; 153: 1067.

Nerantzoulis I, et al: Genital lichen sclerosus in childhood and adolescence. Eur J Pediatr 2017; 176: 1429.

Tausch TJ, Peterson AC: Early aggressive treatment of lichen sclerosus may prevent disease progression. J Urol 2012; 187: 2101.

Tchernev G, et al: Penile melanosis associated with lichen sclerosus et atrophicus. Open Acess Maced J Med Sci 2017; 5: 692.

Thomas LJ, et al: Male genital lichen sclerosus in recipients of bone marrow transplants. Clin Exp Dermatol 2016; 41: 495.

Tomo S, et al: Uncommon oral manifestation of lichen sclerosus. Oral Patol Oral Cir Bucal 2017; 22: 410.

van der Meijden WI, et al: 2016 European guideline for the management of vulval conditions. J Eur Acad Dermatol Venereol 2017; 31: 925.

Ventolini G, et al: Lichen sclerosus. J Low Genit Tract Dis 2012; 16: 271.

West DS, et al: Dermatopathology of the foreskin. J Cutan Pathol 2013; 40: 11.

Weyers W: Hypertrophic lichen sclerosus sine sclerosis. J Cutan Pathol 2015; 42: 118.

Zavras N, et al: Infantile perianal pyramidal protrusion. Case Rep Dermatol 2012; 4: 202.

13 Acne

ACNE VULGARIS

Clinical Features

Acne vulgaris is a chronic inflammatory disease of the pilosebaceous follicles, characterized by comedones, papules, pustules, nodules, and often scars. The comedo is the primary lesion of acne. It may be seen as a flat or slightly elevated papule with a dilated central opening filled with blackened keratin (open comedo or blackhead) (Fig. 13.1). Closed comedones (whiteheads) are usually 1-mm yellowish papules that may require stretching of the skin to visualize. Macrocomedones, which are uncommon, may reach 3–4 mm in size. The papules and pustules are 1–5 mm in size and are caused by inflammation, so erythema and edema occur (Fig. 13.2). They may enlarge, become more nodular (Fig. 13.3), and coalesce into plaques of several centimeters that are indurated or fluctuant, contain sinus tracts, and discharge serosanguineous or yellowish pus.

Patients typically have a variety of lesions in various states of formation and resolution. In light-skinned patients, lesions often resolve with a reddish purple macule that is short lived. In dark-skinned individuals, macular hyperpigmentation results and may last several months (Fig. 13.4). Acne scars are heterogeneous in appearance. Morphologies include deep, narrow, ice pick scars seen most often on the temples and cheeks; canyon-type atrophic lesions on the face (Fig. 13.5); whitish yellow papular scars on the trunk and chin; anetoderma-type scars on the trunk; and hypertrophic and keloidal elevated scars on the neck and trunk.

Acne affects primarily the face, neck, upper trunk (Fig. 13.6), and upper arms. On the face, acne occurs most frequently on the cheeks and to a lesser degree on the nose, forehead, and chin. The ears may be involved, with large comedones in the concha, cysts in the lobes, and sometimes preauricular and retroauricular comedones and cysts. On the neck, especially in the nuchal area, large cystic lesions may predominate.

Acne typically begins at puberty and is often the first sign of increased sex hormone production. When acne begins at age 8–12 years, it is frequently comedonal in character, affecting primarily the forehead and cheeks. It may remain mild in its expression, with only an occasional inflammatory papule. However, as hormone levels rise into the middle teenage years, more severe inflammatory pustules and nodules occur, with spread to other sites. Young men tend to have an oilier complexion and more severe widespread disease than young women. Women may experience a flare of their papulopustular lesions about 1 week before menstruation. Acne may also begin in 20- to 35-year-old women who have not experienced teenage acne. This acne frequently manifests as papules, pustules, and deep, painful, persistent nodules on the jawline, chin, and upper neck.

Acne is primarily a disease of the adolescent, with 85% of all teenagers being affected to some degree. It occurs with greatest frequency between ages 15 and 18 in both genders. Generally, involution of the disease occurs before age 25; however, great variability in age at onset and of resolution occurs. About 12% of women and 3% of men will continue to have clinical acne until age 44. A few will have inflammatory papules and nodules into late adulthood.

Neonatal acne is a common condition that develops a few days after birth, has male preponderance, and is characterized by transient facial papules or pustules that usually clear spontaneously in a few days or weeks (Fig. 13.7). Neonatal cephalic pustulosis (infantile acne) includes cases that persist beyond the neonatal period or that have an onset after the first 6 weeks of life. Most patients' disease remits by age 1 year, although occasionally cases extend into childhood and through puberty. In prolonged cases, topical benzoyl peroxide, erythromycin, or the retinoids may be effective. With more inflammatory disease, oral erythromycin, 125 mg twice daily, or trimethoprim, 100 mg twice daily, may be added to topical medications. Oral isotretinoin has been used in the infantile period and is effective. Midchildhood acne may evolve from persistent infantile acne or begin after age 1 year. It is uncommon and has a male predominance. Grouped comedones, papules, pustules, and nodules can occur alone or in any combination, usually limited to the face (Fig. 13.8). The duration is variable, from a few weeks to several years, and occasionally extends into more severe pubertal acne. Often, there is a strong family history of moderately severe acne. A pediatric endocrinology workup is indicated for midchildhood acne and for earlier-onset patients with physical findings suggestive of a hormonal disorder, such as sexual precocity, virilization, or growth abnormality. Acne onset from age 7–12 is categorized as preadolescent acne. This is the time of adrenarche, and unless there are signs of androgen excess, no workup is needed.

Pathogenesis

Acne vulgaris is exclusively a follicular disease, with the principal abnormality being comedo formation. It is produced by the impaction and distention of the follicles with a keratinous plug in the lower infundibulum. The keratinous plug is caused by hyperproliferation and abnormal differentiation of keratinocytes. Androgens, alterations in lipid composition, and an abnormal response to local cytokines are all hypothesized to be causally important. Androgen stimulation of the sebaceous glands is critical. Acne begins after sebum secretion increases, and women with hyperandrogenic states often manifest acne, along with hirsutism and menstrual abnormalities. Treatment directed at reducing sebaceous secretion, such as isotretinoin, estrogens, or antiandrogens, is effective in clearing acne.

As the retained cells block the follicular opening, the lower portion of the follicle is dilated by entrapped sebum. Disruption of the follicular epithelium permits discharge of the follicular contents into the dermis. The combination of keratin, sebum, and microorganisms, particularly *Propionibacterium acnes*, leads to the release of proinflammatory mediators and the accumulation of lymphocytes, neutrophils, and foreign body giant cells. This in turn causes the formation of inflammatory papules, pustules, and nodulocystic lesions.

Additional factors may exacerbate acne or, in a predisposed patient, cause the onset of acne. Comedogenic greasy or occlusive products such as hair pomades may induce closed comedones and at times inflammatory lesions. Other types of cosmetics may initiate or worsen acne, but acne cosmetica is uncommon because most cosmetics are tested for comedogenicity.

Many types of mechanical or frictional forces can aggravate existing acne. A common problem is the overexuberant washing some patients think may help rid them of their blackheads or oiliness. A key feature of mechanical or frictional acne is an unusual

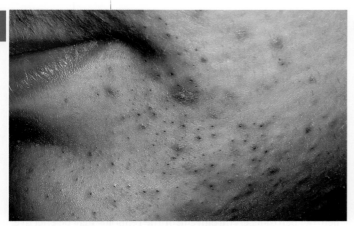

Fig. 13.1 Acne vulgaris, with comedones, on the chin.

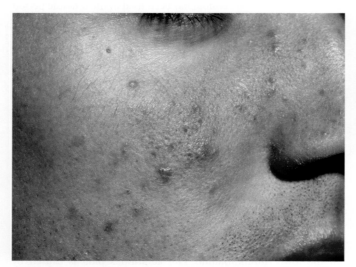

Fig. 13.2 Acne vulgaris, with papules and pustules, on the cheek.

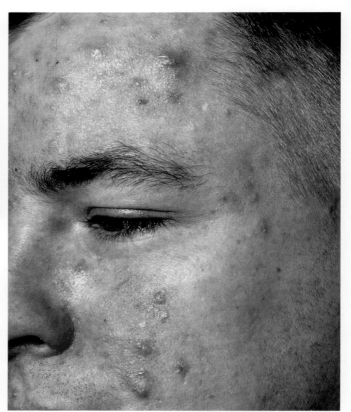

Fig. 13.3 Inflammatory acne with papules and nodules.

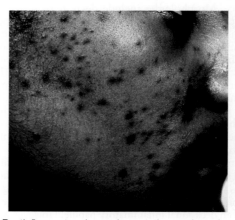

Fig. 13.4 Postinflammatory hyperpigmentation at sites of acne lesions.

distribution of the acne lesions. Provocative factors include chin straps, violins, hats, collars, surgical tape, orthopedic casts, chairs, and seats. One acne patient who had laser hair removal developed flares of inflammatory lesions localized to the acne-prone sites after each laser session; the legs and abdomen were spared. All these factors are likely to irritate the follicular epithelium and exacerbate the changes that lead to comedogenesis and follicular rupture. Prophylactic measures designed to interdict these various mechanical forces are beneficial.

The role of diet in causing or exacerbating acne is being actively investigated. A high-glycemic diet, skim milk, and whey protein may negatively influence acne. Dietary regimens used for therapeutic intervention have yet to be defined, however.

In all women or children with acne, the possibility of a hyperandrogenic state should be considered. In women, the presence of irregular menses, hirsutism, seborrhea, acanthosis nigricans, or androgenic alopecia increases the likelihood of finding clinically significant hyperandrogenism. Additionally, gynecologic endocrine evaluation may be indicated in women who have acne resistant to conventional therapy, who relapse quickly after a course of isotretinoin, or who experience sudden onset of severe acne. Screening tests to exclude a virilizing tumor include serum dehydroepiandrosterone sulfate (DHEAS) and testosterone, obtained 2 weeks before the onset of menses. DHEAS levels may be very high in adrenal tumors (>800 µg/dL) or less dramatic in

congenital adrenal hyperplasia (400–800 µg/dL). Ovarian tumor is suggested by testosterone levels greater than 200 ng/dL. Many patients with late-onset 21-hydroxylase deficiency congenital adrenal hyperplasia will have normal levels of DHEAS. Although 17-hydroxyprogesterone and adrenocorticotropic hormone (ACTH) stimulation tests have been used in this setting, the baseline 17-hydroxyprogesterone may be normal and ACTH stimulation may result in overdiagnosis of the syndrome. It is not clear that screening for adult-onset 21-hydroxylase deficiency improves patient outcome. Cushing syndrome is also to be considered in the differential diagnosis.

The diagnosis of polycystic ovarian syndrome (PCOS) requires that two of three of the following criteria be present: oligoovulation

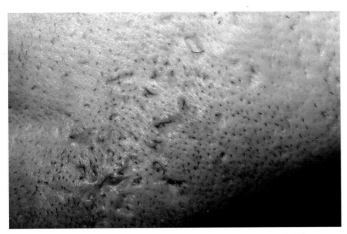

Fig. 13.5 Acne scarring. (Courtesy Steven Binnick, MD.)

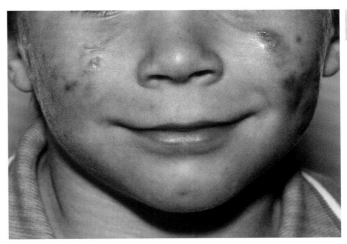

Fig. 13.8 Childhood acne.

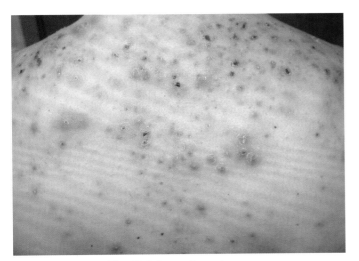

Fig. 13.6 Severe truncal acne.

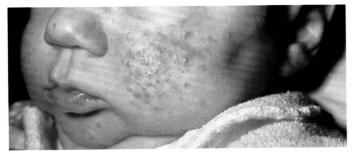

Fig. 13.7 Neonatal cephalic pustulosis (infantile acne).

(with chronic anovulation), and psychiatric disease. Nearly half of PCOS patients have metabolic syndrome. In women with hirsutism of the chest and acanthosis nigricans of the axillae, PCOS is frequently found. Suggested biochemical investigation includes total testosterone, free testosterone, dehydroepiandrosterone (DHEAS), androstenedione, luteinizing hormone, and follicle-stimulating hormone. PCOS is a complex disorder and referral for investigation for ovarian cysts, interpretation of abnormal results, consideration of other testing such as thyroid-stimulating hormone and prolactin, and management of any associated disorders is recommended.

Acne neonatorum is explained by infantile production of androgens, which wanes at 6–12 months. Occasional patients have persistent acne, although acne developing after age 1 and before age 7 (with onset of adrenarche) may be a form of acne cosmetica, acne venenata, drug-induced acne or part of an endocrinologic disorder. A workup should be initiated if acne develops between ages 1 and 7 and no obvious external factor is present. In the absence of any discovered abnormalities, the qualitative or quantitative alteration of cutaneous androgen, metabolism, and increased end-organ sensitivity could be postulated as pathogenic mechanisms for preadolescent acne.

Pathology

Comedones reveal a thinned epithelium and a dilated follicular canal filled with lamellar lipid-impregnated keratinous material. In pustular cases, there are folliculocentric abscesses surrounded by a dense inflammatory exudate of lymphocytes and polymorphonuclear leukocytes. In addition to these findings, indolent nodular lesions frequently show plasma cells, foreign body giant cells, and proliferation of fibroblasts. Epithelial-lined sinus tracts may form.

Treatment

General Principles

It is important to take a complete historical record of prior therapies, including all over-the-counter (OTC) products. The dose, timing, combinations, side effects, and response to interventions should be obtained. Corticosteroids, anabolic steroids, neuroleptics, epidermal growth factor inhibitors, lithium, and cyclosporine may worsen acne. A family history of acne and, if present, its tendency to scarring should be noted. Women should be queried regularly about menstrual irregularities and hair growth in a male pattern, as well as use of cosmetics.

or anovulation, biochemical or clinical signs of hyperandrogenism, and echographic polycystic ovaries. Thus the diagnosis of PCOS may be made clinically by the presence of anovulation (<9 periods per year or periods >40 days apart) and signs of hyperandrogenism, such as acne and hirsutism. Approximately 15% of women of childbearing age will meet the criteria for PCOS. This diagnosis has important implications for affected patients. Systemic disease such as insulin resistance (which may manifest as acanthosis nigricans), obesity, cardiovascular disease, obstructive sleep apnea, nonalcoholic steatohepatitis, endometrial cancer and infertility

Treatment may fail because of drug interactions, coexisting conditions, or antibiotic resistance, but the most common and important cause is lack of adherence to the treatment plan. Utilizing medications that are well tolerated, have convenient dosing regimens, and are cosmetically acceptable will help. Thorough patient education is essential: explain how lesions form, define the expected response to and the duration and side effects of treatment, and give clear, unambiguous instructions. Patients should know the difference between active inflammatory lesions and the purplish red or hyperpigmented macules of inactive resolved lesions. Topical application should be to the entire affected area rather than to specific lesions, and oral and topical medications should be used daily as preventive treatment.

A high-glycemic diet may worsen acne, although the strength of its influence is unknown. The authors in general do not counsel patients to alter their diets unless large quantities of skim milk are being ingested or obesity is present. A trial lessening skim milk intake is worthwhile, with appropriate calcium and vitamin D supplementation given. In obese patients, dietary counseling is recommended, especially if PCOS, or other syndromes known to be associated with insulin resistance and metabolic syndrome (e.g., HAIR-AN syndrome) are present. For some patients who want a more "natural" approach to therapy and a change in diet, a low-glycemic diet may be recommended. Scrubbing of the face increases irritation and may worsen acne. Use of only prescribed medications and avoidance of potentially drying OTC products, such as astringents, harsh cleansers, and antibacterial soaps, should be emphasized. Noncomedogenic cosmetics are recommended, and pressed powders and oil-based products should be avoided.

Medical Therapy

Systemic and topical retinoids, systemic and topical antimicrobials, and systemic hormonal therapy are the main therapeutic classes of treatment available. Treatment guidelines are outlined in Box 13.1. Pregnancy and lactation labeling is undergoing significant changes which will allow a better understanding of the potential risks. This will likely result in less stringent recommendations regarding topical therapies. Such changes are ongoing and in this section pregnancy categories will still be referenced.

Topical Treatment. All topical treatments are preventive, and use for 8–12 weeks is required to judge their efficacy. The entire acne-affected area is treated, not just the lesions, and long-term use is the rule. In many patients, topical therapy may be effective as maintenance therapy after initial control is achieved with a combination of oral and topical treatment.

Topical Retinoids. It has long been appreciated that topical retinoids are especially effective in promoting normal desquamation of the follicular epithelium, reducing comedones and inhibiting the development of new lesions. Additionally, they have a marked antiinflammatory effect, inhibiting the activity of leukocytes, the release of proinflammatory cytokines and other mediators, and the expression of transcription factors and toll-like receptors involved in immunomodulation. These agents also help penetration of other active agents. Thus the topical retinoids should be used in most patients with acne and are the preferred agents in maintenance therapy.

Tretinoin was the first of this group of agents to be used for acne. Popular forms of tretinoin are 0.025% and 0.05% in a cream base and the micronized gels because these are less irritating than standard gels and liquids. Its incorporation into microspheres and a polyolprepolymer also helps limit irritation and make the product more stable in the presence of light and oxidizers. Tretinoin treatment may take 8–12 weeks before improvement occurs. When patients are tolerating the medication and are slow to respond, retinoic acid gel or solution may be used. Tretinoin should be applied at night and is in pregnancy category C.

BOX 13.1 Acne Treatment

MILD
1. Comedonal
   - Topical retinoid ± physical extraction (first line)
   - Alternate retinoid, benzoyl peroxide, salicylic acid, azelaic acid (second line)
2. Papular/pustular
   - Benzoyl peroxide or topical antimicrobial combination + topical retinoid, benzoyl peroxide wash if mild truncal lesions (first line)
   - Alternate antimicrobial combination + alternate topical retinoid, azelaic acid, sodium sulfacetamide–sulfur (second line)

MODERATE
1. Papular/pustular
   - In men, oral antibiotic + topical retinoid + benzoyl peroxide (first line)
   - Alternate antibiotic, alternate topical retinoid (second line); if moderately severe, isotretinoin
   - In women, spironolactone and/or oral contraceptive + topical retinoids ± benzoyl peroxide; oral antibiotic + topical retinoid + benzoyl peroxide (alternative)
   - Isotretinoin if relapses quickly off oral antibiotics, does not clear, or scars

SEVERE
1. Nodular/conglobate
   - Isotretinoin
   - Oral antibiotic + topical retinoid + benzoyl peroxide
   - In women, spironolactone + oral contraceptive + topical retinoid ± topical or oral antibiotics and/or benzoyl peroxide

---

Adapalene is a well-tolerated retinoid-like compound that has efficacy equivalent to the lower concentrations of tretinoin. Because it is light stable, adapalene may be applied in either the morning or the evening. It is in pregnancy category C.

Tazarotene is comparatively strong in its action, but also relatively irritating. It should be applied once at night or every other night, and as it is in pregnancy category X, contraceptive counseling should be provided.

Initially using retinoids every other night or adding a moisturizer with their use may lessen their irritant effects. They are also particularly useful in patients of color because retinoids may lighten postinflammatory hyperpigmentation.

Benzoyl Peroxide. Benzoyl peroxide has a potent antibacterial effect. *Propionibacterium acnes* resistance does not develop during use. Its concomitant use during treatment with antibiotics will limit the development of resistance, even if only given for short 2- to 7-day pulses. Although benzoyl peroxide is most effective in inflammatory acne, some studies have shown it to be comedolytic as well. The wash formulations may be used for mild truncal acne when systemic therapies are not required. These need to be in place 2 minutes to be effective.

Treatment is usually once or twice daily. Benzoyl peroxide may irritate the skin and produce peeling. Water-based formulations of lowest strength are least irritating and do not compromise efficacy. Application limited to once a day or every other day will also help. Allergic contact dermatitis will rarely develop, suggested by the complaint of itch rather than stinging or burning. Benzoyl peroxide is in pregnancy category C.

Topical Antibacterials. Topical clindamycin and erythromycin are available in a number of formulations. In general, they are well tolerated and are effective in mild inflammatory acne. These topical products are in pregnancy category B. Use of these topical antibiotics alone, however, is not recommended because they may induce antibiotic resistance. As mentioned, concurrent therapy with benzoyl peroxide will limit this problem. Concomitant use with a topical retinoid will hasten the response and allow for more rapid discontinuance of the antibiotic.

Dapsone is available topically in a gel formulation. Hemolytic anemia may occur, and skin discoloration is possible when benzoyl peroxide is applied after topical dapsone. Additionally, concomitant oral use of trimethoprim-sulfamethoxazole will increase the systemic absorption of topical dapsone. Dapsone is in pregnancy category C. A topical minocycline product is being actively investigated.

Sulfur, Sodium Sulfacetamide, Resorcin, and Salicylic Acid. Although benzoyl peroxide, retinoids, and topical antibiotics have largely supplanted these older medications, sulfur, resorcin, and salicylic acid preparations are still useful and moderately helpful if the newer medications are not tolerated. They are frequently found in OTC preparations. Sulfacetamide-sulfur combination products are mildly effective in both acne and rosacea, but should be avoided in patients with known hypersensitivity to sulfonamides.

Azelaic Acid. This dicarboxylic acid is usually well tolerated and has mild efficacy in both inflammatory and comedonal acne. Azelaic acid may help to lighten postinflammatory hyperpigmentation and is in pregnancy category B.

Combination Topical Therapy. Several products are available that combine antibiotics such as clindamycin and benzoyl peroxide or combine retinoids and either antibiotics or benzoyl peroxide. In general, these medications increase adherence because they require less frequent application, and they may also limit irritation compared with the cumulative topical application of each product separately. However, combination topical therapy limits flexibility and may cause more irritation than a single product used alone.

Oral Antibiotics. Oral antibiotics are indicated for moderate to severe acne; in patients with inflammatory disease who do not tolerate or respond to topical combinations; for the treatment of chest, back, or shoulder acne; and in patients for whom absolute control is deemed essential, such as those who scar with each lesion or who develop inflammatory hyperpigmentation. It generally takes 8–12 weeks to judge efficacy. Starting at a high dose and stopping it after achieving control is preferred. Limitation on the use of antibiotics is best. Working to maintain control eventually with topical retinoids or retinoid–benzoyl peroxide combination therapy is ideal. A subset of patients will require longer term use if alternate therapies such as isotretinoin or hormonal agents are inappropriate. In these patients reevaluation at regular intervals to judge continued need is recommended.

There is concern that oral antibiotics may reduce the effectiveness of oral contraceptives (OCs). It is appropriate for this as-yet unproved (except with rifampin, which is not used for acne) association be discussed with patients and a second form of birth control offered.

Tetracycline. Tetracycline's availability and utility are limited.

Doxycycline. The usual dose of doxycycline is 50–100 mg once or twice a day, depending on the disease severity. Photosensitivity reactions can occur with this form of tetracycline and can be dramatic. Vaginitis or perianal itching may result and occurs in about 5% of patients, with *Candida albicans* usually present in the involved site. The only other common side effects are gastrointestinal (GI) symptoms such as nausea. To reduce the incidence of esophagitis, tetracyclines should not be taken at bedtime. An enteric-coated formulation is available and limits the GI side effects. Staining of growing teeth occurs, precluding use of tetracyclines in pregnant women and in children under age 9 or 10. The tetracyclines should also be avoided when renal function is impaired.

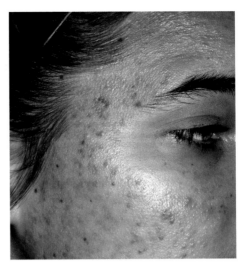

Fig. 13.9 Minocycline hyperpigmentation.

Sub–antimicrobial-dose doxycycline hyclate, given as 20 mg twice daily or as a sustained-release 40-mg once-daily dose, will also serve to limit antibiotic use, as antiinflammatory activity is being utilized, but no antibiotic resistance results because of the low dose. A sustained-release 40-mg formulation of doxycycline monohydrate is also available.

Minocycline. Minocycline is effective in treating acne vulgaris. The usual dose is 50–100 mg once or twice daily, depending on the severity of disease. Its absorption is less affected by milk and food than is doxycycline. Vertigo may occur, and beginning minocycline therapy with a single dose in the evening is prudent. An extended-release preparation is also available, which limits the vestibular side effects. Pigmentation in areas of inflammation, of oral tissues, in postacne osteoma or scars, in a photodistributed pattern, on the shins, or in the sclera, nail bed, ear cartilage, or teeth or in a generalized pattern may also be seen (Fig. 13.9). Additionally, lupus-like syndromes, a hypersensitivity syndrome (fever, hepatitis, and eosinophilia), serum sickness, pneumonitis, and hepatitis are uncommon but potentially serious adverse effects of minocycline.

Amoxicillin. For those who cannot take tetracyclines because of side effects, or in pregnant women requiring oral antibiotic therapy, amoxicillin may be useful. Amoxicillin and the much less effective erythromycin are in pregnancy category B. Amoxicillin can be given in doses ranging from 250 mg daily to 500 mg three times daily. Side effects are allergic reactions, which may be serious, and GI upset. Many patients of acne age have taken amoxicillin in the past and are aware of their allergy status.

Clindamycin. Past experience has shown that clindamycin provides an excellent response in the treatment of acne. However, the potential for the development of pseudomembranous colitis and the availability of isotretinoin have limited its use. The initial dose of clindamycin is 150 mg three times daily, reduced gradually as control is achieved.

Other Antibiotics. Sulfonamides may be effective in many cases unresponsive to other antibiotics; however, the potential for severe drug eruptions limits their use by dermatologists. Trimethoprim-sulfamethoxazole (TMP-SMX; Bactrim, Septra), in double-strength dose twice daily, is recommended initially when given to moderately to severely affected patients who have failed other oral medication. Trimethoprim alone, 300 mg twice daily, is also useful. Oral dapsone has been used in severe acne conglobata (AC) but is rarely used today. Isotretinoin is favored.

Bacterial Resistance. *Propionibacterium acnes* antimicrobial resistance has been a clinically relevant problem. However, with the limited use of erythromycin, clindamycin, and tetracycline, this consideration is less problematic. Doxycycline resistance may occur, and minocycline is a suitable alternative if this problem is suspected. Although concomitant use of benzoyl peroxide will help limit cutaneous drug resistance problems, *Staphylococcus aureus* in the nares, streptococci in the oral cavity, and enterobacteria in the gut may also become resistant. Also, close contacts, including treating dermatologists, may harbor such drug-resistant bacteria. Strategies to prevent antibiotic resistance include limiting the duration of treatment, stressing the importance of adherence to the treatment plan, restricting the use of antibiotics to inflammatory acne, encouraging repeat treatment with the same antibiotic unless it has lost its efficacy, avoiding the use of dissimilar oral and topical antibiotics at the same time, and using isotretinoin if unable to maintain clearance without oral antibacterial therapy.

Hormonal Therapy. Hormonal interventions in women may be beneficial even in the absence of abnormal laboratory tests. The workup for the woman with signs of hyperandrogenism, such as acne, menstrual irregularities, hirsutism, or androgenic alopecia, is presented earlier. Women with normal laboratory values respond to hormonal therapy. Results take longer to be seen with these agents, with first evidence of improvement often not apparent for 3 months and continued improved response seen for at least 6 months. Excellent candidates for hormonal treatment include women with PCOS, late-onset adrenal hyperplasia, or another identifiable endocrinologic condition and women with late-onset moderate to severe acne, acne unresponsive to other oral and topical therapies, or acne that has relapsed quickly after isotretinoin treatment. Women with acne primarily located on the lower face and neck and with deep-seated nodules that are painful and long-lasting (Fig. 13.10) are often quite responsive to hormonal intervention. As emphasis is placed on limiting antibiotic therapy, hormonal treatment may considered a first-line therapy in most women needing an oral intervention.

Oral Contraceptives. The OCs block both adrenal and ovarian androgens. Ortho Tri-Cyclen, Estrostep Fe, Alesse, Yasmin, Beyaz, and Yaz are examples of OCs that have beneficial effects on acne. The progestins that these contain have either low androgenic activity or antiandrogenic activity. Both the physician and the patient should be familiar with the adverse reactions associated with OCs, such as nausea, vomiting, abnormal menses, melasma, weight gain, breast tenderness, and rarely thrombophlebitis, pulmonary embolism, and hypertension.

Spironolactone. Antiandrogen treatment during pregnancy will result in feminization of a male fetus, and thus spironolactone is usually prescribed in combination with OCs. It may be effective

in doses from 25–200 mg/day. Most women will tolerate a starting dose of 100 mg at night. Most also tolerate 150 mg/day (50 in the AM, 100 at night), but many will have side effects at 200 mg/day (100 twice daily). Side effects include irregular menstrual periods, breast tenderness, headache, dizziness, lightheadedness, fatigue, and occasionally diuresis; the non–central nervous system (CNS) effects are dose dependent. Four large recent retrospective studies of over 700 patients confirm the majority experience significant improvement, and many cleared with combination oral and/or topical intervention. Its use during pregnancy will result in feminization of a male fetus. Combination use with OCs serves to limit this problem and improve results. Several months of treatment are usually required to see benefit.

Dexamethasone. Dexamethasone, 0.125–0.5 mg given once at night, reduces androgen excess and may alleviate cystic acne. Although corticosteroids are effective in the treatment of adult-onset adrenal hyperplasia, antiandrogens are often used in this setting.

Prednisone. Although corticosteroids may produce steroid acne, they are also effective antiinflammatory agents in severe and intractable acne vulgaris. In severe cystic acne and AC, corticosteroid treatment is effective; however, side effects restrict its use. Prednisone is generally only given to patients with severe inflammatory acne during the first 1 or 2 months of treatment with isotretinoin, for initial reduction of inflammation, and to reduce isotretinoin-induced flares.

Other Hormonal Agents. Finasteride, flutamide, estrogen, gonadotropin-releasing agonists, and metformin (by decreasing testosterone levels) have all showed a beneficial effect on acne. Because of side effects, expense, and other considerations, however, these agents are not typically used.

Oral Retinoid Therapy

Isotretinoin. Isotretinoin is approved only for severe cystic acne. However, it is useful in less severe forms of acne to prevent the need for continuous treatment and the repeated office visits required. A consensus of experts found that oral isotretinoin is warranted for severe acne, poorly responsive acne that improves by less than 50% after 3 months of therapy with combined oral and topical antibiotics, acne that relapses after oral treatment, scars, and acne that induces psychological distress. Other indications are gram-negative folliculitis, inflammatory rosacea, pyoderma faciale, acne fulminans, and AC.

This retinoid is a reliable remedy in almost all acne patients (Fig. 13.11). The dose of isotretinoin is 0.5–1 mg/kg/day in one or two daily doses. For severe truncal acne in patients who tolerate higher doses, up to 2 mg/kg/day may be given. In practice, most patients are started at 20–40 mg to avoid an early flare, then increased to 40–80 mg/day to limit side effects, which generally are dose related. Doses as low as 0.1 mg/kg/day are almost as effective as the higher doses in clearing acne; the disadvantage is that lower doses are less likely to produce a prolonged remission, even after 20 weeks of treatment. To achieve potentially prolonged remission, patients should receive 120–150 mg/kg over the treatment course. An easy way to calculate the total isotretinoin dose needed is to multiply the patient's weight in kilograms by 3. The product is the total number of 40-mg capsules needed to reach the low end of the dosage spectrum. Two groups reported treating patients with 1.5–2 mg/kg for a total dose of approximately 300 mg/kg. These patients had a low relapse rate, although side effects often limit tolerance of such dosages.

The major advantage of isotretinoin is that it is the only acne therapy that is not open ended (i.e., leads to a remission that may last many months or years). Approximately 40%–60% of patients remain acne free after a single course of isotretinoin. Approximately one half of the relapsing patients will need only topical therapy, with the others requiring oral treatments. Many patients in the latter category prefer to be retreated with isotretinoin because of

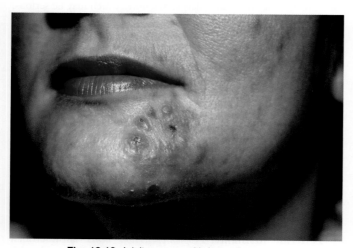

Fig. 13.10 Adult woman with lower face acne.

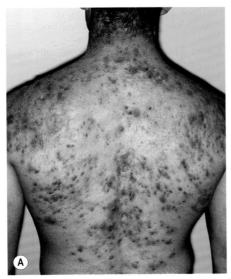 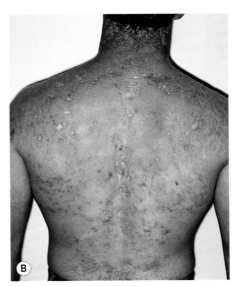

Fig. 13.11 (A) Severe back acne before isotretinoin. (B) Response to treatment.

its reliable efficacy and predictable side effects, which will be similar to those experienced in the first course. Many treated patients will require at least a second course of isotretinoin in 2 years.

Some subsets of patients tend to relapse more often. In patients under age 16 years, 40% need a second course of isotretinoin within 1 year and 73% within 2 years. Adult women and patients with mild acne tend to relapse more often and more quickly than severely affected 17- to 22-year-olds. Although patients' tolerance and response to repeated courses are similar to their experience with the first course, adult women who relapse may be better managed with hormonal therapies and mild acne treated with standard therapy.

In adult acne patients, who frequently tolerate the side effects of isotretinoin less well, lower doses and intermittent therapy are possible. In 80 adult acne patients treated with 0.5 mg/kg/day for 1 week in every 4 weeks over 6 months, acne resolved in 88%, and 39% relapsed after 1 year. In nine patients age 56–75 treated with 0.25 mg/kg/day for 6 months, all cleared and all except one remained clear 36 months later.

Patient education is critical in isotretinoin therapy. Its most serious adverse effect is the risk of severe damage to the fetus if given during pregnancy. Retinoid embryopathy is a well-defined syndrome characterized by craniofacial, cardiovascular, CNS, and thymus abnormalities. It is crucial that a woman of childbearing potential follow closely the manufacturer's recommendations. The use of consent forms, contraception education, and unequivocal documentation of the absence of pregnancy through monthly laboratory testing are important components of a U.S. Food and Drug Administration (FDA)–mandated verification program designed to prevent pregnancy during treatment. Women should not become pregnant until stopping medication for at least 1 month. Isotretinoin is not mutagenic, and there is no risk to a fetus while the male partner is taking the drug.

A second major area of educational emphasis concerns the psychological effects of the medication. Reports of depression, psychosis, suicidal ideation, suicide, and attempted suicide have prompted numerous studies of the mental health of patients taking isotretinoin. Although the usual outcome is improved mood because the disease clears, and a systematic review and meta-analysis found treatment did not appear to be associated with an increased risk of depression, a small number of patients have developed depression and have positive dechallenge and rechallenge tests. Close monitoring for depression, fully educating the patient, and enlisting the help of a roommate or family member to look for changes in mood are methods used to assess the psychological status of the patient taking isotretinoin.

Inflammatory bowel disease (IBD) is a third concern. Patients with IBD have been successfully treated with isotretinoin without flaring, but new-onset IBD in patients exposed to isotretinoin has been a concern. The age of onset of IBD overlaps with the age when acne will frequently be treated with isotretinoin and antibiotics. A meta-analysis has concluded that there was no increased risk of IBD or the subtypes. Long-term use of tetracycline medications and severe acne itself may be predisposing factors for IBD. Due to the past controversy, patients should be educated and monitored appropriately.

Other side effects of isotretinoin are dose dependent and generally not serious. Dry lips, skin, eyes, and oronasal mucosa occur in up to 90% of patients. These effects can be treated with moisturization. Dryness of the nasal mucosa leads to colonization by *S. aureus* in 80%–90% of treated patients. Skin abscesses, staphylococcal conjunctivitis, impetigo, facial cellulitis, and folliculitis may result. Such colonization can be avoided by the use of bacitracin ointment applied to the anterior nares twice daily during isotretinoin therapy. Arthralgias may occur but, as with other side effects, do not require interruption of therapy unless severe. Monitoring of serum lipids is done when initiating and increasing the dose because some patients will develop hypertriglyceridemia. This may be controlled by avoiding smoking and alcohol and following a low-fat diet. It should be emphasized that patients who develop this complication, as well as their family, are at risk for the development of the metabolic syndrome.

Liver function tests should be checked at regular intervals when initiating and increasing the dose. Isotretinoin should be taken with a high-fat meal to ensure excellent absorption. A formulation not requiring this type of meal is available.

Tumor Necrosis Factor Inhibitors. Adalimumab, etanercept, and infliximab have been reported in individual patients to improve or clear severe resistant acne. Some cases have been part of an inflammatory syndrome (e.g., SAPHO, PAPA, PASS) or found in patients with IBD. Paradoxically, acne has also been reported as an adverse reaction to these medications.

Intralesional Corticosteroids. Intralesional corticosteroids are especially effective in reducing inflammatory nodules. Triamcinolone acetonide at 10 mg/mL (Kenalog-10) is best diluted with sterile normal saline solution to 2.5 mg/mL. Injecting less than 0.1 mL directly into the center of the nodule will help safeguard against atrophy and hypopigmentation.

Physical Modalities

Local surgical treatment is helpful in quickly resolving the comedones, although many clinicians wait until after 2 or more months of topical retinoid therapy to extract the remaining comedones. The edge of the follicle is nicked with a No. 11 scalpel blade, and the contents are expressed with a comedo extractor. Scarring is not produced by this procedure. Light electrode desiccation is an alternative. In isotretinoin-treated patients, macrocomedones present at weeks 10–15 may be expressed, because they tend to persist throughout therapy.

The use of photodynamic therapy and various forms of light, laser, or radiofrequency energy is under investigation. Such interventions clearly are capable of destroying sebaceous glands and killing *P. acnes*, but the methods to deliver such treatment in an efficient, cost-effective, safe, relatively pain free, and practical manner are still evolving. These treatments will be a welcome addition with the potential to provide care without the concerns associated with systemic drugs. More studies of larger patient populations with appropriate controls are needed to evaluate the role of light and related energy in the spectrum of acne therapy.

Complications

Even with the excellent treatment options available, scarring may occur. This may be quite prominent and often results from the cystic type of acne, although smaller lesions may produce scarring in some individuals. Pitted scars, wide-mouthed depressions, and keloids, primarily seen along the jawline and chest, are common types of scarring. These may improve spontaneously over 1 year or longer. Many treatment options are available. Procedures reported to be effective in improving appearance include chemical peeling; ablative, nonablative, and vascular laser therapy; skin needling or rolling; dermabrasion; scar excision; subcision; punch grafts alone or followed by dermabrasion or laser smoothing; intralesional corticosteroids or fluorouracil; fractionated laser resurfacing; fat transfer; and use of filler substances.

Other complications from acne are prominent residual hyperpigmentation, especially in darker-skinned patients (Fig. 13.12); pyogenic granuloma formation, which is more common in acne fulminans and in patients treated with high-dose isotretinoin; osteoma cutis, which consists of small, firm papules resulting from long-standing acne vulgaris; and solid facial edema. The latter is a persistent, firm facial swelling that is an uncommon but distressing

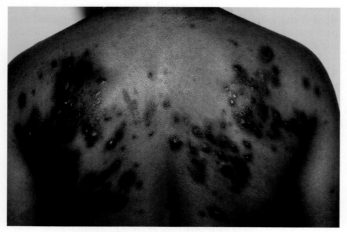

Fig. 13.12 Severe truncal acne with hyperpigmentation.

result of acne vulgaris or acne rosacea. Both corticosteroids and isotretinoin have been reported to be effective treatments.

Abdel Hay R, et al: Interventions for acne scars. Cochrane Database Syst Rev 2016; 4: CD011946.

Asai Y, et al: Management of acne. CMAJ 2016; 188: 118.

Awan SZ, Lu J: Management of severe acne during pregnancy. Int J Womens Dermatol 2017; 13: 145.

Azoulay L, et al: Isotretinoin therapy and the incidence of acne relapse. Br J Dermatol 2007; 157: 1240.

Baldwin H: Treating acne during pregnancy and lactation. Cutis 2015; 96: 11.

Barbieri JS, et al: Approaches to limit systemic antibiotics in acne. J Am Acad Dermatol 2018; Oct 5.

Berard A, et al: Isotretinoin, pregnancies, abortions and birth defects. Br J Clin Pharmacol 2007; 63: 196.

Blasiak RC, et al: High-dose isotretinoin treatment and the rate of retrial, relapse, and adverse effects in patients with acne vulgaris. JAMA Dermatol 2013; 149: 1392.

Brown RJ, et al: Minocycline-induced drug hypersensitivity syndrome followed by multiple autoimmune sequelae. Arch Dermatol 2009; 145: 63.

Buzney E, et al: Polycystic ovary syndrome. J Am Acad Dermatol 2014; 71: 859.e1.

Çerman AA, et al: Dietary glycemic factors, insulin resistance, and adiponectin levels in acne vulgaris. J Am Acad Dermatol 2016; 75: 155.

Charney JW, et al: Spironolactone for the treatment of acne in women, a retrospective study of 110 patients. Int J Womens Dermatol 2017; 3: 111.

Chen W, et al: Acne-associated syndromes. J Eur Acad Dermatol Venereol 2011; 25: 637.

Cyrulnik AA, et al: High-dose isotretinoin in acne vulgaris. Int J Dermatol 2012; 51: 1123.

Dréno B: What is new in the pathophysiology of acne, an overview. J Eur Acad Dermatol Venereol 2017; 31 Suppl 5: 8.

Dréno B, et al: Acne in pregnant women. Acta Derm Venereol 2014; 94: 82.

Dressler C, et al: How much do we know about maintaining treatment response after successful acne therapy? Systematic review of the efficacy and safety of acne maintenance therapy. Dermatology 2016; 232: 371.

Eichenfield LF, et al: Evidence-based recommendations for the diagnosis and treatment of pediatric acne. Pediatrics 2013; 131: S163.

Fitzpatrick L, et al: Oral contraceptives for acne treatment. Cutis 2017; 99: 195.

Grandhi R, Alikhan A: Spironolactone for the treatment of acne. Dermatology 2017; 233: 141.

Hansen TJ, et al: Standardized laboratory monitoring with use of isotretinoin in acne. J Am Acad Dermatol 2016; 75: 323.

Hassoun LA, et al: The use of hormonal agents in the treatment of acne. Semin Cutan Med Surg 2016; 35: 68.

Housman E, Reynolds RV: Polycystic ovary syndrome. J Am Acad Dermatol 2014; 71: 847.e1.

Hu S, et al: Fractional resurfacing for the treatment of atopic facial acne scars in Asian skin. Dermatol Surg 2009; 35: 826.

Huang YC, Cheng YC: Isotretinoin treatment for acne and risk of depression. J Am Acad Dermatol 2017; 76: 1068.

Isvy-Joubert A, et al: Adult female acne treated with spironolactone. Eur J Dermatol 2017; 27: 393.

Jacobs A, et al: Systemic review of the rapidity of the onset of action of topical treatments in the therapy of mild-to-moderate acne vulgaris. Br J Dermatol 2014; 170: 557.

James WD: Clinical practice: acne. N Engl J Med 2005; 352: 1463.

Lee SY, et al: Does exposure to isotretinoin increase the risk for the development of inflammatory bowel disease? Eur J Gastroenterol Hepatol 2016; 28: 210.

Lee YH, et al: Laboratory monitoring during isotretinoin therapy for acne. JAMA Dermatol 2016; 152: 35.

Leyden JJ, et al: The use of isotretinoin in the treatment of acne vulgaris. J Clin Aesthet Dermatol 2014; 7: S3.

Lortscher D, et al: Hormonal contraceptives and acne. J Drugs Dermatol 2016; 15: 670.

Manolache L, et al: A case of solid facial oedema successfully treated with isotretinoin. J Eur Acad Dermatol Venereol 2009; 23: 965.

Margolis D, et al: Potential association between the oral tetracycline class of antimicrobials used to treat acne and inflammatory bowel disease. Am J Gastroenterol 2010; 105: 2610.

McCarty M: Evaluation and management of refractory acne vulgaris in adolescent and adult men. Dermatol Clin 2016; 34: 203.

Morrone A, et al: Clinical features of acne vulgaris in 444 patients with ethnic skin. J Dermatol 2011; 38: 405.

Nast A, et al: European evidence-based guidelines for the treatment of acne. J Eur Acad Dermatol Venereol 2012; 26: S1.

Rademaker M: Making sense of the effects of the cumulative dose of isotretinoin in acne vulgaris. Int J Dermatol 2016; 55: 518.

Rademaker M, et al: Isotretinoin 5 mg daily for low-grade adult acne vulgaris. J Eur Acad Dermatol Venereol 2014; 28: 747.

Rashtak S, et al: Isotretinoin exposure and risk of inflammatory bowel disease. JAMA Dermatol 2014; 150: 1322.

Schmidt TH, et al: Cutaneous findings and systemic associations in women with polycystic ovary syndrome. JAMA Dermatol 2016; 152: 391.

Spring LK, et al: Isotretinoin and timing of procedural interventions. JAMA Dermatol 2017; 153: 802.

Strahan JE, et al: Cyclosporine-induced infantile nodulocystic acne. Arch Dermatol 2009; 145: 797.

Tan J, et al: Oral isotretinoin. Dermatol Clin 2016; 34: 175.

Thiboutot DM, et al: Practical management of acne for clinicians. J Am Acad Dermatol 2018;78: S1.

Zaenglein AL, et al: Guidelines of care for the management of acne vulgaris. J Am Acad Dermatol 2016; 74: 945.

ACNE CONGLOBATA

Cystic acne is the mildest form of AC, an unusually severe type of acne. This form is characterized by numerous comedones (many of which are double or triple) and large abscesses with interconnecting sinuses, cysts, and grouped inflammatory nodules (Fig. 13.13). The cysts occur on the back, buttocks, chest, forehead, cheeks, anterior neck, and shoulders (Fig. 13.14). They contain a thick, yellowish, viscid, stringy, blood-tinged fluid. After incision and drainage, there is frequently a prompt refilling with the same type of material. Pronounced scars remain after healing.

Dissecting cellulitis of the scalp and hidradenitis suppurativa (HS) may be seen with AC, an association known as the "follicular occlusion triad." Gamma-secretase gene mutations may be responsible for familial cases of HS; one family with dominantly inherited AC also has expressed this trait. Additionally patients may present with the combination of pyoderma gangrenosum, AC, and suppurative hidradenitis (PASH) alone or with coexisting axial spondyloarthritis (PASS syndrome).

This severe and painful disease occurs most frequently in young men; it may extend and persist into adulthood and even into the fifth decade of life, especially over the posterior neck and back. Women are less frequently affected. Athletes and bodybuilders should be questioned about the use of anabolic steroids, which may induce such aggressive acne.

The therapy of choice is isotretinoin, 0.5–1 mg/kg/day to a total dose of 150 mg/kg, with a second course if resolution does not occur after a rest period of 2 months. Pretreatment with

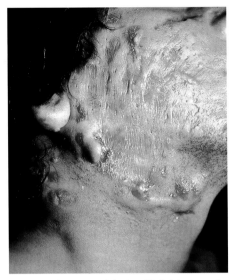

Fig. 13.13 Acne conglobata with fistula formation.

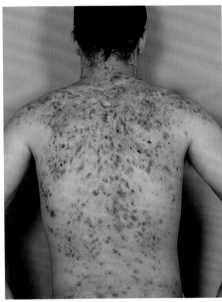

Fig. 13.14 Acne conglobata of the back. (Courtesy Dr. Don Adler.)

prednisone and low initial doses of isotretinoin, as described for acne fulminans, are recommended to avoid flaring of disease. Adalimumab, infliximab, and external beam radiation are other reported therapies. Four patients with PASH syndrome responded to intravenous combination antibiotic therapy given for 3–6 weeks followed by 4–6 week cycles of combined oral antibiotic therapy.

Join-Lambert O, et al: Remission of refractory pyoderma gangrenosum, severe acne, and hidradenitis suppurativa (PASH) syndrome using targeted antibiotic therapy in 4 patients. J Am Acad Dermatol 2015; 73: S66.

Myers JN, et al: Treatment of acne conglobata with modern external beam radiation. J Am Acad Dermatol 2010; 62: 861.

Ratnamala U, et al: Expanding the spectrum of γ-secretase gene mutation-associated phenotypes. Exp Dermatol 2016; 25: 314.

Yiu ZZ, et al: Acne conglobata and adalimumab. Clin Exp Dermatol 2015; 40: 383.

ACNE FULMINANS

Acne fulminans is a rare form of extremely severe cystic acne that occurs primarily in teenage boys. It is characterized by highly inflammatory nodules and plaques that undergo swift suppurative degeneration, leaving ragged ulcerations with hemorrhagic crusts, mostly on the chest and back. The face is usually less severely involved. Isotretinoin, especially when given in high initial doses, or anabolic steroids, may induce this condition.

Less commonly systemic signs and symptoms may accompany acne fulminans. Fever, polyarthralgia and polymyalgia, destructive arthritis, erythema nodosum, and myopathy have been reported. Leukocytosis, anemia, and focal lytic bone lesions often affecting the sternum, clavicles, hips and sacroiliac joints may be seen.

Prednisone is necessary during the initial 4–8 weeks to heal the dramatic lesions of acne fulminans. If isotretinoin induced the flare, it must be discontinued during this phase. After resolution of the inflammation 10–20 mg daily of isotretinoin is added. This should be slowly increased to standard doses and continued for a full 120–150 mg/kg cumulative course. Large cysts may be opened and the contents expressed. Intralesional corticosteroids will aid their resolution. Infliximab, etanercept, cyclosporine and dapsone are alternatives if isotretinoin is contraindicated.

Alakeel A, et al: Acne fulminans. Pediatr Dermatol 2016; 33: e388.

Greywal T, et al: Evidence-based recommendations for the management of acne fulminans and its variants. J Am Acad Dermatol 2017; 77: 109.

Lages RB, et al: Acne fulminans successfully treated with prednisone and dapsone. An Bras Dermatol 2012; 87: 612.

Perez M, et al: When strength turns into disease: acne fulminans in a bodybuilder. An Bras Dermatol 2016; 91: 706.

SAPHO AND RELATED SYNDROMES

The SAPHO syndrome is characterized by synovitis, acne, pustulosis, hyperostosis, and osteitis. Skin findings may include acne fulminans, AC, pustular psoriasis, hidradenitis suppurativa, dissecting cellulitis of the scalp, Sweet syndrome, Sneddon-Wilkinson disease, and palmoplantar pustulosis. These may be present at the outset of the skeletal changes, but most often precede bone findings, or in 15% of adult cases and 70% of childhood cases, do not occur at all. The chest wall and mandible are the most common sites for musculoskeletal complaints in adults; the long bones, particularly the tibia, predominate in children. Bone changes of the anterior chest wall on nuclear scans are the most specific diagnostic findings.

Acquired hyperostosis syndrome (AHYS) and, in a familial setting of a dominantly inherited disorder, pyogenic sterile arthritis, pyoderma gangrenosum, and acne (PAPA syndrome) present with similar clinical scenarios. PAPA syndrome is caused by mutations in the gene for proline-serine-threonine-phosphatase interacting protein 1.

Systemic retinoids and tumor necrosis factor (TNF) antagonists, particularly infliximab, have been successful in treating these patients. If isotretinoin is used, it should be initiated at a low dosage, such as 10 mg/day, in combination with prednisone for the first month to prevent flaring of the disease. Anakinra, ustekinumab, methotrexate, sulfasalazine, and cyclosporine are other, less well-documented but likely effective choices. Pamidronate and other bisphosphonates such as ibandronate, alendronate, and zoledronic acid, are effective in treating the osteoarticular manifestations.

Aljuhani F, et al: The SAPHO syndrome. J Rheumatol 2015; 42: 329.

Anić B, et al: Clinical features of the SAPHO syndrome and their role in choosing the therapeutic approach. Acta Dermatovenerol Croat 2014; 22: 180.

Chen W, et al: Acne-associated syndromes. J Eur Acad Dermatol Venereol 2011; 25: 637.

Firinu D, et al: SAPHO syndrome. Curr Rheumatol Rep 2016; 18: 35.

Galadari H, et al: Synovitis, acne, pustulosis, hyperostosis, and osteitis syndrome treated with a combination of isotretinoin and pamidronate. J Am Acad Dermatol 2009; 61: 123.

Witt M, et al: Disease burden, disease manifestations and current treatment regimen of the SAPHO syndrome in Germany. Semin Arthritis Rheum 2014; 43: 745.

OTHER ACNE VARIANTS

Tropical Acne

Tropical acne is unusually severe acne occurring in the tropics during the seasons when the weather is hot and humid. Nodular, cystic, and pustular lesions occur chiefly on the back, buttocks, and thighs (Fig. 13.15). Characteristically, the face is spared. Conglobate abscesses occur often, especially on the back. Comedones are sparse. Acne tropicalis usually occurs in young adults who may have had acne vulgaris at an earlier age. This is especially true of those in the armed forces stationed in the tropics and carrying backpacks. Treatment is that for cystic acne, but acne tropicalis may persist until the patient moves to a cooler, less humid climate.

Acne Estivalis

Also known as Mallorca acne, this rare form of acne starts in the spring, progresses during the summer, and resolves completely in the fall. Acne estivalis affects almost exclusively women age 25–40. Dull-red, dome-shaped, hard, small papules, usually not larger than 3–4 mm, develop on the cheeks and usually extend on to the sides of the neck, chest, shoulders, and characteristically the upper arms. Comedones and pustules are notably absent or sparse. Acne estivalis does not respond to antibiotics but benefits from application of retinoic acid.

Excoriated Acne

Also known as picker's acne and acne excoriée des jeunes filles, excoriated acne is seen primarily in young women with a superficial type of acne. The primary lesions are trivial or even nonexistent, but the compulsive habit of picking the face and squeezing minute

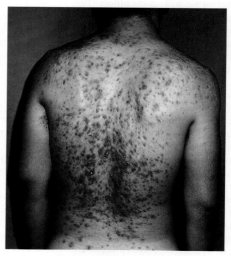

Fig. 13.15 Tropical acne.

comedones produces secondary lesions that crust and may leave scars.

Excoriated acne may be a sign of depression or anxiety. If the patient admits to picking but being unable to stop this habit, improvement may follow support and acne therapy. However, most patients will require interventions with selective serotonin reuptake inhibitors, behavior modification, or psychotherapy. Other pharmacologic treatments that have been successful in case reports include doxepin, clomipramine, naltrexone, pimozide, and olanzapine.

Galdyn IA, et al: The reconstructive challenges and approach to patients with excoriation disorder. J Craniofac Surg 2015; 26: 824.

Hjorth N, et al: Acne aestivalis: Mallorca acne. Acta Dermatol Venereol 1972; 2: 61.

Wells JM: Tropical acne—one hundred cases. J R Army Med Corps 1981; 127: 55.

ACNEIFORM ERUPTIONS

Acneiform eruptions are follicular eruptions characterized by papules and pustules resembling acne. Breaks in the epithelium and spillage of follicular contents into the dermis lead to the lesions. Eruptions are not necessarily confined to the usual sites of acne vulgaris, often have a sudden onset, are monomorphous, and usually appear in a patient well past adolescence. If secondary to a drug, an eruption begins within days of initiation of the medication, may be accompanied by fever and malaise, and resolves when the drug is stopped.

Acneiform eruptions may originate from skin exposure to various industrial chemicals, such as fumes generated in the manufacture of chlorine and its byproducts. These chlorinated hydrocarbons may cause chloracne, consisting of cysts, pustules, folliculitis, and comedones. The most potent acneiform-inducing agents are the polyhalogenated hydrocarbons, notably dioxin (2,3,7,8-tetrachlorodibenzo-p-dioxin). Cutting and lubricating oils, pomades, crude coal tar applied to the skin for medicinal purposes, heavy tar distillates, coal tar pitch, and asbestos are known to cause acneiform eruptions. Acne venenata or contact acne is another term applied to this process. Topical steroids, especially the fluorinated types or when applied under occlusion, topical tacrolimus and pimecrolimus may all induce a papulopustular eruption.

Acneiform eruptions are also induced by systemic medications such as iodides from radiopaque contrast media or potassium iodide, bromides in drugs such as propantheline bromide, testosterone, cyclosporine, antiepileptic medications, lithium, TNF-α antagonists, epidermal growth factor inhibitors, inhibitors of the RAS/RAF/MEK/ERK pathway, and systemic corticosteroids. When medium or high doses of corticosteroids are taken for as briefly as 3–5 days, a distinctive eruption may occur, known as steroid acne. It is a sudden outcropping of inflamed papules, most numerous on the upper trunk and arms (Fig. 13.16) but also seen on the face. The lesions typically present as papules rather than comedones; however, a histologic study confirmed they begin follicularly with microcomedone formation. Tretinoin 0.05% cream applied once or twice daily, may clear the lesions within 1–3 months despite the continuation of high doses of corticosteroid. Oral antibiotics and other typical acne medications are also effective. Epidermal growth factor inhibitors, including monoclonal antibodies and tyrosine and multikinase inhibitors used in cancer therapy, produce a folliculitis in the majority of treated patients as do inhibitors of the downstream signaling pathway. Often, oral minocycline and topical benzoyl peroxide are given prophylactically at the outset of the cancer therapy to prevent what may be a dose-limiting reaction. Radiation therapy for malignancy also can induce acne in the radiation port.

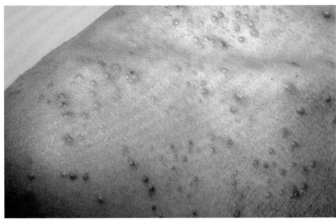

Fig. 13.16 Steroid acne.

Comedonal lesions may be limited to the nasal crease, in the flexural areas in children and on the temple and malar skin in Favre-Racouchot syndrome.

Cho SB, et al: A new case of childhood flexural comedones. J Eur Acad Dermatol Venereol 2009; 23: 366.

Dessinioti C, et al: Acneiform eruptions. Clin Dermatol 2014; 32: 24.

Hubiche T, Sibaud V: Localized acne induced by radiation therapy. Dermatol Online J 2014; 20: 12.

Kashat M, et al: Etanercept-induced cystic acne. Cutis 2014; 94: 31.

Li JC, et al: Facial acne during topical pimecrolimus therapy for vitiligo. Clin Exp Dermatol 2009; 34: e489.

Melnik B, et al: Abuse of anabolic-androgenic steroids and bodybuilding acne. J Dtsch Dermatol Ges 2007; 5: 110.

Pelclova D, et al: Adverse health effects in humans exposed to 2,3,7,8-tetrachlorodibenzo-p-dioxin (TCDD). Rev Environ Health 2006; 21: 119.

Saurat JH, et al: The cutaneous lesions of dioxin exposure. Toxicol Sci 2012; 125: 310.

Sheu J, et al: Papulopustular acneiform eruptions resulting from trastuzumab, a HER2 inhibitor. Clin Breast Cancer 2015; 15: e77.

Turrion Merino L, et al: Localized acneiform eruption following radiotherapy in a patient with breast carcinoma. Dermatol Online J 2014; 20: 13.

Waller B, et al: Transverse nasal crease and transverse nasal milia. Arch Dermatol 2012; 148: 1037.

GRAM-NEGATIVE FOLLICULITIS

Gram-negative folliculitis occurs in patients who have had moderately inflammatory acne for long periods and have been treated with long-term antibiotics, mainly tetracyclines. During antibiotic treatment, patients develop either superficial pustules 3–6 mm in diameter, flaring out from the anterior nares, or fluctuant, deep-seated nodules (Fig. 13.17). Culture of these lesions usually reveals a species of *Klebsiella, Escherichia coli, Enterobacter*, or, from the deep cystic lesions, *Proteus*.

With long-term, broad-spectrum antibiotic therapy, the anterior nares may become colonized with these gram-negative organisms. As the use of long-term antibiotic therapy declines, this disease has become less common.

Isotretinoin is very effective and is the treatment of choice in gram-negative folliculitis. This treatment not only clears the acne component of the disease but also eliminates the colonization of

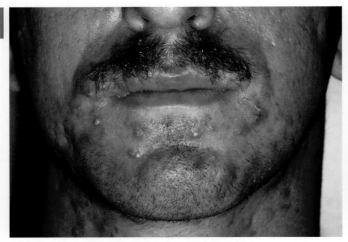

Fig. 13.17 Gram-negative folliculitis.

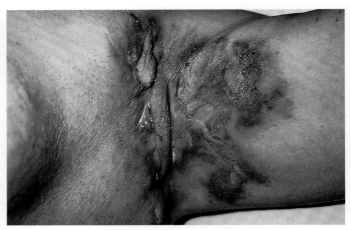

Fig. 13.19 Hidradenitis of the axilla.

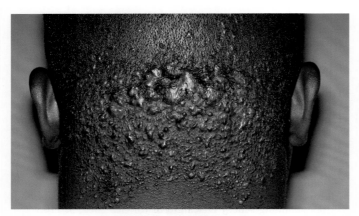

Fig. 13.18 Acne keloidalis nuchae.

the anterior nares with gram-negative organisms. If isotretinoin cannot be tolerated or is contraindicated, amoxicillin or TMP-SMX may be effective in suppressing the disease.

Boni R, et al: Treatment of gram-negative folliculitis in patients with acne. Am J Clin Dermatol 2003; 4: 273.
Del Rosso JQ, et al: When acne is not acne. Dermatol Clin 2016; 34: 225.

ACNE KELOIDALIS

Acne keloidalis is most frequently encountered in young adult black, Hispanic, or Asian men who otherwise are in excellent health. It is not associated with acne vulgaris and is a primary cicatricial alopecia variant. There is a persistent folliculitis and perifolliculitis of the back of the neck that presents as inflammatory papules and pustules. Over time, fibrosis ensues with coalescence of firm papules into keloidal plaques, as on the neck (Fig. 13.18). At times, sinus tract formation results.

Histologically, acne keloidalis is characterized by perifollicular, chronic lymphocytic and plasmacytic inflammation, and lamellar fibroplasia most intense at the level of the isthmus and lower infundibulum of terminal hairs. In the keloidal masses the connective tissue becomes sclerotic, forming hypertrophic scars or keloids. Persistent free hairs in the dermis may be responsible for the prolonged inflammation and eventual scarring.

Topical therapy with potent steroid ointments or foams alone, or following twice-daily tretinoin gel, is useful for the follicular papules. Oral antibiotics of the tetracycline group may be added and are helpful in suppressing the inflammatory response. Ultraviolet B may improve it. Triamcinolone acetonide by intralesional injection, using 5–10 mg/mL into the inflammatory follicular lesions and 40 mg/mL into the hypertrophic scars and keloids, is useful in reducing inflammation and fibrosis. Smaller lesions may be excised to a level below the hair follicle and closed. This may be followed by 40 mg/mL triamcinolone by intralesional injection every 3 weeks. For larger lesions, deep excision or CO_2 laser ablation left to heal by primary intention may be necessary. Laser hair removal with the neodymium:yttrium-aluminum-garnet (Nd:YAG) laser may be used as a preventive measure against acne keloidalis.

Alexis A, et al: Folliculitis keloidalis nuchae and pseudofolliculitis barbae. Dermatol Clin 2014; 32: 183.
Bajaj V, et al: Surgical excision of acne keloidalis nuchae with secondary intention healing. Clin Exp Dermatol 2008; 33: 53.
Dragoni F, et al: Successful treatment of acne keloidalis nuchae resistant to conventional therapy with 1064-nm ND:YAG laser. G Ital Dermatol Venereol 2013; 148: 231.
Okoye GA, et al: Improving acne keloidalis nuchae with targeted ultraviolet B treatment. Br J Dermatol 2014; 171: 1156.

HIDRADENITIS SUPPURATIVA

Clinical Features

Hidradenitis suppurativa is a chronic disease characterized by recurrent abscess formation, primarily within the folded areas of skin that contain both terminal hairs and apocrine glands. The primary site of inflammation is not the gland but the terminal hair. Plewig uses the term *dissecting terminal folliculitis* to unify diseases primarily affecting the terminal hair follicle, such as hidradenitis suppurativa, acne keloidalis nuchae, pilonidal sinus, and dissecting cellulitis of the scalp. The axilla is the most frequently affected site (Fig. 13.19). The inguinal and submammary areas are favored in women (Fig. 13.20), with the buttock, perianal area, and atypical areas (e.g., retroauricular, trunk) more often affected in men, although any and all areas may be involved in either gender. This postpubertal process has a prevalence of 0.1% in the United States. It disproportionately affects women, African Americans, and young people in the 18- to 29-year-old age range. Pediatric cases are uncommon; a hormonal investigation is essential in such patients.

The disease is characterized by the development of tender, red nodules, which at first are firm but soon become fluctuant and

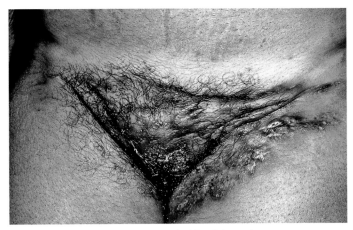

Fig. 13.20 Hidradenitis of the groin.

painful. Rupture of the lesion, suppuration, formation of sinus tracts, and extensive scarring are distinctive. As one area heals, recurrent lesions form, so that the course of the disease is protracted. It may eventually lead to the formation of honeycombed, fistulous tracts with chronic infection. When a probe is used to explore the suppurating nodule, a burrowing sinus tract is usually detected that may extend for many centimeters, running horizontally just underneath the skin surface.

Disease severity varies, as does the impact on quality of life from this chronic, recurrent, painful, odiferous, messy condition. The majority affected by HS are mildly affected. Severe debilitation occurs more often in men than in women. Men also more often have a history of acne and pilonidal cysts. Squamous cell carcinoma (SCC, after an average 19 years of active disease), interstitial keratitis, spondyloarthropathy, urethral vesical and rectal fistulas, anemia, hypoproteinemia, pyoderma gangrenosum (PG), and amyloidosis have been reported to complicate hidradenitis suppurativa, but are rare. The diagnosis of PG is dependent on the presence of a rapidly expanding, painful ulcer with undermined edges. It occurs a median of 19 years after the onset of hidradenitis and may be at sites distant from or within the area of hidradenitis. Some of these patients may have associated conglobate acne (PASH) or PASS syndrome (see under Acne Conglobata). Significant lymphedema of the penis and groin, along with alteration of the anatomy because of surgical intervention, often makes physical examination of these sites difficult. The risk of SCC occurring as an ulceration or thickening in a skin crease, which can metastasize and cause death, requires attention to detail in this regard.

Etiology

Detailed histologic studies of HS reveal that terminal follicle hyperkeratosis is followed by rupture of the follicular epithelium and release of keratin, sebum, bacteria, and hairs into the dermis. The resulting inflammatory process leads to the characteristic clinical findings. The microbiome is altered and secondary bacterial infection with *S. aureus*, *Streptococcus pyogenes*, and various gram-negative organisms may occur. The initiating event is unknown. Comorbidities include inflammatory joint disorders, psychological disorders (anxiety and depression), obesity, metabolic syndrome, hypertension, dyslipidemia, diabetes, inflammatory bowel disease, and polycystic ovarian syndrome. Mechanical friction, often worsened by obesity, is an exacerbating factor, as is bacterial infection. There is an autosomal dominant inherited form of this disease. Mutations in the gamma-secretase genes *NCSTN*, *PSENEN*, and *PSEN1* have been identified. Mutation-positive

patients have severe and extensive disease, and may have onset before age 13.

Differential Diagnosis

Hidradenitis is to be differentiated from common furuncles, which are typically unilateral. Hidradenitis must also be differentiated from Bartholin abscess, scrofuloderma, actinomycosis, granuloma inguinale, and lymphogranuloma venereum.

Treatment

Daily cleansing with chlorhexidine gluconate (Hibiclens) solution or benzoyl peroxide wash is an important preventive measure. Additionally, laser hair removal, if performed, should be done in unaffected sites as a preventive therapy. Other general preventive strategies include reduction of friction by wearing loose-fitting clothing and weight loss, if needed, avoidance of excessive sweating through the use of topical aluminum chloride or botulinum toxin A injections, smoking cessation, and heat avoidance. The recognition and treatment of any comorbid condition or complication is essential.

The earliest lesions often heal quickly with intralesional steroid therapy, which may be used initially in combination with topical clindamycin or oral doxycycline or minocycline. The disease itself causes sterile abscesses, but culture of the pus may reveal *S. aureus* or gram-negative organisms. The latter are usually cultured in patients with chronic disease given long-term antibiotic therapy; antibiotics should be selected based on sensitivities of the cultured organism for as short a time as practical to limit resistance. Antibiotics that may be useful in suppressing the disease include the tetracyclines, amoxicillin, TMP-SMX DS, or dapsone. The combination of clindamycin and rifampin, both given in doses of 300 mg twice daily, has been extensively studied in Europe and found to be quite effective. In severely affected patients, admission and treatment with intravenous ertapenem was reported to calm the disease so outpatient oral management might be effective. Incision and drainage is strongly discouraged.

The TNF antagonists have all been used; adalimumab is FDA approved following two large prospective trial that showed efficacy when dosed at 40 mg per week. Infliximab is also quite effective and may clear the condition during use. Isotretinoin is most effective in young women with mild to moderate disease, but a remission seldom follows their use. Secondary infection with *S. aureus* often occurs. Cyclosporine, acetretin, anakinra, or ustekinumab may work well in select cases. In women, spironolactone and OCs and finasteride in men or postmenopausal women may be a helpful adjuvant. Oral prednisone is uncommonly used to improve response to a primary agent when acute flares intervene; it should be given only in limited duration.

Photodynamic therapy and lasers have also been investigated to various degrees in hidradenitis. Methyl-aminolevulinate or 5-aminolevulinic acid given before blue or red light activation (photodynamic therapy) has had reports of success in some cases, but also anecdotal reports of lack of efficacy. It is inconvenient, costly, and often painful and does not produce remission, so further studies are required before such treatment can be recommended. Nd:YAG laser treatment has been reported to be effective in a prospective, randomized controlled trial of 22 severely affected patients. After a series of three monthly sessions, significant improvement was seen.

Once inflammation is controlled residual fibrosis is best addressed by excision of the affected areas. Wide surgical excision, using intraoperative color marking of sinus tracts, is most effective at limiting recurrence and has been shown to improve quality of life; however, it has moderate morbidity, especially in the groin and perianal areas with pain and symptomatic scarring being the most common complication. The recurrence rate is low in the axillary and perianal areas; however, the inguinal folds and especially the submammary sites more often recur so that excision of the latter site is uncommonly recommended. CO_2 laser may also destroy lesions and sinus tracts. The open areas may be closed or left to heal secondarily.

Management in special situations such as pediatric cases and in pregnancy are addressed in excellent reviews by Liy-Wong et al. and Perng et al., respectively.

Andersen RK, Jemec GB: Treatments for hidradenitis suppurativa. Clin Dermatol 2017; 35: 218.

Bettoli V, et al: Oral clindamycin and rifampicin in the treatment of hidradenitis suppurativa-acne inversa. G Ital Dermatol Venereol 2016; 151: 216.

Boer J, et al: The role of mechanical stress in hidradenitis suppurativa. Dermatol Clin 2016; 34: 37.

Bruzzese V: Pyoderma gangrenosum, acne conglobata, suppurative hidradenitis, and axial spondyloarthritis. J Clin Rheumatol 2012; 18: 413.

Dauden E, et al: Recommendations for the management of comorbidity in hidradenitis suppurativa. J Eur Acad Dermatol Venereol 2018; 32: 129.

de Vasconcelos PT, et al: Scrotal elephantiasis secondary to recalcitrant hidradenitis suppurativa. Indian J Dermatol Venereol Leprol 2015; 81: 524.

Deckers IE, et al: Correlation of early-onset hidradenitis suppurativa with stronger genetic susceptibility and more widespread involvement. J Am Acad Dermatol 2015; 72: 485.

Deckers IE, et al: Inflammatory bowel disease is associated with hidradenitis suppurativa. J Am Acad Dermatol 2017; 76: 49.

Egeberg A, et al: Risk of major adverse cardiovascular events and all-cause mortality in patients with hidradenitis suppurativa. JAMA Dermatol 2016; 152: 429.

Egeberg A, et al: Prevalence and risk of inflammatory bowel disease in patients with hidradenitis suppurativa. J Invest Dermatol 2017; 137: 1060.

Fischer AH, et al: Patterns of antimicrobial resistance in lesions of hidradenitis suppurativa. J Am Acad Dermatol 2017; 76: 309.

Garg A, et al: Incidence of hidradenitis suppurativa in the United States. J Am Acad Dermatol 2017; 77: 118.

Garg A, et al: Sex- and age-adjusted population analysis of prevalence estimates for hidradenitis suppurativa in the United States. JAMA Dermatol 2017; 153: 760.

Horváth B, et al: Pain management in patients with hidradenitis suppurativa. J Am Acad Dermatol 2015; 73: S47.

Huang C, et al: Successful surgical treatment for squamous cell carcinoma arising from hidradenitis suppurativa. Medicine (Baltimore) 2017; 96: e5857.

Huang CM, Kirchhof MG: A new perspective on isotretinoin treatment of hidradenitis suppurativa. Dermatology 2017; 233: 120.

Humphries LS, et al: Wide excision and healing by secondary intent for the surgical treatment of hidradenitis suppurativa. J Plast Reconstr Aesthet Surg 2016; 69: 554.

Ingram JR: The genetics of hidradenitis suppurativa. Dermatol Clin 2016; 34: 23.

Ingram JR, et al: Interventions for hidradenitis suppurativa. JAMA Dermatol 2017; 153: 458.

John H, et al: A systematic review of the use of lasers for the treatment of hidradenitis suppurativa. J Plast Reconstr Aesthet Surg 2016; 69: 1374.

Join-Lambert O, et al: Remission of refractory pyoderma gangrenosum, severe acne, and hidradenitis suppurativa (PASH) syndrome using targeted antibiotic therapy in 4 patients. J Am Acad Dermatol 2015; 73: S66.

Join-Lambert O, et al: Efficacy of ertapenem in severe hidradenitis suppurativa. J Antimicrob Chemother 2016; 71: 513.

Karagiannidis I, et al: Endocrinologic aspects of hidradenitis suppurativa. Dermatol Clin 2016; 34: 45.

Kimball AB, et al: Two phase 3 trials of adalimumab for hidradenitis suppurativa. N Engl J Med 2016; 375: 422.

Kohorst JJ, et al: Surgical management of hidradenitis suppurativa. Dermatol Surg 2016; 42: 1030.

Kohorst JJ, et al: Patient satisfaction and quality of life following surgery for hidradenitis suppurativa. Dermatol Surg 2017; 43: 125.

Lee A, Fischer G: A case series of 20 women with hidradenitis suppurativa treated with spironolactone. Australas J Dermatol 2015; 56: 192.

Liy-Wong C, et al: Hidradenitis suppurativa in the pediatric population. J Am Acad Dermatol 2015; 73: S36.

Makris GM, et al: Vulvar, perianal and perineal cancer after hidradenitis suppurativa. Dermatol Surg 2017; 43: 107.

Mehdizadeh A, et al: Recurrence of hidradenitis suppurativa after surgical management. J Am Acad Dermatol 2015; 73: S70.

Mikkelsen PR, et al: Recurrence rate and patient satisfaction of CO_2 laser evaporation of lesions in patients with hidradenitis suppurativa. Dermatol Surg 2015; 41: 255.

Paul S, et al: Successful use of brachytherapy for a severe hidradenitis suppurativa variant. Dermatol Ther 2016; 29: 455.

Perng P, et al: Management of hidradenitis suppurativa in pregnancy. J Am Acad Dermatol 2017; 76: 979.

Posch C, et al: The role of wide local excision for the treatment of severe hidradenitis suppurativa (Hurley grade III). J Am Acad Dermatol 2017; 77: 123.

Randhawa HK, et al: Finasteride for the treatment of hidradenitis suppurativa in children and adolescents. JAMA Dermatol 2013; 149: 732.

Ratnamala U, et al: Expanding the spectrum of γ-secretase gene mutation-associated phenotypes. Exp Dermatol 2016; 25: 314.

Riis PT, et al: Intralesional triamcinolone for flares of hidradenitis suppurativa. J Am Acad Dermatol 2016; 75: 1151.

Ring HC, et al: The follicular skin microbiome in patients with hidradenitis suppurativa and healthy controls. JAMA Dermatol 2017; 153: 897.

Schrader AM, et al: Hidradenitis suppurativa. J Am Acad Dermatol 2014; 71: 460.

Shalom G, et al: Hidradenitis suppurativa and metabolic syndrome. Br J Dermatol 2015; 173: 464.

Shlyankevich J, et al: Hidradenitis suppurativa is a systemic disease with substantial comorbidity burden. J Am Acad Dermatol 2014; 71: 1144.

Tzanetakou V, et al: Safety and efficacy of anakinra in severe hidradenitis suppurativa. JAMA Dermatol 2016; 152: 52.

Utrera-Busquets M, et al: Severe hidradenitis suppurativa complicated by renal AA amyloidosis. Clin Exp Dermatol 2016; 41: 287.

van Straalen KR, et al: Current and future treatment of hidradenitis suppurativa. Br J Dermatol 2018; Jul 7

Wong D, et al: Low-dose systemic corticosteroid treatment for recalcitrant hidradenitis suppurativa. J Am Acad Dermatol 2016; 75: 1059.

Zouboulis CC, et al: European S1 guideline for the treatment of hidradenitis suppurativa. J Eur Acad Dermatol Venereol 2015; 29: 619.

DISSECTING CELLULITIS OF THE SCALP

Also known as perifolliculitis capitis abscedens et suffodiens, this is an uncommon chronic suppurative disease of the scalp characterized by numerous follicular and perifollicular inflammatory nodules. These nodules suppurate and undermine to

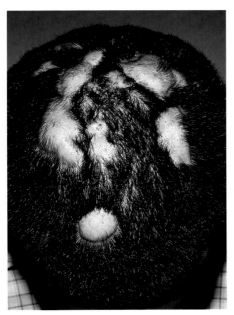

Fig. 13.21 Dissecting folliculitis. (Courtesy Curt Samlaska, MD.)

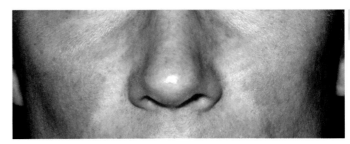

Fig. 13.22 Erythrotelangiectatic rosacea.

ACNE MILIARIS NECROTICA (ACNE VARIOLIFORMIS)

Acne miliaris necrotica consists of follicular vesicopustules, sometimes occurring as solitary lesions that usually are extremely itchy. They appear anywhere in the scalp or adjacent areas, rupture early, and dry up after a few days. In some patients, especially those who manipulate the lesions, *S. aureus* may be cultured. If the lesions leave large scars, the term acne varioliformis is used; they are not separate diseases.

Treatment is with culture-directed antibiotics, or if the culture is negative, oral doxycycline. Doxepin is helpful if patients manipulate their lesions.

Fisher DA: Acne necroticans and *Staphylococcus aureus*. J Am Acad Dermatol 1988; 18: 1136.

Zirn JR, et al: Chronic acneiform eruption with crateriform scars. Arch Dermatol 1996; 132: 1365.

ROSACEA

Clinical Features

Rosacea is characterized by a persistent erythema of the convex surfaces of the face, with the cheeks and nose most frequently affected, followed by involvement of the brow and chin. There is a tendency to spare the periocular skin. Rosacea occurs most often in light-skinned women age 30–50. However, the severe type with phymatous changes occurs almost exclusively in men. Additional common features include telangiectasia, flushing, erythematous papules, and pustules. These tend to cluster in patterns, allowing for the identification of several subsets of patients. Although therapeutic decisions generally depend on individual signs and symptoms manifested, understanding the polar subtypes of erythrotelangiectatic (ETR) and glandular rosacea also has treatment-related implications. Whereas ETR patients are easily irritated and at times reveal a dermatitis surface, glandular patients are generally tolerant of interventions such as benzoyl peroxide and tretinoin.

The erythrotelangiectatic type is characterized by a prominent history of a prolonged (>10 minutes) flushing reaction to various stimuli, such as emotional stress, hot drinks, alcohol, spicy foods, exercise, cold or hot weather, or hot baths and showers (Fig. 13.22). Often, a burning or stinging sensation accompanies the flush, but with no sweating, lightheadedness, or palpitations. The skin is finely textured, may have a roughness and scaling of the affected central facial sites, and is easily irritated. Over time, a purplish suffusion and prominent telangiectasia may result.

The papulopustular subset of patients manifests a strikingly red central face accompanied by erythematous papules often surmounted by a pinpoint pustule (Fig. 13.23). The history of flushing is also present in most patients, but usually symptoms of irritancy are not prominent. The skin is of normal or at times slightly sebaceous quality, and edema of the affected sites may be present. Such edema may dominate the clinical presentation, with

---

form intercommunicating sinuses as long as 5 cm (Fig. 13.21). Scarring and alopecia ensue, although seropurulent drainage may last indefinitely. Adult black men are most often affected, and the vertex and occiput of the scalp are the favored sites.

The primary lesions are follicular and perifollicular erythematous papules that progress to abscesses. This disease is a variant of dissecting terminal hair folliculitis, along with hidradenitis suppurativa, acne keloidalis nuchae, and pilonidal sinus. Coagulase-positive *S. aureus* may be found in the lesions. Care to rule out tinea capitis, which may mimic this condition, is necessary.

Treatment with oral antibiotics such as the tetracyclines, TMP-SMX, or the quinolones may produce good results. If *S. aureus* is cultured, the combination of oral rifampin and clindamycin has produced excellent results. The combination of intralesional steroid injections and isotretinoin at a dose of 0.5–1.5 mg/kg/day for 6–12 months may be successful. Starting at a lower dose, such as 10 mg/day, for the first month or two may prevent a flare of the condition. The length of remission with isotretinoin is variable, but treatment may be repeated with similar results expected. The anti-TNF medications infliximab and adalimumab and the retinoid alitretinoin have been helpful in individual cases.

A surgical approach is sometimes necessary. Marsupialization or excision of sinus tracts may help limit inflammation. The Nd:YAG laser used to remove hair has led to long-term improvement. Excision of the entire scalp has been necessary in select patients.

Badaoui A, et al: Dissecting cellulitis of the scalp. Br J Dermatol 2016; 174: 421.

Housewright CD, et al: Excisional surgery (scalpectomy) for dissecting cellulitis of the scalp. Dermatol Surg 2011; 37: 1189.

Madu P, Kundu RV: Follicular and scarring disorders in skin of color. Am J Clin Dermatol 2014; 15: 307.

Miletta NR, et al: Tinea capitis mimicking dissecting cellulitis of the scalp. J Cutan Pathol 2014; 41: 2.

Prasad SC, et al: Successful treatment with alitretinoin of dissecting cellulitis of the scalp in keratitis-ichthyosis-deafness syndrome. Acta Derm Venereol 2013; 93: 473.

Scheinfeld N: Dissecting cellulitis (perifolliculitis capitis abscedens et suffodiens). Dermatol Online J 2014; 20: 22692.

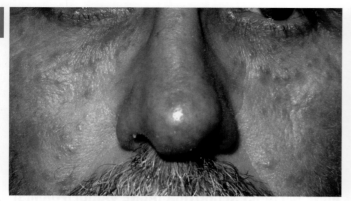

Fig. 13.23 Papulopustular rosacea.

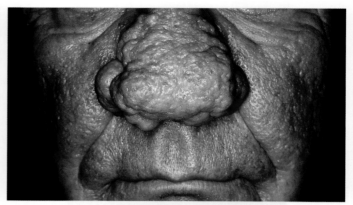

Fig. 13.25 Rhinophyma.

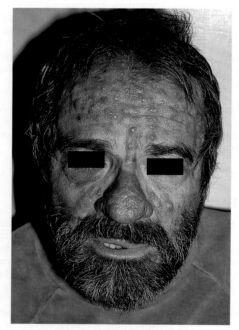

Fig. 13.24 Glandular rosacea.

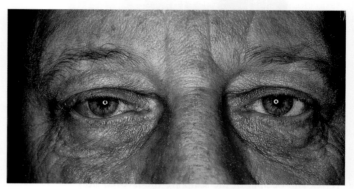

Fig. 13.26 Ocular rosacea.

Etiology

The cause of rosacea remains unknown. Many patients have an abnormal vasomotor response to thermal and other stimuli, as previously described. Early in the process, dysregulation of the innate immune system and neurovascular control is documented. Additionally, chronic solar damage is an important contributor in producing damage to the dermal matrix and ground substance, especially in the erythrotelangiectatic subtype. Chronic vasodilation, edema, and compromise of lymphatic drainage occur and lead to telangiectasia and fibrosis. Pilosebaceous unit abnormalities or androgen influences are not typically thought to be part of the pathogenesis of this condition; however, some evidence points to abnormalities being present in the patients with the glandular type. As expected, the pathogenic factors will vary among the subsets of patients. *Demodex* and *Helicobacter pylori* have been extensively investigated and do not appear to be central to the etiology of rosacea.

Other Clinical Considerations

Ocular Findings

Blepharitis, recurrent chalazion, and conjunctivitis may be seen in all subsets of rosacea (Fig. 13.26). The eye itself may be affected, with keratitis, iritis, and episcleritis. An abnormal Schirmer test occurs in 40% of rosacea patients. Complaints are often of a gritty, stinging, itchy, or burning sensation in the eye. Light sensitivity and a foreign body sensation are also present at times. Ocular rosacea occurs equally in men and women. Such eye findings may occur before the skin disease. These findings have therapeutic implications, and patients will not always complain of them to

the forehead, eyelids, and cheeks variably affected. This has been termed Morbihan disease and is most likely to complicate the papulopustular and glandular types.

In the glandular type of rosacea, men with thick, sebaceous skin predominate. The papules are edematous, the pustules are often 0.5–1.0 cm in size, and nodulocystic lesions may be present (Fig. 13.24). They tend to cluster in the central face, but in affected women the chin is favored. There is frequently a history of adolescent acne, and typical scars may be seen. Flushing is less common, as is telangiectasia, but persistent edema may be problematic. Rhinophyma most often occurs in this glandular subtype (Fig. 13.25). Large, hypertrophic, hyperemic nodular masses are centered over the distal half of the nose. Differentiation of this hypertrophic tissue from a basal cell skin cancer or a cutaneous B-cell lymphoma is at times difficult. Rarely, such soft tissue overgrowth can affect the chin, ears, or forehead. Hugely dilated follicles contain long, vermicular plugs of sebum and keratin. The histologic features are pilosebaceous gland hyperplasia with fibrosis, inflammation, and telangiectasia.

their dermatologist, so these signs and symptoms should be actively sought when evaluating rosacea patients.

Extrafacial Lesions

Flushing may involve the ears, lateral facial contours, neck, upper chest, and scalp. Papules and pustules may be present in persistent erythema of the scalp or the earlobes.

Topical Corticosteroid Use

Long-term use of topical corticosteroids on the face may result in persistent erythema, papules, and pustules. The sites involved in steroid-induced rosacea correspond to the areas of application and are not necessarily limited to the central convexities. Treatment is discontinuance of the corticosteroid and institution of topical tacrolimus in combination with short-term doxycycline or minocycline. Topical tacrolimus itself has paradoxically been reported to induce a rosacea-like reaction, so coverage with an oral antibiotic while discontinuing topical steroids is necessary. Resolution with discontinuance of treatment is expected within 2 months. Additionally, drinking alcohol after application of tacrolimus or pimecrolimus may induce flushing, which may be confused with new-onset flushing related to rosacea.

Perioral Dermatitis

Although perioral dermatitis has been classified with rosacea variants, its distribution, signs, and symptoms vary such that it is discussed separately later in this chapter.

Granulomatous Lesions

Some patients with persistent facial erythema of the convexities, on biopsy of an erythematous papule, show a granulomatous response closely resembling sarcoidosis or a necrotizing granuloma. Many experienced clinicians will accurately predict such findings from the clinical examination. The most important consideration in this case is that the patient's response to treatment may be slower. When involvement of granulomatous facial papules includes the eyelids and upper lip and is not associated with vascular manifestations, such as flushing, erythema, or telangiectasia, the term *granulomatous facial dermatitis* is preferred. This condition is discussed separately.

Differential Diagnosis

The persistent erythema of the central face should be differentiated from that seen in polycythemia vera, carcinoid, mastocytosis, and connective tissue disease (lupus erythematosus, dermatomyositis, mixed connective tissue disease). These conditions do not have associated papules and pustules and will manifest a variety of systemic symptoms and extrafacial signs, and specific laboratory markers are available to confirm clinical suspicions. Haber syndrome is a genodermatosis characterized by a rosacea-like facial dermatosis and multiple verrucous lesions on non–sun-exposed skin. Onset of the facial lesions is in the first two decades of life, in contrast to the later onset of rosacea. Whereas rosacea may occur in human immunodeficiency virus (HIV) disease, a papulonodular eruption of the face that may simulate rosacea also occurs in patients with acquired immunodeficiency syndrome (AIDS) or other immunodeficiency states. On expressing the contents of hair follicles with a comedo extractor, numerous *Demodex* mites are seen. In such cases, success with permethrin cream and lindane has been reported. Lotions containing 5% benzoyl peroxide and 5% precipitated sulfur (Sulfoxyl) are also reported to be helpful.

Treatment

Treatments are directed at specific findings manifested by rosacea patients. Because erythema, telangiectases, papules and pustules, phymas, flushing, ocular symptoms, and skin sensitivity are variably present in the three subsets of disease, the specific approach used will differ according to the phenotypic findings. Some treatments, however, are useful in all patients.

General Nonpharmacologic and Nonsurgical Interventions

Sunscreens are an important component of therapy for all rosacea patients and should be applied each morning. Sunscreens containing physical blockers in a dimethicone or cyclomethicone vehicle generally are better tolerated, especially by the erythrotelangiectatic patients, than those with chemical agents and may be beneficial by strengthening the barrier function of the skin. General avoidance of irritants such as astringents, peeling or acidic agents, and abrasive or exfoliant preparations is recommended. Cosmetic coverage of the erythema and telangiectases is best with a light-green or yellow-tinted foundation set with powder.

If flushing is induced by specific trigger factors, these should be avoided as much as possible. The central face may be predisposed to rosacea because the edema and lack of movement of tissues with muscular movement may lead to lymphedema and inflammation. Circular massage for several minutes a day has led to impressive improvement. Custom-made compressive masks may also be helpful. This benign intervention may be considered and should be studied. Artificial tears and cleansing the lids with warm water twice daily will help ocular symptoms.

Topical Therapy

Metronidazole, sodium sulfacetamide and sulfur cleansers and creams, ivermectin, and azelaic acid are utilized in rosacea. These are the most commonly prescribed medications, are available in a variety of vehicles and are especially useful in treating the inflammatory papules in papulopustular patients. Benzoyl peroxide is a better choice in the papules and nodules seen in the glandular subset of rosacea patients. It is well tolerated by them. If oral antibiotics are needed, the topical products may be used to maintain remission after discontinuance of oral preparations.

Pimecrolimus or tacrolimus may also improve select patients' erythema, especially those with an accompanying roughness or scaling of the skin surface. Both agents help the irritated erythrotelangiectatic and at times the papulopustular patients but are not effective in the glandular type, and tacrolimus in its ointment base may exacerbate the inflammatory component in these patients. These drugs calm inflammation and abate symptoms but require brief (no longer than 1 week) pretreatment with a potent topical corticosteroid to be tolerated initially. The role of topical retinoids requires study. Many rosacea patients may tolerate a nighttime application of tretinoin if Cetaphil lotion is used immediately before use. Retinoids may help repair sun-damaged skin and normalize some of the abnormalities present. The α_2-adrenergic receptor agonist brimonidine is available as a gel for the treatment of facial redness. It is applied once in the morning, which induces vasoconstriction for up to 12 hours. Irritation, exacerbation of flushing, and allergy is not uncommon. Oxymetazoline, an alpha1A-adrenoceptor agonist, is a cream applied once in the morning to treat persistent erythema. It may also induce dermatitis or worsening of the disease.

Oral Therapy

Oral antibiotics, particularly doxycycline, in a subantimicrobial dose of 40-mg extended-release formulation, or 50–100 mg once or twice daily, usually controls more aggressive papular and pustular lesions and helps treat ocular lesions. Oral antibiotics should be discontinued once clearance of the inflammatory lesions is obtained; usually, 2 or 3 months is necessary. The topical approved preparations listed earlier should be used as long-term maintenance after clearance with the oral medications, because the disease will recur in most patients if all therapy is stopped. If significant ocular symptoms are present, oral antibiotics are an effective and convenient method of relieving both the skin and the eye concerns. Cyclosporine ophthalmic emulsion is an effective topical for ocular rosacea. Isotretinoin given in lower doses than in acne vulgaris (0.3 mg/kg), and at times as a long-term suppressant, may be necessary for management of more resistant disease, including patients with a granulomatous histology. Isotretinoin produces dramatic improvement even in cases resistant to other forms of therapy, but relapse often occurs in a few weeks or months. The authors rarely use oral metronidazole (side effects) or the macrolides (lack of efficacy) despite their reported utility in rosacea.

Oral medications for reduction of flushing are infrequently helpful. Occasionally, an escalating dose of propranolol, carvedilol, or clonidine is helpful in reducing symptomatic flushing, but many affected patients find the side effects occur before the beneficial effects are evident. One method is to start propranolol at 10 mg three times daily, and if no response is seen in 2 weeks, to increase the dose by 10 mg at one dose, then again every 2 weeks until side effects require discontinuation or response occurs. Responses are mostly seen at a dose of 20–40 mg three times daily. Carvedilol is started at 3.125 mg twice daily with slow titration to 12.5 mg twice daily depending on tolerance and response.

Surgical Intervention

Surgical approaches to the reshaping of rhinophyma have included the use of a heated scalpel, electrocautery, dermabrasion, laser ablation, tangential excision combined with scissors sculpting, and radiofrequency. Often, a combination of these approaches is used to obtain the best esthetic result. Lasers and light devices are useful for treating the erythema and telangiectases, but the cost is not covered by insurance, which limits their availability. In a comparative study, the pulsed dye laser and intense pulsed-light device both significantly reduced erythema, telangiectasia, and patient-reported symptoms and performed similarly well. Some vascular and CO_2 fractionated lasers may also help in dermal collagen remodeling and nonablative rejuvenation, such that the dermal matrix may be strengthened. For the patient incapacitated by flushing, burning, and stinging, endoscopic transthoracic sympathectomy may be considered, but this extreme measure should only rarely be considered because serious complications may result. An approach to these patients should include not only the medications previously discussed, but for those with significant dysesthesia, treatment with neuroleptics (e.g., gabapentin), tricyclic antidepressants, and pain-modifying antidepressants (e.g., duloxetine) may be necessary.

Other Considerations

Many articles investigating possible associated conditions have been published. Research methods differ, there are conflicting results in some cases, or the findings are yet to be confirmed. Continued research in this area is needed. There is a genetic predisposition to rosacea, with approximately half of the severity score accounted for by genetics and half by the environment. An advocacy group that supports research and education in rosacea, the National Rosacea Society, is an excellent resource for patients.

Aldrich N, et al: Genetic vs environmental factors that correlate with rosacea. JAMA Dermatol 2015; 151: 1213.

Asai Y, et al: Canadian clinical practice guidelines for rosacea. J Cutan Med Surg 2016; 20: 432.

Awais M, et al: Rosacea—the ophthalmic perspective. Cutan Ocul Toxicol 2015; 34: 161.

Bangsgaard N, et al: Sensitization to and allergic contact dermatitis caused by Mirvaso (brimonidine tartrate) for treatment of rosacea—2 cases. Contact Dermatitis 2016; 74: 378.

Barzilai A, et al: Cutaneous B-cell neoplasms mimicking granulomatous rosacea or rhinophyma. Arch Dermatol 2012; 148: 824.

Egeberg A, et al: Prevalence and risk of migraine in patients with rosacea. J Am Acad Dermatol 2017; 76: 454.

Gallo RL, et al: Standard classification and pathophysiology of rosacea: the 2017 update by the National Rosacea Society Expert Committee. J Am Acad Dermatol 2018; 78: 148.

Garg G, et al: Clinical efficacy of tacrolimus in rosacea. J Eur Acad Dermatol Venereol 2009; 23: 239.

Helfrich YR, et al: Clinical, histologic, and molecular analysis of differences between erythematotelangiectatic rosacea and telangiectatic photoaging. JAMA Dermatol 2015; 151: 825.

Hofmann MA, Lehmann P: Physical modalities for the treatment of rosacea. J Dtsch Dermatol Ges 2016; 14 Suppl 6: 38.

Hsu CC, Lee JY: Pronounced facial flushing and persistent erythema of rosacea effectively treated by carvedilol, a nonselective β-adrenergic blocker. J Am Acad Dermatol 2012; 67: 491.

Kabuto M, et al: Successful treatment with long-term use of minocycline for Morbihan disease showing mast cell infiltration. J Dermatol 2015; 42: 827.

Kim MB, et al: Pimecrolimus 1% cream for the treatment of rosacea. J Dermatol 2011; 38: 1135.

Kim SJ, et al: Comparative efficacy of radiofrequency and pulsed dye laser in the treatment of rosacea. Dermatol Surg 2017; 43: 204.

Lee GL, Zirwas MJ: Granulomatous rosacea and periorificial dermatitis. Dermatol Clin 2015; 33: 447.

Lee WJ, et al: Clinical evaluation of 368 patients with nasal rosacea. Dermatology 2015; 230: 177.

Lee WJ, et al: Clinical evaluation of 30 patients with localized nasal rosacea. J Dermatol 2016; 43: 200.

Lee WJ, et al: Histopathological analysis of 226 patients with rosacea according to rosacea subtype and severity. Am J Dermatopathol 2016; 38: 347.

Lee WJ, et al: Prognosis of 234 rosacea patients according to clinical subtype. J Dermatol 2016; 43: 526.

Lowe E, Lim S: Paradoxical erythema reaction of long-term topical brimonidine gel for the treatment of facial erythema of rosacea. J Drugs Dermatol 2016; 15: 763.

Parkins GJ, et al: Neurogenic rosacea. Clin Exp Dermatol 2015; 40: 930.

Pietschke K, Schaller M: Long-term management of distinct facial flushing and persistent erythema of rosacea by treatment with carvedilol. J Dermatolog Treat 2017 Aug 11: 1.

Rallis E, et al: Isotretinoin for the treatment of granulomatous rosacea. J Cutan Med Surg 2012; 16: 438.

Sadeghian A, et al: Etiologies and management of cutaneous flushing. J Am Acad Dermatol 2017; 77: 391.

Schaller M, et al: Rosacea management. J Dtsch Dermatol Ges 2016; 14 Suppl 6: 29.

Schaller M, et al: Rosacea treatment update. Br J Dermatol 2017; 176: 465.

Schaller M, et al: State of the art: systemic rosacea management. J Dtsch Dermatol Ges 2016; 14 Suppl 6: 29.

Tan J, et al: Shortcomings in rosacea diagnosis and classification. Br J Dermatol 2017; 176: 197.

Teraki Y, et al: Tacrolimus-induced rosacea-like dermatitis. Dermatology 2012; 224: 309.

Two AM, et al: Rosacea: part I. J Am Acad Dermatol 2015; 72: 749.

Two AM, et al: Rosacea: part II. J Am Acad Dermatol 2015; 72: 761.

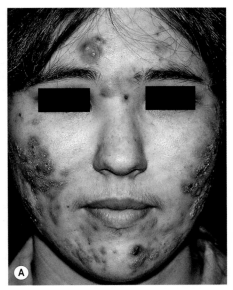 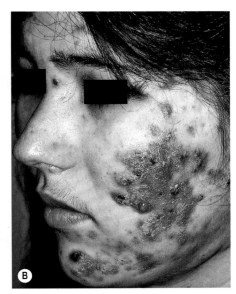

Fig. 13.27 (A and B) Pyoderma faciale. (Courtesy Curt Samlaska, MD.)

Uslu M, et al: Rosacea treatment with intermediate-dose isotretinoin. Acta Derm Venereol 2013; 92: 73.

Van Zuuren E, et al: Interventions for rosacea. Cochrane Database Syst Rev 2015; 4: CD003262.

PYODERMA FACIALE (ROSACEA FULMINANS)

Pyoderma faciale is an uncommon eruptive facial disorder consisting of a dramatically fulminant onset of superficial and deep abscesses, cystic lesions (Fig. 13.27), and sometimes sinus tracts. Edema and at times an intense reddish or cyanotic erythema accompany this pustular process. The lesions often contain greenish or yellowish purulent material. The condition occurs mostly in postadolescent women. It is distinguished from acne by the absence of comedones, rapid onset, fulminating course, and absence of acne on the back and chest. Pyoderma faciale is differentiated from rosacea by the inconsistent history of flushing and of preexisting erythema or telangiectases of the convex portions of the face, and the large abscesses and nodules. After therapy, a residual erythema often persists.

Treatment is similar to that of acne fulminans. Oral steroids are given for several weeks, followed by the addition of isotretinoin, 10–20 mg daily, increasing to 0.5–1 mg/kg only after the acute inflammatory component is under control. Steroids may usually be discontinued after several weeks of isotretinoin, but the latter should be given for a full 120–150 mg/kg total dose. Because patients are predominantly women of childbearing age, pregnancy issues require full discussion. Indeed, four of Plewig et al.'s patients were pregnant and thus could not use isotretinoin. In such patients, amoxicillin, erythromycin, azithromycin, or clindamycin, all pregnancy category B drugs, may be considered.

D'Erme AM, et al: Successful treatment of rosacea fulminans in a 59-year-old woman with macrolide antibiotics and prednisone. Int J Dermatol 2016; 55: e470.

Greywal T, et al: Evidence-based recommendations for the management of acne fulminans and its variants. J Am Acad Dermatol 2017; 77: 109.

Koh HY, et al: Rosacea fulminans. Indian J Dermatol Venereol Leprol 2014; 80: 272.

Mantovani L, et al: Rosacea fulminans or acute rosacea? G Ital Dermatol Venereol 2016; 151: 553.

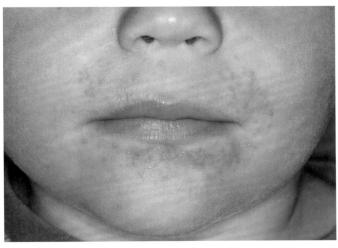

Fig. 13.28 Perioral dermatitis.

Plewig G, et al: Pyoderma faciale. Arch Dermatol 1992; 128: 1611.

Walsh RK, et al: Diagnosis and treatment of rosacea fulminans. Am J Clin Dermatol 2017; ePub ahead of print.

PERIORAL DERMATITIS

Perioral dermatitis is a common eruption consisting of discrete papules and pustules on an erythematous and at times scaling base. It is a distinctive dermatitis confined symmetrically around the mouth, with a clear zone of about 5 mm between the vermilion border and the affected skin (Fig. 13.28). There is no itching, although an uncomfortable burning sensation may be present. It occurs in women age 20–35, however children are also commonly affected. The use of fluorinated topical corticosteroids is the most frequently identified cause. Exposure may be in the form of creams, ointments, or inhalers.

Treatment of perioral dermatitis includes discontinuing topical corticosteroids or protecting the skin from the inhaled product. Tacrolimus ointment 0.1% or pimecrolimus cream will prevent flaring after stopping steroid use. In patients without steroid exposure, oral or topical antibiotics such as doxycycline in adults and erythromycin in children, and topical adapalene, azelaic acid, ivermectin, and metronidazole have all been successful in clearing the eruption.

Periorbital Dermatitis

Periorbital (periocular) dermatitis is a variant of perioral dermatitis occurring on the lower eyelids and skin adjacent to the upper and lower eyelids. Fluorinated topical corticosteroids have been implicated as the cause. If intranasal inhaled corticosteroids are used, a perinasal distribution may be seen. Prompt response to the same treatment employed in the perioral site is expected.

Goel NS, et al: Pediatric periorificial dermatitis. Pediatr Dermatol 2015; 32: 333.
Hall CS, et al: Evidence based review of perioral dermatitis therapy. G Ital Dermatol Venereol 2010; 145: 433.
Lee GL, Zirwas MJ: Granulomatous rosacea and periorificial dermatitis. Dermatol Clin 2015; 33: 447.
Lipozenčić J, Hadžavdić SL: Perioral dermatitis. Clin Dermatol 2014; 32: 125.
Mokos ZB, et al: Perioral dermatitis. Acta Clin Croat 2015; 54: 179.
Poulos GA, et al: Perioral dermatitis associated with an inhaled corticosteroid. Arch Dermatol 2007; 142: 1460.
Schwarz T, et al: A randomized, double-blind, vehicle-controlled study of 1% pimecrolimus cream in adult patients with perioral dermatitis. J Am Acad Dermatol 2008; 59: 34.
Tempark T, et al: Perioral dermatitis. Am J Clin Dermatol 2014; 15: 101.

GRANULOMATOUS FACIAL DERMATITIS

Several dermatoses of the face characterized by granulomas are included in this category. Patients with persistent facial erythema involving one or more convex surfaces of the face may have lesions that show a granulomatous reaction histologically, and they are included within rosacea. Some patients have no other stigmata of rosacea, and their nosology is unclear. These other entities, which meet no other criteria for rosacea other than having pink papules on the face, are included here. Skowron et al. proposed the term *facial idiopathic granulomas with regressive evolution* (FIGURE).

Lupus Miliaris Disseminatus Faciei

Firm, yellowish-brown or red, 1–3 mm, monomorphous, smooth-surfaced papules are present not only on the butterfly areas but also on the lateral areas, below the mandible, periorificially, and rarely in the axillae. The eyelid skin is characteristically involved in patients with lupus miliaris disseminatus faciei (LMDF) (Fig. 13.29). The discrete papules appear as yellowish brown lesions on diascopy and as caseating epithelioid cell granulomas histologically. Patients usually lack a history of flushing, do not have persistent erythema or telangiectasia, have involvement of the eyelids, and heal with scarring, as opposed to rosacea patients. Long-term therapy with minocycline or isotretinoin may be used, often with gratifying results. Eventually, self-involution is expected but may take several years. Tranilast, cyclosporine and nonablative fractionated laser resurfacing are other reported treatments.

Granulomatous Perioral Dermatitis in Children

In otherwise healthy prepubertal children, a profusion of grouped papules may develop on the perioral, periocular, and perinasal

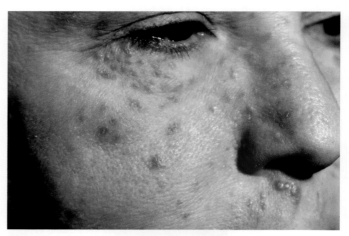

Fig. 13.29 Lupus miliaris.

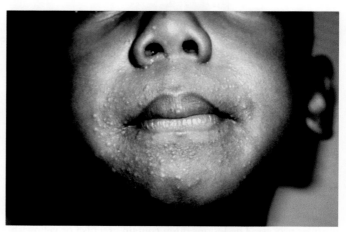

Fig. 13.30 Granulomatous facial dermatitis. (Courtesy Ken Greer, MD.)

areas (Fig. 13.30). Eight of the initial 59 reported patients also had generalized lesions. Besides extremity and truncal lesions, several girls had dramatic lesions of the labia majora. Both genders are affected equally. Children with skin of color (Afro-Caribbean, African American, and Asian) dominate the reports, but white patients are also susceptible. Because the histologic appearance is granulomatous, sarcoidosis is often considered. Topical corticosteroids, however, may worsen the condition, and systemic involvement is not present. Topical metronidazole, ivermectin, erythromycin, sulfacetamide-sulfur combinations, and an oral macrolide or tetracycline-type antibiotic all are often effective. In some patients, the combination of prednisone and dapsone has proved beneficial.

Amiruddin D, et al: Clinical evaluation of 35 cases of lupus miliaris disseminatus faciei. J Dermatol 2010; 37: 618.
Beleznay K, et al: Lupus miliaris disseminatus faciei treated with 1,565 nm nonablative fractionated laser resurfacing. Lasers Surg Med 2014; 46: 663.
Gutte R, et al: Childhood granulomatous periorificial dermatitis in children with extrafacial involvement. Indian J Dermatol Venereol Leprol 2011; 77: 703.
Kim WB, Mistry N: Lupus miliaris disseminatus faciei with isolated axillary involvement. J Cutan Med Surg 2016; 20: 153.
Koike Y, et al: Lupus miliaris disseminatus faciei successfully treated with tranilast. J Dermatol 2011; 38: 588.

Lucas CR, et al: Granulomatous periorificial dermatitis. J Cutan Med Surg 2009; 13: 115.

Noguera-Morel L, et al: Ivermectin therapy for papulopustular rosacea and periorificial dermatitis in children. J Am Acad Dermatol 2017; 76: 567.

Sardana K, et al: Lupus miliaris disseminatus faciei: a resistant case with response to cyclosporine. Dermatol Ther 2017; 30: ePub 2017 Apr 26.

Schaarschmidt ML, et al: Lupus miliaris disseminatus faciei. Acta Derm Venereol 2017; 97: 655.

Skowron F, et al: FIGURE: facial idiopathic granulomas with regressive evolution. Dermatology 2000; 201: 289.

Bacterial infections in the skin often have distinct morphologic characteristics that should alert the clinician that a potentially treatable and reversible condition exists. These cutaneous signs may be an indication of a generalized systemic process or simply an isolated superficial infection. Patients who have immunodeficiencies or are immunosuppressed may acquire severe or refractory pyogenic infections. Patients with atopic dermatitis are also predisposed to bacterial infections due to down regulation of antimicrobial peptides. The categorization of bacterial infections in this chapter first addresses diseases caused by gram-positive bacteria, followed by those caused by gram-negative bacteria, and then several miscellaneous diseases caused by the *Rickettsiae*, mycoplasmas, *Chlamydiae*, and spirochetes.

Chon SY, et al: Antibiotic overuse and resistance in dermatology. Dermatol Ther 2012; 25: 55.

Dawson AL, et al: Infectious skin diseases. Dermatol Clin 2012; 30: 141.

Dumville JC, et al: Preoperative skin antiseptics for preventing surgical wound infections after clean surgery. Cochrane Database Syst Rev 2013; 3: CD003949.

Grice EA, et al: Topographical and temporal diversity of the human skin microbiome. Science 2009; 324: 1190.

Holmes AH, et al: Understanding the mechanisms and drivers of antimicrobial resistance. The Lancet 2016; 387: 176.

Mistry RD: Skin and soft tissue infections. Pediatr Clin North Am 2013; 60: 1063.

Nakatsuji T, et al: Antimicrobials from human skin commensal bacteria protect against *Staphylococcus aureus* and are deficient in atopic dermatitis. Science Translational Medicine 2017; 9.

■ INFECTIONS CAUSED BY GRAM-POSITIVE ORGANISMS

STAPHYLOCOCCAL INFECTIONS

The skin lesions induced by the gram-positive staphylococci usually appear as pustules, furuncles, or erosions with honey-colored crusts. However, bullae, widespread erythema and desquamation, or vegetating pyodermas may also be due to *Staphylococcus aureus* infection. Purulent purpura may indicate bacteremia or endocarditis that can be caused by *S. aureus* or, in immunocompromised patients, *S. epidermidis*. Two distinctive cutaneous lesions that occur with endocarditis are the Osler node and Janeway lesion or spot. The Osler node is a painful, erythematous nodule with a pale center located on the fingertips. The Janeway spot is a nontender, angular hemorrhagic lesion of the soles and palms (Fig. 14.1). These lesions are likely caused by septic emboli leading to clogging of the distal vessels.

From 20%–40% of adults are colonized with *S. aureus* in the nares but the bacteria can also colonize hands and perineum, so this estimate is likely underestimating staphylococcal colonization. One study found that if only nares were cultured, 40% of carriage was missed and perineal colonization correlated better with the strain isolated from the abscess. Carriers are particularly prone to infections with *S. aureus* because of its continuous presence on the skin and nasal mucosa. Spread of infection in the hospital setting is frequently traced to the hands of a health care worker. Proper handwashing or sanitizing technique is essential in preventing spread of infection. Human immunodeficiency virus (HIV)–infected patients are at least twice as often nasal carriers, and they tend to harbor *S. aureus* in higher frequency and density at other sites of the body, thus predisposing them to skin and systemic infection.

Antibiotic resistance has become more common in *S. aureus*. Methicillin-resistant *S. aureus* (MRSA) is an important pathogen in nosocomial and community-acquired skin infections. MRSA infection may be suspected from knowledge of local patterns of resistance, lack of response to initial methicillin-sensitive *S. aureus* (MSSA)–directed therapy (e.g., cephalexin), and factors predisposing to colonization and infection with this organism. Predisposing factors for MRSA include age (>65), exposure to others with MRSA infection, prior antibiotic therapy, trauma to the skin, rectal or nasal colonization, crowded households, child care attendance, contact sports, chronic skin disease, pets, and recent hospitalization or chronic illness. The bacteria can be found on bed linens, remote controls, hand towels, and other inanimate objects, making decolonization very challenging. The primary treatment for an abscess remains drainage although newer literature suppports the addition of oral antibioitcs that may help lessen recurrence. Ideally, antibiotic choice is guided by culture and sensitivities. Often clindamycin, trimethoprim-sulfamethoxazole (TMP-SMX, alone or combined with rifampin), and doxycycline are effective. TMP-SMX and doxycycline do not cover group A streptococci; therefore if a mixed infection is suspected, adding cephalexin or penicillin is necessary, or clindamycin alone may treat both pathogens. Complicated infections with the most resistant strains may require antibiotics that nearly universally cover *S. Aurues* such as vancomycin, linezolid or tedizolid. Bacterial culture is the gold standard for establishing antibiotic susceptibility profiles and is increasingly necessary as resistance becomes more common. Superficial and localized infections may only require topical antibiotic therapy. Systemic antibiotics combined with topical therapy are recommended for patients with more widespread and deeper infections. A semisynthetic penicillin or a first-generation cephalosporin is recommended, unless MRSA is suspected, as detailed earlier. Treatment should generally be given for 7–10 days, although longer courses may sometimes be necessary

Primary Cutaneous Staphylococcal Infections

Staphylococcus can affect the skin locally and the therapy and prevention are similar so will be discussed together at the end of the section.

Impetigo

The bullous variety of impetigo caused by *S. aureus* occurs characteristically in newborns and young children, although it may occur at any age. The majority is caused by phage types 71 or 55 coagulase-positive *S. aureus* or a related group 2 phage type. Bullous impetigo may be an early manifestation of HIV infection. The neonatal type is highly contagious and can spread rapidly nurseries and day cares. In most cases, the disease begins between the fourth and tenth days of life with the appearance of bullae, which may appear on any part of the body but have a predilection for the face and perineum. Sources of the primary

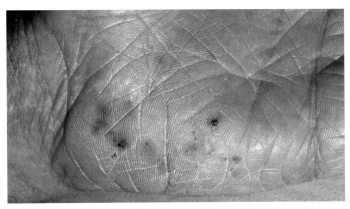

Fig. 14.1 Janeway lesion in subacute bacterial endocarditis.

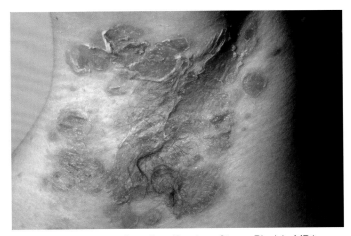

Fig. 14.2 Bullous impetigo. (Courtesy Steven Binnick, MD.)

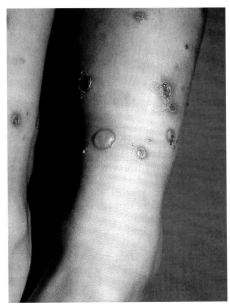

Fig. 14.3 Bullous impetigo.

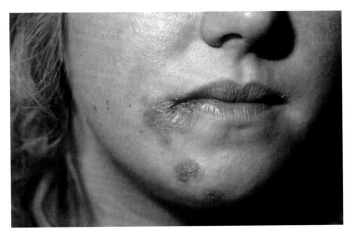

Fig. 14.4 Impetigo.

infection may be the umbilical stump, circumcision, or other area of skin breakdown. Constitutional symptoms are absent at first, but staphylococcal scalded skin or more rarely disseminated infection can occur in neonates. Bacteremia, pneumonia, or meningitis rarely may develop. Any infection in a neonate under 6 weeks should be treated more aggressively, with strong consideration given for oral antibiotics. Herpes simplex infections in neonates can be lethal, so if there is any suspicion for herpes simplex virus (HSV), polymerase chain reaction (PCR) should be done to rule this out.

In warm climates particularly, adults may have bullous impetigo, most often in the axillae or groins, but also on the hands. The lesions are strikingly large, fragile bullae, suggestive of pemphigus and intact bullae may not be present (Fig. 14.2). When these rupture, they leave circinate, weepy, or crusted lesions, and in this stage it may be called impetigo circinata. Children with bullous impetigo (Fig. 14.3) may give a history of an insect bite at the site of onset of lesions. Smaller vesicles can be seen with streptococcal infections or herpes simplex. *Impetigo contagiosa* is a term used to encompass vesicles that might be from a staphylococcal, streptococcal, or combined infection (Fig. 14.4). It is characterized by discrete, thin-walled vesicles that rapidly become pustular and then rupture especially in the setting of atopic dermatitis. Impetigo on the scalp is a frequent complication of pediculosis capitis. In streptococcal-induced impetigo, regional lymphadenopathy is common, but not serious.

Most studies find that 50%–70% of cases are caused by *S. aureus*, with the remainder from either *S. pyogenes* or a combination of these two organisms. Streptococci may represent an early pathogen in the development of impetigo, with staphylococci replacing streptococci as the lesion matures. Group B streptococci are associated with newborn impetigo, and groups C and G are rarely isolated from impetigo, unlike the usual group A.

Impetigo occurs most frequently in early childhood, although all ages may be affected. It occurs in the temperate zone, mostly during the summer in hot, humid weather. Common sources of infection for children are pets, dirty fingernails, and other children in schools, day care centers, or crowded housing areas; sources for adults include infected children and self-inoculation from nasal or perineal carriage. Impetigo often complicates pediculosis capitis, scabies, HSV, insect bites, poison ivy, eczema, and other exudative, pustular, or itching skin diseases.

Group A β-hemolytic streptococcal skin infections (but not those from *S. aureus*) are sometimes followed by acute glomerulonephritis (AGN). Nephritogenic streptococci are generally associated with impetigo rather than with upper respiratory tract infections. The important factor predisposing to AGN is the serotype of the streptococcus producing the impetigo. Type 49, 55, 57, and 60 strains and strain M-type 2 are related to nephritis.

The incidence of AGN with impetigo varies from about 2%–5% (10%–15% with nephritogenic strains of streptococcus) and occurs most frequently in childhood, generally before age 6. The prognosis in children is mostly excellent, but in adults it is not as good. Treatment, however early and appropriate, is not believed to reduce the risk of AGN.

Impetigo may simulate several diseases. The circinate patches can be mistaken for tinea, but clinically are more crusted and eroded whereas tinea is scaling. Impetigo may be mistaken for *Toxicodendron* contact dermatitis due to the vesicles and bullae seen in both. Contact dermatitis is often in linear patterns and on exposed areas whereas impetigo tends to be discrete individual round bullae and erosions. Impetigo is also not associated with the eyelid puffiness, the linear lesions, or the itchiness typically present in dermatitis. In ecthyma, the lesions are crusted ulcers.

When treating impetigo, it is necessary to soak off the crusts frequently, after which an antibacterial ointment should be applied. Applying antibiotic ointment as a prophylactic to sites of skin trauma will prevent impetigo in high-risk children attending day care centers. In one study, infections were reduced by 47% with antibiotic ointment versus 15% with placebo. Additionally, if recurrent staphylococcal impetigo develops, a culture of the anterior nares may yield this organism. Such carrier states may be treated by application of mupirocin ointment to the anterior nares twice daily or by a 10-day course of rifampin, combined with dicloxacillin (for MSSA) or TMP-SMX (for MRSA).

Folliculitis

Folliculitis is the infection of hair follicles. *S. aureus* is the most common cause of folliculitis.

Superficial pustular folliculitis (impetigo of Bockhart) is a superficial folliculitis with thin-walled pustules at the follicle orifices. Susceptible locations are the extremities and scalp, although it is also seen on the face, especially periorally. These fragile, yellowish white, domed pustules develop in crops and heal in a few days.

Staphylococcal folliculitis can affect any hair-bearing areas, often on the trunk and extremities, but may affect areas such as the eyelashes, axillae, pubis, and thighs (Figs. 14.5 and 14.6). On the pubis, it may be transmitted among sexual partners, and "mini" epidemics of folliculitis and furunculosis of the genital and gluteal areas may be considered a sexually transmitted disease (STD). In the beard area, it is called sycosis vulgaris (sycosis barbae).

Sycosis vulgaris, also known as "barber's itch" or sycosis barbae, is a perifollicular, chronic, pustular staphylococcal infection of the bearded region characterized by inflammatory papules and pustules, and a tendency to recurrence (Fig. 14.7). The disease begins with erythema and burning or itching, usually on the upper lip near the nose. In 1 or 2 days, one or more pinhead-sized pustules, pierced by hairs, develop. These rupture after shaving or washing

and leave an erythematous spot, which is later the site of a fresh crop of pustules. In this manner, the infection persists and gradually spreads, at times extending deep into the follicles. A hairless, atrophic scar bordered by pustules and crusts may result. Marginal blepharitis with conjunctivitis is usually present in severe cases of sycosis.

Sycosis vulgaris is to be distinguished from tinea, acne vulgaris, pseudofolliculitis barbae, and herpetic sycosis. Tinea barbae rarely affects the upper lip, which is a common location for sycosis. In tinea barbae, involvement is usually in the submaxillary region or on the chin, and spores and hyphae are found in the hairs. Pseudofolliculitis barbae manifests torpid papules at sites of ingrowing beard hairs in black men. In HSV infection, duration is usually only a few days, and even in persistent cases there are vesicles, which help to differentiate HSV from sycosis vulgaris.

Staphylococcal folliculitis has also been reported frequently in patients with acquired immunodeficiency syndrome (AIDS) and may be a cause of pruritus. An atypical, plaquelike form has been reported. Treatment of folliculitis is addressed later in this chapter.

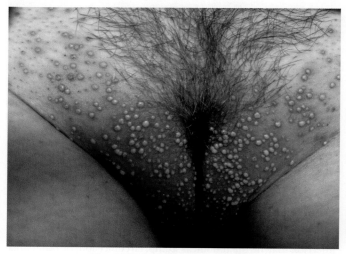

Fig. 14.6 Staphylococcal folliculitis.

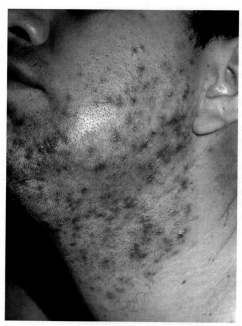

Fig. 14.7 Sycosis barbae. (Courtesy Steven Binnick, MD.)

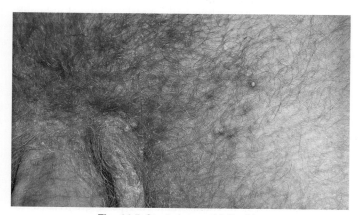

Fig. 14.5 Staphylococcal folliculitis.

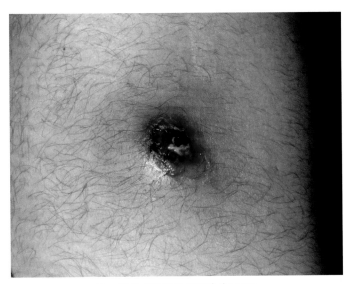

Fig. 14.8 Staphylococcal abscess.

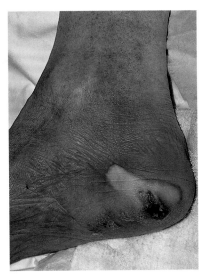

Fig. 14.9 Staphylococcal abscess in a diabetic patient.

Furunculosis

A furuncle, or boil, is an acute, round, tender, circumscribed, perifollicular staphylococcal abscess that generally ends in central suppuration (Fig. 14.8). A carbuncle is merely two or more confluent furuncles, with separate heads.

The lesions begin in hair follicles and often continue for a prolonged period by autoinoculation. Some lesions disappear before rupture, but most undergo central necrosis and rupture through the skin, discharging purulent, necrotic debris. Sites of predilection are the nape, axillae, and buttocks, but furuncles may occur anywhere. The integrity of the skin surface may be impaired by irritation, pressure, friction, hyperhidrosis, dermatitis, dermatophytosis, shaving, and other factors. Local barrier compromise predisposes to infection by providing a portal of entry for the ubiquitous *S. aureus.* The proximate cause is either contagion or autoinoculation from a carrier focus, usually in the nose or perineum. Furuncles are caused by invasion deeper into the skin and are commonly associated with MRSA. Hospital-acquired MRSA is often more resistant to antibiotics, although in recent years multidrug-resistant strains have been seen in patients who seemingly have no risk factors.

Certain systemic disorders may predispose to furunculosis: alcoholism; malnutrition; blood dyscrasias; disorders of neutrophil function; iatrogenic or other immunosuppression (e.g., AIDS); and diabetes (Fig. 14.9). Patients with several of these diseases, as well as those receiving renal dialysis or isotretinoin or acitretin therapy, are often nasal carriers of *S. aureus.* Additionally, atopic dermatitis also predisposes to the *S. aureus* carrier state, which helps explain the observed increases in the incidence of infections in these diseases. Epidemics of staphylococcal infections occur in hospitals. Marked resistance to antibacterial agents in these cases is common. Attempts to control these outbreaks center on meticulous handwashing. In nurseries, a fall in neonatal colonization and infections with *S. aureus* and non–group A streptococci may be achieved by using a 4% solution of chlorhexidine for skin and umbilical cord care.

Folliculitis may be treated with topical therapy or antibacterial washes. Topical antibiotics such as bacitracin, mupirocin, retapamulin ointment, and topical clindamycin are topical antistaphylococcal antibiotics. In addition to treating the individual pustules, benzoyl peroxide washes, dilute sodium hypochlorite baths (½ US cup bleach added to a 40-gallon tub of bathwater), and chlorhexadine washes are antimicrobials that can be helpful to decolonize the skin surface. Skin surface staphylococcal carriage in abrasions and eczematous areas may be addressed with these topical antibiotics, topical chlorhexidine washes, or dilute sodium hypochlorite (bleach) baths. Mupirocin ointment applied to the anterior nares daily for 5 days along with bleach baths may help prevent recurrence.

Early furuncles are incipient and acutely inflamed, and incision may not be possible because the abscess may not have collected yet; warm compresses and oral antibiotics are administered. When a furuncle has become localized and shows definite fluctuation, incision with drainage is indicated. When the inflammation is acute, hot wet soaks with aluminum acetate solution diluted 1 : 20 are beneficial. An anhydrous formulation of aluminum chloride (Drysol, Xerac-AC) is effective when used once nightly for chronic folliculitis, especially of the buttocks. Although drainage alone is effective for many lesions, a recent randomized trial showed that even in abscesses smaller than 5 cm antibiotic therapy with either clindamycin or TMP-SMX in addition to incision and drainage both increased initial cure rate and decreased rebound rate. In furuncles of the external auditory canal, upper lip, and nose, spontaneous drainage is common and a trial of antibiotic therapy may be attempted before surgical incision and drainage. In these patients, antibiotic ointment should be applied and antibiotics given internally. Warm saline-solution compresses should be applied liberally.

For folliculitis, a first-generation cephalosporin or penicillinase-resistant penicillin (e.g., dicloxacillin) is indicated, unless MRSA is suspected (see earlier). Methicillin-resistant and in some parts of the world vancomycin-resistant strains occur and, if suspected, are treated with trimethoprim-sulfamethoxazole, clindamycin, doxycycline, minocycline or linezolid based on cultures. In patients with staphylococcal infections unresponsive to empiric therapy, antibiotic-resistant strains should be suspected and sensitivities checked.

Despite treatment, recurrences of some boils may be anticipated. Usually, no underlying predisposing disease is present; rather, autoinoculation and intrafamilial spread among colonized individuals are responsible.

One of the most important factors in prevention is to avoid autoinoculation. It is important to emphasize that the nasal carrier state predisposes to chronic furunculosis. The skin surface in the region of the furuncles may be a source of colonization, especially if there are cuts, excoriation, or eczematous changes. In addition, the hazard of contamination from the perianal and intertriginous areas must be considered. In general, indications for elimination of the carriage state are recurrent infection, evidence of spread to others, and high-risk individuals in the household. In addition the tubs of moisturizer used by atopic dermatitis patients can be a source of re-inoculation.

Routine precautions to take in attempting to break the cycle of recurrent folliculitis and furunculosis include a daily 4% for a week chlorhexidine wash, with special attention to the axillae, groin, and perianal area; laundering of bedding and clothing on a daily basis initially; use of bleach baths; and frequent handwashing. Additionally, the application of mupirocin ointment twice daily to the nares of patients and family members every fourth week has been found to be effective. Rifampin for 10 days, combined with dicloxacillin for MSSA or TMP-SMX for MRSA, or low-dose clindamycin for 3 months may also be effective in eradicating the nasal carriage state. The use of bacitracin ointment inside the nares twice daily throughout the course of isotretinoin therapy eliminates, or greatly reduces, the risk of inducing nasal carriage of *S. aureus* and thus staphylococcal infections.

Pyogenic Paronychia

Paronychia is an inflammatory reaction involving the folds of the skin surrounding the fingernail (Fig. 14.10). It is characterized by acute or chronic tender, and painful swelling of the tissues around the nail that at first will be red and then pustular, caused by an abscess in the nailfold. When the infection becomes chronic, horizontal ridges appear at the base of the nail. With recurrent bouts, new ridges appear.

The primary predisposing factor that is identifiable is separation of the eponychium (cuticle) from the nail plate. The separation is usually caused by trauma as a result of moisture-induced maceration of the nailfolds from frequent wetting of the hands. The relationship is close enough to justify treating chronic paronychia as a work-related condition in bartenders, food servers, nurses, and others who often wet their hands. The moist grooves of the nail and nailfold become secondarily invaded by pyogenic cocci and yeasts. Alternatively children with atopic dermatitis can inoculate bacteria under the nail by scratching infected atopic dermatitis resulting in a paronychia of the distal finger under the nail. The causative bacteria are usually *S. aureus*, *Streptococcus pyogenes*, *Pseudomonas* species, *Proteus* species, or anaerobes. The pathogenic yeast is most frequently *Candida albicans*.

The bacteria usually cause acute abscess formation (*Staphylococcus*), or erythema and swelling (*Streptococcus*), and *C. albicans* most frequently causes a chronic swelling. If an abscess is suspected, applying light pressure with the index finger against the distal volar aspect of the affected digit will better demonstrate the extent of the collected pus by inducing a well-demarcated blanching. Smears of purulent material will help confirm the clinical impression and drain the abscess allowing more rapid improvement. Myrmecial warts may mimic paronychia. Subungual black macules, followed by edema, pain, and swelling, have been reported as a sign of osteomyelitis caused by *S. aureus* or *Streptococcus viridans*, in children with atopic dermatitis.

Treatment of pyogenic paronychia consists mostly of protection against trauma and concentrated efforts to keep the affected fingernails meticulously dry. Rubber or plastic gloves over cotton gloves should be used whenever the hand must be placed in water. Acutely inflamed pyogenic abscesses should be incised and drained. The abscess may often be opened by pulling the nailfold away from the nail plate but sometime the area must be cleansed with alcohol and a needle or blade be used to drain the abscess. In acute suppurative paronychia, especially if stains show pyogenic cocci, a semisynthetic penicillin or a cephalosporin with excellent staphylococcal activity should be given orally. If these are ineffective, MRSA or a mixed–anaerobic bacteria infection should be suspected. Treatment dictated by the sensitivity of the cultured organism will improve cure rates. Rarely, long-term antibiotic therapy may be required.

Although *Candida* is the most frequently recovered organism in chronic paronychia, topical or oral antifungals lead to cure in only about 50% of cases. If topical corticosteroids are used to decrease inflammation and allow for tissue repair, there may be a higher cure rate. Often, an antifungal liquid such as miconazole is combined with a topical corticosteroid cream or ointment in candidal chronic paronychia.

Botryomycosis

Botryomycosis is an uncommon, chronic, indolent disorder characterized by nodular, crusted, purulent lesions (Fig. 14.11). Sinuses that discharge sulfur granules are present. These heal with atrophic scars. The granules most frequently yield *S. aureus* on culture, although cases caused by *Pseudomonas aeruginosa*, *Escherichia coli*, *Proteus*, *Bacteroides*, and *Streptococcus* have been reported.

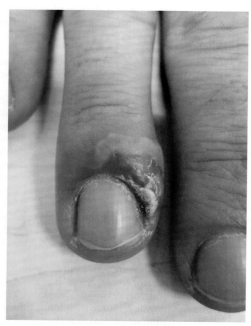

Fig. 14.10 Acute paronychia.

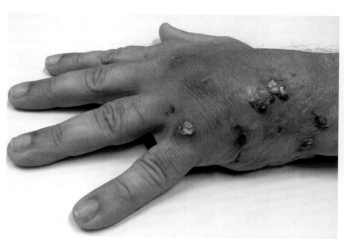

Fig. 14.11 Botyromycosis. (Courtesy Dermatology Division, University of Campinas, Brazil.)

Botryomycosis often occurs in patients with altered immune function, such as those with neutrophilic defects. Other predisposing factors include diabetes, HIV infection, alcoholism, and Job syndrome. Appropriate antibiotics, surgical drainage, and surgical excision are methods used to treat botryomycosis.

Blastomycosis-like Pyoderma

Large, verrucous plaques with elevated borders and multiple pustules occur. Most patients with blastomycosis-like pyoderma have some underlying systemic or local host compromise. Bacteria such as *S. aureus, P. aeruginosa, Proteus, E. coli,* or streptococci may be isolated. Antibiotics appropriate for the organism isolated are curative; however, response may be delayed and prolonged therapy required. Acitretin may also be useful.

Invasive and Systemic Staphylococcal Infections

Pyomyositis

S. aureus abscess formation within the deep, large, striated muscles usually presents with fever and muscle pain and is called pyomyositis. It is typically hematogenous in origin. Pyomyositis is more common in the tropics, where it may affect adults but most frequently occurs in children. In temperate climates, it occurs in children and patients with AIDS. The most frequent site in tropical disease is the thigh, whereas in HIV-infected patients, the deltoid muscle is most often involved, followed closely by the quadriceps. Swelling and occasionally erythema or yellow or purplish discoloration are visible signs of pyomyositis, but these are late findings. Non–*S. aureus* infections may also cause this same clinical picture. Magnetic resonance imaging (MRI) with gadolinium injection will help delineate the extent of disease. Drainage of the abscess and appropriate systemic antibiotics are the recommended treatment.

Staphylococcal Scalded Skin Syndrome

Staphylococcal scalded skin syndrome (SSSS) is a generalized, confluent, superficially exfoliative disease, occurring most often in neonates and children under 5 years of age. It occurs rarely in adults, usually with renal compromise or immunosuppression as a predisposing factor. SSSS is a febrile, rapidly evolving, desquamative infectious disease in which the skin exfoliates in sheets. SSSS is differentiated from Stevens-Johnson syndrome (SJS)/toxic epidermal necrolysis (TEN) based on the level of the epidermal separation and the fact that SSSS does not affect mucous membranes. The skin does not separate at the dermoepidermal junction, as in toxic (drug-induced) TEN, but within the granular layer. The lesions are thus much more superficial and less severe than in TEN, and healing is much more rapid. SSSS is caused by exfoliative exotoxins types A and B, elaborated by the staphylococcus in remote sites. Usually, staphylococci are present at a distant focus, such as the pharynx, nose, ear, or conjunctiva. Septicemia or a cutaneous infection may also be the causative focus.

Clinical manifestations of SSSS begin abruptly with skin redness and tenderness concentrated in the perioroficial areas of the face along with the intertriginous areas (neck, groin, axillae and inguinal folds). Fever is variable and the peeling first starts usually around the eyes, nose and mouth. The redness is often described as simulating a sunburn. The areas of red eventually slough with large sheets of skin being lost (Fig. 14.12). There is sparing of the palms, soles, and mucous membranes. Nikolsky sign is positive and blisters will often form where children are picked up or where electrocardiogram leads are attached and removed. Generalized exfoliation follows within the next hours to days, with large sheets of epidermis separating. Rarely true bullae can form if the sloughing skin is not disrupted. Group 2 *S. aureus*, usually phage types 71 or 55, is

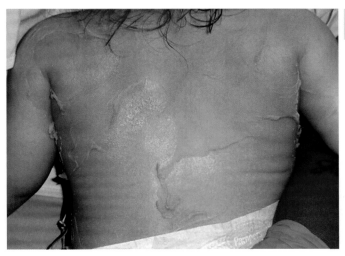

Fig. 14.12 Staphylococcal scalded skin syndrome.

the causative agent in most cases. If taken, cultures should be obtained from a primary site of infection if one can be identified or the nares, perianal area or periocular areas. The red skin and desquamation are sterile because the split is caused by the distant effects of the exfoliative toxins, unlike in bullous impetigo, where *S. aureus* is present in the lesions.

Rapid diagnosis of SSSS can be made by examining frozen sections of a blister roof and observing that the full thickness of the epidermis is not necrotic, as in TEN, but rather is cleaved below the granular layer. The exfoliative toxins A, B, and D specifically cleave desmoglein 1, the antigenic target of autoantibodies in pemphigus foliaceus, thus accounting for the clinical and histologic similarity to pemphigus observed in SSSS and bullous impetigo. In mucous membranes, desmoglein 3 is more prominent than desmoglein 1 and thus because the toxin only targets desmoglien 1 mucous membranes are characteristically spared in SSSS. Treatment of choice is a penicillinase-resistant penicillin such as dicloxacillin combined with fluid therapy and general supportive measures. Addition of clindamycin may help target the bacteria's ability to form the toxin due to its antiribosomal mechanism but as clindamycin resistance is becoming more common, clindamycin should not be used alone without cultures that prove susceptibility to clindamycin. Recent studies have shown SSSS is more commonly caused by MSSA. If MRSA is cultured and response is sluggish, antibiotics directed according to the susceptibility of the recovered organism are needed. The prognosis is excellent in children, but mortality rates in adults can reach 60%.

Gram-Positive Toxic Shock Syndromes

Toxic shock syndrome (TSS) is an acute, febrile, multisystem illness, with one of its major diagnostic criteria being a widespread macular erythematous eruption. It is usually caused by toxin-producing strains of *S. aureus*, most of which were initially isolated from the cervical mucosa in menstruating young women. Patients who don't have TSST-1 toxin antibodies are more susceptible to TSS. Currently, cases are most often caused by infections in wounds, catheters, contraceptive diaphragms, infections of bone, lung, or soft tissue or nasal packing. Mortality in these nonmenstrual cases is higher (up to 20%) compared with menstrual-related cases (<5%), probably as a result of delayed diagnoses. Also, a similar syndrome has been defined in which the cause is group A, or rarely group B, streptococci. This latter multiorgan disease has

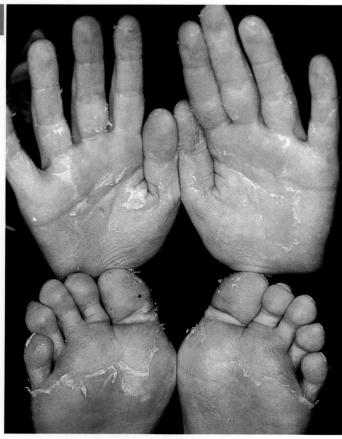

Fig. 14.13 Desquamation of the palms and soles.

systemic components similar to classic staphylococcal TSS; however, the infection is usually a rapidly progressive, destructive soft tissue infection such as necrotizing fasciitis. Underlying chronic illness, recent varicella, and use of nonsteroidal antiinflammatory drugs (NSAIDs) may predispose to TSS. It has a case-fatality rate of 30%. The streptococci are usually of M-types 1 and 3, with 80% of the isolates producing pyrogenic exotoxin A.

The Centers for Disease Control and Prevention (CDC) case definition of staphylococcal TSS includes a temperature of 38.9°C (102°F) or higher, an erythematous eruption, desquamation of the palms and soles 1–2 weeks after onset (Fig. 14.13), hypotension, and involvement of three or more other systems: gastrointestinal (GI; vomiting, diarrhea), muscular (myalgias, increased creatinine kinase level), mucous membrane (hyperemia), renal (pyuria without infection or raised creatinine or blood urea nitrogen levels), hepatic (increased bilirubin/serum glutamic oxaloacetic transaminase/serum glutamic pyruvic transaminase), hematologic (platelets <100 000/mm³), or central nervous system (CNS; disorientation). In addition, serologic tests for Rocky Mountain spotted fever, leptospirosis, and rubeola, and cultures of blood, urine, and cerebrospinal fluid (CSF) should be negative. Procalcitonin, an indicator of severe bacterial infection, may be a biologic marker for the toxic shock syndromes. Bulbar conjunctival hyperemia and palmar edema are two additional clinical clues. Streptococcal TSS is defined by isolation of group A β-hemolytic streptococci, hypotension, and two or more of the following: renal impairment, coagulopathy, hepatic involvement, acute respiratory distress syndrome, a generalized erythematous macular eruption that may desquamate, and soft tissue necrosis, myositis, or gangrene.

Histologic findings are spongiosis and neutrophils scattered throughout the epidermis, individual necrotic keratinocytes, perivascular and interstitial infiltrates composed of lymphocytes and neutrophils, and edema of the papillary dermis. TSS must be differentiated from viral exanthems, Kawasaki disease, scarlet fever, recurrent toxin-mediated perianal erythema, drug eruptions, Rocky Mountain spotted fever, systemic lupus erythematosus (SLE), TEN, and SSSS.

Treatment of TSS consists of systemic antibiotics such as vancomycin, which may be combined with nafcillin, in critically ill adult patients; vigorous fluid therapy to treat shock; and drainage of the *S. aureus*–infected site.

Agarwal V, et al: Pyomyositis. Neuroimaging Clin North Am 2011; 21: 975.

Albrecht VS, et al: *Staphylococcus aureus* colonization and strain type at various body sites among patients with a closed abscess and uninfected controls at U.S. emergency departments. J Clin Microbiol 2015; 53: 3478.

Al-Najar M, et al: Primary extensive pyomyositis in an immunocompetent patient. Clin Rheumatol 2010; 29: 1469.

Antoniou T, et al: Prevalence of community-associated methicillin-resistant *Staphylococcus aureus* colonization in men who have sex with men. Int J STD AIDS 2009; 20: 180.

Atanaskova N, et al: Innovative management of recurrent furunculosis. Dermatol Clin 2010; 28: 479.

Berk DR, et al: MRSA, staphylococcal scalded skin syndrome, and other cutaneous bacterial emergencies. Pediatr Ann 2010; 39: 627.

Braunstein I, et al: Antibiotic sensitivity and resistance patterns in pediatric staphylococcal scalded skin syndrome. Pediatr Dermatol 2014; 31: 305.

Burdette SD, et al: *Staphylococcus aureus* pyomyositis compared with non–*Staphylococcus aureus* pyomyositis. J Infect 2012; 64: 507.

Caum RS, et al: Skin and soft-tissue infections caused by methicillin-resistant *Staphylococcus aureus*. N Engl J Med 2007; 357: 380.

Datta R, et al: Risk of infection and death due to methicillin-resistant *Staphylococcus aureus* in long-term carriers. Clin Infect Dis 2008; 47: 176.

Daum RS, et al: A placebo-controlled trial of antibiotics for smaller skin abscesses. New England Journal of Medicine. 2017 Jun 29; 376(26): 2545-55.

Demos M, et al: Recurrent furunculosis. Br J Dermatol 2012; 167: 725.

Durupt F, et al: Prevalence of *Staphylococcus aureus* toxins and nasal carriage in furunculosis and impetigo. Br J Dermatol 2007; 157: 43.

Elliott DJ, et al: Empiric antimicrobial therapy for pediatric skin and soft-tissue infections in the era of methicillin-resistant *Staphylococcus aureus*. Pediatrics 2009; 123: e959.

Elston DM: How to handle a CA-MRSA outbreak. Dermatol Clin 2009; 27: 43.

Forcade NA, et al: Antibacterials as adjuncts to incision and drainage for adults with purulent methicillin-resistant *Staphylococcus aureus* (MRSA) skin infections. Drugs 2012; 72: 339.

Fritz SA, et al: Contamination of environmental surfaces with *Staphylococcus aureus* in households with children infected with methicillin-resistant *S. aureus*. JAMA Pediatr 2014; 168: 1030.

Garcia C, et al: *Staphylococcus aureus* causing tropical pyomyositis, Amazon Basin, Peru. Emerg Infect Dis 2013; 19: 123.

Gutierrez K, et al: Staphylococcal infections in children, California, USA, 1985–2009. Emerg Infect Dis 2013; 19: 10.

Kato M, et al: Procalcitonin as a biomarker for toxic shock syndrome. Acta Derm Venereol 2010; 90: 441.

Kirkland EB, et al: Methicillin-resistant *Staphylococcus aureus* and athletes. J Am Acad Dermatol 2008; 59: 494.

Lappin E, et al: Gram-positive toxic shock syndromes. Lancet Infect Dis 2009; 9: 281.

Le Bihan C, et al: *Staphylococcus aureus* transmission in the intensive care unit. Ann Infect 2017; 1: 3.

Low DE: Toxic shock syndrome. Crit Care Clin 2013; 29: 651.

Mitsionis GI, et al: Pyomyositis in children. J Pediatr Surg 2009; 44: 2173.

Neylon O, et al: Neonatal staphylococcal scalded skin syndrome. Eur J Pediatr 2010; 169: 1503.

Otto M: *Staphylococcus aureus* toxins. Curr Opin Microbiol 2014; 17: 32.

Ouchi T, et al: A case of blastomycosis-like pyoderma caused by mixed infection of *Staphylococcus epidermidis* and *Trichophyton rubrum*. Am J Dermatopathol 2011; 33: 397.

Patel GK, et al: Staphylococcal scalded skin syndrome. Am J Med 2010; 123: 505.

Patrizi A, et al: Recurrent toxin-mediated perineal erythema. Arch Dermatol 2008; 144: 239.

Piechowicz L, et al: Outbreak of bullous impetigo caused by *Staphylococcus aureus* strains of phage type 3C/71 in a maternity ward linked to nasal carriage of a healthcare worker. Eur J Dermatol 2012; 22: 252.

Rertveit S, et al: Impetigo in epidemic and nonepidemic phases. Br J Dermatol 2007; 157: 100.

Ritting AW, et al: Acute paronychia. J Hand Surg Am 2012; 37: 1068.

Rubenstein E, et al: Botryomycosis-like pyoderma in the genital region of a human immunodeficiency virus (HIV)–positive man successfully treated with dapsone. Int J Dermatol 2010; 49: 842.

Scheinpflug K, et al: Staphylococcal scalded skin syndrome in an adult patient with T-lymphoblastic non-Hodgkin's lymphoma. Oncologie 2008; 31: 616.

Sica RS, et al: Prevalence of methicillin-resistant *Staphylococcus aureus* in the setting of dermatologic surgery. Dermatol Surg 2009; 35: 420.

Van Rijen M, et al: Mupirocin ointment for preventing *Staphylococcus aureus* infections in nasal carriers. Cochrane Database Syst Rev 2008; 4: CD006216.

Wilkins AL, et al: Toxic shock syndrome. J Infect 2017; 74: S147.

STREPTOCOCCAL SKIN INFECTIONS

Specific diseases caused by direct infection with *Streptococcus pyogenes* and its toxins, as discussed in this chapter, also have immune-mediated consequences, including acute rheumatic fever, chronic rheumatic heart disease, guttate psoriasis and acute poststreptococcal glomerulonephritis. The first two only occur after pharyngitis or tonsillitis but guttate psoriasis can occur after perianal streptococcal infection especially in younger children. Although most of such complications occur in resource-poor countries, the global burden of these sequelae is significant.

Ecthyma

Ecthyma is an ulcerative streptococcal or less commonly staphylococcal pyoderma. The disease begins with a vesicle or vesico-pustule, which enlarges and in a few days becomes thickly crusted. The vesicles of streptococcal ecthyma can mimic HSV especially in the setting of atopic dermatitis. When the crust is removed, there is a superficial, saucer-shaped ulcer with a raw base and elevated edges (Fig. 14.14). In urban areas, these lesions are caused by *S. aureus* and are seen in intravenous drug users and HIV-infected patients.

The lesions tend to heal after a few weeks, leaving scars, but rarely may proceed to gangrene when resistance is low. Debilitated patients often have a focus of pyogenic infection elsewhere. Local adenopathy may be present. Uncleanliness, malnutrition, and trauma are predisposing causes.

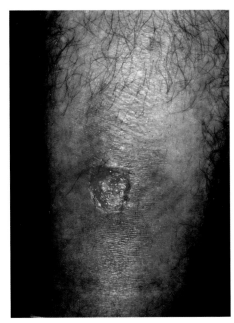

Fig. 14.14 Ecthyma.

Treatment includes cleansing with soap and water after soaking off the crust with compresses, followed by the application of mupirocin, retapamulin, or bacitracin ointment, twice daily. Oral dicloxacillin or a first-generation cephalosporin is also indicated, with adjustments made according to the cultured organism's susceptibilities.

Scarlet Fever

Scarlet fever is a diffuse, erythematous exanthem that occurs during the course of streptococcal pharyngitis. It affects primarily children, who develop the eruption 24–48 hours after onset of pharyngeal symptoms. The tonsils are red, edematous, and covered with exudate. The tongue has a white coating through which reddened, hypertrophied papillae project, giving the so-called white strawberry tongue appearance (as opposed to the red strawberry tongue of Kawasaki that lacks an exudate). By the fourth or fifth day the coating disappears, the tongue is bright red, and the red strawberry tongue remains.

The cutaneous eruption begins on the neck, then spreads to the trunk and finally the extremities (Fig. 14.15). Within the widespread erythema are 1–2 mm papules, which give the skin a rough, sandpaper quality. There is accentuation over the skinfolds, and a linear petechial eruption, called Pastia lines, is often present in the antecubital and axillary folds. There is facial flushing and circumoral pallor. A branny desquamation occurs as the eruption fades, with peeling of the palms and soles taking place about 2 weeks after the acute illness. The latter may be the only evidence that the disease has occurred.

The eruption is produced by erythrogenic exotoxin-producing group A streptococci. Cultures of the pharynx will recover these organisms. Rarely, scarlet fever may be related to a surgical wound or burn infection with streptococci. An elevated antistreptolysin O or DNase B titer may provide evidence of recent infection if cultures are not taken early. A condition known as staphylococcal scarlatina has been described that mimics scarlet fever; however, the strawberry tongue is not seen.

Penicillin, erythromycin, or dicloxacillin treatment is curative for scarlet fever, and the prognosis is excellent.

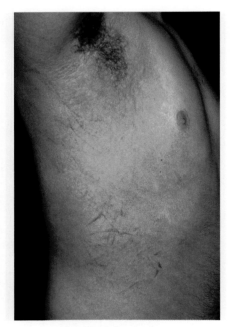

Fig. 14.15 Scarlet fever.

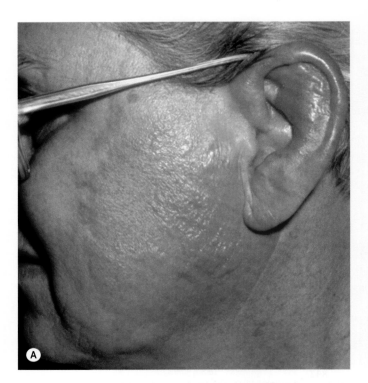

Recurrent Toxin-Mediated Perineal Erythema

This condition manifests as a perineal, erysipelas-like erythema that resolves with desquamation. Strawberry tongue, erythema of the hands with desquamation, and a mild fever 1 or 2 days before the eruption are other signs. In some patients, a staphylococcal or streptococcal pharyngitis, impetigo, or perianal streptococcal dermatitis is present. There may be recurrences in individual patients. Streptococcal pyrogenic exotoxins A and B or TSS toxin 1 may be responsible for the skin findings.

Erysipelas

Also once known as St. Anthony's fire and ignis sacer, erysipelas is an acute β-hemolytic group A streptococcal infection of the skin involving the superficial dermal lymphatics. Occasional cases caused by streptococci of group C or G are reported in adults. Group B *streptococcus* is often responsible in the newborn and may be the cause of abdominal or perineal erysipelas in postpartum women. It is characterized by local redness, heat, swelling, and a highly characteristic raised, indurated border (Fig. 14.16A). The onset is often preceded by prodromal symptoms of malaise for several hours, which may be accompanied by a severe constitutional reaction with chills, high fever, headache, vomiting, and joint pains. There is usually a polymorphonuclear leukocytosis of 20,000 cells/mm³ or more. However, many cases present solely as an erythematous lesion without associated systemic complaints.

The skin lesions may vary from transient hyperemia followed by slight desquamation to intense inflammation with vesicles or bullae. The eruption begins at any one point as an erythematous patch and spreads by peripheral extension. In the early stages, affected skin is bright red, hot to the touch, branny, and swollen. A distinctive feature of the inflammation is the advancing edge of the patch. This is raised and sharply demarcated and feels like a wall to the palpating finger. In some cases, vesicles or bullae that contain seropurulent fluid occur and may result in local gangrene.

The legs and face are the most common sites affected. On the face, the inflammation generally begins on the cheek near the nose or in front of the lobe of the ear and spreads upward to the scalp, with the hairline sometimes acting as a barrier against

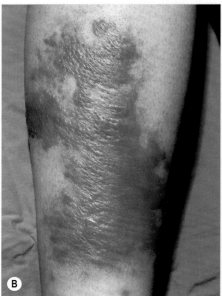

Fig. 14.16 (A and B) Erysipelas.

further extension. On the legs, edema and bullous lesions are prominent features in many patients (Fig. 14.16B). Septicemia, deep cellulitis, necrotizing fasciitis, and abscess formation may be complications, especially in obese patients and those with chronic alcohol abuse. Predisposing causes are surgical wounds, which may lead to gluteal and thigh involvement; fissures in the nares, in the auditory meatus, under the earlobes, on the anus or penis, and between or under the toes, usually the little toe; abrasions or scratches; venous insufficiency; obesity; lymphedema; and chronic leg ulcers.

Recognition of erysipelas generally is not difficult. It may be confused with contact dermatitis from plants, drugs, or dyes and with angioneurotic edema, but with each of these, fever, pain, and tenderness are absent and itching is severe. A butterfly pattern on the face may mimic lupus erythematosus, and ear involvement may suggest relapsing polychondritis.

Systemic penicillin is rapidly effective although since *S. Aureus* cellulitis maybe in the differnetial diagnosis, use of an antibiotic that will cover both is often indicated. Improvement in the general condition occurs in 24–48 hours, but resolution of the cutaneous lesion may require several days. Vigorous treatment with antibiotics should be continued for at least 10 days. Locally, ice bags and cold compresses may be used. Leg involvement, especially when bullae are present, will more likely require hospitalization with intravenous antibiotics. Elderly patients, those with underlying immunocompromise, a longer duration of illness before presentation, and patients with leg ulcers will require longer inpatient stays. A small group will have recurrent disease, in whom long-term antibiotic prophylaxis may be beneficial.

Cellulitis

Cellulitis is a suppurative inflammation involving the subcutaneous tissue. Often, cellulitis follows a wound. On the leg, tinea pedis is a common portal of entry. Mild local erythema and tenderness, malaise, fever and chills may be present but are not necessary for diagnosis. The erythema rapidly becomes intense and spreads (Fig. 14.17). The area may infiltrated and pit on pressure. The central part may become nodular and surmounted by a vesicle that ruptures and discharges pus and necrotic material. Streaks of lymphangitis may spread from the area to the neighboring lymph glands (Fig. 14.18). Gangrene, metastatic abscesses, and

severe sepsis may follow. These complications are unusual in immunocompetent adults, but children and immunocompromised adults are at higher risk.

The diagnosis of bacterial cellulitis is usually made on clinical grounds. It is uncommon for blood studies, including cultures, and skin biopsies or aspirates to be positive. If, however, an open wound is present, a culture may be positive. Streptococci continue to cause approximately 75% of cases and staphylococci the majority of the remainder. Stasis dermatitis may mimic cellulitis. It does not hurt or cause fever, may be circumferential or centered over the medial malleoli, and is usually bilateral. Allergic contact dermatitis is itchy but not painful. Eosinophilic cellulitis is an exuberant response to an insect bite and can simulate cellulitis but typically has less pain and instead of neutrophilia, there is often an eosinophilia. Erythema migrans (Lyme disease) can also present with a red patch but is typically less painful than cellulitis.

Patients with cellulitis without systemic toxicity can be managed as outpatients. Initial empiric therapy with dicloxacillin or cephalexin for 5 days will usually suffice. If MRSA is strongly suspected because of risk factors, treatment strategies are as outlined for staphylococcal infections at the start of this chapter.

Chronic Recurrent Erysipelas, Chronic Lymphangitis

Erysipelas or cellulitis may be recurrent. Predisposing factors include alcoholism, diabetes, immunodeficiency, tinea pedis, venous stasis, lymphedema with or without lymphangiectasias, prosthetic surgery of the knee, a history of saphenous phlebectomy, lymphadenectomy, or irradiation. Chronic lymphedema is the end result of recurrent bouts of bacterial lymphangitis and obstruction of the major lymphatic channels of the skin. The final result is a permanent hypertrophic fibrosis called elephantiasis nostras. It must be differentiated from lymphangioma, acquired lymphangiectasia, and other causes such as neoplasms or filariasis.

During periods of active lymphangitis, antibiotics in large doses are beneficial, and their use must be continued in smaller maintenance doses, for long periods to achieve their full benefits. Compression therapy to decrease lymphedema may aid in the prevention of recurrence.

Necrotizing Fasciitis

Necrotizing fasciitis is an acute necrotizing infection involving the fascia. It may follow surgery, perforating trauma or may occur de novo. In young children, there are peaks of incidence in the neonatal period and children 1–2 years of age and the fasciitis was more often truncal and caused by one pathogen than in older patients. Within 24–48 hours, redness, pain, and edema quickly progress to central patches of dusky-blue discoloration, with or

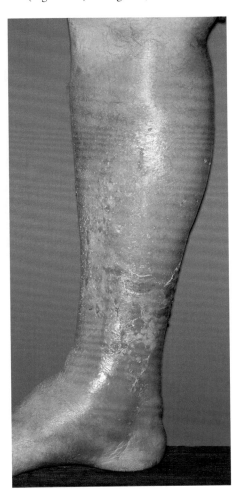

Fig. 14.17 Cellulitis.

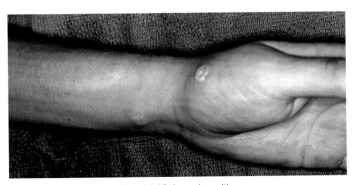

Fig. 14.18 Lymphangitis.

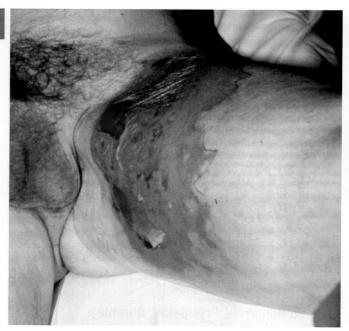

Fig. 14.19 Necrotizing fasciitis.

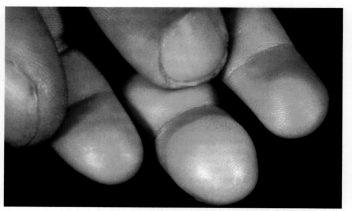

Fig. 14.20 Blistering dactylitis.

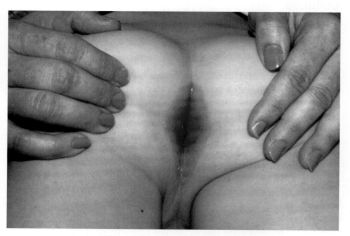

Fig. 14.21 Perianal dermatitis.

without serosanguineous blisters (Fig. 14.19). Anesthesia of the involved skin is characteristic. By the fourth or fifth day, these purple areas become gangrenous. Many forms of virulent bacteria have been cultured from necrotizing fasciitis and it may be polymicrobial. Pathogens isolated include microaerophilic β-hemolytic streptococci, hemolytic staphylococcus, coliforms, enterococci, *Pseudomonas*, and *Bacteroides*. Both aerobic and anaerobic cultures should always be taken.

Early surgical debridement is an essential component of successful therapy. Laboratory studies may help in assessing the risk of a patient having necrotizing fasciitis. One scoring system gives points for abnormalities in C-reactive protein, white blood cell count, hemoglobin, sodium, creatinine, and glucose. Based on the total score, patients are stratified into low-risk, medium-risk, and high-risk categories. Aside from direct surgical visualization, the most definitive confirmatory test is MRI. At the bedside, the clinician may infiltrate the site with anesthetic, make a 2-cm incision down to the fascia, and probe with the finger. Lack of bleeding, a murky discharge, and lack of resistance to the probing finger are ominous signs. If done, a biopsy should be obtained from normal-appearing tissue near the necrotic zone. Treatment should include early surgical debridement, appropriate IV antibiotics, and supportive care. Intravenous immune globulin (IVIG) has not been shown to improve mortality rates. Mortality rate may be 20% even in the best of circumstances. Poor prognostic factors are age over 50, underlying diabetes or atherosclerosis, delay of more than 7 days in diagnosis and surgical intervention, and infection on or near the trunk rather than the more often involved extremities. Neonatal necrotizing fasciitis most frequently occurs on the abdominal wall and has a higher mortality rate than in adults.

Blistering Distal Dactylitis

Blistering distal dactylitis is characterized by tense superficial blisters occurring on a tender erythematous base over the volar fat pad of the phalanx of a finger or thumb or occasionally a toe (Fig. 14.20). The typical patient is age 2–16 years. Group A β-hemolytic streptococci is most typical although if more purulent Bullous impetigo from *S. aureus* can have a similar appearance. These organisms may be cultured from blister fluid.

Perianal Dermatitis

Clinically, perineal dermatitis presents most often as a superficial, perianal, well-demarcated rim of erythema (Fig. 14.21); fissuring may also be seen. Pain or tenderness, especially prominent on defecation, may lead to fecal retention in affected patients, who are usually between ages 1 and 8. It may not resemble cellulitis, but rather dermatitis. It may also affect the vulvar and penile tissues. Group A streptococci are most often the cause; however, *S. aureus* may be recovered rarely, and when this occasionally occurs in adults, the usual cause is group B streptococci. The vast majority of infections are caused by streptococci, so a systemic penicillin or erythromycin combined with a topical antiseptic or antibiotic is the treatment of choice. Perianal streptococcal infections can lead to flares of guttate psoriasis especially in young children who are less likely to get streptococcal pharyngitis. The duration should be 14–21 days, depending on clinical response. Posttreatment swabs and urinalysis to monitor for poststreptococcal glomerulonephritis are recommended.

Streptococcal Intertrigo

Infants and young children may develop a fiery-red erythema and maceration in the neck, axillae, or inguinal folds. There are no satellite lesions. It may be painful and have a foul odor. Streptococcal intertrigo can be mistaken for candidal intertrigo but streptococcal infections are generally more painful and macerated and lack the satellite pustules of candida infections. Group A β-hemolytic streptococci are the cause, and topical antibiotics and oral penicillin are curative in streptococcal intertrigo.

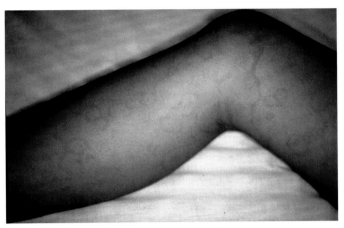

Fig. 14.22 Erythema marginatum.

Erythema Marginatum

Delayed nonsuppurative sequelae of streptococcal infections include erythema nodosum, poststreptococcal glomerulonephritis, and rheumatic fever. The latter only follows pharyngitis or tonsillitis, but two skin signs are among the diagnostic criteria of rheumatic fever: erythema marginatum and subcutaneous nodules. The remaining major signs making up the revised Jones criteria are carditis, polyarthritis, and chorea. Erythema marginatum appears as a spreading, patchy erythema that migrates peripherally and often forms polycyclic configurations (Fig. 14.22). It is evanescent, appearing for a few hours or days on the trunk or proximal extremities and typically spares the face. Heat may make it more visible, and successive crops may appear over several weeks. It is usually part of the early phase of the disease, coexisting with carditis but usually preceding the arthritis. Children younger than 5 years are more likely to manifest the eruption than older patients. A skin biopsy will show a perivascular and interstitial polymorphonuclear leukocyte predominance. In contrast, the subcutaneous nodules occur over bony prominences and appear as a late manifestation. The lesions of erythema marginatum usually are asymptomatic and resolve spontaneously.

Group B Streptococcal Infection

Streptococcus agalactiae is the major cause of bacterial sepsis and meningitis in neonates. It may cause any type of cellulitis including orbital cellulitis or facial erysipelas in these patients. Up to 25% of healthy adults harbor group B streptococci in their genital or GI tract. A guideline by Money et al. emphasizes prevention of such disastrous infections in the newborn through culture identification of mothers at risk and prophylactic antibiotics before delivery in culture-positive women. Skin and soft tissue infections caused by *Strep. agalactiae* in adult commonly can lead to invasive disease and bacteremia. *S. agalactiae* has been reported to cause balanitis, vulvar pain due to fine fissures with minimal erythema, toxic shock–like syndrome, cellulitis, perianal dermatitis, recurrent erysipelas, or blistering dactylitis in adults. Diabetes mellitus, neurologic impairment, cirrhosis, and peripheral vascular disease predispose patients to infection with *S. agalactiae*. In the postpartum period, abdominal or perineal erysipelas may be caused by this organism.

Streptococcus iniae Infections

Cellulitis of the hands may be caused by the fish pathogen *Streptococcus iniae*. The bacteria is inoculated when punctures and cuts occur while cleaning freshly killed fish before cooking. Freshwater dolphins and farm-raised fish both can carry the bacteria. Preparation of other raw seafood may also lead to *S. iniae* infection. Within 24 hours, fever, lymphangitis, and cellulitis without skin necrosis or bulla formation occur. Treatment with penicillin is curative. A similar scenario occurred with a newly described species, *Streptococcus hongkongensis* sp nov. Amoxicillin-clavulanate was effective in the one reported case.

Bachmeyer C, et al: Relapsing erysipelas of the buttock due to *Streptococcus agalactiae* in an immunocompetent woman. Clin Exp Dermatol 2009; 34: 267.

Buckland GT 3rd, et al: Persistent periorbital and facial lymphedema associated with group A beta-hemolytic streptococcal infection. Ophthalm Plast Reconstr Surg 2007; 23: 161.

Carvalho SM, et al: Rheumatic fever. Rev Bras Rheumatol 2012; 52: 241.

Del Giudice P, et al: Severe relapsing erysipelas associated with chronic *Streptococcus agalactiae* vaginal colonization. Clin Infect Dis 2006; 43: e67.

Diaz JH: Skin and soft tissue infections following marine injuries and exposures in travelers. J Travel Med 2014; 21: 207.

El Bouch R, et al: A case of recurrent toxin-mediated perineal erythema. Arch Dis Child 2013; 98: 776.

Fretzayas A, et al: MRSA blistering distal dactylitis and review of reported cases. Pediatr Dermatol 2011; 28: 433.

Glatz M, et al: Erysipelas of the thigh and gluteal region. Dermatology 2012; 225: 277.

Gunderson CG, et al: A systematic review of bacteremias in cellulitis and erysipelas. J Infect 2012; 64: 148.

Hakkarainen TW, et al: Necrotizing soft tissue infections. Curr Probl Surg 2014; 51: 344.

Hirschmann JV, et al: Lower limb cellulitis and its mimics. J Am Acad Dermatol 2012; 67: 163. e1.

Jamal N, et al: Necrotizing fasciitis. Pediatr Emerg Care 2011; 27: 1195.

Kadri SS, et al: Impact of intravenous immunoglobulin on survival in necrotizing fasciitis with vasopressor-dependent shock. 2016; 64: 877.

Kahlke V, et al: Perianal streptococcal dermatitis in adults. Colorectal Dis 2013; 15: 602.

Kilburn SA, et al: Interventions for cellulitis and erysipelas. Cochrane Database Syst Rev 2010; 6: CD004299.

Krasagakis K, et al: Local complications of erysipelas. Clin Exper Dermatol 2010; 36: 351.

Kutsuna S, et al: Scarlet fever in an adult. Intern Med 2014; 53: 167.

Lau SK, et al: *Streptococcus hongkongensis* sp. nov., isolated from a patient with an infected puncture wound and from a marine flatfish. Int J Syst Evol Microbiol 2013; 63: 2570.

Laucerotto L, et al: Necrotizing fasciitis. J Trauma 2012; 72: 560.

Mirowski GW, et al: Cutaneous vulvar streptococcal infection. J Low Genit Tract Dis 2012; 16: 281.

Mittal MK, et al: Group B streptococcal cellulitis in infancy. Pediatr Emerg Care 2007; 23: 324.

Money D, et al: The prevention of early-onset neonatal group B streptococcal disease. J Obstet Gynaecol Can 2013; 35: 939.

Picard D, et al: Risk factors for abscess formation in patients with superficial cellulitis (erysipelas) of the leg. Br J Dermatol 2012; 168: 859.

Raff AB, Kroshinsky D: Cellulitis. JAMA 2016; 316: 325.

Ralph AP, et al: Group A streptococcal diseases and their global burden. Curr Top Microbiol Immunol 2013; 368: 1.

Ruppen C, et al: Osteoarticular and skin and soft-tissue infections caused by *Streptococcus agalactiae* in elderly patients are frequently associated with bacteremia. Diagn Microbiol Infect Dis 2018; 90: 55.

Silverman RA, et al: Streptococcal intertrigo of the cervical folds in a five-month-old infant. Pediatr Infect Dis J 2012; 31: 872.

Singer AJ, et al: Management of skin abscesses in the era of methicillin-resistant *Staphylococcus aureus*. N Engl J Med 2014; 370: 1039.

Sun JR, et al: Invasive infection with *Streptococcus iniae* in Taiwan. J Med Microbiol 2007; 56: 1246.

Thomas K, et al: Prophylactic antibiotics for the prevention of cellulitis (erysipelas) of the leg. Br J Dermatol 2012; 166: 169.

Thomas KS, et al: Penicillin to prevent recurrent leg cellulitis. N Engl J Med 2013; 368: 1695.

Wasserzug O, et al: A cluster of ecthyma outbreaks caused by a single clone of invasive and highly infective *Streptococcus pyogenes*. Clin Infect Dis 2009; 48: 1213.

Zundel S, et al: Diagnosis and treatment of pediatric necrotizing fasciitis. Eur J Pediatr Surg 2017; 27: 127.

MISCELLANEOUS GRAM-POSITIVE SKIN INFECTIONS

Erysipeloid of Rosenbach

The most frequent form of erysipeloid is a sharply marginated and often polygonal patch of purplish erythema (Fig. 14.23). The first symptom is pain at the site of inoculation, followed by swelling and erythema. The erythema slowly spreads to produce a sharply defined, slightly elevated zone that extends peripherally as the central portion fades away. If the finger is involved, the swelling and tenseness make movement difficult. Vesicles frequently occur.

Another characteristic of the disease is its migratory nature; new purplish red patches appear at nearby areas. If the infection originally involved one finger, eventually all the fingers and the dorsum of the hand, the palm, or both may become infected, with the erythema appearing and disappearing; or extension may take place by continuity. The disease involutes without desquamation or suppuration. A diffuse or generalized eruption in regions remote from the site of inoculation may occur, with fever and arthritic symptoms. Rarely, septicemia may eventuate in endocarditis, with prolonged fever and constitutional symptoms.

The infection is caused by *Erysipelothrix rhusiopathiae*. *E. rhusiopathiae* is present on dead matter of animal origin. Swine are more frequently infected than any other animal. Turkeys are also often infected, and the disease may arise from handling contaminated dressed turkeys. It is also present in the slime of saltwater fish, on crabs, and on other shellfish. The disease is widespread along the entire Atlantic seacoast among commercial fishermen. The infection also occurs among veterinarians and in the meatpacking industry, principally from handling pork

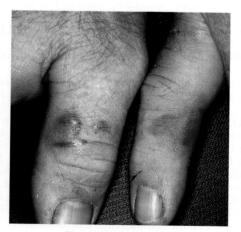

Fig. 14.23 Erysipeloid.

products. *E. rhusiopathiae* is a rod-shaped, nonmotile, gram-positive organism that tends to form long-branching filaments. The organism is cultured best on media fortified with serum, at room temperature.

Treatment

The majority of the mild cases of erysipeloid run a self-limited course of about 3 weeks. In some patients, after a short period of apparent cure, the eruption reappears either in the same area or, more likely, in an adjacent, previously uninvolved area. Penicillin, 1 g/day for 5–10 days, or ampicillin, 500 mg four times daily, is the best treatment for localized disease. If penicillin cannot be used, imipenem or piperacillin-tazobactam are effective. For systemic forms, 12–20 million units/day of IV penicillin for up to 6 weeks may be necessary.

Veraldi S, et al: Erysipeloid. Clin Exp Dermatol 2009; 34: 859.

Werner K, et al: Erysipeloid (*Erysipelothrix rhusiopathiae* infection) acquired from a dead kakapo. Arch Dermatol 2011; 147: 1456.

Pneumococcal Cellulitis

Cellulitis may be caused by *Streptococcus pneumoniae*. Children present with facial or periorbital cellulitis, which may manifest a violaceous hue or bullae. Most patients under 36 months of age are previously healthy. Fever, leukocytosis, and septicemia are almost universal. Response to treatment with penicillin or, in resistant cases, vancomycin is excellent. Most responsible strains are included in the pneumococcal vaccine, so this condition has become rare, as has *Haemophilus influenzae* cellulitis. Chronically ill or immunosuppressed adults may develop pneumococcal cellulitis or other soft tissue infections, such as abscesses or pyomyositis. In patients with diabetes or substance abuse, extremity involvement is the rule, whereas in those with SLE, nephritic syndrome, hematologic disorders, or HIV disease, the head, neck, and upper torso are typically affected. Skin involvement may also be seen as a surgical wound infection. Because septicemia, tissue necrosis, and suppurative complications are common, aggressive management is crucial, with surgical drainage and IV antibiotics directed at the susceptibility of the cultured organism.

Garcia-Lechuz JM, et al: *Streptococcus pneumoniae* skin and soft tissue infections. Eur J Clin Microbiol Infect Dis 2007; 26: 247.

Khan T, Martin DH: *Streptococcus pneumoniae* soft tissue infections in human immunodeficiency virus. Am J Med Sci 2011; 342: 235.

Anthrax

Cutaneous anthrax is uncommon in much of the world; human infection generally results from contact with infected animals or the handling of hides or other animal products from stock that has died from splenic fever. Cattlemen, woolsorters, tanners, butchers, and workers in the goat-hair industry are most liable to infection. Human-to-human transmission has occurred from contact with dressings from lesions. The spores of *Bacillus anthracis* persist and may be aerosolized, so it is a bioterrorism threat.

Anthrax is an acute infectious disease characterized by a rapidly necrosing, painless eschar with associated edema and suppurative regional adenitis (Fig. 14.24). Four forms of the disease occur in humans: *cutaneous*, accounting for 95% of cases worldwide and almost all U.S. cases; *inhalational*, known as woolsorter's disease; *gastrointestinal*, the first case of which occurred in the United States in 2010; and *injectional*, more than 50 cases of which occurred in the United Kingdom and Germany. It is a complication of IV drug use, primarily in heroin addicts.

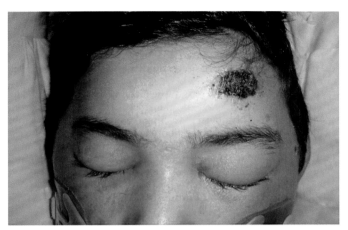

Fig. 14.24 Anthrax with severe edema. (Courtesy Steve Krivda, MD.)

The first clinical manifestation of the cutaneous form is an inflammatory papule, which begins about 3–7 days after inoculation, usually on an exposed site. The inflammation develops rapidly, and a bulla surrounded by intense edema and infiltration forms within another 24–36 hours. It then ruptures spontaneously, and a black eschar is visible, surrounded by vesicles situated on a red, hot, swollen, and indurated area. The lesion is neither tender nor painful. This is of diagnostic importance. Pustules are almost never present. The regional lymph glands become tender and enlarged and frequently suppurate.

In patients with severe disease, the inflammatory signs increase; there is extensive edematous swelling, and other bullae and necrotic lesions develop, accompanied by a high temperature and prostration, terminating in death in a few days or weeks. This may occur in up to 20% of untreated patients. In mild cases, the constitutional symptoms are sometimes slight; the gangrenous skin sloughs, and the resulting ulcer heals.

Internally, inhalational anthrax and GI infection are manifested as necrotic hemorrhagic lesions followed by bacteremia, always ending in death. Patients with injectional disease present with fever and swelling of an extremity.

The disease is produced by *Bacillus anthracis*, a large, square-ended, rod-shaped gram-positive organism that occurs singly or in pairs in smears from the blood or in material from the local lesion, or in long chains on artificial media, where it tends to form spores. The bacillus possesses three virulence factors: a polyglutamate acid capsule inhibiting phagocytosis; an edema toxin, composed of edema factor and a transport protein termed protective antigen; and lethal toxin, composed of lethal factor plus protective antigen.

A biopsy should be obtained. This allows for immunohistochemical and PCR studies, as well as routine histology and tissue Gram stain. Microscopically, there is loss of the epidermis at the site of the ulcer, with surrounding spongiosis and intraepidermal vesicles. Leukocytes are abundant in the epidermis. The dermis is edematous and infiltrated with abundant erythrocytes and neutrophils. Vasodilation is marked. The causative organisms are numerous and are easily seen, especially with Gram stain.

The diagnosis is made by demonstration of the causative agent in smears and cultures of the local material. The characteristic gangrenous lesion, surrounded by vesiculation, intense swelling and redness, lack of pain, and the patient's occupation are accessory factors. PCR identification is readily available due to its bioterrorism threat. Staphylococcal carbuncle is the most easily confused entity, but here tenderness is prominent.

Early diagnosis and prompt treatment with ciprofloxacin (500 mg) or doxycycline (100 mg), twice daily for 60 days, are curative in the cutaneous form when there are no systemic symptoms, lesions are not on the head or neck and are without significant edema, and the patient is not a child younger than 2 years. In these latter conditions, more aggressive IV therapy is required, as outlined in the CDC management guidelines available at the CDC website. Asymptomatic exposed individuals should be given prophylactic treatment with a 6-week course of doxycycline or ciprofloxacin. A vaccine is available.

Aquino LL, et al: Cutaneous manifestations of category A bioweapons. J Am Acad Dermatol 2011; 65: 1213.

Booth M, et al: Confirmed Bacillus anthracis infection among persons who inject drugs, Scotland, 2009-2010. Emerg Infect Dis 2014; 20: 1452.

Denk A, et al: Cutaneous anthrax. Cutan Ocul Toxicol 2016; 35: 177.

Doganay M, Demiraslan H: Human anthrax as a re-emerging disease. Recent Pat Antiinfect Drug Discov 2015; 10: 10.

Listeriosis

Listeria monocytogenes is a gram-positive bacillus with rounded ends that may be isolated from soil, water, animals, and asymptomatic individuals. Human infection probably occurs through the GI tract; in the majority of patients, however, the portal of entry is unknown. Infections in humans usually produce meningitis or encephalitis with monocytosis. Risk factors include alcoholism, advanced age, pregnancy, and immunosuppression.

Cutaneous listeriosis is a rare disease. Veterinarians may contract cutaneous listeriosis from an aborting cow. The organism in the skin lesions is identical to that isolated from the fetus. The eruption consists of erythematous tender papules and pustules scattered over the hands and arms. There may be axillary lymphadenopathy, fever, malaise, and headache.

Neonates are also at risk. Endocarditis, meningitis, and encephalitis caused by *Listeria* may be accompanied by petechiae, pustules, and papules in the skin.

Cases of listeriosis may easily be missed on bacteriologic examination, because the organism produces few colonies on original culture and may be dismissed as a streptococcus or as a contaminant diphtheroid because of the similarity in gram-stained specimens. Serologic tests help to make the diagnosis.

Listeria monocytogenes is sensitive to most antibiotics. Ampicillin combined with gentamicin is the treatment of choice, and TMP-SMX is an effective alternate.

Godshall CE, et al: Cutaneous listeriosis. J Clin Microbiol 2013; 51: 3591.

Zelenik K, et al: Cutaneous listeriosis in a veterinarian with evidence of zoonotic transmission. Zoonoses Public Health 2014; 61: 238.

Cutaneous Diphtheria

Cutaneous diphtheria is common in tropical areas. Most of the U.S. cases are in nonimmunized migrant farmworker families and in elderly alcoholics. Travelers to developing countries may also import disease.

Skin lesions are caused by infection with *Corynebacterium diphtheria* or *ulcerans*, usually in the form of ulcerations. The ulcer is punched out and has hard, rolled, elevated edges with a pale-blue tinge. Often, the lesion is covered with a leathery, grayish membrane. Regional lymph nodes may be affected. Other types of skin involvement include eczematous, impetiginous, vesicular, and pustular lesions. Postdiphtherial paralysis and potentially fatal cardiac complications may occur. These are mediated by a potent exotoxin, which stops protein production at the ribosome level.

Treatment consists of intramuscular (IM) injections of diphtheria antitoxin, 20,000–40,000 U, after a conjunctival test has been performed to rule out hypersensitivity to horse serum. Erythromycin, 2 g/day, is the drug of choice, unless large proportions of resistant organism are known in the area. In severe cases, IV penicillin G, 600,000 U/day for 14 days, is indicated. Rifampin, 600 mg/day for 7 days, will eliminate the *C. diphtheria* carrier state. The reservoir for *C. ulcerans* is thought to be animals.

Abdul Rahim NR, et al: Toxigenic cutaneous diphtheria in a returned traveler. Commun Dis Intell Q Rep 2014; 38: E298.
Lowe CF, et al: Cutaneous diphtheria in the urban poor populations of Vancouver, British Columbia. J Clin Microbiol 2011: 49: 2664.
Moore LSP, et al: *Corynebacterium ulcerans* cutaneous diphtheria. Lancet Infect Dis 2015; 15: 1100.

Corynebacterium jeikeium Sepsis

Corynebacterium jeikeium colonizes the skin of healthy individuals, with the highest concentration being in the axillary and perineal areas. Hospitalized patients are more heavily colonized. Patients with granulocytopenia, indwelling catheters, prosthetic devices, exposure to multiple antibiotics, and valvular defects are at highest risk for the development of sepsis or endocarditis. A papular eruption, cellulitis, subcutaneous abscesses, tissue necrosis, hemorrhagic pustules, and palpable purpura may be seen on the skin. Vancomycin is the drug of choice. Mortality rate is greater than 30% in those with leukopenia.

Olson JM, et al: Cutaneous manifestations of *Corynebacterium jeikeium* sepsis. Int J Dermatol 2009; 48: 886.

Erythrasma

Erythrasma is characterized by sharply delineated, dry, brown, slightly scaling patches occurring in the intertriginous areas (Fig. 14.25), especially the axillae, the genitocrural crease, and the webs between the fourth and fifth toes and less often the third and fourth toes. There may also be patches in the intergluteal cleft, perianal skin, and inframammary area. The vulvar mucosa can be affected by thick, desquamating, yellowish hyperkeratosis. Rarely, widespread eruptions with lamellated plaques occur. The lesions are asymptomatic except in the groin, where there may be some itching and burning. Patients with extensive erythrasma have been found to have diabetes mellitus or other debilitating diseases.

Erythrasma is caused by the diphtheroid *Corynebacterium minutissimum*. This non–spore-forming, rod-shaped, gram-positive organism may occasionally cause cutaneous granulomas or bacteremia in immunocompromised patients. Two other diseases caused by *Corynebacterium*, pitted keratolysis and trichomycosis axillaris, may occur as a triad with erythrasma. In the differential diagnosis, tinea cruris caused by fungi, intertrigo, seborrheic dermatitis, inverse psoriasis, candidiasis, and lichen simplex chronicus must be considered.

The Wood's light is the diagnostic medium for erythrasma. The affected areas show a coral-red fluorescence, which results from the presence of a porphyrin. Washing of the affected area before examination may eliminate the fluorescence. Topical erythromycin solution or topical clindamycin is easily applied and rapidly effective. Oral erythromycin (250 mg four times daily for 2 weeks) and clarithromycin (single 1-g dose) are equally effective.

Chodkiewicz HM, et al: Erythrasma. Int J Dermatol 2013; 52: 516.
Polat M, Ilhan MN: The prevalence of interdigital erythrasma. J Am Podiatr Med Assoc 2015; 105: 121.
Rho NK, Kim BJ: A corynebacterial triad. J Am Acad Dermatol 2008; 58: S57.

Arcanobacterium haemolyticum Infection

This pleomorphic, nonmotile, non–spore-forming, β-hemolytic, gram-positive bacillus causes pharyngitis and an exanthem in young adults. Acute pharyngitis in the 10- to 30-year-old age group is only caused by group A streptococci in 10%–25% of cases. Some of the remainder is caused by *Arcanobacterium haemolyticum*.

The exanthem is an erythematous morbilliform or scarlatiniform eruption involving the trunk and extremities. Although it usually spares the face, palms, and soles, atypical acral involvement has been reported. The general clinical presentation may include mild pharyngitis, severe diphtheria-like illness, or even septicemia. It may also cause cellulitis or ulcerations in the elderly.

Cultures for *A. haemolyticum* should be done on 5% blood agar plates and observed for 48 hours. The diagnostic features are enhanced by a 5%–8% CO_2 atmosphere during incubation at 37°C. Routine pharyngeal specimens are done on sheep blood agar and will miss the growth of this organism because of its slow hemolytic rate and growth of normal throat flora. The treatment of choice is erythromycin, or in the case of severe infection, high-dose penicillin G.

Mehta CL: *Arcanobacterium haemolyticum.* J Am Acad Dermatol 2003; 48: 298.
Miyamoto H, et al: Bacteriological characteristics of *Arcanobacterium haemolyticum* isolated from seven patients with skin and soft-tissue infections. J Med Microbiol 2015; 64: 369.

Intertrigo

Intertrigo is a superficial inflammatory dermatitis occurring where two skin surfaces are in apposition. It is discussed here because of its clinical association with several bacterial diseases in this chapter. As a result of friction (skin rubbing skin), heat, and moisture, the affected fold becomes erythematous, macerated, and secondarily infected. There may be erosions, fissures, and exudation, with symptoms of burning and itching. Intertrigo is most frequently seen during hot and humid weather, chiefly in obese persons. Children and elderly persons are also predisposed. This type of dermatitis may involve the retroauricular areas; the folds of the upper eyelids; the creases of the neck, axillae, and antecubital areas; finger webs; inframammary area; umbilicus; inguinal, perineal, and intergluteal areas; popliteal spaces; and toe webs.

As a result of the maceration, a secondary infection by bacteria or fungi is induced. The inframammary area in obese women is most frequently the site of intertriginous candidiasis. The groin is also frequently affected by fungal (yeast or dermatophyte)

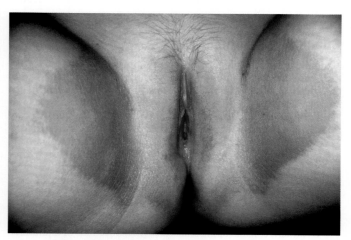

Fig. 14.25 Erythrasma. (Courtesy Steven Binnick, MD.)

infection. Bacterial infection may be caused by streptococci, staphylococci, *Pseudomonas*, or *Corynebacterium*. If *Pseudomonas* is involved, it may stain the underwear bluish green. Streptococcal intertrigo favors the neck, axillary, and inguinal folds of young children. There is a well-demarcated, fiery-red, moist, shiny surface and a foul smell, with an absence of satellite lesions.

The differential diagnosis includes seborrheic dermatitis, intertriginous psoriasis, erythrasma, and if the groin lesions are fissured, Langerhans cell histiocytosis.

Treatment of intertrigo is directed at elimination of maceration. Appropriate antibiotics or fungicides are applied locally. Separating the apposing skin surfaces with gauze or InterDry Ag textile is helpful. The latter has an antimicrobial silver complex impregnated within the fabric that when placed in the folded area not only wicks away moisture, but also retains the activity against fungi and bacteria for up to 5 days. Botulinum toxin type A has been used to dry out areas predisposed to recurrent disease. Castellani paint is also useful, as is an antibacterial ointment. Low-potency topical corticosteroids and topical tacrolimus are helpful to reduce inflammation, but these should always be used in conjunction with a topical antifungal or antimicrobial agent.

Kaya TI, et al: Blue underpants sign. J Am Acad Dermatol 2005; 53: 869.
Muller N: Intertrigo in the obese patient. Ostomy Wound Manage 2011; 57: 16.
Neri I, et al: Streptococcal intertrigo. J Pediatr 2015; 166: 1318.
Santiago-et-Sánchez-Mateos JL, et al: Botulinum toxin type A for the preventative treatment of intertrigo in a patient with Darier's disease and inguinal hyperhidrosis. Dermatol Surg 2008; 34: 1733.

Pitted Keratolysis

In pitted keratolysis, a bacterial infection of the plantar stratum corneum, the thick, weight-bearing portions of the soles become gradually covered with shallow, asymptomatic, discrete round pits 1–3 mm in diameter, some of which become confluent, forming furrows (Fig. 14.26). Men with very sweaty feet during hot, humid weather are most susceptible. Rarely, palmar lesions may occur. No discomfort is produced, although the lesions are often malodorous.

Most disease is caused by *Kytococcus sedentarius*. It produces two serine proteases that can degrade keratin. Clinical diagnosis is not difficult, based on its unique appearance. Histologic examination generally demonstrates keratin pits lined by small cocci as well as filamentous bacteria.

Topical erythromycin, mupirocin, or clindamycin is curative in pitted keratolysis. Miconazole or clotrimazole cream and Whitfield ointment are effective alternatives. Both 5% benzoyl peroxide gel and a 10%–20% solution of aluminum chloride may be used. Botulinum toxin helps if there is associated hyperhidrosis.

Bristow IR, Lee YL: Pitted keratolysis. J Am Podiatr Med Assoc 2014; 104: 177.
de Almeida HL Jr, et al: Pitted keratolysis. An Bras Dermatol 2016; 91: 106.
Pranteda G, et al: Pitted keratolysis, erythromycin, and hyperhidrosis. Dermatol Ther 2014; 27: 101.

CLOSTRIDIAL INFECTIONS AND GANGRENE OF THE SKIN

Gangrene of the skin results from loss of the blood supply of a particular area and, in some cases, from bacterial invasion that promotes necrosis and sloughing of the skin. The various forms of bacterial infection causing gangrene are discussed here. The infectious causes are often severe and acute and may involve deep tissues; MRI may delineate the depth of involvement. Vascular gangrene, purpura fulminans, and diabetic gangrene are covered in Chapter 35 and necrotizing fasciitis earlier in this chapter.

Gas Gangrene (Clostridial Myonecrosis)

Gas gangrene is the most severe form of infectious gangrene (Fig. 14.27); it develops in deep lacerations of muscle tissue. The incubation period is only a few hours. Onset is usually sudden and is characterized by a chill, a rise in temperature, marked prostration, and severe local pain. Gas bubbles (chiefly hydrogen) produced by the infection cause crepitation when the area is palpated. A mousy odor is characteristic. A plain radiograph will demonstrate the air. Gas gangrene is caused by a variety of *Clostridium* species, most frequently *Clostridium perfringens*, *C. oedematiens*, *C. septicum*, *C. difficile*, and *C. haemolyticum*. These are thick, gram-positive rods. *Clostridium* spores are resistant to skin sterilization chemicals; if injecting a site that is being soiled by stool incontinence, a mechanical wash before the sterile procedure, followed by an occlusive sterile dressing, is recommended.

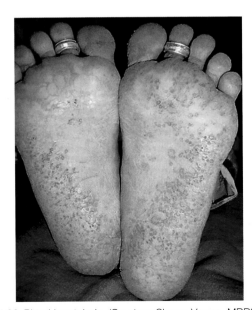

Fig. 14.26 Pitted keratolysis. (Courtesy Shyam Verma, MBBS, DVD.)

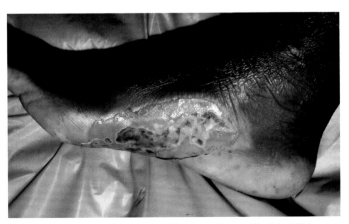

Fig. 14.27 Clostridial ulcer. (Courtesy Steven Binnick, MD.)

A subacute variety of gas gangrene may be caused by an anaerobic streptococcus (peptostreptococcus), *Bacteroides,* or *Prevotella.* This nonclostridial myositis may be clinically similar, but with delayed onset (several days). The purulent exudate has a foul odor, and gram-positive cocci in chains are present. It is important to distinguish these two entities, because involved muscle may recover in nonclostridial myositis, and debridement may safely be limited to removal of grossly necrotic muscle. Infections with both clostridial and nonclostridial organisms such as *Streptococcus faecalis, S. anginosus, Proteus, E. coli, Bacteroides,* and *Klebsiella* species may also cause crepitant cellulitis, when the infection is limited to the subcutaneous tissue. Treatment of all clostridial infections is wide surgical debridement and intensive antibiotic therapy with IV penicillin G and clindamycin. In occasional cases of clindamycin-resistant *C. perfringens,* vancomycin may be an effective alternative. Hyperbaric oxygen therapy may be of value if immediately available. Infected patients with cirrhosis and diabetes have a poorer prognosis.

Chronic Undermining Burrowing Ulcers (Meleney Gangrene)

Chronic burrowing ulcer was first described by Meleney as postoperative progressive bacterial synergetic gangrene. It usually follows drainage of peritoneal abscess, lung abscess, or chronic empyema. After 1 or 2 weeks, the wound markings or retention suture holes assume a carbunculoid appearance, finally differentiating into three skin zones: outer, bright red; middle, dusky purple; and inner, gangrenous with a central area of granulation tissue. The pain is excruciating. In Meleney postoperative progressive gangrene, the essential organism is a microaerophilic, nonhemolytic streptococcus (peptostreptococcus) in the spreading periphery of the lesion, associated with *S. aureus* or Enterobacteriaceae in the zone of gangrene.

This disease is differentiated from ecthyma gangrenosum, which begins as vesicles, rapidly progressing to pustulation and gangrenous ulceration in debilitated patients, and is caused by *P. aeruginosa.* Pyoderma gangrenosum occurs in a different setting, lacks the bacterial findings, and does not respond to antibiotic therapy. Fusospirochetal gangrene occurs after a human bite.

Wide excision and grafting are primary therapy for Meleney gangrene. In polymicrobial infections imipenem or meropenem should be given as adjunctive therapy.

Fournier Gangrene of the Penis or Scrotum

Fournier syndrome is a gangrenous infection of the penis, scrotum, or perineum that may be caused by infection with group A streptococci or with mixed enteric bacilli and anaerobes. This is usually considered a form of necrotizing fasciitis because it spreads along fascial planes. Peak incidence is between ages 20 and 50, although cases have been reported in children. Diabetes mellitus, obesity, poor personal hygiene, long-standing oral corticosteroid therapy, and chronic alcoholism are predisposing factors. Culture for aerobic and anaerobic organisms should be carried out, and appropriate antibiotics started; surgical debridement and general support should be instituted.

Huang CS: Fournier's gangrene. N Engl J Med 2017; 376: 1158.

Kaafarani HM, et al: Necrotizing skin and soft tissue infections. Surg Clin North Am 2014; 94: 155.

Rubegni P, et al: Treatment of two cases of Fournier's gangrene and review of the literature. J Dermatolog Treat 2014; 25: 189.

Takazawa T, et al: A case of acute onset postoperative gas gangrene caused by *Clostridium perfringens.* BMC Res Notes 2016; 9: 385.

Yang Z, et al: Interventions for treating gas gangrene. Cochrane Database Syst Rev 2015; 12: CD010577.

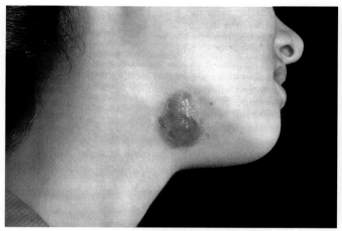

Fig. 14.28 Actinomycosis.

Actinomycosis

Actinomyces are anaerobic, gram-positive, filamentous bacteria that colonize the mouth, colon, and urogenital tract. Infections are seen most often in the cervicofacial area but also on the abdominal region, thoracic area, or pelvis. Middle-aged men are affected most often. Diabetic and immunosuppressed patients and alcoholics with poor dental hygiene are particularly at risk. The lesions begin as firm nodules or plaques and develop draining sinuses. Grains or sulfur granules may be present in the exudate, as in fungal mycetomas. In the cervicofacial region, the infection is known as lumpy jaw. The underlying bone may be involved with periostitis or osteomyelitis. Mandibular infection is seen four times as often as maxillary involvement (Fig. 14.28). The abdomen may be involved after a ruptured appendix or GI surgical procedure. Extension of the infection into the abdominal wall may produce draining sinuses on the abdominal skin. In the thoracic region, lung infection may spread to the thoracic wall.

Oropharyngeal actinomycosis is usually caused by *Actinomyces israelii* and *A. gerencseriae.* The condition is often clinically misdiagnosed as a malignancy; the histologic appearance of the characteristic granules allows diagnosis. Sulfur granules consist of fine, delicate branching filaments. Eosinophilic clubs composed of immunoglobulin are seen at the periphery of the granule (Splendore-Hoeppli phenomenon). They resemble rays; hence the name, ray fungus (*Actinomyces*). Gram stain demonstrates long, gram-positive filaments.

The crushed granule is used for inoculating cultures containing brain-heart infusion blood agar, incubated under anaerobic conditions at 37°C. Culture is difficult; therefore direct microscopy is important.

Penicillin G in large doses, 10–20 MU/day for 1 month, followed by 4–6 g/day of oral penicillin for another 2 months, may produce successful and lasting results. Other effective medications have been ampicillin, erythromycin, tetracyclines, ceftriaxone, and clindamycin. Surgical incision, drainage, and excision of devitalized tissue are important.

Bonnefond S, et al: Clinical features of actinomycosis. Medicine (Baltimore) 2016; 95: e3923.

Boyanova L, et al: Actinomycosis. Future Microbiol 2015; 10: 613.

Cataño JC, Gómez Villegas SI: Cutaneous actinomycosis. N Engl J Med 2016; 374: 1773.

Kolm I, et al: Cervicofacial actinomycosis. Dermatol Online J, 2014: 20: 22640.

Nocardiosis

Nocardiosis usually begins as a pulmonary infection from which dissemination occurs. Dissemination occurs most frequently in association with debilitating conditions, such as Hodgkin disease, periarteritis nodosa, leukemia, AIDS, organ transplants, or SLE. Skin involvement is seen in 10% of disseminated cases in the form of abscesses, erosions, or vesiculopustular lesions (Fig. 14.29). Primary cutaneous disease also occurs in healthy individuals in the form of a draining abscess or lymphangitic nodules after a cutaneous injury.

Nocardia asteroides is usually responsible for the disseminated form of nocardiosis. *Nocardia brasiliensis* is the most common cause of primary cutaneous disease. A prick by a thorn or briar, other penetrating injury, or an insect bite or sting may be the inciting event.

Nocardia are gram-positive, partially acid-fast, aerobic, filamentous bacteria. Some are branched, but filaments tend to be shorter and more fragmentary than those of *Actinomyces*. Biopsy reveals fine filamentous bacteria surrounded by neutrophilic abscesses. Only in mycetoma (see Chapter 15) are sulfur granules present. On Sabouraud dextrose agar, without antibacterial additives, there are creamy or moist, white colonies, which later become chalky and orange colored.

The drug of first choice for cutaneous nocardial infection is TMP-SMX, 5–10 mg/kg/day in two to four divided doses for 3

months, or 6 months if immunocompromised. Minocycline is an alternative. Linezolid is active, but potential adverse effects limit its use. Imipenem plus TMP-SMX or amikacin are effectively used in combination for disseminated infection.

Pai S, et al: Cutaneous nocardiosis. BMJ Case Rep 2015; 2015: 10.1136/bcr-2014-208713.

Shannon K, et al: Nocardiosis following hematopoietic stem cell transplantation. Transpl Infect Dis 2016; 18: 169.

Sheffer S, et al: Lymphocutaneous nocardiosis caused by *Nocardia brasiliensis* in an immunocompetent elderly woman. Int J Dermatol 2016; 55: e45.

Wang HL, et al: Nocardiosis in 132 patients with cancer. Am J Clin Pathol 2014; 142: 513.

■ INFECTIONS CAUSED BY GRAM-NEGATIVE ORGANISMS

PSEUDOMONAS INFECTIONS

Ecthyma Gangrenosum

In the severely ill patient with ecthyma gangrenosum, opalescent, tense vesicles or pustules are surrounded by narrow, pink to violaceous halos. These lesions quickly become hemorrhagic and violaceous and rupture to become round ulcers with necrotic black centers (Fig. 14.30). They are usually on the buttocks and extremities and are often grouped closely together. Ecthyma gangrenosum occurs in debilitated persons who may be suffering from leukemia, in the severely burned patient, in pancytopenia or neutropenia, or in patients with a functional neutrophilic defect, terminal carcinoma, or other severe chronic disease. Healthy infants may develop lesions in the perineal area after antibiotic therapy in conjunction with maceration of the diaper area.

The classic vesicle suggests the diagnosis. The contents of the vesicles or hemorrhagic pustules will show gram-negative bacilli on Gram staining, and cultures will be positive for *P. aeruginosa*. Because this is usually a manifestation of sepsis, the blood culture will also show *P. aeruginosa*. However, in healthy infants with diaper-area lesions, in patients with HIV infection, and in other occasional cases, early lesions may occur at a portal of entry, allowing for diagnosis and treatment before evolution into sepsis occurs. Although ecthyma gangrenosum is classically associated with *P. aeruginosa* infection, similar hemorrhagic pustules may occur from a variety of other gram-negative organisms (e.g., *Serratia marcescens, Klebsiella pneumoniae, Aeromonas hydrophilia, Xanthomonas maltophilia,*

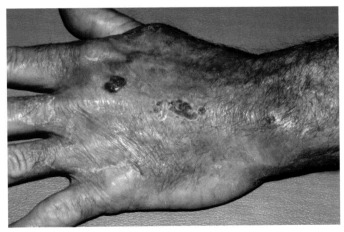

Fig. 14.29 Nocardia.

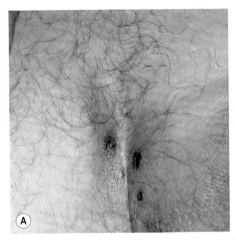

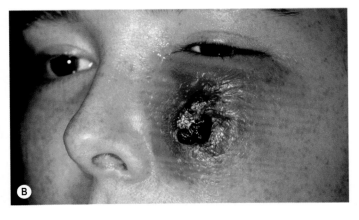

Fig. 14.30 (A and B) Ecthyma gangrenosum.

Morganella morganii, E. coli, Citrobacter freundii), fungal infections (e.g., *Candida albicans, Aspergillus fumigatus, Fusarium solani, Scytalidium dimidiatum*), and at times, *S. aureus.*

Recommended treatment is the immediate institution of IV antipseudomonal penicillin. The addition of granulocyte-macrophage colony-stimulating factor to stimulate both proliferation and differentiation of myeloid precursors is an adjunct in a patient with myelodysplasia or treatment-induced neutropenia. Patients have a poorer prognosis if there are multiple lesions, if there is a delay in diagnosis and institution of appropriate therapy, and if neutropenia does not resolve by the end of a course of antibiotics. Instrumentation or catheterization increases the risk of this infection.

Other lesions also seen with *Pseudomonas* septicemia include sharply demarcated areas of cellulitis, macules, papules, plaques, and nodules, characteristically found on the trunk. *Pseudomonas mesophilica, Burkholderia cepacia, Citrobacter freundii,* and *Stenotrophomonas maltophilia* may also produce such skin lesions in immunocompromised individuals.

Green Nail Syndrome

Green nail syndrome is characterized by onycholysis of the distal portion of the nail and a striking greenish discoloration in the separated areas (Fig. 14.31). It is frequently associated with paronychia in persons who do wet work. Overgrowth of *P. aeruginosa* accounts for the pigment. Soaking the affected finger in a 1% acetic acid solution twice a day has been found to be helpful. Trimming the onycholytic nail plate, followed by application of Neosporin solution twice a day, is also effective.

Green foot syndrome results from colonization of rubber sports shoes with *P. aeruginosa.* The organism produces pyoverdin, which stains the foot and toenails.

Gram-Negative Toe Web Infection

Toe web infection often begins with dermatophytosis. With increasing inflammation and maceration, dermatophytosis may progress to dermatophytosis complex, in which many types of gram-negative organisms may be recovered as it becomes more difficult to culture dermatophytes. Eventually, denudation with purulent or serous discharge and marked edema and erythema of the surrounding tissue may be seen (Fig. 14.32). Prolonged immersion may also cause hydration and maceration of the interdigital spaces, with overgrowth of gram-negative organisms. *P. aeruginosa* is the most prominent, but frequently a mixture of other gram-negative organisms, such as *E. coli* and *Proteus,* are present. Patients may have red, painful nodules of the calf that do not drain, spontaneously involute, then reappear 1–2 weeks later. Culture of these subcutaneous abscesses will reveal *Pseudomonas* or other gram-negative bacteria, which likely originate in the macerated toe webs.

Early dermatophytosis may simply be treated with topical antifungal agents. However, once the scaling and peeling progress to white maceration, soggy scaling, bad odor, edema, and fissuring, treatment must also include topical antibiotics or acetic acid compresses. Drying of the interdigital spaces with a fan is a helpful adjunct. Full-blown gram-negative toe web infection with widespread denudation and erythema, purulence, and edema requires systemic antibiotics. A third-generation cephalosporin or a fluoroquinolone is recommended.

Blastomycosis-like Pyoderma

Large verrucous plaques with elevated borders and multiple pustules may occur as a chronic vegetating infection. Most patients have an underlying systemic or local host compromise. Bacteria such as *P. aeruginosa, S. aureus, Proteus, E. coli,* and streptococci may be isolated. Appropriate antibiotics for the cultured organism may be augmented by acitretin.

Pseudomonas aeruginosa Folliculitis (Hot Tub Folliculitis)

Pseudomonal folliculitis is characterized by pruritic follicular, maculopapular, vesicular, or pustular lesions occurring within 1–4 days after bathing in a hot tub, whirlpool, or public swimming pool (Fig. 14.33). As the water temperature rises, free chlorine levels fall, even though total chlorine levels appear adequate. This

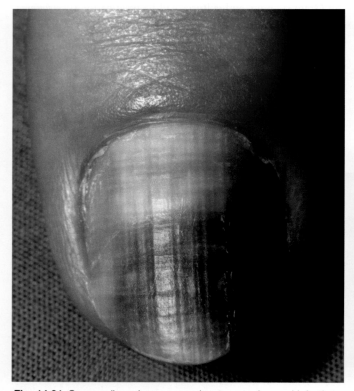

Fig. 14.31 Green nail syndrome secondary to pseudomonal infection. (Courtesy Steven Binnick, MD.)

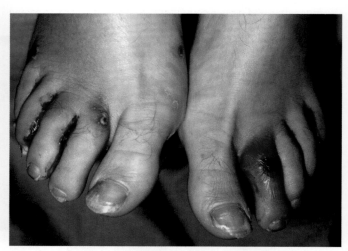

Fig. 14.32 Gram-negative toe web infection. (Courtesy Ken Geer, MD.)

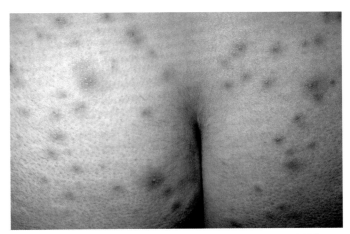

Fig. 14.33 Hot tub folliculitis. (Courtesy Steven Binnick, MD.)

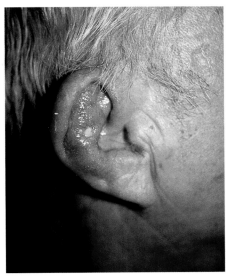

Fig. 14.34 Pseudomonas external otitis after shave biopsy.

allows the bacteria to proliferate. Diving suits may become colonized, and wearing them may result in *P. aeruginosa* folliculitis. One case occurred limited to the hand and wrist occluded under colonized rubber gloves.

Most lesions occur on the sides of the trunk, axillae, breasts, buttocks, and proximal extremities. Associated complaints may include earache, sore throat, headache, fever, and malaise. Rarely, systemic infection may result; breast abscess and bacteremia have been reported. Large community outbreaks have occurred associated with public pools, and 27 employees of a cardboard manufacturing facility who were exposed to wet work developed *Pseudomonas* folliculitis of the extremities as an occupational disorder. *Aeromonas hydrophilia* was found to be responsible for a clinically similar folliculitis that affected two siblings playing in an inflatable swimming pool.

The folliculitis involutes usually within 7–14 days without therapy, although multiple prolonged recurrent episodes have occasionally been reported. In patients with fever, constitutional symptoms, or prolonged disease, a third-generation oral cephalosporin or a fluoroquinolone such as ciprofloxacin or ofloxacin may be useful. Preventive measures have been water filtration, automatic chlorination to maintain a free chlorine level of 1 ppm, maintenance of water at pH 7.2–7.8, and frequent changing of the water. Bromination of the water and ozone ionization are other options.

Pseudomonas hot foot syndrome was reported in a group of 40 children who developed painful, erythematous plantar nodules or pustules after wading in a community pool whose floor was coated with abrasive grit. One biopsy showed neutrophilic eccrine hidradenitis; another revealed dermal microabscesses. Most were treated symptomatically, and resolution occurred within 2 weeks. Other patients have developed it after exposure to sauna and hot tubs.

External Otitis

Swelling, maceration, and pain may be present. In up to 70% of cases, *P. aeruginosa* may be cultured. External otitis is especially common in swimmers. Local application of antipseudomonal and antiinflammatory Cortisporin otic solution or suspension, or 2% acetic acid compresses with topical corticosteroids, will help clear this infection. In patients with otorrhea or pus emanating from the canal, if the symptoms have been present for 1 week or more, or if diabetes or an immunologic defect is present, cleansing the canal, visualizing the tympanic membrane for perforation, and other precautions will be most readily handled by an otolaryngology consultation. Application of otic Domeboro solution after swimming will help prevent recurrence. Fungi such as *Candida* and *Aspergillus*

are other causes. Antifungal solutions (e.g., ciclopiroxolamine) combined with corticosteroid solutions are effective in otomycosis. There is also a threat of external otitis occurring after ear surgery (Fig. 14.34). If the patient is a swimmer or has diabetes, acetic acid compresses for 1 or 2 days before surgery may prevent this complication.

External otitis must be distinguished from allergic contact dermatitis due to neomycin in Cortisporin otic suspension. Allergic contact dermatitis produces severe pruritus, although tenderness may also be noted. Dermatitis may extend down the side of the cheek in a pattern suggesting drainage of the suspension.

A severe type, referred to as malignant external otitis, occurs in elderly patients with diabetes or in those immunocompromised with HIV infection, receiving chemotherapy, or living with organ transplants. The swelling, pain, and erythema are more pronounced, with purulence and a foul odor. Facial nerve palsy develops in 30% of patients, and cartilage necrosis may occur. This is a life-threatening infection in these older, compromised individuals and requires swift institution and prolonged administration (4–6 weeks) of oral quinolone antibiotics.

Lastly, commercial ear piercing of the upper ear cartilage may lead to infection with *Pseudomonas*, with resulting cosmetic deformity.

Gram-Negative Folliculitis

Although gram-negative folliculitis is usually caused by Enterobacteriaceae, *Klebsiella*, *Escherichia*, *Proteus*, or *Serratia*, occasional cases caused by *Pseudomonas* have been seen. They differ from gram-negative infection in patients with acne in that the site of *Pseudomonas* colonization is the external ear, and topical therapy alone to the face and ears is sufficient for cure. Also, an outbreak of gram-negative pustular dermatitis on the legs, arms, torso, and buttocks occurred in a group of college students who hosted a mud-wrestling social event.

Bae JM, et al: Green foot syndrome. J Am Acad Dermatol 2013; 69: e198.

Biscaye S, et al: Ecthyma gangrenosum, a skin manifestation of *Pseudomonas aeruginosa* sepsis in a previously healthy child. Medicine (Baltimore) 2017; 96: e5507.

Chiriac A, et al: Chloronychia. Clin Interv Aging 2015; 10: 265.

Cho SB, et al: Green nail syndrome associated with military footwear. Clin Exp Dermatol 2008; 33: 791.

Corsello G, Vecchio D: Green nail syndrome. Pediatr Int 2014; 56: 801.

Guidry JA, et al: Deep fungal infections, blastomycosis-like pyoderma, and granulomatous sexually transmitted infections. Dermatol Clin 2015; 33: 595.

Keene WE, et al: Outbreak of *Pseudomonas aeruginosa* infections caused by commercial piercing of the upper ear cartilage. JAMA 2004; 291: 981.

Lambor DV, et al: Necrotising otitis externa. J Laryngol Otol 2013; 127: 1071.

Lu XL, et al: Good response of a combined treatment of acitretin and antibiotics in blastomycosis-like pyoderma. Eur J Dermatol 2009; 19: 261.

Michl RK, et al: Outbreak of hot-foot syndrome caused by *Pseudomonas aeruginosa*. Klin Paediatr 2012; 224: 252.

Mouna K, et al: Ecthyma gangrenosum caused by *Escherichia coli* in a previously healthy girl. Pediatr Dermatol 2015; 32: e179.

Nieves D, et al: Smoldering gram-negative cellulitis. J Am Acad Dermatol 1999; 41: 319.

Prindaville B, et al: Chronic granulomatous disease presenting with ecthyma gangrenosum in a neonate. J Am Acad Dermatol 2014; 71: e44.

Rosenfeld RM, et al: Clinical practice guideline: acute otitis externa. Otolaryngol Head Neck Surg 2014; 150: S1.

Roser DJ, et al: *Pseudomonas aeruginosa* dose response and bathing water infection. Epidemiol Infect 2014; 142: 449.

Saegeman V, Van Meensel B: *Aeromonas* associated with swimming pool folliculitis. Pediatr Infect Dis J 2016; 35: 118.

Segna KG, et al: "Hot tub" folliculitis from a nonchlorinated children's pool. Pediatr Dermatol 2011; 28: 590.

MALACOPLAKIA (MALAKOPLAKIA)

This rare granuloma was originally reported only in the genitourinary tract of immunosuppressed renal transplant recipients, but malacoplakia may also occur in the skin and subcutaneous tissues of other immunocompromised patients, as with HIV infection. Patients are unable to resist infections with S. *aureus*, *P. aeruginosa*, and *E. coli*. There is defective intracellular digestion of the bacteria once they have been phagocytosed.

The granulomas may arise as masslike lesions or nodules, abscesses, or ulcerations. They favor the perineum but also affect the abdominal wall, thorax, extremities, and axilla. The tongue is also a site of appearance, usually presenting as a mass lesion. Histologically, foamy eosinophilic Hansemann macrophages contain calcified, concentrically laminated, intracytoplasmic bodies (Michaelis-Gutmann). Scattered immunoblasts, neutrophils, and lymphocytes are found in the dermis.

Successful treatment of malacoplakia depends on the isolated organism; a fluoroquinolone such as ciprofloxacin or ofloxacin typically is useful.

Archer SR, et al: Malakoplakia and primary immunodeficiency. J Pediatr 2014; 165: 1053.

Coates M, et al: A case of cutaneous malakoplakia in the head and neck region and review of the literature. Head Neck Pathol 2016; 10: 444.

Diapera MJ, et al: Malacoplakia of the tongue. Am J Otolaryngol 2009; 30: 101.

Flann S, et al: Cutaneous malakoplakia in an abdominal skin fold. J Am Acad Dermatol 2010; 62: 896.

Verma SB: Cutaneous malakoplakia. Int J Dermatol 2011; 50: 184.

HAEMOPHILUS INFLUENZAE CELLULITIS

Haemophilus influenzae type B causes a distinctive bluish or purplish red cellulitis of the face, accompanied by fever in children younger than 2 years. This condition is rarely seen in countries where the vaccination is available. The importance of recognizing H. *influenzae* cellulitis is related to the bacteremia that often accompanies the cellulitis. The bacteremia may lead to meningitis, orbital cellulitis, osteomyelitis, or pyarthrosis. Cultures of the blood and needle aspirates of the cellulitis should yield the organism. Cefotaxime or ceftriaxone is effective. In a family with children under age 4, the index case, both parents, and children at risk (unvaccinated) should be given rifampin to clear the nasal carriage state and prevent secondary cases. H. *influenzae* type A not covered by the vaccine. Reports of this organism and nontypable H. *influenzae* causing invasive infection, including cellulitis in sites such as the leg and neck in immunocompromised adults are increasing.

Bruce MG, et al: *Haemophilus influenzae* serotype A invasive disease, Alaska, USA, 1983–2011. Emerg Infect Dis 2013; 19: 932.

Sharma A, et al: Pediatric orbital cellulitis in the *Haemophilus influenzae* vaccine era. J AAPOS 2015; 19: 206.

Singh V, et al: Invasive *Haemophilus influenzae* infection in patients with cancer. Cancer Control 2017; 24: 66.

Usui Y, et al: Adult-onset invasive *Haemophilus influenzae* type F caused by acute lower leg cellulitis. Intern Med 2016; 55: 1811.

CHANCROID

Chancroid (soft chancre) is an infectious, ulcerative STD caused by the gram-negative bacillus *Haemophilus ducreyi* (the Ducrey bacillus). One or more tender ulcers on the genitalia and painful inguinal adenitis that may suppurate, are characteristic of the disease. Men outnumber women manyfold. The incidence of chancroid is decreasing worldwide. *H. ducreyi* is now increasingly recognized as a cause of chronic limb ulceration in the South Pacific region.

Chancroid begins as an inflammatory macule or pustule 1–5 days, or rarely as long as 2 weeks, after intercourse. It generally appears on the distal penis or perianal area in men or on the vulva, cervix, or perianal area in women. However, many cases of extragenital infection on the hands, eyelids, lips, or breasts have been reported. Autoinoculation frequently forms kissing lesions on the genitalia, and women are apt to have more numerous lesions. The pustule ruptures early with the formation of a ragged ulcer that lacks the induration of a chancre, usually being soft with an indefinite inflammatory thickening. The ulcers appear punched out or have undermined, irregular edges surrounded by mild hyperemia (Fig. 14.35). The base is covered with a purulent, dirty exudate. The ulcers bleed easily and are very tender.

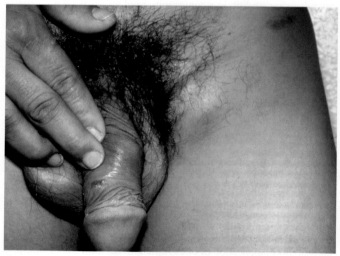

Fig. 14.35 Chancroid.

A number of clinical variants have been described, including granuloma inguinale–like, giant ulcers, serpiginous ulcers, transient chancroid, and follicular and papular variants.

About half the cases of genital chancroid manifest inguinal adenitis. Suppuration of the bubo (inguinal lymph node) may occur despite early antibiotic therapy. The lymphadenitis of chancroid, mostly unilateral, is tender and may rupture spontaneously. Left untreated, the site of perforation of the broken-down bubo will progress to a destructive painful ulcer.

As a result of mixed infection, phagedenic and gangrenous features may develop. Chronic, painful, destructive ulcers, which begin on the prepuce or glans and spread by direct extension along the shaft of the penis, are present. They may sometimes attack the scrotum or pubes. The edges of the ulcer are likely to be elevated, firm, and undermined. The granulating base, which bleeds easily, is covered with a thick, purulent exudate and dirty, necrotic detritus. The neighboring skin may be edematous and dusky red, and the regional lymph glands may be swollen, although this is not necessarily a marked feature. There is severe mutilation as a result of sloughing, with no evidence of spontaneous healing. Complications such as penile amputation from a deep, transverse ulcer may result.

This type of phagedena (spreading and sloughing ulceration) is a rare complication of chancroidal infections together with secondary bacterial infection. Treatment is by the use of antibiotics locally and internally, directed against secondary bacteria, as well as the primary process. Multiple infections may be present, such as chancroid, syphilis, HIV, or granuloma inguinale.

On histologic investigation, the ulcer may include a superficial necrotic zone with an infiltrate consisting of neutrophils, lymphocytes, and red blood cells. Deep to this, new vessel formation is present, with vascular proliferation. Deeper still is an infiltrate of lymphocytes and plasma cells. Ducrey bacilli may or may not be seen in the sections.

The definitive diagnosis of chancroid requires identification by culture. Solid-media culture techniques have allowed definitive diagnosis and sensitivity testing; however, culture is unavailable in many settings, and recovery is only about 80% successful. Specimens for culture should be taken from the purulent ulcer base and active border without extensive cleaning. They should be inoculated in the clinic; transport systems have not been evaluated. The selective medium contains vancomycin, and cultures are done in a water-saturated environment with 1%–5% CO_2, at a temperature of 33°C. Occasional outbreaks are caused by vancomycin-sensitive strains. In these cases, culture will only be successful using vancomycin-free media.

Smears are only diagnostic in 50% of cases in the best hands. A probable diagnosis is made by a clinically compatible examination and negative testing for conditions that may mimic chancroid such as herpes progenitalis. A history of recurrent grouped vesicles at the same site should help eliminate the chance of a misdiagnosis. Traumatic ulcerations should also be ruled out; these occur mostly along the frenulum or as multiple erosions on the prepuce. Adenopathy is absent, and some degree of phimosis is present.

The clinical features that differentiate chancroid from a syphilitic chancre are described in Chapter 18. However, the diagnosis of chancroid does not rule out syphilis. Either the lesion may already be a mixed sore or the subsequent development of syphilis should be anticipated, because the incubation period of the syphilis is much longer than that of chancroid. Serologic tests for syphilis should be obtained initially, then monthly for the next 3 months, and serologic testing for HIV infection should also be done. Chancroidal genital ulcer disease facilitates the transmission of HIV infection. In HIV-infected patients, chancroid may have a prolonged incubation period, the number of ulcers may be increased, extragenital sites are more frequently affected, antibiotic therapy fails more often, and healing is slower when it does occur.

Treatment

The treatment of choice for chancroid is azithromycin, 1 g orally in a single dose or ceftriaxone, 250 mg intramuscularly in a single dose. Erythromycin, 500 mg four times a day for 7 days and ciprofloxacin, 500 mg orally twice a day for 3 days, are also recommended treatments. Ciprofloxacin should not be used in pregnant or lactating women or in children younger than 17 years. Partners who have had sexual contact with the patient within the 10 days before the onset of symptoms should be treated with a recommended regimen.

Phimosis that does not subside after irrigation of the preputial cavity may have to be relieved by a dorsal slit. Circumcision should be deferred for at least 2 or 3 months. If frank pus is already present, repeated aspirations (not incisions) may be necessary.

Canhoto M, et al: *Haemophilus ducreyi* and *Treponema pallidum* co-infection in an HIV-negative male presenting with anal ulceration. Colorectal Dis 2012; 14: e749.

González-Beiras C, et al: Epidemiology of *Haemophilus ducreyi* infections. Emerg Infect Dis 2016; 22: 1.

Lewis DA, Mitjà O: *Haemophilus ducreyi.* Curr Opin Infect Dis 2016; 29: 52.

Roberts SA, Taylor SL: *Haemophilus ducreyi.* Lancet Global Health 2014; 2: e187.

Smith L, Angarone MP: Sexually transmitted infections. Urol Clin North Am 2015; 42: 507.

Spinola SM: *Haemophilus ducreyi* as a cause of skin ulcers. Lancet Glob Health 2014; 2: e387.

GRANULOMA INGUINALE (GRANULOMA VENEREUM, DONOVANOSIS)

Granuloma inguinale is a mildly contagious, chronic, granulomatous, locally destructive disease characterized by progressive, indolent, serpiginous ulcerations of the groins, pubes, genitalia, and anus. The disease begins as single or multiple subcutaneous nodules, which erode through the skin to produce clean, sharply defined lesions, which are usually painless (Fig. 14.36A). More than 80% of cases demonstrate hypertrophic, vegetative granulation tissue, which is soft, has a beefy-red appearance, and bleeds readily. Approximately 10% of cases have ulcerative lesions with overhanging edges and a dry or moist floor (Fig. 14.36B). A membranous exudate may cover the floor of fine granulations, and the lesions are moderately painful. Occasional cases are misdiagnosed as carcinoma of the penis. The lesions enlarge by autoinoculation and peripheral extension with satellite lesions and by gradual undermining of tissue at the advancing edge.

The genitalia are involved in 90% of cases, inguinal region in 10%, anal region in 5%–10%, and distal sites in 1%–5%. Lesions are limited to the genitalia in approximately 80% of patients and to the inguinal region in less than 5%. They most frequently occur on the prepuce or glans in men and on the labia in women. The incubation period is unknown; it may vary between 8 and 80 days, with a 2- to 3-week period being most common.

Persisting sinuses and hypertrophic scars, devoid of pigment, are fairly characteristic of granuloma inguinale. The regional lymph nodes are usually not enlarged. In later stages, as a result of cicatrization, the lymph channels are sometimes blocked, and pseudoelephantiasis of the genitals (esthiomene) may occur. Mutilation of the genitals and destruction of deeper tissues are observed in some patients. Dissemination from the inguinal region may be by hematogenous or lymphatic routes. There may be involvement of liver, other organs, eyes, face, lips, larynx, chest, and, rarely, bones. During childbearing, the cervical lesions may extend to the internal genital organs. Squamous cell carcinoma may rarely supervene.

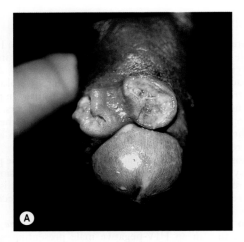

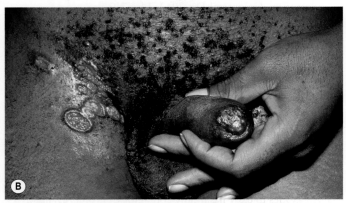

Fig. 14.36 (A and B) Granuloma inguinale.

Granuloma inguinale is caused by the gram-negative bacterium *Klebsiella granulomatis*. It is sexually transmitted in the majority of cases, with conjugal infection occurring in 12%–52% of marital or steady sexual partners. Also, it is speculated that *K. granulomatis* is an intestinal inhabitant that leads to granuloma inguinale through autoinoculation, or sexually through vaginal intercourse if the vagina is contaminated by enteric bacteria, or through rectal intercourse, heterosexual or homosexual. *K. granulomatis* probably requires direct inoculation through a break in the skin or mucosa to cause infection. Those affected are generally young adults.

On histologic investigation, in the center of the lesion, the epidermis is replaced by serum, fibrin, and polymorphonuclear leukocytes. At the periphery, the epidermis demonstrates pseudo-epitheliomatous hyperplasia. In the dermis, there is a dense granulomatous infiltration composed chiefly of plasma cells and histiocytes, and scattered throughout are small abscesses containing polymorphonuclear leukocytes. Characteristic pale-staining macrophages that have intracytoplasmic inclusion bodies are found. The parasitized histiocytes may measure 20 μm or more in diameter. The ovoid Donovan bodies measure 1–2 μm and may be visualized by using Giemsa or silver stains. The best method, however, is toluidine blue staining of semithin, plastic-embedded sections. Crushed smears of fresh biopsy material stained with Wright or Giemsa permit the demonstration of Donovan bodies and provide rapid diagnosis.

Granuloma inguinale may be confused with ulcerations of the groin caused by syphilis or carcinoma, but it is differentiated from these diseases by its long duration and slow course, by the absence of lymphatic involvement, and in the case of syphilis, by a negative test for syphilis and failure to respond to antisyphilitic treatment. It should not be overlooked that other venereal diseases, especially syphilis, often coexist with granuloma inguinale. Additionally, all patients presenting with STDs should be tested for HIV infection and their sexual partners evaluated. Lymphogranuloma venereum (LGV) at an early stage would most likely be accompanied by inguinal adenitis. In later stages, when stasis, excoriations, and enlargement of the outer genitalia are common to granuloma inguinale and LGV, the absence of a positive LGV complement fixation test and the presence of Donovan bodies in the lesions permit the diagnosis of granuloma inguinale.

Treatment

Azithromycin, 1 g once weekly, all for at least 3 weeks is the recommended regimen. Therapy should be continued until all lesions have healed completely. Alternative regimens are TMP-SMX (1 double-strength tablet), ciprofloxacin, 750 mg, or doxycycline (100 mg) twice daily or erythromycin 500 mg four times daily all for a minimum of 3 weeks. The addition of an IV aminoglycoside such as gentamicin, 1 mg/kg every 8 hours, should be considered if lesions do not respond within the first few days and in HIV-infected patients.

Basta-Juzbašić A, Čeović R: Chancroid, lymphogranuloma venereum, granuloma inguinale, genital herpes simplex infection, and molluscum contagiosum. Clin Dermatol 2014; 32: 290.
Narang T, et al: Genital elephantiasis due to donovanosis. Int J STD AIDS 2013; 23: 835.
O'Farrell N, Moi H: 2016 European guideline on donovanosis. Int J STD AIDS 2016; 27: 605.
Ornelas J, et al: Granuloma inguinale in a 51-year-old man. Dermatol Online J 2016; 22.

GONOCOCCAL DERMATITIS

Primary gonococcal dermatitis is a rare infection that occurs after primary inoculation of the skin from an infected focus. It may present as grouped pustules on an erythematous base on the finger, simulating herpetic whitlow, with or without an ascending lymphangitis. Scalp abscesses in infants may occur secondary to direct fetal monitoring in mothers with gonorrhea. It may also cause an inflammation of the median raphe or a lymphangitis of the penis with or without accompanying urethritis. Treatment is the same as that of gonorrheal urethritis. Ceftriaxone as a 125-mg single IM dose together with a single dose of azithromycin 1 g orally is recommended.

Gonococcemia

Gonococcemia is characterized by a hemorrhagic vesiculopustular eruption, bouts of fever, and arthralgia or actual arthritis of one or several joints. The skin lesions begin as tiny sparse erythematous macules (Fig. 14.37). They evolve into either tender vesicopustules on an erythematous or hemorrhagic base, or purpuric macules that may be as large as 2 cm in diameter. These purpuric lesions occur acrally, mostly on the palms and soles, and over joints. They are accompanied by fever, chills, malaise, migratory polyarthralgia, myalgia, and tenosynovitis. Involution of the lesions takes place in about 4 days.

Many patients are women with asymptomatic anogenital infections in whom dissemination occurs during pregnancy or menstruation. Liver function abnormalities, myocarditis, pericarditis, endocarditis, and meningitis may complicate this infection. In severe or recurrent cases, complement deficiency, especially of the late (C5, C6, C7, or C8) components, should be investigated.

The causative organism is *Neisseria gonorrhoeae*. These organisms can at times be demonstrated in the early skin lesion histologically, by smears, and by cultures. Gonococci may be found in the blood, genitourinary tract, pharynx, joints, and skin. The skin lesions of

14

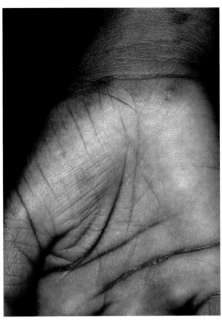

Fig. 14.37 Gonococcemia.

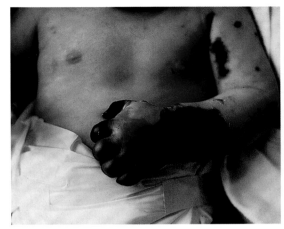

Fig. 14.38 Meningococcemia.

gonococcemia may be identical to those seen in meningococcemia, nongonococcal bacterial endocarditis, rheumatoid arthritis, the rickettsial diseases, SLE, periarteritis nodosa, Haverhill fever, and typhoid fever. Septic emboli with any gram-negative organism or *Candida* classically manifest as hemorrhagic pustules.

The treatment of choice for disseminated gonococcal infection is ceftriaxone, 1 g/day intravenously plus azithromycin 1 g orally for a minimum of 1 week. Serologic testing for HIV infection should also be done, as well as screening for syphilis. Sex partners within 30 days for symptomatic infection and 60 days for asymptomatic infection should be referred for treatment.

Dutertre M, et al: Gonococcemia mimicking a lupus flare in a young woman. Lupus 2014; 23: 81.
Mahendran SM: Disseminated gonococcal infection presenting as cutaneous lesions in pregnancy. J Obstet Gynecol 2007; 27: 617.
Skerlev M, Čulav-Košćak I: Gonorrhea. Clin Dermatol 2014; 32: 275.

MENINGOCOCCEMIA

Acute meningococcemia presents with fever, chills, hypotension, and meningitis. Half to two thirds of patients develop a petechial eruption, most frequently on the trunk and lower extremities, which may progress to ecchymoses, bullous hemorrhagic lesions, and ischemic necrosis (Fig. 14.38). Often, acral petechiae are present, and petechiae may be noted on the eyelids. Angular infarctive lesions with an erythematous rim and gun-metal gray interior are characteristic of meningococcal sepsis. Occasionally, a transient, blanchable, morbilliform eruption is the only cutaneous finding. The oral and conjunctival mucous membranes may be affected.

Meningococcemia primarily affects young children, males more frequently than females. Patients with asplenia, immunoglobulin deficiencies, or inherited or acquired deficiencies of the terminal components of complement or properdin are predisposed to infection.

A rare variant is chronic meningococcemia. There are recurrent episodes of fever, arthralgias, and erythematous macules that may evolve into lesions with central hemorrhage. Acral hemorrhagic pustules, similar to those found in gonococcal sepsis, may be seen. Patients are generally young adults with fevers lasting 12 hours interspersed with 1–4 days of well-being.

Meningococcemia is caused by the fastidious gram-negative diplococcus *Neisseria meningitidis*. It has a polysaccharide capsule that is important in its virulence and serotyping. The human nasopharynx is the only known reservoir, with carriage rates in the general population estimated to be 5%–10%.

IV ceftriaxone, 2 g twice daily, or penicillin G, 300,000 units/kg/day up to 24 MU/day for 7 days, is the treatment of choice. One dose of ciprofloxacin, 500 mg, is given after the initial course of antibiotics to clear nasal carriage. Household members and day care and close school contacts should receive prophylactic therapy. Rifampin, 600 mg every 12 hours for 2 days, is an alternative prophylactic therapy for children and ceftriaxone as a single IM dose of 250 mg for pregnant women. A polyvalent vaccine is effective against groups A, C, Y, and W-135 and is recommended for high-risk groups.

Abbas A, Mujeeb AA: Purpura fulminans caused by meningococcemia in an infant. BMJ Case Rep 2013 Aug 6; 2013.
Takada S, et al: Meningococcemia in adults. Intern Med 2016; 55: 567.

VIBRIO VULNIFICUS INFECTION

Infection with *Vibrio vulnificus*, a gram-negative rod of the non-cholera group of vibrios, may produce either a rapidly expanding cellulitis or a life-threatening septicemia in patients exposed to the organism. This infection mainly occurs along the Atlantic seacoast. It may be acquired through the GI tract; after being ingested with raw oysters or other seafood, the bacterium enters the bloodstream at the level of the duodenum. Pulmonary infection by the aspiration of seawater has been reported. Localized skin infection may result after exposure of an open wound to seawater.

Skin lesions characteristically begin within 24–48 hours of exposure, with localized tenderness followed by erythema, edema, and indurated plaques. Lesions occur in almost 90% of patients and are most common on the lower extremities. A purplish discoloration develops centrally and then undergoes necrosis, forming hemorrhagic bullae or ulcers (Fig. 14.39). Other reported lesions include hemorrhagic bullae, pustules, petechiae, generalized macules or papules, and gangrene.

If the skin is invaded primarily, septicemia may not develop, but the lesions may be progressive, and at times, limb amputation

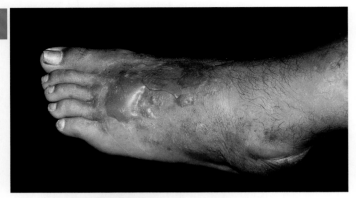

Fig. 14.39 *Vibrio vulnificus* infection. (Courtesy Curt Samlaska, MD.)

may be necessary. With septicemia, cellulitic lesions are the result of seeding of the subcutaneous tissue during bacteremia. Patients with advanced liver disease are at particular risk for developing septicemia. Other predisposing disorders are immunosuppression, alcoholism, adrenal insufficiency, diabetes, renal failure, male gender, and iron-overload states. The virulence of the bacterium is related to the production of exotoxin and various other factors. The mortality in patients with septicemia is greater than 50%.

Treatment of this fulminant infection, which rapidly produces septic shock, includes antibiotics, surgical debridement, and appropriate resuscitative therapy. Doxycycline together with ceftriaxone is the treatment of choice. In patients with preexisting hepatic dysfunction or immunocompromise and whose wounds are exposed to or acquired in saltwater, prophylactic antibiotic coverage with doxycycline, 100 mg every 12 hours, and cleansing with 0.025% sodium hypochlorite solution may prevent progressive infection.

Cazorla C, et al: Fatal *Vibrio vulnificus* infection associated with eating raw oysters, New Caledonia. Emerg Infect Dis 2011; 17: 136.
Huang KC, et al: Distribution of fatal *Vibrio vulnificus* necrotizing skin and soft-tissue infections. Medicine (Baltimore) 2016; 95: e2627.
Matsuoka Y, et al: Accurate diagnosis and treatment of *Vibrio vulnificus* infection. Braz J Infect Dis 2013; 17: 7.
Menon MP, et al: Pre-existing medical conditions associated with *Vibrio vulnificus* septicaemia. Epidemiol Infect 2014; 142: 878.

CHROMOBACTERIOSIS AND *AEROMONAS* INFECTIONS

Chromobacterium is a genus of gram-negative rods that produce various discolorations on gelatin broth. Chromobacteria have been shown to be common water and soil saprophytes of the southeastern United States and Australia. Several types of cutaneous lesions are caused by chromobacteria, ranging from fluctuating abscesses and local cellulitis to anthrax-like carbuncular lesions with lymphangitis and fatal septicemia. *Chromobacterium violaceum*, the most common species, produces a violet pigment. Patients with chronic granulomatous disease may be at particular risk. A fluoroquinolone in combination with an aminoglycoside is best for treatment. After several weeks of parenteral antimicrobial therapy, an oral agent (e.g., TMP-SMX, tetracycline, fluoroquinolone) is given for 2 or 3 months.

A gram-negative bacterium, *Aeromonas hydrophilia*, another typical soil and water saprophyte, may cause similar skin infections as *C. violaceum*, manifesting as cellulitis, pustules, furuncles, gas gangrene, or ecthyma gangrenosum–like lesions, after water-related

trauma and abrasions. Folliculitis caused by *A. hydrophilia* may mimic *Pseudomonas* folliculitis. The treatment of choice is ciprofloxacin.

Edwardsiella tarda and *Shewanella* species are two other rare causes of gram-negative infections caused by marine exposures and injuries.

Chao CM, et al: Comparison of skin and soft tissue infections caused by *Vibrio* and *Aeromonas* species. Surg Infect (Larchmt) 2014; 15: 576.
Diaz JH: Skin and soft tissue infections following marine injuries and exposures in travelers. J Travel Med 2014; 21: 207.
Saegeman V, et al: *Aeromonas* associated with swimming pool folliculitis. Ped Infect Dis 2016: 35: 118.
Yang CH, et al: *Chromobacterium violaceum* infection. J Chin Med Assoc 2011; 74: 435.

SALMONELLOSIS

Salmonella is a genus of gram-negative rods that exist in humans either in a carrier state or as a cause of active enteric or systemic infection. Most cases of typhoid fever caused by *Salmonella typhi* are acquired by ingestion of contaminated food or water. Pets such as lizards, snakes, and turtles carry salmonellae, and acquisition of the organism in petting zoos has also been reported. Poultry and poultry products are the most important sources and are believed to be the cause in about half of common-source epidemics. Handwashing and thorough cooking of meats are recommended preventive measures.

After an incubation period of 1–2 weeks, there is usually an acute onset of fever, chills, headache, constipation, and bronchitis. After 7–10 days of fever and diarrhea, skin lesions, rose-colored macules or papules ("rose spots") 2–5 mm in diameter, appear on the anterior trunk, between the umbilicus and nipples. They occur in crops, each group of 10–20 lesions lasting 3–4 days, the total duration of the exanthem being 2–3 weeks in untreated cases. Rose spots occur in 50%–60% of patients. A more extensive erythematous eruption occurring early in the course, erythema typhosum, is rarely reported, as are erythema nodosum, urticaria, and ulcers or subcutaneous abscesses.

The diagnosis is confirmed by culturing the organism from blood, stool, skin, or bone marrow. If the organism is not grown on *Shigella-Salmonella* medium or is not analyzed correctly, *S. typhi* may be erroneously reported as a coliform. The preferred antibiotic for therapy is ciprofloxacin or ceftriaxone.

Occasionally, *S. typhi* may cause skin lesions without systemic infection. Also, infection with nontyphoid *Salmonella*, such as *S. enterica*, may cause enteric fever with rose spots.

Chiao HY, et al: *Salmonella* abscess of the anterior chest wall in a patient with type 2 diabetes and poor glycemic control. Ostomy Wound Manage 2016; 62: 46.
Coburn B, et al: *Salmonella*, the host and disease. Immunol Cell Biol 2007; 85: 112.
Nishie H, et al: Non-typhoid *Salmonella* infection associated with rose spots. Br J Dermatol 1999; 140: 558.

SHIGELLOSIS

Shigellae are small, gram-negative rods that cause bacillary dysentery, an acute diarrheal illness. Most cases are a result of person-to-person transmission; however, widespread epidemics have resulted from contaminated food and water. Small, blanchable, erythematous macules on the extremities, as well as petechial or morbilliform eruptions, may occur. Men who have sex with men (MSM) may develop a furuncle on the penis caused by *Shigella flexneri*. Shigellosis may then occur as a purely cutaneous form of STD. *Shigella* and *Salmonella* are among the organisms reported to induce the postdysenteric form of Reiter syndrome. Therapy with a fluoroquinolone is curative.

Carter JD, et al: Reactive arthritis. Rheum Dis Clin North Am 2009; 35: 21.

HELICOBACTER CELLULITIS

Fever, bacteremia, cellulitis, and arthritis may all be caused by *Helicobacter cinaedi* or *H. canis*. Generally, these manifestations occur in HIV-infected patients; however, malignancy, diabetes, and alcoholism are other predisposing conditions. Occasionally, *Helicobacter* has been reported to cause postsurgical wound infections and sepsis in otherwise healthy individuals. The cellulitis may be multifocal and recurrent and may have a distinctive red-brown or copper color with minimal warmth. Ciprofloxacin is generally effective for treatment.

Adachi Y, et al: Recurrent superficial cellulitis-like erythema associated with *Helicobacter cinaedi* bacteremia. J Dermatol 2016; 43: 844.
Shimizu S, et al: Cutaneous manifestations of *Helicobacter cinaedi* infection. Acta Derm Venereol 2013; 93: 165.

RHINOSCLEROMA

Rhinoscleroma is a chronic, inflammatory, granulomatous disease of the upper respiratory tract characterized by sclerosis, deformity, remission, and eventual debility. Death resulting from obstructive sequelae may occur. The infection is limited to the nose, pharynx, and adjacent structures. The disease begins insidiously with nasal catarrh, increased nasal secretion, and subsequent crusting. Gradually, there ensues a nodular or rather diffuse sclerotic enlargement of the nose, upper lip, palate, or neighboring structures (Fig. 14.40). The nodules at first are small, hard, subepidermal, and freely movable, but they gradually fuse to form sclerotic plaques that adhere to the underlying parts. Ulceration is common. The lesions have a distinctive stony hardness, are insensitive, and are of a dusky purple or ivory color. Hyperpigmentation can be expected in dark-complexioned individuals. In the more advanced stages of rhinoscleroma, the reactive growth produces extensive mutilation of the face and marked disfigurement. Complete obstruction of the nares, superficial erosions, and seropurulent exudation may occur.

A microorganism, *Klebsiella pneumoniae*, ssp. *rhinoscleromatis*, first isolated by von Frisch, is the causative agent. The rhinoscleroma bacillus is a gram-negative rod, short, nonmotile, round at the ends, always encapsulated in a gelatinous capsule, and measuring 2–3 μm. It is found in the throats of scleroma patients only.

The disease occurs in both genders and is most common during the third and fourth decades of life. Although endemic in tropical countries in Africa and Central America, it is occasionally found in the United States. Rare familial cases have been reported, in which the condition may present in childhood.

In the primary stage of nasal catarrh, the histologic picture is that of a mild, nonspecific inflammation. When proliferation and tumefaction develop, the granulomatous tumor consists largely of plasma cells, Mikulicz cells, an occasional hyaline degenerated plasma cell (Russell body), a few spindle cells, and fibrosis. The bacilli are found within foamy macrophages (Mikulicz cells) and are best visualized with the Warthin-Starry silver stain.

Rhinoscleroma has such distinctive clinical and histologic features that the diagnosis is not difficult. Heat-killed antigen gives a confirmatory positive complement fixation reaction with scleroma patients' serum. Clinically, rhinoscleroma can be confused with syphilitic gumma, sarcoid, leishmaniasis, frambesia (yaws), keloid, lepra, hypertrophic forms of tuberculosis, and rhinosporidiosis.

Treatment

Rhinoscleroma is usually progressive and resistant to therapy. However, it may respond well to the fluoroquinolones, although therapy should be prolonged, lasting at least 3 or 4 months, to limit the chance of relapse. Corticosteroids are useful in the acute phase. Surgical intervention or CO_2 laser treatments may be needed to prevent airway obstruction or to correct deformities.

Cataño JC, Gallego S: Rhinoscleroma. Am J Trop Med Hyg 2015; 92: 3.
Castanedo Cázares JP, Martinez Rosales KI: Rhinoscleroma. N Engl J Med 2015; 372: e33.
Mukara BK, et al: Rhinoscleroma. Eur Arch Otorhinolaryngol 2014; 271: 1851.

PASTEURELLOSIS

Primary cutaneous (ulceroglandular) *Pasteurella haemolytica* (*Mannheimia haemolytica*) infection may occur in patients with skin injury and exposure to this organism. *P. haemolytica* is a common pathogen of domestic animals associated with shipping fever in cattle and septicemia in lambs and newborn pigs. The open sites become inflamed, lymphangitis and fever develop, and axillary lymph nodes become enlarged. Diagnosis is based on demonstration of the bacteria on culture of the lesions.

Pasteurella multocida is a small, nonmotile, gram-negative, bipolar-staining bacterium. It is known to be part of the normal oral and nasal flora of cats and dogs, but it may also be an animal pathogen. The most common type of human infection follows injuries from animal bites, principally cat and dog bites, but also cat scratches. After animal trauma, erythema, swelling, pain, and tenderness develop within a few hours of the bite, with a gray-colored serous or sanguinopurulent drainage from the puncture wounds (Fig. 14.41). There may or may not be regional lymphadenopathy or evidence of systemic toxicity such as chills and fever. Septicemia may follow the local infection in rare cases, and tenosynovitis and osteomyelitis appear with some frequency.

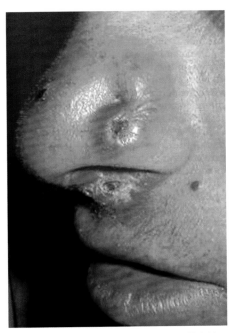

Fig. 14.40 Rhinoscleroma. (Courtesy Jason Robbins, MD.)

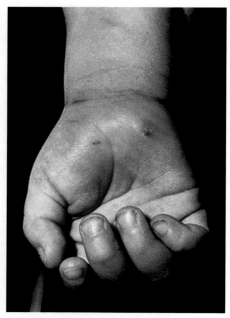

Fig. 14.41 *Pasteurella multocida* infection.

Treatment is with amoxicillin-clavulanate 875/125 mg twice daily in addition to careful cleansing and tetanus prophylaxis.

Blasiak RC, et al: *Pasteurella multocida* cellulitis in a 15-year-old male with chronic lymphedema. J Am Acad Dermatol 2013; 68: e183.
Christenson ES, et al: *Pasteurella multocida* infection in solid organ transplantation. Lancet Infect Dis 2015; 15: 235.
Guilbart M, et al: Fatal multifocal *Pasteurella multocida* infection. BMC Res Notes 2015; 8: 287.

DOG AND HUMAN BITE PATHOGENS

It is recommended that all cat bites and scratches, all sutured wounds of any animal source, and any other animal injuries of an unusual type or source be treated with antibiotics in addition to careful cleansing and tetanus prophylaxis. Although *Pasteurella* species (*P. canis* in dogs and *P. multocida* in cats) are usually present in bite site cultures, a complex mix of various other pathogens, such as streptococci, staphylococci, *Moraxella*, *Neisseria*, *Fusobacterium*, *Bacteroides*, and those individually discussed next, make the combination amoxicillin-clavulanate the best choice of initial therapy.

Capnocytophaga canimorsus is a gram-negative rod that is part of the normal oral flora of dogs and cats. It is associated with severe septicemia after dog bites. Patients who have undergone splenectomy are at particular risk. Alcoholism, chronic respiratory disease, and other medical conditions also predispose to infection; only one quarter of patients were healthy before infection with *C. canimorsus*. A characteristic finding is a necrotizing eschar at the site of the bite. Fever, nausea, and vomiting occur abruptly within 1–3 days, and the eschar develops soon thereafter. Disseminated intravascular coagulation and extensive dry gangrene may complicate the course. Sepsis after a dog bite is another hazard faced by splenectomized patients, in addition to their particular problems with pneumococcus, *Haemophilus influenzae* group B, babesiosis, *Neisseria meningitidis*, and group A streptococcus. *C. canimorsus* is difficult to identify by conventional cultures. Laboratory personnel need to be aware of the clinical suspicion of infection with this organism. A false-positive latex agglutination test for cryptococcal antigen in the CSF may occur. Treatment is

with intensive IV antibiotics. In less severely affected patients, amoxicillin-clavulanate may be effective.

Neisseria species and *Bergeyella zoohelcum* are other oral and nasal commensals in dogs; thus most reports of human disease follow animal bites. *Eikenella corrodens*, a facultative gram-negative bacillus, is a normal inhabitant of the human mouth. Most infections are caused by human bites or fist fights and are often accompanied by *Streptococcus* and *Staphylococcus* organisms. Early prophylactic treatment is with amoxicillin-clavulanate; IV antibiotics are required once clinical infection is present.

Aziz H, et al: The current concepts in management of animal (dog, cat, snake, scorpion) and human bite wounds. J Trauma Acute Care Surg 2015; 78: 641.
Gaastra W, Lipman LJ: *Capnocytophaga canimorsus*. Vet Microbiol 2010; 140: 339.
Howell RD, Sapienza A: The management of domestic animal bites to the hand. Bull Hosp Jt Dis (2013) 2015; 73: 156.
Lohiya GS, et al: Human bites. J Natl Med Assoc 2013; 10: 92.
Rothe K, et al: Animal and human bite wounds. Dtsch Arztebl Int 2015; 112: 433.

GLANDERS

Once known as equinia, farcy, and malleus, glanders is a rare, usually fatal infectious disease that occurs in humans by inoculation with *Burkholderia mallei*. It is encountered in those who handle horses, mules, or donkeys. The distinctive skin lesion is an inflammatory papule or vesicle that arises at the site of inoculation, rapidly becomes nodular, pustular, and ulcerative, and forms an irregular excavation with undermined edges and a base covered with a purulent and sanguineous exudate. In a few days or weeks, other nodules (called "farcy buds") develop along the lymphatics in the adjacent skin or subcutaneous tissues and subsequently break down. In the acute form, the skin involvement may be severe and accompanied by extreme diarrhea. Patients with the chronic form have few skin lesions and milder constitutional symptoms, but repeated cycles of healing and breakdown of nodules may occur for weeks.

The respiratory mucous membranes are especially susceptible to glanders. After accidental inhalation, catarrhal symptoms are first present, and there may be epistaxis or a mucoid nasal discharge, which is a characteristic feature of the disease. The diagnosis is established by finding the gram-negative organism in this discharge or in the skin ulcers and should be confirmed by serum agglutination. This organism has been fatal to many laboratory workers, and exposure in this setting is increasing, with *B. mallei* as well as *B. pseudomallei* considered bioterrorism threats.

Treatment is chiefly by immediate surgical excision of the inoculated lesions and antibiotics. Amoxicillin-clavulanate, doxycycline, or TMP-SMX for up to 5 months may be effective in disease limited to the skin, whereas parenteral ceftazidime can be used for severe or septic infection. Imipenem and doxycycline in combination cured an infected laboratory worker.

Bovine farcy also occurs and is caused by *Mycobacterium farcinogenes* and *M. senegalense*. It is present mostly in sub-Saharan Africa and presents as a suppurative granulomatous inflammation of the skin and lymphatics.

Anderson PD, et al: Bioterrorism. J Pharm Pract 2012; 25: 521.
Dvorak GD, et al: Glanders. J Am Vet Med Assoc 2008; 233: 570.
Hamid ME: Epidemiology, pathology, immunology and diagnosis of bovine farcy. Prev Vet Med 2012; 105: 1.
Whitlock GC, et al: Glanders. FEMS Microbiol Lett 2007; 277: 115.

MELIOIDOSIS

Melioidosis (Whitmore disease) is a specific infection caused by a glanders-like bacillus, *Burkholderia pseudomallei*. The disease has an acute pulmonary and septicemic form in which multiple miliary abscesses in the viscera occur, resulting in rapid death. Less often, it runs a chronic course, with subcutaneous abscesses and multiple sinuses of the soft tissues. Its clinical characteristics are similar to glanders, disseminated fungal infections, and tuberculosis. Severe urticaria and necrotizing fasciitis are uncommon complications.

Melioidosis is endemic in India, Southeast Asia, and northern Australia and should be suspected in military personnel and travelers who have characteristic symptoms of a febrile illness and have been in that region. Patients with diabetes and chronic renal failure are at high risk of severe disease. Recrudescence of disease after a long latency period may occur. Diagnosis is made from the recovery of the bacillus from the skin lesions or sputum and by serologic tests.

Effective therapy is guided by the antibiotic sensitivity of the specific strain. For the acute septicemic phase, ceftazidime, meropenem, or imipenem is indicated for 2 weeks, followed by maintenance oral therapy with TMP-SMX. The majority of chronic cutaneous infections respond well to oral treatment alone. Maintenance oral therapy in both situations should continue for 3 to 6 months.

Benoit TJ, et al: A review of melioidosis cases in the Americas. Am J Trop Med Hyg 2015; 93: 1134.
Currie BJ: Melioidosis. Semin Respir Crit Care Med 2015; 36: 111.
Dan M: Melioidosis in travelers. J Travel Med 2015; 22: 410.
Foong YC, et al: Melioidosis. Rural Remote Health 2014; 14: 2763.
Perumal Samy R, et al: Melioidosis. PLoS Negl Trop Dis 2017; 11: e0004738.

INFECTIONS CAUSED BY *BARTONELLA*

Bartonellae are aerobic, fastidious, gram-negative bacilli. Several species cause human diseases, including *Bartonella henselae* (cat-scratch disease and bacillary angiomatosis), *B. quintana* (trench fever and bacillary angiomatosis), *B. bacilliformis* (verruga peruana and Oroya fever), and *B. grahamii* (cat-scratch disease). These agents are transmitted by arthropod vectors in some cases. Unique to this genus is the ability to cause vascular proliferation, as seen in bacillary angiomatosis and verruga peruana. The bartonellae in affected tissue stain poorly with tissue Gram staining and are usually identified in tissue using modified silver stains such as Warthin-Starry. They are difficult to culture, making tissue identification of characteristic bacilli an important diagnostic test. Electron microscopy and PCR can be used if routine staining is negative.

Cat-Scratch Disease

Cat-scratch disease is relatively common. About 12,000 cases are reported annually in the United States, with the majority occurring in children and young adults. Cat-scratch disease is the most frequent cause of chronic lymphadenopathy in children and young adults.

Bartonella henselae is the primary cause of cat-scratch disease. The infectious agent is transmitted from cat to cat by fleas and from cats to humans by cat scratches or bites. Rarely, dog bites may transmit this infection. *B. henselae* can be found in the primary skin and conjunctival lesions, lymph nodes, and other affected tissues. In geographic areas where cat fleas are present, about 40% of cats are asymptomatically bacteremic with this organism. An immunocompromised patient with typical cat-scratch disease caused

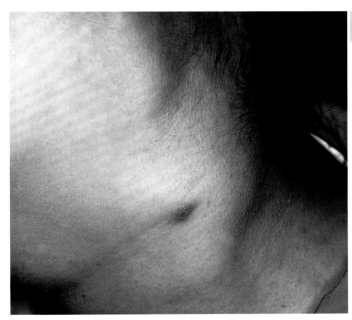

Fig. 14.42 Primary cat-scratch lesion with lymphadenopathy.

by *Bartonella grahamii* has been reported. This organism infects rodents and is likely acquired by cats through hunting.

The primary skin lesion appears within 3–5 days after the cat scratch and may last for several weeks (Fig. 14.42). It is present in 50%–90% of patients. The primary lesion is not crusted, and lymphangitis does not extend from it. The primary lesion may resemble an insect bite but is not pruritic. It heals within a few weeks, usually with no scarring.

Lymphadenopathy, the hallmark of the disease, appears 1 or 2 weeks after the primary lesions or 10–50 days (average 17) after inoculation. Usually, the lymphadenopathy is regional and unilateral. Because most inoculations occur on the upper extremities, epitrochlear and axillary lymphadenopathy is most common (50%), followed by cervical (25%) or inguinal (18%). Generalized lymphadenopathy does not occur, but systemic symptoms such as fever, malaise, and anorexia may be present. Without treatment, the adenopathy resolves over a few weeks to months, with spontaneous suppuration occurring in 10%–50% of patients. If the primary inoculation is in the conjunctiva, there is chronic granulomatous conjunctivitis and preauricular adenopathy—the so-called oculoglandular syndrome of Parinaud. Infrequently, acute encephalopathy, osteolytic lesions, hepatic and splenic abscesses, hypercalcemia, and pulmonary manifestations have been reported. In addition, erythema nodosum and a diffuse exanthem may accompany cat-scratch disease.

Diagnosis is made largely on clinical features. The primary skin lesion or lymph node may be biopsied and the infectious agent identified. Involved lymph nodes and skin lesions demonstrate granulomatous inflammation with central "stellate" necrosis. A serologic test is available, and although not reproducibly positive early in the disease, a titer of more than 1:256 is considered diagnostic of acute infection. A PCR test is becoming increasingly available. Other infectious and neoplastic causes of localized lymphadenopathy, such as tularemia, sporotrichosis, atypical mycobacterial infection, and Hodgkin disease, may need to be excluded.

The vast majority of cases of cat-scratch disease resolve spontaneously without antibiotic therapy. Fluctuant lymph nodes should be aspirated, not incised and drained. The treatment of choice is azithromycin 500 mg the first day followed by 250 mg

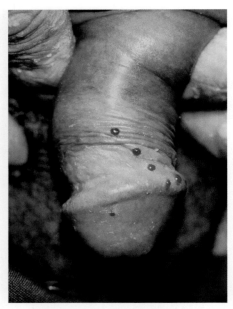

Fig. 14.43 Bacillary angiomatosis.

for 4 days in adults, in children the dose is weight based and given as a liquid.

Trench Fever

Trench fever is caused by *Bartonella quintana*, which is spread from person to person by the body louse. Urban cases of trench fever caused by this agent are now most often seen in louse-infested homeless persons. Patients present with fever that initially lasts about 1 week and then recurs about every 5 days. Other symptoms are headache and neck, shin, and back pain. Endocarditis may occur. There are no skin lesions. Treatment has not been studied systematically. Combination IV gentamicin and oral doxycycline is recommended.

Bacillary Angiomatosis

Bacillary angiomatosis describes a clinical condition characterized by vascular skin lesions resembling pyogenic granulomas (Fig. 14.43). Only two organisms have been proven to cause bacillary angiomatosis: *Bartonella henselae* (cause of cat-scratch disease) and *B. quintana* (cause of trench fever). The skin lesions caused by these two organisms are identical. If bacillary angiomatosis is caused by *B. henselae*, there is usually a history of cat exposure, and the same *Bartonella* can also be isolated from the blood of the source cat. Bacillary angiomatosis caused by *B. quintana* is associated with homelessness and louse infestation. The incubation period is unknown but may be years.

Bacillary angiomatosis occurs primarily in the setting of immunosuppression, especially AIDS, and may be the presenting sign of this condition. The helper T-cell count is usually less than 50 cells/mL. Other immunosuppressed patients, such as those with leukemia or transplant, may acquire the condition. Rarely, bacillary angiomatosis can occur in HIV-negative patients with no apparent immune impairment. In immunoincompetent hosts, the bacteria proliferate locally and are frequently blood-borne. The local proliferation of bacteria produces the angiogenic vascular endothelial growth factor (VEGF), leading to endothelial cell proliferation and the characteristic skin lesions. Immunocompetent hosts generally resist this bacterial proliferation, resulting in granulomatous and necrotic, rather than angiomatous, lesions.

Several different forms of cutaneous lesions occur. The most common form resembles pyogenic granuloma, which may exhibit a surrounding collarete of scale. Less often, subcutaneous masses, plaques, and ulcerations may occur. A single patient may exhibit several of these morphologies. Lesions are tender and bleed easily. Subcutaneous nodules may be poorly marginated. Lesions may number from one to thousands, usually with the number gradually increasing over time if the patient is untreated.

In the setting of bacillary angiomatosis, the infection must be considered disseminated. Bacteremia is detected in about 50% of affected AIDS patients, leading to involvement of many visceral sites, most frequently the lymph node, liver and spleen, and bone. Less frequently, pulmonary, GI, muscle, oral, and brain lesions can occur. *B. henselae* is usually associated with lymph node and liver and spleen involvement, whereas *B. quintana* more often causes bone disease and subcutaneous masses. Visceral disease can be confirmed by appropriate radiologic or imaging studies. Bone lesions are typically lytic, resembling osteomyelitis. In the liver and spleen, "peliosis" occurs. Liver function tests characteristically demonstrate a very elevated lactic dehydrogenase level, an elevated alkaline phosphatase level, slight elevation of the levels of hepatocellular enzymes, and a normal bilirubin level. Lesions on other epithelial surfaces, in muscle, and in lymph nodes are usually angiomatous.

Biopsies of bacillary angiomatosis skin lesions have the same low-power appearance as a pyogenic granuloma, with the proliferation of endothelial cells, forming normal small blood vessels. It is distinguished from pyogenic granuloma by the presence of neutrophils throughout the lesion, not just on the surface, as seen in a pyogenic granuloma. The neutrophils are sometimes aggregated around granular material that stains slightly purple. This purple material represents clusters of organisms, which can often be confirmed by a modified silver stain such as Steiner. Tissue Gram stain does not routinely stain the bacteria in bacillary angiomatosis lesions. Bacillary angiomatosis is easily distinguished histologically from Kaposi sarcoma. In patch or plaque lesions of Kaposi sarcoma, the new blood vessels are abnormal in appearance, being angulated. Endothelial proliferation in Kaposi sarcoma is seen in the dermis around the eccrine units, follicular structures, and existing normal vessels. Nodular Kaposi sarcoma is a spindle cell tumor with slits rather than well-formed blood vessels. Neutrophils and purple granular material are not found in Kaposi sarcoma, but intracellular hyaline globules are present.

The natural history of bacillary angiomatosis is extremely variable. In most patients, however, lesions remain stable or the size or number of lesions gradually increases over time. The initial lesions are usually the largest, and multiple satellite or disseminated smaller lesions occur, representing miliary spread. Untreated bacillary angiomatosis can be fatal, with patients dying of visceral disease or respiratory compromise from obstructing lesions.

The diagnosis of bacillary angiomatosis is virtually always made by identifying the infectious agent in affected tissue. The organisms can also be cultured from the lesions and the patient's blood. However, these organisms grow very slowly, so cultures may not be positive for more than 1 month. Thus tissue and blood cultures are usually confirmatory in nature. Antibodies to *Bartonella* can be detected in most patients but background positivity in the general population of cat owners, this test is not generally useful. PCR is becoming increasingly available.

Treatment

Bacillary angiomatosis is dramatically responsive to clarithromycin 500 mg twice daily or azithromycin 250 mg daily. Treatment should continue for at least 6 months after the treated HIV patient's CD count is above 200 cells/microliter. Once treatment is begun, symptoms begin to resolve within hours to days. A Jarisch-Herxheimer reaction may occur with the first dose of antibiotic.

If patients relapse after an apparently adequate course of treatment, chronic suppressive antibiotic therapy should be considered. Erythromycin and doxycycline may also be effective. TMP-SMX, ciprofloxacin, penicillins, and cephalosporins are not effective. Prophylactic regimens containing a macrolide antibiotic or rifampin prevent the development of bacillary angiomatosis.

Oroya Fever and Verruga Peruana

Oroya fever and verruga peruana represent two stages of the same infection. Oroya fever (Carrión disease) is the acute febrile stage, and verruga peruana the chronic delayed stage. These conditions are limited to and endemic in Peru and a few neighboring countries in the Andes and are restricted to valleys 500–3200 m above sea level. Both these conditions are caused by *Bartonella bacilliformis*, which is transmitted by a sandfly, usually *Lutzomyia verrucarum*. Humans represent the only known reservoir. Men represent about three quarters of cases, and all ages may be affected.

After an incubation period averaging 3 weeks, the acute infection, Oroya fever, develops. Symptomatology is highly variable. Some patients have very mild symptoms. Others may have high fever, headache, and arthralgias. Severe hemolytic anemia can develop, sometimes with leukopenia and thrombocytopenia. Untreated, the fatality rate is 40%–88%, and with antibiotic treatment, is still 8%. After the acute infection resolves, a latency period follows, lasting from weeks to months. The verruga peruana eruptions then occur; these are angiomatous, pyogenic granuloma–like lesions, virtually identical clinically and histologically to the lesions of bacillary angiomatosis (Fig. 14.44). The lesions may be large and few in number (mular form), small and disseminated (miliary form), or nodular and deep. Visceral disease has not been found in verruga peruana, which is rarely fatal. Lesions usually heal spontaneously over several weeks to months without scarring. A lasting immunity results from infection.

The diagnosis of Oroya fever is made by identifying the bacteria within or attached to circulating erythrocytes using a Giemsa stain. Verruga peruana can be diagnosed by skin biopsy, showing the same features as bacillary angiomatosis, but with the organisms staining with Giemsa.

The antibiotic treatment of choice for Oroya fever is chloramphenicol, 2 g/day, because *Salmonella* coinfection is the most

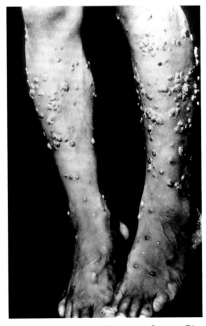

Fig. 14.44 Verruga peruana. (Courtesy Steven Binnick, MD.)

frequent cause of death. Protection from sandfly bites is all important.

Al-Thunayan A, et al: Bacillary angiomatosis presenting as a pyogenic granuloma of the hand in an otherwise apparently healthy patient. Ann Plast Surg 2013; 70: 652.

Anstead GM: The centenary of the discovery of trench fever, an emerging infectious disease of World War 1. Lancet Infect Dis 2016; 16: e164.

Chomel BB, et al: Bartonellosis, an increasingly recognized zoonosis. J Appl Microbiol 2010; 109: 743.

Gai M, et al: Cat-scratch disease. Transplant Proc 2015; 47: 2245.

Mejia F, et al: Bacillary angiomatosis. Am J Trop Med Hyg 2014; 91: 439.

Minnick MF, et al: Oroya fever and verruga peruana. PLoS Negl Trop Dis 2014; 8: e2919.

Pierad-Franhimont C, et al: Skin disease associated with *Bartonella* infection. Clin Dermatol 2010; 28: 483.

Zangwill KM: Cat scratch disease and other *Bartonella* infections. Adv Exp Med Biol 2013; 764: 159.

PLAGUE

Plague normally involves an interaction among *Yersinia pestis*, wild rodents, and fleas parasitic on the rodents. Infection in humans with *Y. pestis* is accidental and usually presents as bubonic plague. Other clinical forms include pneumonic and septicemic plague. In the milder form, the initial manifestations are general malaise, fever, and pain or tenderness in areas of regional lymph nodes, most often in the inguinal or axillary regions. In more severe infections, findings of toxicity, prostration, shock, and occasionally hemorrhagic phenomena prevail. Less common symptoms include abdominal pain, nausea, vomiting, constipation followed by diarrhea, generalized macular erythema, and petechiae. Rarely, vesicular and pustular skin lesions occur.

Plague is caused by *Y. pestis*, a pleomorphic, gram-negative bacillus. The principal animal hosts involved have been rock squirrels, prairie dogs, chipmunks, marmots, skunks, deer mice, wood rats, rabbits, and hares. Transmission occurs through contact with infected rodent fleas or rodents, pneumonic spread, or infected exudates. *Xenopsylla cheopis* (Oriental rat flea) has traditionally been considered the vector in human outbreaks, but *Diamanus montanus*, *Thrassis bacchi*, and *Opisocrostis hirsutus* are species of fleas on wild animals responsible for spreading sylvatic plague in the United States. Rodents carried home by dogs or cats are a potential source—and an important one in veterinarians—of infection. The bites, scratches, or contact with other infectious material while handling infected cats are important factors as residential development continues in areas of plague foci in the western United States. Most U.S. cases occur in the Rocky Mountain states.

Blood, bubo or parabubo aspirates, exudates, and sputum should be examined by smears with Gram stain or specific fluorescent antibody techniques, culture, and animal inoculation. A retrospective diagnosis can be made by serologic analysis.

The most effective drugs against *Y. pestis* are gentamicin and streptomycin, which should be given intravenously. Almost all cases are fatal if not treated promptly.

Anderson PD, et al: Bioterrorism. J Pharm Pract 2012; 25: 521.

Prentice MB, et al: Plague. Lancet 2007; 369: 1196.

Zeppelini CG, et al: Zoonoses as ecological entities. PLoS Negl Trop Dis 2016; 10: e0004949.

RAT-BITE FEVER

Rat-bite fever is a systemic illness usually acquired by direct contact with rats or other small rodents, which carry the gram-negative organisms *Spirillum minor* and *Streptobacillus moniliformis* among their oropharyngeal flora. *S. moniliformis* is the principal cause in the United States, whereas *S. minor* is seen mostly in Asia. Crowded living conditions, homelessness, working with rats in medical research or in pet shops, or having one as a pet are predisposing factors in some infected patients. Although it usually follows a rat bite, infection may follow the bites of squirrels, cats, weasels, pigs, and a variety of other carnivores that feed on rats.

There are at least two distinct forms of rat-bite fever: "sodoku," caused by *Spirillum minor*; and septicemia, caused by *Streptobacillus moniliformis*, otherwise known as epidemic arthritic erythema or Haverhill fever. The latter usually follows the bite of a rat, but some cases have been caused by contaminated milk. The clinical manifestations of these two infections are similar in that both produce a systemic illness characterized by fever, rash, and constitutional symptoms. However, clinical differentiation is possible.

In the streptobacillary form, incubation is brief, usually lasting 10 days after the bite, when chills and fever occur. Within 2–4 more days, the generalized morbilliform eruption appears and spreads to include the palms and soles. It may become petechial. Arthralgia is prominent, and pleural effusion may occur. Endocarditis, pneumonia, and septic infarcts often follow, and 10% of untreated patients may die of these causes.

Although infection with *S. minor* also begins abruptly with chills and fever, the incubation period is longer, 1–4 weeks. The bite site is often inflamed and may become ulcerated. Lymphangitis may be present. The eruption begins with erythematous macules on the abdomen, resembling rose spots, which enlarge, become purplish red, and form extensive indurated plaques. Arthritis may rarely occur. Endocarditis, nephritis, meningitis, and hepatitis are potential complications. About 6% of untreated patients die.

In both types of rat-bite fever, a leukocytosis of 15,000–30,000 cells/mm^3 is present, sometimes with eosinophilia. A biologic false-positive Venereal Disease Research Laboratories (VDRL) test is found in 25%–50% of patients. The course of *S. minor* infection without treatment is generally from 1–2 weeks, though relapses may occur for months.

The diagnosis is confirmed by culturing the causative organism from the blood or joint aspirate, or demonstration of an antibody response in the streptobacillary form. *S. minor* is demonstrable by animal inoculation with the patient's blood, usually in the guinea pig or mouse. Their blood will show large numbers of organisms in Wright-stained smears. Demonstration of *S. minor* in a darkfield preparation of exudate from an infected site establishes the diagnosis.

Rat-bite fever must be differentiated from erysipelas, pyogenic cellulitis, viral exanthems, gonococcemia, meningococcemia, and Rocky Mountain spotted fever.

Prompt cauterization of bites by nitric acid may prevent the disease. Cleansing of the wound, tetanus prophylaxis, and amoxicillin-clavulanate 875/125 mg are recommended for patients seen shortly after a bite. Both types respond readily to penicillin or doxycycline therapy.

Adam JK, et al: Notes from the field: fatal rat-bite fever in a child—San Diego County, California, 2013. MMWR Morb Mortal Wkly Rep. 2014 Dec 19;63(50):1210-1.

Chean R, et al: Rat bite fever as a presenting illness in a patient with AIDS. Infection 2012; 40: 319.

Kawakami Y, et al: A case of *Streptobacillus moniliformis* infection with cutaneous leukocytoclastic vasculitis. Acta Med Okayama 2016; 70: 377.

Lewis BK, et al: Rat bite fever. Pediatr Dermatol 2012; 29: 767.

TULAREMIA

Tularemia, also known as Ohara disease or deer fly fever, is a febrile disease caused by *Francisella tularensis*, a short, nonmotile, non-spore-forming, gram-negative coccobacillus. Tularemia is

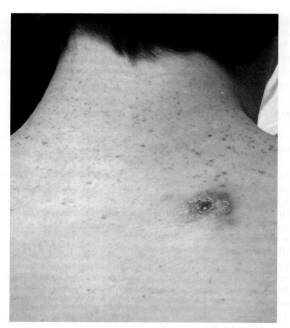

Fig. 14.45 Tularemia. (Courtesy Stephen D. Hess, MD, PhD.)

characterized by sudden onset, with chills, headache, and leukocytosis, after an incubation period of 2–7 days. Its clinical course is divided into several general types. The causative organism poses a bioterrorism threat.

The vast majority of tularemia cases are the ulceroglandular type, which begins with a primary papule or nodule that rapidly ulcerates at the site of infection. This usually occurs through contact with tissues or body fluids of infected mammals from an abrasion or scratch (Fig. 14.45), usually on the fingers, neck, or conjunctiva. The bites of a tick, *Dermacentor andersoni* or *Amblyomma americanum*, and of a deer fly, *Chrysops discalis*, also transmit this disease, and in such cases, primary lesions are usually found on the legs or the perineum. The primary ulcer is tender, firm, indolent, and punched out, with a necrotic base that heals with scar formation in about 6 weeks. A lymphangitis spreads from the primary lesion; the regional lymph glands become swollen, painful, and inflamed, and tend to break down, forming suppurative subcutaneous nodules resembling those of sporotrichosis. The ulcers extend in a chain from the ulcer to the enlarged lymphatic glands.

The course of the ulceroglandular type is marked in the early stages by headache, anorexia, and vomiting, as well as articular and muscular pains. The fever is at first continuous, varying between 102°F and 104°F (38.8°C and 40°C), and later shows morning remissions, then falls by lysis to normal. Other skin lesions encountered in the disease course are not characteristic and are probably of a toxic or reactive nature. A macular, papular, vesicular, or petechial exanthem may occur. Erythema multiforme and erythema nodosum often occur.

In the typhoidal type, the site of inoculation is not known, and there is no local sore or adenopathy. This form of tularemia is characterized by persistent fever, malaise, GI symptoms, and the presence of specific agglutinins in the blood serum after the first week. Other, uncommon types include an oculoglandular form, in which primary conjunctivitis is accompanied by enlargement of the regional lymph nodes. The pneumonic type occurs rarely in laboratory workers and is most severe. The oropharyngeal form may occur after ingestion of infected and inadequately cooked meat. In the glandular type, there is no primary lesion at the site of infection, but there is enlargement of regional lymph glands followed by generalized involvement. Several cases, mostly in children, have been acquired from cat bites, the cats having previously bitten infected rabbits.

The most frequent sources of human infection are the handling of wild rabbits and the bite of deer flies or ticks. Outbreaks of tularemia occur chiefly at times of the year when contact with these sources of infection is likely. No instance of the spread of the infection from person to person by contact has been reported. The disease occurs most often in the western and southern United States, although cases have been reported in almost all states and in Japan. In Russia and other countries in the Northern Hemisphere, tularemia may be contracted from polluted water contaminated by infected rodent carcasses.

A definite diagnosis is made by staining smears obtained from the exudate with specific fluorescent antibody. *F. tularensis* can be cultured only on special media containing cystine glucose blood agar or other selective media. Routine culture media do not support growth. The bacilli can be identified by inoculating guinea pigs intraperitoneally with sputum or with bronchial or gastric washings, exudate from draining lymph nodes, or blood. The agglutination titer becomes positive in the majority of patients after 2 weeks of illness. A fourfold rise in titer is diagnostic; a single convalescent titer of 1:160 or greater is diagnostic of past or current infection. PCR is also successful in identifying the infectious agent.

The main histologic feature of tularemia is that of a granuloma; the tissue reaction consists primarily of endothelial cells and the formation of giant cells. Central necrosis and liquefaction occur, accompanied by polymorphonuclear leukocyte infiltration. Surrounding this is a tuberculoid granulomatous zone, and peripherally lymphocytes form a third zone. Small secondary lesions may develop. These pass through the same stages and tend to fuse with the primary lesion.

All butchers, hunters, cooks, and others who dress rabbits should wear protective gloves. Thorough cooking destroys the infection in a rabbit, thus rendering an infected animal harmless as food. Ticks should be removed promptly, and tick repellents may be of value for people with occupations that require frequent exposure.

Streptomycin given intravenously is the treatment of choice. IV gentamicin, or oral doxycycline or ciprofloxacin are alternatives.

Baggett MV, et al: A 58-year-old woman with a skin ulcer, fever, and lymphadenopathy. N Engl J Med 2016; 374: 573.
Carvalho CL, et al: Tularaemia. Comp Immunol Microbiol Infect Dis 2014; 37: 85.
Joseph B, et al: Current concepts in the management of biologic and chemical warfare causalities. J Trauma Acute Care Surg 2013; 75: 582.
Senel E, et al: Dermatologic manifestations of tularemia. Int J Dermatol 2015; 54: e33.
Ulu-Kilic A, Doganay M: An overview: tularemia and travel medicine. Travel Med Infect Dis 2014; 12: 609.

BRUCELLOSIS

Brucellosis is also known as undulant fever. *Brucellae* are gram-negative rods that produce an acute febrile illness with headache, or at times an indolent chronic disease characterized by weakness, malaise, and low-grade fever. Brucellosis is acquired primarily by contact with infected animals or animal products. Workers in the meatpacking industry are mainly at risk; however, veterinarians, pet owners, and travelers who consume unpasteurized milk or cheese may also contract the disease. Approximately 5%–10% of patients develop skin lesions. The large variety of cutaneous manifestations reported include erythematous papules, diffuse erythema, abscesses, erysipelas-like lesions, leukocytoclastic vasculitis, thrombocytopenic purpura, SJS, and erythema nodosum–like lesions. Biopsy may reveal noncaseating granulomas. Diagnosis is by culture of blood, bone marrow, or granulomas and may be confirmed by a rising serum enzyme-linked immunosorbent assay

(ELISA) or agglutination titer. PCR is available as well. Treatment is with doxycycline and gentamicin in combination.

Albayrak A, et al: Two brucellosis cases with vasculitic skin lesions. Rheumatol Int 2014; 34: 575.
Buzgan T, et al: Clinical manifestations and complications in 1028 cases of brucellosis. Int J Infect Dis 2010; 14: e469.
Norman FF, et al: Imported brucellosis. Travel Med Infect Dis 2016; 14: 182.
Ulu-Kilic A, et al: Clinical presentations and diagnosis of brucellosis. Recent Pat Antiinfect Drug Discov 2013; 8: 34.

■ RICKETTSIAL DISEASES

Rickettsiae are obligate, intracellular, gram-negative bacteria. The natural reservoirs of these organisms are the blood-sucking arthropods; when transmitted to humans through insect inoculation, the rickettsiae may produce disease. Most of the human diseases incurred are characterized by skin eruptions, fever, headache, malaise, and prostration. Diagnosis is usually made on a clinical basis and is confirmed by indirect fluorescence antibody testing, which may be verified by Western blot or PCR. Therapy is with doxycycline, 100 mg twice daily for 7 days. In addition to the diseases discussed in the following sections, Q fever, caused by *Coxiella burnetii*, is an acute febrile illness from this general class that infrequently has skin manifestations, but these are nonspecific and nondiagnostic in nature.

TYPHUS GROUP

Louse-borne epidemic typhus, caused by *Rickettsia prowazekii*; mouse, cat, or rat flea-borne endemic typhus, caused by *Rickettsia typhi*; and scrub typhus, a mite-borne infection caused by *Rickettsia tsutsugamushi*, constitute the typhus group.

Epidemic Typhus

Humans contract epidemic typhus from an infestation by body lice (*Pediculus humanus* var. *corporis*), which harbor the rickettsiae. *R. prowazekii* is not transmitted transovarially because it kills the louse 1–3 weeks after infection. For many years, humans were the only known vector, but several cases of sporadic disease have been reported involving direct or indirect contact with the flying squirrel, and a reservoir exists in this animal. While the louse feeds on the person's skin, it defecates. The organisms in the feces are scratched into the skin. Some 2 weeks after infection, the prodromal symptoms of chills, fever, aches, and pains appear. After 5 days, a pink macular eruption appears on the trunk and axillary folds and rapidly spreads to the rest of the body, but usually spares the face, palms, and soles. These macules may later become hemorrhagic (Fig. 14.46), and gangrene of the fingers, toes, nose, and earlobes may occur.

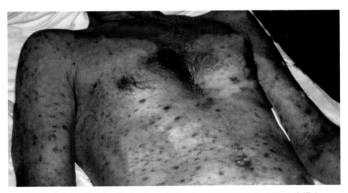

Fig. 14.46 Epidemic typhus. (Courtesy Richard DeVillez, MD.)

Mortality rate is 6%–30% in epidemics, with the highest death and complication rates occurring in patients over age 60.

Serologic testing using immunofluorescent antibody (IFA) and Western blot for specificity becomes positive after the 8th–12th day of illness. Doxycycline, 100 mg twice daily for 7 days, is curative. Prophylaxis is by vaccination and delousing; people who succumb are usually living under miserable sanitary conditions, as occur during war and after natural disasters. Vaccination is suggested only for special high-risk groups.

Brill-Zinsser disease may occur as a recrudescence of previous infection, with a similar but milder course of illness that more closely resembles endemic typhus.

Endemic Typhus

Endemic (murine) typhus is a natural infection of rats and mice by *R. typhi*, sporadically transmitted to humans by the rat flea, *Xenopsylla cheopis*. In south Texas, the disease is transmitted by the cat flea, *Ctenocephalides felis*, with opossums as the natural reservoir of disease. Endemic typhus has the same skin manifestations as epidemic typhus, but these are less severe, and gangrene does not supervene. Approximately 50% of patients with murine typhus have a skin eruption. Serologic testing using IFA and Western blot for specificity becomes positive in 50% of patients at 1 week and almost all by 2 weeks. Fever and severe headache are suggestive early symptoms. Endemic typhus occurs worldwide. In the United States the southeastern states bordering the Gulf of Mexico, especially Texas, and California and Hawaii have been the most common sites of incidence. It most often occurs in urban settings, with peak incidence in the summer and fall. Treatment is the same as that for louse-borne (epidemic) typhus.

Scrub Typhus

Also known as tsutsugamushi fever, scrub typhus is characterized by fever, chills, intense headache, skin lesions, and pneumonitis. The primary lesion is an erythematous papule at the site of a mite bite, most often on the scrotum, groin, or ankle. It becomes indurated, and a multilocular vesicle rests atop the papule. Eventually, a necrotic ulcer with eschar and surrounding indurated erythema develops, and there is regional lymphadenopathy. About 10 days after a mite bite, fever, chills, and prostration develop, and within another 5 days, pneumonitis and the skin eruption evolve. The erythematous macular eruption begins on the trunk, extends peripherally, and fades in a few days. Deafness and tinnitus occur in about one fifth of untreated patients.

Scrub typhus is caused by *R. tsutsugamushi*. The vector is the trombiculid red mite (chigger), which infests wild rodents in scrub or secondary vegetation in transitional terrain between forests and clearings in Far Eastern countries such as Japan, Korea, Southeast Asia, and Australia. Serologic diagnosis and treatment are as for other forms of rickettsias; however, in areas of the world where there is reduced susceptibility to tetracyclines, such as Thailand, rifampin is more reliable.

SPOTTED FEVER GROUP

The spotted fever group includes Rocky Mountain spotted fever, caused by *Rickettsia rickettsii*; Mediterranean (boutonneuse) fever, which when seen in Africa has been called Kenyan or South African tick-bite fever, caused by *R. conorii*; North Asian tick-borne rickettsiosis, caused by *R. sibirica*; Queensland tick typhus, caused by *R. australis*; African tick-bite fever, caused by *R. africae*; Flinders Island spotted fever, caused by *R. honei*; Yucatan spotted fever, caused by *R. felis* carried by the cat flea vector *Ctenocephalides felis*; Japanese spotted fever, caused by *R. japonica*; a spotted fever in the United States caused by *R. parkeri* and one in California caused by *Rickettsia* 364D; Russian vesicular

rickettsiosis, caused by *R. akari* and a novel case in Brazil caused by *Rickettsia* sp. in the Atlantic rainforest. Additionally, tick-borne lymphadenopathy (TIBOLA) and *Dermacentor*-borne necrosis–eschar–lymphadenopathy (DEBONEL) are linked to a disease transmitted by the *Dermacentor* tick; they have distinctive features. The tick usually attaches to the scalp and will cause an eschar and sometimes alopecia. Adenopathy, fever, and a spotted eruption occur.

Only the first two types of spotted fever listed, Rocky Mountain and Mediterranean, are discussed here in detail. All spotted fevers are characterized by headache, fever, and a rash, the latter most frequently being a pink papular eruption, which may have petechiae, and in the case of African tick-bite fever, eschars. All are treated with doxycycline, 100 mg twice daily for 7 days. Most patients respond well, and complications are minimal. Ticks are the vectors of all except Yucatan spotted fever. Tick prevention strategies are outlined in Chapter 20.

Rocky Mountain Spotted Fever

At 1–2 weeks after the tick bite, chills, fever, and weakness occur. An eruption appears, but unlike typhus, it begins on the ankles, wrists, and forehead rather than the trunk. The initial lesions are small, red macules, which blanch on pressure and rapidly become papular in untreated patients. Spread to the trunk occurs over 6–18 hours, and the lesions become petechial and hemorrhagic over 2–4 days (Fig. 14.47).

A vasculitis of the skin is the pathologic process, and *R. rickettsii* can be found in these initial macules by applying a fluorescent antibody technique to frozen sections. This is a very specific, but not very sensitive, method. In the 10%–20% of patients without a rash, the risk of a delay in diagnosis and a fatal outcome is greatest, with the case-fatality rate rising precipitously if antibiotics are not initiated before the fifth day. An eschar is occasionally present at the tick-bite site and is a subtle clue to the diagnosis. In untreated patients with severe disease, a multisystem disorder appears, with renal, pulmonary, CNS, and peripheral nervous system abnormalities and hepatomegaly most often found. Mortality in older patients approaches 60%, but is much lower in younger patients.

Ticks spread the causative organism, *R. rickettsii*. Principal offenders are the wood tick (*Dermacentor andersoni*), the dog tick (*D. variabilis* and *R. sanguineus* in Arizona), and the Lone Star tick (*Amblyomma americanum*). Antibodies become positive in the second or third week of illness, too late to be of help when the decision to institute therapy is necessary. This decision is made by clinical considerations. A clue may be the recent illness of a pet dog, because *R. rickettsii* will cause symptomatic illness in infected dogs. Treatment is with doxycycline, 100 mg twice daily for 7 days.

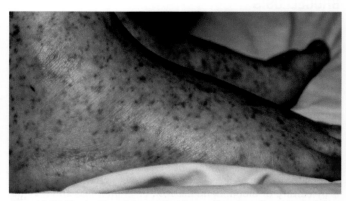

Fig. 14.47 Rocky Mountain spotted fever. (Courtesy Paul Honig, MD.)

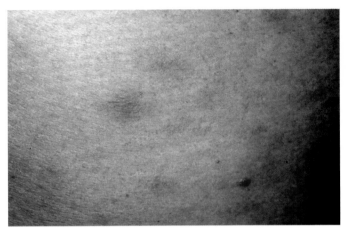

Fig. 14.48 Boutonneuse fever.

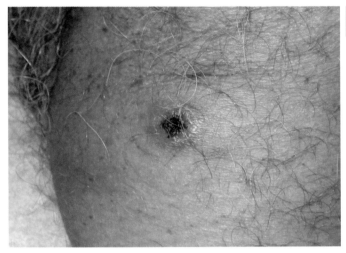

Fig. 14.49 Rickettsialpox.

Mediterranean Spotted Fever

Boutonneuse fever, or Mediterranean fever, is an acute febrile disease endemic in southern Europe and northern Africa; it is the prototype of the spotted fever group of diseases. It affects primarily children and is characterized by a sudden onset with chills, high fever, headache, and lassitude. The tick bite produces an indurated papule known as tache noire, which becomes a necrotic ulcer. The erythematous macular and papular eruption develops on the trunk, palms, and soles (Fig. 14.48).

The causative organism is *Rickettsia conorii*, transmitted by the dog tick, *Rhipicephalus sanguineus*. As with all rickettsial diseases, the diagnosis is confirmed with serology and treatment is with doxycycline. Even without therapy, the prognosis is good, and complications are rare with Mediterranean fever.

RICKETTSIALPOX

First recognized in New York in 1946, rickettsialpox has been found in other U.S. cities and in Russia. It is an acute febrile disease characterized by the appearance of an initial lesion at the site of the mite bite about a week before the onset of the fever. This firm, 5–15 mm, round or oval vesicle persists for 3–4 weeks and heals with a small, pigmented scar. Regional lymphadenitis is present. The fever is remittent and lasts about 5 days. Chills, sweats, headache, and backache accompany the fever. A rash resembling varicella develops 3 or 4 days after onset of fever (Fig. 14.49). This secondary eruption is papulovesicular, numbers about 5 up to 50 lesions, and is generalized in distribution. It fades in about 1 week.

The rodent mite, *Allodermanyssus (Liponyssoides) sanguineus*, transmits the causative organism, *Rickettsia akari*. The house mouse, *Mus musculus*, is the reservoir. All cases have occurred in neighborhoods infested by mice, on which the rodent mite has been found. Diagnosis is confirmed by serologic testing. The disease is self-limited, and complete involution occurs in, at most, 2 weeks. Doxycycline is the agent of choice for treatment of rickettsialpox.

Badiaga S, Brouqui P: Human louse-transmitted infectious diseases. Clin Microbiol Infect 2012; 18: 332.

Badiaga S, et al: Murine typhus in the homeless. Comp Immunol Microbiol Infect Dis 2012; 35: 39.

Buckingham SC: Tick-borne diseases of the USA. J Infect 2015; 71: S88.

Channick RN, et al: A 60-year-old man with weakness, rash and renal failure. N Engl J Med 2012; 366: 1434.

Couto DV, et al: Brazilian spotted fever. An Bras Dermatol 2015; 90: 248.

Faucher JF, et al: Brill-Zinsser disease in a Moroccan man. Emerg Infect Dis 2012; 18: 171.

Lee CS, Hwang JH: Scrub typhus. N Engl J Med 2015; 373: 2455.

Maya RM, et al: Rocky Mountain spotted fever in a patient treated with anti-TNF-α inhibitors. Dermatol Online J 2013; 19: 7.

Mukkada S, Buckingham SC: Recognition of and prompt treatment for tick-borne infections in children. Infect Dis Clin North Am 2015; 29: 539.

Pieracci EG, et al: Fatal flea-borne typhus in Texas. Am J Trop Med Hyg 2017; 96: 1088.

Portillo A, et al: Rickettsioses in Europe. Microbes Infect 2015; 17: 834.

Silva-Pinto A, et al: Tick-borne lymphadenopathy, an emerging disease. Ticks Tick Borne Dis 2014; 5: 656.

Sivarajan S, et al: Clinical and paraclinical profile, and predictors of outcome in 90 cases of scrub typhus, Meghalaya, India. Infect Dis Poverty 2016; 5: 91.

Tsioutis C, et al: Murine typhus in elderly patients. Scand J Infect Dis 2014; 46: 779.

Walker DH: Scrub typhus—scientific neglect, ever-widening impact. N Engl J Med 2016; 375: 913.

Walter G, et al: Murine typhus in returned travelers. Am J Trop Med Hyg 2012; 86: 1049.

Woods CR: Rocky Mountain spotted fever in children. Pediatr Clin North Am 2013; 60: 455.

EHRLICHIOSIS

The tick-borne ehrlichial organisms, which affect phagocytic cells, manifest as a febrile illness accompanied by headache and a rash. Human monocytic ehrlichiosis (HME) is caused by *Ehrlichia chaffeensis;* human granulocytic anaplasmosis (HGA) by *Anaplasma phagocytophilia* groups; Sennetsu fever, a mononucleosis-type illness, by *Ehrlichia sennetsu;* and *Ehrlichia ewingii* all produce a similar symptomatic illness. HME is transmitted by *Amblyomma americanum* or *Dermacentor variabilis*. It is most common in men age 30–60. The predominant U.S. regions reporting ehrlichiosis are the south-central, southeastern, and mid-Atlantic states. The same *Ixodes* ticks that transmit Lyme disease and babesiosis transmit HGA, and the infection occurs in the same geographic areas, the northeast and Pacific northwestern United States. Coinfection with these agents occurs.

Skin eruptions are present in only about one third of HME patients and 10% of HGA patients. The lesions are usually present on the trunk and are nondiagnostic. A mottled or diffuse erythema, a fine petechial eruption, lower extremity vasculitis, and a macular, papular, vesicular, or urticarial morphology have all been seen. Acral edema with desquamation and petechiae of the palate may be present. Involvement of the kidneys, lungs, and CNS occurs in severe cases.

If the diagnosis is suspected, a complete blood count will usually show thrombocytopenia and leukopenia. The leukocytes should be inspected microscopically for intracytoplasmic microcolonies called morulae, seen more frequently in HGA than HME. IFA testing and PCR analysis are positive, but asymptomatic infection is common, and seroprevalence rates are high in endemic areas. Culture of the organism is diagnostic. Doxycycline is the treatment of choice, 100 mg twice daily for 7 days. Life-threatening disease is usually seen in the immunosuppressed population.

Choi E, et al: Tick-borne illnesses. Curr Sports Med Rep 2016; 15: 98.

Ismail N, et al: Human ehrlichiosis and anaplasmosis. Clin Lab Med 2010; 30: 261.

Shah RG, et al: Clinical approach to known and emerging tick-borne infections other than Lyme disease. Curr Opin Pediatr 2013; 25: 407.

LEPTOSPIROSIS

Leptospirosis is a systemic disease caused by many strains of the genus *Leptospira*. After an incubation period of 8–12 days, Weil disease (icteric leptospirosis) starts with an abrupt onset of chills, followed by high fever, intense jaundice, petechiae, and purpura on both skin and mucous membranes, and renal disease, manifested by proteinuria, hematuria, and azotemia. Death may occur in 5%–10% of patients as a result of renal failure, vascular collapse, or hemorrhage. Leukocytosis of 15,000–30,000 cells/mm^3 and lymphocytosis in CSF are usually present.

Pretibial fever (Fort Bragg fever, anicteric leptospirosis) has an associated acute exanthematous infectious erythema, generally most marked on the shins. High fever, conjunctival suffusion, nausea, vomiting, and headache characterize the septicemic first stage. This lasts 3–7 days, followed by a 1- to 3-day absence of fever. During the second stage, when immunoglobulin M (IgM) antibody develops, headache is intense, fever returns, and ocular manifestations, such as conjunctival hemorrhage and suffusion, ocular pain, and photophobia, are prominent. At this time, the eruption occurs. It consists of 1–5 cm erythematous patches or plaques that histologically show only edema and nonspecific perivascular infiltrate. The skin lesions resolve spontaneously after 4–7 days. There may be different clinical manifestations from identical strains of *Leptospira*.

Leptospira interrogans, serotype *icterohaemorrhagiae*, has been the most common cause of Weil disease, whereas pretibial fever is most often associated with serotype *autumnalis*. Humans acquire both types accidentally from urine or tissues of infected animals or indirectly from contaminated soil or from drinking or swimming in contaminated water. Travelers to the tropics who engage in water sports are at risk. In the continental United States, dogs and cats are the most common animal source; worldwide, rats are more often responsible. Leptospira enter the body through abraded or diseased skin and the GI or upper respiratory tract.

Leptospirosis may be diagnosed by finding the causative spirochetes in the blood by darkfield microscopy during the first week of illness, as well as by blood cultures, guinea pig inoculation, and the demonstration of rising antibodies during the second week of the disease. The microagglutination serologic test is the test of choice, but PCR and ELISA testing are also available.

Treatment with tetracyclines and penicillin shortens the disease duration if given early. Doxycycline, 100 mg/day for 1 week, is effective in mild disease; however, IV penicillin is necessary in severely affected patients. A dose of 200 mg once weekly may help prevent infection while visiting a hyperendemic area.

Brett-Major DM, et al: Antibiotic prophylaxis for leptospirosis. Cochrane Database Syst Rev 2009; CD007342.

Haake DA, Levett PN: Leptospirosis in humans. Curr Top Microbiol Immunol 2015; 387: 65.

Picardeau M: Diagnosis and epidemiology of leptospirosis. Med Mal Infect 2013; 43: 1.

Rajapakse S, et al: Current immunological and molecular tools for leptospirosis. Ann Clin Microbiol Antimicrob 2015; 14: 2.

BORRELIOSIS

Spirochetes of the genus *Borrelia* are the cause of Lyme disease. This multisystem infection first presents with skin findings, and over time, multiple cutaneous signs may occur. These microorganisms are also the cause of relapsing fever, an acute illness characterized by paroxysms of fever. The more common type of relapsing fever is tick-borne, occasionally being reported in the United States. A louse-borne type is endemic only in Ethiopia. The nonspecific macular or petechial eruption occurs near the end of the 3- to 5-day febrile crisis.

Lyme Disease

Borrelia burgdorferi sensu lato species complex are responsible for inducing Lyme disease. These spirochetes are transmitted to humans by various members of the family of hard ticks, Ixodidae. Thirteen genomic strains are recognized to be geographically prominent and cause varying skin and systemic disease manifestations. *Borrelia burgdorferi* sensu stricto causes Lyme disease in the United States. *Borrelia lonestari* (a relapsing fever type of *Borrelia*, not in the *B. burgdorferi* sensu lato complex) causes disease in the southern states. It is transmitted by the bite of the Lone Star tick (*Amblyomma americanum*), is the cause of southern tick-associated rash illness (STARI), or Masters disease, a condition characterized by erythema migrans, headache, stiff neck, myalgia, and arthralgia. *Borrelia garinii* and *Borrelia afzelii* are two major strains present in Europe, with *B. garinii* the principal agent of Lyme neuroborreliosis and *B. afzelii* associated with acrodermatitis chronica atrophicans, lymphocytoma, and in some cases, morphea and lichen sclerosis et atrophicus. If disease is not treated in the early stage, chronic arthritis and neurologic and cardiac complications frequently develop. Other strains are present in Europe and Asia, with a few reports implicating them in rare cases of Lyme disease.

Diagnosing early Lyme disease depends on recognition of the skin eruption. Approximately 50% of patients recall a tick bite, which leaves a small, red macule or papule at the site. The sites most often involved are the legs, groin, and axilla, with adults having lower extremity lesions most often and children more likely to manifest erythema migrans on the trunk. Between 3 and 32 days (median 7) after the bite, there is gradual expansion of the redness around the papule (Fig. 14.50A). The advancing border is usually slightly raised, warm, red to bluish red, and free of any scale. Centrally, the site of the bite may clear, leaving only a ring of peripheral erythema, or it may remain red, becoming indurated, vesicular, or necrotic. In Europe, the large annular variety is most common, whereas in the United States the lesions are usually homogeneous or have a central redness. The annular erythema usually grows to a median diameter of 15 cm but may range from 3–68 cm (Fig. 14.50B). It is accompanied by a burning sensation in half of patients; rarely is it pruritic or painful. Localized alopecia may develop at the site of erythema migrans.

period. Malaise, fever, fatigue, headaches, stiff neck, arthralgia, myalgia, lymphadenopathy, anorexia, and nausea and vomiting may accompany early signs and symptoms of infection. Nonspecific findings include an elevated erythrocyte sedimentation rate in 50% and an elevated IgM level, mild anemia, and elevated liver function tests in 20% of patients. Usually, the symptoms are of mild severity, mimicking a slight flulike illness, except in patients coinfected with babesiosis, as in approximately 10% of cases in southern New England. *Ehrlichia* coinfections may also occur, because the latter two diseases are also tick-transmitted infections.

Males and females are equally affected, and the age range most often affected is of bimodal type, with an early peak at 5–19 and a later peak at 55–69 years. Onset of illness is generally between May and November, with more than 80% of cases in the Northern Hemisphere identified in June, July, or August. In the United States tick transmission of Lyme disease is by *Ixodes scapularis* in the Northeast and Midwest, and *Ixodes pacificus* is incriminated in the West. European cases are transmitted by the ticks *Ixodes ricinus* and *I. persulcatus*, and in Asia by *I. ovatus* and *I. persulcatus*.

The different subtypes of *Borrelia* present in Europe account for the clinical illness resulting from infection being somewhat different from that seen in the United States. In Europe a wider array of skin manifestations occur. There, erythema migrans occurs more often in females, is less likely to have multiple lesions, and the lesions last longer if untreated. European cases may also manifest *Borrelia*-induced lymphocytoma. It occurs from the time of erythema migrans until 10 months later. These are B-cell proliferations and present as red, indurated papules and plaques, which occur most often on the areola or earlobe. Acrodermatitis chronica atrophicans (see below) and some cases of morphea, atrophoderma of Pasini and Pierini, anetoderma, and lichen sclerosus et atrophicus are late cutaneous sequelae *of Borrelia afzelii* or *B. garinii* infection in Europe. Some patients with morphea-type lesions may have histopathologic features of an interstitial granulomatous dermatitis with histiocytic pseudorosettes present.

About 10% of untreated U.S. patients eventually develop a chronic arthritis of the knees, which in half of patients leads to severe disability. The arthritis symptoms are unusual in Europe. Cardiac involvement occurs most often in young men, with fluctuating degrees of atrioventricular block or complete heart block occurring over a brief time, 3 days to 6 weeks, early in the course of the illness. In European cases, a dilated cardiomyopathy may eventuate. Neurologic findings include stiff neck, headache, meningitis, cognitive deficits, paresthesias and radiculopathy, Bell palsy, optic neuritis, vestibular neuronitis, oculomotor palsy, and cranial and peripheral neuropathies and are much more frequently manifested in European patients. In Europe, infection may lead to Bannwarth syndrome, which is characterized by focal, severe, radicular pains; lymphocytic meningitis; and cranial nerve paralysis.

Several cases of transplacental transmission of *Borrelia* resulting in infant death have been reported. However, studies of Lyme disease in pregnancy have generally failed to implicate an association with fetal malformations directly.

Biopsy of erythema migrans reveals a superficial and deep perivascular and interstitial mixed-cell infiltrate. Lymphocytes, plasma cells, and eosinophils may be seen, the latter especially prominent when the center of the lesion is biopsied. Warthin-Starry staining may reveal spirochetes in the upper dermis.

The clinical finding of erythema migrans is the most sensitive evidence of early infection. Serologic conversion in U.S. patients is as follows: 27% when symptoms present for fewer than 7 days, 41% with symptoms for 7–14 days, and 88% with symptoms longer than 2 weeks. For this reason, the diagnosis should be made through recognition of erythema migrans. Although culture with PCR analysis is specific, it is not sensitive and is not available in most areas. Serologic testing is then the confirmatory test. The

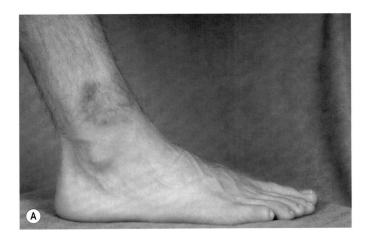

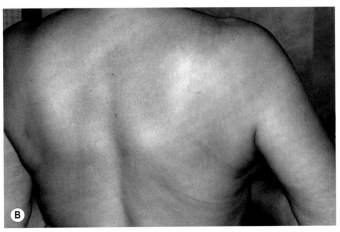

Fig. 14.50 (A and B) Erythema migrans.

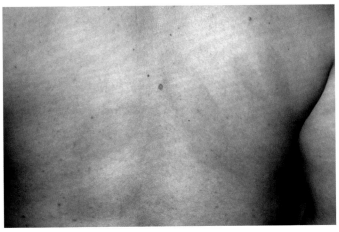

Fig. 14.51 Erythema migrans.

From 25%–50% of patients will develop multiple secondary annular lesions, similar in appearance to the primary lesion, but without indurated centers and generally of smaller size (Fig. 14.51). The lesions, 2–100 in number, spare the palms and soles. Without treatment, erythema migrans and the secondary lesions fade in a median of 28 days, although some may be present for months. Of untreated patients, 10% experience recurrences of erythema migrans over the following months. Diffuse urticaria, malar erythema, and conjunctivitis may be present during this early screening examination is ELISA, which is 89% sensitive and 72% specific. Western blot is used to confirm the result. There are three antigenic bands used in the IgM test and 10 in the IgG test. Two of three in the IgM and 5 of 10 in the IgG must be positive to diagnose Lyme disease. False-positive tests occur in syphilis, pinta, yaws, leptospirosis, relapsing fever, infectious mononucleosis, and disease associated with autoantibody formation. The VDRL is negative in *B. burgdorferi* infection. Patients with erythema migrans secondary to STARI usually have negative serology for Lyme disease.

Treatment

The treatment of choice in adults with Lyme disease is doxycycline, 100 mg twice daily for 3 weeks. Amoxicillin, 500 mg thrice daily for 21 days, or cefuroxime axetil, 500 mg twice daily for 21 days, is also effective. Doxycycline is also effective against *Ehrlichia*, but the β-lactams are not. Children under age 9 should be treated with amoxicillin, 20 mg/kg/day in divided doses. Pregnant women with localized early Lyme disease should take amoxicillin; however, if disseminated disease is present, parenteral penicillin G or ceftriaxone is used. Immunodeficient patients may also benefit from IV penicillin or ceftriaxone, although the data are not robust for this recommendation.

More aggressive regimens are necessary for carditis and neurologic and arthritic involvement, with parenteral dosing regimens often indicated.

Tick control environmental measures and personal avoidance strategies are worthwhile when outdoor activities are planned in tick-infested areas. Inspecting for ticks after returning from outdoor activity is a good preventive measure. The tick needs to be attached for more than 24 hours to transmit disease in the United States. Nymphs are small and may be difficult to see; be aware of the freckle that moves. Prophylactic antibiotic therapy, with one dose of 200-mg doxycycline after a known tick bite with a partially engorged *Ixodes scapularis* in high-incidence areas, is 87% effective. An effective vaccine was withdrawn from the market because of poor sales.

Acrodermatitis Chronica Atrophicans

Also known as primary diffuse atrophy, acrodermatitis chronica atrophicans (ACA) is characterized by the appearance on the extremities of diffuse reddish or bluish red, paper-thin skin. The underlying blood vessels are easily seen through the epidermis. It occurs almost exclusively in Europe. The disease begins on the backs of the hands and feet, then gradually spreads to involve the forearms, the arms, and the lower extremities, knees, and shins. Occasionally, even the trunk may become involved. In the beginning, the areas may be slightly edematous and scaly, but generally they are level with the skin and smooth. After several weeks to months, the skin has a smooth, soft, thin, velvety feel and may easily be lifted into fine folds. It may have a peculiar pinkish gray color and a crumpled-cigarette-paper appearance. Well-defined, smooth, edematous, bandlike thickenings develop and may extend from a finger to the elbow (ulnar bands) or may develop in the skin over the shins. With progression of ACA, marked atrophy of the skin occurs.

Subcutaneous fibrous nodules may form, chiefly over the elbows, wrists, and knees. Nodules may be single or multiple and are firm and painless. Diffuse extensive calcification of the soft tissues may be revealed by radiographic examination. Xanthomatous tumors may occur in the skin. Hypertrophic osteoarthritis of the hands is frequently observed. Occasionally, atrophy of the bones of the involved extremities is encountered. Ulcerations and carcinoma may supervene on the atrophic patches. ACA is slowly progressive but may remain stationary for long periods. Patches may change slightly from time to time, but complete involution never occurs.

A spirochetosis, ACA is a late sequel of infection with *Borrelia afzelii*, transmitted by the tick *Ixodes ricinus*. Almost all patients with ACA have a positive test for antibodies to the spirochete, and Warthin-Starry stains demonstrate *B. afzelii* in tissue in some cases. The organism has been cultured from skin lesions of ACA.

Histologically, there is marked atrophy of the epidermis and dermis without fibrosis. The elastic tissue is absent, and the cutaneous appendages are atrophic. In the dermis, a bandlike lymphocytic infiltration is seen, which varies in abundance according to the stage of the disease. The epidermis is slightly hyperkeratotic and flattened, and beneath it, there is a distinctive narrow zone of connective tissue in which the elastic tissue is intact.

Antibiotic therapy, as for other forms of borreliosis, cures most patients with ACA.

Bhate C, et al: Lyme disease. J Am Acad Dermatol 2011; 64: 619.

Borchers AT, et al: Lyme disease. J Autoimmun 2015; 57: 82.

Caulfield AJ, Pritt BS: Lyme disease coinfections in the United States. Clin Lab Med 2015; 35: 827.

Cutler SJ: Relapsing fever. J Appl Microbiol 2010; 108: 1115.

Glatz M, et al: Clinical spectrum of skin manifestations of Lyme borreliosis in 204 children in Austria. Acta Derm Venereol 2015; 95: 565.

Goddard J: Not all erythema migrans lesions are Lyme disease. Am J Med 2017; 130: 231.

Mead PS: Epidemiology of Lyme disease. Infect Dis Clin North Am 2015; 29: 187.

Nguyen AL, et al: Asymmetric red-bluish foot due to acrodermatitis chronica atrophicans. BMJ Case Rep 2016; bcr2016216033.

O'Connell S, Wolfs TF: Lyme borreliosis. Pediatr Infect Dis J 2014; 33: 407.

Sanchez E, et al: Diagnosis, treatment, and prevention of Lyme disease, human granulocytic anaplasmosis, and babesiosis. JAMA 2016; 315: 1767.

Schriefer ME: Lyme disease diagnosis. Clin Lab Med 2015; 35: 797.

Shapiro ED: Clinical practice. Lyme disease. N Engl J Med. 2014; 370: 1724.

Sood SK: Lyme disease in children. Infect Dis Clin North Am 2015; 29: 281.

Stinco G, et al: Clinical features of 705 *Borrelia burgdorferi* seropositive patients in an endemic area of northern Italy. Scientific World Journal 2014; 2014: 414505.

Walsh CA, et al: Lyme disease in pregnancy. Obstet Gynecol Surv 2007; 62: 41.

MYCOPLASMA

Mycoplasma organisms are distinct from true bacteria in that they lack a cell wall and differ from viruses in that they grow on cell-free media. *Mycoplasma pneumoniae* (Eaton agent) is an important cause of acute respiratory disease in children and young adults. In the summer, it may account for an estimated 50% of pneumonias. Skin eruptions occur during the course of infection in approximately 25% of patients. The most frequently reported is a Stevens-Johnson–like syndrome. Although the skin lesions in these cases may be vesiculobullous or targetoid, a wide variety of eruptions occur, including urticarial, vesiculopustular, maculopapular, scarlatiniform, petechial, purpuric, and morbilliform lesions. These are distributed primarily on the trunk, arms, and legs. Ulcerative stomatitis, conjunctivitis, urogenital, anal or esophageal erosions may be present. Erythema nodosum, acute hemorrhagic edema of infancy, subcorneal pustular dermatosis, and Gianotti-Crosti syndrome have been occasionally reported, as well as isolated mucositis without skin lesions (Fuchs syndrome).

The diagnosis of *M. pneumoniae* infection is made in the acute situation by clinical means, but definitive diagnosis is made by enzyme immunoassay, PCR, or complement fixation techniques. Cold agglutinins with a titer of 1 : 128 or more are usually caused by *M. pneumoniae* infection. Occasionally, acrocyanosis may occur secondary to cold agglutinin disease, which clears with antibiotic therapy. Treatment is with either a macrolide (erythromycin, azithromycin, or clarithromycin) or doxycycline for 7 days.

Canavan TN, et al: *Mycoplasma pneumoniae*-induced rash and mucositis as a syndrome distinct from Stevens-Johnson syndrome and erythema multiforme. J Am Acad Dermatol 2015; 72: 239.

Di Lernia V: *Mycoplasma pneumoniae*. Australas J Dermatol 2014; 55: e69.

Lombart F, et al: Subcorneal pustular dermatosis associated with *Mycoplasma pneumoniae* infection. J Am Acad Dermatol 2014; 71: e85.

Vujic I, et al: *Mycoplasma pneumoniae*-associated mucositis—case report and systematic review of literature. J Eur Acad Dermatol Venereol 2015; 29: 595.

CHLAMYDIAL INFECTIONS

Two species of *Chlamydiae*, *Chlamydia trachomatis* and *Chlamydia psittaci*, have been recognized. The two species share a major common antigen, and there are numerous serotypes within each species. In humans, *Chlamydia* causes trachoma, inclusion conjunctivitis, nongonococcal urethritis, cervicitis, epididymitis, proctitis, endometritis, salpingitis, pneumonia in the newborn, psittacosis (ornithosis), and lymphogranuloma venereum.

LYMPHOGRANULOMA VENEREUM

LGV is an STD caused by microorganisms of the *Chlamydia trachomatis* group and characterized by suppurative inguinal adenitis with matted lymph nodes, inguinal bubo with secondary ulceration, and constitutional symptoms. After an incubation period of 3–20 days, a primary lesion consisting of a 2–3 mm herpetiform vesicle or erosion develops on the glans penis, prepuce, or coronal sulcus, or at the meatus. In MSM, the lesion may be in the rectum. In women, it occurs on the vulva, vagina, or cervix. The lesion is painless and soon becomes a shallow ulceration. The initial symptom may be urethritis or proctitis. Extragenital primary infections of LGV are rare. An ulcerating lesion may appear at the site of infection on the fingers, lips, or tongue. In patients with HIV infection, a painful perianal ulcer may occur. Primary lesions heal in a few days.

About 2 weeks after the appearance of the primary lesion, enlargement of the regional lymph nodes occurs (Fig. 14.52). In one third of patients, the lymphadenopathy is bilateral. In the rather characteristic inguinal adenitis of LGV in men, the nodes in a chain fuse together into a large mass. The color of the skin overlying the mass usually becomes violaceous, the swelling is tender, and the bubo may break down, forming multiple fistulous openings. Adenopathy above and below the Poupart ligament produces the characteristic, but not diagnostic, groove sign. Along with the local adenitis, there may be systemic symptoms of malaise, joint pains, conjunctivitis, loss of appetite, weight loss, and fever, which may persist for several weeks. Patients with septic temperatures, enlarged liver and spleen, and even encephalitis have occasionally been observed.

Primary lesions of LGV are rarely observed in female patients or in MSM; they also have a lower incidence of inguinal buboes. Their bubo is typically pararectal in location. The diagnosis is recognized only much later, when the patient presents with an increasingly pronounced inflammatory stricture, which may be annular or tubular, of the lower rectal wall. Because most of the

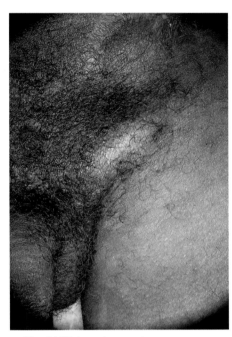

Fig. 14.52 Lymphogranuloma venereum.

lymph channels running from the vulva drain into the nodes around the lower part of the rectum, an inflammatory reaction in these nodes results in secondary involvement of the rectal wall. The iliac nodes may also be involved. LGV may start in the rectum as proctitis, which may then progress to the formation of a stricture. The clinical hallmark is bloody, mucopurulent rectal discharge. Untreated rectal strictures in men and women may eventually require colostomy. With or without rectal strictures, patients in later stages of the disease may show elephantiasis of the genitals with chronic ulcerations and scarring of the vulva or penis (esthiomene).

Cutaneous eruptions take the form of erythema nodosum, erythema multiforme, photosensitivity, and scarlatiniform eruptions. Arthritis associated with LGV involves the finger, wrist, ankle, knee, or shoulder joints. Marked weight loss, pronounced secondary anemia, weakness, and mental depression are often encountered in the course of the anorectal syndrome. Colitis resulting from LGV is limited to the rectum and rectosigmoid structures. Perianal fistulas or sinuses are often seen in cases of anorectal LGV. The various extragenital manifestations include glossitis with regional adenitis, unilateral conjunctivitis with edema of the lids caused by lymphatic blockage with lymphadenopathy, acute meningitis, meningoencephalitis, and pneumonia.

The diagnosis by nucleic acid amplification tests identifies *C. trachomatis* in a wide variety of specimens, including urine; urethral, rectal, and ulcer swabs; bubo aspirates; and biopsy specimens. In the complement fixation test a titer of 1 : 64 is highly suggestive. Microhemagglutination inhibition assays are also available and not only confirm the diagnosis, but also identify the strain. Three serotypes, designated L1, L2, and L3, are known for the LGV chlamydia. Characteristic surface antigens allow separation of the LGV chlamydia from the agents that cause trachoma, inclusion conjunctivitis, urethritis, and cervicitis, which also belong to the *C. trachomatis* group.

LGV occurs in all races, and the highest incidence is found in the 20- to 40-year-old age-group. Asymptomatic female contacts who shed *C. trachomatis* from the cervix are an important reservoir of infection. The classic disease in men is uncommon in the United States, whereas anorectal LGV continues to increase in MSM.

The characteristic changes in the lymph nodes consist of an infectious granuloma with the formation of stellate abscesses. There is an outer zone of epithelioid cells with a central necrotic core composed of debris of lymphocytes and leukocytes. In lesions of long duration, plasma cells may be present. Stellate abscess also occurs in cat-scratch disease, atypical mycobacterial infection, tularemia, and sporotrichosis.

Treatment

The recommended treatment of LGV is doxycycline, 100 mg twice daily for 3 weeks. An alternative is erythromycin, 500 mg four times daily for 21 days. Sexual partners within the prior 30 days should also be treated. The fluctuant nodules are aspirated from above through healthy, adjacent, normal skin to prevent rupture.

It should be emphasized again that all venereal infections may be mixed infections and that observation for simultaneous or subsequent development of another venereal disease should be unrelenting. This includes serologic testing for HIV disease.

Basta-Juzbašić A, Čeović R: Chancroid, lymphogranuloma venereum, granuloma inguinale, genital herpes simplex infection, and molluscum contagiosum. Clin Dermatol 2014; 32: 290.

Borsje A, et al: Lymphogranumola venereum presenting with erythema nodosum. Int J STD AIDS 2016; 27: 1354.

de Vrieze NH, de Vries HJ: Lymphogranuloma venereum among men who have sex with men. Expert Rev Anti Infect Ther 2014; 12: 697.

Macdonald N, et al: Risk factors for rectal lymphogranuloma venereum in gay men. Sex Transm Infect 2014; 90: 262.

Patel S, Hay P: Lymphogranuloma venereum and HIV infection. BMJ Case Rep 2010; bcr0220102771.

Stoner BP, Cohen SE: Lymphogranuloma venereum 2015. Clin Infect Dis 2015; 61: S865.

15 Diseases Resulting From Fungi and Yeasts

■ SUPERFICIAL AND DEEP MYCOSES

Fungal infections, including dermatophytes and candida, are the most common type of infection worldwide. Cutaneous infections are divided into superficial (those that affect mostly the skin) and deep (those that are typically more invasive) mycoses. In addition immunosuppressed patients are at high risk for opportunistic fungal infections, including from molds and other saprophytic fungi that are not typically pathogens in normal hosts.

Most mycotic infections are superficial and are limited to the stratum corneum, hair, and nails. In contrast, most deep mycoses are evidence of disseminated infection, typically with a primary pulmonary focus. Although blastomycosis, histoplasmosis, and coccidioidomycosis generally present as skin lesions, they are almost always evidence of a systemic infection. A few deep mycoses result from direct inoculation into the skin by a thorn or other foreign body, including cutaneous lymphangitic sporotrichosis, primary cutaneous phaeohyphomycosis, and chromomycosis. Phaeohyphomycosis may begin as a skin infection, but similar to all nondermatophyte fungi, immunosuppressed patients are at great risk of dissemination and death. Even cutaneous sporotrichosis may occasionally disseminate. Cutaneous aspergillosis can occur due to cutaneous embolization from a systemic (often a pulmonary) focus, but in immunosuppressed populations, direct inoculation of any saprophytic infection can lead to severe infection and then disseminate. In burn victims, *Aspergillus* can colonize the burn eschar. This colonization may often be treated with debridement alone. Deep incisional biopsies are required to determine whether viable tissue has been invaded beneath the eschar. Evidence of viable tissue invasion suggests a likelihood of systemic dissemination and is usually an indication for systemic antifungal therapy.

The major fungi that cause only stratum corneum, hair, and nail infection are the dermatophytes. They are classified in three genera: *Microsporum*, *Trichophyton*, and *Epidermophyton*. The identity of the pathogen may be important for determining a zoonotic reservoir of infection (e.g., cats or dogs for *Microsporum canis* infections, cattle for *Trichophyton verrucosum*, and rats for granular zoophilic *Trichophyton mentagrophytes*).

Susceptibility and Prevalence

Local immunosuppression from a potent topical corticosteroid or calcineurin inhibitor may promote larger lesions of cutaneous spread of dermatophyte infection. A defective cutaneous barrier, as in patients with ichthyosis, can also predispose to widespread tinea infection. Close contact with other infected individuals can lead to local breakouts of tinea especially tinea capitis. Maceration of the feet due to sweating, athletics, and swimming can increase the risk of tinea pedis.

Dermatophytes almost exclusively infect the skin. Patients with blood type A are somewhat more prone to chronic disease, and those with autosomal recessive CARD9 deficiency are susceptible to invasive dermatophyte fungal infection with dissemination to lymph nodes and the central nervous system (CNS). Many individuals will carry *Trichophyton rubrum* asymptomatically, which may be an autosomal dominant inherited tendency. When they are

exposed to a hot, humid climate or occlusive footwear, these patients often become symptomatic. Reported prevalence rates are therefore greatly affected by climate, footwear, and lifestyle.

Antifungal Therapy

Specific therapeutic recommendations will be made in each section; the following is an overview of available options. Topical agents provide safe, cost-effective therapy for limited superficial fungal infections. When considering the use of an oral antifungal agent, factors include the type of infection, organism, spectrum, pharmacokinetic profile, safety, compliance, age, and cost. Laboratory monitoring recommendations for systemic antifungals change frequently so the reader is advised to read the latest guidelines before prescribing systemic therapy. Griseofulvin has a long safety record but requires longer courses of therapy than newer agents. Topical antifungals remain very cost-effective for limited cutaneous disease. Dermatophyte infection involving hair-bearing areas (scalp, beard, thick hair on arms or legs) often requires oral therapy due to infection of the hair follicle. Infants may respond to topical therapy even in hair-bearing areas due to immature hair follicles. Lesions accidentally pretreated with topical steroids or calcineurin inhibitors may also require systemic therapy.

Various classes of antifungals are in use. The imidazoles include clotrimazole, miconazole, econazole, sulconazole, oxiconazole, voriconazole, efinaconazole, fenticonazole, and ketoconazole. They work by inhibition of cytochrome P450 14α-demethylase, an essential enzyme in ergosterol synthesis. Nystatin is a polyene that works by irreversibly binding to ergosterol, an essential component of fungal cell membranes but is used for *Candida* infections and is not effective for treating dermatophytes. Naftifine, terbinafine, and butenafine are allylamines, and their mode of action is inhibition of squalene epoxydation. The triazoles include itraconazole and fluconazole, which affect the CYP450 system.

For both itraconazole and griseofulvin, fatty food increases absorption. For itraconazole and ketoconazole, antacids, H2 antagonists, and proton pump inhibitors lower absorption. Terbinafine is less active against *Candida* and *Microsporum* species (spp.) in vitro. In vivo, adequate doses can be effective against these organisms. Terbinafine has limited efficacy in the oral treatment of tinea versicolor but is effective topically. Although few drug interactions have been reported with terbinafine, and the bioavailability is unchanged in food, hepatotoxicity, leukopenia, toxic epidermal necrolysis, and taste disturbances occur infrequently. Ketoconazole has a wide spectrum of action against dermatophytes, yeasts, and some systemic mycoses, but has the potential for hepatotoxicity. The U.S. Food and Drug Administration (FDA) has advised that systemic ketoconazole should not be used for skin and nail infections and should only be used for systemic fungal infections when no other medication is available (http://www.fda.gov/Drugs/DrugSafety/ucm500597.htm).

Fluconazole is mainly used to treat *Candida* infections, but has shown efficacy in the treatment of dermatophytoses both in daily and in weekly doses. It also has benefit in infants and young children because fluconazole has approval for candidal infections in infants and therefore is a reasonable off-label option for dermatophyte infections when needed in this population. Griseofulvin is FDA approved for tinea capitis in children over 2 and terbinafine only over age 4 years, but fluconazole has approval in infancy for various fungal infections. Although pulse therapy with fluconazole has been shown effective, patients may have trouble remembering intermittent dosing schedules. Both terbinafine and itraconazole have been shown to be effective and well tolerated in several studies of the treatment of tinea capitis and onychomycosis in children. However, itraconazole has been associated with reports of heart failure.

Voriconazole has exceptional activity against a wide variety of yeasts, as well as many other fungal pathogens, but has been associated with photosensitivity, premature photoaging, actinic keratoses, squamous cell carcinoma, melanoma, and porphyria. Posaconazole has significant in vitro activity against *Candida* spp., although some resistance has been reported to this drug.

The echinocandins inhibit β-(1,3)-glucan synthesis, thus damaging fungal cell walls. These drugs are active against most *Candida* spp. and fungistatic against *Aspergillus* spp. The echinocandins have limited activity against zygomycetes, *Cryptococcus neoformans*, or *Fusarium* spp. Caspofungin was the first drug in this class to be marketed in the United States for refractory invasive aspergillosis. Micafungin also belongs to this antifungal class. Adverse events are uncommon but include phlebitis, fever, elevated liver enzymes, and mild hemolysis. The drugs must be given intravenously. Metabolism is mainly hepatic. In the setting of *Candida* sepsis, results are similar to those achieved with amphotericin B, with substantially lower toxicity. The echinocandins may be used together with other antifungal agents in the treatment of life-threatening systemic fungal infections, such as disseminated aspergillosis refractory to other regimens.

■ THE SUPERFICIAL MYCOSES

TINEA CAPITIS

Tinea capitis, known colloquially as scalp "ringworm," can be caused by all of the pathogenic dermatophytes. In the United States most cases are caused by *Trichophyton tonsurans*. Pet exposure (especially cat) is associated with tinea capitis caused by *Microsporum canis*. As people travel and emigrate from other countries, the diversity of fungi causing tinea capitis in a region can rise.

Tinea capitis occurs mainly in children, although it may be seen at all ages. Boys have tinea capitis more frequently than girls; however, in epidemics caused by *T. tonsurans*, both genders are often affected equally. African American children have a higher incidence of *T. tonsurans* infections than other groups. The infection is also common among Latin American children.

Trichophyton tonsurans can produce black dot tinea (Fig. 15.1), scaling alopecic plaques, subtle seborrheic-like scaling, and/or inflammatory kerion. Black dot tinea occurs due to the fungi invading the follicle (endothrix) and may also be caused by *Trichophyton violaceum*, an organism rarely seen in the United States. Both of these organisms produce chains of large spores within the hair shaft (large-spore endothrix). They do not fluoresce with Wood's light.

The *Microsporum canis* complex includes a group of organisms that produce small spores visible on the outside of the hair shaft (small-spore ectothrix). These fungi fluoresce under Wood's light examination. The *M. canis* complex includes *M. canis*, *M. canis distortum*, *Microsporum ferrugineum*, and *M. audouinii*. *M. canis* infections begin as scaly, erythematous, papular eruptions with loose and broken-off hairs. The lesions typically become highly inflammatory, although *M. audouinii* produces less inflammatory lesions. Deep, tender, boggy plaques exuding pus are known as kerion celsii (Fig. 15.2). Kerion may be followed by scarring and permanent alopecia in the areas of inflammation and suppuration, although with early treatment hair regrowth is common. Prompt administration of oral antifungals is most important but systemic corticosteroids for a short period, along with appropriate antifungal therapy, can greatly diminish the inflammatory response and reduce the risk of scarring, and this therapy should be considered in the patient with highly inflammatory lesions.

Many children are asymptomatic carriers of *T. tonsurans* and represent a source of infection for classmates and siblings. Numerous studies have shown that 5%–15% of urban children in Western countries have positive scalp dermatophyte cultures. In one study, 60% of African American children with a positive scalp culture were asymptomatic.

The prevalence of dermatophytes varies throughout the world. Where animal herding is an important part of the economy, zoonotic fungi account for a significant proportion of cases of tinea. In south-central Asia, *T. violaceum* is the most common dermatophytic species isolated, with *M. audouinii* a close second. Other common organisms include *Trichophyton schoenleinii*, *T. tonsurans*, *Microsporum gypseum*, *T. verrucosum*, and *T. mentagrophytes*. In East Asia, *T. violaceum* and *M. ferrugineum* are important pathogens. In Europe, African and Caribbean immigrants account for a large proportion of new patients with tinea capitis. Important

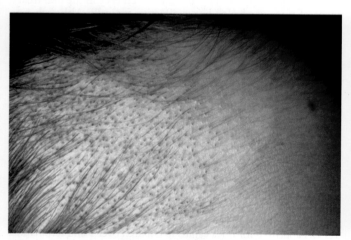

Fig. 15.1 Tinea capitis.

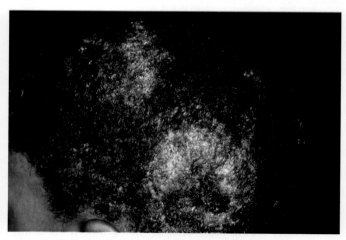

Fig. 15.2 Kerion. (Courtesy Steven Binnick, MD.)

pathogens include *T. tonsurans, M. audouinii* var. *langeronii, Trichophyton soudanense,* and *T. violaceum. Trichophyton megninii* is a rare cause of tinea capitis largely restricted to southwestern Europe. In Africa, large-scale epidemics are associated with *T. soudanense, T. violaceum, T. schoenleinii,* and *Microsporum* spp. In Australia, the predominantly Caucasian population experiences infections, mostly with *M. canis,* but *T. tonsurans* is now equal in prevalence in some areas of the continent. Recent immigrants have a high incidence of tinea capitis with organisms common in their regions of origin. Among African and Arab immigrants, *T. soudanense, T. violaceum,* and *M. audouinii* are particularly common.

Favus

Favus, which is extremely rare in the United States, appears chiefly on the scalp but may affect the glabrous skin and nails. On the scalp, concave sulfur-yellow crusts form around loose, wiry hairs. Atrophic scarring ensues, leaving a smooth, glossy, thin, paper-white patch. On the glabrous skin, the lesions are pinhead to 2 cm in diameter with cup-shaped crusts called scutulae, usually pierced by a hair as on the scalp. The scutulae have a distinctive mousy odor. When the nails are affected, they become brittle, irregularly thickened, and crusted under the free margins. Other types of dermatophytes such as *T. rubrum* may appear similar clinically.

Favus is prevalent in the Middle East, southeastern Europe, South Africa and the countries bordering the Mediterranean Sea.

Pathogenesis and Natural History

The incubation period of anthropophilic (affecting humans) tinea capitis is 2–4 days, although the period is highly variable, and asymptomatic carriers are common. The hyphae grow downward into the follicle, on the hair's surface, and the intrafollicular hyphae break up into chains of spores. There is a period of spread (4 days to 4 months) during which the lesions enlarge and new lesions appear. At about 3 weeks, hairs break off a few millimeters above the skin surface. Within the hair, hyphae descend to the upper limit of the keratogenous zone and here form Adamson "fringe" on about the 12th day. During a refractory period (4 months to several years) fewer new lesions develop. The clinical appearance is constant, with the host and parasite at equilibrium. This may be followed by a period of involution in which the formation of spores gradually diminishes. Zoonotic (from animals) fungal infections often are more highly inflammatory but undergo similar phases of evolution.

Diagnosis

Wood's Light

Ultraviolet (UV) light of 365-nm wavelength commonly known as the Wood's light, is used to demonstrate fungal fluorescence. Infections caused by *M. audouinii, M. canis, M. ferrugineum, M. distortum,* and *T. schoenleinii* will fluoresce. In a darkroom, the skin under this light fluoresces faintly blue, and dandruff usually is bright blue-white. Infected hair fluoresces bright green or yellow-green due to the presence of pteridine. Large-spore endothrix organisms (e.g., *T. tonsurans, T. violaceum*) and *T. verrucosum* (a cause of large-spore ectothrix) do not fluoresce making woods light less helpful because *T. tonsurans* is the most common type of tinea capitis.

Laboratory Examination

Tinea capitis can be a clinical diagnosis if the classic scaling, alopecic plaques with nuchal or posterior cervical lymphadenopathy are seen in a child. In one study 97% percent of children with tinea capitis demonstrated posterior cervical or nuchal lymphadenopathy, making this a very useful negative predictor if absent. For more diffuse "seborrheic" patterns or without significant alopecia or if another diagnosis is being considered, a culture can prove the diagnosis. Cultures from a kerion (inflammatory tinea capitis) may be false negative due to the exuberant inflammatory response so treatment is typically empiric. For demonstration of the fungus in a highly inflammatory plaque, two or three loose hairs are carefully removed with epilating forceps from the suspected areas. If fluorescence occurs, it is important to choose these hairs. Bear in mind that hairs infected with *T. tonsurans* do not fluoresce. In black dot ringworm or in patients with seborrheic scale, small broken fragments of infected hair or scaling can be scraped or brushed off with a sterile toothbrush. The hairs are placed on a slide and covered with a drop of a 10%–20% potassium hydroxide (KOH) solution. A coverslip is then applied, and the specimen is warmed until the hairs are macerated. Dimethyl sulfoxide (DMSO) can be added to the KOH solution in concentrations of up to 40%. This additive allows for rapid clearing of keratin without heating. Once the keratin in the hairs has dissolved somewhat, they can be examined first with a low-power objective and then with a high-power objective for detail. The mycelia may be seen under low-power microscopy, but better observation of both hyphae and spores is obtained by the 10× objective with the condenser lowered down or the light aperture closed by two thirds. A staining method using 100 mg of chlorazol black E dye in 10 mL of DMSO and adding it to a 5% aqueous solution of KOH can be helpful. Toluidine blue 0.1% can also be used on thin specimens, but contains no clearing agent to dissolve keratin. The patterns of endothrix and ectothrix involvement described earlier, together with local prevalence data, allow for identification of the organism.

Exact identification of the causative fungus is generally determined by culture, although molecular sequencing offers a more rapid alternative. For culture, several infected hairs are plated on Sabouraud dextrose agar, Sabouraud agar with chloramphenicol, Mycosel agar, or dermatophyte test medium (DTM). Laboratories differ in how they prefer the sample to be collected, but using a toothbrush to gently remove scale and loose hairs and transfer to the laboratory in a sterile container or a bacterial culturette moistened with sterile saline and then rubbed on the affected areas are the most common methods. On the first three media, a distinctive growth appears within 1–2 weeks. Most frequently, the diagnosis is made by the gross appearance of the culture growth, together with the microscopic appearance. With *Trichophyton* spp., growth on different nutrient agars is often required to identify the organisms beyond genus. DTM not only contains antibiotics to reduce growth of contaminants, but also contains a colored pH indicator to denote the alkali-producing dermatophytes although laboratory regulations have limited this use in academic centers. A few nonpathogenic saprophytes will also produce alkalinization, and in the occasional case of onychomycosis of toenails caused by airborne molds, a culture medium containing an antibiotic may inhibit growth of the true pathogen.

Differential Diagnosis

Tinea capitis must be differentiated clinically from chronic staphylococcal folliculitis, pediculosis capitis (head lice), psoriasis, seborrheic dermatitis, secondary syphilis, trichotillomania, alopecia areata, lupus erythematosus (LE), lichen planus, lichen simplex chronicus, and various inflammatory follicular conditions. The distinctive clinical features of tinea capitis are broken-off stumps of hairs, often in rounded patches in which there are crusts or pustules and few hairs. The broken-off hairs are loose. Diffuse seborrheic scaling with hair loss is a common presentation of *T. tonsurans* infections. Dermoscopy can reveal comma-shaped and corkscrew hairs. Horizontal bands and translucent hairs in *M. canis* infections have been demonstrated on high-power dermoscopy.

In alopecia areata, the affected patches are bald, the skin is smooth and shiny without signs of inflammation or scaling, and exclamation point hairs can be seen on dermoscopy. Stumps of broken-off hairs are infrequently found, and no fungi are demonstrable. In seborrheic dermatitis, the involved areas are covered by fine, dry, or greasy scales. Hair may be lost, but the hairs are not broken and lymphadenopathy is generally absent. Atopic dermatitis can affect the scalp but is rarely only localized to the scalp. In psoriasis, well-demarcated, sometimes diffuse, areas of erythema and white or silver scaling are noted. Although in children psoriasis may first manifest in the scalp, there is usually some evidence of psoriasis elsewhere. Lichen simplex chronicus is frequently localized to the inferior margin of the occipital scalp. In trichotillomania, as in alopecia areata, inflammation and scaling are absent and the patterns of hair loss are unusual clinically. Serologic testing, scalp biopsies, and immunofluorescent studies may be indicated if the alopecia of secondary syphilis or LE is a serious consideration. It should be noted that adult patients with LE are susceptible to tinea capitis, which may be photosensitive and difficult to distinguish from LE plaques without biopsy and KOH examinations.

Treatment

Numerous clinical trials have demonstrated the effectiveness of itraconazole, terbinafine, and fluconazole. Griseofulvin remains the most frequently used antifungal agent in children, but because there are data that terbinafine may be more effective in *T. tonsurans* infections and the course of therapy is shorter, terbinafine is gaining favor, and both are considered first line. Griseofulvin has a long safety record. A meta-analysis of published studies shows mean efficacy for griseofulvin treatment of about 68% for *Trichophyton* spp. and 88% for *Microsporum*. For the ultramicronized form, doses start at 10 mg/kg/day. Griseofulvin must be given with a fatty food to ensure absorption. The ultramicrosized form absorbs more easily so doses are lower. The dose of micronized is 20 mg/kg/day (not to exceed 500 mg twice a day), although some advocate up to 25 mg/kg/day in recalcitrant cases. Treatment should continue for 6–8 weeks, or for at least 2 weeks after clinical or laboratory determined cure. For *Trichophyton* infections, terbinafine is usually effective in doses of 3–6 mg/kg/day for 3–6 weeks. In the United States it is FDA approved over 4 years of age, but some authors advocate for its use in younger children. Published dosing guidelines are based on the terbinafine granules, which can be difficult to obtain. Similar dosing that is used for onychomycosis in children based on the tablets is reasonable: 250-mg tablet for patients over 40 kg, 125 mg (½ tablet) for those 20–40 kg, and 62.5 mg (¼ tablet) for those under 20 kg. Terbinafine should not be mixed with acidic foods such as apple sauce because they may limit absorption. *Microsporum* infections require higher doses and longer courses of therapy with terbinafine, so griseofulvin is preferred in these infections.

Second-line agents include fluconazole (not to exceed adult dose) at doses of 3–6 mg/kg/day for 3–6 weeks lower doses lead to lower cure rates. Fluconazole 6mg/kg/week for 8–12 weeks has also been reported. Itraconazole has been shown to be effective in doses of 5 mg/kg/day (not to exceed adult dose) for 2–3 weeks, but reports of heart failure with itraconazole have limited its use. In neonates and children under 2 topical therapy is occasionally effective, likely due to the less mature hair follicles, but oral antifungals are recommended by a recent review.

Selenium sulfide shampoo or ketoconazole shampoo left on the scalp for 5 minutes three times a week can be used as adjunctive therapy to oral antifungal agents to reduce the shedding of fungal spores. Combs, brushes, and hats should be cleaned carefully, and natural bristle brushes must be discarded.

Prognosis

Recurrence is uncommon when adequate amounts of griseofulvin, fluconazole, or terbinafine have been taken, although exposure to infected persons, asymptomatic carriers, or contaminated fomites will increase the relapse rate. Without medication, there may be spontaneous clearing at about age 15 years, except with *T. tonsurans*, which often persists into adult life.

DERMATOPHYTIDS

In cases of inflammatory tinea capitis, widespread "id" eruptions may appear concomitantly on the trunk and extremities. These are vesicular, lichenoid, papulosquamous, or pustular and represent a systemic reaction to fungal antigens either during the infection or therapy for the infection. Although the eruptions are usually refractory to topical corticosteroids, they typically clear rapidly after treatment of the fungal infection.

An id reaction can be seen on the hands and sides of the fingers when there is an acute fungus infection of the feet. These lesions are mostly vesicular and are extremely pruritic and even tender. Secondary bacterial infection may occur; however, fungus is not demonstrable in the hand lesions. The onset can be accompanied by fever, anorexia, generalized adenopathy, spleen enlargement, and leukocytosis. Dermatophytid reactions from inflammatory tinea capitis may occasionally present as widespread eruption, usually follicular, lichenoid, or papulosquamous. An id reaction characterized by fine papules on the trunk, face, ears and extremities can occur during systemic therapy especially with griseofulvin for tinea capitis. Rarely, the eruption may be morbilliform or scarlatiniform. The erysipelas-like dermatophytid has been reported on the shin but must be differentiated from cellulitis that occurs as a result of skin breaks from tinea pedis.

The histologic picture of an id is characterized by spongiotic vesicles and a superficial, perivascular, predominantly lymphohistiocytic infiltrate. Eosinophils may be present. Diagnosis of a dermatophytid reaction depends on the demonstration of a fungus at some site remote from the suspect lesions of the dermatophytid, the absence of fungus in the id lesion, and involution of the lesion as the fungal infection subsides.

TINEA BARBAE

Ringworm of the beard, also known as tinea sycosis and barber's itch, is more common among those in agricultural pursuits, especially those in contact with farm animals, but may also be seen in wrestlers and through incidental contact. The involvement is mostly one sided on the neck or face. Typical scaling alopecic patches can occur in addition to a more inflammatory superficial, crusted, partially bald patches with folliculitis (Fig. 15.3) or deep, nodular, suppurative lesions possibly indicating a zoonotic infection.

The deep type develops slowly and produces nodular thickenings and kerion-like swellings, usually caused by *T. mentagrophytes* or *T. verrucosum*. As a rule, the swellings are confluent and form diffuse, boggy infiltrations with abscesses. The overlying skin is inflamed, the hairs are loose or absent, and pus may be expressed through the remaining follicular openings. Generally, the lesions are limited to one part of the face or neck in men. The superficial crusted type is characterized by a less inflammatory pustular folliculitis and may be associated with *T. violaceum* or *T. rubrum*. The affected hairs can sometimes be easily extracted. Rarely, *Epidermophyton floccosum* may cause widespread verrucous lesions known as verrucous epidermophytosis.

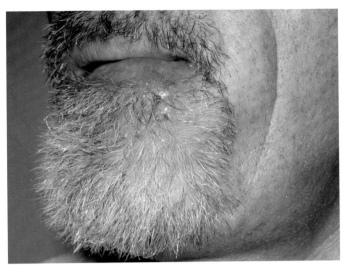

Fig. 15.3 Tinea barbae.

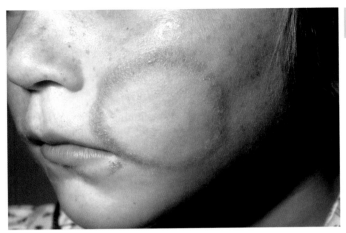

Fig. 15.4 Tinea faciei.

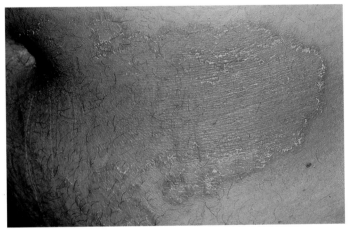

Fig. 15.5 Tinea corporis.

Diagnosis

The clinical diagnosis of tinea barbae is confirmed by the microscopic mounts of extracted hairs or a biopsy and culture of the tissue specimen.

Differential Diagnosis

The differential diagnosis includes staphylococcal folliculitis (sycosis vulgaris) and herpetic infections. Tinea barbae differs from sycosis vulgaris by usually sparing the upper lip and by often being unilateral. In sycosis vulgaris, the lesions are pustules and papules, pierced in the center by a hair, which is loose and easily extracted after suppuration has occurred. Herpetic infections usually demonstrate umbilicated vesicles. Tzanck preparations have a low diagnostic yield, but viral culture or direct fluorescent antibody is virtually always positive.

Treatment

As in tinea capitis, oral antifungal agents are required to cure tinea barbae. Topical agents are only helpful as adjunctive therapy. Oral agents are used in the same doses and for the same durations as in tinea capitis.

TINEA FACIEI

Fungal infection of the face is frequently misdiagnosed (Fig. 15.4). Typical annular rings are usually lacking, and the lesions are exquisitely photosensitive. Frequently, a misdiagnosis of LE is made. Biopsies for direct immunofluorescence often demonstrate some reactants on sun-exposed skin, adding to the possible diagnostic confusion. Erythematous, slightly scaling, indistinct borders may be present at the periphery of the lesions and are the best location for KOH examination. If topical corticosteroids have been used, the lesions will expand and fungal folliculitis is a frequent finding. A biopsy may be required to establish the diagnosis. A high index of suspicion is required, because fungal hyphae may be few in number or confined to hair follicles. The inflammatory pattern may be psoriasiform spongiotic or vacuolar interface. The latter pattern has the potential to perpetuate confusion with LE.

Usually, the infection is caused by *T. rubrum, T. mentagrophytes,* or *M. canis.* Tinea faciei caused by *Microsporum nanum* has been described in hog farmers. If hair follicles are infected such as long the eyebrow or beard area in older children or the infection is widespread, oral medication is required. Otherwise, the infection generally responds well to topical therapy.

TINEA CORPORIS (TINEA CIRCINATA)

Tinea corporis includes all superficial dermatophyte infections of the skin other than those involving the scalp, beard, face, hands, feet, and groin. This form of ringworm is characterized by one or more circular, sharply circumscribed, slightly erythematous, dry, scaly, sometimes hypopigmented patches. An advancing scaling edge is usually prominent (Fig. 15.5). Progressive central clearing produces annular outlines that give them the name "ringworm." Lesions may widen to form rings many centimeters in diameter. In some cases, concentric circles or polycyclic lesions form, making intricate patterns. Although more common on the feet, lesions of tinea corporis can also form vesicles and bullae (bullous tinea). Widespread tinea corporis may be the presenting sign of acquired immunodeficiency syndrome (AIDS) or may be related to the use of a topical corticosteroid or calcineurin inhibitor.

In the United States *T. rubrum, M. canis,* and *T. mentagrophytes* are common causes, although infection can be caused by any of the dermatophytes. Multiple small lesions are usually caused by exposure to a pet with *M. canis.* Other zoonotic fungi, such as granular zoophilic *T. mentagrophytes* related to Southeast Asian bamboo rats, can cause widespread epidemics of highly inflammatory tinea corporis.

Tinea gladiatorum is a common problem for wrestlers. Opponents, equipment, and mats represent potential sources of infection.

Diagnosis

The diagnosis of tinea corporis is by finding the fungus by KOH examination of skin scrapings under the microscope as described earlier. When evaluating tinea corporis, the lines of juncture of normal keratinocytes dissolve into a branching network that may easily be mistaken for fungus structures ("mosaic false hyphae"). This is the most common artifact misinterpreted as a positive KOH examination. Cotton and synthetic fibers from socks may also mimic hyphae. In addition, skin scrapings can be cultured on a suitable medium as described earlier for tinea capitis. Growth of the fungus on culture medium is apparent within 1 week or 2 weeks at most, and in most cases is identifiable to the genus level by the gross and microscopic appearance of the culture. (Biopsy of a chronic refractory dermatosis often reveals tinea incognito.)

Other diseases that may closely resemble tinea corporis are pityriasis rosea, impetigo, nummular dermatitis, secondary and tertiary syphilids, seborrheic dermatitis, and psoriasis. These are distinguished by KOH examination and culture.

Treatment

Localized disease without fungal folliculitis may be treated with topical therapy. Sulconazole (Exelderm), oxiconazole (Oxistat), miconazole (Monistat cream or lotion, or Micatin cream), clotrimazole (Lotrimin or Mycelex cream), econazole (Spectazole), naftifine (Naftin), ketoconazole (Nizoral), ciclopirox olamine (Loprox), terbinafine (Lamisil), efinaconazole, and butenafine (Mentax) are currently available and effective and therapy should be guided based on cost effectiveness. Most treatment times are between 2 and 4 weeks with twice-daily use. Econazole, ketoconazole, oxiconazole, and terbinafine may be used once a day. With terbinafine, the course can be shortened to 1 week. Combination products with a potent corticosteroid such as clotrimazole/betamethasone frequently produce widespread tinea and fungal folliculitis. Their use should be avoided.

Extensive disease or infection of hair follicles requires systemic antifungal treatment. When tinea corporis is caused by *T. tonsurans*, *T. mentagrophytes*, or *T. rubrum*, griseofulvin, terbinafine, itraconazole, and fluconazole are all effective.

Trichophyton species generally respond to shorter courses of terbinafine and Microsporum species respond better to griseofulvin.

Other Forms of Tinea Corporis

Fungal Folliculitis Tinea Incognita and Majocchi Granuloma

Tinea incognita is a term applied to lesions of tinea that have an atypical appearance due to therapy with topical steroids or calcineurin inhibitors. The lesions are often widespread and may lack an advancing, raised, scaly border. Alternatively multiple edges may be present and there may be a lack of central clearing, rather the center may be eczematous (Fig. 15.6). The diagnosis may be established by KOH examination or biopsy.

Treatment of tinea with a topical steroid or calcineurin inhibitor can lead to deeper, more inflammatory infections of the hair follicles. It presents as a circumscribed, annular, raised, crusty, and boggy granuloma in which the follicles are distended with viscid purulent material. These occur most frequently on the shins or wrists. The lesions are often seen in areas of occlusion or shaving,

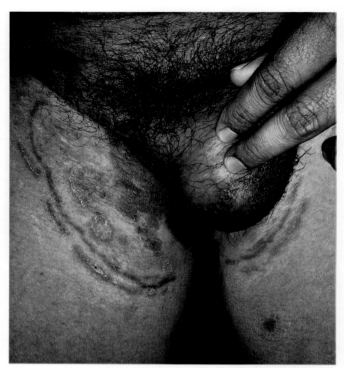

Fig. 15.6 Double-edged border in steroid-modified tinea.

or when a topical corticosteroid has been used. In immunosuppressed patients, the lesions may be deep and nodular. Often, patients have been treated with both topical corticosteroids and antifungal agents. If a topical antifungal has been used recently, KOH examination and culture may be negative. A biopsy may be required to establish the diagnosis. Oral therapy is necessary to cure the lesions. Occasionally, a deep, pustular type of tinea circinata resembling a carbuncle or kerion is observed on the glabrous skin (Fig. 15.7). This type of lesion is a fungal folliculitis caused most often by *T. rubrum* or *T. mentagrophytes* infecting hairs at the site of involvement.

Tinea Imbricata (Tokelau)

Tinea imbricata is a superficial fungal infection limited to southwest Polynesia, Melanesia, Southeast Asia, India, and Central America. It is characterized by concentric rings of scales forming extensive patches with polycyclic borders. Erythema is typically minimal. The eruption begins with one or several small, rounded macules on the trunk and arms. The small macular patch splits in the center and forms large, flaky scales attached at the periphery. As the resultant ring spreads peripherally, another brownish macule appears in the center and undergoes the process of splitting and peripheral extension. This cycle is repeated over and over again. When fully developed, the eruption is characterized by concentrically arranged rings or parallel, undulating lines of scales overlapping each other like shingles on a roof (*imbrex* means "shingle").

The causative fungus is *Trichophyton concentricum*, although a similar pattern may be produced by *T. mentagrophytes* and *T. tonsurans*. Microscopically, the scrapings show interlacing, septate, mycelial filaments that branch dichotomously. Polyhedral spores are also present. Terbinafine has been shown to be very effective while the recurrence rate may be high with griseofulvin.

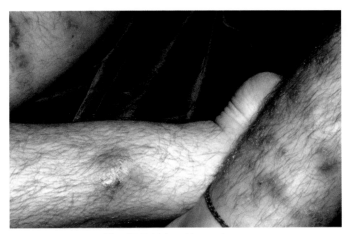

Fig. 15.7 Majocchi granuloma.

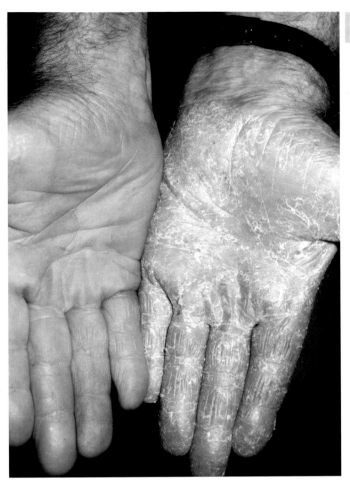

Fig. 15.8 One-hand involvement with tinea. Patient had both feet involved. (Courtesy Steven Binnick, MD.)

Tinea Cruris

Tinea cruris, also known as "jock itch" and "crotch itch," occurs more commonly in men on the upper and inner surfaces of the thighs, especially during the summer when the humidity is high. It begins as a small, erythematous, and scaling or vesicular and crusted patch that spreads peripherally and partly clears in the center, so that the patch is characterized chiefly by its curved, well-defined border, particularly on its lower edge. The border may have vesicles, pustules, or papules. It may extend downward on the thighs and backward on the perineum or about the anus. The scrotum is rarely involved.

Etiology and Differential Diagnosis. Dermatophyte infection of the groin is usually caused by *T. rubrum*, *T. mentagrophytes*, or *E. floccosum*. Infection with *Candida albicans* may closely mimic tinea cruris, but is usually moister, more inflammatory, and associated with satellite macules and can involve the scrotum. *Candida* often produces collarette scales and satellite pustules.

The crural region is also a common site for erythrasma, seborrheic dermatitis, pemphigus vegetans, and intertriginous psoriasis. Erythrasma often has a copper color and is diagnosed by Wood's light examination, which produces coral-red fluorescence. Seborrheic dermatitis generally involves the central chest and axillae in addition to the groin. Pemphigus vegetans produces macerated and eroded lesions. Diagnosis of tinea cruris is established by KOH examination, fungal culture, biopsy or (if caused by a fluorescent fungus) immunofluorescence. Inverse psoriasis may be associated with collarette scales or with serpiginous arrays of pustules at the border of inflammatory lesions. When more typical lesions of psoriasis are lacking, a biopsy may be required to establish the diagnosis.

Treatment. The reduction of perspiration and enhancement of evaporation from the crural area are important prophylactic measures. The area should be kept as dry as possible by the wearing of loose underclothing and trousers. Plain talcum powder or antifungal powders are helpful. Specific topical and oral treatment for tinea cruris is the same as that described earlier for tinea corporis.

TINEA OF HANDS AND FEET

Dermatophytosis of the feet, "athlete's foot," is the most common fungal disease. *T. rubrum* causes the majority of infections although

it can be caused by many other dermatophytes, including *T. tonsurans*. There may be an autosomal dominant predisposition to this form of infection or it may just be being spread within families. *T. rubrum* typically produces a relatively noninflammatory type of dermatophytosis characterized by a dull erythema and pronounced silvery scaling that may involve the entire sole and sides of the foot, giving a moccasin or sandal appearance. The eruption may also be limited to a small patch adjacent to a fungus-infected toenail or to a patch between or under the toes. In some patients, an extensive patchy, scaly eruption covers most of the trunk, buttocks, and extremities. Rarely, there is a patchy hyperkeratosis.

Generally, dermatophyte infection of the hands is of the dry, scaly, and erythematous type suggestive of *T. rubrum* infection. Other areas are frequently affected at the same time, especially the combination of both feet and one hand (Fig. 15.8). Tinea pedis caused by anthropophilic *T. mentagrophytes (interdigitale)* presents with three distinct appearances: (1) multilocular bullae involving the thin skin of the plantar arch and along the sides of the feet and heel, (2) erythema and desquamation between the toes, and (3) white superficial onychomycosis. In the human immunodeficiency virus (HIV)–positive population, this latter syndrome is usually caused by *T. rubrum*. Interdigital tinea must be distinguished from simple maceration caused by a closed web

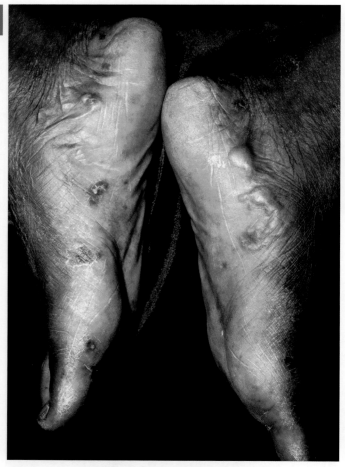

Fig. 15.9 Bullous tinea pedis.

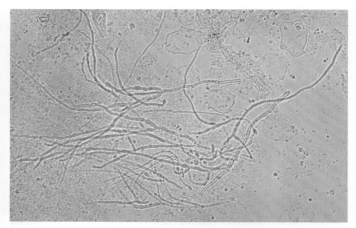

Fig. 15.10 Positive KOH examination.

space, which does not respond to antifungal therapy. Interdigital tinea must also be distinguished from gram-negative toe web infection and candidal infection. Diabetic patients develop interdigital fungal infections at a younger age than patients without diabetes.

T. mentagrophytes often produces acutely inflammatory multilocular bullae (Fig. 15.9). The burning and itching that accompany the formation of the vesicles may cause great discomfort, which is relieved by opening the tense vesicles. They contain a tenacious, clear, straw-colored fluid. Extensive or acute eruptions on the soles may be incapacitating. The fissures between the toes, as well as the vesicles, may become secondarily infected with pyogenic cocci, which may lead to recurrent attacks of lymphangitis and inguinal adenitis. Gram-negative toe web infections may also supervene. Hyperhidrosis is frequently present in this type of dermatophytosis. The sweat between the toes and on the soles has a high pH, and damp keratin is a good culture medium for the fungi.

Dermatophytid of the hands may be associated with inflammatory tinea of the feet and begins with the appearance of groups of minute, clear vesicles on the palms and fingers and sometimes the sides and tops of the feet. The itching may be intense. Typically, both hands are involved, and the eruption tends to be symmetric.

Diagnosis

Demonstration of the fungus by KOH microscopic examination (Fig. 15.10) as described for tinea capitis and corporis earlier establishes the diagnosis. For bullous tinea, bullae should be unroofed, and either the entire roof is mounted intact or scrapings are made from the underside of the roof.

Material may also be placed on Sabouraud dextrose agar, Sabouraud agar with chloramphenicol, Mycosel agar, or DTM. The last three agars inhibit growth of bacterial or saprophytic contaminants. The last two may inhibit some pathogenic nondermatophytes. The alkaline metabolites produced by growth of dermatophytes change the color of the pH indicator in DTM medium from yellow to red.

Prophylaxis

Hyperhidrosis is a predisposing factor for tinea infections. Because the disease often starts on the feet, the patient should be advised to dry the toes thoroughly after bathing. Cold water laundering does not inactivate fungal elements in socks, which may serve as a source of recolonization. Dryness is essential to reduce the incidence of symptomatic reinfection.

The use of a antiseptic powder on the feet after bathing, particularly between the toes, is strongly advised for susceptible persons. Tolnaftate powder (Tinactin) or Zeasorb medicated powder is an excellent dusting powder for the feet. Plain talc, cornstarch, or rice powder may be dusted into socks and shoes to keep the feet dry. Periodic use of a topical antifungal agent may be required, especially when hot occlusive footwear is worn.

Treatment

Clotrimazole, miconazole, sulconazole, oxiconazole, ciclopirox, econazole, ketoconazole, naftifine, terbinafine, flutrimazole, bifonazole, efinaconazole, and butenafine are effective topical antifungal agents but especially in tinea manuum or exuberant tinea pedis, an oral agent may be necessary. When there is significant maceration between the toes, the toes may be separated by foam or cotton inserts in the evening. Aluminum chloride 10% solution or aluminum acetate, 1 part to 20 parts of water, can be beneficial. Interdigital tinea can also be treated with antifungal-impregnated socks. Topical antibiotic ointments, such as gentamicin (Garamycin), that are effective against gram-negative organisms are helpful additions in some moist interdigital lesions. In the ulcerative type of gram-negative toe web infections, systemic antibiotic therapy is necessary (see Chapter 14). Keratolytic agents containing salicylic acid, resorcinol, lactic acid, and urea may be useful in some cases, although all may lead to maceration if occluded.

Treatment of fungal infection of the skin of the feet and hands with griseofulvin, 500–1000 mg/day, can be effective. Dosage for children is 10–20 mg/kg/day. The period of therapy depends on the response of the lesions. Repeated KOH scrapings and cultures should be negative. Shorter courses are possible with other antifungal agents. Recommended adult dosing for terbinafine is 250 mg/day for 1–2 weeks; for itraconazole, 200 mg twice daily for 1 week; and for fluconazole, 150 mg once weekly for 4 weeks.

TINEA NIGRA

Hortaea werneckii (formerly *Phaeoannellomyces werneckii*) is a black, yeastlike hyphomycete that is widely distributed in hot, humid environments. The organism is common in the tropics. In the United States the infection is seen along the Gulf Coast. New taxonomic analysis has led some to classify *Cladosporium castellanii* as the etiologic agent of tinea nigra in humans and confirmed that this fungus is the same as *Stenella araguata*.

Tinea nigra presents as one or several brown or black spots on the palms or soles. The lesions may be mistaken for nevi, melanoma or talon noir hemorrhage under the skin. The pigment is confined to the stratum corneum and scrapes off easily. Dermoscopy has also been used to differentiate the lesions from melanocytic tumors although a case of tinea nigra with a parallel ridge pattern simulating melanoma was reported. The fungus can easily be demonstrated by means of KOH or culture. In KOH preparations, the hyphae appear brown or golden in color. The pigment produced by the fungal hyphae is melanin. Culture will identify the organism, and polymerase chain reaction (PCR) can be useful for rapid identification of *H. werneckii*.

Topical imidazoles and allylamines, such as clotrimazole, miconazole, ketoconazole, sulconazole, econazole, and terbinafine, have been reported as effective. Griseofulvin is not effective. Simply shaving away the superficial epidermis with a blade is frequently both diagnostic and curative of tinea nigra.

Onychomycosis (Tinea Unguium)

Onychomycosis is defined as the infection of the nail plate by fungus and represents up to 30% of diagnosed superficial fungal infections. *T. rubrum* accounts for most cases, but many fungi may be causative. Other etiologic agents include *E. floccosum* and various species of *Microsporum* and *Trichophyton* fungi. It may also be caused by yeasts and nondermatophytic molds.

The four classic types of onychomycosis are as follows:

1. Distal subungual onychomycosis primarily involves the distal nail bed and the hyponychium, with secondary involvement of the underside of the nail plate of fingernails and toenails (Fig. 15.11). It is usually caused by *T. rubrum* although *T. tonsurans* is growing in prevalence in children.
2. White superficial onychomycosis (leukonychia trichophytica) is an invasion of the toenail plate on the surface of the nail. It is produced by *T. mentagrophytes*, *Cephalosporium*, *Aspergillus*, and *Fusarium oxysporum* fungi. In the HIV-positive population, it is typically caused by *T. rubrum*.
3. Proximal subungual onychomycosis involves the nail plate mainly from the proximal nailfold, producing a specific clinical picture (Fig. 15.12). It is produced by *T. rubrum* and *Trichophyton megninii* and may be an indication of HIV infection.
4. *Candida* onychomycosis produces destruction of the nail and massive nail bed hyperkeratosis. It is caused by *C. albicans* and

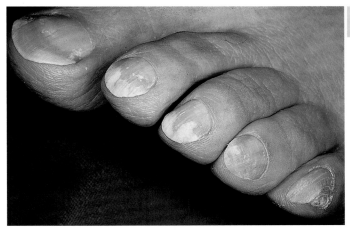

Fig. 15.11 Distal subungual onychomycosis.

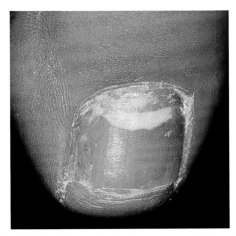

Fig. 15.12 White proximal subungual onychomycosis.

is seen in patients with chronic mucocutaneous candidiasis and other forms of immunodeficiency.

Onychomycosis caused by *T. rubrum* usually starts at the distal corner of the nail and involves the junction of the nail and its bed. A yellowish discoloration occurs, which spreads proximally as a streak in the nail. Later, subungual hyperkeratosis becomes prominent and spreads until the entire nail is affected. Gradually, the entire nail becomes brittle and separated from its bed as a result of the piling up of subungual keratin. Fingernails and toenails present a similar appearance, and the skin of the soles is likely to be involved, with characteristic branny scaling and erythema.

Onychomycosis caused by *T. mentagrophytes* is usually superficial, and there is no paronychial inflammation. The infection generally begins with scaling of the nail under the overhanging cuticle and remains localized to a portion of the nail. In time, however, the entire nail plate may be involved. White superficial onychomycosis is the name given to one type of superficial nail infection caused by this fungus in which small, chalky white spots appear on or in the nail plate. These are so superficial that they may be easily shaved off. *T. violaceum*, *T. schoenleinii*, and *T. tonsurans* occasionally invade the nails, as does *Trichosporon beigelii*.

Scopulariopsis brevicaulis and other nondermatophyte molds are infrequently isolated from onychomycosis. Infection usually begins at the lateral edge of the nail, burrows beneath the plate, and produces large quantities of cheesy debris. *Nattrassia mangiferae*

(*Hendersonula toruloidea*) and *Scytalidium hyalinum* have been reported to cause onychomycosis, as well as a moccasin-type tinea pedis. Other common causes of nondermatophyte molds are *Aspergillus* species, *Fusarium*, and *Acremonium*. In addition to the more common features of onychomycosis, such as nail plate thickening, opacification, and onycholysis, features of infection with these fungi include lateral nail invasion alone, paronychia, and transverse fracture of the proximal nail plate. When these agents are suspected, culture must be done with a medium that does not contain cycloheximide (found in Mycosel agar). Oral griseofulvin is not effective in the treatment of these organisms.

The pathogen is heavily influenced by heredity, geography, and footwear. In the United States most tinea pedis and onychomycosis are caused by *T. rubrum*.

Diagnosis

The demonstration of fungus is made by microscopic examination or by culture. The submitted clippings or curettings must include dystrophic subungual debris. Samples obtained by a drilling technique may have a higher yield than those obtained by curettage. Immediate examination may be made if very thin shavings or curettings are taken from the diseased nail bed and examined with KOH solution with or without an added stain. Histologic examination, PCR, and calcofluor white microscopy and culture have also been used.

Histopathologic examination with periodic acid–Schiff (PAS) stain has been found to be 41%–93% sensitive in various studies. It has proved more sensitive than either KOH or culture in several studies. Immunofluorescent microscopy without calcofluor white is comparable to PAS staining, but high background eosin fluorescence can make the sections difficult to read. Studies have shown the sensitivity of culture to be 30%–70%. Combining KOH and culture has yielded sensitivities in the range of 80%–85%.

DTM can also be used with approximately 50% sensitivity but laboratory regulations have limited its use in the United States. PCR is emerging as an alternative method of detection.

Because no single method offers 100% sensitivity, a variety of methods are still in use. KOH has the advantage of being performed rapidly in the office. Histologic examination usually provides results within 24 hours, whereas culture can take days to weeks. Identification of genus and species is only possible with culture or PCR.

Differential Diagnosis

Dystrophic nails can be caused by psoriasis, lichen planus, eczema, and contact dermatitis and may be clinically indistinguishable from fungal nails. Confirmatory tests to identify the fungus are mandatory to establish a diagnosis. Psoriasis may involve other nails with pitting, onycholysis, oil spots, and salmon patches or by heaped-up subungual keratinization. Typical features of psoriasis may be present on other areas of skin. Lichen planus may produce rough nails or pterygium formation and may involve the oral mucosa or skin. Eczema and contact dermatitis affect the adjacent nailfold. Langerhans cell histiocytosis can also lead to subungual debris and hemorrhage and may be a marker for systemic disease. Hyperkeratotic ("Norwegian") scabies can also produce dystrophic nails, but this is associated with generalized hyperkeratosis.

Onychomycosis among psoriasis patients is reported with varying prevalence but occurs in about 22%, compared with 13% for patients with other skin diseases. Onychomycosis occurs more frequently in men than in women with psoriasis.

Treatment

Many patients with onychomycosis are not symptomatic and may not seek treatment. Patients with diabetes or peripheral neuropathy may be at higher risk for bacterial cellulitis related to onychomycosis, and the benefits of treatment may be greater in this population. These factors, as well as cost, risk of recurrence, and spread to other family members should be considered as part of the decision to treat onychomycosis.

The topical management of onychomycosis has improved with the introduction of ciclopirox, efinazole, and amorolfine nail lacquers. These agents are modestly effective at moderate cost. Efinazole and ciclopirox must be used for 48 weeks. Topical therapy with ciclopirox achieved a 71% effective cure rate and 77% mycologic cure rate in children, possibly due to thinner nail plates or increased compliance. Efinazole has a complete cure rate of 15%–17% but mycologic cure rate of 55%. No topical agent achieves the cure rates possible with oral therapy, but topical agents have lower risk of side effects because they are not systemic. Neodymium:yttrium-aluminum-garnet (Nd:YAG) laser therapy was recently reported to have a 50%–60% cure rate after multiple therapies.

For adults with disease involving fingernails, terbinafine is given in doses of 250 mg/day for 6 weeks; the dose for children is 250 mg daily for patients over 40 kg, 125 mg ($\frac{1}{2}$ tablet) for those 20–40 kg, and 62.5 mg ($\frac{1}{4}$ tablet) for those under 20 kg. For toenails, the course of treatment is generally 12 weeks. In adults, Itraconazole is generally given as pulsed dosing, 200 mg twice daily for 1 week of each month, for 2 months when treating fingernails and for 3–4 months when treating toenails. Fluconazole, 150–300 mg once weekly for 6–12 months, appears to be effective. About 20% of patients will not respond to treatment. The presence of a dermatophytoma within the nail may be associated with a higher risk of failure. Dermatophytomas present as yellow streaks within the nail and may respond to unroofing and curettage. Recurrence rates may be lower with itraconazole than with terbinafine monotherapy, and combined therapy does not result in a lower rate of recurrence. See monitoring recommendations earlier in this chapter.

Several studies suggest that continuous therapy with terbinafine for 4 months is cost-effective compared with other possible agents and regimens. Most clinical trials have been industry sponsored, however, and little independent research is available for review. Terbinafine, itraconazole, and fluconazole have all been shown to be effective. Dosage depends on body weight, as previously indicated. Duration of treatment is the same as for adults.

Although data are limited, treatment with systemic antifungals is generally effective in onychomycosis caused by *Aspergillus* spp. *Scopulariopsis brevicaulis* and *Fusarium* spp. Infection may be difficult to eradicate, and treatment with both systemic antifungals and topical nail lacquers may be appropriate. Nail avulsion represents another option but is more painful and recurrence can still occur.

Candida onychomycosis is a sign of immunosuppression but can be seen infants as well. Systemic treatment with itraconazole or fluconazole is usually effective, but relapses are the rule. When treating *Candida* infections, combinations of topical and systemic treatment can be used for synergistic effect. The combination of topical amorolfine and oral itraconazole, which interferes with different steps of ergosterol synthesis, has been shown to exhibit substantial synergy in this setting. Combination treatment with topical amorolfine and two pulses of itraconazole may be as effective as three pulses of itraconazole, with lower cost.

Itraconazole pulsed treatment has been shown to have a low incidence of liver function abnormalities (alanine transaminase [ALT], aspartate transaminase [AST], alkaline phosphatase, total bilirubin). Product labeling recommends liver function tests (LFTs) for patients receiving continuous itraconazole for periods exceeding 1 month. Monitoring is required for the pulsed regimen if the patient has a history of hepatic disease, has abnormal baseline LFTs, or development of signs or symptoms suggestive of liver dysfunction.

Molds are sensitive to ozone gas, UV light, and visible light. *T. rubrum* in culture has been shown to be susceptible to UVC radiation, photodynamic therapy (PDT), psoralen with UVA (PUVA), and various forms of laser light. However, the mechanism of action and degree of effectiveness of these therapies require further study. For PDT with broad-band white light, the phthalocyanines and Photofrin displayed a fungistatic effect, whereas porphyrins caused photodynamic killing of the dermatophyte. 5,10,15-*Tris*(4-methylpyridinium)-20-phenyl-(21H,23H)-porphine trichloride and deuteroporphyrin monomethylester showed superior results in vitro. Further study of various methods of phototherapy is warranted.

Barot BS, et al: Drug delivery to the nail: therapeutic options and challenges for onychomycosis. Crit Rev Ther Drug Carrier Syst 2014; 31: 459.

Becker C, et al: Lasers and photodynamic therapy in the treatment of onychomycosis. Dermatol Online J 2013; 19:19611.

Bonifaz A, et al: Dermatophyte isolation in the socks of patients with tinea pedis and onychomycosis. J Dermatol 2013; 40: 504.

Boyd AS: Tinea capitis caused by Trichophyton rubrum mimicking favus. Cutis 2016; 98: 389.

Bristow IR: The effectiveness of lasers in the treatment of onychomycosis. J Foot Ankle Res 2014; 7: 34.

Carney C, et al: Treatment of onychomycosis using a submillisecond 1064-nm neodymium:yttrium-aluminum-garnet laser. J Am Acad Dermatol 2013; 69: 578.

Eichenfield LF, Friedlander SF: Pediatric onychomycosis. J Drugs Dermatol 2016; 16: 105.

Elewski BE, et al: Onychomycosis. J Drugs Dermatol 2013; 12: s96.

El-Gohary M, et al: Topical antifungal treatments for tinea cruris and tinea corporis. Cochrane Database Syst Rev 2014; 8: CD009992.

Friedlander SF, et al: Onychomycosis does not always require systemic treatment for cure. Pediatr Dermatol 2013; 30: 316.

Fuller LC, et al: British Association of Dermatologists' guidelines for the management of tinea capitis 2014. Br J Dermatol 2014; 171: 454.

Ghannoum MA, et al: Molecular analysis of dermatophytes suggests spread of infection among household members. Cutis 2013; 91: 237.

Gupta AK, et al: Medical devices for the treatment of onychomycosis. Dermatol Ther 2012; 25: 574.

Gupta AK, et al: Recurrences of dermatophyte toenail onychomycosis during long-term follow-up after successful treatments with mono- and combined therapy of terbinafine and itraconazole. J Cutan Med Surg 2013; 17: 201.

Ilkit M, et al: Tinea pedis. Crit Rev Microbiol 2015; 41: 374.

Kumar V, et al: Extensive nail changes in a toddler with multisystemic Langerhans cell histiocytosis. Pediatr Dermatol 2017; 34: 732.

Lacarrubba F, et al: Newly described features resulting from high-magnification dermoscopy of tinea capitis. JAMA Dermatol 2015; 151: 308.

Lanternier F, et al: Deep dermatophytosis and inherited CARD9 deficiency. N Engl J Med 2013; 369: 1704.

Miyajima Y, et al: Rapid real-time diagnostic PCR for *Trichophyton rubrum* and *Trichophyton mentagrophytes* in patients with tinea unguium and tinea pedis using specific fluorescent probes. J Dermatol Sci 2013; 69: 229.

Motamedi M, et al: Growing incidence of non-dermatophyte onychomycosis in Tehran, Iran. Jundishapur J Microbiol. 2016; 9: e40543.

Neri I, et al: Corkscrew hair. JAMA Dermatol 2013; 149: 990.

Noguchi H, et al: Tinea nigra showing a parallel ridge pattern on dermoscopy. J Dermatol 2015; 42: 518.

Shemer A: Update: medical treatment of onychomycosis. Dermatol Ther 2012; 25: 582.

Shemer A, et al: Increased risk of tinea pedis and onychomycosis among swimming pool employees in Netanya area, Israel. Mycopathologia 2016; 181: 851.

Shemer A, et al: Treatment of tinea capitis—griseofulvin versus fluconazole—a comparative study. J Dtsch Dermatol Ges 2013; 11: 737.

Solís-Arias MP, Garcia-Romero MT: Onychomycosis in children. Int J Dermatol 2017; 56: 123.

Tietz HJ, et al: Efficacy of 4 weeks topical bifonazole treatment for onychomycosis after nail ablation with 40% urea. Mycoses 2013; 56: 414.

Verma SB: Steroid modified tinea. BMJ 2017; 356: j973.

Wanitphakdeedecha R, et al: Efficacy and safety of 1064-nm Nd:YAG laser in treatment of onychomycosis. J Dermatol Treat 2016; 27: 75.

Yuen CW, et al: Treatment of interdigital-type tinea pedis with a 2-week regimen of wearing hygienic socks loaded with antifungal microcapsules. J Am Acad Dermatol 2013; 69: 495.

Zampella JG, et al: Tinea in tots. J Pediatr 2017; 183: 12.

CANDIDIASIS

Candidiasis is also known as candidosis or moniliasis. *Candida albicans* is a common inhabitant of the human gastrointestinal (GI) tract, genitourinary tract, and skin. Under the right conditions, *C. albicans* becomes a pathogen, and can infect the skin, nails, and mucous membranes. *Candida albicans* is an opportunistic organism, acting as a pathogen in the presence of impaired immune response, or where local conditions favor growth. Warmth and moisture favor candidal growth, as can reductions in competing flora during antibiotic therapy. The intertriginous areas, including perianal and inguinal folds, abdominal creases, inframammary creases, interdigital areas, nailfolds, and axillae, are at especially high risk. Higher skin pH can occur due to occlusion from diapers and underwear liners also favor candidal growth.

Diagnosis

Candida is often a clinical diagnosis based on red maceration in skin folds with pustules and peeling at the edges of the red patch (satellite pustules). A KOH preparation will show spores and pseudohyphae. On Gram stain the yeast forms dense, gram-positive, ovoid bodies, 2–5 μm in diameter. A combination of Gomori methenamine silver (GMS) and Congo red staining can be helpful in the differential diagnosis of fungal infections. *Blastomyces* and *Pityrosporum* are positive for both, whereas *Candida* and *Histoplasma* are GMS positive and Congo red negative.

Candida proliferates in both budding and mycelial forms in the stratum corneum or superficial mucosa. Budding yeast and pseudohyphae are easier to detect in histologic section with a PAS stain. Whereas dermatophyte hyphae tend to run parallel to the skin surface, *Candida* pseudohyphae are more prone to vertical orientation.

Topical Anticandidal Agents

Most of the topical agents marketed for tinea are also effective for candidiasis. These include clotrimazole, econazole, ketoconazole, miconazole, oxiconazole, sulconazole, naftifine, terconazole, ciclopirox olamine, butenafine, terbinafine, nystatin, and topical amphotericin B lotion. Older agents, such as gentian violet, Castellani paint, and boric acid, are still sometimes used. Mupirocin has been show in a large study to have excellent candida coverage. Oral nystatin is as effective as intravenous (IV) fluconazole at preventing invasive *Candida* infections in preterm neonates. The oral preparation is more easily administered and is lower in cost.

Other Agents

Fluconazole can be used for acute infections or more chronically for prevention in *Candida* related to genodermatoses. Posaconazole, itraconazole, voriconazole, echinocandins, anidulafungin, and amphotericin B are also used in various settings. Various flavonoid compounds, including apigenin and kaempferol, alkaloid ibogaine (an indole), and the protoberberine alkaloid berberine, have been studied for their inhibitory effects. Topical application of each of these agents accelerated elimination from cutaneous sites of inoculation.

Candidal Intertrigo

The pruritic intertriginous eruptions caused by *C. albicans* may arise between the folds of the genitals; in groins or armpits; between the buttocks (Fig. 15.13); under large, pendulous breasts; under overhanging abdominal folds; or in the umbilicus. The pink to red, intertriginous moist patches are surrounded by a thin, overhanging fringe of somewhat macerated epidermis ("collarette" scale). Some eruptions in the inguinal region may resemble tinea cruris, but usually there is less scaliness and a greater tendency to fissuring. Persistent excoriation and subsequent lichenification and drying may modify the original appearance over time. Often, tiny, superficial, white pustules are observed closely adjacent to the patches. When present, *Candida* can cause flares of inverse psoriasis, although prevalence of *Candida* is not increased in the intertriginous areas of patients with either psoriasis or atopic dermatitis.

Topical anticandidal preparations are usually effective, but recurrence is common. Combinations of a topical anticandidal agent with a midstrength corticosteroid may lead to more rapid relief. Castellani paint may also be helpful. Patients often prefer colorless paint.

Diaper Candidiasis

The diagnosis of candidiasis may be suspected from involvement of the folds and occurrence of many small, erythematous desquamating "satellite" or "daughter" lesions scattered along the edges of the larger macules. Topical anticandidal agents are effective, sometimes compounded in zinc oxide ointment to act as a barrier against the irritating effect of urine. Recurrent diaper candidiasis may be associated with oral and gut colonization and may respond to the addition of oral nystatin suspension.

Oral Candidiasis (Thrush)

The mucous membrane of the mouth may be involved in healthy infants. In the newborn, colonization may be acquired from contact with the vaginal tract of the mother. In older children and adults, thrush is often seen after antibiotic therapy but can be a sign of immunosuppression.

The most common presentations of candida in the mouth are grayish white membranous plaques found on the surface of the tongue and buccal mucosa and maceration at the angle of the mouth (perlèche). On the mucous membranes, the base of these plaques is moist, reddish, and macerated (Fig. 15.14).

In adults, the appearance may resemble that seen in children or may be drier and more erythematous. A dry mouth predisposes to candidal growth because innate immunity molecules in the saliva inhibit candida. Broad-spectrum antibiotics also predispose to candidiasis. The papillae of the tongue may appear atrophic, with the surface smooth, glazed, and bright red. Frequently, the infection extends onto the angles of the mouth to form perlèche. This appearance is common in elderly, debilitated, and malnourished patients and in patients with diabetes. It is often the first manifestation of AIDS and is present in almost all untreated patients with

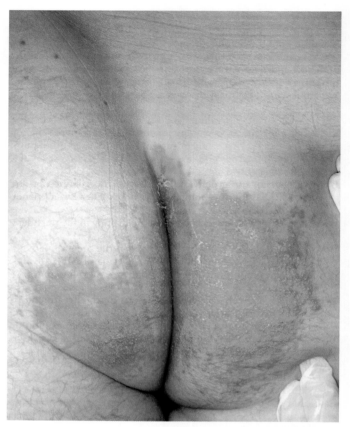
Fig. 15.13 Candidiasis.

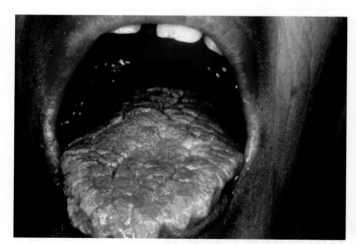
Fig. 15.14 Thrush in chronic mucocutaneous candidiasis.

advanced AIDS. The observation of oral "thrush" in an adult with no known predisposing factors warrants a search for other evidence of infection with HIV, such as lymphadenopathy, leukopenia, or HIV antibodies in the serum.

Various treatment options for oral candidiasis are available. Infants are usually treated with oral nystatin suspension. An adult can let clotrimazole troches dissolve in the mouth. A single, 150-mg dose of fluconazole is effective for many mucocutaneous infections in adults. In immunosuppressed patients, higher doses may be needed. Itraconazole, can also be effective. Although terbinafine may be ineffective in vitro, there is often adequate in vivo activity.

Perlèche

Perlèche, or angular cheilitis, is characterized by maceration and transverse fissuring of the oral commissures. The earliest lesions are poorly defined, grayish white, thickened areas with slight erythema of the mucous membrane at the oral commissure. When more fully developed, this thickening has a bluish white or mother-of-pearl color and may be contiguous with a wedge-shaped, erythematous scaling dermatitis of the skin portion of the commissure. Fissures, maceration, and crust formation ensue. Soft, pinhead-sized papules may appear. Involvement is usually bilateral. Perlèche is frequently caused by *C. albicans* but superinfection with *Staphylococcus aureus* and gram-negative bacteria may occur. Similar changes may occur in riboflavin deficiency or other nutritional deficiency.

Identical fissuring occurs at the mucocutaneous junction from drooling in persons with malocclusion caused by poorly fitting dentures and in older patients in whom atrophy of the alveolar ridges ("closing" the bite) has caused the upper lip to overhang the lower at the commissures.

If infection is caused by *C. albicans* and there is an inflammatory response, anticandidal can be combined with low to midstrength topical corticosteroids to speed healing. If the perlèche is caused by vertical shortening of the lower third of the face, dental or oral surgical intervention may be helpful. Injection of collagen into the depressed sulcus at the oral commissure can be beneficial.

Candidal Vulvovaginitis

Candida albicans is a common inhabitant of the vaginal tract. Overgrowth can cause severe pruritus, burning, and discharge. The labia may be erythematous, moist, and macerated and the cervix hyperemic, swollen, and eroded, showing small vesicles on its surface. The vaginal discharge is not usually profuse and varies from watery, to thick and white or curdlike.

Candidal infection may develop during pregnancy, in diabetes, or secondary to therapy with broad-spectrum antibiotics. Among diabetic patients, candidal overgrowth is related to the degree of hyperglycemia. Recurrent vulvovaginal candidiasis has also been associated with long-term tamoxifen treatment. Candidal balanitis may be present in an uncircumcised sexual partner. Diagnosis is established by the clinical symptoms and findings, as well as the demonstration of the fungus by KOH microscopic examination and culture. PCR is available and is the gold standard.

Oral fluconazole, is often effective. In some patients with predisposing factors, longer courses of fluconazole, or itraconazole, for 5–10 days may be needed. Topical options include miconazole, nystatin, clotrimazole, and terconazole. Clotrimazole exerts antiinflammatory as well as anticandidal effects. Probiotic, anti-candidal bacteria and yogurt have demonstrated some ability to decrease *Candida* colonization.

Non-*albicans* types of *Candida* may be responsible for recalcitrant infections. *Candida glabrata* vaginitis may be refractory to azole drugs and can be difficult to eradicate. Topical boric acid, amphotericin B, and flucytosine may be helpful.

Congenital Cutaneous Candidiasis

Premature rupture of membranes together with a birth canal infected with *C. albicans* may lead to congenital cutaneous candidiasis. The eruption is usually noted within a few hours of delivery. Erythematous macules and patches progress to thin-walled pustules, which rupture, dry, and desquamate within about 1 week. Lesions are usually widespread, involving the trunk, neck, and head and sometimes the palms and soles, including the nailfolds. The oral cavity and diaper area are spared, in contrast to the usual type of acquired neonatal infection. The differential diagnosis includes other neonatal vesiculopustular disorders, including infections such as listeriosis, syphilis, staphylococcal and herpes infections, as well as noninfectious pustulosis including erythema toxicum neonatorum, transient neonatal pustular melanosis, miliaria rubra, and congenital ichthyosiform erythroderma. If infection is suspected early, the amniotic fluid, placenta, and cord should be examined for evidence of infection.

Infants with candidiasis limited to the skin have favorable outcomes; however, systemic involvement may occur. Disseminated infection is suggested by evidence of respiratory distress or other laboratory or clinical signs of neonatal sepsis. Dissemination is more common in infants who weigh less than 1500 g. In these preterm infants the *Candida* can disseminate, and congenital candidiasis is a medical emergency requiring systemic therapy. Treatment with broad-spectrum antibiotics and altered immune responsiveness can also predispose to dissemination. Infants with congenital cutaneous candidiasis should be considered for systemic therapy, especially if any risk factors for dissemination.

Perianal Candidiasis

Infection with *C. albicans* may present as pruritus ani. Perianal dermatitis with erythema, oozing, and maceration is present. Pruritus and burning can be extremely severe. Satellite lesions may be present, but their absence does not exclude candidiasis. Perianal streptococcal disease can present with similar erythema and a culture can help differentiate. Mupirocin has shown benefit in perianal candida in addition to its indication for gram-positive organisms such as *Streptococcus* and can be used while awaiting cultures if the diagnosis is not clear. *Candida* growth is also enhanced on abnormal tissue, such as extramammary Paget disease. If the tissue does not return to normal after the candidiasis is treated, a biopsy may be warranted.

Candidal Paronychia

Inflammation of the nailfold produces redness, edema, and tenderness of the proximal nailfolds and gradual thickening and brownish discoloration of the nail plates. Usually, only the fingernails are affected.

Although acute paronychia is usually staphylococcal in origin, chronic paronychia is typically multifactorial. Irritant dermatitis can lead to broken skin and maceration, which predisposes to Candida infection. Anticandidal agents may be helpful and may be used in combination with a topical corticosteroid to heal the preceding dermatitis.

Candidal paronychia is frequently seen in diabetic patients, and part of the treatment is bringing the diabetes under control. The avoidance of chronic exposure to moisture and irritants is also essential in these patients. If topical treatment fails, oral fluconazole once a week or itraconazole in pulsed dosing can be effective.

Repetitive contact urticaria or allergic contact dermatitis to foods and spices may mimic candidal paronychia. Patch and radioallergosorbent testing (RAST) may be of value.

Erosio Interdigitalis Blastomycetica

A form of candidiasis, erosio interdigitalis blastomycetica is seen as an oval-shaped area of macerated white skin on the web between and extending onto the sides of the fingers or toes. Usually, at the center of the lesion, there are one or more fissures with raw, red bases. As the condition progresses, the macerated skin peels off, leaving a painful, raw, denuded area surrounded by a collar of overhanging white epidermis. On the hand, it is almost always the third web, between the middle and ring fingers, that is affected. The moisture beneath the ring macerates the skin and predisposes to infection. On the feet, it is the fourth interspace that is most often involved, but the areas are apt to be multiple. Clinically, this may be indistinguishable from tinea pedis. Usually, the white, sodden epidermis is thick and does not peel off freely. The disease is also seen in patients with diabetes and those who do wet work.

Diagnosis of erosio interdigitalis blastomycetica is made by culture. Lesions may respond to drying, topical anticandidal agents, or application of filter paper soaked with Castellani paint.

Candidid

As in dermatophytosis, patients with candidiasis may develop secondary id reactions (candidid). These are much less common than the reactions seen with acute inflammatory dermatophytosis. The reactions, which have been reported to clear with treatment of candidal infection, are usually of the erythema annulare centrifugum or chronic urticaria type.

Antibiotic (Iatrogenic) Candidiasis

The use of oral antibiotics, such as the tetracyclines and their related products, may induce clinical candidiasis involving the mouth, GI tract, or perianal area. In addition, vulvovaginitis may occur bacterial flora in the GI system are likely changed by suppression of some of the antibiotic-sensitive bacteria, thereby permitting other organisms such as *Candida* to flourish. Fluconazole, will treat this adequately if antibiotic therapy is given for a limited time. For more prolonged courses of antibiotic therapy, the dose of fluconazole may have to be repeated, or a longer course of a topical agent may be used.

Chronic Mucocutaneous Candidiasis

The term chronic mucocutaneous candidiasis (CMCC) designates a group of patients with heterogeneous disorders whose infection with *Candida* is chronic but limited to mucosal surfaces, skin, and nails. Onset is typically before age 6 years. Onset in adult life may herald the occurrence of thymoma. These cases may be either inherited or sporadic. Inherited types may be associated with endocrinopathy. Oral lesions are diffuse, and perlèche and lip fissures are common. The nails become thickened and dystrophic, with associated paronychia that may be the presenting sign. Hyperkeratotic, hornlike, or granulomatous lesions are often seen on the skin (Figs. 15.15 and 15.16).

Chronic mucocutaneous candidiasis occurs in a number of syndromes. Autosomal dominant signal transducer and activator of transcription 1 *(STAT1)* gain-of-function mutation, impairing interleukin-17 (IL-17)–producing T-cell development, is the best described abnormality. Autosomal recessive IL-17RA, and autosomal dominant IL-17F and IL-17RC deficiencies have been reported in CMCC patients. Autosomal dominant hyper-IgE syndrome is related to *STAT3* mutations, resulting in low IL-17 T-cell numbers. Dectin 1 and IL-22 encoding genes modulate the response to *Candida* infections through a T-helper cell type 17 (Th17) mechanism, although dectin 1 does not appear to be critical in some models of mucosal candidiasis. CARD9 deficiency predisposes to invasive candidiasis as well as invasive and disseminated dermatophytosis. Autoimmune polyendocrinopathy candidiasis ectodermal dystrophy is an autosomal recessive syndrome caused by mutations of the autoimmune regulator gene *(AIRE)*, resulting in failure of T-cell tolerance within the thymus, with decreased numbers of IL-17 T cells. Hallmarks of the syndrome include CMCC, chronic hypoparathyroidism, hypothyroidism, and Addison disease.

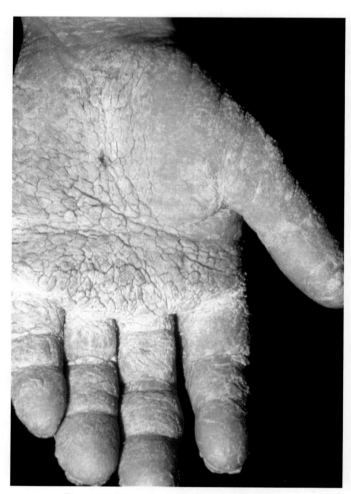

Fig. 15.15 Chronic mucocutaneous candidiasis.

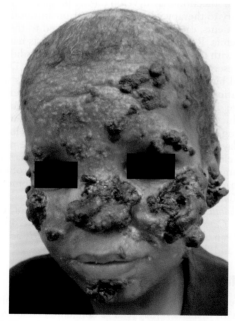

Fig. 15.16 Chronic mucocutaneous candidiasis. (Courtesy Leslie Castelo-Soccio, MD.)

Abnormalities of type 1 cytokine production in response to *Candida* have been reported. Specifically, there may be greatly impaired IL-12 production and dramatically increased levels of IL-6 and IL-10. Reductions in natural killer (NK) cells have also been noted. In a five-generation Italian family with CMCC affecting only the nails, low serum intercellular adhesion molecule 1 (ICAM-1) was noted. The defect was linked to a 19 cM pericentromeric region on chromosome 11.

Systemic fluconazole, itraconazole, or ketoconazole is necessary to control CMCC although the FDA warns against the use of systemic ketoconazole for skin infections. Courses are typically prolonged, repeated, and given at higher doses than the usual recommended dose. Patients with achlorhydria may have problems with absorption of itraconazole and ketoconazole. Cimetidine was reported to restore deficient cell-mediated immunity in four adults from one family, at a dose of 300 mg four times daily. One patient with alopecia areata (AA) and CMCC due to a mutation in STAT-1 responded to ruxolitinib being given for their AA. Granulocyte colony-stimulating factor (G-CSF) infusion has been reported to restore IL-17 secretion, with subsequent clinical remission.

Systemic Candidiasis

Candida albicans is capable of causing disseminated disease and sepsis, invariably when host defenses are compromised. Patients at high risk include those with malignancies, especially leukemia and lymphoma, who may have impaired immune defenses; premature neonates; AIDS patients; debilitated and malnourished patients; those with a transplant who require prolonged immunosuppressive therapy; patients receiving oral cortisone; those who have had multiple surgical operations, especially cardiac surgery; and patients with indwelling IV catheters. IV drug users also are at high risk.

The initial sign of systemic candidiasis may be fever of unknown origin, pulmonary infiltration, GI bleeding, endocarditis, renal failure, meningitis, osteomyelitis, endophthalmitis, peritonitis, proximal muscle weakness and tenderness, or a disseminated macular exanthema. The cutaneous lesions begin as erythematous macules that may become papular, pustular, hemorrhagic, or ulcerative. Deep abscesses may occur. The trunk and extremities are the usual sites of involvement. Proximal muscle tenderness frequently accompanies the exanthema and may be a valuable clue to the correct diagnosis.

The demonstration of microorganisms or a positive culture will substantiate a diagnosis of candidiasis only if the microorganism is found in tissues or fluids ordinarily sterile for *Candida* and if the clinical picture is compatible. *Candida* colonization of endotracheal tubes used in supporting low-birth-weight neonates predisposes to systemic disease. If *Candida* is cultured within the first week of life, there is a high rate of systemic disease.

The mortality rate attributed to systemic candidiasis has declined because of early empiric antifungal treatment and better prophylaxis. Data in children are similar to those in adults. Although amphotericin B remains the gold standard of treatment in systemic candidiasis, other, safer options such as liposomal amphotericin are available. Fluconazole has been effective as prophylaxis with bone marrow transplantation, as well as in the treatment of oropharyngeal candidosis and candidemia in nonneutropenic patients. At high doses, fluconazole is sometimes used for *Candida* in neutropenic patients. Voriconazole, a triazole antifungal, acts by inhibiting synthesis of ergosterol in the fungal cell membrane but leads to extreme photosensitivity. Voriconazole has produced liver abnormalities, rash, and visual disturbances, and these must be monitored during therapy. Posaconazole is a triazole active against *Candida*, although some problems with resistance have been reported. Caspofungin is an echinocandin antifungal that inhibits β-1,3-D-glucan synthesis in the cell wall. Micafungin and

anidulafungin are echinocandins. The newer triazoles and echinocandins have broad spectrums and are effective against invasive *Aspergillus* and *Candida* infections. A meta-analysis of studies of *Candida* sepsis concluded that clinical efficacy was similar among the agents studied, but microbiologic failure was more common with fluconazole than with amphotericin B or anidulafungin. Amphotericin B had a higher rate of adverse events than fluconazole or the echinocandins. Some data favor caspofungin or micafungin over anidulafungin in neutropenic patients. The antiarrhythmic drug amiodarone has some fungicidal activity, and low doses of amiodarone produced a synergistic effect with fluconazole in fluconazole-resistant *C. albicans*.

Despite advances in treatment, the mortality rate associated with systemic candidiasis remains high.

Al Rushood M, et al: Autosomal dominant cases of chronic mucocutaneous candidiasis segregates with mutations of signal transducer and activator of transcription 1, but not of toll-like receptor 3. J Pediatr 2013; 163: 277.

Autmizguine J, et al: Pharmacokinetics and pharmacodynamics of antifungals in children: clinical implications. Drugs 2014; 74: 891.

Dias MF, et al: Treatment of superficial mycoses. An Bras Dermatol 2013; 88: 937.

Dias MF, et al: Update on therapy for superficial mycoses. An Bras Dermatol 2013; 88: 764.

Griffin AT, Hanson KE: Update on fungal diagnostics. Curr Infect Dis Rep 2014; 16: 415.

Ling Y, et al: Inherited IL-17RC deficiency in patients with chronic mucocutaneous candidiasis. J Exp Med 2015; 212: 619.

Mintz JD, Martens MG: Prevalence of non-albicans candida infections in women with recurrent vulvovaginal symptomatology. Adv Infect Dis 2013; 3: 238.

Salvatori O, et al: Innate immunity and saliva in *Candida albicans*–mediated oral diseases. J Dent Res 2016; 95: 365.

Schimke LF, et al: A novel gain-of-function *IKBA* mutation underlies ectodermal dysplasia with immunodeficiency and polyendocrinopathy. J Clin Immunol 2013; 33: 1088.

Sobel JD, Akins RA: The role of PCR in the diagnosis of *Candida* vulvovaginitis. Curr Infect Dis Rep 2015; 17: 33.

Wildbaum G, et al: Continuous G-CSF therapy for isolated chronic mucocutaneous candidiasis. J Allergy Clin Immunol 2013; 132: 761.

Wilson D, et al: Clotrimazole dampens vaginal inflammation and neutrophil infiltration in response to *Candida albicans* infection. Antimicrob Agents Chemother 2013; 57: 5178.

GEOTRICHOSIS

Geotrichum candidum is an ascomycetous anamorph, yeastlike fungus found as part of the natural flora of milk. It is also found on fruit and tomatoes and in soil. It is used commercially as a maturing agent for cheese. Individual strains may be more moldlike or yeastlike. Substantial genetic polymorphism has been noted in *G. candidum.*

In immunosuppressed individuals, *G. candidum* or *Geotrichum capitatum (Blastoschizomyces capitatus)* may act as an opportunistic pathogen, causing disseminated or mucocutaneous geotrichosis. Mucocutaneous disease is characterized by erythema, pseudomembranes, and mucopurulent sputum similar to that seen in thrush. The intestinal, bronchial, and pulmonary forms are similar to candidal infection. *G. candidum* is usually isolated as a saprophyte. If cultured repeatedly from diseased tissue, it should be assumed to be acting as a pathogen.

The diagnosis is made by the repeated demonstration of the organism by KOH microscopic examination and by its culture from sputum on Sabouraud dextrose agar. Direct examination shows branching septate mycelium and chains of rectangular cells.

In culture, there is a mealy growth at room temperature. The hyphae form rectangular arthrospores.

Treatment of mucocutaneous disease can be accomplished with oral nystatin, or nystatin (Mycostatin) suspension in some cases. For more severe or disseminated disease, liposomal amphotericin B, caspofungin, voriconazole, itraconazole, flucytosine, or combinations of these agents have been effective.

Martins N, et al: Candidiasis. Mycopathologia 2014; 177: 223.

PIEDRA

Piedra is a superficial infection of the outside of the hair shaft. In black piedra, dark, pinhead- to pebble-sized formations occur on the hairs of the scalp, brows, lashes, or beard. These nodules are distributed irregularly along the length of the shaft. Black piedra, usually caused by *Piedraia hortai*, occurs mostly in the tropics, especially in South America and Asia. The nodelike masses in KOH preparations show numerous oval asci containing two to eight ascospores and mycelium. Cultures produce black colonies composed of hyphae and chlamydospores.

White piedra is typically caused by *Trichosporon (Trichosporum) beigelii* or *Trichosporon inkin* and occurs more often in temperate climates. Based on molecular analysis, the taxon *T. beigelii* has been replaced by several species. A synergistic corynebacterial infection is often present in white piedra, as demonstrated by culture and electron microscopy. *T. beigelii* has also been implicated as a cause of onychomycosis. *T. inkin* is implicated as an etiologic agent of pubic white piedra. *Trichosporon asahii* causes white piedra and onychomycosis and has been isolated from black piedra. *Trichosporon* spp. can also cause disseminated disease in immunosuppressed patients, and *T. asahii* has produced disseminated cutaneous infections in immunocompetent hosts. In white piedra, patients present with yellow or beige-colored, soft, slimy sheaths coating the hair shafts (Fig. 15.17). The sheaths are composed of hyphae, arthrospores, and bacteria. The culture shows soft, cream-colored colonies composed of blastospores and septate hyphae, which fragment into arthrospores.

Treatment of piedra involves cutting or shaving the hair, but this may not be acceptable to the patient. Oral and topical terbinafine have been effective in black piedra. For white piedra, oral itraconazole, topical imidazoles, ciclopirox olamine, 2% selenium sulfide, 6% precipitated sulfur in petrolatum, chlorhexidine solutions, Castellani paint, zinc pyrithione, amphotericin B lotion, and 2%–10% glutaraldehyde have all been used successfully.

Essential oils derived from *Cymbopogon winterians, Mentha piperita, Cinnamomum zeylanicum, Melaleuca alternifolia,* and *Eucalyptus globulus* have demonstrated efficacy against *Trichosporon ovoides.*

Richini-Pereira VB, et al: White piedra. Rev Soc Bras Med Trop 2012; 45: 402.
Saxena S, et al: Inhibitory effect of essential oils against *Trichosporon ovoides* causing piedra hair infection. Braz J Microbiol 2012; 43: 1347.
Uniyal V, et al: Screening of some essential oils against *Trichosporon* species. J Environ Biol 2013; 34: 17.

TINEA VERSICOLOR (PITYRIASIS VERSICOLOR)

Tinea versicolor is caused by *Malassezia* spp. The major implicated species is *Malassezia globosa*, although *M. restricta, M. sympodialis, M. furfur, M. obtusa,* and *M. slooffiae* have also been implicated. Tinea versicolor typically presents as hypopigmented or hyperpigmented, coalescing scaly macules on the trunk and upper arms (Fig. 15.18). Pink, atrophic, and trichrome variants exist and can produce striking clinical pictures. The eruption is more common

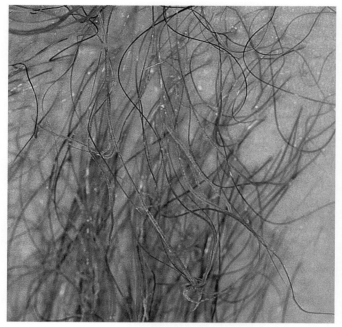
Fig. 15.17 White piedra.

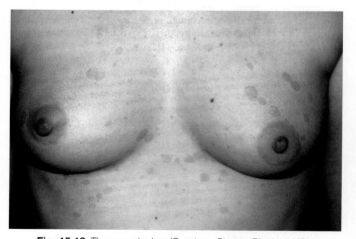
Fig. 15.18 Tinea versicolor. (Courtesy Steven Binnick, MD.)

during the summer months and favors oily areas of skin. Sites of predilection are the sternal region and the sides of the chest, abdomen, back, pubis, neck, and intertriginous areas such as antecubital and popliteal fossae. The disease may also occur on the scalp, palms, and soles. The face may be involved in infants and immunocompromised patients. Penile lesions may develop as well, and the organism is commonly isolated from patients with balanoposthitis. Mild itching and inflammation around the patches may be present. In some patients, many follicular papules are present.

In hypopigmented tinea versicolor, abnormally small and poorly melanized melanosomes are produced and are not transferred to keratinocytes properly. This becomes most conspicuous in dark-skinned people. This hypopigmentation may persist for weeks or months after the fungal disease is cured. UV exposure may speed normalization of the pigment.

Diagnosis

The *Malassezia* fungus is easily demonstrated in scrapings of the profuse scales that cover the lesions. Tape stripping of the lesions can also be performed. Microscopically, there are short, thick fungal hyphae and large numbers of variously sized spores. This combination of strands of mycelium and numerous spores is commonly referred to as "spaghetti and meatballs." The fungus can be highlighted by a variety of stains, including Parker blue-black ink (mixed 1:1 with 20% KOH), 1% Chicago sky blue 6B with 8% KOH, and Gram stain. Identification by culture requires lipid enrichment of the media and is rarely done to establish the diagnosis unless there is resultant malassezia sepsis as can be seen in patients on lipid rich hyperalimentation. Wood's light examination accentuates pigment changes and may demonstrate yellow-green fluorescence of the lesions in adjacent follicles. Biopsy will demonstrate a thick basket-weave stratum corneum with hyphae and spores. In the atrophic variant, epidermal colonization with hyphae and spores is accompanied by effacement of the rete ridges, subepidermal fibroplasia, pigment incontinence, and elastolysis.

Differential Diagnosis

Tinea versicolor must be differentiated from seborrheic dermatitis, pityriasis rosea, pityriasis rubra pilaris, pityriasis alba, Hansen disease, syphilis, confluent and reticulated papillomatosis and vitiligo. In the atrophic variant of tinea versicolor, the lesions may suggest parapsoriasis, mycosis fungoides, anetoderma, LE, or steroid atrophy. The diagnosis in all forms of tinea versicolor is generally easily established by KOH examination. In seborrheic dermatitis, the patches have an erythematous yellowish tint, and the scales are soft and greasy and typical locations along the glabella, nasolabial folds and scalp are involved. In tinea versicolor the scales are furfuraceous (fluffy). Macular syphilid consists of faint pink lesions, less than 1 cm in diameter, irregularly round or oval, which are distributed principally on the nape, sides of the trunk, and flexor aspects of the extremities. The lesions are slightly indurated, with a peripheral scale, and may be copper colored. General adenopathy may be present. Serologic tests are positive in this phase of syphilis, but prozone reactions may occur, and the serum may require dilution.

Treatment

Imidazoles, triazoles, selenium sulfide, ciclopirox olamine, zinc pyrithione, sulfur preparations, salicylic acid preparations, propylene glycol, and benzoyl peroxide have been used successfully as topical agents. Selenium sulfide lotion is very cost-effective and can be applied daily for a week; it is washed off after 10 minutes and is also effective in a single, overnight application, which can be repeated monthly as prophylaxis. The scalp and trunk can be shampooed monthly with selenium sulfide to reduce scalp colonization. Zinc pyrithione soap is also cost-effective and well tolerated for treatment and prophylaxis.

In adults, Oral itraconazole, 200 mg once daily for 7 days or 400 mg single dose has been used. Fluconazole, 400 mg once, may also be effective and can be repeated monthly. Although oral terbinafine has been ineffective, it is effective topically. Twice-daily applications are superior to once-daily applications. Alternatively, 5-aminolevulinic acid PDT has been reported as effective.

Patients should be informed that the hypopigmentation or hyperpigmentation will take time to resolve and is not a sign of treatment failure. Relapse is likely if prophylactic therapy is not given occasionally, but many prophylactic options are available.

After initial therapy, patients may prefer weekly washing with a topical zinc pyrithione bar or single, overnight applications of selenium sulfide, ketoconazole, econazole, or bifonazole shampoo every 30–60 days, or monthly oral therapy.

Pityrosporum Folliculitis

Pityrosporum folliculitis has been a controversial entity, but its prompt response to antifungal agents suggests that *Pityrosporum* yeast (the yeast phase of *Malassezia* spp.) are indeed pathogenic. Criteria for diagnosis include characteristic morphology, demonstration of yellow-green Wood's light fluorescence of the papules or identification of *Pityrosporum* yeast in smears or biopsies, and prompt response to antifungal treatment. Fungal stains, Gram stain, and May-Grünwald-Giemsa stain have been used. Lesions tend to be chronic, moderately itchy, monomorphic dome-shaped follicular papules and tiny pustules involving the upper back and adjacent areas. The face and scalp may be involved, and the lesions are sometimes found in association with either tinea versicolor or seborrheic dermatitis. *Pityrosporum* folliculitis is more common in organ or marrow transplant recipients and after antibiotic therapy especially for acne. *Pityrosporum* yeast is a normal part of the follicular flora, so alterations in flora may favor uncontrolled growth of the yeast. Such a case occurs when *Propionibacterium acnes* is suppressed by tetracycline therapy.

The eruption responds to oral fluconazole, 400 mg once; or itraconazole, 200 mg/day for 5–7 days. As previously noted, the FDA warns against using oral ketoconazole for skin and nail infections. Topical therapy with 2.5% selenium sulfide applied overnight is also generally effective. Other treatments include 30%–50% propylene glycol in water and topical imidazole creams. PDT may be considered in refractory disease. Topical clioquinol combined with narrow band UVB was also successful in a small trial. Relapses are common, but prophylaxis may be successful with monthly applications of selenium sulfide or maintenance doses of topical econazole.

Akaza N, et al: *Malassezia globosa* tends to grow actively in summer conditions more than other cutaneous *Malassezia* species. J Dermatol 2012; 39: 613.

Gupta AK, Lyons DC: Pityriasis versicolor. Expert Opin Pharmacother 2014; 15: 1707.

Gupta AK, et al: Systematic review of systemic treatments for tinea versicolor and evidence-based dosing regimen recommendations. J Cutan Med Surg 2014; 18: 79.

Jiang Y: Efficacy observation of clioquinol cream combined with NB-UVB in treatment of pityrosporum folliculitis. Evaluatin and analysis of drug-use in hospitals of China. 2015; 15: 1585.

Mostafa WZ, et al: Hair loss in pityriasis versicolor lesions. J Am Acad Dermatol 2013; 69: e19.

Prindaville B, et al: *Pityrosporum* folliculitis. J Am Acad Dermatol 2017 Nov 11. ePub ahead of print.

Saad M, et al: Molecular epidemiology of *Malassezia globosa* and *Malassezia restricta* in Sudanese patients with pityriasis versicolor. Mycopathologia 2013; 175: 69.

Spence-Shishido A, et al: In vivo Gram staining of tinea versicolor. JAMA Dermatol 2013; 149: 991.

Varada S, et al: Uncommon presentations of tinea versicolor. Dermatol Pract Concept 2014; 4: 93.

■ THE DEEP MYCOSES

Most deep cutaneous fungal infections are a manifestation of systemic infection from inhalation of aerosolized fungus. When primary infection is introduced directly into the skin from puncture wounds, abrasions, or other trauma, a chancriform or verrucous lesion will form that may be accompanied by secondary lymphangitis. Chest radiographs should be taken when investigating patients with deep mycoses, except for the classic inoculation types, such as sporotrichosis, mycetoma, chromoblastomycosis, and phaeohyphomycosis.

COCCIDIOIDOMYCOSIS

Coccidioidomycosis is also known as coccidioidal granuloma, valley fever, and San Joaquin Valley fever.

Primary Pulmonary Coccidioidomycosis

Inhalation of *Coccidioides immitis* or *C. posadasii*, followed by an incubation period of 10 days to several weeks, produces a respiratory infection that may be mild, with only a low-grade fever resembling a flulike illness. Approximately 60% of infected persons are entirely asymptomatic. Severe symptoms of chills, high fever, night sweats, severe headache, backache, and malaise may ensue in a minority. A large percentage of patients show lung changes on radiographic examination. These include hilar adenopathy, peribronchial infiltration, or an infiltrate compatible with bronchopneumonia. At the time of onset, a generalized maculopapular eruption may be present, which may be confused with a drug eruption, viral exanthem, or scarlet fever.

Within a few weeks, the pulmonary symptoms subside. In about 30% of women and in 15% of men, skin manifestations appear in the form of erythema nodosum over the shins and sometimes over the thighs, hips, and buttocks. These tender lesions may become confluent, gradually turn from purple to brown, and then disappear in about 3 weeks. Erythema nodosum is a favorable prognostic sign and occurs mostly in white individuals with transient self-limited disease. Sometimes, erythema multiforme may develop in a similar clinical setting.

Although valley fever is usually self-limited and patients recover spontaneously, a small percentage steadily progress into the chronic, progressive, disseminated form. The propensity for disseminated disease is several-fold higher in Hispanics and Native Americans and many times higher for African Americans, Filipinos, and Vietnamese. In women, pregnancy may predispose to systemic disease. Infants, the elderly population, persons with blood types B or AB, and immunosuppressed patients, such as those with AIDS, a history of organ transplantation, or a hematogenous malignancy or those receiving immunosuppressive therapy, are also at increased risk for severe disease. Donor-derived organ transplant transmission has been documented many times; risk is primarily in the first year after transplant. Autosomal dominant interferon-γ receptor 1 deficiency also may predispose to disseminated disease.

Disseminated Coccidioidomycosis (Coccidioidal Granuloma)

Dissemination occurs in less than 1% of infections, but its incidence is heavily influenced by the factors previously listed. Target organs include the bones, joints, viscera, brain, meninges, and skin. A single organ or multiple organs may be involved. Skin lesions occur in 15%–20% of patients (Fig. 15.19) with disseminated disease and may appear as verrucous nodules, as pink papules resembling basal cell carcinoma, or as subcutaneous abscesses. The face is frequently involved. Some chronic lesions develop into plaques that resemble mycosis fungoides or North American blastomycosis. In AIDS patients, umbilicated papules may mimic molluscum contagiosum. Umbilicated papules are more often associated with cryptococcosis but can occur with a variety of fungi.

Primary Cutaneous Coccidioidomycosis

The primary form occurs rarely, and skin disease should be considered a manifestation of disseminated disease unless there

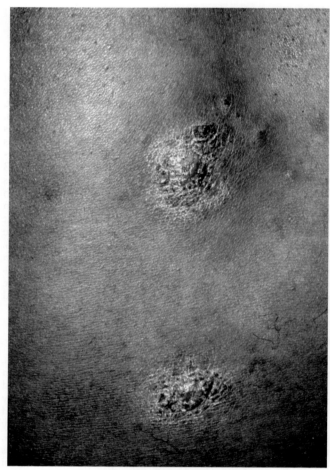

Fig. 15.19 Coccidioidomycosis.

is a definite history of inoculation, or a colonized splinter is found in the lesion. Between 1 and 3 weeks after inoculation, an indurated nodule develops that may ulcerate. Later, nodules appear along the lymphatic vessels. Spontaneous recovery may result after several weeks, although most patients are treated with systemic agents.

Etiology and Pathology

The causative organism, *C. immitis*, has been isolated from the soil and from vegetation. It is commonly found in the burrows of rodents, often at a depth of about 20 cm. Epidemics occur when the soil is disrupted to a depth of 20 cm or more. This can occur as a result of road work, laying of telephone or electric cable, dust storms, and earthquakes. Outbreaks occur sporadically in California and Arizona.

Coccidioides immitis is dimorphous, reproducing brittle mycelia at room temperature, and spherules in tissue. Spherules are unencapsulated with a thick, refractile wall and a granular interior. They measure 5–200 μm in diameter but average 20 μm. Endosporulation can occur, and although the organism can resemble *Rhinosporidium*, *Coccidioides* is typically much smaller and more uniform in size. It also lacks the small, central nucleus that is uniformly present in nonsporulating *Rhinosporidium*.

Culture

Coccidioides is readily grown at room temperature and is highly infectious. For this reason, culture of deep fungi should be performed only in laboratories with biocontainment hoods. PCR primers and a DNA hybridization probe test that targets organism-specific ribosomal RNA are available for rapid identification.

Epidemiology

Coccidioidomycosis principally occurs in limited areas in the Western Hemisphere. It is endemic in northern Mexico, Argentina, Venezuela, and the southwestern United States (lower Sonoran Life Zone). In highly endemic areas, most residents will have been infected, and new residents have a good chance of becoming infected within 6 months. Very few will develop disseminated disease, although the attack rate has recently increased in both California and Arizona.

Differential Diagnosis

Clinically, it is extremely difficult to differentiate coccidioidomycosis from blastomycosis, which it closely resembles. Definite diagnosis depends on serologic testing and the demonstration of *C. immitis* or *C. posadasii* microscopically, culturally, or by PCR. A positive reaction of the delayed tuberculin type develops early on skin testing and remains high in those who resist the disease well. A negative skin test occurs with dissemination.

Immunology

Precipitin, latex agglutination, immunodiffusion, a widely used nuclei acid hybridization test, and complement fixation serologic tests have been developed. The precipitin, immunodiffusion, enzyme-linked immunosorbent assay (ELISA), and latex agglutination tests are useful in recent infection because a maximum titer is reached in 1–2 weeks. They permit detection of coccidioidal immunoglobulin M (IgM) in early coccidioidomycosis. In later infections, the complement fixation test is useful. In primary coccidioidomycosis, the titer is low, whereas in subsequent dissemination, there is a rapid rise in titer. Titers greater than 1:32 indicate disseminated disease is present and correlate with severity. They are used to follow progress in treatment and relapse after therapy. When the disease has disseminated, cerebrospinal, synovial, and peritoneal fluid can be tested for coccidioidal antibody. The *Coccidioides*-specific ELISA detects antigenuria in about 70% of patients with coccidioidomycosis and is negative in more than 99% of controls without fungal infections. Cross-reactions with other systemic mycoses occur in 10% of patients. An isolated positive enzyme immunoassay (EIA) IgM test usually means disseminated disease. Serologic titers may be falsely negative in patients receiving immunosuppressive therapy.

Treatment

Both fluconazole, 400 mg/day, and itraconazole solution, 200 mg daily, have similar efficacy in mild to moderate nonmeningeal disease. Treatment must be continued for 3–12 months. Many patients will require ongoing suppressive therapy. In patients infected with HIV, lifetime suppressive doses of 200 mg/day are advised, and potent antiretroviral therapy is associated with improved outcomes. In coccidioidomycotic meningitis or severe disseminated disease, a combination of amphotericin B and fluconazole is used. Posaconazole is a second-line agent. Voriconazole has been used successfully in meningeal disease. Azole resistance has been reported and should be suspected in patients with refractory disease. Surgical debridement of abscesses may be necessary. For primary inoculation, itraconazole 400 mg daily for 6 months is usually effective.

Carpenter JB, et al: Clinical and pathologic characteristics of disseminated coccidioidomycosis. J Am Acad Dermatol 2010; 62: 831.

Cummings KC, et al: Point-source outbreak of coccidioidomycosis in construction workers. Epidemiol Infect 2010; 138: 507.
DiCaudo DJ: Coccidioidomycosis. Semin Cutan Med Surg 2014; 33: 140.
Fernandez-Flores A, et al: Morphological findings of deep cutaneous fungal infections. Am J Dermatopathol 2014; 36: 531.
Garcia Garcia SC, et al: Coccidioidomycosis and the skin. An Bras Dermatol 2015; 90: 610.
Langelier C, et al: Beyond the superficial: *Coccidioides immitis* fungaemia in a man with fever, fatigue and skin nodules. BMJ Case Rep 2014 Sep 16; 2014.
Miller SS, et al: Disseminated coccidioidomycosis in a patient managed with adalimumab for Crohn's disease. Nat Rev Gastroenterol Hepatol 2010; 7: 231.
Rodríguez-Cerdeira C, et al: Systemic fungal infections in patients with human immunodeficiency virus. Actas Dermosifiliogr 2014; 105: 5.
Tortorano AM, et al: Primary cutaneous coccidioidomycosis in an Italian nun working in South America and review of published literature. Mycopathologia 2015; 180: 229.
Vin DC, et al: Refractory disseminated coccidioidomycosis and mycobacteriosis in interferon-gamma receptor 1 deficiency. Clin Infect Dis 2009; 49: e62.

HISTOPLASMOSIS

Histoplasmosis is caused by inhalation of airborne spores. It may be asymptomatic or may cause limited lung disease. Dissemination to other organs, including the skin, occurs in about 1 in 2000 patients with acute infection. Immunodeficiency, old age, and systemic corticosteroids predispose to widespread disease. Donor-derived organ transplant transmission has often been documented. Cases misdiagnosed as sarcoidosis and treated with corticosteroids have disseminated widely. In disseminated disease, mucous membranes are involved much more frequently than skin. Primary cutaneous disease is exceedingly rare.

Primary Pulmonary Histoplasmosis

Primary pulmonary histoplasmosis is usually a benign, self-limited form of acute pneumonitis characterized by fever, malaise, night sweats, chest pain, cough, and hilar adenopathy. Resolution of the pneumonitis occurs rapidly, and the only residua may be calcifications in the lung and a positive skin test to histoplasmin. However, serious pneumonitis caused by histoplasmosis does occur. Such cases have been reported among cave workers in Mexico and travelers returning from Central America. A chronic pulmonary form may occur in patients with emphysema.

Approximately 10% of patients with acute symptomatic infection develop arthritis and erythema nodosum. During a large Midwestern U.S. epidemic, about 4% of patients diagnosed with histoplasmosis presented with erythema nodosum. Erythema multiforme has also been described.

Progressive Disseminated Histoplasmosis

Most patients who develop this severe, progressive, disseminated form are immunocompromised or taking systemic corticosteroids. Leukemia, lymphoma, lupus erythematosus, renal transplantation, or AIDS are frequent predisposing diseases. Cases have also been reported in patients receiving low-dose methotrexate for psoriasis and in patients receiving anti–tumor necrosis factor (TNF) therapy. Approximately 20% have no identifiable risk factor.

The reticuloendothelial system, genitourinary tract, adrenals, GI tract, adrenal glands, and heart may be involved. Ulcerations and granulomas of the oronasopharynx are the most common mucocutaneous lesions, occurring in about 20% of patients with disseminated histoplasmosis (Fig. 15.20). Beginning as solid, indurated plaques, the lesions ulcerate and become deep-seated, painful, and secondarily infected. Perianal lesions may also occur.

Skin lesions are present in approximately 6% of patients with dissemination but may occur in 10%–25% of patients with AIDS and in renal transplant recipients. The morphologic patterns are nonspecific and protean, including umbilicated nodules, papules, plaques (Fig. 15.21), ulcers, cellulitis, abscesses, pyoderma, pustules, and furuncles. Demonstration of the organisms is readily made from histologic sections and cultures of the exudate. The most common manifestation in children is purpura, which usually appears a few days before death and is probably caused by severe involvement of the reticuloendothelial system, with emaciation, chronic fever, and severe GI symptoms. In the HIV-positive population, dyspnea, platelet count less than 100,000/mm^3, and lactate dehydrogenase level more than twofold the upper limit of normal are poor prognostic factors and independently associated with death during the first 30 days of antifungal treatment.

Primary Cutaneous Histoplasmosis

The rare primary cutaneous form is characterized by a chancre-type lesion with regional adenopathy.

African Histoplasmosis

African histoplasmosis is caused by *Histoplasma capsulatum* var. *duboisii*. Skin lesions are much more common and include superficial cutaneous granulomas, subcutaneous granulomas, and osteomyelitic lesions with secondary involvement of the skin (cold abscesses). Papular, nodular, circinate, eczematoid, and psoriasiform lesions may be seen. The granulomas are dome-shaped nodules, painless but slightly pruritic. There may be skin and mucous membrane manifestations such as ulcerations of the nose, mouth, pharynx, genitals, and anus. These ulcers are chronic, superficial lesions with no induration or noticeable inflammatory reaction. Erythema nodosum occurs frequently. Emaciation and chronic fevers are common systemic signs. Late occurrence many years after exposure may occur.

Etiology and Pathology

Histoplasmosis is caused by *H. capsulatum*, a dimorphic fungus that exists as a soil saprophyte. The organism is frequently found in bat and bird feces.

In tissue, there are 2–3 μm round bodies within the cytoplasm of large macrophages or the cytoplasm of keratinocytes. A pseudocapsule surrounds each organism. The organisms bear a striking resemblance to those of leishmaniasis but lack a kinetoplast and are distributed evenly throughout the cytoplasm, whereas leishmanial organisms often line up at the periphery of the cell. Budding forms may rarely be present, and mycelial and pleomorphic budding forms are sometimes seen in cavitary pulmonary disease, endocardial disease, aortic plaques, or skin lesions. Morphologically, these forms resemble *Candida* more than typical intracellular *Histoplasma*. On direct examination, the organism may be demonstrated in the peripheral blood, sputum, bronchial washings, cerebrospinal fluid, sternal marrow, lymph node touch smears, or ulcers when stained with Giemsa, PAS, or GMS. In African histoplasmosis, the organisms are 10–13 μm in diameter and are typically found within multinucleated giant cells.

In disseminated disease, the bone marrow is frequently involved. Blood, urine, and tissue from oral and skin lesions should also be cultured. PCR probes are available for rapid culture confirmation.

Epidemiology

Although histoplasmosis occurs throughout the world, it is most common in North America, especially in the central U.S.

states along the Mississippi River basin. It is also found along the Potomac, Delaware, Hudson, and St. Lawrence rivers. It has been reported in the major river valleys of South America, Central Africa, China, and Southeast Asia but seems to spare the Nile River Valley. The disease is heavily endemic in Puerto Rico and Nicaragua.

Transmission of the disease does not occur between individuals; instead, the infection is contracted from the soil by inhalation of the spores, especially in a dusty atmosphere. The spores have been demonstrated in the excreta of starlings, chickens, turkeys,

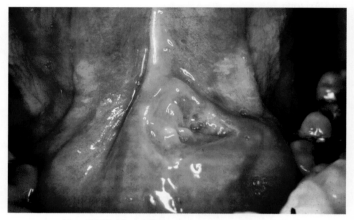

Fig. 15.20 Ulcer of disseminated histoplasmosis.

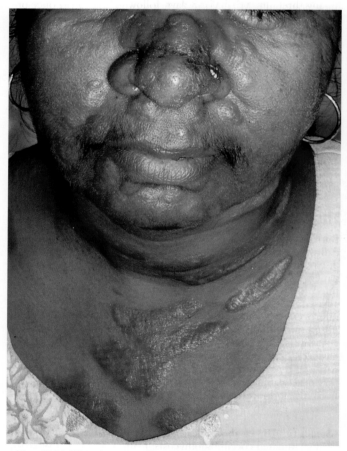

Fig. 15.21 Histoplasmosis. (Courtesy Shyam Verma, MBBS, DVD.)

and bats. The disease may be contracted by persons who enter caves inhabited by bats or birds. Epidemics have been reported from exposure to silos, abandoned chicken houses, and storm cellars.

In the 1978 histoplasmosis outbreak in Indianapolis, Indiana, 488 clinically recognized cases occurred, and 55 had disseminated disease. The actual number infected persons was probably well over 100,000. Nineteen died, none of whom was under age 1 year. Fatal or disseminated infections occurred in 74% of immunosuppressed persons, compared with 6.5% of those not immunosuppressed. Age over 54 was a worse prognostic factor than chronic lung disease in nonimmunosuppressed persons. Disseminated histoplasmosis is seen as an opportunistic infection in HIV-infected patients.

Immunology

The best diagnostic test for histoplasmosis has been urinary ELISA, but PCR assays are available and demonstrate excellent sensitivity. Serologic testing for antibodies requires that the patient has normal immune responsiveness (false negatives) and is further limited by a high rate of false-positive results, especially cross-reactions with blastomycosis. False positives also occur in the latter situation when measuring polysaccharide antigen in the serum or urine, the most sensitive and rapid test. The complement fixation test, when positive at a titer of 1:32 or greater, indicates active or recent infection. Because of the limitations of serologic studies, culture remains the gold standard.

Treatment

For mild to moderate progressive disseminated disease itraconazole, 200 mg three times daily for 3 days, followed by 200 mg once or twice daily for 12 months is given. Amphotericin B is the treatment of choice in severely ill patients and immunocompromised patients. A suppressive dose of itraconazole, 200 mg/day, follows the IV amphotericin and may be needed as lifelong treatment.

Akin L, et al: Oral presentation of disseminated histoplasmosis. J Oral Maxillofac Surg 2011; 69: 535.

Buitrago MJ, et al: A case of primary cutaneous histoplasmosis acquired in the laboratory. Mycoses 2011; 54: e859.

Chang P, et al: Skin lesions of histoplasmosis. Clin Dermatol 2012; 30: 592.

Galandiuk S, et al: Infliximab-induced disseminated histoplasmosis in a patient with Crohn's disease. Nat Clin Pract Gastroenterol Hepatol 2008; 5: 283.

Honarpisheh HH, et al: Cutaneous histoplasmosis with prominent parasitization of epidermal keratinocytes. J Cutan Pathol 2016; 43: 1155.

Régnier-Rosencher E, et al: Late occurrence of *Histoplasma duboisii* cutaneous and pulmonary infection 18 years after exposure. J Mycol Med 2014; 24: 229.

Rodríguez-Cerdeira C, et al: Systemic fungal infections in patients with human immunodeficiency virus. Actas Dermosifiliogr 2014; 105: 5.

Sun NZ, et al: Cutaneous histoplasmosis in renal transplant recipients. Clin Transplant 2014; 28: 1069.

CRYPTOCOCCOSIS

Cryptococcosis generally begins as a pulmonary infection and remains localized to the lung in 90% of patients. In the remaining 10%, the organisms hematogenously disseminate to other organs, with the CNS and the skin the two most common secondary sites. Patients in the 10% group are usually immunocompromised or debilitated. The incidence of dissemination is much higher in patients with AIDS, occurring in up to 50% of this population.

Primary pulmonary cryptococcosis infection may be so mild that the symptoms of fever, cough, and pain may be absent. On the other hand, some cases may be severe enough to cause death. Radiographic studies will reveal disease at this stage.

When dissemination occurs, the organism has a special affinity for the CNS. Cryptococcosis is the most common cause of mycotic meningitis. The patient may have restlessness, hallucinations, depression, severe headache, vertigo, nausea and vomiting, nuchal rigidity, seizures, and symptoms of intraocular hypertension. Other organs, such as the liver, skin, spleen, myocardium, and skeletal system, as well as the lymph nodes, may be involved. Disseminated cryptococcosis can present in many organ systems; hepatitis, osteomyelitis, prostatitis, pyelonephritis, peritonitis, and skin involvement have all been reported as initial manifestations of disease. The incidence of skin involvement in patients with cryptococcosis is 10%–15%, although it is lower in the HIV-infected population. Cutaneous lesions may precede overt systemic disease by 2–8 months.

Skin infection with cryptococcosis occurs most frequently on the head and neck. A variety of morphologic lesions have been reported, including subcutaneous swellings, abscesses, blisters, tumor-like masses, molluscum contagiosum–like lesions (Fig. 15.22), draining sinuses, ulcers, eczematous plaques, granulomas, papules, nodules, pustules, acneiform lesions, plaques, and cellulitis. Approximately 50% of patients with HIV and disseminated cryptococcosis will develop molluscum contagiosum–like lesions. In these patients, there is often a central hemorrhagic crust. Lesions may first become evident in HIV-infected patients during highly active antiretroviral therapy (HAART), as they may with histoplasmosis and coccidioidomycosis. Solitary cutaneous lesions and indolent cellulitis may be the presenting signs of disseminated disease.

Primary inoculation cryptococcosis is a rare disease. To establish the diagnosis, there should be a clear history of implantation or a foreign body found in association with the organism. Usually, primary inoculation disease presents as a solitary skin lesion on an exposed area, frequently in the form of a whitlow. Risk factors include outdoor activities and exposure to bird droppings. *Cryptococcus neoformans* serotype D is more often associated with primary cutaneous disease. Although primary cutaneous disease exists, for all practical purposes, identification of cryptococci in the skin

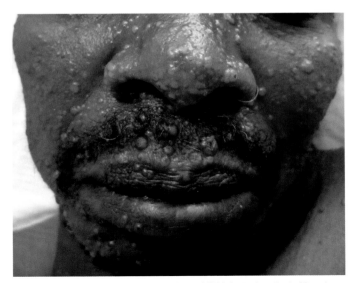

Fig. 15.22 Cryptococcal infection in an HIV-infected patient. (Courtesy Michelle Weir, MD.)

indicates disseminated disease with a poor prognosis, and it requires a search for other sites of involvement.

Etiology and Pathology

The causative organism is *C. neoformans* or in subtropical or tropical areas, *Cryptococcus gattii*. It appears in tissue as a pleomorphic budding yeast. The organisms vary greatly in size and shape, in contrast to most other fungal organisms. The capsule is usually prominent, although it is inversely proportional to the extent of the granulomatous reaction. Generally, the capsule is easily identified in hematoxylin and eosin (H&E) sections, although mucicarmine, methylene blue, or alcian blue staining can also be used. Usually, multiple yeast share a common capsule. *Cryptococcus* stains well with the Fontana-Masson stain for melanin.

Epidemiology

Cryptococcosis has a worldwide distribution and affects both humans and animals. The organism has been recovered from human skin, soil, dust, and pigeon droppings; when deposited on window ledges in large cities, pigeon droppings are a source of infection. The patient with disseminated cryptococcosis usually has a concomitant debilitating disease, such as AIDS, cancer, leukemia, lymphoma, renal failure, hepatitis, alveolar proteinosis, severe diabetes mellitus, sarcoidosis, tuberculosis, or silicosis. Long-term oral prednisone or immunosuppressive therapy for chronic illnesses, such as renal transplantation, sarcoidosis, or connective tissue disease, may also be a factor. Males outnumber females 2:1. Cryptococcosis is most frequent in persons age 30–60 years.

Patients with AIDS are particularly at risk for disseminated disease. Cryptococcosis is the fourth leading cause of opportunistic infection and the second most common fungal opportunist, with 5%–9% of patients manifesting symptomatic disease. Dissemination occurs in 50% of patients with AIDS, with skin involvement reported in 6%.

Immunology

The latex slide agglutination test is sensitive and specific. It may give false-positive results in the presence of rheumatoid factor. Direct microscopic examination and latex agglutination have been used with lesional skin scrapings to aid in rapid diagnosis. The complement fixation test for cryptococcal polysaccharide, indirect fluorescence test, and ELISA for cryptococcal antigen detection are all helpful, although ELISA is capable of detecting the presence of antigen earlier and at a lower concentration than the other two tests.

Mycology

For direct examination, a drop of serum or exudate is placed on a slide and a coverslip inserted. If examination shows yeast, 1 drop of 10% KOH can be added to half the coverslip and 1 drop of India ink to the other half to demonstrate the capsule. The skin biopsy specimen should be cultured. A commercially available DNA probe detection assay allows rapid culture confirmation.

Treatment

For mild to moderately ill non-AIDS patients, fluconazole, 400 mg/day for 8–24 weeks, may be effective. In seriously ill non-HIV patients, amphotericin B intravenously initially, followed by fluconazole orally, is standard treatment. In non-AIDS meningitis and all HIV-positive patients, flucytosine is given after initial amphotericin B treatment, and in patients infected with HIV, fluconazole is given indefinitely at a suppressive dose of 200 mg/day. For primary inoculation cases, surgical treatment alone or with fluconazole or itraconazole for 3–6 months is generally effective.

Du L, et al: Systemic review of published reports on primary cutaneous cryptococcosis in immunocompetent patients. Mycopathologia 2015; 180: 19.

Hoang JK, et al: Localized cutaneous *Cryptococcus albidus* infection in a 14-year-old boy on etanercept therapy. Pediatr Dermatol 2007; 24: 285.

Ikeda T, et al: Disseminated cryptococcosis-induced skin ulcers in a patient with autoimmune hepatitis. Case Rep Dermatol 2014; 6: 98.

Lenz D, et al: Primary cutaneous cryptococcosis in an eight-year-old immunocompetent child. Klin Pediatr 2015; 227: 41.

Luo FL, et al: Clinical study of 23 pediatric patients with cryptococcosis. Eur Rev Med Pharmacol Sci 2015; 19: 3801.

Negroni R: Cryptococcosis. Clin Dermatol 2012; 30: 599.

Rodríguez-Cerdeira C, et al: Systemic fungal infections in patients with human immunodeficiency virus. Actas Dermosifiliogr 2014; 105: 5.

Wilson ML, et al: Primary cutaneous cryptococcosis during therapy with methotrexate and adalimumab. J Drugs Dermatol 2008; 7: 53.

Zhu TH, et al: Cryptococcal cellulitis on the shin of an immunosuppressed patient. Dermatol Online J 2016 Jun 15; 22.

NORTH AMERICAN BLASTOMYCOSIS

Most cutaneous North American blastomycosis is the result of dissemination from a primary pulmonary focus. The lesions are chronic, slowly progressive, verrucous, and granulomatous and are characterized by thick crusts, warty vegetations, discharging sinuses, and pustules along the advancing edge (Fig. 15.23). The lesions are often multiple and are located mostly on exposed skin. Papillomatous proliferation is most pronounced in lesions on the hands and feet, where the patches become very thick. The patches tend to involute centrally and to form white scars as they spread peripherally. The crusts are thick and dirty gray or brown. Beneath the crusts, exuberant granulations are covered with a seropurulent exudate, which oozes out of small sinuses that extend down to indolent subcutaneous abscesses. Lower extremity nodules and plaques clinically and histologically suggestive of Sweet syndrome have also been described.

The primary infection is almost always in the upper or middle lobes of the lungs, and most cases never develop cutaneous dissemination. When dissemination does occur, the most common site is the skin, accounting for at least 80% of cases of disseminated disease. It also frequently disseminates to bone, especially the ribs and vertebrae. Other targets are the CNS, liver, spleen, and genitourinary system.

Cutaneous blastomycosis rarely occurs as a result of primary cutaneous inoculation. Such patients have a clear history of inoculation and present with a small primary nodule and subsequent secondary nodules along the draining lymphatics, creating a picture similar to sporotrichosis. Healing takes place within several months.

Etiology and Pathology

The fungus *Blastomyces dermatitidis* causes North American blastomycosis. It is frequently found in soil and animal habitats. *B. dermatitidis* is a dimorphic fungus with a mycelial phase at room temperature and a yeast phase at 37°C. Direct microscopic examination of a KOH slide of the specimen should always be made, because culture of the fungus is difficult and the organism may be found in purulent exudates obtained from skin lesions. The specimen should be cultured. A DNA probe detection assay is available for rapid culture confirmation.

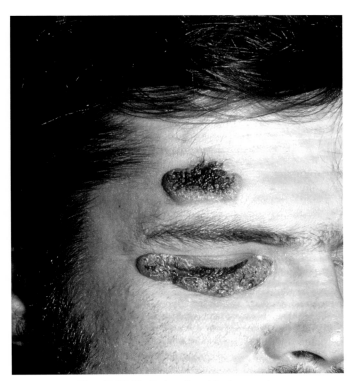

Fig. 15.23 North American blastomycosis.

Cutaneous blastomycosis usually demonstrates marked pseudoepitheliomatous hyperplasia of the epidermis with neutrophilic abscesses. Giant cells are frequently present in the dermal infiltrate. Organisms are typically few in number and are most frequently found within giant cells or intraepidermal abscesses. The organism is a thick-walled yeast, usually 5–7 μm in diameter, although giant forms have been reported in tissue. *B. dermatitidis* lacks a capsule but has a thick and distinctly asymmetric refractile wall. Broad-based budding may occasionally be noted. Rarely, acute skin lesions may lack pseudoepitheliomatous hyperplasia and demonstrate a diffuse neutrophilic dermal infiltrate. They may present as cutaneous nodules, sometimes with a localized distribution.

Primary cutaneous blastomycosis demonstrates a neutrophilic infiltrate with many budding cells of blastomycetes. In later lesions, a granulomatous infiltrate is found. The lymph nodes may show marked inflammatory changes, giant cells containing the organisms, lymphocytes, and plasma cells. Lung involvement may show many changes that are suggestive of tuberculosis with tubercle formation. Purulent abscesses may occur in the lungs and bone.

Epidemiology

North American blastomycosis is prevalent in the southeastern United States and the Ohio and Mississippi river basins, reaching epidemic proportions in Kentucky and Mississippi; the latter has the highest prevalence of blastomycosis in North America. There is a male/female ratio of approximately 6:1, and most patients are over age 60. Often, the cutaneous form occurs in patients without a known history of pulmonary lesions.

Outdoor activity after periods of heavy rain is a risk factor for acute pulmonary disease. Beaver lodges are a common site for the fungus, and some reports have linked outbreaks of disease with outings near a beaver lodge. Blastomycosis has also been reported from the bite of a dog with pulmonary blastomycosis. Transmission

has been reported between men with prostatic involvement and their sexual partners.

Risk factors for symptomatic disease include preexisting illness. In one study, one quarter of patients with blastomycosis had underlying immunosuppression, including those with organ transplantation, and 22% had diabetes mellitus. In the southern states, blacks have a higher incidence than whites, and the mortality rate is also higher among African Americans.

Immunology

Serologic tests are performed by immunodiffusion or ELISA. Commercial antigen test kits are available for rapid diagnosis.

Differential Diagnosis

Blastomycosis may closely resemble halogenoderma, blastomycosis-like pyoderma, pemphigus vegetans, tuberculosis verrucosa cutis, syphilis, granuloma inguinale, drug eruptions, and trichophytic granuloma. The diagnosis is established by demonstration of *B. dermatitidis* or serologic testing.

Treatment

In mild to moderate disease itraconazole 200 mg thrice daily for 3 days, then twice daily for 6–12 months is the treatment of choice. Amphotericin B given for 1–2 weeks followed by itraconazole 6–12 months for more severe disease is indicated.

Berg AS, et al: Giant periorbital verrucoid plaque. Am J Dermatopathol 2016; 38: 758.

Brick KE, et al: Cutaneous and disseminated blastomycosis. Pediatr Dermatol 2013; 30: 23.

Castillo CG, et al: Blastomycosis. Infect Dis Clin North Am 2016; 30: 247.

Lopez-Martinez R, et al: Blastomycosis. Clin Dermatol 2012; 30: 565.

Rucci J, et al: Blastomycosis of the head and neck. Am J Otolaryngol 2014; 35: 390.

SOUTH AMERICAN BLASTOMYCOSIS

Mucocutaneous involvement in South American blastomycosis, also known as paracoccidioidomycosis, is almost always a sign of disseminated disease, primarily in the lungs. Rare cases may arise from inoculation. In Brazil, the disease causes about 200 deaths per year.

The mucocutaneous type usually begins in the mouth, where small papules and ulcerations appear. Gingival lesions are most common, followed by lesions of the tongue and lips. With time, adjacent tissues are affected, and extensive ulcerations eventually destroy the nose, lips, and face. Skin lesions may show ulcerations (Fig. 15.24), pseudoepitheliomatous hyperplasia, and microabscesses. The lymphangitic type manifests itself by enlargement of the regional lymph nodes soon after the appearance of the initial lesions about the mouth. The adenopathy may extend to the supraclavicular and axillary regions. Nodes may become greatly enlarged and break down with ulcerations that secondarily involve the skin, causing severe pain and dysphagia with progressive cachexia and death. Primary skin lesions are less common. The infection may closely simulate Hodgkin disease, especially when the suprahyoid, preauricular, or retroauricular groups of lymph nodes are involved.

There is a visceral type, caused by hematogenous spread of the disease to the liver, adrenal glands, spleen, intestines, and other organs. There is also a mixed type that has the combined symptomatology of the mucocutaneous, lymphangitic, and visceral types. South American blastomycosis may present as a rapidly progressive

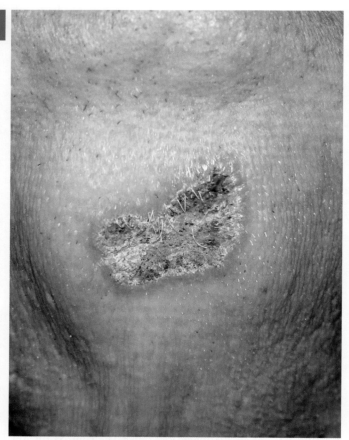

Fig. 15.24 Paracoccidioidomycosis. (Courtesy Lauro de Souza Lima Institute, Brazil.)

acute disease or follow a subacute course, or it may occur as a chronic, slowly advancing form.

Etiology and Pathology

South American blastomycosis is caused by the fungus *Paracoccidioides brasiliensis*. Biopsies may demonstrate pseudoepitheliomatous hyperplasia, abscess formation, or ulceration. A granulomatous inflammatory infiltrate is frequently present, consisting of lymphocytes, epithelioid cells, and Langerhans giant cells. The organism appears as a round cell, 10–60 μm in diameter, with a delicate wall. Multiple buds may be present, creating a resemblance to a mariner's wheel.

This chronic granulomatous disease is endemic in Brazil and also occurs in Argentina and Venezuela. Occasional cases have been reported in the United States, Mexico, Central America, Europe, and Asia. Most of these patients have a travel history to endemic areas. The disease is generally found among laborers, mostly in men. Although the initial infection is usually respiratory, some individuals may become infected by picking their teeth with twigs or from chewing leaves.

South American blastomycosis is 15 times more common in men, which is of particular interest because it has been shown that 17β-estradiol inhibits transition from the mycelial to the tissue-invasive yeast form. *P. brasiliensis* can lodge in periodontal tissues and some cases start after extraction of teeth. Many cases have been reported in patients with AIDS or organ transplant recipients, in whom the course is usually acute and severe.

Immunology

Complement fixation tests are positive in 97% of severe cases, and the titer rises as the blastomycosis becomes more severe. With improvement, the titer decreases. Immunodiffusion tests are often used for diagnosis and posttherapy follow-up. The test is highly specific but only about 90% sensitive.

Treatment

Itraconazole, 200 mg/day for 6–9 months for mild disease and 12–18 months for moderate disease, is indicated. For severe disease initial amphotericin followed by itraconazole as in North American blastomycosis should be given. Ketoconazole and trimethoprim-sulfamethoxazole (TMP-SMX) are alternative treatments. When HIV patients are infected, lifelong therapy with TP-SMX is the rule.

Cataño JC, Morales M: Cutaneous paracoccidioidomycosis. Am J Trop Med Hyg 2015; 93: 433.
López-Martínez R, et al: Paracoccidioidomycosis in Mexico. Mycoses 2014; 57: 525.
Marques SA: Paracoccidioidomycosis. An Bras Dermatol 2013; 88: 700.
Safe IP, et al: Extra-pulmonary manifestations of paracoccidioidomycosis associated with acquired immunodeficiency syndrome. An Bras Dermatol 2014; 89: 150.
Zavascki AP, et al: Paracoccidioidomycosis in organ transplant recipient. Rev Inst Med Trop São Paulo 2004; 46: 279.

SPOROTRICHOSIS

Sporotrichosis usually results from direct inoculation by a thorn, cat's claw, or other minor penetrating injury. The earliest manifestation may be a small nodule that may heal and disappear before the onset of other lesions. In the course of a few weeks, nodules generally develop along the draining lymphatics (Fig. 15.25). These lesions are at first small, dusky red, painless, and firm. In time, the overlying skin becomes adherent to them and may ulcerate. When the lesions occur on the face, the lymphatic drainage is radial, rather than linear, and secondary nodules occur as rosettes around the primary lesion.

Regional lymphangitic sporotrichosis is the common type, accounting for 75% of cases. Fixed cutaneous sporotrichosis is seen in 20% of cases and is characterized by a solitary ulcer, plaque, or crateriform nodule without regional lymphangitis (Fig. 15.26). It may also present as localized rosacea-like lesions of the face without regional lymphangitis. Increased host resistance, a smaller inoculum, facial location, and variations in strain pathogenicity have all been suggested as triggers for the fixed cutaneous form. The distribution in children is similar to that in adults.

Disseminated sporotrichosis is the least common form. Factors that predispose to extracutaneous disease include oral prednisone therapy, other immunosuppressive drugs (including TNF-α inhibitors), chronic alcoholism, diabetes mellitus, hematologic malignancies, and AIDS. Systemic invasion may produce cutaneous, pulmonary, GI, articular, and brain lesions. Arthritis or bone involvement occurs in most patients. The cutaneous lesions are reddish, tender nodules, which soften, form cold abscesses, and eventually suppurate, leaving chronic ulcers or fistulas. These are usually around arthritic joints and the face and scalp, but may occur anywhere on the skin. At times, only internal involvement is apparent.

Etiology and Pathology

Sporotrichosis is caused by the *Sporothrix schenckii* complex, with more than six species identified by molecular techniques. These

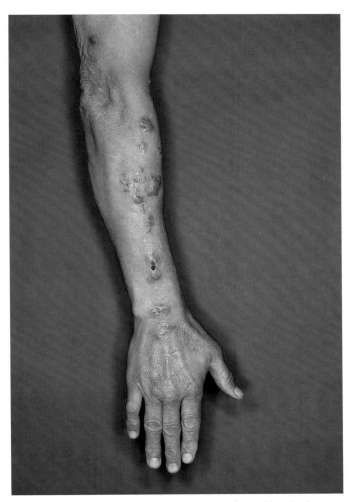

Fig. 15.25 Sporotrichosis. (Courtesy Lauro de Souza Lima Institute, Brazil.)

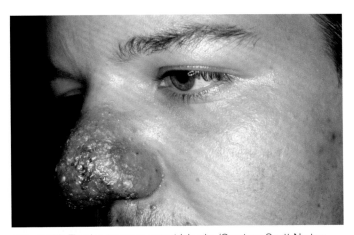

Fig. 15.26 Fixed cutaneous sporotrichosis. (Courtesy Scott Norton, MD.)

fungi are dimorphic in that they grow in a yeast form at 37°C and in a mycelial form at room temperature. Cutaneous disease typically presents with palisading granulomatous dermatitis surrounding a stellate suppurative abscess. Organisms appear as cigar-shaped yeast in tissue but are rarely seen in North American cases. In Asian cases of sporotrichosis, the organisms are frequently more numerous. Asteroid bodies and mycelial elements are prevalent in regional lymphangitic sporotrichosis. PCR methods of detection are available.

Epidemiology

There seems to be no geographic limitation to the occurrence of sporotrichosis. Most often, the primary invasion is seen as an occupational disease in gardeners, florists, and laborers after injuries by thorns, straw, or sphagnum moss. The pathogen typically lives as a saprophyte on grasses, shrubs, and other plants. Carnations, rose bushes, barberry shrubs, and sphagnum moss are common sources. High humidity and high temperature favor infection. Experimentally, it has been produced in many laboratory animals, and spontaneous cases have been observed in horses, mules, dogs, cats, mice, and rats. In cats, sporotrichosis usually produces disseminated disease. The organism may be found on the claws and may be transmitted to humans through cat scratches. This is becoming the most common mode of transmission in many areas of the world. Multiple family members or veterinary workers may be infected by a single cat.

Immunology

Although skin testing and agglutination tests may be done, the clinical findings, biopsy, and culture remain the most common means of establishing a diagnosis.

Differential Diagnosis

Demonstration by culture establishes the diagnosis, and it is important to differentiate sporotrichosis from other lymphangitic infections. Atypical mycobacteriosis (especially *Mycobacterium marinum*), leishmaniasis, and nocardiosis all produce lymphangitic spread. In contrast, tuberculosis, cat-scratch disease, tularemia, glanders, melioidosis, lymphogranuloma venereum, and anthrax produce ulceroglandular syndromes (ulcer with regional lymphadenopathy rather than ulcer with nodules along lymphatic vessels).

Treatment

Itraconazole is effective for cutaneous and lymphocutaneous sporotrichosis at a dose of 200 mg/day for 2–4 weeks after all lesions have resolved, usually 3–6 months. If there is no response, the dose may be doubled, or terbinafine, 500 mg two times daily, is a further option.

For cutaneous forms, potassium iodide, 3–6 g/day, remains an effective and inexpensive therapeutic option and may be effective when itraconazole therapy fails. Decades of experience demonstrate the effectiveness of potassium iodide despite the absence of published high-level evidence. Iodide therapy usually requires 6–12 weeks of treatment. Generally, it is best to begin with 5 drops of the saturated solution in grapefruit or orange juice three times daily after meals. The drops can also be put in milk, but strong-flavored citrus juices are better at masking the taste. The dose should be gradually increased up to 40–50 drops three times daily. Potassium iodide is not suitable for pregnant women. Adverse effects of iodide therapy include nausea, vomiting, parotid swelling, acneiform rash, coryza, sneezing, swelling of the eyelids, hypothyroidism, a brassy taste, increased lacrimation and salivation, flares of psoriasis, and occasionally depression. Most of the side effects can be controlled by stopping the drug for a few days and reinstituting therapy at a reduced dosage.

Application of local hot compresses, hot packs, or a heating pad twice a day has been advocated as a useful adjunct, because *S. schenckii* is intolerant to temperatures above 38.5°C (101°F).

In adult disseminated sporotrichosis, amphotericin B, given as a lipid formulation at 3–5 mg/kg daily, is recommended, followed by itraconazole 200 mg twice daily for at least 1 year. In immunocompromised patients, treatment with 200 mg/day may need to be lifelong.

Bonifaz A, et al: Sporotrichosis in childhood. Pediatr Dermatol 2007; 24: 369.

Bonifaz A, et al: Cutaneous disseminated sporotrichosis. J Eur Acad Dermatol Venereol 2017; ePub ahead of print.

De Lima Barros MB, et al: Treatment of cutaneous sporotrichosis with itraconazole: study of 645 patients. Clin Infect Dis 2011; 52: e200.

Freitas DF, et al: Sporotrichosis in HIV-infected patients. Med Mycol 2012; 50: 170.

Gewehr P, et al: Sporotrichosis in renal transplant patients. Can J Infect Dis Med Microbiol 2013; 24: e47.

Gremião ID, et al: Feline sporotrichosis. Med Mycol 2015; 53: 15.

Schubach A, et al: Epidemic sporotrichosis. Curr Opin Infect Dis 2008; 21: 129.

Sharon VR, et al: Disseminated cutaneous sporotrichosis. Lancet Infect Dis 2013; 13: 95.

Vásquez-del-Mercado E, et al: Sporotrichosis. Clin Dermatol 2012; 30: 437.

Yamada K, et al: Cutaneous sporotrichosis treatment with potassium iodide. Rev Inst Med Trop São Paulo 2011; 53: 89.

CHROMOBLASTOMYCOSIS

Chromoblastomycosis usually affects one of the lower extremities (Fig. 15.27). It occurs as a result of direct inoculation of the organism into the skin. As a rule, lesions begin as a small, pink, scaly papule or warty growth on some part of the foot or lower leg, then slowly spread through direct extension and satellite lesions. With time, they develop a verrucous or nodular border and central atrophy and scarring. Small lesions may resemble common warts. Regional lymphadenitis may result from secondary bacterial infection, and a lymphangitic pattern of infection has been reported. In rare cases, the disease begins on an upper extremity or the face. Rarely, CNS involvement has been reported, both with and without associated skin lesions.

There is a 4:1 male predominance, and farmers account for almost 75% of patients with chromoblastomycosis. The disease is slowly progressive, and the average time between the appearance of lesions and diagnosis is almost 15 years. Lesions occur at sites of minor trauma. Squamous cell carcinoma may occur in long-standing cases.

Etiology and Pathology

Most cases are caused by one of several dematiaceous fungi. *Fonsecaea pedrosoi* is the most common cause and accounts for 90% or more of the cases reported in South America and is also the most common cause in other parts of the world. Other agents include *Phialophora verrucosa*, *Fonsecaea compacta*, *Cladosporium carrionii*, and *Rhinocladiella aquaspersa*. *Exophiala spinifera* and *Exophiala jeanselmei* have been reported in isolated cases. Patients may have more than one organism, and cutaneous lesions caused by both paracoccidioidomycosis and chromoblastomycosis have been reported in the same patient. Patients may also have chromoblastomycosis concurrently with mycetoma or invasive phaeohyphomycosis.

Histopathologically, lesions are characterized by pseudoepitheliomatous hyperplasia with intraepidermal abscess, a dermal granulomatous reaction, and the presence of pigmented fungal sclerotic bodies. The fungi often appear in clusters that reproduce by equatorial septation, rather than by budding. The presence of

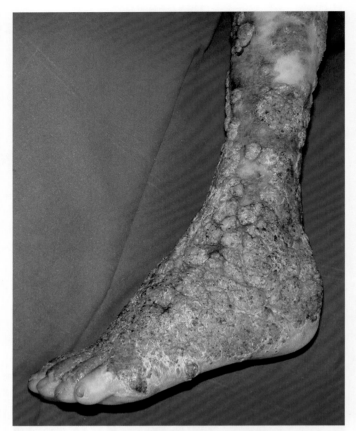

Fig. 15.27 Chromomycosis. (Courtesy Lauro de Souza Lima Institute, Brazil.)

sclerotic bodies (Medlar bodies, "copper pennies") rather than hyphae distinguishes the infection from invasive phaeohyphomycosis. The organisms are often seen in association with an embedded splinter. Medlar bodies are usually easily identified as they produce melanin and are pigmented, but Ziehl-Neelsen and Wade-Fite stains have also been used to identify the pathogenic organisms, as has duplex PCR.

Epidemiology

Chromoblastomycosis was first recognized in Brazil but has been found in other parts of South America and the Caribbean, Madagascar, South Asia, East Asia, the United States, Russia, and many other countries. Barefooted farm workers bear the largest burden of infection. Trauma from wood products and soil exposure results in implantation of the organism, and dissemination is rare.

Treatment

Treatment is difficult, and chromoblastomycosis often affects those who cannot afford medication. In some series, only about 30% of patients were cured, although almost 60% improved. About 10% fail therapy, and recrudescence of the disease is noted in more than 40% of patients. Smaller lesions are best treated by surgical excision or cryotherapy. In one study of 22 patients, the number of cryosurgeries varied from 1 to 22, and treatment lasted for up to 126 months. Only three patients did not respond. If the lesions are extensive, chronic, or burrowing, itraconazole 200–400 mg/day, is given for 6–12 months or until there is a response. Terbinafine, 500–1000 mg/day, alone or in combination with itraconazole, 200–400 mg/day, has been effective in some patients, as has posaconazole, 800 mg/day. Cryotherapy, CO_2 laser vaporization, PDT, and local hyperthermia are adjuncts. Combination amphotericin B and itraconazole has been used in resistant cases, as has isolated limb infusion with melphalan and actinomycin D. Despite these options, some lesions remain resistant, and amputation may be unavoidable in some patients.

Khan S, et al: Chromoblastomycosis due to *Fonsecaea pedrosoi.* J Infect Dev Ctries 2015; 9: 325.
Queiroz-Telles F: Chromoblastomycosis. Rev Inst Med Trop Sao Paulo 2015; 57 Suppl 19: 46.
Queiroz-Telles F, et al: Challenges in the therapy of chromoblastomycosis. Mycopathologia 2013; 175: 477.
Spiker A, Ferringer T: Chromoblastomycosis. Cutis 2015; 96: 224.
Torres E, et al: Chromoblastomycosis associated with lethal squamous cell carcinoma. An Bras Dermatol 2010; 85: 267.
Torres-Guerrero E, et al: Chromoblastomycosis. Clin Dermatol 2012; 30: 403.

PHAEOHYPHOMYCOSIS

This heterogeneous group of mycotic infections is caused by dematiaceous fungi with morphologic characteristics in tissue that include hyphae, yeastlike cells, or a combination of these. This contrasts with chromomycosis, in which the organism forms round, sclerotic bodies.

There are many types of clinical lesions caused by these organisms. Tinea nigra is an example of superficial infection. Alternariosis can also present as a superficial pigmented fungal infection in immunocompetent patients. Subcutaneous disease occurs most frequently as indolent abscesses at the site of minor trauma (so called "phaeomycotic cyst") (Fig. 15.28). *Exophiala jeanselmei* is the most common cause of this presentation in temperate climates. Systemic phaeohyphomycosis is largely a disease of immunocompromised patients, including solid-organ transplant recipients and patients with CARD9 deficiency, although primary cerebral forms occur in immunocompetent patients. Localized forms generally result from primary inoculation of the organism into the skin. Disseminated disease may also begin as a skin infection. The lesions usually appear as dry, black, leathery eschars with a scalloped, erythematous, edematous border. *Bipolaris spicifera* is the most common cause of disseminated disease, although *Scedosporium prolificans* has been reported as the most common organism in some areas. The presence of melanin in the cell wall may be a virulence factor for these fungi. Eosinophilia is noted in about 10% of patients with disseminated disease. Phaeohyphomycosis often disseminates to many organs. In some series, the mortality rate from disseminated disease is about 80%.

Etiology and Pathology

Many black molds are capable of causing phaeohyphomycosis, including *E. jeanselmei, B. spicifera, Alternaria* spp., *Dactylaria gallopava, Phialophora parasitica, Cladosporium sphaerospermum, Wangiella dermatitidis, Exserohilum rostratum, Cladophialophora bantiana, Wallemia sebi,* and *Chaetomium globosum.* Some fungi, such as *Phialophora verrucosa,* can cause both phaeohyphomycosis and chromoblastomycosis. Some fungi, such as *E. jeanselmei,* may cause mycetoma (characterized by grain formation) in some patients and phaeohyphomycosis or chromoblastomycosis in others.

All these organisms produce pigmented hyphae in tissue and culture, although the pigment may only be visible focally in some histologic sections. Melanin can be stained by the Fontana-Masson method, but many molds produce enough melanin to stain positive, and a positive stain should not be misinterpreted as proof of phaeohyphomycosis. Organisms as diverse as zygomycetes and dermatophytes can stain with Fontana-Masson. When hyphae

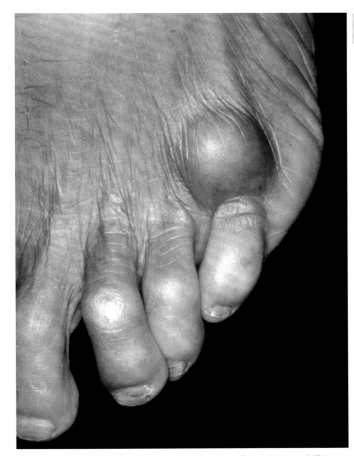

Fig. 15.28 Phaeohyphomycosis. (Courtesy Scott Norton, MD.)

appear brown in tissue, there is little question as to the diagnosis, but when the organism appears hyaline in tissue, the presence of melanin staining must be interpreted in the context of the fungal morphology. Most organisms of phaeohyphomycosis produce thick, refractile walls and have prominent bubbly cytoplasm. This contrasts with the thin, delicate walls of organisms such as *Aspergillus, Fusarium,* and dermatophytes. Zygomycetes are aseptate and usually appear hollow in tissue sections. Their thick, refractile wall usually stains intensely red with H&E, contrasting with the pale wall of a phaeomycotic organism. Some organisms, such as *Bipolaris,* produce round, dilated structures that resemble spores in tissue. The mix of round structures and hyphae is a helpful clue to the presence of a black mold in tissue.

Treatment

Phaeomycotic cysts are best treated with excision. Superficial phaeohyphomycosis may respond to topical antifungal agents and superficial debridement. For invasive and disseminated disease, surgical excision should generally be combined with antifungal therapy. Itraconazole has the best record of treating this group of infections, and doses of 400 mg/day are usually needed for at least 6 months. Case reports indicate success with voriconazole and posaconazole so they are alternatives. In widely disseminated disease, excision of lesions becomes impractical, but debulking of skin disease may be of some value.

ALTERNARIOSIS

Alternaria is a genus of molds recognized as common plant pathogens but also as a cause of human infection. As a pigmented fungus, it is one cause of phaeohyphomycosis. Most reported cases of invasive infection have occurred in immunocompromised patients, with the most frequent risk factors being solid-organ transplantation and Cushing syndrome. Cutaneous alternariosis usually presents as focal ulcerated papules and plaques or pigmented patches on exposed skin of the face, forearms and hands, or knees of immunocompetent patients. Topical corticosteroids may predispose to local infection. Localized disease in immunocompetent patients may respond to local debridement, hyperthermia, wide surgical excision, or Mohs micrographic surgery. Itraconazole has been successful, although resistance has also been reported. Terbinafine, posaconazole, voriconazole, ketoconazole, caspofungin, and intralesional miconazole have also been used successfully in individual cases.

Coutinho I, et al: Cutaneous alternariosis—a case series of an increasing phaeohyphomycosis. J Eur Acad Dermatol Venereol 2015; 29: 2053.

Fukai T, et al: A case of phaeohyphomycosis caused by *Exophiala oligosperma* successfully treated with local hyperthermia. Med Mycol J 2013; 54: 297.

Hsu CC, et al: Cutaneous alternariosis in a renal transplant recipient. Asian J Surg 2015; 38: 47.

Isa-Isa R, et al: Subcutaneous phaeohyphomycosis (mycotic cyst). Clin Dermatol 2012; 30: 425.

Kollipara R, et al: Emerging infectious diseases with cutaneous manifestations. J Am Acad Dermatol 2016; 75: 19.

Lanternier F, et al: Inherited CARD9 deficiency in 2 unrelated patients with invasive *Exophiala* infection. J Infect Dis 2015; 211: 1241.

Lyskova P, et al: Successful posaconazole therapy of disseminated alternariosis due to *Alternaria infectoria* in a heart transplant recipient. Mycopathologia 2017; 182: 297.

McCarty TP, et al: Phaeohyphomycosis in transplant recipients. Med Mycol 2015; 53: 440.

Simpson CL, et al: Refractory cutaneous alternariosis successfully treated with Mohs surgery and full-thickness skin grafting. Dermatol Surg 2016; 42: 426.

MYCETOMA

Mycetoma, also known as Madura foot and maduromycosis, is a chronic, granulomatous, subcutaneous, inflammatory disease caused by filamentous bacteria (actinomycetoma) or true fungi (eumycetoma). The organisms enter the skin by traumatic inoculation. Both forms of mycetoma present as a triad of progressive subcutaneous swelling with sinus tracts that discharge grains (Fig. 15.29).

The disease progresses slowly. Mycetomas generally begin on the instep or the toe webs. The lesion usually is relatively painless, nontender, and firm. The overlying skin may be normal or attached to the underlying nodularity. Mature lesions often have draining sinuses. Not only the skin and subcutaneous tissues, but also the underlying fascia and bone are involved. Other parts of the body, such as the hands, arms, chest, jaw, and buttocks, may be involved. Exposed sites are most common, and lesions in covered areas are almost always actinomycetomas.

Etiology and Pathology

Mycetoma is divided into actinomycetoma, produced by bacteria, and eumycetoma, produced by fungi. Actinomycetomas are caused by *Nocardia asteroides, N. brasiliensis, N. caviae, N. otitidiscaviarum, Actinomadura madurae, Actinomadura pelletieri, Actinomyces israelii*

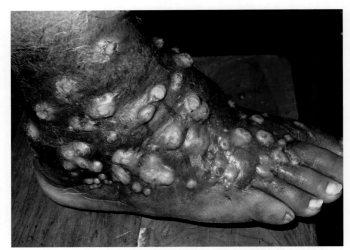

Fig. 15.29 Mycetoma. (Courtesy Debabrata Bandyopadhyay, MD.)

(the major cause of lumpy jaw), and *Streptomyces somaliensis*. Eumycetomas are caused by fungi, including pigmented fungi such as *Madurella* spp., and hyaline fungi such as *Pseudallescheria*. Causative dematiaceous organisms include *Madurella grisea, M. mycetomatis, Leptosphaeria senegalensis, L. tompkinsii, Exophiala jeanselmei, Pyrenochaeta romeri, Phialophora verrucosa, Curvularia lunata*, and *C. geniculate*. The hyaline or white fungi that cause mycetoma include *Pseudallescheria boydii* (which may occasionally disseminate as the asexual form, *Scedosporium apiospermum*), *Acremonium falciforme, A. recifei, Fusarium moniliform, F. solanii, Aspergillus nidulans*, and *Neotestudina rosatii*.

Almost all actinomycetomas produce light-colored grains, as do hyaline fungi. Red grains are usually produced by *A. pelletieri*. Pigmented fungi produce dark grains.

Histologic sections demonstrate stellate abscesses containing grains. Gram stain of an actinomycotic grain shows gram-positive, thin filaments, 1–2 μm thick, embedded in a gram-negative amorphous matrix. Club formation in the periphery of a grain may be seen. In eumycotic grains special stains such as PAS and GMS, will clearly show hyphae of 2–5 μm thickness and other fungal structures. When obtaining a specimen for culture it should be taken from deep tissue, at the base of the biopsy.

Epidemiology

The mycetoma belt stretches between the latitudes of 15° south and 30° north. Relatively arid areas have higher rates of infection than humid areas. In the Western Hemisphere, the incidence is highest in Mexico, followed by Venezuela and Argentina. In Africa, it is found most frequently in Senegal, Sudan, and Somalia. Mycetomas are also reported in large numbers in India. Actinomycetomas outnumber eumycetomas by 3:1, which is fortunate because actinomycetomas are much more responsive to therapy. The male/female ratio varies from 2:1 to 5:1.

Diagnosis

Mycetoma may be diagnosed when the triad of signs, tumefaction, sinuses, and granules, are present. Pus gathered from a deep sinus will show the granules when examined microscopically. The slide containing the specimen should have 1 drop of 10% NaOH added and a coverslip placed on top. A biopsy may be required. Radiographs will show the bone involvement, and magnetic resonance images may show the "dot in a circle" sign, corresponding to grains.

Treatment

Actinomycetomas generally respond to antibiotic therapy, although patients with advanced disease may also need surgery. In *A. israelii* infection, penicillin in large doses is curative. *N. asteroides* or *N. brasiliensis* is usually treated with sulfonamides. Severe refractory disease may respond to imipenem.

Patients in the early stage of eumycetoma may be successfully treated by surgical removal of the area. In the more advanced stages, a combination of antifungal therapy and surgery may be successful. In some patients with eumycetoma, amputation will be necessary. Posaconazole alone or combined with surgical excision is the treatment of choice for cases caused by *P. boydii*.

Castro LG, et al: Clinical and mycologic findings and therapeutic outcome of 27 mycetoma patients from São Paulo, Brazil. Int J Dermatol 2008; 47: 160.
Mestre T, et al: Mycetoma of the foot—diagnosis of the etiologic agent and surgical treatment. Am J Trop Med Hyg 2015; 93: 1.
Nenoff P, et al: Eumycetoma and actinomycetoma—an update on causative agents, epidemiology, pathogenesis, diagnostics and therapy. J Eur Acad Dermatol Venereol 2015; 29: 1873.
Reis LM, et al: Dermoscopy assisting the diagnosis of mycetoma. An Bras Dermatol 2014; 89: 832.
Van de Sande WW: Global burden of human mycetoma. PLoS Negl Trop Dis 2013; 7: e2550.
Zijlstra EE, et al: Mycetoma. Lancet Infect Dis 2016; 16: 100.

KELOIDAL BLASTOMYCOSIS (LOBOMYCOSIS OR LACAZIOSIS)

Keloidal blastomycosis was originally described by Jorge Lobo in 1931. Most cases have occurred in countries in Central and South America. One case occurred in an aquarium attendant in Europe who cared for an infected dolphin; and another in an American who had walked under the pounding water of Angel Falls on a trip to South America.

Keloidal blastomycosis may involve any part of the body, and the lesions appear characteristically keloidal (Fig. 15.30). Fistulas may occur. The nodules gradually increase in size by invasion of the surrounding normal skin or through the superficial lymphatics. Long-standing cases may involve the regional lymph nodes. A common location is the ear, which may resemble the cauliflower ear of a boxer. Disseminated disease has also been described.

The fungus is probably acquired from water, soil, or vegetation in forested areas where the disease is prevalent. Agricultural laborers have been most frequently affected, with 90% of cases occurring in men.

The causative organism, *Lacazia loboi*, is an obligate parasite. Culture has not been successful, but the organism can grow in mouse footpads. Histologically, the epidermis is atrophic. The organisms are thick-walled, refractile spherules, larger than those of *P. brasiliensis*. One or two buds may be seen, but never multiple budding as in *P. brasiliensis*. The organisms are typically numerous and appear in chains of spheres connected by short, narrow tubes. The cellular infiltrate is composed of histiocytes, giant cells, and lymphocytes.

Surgical excision of the affected areas may be curative when the lesions are small, but recurrence is common. Complete resolution of keloidal blastomycosis has been reported in a patient treated for 1 year with a combination of itraconazole, 100 mg/day, and clofazimine, 100 mg/day. Posaconazole 400 mg twice daily for 27 days was effective in another report. Cryotherapy may be a useful adjuvant.

Carvalho KA, et al: Jorge Lobo's disease. An Bras Dermatol 2015; 90: 586.

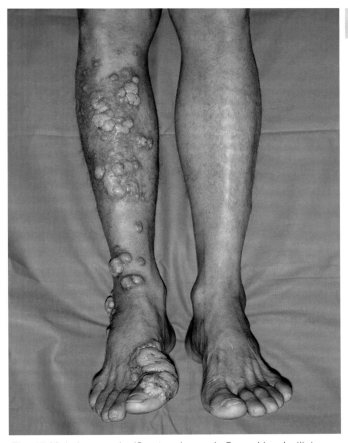

Fig. 15.30 Lobomycosis. (Courtesy Lauro de Souza Lima Institute, Brazil.)

de Souza MN, et al: Lobomycosis of the lower limb in an Amazonian patient. Am J Trop Med Hyg 2015; 93: 675.
Francesconi F, Francesconi V: Lobomycosis. N Engl J Med 2011; 364: e2.
Francesconi VA, et al: Lobomycosis. Ther Clin Risk Manag 2014; 10: 851.

RHINOSPORIDIOSIS

Rhinosporidiosis is a polypoid disease usually involving mucosal surfaces, especially the nasal mucosa (Fig. 15.31). Conjunctival, lacrimal, oral, and urethral tissues may also be involved, and genital lesions may resemble condylomata. The lesions begin as small papillomas and develop into pedunculated tumors with fissured and warty surfaces. Grayish white flecks may be noted on the tissue, corresponding to transepithelial elimination of large sporangia. Bleeding occurs easily. Widespread cutaneous lesions are rare. Conjunctival lesions begin as small, pinkish papillary nodules, which later become larger, dark, and lobulated. Rectal and vaginal lesions have been reported. As with penile lesions, they may resemble condylomata or polyps. Dissemination rarely occurs, and bone involvement has been described. The disease is endemic in Sri Lanka and India but also occurs in parts of East Asia, Latin America, the southern United States, the United Kingdom, and Italy.

Rhinosporidium seeberi, a lower aquatic fungus found in stagnant water, is the causative organism. The organisms appear as spherules 7–10 μm in diameter, which are contained within large, cystic sporangia that may be as large as 300 μm in diameter. When the organism does not form endospores, it resembles *Coccidioides immitis* spherules, but differs by the regular presence of a central nucleus

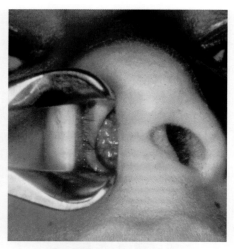

Fig. 15.31 Rhinosporidiosis.

within each organism. The organisms are usually present within a polypoid structure. A granulomatous response is seen in about 50% of patients, and gigantic foreign body giant cells can rarely be noted filled with organisms.

Suppurative inflammation may be observed at the site of rupture of sporangia. Transepithelial elimination of sporangia is common. Destruction of the involved area by excision or electrosurgery is the most common method of treatment. Antifungal agents have been of little value. Dapsone is the only medication to have shown much benefit.

Chatterjee K, et al: A curious ulcer on the pinna: rhinosporidiosis at an unusual place. Int J Dermatol 2015; 54: e277.
Sudarshan V, et al: Rhinosporidiosis in Raipur, Chhattisgarh. Indian J Pathol Microbiol 2007; 50: 718.
Tubachi P, et al: Primary cutaneous rhinosporidiosis. BMJ Case Rep 2015 Apr 1, 2015.

ZYGOMYCOSIS (PHYCOMYCOSIS)

There are a number of important pathogens in the class Zygomycetes. The two orders within this class that cause cutaneous infection most often are the Entomophthorales and Mucorales.

Entomophthoromycosis

Infections caused by the order Entomophthorales have been named entomophthoromycosis, rhinoentomophthoromycosis, conidiobolomycosis, or basidiobolomycosis. Infection occurs usually in healthy individuals, and unlike mucormycosis, often runs an indolent course. The infections may be classified as cutaneous, subcutaneous, visceral, or disseminated. Subcutaneous lesions occur in two basic types, each involving different anatomic sites, either as well-circumscribed subcutaneous masses involving the nose, paranasal tissue, and upper lip, or as nodular, subcutaneous lesions located on the extremities, buttocks, and trunk.

Etiology

Conidiobolus coronatus typically causes the perinasal disease, whereas *Basidiobolus ranarum* causes the type of subcutaneous disease seen on the face.

Epidemiology

Occurrence is worldwide. Entomophthoromycosis was first reported in Indonesia, where it is prevalent. Since then, reports have come from Africa, Asia, and the Americas. Generally, infection occurs in a belt between 15° north and 15° south of the equator.

Diagnosis

Isolation and identification of the causative fungus are fundamental to the diagnosis. Culture on Sabouraud dextrose agar is made of nasal discharge, abscess fluid, or biopsy specimens. Biopsy specimens will show fibroblastic proliferation and an inflammatory reaction with lymphocytes, plasma cells, histiocytes, eosinophils, and giant cells. The organisms appear as broad hyphae that are generally aseptate and may be branched at right angles. The Splendore-Hoeppli phenomenon is common and appears as eosinophilic sleeves around the hyphae. Pythiosis, caused by *Pythium insidiosum*, a primitive aquatic hyphal organism that acts as a zoonotic pathogen, may affect humans and has a similar appearance.

Treatment

Potassium iodide has been the drug of choice for entomophthoromycosis, although amphotericin B, cotrimoxazole, ketoconazole, itraconazole, and fluconazole have also been used successfully. Excision of small lesions is an alternative method of management, but the recurrence rate is significant. Rare human cases of pythiosis have responded to amphotericin B.

Mucormycosis

Mucormycosis refers to infections caused by the order Mucorales of the class Zygomycetes. When invasive, infections characteristically are acute, rapidly developing, and often fatal. In some series the mortality rate is about 80%. Most infections occur in keto-acidotic patients with diabetes, but leukemia, lymphoma, AIDS, iatrogenic immunosuppression in transplant patients, chronic renal failure, and malnourishment all predispose to these infections. Infection has also been associated with methotrexate, prednisone, and infliximab therapy. Healthy individuals may also develop these infections. In them, primary cutaneous disease occurs often after trauma, burns, or as a result of contaminated surgical dressings.

The five major clinical forms of mucormycosis (rhinocerebral, pulmonary, cutaneous, GI, disseminated) all demonstrate vasculotropism of the organisms. This leads to infarction, gangrene, and the formation of black, necrotic, purulent debris. Ulceration, cellulitis, ecthyma gangrenosum–like lesions, and necrotic abscesses may occur. The infection may involve the skin through traumatic implantation or by hematogenous dissemination.

Etiology

The fungi that cause this infection are ubiquitous molds common in the soil, on decomposing plant and animal matter, and in the air. The pathogenic genera include *Rhizopus, Absidia, Mucor, Cunninghamella, Apophysomyces, Rhizomucor, Saksenaea, Mortierella,* and *Cokeromyces.*

Diagnosis

Tissue obtained by biopsy or curettage is examined microscopically and cultured. Prompt diagnosis of mucormycosis is essential in this rapidly fatal infection. Histologically, the organism generally appears as eosinophilic, thick-walled hyphae that look hollow in cross section. The organism is quite irregular in outline, and right-angle branching is common. The organisms are highly vasculotropic and dissect along the media of muscular vessels, resulting in infarction of tissue. Fungal stains, such as GMS, have been used, but zygomycetes show variable staining with fungal stains. Often H&E is the optimal stain, and the organisms may stain avidly with a tissue Gram stain.

Treatment

A combination of excision of affected tissue and antifungal therapy, usually with liposomal amphotericin B, is necessary in most patients with mucormycosis. Alternatives include posaconazole, 400 mg twice daily with meals, or isavuconazole. Primary cutaneous disease in an immunocompetent patient may be treated with excision or Mohs surgery alone.

Chander J, et al: Changing epidemiology of mucoralean fungi. Mycopathologia 2015; 180: 181.

Chander J, et al: *Saksenaea erythrospora*, an emerging mucoralean fungus causing severe necrotizing skin and soft tissue infection. Infect Dis (Lond) 2017; 49: 170.

Cheng VCC, et al: Hospital outbreak of pulmonary and cutaneous zygomycosis due to contaminated linen items from substandard laundry. Clin Infect Dis 2016; 62: 714.

Davuodi S, et al: Fatal cutaneous mucormycosis after kidney transplant. Exp Clin Transplant 2015; 13: 82.

El-Shabrawi MH, et al: Entomophthoromycosis. Mycoses 2014; 57 Suppl 3: 132.

Hawkes JE, et al: Chronic, painful, nonhealing ulcer on the right arm following minor trauma. JAMA Dermatol 2015; 151: 787.

Kollipara R, et al: Emerging infectious diseases with cutaneous manifestations. J Am Acad Dermatol 2016; 75: 19.

Krajaejun T, et al: Clinical and epidemiological analyses of human pythiosis in Thailand. Clin Infect Dis 2006; 43: 569.

Kucinskiene V, et al: Cutaneous fungal infection in a neonatal intensive care unit patient. Pediatr Dermatol 2014; 31: 267.

Pana ZD, et al: Invasive mucormycosis in children. BMC Infect Dis 2016; 16: 667.

Peixoto D, et al: Isavuconazole treatment of a patient with disseminated mucormycosis. J Clin Microbiol 2014; 52: 1016.

Rodríguez-Lobato E, et al: Primary cutaneous mucormycosis caused by *Rhizopus oryzae*. Mycopathologia 2017; 182: 387.

Skiada A, et al: Global epidemiology of cutaneous zygomycosis. Clin Dermatol 2012; 30: 628.

HYALOHYPHOMYCOSIS

The term *hyalohyphomycosis* contrasts with *phaeohyphomycosis* and refers to opportunistic mycotic infections caused by nondematiaceous molds. Most of these organisms are septate, and compared with black molds, most have delicate walls. Organisms include *Penicillium, Acremonium, Trichoderma, Scedosporium, Fusarium, Aspergillosis, Scedosporium apiospermum*, and *Paecilomyces*. The two most important of this group, *Fusariosis* and *Aspergillosis*, will be discussed separately.

These organisms are ubiquitous; they occur as saprophytes in soil or water or on decomposing organic debris. They generally do not cause disease except in immunocompromised patients. *Fusarium solani* (keratomycosis) and *Fusarium oxysporum* (white superficial onychomycosis) are exceptions. Localized hyalohyphomycosis has also occurred in immunocompetent patients after traumatic implantation. There is no classic clinical morphology to the lesions, but keratotic masses, ulcerations, ecthyma gangrenosum–like lesions, erythematous nodules, dark eschars, and disseminated erythema have been described (Fig. 15.32).

Penicillium marneffei infection is an indicator of HIV disease, especially in Southeast Asia. This organism is dimorphic and appears in tissue as small, intracellular organisms within histiocytes. The histologic similarity to histoplasmosis is striking.

Most of these infections are treated with a combination of excision and amphotericin B. *Scedosporium* and *Paecilomyces* respond in some cases to voriconazole or posaconazole. In *Penicillium* infections in HIV patients, itraconazole is used indefinitely after initial therapy with amphotericin B.

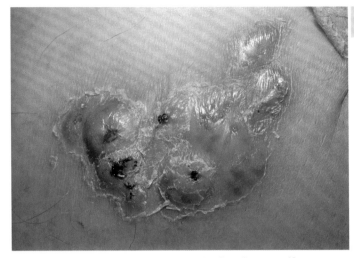

Fig. 15.32 Hyalohyphomycosis caused by *Paecilomyces*. (Courtesy Dan Loo, MD.)

PNEUMOCYSTOSIS

Pneumocystis jiroveci (formerly *P. carinii*) is an opportunistic infection, occurring primarily as a pulmonary infection in AIDS patients. Extrapulmonary involvement is uncommon and usually occurs in the reticuloendothelial system. Skin findings may occur. At least half of reported cases are of nodular growths in the auditory canal, with the remainder having nonspecific, pink to skin-colored papules and nodules that may ulcerate. On biopsy, the dermis contains foamy material within which Giemsa-positive organisms are identified. Mixed cutaneous infection with *Cryptococcus* has been reported; the skin lesions appeared xanthomatous. Cutaneous botryomycosis caused by combined *Staphylococcus aureus* and *P. jiroveci* has been reported in patients with HIV infection. A 3-week course of trimethoprim-sulfamethoxazole is the treatment of choice. In combined infections, all pathogens require treatment. Dapsone prophylaxis has been associated with acute generalized exanthematous pustulosis.

Peña ZG, et al: Mixed *Pneumocystis* and *Cryptococcus* cutaneous infection histologically mimicking xanthoma. Am J Dermatopathol 2013; 35: e6.

Vas A, et al: Acute generalised exanthematous pustulosis induced by *Pneumocystis jirovecii* pneumonia prophylaxis with dapsone. Int J STD AIDS 2013; 24: 745.

FUSARIOSIS

Fusarium has emerged as an important pathogen, especially in patients with hematologic malignancy, neutropenia, and T-cell immunodeficiency, particularly those with hematopoietic stem cell transplants and graft-versus-host disease (GVHD). Skin involvement is present in about 70% of patients, and the infection may begin in the skin and then disseminate. Many cases begin in the lungs or sinuses, then disseminate to the skin. Blood cultures usually are positive, but skin biopsies provide the highest diagnostic yield. Contaminated hospital plumbing may be a source of fusariosis. *Fusarium* has been cultured from drains, water tanks, sink faucet aerators, and shower heads. Aerosolization of *Fusarium* spp. by shower heads has been documented.

The mortality rate is high but has improved with the availability of new antifungal agents. Neutropenia, a factor predicting mortality, must be controlled with colony-stimulating factors. Liposomal amphotericin B is the drug of choice; voriconazole and posaconazole are second-line drugs. Posaconazole can raise calcineurin inhibitor levels in the blood, and these must be closely monitored during therapy.

ASPERGILLOSIS

Aspergillosis is second only to candidiasis in frequency of opportunistic fungal disease in patients with leukemia and other hematologic neoplasia. Neutropenia remains the key risk factor for invasive aspergillosis in this population. Risk factors include prolonged corticosteroid therapy, other immunosuppressive therapy, GVHD, and cytomegalovirus infection. Solid-organ transplant patients are predisposed to *Aspergillus* infections. Pulmonary involvement is usually present in invasive disease; skin lesions are present in only about 10% of patients. Biopsy of a skin lesion may establish the diagnosis when other studies have failed. Blood culture is an insensitive method of diagnosis.

Aspergillus fumigatus is the most common cause of disseminated aspergillosis with cutaneous involvement. The organism grows on media without cycloheximide in 24 hours or longer. In tissue, the organisms appear as slender hyphae with delicate walls and bubbly cytoplasm. The appearance is identical to that of *Fusarium*, except for the lack of vesicular swellings along hyphae. The hyphae in both are septate with 45-degree branching. Both tend to be vasculotropic and are associated with cutaneous necrosis. *Aspergillus flavus* rarely causes fungus balls in the lungs but is a common cause of fungal sinusitis and skin lesions. *Aspergillus niger* is a rare cause of disseminated infection with skin lesions. In third-degree burns, *Aspergillus* often colonizes the eschar. Deep incisional biopsies are required to distinguish invasive disease from colonization.

Primary Cutaneous Aspergillosis

Primary cutaneous aspergillosis is a rare disease. Most cases occur at the site of IV cannulas in immunosuppressed patients. Hemorrhagic bullae and necrotic ulcers may be present (Fig. 15.33). *A. flavus* is most frequently associated with this form of infection. Patients must be treated aggressively because the fungus may disseminate from the skin lesion.

Aspergillus is a frequent contaminant in cultures from thickened, friable, dystrophic nails, and various *Aspergillus* spp. have been implicated as true etiologic agents of onychomycosis. Nail infection may respond to itraconazole.

Otomycosis

The ear canal may be infected by *Aspergillus fumigatus*, *A. flavus*, and *A. niger*. Pathogenic bacteria, especially *Pseudomonas aeruginosa*, are often found concurrently. The colonization may be benign, but malignant otitis may occasionally occur, especially in diabetic or iatrogenically immunosuppressed patients. Invasive disease must be treated with systemic agents. Topical clotrimazole ear drops are effective in immunocompetent patients.

Treatment

Voriconazole is the treatment of choice for invasive aspergillosis, although visual disturbances, photosensitivity, skin cancer, and skin eruptions can be a problem with this drug. Liposomal amphotericin B, caspofungin, micafungin, posaconazole, and isavuconazole are alternate therapies.

Bernardeschi C, et al: Cutaneous invasive aspergillosis. Medicine (Baltimore) 2015; 94: e1018.
Das S, et al: *Acremonium* species. Mycopathologia 2010; 170: 361.
Delia M, et al: Fusariosis in a patient with acute myeloid leukemia. Mycopathologia 2016; 181: 457.

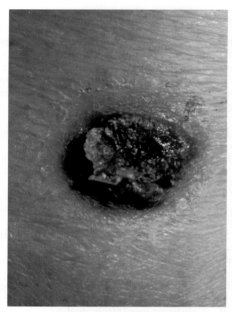

Fig. 15.33 Primary aspergillosis.

Hsu CC, et al: Cutaneous alternariosis in a renal transplant recipient. Asian J Surg 2015; 38: 47.
Kepenekli E, et al: Refractory invasive aspergillosis controlled with posaconazole and pulmonary surgery in a patient with chronic granulomatous disease. Ital J Pediatr 2014; 40: 2.
Kluger N, Saarinen K: *Aspergillus fumigatus* infection on a home-made tattoo. Br J Dermatol 2014; 170: 1373.
Maertens JA, et al: Isavuconazole versus voriconazole for primary treatment of invasive mould disease caused by *Aspergillus* and other filamentous fungi (SECURE). Lancet 2016; 387: 760.
Schwartz KL, et al: Invasive fusariosis. J Pediatric Infect Dis Soc. 2015; 4: 163.
Tatara AM, et al: Factors affecting patient outcome in primary cutaneous aspergillosis. Medicine (Baltimore) 2016; 95: e3747.
Varon AG, et al: Superficial skin lesions positive for *Fusarium* are associated with subsequent development of invasive fusariosis. J Infect 2014; 68: 85.
Vennewald I et al: Otomycosis. Clin Dermatol 2010; 28: 202.
Yang YS, et al: A rare skin presentation of *Penicillium marneffei* infection in an AIDS patient. Int J STD AIDS 2012; 23: 64.

■ DISEASE CAUSED BY ALGAE (PROTOTHECOSIS)

Protothecosis is caused by the *Prototheca* genus of saprophytic, achloric (nonpigmented) algae. These organisms reproduce asexually by internal septation or morulation. This reproductive method, along with the absence of glucosamine and muramic acid in the cell wall, separates the genus from the bacteria and fungi. Two *Prototheca* species cause disease in humans, *Prototheca wickerhamii* and *Prototheca zopfii*. Stagnant water, tree slime, and soil appear to be the source of infection in most cases.

Skin lesions may present as verrucous lesions, ulcers, papulonodular lesions, or crusted papules with umbilication. Protothecosis of the olecranon bursa is usually seen in healthy individuals, but cutaneous infections have been most often reported in patients receiving immunosuppressive therapy and in those with renal failure, liver disease, AIDS, hematologic malignancy, or diabetes mellitus. Neutropenia is not a common risk factor.

Prototheca spp. are easily recognized in PAS-stained tissue specimens when the characteristic morulating cells are visible.

These are more common in *P. wickerhamii*. The organism also appears with a single, black nucleus and a thick, slightly asymmetric, refractile wall. It grows on most routine mycologic media, but cycloheximide will suppress growth of *Prototheca* spp. The use of fluorescent antibody reagents permits the rapid and reliable identification of *Prototheca* spp. in culture and tissue.

IV amphotericin B remains the most effective agent for disseminated *Prototheca* infections. Voriconazole, posaconazole, itraconazole, and fluconazole have been successful in individual cases. Surgery and topical amphotericin B have been used for isolated cutaneous disease.

Figueroa CJ, et al: A case of protothecosis in a patient with multiple myeloma. J Cutan Pathol 2014; 41: 409.

Fong K, et al: Cutaneous protothecosis in a patient with previously undiagnosed HIV infection. Australas J Dermatol 2015; 56: e71.

Kovalyshyn I, et al: Erythematous and edematous plaques on the bilateral extremities in an immunocompromised patient. Int J Dermatol 2016; 55: e59.

Murata M, et al: Disseminated protothecosis manifesting with multiple, rapidly-progressing skin ulcers. Eur J Dermatol 2015; 25: 208.

16   Mycobacterial Diseases

TUBERCULOSIS

No ideal classification scheme exists for cutaneous tuberculosis (TB), but the system listed here is logical and takes into account the mechanism of disease acquisition. Unfortunately, unlike in Hansen disease, these categories do not correlate perfectly to host immunity. The four major categories of cutaneous TB are as follows:

1. Inoculation from an exogenous source (primary inoculation TB, TB verrucosa cutis)
2. Endogenous cutaneous spread contiguously or by autoinoculation (scrofuloderma, TB cutis orificialis)
3. Hematogenous spread to the skin (lupus vulgaris; acute miliary TB; TB ulcer, gumma, or abscess; tuberculous cellulitis) (Lupus vulgaris can also occur adjacent to lesions of scrofuloderma, suggesting that both hematogenous spread and local spread are capable of triggering this reaction pattern.)
4. Tuberculids (erythema induratum [Bazin disease], papulonecrotic tuberculid, lichen scrofulosorum)

The finding of mycobacterial deoxyribonucleic acid (DNA) by polymerase chain reaction (PCR) in tuberculids suggests that tuberculids also represent hematogenous dissemination of TB, which is quickly controlled by the host, usually resulting in the absence of detectable organisms by culture and histologic methods. Miliary TB is the form with least effective host immunity. Tuberculous ulcer/abscess/cellulitis and TB cutis orificialis are conditions of poor host immunity against *Mycobacterium tuberculosis*. Bacilli are prominent in these forms of cutaneous TB, and histologic and microbiologic confirmation is usually straightforward. This is fortunate, because cellular-based diagnostic modalities (purified protein derivative [PPD], interferon-γ release assay [IGRA]) may be negative. TB verrucosa cutis and lupus vulgaris are conditions of high host immunity to TB, and tuberculin skin tests and IGRA for TB will usually be positive. Scrofuloderma is usually associated with a positive PPD, and identification by culture and histologic methods is positive in only 20% and 40% of cases, respectively. In its initial stage, primary inoculation TB will be multibacillary and culture positive. As host immunity develops, the skin test becomes positive, and the number of organisms on biopsy diminishes. The tuberculids also represent high host immune response manifestations of TB, and bacilli are rarely found.

Epidemiology

The increase in the numbers of cases of TB that started in the mid-1980s in the United States was associated with three phenomena: large numbers of immigrants from high-prevalence countries, the human immunodeficiency virus/acquired immunodeficiency syndrome (HIV/AIDS) epidemic, and an increasing number of persons in congregative facilities (shelters for homeless persons, prisons). Asians, African Americans, and Hispanics have the greatest risk for developing TB in the United States. Aggressive diagnosis and treatment programs have led to a reduction in new U.S. cases of TB. The infection rate in the U.S.-born population of adults is now 3 cases per 100,000 population. However, local pockets of TB are still found in U.S. regions of otherwise very low incidence. This is partly attributable to the persistently high infection rate in the foreign-born U.S. population, which has also fallen dramatically over the years, but is still at 15 cases per 100,000.

In the developing world, TB is the number one cause of death resulting from a single infectious agent. The increasing number of infections has been driven largely by the HIV/AIDS epidemic. One third or more of HIV-infected persons in Africa are also infected with *M. tuberculosis*. Latent TB is 100 times more likely to reactivate in persons with HIV infection, and HIV-infected persons are much more likely to acquire new tuberculous infection. Countries such as India still account for a quarter of the total global TB burden, although great progress has been made. Hematopoietic stem cell transplantation and solid organ transplant recipients are particularly prone to TB, at a rate of 10 to 70 times the general population.

TB has increasingly become resistant to first-line treatments. Strains classified as *multidrug-resistant tuberculosis* (MDR-TB) are resistant to at least isoniazid and rifampin. *Extensively drug-resistant tuberculosis* (XDR-TB) is, in addition, resistant to any fluoroquinolone and at least one of the following: capreomycin, kanamycin, or amikacin. The emergence of these resistant strains of TB has made treatment more costly and more difficult. However, aggressive treatment protocols using multiple drugs for up to 2 years and, when indicated, surgical techniques can cure up to 60% of even XDR-TB patients.

Cutaneous TB is an uncommon complication of tuberculous infection, with less than 2% of TB patients having skin lesions, even in highly endemic areas. The types of cutaneous lesion that the patient will develop depend on the following host factors:

1. *Age:* About 25% of scrofuloderma cases and most cases of lichen scrofulosorum occur in children.
2. *Gender:* Women are 10 times more likely to develop erythema induratum, but men are two to three times more likely to have other forms of cutaneous TB.
3. *Anatomic location:* Lupus vulgaris occurs on the face and extremities, whereas TB verrucosa cutis occurs predominantly on the hands.
4. *Nutritional status:* Tuberculous abscesses and scrofuloderma are associated with malnutrition.

The pattern of cutaneous TB has been changing over the last few decades and is different in developed than in developing nations. The average age of patients with cutaneous TB has increased in developed countries, and tuberculids, especially erythema induratum, represent a larger proportion of cases. In Hong Kong 85% of cases of cutaneous TB are tuberculids. This suggests that most cutaneous TB in adults will be found in patients infected in the distant past who are reactivating their disease, not recently infected persons. Cutaneous TB is uncommon in immunosuppressed hosts; when they acquire new TB or reactivate their TB, it usually reactivates at a noncutaneous site and is diagnosed before skin disease occurs. Miliary TB is the most frequently reported form of cutaneous TB in the HIV-infected patient. In areas of high TB endemicity in the developing world, cutaneous TB is still common. More than 50% of cases will occur before age 19. The likelihood of finding associated systemic TB is higher in children than adults. Nonetheless, unlike in all other forms of extrapulmonary TB, failure to find an underlying focus of TB in patients with cutaneous TB can occur. Between 3% and 12% of patients with cutaneous TB will have an abnormal chest radiograph. Most often, TB of the lymph nodes will be found.

Tuberculin Testing

The tuberculin skin test (TST) is designed to detect a memory cell–mediated immune response to *M. tuberculosis*. The test becomes positive 2–10 weeks after infection and remains positive for many years, although it may wane with age. PPD preparations are currently used for testing in the United States and Canada at a dose of 5 tuberculin units (TU). The intradermal, or Mantoux, test is the standard and offers the highest degree of consistency and reliability. The test is read 48–72 hours after intradermal injection. Induration measuring 5 mm or more is considered positive in HIV-infected patients, in solid organ transplantation patients, in those with risk factors for developing TB (e.g., patients who will receive or are receiving anti–tumor necrosis factor [TNF] therapy), in those on greater than 15 mg/day of prednisone for over 1 month, in patients on current cancer chemotherapy, in recent close contacts, or in those with chest x-ray findings consistent with healed TB. Because children are at increased risk of developing active TB after exposure, a 5-mm or larger reaction in contact investigations is considered positive. If the PPD measures more than 10 mm, it is considered positive in injection (intravenous) drug users (IDUs), HIV-negative IDUs, those born in foreign countries of high TB prevalence, health care workers, residents and employees in high-risk congregate facilities, and those with medical conditions that predispose to TB. If induration is more than 15 mm, it is positive in all others; 0- to 4-mm induration is negative.

The lower the threshold for positivity for the TST, the less this represents true positivity (the higher number of false positives). This is why a TST of less than 15 mm is considered positive only in patients at higher risk for having latent TB. Conversely, as the cutoff for true positivity is raised, the number of infected persons the TST detects will decrease (the number of false negatives increases). A TST of over 6 mm will detect 89% of persons with latent TB, over 10 mm will detect 75%, and over 15 mm will detect only 47% of latently infected patients. At least 7% of patients with latent TB will have a completely negative TST. Many intermediate TST responses may represent cross-reaction with atypical mycobacteria. Bacillus (bacille) Calmette-Guérin (BCG) immunization leads to a positive tuberculin result in immunized children, but this reaction usually does not persist beyond 10 years. Repeated BCG immunization or BCG administration after age 2 years is more likely to result in a persistently positive TST on this basis. However, positive reactions in adults should not automatically be attributed to childhood BCG administration.

Reactivity to the tuberculin protein is impaired in certain conditions in which cellular immunity is impaired. Lymphoproliferative disorders, sarcoidosis, corticosteroid and immunosuppressive drugs (including TNF inhibitors), severe protein deficiency, chronic renal failure, and numerous infectious illnesses, including HIV infection, are capable of diminishing tuberculin reactivity. In overwhelming TB (miliary disease), more than 50% of patients have a negative skin test before beginning therapy. A negative or doubtful reaction to a PPD preparation does not rule out TB infection, particularly in the patient with suggestive symptoms and signs.

TST then has significant limitations, which also include negative tests in a substantial number of patients with active TB (sensitivity only 77%), repeat visits to interpret, technical competence of person applying the test, booster effect of repeat testing creating potential false-positive results, and false-positive tests in persons with prior BCG vaccination. To overcome these obstacles, antigen-specific in vitro assays have been developed. These assays measure the amount of interferon (IFN)–γ released by peripheral blood T cells (IGRAs; e.g., QuantiFERON-TB Gold, ELISpot^PLUS, T-SPOT). Results are variable with respect to the sensitivity and specificity of these assays, but they are valuable in certain settings. They are considerably more specific in the BCG-vaccinated population, in whom the TST is only 60% specific, whereas IGRAs are 93% specific. In addition, in HIV-infected patients and those receiving corticosteroids, IGRAs are much more likely to be positive than a TST in those with *M. tuberculosis* infection. In children under age 5 the TST is preferred, as it is in those requiring serial testing. In other settings either TST or IGRAs may be used. If the TST is combined with an IGRA and the tests are concordant, false-negative results are 2% and false-positive tests only 1%. Therefore a combination of TST and IGRA may be used to clarify a TST result. In such cases the two tests should be done simultaneously, as the IGRA results may be boosted in a patient who has had a TST within the prior 3 months.

Appropriate screening before initiating anti-TNF therapy or immunosuppression in a dermatology patient would include the following:

1. Screen for active TB by history and physical examination (and chest x-ray where suspicion for TB is elevated).
2. Administer a TST or an IGRA.
3. Interpret the test results with caution in patients already on significant iatrogenic immunosuppressive or anti-TNF treatments.
4. Regularly monitor patients on anti-TNF agents for the development of TB with appropriate history, physical examination, and laboratory testing; and suspect and screen for TB if clinical symptoms may indicate infection.
5. Rescreen with a TST or IGRA annually.

Bacille Calmette-Guérin Vaccination

BCG is a live attenuated strain of *Mycobacterium bovis* used in most parts of the world (except North America and Western Europe) to immunize infants. It enhances immunity to TB and is effective in reducing childhood TB, especially if given to neonates. Once the patient has been vaccinated, the TST becomes positive and remains so for a period of less than 10 years (unless the person is BCG immunized after age 2 or repeatedly immunized). In an adult who was vaccinated as a child in a foreign country with a high prevalence of TB and whose TST measures more than 10 mm, active TB should be assumed. The use of BCG instillation in the bladder to treat bladder cancer has been associated with disseminated disease, usually pneumonitis, hepatitis, prostatitis, and abdominal aneurysms.

Dermatologic complications of BCG vaccination are rarely seen. Localized abscesses and regional suppurative adenitis occur at a rate of about 0.4 per 1000 vaccines. Excessive ulceration may occur if the BCG is inoculated too deeply. Scrofuloderma is rare. Disseminated infection is seen in 1–4 cases per 1 million infants vaccinated and is associated with high mortality. Disseminated BCG develops only in the setting of immunodeficiency. Lupus vulgaris can occur rarely at the vaccination site or at a distant site and will respond to appropriate antituberculous treatment. Papular and papulonecrotic tuberculids, as well as erythema induratum, can occur after BCG immunization, appearing 10 days to several months after vaccination. Treatment may not be necessary for the BCG-induced tuberculids; they frequently heal in a few months with no treatment.

Inoculation Cutaneous Tuberculosis From Exogenous Source

Primary Inoculation Tuberculosis (Primary Tuberculous Complex, Tuberculous Chancre)

Primary inoculation TB develops at the site of inoculation of tubercle bacilli into a TB-free individual (Fig. 16.1). Regional lymphadenopathy usually occurs, completing the "complex." It

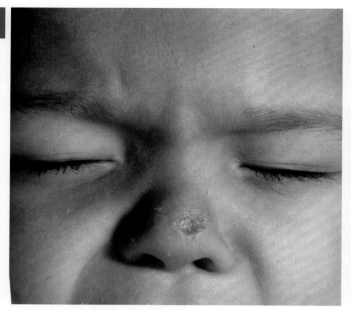

Fig. 16.1 Primary inoculation tuberculosis.

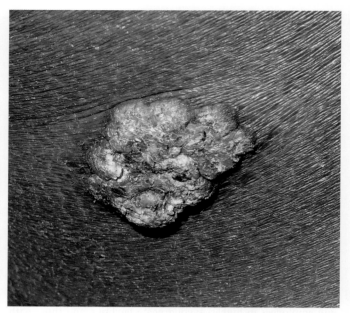

Fig. 16.2 Tuberculosis verrucosa cutis. (Courtesy Debabrata Bandyopadhyay, MD.)

occurs chiefly in children and affects the face or extremities. The inoculation can occur during tattooing, medical injections, nose piercing, or external physical trauma. The earliest lesion, appearing 2–4 weeks after inoculation, is a painless brown-red papule that develops into an indurated nodule or plaque that may ulcerate. This is the tuberculous chancre. Prominent regional lymphadenopathy appears 3–8 weeks after infection and, occasionally, suppurative and draining lesions may appear over involved lymph nodes. Primary tuberculous complex occurs on the mucous membranes in about one third of patients. Spontaneous healing usually occurs within 1 year, with the skin lesion healing first, then the lymph node, which is often persistently enlarged and calcified. Delayed suppuration of the affected lymph node, lupus vulgaris overlying the involved node, and occasionally dissemination may follow this form of cutaneous TB.

Histologically, there is a marked inflammatory response during the first 2 weeks, with many polymorphonuclear leukocyte neutrophils (PMNs) and tubercle bacilli. During the next 2 weeks, the picture changes. Lymphocytes and epithelioid cells appear and replace the PMNs. Distinct tubercles develop within 3 or 4 weeks of inoculation. Simultaneously, with the appearance of epithelioid cells, the number of tubercle bacilli decreases rapidly.

The differential diagnosis of primary inoculation TB extends over the spectrum of chancriform conditions of deep fungal or bacterial origin, such as sporotrichosis, blastomycosis, histoplasmosis, coccidioidomycosis, nocardiosis, syphilis, leishmaniasis, yaws, tularemia, and atypical mycobacterial disease. Pyogenic granuloma and cat-scratch disease must also be considered.

Paucibacillary Cutaneous Tuberculosis From Exogenous or Endogenous Source in Persons With High Immunity

Tuberculosis Verrucosa Cutis. TB verrucosa cutis occurs from exogenous inoculation of bacilli into the skin of a previously sensitized person with strong immunity against *M. tuberculosis*. The tuberculin test is strongly positive. The prosecutor's wart resulting from inoculation during an autopsy is the prototype of TB verrucosa cutis.

Clinically, the lesion begins as a small papule, which becomes hyperkeratotic, resembling a wart. The lesion enlarges by peripheral expansion, with or without central clearing, sometimes reaching several centimeters or more in diameter (Fig. 16.2). Fissuring of the surface may occur, discharging purulent exudate. Lesions are almost always solitary, and regional adenopathy is usually present only if secondary bacterial infection occurs. Frequent locations for TB verrucosa cutis are on the dorsa of the fingers and hands in adults and the ankles and buttocks in children. The lesions are persistent but usually superficial and limited in extent. Local scarring, as seen in lupus vulgaris, can occur. Although sometimes separated by exudative or suppurative areas, the lesions seldom ulcerate and may heal spontaneously.

Histologically, there is pseudoepitheliomatous hyperplasia of the epidermis and hyperkeratosis. Suppurative and granulomatous inflammation is seen in the upper and middle dermis, sometimes perforating through the epidermis. Caseation is rare. The number of acid-fast bacilli (AFB) is usually scant, and failure to find AFB should not be used to exclude the diagnosis. Culture will be positive in slightly more than 50% of cases.

TB verrucosa cutis is differentiated only by culture from atypical mycobacteriosis caused by *Mycobacterium marinum*. It must also be distinguished from North American blastomycosis, chromoblastomycosis, verrucous epidermal nevus, hypertrophic lichen planus, halogenoderma, and verruca vulgaris.

Lupus Vulgaris. Lupus vulgaris may appear at sites of inoculation, in scrofuloderma scars, or most frequently at distant sites from the initial infectious focus, probably by hematogenous dissemination. Approximately half of such cases will have evidence of TB elsewhere, so a complete evaluation is mandatory. Because lupus vulgaris is associated with moderately high immunity to TB, most patients will have a positive tuberculin test.

Lupus vulgaris typically is a single plaque composed of grouped red-brown papules, which, when blanched by diascopic pressure, have a pale, brownish yellow or "apple jelly" color. On dermoscopy a yellowish-orange patch may indicate the presence of dermal granulomas secondary to lupus vulgaris, sarcoidosis, a foreign body reaction, or cutaneous leishmaniasis. The papules, called lupomas, tend to heal slowly in one area and progress in another. They are minute, translucent, and embedded deeply and diffusely in the infiltrated dermis, expanding by the development of new papules at the periphery, which coalesce with the main

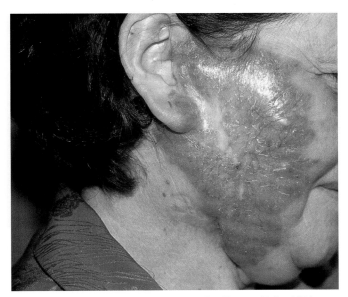

Fig. 16.3 Lupus vulgaris. (Courtesy Dr. Tavares-Bello, MD.)

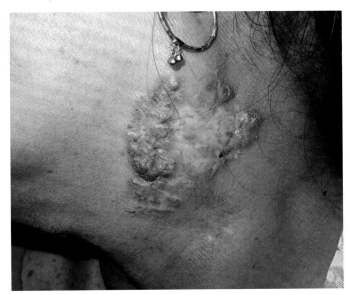

Fig. 16.4 Lupus vulgaris. (Courtesy Debabrata Bandyopadhyay, MD.)

plaque (Figs. 16.3 and 16.4). The plaques are slightly elevated. The disease is destructive, frequently causes ulceration, and on involution leaves deforming scars as it slowly spreads peripherally over the years. Lupus vulgaris lesions of the head and neck can be associated with lymphangitis or lymphadenitis in some cases. If lesions involve the nose or the earlobes, these structures are shrunken and scarred, as if nibbled away. Atrophy is prominent, and ectropion and eclabion may occur. The tip of the nose may be sharply pointed and beaklike, or the whole nose may be destroyed, with only the orifices and the posterior parts of the septum and turbinates visible. The upper lip, a site of predilection, may become diffusely swollen and thickened, with fissures, adherent thin crusts, and ulcers. On the trunk and extremities, lesions may be annular or serpiginous or may form gyrate patterns. On the hands and feet and around the genitals or buttocks, lesions may cause mutilation by destruction, scar formation, warty thickenings, and elephantiasic enlargement.

An unusual form of lupus vulgaris may follow measles or another significant febrile illness. The window of immune deficiency caused by the acute illness results in dissemination of the TB hematogenously from a single focus of lupus vulgaris. Multiple erythematous papules in a generalized distribution appear a month or more after the illness. These lesions evolve to small papules and plaques, clinically and histologically resembling lupus vulgaris. The TST is negative during the immediate period after the febrile illness, then rapidly reverts to strongly positive. This is called "lupus vulgaris postexanthematicus."

Although classically considered a scarring and atrophying process, lesions of the lips and ears may be quite hyperplastic. The lips may resemble cheilitis granulomatosis clinically and histologically. Uniform hyperplasia of the ear pinna and lobe may closely mimic "turkey ear," as described in sarcoidosis. When the mucous membranes are involved, the lesions become papillomatous or ulcerative. They may appear as circumscribed, grayish, macerated, or granulating plaques. On the tongue, irregular, deep, painful fissures occur, sometimes associated with microglossia to the degree that nutrition is compromised.

The rate of progression of lupus vulgaris is slow, and a lesion may remain limited to a small area for several decades. The onset may be in childhood and persist throughout life. It may slowly spread, and new lesions may develop in other regions. In some patients, the lesions become papillomatous, vegetative, or thickly crusted, with a rupioid appearance. Squamous cell carcinoma may develop in long-standing lesions.

Histologically, classic tubercles are the hallmark of lupus vulgaris. Caseation within the tubercles is seen in about half the cases and is rarely marked. Sarcoidosis may be simulated. The epidermis is affected secondarily, sometimes flattened and at other times hypertrophic. AFB are found in 10% or less of cases with standard acid-fast stains. PCR may only be positive in the minority of cases of paucibacillary forms of cutaneous TB. Cultures of the skin lesions grow *M. tuberculosis* in about half the cases.

Colloid milia, acne vulgaris, sarcoidosis, and rosacea may simulate lupus vulgaris. Differentiation from tertiary syphilis, chronic discoid lupus erythematosus, Hansen disease, systemic mycoses, and leishmaniasis may be more difficult, and biopsy and tissue cultures may be required.

Cutaneous Tuberculosis From Endogenous Source by Direct Extension (Scrofuloderma and Periorificial Tuberculosis)

Scrofuloderma is tuberculous involvement of the skin by direct extension from an underlying focus of infection. It occurs most frequently over the cervical lymph nodes but also may occur over bone or around joints if these are involved. Clinically, the lesions begin as subcutaneous masses, which enlarge to form nodules. Suppuration occurs centrally. They may be erythematous or skin colored, and usually the skin temperature is not increased over the mass. Lesions may drain, forming sinuses, or they may ulcerate with reddish granulation at the base (Figs. 16.5 and 16.6). Surgical procedures may incite lesions of scrofuloderma over joints or the abdominal cavity, apparently by releasing the loculated focus and contaminating the track along which instruments are inserted. Scrofuloderma heals with characteristic cordlike scars, frequently allowing the diagnosis to be made many years later.

Perianal TB is characterized by a chronic anal fistula characteristically in men age 30–60. The intestinal tract, especially the rectum, is involved in most of these cases. Anal strictures and involvement of the scrotum may occur if disease is untreated.

Histologically, in scrofuloderma, the tuberculous process begins in the underlying lymph node or bone and extends through the deep dermis. Necrosis occurs with formation of a cavity filled with liquefied debris and PMNs. At the periphery, more typical

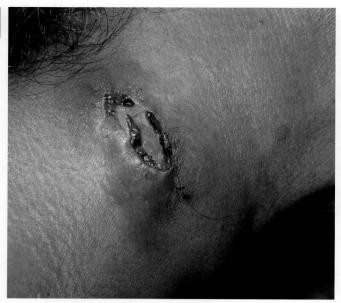

Fig. 16.5 Scrofuloderma. (Courtesy Debabrata Bandyopadhyay, MD.)

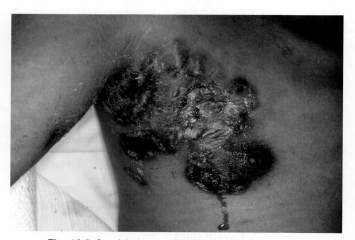

Fig. 16.6 Scrofuloderma. (Courtesy Scott Norton, MD.)

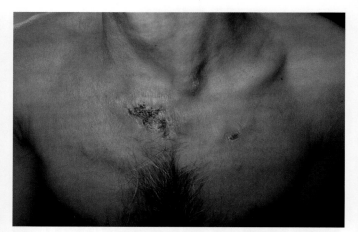

Fig. 16.7 Metastatic tuberculosis. (Courtesy Debabrata Bandyopadhyay, MD.)

Cutaneous Tuberculosis From Hematogenous Spread

Miliary (Disseminated) Tuberculosis

Miliary TB appears in the setting of fulminant TB of the lung or meninges. Generally, patients have other unmistakable signs of severe disseminated TB. It is most common in children but may occur in adults. Most reported cases of cutaneous TB seen in patients with AIDS are of this type. Miliary TB may also follow infectious illnesses that reduce immunity, especially measles. Because this represents uncontrolled hematogenous infection, the TST is negative. Lesions are generalized and may appear as erythematous macules or papules, pustules, subcutaneous nodules, and purpuric "vasculitic" lesions. Ulceration may occur, and the pain in the infarcted lesions may be substantial. The prognosis is guarded.

Skin biopsies show diffuse suppurative inflammation of the dermis or subcutis with predominantly PMNs, at times forming abscesses. Caseating granulomas may be seen. AFB are abundant.

Metastatic Tuberculous Abscess, Ulceration, or Cellulitis

The hematogenous dissemination of mycobacteria from a primary focus may result in firm, nontender, erythematous plaques (resembling cellulitis) or nodules (Fig. 16.7). The nodules can evolve to form abscesses, ulcers, or draining sinus tracts. This form of cutaneous TB is usually seen in children, and most patients have decreased immunity from malnutrition, infection, or an immunodeficiency state. Patients presenting with tuberculous skin ulcers may or may not have other foci of TB identified. Aerosolization of mycobacteria may occur during incision and drainage and during dressing changes, leading to secondary cases among surgical and nursing staff treating these ulcers. Histologically, abscess formation and numerous AFB are seen.

Sporotrichoid Tuberculosis

Although TB is usually thought to be spread either by direct extension or hematogenously, in about 3% of patients with cutaneous TB, the lesions occur in a sporotrichoid pattern, suggesting lymphatic spread (Fig. 16.8). Classically, this begins with a distal lesion, and new lesions appearing more proximally. Less often, a proximal lesion is present initially, and new lesions appear distally (retrograde lymphatic spread). The draining proximal lymph nodes may be enlarged. The individual lesions have the same morphology

granulomatous inflammation is seen, along with AFB observed in slightly less than half of cases.

Scrofuloderma should be differentiated from atypical mycobacterial infection, sporotrichosis, actinomycosis, coccidioidomycosis, and hidradenitis suppurativa. Lymphogranuloma venereum (LGV) favors the inguinal and perineal areas, with positive serologic tests for LGV.

TB cutis orificialis is a form of cutaneous TB that occurs at the mucocutaneous borders of the nose, mouth, anus, urinary meatus, and vagina and on the mucous membrane of the mouth or tongue. It is caused by autoinoculation from underlying active visceral TB, particularly of the larynx, lungs, intestines, and genitourinary tract. It indicates failing resistance to the disease. Consequently, tuberculin positivity is variable but usually positive. Lesions ulcerate from the beginning and extend rapidly, with no tendency to spontaneous healing. The ulcers are usually soft and punched out and have undermined edges. Histologically, the ulcer base is usually composed largely of granulation tissue infiltrated with PMNs. Deep and lateral to the ulcer, granulomatous inflammation may be found, and AFB are numerous.

Tuberculous Mastitis

Rarely, TB will present as subcutaneous nodules on the breast. The lesions can suppurate, forming abscesses, or break down, forming sinus tracts. The condition favors women of childbearing age but can also affect men. Tuberculous mastitis may closely resemble breast cancer, so biopsies are frequently done. Abscesses may be incised and drained. The consequence of the ongoing inflammation, destroying the fat of the breast, and the surgical procedures can be a severely disfigured breast. An underlying focus of TB may be present in the underlying bone or at a distant site in some cases. TST is positive. Histology shows granulomatous inflammation with negative AFB stains. Culture is usually negative. The diagnosis of tuberculous mastitis should be considered in all patients with granulomatous mastitis from endemic areas of TB.

Tuberculids

Tuberculids are a group of skin eruptions associated with an underlying or silent focus of TB. They are diagnosed by their characteristic clinical features, histologic findings, a positive TST or IGRA, sometimes by the finding of TB at a distant site, and resolution of the eruption with antituberculous therapy. Tuberculids represent cutaneous lesions induced by hematogenous dissemination of tubercle bacilli to the skin. Lupus vulgaris may develop at the sites of tuberculids, and *M. tuberculosis* DNA may be found in tuberculid lesions by PCR. Tuberculids usually occur in persons with a strong immunity to TB (and thus a positive PPD). This results in rapid destruction of the bacilli and autoinvolution of individual lesions in many cases. New lesions continue to appear, however, because hematogenous dissemination from the underlying focus continues. Tuberculids tend to be bilaterally symmetric eruptions because they result from hematogenous dissemination.

Papulonecrotic Tuberculid

Papulonecrotic tuberculid is usually an asymptomatic, chronic disorder, presenting in successive crops. Lesions are symmetrically distributed on the extensor extremities, especially on the tips of the elbows and on the knees; dorsal surfaces of the hands and feet; buttocks; face and ears; and glans penis. Lesions may favor pernio-prone sites and may be worse during winter months. Two thirds of cases occur before age 30, and females are affected 3:1 over males. Evidence of prior or active TB is found in one third to two thirds of patients, especially in the lymph nodes. The TST is positive and may generate a necrotic reaction.

Typical lesions vary in size from 2–8 mm and are firm, inflammatory papules that become pustular or necrotic (Fig. 16.9). Lesions resolve slowly over several weeks, but occasional ulcers persist longer. Varioliform scarring follows the lesions. Crops recur over months to years.

Papulonecrotic tuberculids may appear in association with other cutaneous manifestations of TB, particularly erythema induratum or scrofuloderma. Associated clinical phenomena have included tuberculous arteritis with gangrene in young adult Africans and development of lupus vulgaris from the lesions. HIV-infected persons may develop papulonecrotic tuberculid.

Histologically, the epidermis is ulcerated in well-developed lesions. A palisaded collection of histiocytes surrounds an ovoid or wedge-shaped area of dermal necrosis. Well-formed tubercles are not seen, except in nonhealing lesions evolving into lupus vulgaris. Vascular changes are prominent, ranging from a mild lymphocytic vasculitis to fibrinoid necrosis and thrombotic occlusion of vessels. This is not a neutrophilic leukocytoclastic vasculitis, but rather a chronic granulomatous, small-vessel vasculitis. Capillaries, venules, and arterioles may be involved. AFB stains are negative, but PCR may detect mycobacterial DNA in up to half of patients with papulonecrotic tuberculid.

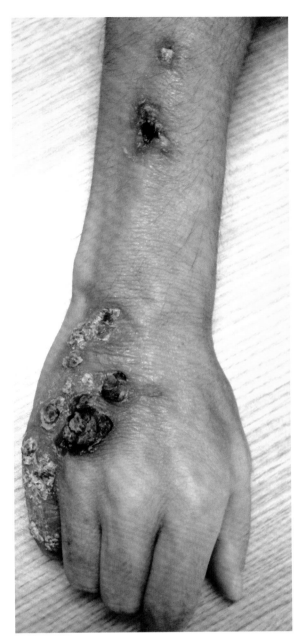

Fig. 16.8 Sporotrichoid tuberculosis. (Courtesy Dr. Juliana Kauge.)

in any given patient, but different patients can have different morphologies. A string of lupus vulgaris–like lesions is most common. Less often, a string of deep nodules may become fluctuant, drain to the surface, or ulcerate, forming linear scrofuloderma-like lesions. The draining lymph node may be enlarged (more often than in sporotrichoid atypical mycobacterial infection). The TST is positive. Underlying foci of systemic TB are often not found. Biopsy of the lesions (and affected lymph nodes) typically shows granulomatous inflammation, but AFB stains are usually negative. Culture may be positive.

This form of TB presents significant diagnostic problems, because sporotrichoid lesions would more often result from atypical mycobacteria or sporotrichosis. Because atypical mycobacteria, especially *M. marinum*, may result in a positive TST, confirming the diagnosis is difficult, even if AFB are found on biopsy. Culture and PCR used to speciate the infecting organism from the biopsy is definitive.

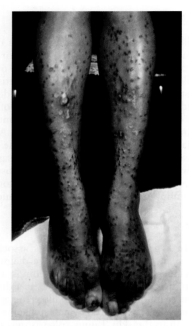

Fig. 16.9 Papulonecrtotic tuberculid. (Courtesy James Steger, MD.)

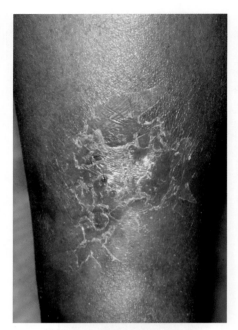

Fig. 16.10 Erythema induratum.

Papulopustular secondary syphilis, pityriasis lichenoides et varioliformis acuta, Churg-Strauss granuloma, lymphomatoid papulosis, perforating granuloma annulare, perforating collagenosis, and necrotizing or septic vasculitis share clinical and histologic features with papulonecrotic tuberculid.

Lichen Scrofulosorum

Lichen scrofulosorum consists of groups of indolent, minute, keratotic discrete papules scattered over the trunk. The lesions are 2–4 mm, follicular or parafollicular, and yellow-pink to reddish brown. They are firm and flat topped or surmounted by a tiny pustule or thin scale. The lesions are arranged in nummular or discoid groups, where they persist unchanged for months and cause no symptoms. They may slowly undergo spontaneous involution, followed at times by recurrence. About 95% of cases of lichen scrofulosorum occur in children and adolescents under age 20. Active TB at a distant site, usually the bones or lymph nodes, is present in about three quarters of patients. The tuberculin test is always positive.

Histologically, lichen scrofulosorum shows noncaseating tuberculoid granulomas just beneath the epidermis, between and surrounding hair follicles. Normally, tubercle bacilli are not seen in the pathologic specimens and cannot be cultured from biopsy material.

Lichen nitidus, lichen planus, secondary syphilis, and sarcoidosis should be considered in the differential diagnosis.

Erythema Induratum and Vascular Reactions Caused by Tuberculosis (Nodular Tuberculid and Nodular Granulomatous Phlebitis)

Erythema induratum (Bazin disease) is chronic and occurs predominantly (80%) in women of middle age. Lesions favor the posterior lower calf, which may also show acrocyanosis. Individual lesions are tender, erythematous or violaceous, 1–2 cm subcutaneous nodules (Fig. 16.10). They resolve spontaneously, with or without ulceration, over several months and can heal with scarring. A clinically similar but less common condition called nodular granulomatous phlebitis also affects women primarily but involves both the lower legs and the thighs, usually along the course of the saphenous vein. Individual lesions evolve over weeks to months but may recur for years in a seasonal pattern. They do not ulcerate or heal with scarring. The TST is positive. Idiopathic nodular vasculitis unassociated with TB may have identical clinical and histologic features, and this diagnosis is made when the PPD is negative.

The primary pathologic changes occur in the subcutaneous fat, which shows lobular panniculitis with fat necrosis. Granulomatous inflammation occurs in two thirds of cases and is noncaseating. In addition, a granulomatous vasculitis of arterioles can be present in the fat and is the apparent cause of the fat necrosis. Biopsies of nodular granulomatous phlebitis show thrombosis of and granulomatous inflammation centered around veins in the deep dermis. AFB are not found on special stains or cultures of the biopsy. PCR may help to confirm these diagnoses; however, the positive PPD obviates the need for it. At times, necrotizing vasculitis is present at the dermohypodermal junction. This reaction has been termed nodular tuberculid. The histology of nodular tuberculid may be identical or very similar to polyarteritis nodosa. More rarely, small-vessel vasculitis (leukocytoclastic vasculitis) or Sweet syndrome–like lesions may be seen as a "reaction" to an underlying focus of TB.

Erythema induratum must be distinguished from erythema nodosum, nodular vasculitis, polyarteritis nodosa, tertiary syphilis, and other infectious and inflammatory panniculitides. Erythema nodosum is of relatively short duration, develops rapidly, and chiefly affects the anterior rather than the posterior calves. It produces tender, painful, scarlet or contusiform nodules that appear simultaneously and do not ulcerate. Histology demonstrates a septal panniculitis. In erythema induratum patients, the pain is less severe, and the lesions tend to evolve serially or in crops. A syphilitic gumma is usually unilateral and single or may appear as a small, distinct group of lesions.

Diagnosis of Cutaneous Tuberculosis

Biopsy with acid-fast staining should be done when the history and physical examination suggest cutaneous TB. PCR is increasingly used to identify mycobacterial DNA in tissue specimens and other biologic samples. It may be positive when both stains and cultures are negative; in paucibacillary disease, however, PCR is not reliably positive. Culture remains the gold standard and provides the means to determine antibiotic sensitivity and response to treatment.

Treatment

Testing for HIV is recommended for all patients diagnosed with TB because HIV-infected patients may require longer courses of therapy, even when antiretroviral therapy is given. In addition, every effort should be made to culture the organism for sensitivity testing because MDR-TB is common in some communities. For all forms of cutaneous TB, multidrug chemotherapy is recommended. The recommendations of the local health clinics that manage other forms of TB should be followed. Three-drug or four-drug regimens are usually recommended for initial empiric treatment. Directly observed therapy is a strategy designed to ensure cure. "Priority patients" are those with prior treatment failure, pulmonary TB with a positive smear, HIV coinfection, current or prior drug use, drug-resistant disease, psychiatric illness, memory impairment, or previous nonadherence to therapy. Surgical excision is useful for the treatment of isolated lesions of lupus vulgaris and TB verrucosa cutis, and surgical intervention also may benefit some patients with scrofuloderma. In many cases of cutaneous TB, the organism has not been identified by either histology or culture, so treatment is inherently empiric. Virtually all forms of cutaneous TB will have begun to respond to treatment by 6 weeks. Failure to respond within this period should result in reconsideration of the diagnosis, assessment for compliance, and concern about drug resistance.

Aguado JM, et al: Tuberculosis and transplantation. Microbiol Spectr 2016; 4.
Ahn CS, et al: To test or not to test? An updated evidence-based assessment of the value of screening and monitoring tests when using systemic biologic agents to treat psoriasis and psoriatic arthritis. J Am Acad Dermatol 2015; 73: 420.
Aliaagaoglu C, et al: Scrofuloderma. Int J Dermatol 2015; 54: 612.
Bombonato C, et al: Orange color. J Am Acad Dermatol 2015; 72: S60.
Cantini F, et al: Guidance for the management of patients with latent tuberculosis infection requiring biologic therapy in rheumatology and dermatology clinical practice. Autoimmun Rev 2015; 14: 503.
Chahar M, et al: Multifocal tuberculosis verrucosa cutis. Dermatol Online J 2015; 21.
Chakraborty PP, et al: Primary *Mycobacterium tuberculosis* infection over insulin injection site. BMJ Case Rep 2016 Nov 8; 2016.
Chirch LM, et al: Proactive infectious disease approach to dermatologic patients who are taking tumor necrosis factor-alfa antagonists: Part II. J Am Acad Dermatol 2014; 71: 11.e1.
Cruz AT, Starke JR: Managing tuberculosis infection in children in the USA. Future Microbiol 2016; 11: 669.
Dhawan AK, et al: Tattoo inoculation lupus vulgaris in two brothers. Indian J Dermatol Venereol Leprol 2015; 81: 516.
Dorman SE, et al: Interferon-γ release assays and tuberculin skin testing for diagnosis of latent tuberculosis infection in healthcare workers in the United States. Am J Respir Crit Care Med 2014; 189: 77.
Elliott C, Hall J: Tuberculosis testing. J Fam Pract 2015; 64: 553.
Gavriilaki E, et al: Disseminated tuberculosis. Hemodial Int 2015; 19: E8.
Gyldenlove M, et al: Cutaneous necrotic ulceration due to BCG re-vaccination. Hum Vaccin Immunother 2012; 8: 424.
Haase O, et al: Recurrent abscesses of the neck. JAMA Dermatol 2014; 150: 909.

Hallensleben ND, et al: Tuberculids. J Eur Acad Dermatol Venereol 2016; 30: 1590.
Heller MM, et al: Fatal case of disseminated BCG infection after vaccination of an infant with in utero exposure to infliximab. J Am Acad Dermatol 2011; 65: 870.
Hill MK, Sanders CV: Cutaneous tuberculosis. Microbiol Spectr 2017; 5.
Joshi HS, et al: Lichen scrofulosorum. BMJ Case Rep 2014 Jan 30; 2014.
Kar S, et al: Scrofuloderma. Indian J Tuberc 2011; 58: 189.
Khullar G, et al: Disseminated cutaneous BCG infection following BCG immunotherapy in patients with lepromatous leprosy. Lepr Rev 2015; 86: 180.
Kim JE, et al: Tuberculous cellulitis as a manifestation of miliary tuberculosis in a patient with malignancy-associated dermatomyositis. J Am Acad Dermatol 2011; 65: 450.
Kumar P, et al: Lichen scrofulosorum Indian Pediatr 2014; 51: 335.
Kumar U, et al: Psoriasiform type of lichen scrofulosorum: Pediatr Dermatol 2011; 28: 532.
Laws PM, et al: Nonhealing vegetating plaque on the finger: Cutis 2011; 87: 30.
Leon-Mateo A, et al: Perianal ulceration. J Eur Acad Dermatol Venereol 2005; 19: 364.
Liu Y, et al: Analysis of 30 patients with acupuncture-induced primary inoculation tuberculosis. PLoS One 2014; 9: e100377.
Ljubenovic MS, et al: Cutaneous tuberculosis and squamous-cell carcinoma. An Bras Dermatol 2011; 86: 541.
McHugh A, et al: Nodular granulomatous phlebitis. Australas J Dermatol 2008; 49: 220.
Mert A, et al: Miliary tuberculosis. Medicine (Baltimore) 2017; 95: e5875.
Pescitelli L, et al: Tuberculosis reactivation risk in dermatology. J Rheumatol Suppl 2014; 91: 65.
Prajapati V, et al: Erythema induratum. J Cutan Med Surg 2013; 17 Suppl 1: S6.
Rajagopala S, Agarwal R: Tuberculosis mastitis in men. Am J Med 2008; 121: 539.
Ramesh V: Sporotrichoid cutaneous tuberculosis. Clin Exp Dermatol 2007; 32: 680.
Ramesh V, et al: Lupus vulgaris postexanthematicus. Clin Exp Dermatol 2005; 30: 187.
Rao AG: Scrofuloderma associated with tuberculosis verrucosa cutis. Indian J Dermatol Venereol Leprol 2014; 80: 76.
Regnier S, et al: Cutaneous military resistant tuberculosis in a patient infected with human immunodeficiency virus. Clin Exp Dermatol 2009; 34: e690.
Rhodes J, et al: Lupus vulgaris. Australas J Dermatol 2013; 54: e53.
Santos JB, et al: Cutaneous tuberculosis. An Bras Dermatol 2014; 89: 219.
Sellami K, et al: Twenty-nine cases of lupus vulgaris. Med Mal Infect 2016; 46: 93.
Sethuraman G, et al: Cutaneous tuberculosis in children. Pediatr Dermatol 2013; 30: 7.
Sharma S, et al: Clinicopathologic spectrum of cutaneous tuberculosis. Am J Dermatopathol 2015; 37: 444.
Sharma SK, Mohan A: Miliary tuberculosis. Microbiol Spectr 2017; 5.
Singal A, et al: Lichen scrofulosorum. Int J Dermatol 2005; 44: 489.
Singal A, et al: Ulcerated lupus vulgaris at the site of bacille Calmette-Guérin vaccination. Pediatr Dermatol 2013; 30: 147.
Striegel AK, et al: Two cases of lupus vulgaris in childhood and review of the clinical challenges. Klin Pediatr 2014; 226: 40.
Tissot C, et al: Life-threatening disseminated tuberculosis as a complication of treatment by infliximab for Crohn's disease: J Crohns Colitis 2012; 6: 946.

Tornheim JA, Dooley KE: Tuberculosis associated with HIV infection. Microbiol Spectr 2017; 5.

Troelsen T, Hilberg O: Tuberculous abscess. N Engl J Med 2014; 371: 161.

van Zyl L, et al: Cutaneous tuberculosis overview and current treatment regimens. Tuberculosis (Edinb) 2015; 95: 629.

Vera-Kellet C, et al: Usefulness of interferon-γ release assays in the diagnosis of erythema induratum. Arch Dermatol 2011; 147: 949.

von Huth S, et al: Two cases of erythema induratum of Bazin—a rare cutaneous manifestation of tuberculosis. Int J Infect Dis 2015; 38: 121.

Wang H, et al: Cutaneous tuberculosis: a diagnostic and therapeutic study of 20 cases. J Dermatol Treat 2011; 22: 310.

Williams C, et al: Turkey ear. Br J Dermatol 2007; 157: 816.

NONTUBERCULOUS MYCOBACTERIOSIS

Many facultative pathogens and saprophytes, which are acid-fast mycobacteria but do not cause TB, are grouped under the designation "nontuberculous mycobacteria." The number of new species has been growing dramatically, with now at least 190 known species. Many of these organisms do not often cause infection and are simply commensals or saprophytes. They exist in a wide variety of natural sources, such as soil, water, and animals; most human disease is acquired from the environment. The number of cases of human infection with these organisms is increasing. This is a result of improved culture and identification techniques, the rising number of cosmetic procedures which may be complicated by infection with rapid growing mycobacteria, and the large immunocompromised population. An increasing number of patients receiving biologic therapy, those with solid-organ or stem cell transplants, and other causes of immunocompromise have been reported with infections. Only select organisms that most frequently affect the skin are discussed in detail here. *M. leprae* and Hansen disease are discussed in Chapter 17.

Classification of Mycobacteria

The clinical care of the patient with nontuberculous mycobacterial infection depends on culturing and identifying the responsible agent from tissue specimens. Identification of specific *Mycobacterium* species is now made using molecular techniques; however, the growth rates have some utility in considering a practical classification. Rapidly growing mycobacteria of the *Mycobacterium fortuitum*, *chelonae*, and *abscessus* group are usually associated with previous surgery, injection, or trauma. The laboratory should be familiar with the special media, necessary incubation times and temperature, and identification characteristics of these organisms. Even with modern techniques, recovery of these organisms from infections is not universal. Granuloma formation may not occur in histologic sections, and AFB stains may be negative. For this reason, if nontuberculous mycobacterial infection is suspected, a biopsy should be done, part of which should be cultured at high and low temperatures and on special media; AFB stains of the tissue should be performed; and in select patients, PCR for specific species from fresh tissue or the paraffin-fixed material should be considered. In some patients, a clinical diagnosis must be made and empiric therapy given.

Fish Tank Granuloma

Mycobacterium marinum is found in fresh and salt water and can infect fish, often killing home aquarium fish. It grows optimally at 30°C. Many infections in the United States and Europe are associated with home aquariums. Fishermen, fish sellers, and persons involved in aquaculture are also at risk. Skin lesions favor males (60%). History of an injury preceding or simultaneous with exposure

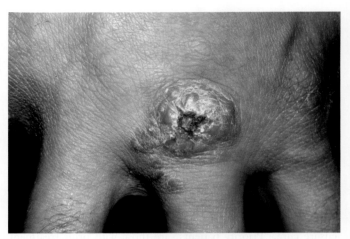

Fig. 16.11 *Mycobacterium marinum* infection. (Courtesy Steven Binnick, MD.)

to contaminated water is usually present. Exposure can be indirect, such as contact with a bucket used to empty an aquarium.

An indolent lesion usually starts about 3 weeks after exposure as a small papule or nodule located on the hands (Fig. 16.11), knees, elbows, or feet. It often has a keratotic or warty surface. A sporotrichoid pattern with a succession of nodules ascending the arm is common. Less often, ulcers and abscesses may be the presentation, especially in immunosuppressed hosts. Tenosynovitis, bursitis, arthritis, and osteitis are the most frequent forms of deep structure involvement. There may be involvement of the tendon sheaths of the dorsal hands and less frequently the palms. This may limit range of motion and result in significant thickening and induration. Such patients may require surgical as well as medical management. The natural history is for slow progression, and lesions may be relatively indolent for years. Spontaneous resolution may occur in 10%–20% of patients with skin lesions after many months. Patients on TNF-α inhibitor therapy and immunosuppressed patients such as those on prednisone may develop widely disseminated lesions that are progressive.

Histopathologically, there is a suppurative and granulomatous reaction with overlying hyperkeratosis and acanthosis. Acid-fast organisms are found in only about 20% of cases. Tissue culture will be positive in about three quarters of cases. The TST and IGRA to *M. tuberculosis* usually become positive in those who have had *M. marinum* infection.

Treatment is determined by the extent of the infection and the patient's immune status. Optimal treatment has not yet been established. Single-agent therapy is often adequate for immunocompetent patients with infections limited to skin and soft tissue, clarithromycin (500 mg twice daily) seems to be the best single agent; minocycline, 100 mg twice daily, doxycycline (100 mg twice daily), or trimethoprim-sulfamethoxazole (TMP-SMX, 160/800 mg twice daily) are alternative choices. In more severe disease or deep tissue involvement, or in an immunocompromised patient combinations of double or triple therapy, including rifampin, is necessary. The sensitivities of the organism isolated can be used in cases failing initial empiric treatment. For localized lesions in the immunocompetent host, treatment is recommended for at least 1–2 months after resolution of lesions, which is usually 3–4 months in total. More than 90% of such patients will be cured. Only about 75% of patients with deep structure infections will be cured with antibiotics, with or without supplemental surgery. In this situation, treatment is often prolonged—many months to years. The wearing of gloves during and personal disinfectant methods after fish tank cleaning are helpful preventative strategies.

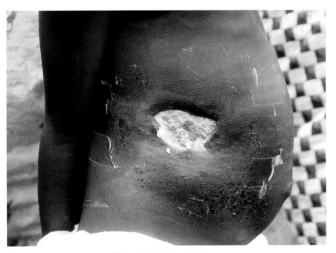

Fig. 16.12 Buruli ulcer.

Buruli Ulcer

Buruli ulcer is the third most common type of mycobacterial skin infection in immunocompetent people. In Africa, 75% of cases occur in children, and elderly persons are disproportionately affected. In endemic areas in Australia, elderly people are seven times more likely to be infected. The lesion usually begins on an extremity as a solitary, hard, painless, subcutaneous nodule called the "preulcerative stage." There can be significant local edema at this point. If untreated, some lesions ulcerate and expand by undermining the surrounding skin (Fig. 16.12). They may become very large, exposing muscle and tendon over a large portion of an affected extremity. Despite their appearance, the lesions are remarkably painless. Persons with hemoglobin SS or SC are as much as five times more likely to develop osteomyelitis from *M. ulcerans*. Histologically, there is extensive coagulative necrosis, minimal cellular infiltrate, and numerous clumps of AFB in the center of the necrotic area.

Mycobacterium ulcerans is the cause of Buruli ulcer. This organism occurs in Australia, numerous African nations (especially in Central and West Africa), Asia, French Guyana, Peru, Suriname, Mexico, and Brazil. The pathogenesis of this infection is now well defined. *M. ulcerans* produces a toxin, mycolactone, responsible for the extensive necrosis and ulceration. In addition to having cellular toxicity, mycolactone is also locally immunosuppressive. Tissue necrosis creates a microaerophilic environment that favors the growth of *M. ulcerans*. Strains of *M. ulcerans* lacking mycolactone are not capable of producing disease. This toxin is also critical in maintaining the life cycle of the organism.

Mycobacterium ulcerans grows under a biofilm on aquatic plants. Snails and other water animals eat the contaminated plants, and carnivorous insects eat the plant-consuming molluscs. *M. ulcerans* moves from the gut of the carnivorous insects to their salivary glands. Only *M. ulcerans* species producing mycolactone are capable of establishing a reservoir in the insect salivary gland. *M. ulcerans* is found in no other tissue in the biting insects and produces no biofilm in the insect salivary gland. When these insects bite a human, they inoculate the mycobacteria into the host and begin the infection. Infection in the human is again associated with the production of the biofilm, which makes treatment difficult. This explains the association between infection and exposure to water, especially swampy water. Interestingly, being repeatedly bitten by these carnivorous insects results in the production of antibodies against the insect salivary contents. This immune response to the insect saliva is protective against *M. ulcerans* infection, explaining why persons working regularly in swampy water are at lower risk

for infection than those visiting the area. In Australia, mosquito bites are associated with the development of *M. ulcerans* infection. Whether the mosquitoes carry the infection by the same mechanism as the carnivorous water insects is unknown.

The diagnosis of Buruli ulcer is often made clinically in areas of endemicity. AFB smears of the edge of ulcerative lesions or of aspirates from the center of preulcerative lesions, culture of the lesion, PCR, and histologic examination all can confirm the diagnosis. AFB stains are positive in up to 80% of lesions. Culture has a similar positivity rate. PCR may be slightly less sensitive. When AFB smears, culture, and PCR were all done on the same lesion, at least one test was positive in 94% of cases. Preulcerative lesions give the highest culture results, because ulcerative lesions contain fewer organisms and are contaminated.

Treatment of Buruli ulcer is daily observed treatment for 8 weeks with streptomycin and rifampin. Healing is slow, with half of lesions healing by 24 weeks (with only 8 weeks of antibiotic treatment) and some requiring more than 9 months to heal. Ciprofloxacin may be substituted for streptomycin therapy as an alternative. Surgical excision with delayed grafting is the standard treatment offered to those refusing or intolerant to antibiotic treatment.

Severe scarring can result from untreated and large lesions, leading to contracture deformity or amputation. If the periocular tissues are affected, enucleation of the eye may be required. Multiple metastatic skin lesions can occur. Bone lesions are uncommon and in three quarters of patients, occur at a site distant from the primary ulcer. Rarely, death may result.

Other Nontuberculous Mycobacterial Infections

Mycobacterium Haemophilum

Mycobacterium haemophilum most often infects immunosuppressed patients with HIV infection, with an organ transplant, those receiving biologic agents, or with leukemia or lymphoma. The reservoir for the organism is unknown but thought to be water. Because *M. haemophilum* grows preferentially at 30°C–32°C, skin lesions at acral sites predominate. Papules, plaques (at times cellulitis-like), and dermal or subcutaneous nodules are the primary lesions. These initial lesions break down in many cases, forming painful, draining ulcers. Cutaneous infections after acupuncture, following application of permanent eyebrow makeup, and within tattoos have been reported in immunocompetent and immunosuppressed patients. Septic arthritis, osteomyelitis, and pulmonary nodules may occur. *M. haemophilum* has specific growth requirements, so isolation is not possible using routine laboratory culture techniques. If *M. haemophilum* infection is suspected, the laboratory should be notified so that it can prepare the special media necessary to isolate it. *M. haemophilum* is sensitive to ciprofloxacin, clarithromycin, and rifabutin. Combination therapy with all three medications has been reported to be effective. Treatment is for 1 year. Adjunctive surgery may be required.

Rapidly Growing Mycobacteria

Mycobacterium fortuitum, *M. chelonae*, and *M. abscessus* usually cause subcutaneous abscesses or cellulitis. These rapidly growing mycobacteria (RGM) are frequently resistant to standard antituberculosis medications. Infections usually occur after trauma in immunocompetent patients. Infections may follow a variety of cosmetic surgery procedures (e.g., laser resurfacing, laser hair removal, injection with dermal fillers or botulinum toxin, mesotherapy, liposuction), skin piercing, injection with biologics, skin biopsy, Mohs surgery, acupuncture, catheterization or within tattoos. Outbreaks of leg abscesses caused by *M. fortuitum* have been acquired in nail salon whirlpool footbaths. Most RGM cases are restricted to the skin and start as small erythematous papules,

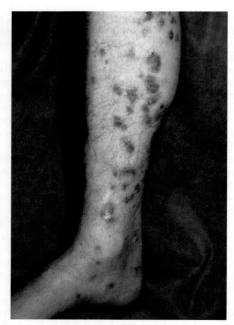

Fig. 16.13 *Mycobacterium fortuitum* infection.

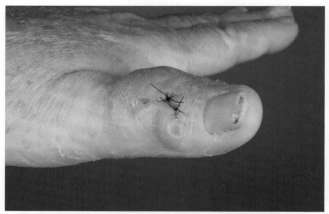

Fig. 16.14 *Mycobacterium avium-intracellulare* complex, primary inoculation in a healthy woman.

many of which spontaneously heal. Others progress to large, fluctuant abscesses, which are quite painful and can ulcerate (Fig. 16.13). Sporotrichoid or disseminated disease may occur in immunocompromised patients, but proximal adenopathy is rarely found. Shaving of the legs before visiting the nail salon appears to be a risk factor for acquiring infection with RGM. In renal transplant patients, tender, nodular lesions of the legs are most common. Deep extension into bone underlying a chronic ulcer can occur. Because these infections on the skin are indolent and the organisms grow rapidly, waiting for susceptibilities can be considered.

Treatment is determined by extent of disease and immune status of the patient. For *M. chelonae* and *abscessus* infections, clarithromycin, 500 mg twice daily for 6 months or more, is effective and well tolerated in many patients with disseminated cutaneous infection. Monotherapy may allow resistance to occur, but this rarely happens in immunocompetent patients with simple skin infections. In severe cases and in the setting of immunosuppression, combination treatment with moxifloxacin and surgical debridement should be used. The optimal regimen for treatment of *M. fortuitum* has not been defined, and combination treatment is recommended. Amikacin plus cefoxitin and probenecid can be recommended for initial therapy for 6 weeks, followed by doxycycline or TMP-SMX for up to 1 year. Surgical excision, debridement, and drainage may reduce duration of therapy.

Mycobacterium Avium-Intracellulare Complex

The *M. avium-intracellulare* complex was an uncommon cause of skin infection before the AIDS epidemic. In patients with AIDS who develop disseminated *M. avium-intracellulare* infections, the skin can be involved by hematogenous dissemination and may present as nodules, ulcers, or pustules or have a cellulitis-like appearance. Immunocompromised children with chronic pulmonary infections are also at risk. Only occasional reports of immunocompetent patients with inoculation-type lesions have been reported (Fig. 16.14). Therapy for disseminated infection is undertaken with at least three agents, most often clarithromycin or azithromycin plus ethambutol, and rifabutin. Adequate antiretroviral therapy should be assured in HIV-infected persons.

Mycobacterium Kansasii

Mycobacterium kansasii rarely causes skin infection, usually after minor trauma. Three quarters of cases occur in immunosuppressed persons. Lesions can be papules, nodules, pustules, cellulitis, or sporotrichoid. Initial treatment with isoniazid, rifampin, and ethambutol until 12 months after clearing, 15 months for HIV patients, is recommended. Surgical removal can be beneficial if practical. In immunosuppressed patients, cutaneous lesions can occur through hematogenous dissemination, and a visceral source, especially pulmonary, should be sought.

Atkins BL, et al: Skin and soft tissue infections caused by nontuberculous mycobacteria. Curr Opin Infect Dis 2014; 27: 137.

Aubry A, et al: *Mycobacterium marinum.* Microbiol Spectr 2017; 5.

Bhargava A, Chandrasekar PH: Gradually worsening tattoo lesion. JAMA 2015; 314: 2071.

Brix SR, et al: Disseminated *Mycobacterium haemophilum* infection in a renal transplant recipient. BMJ Case Rep 2016 Oct 31; 2016.

Caron J, et al: Aggressive cutaneous infection with *Mycobacterium marinum* in two patients receiving anti–tumor necrosis factor-alfa agents. J Am Acad Dermatol 2011; 65: 1060.

Chatzikokkinou P, et al: Disseminated cutaneous infection with *Mycobacterium chelonae* in a renal transplant recipient. Cutis 2015; 96: E6.

Cheung JP, et al: *Mycobacterium marinum* infection on the hand and wrist. J Orthop Surg 2012; 20: 214.

Cho SY, et al: *Mycobacterium chelonae* infections associated with bee venom acupuncture. Clin Infect Dis 2014; 58: e110.

Collins CS, et al: Disseminated *Mycobacterium haemophilum* infection in a 72-year-old patient with rheumatoid arthritis on infliximab. BMJ Case Rep 2013 Mar 15; 2013.

Drage LA, et al: An outbreak of *Mycobacterium chelonae* infections in tattoos. J Am Acad Dermatol 2010; 62: 501.

Dyer J, et al: Primary cutaneous *Mycobacterium avium* complex infection following squamous cell carcinoma excision. Cutis 2016; 98: E8.

Eberst E, et al: Epidemiological, clinical, and therapeutic pattern of *Mycobacterium marinum* infection. J Am Acad Dermatol 2012; 66: e15.

Fowler J, et al: Localized cutaneous infections in immunocompetent individuals due to rapidly growing mycobacteria. Arch Pathol Lab Med 2014; 138: 1106.

Giulieri S, et al: Outbreak of *Mycobacterium haemophilum* infections after permanent makeup of the eyebrows. Clin Infect Dis 2011; 52: 488.

Gonzalez-Santiago TM, Drage LA: Nontuberculous mycobacteria. Dermatol Clin 2015; 33: 563.

Jacobs S, et al: Disseminated *Mycobacterium marinum* infection in a hematopoietic stem cell transplant recipient. Transpl Infect Dis 2012; 14: 410.

Johnson MG, Stout JE: Twenty-eight cases of *Mycobacterium marinum* infection. Infection 2015; 43: 655.

Kay MK, et al: Tattoo-associated *Mycobacterium haemophilum* skin infection in immunocompetent adult. Emerg Infect Dis 2011; 17: 1734.

Kim MJ, et al: *Mycobacterium chelonae* wound infection after liposuction. Emerg Infect Dis 2010; 16: 1173.

Kollipara R, et al: Disseminated *Mycobacterium avium* complex with cutaneous lesions. J Cutan Med Surg 2016; 20: 272.

Kumar S, et al: The Buruli ulcer. Int J Low Extrem Wounds 2015; 14: 217.

Kump PK, et al: A case of opportunistic skin infection with *Mycobacterium marinum* during adalimumab treatment in a patient with Crohn's disease. J Crohns Colitis 2013; 7: e15.

Lage R, et al: *Mycobacterium chelonae* cutaneous infection in a patient with mixed connective tissue disease. An Bras Dermatol 2015; 90: 104.

Lamb RC, Dawn G: Cutaneous non-tuberculous mycobacterial infections. Int J Dermatol 2014; 53: 1197.

Lan NP, et al: *Mycobacterium fortuitum* skin infections after subcutaneous injections with Vietnamese traditional medicine. BMC Infect Dis 2014; 14: 550.

Landriscina A, et al: A surprising case of *Mycobacterium avium* complex skin infection in an immunocompetent patient. J Drugs Dermatol 2014; 13: 1491.

Lee SR, et al: *Mycobacterium abscessus* complex infections in humans. Emerg Infect Dis 2015; 21: 1638.

Lindeboom JA, et al: Clinical manifestations, diagnosis, and treatment of *Mycobacterium haemophilum* infections. Clin Microbiol Rev 2011; 24: 701.

Lo Schiavo A, et al: Sporotrichoid cutaneous infection by *Mycobacterium abscessus*. Int J Dermatol 2014; 53: e291.

Merritt RW, et al: Ecology and transmission of Buruli ulcer disease. PLoS Negl Trop Dis 2010: 4: e911.

Murback ND, et al: Disseminated cutaneous atypical mycobacteriosis by *M. chelonae* after sclerotherapy of varicose veins in a immunocompetent patient. An Bras Dermatol 2015; 90: 138.

O'Brien DP, et al: *Mycobacterium ulcerans* in the elderly. PLoS Negl Trop Dis 2015; 9: e0004253.

Oh CC, et al: *Mycobacterium haemophilum* in an elderly Chinese woman. Int J Dermatol 2014; 53: 1129.

Quinones C, et al: An outbreak of *Mycobacterium fortuitum* cutaneous infection associated with mesotherapy. J Euro Acad Dermatol Venereol 2010; 24: 604.

Rodriguez JM, et al: *Mycobacterium chelonae* facial infections following injection of dermal filler. Aesthet Surg J 2013; 33: 265.

Shibayama Y, et al: A case of *Mycobacterium abscessus* infection presenting as a cystic lesion in an insulin injection site in a diabetic patient. J Dermatol 2014; 41: 469.

Sinagra JL, et al: *Mycobacterium abscessus* hand-and-foot disease in children. Pediatr Dermatol 2014; 31: 292.

Sousa PP, et al: *Mycobacterium abscessus* skin infection after tattooing. An Bras Dermatol 2015; 90: 741.

Spiliopoulou I, et al: *Mycobacterium kansasii* cutaneous infection in a patient with sarcoidosis treated with anti-TNF agents. Acta Clin Belg 2014; 69: 229.

Sprague J, et al: Cutaneous infection with *Mycobacterium kansasii* in a patient with myelodysplastic syndrome and Sweet syndrome. Cutis 2015; 96: E10.

Thanou-Stravraki A, et al: Noodling and *Mycobacterium marinum* infection mimicking seronegative rheumatoid arthritis complicated by anti–tumor necrosis factor α therapy. Arthritis Care Res 2011; 63: 160.

Wu TS, et al: Fish tank granuloma caused by *Mycobacterium marinum*. PLoS One 2012; 7: e41296.

Yotsu RR, et al: Revisiting Buruli ulcer. J Dermatol 2015; 42: 1033.

17 Hansen Disease

EPIDEMIOLOGY

The World Health Organization (WHO) has committed itself to eliminating Hansen disease as a public health problem, but the disease remains endemic in certain regions, with 95% of cases reported from 16 countries. Brazil, India, and Indonesia account for 80% of all cases worldwide. Although 90% of diagnosed U.S. cases are imported, Hansen disease is endemic in the coastal southeastern United States and in Hawaii. In the southeastern states, cases may be related to exposure to armadillos, a natural host for the infectious agent.

It is believed that more than 90% of persons exposed to *Mycobacterium leprae* are able to resist infection. In endemic areas, between 1.7% and 31% of the population is seropositive for antibodies to leprosy-specific antigens, suggesting widespread exposure to the bacillus. About 17% of household contacts of multibacillary patients have *M. leprae*, which is detectable by polymerase chain reaction (PCR) on skin swabs, with 4% detectable in nasal swabs. This clears after the multibacillary patient has been treated with multidrug therapy (MDT) for 2 months. Thus although many persons can be transiently infected, they apparently are able to resist overt clinical infection.

There appears to be a genetic basis for susceptibility to acquire Hansen disease. Monozygotic twins have concordant disease in 60%–85% of cases, and dizygotic twins in only 15%–25%. Numerous genes have been identified as possibly conferring susceptibility to infection with *M. leprae*. Different genes have been identified in different populations, suggesting that multiple genetic causes of susceptibility to infection are possible with *M. leprae*. Tight genetic linkage with the PARK2/PACRG regulatory region, HLA-DRB1, and lymphotoxin A (LTA+80) has been detected. *PARK2* is a gene involved in the development of Parkinson disease, and LTA+80 is a low-production lymphotoxin A allele associated with malaria parasitemia. Interleukin (IL)–17F single nucleotide polymorphism (SNP) is associated with an increased susceptibility to Hansen disease, and type 1 reactions in paucibacillary patients. In Chinese patients, susceptibility was linked to multiple genes, including *CCDC12*, *C13orf31*, and a series of genes known to be associated with susceptibility to other mycobacterial diseases, including *NOD2*, *IL12B*, *RIP2K*, and *TNFSF15*.

In adult cases, men outnumber women 1.5:1. Although Hansen disease occurs at all ages, most cases appearing or acquired in endemic areas present before age 35. Patients exposed to armadillos present on average at age 50. The latency period between exposure and overt signs of disease is usually 5 years for paucibacillary cases and an average of 10 years in multibacillary cases. Infected women are likely to present during or immediately after pregnancy.

The mode of transmission remains controversial. Except for cases associated with armadillo exposure, other patients with Hansen disease are thought to be the only possible source of infection. Rarely, tattooing or other penetrating injury to the skin can be the route of infection. Multibacillary cases are much more infectious than paucibacillary cases, so the nature of the source case is the most important factor in transmission. Contact is associated with acquiring infection. Household contacts represent 28% of new Hansen disease patients; there is an 8–10 times greater risk of acquiring disease if the household contact has lepromatous disease, versus only 2–4 times if the contact has tuberculoid leprosy. In 80% of all new cases of Hansen disease, there is a clear history of social contact with an untreated patient with Hansen disease. PCR can detect *M. leprae* on the intact skin by saline washings in up to 90% of multibacillary patients with a high bacterial load (bacterial index [BI] >3). Up to 70% of nasal swabs are similarly positive. Whereas the swabs from the patients remain positive after 3 months of MDT, the swabs of household contacts become negative, suggesting that the bacilli seen in patients are nonviable, and that the risk of transmission is substantially reduced after the index patient is treated. Unfortunately, persons may be infectious from their skin or nasal secretions, with no clinical evidence of Hansen disease (multibacillary patients who are not yet symptomatic and without identifiable skin lesions). This may make strategies relying on treatment of contacts of known Hansen disease patients ineffective in eradicating the disease. In nonendemic areas, transmission to contacts is rare, a reassuring fact for the families of patients diagnosed in areas where Hansen disease is uncommon. The last case of secondary transmission of Hansen disease in the United Kingdom was in 1923.

THE INFECTIOUS AGENT

Until recently, it had been thought that all cases of human and animal leprosy are caused by the same organism, *Mycobacterium leprae*. This is a weakly acid-fast organism that has not been successfully cultured in vitro. *M. leprae* grows best at temperatures (30°C) below the core body temperature of humans. This explains the localization of Hansen disease lesions to cooler areas of the body and the sparing of the midline and scalp. The organism may be cultivated in mouse footpads and most effectively in armadillos, whose lower body temperature is more optimal for growth of *M. leprae*. Phenolic glycolipid 1 (PGL-1) is a surface glycolipid unique to the leprosy bacillus. In infected tissues, the leprosy bacillus favors intracellular locations, within macrophages and nerves. The genome of the leprosy bacillus has been sequenced and compared with its close relative, the tuberculous bacillus. The genome of *M. leprae* contains only 50% functional genes, apparently the result of significant reductive evolution. As with other intracellular parasites, and in the absence of the ability to share DNA with other bacteria, *M. leprae* has lost many nonessential genes, including those involved in energy metabolism, making it dependent on the intracellular environment for essential nutrients. This may explain the extremely long generation time, 12–14 days, and the inability to culture *M. leprae* in vitro.

A second organism, *Mycobacterium lepromatosis*, has been isolated from Hansen disease patients in Mexico and reported as the major cause of leprosy in some regions. Some patients are infected with both *M. leprae* and *M. lepromatosis*. This second mycobacterium is specifically associated with the diffuse type of lepromatous leprosy (DLL), also known as "Lucio leprosy." These are the patients who develop Lucio phenomenon. Invasion of the endothelial cells characterizes infection with the new organism. Although not all researchers accept *M. lepromatosis* as a second, separate species capable of causing Hansen disease, it does suggest more than one causative organism for leprosy.

DIAGNOSIS

A diagnosis of Hansen disease must be considered in any patient with neurologic and cutaneous lesions. The diagnosis is frequently

TABLE 17.1 Spectrum of Host-Parasite Relationship in Hansen Disease

	High Resistance		Unstable Resistance		No Resistance
	Tuberculoid (TT)	Borderline Tuberculoid (BT)	Borderline (BB)	Borderline Lepromatous (BL)	Lepromatous (LL)
Lesions	1–3	Few	Few or many asymmetric	Many	Numerous and symmetric
Smear for bacilli	0	1+	2+	3+	4+
Lepromin test	3+	2+	2	2	0
Histology	Epithelioid cells decreasing ⟶ Nerve destruction, sarcoid-like granuloma			Increasing histiocytes, foam cells, granuloma, xanthoma-like	

Modified from Dr. J. H. Petit.

delayed in the developed world; clinicians do not readily think of Hansen disease because they may never have seen it. In the United States this diagnostic delay averages $1\frac{1}{2}$–2 years. In the United Kingdom, in more than 80% of patients with Hansen disease, the correct diagnosis was not suspected during the initial medical evaluation.

Hansen disease is diagnosed, as with other infectious diseases, by identifying the infectious organism in affected tissue. Because the organism cannot be cultured, this may be very difficult. Biopsies from skin or nerve lesions, stained for the bacillus with Fite-Faraco stain, are usually performed in the developed world. In some Hansen disease clinics, and in the developing world where the disease is endemic, organisms are identified in slit smears of the skin. Smears are very specific, but 70% of all patients with Hansen disease have negative smears. Smears are taken from lesions and cooler areas of the skin, such as the earlobes, elbows, and knees. If organisms are found on skin smears, the patient is said to be multibacillary. If the results of skin smears are negative (and there are five or fewer lesions), the patient is called paucibacillary.

Nerve involvement is detected by enlargement of peripheral nerves and lesional loss of sensation. Enlarged nerves are found in more than 90% of patients with multibacillary Hansen disease and in 75%–85% of patients with paucibacillary disease. About 70% of lesions have reduced sensation, but lesional dysesthesia is not detected in patients with multibacillary Hansen disease, the most infectious form.

Serologic tests to detect antibodies against *M. leprae*–unique antigens have limitations in the diagnosis of leprosy and reactional states. They are universally positive in patients with multibacillary disease, in whom the diagnosis is not difficult. In paucibacillary patients, these tests are often negative, and in endemic areas there is a high background rate of positivity of serologic tests. In pure neural Hansen disease, however, about 50% of patients are seropositive, and serologic testing might be of use. Based on the technology of the T-cell interferon-γ (IFN-γ) production–based assays for *M. tuberculosis* infection, researchers have identified unique peptides of *M. leprae* and developed a research IFN-γ release assay (IGRA). This was able to detect all paucibacillary cases in a Hansen disease cohort. In addition, 13 of 14 household contacts of Hansen disease patients were positive with IGRA. Ideally, in endemic areas, both serologic and cell-based assays can be used to detect all patients with Hansen disease.

In endemic areas, active surveillance of contacts is recommended. In Brazil, about 2% of both in-domicile and extradomiciliary contacts are found to have Hansen disease. Most cases are associated with patients who have multibacillary Hansen disease.

CLASSIFICATION

Hansen disease may present with a broad spectrum of clinical diseases. The Ridley and Jopling scale classifies cases based on clinical, bacteriologic, immunologic, and histopathologic features

(Table 17.1). In many exposed patients, the infection apparently clears spontaneously, and no clinical lesions develop. Patients who do develop clinical disease are broadly classified into two groups for the purposes of treatment and for trials that compare treatment strategies. Paucibacillary patients have few or no organisms in their lesions and usually have three to five lesions or fewer (for treatment purposes, the finding of acid-fast bacilli by stains or smears classifies a patient as having multibacillary Hansen disease). Multibacillary patients have multiple, symmetric lesions and organisms detectable by biopsy or smears. The individual's cell-mediated immune response to the organism determines the form that Hansen disease will take in the individual. If the cell-mediated immune response against *M. leprae* is strong, the number of organisms will be low (paucibacillary), and conversely, if this response is inadequate, the number of organisms will be high (multibacillary).

The most common outcome after exposure is probably spontaneous cure. If skin disease does appear, the initial clinical lesion may be a single, hypopigmented patch, perhaps with slight anesthesia. This is called indeterminate disease, because the course of the disease cannot be predicted at this stage. The lesion may clear spontaneously or may progress to any other form of Hansen disease.

The spectrum of Hansen disease has two stable poles, the tuberculoid and lepromatous forms (see Table 17.1). These so-called polar forms do not change; the patient remains in one or the other form throughout the course of the disease. The polar tuberculoid form (called TT), the type with high cell-mediated immunity, is characterized by less than five lesions (often only one) and very few organisms (paucibacillary disease). The patient has strong cell-mediated immunity against the organism. The natural history of many TT leprosy patients is for spontaneous cure over several years. The polar lepromatous form (LL) has very limited cell-mediated immunity against the organism; lesions are numerous and contain many organisms (multibacillary). Between these two poles is every possible degree of infection, forming the borderline spectrum. Cases near the tuberculoid pole are called borderline tuberculoid (BT), those near the lepromatous pole are called borderline lepromatous (BL), and those in the middle are called borderline borderline (BB). Borderline Hansen disease is characteristically unstable, and with time, cases move from the TT to the LL pole, a process called downgrading.

Hansen disease may involve only the nerves. This pure neural disease may be indeterminate, tuberculoid, or lepromatous (paucibacillary or multibacillary) and is so classified. In Nepal and India, pure neural Hansen disease may represent as much as 5% of all new cases.

Early and Indeterminate Hansen Disease

Usually, the onset of Hansen disease is insidious. Prodromal symptoms are generally so slight that the disease is not recognized until the appearance of a cutaneous eruption. Actually, the first clinical manifestation in 90% of patients is numbness, and years may elapse before skin lesions or other signs are identified. The earliest sensory changes are loss of the senses of temperature and light touch, most often in the feet or hands. The inability to discriminate hot from cold may be lost before pinprick sensibility. Such dissociation of sensibility is especially suspicious. The distribution of these neural signs and their intensity will depend on the type of disease that is evolving.

Often, the first lesion noted is a solitary, poorly defined, hypopigmented macule that merges into the surrounding normal skin. Less often, erythematous macules may be present. Such lesions are most likely to occur on the cheeks, upper arms, thighs, and buttocks. Examination reveals that sensory functions are either normal or minimally altered. Peripheral nerves are not enlarged, and plaques and nodules do not occur. Histologically, a variable lymphocytic infiltrate (without granulomas) is seen, sometimes with involvement of the cutaneous nerves. Usually, no bacilli, or only a few, are seen on biopsy of this indeterminate form. It is the classification, not the diagnosis, that is indeterminate. Few cases remain in this state; they evolve into lepromatous, tuberculoid, or borderline types, or (if cell-mediated immunity is good) often spontaneously resolve and never develop other signs or symptoms of Hansen disease.

Tuberculoid Leprosy

Tuberculoid lesions are solitary or few in number (five or less) and asymmetrically distributed. Lesions may be hypopigmented or erythematous and are usually dry, scaly, and hairless (Fig. 17.1). The typical lesion of tuberculoid leprosy is the large, erythematous plaque with a sharply defined and elevated border that slopes down to a flattened atrophic center. This has been described as having the appearance of "a saucer right side up." Lesions may also be macular and hypopigmented or erythematous, resembling clinically indeterminate lesions. The presence of palpable induration and neurologic findings distinguish tuberculoid lesions from indeterminate lesions clinically. The most common locations are the face, limbs, or trunk; the scalp, axillae, groin, and perineum are not involved.

A tuberculoid lesion is anesthetic or hypesthetic and anhidrotic, and superficial peripheral nerves serving or proximal to the lesion are enlarged, tender, or both. The greater auricular nerve and the superficial peroneal nerve may be visibly enlarged. Nerve involvement is early and prominent in tuberculoid leprosy, leading to characteristic changes in the muscle groups served. There may be atrophy of the interosseous muscles of the hand, with wasting of the thenar and hypothenar eminences, contracture of the fingers,

paralysis of the facial muscles, and footdrop. Facial nerve damage dramatically increases the risk for ocular involvement and vision loss.

The evolution of the lesions is generally slow. There is often spontaneous remission of the lesions in about 3 years, or remission may result sooner with treatment. Spontaneous involution may leave pigmentary disturbances.

Borderline Tuberculoid (BT) Leprosy

BT lesions are similar to tuberculoid lesions, except that they are smaller and more numerous (Fig. 17.2). Satellite lesions around large macules or plaques are characteristic.

Borderline Borderline (BB) Leprosy

In BB leprosy, the skin lesions are numerous (but countable) and consist of red, irregularly shaped plaques. Small satellite lesions may surround larger plaques. Lesions are generalized but asymmetric. The edges of lesions are not as well defined as the ones seen at the tuberculoid pole. Nerves may be thickened and tender, but anesthesia is only moderate in the lesions.

Borderline Lepromatous (BL) Leprosy

In BL leprosy, the lesions are symmetric and numerous (too many to count) and may include macules, papules, plaques, and nodules (Fig. 17.3). The number of small, lepromatous lesions outnumbers the larger, borderline-type lesions. Nerve involvement appears later; nerves are enlarged, tender, or both, and it is important to note that involvement is symmetric. Sensation and sweating over individual lesions are normal. Patients usually do not show the features of full-blown lepromatous leprosy, such as madarosis (loss of the eyebrows), keratitis, nasal ulceration, and leonine facies.

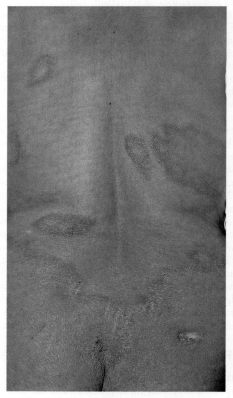

Fig. 17.2 Borderline tuberculoid leprosy.

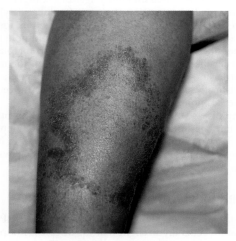

Fig. 17.1 Tuberculoid leprosy.

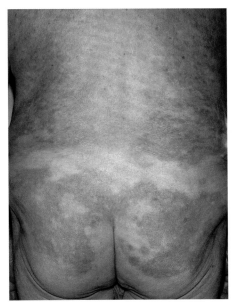

Fig. 17.3 Borderline lepromatous leprosy.

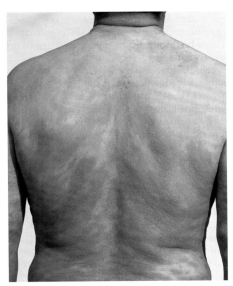

Fig. 17.4 Lepromatous leprosy.

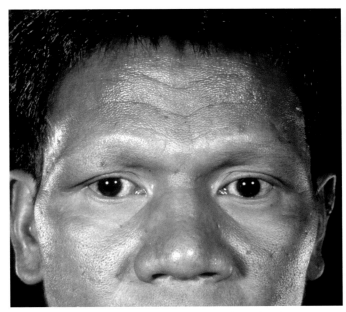

Fig. 17.5 Diffuse leprosy of Lucio. Note loss of eyebrows.

Lepromatous Leprosy

Lepromatous leprosy may begin as such or develop after indeterminate leprosy or from downgrading of borderline leprosy. The cutaneous lesions of lepromatous leprosy consist mainly of pale macules (Fig. 17.4) or diffuse infiltration of the skin. There is a tendency for the disease to become progressively worse without treatment. Lepromatous leprosy may be divided into a polar form (LLp) and a subpolar form (LLs); these forms may behave differently.

Macular lepromatous lesions are diffusely and symmetrically distributed over the body. Tuberculoid macules are large and few in number, whereas lepromatous macules are small and numerous. Lepromatous macules are poorly defined, show no change in skin texture, and blend imperceptibly into the surrounding skin. There is minimal or no loss of sensation over the lesions, no nerve thickening, and no change in sweating. A slow, progressive loss of hair takes place from the outer third of the eyebrows, then the eyelashes, and finally the body; however, the scalp hair usually remains unchanged.

Lepromatous infiltrations may be divided into the diffuse, plaque, and nodular types. The diffuse type is characterized by the development of a diffuse infiltration of the face, especially the forehead, madarosis, and a waxy, shiny appearance of the skin, sometimes described as "varnished." Diffuse leprosy of Lucio (DLL) is a striking form, uncommon except in western Mexico and certain other Latin American areas, where almost one third of lepromatous cases may be of this type. This form of lepromatous leprosy is characterized by diffuse lepromatous infiltration of the skin (Fig. 17.5); localized lepromas do not form. A unique complication of this subtype is the reactional state referred to as Lucio phenomenon (erythema necroticans).

The infiltrations may be manifested by the development of nodules called lepromas (Fig. 17.6). The early nodules are poorly defined and occur most often in acral parts: ears, brows, nose, chin, elbows, hands, buttocks, or knees.

Nerve involvement invariably occurs in lepromatous leprosy but develops very slowly. As with the skin lesions, nerve disease is bilaterally symmetric, usually in a stocking-glove pattern. This is frequently misdiagnosed as diabetic neuropathy in the United States if it is the presenting manifestation.

Histoid Leprosy

Histoid leprosy is an uncommon form of multibacillary Hansen disease in which skin lesions appear as large, yellow-red, shiny papules and nodules in the dermis or subcutaneous tissue. Lesions appear on a background of normal skin. They vary in size from 1–15 mm in diameter, and may appear anywhere on the body but favor the buttocks, lower back, face, and bony prominences. They may closely resemble molluscum contagiosum. This pattern may appear de novo but has mostly been described in patients with resistance to dapsone.

NERVE INVOLVEMENT

Nerve involvement is characteristic and unique to Hansen disease. This neural predilection or neurotropism is a histopathologic hallmark of Hansen disease. Nerve involvement is responsible for

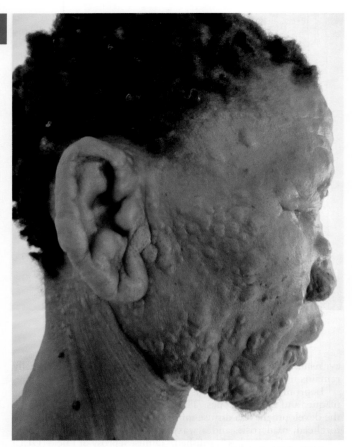

Fig. 17.6 Lepromatous leprosy. (Courtesy Michelle Weir, MD.)

enter resident macrophages or selectively enter Schwann cells. Damage to the nerves could then occur by the following mechanisms:

1. Obstruction of neural vessels
2. Vasculitis of neural vessels
3. Interference with metabolism of the Schwann cell, making it unable to support the neuron
4. Immunologic attack on endothelium or nerves
5. Infiltration and proliferation of *M. leprae* in the closed and relatively nonexpandable endoneural and perineural spaces

Different and multiple mechanisms may occur in different forms of Hansen disease and in the same patient over time. The selective ability of *M. leprae* to enter Schwann cells is unique among bacteria. *M. leprae*–unique PGL-1, expressed abundantly on the surface of leprosy bacilli, binds selectively to the α2 G module of laminin 2. This α2 chain is tissue restricted and specifically expressed on peripheral nerve Schwann cells. Other accessory binding molecules may facilitate the binding and endocytosis. The nerves become immunologic targets when they present *M. leprae* antigens on their surface in the context of major histocompatibility complex (MHC) class II molecules. Schwann cells and thus nerves are usually protected from immunologic attack mediated by the adaptive immune system because they rarely present MHC class II antigens on their surface. In Hansen disease, expression of these immunologic molecules occurs on the surface of Schwann cells, making them potential targets for CD4+ cytotoxic T cells. This mechanism may be important in the nerve damage that occurs in type 1 (reversal) reactions.

Schwann cells have been infected with *M. leprae* in vitro. Infected Schwann cells with high bacterial load are reprogrammed into mesenchymal stem cell–like cells. In association with Schwann cells, these dedifferentiated cells attract histiocytes and form granulomas. The attracted histiocytes are infected by the mycobacteria-containing Schwann cells and are released from the granulomas. If this process also occurs in vivo, it may be the mechanism by which multibacillary disease is spread throughout the body from a reservoir of infected nerves.

The neural signs in Hansen disease are dysesthesia, nerve enlargement, muscular weakness and wasting, and trophic changes. The lesions of the vasomotor nerves accompany the sensory disturbances or may precede them. Dysesthesia develops in a progressive manner. The first symptom is usually an inability to distinguish hot and cold. Subsequently, the perception of light touch is lost, then that of pain, and last the sense of deep touch. At times, the sensory changes in large Hansen disease lesions are not uniform because of the variation in the involvement of the individual neural filaments supplying the area. Therefore the areas of dysesthesia may not conform to the distribution of any particular nerve and, except in lepromatous cases, are not symmetric.

Nerve involvement mainly affects (and is most easily observed in) the more superficial nerve trunks, such as the ulnar, median, radial, peroneal, posterior tibial, fifth and seventh cranial, and especially the great auricular nerve. Beaded enlargements, nodules, or spindle-shaped swellings may be found, which at first may be tender. Neural abscesses may form. The ulnar nerve near the internal condyle of the humerus may be as thick as the little finger, round, and stiff and is often easily felt several centimeters above the elbow.

Because the presentation of neural involvement in Hansen disease is variable, the diagnosis is often not suspected, especially in nonendemic areas. Even in endemic areas, the diagnosis may be delayed. Between one half and one third of patients with pure neural Hansen disease, a biopsy of hypesthetic skin can show specific leprotic skin changes, and if nonspecific inflammation is considered confirmatory, the positivity of such biopsies is greater than 50%. Therefore skin biopsy of a hypesthetic skin site should

the clinical findings of anesthesia within lesions (paucibacillary and borderline leprosy) and of a progressive stocking-glove peripheral neuropathy (lepromatous leprosy). The neuropathy is termed *primary impairments* (WHO grade 1). Secondary (or visible) impairments (WHO grade 2) are a consequence of the neuropathy and include skin fissures, wounds, clawing of digits, contractures, shortening of digits, and blindness. Neural damage leads to deformities and in endemic regions results in Hansen disease being a major cause of "limitations of activity" (formerly called disability) and "restrictions in social participation" (formerly called handicap). Neuropathy is present in 1.3%–3.5% of paucibacillary patients and 7.5%–24% of multibacillary patients undergoing MDT. Secondary impairments occur in 33%–56% of multibacillary patients. Neuropathy may progress, even after effective MDT, and secondary impairments may continue to appear for years as a consequence of the neuropathy. This requires patients with neuropathy to be constantly monitored, even though they are "cured" of their infection.

Nerve enlargement is rare in other skin diseases, so the finding of skin lesions with enlarged nerves should suggest Hansen disease. Nerve involvement tends to occur with skin lesions, and the pattern of nerve involvement parallels the skin disease. Tuberculoid leprosy is characterized by asymmetric nerve involvement localized to the skin lesions. Lepromatous nerve involvement is symmetric and not associated with skin lesions. Nerve involvement without skin lesions, called pure neural leprosy, can occur and may be either tuberculoid (paucibacillary) or lepromatous (multibacillary). Nerve disease can be symptomatic or asymptomatic.

Leprosy bacilli may be delivered to the nerves through the perineural and endoneural blood vessels. Once the bacilli transgress the endothelial basal lamina and are in the endoneurium, they

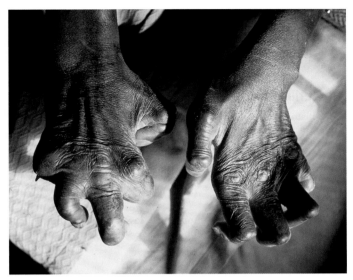

Fig. 17.7 Claw hand of Hansen disease.

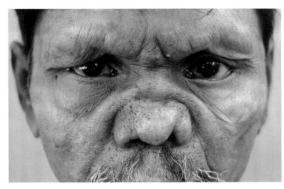

Fig. 17.8 Lepromatous leprosy. (Courtesy Shyam Verma, MBBS, DVD.)

be considered before nerve biopsy when pure neural Hansen disease is a possibility.

As a result of the nerve damage, areas of anesthesia, paralysis, and trophic disorders in the peripheral parts of the extremities gradually develop. Muscular paralysis and atrophy generally affect the small muscles of the hands and feet or some of the facial muscles, producing weakness and progressive atrophy. Deeper motor nerves are only rarely involved. The fingers develop contractures, with the formation of a clawhand (Fig. 17.7). Also, as the result of resorption of phalangeal bones, fingers and toes become shorter. Ptosis, ectropion, and a masklike appearance occur from damage to the fifth and seventh cranial nerves.

Subsequent to nerve damage, ulceration, hyperkeratosis, bullae, alopecia, anhidrosis, and mal perforans pedis can develop. Trophic ulceration usually manifests as a perforating ulcer on the ball or heel of the foot.

OCULAR INVOLVEMENT

Corneal erosions, exposure keratitis, and ulcerations may result from involvement of the seventh cranial nerve in Hansen disease patients. Specific changes may include corneal opacity, avascular keratitis, pannus formation, interstitial keratitis, and corneal lepromas. The corneal opacities enlarge and finally form visible white flecks called "pearls." When (in BL or lepromatous cases only) the iris and the ciliary body become involved, miliary lepromas (iris pearls), nodular lepromas, chronic granulomatous iritis, and acute diffuse iridocyclitis may result. Of multibacillary patients, 2.8%–4.6% are blind at diagnosis, and 11% will have a potentially blinding process.

MUCOUS MEMBRANE INVOLVEMENT

The mucous membranes may also be affected, especially in the nose, mouth, and larynx. The nasal mucosa is most frequently involved, and lepromatous patients frequently complain of chronic nasal congestion. By far the most common lesions in the nose are infiltrations and nodules. Perforation of the nasal septum may occur in patients with advanced Hansen disease, with collapse of the nasal bridge (Fig. 17.8). Saddle-nose deformities and loss of the upper incisor teeth can occur.

Nodules occurring on the vocal cords will produce hoarseness.

VISCERAL INVOLVEMENT

In lepromatous leprosy, the body is diffusely involved and bacteremia occurs. Except for the gastrointestinal tract, lungs, and brain, virtually every organ can contain leprosy bacilli. The lymph nodes, bone marrow, liver, spleen, and testicles are most heavily infected. Visceral infection is restricted mostly to the reticuloendothelial system, which despite extensive involvement rarely produces symptoms or findings. Testicular atrophy with loss of androgens can result in gynecothelia (hypertrophy of nipple) and/or gynecomastia, or premature osteoporosis. Secondary amyloidosis with renal impairment may complicate multibacillary leprosy. Glomerulonephritis occurs in more than 5% and perhaps as many as 50% of Hansen disease patients and is not correlated with bacillary load or the presence of erythema nodosum leprosum.

SPECIAL CLINICAL CONSIDERATIONS AND HANSEN DISEASE
Pregnancy

Hansen disease may be complicated in several ways by pregnancy. As a state of relative immunosuppression, pregnancy may lead to an exacerbation or reactivation after apparent cure. In addition, pregnancy or, more often, the period immediately after delivery may be associated with the appearance of reactional states in patients with Hansen disease. Pregnant patients with Hansen disease cannot be given certain medications used to treat the disease, such as thalidomide, ofloxacin, and minocycline. MDT is tolerated by pregnant women if these restricted agents are avoided.

Human Immunodeficiency Virus

Human immunodeficiency virus (HIV) infection, although a cause of profound immunosuppression of the cell-mediated immune system, does not seem to have an adverse effect on the course of Hansen disease. Patients are treated with the same agents and can be expected to have similar outcomes in general. Duration of treatment with MDT may need to be extended in patients with HIV infection. Treatment of HIV-infected patients with Hansen disease using effective antiretroviral drugs may be associated with the appearance of reactional states (usually type 1) as part of the immune reconstitution syndrome. This virtually always occurs in the first 6 months of antiviral therapy.

Organ Transplantation

Hansen disease has been reported in organ transplant recipients (renal, liver, heart, and bone marrow). If the disease has been treated and the patient is then given a transplant, Hansen disease can recur, apparently as a result of the immunosuppressive regimen. In addition, transplant patients may present with new Hansen disease, most frequently toward the lepromatous pole (BL or LL). Erythema nodosum leprosum (ENL) may occur. The correct management of the organ transplant recipient with Hansen disease is not known, but MDT with highly active agents is usually given.

Patients with Hansen disease may also acquire a second cutaneous mycobacterial infection. This may occur as a complication of corticosteroid treatment for reactional states. *Mycobacterium fortuitum* has been reported in one case, and one of the authors has seen coinfection with *M. haemophilum*. In these patients, the MDT plan should include agents effective against both Hansen disease and the second mycobacterial infection.

IMMUNOPATHOGENESIS

The patient's immune reaction to the leprosy bacillus and ongoing exposure are critical elements in determining the outcome of infection. Continuous exposure downregulates the cellular immune response against the pathogen and favors lepromatous disease. Tuberculoid patients make well-formed granulomas that contain helper T cells, whereas lepromatous patients have poorly formed granulomas, and suppressor T cells predominate. The cytokine profile in tuberculoid lesions is good cell-mediated immunity, with IFN-γ and interleukin-2 (IL-2) present. In lepromatous patients, these cytokines are reduced, and IL-4, IL-5, and IL-10, cytokines that downregulate cell-mediated immunity and enhance suppressor function and antibody production, are prominent. Lepromatous leprosy thus represents a classic T-helper cell type 2 (Th2) response to *M. leprae*. Lepromatous patients have polyclonal hypergammaglobulinemia and high antibody titers to *M. leprae*–unique antigens and may have false-positive syphilis serology, rheumatoid factor, and antinuclear antibodies. Although the cell-mediated immune response of lepromatous patients to *M. leprae* is reduced, these patients are not immunosuppressed for other infectious agents. Tuberculosis behaves normally in patients with lepromatous leprosy.

HISTOPATHOLOGY

Ideally, biopsies should be performed from the active border of typical lesions and should extend into the subcutaneous tissue. Punch biopsies are usually adequate. Fite-Faraco stain is optimal for demonstrating *M. leprae*. Because the diagnosis of Hansen disease is associated with significant social implications, evaluation must be complete, including evaluation of multiple sections in paucibacillary cases. Consultation with a pathologist experienced in the diagnosis of Hansen disease can be helpful if the diagnosis is suspected, but organisms cannot be identified in the affected tissue, especially in paucibacillary disease and reactional states. PCR has not been very useful; it is positive in only 50% of paucibacillary cases. The histologic features of Hansen disease correlate with the clinical pattern of disease. Nerve involvement is characteristic, and histologic perineural and neural involvement should suggest Hansen disease.

Tuberculoid Leprosy

Dermal tuberculoid granulomas, consisting of groups of epithelioid cells with giant cells, are found in tuberculoid leprosy. The granulomas are elongated and generally run parallel to the surface, following neurovascular bundles. The epithelioid cells are not vacuolated or lipidized. The granulomas extend up to the epidermis, with no grenz zone. Lymphocytes are found at the periphery of the granulomas. Acid-fast bacilli are rare. The most important specific diagnostic feature, besides finding bacilli, is selective destruction of nerve trunks and the finding of perineural concentric

fibrosis. An S-100 stain may show this selective neural destruction by demonstrating unrecognizable nerve remnants in the inflammatory foci. Bacilli are most frequently found in nerves, but the subepidermal zone and arrector pili muscles are other fruitful areas.

Borderline Tuberculoid Leprosy

The histopathology of BT leprosy is similar to that seen in the tuberculoid variety. However, epithelioid cells may show some vacuolation, bacilli are more abundant, and a grenz zone separates the inflammatory infiltrate from the overlying epidermis in BT leprosy.

Borderline Leprosy

In borderline leprosy, granulomas are less well organized, giant cells are not seen, the macrophages have some foamy cytoplasm, and organisms are abundant.

Borderline Lepromatous Leprosy

In BL lesions, foamy histiocytes, rather than epithelioid cells, make up the majority of the granuloma. Lymphocytes are still present and may be numerous in the granulomas but are dispersed diffusely within them, not organized at the periphery. Perineural involvement with lymphocyte infiltration may be present. Organisms are abundant and may be found in clumps.

Lepromatous Leprosy

In lepromatous leprosy, granulomas are composed primarily of bacilli-laden and lipid-laden histocytes. These are the so-called lepra cells or foam cells of Virchow. The infiltrate is localized in the dermis and may be purely perivascular or sheetlike and separated from the epidermis by a well-defined grenz zone. Acid-fast bacilli are typically abundant and appear as round clumps (globi). Pure polar lepromatous leprosy differs from the subpolar type primarily in the paucity of lymphocytes in the pure polar form.

REACTIONAL STATES

Reactions are a characteristic and clinically important aspect of Hansen disease. The majority of reactions occur after initiation of therapy, with an incidence of about 50% in patients starting MDT. In addition to antibiotic therapy, intercurrent infections, vaccination, pregnancy, vitamin A, iodides, and bromide may trigger reactions. Reactions can be severe and are an important cause of permanent nerve damage in borderline patients. Reactional states frequently appear abruptly, unlike Hansen disease itself, which changes slowly. A reaction is therefore a common reason why patients seek consultation. In addition, if a patient believes that the chemotherapy is triggering the reaction, the patient will tend to discontinue the treatment, leading to treatment failure.

Reactional states are divided into two forms, called type 1 and type 2 reactions. Type 1 reactions are caused by cell-mediated immune inflammation within existing skin lesions. These generally occur in patients with borderline leprosy (BT, BB, BL). Type 2 reactions are mediated by immune complexes and occur in lepromatous patients (BL, LL).

Type 1 Reactions (Reversal, Lepra, and Downgrading Reactions)

Type 1 reactions represent an enhanced cell-mediated immune response to *M. leprae* and usually occur after treatment is initiated. If the reactions occur with antibiotic chemotherapy, they are called reversal reactions, and if they occur as borderline disease shifts

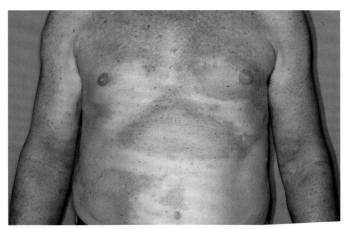

Fig. 17.9 Type 1 reactional leprosy. (Courtesy Laura de Souza Lima Institute, Brazil.)

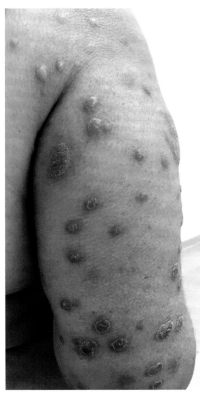

Fig. 17.10 Type 2 reactional leprosy. (Courtesy Aileen Chang, MD.)

toward the lepromatous pole (downgrading), they are called downgrading reactions. These two reaction types are clinically identical. Patients in all parts of the borderline spectrum may be affected by type 1 reactions, but these are most severe in patients with BL leprosy who have a large amount of *M. leprae* antigen and therefore have prolonged and repeated reactions during treatment.

Type 1 reactions clinically present with inflammation of existing lesions (Fig. 17.9). The patient has no systemic symptoms, such as fever, chills, or arthralgias. Lesions swell, become erythematous, and are sometimes tender, simulating cellulitis. In severe cases, ulceration can occur.

Patients may state that new lesions appeared with the reaction, but these probably represent subclinical lesions that were highlighted by the reaction. The major complication of type 1 reactions is nerve damage. As the cell-mediated inflammation attacks *M. leprae* antigen, any infected tissue compartment can be damaged. Because bacilli are preferentially in nerves, neural symptoms and findings are often present. Reversal reaction occurring within a nerve may lead to sudden loss of nerve function and permanent damage to that nerve. This makes type 1 reactions an emergency. In this setting, affected nerves are enlarged and tender. In other patients, the neuritis may be subacute or chronic and of limited acute symptomatology, but may still result in severe nerve damage. Histologically, skin lesions show perivascular and perineural edema and large numbers of lymphocytes. Severe reactions may demonstrate tissue necrosis. Bacilli are reduced.

Type 2 Reactions (Erythema Nodosum Leprosum)

ENL occurs in half of patients with BL or lepromatous leprosy, 90% of the time within a few years of institution of antibiotic treatment for Hansen disease or during pregnancy. ENL represents immune complex–mediated vasculitis, with most of the complexes forming locally rather than circulating. Nerve damage in leprosy is related to in situ generation of the membrane attack complex, and higher levels are found in ENL. Increased levels of tumor necrosis factor–α (TNF-α) and other proinflammatory cytokines are found along with an increased CD4(+)/CD8(+) ratio in both skin and peripheral blood.

In contrast to type 1 reactions, type 2 (ENL) can result in multisystem involvement and is usually accompanied by systemic symptoms (fever, myalgias, arthralgias, anorexia). Skin lesions are characteristically erythematous, subcutaneous, and dermal nodules that are widely distributed (Fig. 17.10). They do not occur at the sites of existing skin lesions. Severe skin lesions can ulcerate. Unlike classic erythema nodosum, lesions of ENL are generalized and favor the extensor arms and medial thighs.

A multisystem disease, ENL can produce conjunctivitis, neuritis, keratitis, iritis, synovitis, nephritis, hepatosplenomegaly, orchitis, and lymphadenopathy. The intensity of the reaction may vary from mild to severe and may last from a few days to weeks, months, or even years. Histologically, ENL demonstrates a leukocytoclastic vasculitis. Laboratory evaluation will reveal an elevated sedimentation rate, increased C-reactive protein, and a neutrophilia.

Lucio Phenomenon

Lucio phenomenon is an uncommon and unusual reaction that occurs in patients with diffuse lepromatous leprosy (DLL) of the "la bonita" type, most often found in western Mexico. Some consider it a subset of ENL, but Lucio's reaction differs in that it lacks neutrophilia and systemic symptoms. It is not associated with institution of antibiotic treatment as is ENL, and Lucio phenomenon is frequently the reason for initial presentation in affected patients. Purpuric macules evolve to bullous lesions that rapidly ulcerate, especially below the knees (Fig. 17.11). These may be painful but may also be relatively asymptomatic. Histologically, bacilli are numerous and, in addition to being in the dermis, are seen within blood vessel walls with thrombosis of middermal vessels, resulting in cutaneous infarction. Fever, splenomegaly, lymphadenopathy, glomerulonephritis, anemia, hypoalbuminemia, polyclonal gammopathy, and hypocalcemia may be associated conditions. If the patient is diagnosed early, before significant metabolic and infectious complications occur, the outcome is favorable.

TREATMENT

Dapsone monotherapy promotes resistance. MDT is now standard. Treatment recommendations are summarized in Tables 17.2 and 17.3.

TABLE 17.2 U.S. Department of Health and Human Services Treatment Guidelines

ADULTS

Tuberculoid (TT and BT) (WHO Classification Paucibacillary, "Pb")

Agent	Dose	Duration
Dapsone	100 mg daily	12 months
Rifampicin	600 mg daily	

ADULTS

Lepromatous (LL, BL, BB) (WHO Classification Multibacillary, "Mb")

Agent	Dose	Duration[a]
Dapsone	100 mg daily	24 months
Rifampicin	600 mg daily	
Clofazimine	50 mg daily	

ALTERNATIVE ANTIMICROBIAL AGENTS

Minocycline, 100 mg daily, substituted for dapsone in individuals who do not tolerate this drug. It can also be used instead of clofazimine, although evidence of antiinflammatory activity against type 2 reactions is not as substantial.

Clarithromycin, 500 mg daily, can be used as a substitute for any of the other drugs in a multiple-drug regimen.

Ofloxacin, 400 mg daily, may be used in place of clofazimine, for adults. This is not recommended for children.

RECOMMENDED LABORATORY TESTS AND FREQUENCY

	Initial visit	Second visit (1–2 Months)	3 Months	6 Months	12 Months	18 Months	24 Months
CBC + platelets	X	X	X	X	X	X	X
AST	X		X	X	X	X	X
ALT	X		X	X	X	X	X
Ca	X						
BUN	X						
Creatinine	X						
Bilirubin	X						
G6PD	X						
Hepatitis B							
Hepatitis C							

ALT, Alanine transaminase; *AST,* aspartate transaminase; *BUN,* blood urea nitrogen; *Ca,* calcium; *CBC,* complete blood count; *G6PD,* glucose-6-phosphate dehydrogenase; *WHO,* World Health Organization.

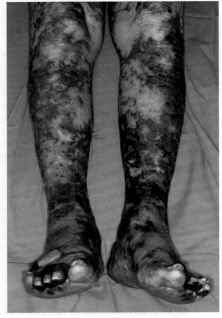

Fig. 17.11 Lucio phenomenon. (Courtesy Laura de Souza Lima Institute, Brazil.)

TABLE 17.3 World Health Organization Treatment Guidelines

ADULTS

Single Skin Lesion Paucibacillary Leprosy

Agent	Dose	Duration
Rifampicin	600 mg	Single dose
Ofloxacin	400 mg	
Minocycline	100 mg	

ADULTS

Tuberculoid (TT and BT) (WHO Classification Paucibacillary, "Pb")

Agent	Dose	Duration
Dapsone	100 mg daily	6 months
Rifampicin	600 mg monthly	

ADULTS

Lepromatous (LL, BL, BB) (WHO Classification Multibacillary, "Mb")

Agent	Dose	Duration
Dapsone	100 mg daily	12 months
Rifampicin	600 mg monthly	
Clofazimine	300 mg monthly and 50 mg daily	

WHO, World Health Organization.

The WHO defines paucibacillary disease as the presence of no bacilli on smears or biopsy and ≤5 lesions. Alternative regimens have been suggested for patients with compromised immunity and in those with multibacillary disease with a very high bacterial load. Therapies consist of an intensive regimen for 6–12 months that can be followed by a continuous phase for another 18 months. Rifapentine, 900 mg, appears superior to rifampin in these combinations. Proposed newer "intensive" drug regimens for rifampin-sensitive multibacillary patients include rifapentine, 900 mg; moxifloxacin, 400 mg; and clarithromycin, 1000 mg (or minocycline, 200 mg), all once monthly for 12 months. For rifampin-resistant patients, moxifloxacin, 400 mg; clofazimine, 50 mg; clarithromycin, 500 mg; and minocycline, 100 mg, are given daily, supervised for 6 months. The continuous phase of treatment could comprise moxifloxacin, 400 mg; clarithromycin, 1000 mg; and minocycline, 200 mg, once monthly, supervised for an additional 18 months.

Drug resistance is widespread and has even recently been reported in the United States. It should be suspected if the patient fails to respond to treatment. There are currently available PCR techniques to detect drug resistance from biopsy specimens based on known mutations such as those DNA gyrase responsible for quinolone resistance.

At the end of treatment, visible skin lesions are often still present, especially with the WHO short-duration treatments. Paucibacillary lesions tend to clear 1–2 years after the 6-month treatment course. In the United States treatment could be continued until skin lesions are clear, even if the recommended duration of treatment has been passed. With short-duration MDT, it is very difficult to distinguish clinical relapse (failure of treatment) from late type 1 reactions causing skin lesions to reappear. Pathologic examination (biopsy) or an empiric trial of prednisone for several months may be considered in these patients.

Significant disagreement surrounds the effectiveness of the 1-year or 2-year WHO-recommended MDT regimens. Relapse rates for multibacillary patients treated with MDT for 1 or 2 years have been reported to be as high as 7%–20% overall, and 13%–39% with BI of 4 or greater at diagnosis. Based on this information, patients with BL/LL disease with a BI of 4 or greater are at highest risk for relapse and should be treated beyond the 1-year recommended period, with treatment continued until smear negativity.

Treatment of Hansen disease patients with effective antibiotic regimens usually does not result in regaining of neurologic deficits. When deficits do recover, it appears to be mostly from elimination of the perineural inflammation, rather than regeneration of the affected nerves. Therefore early treatment of patients when neurologic defects are minimal and aggressive treatment of type 1 reactions are the key to limiting neural damage in Hansen disease.

Adjunctive Treatments

Once neurologic complications have occurred, patients with Hansen disease should be offered occupational therapy. This should include training on how to avoid injury to insensitive skin of the hands and feet. Special shoes may be required. Ocular complications are common, and an ophthalmologist with specific skill in treating patients with Hansen disease is an invaluable member of the treatment team.

MANAGEMENT OF REACTIONS

Even though reactions may appear after drug treatment is instituted, it is not advisable to discontinue or reduce antileprosy medication because of these. In mild reactions—those without neurologic complications or severe systemic symptoms or findings—treatment may be supportive. Bed rest and administration of aspirin or nonsteroidal antiinflammatory drugs may be used.

Type 1 reactions are usually managed with systemic corticosteroids. Prednisone is given orally, starting at a dose of 40–60 mg/day. Neuritis and eye lesions are urgent indications for systemic steroid therapy. Nerve abscesses may also need to be surgically drained immediately to preserve and recover nerve function. The corticosteroid dose and duration are determined by the clinical course of the reaction. Once the reaction is controlled, the prednisone may need to be tapered slowly, over months to years. The minimum dose required and alternate-day treatment should be used in corticosteroid courses more than 1 month in duration. Clofazimine appears to have some activity against type 1 reactions and may be added to the treatment in doses of up to 300 mg/day if tolerated. Cyclosporine can be used if steroids fail or as a steroid-sparing agent. The starting dose would be 5–10 mg/kg. If during treatment the function of some nerves fails to improve while the function of others normalizes, the possibility of mechanical compression should be evaluated by surgical exploration. Transposition of the ulnar nerve does not seem to be more effective than immunosuppressive treatment for ulnar nerve dysfunction.

Thalidomide has been demonstrated to be uniquely effective against ENL and is the treatment of choice. The initial recommended dosage is up to 400 mg/day in patients weighing more than 50 kg. This dose is highly sedating in some patients, and patients may complain of central nervous system side effects, even at doses of 100 mg/day. For this reason, such a high dose should be used for only a brief period, or in milder cases, treatment may be started at a much lower dose, such as 100–200 mg/day. In patients with an acute episode of ENL, the drug may be discontinued after a few weeks to months. In chronic type 2 reactions, an attempt to discontinue the drug should be made every 6 months. Thalidomide is a potent teratogen and should not be given to women of childbearing age. Long-term use is associated with predominantly sensory neuropathy, and even short-term use is associated with a risk of thromboembolic phenomena, as well as constipation. Systemic corticosteroids are also effective in type 2 reactions, but long-term use may lead to complications. Clofazimine in higher doses, up to 300 mg/day, is effective in ENL and may be used alone or to reduce corticosteroid or thalidomide doses. The combination of pentoxifylline, 400–800 mg twice daily, and clofazimine, 300 mg/day, can be given to patients with ENL when thalidomide cannot be used or to avoid the use of systemic steroids to manage severe ENL. Pentoxifylline alone is inferior to steroids and thalidomide but can be considered in milder cases. TNF inhibitors have been reported to be effective in treating recurrent ENL.

Lucio phenomenon is poorly responsive to both corticosteroids and thalidomide. Effective antimicrobial chemotherapy for lepromatous leprosy is the only recommended treatment, combined with wound management for leg ulcers.

PREVENTION

Because a defect in cell-mediated immunity is inherent in the development of Hansen disease, vaccine therapies are being tested. Bacille Calmette-Guérin (BCG) vaccination alone provides about 34%–80% protection against *M. leprae* infection. Other vaccines have been produced, but it is unclear if vaccine will be needed except in the areas of highest endemicity, because MDT has been effective in reducing the prevalence of Hansen disease. Because 80% of patients have contact with multibacillary patients, prevention depends on treating active multibacillary patients and examining exposed persons on an annual basis to detect early evidence of infection. Prophylactic antibiotic regimens have been used in such exposed patients and demonstrate a reduction in new Hansen disease cases by more than 50% in the first 2 years. Patients who had less contact with the source patient benefited more. In the United Kingdom, close contacts under age 12 whose source case was lepromatous are given rifampin, 15 mg/kg once monthly for

6 months. Several trials of chemoprophylaxis in whole endemic regions (once-yearly MDT with single-dose rifampin, minocycline, and clofazimine) have shown early promise and may be useful in hyperendemic regions.

Antunes DE, et al: Number of leprosy reactions during treatment: clinical correlations and laboratory diagnosis. Rev Soc Bras Med Trop 2016; 49: 741.

Bahia El Idrissi N, et al: In situ complement activation and T-cell immunity in leprosy spectrum. PLoS One 2017; 12: e0177815.

Balamayooran G, et al: The armadillo as an animal model and reservoir host for *Mycobacterium leprae*. Clin Dermatol 2015; 33: 108.

Cruz RCDS: Leprosy: current situation, clinical and laboratory aspects, treatment history and perspective of the uniform multidrug therapy for all patients. An Bras Dermatol. 2017 Nov-Dec;92(6):761-773. doi: 10.1590/abd1806-4841.20176724. Review. PubMed PMID: 29364430; PubMed Central PMCID: PMC5786388.

de Carvalho FM, et al: Interruption of persistent exposure to leprosy combined or not with recent BCG vaccination enhances the response to *Mycobacterium leprae* specific antigens. PLoS Negl Trop Dis 2017; 11: e0005560.

Dogra S, et al: Clinical characteristics and outcome in multibacillary (MB) leprosy patients treated with 12 months WHO MDT-MBR. Lepr Rev 2013; 84: 65.

Hossain D: Using methotrexate to treat patients with ENL unresponsive to steroids and clofazimine. Lepr Rev 2013; 84: 105.

Manickam P, et al: International open trial of uniform multidrug therapy regimen for leprosy patients. Indian J Med Res 2016; 144: 525.

Massone C, et al: Histopathology of the lepromatous skin biopsy. Clin Dermatol 2015; 33: 38.

Mathur M, et al: Histoid leprosy. Int J Dermatol. 2017; 56: 664.

Muthuvel T, et al: Leprosy trends at a tertiary care hospital in Mumbai, India, from 2008 to 2015. Glob Health Action 2016; 9: 32962.

Nath I, et al: Immunology of leprosy and diagnostic challenges. Clin Dermatol 2015; 33: 90.

Polycarpou A, et al: A systematic review of immunological studies of erythema nodosum leprosum. Front Immunol 2017; 8: 233.

Saunderson PR: Uniform multidrug therapy for leprosy—time for a rethink? Indian J Med Res 2016; 144: 499.

Silva BJ, et al: Autophagy is an innate mechanism associated with leprosy polarization. PLoS Pathog 2017; 13: e1006103.

Tatipally S: Polymerase Chain Reaction (PCR) as a Potential Point of Care Laboratory Test for Leprosy Diagnosis-A Systematic Review. Trop Med Infect Dis. 2018 Oct 1;3(4). pii: E107. doi: 10.3390/tropicalmed3040107. Review. PubMed PMID: 30275432.

Vieira MCA: Leprosy in children under 15 years of age in Brazil: A systematic review of the literature. PLoS Negl Trop Dis. 2018 Oct 2;12(10):e0006788. doi: 10.1371/journal.pntd.0006788. eCollection 2018 Oct. PubMed PMID: 30278054.

Williams DL, et al: Primary multi-drug resistant leprosy, United States. Emerg Infect Dis 2013; 19: 179.

Yamaguchi T, et al: Quinolone resistance-associated amino acid substitutions affect enzymatic activity of *Mycobacterium leprae* DNA gyrase. Biosci Biotechnol Biochem 2017; 81: 1343.

18   Syphilis, Yaws, Bejel, and Pinta

SYPHILIS

Syphilis, also known as lues, is a contagious, sexually transmitted disease caused by the spirochete *Treponema pallidum* subspecies *pallidum*. The only known host is the human. The spirochete enters through the skin or mucous membranes, where the primary manifestations are seen. In congenital syphilis, the treponeme crosses the placenta and infects the fetus. The risk of acquiring infection from sexual contact with an infected partner in the previous 30 days is 16%–30%. Syphilis results in multiple patterns of skin and visceral disease and can be lifelong.

Syphilis, yaws, pinta, and endemic syphilis are closely related infectious conditions caused by "genetically monomorphic bacteria," with less than 2% difference in the genomes of the treponemes (treponemas) that cause these infections. Historically, yaws first arose with humans in Africa and spread with human migrations to Europe and Asia. Endemic syphilis evolved from yaws and became endemic in the Middle East and the Balkans at some later date. Yaws moved with human migration to the New World and became endemic in South America. Syphilis, *T. pallidum pallidum*, may have originated in the New World from *T. pallidum pertenue*, the organism causing yaws, much as human immunodeficiency virus (HIV) evolved in Africa from simian immunodeficiency virus (SIV). A tribe in Guyana with a spirochetal infection with features of both yaws and syphilis was identified. Sequencing the genome of this spirochete suggested that it was the ancestor of *T. pallidum pallidum*. This lends support to the theory that syphilis originated more recently in the New World and was brought back to Europe by sailors who went to the New World with Christopher Columbus. Exactly how and when it became primarily a venereally transmitted disease is unclear, but apparently this happened toward the end of the 15th century.

Treponema pallidum is a delicate, spiral spirochete that is actively motile. The number of spirals varies from 4 to 14, and the entire length is 5–20 μm. It can be demonstrated in preparations from fresh primary or secondary lesions by darkfield microscopy or by fluorescent antibody techniques. The motility is characteristic, consisting of three movements: a projection in the direction of the long axis, a rotation on its long axis, and a bending or twisting from side to side. The precise uniformity of the spiral coils is not distorted during these movements. Microscopic characteristics of *T. pallidum* cannot be distinguished from commensal oral treponemes, so darkfield examination of oral lesions is unreliable. Direct fluorescent antibody testing can be used for confirmation.

The genome of *T. pallidum* has been sequenced and contains about one quarter of the number of genes of most bacteria. It lacks significant metabolic capacity. It is very sensitive to temperature, with some enzymes working poorly at typical body temperature (perhaps explaining why fever therapy was effective). These two factors may contribute to the inability to culture the organism in vitro. *T. pallidum* is an effective pathogen because it disseminates widely and rapidly after infection. It is in the bloodstream within hours of intratesticular injection and in numerous organs, including the brain, within 18 hours after inoculation. Once the organisms reach a tissue, they are able to persist for decades. In each tissue, the number of organisms is very low, perhaps below a "critical antigenic mass." In addition, *T. pallidum* expresses very few antigenic targets on its surface (only about 1% as many as *Escherichia coli*). The outer membrane proteins of *T. pallidum* also undergo rapid mutation, so that during an infection, the host accumulates numerous subpopulations of organisms with different surface antigens. This low infection load, widespread dissemination, poor surface antigen expression, and rapid evolution of antigenically distinct subpopulations may allow the infection to persist despite the development by the host of antigen-specific antibodies and immune cells.

Syphilis remains a major health problem worldwide, despite a highly effective and economical treatment for more than 50 years. The story of the U.S. and world epidemiology of syphilis illustrates a movement of infection from one population to another due to changing social conditions and behaviors. Just as the health systems respond to one epidemic, another appears. Using serologic testing, contact tracing, and penicillin treatment, U.S. health departments reduced the incidence of syphilis dramatically from the turn of the 20th century through the mid-1950s. The incidence then gradually increased through the next two decades and into the 1980s. In the early 1980s half the cases of syphilis diagnosed were in men who have sex with men (MSM). Changes in sexual behavior patterns among gay men in response to the acquired immunodeficiency syndrome (AIDS) epidemic reduced the number of these cases, but in the late 1980s syphilis again began to increase dramatically, associated with drug use, especially crack cocaine. The incidence of syphilis increased disproportionately among socioeconomically disadvantaged minority populations, especially in major cities. Throughout the 1990s the rate of syphilis fell in the United States, so that by 1999 the national rate of 2.6 cases in 100,000 population was the lowest level ever recorded. In addition, half of new cases were concentrated in 28 counties, mainly in the southeastern United States and in select urban areas. With the advent of effective antiretroviral therapy for HIV, there was a change in sexual behavior in MSM, including those with HIV infection. Epidemics of syphilis in this group have now occurred in many major North American, European, and Asian cities. This epidemic is characterized by an older average age, anonymous sex partners (often met on the Internet), use of amphetamines and sildenafil citrate (Viagra), HIV-positive status, and oral sex as the sole sexual exposure. In addition, there was a syphilis epidemic in Russia and the newly independent states starting in the late 1990s, with rates of syphilis 34 times that of Western Europe. Beginning in the mid-1990s, China had a syphilis epidemic affecting primarily unmarried men, female sex workers, and MSM, so that in 2008 one province in China (Guangdong) had more syphilis cases than the whole European Union.

Worldwide, an estimated 12 million persons are infected annually with syphilis, 2 million of whom are pregnant women. The U.S. Centers for Disease Control and Prevention (CDC) and the World Health Organization (WHO) have undertaken campaigns to eradicate syphilis. The shifting epidemiology of syphilis over more than five decades suggests it will not be an easy task without an effective vaccine. Until then, reporting of all cases to public health departments for tracing and treatment of contacts should be continued, along with widespread screening of persons at risk, including all pregnant women, female sex workers, MSM, and men with HIV infection.

Serologic Tests

Serologic testing for infection with *T. pallidum*, as in tuberculosis, is undergoing changes that incorporate newer technologies into establishing the diagnosis. Tests are considered either "treponemal" or "nontreponemal." Treponemal tests detect specific antitreponemal antibodies by enzyme immunoassay (EIA) or *T. pallidum* particle assay (TPPA). These new treponemal tests have specificity and sensitivity exceeding 95%, even in patients with primary syphilis. These generate more positive tests that require further testing than do older strategies. Nontreponemal tests are based on the fact that serum of persons with syphilis aggregates a cardiolipin-cholesterol-lecithin antigen. This aggregation can be viewed directly in tubes or on cards or slides, or it can be examined in an autoanalyzer. Because these tests use lipoidal antigens rather than *T. pallidum* or its components, they are called nontreponemal antigen tests. The most widely used nontreponemal tests are the rapid plasma reagin (RPR) and Venereal Disease Research Laboratories (VDRL) tests. These nontreponemal tests are the standard tests used in the United States and generally become positive within 5–6 weeks of infection, shortly before the chancre heals. Tests are usually strongly positive throughout the secondary phase, except in rare patients with AIDS, whose response is less predictable, and usually become negative during therapy, especially if therapy is begun within the first year of infection. Results may also become negative after a few decades, even without treatment. EIA tests are available that detect both immunoglobulin G (IgG)– and immunoglobulin M (IgM)–specific antibodies against *T. pallidum*. The IgM becomes detectable 2–3 weeks after infection, about the time the chancre appears. The IgG test becomes positive at 4–5 weeks; thus the IgM test is much more useful in diagnosing primary syphilis. The "treponemal" tests used in the United States are the microhemagglutination assay for *T. pallidum* (MHA-TP) or the fluorescent treponemal antibody absorption (FTA-ABS) test. These specific treponemal tests are also positive earlier than the nontreponemal tests and may be used to confirm the diagnosis of primary syphilis in a patient with a negative RPR/VDRL. The EIA, TPPA, FTA-ABS, and MHA-TP remain positive for life in the majority of patients, although in 13%–24% of patients these tests will become negative with treatment, regardless of stage and HIV status. The IgM EIA test, however, becomes negative after treatment in early syphilis, so that at 1 year 92% of these patients are negative on the IgM EIA.

All these tests can have false-positive results, so all positive results are confirmed by another test. In most U.S. cities, this involves screening the patient with a nontreponemal test, usually an RPR, and confirming all positives with a specific treponemal test, usually an MHA-TP. If a treponemal test, such as the TPPA or EIA, is used for initial screening, either a nontreponemal test or the other, specific treponemal test should be used to confirm the first test. A nontreponemal RPR/VDRL is also performed on all positives to determine the titer and monitor treatment success. If the initial screening treponemal-specific test is positive, but the nontreponemal test is negative, a history of prior syphilis and treatment should be sought. If prior syphilis and adequate treatment can be documented, and if examination shows no evidence of either primary or late syphilis, the patient is followed and considered serofast after treatment. If the nontreponemal test is negative, but a second treponemal test is positive, and if no prior history of syphilis and its treatment can be found, the patient is considered to have late latent syphilis (less likely, recent infection) and is treated appropriately. This patient is considered noninfectious. If the two treponemal tests are discordant, one positive and the other negative, a third treponemal-specific test can be ordered, or the case can be referred to a public health department for expert consultation. Because the nontreponemal tests are falsely negative in 25% or more of patients with primary syphilis and in up to 40% with late syphilis, in these patients a specific treponemal test should also be performed as a screening test.

In resource-poor countries, serologic testing for syphilis is largely unavailable because reagents require refrigeration or the tests require electrical equipment for processing. In Bangladesh and in some countries in sub-Saharan Africa and South America, more than 75% of women receive prenatal care, but only about 40% receive prenatal syphilis screening. Syphilis is endemic in these regions, with infection rates in pregnant women exceeding 1%, and thus millions of pregnant women with syphilis go undiagnosed. More than half a million babies die of congenital syphilis in sub-Saharan Africa every year. New, rapid treponemal-specific tests that can be used in these resource-poor countries have been developed. They cost only $0.31–$0.41 (U.S.) per test and await available funding to be put into use.

Nontreponemal tests are very valuable in following the efficacy of treatment in syphilis. By diluting the serum serially, the strength of the reaction can be stated in dilutions; the number given is the highest dilution giving a positive test result. In primary infection, the titer may be only 1:2; in secondary syphilis, it is regularly high, 1:32 to 1:256, or higher; in late syphilis, generally much lower, perhaps 1:4 or 1:8. The rise of titer in early infection is of great potential diagnostic value, as is the fall after proper treatment or the rise again if there is reinfection or relapse. Patients with very high antibody titers, as occur in secondary syphilis, may have a false-negative result when undiluted serum is tested. This "prozone" phenomenon will be overcome by diluting the serum.

Biologic False-Positive Test Results

"Biologic false-positive" (BFP) test result is used to denote a positive serologic test for syphilis in persons with no history or clinical evidence of syphilis. The term *BFP* is usually applied to the situation of a positive nontreponemal test and a negative treponemal test. About 90% of BFP test results are of low titer (<1:8). "Acute" BFP reactions are defined as those that revert to negative in less than 6 months; those that persist for more than 6 months are categorized as "chronic." Acute BFP reactions may result from vaccinations, infections (infectious mononucleosis, hepatitis, measles, typhoid, varicella, influenza, lymphogranuloma venereum, malaria), and pregnancy. Chronic BFP reactions are seen in connective tissue diseases, especially systemic lupus erythematosus (SLE) (44%), chronic liver disease, multiple blood transfusions/intravenous drug use, and advancing age.

False-positive results to specific treponemal tests are less common but have been reported to occur in lupus erythematosus, drug-induced lupus, scleroderma, rheumatoid arthritis, smallpox vaccination, pregnancy, other related treponemal infections (see next), and genital herpes simplex infections. A pattern of beaded fluorescence associated with FTA-ABS testing may be found in the sera of patients without treponemal disease who have SLE. The beading phenomenon, however, is not specific for SLE or even for connective tissue diseases.

Cutaneous Syphilis

Chancre (Primary Stage)

The chancre is usually the first cutaneous lesion, appearing 18–21 days after infection. The typical incipient chancre is a small red papule or a crusted superficial erosion. In a few days to weeks, it becomes a round or oval, indurated, slightly elevated papule, with an eroded but not ulcerated surface that exudes a serous fluid (Fig. 18.1). On palpation, it has a cartilage-like consistency. The lesion is usually, but not invariably, painless. This is the uncomplicated or classic hunterian chancre. The regional lymph nodes on one or both sides are usually enlarged, firm, and nontender and do not suppurate. Adenopathy begins 1 or 2 weeks after the

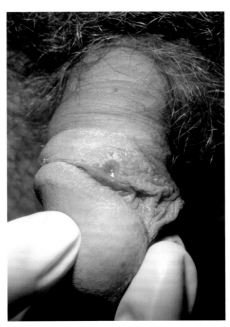

Fig. 18.1 Primary syphilis.

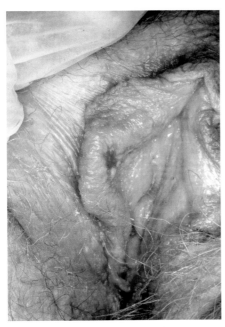

Fig. 18.2 Primary syphilis.

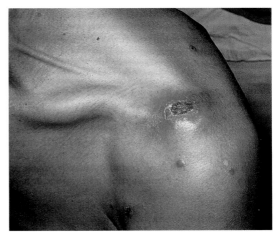

Fig. 18.3 Primary syphilis, chancre on shoulder with secondary lesions present.

chancre appears. The hunterian chancre leaves no scar when it heals.

Chancres generally occur singly, although they may be multiple, especially on the penis in MSM who are infected through oral intercourse. The lesions vary in diameter from a few millimeters to several centimeters. The genital chancre is less often observed in women because of its location within the vagina or on the cervix (Fig. 18.2). Extensive edema of the labia or cervix may occur. In men, the chancre is commonly located in the coronal sulcus or on either side of the frenum. A chancre in the prepuce, being too hard to bend, will flip over all at once when the prepuce is drawn back, a phenomenon called a "dory flop" (resembling a broad-beamed skiff or dory being turned upside down). Untreated,

the chancre tends to heal spontaneously in 1–4 months. About the time it disappears, or slightly before, constitutional symptoms and objective signs of generalized (secondary) syphilis occur (Fig. 18.3).

Extragenital chancres may be larger than those on the genitalia. They affect the lips, tongue, tonsil, female breast, index finger, and, especially in MSM, the anus. Oral chancres form firm, eroded papules on the lip, tongue, uvula, or tonsillar pillar and are associated with a history of oral sex. Unilateral cervical adenopathy can be present. The presenting complaints of an anal chancre include an anal sore or fissure and irritation or bleeding on defecation. Anal chancre must be ruled out in any anal fissure not at the 6 or 12 o'clock positions. When there is a secondary eruption, no visible chancre, and the glands below Poupart ligament are greatly enlarged, anal chancre should be suspected.

Atypical chancres are common. Simultaneous infection by a spirochete and another microbial agent may produce an atypical chancre. The mixed chancre caused by infection with *Haemophilus ducreyi* and *Treponema pallidum* will produce a lesion that runs a course different from either chancroid or primary syphilis alone. Such a sore begins a few days after exposure, because the incubation period for chancroid is short, and later the sore may transform into an indurated syphilitic lesion. A phagedenic chancre results from the combination of a syphilitic chancre and contaminating bacteria that may cause severe tissue destruction and result in scarring. Edema indurativum, or penile venereal edema, is marked solid edema of the labia or the prepuce and glans penis accompanying a chancre. Chancre redux is relapse of a chancre with insufficient treatment, accompanied by enlarged lymph nodes. Pseudochancre redux is a gumma occurring at the site of a previous chancre; it is distinguished from relapsing chancre by the absence of lymphadenopathy and a negative darkfield examination. Syphilitic balanitis of Follmann may occur in the absence of a chancre. The lesions may be exudative, circinate, or erosive.

Histologic evaluation of a syphilitic chancre reveals an ulcer covered by neutrophils and fibrin. Subjacent, there is a dense infiltrate of lymphocytes and plasma cells. Blood vessels are prominent with plump endothelial cells. Spirochetes are numerous in untreated chancres and can be demonstrated with an appropriate silver stain, such as the Warthin-Starry, Levaditi, or Steiner methods, or by immunoperoxidase staining. Spirochetes are best found in the overlying epithelium or adjacent or overlying blood vessels in the upper dermis.

In a patient who presents with an acute genital ulceration, darkfield examination should be performed if available. The finding of typical *T. pallidum* in a sore on the cutaneous surface establishes a diagnosis of syphilis. *Treponema pertenue*, which causes yaws, and *Treponema carateum*, which causes pinta, are both indistinguishable morphologically from *T. pallidum*, but the diseases that they produce are usually easy to recognize. Commensal spirochetes of the oral mucosa are indistinguishable from *T. pallidum*, making oral darkfield examinations unreliable. If the darkfield examination results are negative, the examination should be repeated daily for several days, especially if the patient has been applying a topical antibacterial agent.

The lesion selected for examination is cleansed with water and dried. It is grasped firmly between the thumb and index finger and abraded sufficiently to cause clear or faintly blood-stained plasma to exude when squeezed. In the case of an eroded chancre, a few vigorous rubs with dry gauze are usually sufficient. If the lesion is made to bleed, it is necessary to wait until free bleeding has stopped to obtain satisfactory plasma. The surface of a clean coverslip is touched to the surface of the lesion so that plasma adheres. Then it is dropped on a slide and pressed down so that the plasma spreads out in as thin a film as possible. Immersion oil forms the interface between the condenser and slide and between the coverslip and objective. The specimen must be examined quickly, before the thin film of plasma dries.

An alternative to darkfield microscopy is the direct fluorescent antibody test (DFAT-TP) for the identification of *T. pallidum* in lesions. Serous exudate from a suspected lesion is collected as just described, placed on a slide, and allowed to dry. Many health departments will examine such specimens with fluorescent antibodies specific to *T. pallidum*. The method, unlike the darkfield examination, can be used for diagnosing oral lesions. Multiplex polymerase chain reaction (PCR) is also an accurate and reproducible method for diagnosing genital ulcerations, with the advantage of being able to diagnose multiple infectious agents simultaneously. In genital ulcer disease outbreaks, PCR should be made available.

The results of serologic tests for syphilis are positive in 75% (nontreponemal tests) to 90% (treponemal tests) of patients with primary syphilis; both these tests should be performed in every patient with suspected primary syphilis. The likelihood of positivity depends on the duration of infection. If the chancre has been present for several weeks, test results are usually positive.

A syphilitic chancre must be differentiated from chancroid. The chancre has an incubation period of 3 weeks; is usually a painless erosion, not an ulcer; has no surrounding inflammatory zone; and is round or oval. The edge is not undermined, and the surface is smooth and at the level of the skin. It has a dark, velvety red, lacquered appearance; it has no overlying membrane; and it is cartilage hard on palpation. Lymphadenopathy may be bilateral and is nontender and nonsuppurative. Chancroid, on the other hand, has a short incubation period of 4–7 days; the ulcer is acutely inflamed, is extremely painful, and has a surrounding inflammatory zone. The ulcer edge is undermined and extends into the dermis. It is covered by a membrane and feels soft. Lymphadenopathy is usually unilateral and tender and may suppurate. Chancroid lesions are usually multiple and extend into each other. Cultures for chancroid on special media confirm the diagnosis. However, because a combination of a syphilitic chancre and chancroid (mixed sores) is indistinguishable from chancroid alone, appropriate direct and serologic testing should be performed to investigate the presence of syphilis. Again, multiplex PCR allows for the simultaneous diagnosis of many infectious agents in genital ulcer diseases.

The primary lesion of granuloma inguinale begins as an indurated nodule that erodes to produce hypertrophic, vegetative granulation tissue. It is soft and beefy-red and bleeds readily. A smear of clean granulation tissue from the lesion stained with Wright or Giemsa reveals Donovan bodies in the cytoplasm of macrophages.

The primary lesion of lymphogranuloma venereum (LGV) is usually a small, painless, transient papule or a superficial nonindurated ulcer. It most often occurs on the coronal sulcus, prepuce, or glans in men or on the fourchette, vagina, or cervix in women. A primary genital lesion is noticed by about 30% of infected heterosexual men, but less frequently in women. Primary lesions are followed in 7–30 days by adenopathy of the regional lymph nodes. LGV is confirmed by serologic tests.

Herpes simplex begins with grouped vesicles, often accompanied or preceded by burning pain. After rupture of the vesicles, irregular, scalloped, tender, soft erosions form.

Secondary Syphilis

Cutaneous Lesions. The skin manifestations of secondary syphilis occur in 80% or more of patients with secondary syphilis. The early eruptions are symmetric, more or less generalized, superficial, nondestructive, exanthematous, transient, and macular; later they are maculopapular or papular eruptions, which are usually polymorphous, and less often, scaly, pustular, or pigmented. The early manifestations tend to be distributed over the face, shoulders, flanks, palms and soles, and anal or genital regions. The severity varies widely. The presence of lesions on the palms and soles is strongly suggestive. However, a generalized syphilid can spare the palms and soles. The individual lesions are generally less than 1 cm in diameter, except in the later secondary or relapsing secondary eruptions.

Macular Eruptions. The earliest form of macular secondary syphilis begins with the appearance of an exanthematous erythema 6–8 weeks after the development of the chancre, which may still be present. The syphilitic exanthem extends rapidly, so that it is usually pronounced a few days after onset. It may be evanescent, lasting only a few hours or days, or it may last several months, or partially recur after having disappeared. This macular eruption appears first on the sides of the trunk, about the navel, and on the inner surfaces of the extremities.

Individual lesions of macular secondary syphilis consist of round, indistinct macules that are nonconfluent and rarely may be slightly elevated or urticarial. The color varies from a light pink or rose to brownish red. The macular eruption may not be noticed on black skin and may be so faint that it is also not recognized on other skin colors. Pain, burning, and itching are usually absent, although pruritus may be present in 10%–40% of patients. Simultaneous with the onset of the eruption, there is a generalized shotty adenopathy, most readily palpable in the posterior cervical, axillary, and epitrochlear areas. Rarely, secondary syphilis may cause livedo reticularis. The macular eruption may disappear spontaneously after a few days or weeks without residua or may result in postinflammatory hyperpigmentation. After a varying interval, macular syphilis may be followed by other eruptions.

Papular Eruptions. Papular eruptions usually arise slightly later than the macular eruption. The fully developed lesions are round and of a raw-ham or coppery shade (Fig. 18.4). Although papules most frequently are 2–5 mm in diameter, nodules coalescing to large plaques can occur. Lesions often are only slightly raised, but a deep, firm infiltration is palpable. The surface is smooth, sometimes shiny, and at other times covered with a thick, adherent scale. When this desquamates, it leaves a characteristic collarette of scales overhanging the border of the papule.

Papules are frequently distributed on the face and flexures of the arms and lower legs and are often distributed all over the trunk (Fig. 18.5). Palmar and plantar involvement characteristically appears as indurated, yellowish red spots (Fig. 18.6). Ollendorf (Buschke-Ollendorff) sign is present; the papule is exquisitely tender to the touch of a blunt probe. Healing lesions frequently leave hyperpigmented spots that, especially on the palms and soles, may persist for weeks or months. Split papules are hypertrophic, fissured papules that form in the creases of the alae nasi and at the oral commissures. These may persist for a long period. The papulosquamous syphilids, in which the adherent scales covering

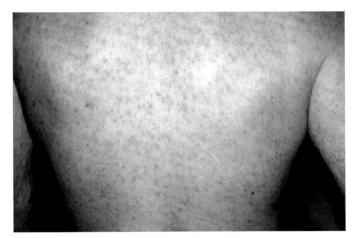

Fig. 18.4 Secondary syphilis.

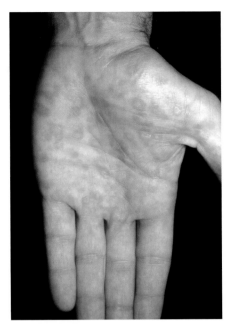

Fig. 18.6 Secondary syphilis.

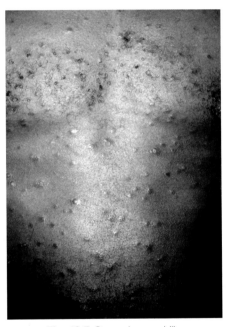

Fig. 18.5 Secondary syphilis.

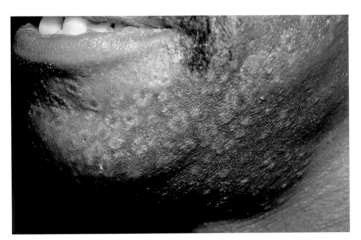

Fig. 18.7 Annular secondary syphilis.

the lesions more or less dominate the picture, may produce a psoriasiform eruption. Follicular or lichenoid syphilids appear as minute, scale-capped papules. If they are at the ostia of hair follicles, syphilids are likely to be conical; elsewhere on the skin, they are domed. Often, syphilids are grouped to form scaling plaques in which the tiny, coalescing papules are still discernible.

As with the other syphilids, papular eruptions tend to be disseminated but may also be localized, asymmetric, configurate, hypertrophic, or confluent. The arrangement may be corymbose or in patches, rings, or serpiginous patterns.

The annular syphilid, as with sarcoidosis, which it may mimic, is more common in blacks (Fig. 18.7). It is often located on the cheeks, especially close to the angle of the mouth, where it may form annular, arcuate, or gyrate patterns of delicate, slightly raised, infiltrated, finely scaling ridges. These ridges are made up of minute, flat-topped papules, and the boundaries between ridges may be difficult to discern. An old term for annular syphilids was "nickels and dimes."

The corymbose syphilid is another infrequent variant, usually occurring late in the secondary stage, in which a large central

papule is surrounded by a group of tiny satellite papules. The pustular syphilids are among the rarer manifestations of secondary syphilis. They occur widely scattered over the trunk and extremities, but they usually involve the face, especially the forehead. The pustule usually arises on a red, infiltrated base. Involution is usually slow, resulting in a small, rather persistent, crust-covered, superficial ulceration. Lesions in which the ulceration is deep are called ecthymatous. Closely related is the rupial syphilid, a lesion in which a relatively superficial ulceration is covered with a pile of terraced crusts resembling an oyster shell. Lues maligna is a rare form of secondary syphilis with severe ulcerations, pustules, or rupioid lesions, accompanied by severe constitutional symptoms. This form of secondary syphilis appears to be more common in HIV-infected men.

Involvement of the palms and soles is a characteristic feature of secondary syphilis. In some cases, instead of discrete lesions, the whole area of the palms and soles can be symmetrically involved, resembling keratoderma blennorrhagicum, hyperkeratotic hand eczema, or even an acquired keratoderma, such as Howel-Evans syndrome. Similarly, cutaneous lesions can be very psoriasiform,

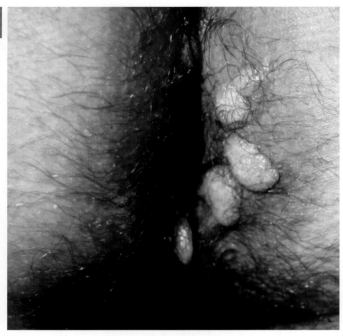

Fig. 18.8 Condylomata lata.

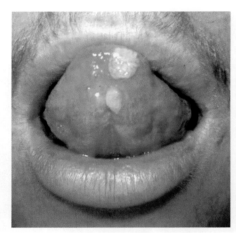

Fig. 18.9 Mucous patches of secondary syphilis.

and if they develop in a person with known psoriasis, lesions can be mistaken for a flare of that disease. Anetoderma may occur after treatment of secondary syphilis.

Condylomata lata are papular lesions, relatively broad and flat, located on folds of moist skin, especially around the genitalia and anus, but also at the angles of the mouth, nasolabial fold, and toe webs. They may become hypertrophic and, instead of infiltrating deeply, protrude above the surface, forming a soft, red, often mushroom-like mass 1–3 cm in diameter, usually with a smooth, moist, weeping, gray surface (Fig. 18.8). Condyloma lata may be lobulated but are not covered by the digitate elevations characteristic of venereal warts (condylomata acuminata). Secondary syphilis may initially present with perianal erosions and plaques that may mimic cutaneous Crohn disease.

Syphilitic alopecia is irregularly distributed so that the scalp has a moth-eaten appearance. It is unusual, occurring in about 5% of patients with secondary syphilis. Smooth, circular areas of alopecia mimicking alopecia areata may occur in syphilis, and an ophiasis pattern may rarely be seen.

Mucous membrane lesions are present in one third of patients with secondary syphilis and may be the only manifestation of the infection. The most common mucosal lesion in the early phase is the syphilitic sore throat, a diffuse pharyngitis that may be associated with tonsillitis or laryngitis. Hoarseness and sometimes complete aphonia may be present. On the tongue, smooth, small or large, well-defined patches devoid of papillae may be seen, most frequently on the dorsum near the median raphe (Fig. 18.9). Ulcerations may occur on the tongue and lips during the late secondary period, at times resembling aphthae or major aphthae. A rare variant of syphilis is one presenting with oral and cutaneous erosions that histologically show the features of pemphigus vulgaris, with a suprabasilar acantholytic blister, as well as positive direct and indirect immunofluorescence findings of pemphigus.

Mucous patches are the most characteristic mucous membrane lesions of secondary syphilis. They are macerated, flat, grayish, rounded erosions covered by a delicate, soggy membrane. These highly infectious lesions are about 5 mm in diameter and teem with treponemas. They occur on the tonsils, tongue, pharynx, gums, lips, and buccal areas or on the genitalia, chiefly in women,

in whom the lesions are most common on the labia minora, vaginal mucosa, and cervix. Such mucous erosions are transitory and change from week to week, or even from day to day. Lesions of the oral mucosa frequently contain plasma cells, so the oral pathologist may not consider syphilis. Because the oral lesions of secondary syphilis are usually teeming with spirochetes, a *T. pallidum*–specific immunoperoxidase stain is useful in confirming the diagnosis.

Relapsing Secondary Syphilis. The early lesions of syphilis undergo involution either spontaneously or with treatment. Relapses occur in about 25% of untreated patients, 90% within the first year. Such relapses may take place at the site of previous lesions, on the skin or in the viscera. Recurrent eruptions tend to be more configurate or annular, larger, and asymmetric.

Systemic Involvement. The lymphatic system in secondary syphilis is characteristically involved. The lymph nodes most frequently affected are the inguinal, posterior cervical, postauricular, and epitrochlear. The nodes are shotty, firm, slightly enlarged, nontender, and discrete.

Acute glomerulonephritis, gastritis or gastric ulceration, proctitis, hepatitis, acute meningitis, unilateral sensorineural hearing loss, iritis, anterior uveitis, optic neuritis, Bell palsy, multiple pulmonary nodular infiltrates, periostitis, osteomyelitis, polyarthritis, and tenosynovitis may all be seen in secondary syphilis.

Histopathology

Lesions of secondary syphilis may demonstrate neutrophils within the stratum corneum, elongation of rete ridges, interface dermatitis with a lymphocyte in every vacuole, an interstitial infiltrate (busy dermis), perivascular plasma cells, lymphocytes with visible amphophilic cytoplasm, and endothelial swelling (plump endothelial cells with absence of a lumen). Plasma cells are absent about 30% of cases, and many cases lack other characteristic features as well. Examples of syphilis with fewer histologic features are more likely to demonstrate effacement of the rete pattern rather than elongation of the rete ridges. A high index of suspicion is required, and any combination of interface dermatitis, interstitial inflammation, endothelial swelling, lymphocytes with visible cytoplasm, or plasma cells should raise the possibility of secondary syphilis. As lesions age, macrophages become more numerous, so that in late secondary lues, granulomatous foci are often present, mimicking sarcoidosis, or less often, a granuloma annulare–like pattern. Condylomata lata show spongiform pustules within areas of papillated epithelial hyperplasia, and spirochetes are numerous.

In early-syphilis skin lesions, spirochetes are most numerous within the epidermis and around superficial vessels. Silver stains are technically difficult, but because the number of organisms is high in early syphilis, the tests are usually positive. PCR and immunoperoxidase assay may identify *T. pallidum* infection when silver stains are negative. However, immunoperoxidase stains may be negative and silver stains positive; therefore if suspicion of early syphilis is high, both silver stains and immunoperoxidase assays may need to be performed.

Diagnosis and Differential Diagnosis

Syphilis has long been known as the "great imitator," because the various cutaneous manifestations may simulate almost any cutaneous or systemic disease. Pityriasis rosea may be mistaken for secondary syphilis, especially because both begin on the trunk. The herald patch, the oval patches with a fine scale at the edge, patterned in the lines of skin cleavage, the absence of lymphadenopathy, and infrequent mucous membrane lesions help to distinguish pityriasis rosea from secondary syphilis. Drug eruptions may produce a similar picture to secondary syphilis but tend to be morbilliform and also pruritic, whereas secondary syphilis is not. Drug eruptions in pityriasis rosea are often pruritic, whereas those in secondary syphilis usually are not.

Lichen planus may resemble papular syphilid. The characteristic papule of lichen planus is flat topped and polygonal, has Wickham striae, and exhibits Koebner phenomenon. Pruritus is severe in lichen planus but is less common and less severe in syphilis. Psoriasis may be distinguished from papulosquamous secondary syphilis by the presence of adenopathy, mucous patches, and alopecia in the latter. Sarcoidosis may produce lesions morphologically identical to secondary syphilis. Histologically, multisystem involvement, adenopathy, and granulomatous inflammation are common to both diseases. Serologic testing and biopsy specimens will distinguish sarcoidosis from syphilis.

The differential diagnosis of mucous membrane lesions of secondary syphilis is of importance. Infectious mononucleosis may cause a biologic false-positive test for syphilis but is diagnosed by serology. Geographic tongue may be confused with the desquamative patches of syphilis or with mucous patches. Lingua geographica occurs principally near the edges of the tongue in relatively large areas, which are often fused and have lobulated contours. It continues for several months or years and changes in extent and degree of involvement from day to day. Recurrent aphthous ulceration produces one or several painful ulcers, 1–3 mm in diameter, surrounded by hyperemic edges, with a grayish covering membrane, on nonkeratinized mucosal epithelium, especially in the gingival sulcus. A prolonged, recurrent history is characteristic. Syphilis of the lateral tongue may resemble oral hairy leukoplakia.

Latent Syphilis

After the lesions of secondary syphilis have involuted, a latent period occurs. This may last for a few months or continue for the remainder of the infected person's life. Between 60% and 70% of untreated infected patients remain latently asymptomatic for life. During this latent period, there are no clinical signs of syphilis, but the serologic tests for syphilis are reactive. During the early latent period, infectivity persists; for at least 2 years, a woman with early latent syphilis may infect her unborn child. For treatment purposes, it is important to distinguish early latency (<1-year duration) from late latency (>1 year or unknown duration).

Late Syphilis

For treatment purposes, late syphilis is defined by the CDC as infection of more than 1 year in duration and by the WHO as more than 2 years in duration. Only about one third of patients with late syphilis will develop complications of their infection.

Tertiary Cutaneous Syphilis

Tertiary syphilids most often occur 3–5 years after infection. About 16% of untreated patients will develop tertiary lesions of the skin, mucous membrane, bone, or joints. Skin lesions tend to be localized, to occur in groups, to be destructive, and to heal with scarring. Treponemas are usually not found by silver stains or darkfield examination but may be demonstrated by immunoperoxidase techniques.

Two main types of cutaneous tertiary syphilis are recognized, the nodular syphilid and the gumma, although the distinction is sometimes difficult to make. The nodular, noduloulcerative, or tubercular type consists of firm, reddish brown or copper-colored papules or nodules, 2 mm in diameter or larger. The individual lesions are usually covered with adherent scales or crusts (Fig. 18.10). The lesions tend to form rings and to undergo involution as new lesions develop just beyond them, producing characteristic circular or serpiginous patterns. A distinctive type is the kidney-shaped lesion, which typically occurs on the extensor surfaces of the arms and on the back. Individual lesions are composed of nodules in different stages of development, so that scars and pigmentation often are found together with fresh as well as ulcerated lesions. On the face, the nodular eruption closely resembles lupus vulgaris. When the disease is untreated, the process may last for years, slowly marching across large areas of skin. The nodules may enlarge and eventually break down to form painless, rounded, smooth-bottomed ulcers a few millimeters deep. These punched-out ulcers arise side by side and form serpiginous syphilitic ulcers, palm sized in aggregate, enduring for many years (Fig. 18.11).

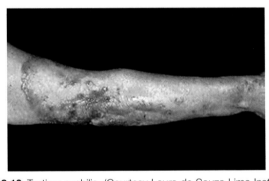

Fig. 18.10 Tertiary syphilis. (Courtesy Laura de Souza Lima Institute, Brazil.)

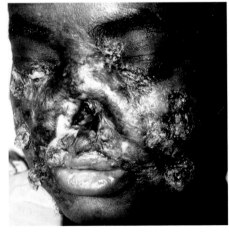

Fig. 18.11 Destruction of the central face in tertiary syphilis.

Gummas may occur as unilateral, isolated, single or disseminated lesions, or in serpiginous patterns resembling those of the nodular syphilid. They may be restricted to the skin or, originating in the deeper tissues, break down and secondarily involve the skin. The individual lesions, which begin as small nodules, slowly enlarge to several centimeters. Central necrosis is extensive and may lead to the formation of a deep, punched-out ulcer with steep sides and a gelatinous, necrotic base. Again, progression may take place in one area while healing proceeds in another. Perhaps the most frequent site of isolated gummas is the lower legs, where deep punched-out ulcers are formed, often in large, infiltrated areas. On the lower extremities, gummas are frequently mistaken for erythema induratum.

Lesions may be isolated to the mucous membranes, often the tongue, on which nonindurated punched-out ulcers occur. A superficial glossitis may cause irregular ulcers, atrophy of the papillae, and smooth, shiny scarring, a condition known as smooth atrophy. In interstitial glossitis, there is an underlying induration. In the advanced stages, tertiary syphilis of the tongue may lead to a diffuse enlargement (macroglossia). Perforation of the hard palate from gummatous involvement is a characteristic tertiary manifestation. It generally occurs near the center of the hard palate. Destruction of the nasal septum may also occur.

Histologically, nodular lesions of late syphilis usually have changes that resemble those of secondary lesions, with the addition of tuberculoid granulomas containing varying numbers of multinucleate giant cells. The epidermis is often atrophic rather than hyperplastic. In gummas, necrosis within granulomas and fibrosis occur as lesions resolve. Spirochetes are scant.

For diagnosis of late syphilis, clinicians rely heavily on specific treponemal tests. The nontreponemal tests, such as the VDRL and RPR, are positive in approximately 60% of patients. When there are mucous membrane lesions, for which a diagnosis of carcinoma must also be considered, histologic examination is performed. Darkfield examination is not indicated, because it is always negative. When not ulcerated, lesions of tertiary syphilis must be distinguished from malignant tumors, leukemids, and sarcoidosis. The ulcerated tertiary syphilids must be differentiated from other infections, such as scrofuloderma, atypical mycobacterial infection, and deep fungal infection. Wegener granulomatosis and ulcerated cutaneous malignancies must be considered. Histology and appropriate cultures may be required.

Late Osseous Syphilis

Occasionally, gummatous lesions involve the periosteum and the bone. Skeletal tertiary syphilis most often affects the head and face and the tibia. Late manifestations of syphilis may produce periostitis, osteomyelitis, osteitis, and gummatous osteoarthritis. Osteocope (bone pain), most often at night, is a suggestive symptom.

Syphilitic joint lesions also occur, with the Charcot joint being the most prevalent manifestation. These are often associated with tabes dorsalis and occur most frequently in men. Although any joint may be involved, the knees and ankles are most often affected. There is hydrops, then loss of the contours of the joint, hypermobility, and no pain. Joint lesion is readily diagnosed by x-ray examination.

Neurosyphilis

Central nervous system (CNS) infection can occur at any stage of syphilis, even the primary stage. Up to 100% of patients with syphilis may develop CNS infection, but in 80% it is spontaneously cleared by the immune system. This explains why most persons with CNS involvement have no symptoms. About one third of patients who do not spontaneously clear their CNS infection will develop symptomatic neurosyphilis. Finding cerebrospinal fluid (CSF) pleocytosis or a positive CSF-VDRL test has been used to confirm the diagnosis of CNS infection by *T. pallidum*. Unfortunately, a significant proportion of patients with CSF infection with *T. pallidum* will have a negative CSF-VDRL (46%) and nondiagnostic CSF pleocytosis (<20 white blood cells/μL) (33%). In patients with a negative CSF-VDRL but pleocytosis, FTA test can be performed on CSF, thought by many to be 100% sensitive but not specific for CNS syphilis. Combining this with flow cytometry to look for B cells in the CSF, which is 100% specific but only 40% sensitive, will allow the confirmation or exclusion of neurosyphilis in most patients with CSF pleocytosis. The likelihood of having CNS infection is 10-fold greater in persons with RPR of 1:32 or greater. HIV-negative persons with negative CSF examinations have almost no risk of developing neurosyphilis. However, CSF evaluations are not routinely performed in asymptomatic persons with early syphilis, so identifying those at risk for symptomatic neurosyphilis is problematic. *T. pallidum* CNS infection may also be strain dependent, and eventually, typing the infecting strain may predict those at highest risk for neurosyphilis.

Because CNS infection is common and the recommended treatments with benzathine penicillin do not reach treponemicidal levels in the CSF, persistent concern surrounds the failure to diagnose and treat asymptomatic neurosyphilis. Apparently, although treatment does not clear the spirochetes from the CSF, most non–HIV-infected persons are able to clear the CNS infection spontaneously. CSF evaluation is recommended in all patients with syphilis with any neurologic, auditory, or ophthalmic signs or symptoms, possibly resulting from syphilis, independent of stage or HIV status. In borderline cases, those with RPR of 1:32 or greater should have CSF evaluation. The indications for lumbar puncture in patients with coexistent HIV infection and early syphilis (<1 or 2 years' duration) remains unclear. The two factors predicting the likelihood of CNS infection are RPR of 1:32 or more and CD4 count of 350 cells/μL or less. Patients with latent syphilis or syphilis of unknown duration should have CSF evaluation if they are HIV positive or fail initial therapy, or if therapy other than penicillin is planned for syphilis of more than 1 year in duration. Patients with tertiary syphilis should have CSF evaluation before treatment to exclude neurosyphilis. An appropriate fall in the serum RPR after treatment for neurosyphilis predicts clearing of the CNS infection, so a repeat lumbar puncture after therapy is not required in HIV-negative or HIV-positive patients adequately treated for neurosyphilis.

Early Neurosyphilis. Early neurosyphilis is mainly meningeal, occurs in the 2 years of infection, and affects 1.4%–6% of untreated persons with syphilis. Meningeal neurosyphilis manifests as meningitis, with fever, headache, stiff neck, nausea, vomiting, cranial nerve disorders (loss of hearing, often unilateral, and facial weakness), photophobia, blurred vision, seizures, and delirium.

Meningovascular Neurosyphilis. Meningovascular neurosyphilis most frequently occurs 5–12 years after infection, affecting about 3% of untreated syphilis patients. It is caused by thrombosis of vessels in the CNS and presents, as in other CNS ischemic events, with acute onset of symptoms. Hemiplegia, aphasia, hemianopsia, transverse myelitis, and progressive muscular atrophy may occur. Cranial nerve palsies may also occur, such as eighth nerve deafness and eye changes. The eyes may show fixed pupils, Argyll Robertson pupils, or anisocoria.

Late (Parenchymatous) Neurosyphilis. Parenchymatous neurosyphilis tends to occur more than 10 years after infection. There are two classic clinical patterns: tabes dorsalis and general paresis.

Tabes dorsalis is the degeneration of the dorsal roots of the spinal nerves and of the posterior columns of the spinal cord. The symptoms and signs are numerous. Gastric crisis with severe pain and vomiting is the most frequent symptom. Other symptoms are lancinating pains, urination difficulties, paresthesias (numbness, tingling, burning), spinal ataxia, diplopia, strabismus, vertigo, and deafness. The signs that may be present are Argyll Robertson pupils, absent or reduced reflexes, Romberg sign, deep tendon tenderness, loss of proprioception and vibratory sensation, atonic bladder, trophic changes, malum perforans pedis, Charcot joints, and optic atrophy.

Paresis has prodromal manifestations of headache, fatigability, and inability to concentrate. Later, personality changes occur, along with memory loss and apathy. Grandiose ideas, megalomania, delusions, hallucinations, and finally dementia may occur.

Late Cardiovascular Syphilis

Late cardiovascular syphilis occurs in about 10% of untreated patients. Aortitis is the basic lesion of cardiovascular syphilis, resulting in aortic insufficiency, coronary artery disease, and ultimately aortic aneurysm.

Congenital Syphilis

Congenital syphilis has reappeared with heterosexual syphilis epidemics. There were 195 cases of congenital syphilis reported in New York City from 2000 to 2009. Cases are also reported from Asia and Europe. In sub-Saharan Africa, where prenatal syphilis testing is not available, even for women with prenatal care, congenital syphilis is common. A total of 21% of all perinatal deaths in sub-Saharan Africa are caused by congenital syphilis. Prenatal syphilis is acquired in utero from the mother, who usually has early syphilis. Infection through the placenta usually does not occur before the fourth month, so treatment of the mother within the first two trimesters will almost always prevent negative outcomes. For this reason, prenatal care with syphilis serologies done in the early second trimester and at delivery (and any time in between if there is clinical suspicion of syphilis or high risk of acquisition of syphilis) is recommended. Common causes for failure to prevent congenital syphilis in mothers who received prenatal care are (1) lack of documented treatment of syphilis diagnosed before pregnancy, (2) absence of serologic testing during pregnancy, (3) late or no maternal treatment, and (4) treatment with a nonpenicillin regimen. If any of these is noted in the maternal history, congenital syphilis should still be suspected.

Recent reports from China suggest that preschool children may acquire syphilis by nonsexual close contact. In all cases, a caregiver had infectious syphilis, but sexual abuse was apparently excluded. This report suggests that the diagnosis of syphilis should be considered whenever the clinical manifestations suggest this possibility.

If the mother has early syphilis and prenatal infection occurs soon after the fourth month, fetal death and miscarriage occur in about 40% of pregnancies. During the remainder of the pregnancy, infection is equally likely to produce characteristic physical developmental stigmata or, after the eighth month, active, infectious congenital syphilis. About 40% of pregnant women with untreated early syphilis will have a syphilitic infant. Infant mortality rate from congenital syphilis can exceed 10%. In utero infection of the fetus is rare when the pregnant mother has had syphilis for 2 or more years. Two thirds of neonates with congenital syphilis are normal at birth and only detected by serologic testing. Lesions occurring within the first 2 years of life are called early congenital syphilis, and those developing thereafter, late congenital syphilis. The clinical manifestations of these two syndromes are different.

Early Congenital Syphilis

Early congenital syphilis describes those cases presenting within the first 2 years of life. Cutaneous manifestations usually appear during the third week of life, but sometimes occur as late as 3 months after birth. Neonates born with findings of congenital syphilis are usually severely affected. They may be premature and are often marasmic, fretful, and dehydrated. The face is pinched and drawn, resembling that of an old man or woman. Multisystem disease is characteristic.

Snuffles, a form of rhinitis, is the most frequent and often the first specific finding. The nose is blocked, often with blood-stained mucus, and a copious discharge of mucus runs down over the lips. The nasal obstruction often interferes with the child's nursing. In persistent and progressive snuffles, ulcerations develop that may involve the bones and ultimately cause perforation of the nasal septum or development of saddle nose, which are important stigmata later in the disease.

Cutaneous lesions of congenital syphilis resemble those of acquired secondary syphilis and occur in 30%–60% of infants with syphilis (Fig. 18.12). Annular lesions resembling those of neonatal lupus erythematosus may be present and may contain dermal mucin. The early skin eruptions are usually morbilliform and more rarely, purely papular. The lesions are at first a bright or violaceous red, later fading to a coppery color. The papules may become large and infiltrated; scaling often is pronounced. There is secondary pustule formation with crusting, especially in lesions that appear 1 year or more after birth. The eruption shows a marked predilection for the face, arms, buttocks, legs, palms, and soles.

Syphilitic pemphigus, a bullous eruption, usually on the palms and soles, is a relatively uncommon lesion. Lesions are present at birth or appear in the first week of life. They are teeming with spirochetes. The bullae quickly become purulent and rupture,

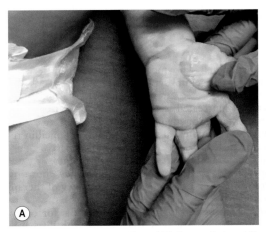
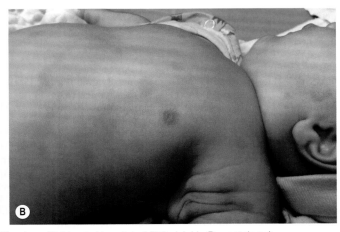

Fig. 18.12 (A and B) Congenital syphilis. (Courtesy Children's Hospital of Philadelphia Dermatology.)

leaving weeping erosions. They are found also on the eponychium, wrists, ankles, and infrequently on other parts of the body. Even in the absence of bullous lesions, desquamation is common, often preceded by edema and erythema, especially on the palms and soles.

Various morphologies of cutaneous lesions occur on the face, perineum, and intertriginous areas. These are usually fissured lesions resembling mucous patches. In these sites, radial scarring often results, leading to rhagades. Condylomata lata, large, moist, hypertrophic papules, are found around the anus and in other folds of the body. They are more common about the first year of life than in the newborn period. In the second or third year, recurrent secondary eruptions are likely to take the papulopustular form. Annular lesions occur, similar to those in adults. Mucous patches in the mouth or on the vulva are seen infrequently.

Bone lesions occur in 70%–80% of infants with early congenital syphilis. Epiphysitis is common and apparently causes pain on motion, leading to the infant refusing to move (Parrot pseudoparalysis). Radiologic features of the bone lesions in congenital syphilis during the first 6 months after birth are quite characteristic, and x-ray films are an important part of the evaluation of a child suspected of having congenital syphilis. Bone lesions occur chiefly at the epiphyseal ends of the long bones. The changes may be classified as osteochondritis, osteomyelitis, and osteoperiostitis.

A general enlargement of the lymph nodes usually occurs, with enlargement of the spleen. Clinical evidence of liver involvement is common, manifested by both hepatomegaly and elevated liver function test results, and interstitial hepatitis is a frequent finding at autopsy. The nephrotic syndrome and less often acute glomerulonephritis have been reported in congenital syphilis.

Symptomatic or asymptomatic neurosyphilis, as demonstrated by a positive CSF serologic test, may be present. Of infants with congenital syphilis diagnosed by clinical and laboratory findings born to mothers with untreated early syphilis, 86% will have CNS involvement, compared with only 8% of those with no clinical or laboratory findings. All infants with early congenital syphilis are treated as if they have neurosyphilis because it is very common, and CSF-VDRL test may be negative, even in documented CNS infection. Clinical manifestations may not appear until the third to sixth month of life and are meningeal or meningovascular in origin. Meningitis, obstructive hydrocephalus, cranial nerve palsies, and cerebrovascular accident (stroke) may all occur.

Late Congenital Syphilis

Although no sharp line can be drawn between early and late congenital syphilis, children who appear normal at birth and develop the first signs of the disease after age 2 years show a different clinical picture. Lesions of late congenital syphilis are of two types: persistent inflammatory foci and malformations of tissue affected at critical growth periods (stigmata).

Inflammatory Lesions. Lesions of the cornea, bones, and CNS are the most important. Interstitial keratitis, which begins with intense pericorneal inflammation and persists to characteristic diffuse clouding of the cornea without surface ulceration, occurs in 20%–50% of children with late congenital syphilis. If persistent, it leads to permanent, partial or complete opacity of the cornea. Syphilitic interstitial keratitis must be differentiated from Cogan syndrome, consisting of nonsyphilitic interstitial keratitis, usually bilateral, associated with vestibuloauditory symptoms, such as deafness, tinnitus, vertigo, nystagmus, and ataxia. It is congenital.

Perisynovitis (Clutton joints), which affects the knees, leads to symmetric, painless swelling. Gummas may also be found in any of the long bones or in the skull. Ulcerating gummas are frequently

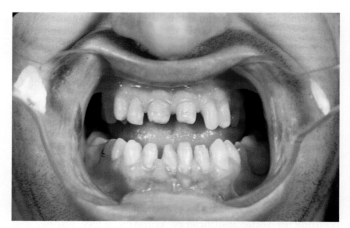

Fig. 18.13 Hutchinson teeth in congenital syphilis.

seen and probably begin more often in the soft parts or in the underlying bone than in the skin itself. When they occur in the nasal septum or palate, ulcerating gummas may lead to painless perforation.

The CNS lesions in late congenital syphilis are, as in late adult neurosyphilis, usually parenchymatous (tabes dorsalis or generalized paresis). Seizures are a frequent symptom in congenital cases.

Malformations (Stigmata). The destructive effects of syphilis in young children often leave scars or developmental defects called stigmata, which persist throughout life and confirm a diagnosis of congenital syphilis. Hutchinson emphasized the diagnostic importance of changes in the incisor teeth, opacities of the cornea, and eighth cranial nerve deafness, which have since become known as the Hutchinson triad. Hutchinson teeth, corneal scars, saber shins, rhagades of the lips, saddle nose, and mulberry molars are of diagnostic importance.

Hutchinson teeth are a malformation of the central upper incisors that appear in the secondary or permanent teeth. The characteristic teeth are cylindrical rather than flattened, the cutting edge is narrower than the base, and in the center of the cutting edge a notch may develop (Fig. 18.13). The mulberry molar, usually the first molar and appearing about age 6 years, is a hyperplastic tooth; its flat occlusal surface is covered with a group of little knobs representing abortive cusps. Nasal chondritis in infancy results in flattening of the nasal bones, forming a so-called saddle nose. The unilateral thickening of the inner third of one clavicle (Higouménaki sign) is a hyperostosis resulting from syphilitic osteitis in individuals who have had late congenital syphilis. The lesion appears typically on the right side in right-handed persons and on the left side in left-handed persons.

Diagnosis

Infants of women who meet the following criteria should be evaluated for congenital syphilis:

1. Maternal untreated syphilis, inadequate treatment, or no documentation of adequate treatment
2. Treatment of maternal syphilis with nonpenicillin regimen
3. Treatment less than 1 month before delivery
4. Inadequate maternal response to treatment
5. Appropriate treatment before pregnancy, but insufficient serologic follow-up to document adequacy of therapy

The results of serologic tests for syphilis for every woman delivering a baby must be known before the discharge of that baby from the hospital. Serologic testing of the mother and child at delivery are recommended. Evaluation of the children as just noted might include the following:

1. A complete physical examination for findings of congenital syphilis
2. Nontreponemal serology of the infant's serum (not cord blood)
3. CNS evaluation
4. Pathologic evaluation of the placenta using specific antitreponemal antibody staining

Treatment

Penicillin remains the drug of choice for treatment of all stages of syphilis. Erythromycin is not recommended for treatment of any stage or form of syphilis. HIV testing is recommended in all patients with syphilis. Treatment for HIV-infected patients is discussed later. Patients with primary, secondary, or early latent syphilis known to be of less than 1 year in duration can be treated with a single intramuscular injection of 2.4 million units (megaunits, MU) of benzathine penicillin G. In nonpregnant, penicillin-allergic, HIV-negative patients, tetracycline, 500 mg orally four times daily, or doxycycline, 100 mg orally twice daily for 2 weeks, is recommended. Ceftriaxone, 1 g intramuscularly or intravenously for 8–10 days, is an acceptable alternative if the patient cannot tolerate the previous options. Azithromycin and erythromycin can no longer be recommended as treatment for syphilis because of the worldwide presence of macrolide resistance, caused by a mutation in the gene encoding part of the ribosome responsible for binding macrolides. Close follow-up is recommended for all patients treated with non–penicillin-based regimens. These alternative agents are not recommended for persons with HIV infection and syphilis.

The recommended treatment of late or late latent syphilis of more than 1-year duration in an HIV-negative patient is benzathine penicillin G, 2.4 MU intramuscularly once weekly for 3 weeks. In a penicillin-allergic, nonpregnant, HIV-negative patient, doxycycline, 100 mg orally twice daily, for 14 days (28 days for latent syphilis) is recommended. Persons with a penicillin allergy whose compliance with therapy cannot be ensured should be desensitized and treated with benzathine penicillin. CSF evaluation is recommended if neurologic or ophthalmologic findings are present, if there is evidence of active late (tertiary) syphilis, if treatment has previously failed, if the nontreponemal serum titer is 1 : 32 or higher, or if any regimen not based on penicillin is planned.

Recommended treatment regimens for neurosyphilis include penicillin G crystalline, 3–4 MU intravenously every 4 hours for 10–14 days, or procaine penicillin, 2.4 MU/day intramuscularly, plus probenecid, 500 mg orally four times daily, both for 10–14 days. These regimens are shorter than those for treatment of late syphilis, so they may be followed by benzathine penicillin G, 2.4 MU intramuscularly, once weekly for 3 weeks. Patients allergic to penicillin should have their allergy confirmed by skin testing. If allergy exists, desensitization and treatment with penicillin are recommended.

Treatment of congenital syphilis in the neonate is complex. Therapy should be undertaken in consultation with a pediatric infectious disease specialist. Management strategies can be found in the CDC *Guidelines for the Management of Sexually Transmitted Diseases.* Older children with congenital syphilis should have a CSF evaluation and may be treated with aqueous crystalline penicillin G, 200,000–300,000 U/kg/day intravenously or intramuscularly (50,000 U every 4–6 hours) for 10–14 days. The CDC also lists benzathine penicillin G 50,000 U/kg intramuscularly, up to the adult dose of 2.4 million units in a single dose.

Pregnant women with syphilis should be treated with penicillin in doses appropriate for the stage of syphilis. A second dose of benzathine penicillin, 2.4 MU intramuscularly, may be administered 1 week after the initial dose in pregnant women with primary, secondary, or early latent syphilis. Sonographic evaluation of the fetus in the second half of pregnancy for signs of congenital infection may facilitate management and counseling. Expert consultation should be sought when evidence of fetal syphilis is found, because fetal treatment failure is increased in this situation. Follow-up quantitative serologic tests should be performed monthly until delivery. Pregnant women who are allergic to penicillin should be skin-tested and desensitized if test results are positive.

Jarisch-Herxheimer or Herxheimer Reaction

A febrile reaction often occurs after the initial dose of antisyphilitic treatment, especially penicillin, is given. Although historically reported to occur in more than 50% of patients treated for early syphilis, a recent report found a rate of only 10%. The reaction generally occurs 6–8 hours after treatment and consists of shaking chills, fever, malaise, sore throat, myalgia, headache, tachycardia, and exacerbation of the inflammatory reaction at sites of localized spirochetal infection. A vesicular Herxheimer reaction can occur. A Herxheimer reaction in pregnancy may induce premature labor and fetal distress. Every effort should be made to avoid this complication. Early in pregnancy, women should rest and take acetaminophen for fever. Women treated after 20 weeks of pregnancy should seek obstetric evaluation if they experience fever, decreased fetal movement, or regular contractions within 24 hours of treatment. Increased inflammation in a vital structure may have serious consequences, as when aneurysm of the aorta or iritis is present. When the CNS is involved, avoiding the Herxheimer reaction is especially important, even though the paralyses that may result are often transitory. It is important to distinguish the Herxheimer reaction from a drug reaction to penicillin or other antibiotics. The reaction has also been described in other spirochetal diseases, such as leptospirosis and louse-borne relapsing fever.

Treatment of Sex Partners

Sexual partners of persons with syphilis should be identified. Persons who are exposed within 90 days of the diagnosis of primary, secondary, or early latent syphilis, even if seronegative, should be treated presumptively. If the exposure occurred before 90 days of diagnosis but follow-up is uncertain, presumptive treatment should be given. If the infectious source has a serologic titer of greater than 1 : 32, the patient should be presumed to have infectious early syphilis, and sexual partners should be treated. At-risk partners are identified as those exposed within 3 months plus the duration of the primary lesions, for 6 months plus the duration of the secondary lesions, or 1 year for latent syphilis. Treatment of sexual partners is based on their clinical and serologic findings. If they are seronegative but had exposures as previously outlined, treatment would be as for early syphilis, with benzathine penicillin, 2.4 MU intramuscularly as one dose.

Serologic Testing After Treatment

Before therapy and then regularly thereafter, quantitative VDRL or RPR testing should be performed on patients who are to be treated for syphilis to ensure appropriate response.

Clinical and serologic evaluation should be performed at 6 and 12 months after treatment. A fourfold increase in serologic titer clearly indicates treatment failure or reinfection. Failure of nontreponemal test titers to decline fourfold within that time period may also indicate treatment failure, but 15%–20% of persons with primary and secondary syphilis will not achieve the fourfold decline at 1 year after treatment. These persons should receive additional clinical and serologic follow-up and be evaluated for HIV infection and CNS infection.

If it is decided to retreat the patient, injection of benzathine penicillin G 2.4 MU weekly for 3 weeks is recommended.

Patients treated for latent or late syphilis may be serofast, so failure to observe a titer fall in these patients does not in itself indicate a need for retreatment. If the titer is less than 1:32, the possibility of a serofast state exists, and retreatment should be planned on an individual basis.

Seroreversion in specific treponemal tests can occur. By 36 months, 24% of patients treated for early syphilis had a negative FTA-ABS and 13% had a negative MHA-TP.

Syphilis and HIV Disease

Syphilis and other genital or anal sexually transmitted diseases enhance the risk of transmission and acquisition of HIV. This may result from early lesions of syphilis containing mononuclear cells with enhanced expression of CCR5, the coreceptor for HIV-1. HIV testing is recommended in all patients with syphilis. Maternal syphilis increases the risk of HIV transmission to the infant.

Most HIV-infected patients with syphilis exhibit the classic clinical manifestations with appropriate serologic titers for that stage of disease. Responses to treatment, both clinical and serologic in HIV-infected patients with syphilis, generally follow the clinical and serologic patterns seen in patients without coexisting HIV infection. In a large study that compared HIV-positive and HIV-negative patients with syphilis, the former were more likely to present with secondary syphilis (53% vs. 33%) and were more likely to have a chancre that persisted when they had secondary syphilis (43% vs. 15%). Unusual clinical manifestations of syphilis in HIV range from florid skin lesions to few atypical ones, but these are exceptions, not the rule. Because most HIV-infected patients in large urban areas in the United States and Western Europe who acquire syphilis are MSM, chancres may be in atypical locations, such as the lips, tongue, or anus.

In general, the nontreponemal tests are of higher titer in HIV-infected persons. Rarely, the serologic response to infection may be impaired or delayed, and seronegative secondary syphilis has been reported. Biopsy of the skin lesions and histopathologic evaluation with special stains will confirm the diagnosis of syphilis in such patients. This approach, along with darkfield examination of appropriate lesions, should be considered if the clinical eruption is characteristic of syphilis and the serologic tests yield negative results.

Neurosyphilis has been frequently reported in HIV-infected persons, even after appropriate therapy for early syphilis. Manifestations have been those of early neurosyphilis or meningeal or meningovascular syphilis. These have included headache, fever, hemiplegia, and cranial nerve (CN) deficits, especially deafness (CN VIII), decreased vision (CN II), and ocular palsies (CNs III and VI). Whether HIV-infected persons are at increased risk for these complications or whether they occur more quickly is unknown. It is known that spirochetes are no more likely to remain in the CSF after treatment in HIV-infected persons than in HIV-negative persons. Whether the impaired host immunity allows these residual spirochetes to cause clinical relapse more frequently or more quickly in the setting of HIV is unknown.

Patients with HIV infection who have primary or secondary syphilis, who are not allergic to penicillin, and who have no neurologic or psychiatric findings should be treated with benzathine penicillin G, 2.4 MU intramuscularly. There is no evidence that additional treatment will reduce the risk of treatment failure. Patients who are allergic to penicillin should be desensitized and treated with penicillin. Following treatment, the patient should have serologic follow-up with quantitative nontreponemal tests at 3, 6, 9, 12, and 24 months. Failure of the titer to fall is an indication for reevaluation, including lumbar puncture. Factors associated with treatment failure in HIV disease include a low initial serologic titer (RPR <1:16), a history of prior syphilis, and a CD4 count less than 350 cells/mL.

Because of the concerns about neurologic relapse in the syphilitic patient with HIV disease, more careful CNS evaluation is advocated. Lumbar puncture is recommended in HIV-infected patients with latent syphilis (of any duration), with late syphilis (even with a normal neurologic examination), and with any neurologic or psychiatric signs or symptoms. If RPR is 1:32 or greater and CD4 count is less than 350 cells/mL, neurosyphilis is more likely, and lumbar puncture can be considered. Treatment in these patients will be determined by the result of their CSF evaluation. HIV-infected patients with primary or secondary syphilis should be counseled about their possible increased risk of CNS relapse.

Benzathine penicillin, 2.4 MU intramuscularly, should be used to treat all HIV-infected contacts of patients with syphilis who are at risk of acquiring infection.

An Q, et al: Syphilis screening and diagnosis among men who have sex with men, 2008-2014, 20 U.S. cities. J Acquir Immune Defic Syndr 2017; 75: S363.

Cid PM, et al: Pathologically confirmed malignant syphilis using immunohistochemical staining. Sex Transm Dis 2014; 41: 94.

Czerninski R, et al: Oral syphilis lesions. Quintessence Int 2011; 42: 883.

de Voux A, et al: State-specific rates of primary and secondary syphilis among men who have sex with men—United States, 2015. MMWR Morb Mortal Wkly Rep 2017; 66: 349.

Flamm A, et al: Histologic features of secondary syphilis. J Am Acad Dermatol 2015; 73: 1025.

Forrest CE, et al: Clinical diagnosis of syphilis. Int J STD AIDS 2016; 27: 1334.

Galvao TF, et al: Safety of benzathine penicillin for preventing congenital syphilis. PLoS One 2013; 8: e56463.

Gulland A: Number of cases of syphilis continue to rise. BMJ 2017; 357: j2807.

Harding AS, Ghanem KG: The performance of cerebrospinal fluid treponemal-specific antibody tests in neurosyphilis. Sex Transm Dis 2012; 39: 291.

Iwahashi M, Kusama Y: Congenital syphilis. Pediatr Int 2017; 59: 746.

John-Stewart G, et al: Prevention of Mother-to-Child Transmission of HIV and Syphilis. In: Holmes KK, Bertozzi S, Bloom BR, Jha P, editors. Major Infectious Diseases. 3rd edition. Washington (DC): The International Bank for Reconstruction and Development / The World Bank; 2017 Nov 3. Chapter 6. PubMed PMID: 30212095.

Katanami Y, et al: Amoxicillin and ceftriaxone as treatment alternatives to penicillin for maternal syphilis. Emerg Infect Dis 2017; 23: 827.

Kinikar A, et al: Maternal syphilis. Sex Transm Dis 2017; 44: 371.

Knaute DF, et al: Serological response to treatment of syphilis according to disease stage and HIV status. Clin Infect Dis 2012; 55: 1615.

Kojima N, et al: An Update on the Global Epidemiology of Syphilis. Curr Epidemiol Rep. 2018 Mar;5(1):24-38. doi: 10.1007/s40471-018-0138-z. Epub 2018 Feb 19. PubMed PMID: 30116697; PubMed Central PMCID: PMC6089383.

Kubanov A, et al: Novel *Treponema pallidum* recombinant antigens for syphilis diagnostics. Biomed Res Int 2017; 2017: 1436080.

Mayer KH. Old Pathogen, New Challenges: A Narrative Review of the Multilevel Drivers of Syphilis Increasing in American Men Who Have Sex With Men. Sex Transm Dis. 2018 Sep;45(9S Suppl 1):S38-S41. doi: 10.1097/OLQ.0000000000000815. PubMed PMID: 30106386; PubMed Central PMCID: PMC6093307.

Ong D, et al: Keeping an eye on syphilis. Aust Fam Physician 2017; 46: 401.

Parker SR, et al: Seronegative syphilis. Int J Infect Dis 2014; 18: 104.

Pham MN, et al: Penicillin desensitization. Ann Allergy Asthma Immunol 2017; 118: 537.

Quilter L, et al: Prevention of sexually transmitted diseases in HIV-infected individuals. Curr HIV/AIDS Rep 2017; 14: 41.

Rosa G, et al: Secondary syphilis in HIV positive individuals. J Cutan Pathol 2016; 43: 847.

Shockman S, et al: Syphilis in the United States. Clin Dermatol 2014; 32: 213.

Stamm LV: Syphilis. Microb Cell 2016; 3: 363.

Tsimis ME, et al: Update on syphilis and pregnancy. Birth Defects Res 2017; 109: 347.

US Preventive Services Task Force, Curry SJ, et al: Screening for Syphilis Infection in Pregnant Women: US Preventive Services Task Force Reaffirmation Recommendation Statement. JAMA. 2018 Sep 4;320(9):911-917. doi: 10.1001/jama.2018.11785. PubMed PMID: 30193283.

White AC Jr: Treatment of early syphilis in HIV. Clin Infect Dis. 2017; 64: 765.

Zhang J, Izzo A: Meningovascular syphilis. Neurohospitalist 2017; 7: 145.

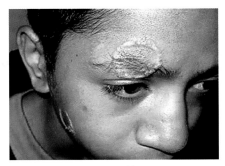

Fig. 18.14 Yaws.

NONVENEREAL TREPONEMATOSES: YAWS, ENDEMIC SYPHILIS, AND PINTA

This group of diseases is called the endemic or nonvenereal treponematoses. They share many epidemiologic and pathologic features. As with venereal syphilis, the clinical manifestations are divided into early and late stages. Early disease is considered infectious and lasts for approximately 5 years. There are periods of latency. The histology is similar in all the diseases and resembles venereal syphilis. Cutaneous manifestations are prominent. The bones and mucosa may also be involved in some cases (except in pinta). Cardiovascular and nervous system involvement and congenital disease are not seen. Children younger than 15 years are primarily affected. Person-to-person contact or sharing of a drinking vessel is the mode of transmission.

The endemic treponematoses are closely related to poverty and a lack of available health services. They are described as occurring "where the road ends." These diseases tend to occur in the tropics, especially yaws, and the wearing of few clothes and a hot, humid climate are associated with higher prevalence. In endemic areas, as hygiene improves, "attenuated" forms of yaws and endemic syphilis appear. A larger percentage of the population is latently infected, and secondary lesions are fewer in number, drier, and limited to moist skinfolds. Instead of several "crops" of eruptions lasting months to years, infected persons have only a single crop. Transmission is thus reduced, although a large percentage of the population may be infected.

Yaws was nearly eradicated during the 1950s through mass-treatment campaigns, but has undergone a resurgence in Cameroon, Fiji, Indonesia, Timor, Papua New Guinea, the Solomon Islands, and Vanuatu. The discovery of treponemal infection with a high genetic similarity to yaws in monkeys in Africa suggests a possible animal reservoir for this infection, and evidence suggests that necrophagous flies can carry and spread the organism, further complicating eradication efforts.

Yaws (Pian, Frambesia, Bouba)

Yaws is caused by *Treponema pallidum* subsp. *pertenue*. It is transmitted nonsexually, by contact with infectious lesions. Yaws predominantly affects children younger than 15 years. The disease has a disabling course, affecting the skin, bones, and joints, and is divided into early (primary and secondary) and late (tertiary) disease.

Early Yaws

A primary papule or group of papules appears at the site of inoculation after an incubation period of about 3 weeks (10 days to 3 months), during which there may be headache, malaise, and other mild constitutional symptoms. The initial lesion becomes crusted and larger (2–5 cm) and is known as the "mother yaw" (maman pian). The crusts are amber-yellow. They may be knocked off, forming an ulcer with a red, pulpy, granulated surface, but quickly reform, so that the typical yaws lesion is crusted. The lesion is not indurated. There may be some regional adenopathy.

Exposed parts are most frequently involved—the extremities, particularly the lower legs, feet, buttocks, and face—although the mother's breasts and trunk may be infected by her child. The lesion is almost always extragenital, and when genital, is a result of accidental contact rather than intercourse. After being present for about 3–6 months, the mother yaw spontaneously disappears, leaving slight atrophy and depigmentation.

Weeks or months after the primary lesion appears, secondary yaws develops. Secondary lesions resemble the mother yaw, but they are smaller and may appear around the primary lesions or in a generalized pattern. The secondary lesions may clear centrally and coalesce peripherally, forming annular lesions (ringworm yaws or tinea yaws) (Fig. 18.14). The palms and soles may be involved, resembling secondary syphilis. In some sites, especially around the body orifices and in the armpits, groins, and gluteal crease, condylomatous lesions may arise, resembling condyloma latum of secondary syphilis. In drier endemic regions and during drier seasons, lesions tend to be fewer, less papillomatous, and more scaly, and instead of being generalized, favor the folds of the axillae, groin, and oral cavity. Yaws in the dry seasons and dry geographic areas closely resembles endemic syphilis. The palms and soles may develop thick, hyperkeratotic plaques that fissure. They are painful, resulting in a crablike gait (crab yaws). At times there is paronychia. Generalized lymphadenopathy, arthralgias, headaches, and malaise are common. With improved nutrition and hygiene, an "attenuated" form, with only scattered, flat, gray lesions in intertriginous areas, has been described.

Over a few weeks or months, the secondary lesions may undergo spontaneous involution, leaving either no skin changes or hypopigmented macules that later become hyperpigmented. However, the eruption may persist for many months as a result of fresh, recurrent outbreaks. The course is slower in adults than in children, in whom the secondary period rarely lasts longer than 6 months. During latency, skin lesions may relapse for as long as 5 years. Painful osteoperiostitis and polydactylitis may present in early yaws as fusiform swelling of the hands, feet, arms, and legs.

Late Yaws

The disease usually terminates with the secondary stage, but in about 10% of patients, it progresses to the late stage, usually 5–10 years after initial infection. The typical late-yaws skin lesions are gummas that present as indolent ulcers with clean-cut or undermined edges. They tend to fuse and form configurate and occasionally serpiginous patterns clinically indistinguishable from those of tertiary syphilis. On healing, these lesions scar, leading to contractures and deformities. Hyperkeratotic palmoplantar plaques and keratoderma frequently recur in the late stage.

Similar processes may occur in the skeletal system and other deep structures, leading to painful nodes on the bones, or destruction of the palate and nasal bone (gangosa). There may be periostitis, particularly of the tibia (saber shin, saber tibia), epiphysitis, chronic synovitis, and juxta-articular nodules. Goundou is a rare proliferative osteitis initially affecting the nasal aspects of the maxilla. Two large, hard tumors form on the lateral aspects of the nose. These can significantly obstruct vision. The process may extend into other bones of the central face, affecting the palate and nose, and resulting in protrusion of the whole central face as a mass. Although yaws is classically thought to spare the eye and nervous system, abnormal CSF findings in early yaws and scattered reports of eye and neurologic findings in patients with late yaws suggest that yaws, like syphilis, has the potential to cause neurologic or ophthalmic sequelae, although rarely.

Histopathology

Early yaws shows epidermal edema, acanthosis, papillomatosis, neutrophilic intraepidermal microabscesses, and a moderate to dense perivascular infiltrate of lymphocytes and plasma cells. Treponemas are usually demonstrable in the primary and secondary stages with the use of the same silver stains employed in diagnosing syphilis. Tertiary yaws shows features identical to the gumma of tertiary syphilis.

Diagnosis

The diagnosis should be suspected from the typical clinical appearance in a person living in an endemic region. The presence of keratoderma palmaris et plantaris in such a person is highly suggestive of yaws. Darkfield demonstration of spirochetes in the early lesions and a reactive VDRL or RPR test can be used to confirm primary and secondary yaws.

Endemic Syphilis (Bejel)

Bejel is a Bedouin term for this nonvenereal treponematosis, which occurs primarily in the seminomadic tribes who live in the arid regions of North Africa, Southwest Asia, and the eastern Mediterranean. The etiologic agent of bejel is *Treponema pallidum* subsp. *endemicum*. It occurs primarily in childhood and is spread by skin contact or from mouth to mouth by kissing or use of contaminated drinking vessels. The skin, oral mucosa, and skeletal system are primarily involved.

Primary lesions are rare, probably occurring undetected in the oropharyngeal mucosa. The most common presentation is with secondary oral lesions resembling mucous patches. These are shallow, relatively painless ulcerations, occasionally accompanied by laryngitis. Split papules, angular cheilitis, condylomatous lesions of the moist folds of the axillae and groin, and a nonpruritic generalized papular eruption may be seen. Generalized lymphadenopathy is common. Osteoperiostitis of the long bones may occur, causing nocturnal leg pains.

Untreated secondary bejel heals in 6–9 months. The tertiary stage can occur between 6 months and several years after the early symptoms resolve. In the tertiary stage, leg pain (periostitis) and gummatous ulcerations of the skin, nasopharynx, and bone occur. Gangosa (rhinopharyngitis mutilans) can result. Rarely reported neurologic sequelae seem to be restricted to the eye, including uveitis, choroiditis, chorioretinitis, and optic atrophy. As with yaws, with improved nutrition, an attenuated form of endemic syphilis

occurs, often presenting with leg pain from periostitis. The diagnosis of bejel is confirmed by the same means as for venereal syphilis.

Pinta

Pinta is an infectious, nonvenereal, endemic treponematosis caused by *Treponema carateum*. The mode of transmission is unknown, but repeated, direct, lesion-to-skin contact is likely. Only skin lesions occur. By contrast with yaws and bejel, pinta affects persons of all ages, favoring those 14–30 years old. It was once prevalent in the forests and rural areas of Central and South America and Cuba, but it is now rarely reported. The manifestations of pinta may be divided into primary, secondary (early), and tertiary (late) stages. Historically, however, patients may describe continuous evolution from secondary dyspigmented lesions to the characteristic achromic lesions of tertiary pinta.

Primary Stage

It is believed that the initial lesion appears 7–60 days after inoculation. The lesion begins as a tiny red papule that becomes an elevated, poorly defined, erythematous, infiltrated plaque up to 10–12.5 cm in diameter over 2–3 months. Expansion of the primary lesion may occur by fusion with surrounding satellite macules or papules. Ultimately, it becomes impossible to distinguish the primary lesion from the secondary lesions. At no time is there erosion or ulceration such as occurs in the syphilitic chancre. Most initial lesions of pinta develop on the legs and other uncovered parts. The RPR and VDRL tests are nonreactive in the primary stage. Darkfield examination may be positive.

Secondary Stage

The secondary stage of pinta appears 5 months to 1 year or more after infection. It begins with small, scaling papules that may enlarge and coalesce, simulating psoriasis, ringworm, eczema, syphilis, or Hansen disease. The papules are located mostly on the extremities and face and frequently are somewhat circinate. Over time, the initially red to violaceous lesions show postinflammatory hyperpigmentation, in shades of gray, blue, or brown, or hypopigmentation. Secondary lesions are classified as erythematous, desquamative, hypochromic, or hyperchromic. Multiple different morphologies may be present simultaneously, giving a very polymorphous appearance. Nontreponemal tests for syphilis are reactive in the secondary stage in about 60% of pinta patients. Darkfield examination may show spirochetes.

Late Dyschromic Stage

Until the 1940s the late pigmentary changes were the only recognized clinical manifestations of pinta. These have an insidious onset, usually in adolescents or young adults, of widespread depigmented macules resembling vitiligo. The lesions are located chiefly on the face, waistline, wrist flexures, and trochanteric region, although diffuse involvement may occur, so that large areas on the trunk and extremities are affected. The lesions are symmetric in more than one third of patients. Hemipinta is a rare variety of the disease in which the pigmentary disturbances affect only half the body. In the late dyschromic stage of pinta, the serologic test for syphilis is positive in nearly all patients.

Histopathology

Skin lesions in early pinta show moderate acanthosis; occasionally, lichenoid changes with basal layer vacuolization; and an upper dermal perivascular infiltrate of lymphocytes and plasma cells.

Melanophages are prominent in the upper dermis. Spirochetes may be demonstrated in the epidermis by special stains in primary, secondary, and hyperpigmented lesions of tertiary pinta. In tertiary pinta, the depigmented skin shows a loss of basal pigment, pigmentary incontinence, and virtually no dermal inflammatory infiltrate. Spirochetes are rarely found in depigmented tertiary lesions.

Treatment

The treatment of choice for all endemic treponematoses is benzathine penicillin G, 1.2–2.4 MU intramuscularly (0.6–1.2 MU for children under age 10). In penicillin-allergic patients, tetracycline, 500 mg four times daily for adults, or erythromycin, 8–10 mg/kg four times daily for children, for 15 days is recommended. Penicillin-resistant yaws has been reported from New Guinea, and a single oral dose of azithromycin (30 mg/kg) has been shown to be noninferior to benzathine penicillin for the treatment of early yaws, supporting the WHO policy for use of oral azithromycin in resource-poor settings. The dose recommended for trachoma is lower than that for yaws, but also lowers the prevalence of yaws infection. In tertiary pinta, the blue color gradually disappears, as do the areas of partial depigmentation. The vitiliginous areas, if present for more than 5 years, are permanent.

Eradication of the endemic treponematoses is possible with persistent and effective treatment strategies, including the following:

1. Screening of the whole population in endemic areas
2. Diagnosis of patients seen at health services and by community outreach
3. Health education
4. Improved hygiene (soap and water)

If more than 10% of the population is affected, the whole population is treated (mass treatment). If 5%–10% of the population is affected, treat all active cases, all children younger than 15, and all contacts (juvenile mass treatment). If less than 5% of the population is infected, treat all active cases and all household and close personal contacts (selective mass treatment). Unfortunately, with the areas affected by the endemic treponematoses also struggling with epidemics of HIV, tuberculosis, and malaria, eradication programs have been largely discontinued.

Ayove T, et al: Sensitivity and specificity of a rapid point-of-care test for active yaws. Lancet Glob Health 2014; 2: e415.

Boock AU, et al: Yaws resurgence in Bankim, Cameroon. PLoS Negl Trop Dis 2017; 11: e0005557.

Cocks N, et al: Community seroprevalence survey for yaws and trachoma in the western division of Fiji. Trans R Soc Trop Med Hyg 2016; 110: 582.

Eckhoff G, et al: Mass treatment with single-dose azithromycin for yaws. N Engl J Med 2016; 375: 1093.

Engelman D, et al: Opportunities for integrated control of neglected tropical diseases that affect the skin. Trends Parasitol 2016; 32: 843.

Giacani L, Lukehart SA: The endemic treponematoses. Clin Microbiol Rev 2014; 27: 89.

Kazadi WM, et al: Epidemiology of yaws. Clin Epidemiol 2014; 6: 119.

Kwakye-Maclean C, et al: A single dose oral azithromycin versus intramuscular benzathine penicillin for the treatment of yaws. PLoS Negl Trop Dis 2017; 11: e0005154.

Marks M, et al: Endemic treponemal diseases. Trans R Soc Trop Med Hyg 2014; 108: 601.

Marks M, et al: Metaanalysis of the performance of a combined treponemal and nontreponemal rapid diagnostic test for syphilis and yaws. Clin Infect Dis 2016; 63: 627.

Marks M, et al: Prevalence of active and latent yaws in the Solomon Islands 18 months after azithromycin mass drug administration for trachoma. PLoS Negl Trop Dis 2016; 10: e0004927.

Mitjà O, et al: Advances in the diagnosis of endemic treponematoses. PLoS Negl Trop Dis 2013; 7: e2283.

Mitjà O, et al: Yaws. Lancet 2013; 381: 763.

Stamm LV: Flies and yaws. EBioMedicine 2016; 11: 9.

19 Viral Diseases

Viruses are obligatory intracellular parasites. The structural components of a viral particle (virion) consist of a central core of nucleic acid, a protective protein coat (capsid), and (in certain groups of viruses only) an outermost membrane or envelope. The capsid of the simplest viruses consists of many identical polypeptides (structural units) that fold and interact with one another to form morphologic units (capsomeres). The number of capsomeres is believed to be constant for each virus with cubic symmetry, and it is an important criterion in the classification of viruses. The protein coat determines serologic specificity, protects the nucleic acid from enzymatic degradation in biologic environments, controls host specificity, and increases the efficiency of infection. The outermost membrane of the enveloped viruses is essential for the attachment to, and penetration of, host cells. The envelope also contains important viral antigens.

Two main groups of viruses are distinguished: deoxyribonucleic acid (DNA) and ribonucleic acid (RNA). The DNA virus types are parvovirus, papovavirus, adenovirus, herpesvirus, and poxvirus. RNA viruses are picornavirus, togavirus, reovirus, coronavirus, orthomyxovirus, retrovirus, arenavirus, rhabdovirus, and paramyxovirus. Some viruses are distinguished by their mode of transmission: arthropod-borne viruses, respiratory viruses, fecal-oral or intestinal viruses, venereal viruses, and penetrating-wound viruses.

HERPESVIRUS GROUP

The herpes viruses are medium-sized viruses that contain double-stranded (ds) DNA and replicate in the cell nucleus. They are characterized by the ability to produce latent but lifelong infection by infecting immunologically protected cells (immune cells and nerves). Intermittently, they have replicative episodes with amplification of the viral numbers in anatomic sites conducive to transmission from one host to the next (genital skin, orolabial region). The vast majority of infected persons remain asymptomatic. Viruses in this group are varicella-zoster virus (VZV; human herpesvirus type 3 [HHV-3]); herpes simplex virus types 1 and 2 (HSV-1 and HSV-2); cytomegalovirus (CMV); Epstein-Barr virus (EBV); human herpesviruses types 6, 7, and 8 (HHV-6, HHV-7, and HHV-8); *Herpesvirus simiae* (B virus); and other viruses of animals.

Herpes Simplex Virus (Human Herpesvirus Types 1 and 2)

Infection with HSV is one of the most prevalent infections worldwide. HSV-1 infection, the cause of most cases of orolabial herpes, is more common than infection with HSV-2, the classical cause of most cases of genital herpes, though rates of HSV-1 in genital herpes has been rising, particularly in younger patients. Between 30% and 95% of adults (depending on the country and group tested) are seropositive for HSV-1, although seroprevalence of HSV-1 has decreased in the United States among adolescents (age 14–19 years) more recently. Seroprevalence for HSV-2 is lower, and it appears at the age of onset of sexual activity. About 2.4% of adults become infected annually with HSV-2 in their third decade of life. In the United States about 25% of adults are infected with HSV-2, with black men and women twice as likely to be HSV-2 infected as whites. In sexually transmitted disease (STD) clinic patients, the infection rate is 30%–50%. In sub-Saharan Africa, infection rates are 60%–95%. Worldwide, the seroprevalence is higher in persons infected with human immunodeficiency virus (HIV). Serologic data show that many more people are infected than give a history of clinical disease. For HSV-1, about 50% of infected persons give a history of orolabial lesions. For HSV-2, 20% of infected persons are completely asymptomatic (latent infection), 20% have recurrent genital herpes they recognize, and 60% have clinical lesions that they do not recognize as genital herpes (subclinical or unrecognized infection). Most persons with HSV-2 infection are symptomatic, but the majority do not recognize that their symptoms are caused by HSV. All persons infected with HSV-1 and HSV-2 are potentially infectious even if they have no clinical signs or symptoms. Routine screening for HSV in asymptomatic patients, including those who are pregnant, is not currently recommended; testing is appropriate in patients with signs or symptoms of the disease.

Herpes simplex infections are classified as either "first episode" or "recurrent." Most patients have no lesions or findings when they are initially infected with HSV. When patients have their first clinical lesion, this is usually a recurrence. Because the initial clinical presentation is not associated with a new infection, the previous terminology of "primary" infection has been abandoned. Instead, the initial clinical presentation is called a first episode and may represent a true primary infection or a recurrence. Persons with chronic or acute immunosuppression may have prolonged and atypical clinical courses.

Infections with HSV-1 or HSV-2 are diagnosed by specific and nonspecific methods. Bedside, in-office diagnosis can be made using the Tzanck smear. It is nonspecific because both HSV and VZV infections result in the formation of multinucleate epidermal giant cells. Although the technique is rapid, its success depends heavily on the skill of the interpreter. The accuracy rate is 60%–90%, with a false-positive rate of 3%–13%. The direct fluorescent antibody (DFA) test is more accurate and will identify virus type; results can be available in hours if a virology laboratory is nearby. Both Tzanck, which is neither sensitive nor specific, and DFA, which is nonspecific, are less useful than viral culture or polymerase chain reaction (PCR) testing. Viral culture is very specific and relatively rapid, compared with serologic tests, because HSV is stable in transport and grows readily and rapidly in culture, and can be used for antiviral sensitivity testing if necessary, though it can be expensive to culture virus. Results are often available in 48–72 hours. PCR is as specific as viral culture but four times more sensitive and can be performed on dried or fixed tissue, and is becoming increasingly viewed as the test of choice. Skin biopsies of lesions can detect viropathic changes caused by HSV, and with specific HSV antibodies, immunoperoxidase (IP) techniques can accurately diagnose infection. The accuracy of various tests depends on lesion morphology. Only acute, vesicular lesions are likely to be positive with Tzanck smears. Crusted, eroded, or ulcerative lesions are best diagnosed by viral culture, DFA, histologic methods, or PCR.

Serologic tests are generally not used in determining whether a skin lesion is caused by HSV infection. A positive serologic test indicates only that the individual is infected with that virus, not that the viral infection is the cause of the current lesion. In addition to determining the infection rate in various populations, serologic tests are most useful in evaluating couples in which only one partner gives a history of genital herpes (discordant couples), in

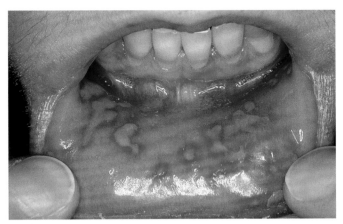

Fig. 19.1 Herpetic gingivostomatitis, extensive erosions of the oral mucosa.

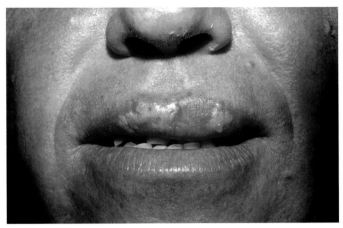

Fig. 19.2 Recurrent herpes simplex infection.

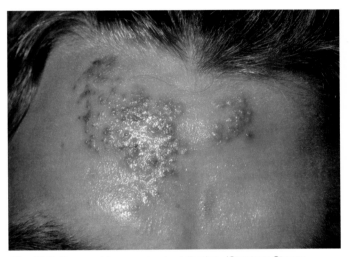

Fig. 19.3 Recurrent herpes simplex infection. (Courtesy Steven Binnick, MD.)

couples (if childbearing) at risk for neonatal herpes infection, and for possible HSV vaccination (when available).

Orolabial Herpes

Orolabial herpes is virtually always caused by HSV-1. In 1% or less of newly infected persons, herpetic gingivostomatitis develops, mainly in children and young adults (Fig. 19.1). The onset is often accompanied by high fever, regional lymphadenopathy, and malaise. The herpetic lesions in the mouth are usually broken vesicles that appear as erosions or ulcers covered with a white membrane. The erosions may become widespread on the oral mucosa, tongue, and tonsils, and the gingival margin is usually eroded. Herpetic gingivostomatitis produces pain, foul breath, and dysphagia. In young children, dehydration may occur. It may cause pharyngitis, with ulcerative or exudative lesions of the posterior pharynx. The duration, untreated, is 1–2 weeks. If the initial episode of herpetic gingivostomatitis or herpes labialis is so severe that intravenous (IV) administration is required, IV acyclovir, 5 mg/kg three times daily, is recommended. Oral therapeutic options include acyclovir suspension, 15 mg/kg five times daily for 7 days; valacyclovir, 1 g twice daily for 7 days; or famciclovir, 500 mg twice daily for 7 days. This therapy reduces the duration of the illness by more than 50%.

The most frequent clinical manifestation of orolabial herpes is the "cold sore" or "fever blister." Recurrent HSV-1 is the cause of 95% or more of cases and typically presents as grouped blisters on an erythematous base. The lips near the vermilion are most frequently involved (Fig. 19.2), although lesions may occur wherever the virus was inoculated or proliferated during the initial episode (Fig. 19.3). Recurrences may be seen on the cheeks, eyelids, and earlobes. Oral recurrent HSV usually affects the keratinized surfaces of the hard palate and attached gingiva. Outbreaks are variable in severity, partly related to the trigger of the outbreak. Some outbreaks are small and resolve rapidly, whereas others may be severe, involving both the upper and the lower lip. In severe outbreaks, lip swelling is often present. Patient symptomatology is variable. A prodrome of up to 24 hours of tingling, itching, or burning may precede the outbreak. Local discomfort, as well as headache, nasal congestion, or mild flulike symptoms, may occur. Ultraviolet (UV) exposure, especially UVB, is a frequent trigger of recurrent orolabial HSV, and severity of the outbreak may correlate with intensity of the sun exposure. Surgical and dental procedures of the lips (or other areas previously affected with HSV) may trigger recurrences, and a history of prior HSV should be solicited in all patients in whom such procedures are recommended (see next section).

In most patients, recurrent orolabial herpes represents more of a nuisance than a disease. Because UVB radiation is a common trigger, use of a sunblock daily on the lips and facial skin may reduce recurrences. All topical therapies for the acute treatment of recurrent orolabial herpes have limited efficacy, reducing disease duration and pain by 1 day or less. Tetracaine cream, penciclovir cream, and acyclovir cream (not ointment) have some limited efficacy. Topical acyclovir ointment and docosanol cream provide minimal to no reduction in healing time or discomfort. The minimal benefit from these topical agents suggests that they should not be recommended for significant symptomatic orolabial herpes outbreaks. If oral therapy is contemplated for patients with severely symptomatic recurrences of orolabial HSV, it must be remembered that much higher doses of oral antivirals are required than for treatment of genital herpes. Intermittent treatment with valacyclovir, 2 g twice daily for 1 day, or famciclovir, 1.5 g as a single dose, starting at the onset of the prodrome, are simple and effective oral, 1-day regimens. Because the patient's own inflammatory reaction against the virus contributes substantially to the severity of lesions of orolabial herpes simplex, topical therapy with a high-potency topical corticosteroid (fluocinonide gel 0.05%, three times daily) in combination with an oral antiviral agent more rapidly reduces pain and reduces maximum lesion area and time to healing. In nonimmunosuppressed patients, if episodic treatment for orolabial HSV is recommended and an oral agent is used, the addition of a high-potency topical corticosteroid should be considered. In patients with six or more outbreaks per year, chronic suppressive daily antiviral therapy can be used. Squaric acid dibutyl ester has been used as an immunosensitizer in one small study to reduce recurrent outbreaks.

Although most patients with orolabial herpes simplex do not require treatment, certain medical and dental procedures may trigger outbreaks of HSV. If the cutaneous surface has been damaged by the surgical procedure (e.g., dermabrasion, chemical peel, laser resurfacing), the surgical site can be infected by the virus and may result in prolonged healing and possible scarring. Prophylaxis is regularly used before such surgeries in patients with a history of orolabial herpes simplex. Famciclovir, 250 mg twice daily, and valacyclovir, 500 mg twice daily, or oral acyclovir 400 mg three times daily, are prophylactic options, to be begun 24 hours before the procedure. Duration of treatment in part depends on severity of the skin insult and rate of healing but should be at least 1 week and could be as long as 14 days. For routine surgeries at sites of HSV recurrences (upper or lower lip), acyclovir, 200 mg five times daily; famciclovir, 250 mg three times daily; or valacyclovir, 1 g twice daily, starting 2–5 days before the procedure and continuing for 5 days, can be considered. Prophylaxis could also be considered before skiing or tropical vacations and before extensive dental procedures, at the same dosages. Reactivation of orolabial herpes has also been associated with hyaluronic acid filler injections in about 1.5% of patients; and extensive facial HSV-1 infection has followed intense inhaled corticosteroid therapy. Kissing of the penis during circumcision can lead to penile HSV-1 infection, which can present acutely, or even years after the initial exposure. Some of these infants have died of disseminated or central nervous system HSV infection.

Herpetic Sycosis

Recurrent or initial herpes simplex infections (usually from HSV-1) may primarily affect the hair follicle. The clinical appearance may vary from a few eroded follicular papules (resembling acne excoriée) to extensive lesions involving the whole beard area in men (Fig. 19.4). Close razor blade shaving immediately before initial exposure

or in the presence of an acute orolabial lesion may be associated with a more extensive eruption. The onset may be acute (over days) or more subacute or chronic. Diagnostic clues include the tendency for erosions, a self-limited course of 2–3 weeks, and an appropriate risk behavior. The diagnosis may be confirmed by biopsy. Although the herpes infection is primarily in the follicle, surface cultures of eroded lesions will usually be positive in the first 5–7 days of the eruption.

Herpes Gladiatorum

Infection with HSV-1 is highly contagious to susceptible persons who wrestle with an infected individual with an active lesion. One third of susceptible wrestlers will become infected after a single match. In tournaments and wrestling camps, outbreaks can be epidemic, affecting up to 20% of all participants. Lesions usually occur on the lateral side of the neck, the side of the face, and the forearm, all areas in direct contact with the face of the infected wrestler (Fig. 19.5). Vesicles appear 4–11 days after exposure, often preceded by 24 hours of malaise, sore throat, and fever. Ocular symptoms may occur. Lesions are frequently misdiagnosed as a bacterial folliculitis. Any wrestler with a confirmed history of orolabial herpes should be taking suppressive antiviral therapy during all periods of training and competition. Rugby players (especially forwards who participate in scrums), mixed–martial arts fighters, and even boxers are also at risk.

Herpetic Whitlow

Herpes simplex infection may occur infrequently on the fingers or periungually. Lesions begin with tenderness and erythema, usually of the lateral nailfold or on the palm. Deep-seated blisters develop 24–48 hours after symptoms begin (Fig. 19.6). The blisters may be tiny, under the thick epidermis, and require careful inspection to detect them. Deep-seated lesions that appear unilocular may be mistaken for a paronychia or other inflammatory process. Lesions may progress to erosions or may heal without ever impairing epidermal integrity because of the thick stratum corneum in this location. Herpetic whitlow may simulate a felon. Swelling of the affected hand can occur. Lymphatic streaking and swelling of the epitrochlear or axillary lymph nodes may occur, mimicking a bacterial cellulitis. Repeated episodes of herpetic lymphangitis may lead to persistent lymphedema of the affected hand. Herpetic whitlow has become much less common among health care workers since the institution of universal precautions and glove use during contact with the oral mucosa. Currently, most cases are seen in persons with herpes elsewhere. Children may be infected while

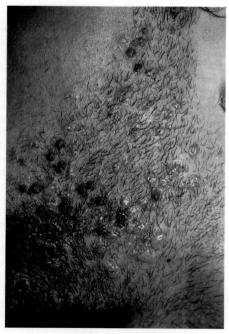

Fig. 19.4 Herpetic sycosis.

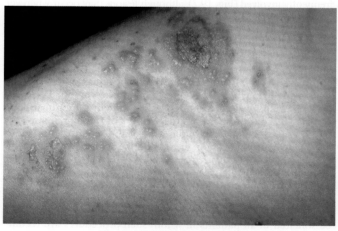

Fig. 19.5 Herpes gladiatorum.

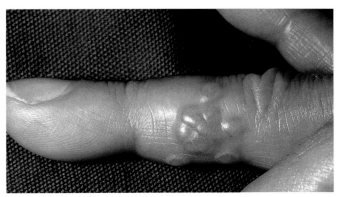

Fig. 19.6 Herpetic whitlow, classic grouped vesicles.

thumb sucking or nail biting during their initial herpes outbreak or by touching an infectious lesion of an adult. Herpetic whitlow is bimodal in distribution, with about 20% of cases occurring in children younger than 10 years and 55% of cases in adults between ages 20 and 40. Virtually all cases in children are caused by HSV-1, and there is often a coexisting herpetic gingivostomatitis. In adults, up to three quarters of cases are caused by HSV-2. Among adults, herpetic whitlow is twice as common in women. Herpetic whitlow in health care workers can be transmitted to patients. In patients whose oropharynx is exposed to the ungloved hands of health care workers with herpetic whitlow, 37% develop herpetic pharyngitis.

Herpetic Keratoconjunctivitis

Herpes simplex infection of the eye is a common cause of blindness in the United States. It occurs as a punctate or marginal keratitis or as a dendritic corneal ulcer, which may cause disciform keratitis and leave scars that impair vision. Topical corticosteroids in this situation may induce perforation of the cornea. Vesicles may appear on the lids, and preauricular nodes may be enlarged and tender. Recurrences are common. Ocular symptoms in any person with an initial outbreak of HSV could represent ocular HSV, and an ophthalmologic evaluation should be performed to exclude this possibility.

Genital Herpes

Genital herpes infection is usually caused by HSV-2. In the mid-1980s the prevalence of genital herpes caused by HSV-1 began to increase because of changes in sexual habits and decreasing prevalence of orolabial HSV-1 infection in developed nations. In women under age 25, HSV-1 represents more than 50% of cases of genital herpes, whereas in women over 25 and in men of all ages, HSV-2 remains the most common cause of genital herpes. HSV-1 in the genital area is much less likely to recur. Only 20%–50% of patients have a recurrence; when it does recur, the average patient experiences only about one outbreak per year.

Genital herpes is spread by skin-to-skin contact, usually during sexual activity. The incubation period averages 5 days. Active lesions of HSV-2 contain live virus and are infectious. Persons with recurrent genital herpes shed virus asymptomatically between outbreaks (asymptomatic shedding). Even persons who are HSV-2 infected but have never had a clinical lesion (or symptoms) shed virus, so everyone who is HSV-2 infected is potentially infectious to a sexual partner. Asymptomatic shedding occurs simultaneously from several anatomic sites (penis, vagina, cervix, rectum) and can occur through normally appearing intact skin and mucosae. In addition, persons with HSV-2 infection may have lesions they do not recognize as being caused by HSV (unrecognized outbreak) or have recurrent lesions that do not cause symptoms (subclinical outbreak). Most transmission of genital herpes occurs during subclinical or unrecognized outbreaks, or while the infected person is shedding asymptomatically.

The risk of transmission in monogamous couples, in which only one partner is infected, is about 5%–10% annually, with women being at much greater risk than men for acquiring HSV-2 from their infected partner. Prior HSV-1 infection does not reduce the risk of being infected with HSV-2 but does make it more likely that initial infection will be asymptomatic. There is no strategy that absolutely prevents herpes transmission. All prevention strategies are more effective in reducing the risk of male-to-female transmission than female-to-male transmission. Condom use for all sexual exposures and avoiding sexual exposure when active lesions are present have been shown to be effective strategies, as has chronic suppressive therapy of the infected partner with valacyclovir.

The symptomatology during acquisition of infection with HSV-2 has a broad clinical spectrum, from totally asymptomatic to severe genital ulcer disease (erosive vulvovaginitis or proctitis). Only 57% of new HSV-2 infections are symptomatic. Clinically, the majority of symptomatic initial herpes lesions are classic, grouped blisters on an erythematous base. At times, the initial clinical episode is that of typical grouped blisters, but with a longer duration of 10–14 days. Although uncommon and representing 1% or fewer of new infections, severe first-episode genital herpes can be a significant systemic illness. Grouped blisters and erosions appear in the vagina, in the rectum, or on the penis, with continued development of new blisters over 7–14 days. Lesions are bilaterally symmetric and often extensive, and the inguinal lymph nodes can be enlarged bilaterally. Fever and flulike symptoms may be present, but in women the major complaint is vaginal pain and dysuria (herpetic vulvovaginitis). The whole illness may last 3 weeks or more. If the inoculation occurs in the rectal area, severe proctitis may occur from extensive erosions in the anal canal and on the rectal mucosa. The initial clinical episode of genital herpes is treated with oral acyclovir, 200 mg five times or 400 mg three times daily; famciclovir, 250 mg three times daily; or valacyclovir, 1000 mg twice daily, all for 7–10 days. It is clinically difficult to distinguish true initial (or primary) HSV-2 infection from a recurrence, so all patients with their initial clinical episode receive the same therapy. Only serology can determine whether the person is totally HSV naïve and experiencing a true primary episode, is partially immune from prior HSV-1 infection, or is already HSV-2 infected with first clinical presentation actually a recurrence. In fact, 25% of "initial" clinical episodes of genital herpes are actually recurrences.

Virtually all persons infected with HSV-2 will have recurrences, even if the initial infection was subclinical or asymptomatic. HSV-2 infection results in recurrences in the genital area six times more frequently than HSV-1. Twenty percent of persons with HSV-2 infection are truly asymptomatic, never having had either an initial lesion or a recurrence. Twenty percent of patients have lesions they recognize as recurrent genital herpes, and 60% have clinical lesions that are culture positive for HSV-2, but that are unrecognized by the patient as being caused by genital herpes. This large group of persons with subclinical or unrecognized genital herpes are infectious, at least intermittently, and represent one factor in the increasing number of new HSV-2 infections.

Typical recurrent genital herpes begins with a prodrome of burning, itching, or tingling. Usually within 24 hours, red papules appear at the site, progress to blisters filled with clear fluid over 24 hours, form erosions over the next 24–36 hours, and heal in another 2–3 days (Fig. 19.7). The average total duration of a typical outbreak of genital herpes is 7 days. Lesions are usually grouped blisters and evolve into coalescent grouped erosions, which characteristically have a scalloped border. Erosions or ulcerations

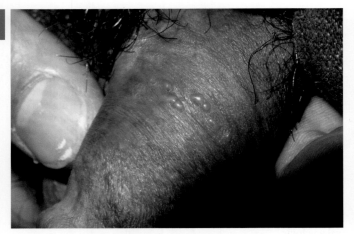

Fig. 19.7 Herpes genitalis. (Courtesy Steven Binnick, MD.)

from genital herpes are usually very tender and not indurated (unlike chancre of primary syphilis). Lesions tend to recur in the same anatomic region, although not at exactly the same site (unlike fixed drug eruption). Less classic clinical manifestations are tiny erosions or linear fissures on the genital skin. Lesions occur on the vulva, vagina, and cervical mucosa, as well as on the penile and vulval skin. The upper buttock is a common site for recurrent genital herpes in both men and women. Intraurethral genital herpes may present with dysuria and a clear penile discharge and is usually misdiagnosed as a more common, nongonococcal urethritis such as *Chlamydia* or *Ureaplasma* infection. Inguinal adenopathy may be present. Looking into the urethra and culturing any erosions will establish the diagnosis. Recurrent genital herpes usually heals without scarring.

The natural history of untreated recurrent genital herpes is not well studied. Over the first few years of infection, the frequency of recurrences usually stays the same. Over periods longer than 3–5 years, the frequency of outbreaks decreases in at least two thirds of patients treated with suppressive antiviral therapy.

Recurrent genital herpes is a problematic disease because of the associated social stigma. Because it is not curable, patients frequently have a significant emotional response when first diagnosed, including anger (at presumed source of infection), depression, guilt, and feelings of unworthiness. During the visit, the health care worker should ask about the patient's feelings and any psychological complications. This psychological component of genital herpes must be recognized, addressed directly with the patient, and managed properly for the therapy of recurrent genital herpes to be successful. Education regarding timing of outbreak and exposure, including potential for initial asymptomatic infection, is important.

Management of recurrent genital herpes should be individualized. A careful history, including a sexual history, should be obtained. Examination should include seeing the patient during an active recurrence so that the infection can be confirmed. The diagnosis of recurrent genital herpes should not be made on clinical appearance alone because of the psychological impact of the diagnosis. The diagnosis is best confirmed by viral culture, PCR, or DFA, allowing for typing of the causative virus. Genital HSV is a risk factor for HIV infection, and patients with genital HSV should be evaluated for and counseled about other STDs.

Treatment depends on several factors, including the frequency of recurrences, severity of recurrences, infection status of the sexual partner, and psychological impact of the infection on the patient. For patients with few or mildly symptomatic recurrences, treatment is often unnecessary. Counseling regarding transmission risk is required. In patients with severe but infrequent recurrences and

in those with severe psychological complications, intermittent therapy may be useful. To be effective, intermittent therapy must be initiated at the earliest sign of an outbreak. The patient must be given the medication before the recurrence so that treatment can be started by the patient when the first symptoms appear. Intermittent therapy only reduces the duration of the average recurrence by about 1 day. However, it is a powerful tool in the patient who is totally overwhelmed by each outbreak. The treatment of recurrent genital herpes is acyclovir, 200 mg five times daily or 800 mg twice daily, or famciclovir, 125 mg twice daily, for 5 days. Shorter regimens that are equally effective include valacyclovir, 500 mg twice daily for 3 days; acyclovir, 800 mg three times daily for 2 days; or famciclovir, 1 g twice daily for 1 day.

For patients with frequent recurrences (>6–12 yearly), suppressive therapy may be more reasonable. Acyclovir, 400 mg twice daily, 200 mg three times daily, or 800 mg once daily, will suppress 85% of recurrences, and 20% of patients will be recurrence free during suppressive therapy. Valacyclovir, 500 mg/day (or 1000 mg/day for those with >10 recurrences/year), or famciclovir, 250 mg twice daily, is an equally effective alternative. Up to 5% of immunocompetent patients will have significant recurrences on these doses, and the dose of the antiviral may need to be increased. Chronic suppressive therapy reduces asymptomatic shedding by almost 95%. After 10 years of suppressive therapy, many patients can stop treatment, with substantial reduction in frequency of recurrences. Chronic suppressive therapy is safe, and laboratory monitoring is not required.

Intrauterine and Neonatal Herpes Simplex

Neonatal herpes infection occurs in 1:3000 to 1:20,000 live births, with an estimate of 14,000 cases annually worldwide and 1500–2200 cases of neonatal herpes annually in the United States. Eighty-five percent of neonatal herpes simplex infections occur at delivery; 5% occur in utero with intact membranes; and 10%–15% occur from nonmaternal sources after delivery. In utero infection may result in fetal anomalies, including skin lesions and scars, limb hypoplasia, microcephaly, microphthalmos, encephalitis, chorioretinitis, and intracerebral calcifications. It is either fatal or complicated by permanent neurologic sequelae.

Seventy percent of neonatal herpes simplex infections are caused by HSV-2 worldwide; however, in the United States recently HSV-1 was reported more frequently than HSV-2. Neonatal HSV-1 infections are usually acquired postnatally through contact with a person with orolabial disease, but can also occur intrapartum if the mother is genitally infected with HSV-1. The clinical spectrum of perinatally acquired neonatal herpes can be divided into the following three forms:

1. Localized infection of the skin, eyes, and/or mouth (SEM)
2. Central nervous system (CNS) disease
3. Disseminated disease (encephalitis, hepatitis, pneumonia, and coagulopathy)

The pattern of involvement at presentation is important prognostically. With treatment, localized disease (skin, eyes, or mouth) is rarely fatal, whereas brain or disseminated disease is fatal in 15%–50% of neonates so affected. In treated neonates, long-term sequelae occur in 10% of infants with localized disease. More than 50% of patients with CNS or disseminated neonatal herpes have neurologic disability.

In 68% of infected babies, skin vesicles are the presenting sign and are a good source for virus recovery. However, 39% of neonates with disseminated disease, 32% with CNS disease, and 17% with SEM disease never develop vesicular skin lesions. Because the incubation period may be as long as 3 weeks and averages about 1 week, skin lesions and symptoms may not appear until the child has been discharged from the hospital.

The diagnosis of neonatal herpes is confirmed by viral culture or preferably immediate DFA staining of material from skin or ocular lesions. CNS involvement is detected by PCR of the cerebrospinal fluid (CSF). PCR of the CSF is negative in 24% of neonatal CNS herpes infections, so pending other testing, empiric therapy may be required. Neonatal herpes infections are treated with IV acyclovir for 14 days for SEM disease and for 21 days for CNS and disseminated disease.

Seventy percent of mothers of infants with neonatal herpes simplex are asymptomatic at delivery and have no history of genital herpes. Thus extended history taking is of no value in predicting which pregnancies may be complicated by neonatal herpes. The most important predictors of infection appear to be the nature of the mother's infection at delivery (first episode vs. recurrent) and the presence of active lesions on the cervix, vagina, or vulvar area. The risk of infection for an infant delivered vaginally when the mother has active recurrent genital herpes infection is 2%–5%, whereas it is 26%–56% if the maternal infection at delivery is a first episode. One strategy to prevent neonatal HSV would be to prevent transmission of HSV to at-risk women during pregnancy, eliminating initial HSV episodes during pregnancy. To accomplish this, pregnant women and their partners would be tested to identify discordant couples for HSV-1 and HSV-2. If the woman is HSV-1 negative and the man is HSV-1 positive, orogenital contact during pregnancy should be avoided and a condom used for all episodes of sexual contact. Valacyclovir suppression of the infected male could also be considered but might have limited efficacy. If the woman is HSV-2 seronegative and her partner is HSV-2 seropositive, barrier protection for sexual contact during gestation is recommended, and valacyclovir suppression of the man could be considered. Abstinence from intercourse during the third trimester would also reduce the chances of an at-risk mother acquiring genital herpes that might first present perinatally. These strategies have not been tested and could not be guaranteed to prevent all cases of neonatal HSV. At a minimum, discordant couples should be informed of the increased risk to the fetus from the mother's acquisition of HSV during pregnancy.

The appropriate management of pregnancies complicated by genital herpes is complex and still controversial. Routine prenatal cultures are not recommended for women with recurrent genital herpes because they do not predict shedding at delivery. Such cultures may be of value in women with primary genital herpes during pregnancy. Scalp electrodes should be avoided in deliveries where cervical shedding of HSV is possible; they can increase the risk of neonatal infection by up to sevenfold (Fig. 19.8). Vacuum-assisted delivery also increases the relative risk of neonatal transmission of HSV 2–27 times. Genital HSV-1 infection appears to be much more frequently transmitted intrapartum than HSV-2. The current recommendation is still to perform cesarean section in the mother with active genital lesions or prodromal symptoms. This will reduce the risk of transmission of HSV to the infant from 8% to 1% for women who are culture positive from the cervix at delivery. However, this approach will not prevent all cases of neonatal herpes, is expensive, and has a high maternal morbidity. Because the risk of neonatal herpes is much greater in mothers who experience their initial episode during pregnancy, antiviral treatment of all initial episodes of genital HSV in pregnancy is recommended (except in the first month of gestation, when there may be an increased risk of spontaneous abortion). Standard acyclovir doses for initial episodes, 400 mg three times daily for 10 days, are recommended. This is especially true for all initial episodes in the third trimester. Chronic suppressive therapy with acyclovir has been used from 36 weeks of gestation to delivery in women with an initial episode of genital HSV during pregnancy, to reduce outbreaks and prevent the need for cesarean section. This approach has been recommended by the American College of Obstetrics and Gynecology and may also be considered for women with recurrent genital herpes.

The condition of extensive congenital erosions and vesicles healing with reticulate scarring may represent intrauterine neonatal herpes simplex. The condition is rare because intrauterine HSV infection is rare and usually fatal. Probably only a few children survive to present later in life with the characteristic widespread reticulate scarring of the whole body. This may explain the associated CNS manifestations seen in many affected children. One author treated a child with this condition who developed infrequent widespread cutaneous blisters from which HSV could be cultured. Modern obstetric practices, which screen for herpes in pregnant women, and prophylactic treatment with acyclovir in the third trimester may prevent the condition, explaining the lack of recent cases.

Eczema Herpeticum (Kaposi Varicelliform Eruption)

Infection with herpesvirus in patients with atopic dermatitis (AD) may result in spread of herpes simplex throughout the eczematous areas, called eczema herpeticum (EH) (Fig. 19.9) or Kaposi varicelliform eruption (KVE). In a large series, development of EH was associated with more severe AD, higher IgE levels, elevated eosinophil count, food and environmental allergies (as defined by radioallergosorbent testing [RAST]), and onset of AD before age 5 years. EH patients are also more likely to have *Staphylococcus aureus* and molluscum contagiosum infections. All these features identify AD patients who have significant T-helper type 2 cell (Th2) shift of their immune system. The use of topical calcineurin inhibitors (TCIs) has been repeatedly associated with EH

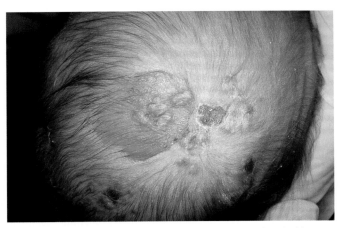

Fig. 19.8 Neonatal herpes; a scalp monitor was associated with infection of this infant.

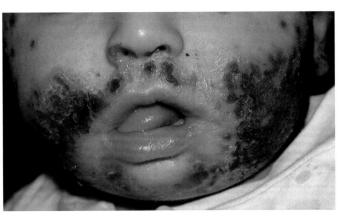

Fig. 19.9 Eczema herpeticum.

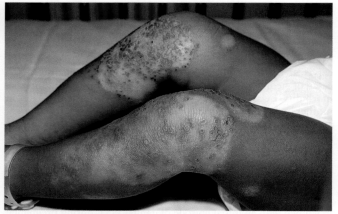

Fig. 19.10 Eczema herpeticum, sudden appearance of uniform erosions, accentuated in areas of active dermatitis.

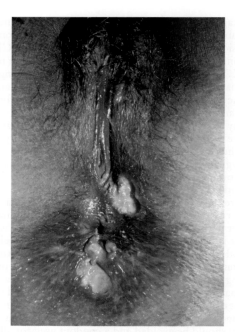

Fig. 19.11 Ulcerative herpes simplex in an HIV-infected patient.

development. Bath or hot tub exposure has been reported as a risk factor. The Th2 shift of the immune system and TCIs are both associated with a decrease in antimicrobial peptides in the epidermis, an important defense against cutaneous HSV infection. Increased interleukin-10 (IL-10)–producing proinflammatory monocytes lead to local expansion of regulatory T cells and may contribute to the development of EH. HLA-B7 and local IL-25 expression are also associated with EH. In Japan, polymorphisms in the gene for IL-19 are associated with EH complicating TCI treatment. The repair of the epidermal lipid barrier with physiologic lipid mixtures reverses some of the negative effects of the TCIs and may reduce the risk of EH. One sequencing study suggested that *IFNGR1* variants may confer susceptibility.

Cutaneous dissemination of HSV-1 or HSV-2 may also occur in severe seborrheic dermatitis, scabies, Darier disease, benign familial pemphigus, pemphigus (foliaceus or vulgaris), pemphigoid, cutaneous T-cell lymphoma, Wiskott-Aldrich syndrome, allergic and photoallergic contact dermatitis, burns, and other states with widespread damage to the epidermis. In its severest form, hundreds of umbilicated vesicles may be present at the onset, with fever and regional adenopathy. Although the cutaneous eruption is alarming, the disease is often self-limited in healthy individuals. Much milder cases are considerably more common and probably go unrecognized and untreated. They present as a few superficial erosions or even small papules (Fig. 19.10). In patients with systemic immunosuppression in addition to an impaired barrier, such as patients with pemphigus and cutaneous T-cell lymphoma, KVE can be fatal, usually from *S. aureus* septicemia, but also from visceral dissemination of herpes simplex.

Psoriasis patients treated with immunosuppressants may develop KVE as well, although this is less common. It usually occurs in the setting of worsening disease or erythroderma. Patients present with erosive lesions in the axilla and erosions of the psoriatic plaques. Lesions extend cephalad to caudad, and the development of large, ulcerated, painful plaques can occur. The lesions are often coinfected with bacteria and yeast. Cultures positive for other pathogens do *not* exclude the diagnosis of KVE, and specific viral culture, DFA, and biopsy should be done if diagnosis of KVE is suspected. Given the limited toxicity of systemic antiviral therapy, treatment should be started immediately, pending the return of laboratory confirmation. Depending on the severity of the disease, either IV or oral antiviral therapy should be given for KVE patients. In children with EH, bacterial superinfection is not uncommon, and early antibiotics in patients with bacteremia are important, though empiric antibiotics are not indicated. Systemic steroids should be avoided, but topical corticosteroids during an eruption do not appear to prolong hospital stay

and in some cases may be helpful, though further study is necessary.

Immunocompromised Patients

In patients with suppression of the cell-mediated immune system by cytotoxic agents, corticosteroids, or congenital or acquired immunodeficiency, primary and recurrent cases of herpes simplex are more severe, persistent, and symptomatic and more resistant to therapy. In some settings, such as in bone marrow transplant recipients, the risk of severe reactivation is so high that prophylactic systemic antivirals are administered. In immunosuppressed patients, any erosive mucocutaneous lesion should be considered to be herpes simplex until proved otherwise, especially lesions in the genital and orolabial regions. Atypical morphologies are also seen. HSV reactivation is common with institution of effective antiretroviral therapy (ART) and can be part of the immune reconstitution inflammatory syndrome (IRIS). Oral antivirals prevent this reactivation and can be considered in the HIV-infected patient who will receive ART.

Typically, lesions appear as erosions or crusts (Fig. 19.11). The early vesicular lesions may be transient or never seen. The three clinical hallmarks of HSV infection are pain, an active vesicular border, and a scalloped periphery. Untreated erosive lesions may gradually expand, but they may also remain fixed and even become papular or vegetative, mimicking a wart or granulation tissue. In the oral mucosa, numerous erosions may be seen, involving all surfaces, unlike the hard, keratinized surfaces usually involved by recurrent oral herpes simplex in the immunocompetent host. The tongue may be affected with geometric fissures on the central dorsal surface (Fig. 19.12). Symptomatic stomatitis associated with cancer chemotherapy may be caused or exacerbated by HSV infection. Herpetic whitlow presents as a painful paronychia that is initially vesicular and involves the lateral or proximal nailfolds. Untreated, it may lead to loss of the nail plate and ulceration of a large portion of the digit.

Despite the frequent and severe skin infections caused by HSV in the immunosuppressed patient, visceral dissemination is unusual. Extension of oral HSV into the esophagus or trachea may develop spontaneously or as a complication of intubation through an infected

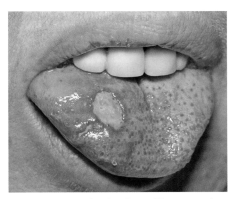

Fig. 19.12 Immunocompromised patient with tongue ulcer and fissures secondary to HSV.

oropharynx. Ocular involvement can occur from direct inoculation, and if lesions are present around the eye, careful ophthalmologic evaluation is required.

In an immunosuppressed host, most herpetic lesions are ulcerative and not vesicular. Viral cultures or PCR from the ulcer margin are positive. At times, these tests are negative, but a skin biopsy will show typical herpetic changes in the epithelium adjacent to the ulceration. If an ulceration does not respond to treatment in 48 hours and cultures are negative, a biopsy is recommended, because it may be the only technique that demonstrates the associated herpesvirus infection.

Therapy often can be instituted on clinical grounds pending confirmatory tests. Acyclovir, 400 mg orally three times daily; famciclovir, 500 mg twice daily; or valacyclovir, 1 g twice daily, all for a minimum of 5–10 days, is used. Therapy should continue until lesions are essentially healed. In severe infection, or in the hospitalized patient with moderate disease, IV acyclovir (5 mg/kg) can be given initially to control the disease. In patients with acquired immunodeficiency syndrome (AIDS) and those with persistent immunosuppression, consideration should be given to chronic suppressive therapy with acyclovir, 400–800 mg two or three times daily, or valacyclovir or famciclovir, 500 mg twice daily.

In the immunosuppressed host (but not in the immunocompetent host), long-term treatment with acyclovir and its analogs, or treatment of large herpetic ulcerations, may be complicated by the development of acyclovir resistance. This resistance may be caused by selection of acyclovir-resistant wild-type virus, which is present in large numbers on the surface of such large herpes lesions. In the immunocompetent host, these acyclovir-resistant mutants are few in number and eradicated by the host's immune system. The immunosuppressed host has much more HSV in the lesions, and the host's immune system is ineffective in killing the virus. These acyclovir-resistant viral strains may be difficult to culture and may be identified only by skin biopsy or PCR of the ulceration. Antiviral resistance is suspected if maximum oral doses of acyclovir, valacyclovir, or famciclovir do not lead to improvement. IV acyclovir, except if given by constant infusion, will also invariably fail in such patients. Resistance to one drug is associated with resistance to all three of these drugs, usually from loss of the viral thymidine kinase. HSV isolates can be tested for sensitivity to acyclovir and some other antivirals. The standard treatment of acyclovir-resistant herpes simplex is IV foscarnet. In patients intolerant of or resistant to foscarnet, IV cidofovir may be used; brincidofovir is being investigated and may be an option in the future. Smaller lesions can sometimes be treated with topical trifluorothymidine (Viroptic) with or without topical or intralesional interferon (IFN) alpha, or topical or intralesional cidofovir. Imiquimod may sometimes be of benefit in healing these lesions,

perhaps through activation of cystatin A. Destruction of small lesions by desiccation, followed by the previous therapies, may also be curative. If an HIV-infected patient with previous acyclovir-resistant genital herpes has a recurrence, at least half will be acyclovir sensitive, as the latent virus within the nerve that is reactivating is usually the initial virus from first infection, so a trial of standard antivirals is acceptable. If an AIDS patient has a nonhealing genital ulcer that harbors HSV, there may be dual infection with cytomegalovirus, and only treatment with an agent active against both HSV and CMV will lead to improvement in those cases.

Histopathology

The vesicles of herpes simplex are intraepidermal. The affected epidermis and adjacent inflamed dermis are infiltrated with leukocytes. Ballooning degeneration of the epidermal cells produces acantholysis. The most characteristic feature is the presence of multinucleated giant cells, which tend to mold together, forming a crude jigsaw puzzle appearance. The steel-gray color of the nucleus and peripheral condensation of the nucleoplasm may be clues to HSV infection, even if multinucleate cells are not seen. IP stains can detect HSV and differentiate from VZV even in paraffin-fixed tissue, allowing the diagnosis to be absolutely confirmed from histologic material.

Differential Diagnosis

Herpes labialis most often must be differentiated from impetigo. Herpetic lesions are composed of groups of tense, small vesicles, whereas in bullous impetigo, the blisters are unilocular, occur at the periphery of a crust, and are flaccid. A mixed infection is not unusual and should especially be suspected in immunosuppressed hosts and when lesions are present in the typical herpetic regions around the mouth. Herpes zoster presents with clusters of lesions along a dermatome, but early on, if the number of zoster lesions is limited, it can be relatively indistinguishable from herpes simplex. In general, herpes zoster will be more painful and over 24 hours will progress to involve more of the affected dermatome.

A genital herpes lesion, especially on the glans or corona, can be mistaken for a syphilitic chancre or chancroid. Darkfield examination, multiplex PCR, and cultures for *Haemophilus ducreyi* on selective media will aid in making the diagnosis, as will diagnostic tests for HSV (Tzanck, culture, or DFA). Combined infections occur in up to 20% of patients, so finding a single pathogen may not complete the diagnostic evaluation, and patients are often empirically treated for multiple ulcer-forming STDs and screened for other STDs when one is diagnosed.

Herpetic gingivostomatitis is often difficult to differentiate from aphthosis, streptococcal infections, diphtheria, coxsackievirus infections, and oral erythema multiforme. Aphthae tend to occur mostly on the buccal and labial mucosae. They usually form shallow, grayish erosions, generally surrounded by a prominent ring of hyperemia. Aphthae typically occur on nonattached mucosa, whereas recurrent herpes of the oral cavity primarily affects the attached gingiva and palate.

Aronson PL, et al: Empiric antibiotics and outcomes of children hospitalized with eczema herpeticum. Pediatr Dermatol 2013; 30: 207.

Aronson PL, et al: Topical corticosteroids and hospital length of stay in children with eczema herpeticum. Pediatr Dermatol 2013; 30: 215.

Ashack KA, et al: Skin infections among US high school athletes. J Am Acad Dermatol 2016; 74: 679.

Beck LA, et al: Phenotype of atopic dermatitis subjects with a history of eczema herpeticum. J Allergy Clin Immunol 2009; 124: 260.

Bernstein DI, et al: Epidemiology, clinical presentation, and antibody response to primary infection with herpes simplex virus type 1 and type 2 in young women. Clin Infect Dis 2013; 56: 344.

Bibbins-Dombingo K, et al: Serologic screening for genital herpes infection. JAMA 2016; 316: 2525.

Bradley H, et al: Seroprevalence of herpes simplex virus types 1 and 2—United States, 1999–2010. J Infect Dis 2014; 209: 325.

Brown ZA, et al: Effect of serologic status and cesarean delivery on transmission rates of herpes simplex virus from mother to infant. JAMA 2003; 289: 203.

Chen CY, Ballard RC: The molecular diagnosis of sexually transmitted genital ulcer disease. Methods Mol Biol 2012; 903: 103.

Chosidow O, et al: Valacyclovir as a single dose during prodrome of herpes facialis. Br J Dermatol 2003; 148: 142.

Corey L, et al: Once-daily valacyclovir to reduce the risk of transmission of genital herpes. N Engl J Med 2004; 354: 11.

De SK, et al: Herpes simplex virus and varicella zoster virus. Curr Opin Infect Dis 2015; 28: 589.

Dickson N, et al: HSV-2 incidence by sex over four age periods to age 38 in a birth cohort. Sex Transm Infect 2014; 90: 243.

Fatahzadeh M, Schwartz RA: Human herpes simplex virus infections. J Am Acad Dermatol 2007; 57: 737.

Gao L, et al: Targeted deep sequencing identifies rare loss-of-function variants in IFNGR1 for risk of atopic dermatitis complicated by eczema herpeticum. J Allergy Clin Immunol 2015; 136: 1591.

Gazzola R, et al: Herpes virus outbreaks after dermal hyaluronic acid filler injections. Aesthet Surg J 2012; 32: 770.

Hirokawa D, et al: Treatment of recalcitrant herpes simplex virus with topical imiquimod. Cutis 2011; 88: 276.

Hollier LM, et al: Third trimester antiviral prophylaxis for preventing maternal genital herpes simplex virus (HSV) recurrences and neonatal infection. Cochrane Database Syst Rev 2008; 1: CD004946.

Jiang YC, et al: New strategies against drug resistance to herpes simplex virus. Int J Oral Sci 2016; 8: 1.

Johnston C, et al: Current concepts for genital herpes simplex virus infection. Clin Microbiol Rev 2016; 29: 149.

Jones CA, et al: Antiviral agents for treatment of herpes simplex virus infection in neonates. Cochrane Database Syst Rev 2009; 3: CD004206.

Kan Y, et al: Imiquimod suppresses propagation of herpes simplex virus 1 by upregulation of cystatin A via the adenosine receptor A_1 pathway. J Virol 2012; 86: 10338.

Katz K: Screening for genital herpes. JAMA Dermatol 2017; 153: 265.

Kim BE, et al: IL-25 enhances HSV-1 replication by inhibiting filaggrin expression, and acts synergistically with Th2 cytokines to enhance HSV-1 replication. J Invest Dermatol 2013; 133: 2678.

Kortekangas-Savolainen O, et al: Epidemiology of genital herpes simplex virus type 1 and 2 infections in southwestern Finland during a 10-year period (2003–2012). Sex Transm Dis 2014; 41: 268.

Kotzbauer D, et al: Clinical and laboratory characteristics of central nervous system herpes simplex virus infection in neonates and young infants. Pediatr Infect Dis J 2014; 33: 1187.

Leas BF, et al: Neonatal HSV-1 infection and Jewish ritual circumcision with oral suction. J Pediatric Infect Dis Soc 2015; 4: 126.

Leung DY: Why is eczema herpeticum unexpectedly rare? Antiviral Res 2013; 98: 153.

Looker KJ, et al: First estimates of the global and regional incidence of neonatal herpes infection. Lancet Glob Health 2017; 5: e300.

Mathais RA, et al: Atopic dermatitis complicated by eczema herpeticum is associated with HLA B7 and reduced interferon-γ-producing CD8+ T cells. Br J Dermatol 2013; 169: 700.

Muluneh B, et al: Successful clearance of cutaneous acyclovir-resistant, foscarnet-refractory herpes virus lesions with topical cidofovir in an allogeneic hematopoietic stem cell transplant patient. J Oncol Pharm Pract 2013; 19: 181.

Palli MA, et al: Immunotherapy of recurrent herpes labialis with squaric acid. JAMA Dermatol 2017; 153: 828.

Pichler M, et al: Premature newborns with fatal intrauterine herpes simplex virus-1 infection. J Eur Acad Dermatol Venereol 2015; 29: 1216.

Robinson JL, et al: Prevention, recognition and management of neonatal HSV infections. Expert Rev Anti Infect Ther 2012; 10: 675.

Rojek NW, Norton SA: Diagnosis of neonatal infection with herpes simplex virus. JAMA 2014; 311: 527.

Schoenfeld J, et al: Cutaneous co-infected cytomegalovirus and herpes simplex virus perigenital ulcers in human immunodeficiency virus patients. J Clin Aesthet Dermatol 2013; 6: 41.

Seang S, et al: Long-term follow-up of HIV-infected patients once diagnosed with acyclovir-resistant herpes simplex virus infection. Int J STD AIDS 2014; 25: 676.

Shenoy R, et al: Eczema herpeticum in a wrestler. Clin J Sport Med 2015; 25: e18.

Takahashi R, et al: Pathological role of regulatory T cells in the initiation and maintenance of eczema herpeticum lesions. J Immunol 2014; 192: 969.

Tobian AA, et al: Reactivation of herpes simplex virus type 2 after initiation of antiretroviral therapy. J Infect Dis 2013; 208: 839.

Wanat KA, et al: Intralesional cidofovir for treating extensive genital verrucous herpes simplex virus infection. JAMA Dermatol 2013; 149: 811.

Wanat KA, et al: Bedside diagnostics in dermatology. J Am Acad Dermatol 2017; 77: 197.

Whitley RJ: Changing epidemiology of herpes simplex virus infections. Clin Infect Dis 2013; 56: 352.

Wollenberg A, et al: Predisposing factors and clinical features of eczema herpeticum. J Am Acad Dermatol 2003; 49: 198.

Workowski KA, et al: Sexually transmitted diseases treatment guidelines, 2015. MMWR Recomm Rep 2015; 64: 1.

Varicella

Varicella, commonly known as chickenpox, is the primary infection with the VZV. In temperate regions, 90% of cases occur in children younger than 10 years, with the highest age-specific incidence in ages 1–4 in unvaccinated children. More than 90% of adults in temperate countries have evidence of prior infection and are "immune" to varicella by age 15. In tropical countries, however, varicella tends to be a disease of teenagers, and only 60% of adults are "immune" serologically. Outbreaks among non–U.S.-born crew members have occurred on cruise ships.

The incubation period of VZV is 10–21 days, usually 14–15 days. Transmission is by the respiratory route and less often by direct contact with the lesions. A susceptible person may develop varicella after exposure to the lesions of herpes zoster. Infected persons are infectious from 5 days before the eruption appears and are most infectious 1–2 days before the rash appears. Infectivity usually ceases 5–6 days after the eruption appears. There is an initial viral replication in the nasopharynx and conjunctiva, followed by viremia and infection of the reticuloendothelial system (liver, spleen) between days 4 and 6. A secondary viremia occurs at days 11–20, resulting in infection of the epidermis and the appearance of the characteristic skin lesions. Low-grade fever, malaise, and headache are usually present but slight. The severity

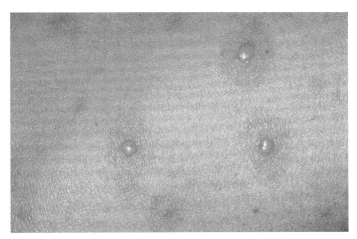

Fig. 19.13 Varicella.

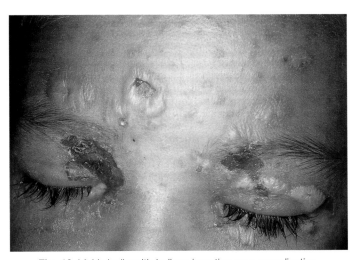

Fig. 19.14 Varicella with bullous impetigo as a complication.

of the disease is age dependent, with adults having more severe disease and a greater risk of visceral disease. In healthy children, mortality from varicella is 1.4 in 100,000 cases; in adults, 30.9 in 100,000 cases. Pregnant women have five times greater risk of an adverse outcome. As with most viral infections, immunosuppression may worsen the course of the disease. Lifelong immunity follows varicella, and second episodes of "varicella" indicate either immunosuppression or another viral infection such as coxsackievirus.

Varicella is characterized by a vesicular eruption consisting of delicate "teardrop" vesicles on an erythematous base (Fig. 19.13). The eruption starts with faint macules that develop rapidly into vesicles within 24 hours. Successive fresh crops of vesicles appear for a few days, mainly on the trunk, face, and oral mucosa. Initially, the exanthem may be limited to sun-exposed areas, the diaper area of infants, or sites of inflammation. The vesicles quickly become pustular and umbilicated, then crusted. Because the lesions appear in crops, lesions of various stages are present at the same time, a useful clue to the diagnosis. Lesions tend not to scar, but larger lesions and those that become secondarily infected may heal with a characteristic round, depressed scar.

Secondary bacterial infection with *S. aureus* or a streptococcus is the most common complication of varicella (Fig. 19.14). Rarely, it may be complicated by osteomyelitis, other deep-seated infections, or septicemia. Other complications are rarer. Pneumonia is uncommon in normal children but is seen in 1 in 400 adults with varicella. It may be bacterial or caused by VZV, a difficult differential diagnosis. Cerebellar ataxia and encephalitis are the most common neurologic complications. VZV can rarely infect cerebral arteries and cause a vasculopathy leading to stroke, sinus thromboses, and giant cell arteritis. VZV may cause stroke in both children and adults. Asymptomatic myocarditis and hepatitis may occur in children with varicella, but rarely are significant and resolve spontaneously with no treatment. Reye syndrome, with hepatitis and acute encephalopathy, is associated with the use of aspirin to treat the symptoms of varicella. Aspirin is absolutely contraindicated in patients with varicella. Any child with varicella and severe vomiting should be referred immediately to exclude Reye syndrome. Symptomatic thrombocytopenia is a rare manifestation of varicella, which can occur either with the exanthem or several weeks after. Purpura fulminans, a form of disseminated intravascular coagulation associated with low levels of proteins C and S, may complicate varicella.

The diagnosis of varicella is easily made clinically. Tzanck smear from a vesicle will usually show characteristic multinucleate giant cells, and DFA can confirm the infection and type the virus. PCR is increasingly used due to high sensitivity and specificity. VZV grows poorly and slowly in the laboratory, so viral culture is rarely indicated.

Treatment

Both immunocompetent children and adults with varicella benefit from acyclovir therapy if started early, within 24 hours of the eruption's appearance. Therapy does not seem to alter the development of adequate immunity to reinfection. Because the complications of varicella are infrequent in children, routine treatment is not recommended; therapeutic decisions are made on a case-by-case basis. Acyclovir therapy appears mainly to benefit secondary cases within a household, which tend to be more severe than the index case. In this setting, therapy can be instituted earlier. Therapy does not return children to school sooner, however, and the impact on parental workdays missed is not known. The dose of acyclovir is 20 mg/kg, maximum 800 mg per dose, four times daily for 5 days. Aspirin and other salicylates should not be used as antipyretics in varicella because their use increases the risk of Reye syndrome. Topical antipruritic lotions, oatmeal baths, dressing the patient in light, cool clothing, and keeping the environment cool may all relieve some of the symptomatology. Children living in warm homes and kept very warm with clothing have anecdotally been observed to have more numerous skin lesions. Children with AD, Darier disease, congenital ichthyosiform erythroderma, diabetes, cystic fibrosis, conditions requiring chronic salicylate or steroid therapy, and inborn errors of metabolism should be treated with acyclovir, because they may have more complications or exacerbations of their underlying illness with varicella.

Varicella is more severe and complications are more common in adults. Between 5% and 14% of adults will have pulmonary involvement. Smokers and those with preexisting lung disease (but not asthma) are at increased risk. The pneumonitis can progress rapidly and be fatal. Adults with varicella and at least one other risk factor should be evaluated with physical examination, pulse oximetry, and chest radiography. Antiviral treatment is recommended in all adolescents and adults (13 and older) with varicella. The dose is 800 mg four or five times daily for 5 days. Severe, fulminant cutaneous disease and visceral complications are treated with IV acyclovir, 10 mg/kg every 8 hours, adjusted for creatinine clearance. If the patient is hospitalized for therapy, strict isolation is required. Patients with varicella should not be admitted to wards with immunocompromised hosts or to pediatric wards, but rather are best placed on wards with healthy patients recovering from acute trauma.

Pregnant Women and Neonates

Maternal VZV infection may result in severe illness in the mother, and if the infection occurs before 28 weeks of gestation, and especially before 20 weeks, a small but significant risk of infection of the fetus (congenital varicella syndrome). In one study, 4 of 31 women with varicella in pregnancy developed varicella pneumonia. The risk for spontaneous abortion by 20 weeks is 3%; in an additional 0.7% of pregnancies, fetal death occurs after 20 weeks. The risk of preterm labor, as reported in various studies, has varied from no increased risk to a threefold increase. Severe varicella and varicella pneumonia or disseminated disease in pregnancy should be treated with IV acyclovir. All varicella in pregnancy should be treated with oral acyclovir, 800 mg five times daily for 7 days, (adjusted for renal function) except perhaps during the first month, when a specialist should be consulted. In all women past 35 weeks of gestation or with increased risk of premature labor, admission and IV acyclovir, 10 mg/kg three times daily, ("adjusted for renal function") should be recommended. The patient should be evaluated for pneumonia, renal function should be carefully monitored, and the patient should be switched to oral therapy once lesions stop appearing (usually in 48–72 hours).

Varicella-zoster immune globulin (VZIG) should not be given once the pregnant woman has developed varicella. VZIG should be given for significant exposures (see next section) within the first 72–96 hours to ameliorate maternal varicella and prevent complications. Its use should be limited to seronegative women because of its cost and the high rate of asymptomatic infection in U.S. patients. The lack of a history of prior varicella is associated with seronegativity in only 20% or fewer of the U.S. population.

Congenital varicella syndrome is characterized by a series of anomalies, including hypoplastic limbs (usually unilateral and lower extremity), cutaneous scars, and ocular and CNS disease. This may not be identified until months after infection. Repeated sonographic examination can be used to monitor at-risk pregnancies. Female fetuses are affected more often than males. The overall risk for this syndrome is about 0.4%; the highest risk, about 2%, is from maternal varicella between weeks 13 and 20. Infection of the fetus in utero may result in zoster occurring postnatally, often in the first 2 years of life. This occurs in about 1% of varicella-complicated pregnancies, and the risk for this complication is greatest in varicella occurring in weeks 25–36 of gestation. The value of VZIG in preventing or modifying fetal complications of maternal varicella is unknown. In one study, however, of 97 patients with varicella in pregnancy treated with VZIG, none had complications of congenital varicella syndrome or infantile zoster, suggesting some efficacy for VZIG. Although apparently safe in pregnancy, acyclovir's efficacy in preventing fetal complications of maternal varicella is unknown.

If the mother develops varicella between 5 days before and 2 days after delivery, neonatal varicella can occur and may be severe because of inadequate transplacental delivery of antivaricella antibody. These neonates develop varicella at 5–10 days of age. In such cases, administration of VZIG is warranted, and IV acyclovir therapy should be considered.

Varicella Vaccine

Live attenuated viral vaccine for varicella is a currently recommended childhood immunization. Two doses are now recommended, one between age 12 and 15 months and the second at 4–6 years. This double-vaccination schedule is recommended because epidemics of varicella still occurred in children ages 9–11 in well-immunized communities, suggesting a waning of immunity by this age. The introduction of widespread vaccination has led to a dramatic decrease in varicella-related hospitalizations. Complications of varicella vaccination are uncommon, and severe complications are rare. A systematic literature review suggested that there were approximately 50–60 breakthrough varicella cases with disseminated infection associated with over 30 million doses of virus. A mild skin eruption from which virus usually cannot be isolated, occurring locally at the injection site within 2 days or generalized 1–3 weeks after immunization, occurs in 6% of children. Many of the breakthrough cases in vaccinated children are mild, and many reported skin lesions were not vesicular (see next section, Modified Varicella-like Syndrome). Prevention of severe varicella is virtually 100%, even when the vaccine is given within 36 hours of exposure. Immunized children with no detectable antibody also have reduced severity of varicella after exposure. Secondary complications of varicella, including scarring, are virtually eliminated by vaccination. One theoretical population-based consequence of widespread vaccination and reduced rates of infection is whether there will be an observed loss of natural "booster" exposures to the virus, and perhaps a changing epidemiology of the disease and increased incidence of zoster (shingles).

Household exposure of immunosuppressed children to recently immunized siblings does not appear to pose a great risk. Children whose leukemia is in remission are also protected by the vaccine but may require three doses. Leukemic children still receiving chemotherapy have a complication rate from vaccination (usually a varicella-like eruption) approaching 50%. They may require acyclovir therapy. Unprotected close contacts develop varicella 15% of the time. In leukemic children, adequate immunization results in complete immunity in some and partial immunity in the others, protecting them from severe varicella. Immunization also reduces the attack rate for zoster in leukemic children. As a live vaccine, administration is contraindicated during pregnancy and in immunosuppressed patients.

Modified Varicella-Like Syndrome. Children immunized with live attenuated varicella vaccine may develop varicella of reduced severity on exposure to natural varicella. This has been called modified varicella-like syndrome (MVLS). The frequency of MVLS is between 0% and 2.7% per year, and children with lower antibody titers are more likely to develop the illness. MVLS occurs an average of 15 days after exposure to varicella and consists primarily of macules and papules with relatively few vesicles. The average number of lesions is about 35–50, compared with natural varicella, which usually has about 300 lesions. The majority of patients are afebrile and the illness is mild, lasting fewer than 5 days on average.

Immunocompromised Patients

Varicella cases can be extremely severe and even fatal in immunosuppressed patients, especially in individuals with impaired cell-mediated immunity. Before effective antiviral therapy, almost one third of children with cancer developed complications of varicella and 7% died. In this setting, varicella pneumonia, hepatitis, and encephalitis are common. Prior varicella does not always protect the immunosuppressed host from multiple episodes. The skin lesions in the immunosuppressed host are usually identical to varicella in the healthy host; however, the number of lesions may be numerous (Fig. 19.15). In an immunosuppressed patient, the lesions more frequently become necrotic, and ulceration may occur. Even if the lesions are few, the size of the lesion may be large, up to several centimeters, and necrosis of the full thickness of the dermis may occur. In patients with HIV infection, varicella may be severe and fatal. Atypical cases of a few scattered lesions without a dermatomal distribution usually represent reactivation disease with dissemination. Chronic varicella may complicate HIV infection, resulting in ulcerative (ecthymatous) or hyperkeratotic (verrucous) lesions. These patterns of infection may be associated with acyclovir resistance.

The degree of immunosuppression likely to result in severe varicella has been debated. There are case reports of severe

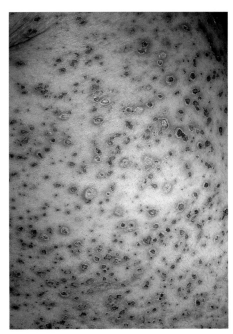

Fig. 19.15 Varicella in a patient with advanced Hodgkin disease.

and even fatal varicella in otherwise healthy children given short courses of oral corticosteroids or even using only inhaled corticosteroids. In a case-control study, however, corticosteroid use did not appear to be a risk factor for development of severe varicella. In the United Kingdom, any patient receiving or having received systemic corticosteroids in the prior 3 months, regardless of dose, is considered at increased risk for severe varicella. Inhaled steroids are not considered an indication for prophylactic antiviral treatment. A "high-risk" or significant exposure is defined as follows:

1. Household contact (i.e., living in same house as a patient with chickenpox or zoster)
2. Face-to-face contact for at least 5 minutes with a patient who has chickenpox
3. Contact indoors for more than 1 hour with a patient who has chickenpox or herpes zoster or, in a hospital setting, a patient with chickenpox or herpes zoster in an adjacent bed or the same open ward

Immunosuppressed children with no prior history of varicella and a high-risk exposure should be treated with VZIG as soon as possible after exposure (within 96 hours). Preengraftment bone marrow transplant patients should receive the same therapy. VZIG treatment does not reduce the frequency of infection, but it does reduce the severity of infection and complications. The value of prophylactic antivirals is unknown. Parents of immunosuppressed children and their physicians should be aware that severe disease can occur and counseled to return immediately after significant exposure or if varicella develops.

An unusual variant of recurrent varicella is seen in elderly patients with a history of varicella in childhood, who have a malignancy of the bone marrow and are receiving chemotherapy. They develop a mild illness with 10–40 widespread lesions and usually no systemic findings. This type of recurrent varicella tends to relapse. It is different from typical varicella because all the lesions are in a single stage of development, and thus it could be easily confused with smallpox.

Ideally, management of varicella in the immunocompromised patient would involve prevention through varicella vaccination

before immunosuppression. Vaccination is safe if the person is more than 1 year from induction chemotherapy, if chemotherapy is halted about the time of vaccination, and if lymphocyte count is higher than 700/mm^3. IV acyclovir, 10 mg/kg three times daily (or 500 mg/m^2 in children) is given as soon as the diagnosis of varicella is suspected. IV therapy is continued until 2 days after all new vesicles have stopped. Oral antivirals are continued for a minimum of 10 days of treatment. VZIG is of no proven benefit once clinical disease has developed, but may be given if the patient has life-threatening disease and is not responding to IV acyclovir.

In HIV-infected adults, treatment is individualized. Persons with typical varicella should be evaluated for the presence of pneumonia or hepatitis. Valacyclovir, 1 g three times daily; famciclovir, 500 mg three times daily; or acyclovir, 800 mg 5 times daily, may be used if no visceral complications are present. Valacyclovir and famciclovir may be preferable to acyclovir because of their enhanced oral bioavailability. Visceral disease mandates IV therapy. If the response to oral antiviral agents is not rapid, IV acyclovir therapy should be instituted. The optimal duration of oral antiviral treatment is unknown but must be at least until all lesions are crusted and have no elevated or active borders. Given the safety and efficacy of oral antivirals, treatment duration of at least 10 days and perhaps longer should be considered. Most cases of chronic or acyclovir-resistant VZV infection are associated with initial inadequate oral doses of acyclovir (too short in duration, too low a dose, or in patients with gastrointestinal [GI] disease, in whom reduced GI absorption may be associated with inadequate blood levels of acyclovir). Patients with atypical disseminated disease must be treated aggressively until all lesions resolve. The diagnosis of acyclovir-resistant VZV infection may be difficult. Acyclovir-resistant VZV strains may be difficult to culture, and sensitivity testing is still not standardized or readily available for VZV. Acyclovir-resistant varicella is treated with foscarnet or, in nonresponsive patients, with cidofovir.

Amlie-Lefond C, et al: Varicella zoster virus. J Stroke Cerebrovasc Dis 2016; 25: 1561.

Bate J, et al: Varicella postexposure prophylaxis in children with cancer. Arch Dis Child 2012; 97: 853.

Baxter R, et al: Long-term effectiveness of varicella vaccine. Pediatrics 2013; 131: e1389.

Bollaerts K, et al: A systematic review of varicella seroprevalence in European countries before universal childhood immunization. Epidemiol Infect 2017; 145: 2666.

Centers for Disease Control and Prevention (CDC): FDA approval of an extended period for administering VariZIG for postexposure prophylaxis of varicella. MMWR Morb Mortal Wkly Rep 2012; 61: 212.

Creed E, et al: Varicella zoster vaccines. Dermatol Ther 2009; 22: 143.

Gabutti G, et al: Varicella-zoster virus. Minerva Pediatr 2016; 68: 213.

Hirose M, et al: The impact of varicella vaccination on varicella-related hospitalization rates. Rev Paul Pediatr 2016; 34: 359.

Kao CM, et al: Child and adolescent immunizations. Curr Opin Pediatr 2014; 26: 383.

Leung J, et al: Severe varicella in persons vaccinated with varicella vaccine. Expert Rev Vaccines 2017; 16: 391.

Marin M, et al: Varicella prevention in the United States. Pediatrics 2008; 122: e744.

Marin M, et al: Global varicella vaccine effectiveness. Pediatrics 2016; 137: e20153741.

Nagel MA, et al: Varicella zoster virus vasculopathy. J Neuroimmunol 2017; 308: 112.

Sauerbrei A: Diagnosis, antiviral therapy, and prophylaxis of varicella-zoster virus infections. Eur J Clin Microbiol Infect Dis 2016; 35: 723.

Sugiura K, et al: Varicella zoster virus-associated generalized pustular psoriasis in a baby with heterozygous IL36RN mutation. J Am Acad Dermatol 2014; 71: e216.

Wilson DA, et al: Should varicella-zoster virus culture be eliminated? A comparison of direct immunofluorescence antigen detection, culture, and PCR with a historical review. J Clin Microbiol 2012; 50: 4120.

Varicella-Zoster Virus (Zoster, Shingles, Herpes Zoster), Human Herpesvirus Type 3

Zoster is caused by reactivation of VZV. Following primary infection or vaccination, VZV remains latent in the sensory dorsal root ganglion cells. The virus begins to replicate at some later time, traveling down the sensory nerve into the skin. Immunosuppression, including use of tumor necrosis factor (TNF) inhibitors, Janus kinase Janus kinase (JAK)-inhibitors, and some cancer therapies, HIV, and age-related deficiency of cell-mediated immunity are some of the most common causes of zoster. A family history of zoster is associated with an increased risk of developing zoster, suggesting a genetic risk component. Patients on hemodialysis and those with comorbidities have increased risk of zoster, possibly related to the association between zoster risk and cholesterol level. Statin use also slightly increases the risk for zoster. Zoster patients are more likely to be subsequently diagnosed with a malignancy, especially a hematologic malignancy, with an absolute risk of any cancer of 0.7%–1.8% at 1 year after zoster.

The incidence of zoster increases with age. Under age 45, the annual incidence is less than 1 in 1000 persons. Among patients older than 75, the rate is more than four times greater. For white persons older than 80, the lifetime risk of developing zoster is 10%–30%. Women appear to have higher risk than men. Overall, about one in three unvaccinated persons will develop herpes zoster. For unknown reasons, being nonwhite reduces the risk for herpes zoster, with African Americans one half to one fourth less likely to develop zoster. Autoimmune diseases, asthma, diabetes, and chronic obstructive pulmonary disease are also associated with increased risk. Immunosuppression, especially hematologic malignancy and HIV infection, dramatically increases the risk for zoster. In HIV-infected patients, annual incidence is 30 in 1000 persons, or an annual risk of 3%. With the universal use of varicella vaccination and decrease in pediatric and adolescent varicella cases, older persons will no longer have periodic boosts of the anti-VZV immune activity. Theoretically this could result in an increase in the incidence of zoster.

Herpes zoster classically occurs unilaterally within the distribution of a cranial or spinal sensory nerve, often with some overflow into the dermatomes above and below. The dermatomes most frequently affected are the thoracic (55%), cranial (20%, with the trigeminal nerve being the most common single nerve involved), lumbar (15%), and sacral (5%). The cutaneous eruption is frequently preceded by one to several days of pain in the affected area, although the pain may appear simultaneously or even after the skin eruption, or the eruption may be painless. The eruption initially presents as papules and plaques of erythema in the dermatome (Fig. 19.16). Within hours the plaques develop blisters. Lesions continue to appear for several days. The eruption may have few lesions or reach total confluence in the dermatome. Lesions may become hemorrhagic, necrotic, or bullous. Rarely, the patient may have pain, but no skin lesions (zoster sine herpete). Pain severity correlates with extent of the skin lesions, and elderly persons tend to have more severe pain. In patients under age 30, the pain may be minimal. Scattered lesions can occur outside the dermatome, usually fewer than 20. In the typical case, new vesicles appear for 1–5 days, become pustular, crust, and heal. The total duration of the eruption depends on three factors: patient age, severity of eruption, and presence of underlying immunosuppression. In younger patients, the total duration is 2–3 weeks, whereas in elderly

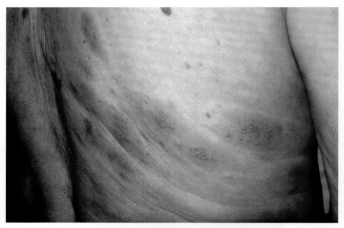

Fig. 19.16 Herpes zoster.

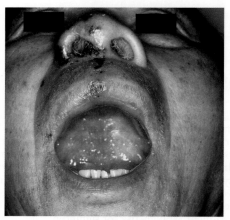

Fig. 19.17 Oral zoster.

patients, the cutaneous lesions of zoster may require 6 weeks or more to heal. Scarring is more common in elderly and immunosuppressed patients. Scarring also correlates with the severity of the initial eruption. Lesions may develop on the mucous membranes within the mouth in zoster of the maxillary division (Fig. 19.17) or mandibular division of the facial nerve, or in the vagina with zoster in the S2 or S3 dermatome. Zoster may appear in recent surgical scars and may follow injections of botulinum toxin.

Zoster may rarely be seen in children under age 1 year. This can result from intrauterine exposure to VZV or exposure to VZV during the first few months of life. The maternal antibodies still present result in muted expression of varicella—subclinical or very mild disease. The immaturity of the infant's immune system results in poor immune response to the infection, allowing for early relapse in the form of zoster.

Disseminated Herpes Zoster

Disseminated herpes zoster is defined as more than 20 lesions outside the affected dermatome. It occurs chiefly in older or debilitated individuals, especially in patients with lymphoreticular malignancy or AIDS. Low levels of serum antibody against VZV are a highly significant risk factor in predicting dissemination of disease. The dermatomal lesions are sometimes hemorrhagic or gangrenous. The outlying vesicles or bullae, which are usually not grouped, resemble varicella and are often umbilicated and may be hemorrhagic. Visceral dissemination to the lungs, liver, and/or CNS may occur in the patient with disseminated zoster.

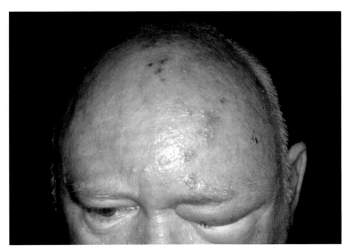

Fig. 19.18 Herpes zoster.

Disseminated zoster requires careful evaluation and systemic antiviral therapy. Initially, IV acyclovir is given, which may be changed to an oral antiviral agent once visceral involvement has been excluded and the patient has received at least 2–3 days of IV therapy.

Ophthalmic Zoster

In herpes zoster ophthalmicus, the ophthalmic division of the fifth cranial nerve is involved. If the external division of the nasociliary branch is affected, with vesicles on the side and tip of the nose (Hutchinson sign), the eye is involved 76% of the time, compared with 34% when it is not involved (Fig. 19.18). Vesicles on the lid margin are virtually always associated with ocular involvement. In any case, the patient with ophthalmic zoster should be seen by an ophthalmologist. Systemic antiviral therapy should be started immediately, pending ophthalmologic evaluation. Ocular involvement is most often in the form of uveitis (92%) and keratitis (50%). Less common but more severe complications include glaucoma, optic neuritis, encephalitis, hemiplegia, and acute retinal necrosis. These complications are reduced from 50% of patients to 20%–30% with effective antiviral therapy. Unlike the cutaneous lesions, ocular lesions of zoster and their complications tend to recur, sometimes as long as 10 years after the zoster episode.

Other Complications

Motor nerve neuropathy occurs in about 3% of patients with zoster and is three times more common if zoster is associated with underlying malignancy. About 75% of patients slowly recover, leaving 25% with some residual motor deficit. Thoracic zoster may be associated with motor neuropathy of the abdominal muscles resulting in a bulge on the flank or abdomen, called a "postherpetic pseudotumor." If the sacral dermatome S3, or less often S2 or S4, is involved, urinary hesitancy or actual urinary retention may occur. Hematuria and pyuria may also be present. The prognosis is good for complete recovery. Similarly, pseudoobstruction, colonic spasm, dilation, obstipation, constipation, and reduced anal sphincter tone can occur with thoracic (T6–T12), lumbar, or sacral zoster. Recovery is complete. Maxillary and mandibular alveolar bone necrosis may occur an average of 30 days after zoster of the maxillary or mandibular branches of the trigeminal nerve. Limited or widespread loss of teeth may result.

Ramsay Hunt syndrome (herpes zoster oticus) results from involvement of the facial and auditory nerves by VZV. Herpetic inflammation of the geniculate ganglion is thought to be the cause of this syndrome. The presenting features include zoster of the external ear or tympanic membrane; herpes auricularis with ipsilateral facial paralysis; or herpes auricularis, facial paralysis, and auditory symptoms. Auditory symptoms include mild to severe tinnitus, deafness, vertigo, nausea and vomiting, and nystagmus.

Herpes zoster can be associated with delayed complications, many of which are caused by vasculopathies affecting the CNS or even the peripheral arteries. There appears to be an increased risk of both ischemic and hemorrhagic stroke within the first 3 months after zoster, which fades by 1 year. Delayed contralateral hemiparesis, simulating cerebrovascular accident (stroke), is a rare but serious complication of herpes zoster that occurs weeks to months (mean 7 weeks) after an episode of zoster affecting the first branch of the trigeminal nerve. By direct extension along the intracranial branches of the trigeminal nerve, VZV gains access to the CNS and infects the cerebral arteries. Patients present with headache and hemiplegia. Arteriography is diagnostic, demonstrating thrombosis of the anterior or middle cerebral artery. This form of vasculopathy can also occur after varicella and may be the cause of up to one third of ischemic strokes in children. The recognized vasculopathic complications of VZV have been expanded to include changes in mental status, aphasia, ataxia, hemisensory loss, and both hemianopia and monocular visual loss. Monocular vision loss can occur up to 6 months after zoster. Aneurysm, subarachnoid or cerebral hemorrhage, carotid dissection, and even peripheral vascular disease are other recognized forms of VZV vasculopathy. The vasculopathy may be multifocal and involve both large and small arteries. In more than one third of cases, VZV vasculopathy occurs without a rash. Magnetic resonance imaging (MRI) is virtually always abnormal. The diagnosis is confirmed by VZV PCR and anti-VZV IgG antibody testing of the CSF. Because this is caused by active viral replication in the vessels, the treatment is IV acyclovir, 10–15 mg/kg three times daily for a minimum of 14 days. In some patients, months of oral antivirals are given if symptoms are slow to resolve. A short burst of systemic corticosteroids is also given in some cases. VZV has been linked to giant-cell arteritis as well, theoretically through similar mechanisms. One recent meta-analysis has also suggested an increased risk of cardiac events associated with herpes zoster as well.

Treatment

Middle-age and elderly patients with herpes zoster are urged to restrict their physical activities or even stay home in bed for a few days. Bed rest may be of paramount importance in the prevention of neuralgia. Younger patients may usually continue with their customary activities. Local applications of heat, as with an electric heating pad or a hot water bottle, are recommended. Simple local application of gentle pressure with the hand or with an abdominal binder often gives great relief.

Antiviral therapy is the cornerstone in the management of herpes zoster. Because antiviral therapy does not reduce the rate of zoster-associated pain (ZAP), clinicians may underappreciate the tremendous benefit that antivirals provide. The main benefit of therapy is reduction of the duration and severity of ZAP. Therefore treatment in immunocompetent patients is indicated for those at highest risk for persistent pain—those over age 50. It is also recommended to treat all patients with painful or severe zoster, ophthalmic zoster, Ramsay Hunt syndrome, immunosuppression, cutaneous or visceral dissemination, and motor nerve involvement. In the most severe cases, especially in ophthalmic zoster and disseminated zoster, initial IV therapy may be considered. Therapy should be started as soon as the diagnosis is suspected, pending laboratory confirmation. It is preferable for treatment to be instituted within the first 3 or 4 days. In immunocompetent patients, the efficacy of starting treatment beyond this time is unknown. Treatment leads to more rapid resolution of the skin lesions and, most importantly, substantially decreases the duration of ZAP. Valacyclovir, 1000 mg, and famciclovir, 500 mg, may be given three times daily. These agents are as effective as or superior to acyclovir, 800 mg five times daily, probably because of better absorption or medication compliance with simpler regimens. Side-by-side trials have demonstrated valacyclovir and famciclovir to be of similar efficacy, but one study from Japan showed famciclovir to result in more rapid reduction in acute zoster pain.

In the immunocompetent host, a total of 7 days of treatment has been as effective as 21 days. These antivirals must be dose-adjusted in patients with renal impairment. In an elderly patient, if the renal status is unknown, the valacyclovir and famciclovir may be started at twice-daily dosing (which is almost as effective), pending evaluation of renal function, or acyclovir can be used. For patients with renal failure (creatinine clearance <25 mL/min), acyclovir is preferable. In the patient with known or acquired renal failure, acyclovir neurotoxicity can occur from IV acyclovir or oral valacyclovir therapy. This can present in the acute setting as hallucinations or with prolonged elevated blood levels, disorientation, dizziness, loss of decorum, incoherence, photophobia, difficulty speaking, delirium, confusion, agitation, and death delusion. Because acyclovir can reduce renal function, the patient's baseline renal function may have been normal, but high doses of acyclovir may have reduced renal function, leading to neurotoxic acyclovir levels.

In the immunosuppressed patient, an antiviral agent should always be given because of the increased risk of dissemination and zoster-associated complications. The doses are identical to those used in immunocompetent hosts. Immunosuppressed patients with ophthalmic zoster, disseminated zoster, or Ramsay Hunt syndrome and those failing oral therapy should receive IV acyclovir, 10 mg/kg three times daily, adjusted for renal function.

Because some of the pain during acute zoster (acute zoster neuritis) may have an inflammatory component, corticosteroids have been used during the acute episode. The use of corticosteroids in this setting is controversial. In selected older patients, corticosteroid use is associated with better quality-of-life measures, reduction in time to uninterrupted sleep, quicker return to usual activities, and reduced analgesic use. A tapering dose of systemic corticosteroids, starting at about 1 mg/kg and lasting 10–14 days, is adequate to achieve these benefits. Systemic corticosteroids should not be used in immunosuppressed patients or when there is a contraindication. All factors considered, the benefits of corticosteroid therapy during acute zoster appear to outweigh the risks in treatment-eligible patients. Reduction in postherpetic neuralgia (PHN) by corticosteroids has never been documented despite multiple studies, but this is also true of antiviral therapy, which reduces the severity and duration but not the prevalence of postherpetic neuralgia.

Zoster-Associated Pain (Postherpetic Neuralgia)

Pain is the most troublesome symptom of zoster; 84% of patients over age 50 will have pain preceding the eruption, and 89% will have pain with the eruption. Various terminologies are used to classify the pain. The simplest approach is to refer to all pain occurring immediately before or after zoster as "zoster-associated pain" (ZAP). Another classification system separates acute pain (within first 30 days), subacute pain (30–120 days), and chronic pain (>120 days).

Two different mechanisms are proposed to cause ZAP: sensitization and deafferentation. Nociceptors (sensory nerves mediating pain) become sensitized after injury, resulting in ongoing discharge and hyperexcitability (peripheral sensitization). Prolonged discharge of the nociceptor enhances the dorsal horn neurons to afferent stimuli and expands the dorsal horn neuron's receptive field (central sensitization), leading to allodynia and hyperalgesia. In addition, neural destruction causes spontaneous activity in deafferented central neurons, generating constant pain. The spinal terminals of mechanoreceptors may contact receptors formerly occupied by C fibers, leading to hyperalgesia and allodynia. The loss of function or death of dorsal horn neurons, which have an inhibitory effect on adjacent neurons, contributes to increased activity transmitted up the spinal cord. The central sensitization is initially temporary (self-limited) but may become permanent.

The quality of the pain associated with herpes zoster varies, but three basic types have been described: the constant, monotonous, usually burning or deep, aching pain; the shooting, lancinating (neuritic) pain; and triggered pain. The last is usually allodynia (pain with normal nonpainful stimuli such as light touch) or hyperalgesia (severe pain produced by a stimulus normally producing mild pain). The character and quality of acute zoster pain are identical to the pain that persists after the skin lesions have healed, although these may be mediated by different mechanisms.

The rate of resolution of pain after herpes zoster is reported over a wide range. The following data are from a prospective study and do not represent selected patients, as are recruited in drug trials for herpes zoster. The tendency to have persistent pain is age dependent, occurring for longer than 1 month in only 2% of persons under age 40. Fifty percent of persons over age 60 and 75% of those over 70 continue to have pain beyond 1 month. Although the natural history is for gradual improvement in persons over age 70, 25% have some pain at 3 months and 10% have pain at 1 year. Severe pain lasting longer than 1 year is uncommon, but 8% of persons over 60 have mild pain and 2% still have moderate pain at 1 year.

The ZAP, especially that of long duration, is very difficult to manage. Adequate medication should be provided to control the pain from the first visit. Once established, neuropathic pain is difficult to control. Every effort should be made to prevent neuronal damage. In addition, chronic pain may lead to depression, complicating pain management. Patients with persistent, moderate to severe pain may benefit from referral to a pain clinic. With this background, the importance of early and adequate antiviral therapy and pain control cannot be overemphasized.

Oral antiviral agents are recommended in all patients over age 50 with pain who still have blisters, even if the drugs are not given within the first 96 hours of the eruption. Oral analgesia should be maximized using acetaminophen, nonsteroidal antiinflammatory drugs (NSAIDs), and opiate analgesia as required. The combination of oral gabapentin and valacyclovir was reported to reduce PHN in one study criticized due to the lack of a control group, but gabapentin alone has not been shown to be highly effective in other zoster trials. Capsaicin applied topically every few hours may reduce pain, but the application itself may cause burning, and the benefits are modest. Local anesthetics, such as 10% lidocaine in gel form, 5% lidocaine-prilocaine, or lidocaine patches (Lidoderm), may acutely reduce pain. Combined topical amitriptyline 4% and ketamine 2% has been reported for PHN and other neuropathic pain conditions. These topical measures may provide some short-term analgesic effect, but do not appear to have any long-term benefit in reducing the severity or prevalence of ZAP. Patients with PHN have lower vitamin C levels than controls, and vitamin C supplementation intravenously (not orally) has been associated with PHN reduction. Sublesional anesthesia, epidural blocks (with or without ketamine), and sympathetic blocks with and without corticosteroids are reported in large series (but rarely studied in controlled trials) to provide acute relief of pain. Although the benefit of nerve blocks in preventing or treating persistent ZAP remains to be proved, these are a reasonable consideration in the acute setting if the patient is having severe pain (unable to eat or sleep) and if oral therapy has yet to be effective. Nerve blocks may also be used in patients who have failed the standard therapies. A transcutaneous electrical nerve stimulation (TENS) unit may be beneficial for persistent neuralgia. Ultrasound-guided spinal nerve radiofrequency treatment has been utilized as well. Botulinum toxin, 100 U, spread out over the affected area in a checkerboard or fanlike pattern with 5 U per route, has dramatically improved PHN in anecdotal reports.

Despite this vast array of medication options, PHN is typically difficult to treat for two reasons. First, the recommended medications are simply often not effective. Second, in elderly patients, who are most severely affected by PHN, these medications have significant and often intolerable side effects, limiting the dose that can be prescribed. If multiple agents are combined to reduce the toxicity of any one agent, their side effects overlap (sedation, depression, constipation) and drug-drug interactions may occur, limiting combination treatment options.

Three classes of medication are used as standard therapies to manage ZAP and PHN: tricyclic antidepressants (TCAs), antiseizure medications, and long-acting opiates. If opiate analgesia is required, it should be provided by a long-acting agent, and the duration of treatment should be limited and the patient transitioned to another class of agent. Constipation is a major side effect in elderly persons. During painful zoster, these patients ingest less fluid and fiber, enhancing the constipating effects of the opiates. Bulk laxatives should be recommended. Tramadol is an option for acute pain control, but drug interactions with the TCAs must be monitored. TCAs such as amitriptyline (or nortriptyline) and desipramine are well tested and documented as effective for the management of PHN and are considered first-line agents. The TCAs are dosed at 25 mg/night (or 10 mg for those over age 65–70). The dose is increased by the same amount nightly until pain control is achieved or the maximum dose is reached. The ultimate dose is between 25 and 100 mg in a single nightly dose. The early use of amitriptyline was able to reduce the pain prevalence at 6 months, suggesting that early intervention is optimal. Venlafaxine (Effexor) may be used in patients who do not tolerate TCAs, at a starting dose of 25 mg/night, gradually titrated upward as required. Gabapentin (Neurontin) and pregabalin (Lyrica) have been documented as helping to reduce ZAP. The starting dose of gabapentin is usually 300 mg three times daily, escalating up to 1800 mg/day. A minimum total dose of 600 mg or more is needed to obtain optimal benefit. One meta-analysis suggests that higher-dose gabapentin (1800 mg/day) can reduce PHN pain, though somnolence, dizziness, and other side effects were common. Pregabalin has improved pharmacokinetics and is given at 300 mg or 600 mg daily, depending on renal function, with better absorption and steadier blood levels. The anticonvulsants diphenylhydantoin, carbamazepine, and valproate; neuroleptics such as chlorprothixene and phenothiazines; and H_2 blockers such as cimetidine cannot be recommended because they have been not been studied critically, many are poorly tolerated by elderly patients, and some are associated with significant side effects. If the patient fails to respond to local measures, oral analgesics (including opiates), TCAs, gabapentin, and venlafaxine, referral to a pain center is recommended.

Immunosuppressed Patients

Immunosuppression increases the risk of zoster, though studies vary as to the impact. The use of TNF inhibitors was initially reported to increase the risk of development of zoster by 1.6 times (or 60%), though a large cohort study suggested no increased risk with monotherapy, only an elevated risk with combination TNF-I and methotrexate. The risk is significant enough that prophylactic immunization should be considered, if not contraindicated, before a patient starts a TNF inhibitor. VZV immunization of patients already receiving TNF inhibition who have had prior varicella has not led to increased zoster or adverse events, and it has reduced the rate of zoster with anti-TNF therapy. This strategy should be considered on a case-by-case basis, perhaps in consultation with an infectious disease specialist. This may be more of a risk with newer classes of drugs, particularly the JAK inhibitors, which appear to carry an elevated risk for zoster.

Patients with malignancy, especially Hodgkin disease and leukemia, are five times more likely to develop zoster than their age-matched counterparts. Patients who also have a higher incidence of zoster include those with deficient immune systems, such as individuals who are immunosuppressed for organ transplantation or by connective tissue disease, or by the agents used to treat these conditions, especially corticosteroids, chemotherapeutic agents, cyclosporine, sirolimus, and tacrolimus. After stem cell transplantation for leukemia, up to 68% of patients will develop herpes zoster in the first 12 months (median 5 months). The cumulative incidence of VZV reactivation in this group may exceed 80% in the first 3 years. Antiviral prophylaxis has been shown to reduce zoster in this population. Because zoster is 30 times more common in HIV-infected persons, the zoster patient under age 50 should be questioned about HIV risk factors. In pediatric patients with HIV infection and in other immunosuppressed children, zoster may rapidly follow primary varicella.

The clinical appearance of zoster in the immunosuppressed patient is usually identical to typical zoster, but the lesions may be more ulcerative and necrotic and may scar more severely. Dermatomal zoster may appear, progress to involve the dermatome, and persist without resolution. Multidermatomal zoster is more common in immunosuppressed patients, including the rare variant "herpes zoster duplex bilateralis," with involvement of two different contralateral dermatomes. Visceral dissemination and fatal outcome are extremely rare in immunosuppressed patients (about 0.3%), but cutaneous dissemination is possible, occurring in 12% of cancer patients, especially those with hematologic malignancies. In bone marrow transplant patients with zoster, 25% develop disseminated zoster and 10%–15%, visceral dissemination. Disseminated zoster may be associated with the syndrome of inappropriate antidiuretic hormone secretion (SIADH) and present with hyponatremia, abdominal pain, and ileus. This later presentation has been reported in stem cell transplant patients. Despite treatment with IV acyclovir, the SIADH can be fatal. In this patient, the number of skin lesions may be small, and the lesions resemble "papules" rather than vesicles. The mortality rate in patients with zoster who have undergone bone marrow transplantation is 5%. VZV IgG serostatus is determined before transplant, and all seropositive patients receive prophylaxis with either acyclovir, 800 mg twice daily, or valacyclovir, 500 mg twice daily, for 1 year or longer if the patient is receiving immunosuppressive therapy. In AIDS patients, ocular and neurologic complications of herpes zoster are increased. Immunosuppressed patients often have recurrences of zoster, up to 25% in patients with AIDS (Fig. 19.19).

Two atypical patterns of zoster have been described in AIDS patients: ecthymatous lesions, which are punched-out ulcerations with a central crust, and verrucous lesions (Fig. 19.20). These patterns were not reported before the AIDS epidemic. Atypical clinical patterns, especially the verrucous pattern, may correlate with acyclovir resistance.

Diagnosis

The same techniques used for the diagnosis of varicella are used to diagnose herpes zoster. The clinical appearance is often adequate to suggest the diagnosis, and an in-office Tzanck smear can rapidly confirm the clinical suspicion. Zosteriform herpes simplex can also have a positive Tzanck smear, but the number of lesions is usually more limited and the degree of pain substantially less than with zoster. Beyond Tzanck preparation, PCR or DFA testing is preferred to a viral culture because it is rapid, types the virus, and has a higher yield than culture. Compared with documented VZV infections, Tzanck smear was 75% positive (with up to 10% false-positives and high variability, depending on skill of examiner), and culture only 44% positive. PCR testing is 97% positive and is generally the test of choice. In atypical lesions, biopsy may be necessary to demonstrate the typical herpes virus cytopathic effects.

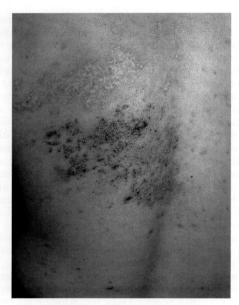

Fig. 19.19 Recurrent zoster in AIDS patient.

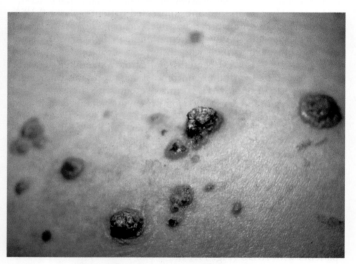

Fig. 19.20 Verrucous zoster in AIDS patient.

IP stain tests can then be performed on paraffin-fixed tissue to identify VZV specifically. When acyclovir fails clinically, viral culture may be attempted and acyclovir sensitivity testing performed. It is not as standardized for VZV as it is for HSV, and availability is limited.

Histopathology

As with herpes simplex, the vesicles in zoster are intraepidermal. Within and at the sides of the vesicle are large, swollen cells called balloon cells, which are degenerated cells of the spinous layer. Acidophilic inclusion bodies similar to those seen in HSV are present in the nuclei of the cells of the vesicle epithelium. Multinucleated keratinocytes, nuclear molding, and peripheral condensation of the nucleoplasm are characteristic and confirmatory of an infection with either HSV or VZV. In the vicinity of the vesicle, there is marked intercellular and intracellular edema. In the upper part of the dermis, vascular dilation, edema, and perivascular infiltration of lymphocytes and polymorphonuclear leukocytes (PMNs) are present. Atypical lymphocytes may also

be found. An underlying leukocytoclastic vasculitis suggests VZV infection over HSV. Inflammatory and degenerative changes are also noted in the posterior root ganglia and in the dorsal nerve roots of the affected nerve. The lesions correspond to the areas of innervation of the affected nerve ganglion, with necrosis of the nerve cells.

Differential Diagnosis

The distinctive clinical picture of zoster permits a diagnosis with little difficulty. A unilateral, painful eruption of grouped vesicles along a dermatome, with hyperesthesia and on occasion regional lymph node enlargement, is typical. Occasionally, segmental cutaneous paresthesias or pain may precede the eruption by 4 or 5 days. In such patients, prodromal symptoms are easily confused with the pain of angina pectoris, duodenal ulcer, biliary or renal colic, appendicitis, pleurodynia, or early glaucoma. The diagnosis becomes obvious once the cutaneous eruption appears. Herpes simplex and herpes zoster are confused if the lesions of HSV are linear (zosteriform HSV), or if the number of zoster lesions is small and localized to one site (not involving whole dermatome). DFA testing or viral culture will distinguish them; DFA is generally preferred because it is rapid and sensitive.

Prevention of Zoster

A vaccine using the same attenuated virus as in the varicella vaccination, but at much higher titers, was licensed for the prevention of herpes zoster (Zostavax), and initially recommended in all persons 60 years or older. This vaccination reduced the incidence of zoster by 50%. In addition, PHN was 67% lower in the vaccine recipients, and duration of ZAP was shortened. Those vaccinated between ages 60 and 69 had a greater reduction in zoster incidence than those over 70, but in both groups, PHN and burden of illness were reduced similarly. Vaccination has led to a reduced rate of ED visits and costs associated with zoster in populations recommended for vaccination. Because it is a live virus vaccine, persons taking antiviral medications must stop them 24 hours before immunization and not take them for 14 days after immunization. Immunosuppressed patients can be safely immunized following specific guidelines. A second zoster vaccine has been developed (Shingrix), which is now recommended for healthy adults 50 years and older, including adults who previously received the first generation shingles vaccine (Zostavax), and is now the preferred vaccine for shingles. This vaccine demonstrated a moderately high rate of side effects, including 81% of subjects with injection-site reactions (pain, myalgia) and 66% with systemic reaction (myalgias), in clinical trials.

Institutionalized patients who develop herpes zoster are infectious to other patients and the health care team. Prior immunization with varicella vaccine and "adequate serologic titers" may not prevent acquiring infection, especially in immunosuppressed patients. Covering the cutaneous lesions specifically with semipermeable dressings (not just gauze bandages) appears to reduce transmission. Patients with active disease should avoid unvaccinated, nonimmunized, immunosuppressed, or pregnant patients if possible.

Inflammatory Skin Lesions after Zoster Infection (Isotopic Response)

Following zoster, inflammatory skin lesions may rarely occur within the affected dermatome. Lesions usually appear within 1 month, or rarely, longer than 3 months, after the zoster. Clinically, the lesions are usually flat-topped or annular papules in the dermatome. Histologically, such papules most frequently demonstrate various patterns of granulomatous inflammation from typical granuloma annulare to sarcoidal reactions or even granulomatous vasculitis

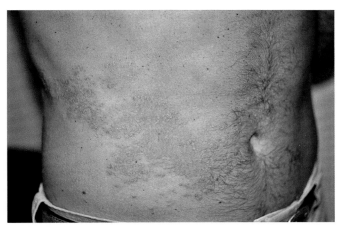

Fig. 19.21 Dermatome previously affected by zoster developed a granulomatous dermatitis histologically consistent with granuloma annulare.

(Fig. 19.21). Persistent viral genome has not been detected in these lesions, suggesting that continued antiviral therapy is not indicated. Persistent VZV glycoproteins may be the triggering antigens. Topical and intralesional therapy with corticosteroids is beneficial, but the natural history of these lesions is generally spontaneous resolution. Less often, other inflammatory skin diseases have been reported in areas of prior zoster, including lichen planus, lichen sclerosus, vitiligo, Kaposi sarcoma (KS), graft-versus-host disease (GVHD), morphea, and benign or even atypical lymphoid infiltrates. Leukemic infiltrates and lymphomas may affect zoster scars, as can metastatic carcinomas (inflammatory oncotaxis) or nonmelanoma skin cancers (NMSCs).

Ansaldi F, et al: Real-world effectiveness and safety of a live-attenuated herpes zoster vaccine. Adv Ther 2016; 33: 1094.

Antoniou T, et al: Statins and the risk of herpes zoster. Clin Infect Dis 2014; 58: 350.

Beal B, et al: Gabapentin for once-daily treatment of post-herpetic neuralgia. Clin Interv Aging 2012; 7: 249.

Cacciapaglia F, et al: Varicella-zoster virus infection in rheumatoid arthritis patients in the anti-tumour necrosis factor era. Clin Exp Rheumatol 2016; 33: 917.

Chakravarty EF: Incidence and prevention of herpes zoster reactivation in patient with autoimmune diseases. Rheum Dis Clin North Am 2017; 43: 111.

Cohen JI: Herpes zoster. N Engl J Med 2013; 369: 255.

Dommasch ED, et al: Trends in nationwide herpes zoster emergency department utilization from 2006-2013. JAMA Dermatol 2017; 153: 874.

Erskine N, et al: A systematic review and meta-analysis on herpes zoster and the risk of cardiac and cerebrovascular events. PLoS One 2017; 12: e0181565.

Fan H, et al: Efficacy and safety of gabapentin 1800 mg treatment for post-herpetic neuralgia. J Clin Pharm Ther 2014; 39: 334.

Fett N: Gabapentin not shown to prevent postherpetic neuralgia. Arch Dermatol 2012; 148: 400.

Friesen KJ, et al: Cost of shingles. BMC Infect Dis 2017; 17: 69.

Gabutti G, et al: Prevention of herpes zoster and its complications. Hum Vaccin Immunother 2017; 13: 391.

Gagliardi AM, et al: Vaccines for preventing herpes zoster in older adults. Cochrane Database Syst Rev 2016; 3: CD008858.

Gilden D, et al: Varicella zoster virus and giant cell arteritis. Curr Opin Infect Dis 2016; 29: 275.

Green CB, Stratman EJ: Prevent rather than treat postherpetic neuralgia by prescribing gabapentin earlier in patients with herpes zoster. Arch Dermatol 2011; 147: 908.

Hadley GR, et al: Post-herpetic neuralgia. Curr Pain Headache Rep 2016; 20: 17.

Hales CM, et al: Update on recommendations for use of herpes zoster vaccine. MMWR Morb Mortal Wkly Rep 2014; 63: 729.

Han Y, et al: Corticosteroids for preventing postherpetic neuralgia. Cochrane Database Syst Rev 2013; 3: CD005582.

Kawai K, et al: Risk factors for herpes zoster. Mayo Clin Proc 2017; 92: 1806.

Keating GM: Shingles (Herpes zoster) vaccine (Zostavax). BioDrugs 2016; 30: 243.

Kim SR, et al: Varicella zoster. Expert Opin Pharmacother 2014; 15: 61.

Lal H, et al: Efficacy of an adjuvanted herpes zoster subunit vaccine in older adults. N Engl J Med 2015; 372: 2087.

Lapolla W, et al: Incidence of postherpetic neuralgia after combination treatment with gabapentin and valacyclovir in patients with acute herpes zoster. Arch Dermatol 2011; 147: 901.

Lian Y, et al: Herpes zoster and the risk of ischemic and hemorrhagic stroke. PLoS One 2017; 12: e0171182.

Neuzil KM, et al: Preventing shingles and its complications in older persons. N Engl J Med 2016; 375: 1079.

Pi ZB, et al: Randomized and controlled prospective trials of ultrasound-guided spinal nerve posterior ramus pulsed radiofrequency treatment for lower back post-herpetic neuralgia. Clin Ter 2015; 166: e301.

Pickering G: Antiepileptics for post-herpetic neuralgia in the elderly. Drugs Aging 2014; 31: 653.

Sawynok J, et al: Topical amitriptyline and ketamine for post-herpetic neuralgia and other forms of neuropathic pain. Expert Opin Pharmacother 2016; 17: 601.

Schmidt SA, et al: Herpes zoster as a marker of occult cancer. J Infect 2017; 74: 215.

Schuster AK, et al: Valacyclovir versus acyclovir for the treatment of herpes zoster ophthalmicus in immunocompetent patients. Cochrane Database Syst Rev 2016; 11: CD011503.

Seo HM, et al: Antiviral prophylaxis for preventing herpes zoster in hematopoietic stem cell transplant recipients. Antiviral Res 2017; 140: 106.

Shalom G, et al: Systemic therapy for psoriasis and the risk of herpes zoster. JAMA Dermatol 2015; 151: 533.

Shreberk-Hassidim R, et al: Janus kinase inhibitors in dermatology. J Am Acad Dermatol 2017; 76: 745.

Snedecor SJ, et al: Systematic review and meta-analysis of pharmacological therapies for pain associated with postherpetic neuralgia and less common neuropathic conditions. Int J Clin Pract 2014; 68: 900.

Tran CT, et al: Herpes zoster. Joint Bone Spine 2017; 84: 21.

Tyring SK: Management of herpes zoster and postherpetic neuralgia. J Am Acad Dermatol 2007; 57: S136.

Vrcek I, et al: Herpes zoster ophthalmicus. Am J Med 2017; 130: 21.

Wise J: Shingles is linked to increased risk for cardiovascular events. BMJ 2015; 351: h6757.

Yamaoka K: Benefit and risk of tofacitinib in the treatment of rheumatoid arthritis. Drug Saf 2016; 39: 823.

Yang SY, et al: Risk of stroke in patients with herpes zoster. J Stroke Cerebrovasc Dis 2017; 26: 301.

Epstein-Barr Virus (Human Herpesvirus Type 4)

Epstein-Barr virus (EBV) is a γ-herpesvirus. It infects human mucosal epithelial cells and B lymphocytes, and infection persists for the life of the host. EBV infection may be latent—not producing virions, but simply spread from mother cell to both daughter cells by copying the viral DNA with each host cell replication. Intermittently, infection may be productive, resulting in production and release of infectious virions. EBV infection may transit between latent and productive infection many times. The ability of EBV to maintain persistent infection is aided by the expression of the EBV nuclear antigen 1 (EBNA-1) viral gene product, which prevents cytotoxic T-lymphocyte response to the virus.

Initial infection with EBV occurs in childhood or early adulthood, so that by their early twenties, 95% of the population has been infected. The virus is shed into the saliva, so contact with oral secretions is the most common route of transmission. Primary infection may be asymptomatic or may produce only a mild, nonspecific febrile illness, especially in younger children. In young adults, primary infection is more likely to be symptomatic and in 50% of cases produces a syndrome termed *infectious mononucleosis* (IM). The incubation period is 3–7 weeks. IM is characterized by a constellation of findings: fever (up to 40°C), headache, lymphadenopathy, splenomegaly, and pharyngitis (sore throat).

Cutaneous and mucous membrane lesions are present in about 10% of IM patients. Exanthems occur in less than 5%, more often in children. Edema of the eyelids and a macular or morbilliform eruption are most common. The eruption is usually on the trunk and upper extremities. Other, less common eruptions are urticarial, vesicular, bullous, petechial, erythema multiforme, and purpuric types. Cold urticaria transiently occurs in 5% of patients with IM. Leukocytoclastic vasculitis and large-vessel arteritis have been seen in chronic EBV infection, often in the setting of immunodeficiency. The mucous membrane lesions consist of distinctive pinhead-sized petechiae, 5–20 in number, at the junction of the soft and hard palate (Forchheimer spots). Gianotti-Crosti syndrome (GCS) and the papular-purpuric glove-and-stocking (or gloves-and-socks) syndrome are two specific viral exanthem patterns that may occur in the patient with asymptomatic primary EBV infection. EBV is now the leading cause of GCS worldwide. EBV reactivation has been infrequently associated with drug-induced hypersensitivity syndrome. EBV is also associated with enhanced insect bite reactions.

Painful genital ulcerations may precede the symptomatic phase of IM, especially in premenarcheal girls. The ulcerations are up to 2 cm in diameter, single or multiple, and may be accompanied by marked swelling of the labia. Lesions last several weeks and heal spontaneously, often as the patient is developing symptoms of IM. Transmission to patients through orogenital sex has been proposed, but the virus may also reach the vulvar mucosa hematogenously. EBV may be the cause of some nonsexually related genital ulcers (Lipschutz ulcers). The lesions closely resemble herpetic ulcerations and fixed drug eruption, which must be considered in the differential diagnosis.

Laboratory evaluation in patients with IM frequently shows an absolute lymphocytosis of greater than 50% and monocytosis with abnormally large, "atypical" lymphocytes. The white blood cell (WBC) count ranges from 10,000–40,000 cells/mm³. Liver function tests (LFTs) may be elevated. Heterophile antibodies will be present in 95% or more of cases. In acute primary EBV infection, immunoglobulin M (IgM) antibodies to early antigen (EA) and viral capsid antigen (VCA) are found in high titer and decrease during recovery. Antibodies to VCA and EBNA appear in the recovering phase and persist for years after primary infection. There is no specific therapy, and in most IM patients, no treatment is required. Acyclovir is not effective in altering the length or severity of IM, although it is active against EBV in doses used for VZV. A recent Cochrane review concluded there is a lack of quality evidence to support antiviral therapy, and treatment decisions depend on the clinical scenario. If patients have severe pharyngeal involvement with encroachment on the airway, or cytopenias or liver failure, oral corticosteroid therapy (40–60 mg/day of prednisone) is useful to induce a prompt response, but are not generally indicated for symptom control in more mild cases. Most patients

recover completely. Patients who participate in contact sports should have abdominal ultrasonography to rule out splenomegaly if planning to participate within 1 month of IM diagnosis.

Almost all patients with IM treated with ampicillin, amoxicillin, or other semisynthetic penicillins typically develop a generalized, pruritic, erythematous to copper-colored macular exanthem on the 7th–10th day of therapy. The eruption starts on the pressure points and extensor surfaces, generalizes, and becomes confluent. The eruption lasts about 1 week and resolves with desquamation. The eruption often does not recur when these medications are given after the acute mononucleosis has resolved, and this is not a true drug allergy.

Oral hairy leukoplakia (OHL) is a distinctive condition initially reported in strong association with HIV, though now has been recognized in patients with other forms of immunocompromise. It appears as poorly demarcated, corrugated white plaques seen on the lateral aspects of the tongue (Fig. 19.22). Lesions on the other areas of the oral mucosa are simply white plaques without the typical corrugations. OHL can be distinguished from thrush by the fact that OHL cannot be removed by firm scraping with a tongue blade. More than one third of patients with AIDS have OHL, but is not restricted to patients with HIV infection; it also occurs in other immunosuppressed hosts, especially renal and bone marrow transplant recipients, and those using inhaled steroids for chronic obstructive pulmonary disease. OHL can be a part of the IRIS. EBV does not establish infection in the basal cell layer of the oral epithelium but is maintained by repeated direct infection of the epithelium by EBV in the oral cavity. Only chronically immunosuppressed patients continuously shed EBV in their oral secretions, thus explaining the restriction of OHL to immunosuppressed hosts. In normal persons, a similar morphologic and histologic picture can be seen (pseudo-OHL), but EBV is not found in these patients' lesions. Thus the finding of OHL warrants immunologic evaluation. A biopsy of the OHL lesions searching for EBV in the epithelium can be useful in this setting. OHL is usually asymptomatic and requires no treatment. If treatment is requested in immunosuppressed patients, podophyllin, applied for 30 seconds to 1 minute to the lesions once each month, is the simplest approach. Tretinoin gel, applied topically twice daily, or oral acyclovir, 400 mg five times daily, is also effective. Lesions recur when treatment is discontinued.

In immunosuppressed and immunocompetent hosts, EBV may be responsible for benign and malignant disorders, some of which can be fatal. These include Kikuchi disease (histiocytic necrotizing lymphadenitis), hydroa vacciniforme (HV) and HV-like lymphoma, hypereosinophilic syndrome, leiomyomas and leiomyosarcomas, lymphomatoid granulomatosis, erythema multiforme, and multiple

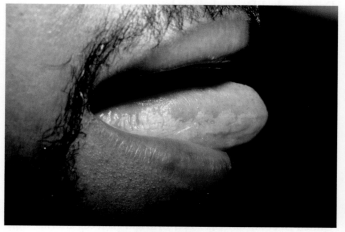

Fig. 19.22 Oral hairy leukoplakia.

types of lymphoma and lymphoproliferative disorders, especially in organ transplant recipients (posttransplant lymphoproliferative disorders, immunosuppression-associated lymphoproliferative disorders). Richter syndrome (development of lymphoma in the patient with chronic lymphocytic leukemia) can present in the skin and may be associated with fludarabine treatment of EBV infection. EBV and other HHV reactivation has been demonstrated in drug reaction with eosinophilia and systemic symptoms (DRESS), and viral replication and host-antiviral response is felt to play a role in the pathophysiology. Ongoing studies are exploring whether there is a connection between EBV and autoimmune disorders, including multiple sclerosis and systemic lupus erythematosus.

Cytomegalovirus (Cytomegalic Inclusion Disease); Human Herpesvirus Type 5

Congenital cytomegalovirus (CMV) infection, as documented by CMV excretion, is found in 1% of newborns, 90% of whom are asymptomatic. Clinical manifestations in infants may include jaundice, hepatosplenomegaly, cerebral calcifications, chorioretinitis, microcephaly, mental retardation, and deafness. Cutaneous manifestations may result from thrombocytopenia, with resultant petechiae, purpura, and ecchymoses. Purpuric lesions, which may be macular, papular, or nodular, may show extramedullary hematopoiesis (dermal erythropoiesis), producing the "blueberry muffin baby." A generalized vesicular eruption may rarely occur. Most symptomatic cases occur within the first 2 months of life. Neonatal disease is more severe and sequelae are more frequent in neonates of mothers with primary rather than recurrent CMV disease in pregnancy.

Between 50% and 80% of immunocompetent adults and up to 100% of HIV-infected men who have sex with men (MSM) are infected with CMV. Infection in adults may be acquired by exposure to infected children, sexual transmission, and transfusion of CMV-infected blood. Symptomatic primary infection in adults is unusual and is identical to IM caused by EBV. An urticarial or morbilliform eruption or erythema nodosum may occur in primary CMV infection in immunocompetent adults. Ampicillin and amoxicillin administration will often result in a morbilliform eruption in acute CMV infection, similar to that seen in acute EBV infection.

Infection with CMV is common in AIDS patients, most frequently causing retinitis (20% of patients), colitis (15%), cholangitis, encephalitis, polyradiculomyopathy, and adrenalitis. It occurs in the setting of very advanced HIV infection, usually with CD4 counts below 50, and has become much less common in the era of highly active antiretroviral therapy (HAART).

CMV infection can manifest in other immunosuppressed hosts. CMV viremia is routinely monitored after stem cell transplant depending on host/donor CMV serostatus, and some cases are treated with prophylactic antivirals or preemptive therapy based on serial CMV PCR testing. Infection will usually affect the GI tract or lungs. Skin disease is rare but may have a wide range of manifestations, from nonspecific morbilliform exanthems that can easily be mistaken for drug reactions, to ulcerated plaques.

Cytomegalovirus infection in tissues is usually identified by the histologic finding of a typical CMV cytopathic effect. In a very small percentage of AIDS patients with CMV infection, skin lesions may occur that contain such cytopathic changes. In most cases, CMV is found in association with another infectious process, and the treatment of that other infection will lead to resolution of the CMV in the skin without its treatment. This is especially true of perianal HSV ulcerations. CMV may even be found in totally normal skin in CMV-viremic AIDS patients, suggesting that finding the CMV cytopathic effect is insufficient alone to imply a causal relationship of the CMV to any cutaneous lesion. Only in the case of perianal and oral ulcerations has the pathogenic

role of CMV been documented. In unusual cases of extremely painful genital ulcerations, only CMV infection is found histologically, or the ulceration persists after effectively treating HSV, with CMV identified histologically. The CMV cytopathic changes may be noted in the nerves at the base of these ulcerations, suggesting that CMV neuritis may be producing the severe pain that characterizes these cases. The diagnosis of CMV ulceration is one of exclusion. CMV cytopathic changes must be seen in the lesion and cultures, and histologic evidence of any other infectious agent must be negative. In these ulcerations, clinically suggested by their location (genital or oral) and painful nature, specific treatment with valganciclovir, foscarnet, or cidofovir will lead to healing of the ulceration and dramatic resolution of the pain.

The CMV infecting endothelial cells may produce a vasculopathy in CMV-viremic or partially reactivating patients. This can lead to prominent vasculopathic changes, including Raynaud phenomenon, deep venous thrombosis, digital gangrene, and reticulated purpura. Anticardiolipin antibodies may be positive. Anti-CMV therapy can reverse the syndrome and clear the anticardiolipin antibodies.

Ascherio A, Munger KL: EBV and autoimmunity. Curr Top Microbiol Immunol 2015; 390: 365.

Chambers AE, et al: Twenty-first-century oral hairy leukoplakia–a non-HIV-associated entity. Oral Surg Oral Med Oral Pathol Oral Radiol 2015; 119: 326.

Chawla JS, et al: Oral valganciclovir versus ganciclovir as delayed pre-emptive therapy for patients after allogeneic hematopoietic stem cell transplant. Transpl Infect Dis 2012; 14: 259.

De Paor M, et al: Antiviral agents for infectious mononucleosis. Cochrane Database Syst Rev 2016; 12: CD011487.

Elqui de Oliveira D, et al: Viral carcinogenesis beyond malignant transformation. Trends Microbiol 2016; 24: 649.

Ferguson NN, et al: Primary cutaneous polymorphic EBV-associated posttransplant lymphoproliferative disorder after a renal transplant and review of the literature. Am J Dermatopathol 2015; 37: 790.

Fernandez-Flores A: Epstein-Barr virus in cutaneous pathology. Am J Dermatopathol 2013; 35: 763.

Gabrib G, et al: Atypical presentation of exophytic herpes simplex virus type 2 with concurrent cytomegalovirus infection: a significant pitfall in diagnosis. Am J Dermatopathol 2013; 35: 371.

Garcia JG, et al: Lipschutz ulcer. Am J Emerg Med 2016; 34: 1326e1.

Klion AD, et al: Chronic active Epstein-Barr virus infection. Blood 2013; 121: 2364.

Lee HY, et al: Primary Epstein-Barr virus infection associated with Kikuchi's disease and hemophagocytic lymphohistiocytosis. J Microbiol Immunol Infect 2010; 43: 253.

Lehloenya R, Meintjes G: Dermatologic manifestations of the immune reconstitution inflammatory syndrome. Dermatol Clin 2006; 24: 549.

Lennon P, et al: Infectious mononucleosis. BMJ 2015; 350: h1825.

Maffini E, et al: Treatment of CMV infection after allogeneic hematopoietic stem cell transplantation. Expert Rev Hematol 2016; 9: 585.

Marty FM, et al: Letermovir prophylaxis for CMV in hematopoietic-cell transplantation. N Engl J Med 2017; 377: 2433.

Milano F, et al: Intensive strategy to prevent CMV disease in seropositive umbilical cord blood transplant recipients. Blood 2011; 118: 5689.

Ozoya OO, et al: EBV-related malignancies, outcomes, and novel prevention strategies. Infect Disord Drug Targets 2016; 16: 4.

Shabani M, et al: Primary immunodeficiencies associated with EBV-induced lymphoproliferative disorders. Crt Rev Oncol Hematol 2016; 108: 109.

Rezk E, et al: Steroids for symptom control in infectious mononucleosis. Cochrane Database Syst Rev 2015; 11: CD004402.

Ryan, C et al: Cytomegalovirus-induced cutaneous vasculopathy and perianal ulceration. J Am Acad Dermatol 2011; 64: 1216.

Tetzlaff MT, et al: Epstein-Barr virus–associated leiomyosarcoma with cutaneous involvement in an African children with human immunodeficiency virus. J Cutan Pathol 2011; 38: 731.

Thompson DF, et al: Antibiotic-induced rash in patients with infectious mononucleosis. Ann Pharmacother 2017; 51: 154.

Human Herpesviruses 6 and 7

Infection with HHV-6 is almost universal in adults, with seropositivity in the 80%–85% range in the United States, and seroprevalence almost 100% in children. There are intermittent periods of viral reactivation throughout life; persistent infection occurs in several organs, particularly in the CNS. Acute seroconversion to HHV-6 and to HHV-7 each appears to be responsible for about one third of roseola cases, and in the remaining third, neither is found. HHV-6 infection occurs earlier than HHV-7, and second episodes of roseola in HHV-6–seropositive children may be caused by HHV-7. Primary infection with HHV-6 is associated with roseola in only 9% of cases, and 18% of children with seroconversion have a rash. Primary infection may occur with only fever and no rash, or rash without fever. Other common findings include otitis media, diarrhea, and bulging fontanelles, sometimes with findings of meningoencephalitis and seizures. Infrequently, hepatitis, intussusception, and even fatal multisystem disease may occur. In adults, acute HHV-6 infection resembles acute mononucleosis. Some have suggested that HHV-6 and HHV-7 may be involved in the development of pityriasis rosea. HHV-6 and HHV-7 reactivation has been demonstrated during DRESS syndrome (along with less commonly EBV and CMV), with many feeling that the drug trigger then allows latent virus replication followed by a host-antiviral response leading to the clinical phenotype observed, which explains the long time course and prolonged treatment required, and the potential for delayed autoimmune sequelae.

As with other herpesviruses, the pattern of disease in HHV-6 may be different in immunosuppressed hosts. HHV-6 reactivation is common after transplantation: 32% after solid-organ and 48% after bone marrow transplantation, peaking on day 21. These patients can be quite ill, with fever, diarrhea, and elevated LFTs, simulating GVHD, with some developing pneumonitis and CNS manifestations as well. Engraftment can be delayed. HHV-6 viremia, detected by PCR, can confirm the diagnosis. Chronic macular erythema has been reported in several cases. Careful histologic evaluation has identified HHV-6–infected lymphocytes and histiocytes in the macular erythema, confirming the diagnosis. Antiviral therapy with ganciclovir, foscarnet, or valganciclovir can lead to improvement, with broad-acting antiviral T cells under investigation.

Roseola Infantum (Exanthem Subitum, Sixth Disease)

Roseola infantum is a common cause of sudden, unexplained high fever in young children between 6 and 36 months of age. Prodromal fever is usually high and may be accompanied by convulsions and lymphadenopathy. Suddenly, on about the fourth day, the fever drops. Coincident with the decrease in temperature, a morbilliform erythema of discrete, rose-colored macules appears on the neck, trunk, and buttocks and sometimes on the face and extremities. Often, there is a blanched halo around the lesions. The eruption may also be papular or rarely even vesicular. The mucous membranes are spared. Complete resolution of the eruption occurs in 1–2 days. A case of spontaneously healing,

generalized eruptive histiocytosis has been reported after exanthem subitum.

Human Herpesvirus 8

A γ-herpesvirus, HHV-8 is most closely related to EBV. HHV-8 has been found in all patients with KS, including those who have AIDS (Fig. 19.23), in African cases; in elderly men from the Mediterranean basin; and in transplant patients. In addition, the seropositivity rate (infection rate) for this virus correlates with the prevalence of KS in a given population.

The background seroprevalence rate of HHV-8 in North America and Northern Europe is near zero. Seroprevalence is highest in KS-endemic areas in sub-Saharan Africa (50%–100%). In the general population in Italy, the seroprevalence is 10%–15% (6%–10% in children under age 16, 22% after age 50). In south-central Italy and in Sardinia, seroprevalence rates are higher, 20%–25% for the general population. In Italy, high rates of HHV-8 seropositivity are also seen in HIV-infected MSM (up to 60%), in female prostitutes (40%), and in heterosexual men who have had sex with prostitutes (40%). Infection with HHV-8 precedes and predicts subsequent development of KS in HIV-infected men. In addition to KS lesions, HHV-8 can be found in saliva and in circulating blood cells in HHV-8–infected patients. HHV-8 is also found in the semen of up to 20% of KS patients. Heterosexual partners of patients with classic KS have high rates of HHV-8 seropositivity (>40%). These epidemiologic features all strongly support sexual transmission as an important mechanism of the spread of HHV-8. The finding of a significant number of infections in prepubertal children, however, suggests that nonsexual methods of transmission also exist. HHV-8 seroprevalence rate in heterosexual IV drug users and persons with HIV infection acquired

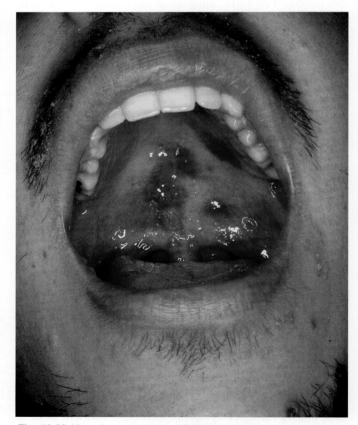

Fig. 19.23 Kaposi sarcoma in an HIV-infected patient; the palate is commonly involved.

through blood transfusion are not increased above that in the general population, suggesting that HHV-8 is poorly transmitted by blood and blood products.

Human herpesvirus 8 is present in a rare type of B-cell lymphoma called body cavity–based B-cell lymphoma or primary effusion lymphoma (PEL), which presents with pleural, pericardial, and peritoneal malignant effusions. Rarely, this form of lymphoma may be associated with skin lesions or may present as an intravascular lymphoma. The cutaneous lesions can resemble a CD30-positive, anaplastic, large T-cell lymphoma. HHV-8 is also found in all patients with multicentric Castleman disease (MCD) associated with HIV infection and in 10%–50% of HIV-negative patients with MCD. Cytokine production, specifically IL-6 from Kaposi syndrome herpesvirus (KSHV)–infected cells (vIL-6) and host inflammatory cells (hIL-6), along with VEGF, appears causal. Exanthems and cutaneous nodules may accompany MCD, and HHV-8 has been identified in the skin lesions. KSHV inflammatory cytokine syndrome (KICS) is an inflammatory syndrome analogous to MCD but lacking the prominent lymphadenopathy. It is also mediated by IL-6 and other cytokines. In HHV-8–associated MCD and KICS, HHV-8 viral loads are much higher than in patients with KS, perhaps aiding in the diagnosis. Kikuchi disease has been linked primarily to EBV, but one study suggests potential association with HHV-8 instead.

Ahluwalia J, et al: Human herpesvirus 6 involvement in paediatric drug hypersensitivity syndrome. Br J Dermatol 2015; 172: 1090.
Auten M, et al: Human herpesvirus 8-related diseases. Semin Diagn Pathol 2017; 34: 371.
Chong Y, et al: Causative agents of Kikuchi-Fujimoto disease. Int J Pediatr Otorhinolaryngol 2014; 78: 1890.
Dittmer DP, et al: Kaposi sarcoma-associated herpesvirus. J Clin Invest 2016; 126: 3165.
El-Ela MA, et al: Is there a link between human herpesvirus infection and Toll-like receptors in the pathogenesis of pityriasis rosea? Acta Dermatovenerol Croat 2016; 24: 282.
Fule Robles JD, et al: Human herpesvirus types 6 and 7 infection in pediatric hematopoietic stem cell transplant recipients. Ann Transplant 2014; 19: 269.
Inazawa N, et al: Virus reactivations after autologous hematopoietic stem cell transplantation detected by multiplex PCR assay. J Med Virol 2017; 89: 358.
Liu AY, et al: Idiopathic multicentric Castleman's disease. Lancet Haematol 2016; 3: e163.
Mohammadpour Touserkani F, et al: HHV-6 and seizure. J Med Virol 2017; 89: 161.
Müzes G, et al: Successful tocilizumab treatment in a patient with human herpesvirus 8–positive and human immunodeficiency virus–negative multicentric Castleman's disease of plasma cell type nonresponsive to rituximab-CVP therapy. APMIS 2013; 121: 668.
Papadopoulou A, et al: Activity of broad-spectrum T cells as treatment for AdV, EBV, CMV, BKV, and HHV6 infections after HSCT. Sci Transl Med 2014; 6: 242ra83.
Roux J, et al: Human herpesvirus-6 cytopathic inclusions. Am J Dermatopathol 2012; 34: e73.
Schlaweck S, et al: Exanthem subitum after autologous stem cell transplantation. Transpl Infect Dis 2016; 18: 255.
Stone RC, et al: Roseola infantum and its causal human herpesviruses. Int J Dermatol 2014; 53: 397.
Wolz MM, et al: Human herpesvirus 6, 7, and 8 from a dermatologic perspective. Mayo Clin Proc 2012; 87: 1004.

B Virus

B virus (*Herpesvirus simiae*) is endemic in Asiatic Old World monkeys (macaques) and may infect other monkeys housed in close quarters with infected monkeys. In macaques, *H. simiae* disease is a recurrent vesicular eruption analogous to HSV in humans, with virus shed from conjunctiva, oral mucosa, and urogenital area. Humans become infected after being bitten, scratched, or contaminated by an animal shedding B virus. Usually, patients are animal handlers or researchers. Rare cases of respiratory or human-to-human contact spread have been reported. Within a few days of the bite, vesicles, erythema, necrosis, or edema appear at the site of inoculation. Regional lymph nodes are enlarged and tender. Fever is typically present. In a substantial number of human infections, rapid progression to neurologic disease occurs. This is initially manifested by peripheral nerve involvement (dysesthesia, paresthesia), then progresses to spinal cord involvement (myelitis and ascending paralysis with hyporeflexia), and finally to brain disease (decreased consciousness, seizures, respiratory depression). Of 22 reported patients, 15 have died, and all survivors of encephalitis had severe neurologic sequelae. Treatment with acyclovir or ganciclovir has been successful in some, but other patients similarly treated have died.

Estep RD, et al: Simian herpesviruses and their risk to humans. Vaccine 2010; 285: 878.
Rohrman M: Macacine herpes virus (B virus). Workplace Health Saf 2016; 64: 9.

INFECTIOUS HEPATITIS

Hepatitis B Virus

Hepatitis B virus (HBV) is a dsDNA virus that is spread by blood and blood products, and sexually in Europe and the Western Hemisphere. In Africa and Asia, infection often occurs perinatally. HBV and hepatitis C virus (HCV) are the primary cause of hepatocellular carcinoma and may also cause liver failure and cirrhosis. Acute infection with HBV is associated with anorexia, nausea, right upper quadrant pain, and malaise. Between 10% and 30% of patients with acute HBV infection have a serum sickness–like illness with urticaria, arthralgias, and occasionally arthritis, glomerulonephritis, or vasculitis. These symptoms appear 1–6 weeks before onset of clinically apparent liver disease and fade as jaundice starts. Immune complexes containing hepatitis B surface antigen (HBsAg) and hypocomplementemia are found in serum and joint fluid. The process spontaneously resolves as antigen is cleared from the blood.

Hepatitis B is associated with polyarteritis nodosa (PAN), with some studies suggesting that more than 30% PAN cases are secondary to HBV. PAN usually occurs within the first 6 months of infection, even during the acute phase, but may occur as long as 12 years after infection. Unlike the urticarial reaction, which is usually associated eventually with development of clinical hepatitis, HBV infection associated with PAN may be silent.

Immunosuppressive treatments can lead to reactivation of silent HBV infection. Before initiating treatment with an immunosuppressive agent (including TNF inhibitors), the patient should be screened for HBV infection by checking hepatitis B antibodies. Only two thirds of patients who receive immunomodulators will be HBsAg positive. Although 75% of HBV-infected patients will remain asymptomatic during immunomodulator treatment, a third will develop severe hepatitis, and more than 10% will die or develop fulminant hepatitis. Rituximab and cyclophosphamide cause reactivation early. Most of these patients would be candidates for preemptive antiviral therapy, so all patients with serologic evidence of HBV infection in whom immunosuppressive treatment or TNF inhibitor therapy is being considered should be referred to a hepatologist before initiating immunosuppressive therapy.

A highly effective vaccine is available to prevent HBV infection. It is recommended as a part of standard childhood immunizations, and all health care workers should be immunized. Patients who will receive TNF inhibitor treatment and who are not immunized may be considered for immunization.

Hepatitis C Virus

Hepatitis C virus (HCV) is a single-stranded (ss) RNA virus that causes most cases of non-A, non-B viral hepatitis. Now that a serologic test is available to screen blood products for HCV infection, the vast majority of new cases of HCV infection are parenterally transmitted by IV drug use. Compared with hepatitis B, sexual transmission is uncommon (<1% transmission/year of exposure). Mother-to-infant spread occurs in 5% of cases. Only about one third of patients are symptomatic during acute infection. Between 55% and 85% of patients will have chronic infection. Although most patients have minimal symptoms for the first one to two decades of infection, cirrhosis and liver failure, as well as hepatocellular carcinoma, are common sequelae. Chronic HCV infection is associated with various skin disorders, either by direct effect or from the associated hepatic damage.

Cutaneous necrotizing vasculitis, which is usually associated with a circulating mixed cryoglobulin, occurs in approximately 1% of patients with chronic HCV infection. In 84%–90% of patients with type II or type III cryoglobulinemia, HCV infection is present. The most common clinical presentation is palpable purpura of the lower extremities (90% of cases). Livedo reticularis, retiform purpura, urticaria, and subcutaneous nodules showing a granulomatous vasculitis may also occur. Arthropathy, glomerulonephritis, and neuropathy frequently accompany the skin eruption. Leg ulcers can occur in 10%–20%. Rheumatoid factor, a type II cryoglobulin, and hypocomplementemia (often isolated low C4 and normal C3) are found in the majority of cases. Histologically, a leukocytoclastic vasculitis is seen in all patients, though some may also show small fibrin thrombi and vasculopathy. In some, the vasculitis may involve small arteries, giving a histologic pattern similar to that seen in PAN. In various studies, 5%–20% of patients with PAN were HCV positive, suggesting that both HBV and HCV can cause PAN. The presence of anti-HCV antibodies should not be used as the sole diagnostic test in patients with PAN, because PAN may cause a false-positive enzyme-linked immunosorbent assay (ELISA) test for HCV. HCV-infected patients with mixed cryoglobulinemia are 35 times more likely to develop non-Hodgkin lymphoma, usually of the B-cell type. In virus-associated vasculitis, treating the underlying virus is essential.

Patients with porphyria cutanea tarda (PCT) often have hepatocellular abnormalities. Depending on the prevalence of HCV infection in the population studied, 10%–95% of sporadic (not familial) PCT cases are HCV associated. Treatment of the HCV infection may lead to improvement of the PCT.

Hepatitis C infection has been associated with lichen planus, with about a fourfold increased risk for its development in the HCV-positive patient. The likelihood of identifying HCV infection in a patient with lichen planus is greatest in geographic regions with high rates of HCV infection. Patients with oral lichen planus are also more likely to be HCV infected. Serologic testing in a patient should be considered if the patient has HCV risk factors or abnormal LFTs or is from a geographic region where, or from population in whom, HCV infection is common. HCV may also be associated with cutaneous B-cell lymphoma. In studies from Japan and Israel, patients with HCV infection were almost twice as likely to develop psoriasis, especially men over 40 years. They were less obese but had higher rates of hypertension and diabetes mellitus. Approximately 15% of patients with HCV infection have pruritus. Pruritus virtually always is associated with advanced liver disease and abnormal LFTs. Patients with pruritus and normal LFTs and no history of hepatitis rarely will be infected with HCV.

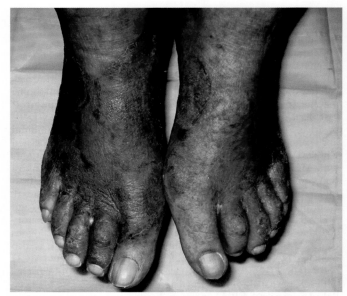

Fig. 19.24 Necrolytic acral erythema. (Courtesy Carrie Kovarik, MD.)

Necrolytic acral erythema (NAE) is a rare condition associated with HCV infection. It affects persons of African origin and occurs in less than 2% of HCV-infected patients in the United States. It resembles the nutritional deficiency dermatoses, except that it has an acral distribution. The clinical lesions are painful or pruritic, keratotic, well-defined plaques with raised red scaly borders or diffuse hyperkeratosis (Fig. 19.24). Erosion and flaccid blisters may occur, contributing to the discomfort. The dorsal feet (less often the dorsal hands) as well as the lower extremities may be involved. Histologically, there is necrosis of the superficial portion of the epidermis, along with hyperkeratosis, papillomatosis, loss of the granular cell layer, and parakeratosis. Intraepidermal spongiotic foci are present, which may be macroscopic at times, with the cleavage plane between the necrotic and viable epidermis. Generally zinc, essential fatty acid, and glucagon levels are normal, unlikely in other "deficiency" dermatoses, but the patients may be hypoalbuminemic and have low serum amino acids because of their liver disease. Some cases of NAE have been described with zinc deficiency, and as responsive to zinc supplementation. Treatment of the associated HCV infection with IFN and ribavirin, IFN plus zinc, and liver transplantation has resulted in resolution. Hyperalimentation was also partially effective in some patients, as was amino acid supplementation with zinc.

The treatment of HCV infection is rapidly evolving. A combination of IFN alpha and ribavirin is the historical treatment for patients with chronic HCV infection, with sustained responses in slightly over 50% of patients. Combined IFN and ribavirin therapy may be complicated by an eczematous eruption with pruritus in about 8% of patients and severe pruritus in about 1%. Eczema typically affects the distal extremities, dorsal hands, face, neck, and less frequently the trunk, axillae, and buttocks. The eruption may be photodistributed and photoexacerbated. These eczematous eruptions typically begin 2–4 months after initiation of treatment. In affected patients, prior treatment with IFN alone was usually not associated with an eczematous eruption. Histologically, the eruptions show a spongiotic dermatitis. The eruption resolves completely if treatment is stopped for 2–3 weeks but will recur when treatment is restarted. Aggressive therapy with antihistamines, emollients, and potent topical corticosteroids will usually control the eczema, allowing uninterrupted continuation of treatment. IFN has also been reported to induce granulomatous reactions, including cutaneous and systemic sarcoidosis, both at injection sites and remotely.

Telaprevir, an HCV protease inhibitor, was introduced as an agent to enhance response of HCV to treatment. This agent, however, was associated with a high rate of adverse skin reactions (60%–80% of patients). Most occurred in the first 10 days of telaprevir administration. More than 90% of telaprevir-associated drug reactions are graded as mild (localized, grade 1) or moderate (diffuse, grade 2) and could be treated with topical agents and oral antipruritics. Over time, numerous severe cutaneous reactions, including high rates of DRESS and Stevens-Johnson syndrome, were observed. Newer agents are available with both better efficacy and substantially reduced adverse event rates, and telaprevir is no longer available in the United States.

Newer "direct-acting antiviral" (DAA) agents include elbasvir-grazoprevir, combination regiments with paritaprevir-ritonavir-ombitasvir, and other novel antiviral agents. Generally regimens are tailored to the patient based on the level of cirrhosis, prior treatment history, and HCV-genotype status.

Alaizari NA, et al: Hepatitis C virus infections in oral lichen planus. Aust Dent J 2016; 61: 282.

Birkenfeld S, et al: A study on the association with hepatitis B and hepatitis C in 1557 patients with lichen planus. J Eur Acad Dermatol Venereol 2011; 25: 436.

Botelho LF, et al: Necrolytic acral erythema. An Bras Dermatol 2016; 91: 649.

Cacoub P, et al: Cryoglobulinemia vasculitis. Am J Med 2015; 128: 950.

Dammacco F, et al: The expanding spectrum of HCV-related cryoglobulinemic vasculitis. Clin Exp Med 2016; 16: 233.

Dammacco F, Sansonno D: Therapy for hepatitis C virus-related cryoglobulinemic vasculitis. N Engl J Med 2013; 369: 1035.

De Virgilio A, et al: Polyarteritis nodosa. Autoimmune Rev 2016; 15: 564.

Gragnani L, et al: Hepatitis C virus-related mixed cryoglobulinemia. World J Gastroenterol 2013; 19: 8910.

Hou YC, et al: Zinc-responsive necrolytic acral erythema in a patient with psoriasis. Int J Low Extrem Wounds 2016; 15: 260.

Jakobsen JC, et al: Direct-acting antivirals for chronic hepatitis C. Cochrane Database Syst Rev 2017; 6: CD012143.

Kishi A, et al: Biphasic skin reactions during telaprevir-based therapy of Japanese patients infected with hepatitis C virus. J Am Acad Dermatol 2014; 70: 584.

Montaudié H, et al: Drug rash with eosinophilia and systemic symptoms due to telaprevir. Dermatology 2010; 221: 303.

Motaparthi K, et al: From the Medical Board of the National Psoriasis Foundation: recommendations for screening for hepatitis B infection prior to initiating anti–tumor necrosis factor-alfa inhibitors or other immunosuppressive agents in patients with psoriasis. J Am Acad Dermatol 2013; 70: 178.

Muchtar E, et al: How I treat cryoglobulinemia. Blood 2017; 129: 289.

Ozen S: The changing face of polyarteritis nodosa and necrotizing vasculitis. Nat Rev Rheumatol 2017; 13: 381.

Rebora A: Skin diseases associated with hepatitis C virus. Clin Dermatol 2010; 28: 489.

Roujeau JC, et al: Telaprevir-related dermatitis. JAMA Dermatol 2013; 149: 2.

Teng GG, et al: Vasculitis related to viral and other microbial agents. Best Pract Res Clin Rheumatol 2015; 29: 226.

Vigano M, et al: HBV-associated cryoglobulinemic vasculitis. Kidney Blood Press Res 2014; 39: 65.

Yost JM, et al: Necrolytic acral erythema. Dermatol Online J 2013; 19: 20709.

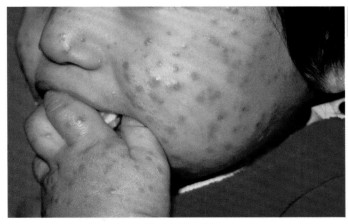

Fig. 19.25 Gianotti-Crosti syndrome.

Gianotti-Crosti Syndrome (Papular Acrodermatitis of Childhood, Papulovesicular Acrolocated Syndrome)

Gianotti-Crosti syndrome (GCS) is a characteristic viral exanthem. It was initially associated with the early anicteric phase of HBV infection. With universal HBV immunization, HBV is now a rare cause of GCS. EBV is now the most common cause of GCS worldwide. Other implicated infectious agents have included adenovirus, CMV, enteroviruses (coxsackie A16, B4, and B5), vaccinia virus, rotavirus, hepatitis A and C, respiratory syncytial virus, parainfluenza virus, parvovirus B19, rubella virus, HHV-6, streptococcus, and *Mycobacterium avium*. Immunizations against poliovirus, diphtheria, tetanus, pertussis, Japanese encephalitis, influenza, and hepatitis B and measles (together) have also caused GCS.

The clinical features are identical, independent of the cause. GCS typically affects children 6 months to 14 years of age (median age 2 years, 90% of cases occurring before the age of 4), more commonly in those with atopy, and may rarely be seen in adults (women primarily, men very rarely). Proposed diagnostic criteria involve the following positive clinical features of GCS:

1. Monomorphous, flat-topped, pink-brown papules or papulovesicles of 1–10 mm in diameter (Figs. 19.25 and 19.26)
2. Any three or all four sites involved—face, buttocks, forearms, and extensor legs
3. Symmetry
4. Duration of at least 10 days

Negative clinical features include the following:

1. Extensive truncal lesions
2. Scaly lesions

The lesions develop over a few days but last longer than most viral exanthems (>10 days and up to many weeks). Lesion numbers may vary from a few to a generalized eruption coalescing to form plaques covering the face, trunk, and upper extremities. Early in the course of the eruption, the lesions will demonstrate a Koebner phenomenon. Pruritus is variable, and the mucous membranes are spared, except when inflamed by the associated infectious agent. Depending on the cause, the lymph nodes, mainly inguinal and axillary, are moderately enlarged for 2–3 months. No treatment appears to shorten the course of GCS, which is self-limited.

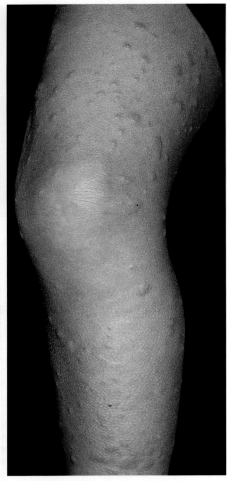

Fig. 19.26 Papules on the leg, Gianotti-Crosti syndrome. (Courtesy Curt Samlaska, MD.)

Brandt O, et al: Gianotti-Crosti syndrome. J Am Acad Dermatol 2006; 54: 136.

Chuh A, et al: Is Gianotti-Crosti syndrome associated with atopy? Pediatr Dermatol 2016; 33: 488.

Chuh A, et al: The diagnostic criteria of pityriasis rosea and Gianotti-Crosti syndrome—a protocol to establish diagnostic criteria of skin diseases. J R Coll Physicians Edinb 2015; 45: 218.

Retrouvey M, et al: Gianotti-Crosti syndrome following childhood vaccinations. Pediatr Dermatol 2013; 30: 137.

Stojkovic-Filipovic J, et al: Gianotti-Crosti syndrome associated with Ebstein-Barr virus and parvovirus B-19 coinfection in a male adult. G Ital Dermatol Venereol 2016; 151: 106.

POXVIRUS GROUP

The poxviruses are DNA viruses of a high molecular weight. The viruses are 200–300 nm in diameter and thus can be seen in routine histologic material. Molluscum contagiosum virus and the now-eliminated variola virus are the only poxviruses for which humans represent the primary host and reservoir. The other poxviruses are primarily infections of animals, from whom humans accidentally become infected. The orthopoxviruses that have infected humans include vaccinia, monkeypox, cowpox, buffalopox, and camelpox. The parapoxviruses causing human disease include orf, bovine papular stomatitis, and sealpox. Many other genera of poxviruses have recently been discovered but are primarily pathogens in wild

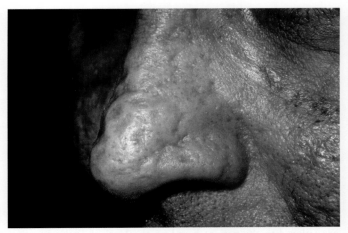

Fig. 19.27 Smallpox scarring. (Courtesy Steven Binnick, MD.)

animals, so human disease is extremely rare or is not yet identified.

Variola Major (Smallpox)

Smallpox was eradicated worldwide in 1977. It continues to be of interest to dermatologists as a potential biologic warfare agent, and some have suggested that wild smallpox may have the potential to reemerge as climate change and global warming thaw previously frozen mass graves from the era when smallpox was rampant. Variola is spread by the respiratory route, with 37%–88% of unvaccinated contacts becoming infected. The incubation period for smallpox is 7–17 days (average 10–12 days). The prodromal phase consists of 2–3 days of high fever (>40°C), severe headache, and backache. The fever subsides, and an exanthem covers the tongue, mouth, and oropharynx. This is followed in 1 day by the appearance of skin lesions, distributed in a centrifugal pattern, with the face, arms, and legs more heavily involved than the trunk. Lesions appear first on the palms and soles and feel like firm "BBs" under the skin. Beginning as erythematous macules (days 1–2), the lesions all in synchrony become 2–3 mm papules (days 2–4) and evolve to 2–5 mm vesicles (days 4–7) and 4–6 mm pustules (days 5–15). The pustules umbilicate, collapse, and form crusts beginning in the second week. The total evolution averages 2 weeks. Lesions on the palms and soles persist the longest. The crusts separate after about 1 more week, leaving scars (Fig. 19.27), which are permanent in 65%–80% of the survivors. Patients are infectious from the onset of the exanthem through the first 7–10 days of the eruption. A variety of complications occur, including pneumonitis, blindness caused by viral keratitis or secondary infection (1% of patients), encephalitis (<1% of patients), arthritis (2% of children), and osteitis. Immunity is lifelong. The mortality rate was 5%–40% in undeveloped countries (and before current intensive care and antiviral management).

Diagnosis is made by electron microscopy, viral culture, and PCR. Special laboratories, usually associated with city and state health departments in the United States, can process these specimens and confirm the diagnosis. The differential diagnosis is primarily varicella, especially the more severe form seen in adults. In varicella, the prodrome lasts for 1–2 days; fever begins with onset of the eruption (not preceding it by 1–3 days, as in variola); the eruption is concentrated on the torso (not centrifugally); and individual lesions of different stages are present and evolve from vesicles to crust within 24 hours. The diagnostic test of choice in these patients is a Tzanck smear, which can rapidly confirm the multinucleated cells of varicella, followed by confirmatory testing with PCR or DFA.

Treatment of smallpox includes strict isolation and protection of health care workers. Only vaccinated persons should treat the patient, and any of those exposed should immediately be vaccinated because this modifies the disease, with ring vaccination of contacts. Cidofovir modifies infections by other orthopoxviruses and may be indicated.

Breman JG, Henderson DA: Diagnosis and management of smallpox. N Engl J Med 2002; 346: 1300.
Centers for Disease Control and Prevention: Smallpox. Retrieved July 12, 2017, from https://www.cdc.gov/smallpox/index.html.
Jahrling PB, Tomori O: Variola virus archives. Lancet 2014; 383: 1525.
Thèves C, et al: The rediscovery of smallpox. Clin Microbiol Infect 2014; 20: 210.

Vaccinia

The vaccinia virus (VACV) has been propagated in laboratories for immunization against smallpox. There are multiple strains used in vaccines, and the rates of complications vary somewhat, depending on the strain used. The available antiviral agents with activity against vaccinia are limited. If a case of vaccinia is encountered, the state health department or the U.S. Centers for Disease Control and Prevention (CDC) should be contacted immediately for optimal management. VACV appears to have been initially isolated by Jenner from horse hooves and is closely related to horsepoxvirus. There have been epidemics of VACV infections on the teats of dairy cattle, the mouths of their calves, and the hands of dairy farmers in Brazil since the 1990s. VACV has also been isolated from wild rodents in Brazil.

Vaccination

Vaccination is inoculation of live VACV into the epidermis and upper dermis by the multiple puncture technique. Between 3 and 5 days after inoculation, a papule forms, which becomes vesicular at days 5–8, then pustular, reaching a maximum size at days 8–10. The pustule dries from the center outward, revealing the pathognomonic umbilicated pustule, and forms a scab that separates 14–21 days after vaccination, resulting in a pitted scar. Formation by days 6–8 of a papule, vesicle, ulcer, or crusted lesion, surrounded by a rim of erythema and induration, is termed a "major reaction" or "take." The rim of erythema averages 3.5–4 cm in diameter in new vaccinees and peaks on days 9–11. Repeat vaccinees have reactions of a similar time course, but the maximum diameter of the erythema is only 1–2 cm. Reactions that do not match this description are considered equivocal, and such persons cannot be considered immune; revaccination should be considered. A large vaccination reaction, or "robust take," is the development of a plaque of erythema and induration greater than 10 cm at the site of inoculation. This occurs in 10% of initial vaccinees. It peaks at days 8–10 and resolves without treatment within 72 hours. Cellulitis secondary to vaccination occurs on days 1–5 after vaccination or after several weeks and progresses without treatment. Management should be expectant, but a bacterial culture may be taken. Vaccinated patients may have fever on days 8–10 after vaccination, so culture is not helpful in separating cellulitis from a "robust take." Rarely, patients will develop lesions at the site of vaccination an average of 2 months later. Their nature is unknown, but these lesions have not been identified as containing live virus and are self-limited.

Vaccination involves the inoculation of a live virus. Complications result from an abnormal response to the vaccination by the host or from inadvertent transmission to another person. Persons with eczema or systemic immunity are at particular risk for adverse outcomes from vaccination. Because some complications

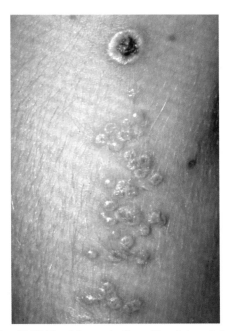

Fig. 19.28 Vaccinia vaccination with autoinoculation.

may be fatal, extremely careful steps must be taken to avoid complications.

Inadvertent Inoculation and Autoinoculation

Inadvertent inoculation of vaccinia may occur by transmission of virus by hands or fomites from the vaccination site to another skin area or the eye, or to another person. Accidental autoinoculation occurs in about 1 in 1000 vaccinees (Fig. 19.28). Autoinoculation most often occurs around the eyes and elsewhere on the face, but the groin and other sites may be involved. These lesions evolve in parallel with the primary vaccination site and, except for ocular lesions, cause no sequelae, except scarring at times. Any evidence of ocular inflammation in a recently vaccinated individual could represent ocular vaccinia infection and requires immediate ophthalmologic evaluation. Transmission to others (secondary transfer) is rare if the vaccination site is kept covered until it heals (7.4 in 100,000 primary vaccinees). It usually occurs within a household or through intimate contact. Serial transmission can occur among male sports partners and has been reported in serial sexual partners. Correct bandaging of the vaccination site using foam or occlusive dressings, not gauze bandages, and treating the inoculation site with povidone-iodine ointment beginning 7 days after immunization both can reduce viral shedding and might reduce autoinoculation and secondary cases.

Generalized Vaccinia

From 6–9 days after vaccination, a generalized vaccinia eruption may occur, in about 81 per 1 million new vaccinees or 32 per 1 million repeat vaccinees. The lesions are papulovesicles that become pustules and involute in 3 weeks, although successive crops may occur within that time. Generalized vaccinia may be accompanied by fever, but patients do not appear ill. Lesions may be generalized or limited to one anatomic region and can number from a few to hundreds. They can be confused with multisite autoinoculation, as well as erythema multiforme. The diagnosis is confirmed by biopsy, viral culture, or PCR. Generalized vaccinia is self-limited and does not require treatment in the immunocompetent host. In the patient with underlying immunodeficiency, early intervention with vaccinia immune globulin intravenous (VIGIV) may be beneficial.

Eczema Vaccinatum

Eczema vaccinatum is analogous to EH, representing VACV infection superimposed on a chronic dermatitis, especially AD. Patients with Darier disease, Netherton syndrome, and other disorders of cornification may also be at risk. Because patients with AD or any past history of AD should not be vaccinated, most cases of eczema vaccinatum represent secondary transfer to an at-risk individual from a recent vaccinee, usually a family member. The vesicles appear suddenly, mostly in areas of active dermatitis. The lesions are sometimes umbilicated and appear in crops, resembling smallpox or chickenpox. The onset is sudden, and fresh vesicles appear for several days. Scarring is common. Often, cervical adenopathy and fever occur, and affected persons are systemically ill (unlike those with generalized vaccinia). Secondary bacterial infection can complicate eczema vaccinatum. The mortality rate for eczema vaccinatum is 30%–40% if untreated. VIGIV reduces the mortality rate to 7%. Multiple doses of VIGIV and perhaps treatment with effective antivirals may be required.

Progressive Vaccinia (Vaccinia Necrosum, Vaccinia Gangrenosum)

Progressive vaccinia is a rare, severe, and often fatal complication of vaccination that occurs in immunodeficient persons. Most cases occur when infants with undiagnosed immunodeficiency are immunized. The initial vaccination site continues to progress and fails to heal after more than 15 days. The vaccination site is characterized by a painless but progressive necrosis and ulceration (Fig. 19.29), with or without metastatic lesions to distant sites (skin, bones, viscera). No inflammation is present at the sites of infection, even histologically. Untreated progressive vaccinia is virtually always fatal. Progressive vaccinia is diagnosed by skin biopsy, viral culture, or PCR. VIGIV should be given, and antiviral antibiotics available from the CDC have been effective in this rare condition.

Cutaneous Immunologic Complications

A spectrum of erythematous eruptions follows vaccination. These eruptions are more common than generalized vaccinia, with which they are often confused. Cases of Stevens-Johnson syndrome after vaccination have been seen in the past, primarily in children, but apparently are rare in adult vaccinees.

Benign Hypersensitivity Reactions to Vaccinia. About 0.08% of vaccinees will develop a diffuse cutaneous eruption during the second week after vaccination, around the peak of the immunization site reaction. These reactions have been classified as exanthematous (by far the most common), urticaria, and erythema multiforme (EM)–like (the most rare). A follicular eruption has also been reported (see next section). All these reaction patterns evolve over 1–2 days and resolve over days. Patients may have mild symptoms but are afebrile. At times, the eruption may evolve from around the inoculation site and generalize, called "roseola vaccinia" in the past. Primary vaccinees are more likely to develop these reactions. Histology is nonspecific, showing features of a viral exanthem (mild spongiotic dermatitis). These reactions are distinguished from generalized vaccinia by a later onset (end of second week vs. days 6–9 after vaccination), prominent erythema, lack of vesicles and pustules, and negative laboratory testing for vaccinia virus. The eruptions described as EM-like lack mucosal involvement and blistering and more closely resemble urticaria multiforme (see Chapter 7). They are distinguished from EM/ Stevens-Johnson syndrome by the absence of atypical purpuric or typical targetoid lesions, lack of mucosal involvement, and histologic evaluation.

Postvaccination Follicular Eruption. A generalized variant of the eruption occurred in 2.7% of new vaccinees and a localized variant in 7.4% during a trial of Aventis Pasteur smallpox vaccine. In the second week, 9–11 days after vaccination, multiple follicular, erythematous papules appeared, primarily on the face, trunk, and proximal extremities. Lesions were mildly pruritic. Over several days, the lesions evolved to pustules, which resolved without scarring. Lesions were simultaneously at different stages of development. The number of lesions was usually limited and rarely exceeded 50. Lesions spontaneously resolved over a few days. Histologic evaluation revealed a suppurative folliculitis. No virus was detected in the lesions by PCR or viral culture.

Other Skin Lesions at Vaccination Scars. Melanomas, basal cell carcinomas (BCCs), and squamous cell carcinomas (SCCs) have all occurred in vaccination scars. Benign lesions with a tendency to occur in scars, such as dermatofibromas, sarcoidosis, and granuloma annulare, also can occur in vaccination scars.

Bessinger GT, et al: Benign hypersensitivity reactions to smallpox vaccine. Int J Dermatol 2007; 4: 460.

Bunick CG, et al: Expanding the histologic findings in smallpox-related post-vaccinial non-viral folliculitis. J Cutan Pathol 2013; 40: 305.

Centers for Disease Control and Prevention: Secondary and tertiary transmission of vaccinia virus after sexual contact with a smallpox vaccine—San Diego, California, 2012. MMWR Morb Mortal Wkly Rep 2013; 62: 145.

Ferguson JL, et al: Rash in a U.S. Marine after predeployment vaccinations. Am Fam Physician 2017; 95: 37.

Hammarlund E, et al: Traditional smallpox vaccination with reduced risk of inadvertent contact spread by administration of povidone iodine ointment. Vaccine 2008; 26: 430.

Hivnor C, James W: Autoinoculation vaccinia. J Am Acad Dermatol 2003; 50: 139.

Gilbert SC: Clinical development of modified vaccinia virus Ankara vaccines. Vaccine 2013; 31: 4241.

Middaugh N, et al: Notes from the field: adverse reaction after vaccinia virus vaccination—New Mexico, 2016. MMWR Morb Mortal Wkly Rep 2016; 65: 1351.

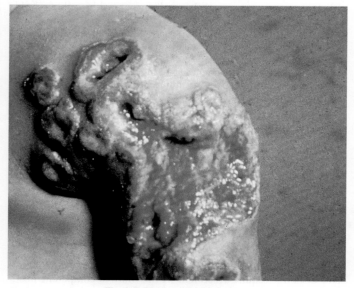
Fig. 19.29 Vaccinia necrosum.

Human Monkeypox

Human monkeypox (virus, MPXV), caused by an orthopoxvirus, is a sporadic zoonosis that occurs in remote areas of the tropical rainforests in central and western Africa, primarily the Democratic Republic of Congo. The mortality rate is 1%–8%. The number of cases has dramatically increased since the 1980s. The main vector for monkeypox is wild African rodents and monkeys. Humans are accidental hosts. Direct contact with an infected animal or person appears to be required to acquire the infection. In Africa, more than 90% of cases occur in children under 15 years of age, in whom the fatality rate is 11%. The secondary attack rate in African households is 10%–12%. An outbreak of 81 cases of monkeypox occurred in the United States. Prairie dogs became infected when housed with infected African rodents. Persons who purchased the prairie dogs became infected, most frequently through bites or scratches or areas of damaged skin. The pattern of monkeypox seen in the U.S. cases was different from that of African cases; transmission was believed to be by inoculation, and many of the affected persons were previously immunized with vaccinia. Primary skin lesions occurred at sites of inoculation and limited spread occurred thereafter, with the appearance of 1–50 additional satellite and disseminated lesions over several days. Patients often had fever, respiratory symptoms, and characteristic lymphadenopathy (67%). About one quarter required hospitalization, and only two children had serious clinical illness, one with encephalitis and one with severe oropharyngeal lesions.

In Africa, monkeypox is clinically similar to smallpox, with an incubation period of 10–14 days. Patients develop headache (100%); fever, sweats, and chills (82%); and lymphadenopathy (90%). Lymphadenopathy is not a feature of smallpox. The prodrome lasts 2 days, followed by the appearance of 2–5 mm papules. The lesions spread centrifugally and progress from papules to vesicles, then pustules all in 14–21 days. In 80% of patients, the lesions are largely monomorphic but are more pleomorphic than smallpox. The distribution is generalized, and the buccal mucosa can be affected. Lesions resolve with hemorrhagic crusts. The disease is self-limited. It is less severe in persons previously vaccinated against smallpox.

Buffalopoxvirus

Buffalopoxvirus (BPXV) is an orthopoxvirus closely related to VACV. It affects buffalo, cows, and humans, and multiple outbreaks have occurred in India. Wild rodents are probably the natural reservoir. Lesions occur on the hands and arms of animal handlers and resemble a milder form of cowpox. Family members may be affected, and children have developed lesions resembling eczema vaccinatum.

Zoonotic Poxvirus Infections

The diagnosis of zoonotic poxvirus infection is usually by epidemiologic history, clinical features, and electron microscopy, which can separate the various poxvirus genera. Laboratory culture is slow, and PCR analysis of the viral DNA allows for speciation. Rarely is antiviral therapy indicated; most diseases are self-limited. Cidofovir would be thought to have activity against the zoonotic poxviruses.

Cowpox

Cowpox (virus, CPXV) is an orthopoxvirus that is geographically restricted to the United Kingdom, Europe, Russia, and adjacent states. It is largely a zoonosis that rarely affects cattle. The domestic cat is the usual source of human infection. Cats acquire infection from wild animal reservoirs (small wild rodents such as mice and voles). Lesions first appear on the head and then on the paws and ears. Feline infection may be asymptomatic, or the cat may be very ill. Most human cases occur in the late summer and in fall. The recent popularity of pet rats in Europe has led to several cases of rat-to-human transmission of CPXV, especially in children too young to have received smallpox vaccination.

The incubation period of CPXV is about 7 days. There is then an abrupt onset of fever, malaise, headache, and muscle pain. Lesions are usually solitary (72%), with coprimary lesions in 25% of cases. Lesions occur on the hands and fingers in half the cases and the face in another third. Pet rats seem to infect children usually on the neck. Secondary lesions are uncommon and generalized disease is rare, usually occurring in patients with AD and Darier disease. The lesion progresses from a macule through a vesicular stage, then a pustule that becomes blue-purple and hemorrhagic. A hard, painful, 1–3 cm, indurated eschar develops after 2–3 weeks and may resemble cutaneous anthrax. In anthrax, however, the eschar forms by day 6. Lesions are always painful, and there is local lymphadenopathy, which is usually tender. The amount of surrounding edema and induration is much more marked than in orf. Patients are systemically ill until the eschar stage. Healing usually takes 6–8 weeks. Scarring is common after cowpox.

Farmyard Pox

Because closely related parapoxviruses of sheep and cattle cause similar disease in humans, orf and milker's nodules have been collectively called farmyard pox. The epidemiologic features are discussed separately, but the clinical and histologic features, which are identical, are discussed jointly. The diagnosis of these infections is based on taking an accurate history and can virtually always be confirmed by routine histologic evaluation.

Bovine-Associated Parapoxvirus Infections: Milker's Nodules, Bovine Papular Stomatitis (BPSV), and Pseudocowpox (PCPV). Bovine-associated parapoxvirus infections cause worldwide occupational disease of milkers or veterinarians, most often transmitted directly from the udders (milker's nodules) or muzzles (bovine papular stomatitis) of infected cows. Lesions are usually solitary or few in number and are confined to the hands or forearms (Fig. 19.30). Numerous lesions have been reported in healing first-degree and second-degree burns in milker's nodules. These cases occurred on farms with infected cattle, but the patients had not had direct contact with the cattle, suggesting indirect viral transmission.

Orf. Also known as ecthyma contagiosum, orf is a common disease in goat-farming and sheep-farming regions throughout the world. Direct transmission from active lesions on lambs is most common,

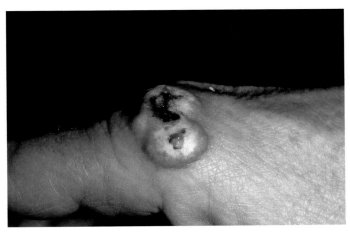

Fig. 19.30 Milker's nodule.

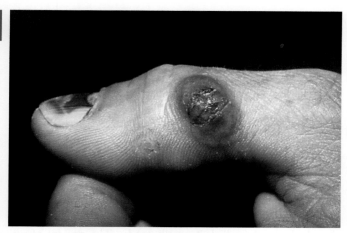

Fig. 19.31 Orf.

but infection from fomites also frequently occurs because the virus is resistant to heat and dryness. Slaughtering of animals for religious feasts can spread the disease, and in Australia, deer was the vector for one case. Once patients are infected, autoinoculation (particularly to the genital area) can occur, but human-to-human transmission is rare. One report detailed orf occurring in skin-graft donor and recipient sites. One patient receiving etanercept developed a giant lesion and progressive disease. He was successfully treated with surgical removal, cryotherapy, and topical imiquimod, with discontinuation of the etanercept.

Clinical Features. The incubation period for farmyard pox is about 1 week. Lesions are usually solitary and occur on the hands, fingers (Fig. 19.31), or face. Lesions evolve through the following six stages:

1. A papule forms, which then becomes a target lesion with a red center surrounded by a white ring and then a red halo.
2. In the acute stage, a red, weeping nodule appears, resembling pyogenic granuloma.
3. In a hairy area, temporary alopecia ensues.
4. In the regenerative stage, the lesion becomes dry with black dots on the surface.
5. The nodule then becomes papillomatous.
6. The nodule finally flattens to form a dry crust, eventually healing.

Lesions are usually about 1 cm in diameter, except in immunosuppressed patients, in whom giant lesions may occur. Dermoscopy likely varies by stage, but a nodule with central crust, white structureless areas, white streaks, surrounded by vessels and peripheral scale has been described. Spontaneous resolution occurs in about 6 weeks, leaving minimal scarring. Mild swelling, fever, pain, and lymphadenitis may accompany the lesions, but these symptoms are milder than those seen in cowpox. Orf may be associated with an EM-like eruption in about 5% of patients. Treatment is supportive, although shave excision may accelerate healing. Topical cidofovir and imiquimod have been effective.

Histologic Features. Histologic features of farmyard pox correlate with the clinical stage. Nodules show a characteristic pseudoepitheliomatous hyperplasia covered by a parakeratotic crust. Keratinocytes always demonstrate viropathic changes of nuclear vacuolization and cytoplasmic, 3–5 μm, eosinophilic inclusions surrounded by a pale halo. The papillary dermis is severely edematous. The dermal infiltrate, which is dense and extends from the interface to the deep dermis, consists of lymphocytes, histiocytes, neutrophils, and eosinophils. Massive capillary proliferation and

dilation are present in the upper dermis. Electron microscopy has been used to identify the viral particles.

Human Tanapox

Tanapox infection is a yatapoxvirus infection endemic to equatorial Africa. It is spread from its natural hosts, nonhuman primates, through minor trauma. Human-to-human transmission is rare. Tanapox infection is manifested by mild fever of abrupt onset lasting 3–4 days, followed by the appearance of one or two pock lesions. Lesions are firm and cheesy, resembling cysts. The disease is self-limited, and smallpox vaccination would not be expected to be protective. Rare cases have been imported into Europe and the United States.

Cann JA, et al: Comparative pathology of smallpox and monkeypox in man and macaques. J Comp Pathol 2013; 148: 6.

Centers for Disease Control and Prevention: Update: multistate outbreak of monkeypox—Illinois, Indiana, Kansas, Missouri, Ohio, and Wisconsin, 2003. Arch Dermatol 2003; 139: 1229.

Dhar AD, et al: Tanapox infection in a college student. N Engl J Med 2004; 350: 361.

Donoghue S, et al: Orf from deer. Australas J Dermatol 2015; 56: 67.

Gallina L, et al: Erythema multiforme after orf virus infection. Epidemiol Infect 2016; 144: 88.

Hsu CH, et al: Unique presentation of Orf virus infection in a thermal-burn patient after receiving an autologous skin graft. J Infect Dis 2016; 214: 1171.

Joseph RH, et al: Erythema multiforme after orf virus infection. Epidemiol Infect 2015; 143: 385.

Koufakis T, et al: Orf disease. Braz J Infect Dis 2014; 18: 568.

Lederman ER, et al: Progressive vaccinia. J Infect Dis 2012; 206: 1372.

McCollum AM, Damon IK: Human monkeypox. Clin Infect Dis 2014; 58: 260.

Peng F, et al: A case of orf identified by transmission electron microscopy. Chin Med J 2016; 129: 108.

Rajkomar V, et al: A case of human to human transmission of orf between mother and child. Clin Exp Dermatol 2016; 41: 60.

Rørdam OM, et al: Giant orf with prolonged recovery in a patient with psoriatic arthritis treated with etanercept. Acta Derm Venereol 2013; 93: 487.

Reynolds MG, Damon IK: Outbreaks of human monkeypox after cessation of smallpox vaccination. Trends Microbiol 2012; 20: 80.

Shcelkunov SN: An increasing danger of zoonotic orthopoxvirus infection. PLoS Pathog 2013; 9: e1003756.

Veraldi S, et al: Presentation of orf after sheep slaughtering for religious feasts. Infection 2014; 42: 767.

Vogel S, et al: The Munich outbreak of cutaneous cowpox infection. Acta Derm Venereol 2012; 92: 126.

Molluscum Contagiosum

Molluscum contagiosum (MC) is caused by up to four closely related types of poxvirus, MCV-1 to MCV-4, and their variants. Although the proportion of infection caused by the various types varies geographically, MCV-1 infections are most common worldwide. In small children, virtually all infections are caused by MCV-1. In contrast to HSV, there is no difference in the anatomic region of isolation with regard to infecting type. In patients infected with HIV, however, MCV-2 causes the majority of infections (60%).

Infection with MCV is worldwide and increasing. Three groups are primarily affected: young children (highest in ages 1–4 years), sexually active young adults (ages 20–29), and immunosuppressed

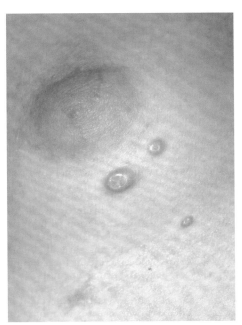

Fig. 19.32 Molluscum contagiosum. (Courtesy Steven Binnick, MD.)

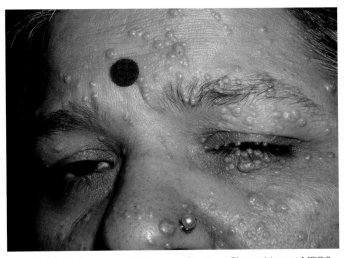

Fig. 19.33 Molluscum contagiosum. (Courtesy Shyam Verma, MBBS, DVD.)

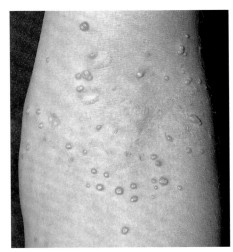

Fig. 19.34 Molluscum contagiosum in child with atopic dermatitis.

persons, especially those with HIV infection. MC is most easily transmitted by direct skin-to-skin contact, especially if the skin is wet. Bathing and swimming pools have been associated with infection although it is not clear how much of this is because of sharing wet towels, kickboards and other swim equipment. Even plantar lesions can be seen.

In all forms of MC infection, the lesions can vary in size and presentation although the most typical is a small smooth-surfaced, firm, dome-shaped, pearly papule, averaging 3–5 mm in diameter (Fig. 19.32 and 19.33). Early lesions can be less than 1 mm and larger "giant" cystic lesions can be over 1 cm. A central umbilication or central white core is characteristic but may not be notable until the lesions get to a certain size. Side lighting can help highlight the opening in the top of the lesion and when the lesions are frozen, often a small circular area is highlighted on top. Irritated lesions may become crusted and even pustular, simulating secondary bacterial infection. The inflammatory response can result in warmth,

surrounding redness and pain that closely simulates and may be indistinguishable from cellulitis. Lesions that rupture into the dermis may elicit a marked suppurative inflammatory reaction that resembles an abscess.

The clinical pattern depends on the risk group affected. In young children, even with normal immunity, the lesions are usually generalized and number from a few to more than 100. Lesions tend to be on the axillae, inguinal areas, popliteal or antecubital fossae and face. Genital lesions, as part of a wider distribution, occur in 10% of childhood cases. When MC is restricted to the genital area in a child, inappropriate sexual contact must be considered but even in this scenario, the infection is usually not from this type of contact. Children with AD, either active or inactive, are four times more likely than nonatopic children to have more than 50 lesions and the course may last longer. Exuberant infection especially in association with other viral infections should raise the possibility of immunodeficiency such as a DOCK-8 mutation. Transmission from the mother's skin can occur during vaginal delivery and may be associated with presentation in the first few months of life especially on the scalp. Immunosuppression, either systemic T-cell immunosuppression (usually HIV, immunosuppressive medications, and malignancies) or abnormal cutaneous immunity (as in AD or topical steroid use), predisposes to infection. In AD patients, lesions tend to be confined to dermatitic skin (Fig. 19.34). The MC virus itself has been shown to cause inhibit NF Kappa B possibly explaining how it avoids the immune system for so long.

Several forms of inflammation occur in children with MC. The most common inflammatory response, seen in 40% of affected children, is "molluscum dermatitis." More common in atopic children, it is a mild, eczematous eruption surrounding the individual lesions. An asymmetric, new dermatitis in an axilla or antecubital or popliteal fossa of a young child should alert the clinician to evaluate for very small molluscum causing the dermatitis. The dermatitis is not associated with more rapid resolution of the MC, and treatment of this dermatitis with low potency topical corticosteroids does not appear to lead to increased MC. Inflamed MC is characterized by erythema and swelling of the individual lesions, sometimes with pustulation or fluctuance. It occurs in 20% of children with MC and usually heralds the resolution of disease. This has been named the "BOTE" sign (beginning of the end) and can be helpful for parents who are concerned about the redness and pain to understand that the infection may be close to resolution. Secondary infection may occur, but most inflamed MC are not infected, but rather undergoing spontaneous involution by the immune response. Rarely, erythema annulare centrifugum may be associated with MC. A Giannotti-Crosti type reaction characterized by minimally pruritic symmetric monomorphic papules on the extensor surfaces including the elbows and knees sparing the trunk can occur as the lesions are starting to resolve occurring in up to 5% of children with MC. The lesions closely resemble individual lesions of molluscum causing parents and clinician to mistakenly think the molluscum is suddenly rapidly spreading.

In adults, MC can be sexually transmitted, and other STDs may coexist. The lesions favor the lower abdomen, upper thighs, and perineum including the penile shaft in men. Pubic hair removal by shaving, clipping, or waxing is a risk factor for acquiring MC by sexual contact or spreading it once the infection has occurred. Mucosal involvement is very uncommon.

Lesions on the eyelid margin or conjunctiva may be associated with a conjunctivitis or keratitis. Rarely, the molluscum lesions may present as a cutaneous horn. Between 10% and 30% of AIDS patients not receiving ART have MC. Virtually all HIV-infected patients with MC already have an AIDS diagnosis and a helper T-cell (Th) count of less than 100. In untreated HIV disease, lesions favor the face (especially the cheeks, neck, and eyelids) and genitalia. Lesions may form confluent plaques and facial disfigurement can occur. Giant lesions can occur and may be confused with a skin cancer. Involvement of the oral and genital mucosa may occur, virtually always indicative of advanced AIDS (Th count <50).

MC has a characteristic histopathology. Lesions primarily affect the follicular epithelium. The lesion is acanthotic and cup shaped. In the cytoplasm of the prickle cells, numerous small, eosinophilic and later basophilic inclusion bodies form, called molluscum bodies or Henderson-Paterson bodies. Eventually, their bulk compresses the nucleus to the side of the cell. In the fully developed lesion, each lobule empties into a central crater. Inflammatory changes are slight or absent. Latent infection has not been found, except in untreated AIDS patients, in whom even normal-appearing skin may contain viral particles. Therefore new appearance of previously undetectable MC may be seen in AIDS patients starting ART as a part of IRIS. Resolving and inflamed lesions may contain a dense inflammatory infiltrate of lymphocytes and neutrophils. Some of the lymphocytes may be large and CD30 positive. MCV contains an IL-18–binding protein. This blocks the host's initial effective Th1 immune response against the virus by reducing local IFN-γ production.

The diagnosis of MC is easily established in most cases because of the distinctive central umbilication of the dome-shaped lesion. Other papules that can also umbilicate and simulate molluscum include the infections *Cryptococcus, Histoplasmosis, coccidioidiomycosis* and *Penicillium marnefii* and the skin tumors keratoacanthoma and desmoplastic trichilemmoma. Lesions that cluster and coalesce in the intergluteal cleft can mimic condyloma accuminatum and especially in a young child, it is vital to differentiate these diagnosis because condyloma is more likely to be transmitted due to inappropriate sexual contact. The central umbilication of molluscum may be enhanced by light cryotherapy, which highlights the round opening of the umbilication. For confirmation, the pasty core of a lesion can be expressed, squashed firmly between two microscope slides (or slide and coverslip with caution not to break the coverslip), and stained with Wright, Giemsa, or Gram, the oval Henderson Patterson bodies can be seen.

Treatment is determined by the clinical setting. In young immunocompetent children, especially those with numerous lesions, because the lesions spontaneously resolve, it is reasonable not to treat. Aggressive treatment may be emotionally traumatic and may lead to scarring. Individual lesions last 2–4 months each; duration of infection is 12–18 months. Because the MC lesions often induce an eczematous reaction around them, just treating this with low-potency topic steroid is reasonable to decrease itch while awaiting resolution.

Simple at home therapies include pressing tape against a lesion and picking it up multiple times per day for a few weeks or continuous application of surgical tape to each lesion daily after bathing for 16 weeks. Topical cantharidin is often used to lesions on the body and extremities though typically the face is avoided as is the perineum in children due to risk of exuberant blisters in these areas. The more that is applied and longer the therapy is left on prior washing, the more vesiculation that occurs. Cantharone mixed with podophyllin should be avoided in molluscum as it is unnecessarily strong. Cantharone is applied by the wooden end of a cotton swab only to the lesion and left on for 1–6 hours before washing. Approximately 20 lesions can be treated per setting. This therapy is well tolerated, has a very high satisfaction rate for patients and their parents, and complications are rare.

If lesions are limited and the child is cooperative, slightly nicking the opening of the lesions with a blade or needle to allow for comedone extraction, squeezing the lesion with a tissue forceps, light cryotherapy, application of trichloroacetic acid (TCA, 35%–100%), and removal by curettage are all alternatives. The application of lidocaine-prilocaine cream for 1 hour before any painful treatments has made the management of MC in children easier but there are reports of systemic toxicity so caution is advised. No controlled trials have confirmed the efficacy of imiquimod, and two large trials have shown that it is no more effective than placebo. Topical tretinoin applied with a toothpick or Q tip in very small amounts to the individual lesions can be used with some benefit especially for lesions on the face to induce some slight irritation and activate the immune system. Intralesional immunotherapy with candidal antigen injections in up to three lesions led to complete resolution of all lesions in 55% of children in one study. Hydrogen peroxide 1% cream, ingenol mebutate, pulse dye laser, povidone iodine, aloe vera and potassium hydroxide 10% are other reported therapies.

Oral cimetidine has been similarly used for its immunomodulatory effects and may have benefit mostly in some patients with atopic patients. In patients with AD, curettage or cryotherapy is most effective while least likely to exacerbate the AD. If cantharone is used, the AD in the area should be treated before therapy to decrease the risk of exuberant response.

In adults with genital molluscum, removal by cryotherapy or curettage is very effective. Neither imiquimod nor podophyllotoxin has been demonstrated to be effective. In fact, the failure of these agents to improve "genital warts" suggests the diagnosis of genital MC. Sexual partners should be examined; screening for coexistent STDs is mandatory.

In immunosuppressed patients, especially those with AIDS, management of MC can be difficult. Treatment of the HIV infection, is predictably associated with a dramatic resolution of the lesions. This response is delayed 6–8 months from the institution of treatment, so reports of resolution with certain agents in the HIV patient is confounded by the coexistent therapy. MC occurs frequently in the beard area, so shaving with a blade razor should be discontinued to prevent its spread. If lesions are few, curettage or core removal with a blade and comedo extractor is most effective. Cantharone or TCA may be applied to individual lesions. Temporary dyspigmentation and slight surface irregularities may occur. Cryotherapy may be effective but must be used with caution in persons of color due to risk of dyspigmentation. When lesions are numerous or confluent, treatment of the whole affected area may be required because of possible latent infection. TCA peels above 35% concentration (medium depth) or daily applications of 5-fluorouracil (5-FU) to the point of skin erosion may eradicate lesions, at least temporarily. In patients with HIV infection, continuous application of tretinoin cream once nightly at the highest concentration tolerated may reduce the rate of appearance of new lesions. Topical 1%–3% cidofovir application and systemic infusion of this agent have been reported to lead to dramatic resolution of molluscum in patients with AIDS.

Arora S, et al: Idiopathic CD4 lymphocytopenia presenting as recurrent giant molluscum contagiosum. Indian J Dermatol Venereol Leprol 2013; 79: 555.

Bansal S, et al: Disseminated molluscum contagiosum in a patient on methotrexate therapy for psoriasis. Indian J Dermatol Venereol Leprol 2014; 80: 179.

Berger EM, et al: Experience with molluscum contagiosum and associated inflammatory reactions in a pediatric dermatology practice. Arch Dermatol 2012; 148: 1257.

Brady G, et al: Molluscum contagiosum virus protein MC005 inhibits NFκB activation by targeting NEMO-regulated IKK activation. J Virol 201; 91: e00545.

Butala N, et al: Molluscum BOTE sign. Pediatrics 2013; 131: e1650.

Can B, et al: Treatment of pediatric molluscum contagiosum with 10% potassium hydroxide solution. J Dermatolog Treat 2014; 25: 246.

Capriotti K, et al: Molluscum contagiosum treated with dilute povidone-iodine. J Clin Aesthet Dermatol 2017; 10: 41.

Cohen PR, Tschen JA: Plantar molluscum contagiosum. Cutis 2012; 90: 35.

Desreuelles F, et al: Pubic hair removal: a risk factor for "minor" STI such as molluscum contagiosum. Sex Transm Infect 2013; 89: 212.

Drain PK, et al: Recurrent giant molluscum contagiosum immune reconstitution inflammatory syndrome (IRIS) after initiation of antiretroviral therapy in an HIV-infected man. Int J STDS AIDS 2014; 25: 235.

Enns LL, Evans MS: Intralesional immunotherapy with *Candida* antigen for the treatment of molluscum contagiosum in children. Pediatr Dermatol 2011; 28: 254.

Foissac M, et al: Efficacy and safety of intravenous cidofovir in the treatment of giant molluscum contagiosum in an immunosuppressed patient. Ann Dermatol Venereol 2014; 141: 620.

Heng YK, et al: Verrucous plaques in a pemphigus vulgaris patient on immunosuppressive therapy. Int J Dermatol 2012; 51: 1044.

Javed S, Tyring SK: Treatment of molluscum contagiosum with ingenol mebutate. J Am Acad Dermatol 2014; 70: e105.

Katz, KA: Imiquimod is not an effective drug for molluscum contagiosum. Lancet 2014; 14: 372.

Kim MS, et al: Atypical molluscum contagiosum accompanied by CD30-positive lymphoid infiltrates. Pediatr Dermatol 2013; 30: 141.

Lao M, et al: Safe and speedy cantharidin application. J Am Acad Dermatol 2013; 69: e47.

McCollum AM, et al: Molluscum contagiosum in a pediatric American Indian population. PLoS One 2014; 9: e103419.

Moye VA, et al: Safety of cantharidin. Pediatr Dermatol 2014; 13: 458.

Navarrete-Dechent C, et al: Desmoplastic trichilemmoma dermoscopically mimicking molluscum contagiosum. J Am Acad Dermatol 2017; 76: S22.

Neri I, et al: Congenital molluscum contagiosum. Paediatr Child Health 2017; 22: 241.

Nguyen HP, et al: Treatment of molluscum contagiosum in adult, pediatric, and immunodeficient populations. J Cutan Med Surg 2014; 18: 299.

Olsen JR, et al: Epidemiology of molluscum contagiosum in children. Fam Pract 2014; 31: 130.

Olsen JR, et al: Time to resolution and effect on quality of life of molluscum contagiosum in children in the UK. Lancet Infect Dis 2015; 15: 190.

Olsen JR, et al: Molluscum contagiosum and associations with atopic eczema in children. Br J Gen Pract 2016; 66: e53.

Pereira de Carvalho CH, et al: Intraoral molluscum contagiosum in a young immunocompetent patient. Oral Surg Oral Med Oral Pathol Oral Radiol 2012; 114: e57.

Pompei DT, et al: Cantharidin therapy. J Am Acad Dermatol 2013; 68: 1045.

Semkova K, et al: Hydrogen peroxide 1% cream under occlusion for treatment of molluscum contagiosum in an 8-month-old infant: an effective and safe treatment option. Clin Exp Dermatol 2014; 39: 560.

Shinkai K, Fox LP: The diagnosis: inflamed molluscum contagiosum as a manifestation of immune reconstitution inflammatory syndrome. Cutis 2012; 89: 219.

Siah TW, et al: Gross generalized molluscum contagiosum in a patient with autosomal recessive hyper-IgE syndrome, which resolved spontaneously after haematopoietic stem-cell transplantation. Clin Exp Dermatol 2013; 38:197.

Sim JH, Lee ES: Molluscum contagiosum presenting as a cutaneous horn. Ann Dermatol 2011; 23: 262.

Van der Wouden JC, et al: Interventions for cutaneous molluscum contagiosum. Cochrane Database Syst Rev 2009; 4: CD004767.

Xiang Y, Moss B: Molluscum contagiosum virus interleukin-18 (IL-18) binding protein is secreted as a full-length form that binds cell surface glycosaminoglycans through the C-terminal tail and a furin-cleaved form with only IL-18 binding domain. J Virol 2003; 77: 2623.

PICORNAVIRUS GROUP

Picornavirus designates viruses that were originally called enteroviruses (polioviruses, coxsackieviruses, and echoviruses), plus the rhinoviruses. The picornaviruses are small, ssRNA, icosahedral viruses varying in size from 24–30 nm. Only the enterovirus types 70, 71 coxsackieviruses (A16, and A6) and echoviruses, and are significant causes of skin disease.

Enterovirus Infections

Person-to-person transmission occurs by the intestinal-oral route, oral-oral or respiratory routes or by direct inoculation from active lesions to broken skin. Enteroviruses are identified by type-specific antigens. Viral cultures obtained from the rectum, pharynx, eye, and nose may isolate the infecting agent and stool will carry the virus for weeks after the cutaneous infection resolves Usually, the diagnosis is by clinical characteristics although with the more exuberant A6 infections, differentiation from HSV is sometimes necessary. Enteroviral infections most frequently occur in children between ages 6 months and 6 years.

Many nonspecific exanthems and enanthems that occur during the summer and early fall are caused by coxsackievirus or echovirus. The exanthemata most typically are diffuse macular or morbilliform erythemas, which sometimes also contain vesicular lesions or petechial or purpuric areas. Each type of exanthem has been associated with many subtypes of coxsackievirus or echovirus (one exanthem, many possible viral causes). Echovirus 9, the most prevalent enterovirus, causes a morbilliform exanthem, initially on the face and neck, then the trunk and extremities. Only occasionally is there an eruption on the palms and soles. Small, red or white lesions on the soft palate may occur. Rarely, Echovirus 9 has caused an eruption resembling acute meningococcemia. The most common specific eruptions caused by enteroviruses are hand-foot-and-mouth disease, herpangina, enterovirus superinfecting AD (eczema coxackium) and a roseola-like illness. Rare reported presentations of enterovirus infection include a unilateral vesicular eruption simulating herpes zoster, caused by echovirus 6; a fatal dermatomyositis-like illness in a patient with hypogammaglobulinemia, caused by echovirus 24. Pleconaril and other antienteroviral agents may be useful in severe enteroviral infections.

Although the cutaneous eruptions caused by these viruses are quite benign, infections with enterovirus 71 can be severe, with the development of brainstem encephalitis and fatal neurogenic pulmonary edema, as well as ascending flaccid paralysis resembling

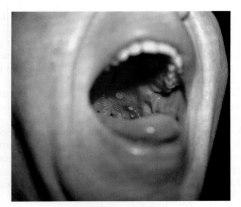

Fig. 19.35 Herpangina.

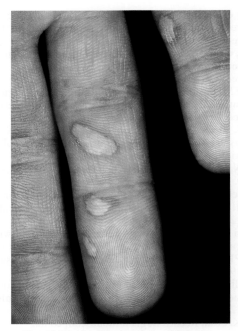

Fig. 19.36 Hand-foot-and-mouth disease.

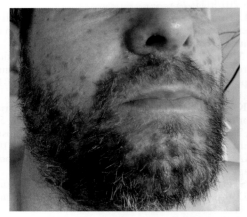

Fig. 19.37 Coxsackie A6 hand-foot-and-mouth disease.

poliomyelitis. Epidemics with severe disease have been reported in Bulgaria, Hungary, Japan, Australia, Malaysia, and Singapore..

Herpangina

Herpangina, a disease of children worldwide, is caused by multiple types of coxsackievirus (most frequently A8, A10, and A16), echoviruses, and enterovirus 71. In the severe outbreaks in Taiwan, 10% of patients with fatal cases had herpangina. It begins with acute onset of fever, headache, sore throat, dysphagia, anorexia, and sometimes, stiff neck. The most significant finding, which is present in all patients, is one or more yellowish white, slightly raised, 2-mm vesicles in the throat, usually surrounded by an intense areola (Fig. 19.35). The lesions are found most frequently on the anterior faucial pillars, tonsils, uvula, or soft palate. The lesions can cluster, ranging in number from one to having the entire visible pharynx may be studded with them. Usually, the individual or coalescent vesicles ulcerate, leaving a shallow, punched-out, grayish yellow crater 2–4 mm in diameter. The lesions disappear in 5–10 days. Coxsackievirus A10 causes acute lymphonodular pharyngitis, a variant of herpangina, characterized by discrete, yellow-white papules in the same distribution as herpangina. Herpangina is differentiated from aphthosis and primary herpetic gingivostomatitis by the location of the lesions in the posterior oropharynx and by isolation of an enterovirus. Treatment of herpangina is supportive, consisting of topical anesthetics and maintain hydration.

Hand-Foot-and-Mouth Disease

Hand-foot-and-mouth disease (HFMD) is usually a mild illness caused primarily by coxsackievirus A16, but also other cocksackie A and B viruses, as well as enterovirus 71. It primarily affects children age 6 months to 10 years, but exposed adults may also develop disease. Infection begins with a fever and sore mouth. In 90% of patients, oral lesions develop; these consist of small (4–8 mm), rapidly ulcerating vesicles surrounded by a red areola on the buccal mucosa, tongue, soft palate, and gingiva. Lesions on the hands and feet are asymptomatic red papules that quickly become small, gray, 3–7 mm vesicles surrounded by a red halo. They are often oval, linear, or crescentic and run parallel to the skin lines on the fingers and toes (Fig. 19.36). They are distributed sparsely on the dorsa of the fingers and toes and more frequently on the palms and soles. Especially in children who wear diapers, vesicles and erythematous, edematous papules may occur on the buttocks. The infection is usually mild and seldom lasts more than 1 week.

Cocksackievirus A6 (CVA6) has become a common cause of "atypical HFMD" in Europe, the United States, and Asia. CVA6 can cause typical HFMD but also a more widespread eruption with numerous lesions on the trunk in addition to the characteristic locations. Perioral lesions suggest CVA6 HFMD, and when severe, can suggest severe impetigo or Stevens-Johnson syndrome. Hospitalization may be required for severe dehydration and pain management. Child-to-adult transmission can occur because most adults are not immune to CVA6 (Fig. 19.37). In adults, numerous widespread purpuric lesions can occur, simulating a vasculitis or the atypical targets of EM major. In children with AD, CVA6 causes a vesicular and erosive eruption concentrated in the areas of dermatitis, similar to EH, called "eczema coxsackium." Treatment is supportive, although therapy for the AD to prevent pruritis can be helpful. Monitoring for secondary bacterial infection is important. Onychomadesis often follows HFMD (especially CVA6), about 1 month after the acute viral syndrome.

The virus may be recovered by PCR from the skin vesicles. Histopathologic findings are those of an intraepidermal blister formed by vacuolar and reticular degeneration of keratinocytes, similar to other viral blisters. Inclusion bodies and multinucleated giant cells are absent. HFMD is distinguished from herpangina by the distribution of the oral lesions and the presence of skin lesions. HFMD usually requires no treatment.

Eruptive Pseudoangiomatosis

Eruptive pseudoangiomatosis has been described in summer in the Mediterranean region and in South Korea. The disorder is characterized by the sudden appearance of 2–4 mm, blanchable red papules that resemble angiomas. The red papules blanch on pressure and are often surrounded by a 1–2 mm pale halo. Lesions often number about 10 but may be much more numerous. Most lesions appear on the exposed surfaces of the face and extremities, but the trunk may also be affected. In children, lesions are short-lived, virtually always resolving within 10 days. Lesions may last slightly longer in adults. Annual recrudescences may occur. Epidemics have been described in adults, and even health care workers caring for patients with eruptive pseudoangiomatosis have developed lesions. Echoviruses 25 and 32 had been implicated in the initial reports. The occurrence in young children and the presence of miniepidemic outbreaks suggest an infectious trigger. This disorder closely resembles "erythema punctatum Higuchi," which is common in Japan and known to be caused by *Culex pipiens pallens* bites. It appears that mosquito bites, viral infection, or enhanced insect bite reaction due to intercurrent viral infection are possible pathogenic causes of eruptive pseudoangiomatosis. In children, it is usually associated with a viral syndrome, but most affected adults have no viral symptoms. In adults, females outnumber males 2:1. Histologically, dilated upper dermal vessels, but not increased numbers of blood vessels, with prominent endothelial cells are seen. There is no known treatment.

Ben-Chetrit E, et al: Coxsackievirus A6–related hand foot and mouth disease. J Clin Virol 2014; 59: 201.

Chung WH, et al: Clinicopathologic analysis of coxsackievirus A6 new variant induced widespread mucocutaneous bullous reactions mimicking severe cutaneous adverse reactions. J Infect Dis 2013; 208: 1968.

Cox JA, et al: Immunopathogenesis and virus-host interactions of enterovirus 71 in patients with hand, foot and mouth disease. Front Microbiol 2017; 8: 2249.

Feder HM, et al: Atypical hand, foot, and mouth disease. Lancet Infect Dis 2014; 14: 83.

He Y, et al: Risk factors for critical disease and death from hand, foot, and mouth disease. Pediatr Infect Dis 2014; 33: 966.

Hubiche T, et al: Dermatological spectrum of hand, foot and mouth disease from classical to generalized exanthema. Pediatr Infect Dis J 2014; 33: e92.

Kaminska K, et al: Coxsackievirus A6 and hand, foot and mouth disease. Case Rep Dermatol 2013; 5: 203.

Kim JE, et al: Clinicopathologic review of eruptive pseudoangiomatosis in Korean adults. Int J Dermatol 2013; 52: 41.

Mathes EF, et al: "Eczema coxsackium" and unusual cutaneous findings in an enterovirus outbreak. Pediatrics 2013; 132: 3149.

Matsuzawa M, et al: Coxsackie A16 virus–associated atypical hand-foot-and-mouth disease. Intern Med 2014; 53: 643.

Oka K, et al: Two cases of eruptive pseudoangiomatosis induced by mosquito bites. J Dermatol 2012; 39: 301.

Sabanathan S, et al: Enterovirus 71 related severe hand, foot and mouth disease outbreaks in South-East Asia. J Epidemiol Community Health 2014; 68: 500.

Shin JY, et al: A clinical study of nail changes occurring secondary to hand-foot-mouth disease. Ann Dermatol 2014; 26: 280.

FILOVIRUS

The viruses in the *Filovirus* genus are single-stranded and on electron micrographs they appear filamentous, hence the name.

Filoviruses are among the most virulent and hazardous pathogens for humans and nonhuman primates and are most closely related to the human viruses that cause measles and rabies. There are two genera, *Marburg virus* (MARV) and *Ebola virus* (EBOV). The incubation period is 1–21 days. The initial symptomatic phase (phase I) is characterized by abrupt onset of fever, headache (usually occipital), myalgias, and arthralgias. Phase II starts 2–4 days after symptom onset and lasts for 7–10 days. Abdominal pain, watery diarrhea, and violent sore throat occur. In phase II a nonpruritic morbilliform eruption resembling measles appears 4–5 days after symptom onset in more than half of patients. The onset of the eruption begins as pinpoint dark red follicular papules. The exanthema may begin acrally and spread centripetally to the trunk or vice versa, beginning proximally and extending centrifugally. By day 8 the skin has a generalized, dark, livid erythema. The eruption resolves over a few days in the survivors, followed by desquamation of the affected skin, especially of the palms and soles. Mucosal lesions are also seen in half of patients with bilateral conjunctival congestion, aphthous-like oral lesions, gingivitis, glossitis, and with extension down the throat, dysphagia. The oral lesions can have a gray exudate or small (tapioca granule) white lesions on the soft palate. Phase III is the terminal phase with shock and multiorgan failure. In this stage, supportive care can maintain the patient until the spontaneous eradication of the virus. Convalescence is prolonged with intense fatigue and migratory arthralgias.

In the nonepidemic setting the initial presentation of the symptoms and skin findings are not specific and can be mistaken for viral or bacterial gastroenteritis, Lassa fever, Dengue, Chikungunya, and even measles, which have overlapping signs and symptoms. In the epidemic setting rapid recognition, establishment of high-quality isolation facilities to treat victims, and absolutely rigid infection control measures to handle infected persons, corpses, and EBOV-infected material are essential.

The animal reservoir for these viruses is four fruit bat species found in Africa. Transmission occurs in humans through contact with female bat blood, infected nonhuman primates and by contact with the bodily fluids of infected humans (including but not limited to blood, urine, sweat, semen, and breast milk). Infected humans can transmit the virus from the time they become febrile. The diagnoses of these agents is by PCR.

The case fatality rate approaches 90% in African outbreaks but appears to be much lower if aggressive supportive medical care is available. Due to the highly contagious nature of these viruses, health care workers are particularly at risk of becoming infected, and special precautions must be taken when managing infected patients.

Neutralizing antibodies from survivors and experimental antivirals are being tested as therapies.

Dixon MG, et al: Ebola viral disease outbreak—West Africa 2014. MMWR Morb Mortal Wkly Rep 2014; 63: 548.

Gatherer D: The 2014 Ebola virus disease outbreak in West Africa. J Gen Virol 2014; 95: 1619.

Nkoghe D, et al: Cutaneous manifestations of *Filovirus* infections. Int J Dermatol 2012; 51: 1037.

PARAMYXOVIRUS GROUP

The most important dermatologic diseases caused by paramyxoviruses are measles (rubeola) and German measles (rubella). Other viruses of this group are mumps virus, parainfluenza virus, Newcastle disease virus, and respiratory syncytial virus.

Measles

Measles is a highly infectious and potentially fatal viral infection. Highly effective two-dose vaccines are available, and when countries reach a rate of 95% vaccination, measles elimination has been achieved. However, measles remains a major health problem in many nations, including developed countries that provide immunizations to their population. Numerous hospitalizations and even deaths from measles are still occurring in developed nations. The majority of cases are in unvaccinated persons, supporting the concept that vaccination (specifically two doses) is protective, and that these measles epidemics and deaths are preventable. Because the children in unvaccinated groups may share common schools, camps, and social networks, they provide a prime breeding ground for epidemics. Some developed European and Asian countries (notably Japan, with 200,000 cases annually) have not been able to achieve high immunization levels, meaning that their populations are still at risk. The lack of "herd" immunity in these nations leaves at particular risk those infants and susceptible children who cannot be immunized because of other medical conditions. Cases of measles continue to be imported into the United States, which have resulted in numerous "outbreaks." Dermatologists and pediatricians in the Americas need to be alert for cases of measles when seeing persons from these countries or unvaccinated persons from the Americas especially if they have traveled to nations known to have ongoing measles outbreaks. In the current epidemics, however, older children, adolescents, and adults can be affected. Measles is spread by respiratory droplets and has an incubation period of 9–12 days.

The prodrome consists of fever, malaise, conjunctivitis, and prominent upper respiratory symptoms (nasal congestion, sneezing, coryza, cough). Koplik spots, which are pathognomonic, appear during the prodrome (Fig. 19.38). The spots appear first on the buccal mucosa nearest to the lower molars as 1-mm white papules on an erythematous base. They may spread to involve other areas of the buccal mucosa and pharynx. They have been less frequently reported in recent outbreaks. After 1–7 days, the exanthem appears, usually as macular or morbilliform lesions on the anterior scalp line and behind the ears. Lesions begin as discrete erythematous papules that gradually coalesce. The rash spreads quickly over the face (Fig. 19.39), then by the second or third day (unlike the more rapid spread of rubella) extends down the trunk to the extremities. By the third day, the whole body is involved. Lesions are most prominent and confluent in the initially involved areas and may be more discrete on the extremities. Purpura may be present, especially on the extremities, and should not be confused with "black measles," a rare, disseminated intravascular coagulation–like complication of measles. After 6–7 days, the exanthem clears, with simultaneous subsidence of the fever. Rubella, scarlet fever, secondary syphilis, enterovirus infections, and drug eruptions are in the differential diagnosis.

Complications include otitis media, pneumonia, encephalitis, and thrombocytopenic purpura. Encephalitis, although rare (<1% of cases), can be fatal. Infection in pregnant patients is associated with fetal death. Complications and fatalities are more common in children who are undernourished or have T-cell deficiencies. In HIV-infected children, the exanthem may be less prominent.

Modified measles occurs in a partially immune host as a result of prior infection, persistent maternal antibodies, or immunization, and this is a milder disease that may be difficult to differentiate from other exanthems. Patients may have only fever, or fever and a rash. The course is shorter, the exanthem less confluent, and Koplik spots may be absent.

A diagnosis of measles is established by the presence of a high fever, Koplik spots, the characteristic conjunctivitis, upper respiratory symptoms, and typical exanthem. Lymphopenia is common, with a decreased WBC count. Biopsies of skin lesions may show syncytial keratinocytic giant cells, similar to those seen in respiratory secretions. Laboratory confirmation can be with acute and convalescent serologic tests or PCR. PCR-based technologies can rapidly detect the measles virus genome in urine, oropharyngeal secretions, and blood and are highly useful in modified and previously vaccinated patients. Identification of virus-specific IgM (5 days after the rash presents) is highly suggestive of infection in an unimmunized individual. If done too early, however, a serum IgM assay may lead to a false-negative result, and the test should be repeated.

Administration of high doses of vitamin A may reduce the morbidity and mortality rates of hospitalized children with measles. Two doses of retinyl palmitate, 200,000 IU 24 hours apart, are recommended for all children 6–24 months of age, immunodeficient children, children with malnutrition or evidence of vitamin A deficiency, and recent immigrants from areas of high measles mortality. Otherwise, treatment is symptomatic, with bed rest, analgesics, and antipyretics.

Live virus vaccination is recommended at age 12 months, with a booster before entering school (age 4–5 years). A faint maculopapular exanthem may occur 7–10 days after immunization. Prophylaxis with vaccination and immune globulin should be offered to exposed susceptible persons. It must be provided within

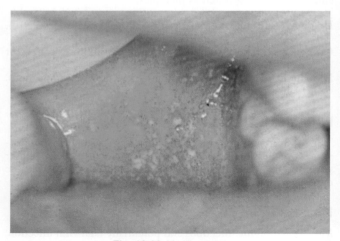

Fig. 19.38 Koplik spots.

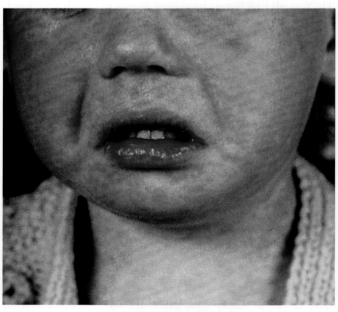

Fig. 19.39 Rubeola (measles).

the first few days after exposure, so identification of susceptible persons is critical. In an Australian outbreak, these strategies prevented 80% of possible secondary cases.

Rubella

Rubella, commonly known as German measles, is caused by a togavirus and probably spreads by respiratory secretions. The incubation period is 12–23 days (usually 15–21). Live virus vaccination is highly effective, providing lifelong immunity.

There is a prodrome of 1–5 days consisting of fever, malaise, sore throat, eye pain, headache, red eyes, runny nose, and adenopathy. Pain on lateral and upward eye movement is characteristic. The exanthem begins on the face and progresses caudad, covering the entire body in 24 hours and resolving by the third day. The lesions are typically pale-pink, morbilliform macules, smaller than those of rubeola. The eruption may resemble roseola or erythema infectiosum. An exanthem of pinhead-sized red macules or petechiae on the soft palate and uvula (Forchheimer sign) may be seen. Posterior cervical, suboccipital, and postauricular lymphadenitis occurs in more than half of cases. Rubella is in general a much milder disease than rubeola. Arthritis and arthralgias are common complications, especially in adult women, lasting 1 month or longer. The diagnosis is confirmed by finding rubella-specific IgM in oral fluids or the serum. This IgM develops rapidly, but 50% of sera drawn on the first day of the rash are negative. The virus is rapidly cleared from the blood, being absent by day 2 of the rash. However, the virus is found in oral secretions for 5–7 days after the rash has appeared. PCR-based techniques to identify virus in oral secretions may detect infection more effectively in earlier samples. The combination of PCR-based virus detection tests and identification of rubella virus–specific IgM will result in rapid confirmation of most cases of rubella within the first few days of appearance of disease symptoms.

Congenital Rubella Syndrome

Infants born to mothers who had rubella during the first trimester of pregnancy may have congenital cataracts, cardiac defects, and deafness. Numerous other manifestations, such as glaucoma, microcephaly, and various visceral abnormalities, may emerge. Among the cutaneous expressions are thrombocytopenic purpura; hyperpigmentation of the navel, forehead, and cheeks; bluish red, infiltrated, 2–8 mm lesions ("blueberry muffin" type), which represent dermal erythropoiesis; chronic urticaria; and reticulated erythema of the face and extremities.

Andersen DV, Jørgensen IM: MMR vaccination of children with egg allergy is safe. Dan Med J 2013; 60: A4573.

Caseris M, et al: French 2010–2011 measles outbreak in adults. Clin Microbiol Infect 2014; 20: O242.

Centers for Disease Control and Prevention (CDC): Recommendations from an ad hoc meeting of the WHO Measles and Rubella Laboratory Network (LabNet) on use of alternative diagnostic samples for measles and rubella surveillance. MMWR Morb Mortal Wkly Rep 2008; 57: 657.

Gahr P, et al: An outbreak of measles in an undervaccinated community. Pediatrics 2014; 134: e220.

Giusti D, et al: Virological diagnosis and management of two cases of congenital measles. J Med Virol 2013; 85: 2136.

Muscat M, et al: Measles in Europe. Lancet 2009; 373: 383.

Nagai M, et al: Modified adult measles in outbreaks in Japan, 2007–2008. J Med Virol 2009; 81: 1094.

Nakayama T: Laboratory diagnosis of measles and rubella infection. Vaccine 2009; 27: 3228.

Ortega-Sanchez IR, et al: The economic burden of sixteen measles outbreaks on United States public health departments in 2011. Vaccine 2014; 32: 1311.

Sammons JS: Ready or not: responding to measles in the poste-limination era. Ann Intern Med 2014; 161: 145.

Sheikine Y, et al: Histopathology of measles exanthem. J Cutan Pathol 2012; 39: 667.

Sheppeard V, et al: The effectiveness of prophylaxis for measles contacts in NSW. NSW Public Health Bull 2009; 20: 81.

Tanne JH: Rise in US measles cases is blamed on unimmunized travelers. BMJ 2014; 348: g3478.

Tapisiz A, et al: Prevention of measles spread on a paediatric ward. Epidemiol Infect 2015; 143: 720.

Tod B, et al: Dermatological manifestations of measles infection in hospitalized paediatric patients observed in the 2009–2011 Western Cape epidemic. S Afr Med J 2012; 102: 356.

Young MK, et al: Post-exposure passive immunization for preventing measles. Cochrane Database Syst Rev 2014; 4: CD010056.

Zipprich J, et al: Notes from the field: measles—California, January 1–April 18, 2014. MMWR Morb Mortal Wkly Rep 2014; 63: 362.

Asymmetric Periflexural Exanthem of Childhood (APEC)

This clinical syndrome, also known as unilateral laterothoracic exanthem, or superimposed lateralized exanthema, occurs primarily in the late winter and early spring and appears to be most common in Europe. It affects girls more often than boys (1.2 : 1 to 2 : 1). It occurs in children 8 months to 10 years of age, but most cases are between 2 and 3 years. Multiple cases have been reported in adults. The cause is unknown, but a viral origin has been proposed because it occurs in young children and is seasonal, and secondary cases in families have been reported. No reproducible viral etiology has been implicated; however, at least three cases attributed to parvovirus B19 have been reported. Adenovirus, parainfluenza virus, HHV-6, HHV-7, and EBV have also been described in association with "superimposed lateralized exanthema." Clinically, two thirds to three quarters of affected children have symptoms of a mild upper respiratory or GI infection, usually preceding the eruption. The lesions are usually discrete, 1-mm erythematous papules that coalesce to poorly marginated morbilliform plaques. Pruritus is usually present but is mild. Lesions begin unilaterally close to a flexural area, usually the axilla (75% of cases). Spread is centrifugal, with new lesions appearing on the adjacent trunk and proximal extremity. Normal skin may intervene between lesions. The contralateral side is involved in 70% of cases after 5–15 days, but the asymmetric nature is maintained throughout the illness. Lymphadenopathy of the nodes on the initially affected side occurs in about 70% of patients. The APEC syndrome lasts 2–6 weeks on average, but may last more than 2 months, and resolves spontaneously. Topical corticosteroids and oral antibiotics are of no benefit, but oral antihistamines may help associated pruritus. Histologically, a mild to moderate lymphocytic (CD8+ T-cell) infiltrate surrounds and involves the eccrine ducts but not the secretory coils. There may be an accompanying interface dermatitis of the upper eccrine duct and adjacent epidermis.

Drago F, et al: Unilateral laterothoracic or asymmetric periflexural exanthema. Clin Exp Dermatol 2015; 40: 570.

Guimera-Martin-Neda G, et al: Asymmetric periflexural exanthem of childhood. J Eur Acad Dermatol Venereol 2006; 20: 461.

Happle R: Superimposed segmental manifestations of polygenic skin disorders. J Am Acad Dermatol 2007; 57: 690.

PARVOVIRUS GROUP

Parvovirus B19 is the most common agent in this *Erythrovirus* genus to cause human disease. Infection is worldwide, occurring in 50% of persons by age 15. The vast majority of elderly adults are

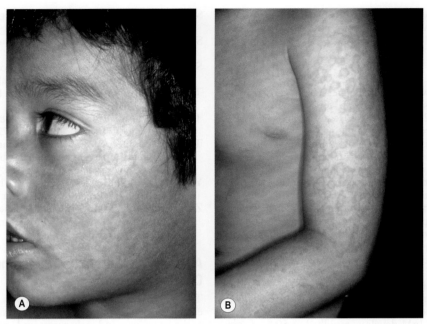

Fig. 19.40 (A and B) Erythema infectiosum.

seropositive. Infections are more common in the spring in temperate climates. Epidemics in communities occur about every 6 years. The virus is spread by the respiratory route, and infection rates are very high within households. Most infections are asymptomatic. The propensity for parvovirus B19 to affect the bone marrow is reflected by the presence of thrombocytopenia or leukopenias during the acute infection. Parvovirus DNA has been found in a wide variety of dermatologic conditions, suggesting the virus may persist in skin but not be pathogenic, casting some doubt on the true association between the virus and some dermatologic diseases. Regardless, parvovirus B19 is the prototype for the concept of "one virus, many exanthems." The patient may have multiple types of exanthems simultaneously or sequentially. Erythema infectiosum and papular-purpuric gloves-and-socks syndrome are both strongly associated with parvovirus B19 infection. Parvovirus B19 may also play a role in some cases of GCS and APEC. Parvovirus B19 has been reported to present with acute generalized exanthematous pustulosis, flagellate erythema, cellulitis-like lesions, microvesicular eruptions, reticulated and annular erythema, and more. Acral, periflexural eruptions with purpuric, annular, or reticulate lesions have been suggested as signs of parvovirus infection. Parvovirus was demonstrated in two pediatric cases of DRESS. Other known complications of this viral infection include arthropathy (especially in middle-age females), aplastic crisis in hereditary spherocytosis and sickle cell disease, and chronic anemia in immunosuppressed patients. Infection of a pregnant woman leads to transplacental infection in 30% of cases and a fetal loss rate of 5%–9%. Acute viral myocarditis and pericarditis are frequently secondary to parvovirus B19 infection.

Erythema Infectiosum (Fifth Disease)

Erythema infectiosum is a worldwide benign infectious exanthem that occurs in epidemics in the late winter and early spring. In normal hosts (but not immunosuppressed or sickle cell patients in crisis), viral shedding has stopped by the time the exanthem appears, making isolation unnecessary. The incubation period is 4–14 days (average 7 days). Infrequently, a mild prodrome of headache, runny nose, and low-grade fever may precede the rash by 1 or 2 days.

Erythema infectiosum has three phases. It begins abruptly with an asymptomatic erythema of the cheeks (Fig. 19.40A), referred to as "slapped cheek." The erythema is typically diffuse and macular, but tiny translucent papules may be present. It is most intense beneath the eyes and may extend over the cheeks in a butterfly-wing pattern. The perioral area, lids, and chin are usually unaffected. After 1–4 days, the second phase begins, consisting of discrete erythematous macules and papules on the proximal extremities and later the trunk. This evolves into a reticulate or lacy pattern (Fig. 19.40B). These two phases typically last 5–9 days. A characteristic third phase is the recurring stage. The eruption is greatly reduced or invisible, only to recur after the patient is exposed to heat (especially when bathing) or sunlight, or in response to crying or exercise. About 7% of children with erythema infectiosum have arthralgias. However, 80% of adults, especially women, have joint involvement, often with little to no rash. Necrotizing lymphadenitis may also occur in the cervical, epitrochlear, supraclavicular, and intraabdominal lymph nodes. Children with aplastic crisis caused by parvovirus B19 usually do not have a rash. However, even healthy children can develop significant bone marrow complications, although transient and self-limited.

Papular-Purpuric Gloves-and-Socks Syndrome

The papular-purpuric gloves-and-socks (or glove-and-stocking) syndrome (PPGSS), which is less common than erythema infectiosum, occurs primarily in teenagers and young adults. Pruritus, edema, and erythema of the hands and feet appear, and a fever is present. The lesions are sharply cut off at the wrists and ankles (Fig. 19.41). Over a few days, they become purpuric. There is a mild erythema of the cheeks, elbows, knees, and groin folds. Oral erosions, shallow ulcerations, aphthous ulcers on the labial mucosa, erythema of the pharynx, Koplik spots, or petechial lesions may be seen on the buccal or labial mucosa. The lips may be red and swollen. Vulvar edema and erythema accompanied by dysuria may be seen. An unusual variant is a unilateral petechial and erythematous eruption of the axilla. The acral erythema may rarely move proximally along lymphatics, simulating a lymphangitis. Transient lymphocytopenia, decreased platelet count, and elevated LFTs may be seen. PPGSS resolves within 2 weeks. Evidence of

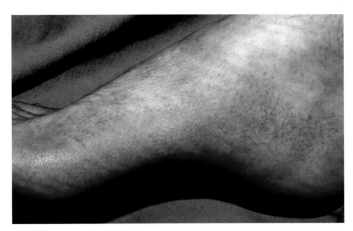

Fig. 19.41 Purpuric glove-sock syndrome.

seroconversion for parvovirus B19 has been found in most reported patients. Histologically, a dermal infiltrate of CD30+ T lymphocytes surrounds the upper dermal vessels. There is an interface component and prominent extravasation of red blood cells in petechial lesions. Parvovirus B19 antigen has been found in the endothelial cells, sweat glands and ducts, and epidermis. Because the antigen is located in the endothelial cells, a leukocytoclastic vasculitis picture both clinically and histologically may be seen. Similarly, a Degos disease–like morphology can occur. In HIV-infected patients who develop PPGSS, the eruption is more persistent, lasting 3 weeks to 4 months, and is associated with anemia.

Not all cases of PPGSS are caused by parvovirus B19. In adults, it may be associated with HBV infection. In children, the syndrome occurs at an average age of 23 months. The eruption lasts an average of 5 weeks. Also in children, CMV and EBV are the most common documented causes in Taiwan, where PPGSS appears to be very common in the last quarter of the year.

Other Skin Findings Attributed to Parvovirus B19

In some patients, the exanthem of parvovirus B19 affects primarily the flexural areas, especially the groin. This may present as APEC (see earlier), petechiae in the groin, or an erythema studded with pustules in the groin and to a lesser degree in the axillae, resembling baboon syndrome. The petechial eruption of PPGSS may also involve the perioral area and has been called the "acropetechial syndrome." An outbreak in Kerala, India, described 50 children, mostly under age 2 years, who presented with high fever and a diffuse, intensely erythematous, tender skin eruption. The children were very irritable and cried when held. Their skin was extremely swollen, and whole-body edema was present. The acute exanthem was followed by diffuse desquamation. There were no secondary cases. IgM for parvovirus B19 was detected in 15 of 24 cases tested. The authors called this "red baby syndrome."

Infection with parvovirus B19 may trigger a hemophagocytic (or macrophage activation) syndrome. This presents with progressive cytopenias, liver dysfunction, coagulopathy, high ferritin level, and hemophagocytosis. Numerous nonspecific eruptions have been described with hemophagocytic syndrome, including nodules, ulcers, purpura, and panniculitis. The diagnostic hemophagocytic cells may occasionally be identified in skin biopsies. Infection with parvovirus B19 may lead to cutaneous necrosis in persons with a hypercoagulable state, such as paroxysmal nocturnal hemoglobinuria. The presence of edema, purpuric lesions, facial erythema, fever, cytopenias, and hypocomplementemia, even with positive antinuclear antibodies, allows for severe cases of parvovirus B19 infection to be confused with systemic lupus erythematosus.

Parvovirus has been associated with the development of autoimmune diseases, potentially through molecular mimicry.

Cooray M, et al: Parvovirus infection mimicking systemic lupus erythematosus. CMAJ 2013; 185: 1342.

Coughlin CC, et al: Drug hypersensitivity syndrome with prolonged course complicated by parvovirus infection. Pediatr Dermatol 2016; 33: e364.

Cugler T, et al: Severe glomerulonephritis and encephalopathy associated with parvovirus B19 infection mimicking systemic lupus erythematosus. Scand J Rheumatol 2012, 41: 79.

Drago F, et al: Atypical exanthems associated with parvovirus B19 infection in children and adults. J Med Virol 2015; 87: 1981.

Drago F, et al: Atypical exanthems associated with parvovirus B19 infection. Infez Med 2015; 23: 283.

Drago F, et al: Exanthems associated with parvovirus B19 infection in adults. J Am Acad Dermatol 2014; 71: 1256.

Dyrsen ME, et al: Parvovirus B19–associated catastrophic endothelialitis with a Degos-like presentation. J Cutan Pathol 2008; 35: 20.

Gutermuth J, et al: Papular-purpuric gloves and socks syndrome. Lancet 2011; 378: 198.

Kerr JR: The role of parvovirus B19 in the pathogenesis of autoimmunity and autoimmune disease. J Clin Pathol 2016; 69: 279.

Landry ML: Parvovirus B19. Microbiol Spectr 2016; 4.

Lee D, et al: Acute generalized exanthematous pustulosis induced by parvovirus b19 infection. Ann Dermatol 2014; 26: 399.

Mage V, et al: Different patterns of skin manifestations associated with parvovirus B19 primary infection in adults. J Am Acad Dermatol 2014; 71: 62.

Martin JM, et al: Parvovirus B19-associated microvesicular eruption. Pediatr Dermatol 2015; 32: e303.

Miguelez A, et al: Flagellate erythema in parvovirus B19 infection. Int J Dermatol 2014; 53: e583.

Neri I, et al: Cellulitis-like lesions. J Pediatr 2016; 175: 239.

Rogo LD, et al: Human parvovirus B19. Acta Virol 2014; 58: 199.

Santonja C, et al: Immunohistochemical detection of parvovirus B19 in "gloves and socks" papular purpuric syndrome. Am J Dermatopathol 2011; 33: 790.

Santonja C, et al: Detection of human parvovirus B19 DNA in 22% of 1815 cutaneous biopsies of a wide variety of dermatological conditions suggests viral persistence after primary infection and casts doubts on its pathogenic significance. Br J Dermatol 2017; 177: 1060.

Soderlung-Venermo M: Clinical significance of parvovirus B19 DNA in cutaneous biopsies. Br J Dermatol 2017; 177: 900.

Tuccio A, et al: Petechnial rash associated with parvovirus B19 in children. Infez Med 2014; 22: 250.

Valentin MN, Cohen PJ: Pediatric parvovirus B19. Cutis 2013; 92: 179.

ARBOVIRUS GROUP (TOGAVIRIDAE)

The arboviruses comprise the numerous arthropod-borne RNA viruses. These viruses multiply in vertebrates, as well as in arthropods. The vertebrates usually act as reservoirs and the arthropods as vectors of the various diseases.

West Nile Fever

West Nile virus (WNV) is a flavivirus that is endemic in East Africa. It first appeared in eastern North America in 1999 and reached California by 2004. It is primarily an infection of the crow family (crows, ravens, magpies, and bluejays). It is spread by *Culex* mosquitoes, though very rarely via transfusion, transplantation, and one report exists of possible sexual transmission. Approximately 80% of infected persons will have no symptoms. After an incubation period of 3–15 days, a febrile illness of sudden onset occurs. Headache, myalgia, arthralgia, conjunctivitis, pharyngitis, cough, adenopathy, abdominal pain, hepatitis, pancreatitis, and myocarditis are recognized clinical manifestations. The primary complications, however, are neurologic disease, including seizures (10% of symptomatic adults), ascending flaccid paralysis (as in poliomyelitis), ataxia, meningitis, encephalitis, myelitis, cranial neuropathies, optic neuritis, and reduced level of consciousness. A significant percentage of affected persons are left with permanent neurologic sequelae. About 20% of hospitalized patients will have an exanthem. The exanthema of WNV is nonpruritic and composed of 50–100 erythematous, poorly defined macules 0.5–1 cm in diameter, primarily on the trunk and proximal extremities, with papular and psoriasiform variants rarely reported. It lasts 5–7 days and resolves without scaling, and one study suggested development of the rash was associated with better prognosis.

Sandfly Fever

Sandfly fever is also known as phlebotomus fever and pappataci fever. The vector, *Phlebotomus papatasii*, is found in the Mediterranean area (Sicilian fever, Naples fever, and Toscana virus), Russia, China, and India. Sicilian and Naples sandfly fever viral infections disappeared or dramatically decreased with mosquito eradication programs, Toscana virus infection is still common. Although most infected persons are asymptomatic, 80% of aseptic meningitis cases in the summer in endemic areas are caused by this agent. Small, pruritic papules appear on the skin after the sandfly bite and persist for 5 days. After an incubation period of another 5 days, fever, headache, malaise, nausea, conjunctival injection, stiff neck, and abdominal pains suddenly develop. The skin manifestations consist of a scarlatiniform eruption on the face and neck. Recovery is slow, with recurring bouts of fever. No specific treatment is available.

Dengue

More than 100 million cases of dengue occur annually worldwide, and the global prevalence is growing. In European hospitals that evaluate patients with fever after trips to the tropics, dengue is the most common febrile illness in travelers returning from Southeast Asia who develop a fever within 1 month of the trip. It is transmitted by *Aedes* mosquitoes, which have adapted well to living around humans in urban environments. It affects primarily tropical regions where temperatures rarely drop below 20°C, favoring the reproduction of the mosquito vector. Southeast Asia and the Western Pacific are the most severely affected regions, but India, Cuba, and the tropical Americas also have numerous cases. There have been several U.S. outbreaks, in Houston, Texas, Hawaii, and Key West, Florida, and many of these cases appear *not* to have been imported, suggesting dengue is potentially endemic in these climates. Climate change has led to an expanded habitat for the *Aedes* vector, including in the southern continental United States. Persons of African ancestry seem to be at much less risk of developing dengue.

Dengue fever begins 2–15 days after the infectious mosquito bite. The clinical features are characteristic and consist of the sudden onset of high fevers accompanied by myalgias, headache, and the skin rash; patients may also have retro-orbital pain, and severe backache (breakbone fever). Common associated laboratory findings include elevated LFTs (about three times normal on average), thrombocytopenia (platelet count <100,000 in 50% of patients), and a leukopenia. These are present during the acute illness and help to suggest dengue as the correct diagnosis. About 50% of patients will develop a characteristic skin eruption. In 90% of patients, the eruption begins between days 3 and 5 of the

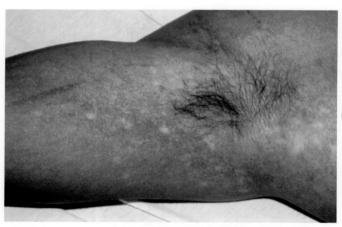

Fig. 19.42 Dengue fever. Linear bleeding points appeared after application of a blood pressure cuff.

illness, often as the fever defervesces. The skin eruption occurs in less than 10% of patients before the onset of fever. The eruption is most often generalized (50%) or involves only the extremities (30%) or the trunk (20%). Lesions are macular or morbilliform and are usually confluent, characteristically sparing small islands of normal skin—"islands of white in a sea of red" (Fig. 19.42). Persistent blanching after pressing the skin can also be seen. A "tourniquet test" involves taking the blood pressure, leaving the cuff inflated for 5 minutes, waiting 2 minutes, and counting petechiae; 10 or more per square inch is considered positive and a clue to dengue. Facial flushing may be prominent. The rash is either asymptomatic or only mildly pruritic. Petechiae may be present, but the finding of cutaneous hemorrhage should raise the suspicion of dengue hemorrhagic fever/dengue shock syndrome (DHF/DSS, severe dengue). Complete recovery occurs in 7–10 days. Biopsy of the exanthem shows minimal findings and is of no value in predicting the severity of the patient's condition or in identifying DHF/DSS/severe dengue. Helpful clues to suggest dengue from other tropical febrile illnesses in one predictive study in Honduras included petechiae, skin rash, myalgia, retro-ocular pain, positive tourniquet test, and gingival bleeding.

There are four serotypes of dengue. After infection with one serotype, the individual is resistant to reinfection with that serotype. However, if that person becomes infected with another serotype, the individual is at risk of developing severe complications from the second episode of dengue. The patient's antidengue antibodies are incapable of preventing infection by or replication of the new dengue virus type. However, antibodies do trigger increased viral phagocytosis by mononuclear cells and amplified cytokine production. The World Health Organization (WHO) 2009 classification system divides cases into dengue without warning signs, dengue with warning signs, and severe dengue. This more objective schema is more sensitive in identifying patients with early, severe dengue. Signs of severe dengue in one systematic review included hepatomegaly, lethargy, abdominal pain, bleeding, and complete blood count abnormalities. The potentially fatal syndromes that can occur in dengue infection are characterized by hemorrhage (dengue hemorrhagic fever/DHF), at times with extensive plasma leakage (dengue shock syndrome/DSS/severe dengue). The fatality rate for severe dengue may be as high as 40%. The diagnosis of dengue is made by detection of dengue-specific IgM in the sera by ELISA, with acute and convalescent serologies demonstrating seroconversion. Some laboratories can detect viral RNA in acute serum samples. An effective vaccine has not been developed; the only preventive strategy for travelers is to avoid mosquito bites. In children, dengue fever and Kawasaki disease have occurred simultaneously. These two syndromes may be almost identical in their presentation, so this differential diagnosis can be extremely difficult. When both diagnoses have been made simultaneously, the patient had persistent fever (>1 week), a reactive thrombocytosis after the initial thrombocytopenia, and in some cases, characteristic cardiac lesions.

Alphavirus

Sindbis Virus

In Finland, Sindbis virus infection is transmitted by the *Culiseta* mosquito. An eruption of multiple, erythematous, 2–4 mm papules with a surrounding halo is associated with fever and prominent arthralgias. The eruption and symptoms resolve over a few weeks. Histologically, the skin lesions show a perivascular lymphocytic infiltrate with large, atypical cells, simulating lymphomatoid papulosis. CD30 does not stain the large cells, however, allowing their distinction.

Chikungunya Virus

Chikungunya virus is transmitted by the *Aedes* mosquito. Derived from the Makonde language of sub-Saharan Africa, *chikungunya* means "that which bends up," describing the characteristic stooped posture resulting from the joint symptoms of the disease. It is endemic in Africa, India, Sri Lanka, Southeast Asia, the Philippines, the islands of the Indian Ocean, and the Caribbean region. The first U.S. cases of chikungunya infection were reported during summer 2014 in southern Florida. More continental U.S. cases have occurred in humid, Southern states, as the climate for the vector expands due to climate change. The incubation period is 2–7 days. The patient presents with abrupt onset of high fever. Significant joint symptoms are characteristic and occur in 40% of infected patients. Most often, there is swelling and pain in the small joints of the hands and feet. The joint symptoms may persist for weeks to months, with about 50% of patients still having some symptoms at 6 months. Patients may develop neuropathic acral findings, including Raynaud phenomenon, erythromelalgia, or severe acral coldness, as late sequelae. Headache occurs in 70% of patients and nausea and vomiting in 60%. Lymphopenia, thrombocytopenia, and elevated LFTs can be observed in the first week of the illness. Although generally a nonfatal and self-limited illness, severe complications can occur with chikungunya infection, causing death in about 1 in 1000 infected patients.

About half to three quarters or more of patients with chikungunya virus infection develop a rash. It is pruritic in 20%–50% of the patients. The most common and characteristic exanthem is described as morbilliform and most frequently affects the arms, upper trunk, and face. It can be confluent, and islands of sparing can be seen. It appears by the second day of the fever in more than half of patients, and in another 20% on the third or fourth day; only about one fifth of patients develop the eruption after the fifth day of the illness. Ecchymoses may appear during the acute illness. Aphthous-like ulcerations can occur in the oral, penoscrotal, and less often the axillary regions. These may be preceded by intense erythema and pain in the affected area. After acute chikungunya infection, striking hyperpigmentation of the skin may occur, including postinflammatory hyperpigmentation, freckling, streaks, and broad areas of hyperpigmentation.

A bullous eruption may occur in acute chikungunya virus infection. About 90% of those with a bullous eruption are under 1 year of age, and most of the severe cases occur before age 6 months. In children, 17% develop a vesiculobullous component to their eruption, compared with only 3% of adults. There is an initial exanthem, followed in hours or days by flaccid or tense nonhemorrhagic blisters that rupture easily. Nikolsky sign is positive. The genitalia, palms, and soles are spared. There is a close resemblance to toxic epidermal necrolysis, and up to 80%

of the total body surface area may become denuded. High titers of virus are recovered from blister fluid (in excess of that present in blood). Biopsy demonstrates an intraepidermal blister with acantholytic cells floating free in the blister cavity. These patients are managed similar to burn patients, and most recover. Skin grafting usually is not required.

The diagnosis of chikungunya virus infection is made by detecting virus-specific IgM in the serum. Confirmation is by seroconversion over the next several months, with development of virus-specific IgG. PCR-based methods may detect viral genome in the blisters or serum during the acute illness.

It may be difficult to differentiate dengue from chikungunya fever, because both are endemic in the same geographic regions, and their clinical symptoms and laboratory findings are similar. Arthralgias occur in a significant percentage of patients with chikungunya virus infection, approaching 100% in those with a rash, but also occur in patients with dengue. Neutropenia is seen in 80% of dengue patients and only 10% of chikungunya patients. A positive tourniquet test does not distinguish these two infections, but thrombocytopenia is more common in dengue (85% or greater) than chikungunya (35%) patients.

Zika Virus

In late 2015 to early 2016 the emergency of Zika virus was recognized as a dangerous pathogen with the potential for devastating consequences during fetal infection. Zika's primary vector is the *A. aegypti* mosquito, though the *Aedes albopictus* may transmit the virus as well; these are found in 30–41 U.S. states. Most cases occur in tropical regions of Central and South America, such as Brazil. Travel associated cases account for the majority of cases in the continental United States, but isolated outbreaks of locally acquired Zika have been reported, and Puerto Rico experienced rapid, extensive spread of the virus. Twenty-five percent of Puerto Rican individuals, including 6000–10,000 pregnant women, were suspected of Zika infection in 2016. Rapid mosquito control efforts, including avoiding standing water, application of insecticides and larvicides, and widespread use of repellant, helped contain the Miami outbreak but are not always as successful in endemic areas. Sexual transmission may occur, and the virus may persist in semen for many months after infection.

Zika infection was rapidly recognized for its potential for serious birth defects, including microcephaly and brain damage. In adults, neurologic diseases such as Guillain-Barré can complicate infection, and severe thrombocytopenia has been reported. The long-term consequences of birth defects and brain damage to babies born with Zika-related birth defects is anticipated to be devastating, with over 1700 cases of microcephaly reported in Northeastern Brazil alone. Pregnant women should avoid travel to areas with Zika, and long-sleeved shirts and insect repellents with DEET are advised. As Zika can persist in semen for months, condom use is recommended for men who have been in Zika-affected areas.

Clinically, patients with Zika infection present with fever, rash, joint pain, and often a conjunctivitis. Hyperemic sclerae appears to be a helpful clue; petechiae on the palate, or elsewhere, occasionally with gingival bleeding, and a diffuse papular eruption, descending in a cranial-caudal fashion, have been described. One model suggests that rash with pruritus or conjunctival hyperemia, without any other signs such as fever, petechiae, or anorexia, may be the best clinical clue to differentiate Zika from other arboviruses.

Anderson RC, et al: Punctate exanthema of West Nile virus infection. J Am Acad Dermatol 2004; 51: 820.

Bandyopadhyay D, et al: Mucocutaneous features of Chikungunya fever. Int J Dermatol 2008; 47: 1148.

Braga JU, et al: Accuracy of Zika virus disease case definition during simultaneous Dengue and Chikungunya epidemics. PLoS One 2017; 12: e0179725.

Bouri N, et al: Return of epidemic dengue in the United States. Public Health Rep 2012; 127: 259.

Del Giudice P, et al: Skin manifestations of West Nile virus infection. Dermatology 2005; 211: 348.

Derrington SM, et al: Mucocutaneous findings and course in an adult with Zika virus infection. JAMA Dermatol 2016; 152: 691.

Farahnik B, et al: Cutaneous manifestations of the Zika virus. J Am Acad Dermatol 2016; 74: 1286.

Fernandez E, et al: A predictive model to differentiate dengue from other febrile illness. BMC Infect Dis 2016; 16: 694.

Frieden TR, et al: Zika virus 6 months later. JAMA 2016; 316: 1443.

Huhn GD, et al: Rash is a prognostic factor in West Nile virus. Clin Inf Dis 2006; 43: 388.

Johnston D, et al: Notes from the field: outbreak of locally acquired cases of Dengue fever—Hawaii, 2015. MMWR Morb Mortal Wkly Rep 2016; 65: 34.

Kaffenberger BH, et al: The effect of climate change on skin disease in North America. J Am Acad Dermatol 2017; 76: 140.

Kenzaka T, Kumabe A: Skin rash from dengue fever. BMJ Case Rep 2013 Nov 25; 2013.

Lupi O, Tyring SK: Tropical dermatology. J Am Acad Dermatol 2003; 49: 979.

Murray KO, et al: Identification of dengue fever cases in Houston, Texas, with evidence of autochthonous transmission between 2003 and 2005. Vector Borne Zoonotic Dis 2013; 13: 835.

Nelwan EJ, et al: Dengue convalescent rash in adult Indonesian patients. Acta Med Indones 2014; 46: 339.

Robin S, et al: Severe bullous skin lesions associated with chikungunya virus infection in small infants. Eur J Pediatr 2010; 169: 67.

Singh RK, et al: A quick review of the cutaneous findings of the Zika virus. Dermatol Online J 2016; 22.

Wakimoto MD, et al: Dengue in children. Expert Rev Anti Infect Ther 2015; 13: 1441.

Yacoub S, et al: Dengue: an update for clinicians working in non-endemic areas. Clin Med (Lond) 2015; 15: 82.

PAPOVAVIRUS GROUP

Papovaviruses are naked dsDNA viruses characterized as slow growing. They replicate inside the nucleus. Because papovaviruses contain no envelope, they are resistant to drying, freezing, and solvents. In addition to the human papillomaviruses, which cause warts, papillomaviruses of rabbits and cattle, polyomaviruses of mice, and vacuolating viruses of monkeys are some of the other viruses in the papovavirus group.

Warts (Verruca)

There are more than 150 types of human papillomavirus (HPV). The genome of HPV consists of early genes ($E1$, $E2$, $E4$, $E5$, $E6$, and $E7$), two late genes ($L1$ and $L2$), and in between an upstream regulatory region (URR). $L1$ and $L2$ code for the major and minor capsid proteins. $L1$ encodes for the major capsid protein and self-assembles into virus-like particles (VLPs). These VLPs are the antigens in currently available HPV vaccines. The $L2$ gene encodes the minor capsid protein and has at least two important functions. L2 protein helps expose the keratinocyte-binding determinant of the L1 protein, allowing for the HPV to bind onto the basal keratinocyte and to be taken into the cell. The processing of HPV surface proteins in the skin takes up to 24 hours, allowing for exposure to anti-HPV antibodies. The L2 protein also is immunomodulatory, downregulating the function of Langerhans cells through the phosphoinositide 3-kinase pathway. A new HPV type is defined when there is less than 90% DNA homology with any other known type in the $L1$ and $E6$ genes.

Viruses with 90%–98% homology are classified as subtypes. The gene sequences from HPVs throughout the world are similar. Most HPV types cause specific types of warts and favor certain anatomic locations, such as plantar warts, common warts, and genital warts. HPVs 1, 2, 27, and 57 cause the vast majority of cutaneous (nongenital) warts. HPV-1 is associated with plantar warts in children younger than 12 years. HPV-2 is more common in hand warts. HPV-27 and HPV-57 are associated with common and plantar warts in adults (>21 years). External genital warts are caused by HPV-6/11 and anogenital dysplasia by HPV-16/18. A large proportion of the HPV types rarely cause warts and appear to be pathogenic only in immunosuppressed patients or those with epidermodysplasia verruciformis. However, many persons may carry, or may be latently infected with, these rare wart types, explaining the uniformity of gene sequence and clinical presentation worldwide. In the immunosuppressed patient, HPV types may cause warty lesions of a different clinical morphology than in an immunocompetent host.

Infection with HPV may be clinical, subclinical, or latent. Clinical lesions are visible by gross inspection. Subclinical lesions may be seen only by aided examination (e.g., acetic acid soaking). Latent infection describes the presence of HPV or viral genome in apparently normal skin. Latent infection is thought to be common, especially in genital warts, and explains in part the failure of destructive methods to eradicate warts.

Infection with HPV is extremely common; most people will experience infection during their lifetime. In Australia 22% and in The Netherlands 33% of schoolchildren were found to have nongenital cutaneous warts. Common warts are found in about 10%–15% of children, plantar warts in 6%–20% (higher in The Netherlands than Australia), and flat warts are only reported in schoolchildren from Australia (2%). White persons have visible cutaneous warts twice as frequently as other ethnicities. Genital warts begin to appear with sexual activity, with 10% of women acquiring HPV infection before they have intercourse, suggesting oral/digital/genital-to-genital contact is capable of transmitting HPV. HPV infection rates, including latent infection, exceed 50% in sexually active populations in many parts of the world.

Human papillomaviruses have coexisted with humans for many millennia, and humans are their primary host and reservoir. HPVs have been successful pathogens of human because they evade the human immune response. This is achieved primarily through avoiding the expression of antigens on the surface of keratinocytes until the keratinocytes are above the level of the antigen-presenting cells in the epidermis. HPVs also reduce Langerhans cells in the vicinity of infection and inactivate them through the L2 protein on their surface. Through $E6$ and $E7$, HPV reduces local production of key immune reactants (e.g., TLR9, IL-8), muting the local immune response. HPVs thus live in equilibrium with their human hosts through a combination of immune evasion and programmed immune suppression (tolerance).

Management of warts is based on their clinical appearance and location and the patient's immune status. In general, warts of all types are more common and more difficult to treat in persons with suppressed immune systems (Fig. 19.43). Except in WHIM syndrome (warts, hypogammaglobulinemia, infection, and myelokathexis: gain-of-function mutation of $CXCR4$), syndromes of reduced immunoglobulin production or B-cell function are not associated with increased HPV infection. Medical conditions or treatments associated with suppression of cell-mediated immunity are associated with high rates of clinical HPV infection and HPV-induced neoplasias. The common clinical scenarios are iatrogenic medications (e.g., in organ transplant recipients), viral infections that result in T-cell deficiency (e.g., HIV), and congenital syndromes of T-cell immunodeficiency. Patients with GATA2 deficiency frequently present with extensive warts. WILD syndrome is the association of primary lymphedema, disseminated warts, and anogenital dysplasia with depressed cell-mediated immunity and probably represents

19

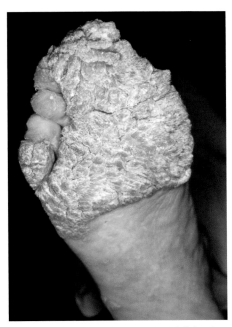

Fig. 19.43 Extensive warts as seen in immunodeficiencies such as WHIM and DOCK8.

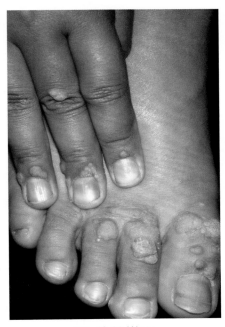

Fig. 19.44 Warts.

GATA2 deficiency. Idiopathic CD4 lymphopenia and autosomal recessive hyper-IgE syndrome caused by DOCK8 deficiency are two other T-cell immunodeficiency states associated with HPV infection. Because warts in some anatomic regions are important cofactors in cancer, histologic evaluation of warty lesions in the immunodeficient patient can be critically important.

Verruca Vulgaris

Common warts are a significant cause of concern and frustration for patients and parents (Fig. 19.44). Social activities can be affected, lesions can be uncomfortable or bleed, and treatment is often painful and frustratingly ineffective. Human papillomavirus types 1, 2, 4, 27, 57, and 63 cause common warts. Common warts occur most commonly between ages 5 and 20, and only 15% occur after age 35. Frequent immersion of hands in water is a risk factor for common warts. Warts often spread from infected close contacts. Public exposures such as swimming pools, public showers, and going barefoot are associated to a lesser degree. Meat handlers (butchers), fish handlers, and other abattoir workers have a high incidence of common warts of the hands. Warts in butchers are caused by HPV-2 and HPV-4; up to 27% of hand warts from butchers are caused by HPV-7, which is found only on the hands where there is direct contact with meat but interestingly not on the slaughtered animals. HPV-7 is rarely found in warts in the general population (<0.3%), although there is a recent report showing HPV-7 in warts in toe web spaces. HPV-57 has been reported to cause dystrophy of all 10 fingernails, with marked subungual hyperkeratosis and destruction of the nail plate without periungual involvement. Clinicians usually do not determine the subtype of HPV when treating warts, but there are certain types of high-risk HPV types, such as 16 and 18, that have a higher risk of SCC.

The natural history of common warts is for spontaneous resolution. Reported clearance rates in children are 23% at 2 months, 30% at 3 months, 50% at 1 year, 65%–78% at 2 years, and 90% over 5 years. Common warts are usually located on the hands, favoring the fingers and palms. Periungual warts are more common in nail biters and may be confluent, involving the proximal and lateral nailfolds. Other sources of maceration can worsen warts including wearing sports gloves and overwashing. Fissuring may lead to bleeding and tenderness. Lesions range in size from pinpoint to more than 1 cm, most averaging about 5 mm. They grow in size for weeks to months and usually present as elevated, rounded papules with a rough, grayish surface, which is so characteristic that it has given us the word "verrucous," used to describe lesions with similar surface character (e.g., seborrheic keratosis). In some cases, a single wart (mother wart) appears and grows slowly for a long time, and then suddenly many new warts erupt. On the surface of the wart, tiny black dots may be visible, representing thrombosed, dilated capillaries. This clinical sign is very useful to differentiate from corns, callus, or other unusual cutaneous growths such as epitheliod sarcoma. Trimming the surface keratin makes the capillaries more prominent and may be used to aid diagnosis. The dermatoglyphics (fingerprint/toeprint folds) will stop at the base of a wart, in contrast to calluses, in which these lines are accentuated.

Common warts may occur anywhere on the skin including the lip margin and face, spreading from the hands by autoinoculation. In nail biters, warts may be seen on the lips and tongue, usually in the middle half or the oral commissures. Digitate or filiform warts tend to occur on the face and scalp and present as single or multiple projection with multiple small spikes at the tip on close inspection.

Pigmented Warts

Pigmented warts have frequently been reported in Japan although likely occurs in any patient with types III to VI skin. They appear on the hands or feet and resemble common warts or plantar warts, except for their hyperpigmentation. They are caused by HPV-4, HPV-60, and HPV-65. The pigmentation is caused by melanocytes in the basal cell layer of the HPV-infected tissue that contain large amounts of melanin. This is proposed to be caused by "melanocyte blockade," or the inability of the melanocytes to transfer melanin to the HPV-infected cells.

Flat Warts (Verruca Plana)

Human papillomavirus types 3, 10, 28, and 41 most often cause flat warts. Children and young adults are primarily affected. Sun

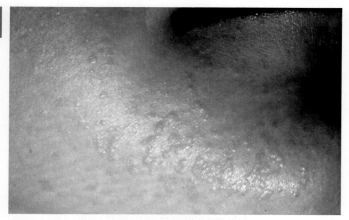

Fig. 19.45 Flat warts.

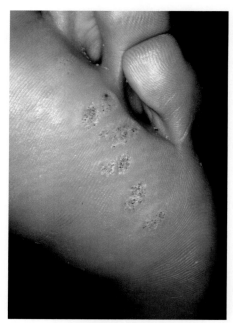

Fig. 19.46 Plantar warts.

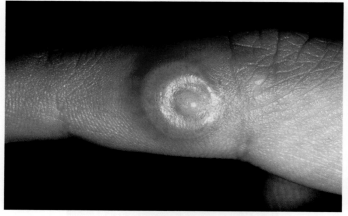

Fig. 19.47 Myrmecia.

exposure appears to be a risk factor for acquiring flat warts. Flat warts present most often as 2–4 mm, flat-topped papules that are slightly erythematous or brown on pale skin and hyperpigmented on darker skin. They occur more commonly on the sun-exposed surfaces likely due to immunosuppression. The face and extremities are most common, especially the forehead, cheeks, nose, and particularly the area around the mouth and the backs of the hands, but the lesions can occur anywhere, including the neck, dorsa of the hands, wrists, elbows, or knees. They are generally multiple and are grouped or in lines induced by koebnerization forming linear, slightly raised, papular lesions (Fig. 19.45). They are more common in swimmers. People with autism spectrum disorders or obsessive compulsive disorders who wash excessively and have dorsal had dermatitis can get exuberant flat warts. In shaved skin, numerous flat warts may develop as a result of autoinoculation. Hyperpigmented lesions occur, and when scarcely elevated, may be confused with lentigines or ephelides. Plaquelike lesions may be confused with verrucous epidermal nevus, lichen planus, lichen striatus, angiofibromas in tuberous sclerosis, and molluscum contagiosum. When lesions occur only on the central face and are erythematous, they can be easily confused with papular acne vulgaris. Of all clinical HPV infections, flat warts have the highest rate of spontaneous remission and are the most challenging to treat because they are so flat to the skin. Topical retinoids are often the treatment of choice because they can be used on the face.

Plantar Warts (Verruca Plantaris)

Human papillomaviruses 1, 2, 27, and 57 cause plantar warts. These warts generally appear at pressure points on the ball of the foot, especially over the midmetatarsal area, but may be anywhere on the sole. Frequently, several lesions develop on one foot (Fig. 19.46). Sometimes they are grouped, or several contiguous warts fuse so that they appear as one "mosaic" wart. The soft, pulpy cores are surrounded by a firm, horny ring. Plantar warts may be confused with corns or calluses but warts have a soft, central core and black or bleeding points from the superficial capillaries when pared down, features that calluses lack.

The myrmecia type of verruca occurs as smooth-surfaced, deep, often inflamed and tender papules or plaques, mostly on the palms or soles, but also beside or beneath the nails, or less often on the pulp of the digits (Fig. 19.47). They are distinctively dome shaped and much bulkier beneath the surface than they appear. Myrmecia are caused by HPV-1. They can be mistaken for a paronychia or digital mucinous cyst.

HPV-60 causes a peculiar type of plantar wart called a ridged wart because of the persistence of the dermatoglyphics across the surface of the lesion. Typically, the warts are slightly elevated, skin-colored, 3–5 mm papules. They occur on non–weight-bearing areas and lack the typical features of plantar warts. HPV-60 also causes plantar verrucous cysts, 1.5–2 cm, epithelium-lined cysts on the plantar surface. These cysts tend to occur on weight-bearing areas, suggesting that HPV-infected epidermis is implanted into the dermis, forming the cyst. It is common to see ridged warts near plantar verrucous cysts.

Histologic Features

Typical nongenital warts rarely require histologic confirmation, although a biopsy may be useful in several settings. Histology can be used to distinguish a wart from a corn and, more important, epithelioid sarcoma that can present as a papule or nodule on the palm or sole. Cytologic atypia and extension into the dermis suggest the diagnosis of an HPV-induced SCC. There is a correlation between HPV type and the histologic features of the wart, allowing identification of the HPV types that cause specific lesions, a useful feature in the diagnosis of epidermodysplasia verruciformis, for example.

Treatment of Common and Plantar Warts

The quality of evidence regarding the efficacy of therapies for warts is low. Studies have not used standard treatment protocols, and until recently, HPV type has not been evaluated along with treatment response. This hinders the development of evidence-based guidelines. The form of therapy used depends on patient preference, the type of wart being treated, the patient's age and immune status, and previous therapies used and their success or failure. With any treatment modality, at least 3 months of sustained management is considered a reasonable therapeutic trial. With immunologic treatments, this may be insufficient to see a response. No treatment should be abandoned too quickly or prolonged too long if not effective. Because many nongenital warts will spontaneously regress, the treatment algorithm should allow for nonaggressive options, and the patient should be offered the option of no treatment. Indications for treatment are pain, interference with function, social embarrassment, and risk of malignancy. The ideal aims of therapy are as follows:

1. Wart resolution
2. Avoidance of scarring or permanent sequelae from the treatment
3. Ideally, to induce lifelong immunity to that HPV type

Because the therapeutic options are similar for common and plantar, the therapies are considered together. In general, plantar warts are more refractory to any form of treatment than are common warts. The exception is HPV-1–induced plantar warts in children under 12 years, which have a high response rate (>50%).

Therapeutic Options

Destructive/Occlusive Therapy. Destructive methods are most often used as initial therapy by most practitioners for all types of warts with the exception of flat warts. Cryotherapy is a reasonable first-line treatment. In plantar warts, no trial has demonstrated cryotherapy to be superior to placebo in treating plantar warts. The cure rate is 20%–50% with repeated applications over several months. The wart should be frozen adequately to produce a blister after 1 or 2 days. This correlates with a thaw time of 30–45 seconds for most common warts. A sustained 10-second freeze with a spray gun was found to be more effective than simply freezing to obtain a 2–3 mm halo around the wart. Liquid nitrogen freezes to a lower temperature than other agents used for cryotherapy and is thus preferred. Aggressive cryotherapy can produce significant blistering and may be complicated by significant postprocedural pain for several days. A single freeze-thaw cycle was found may be as effective as two cycles. The ideal frequency of treatment is every 2 or 3 weeks, just as the old blister peels off to avoid regrowth in between treatments. No device used to apply liquid nitrogen should be allowed to touch multiple patients due to risk of spread. Children may be frightened by a spray device, so a cotton-tipped swab is an option for them. Cryotherapy can be effective for periungual warts. Damage to the matrix is unusual or rare, because periungual warts usually affect the lateral nailfolds, not the proximal one. Complications of cryotherapy include hypopigmentation, depigmentation, scarring (infrequent), and, rarely, damage to the digital nerve from freezing too deeply on the side of the digit. Patients with Fanconi anemia, cryoglobulinemia, poor peripheral circulation, and Raynaud phenomenon may develop severe blisters when cryotherapy is used to treat their warts. Doughnut warts, with central clearing and an annular recurrence, may complicate cryotherapy or more typically cantharone (see later discussion).

Topical salicylic acid in concentrations ranging from 10%–26% over the counter is an effective patient-applied treatment. Results have been conflicting, with some studies showing equal efficacy with cryotherapy and others showing marked inferiority to cryotherapy. To optimize salicylic acid treatment, the following treatment approach is suggested. After the wart-affected area is soaked in water for 5–10 minutes, the topical medication is applied, allowed to dry, and covered with a strip bandage for 24 hours. This is repeated daily. The superficial keratinous debris may be removed by scraping with a table knife, pumice stone, or emery board (each of which should be washed or discarded between therapies).

Silver nitrate has been used in limited studies with cure rates higher than placebo but caution is advised due to risk of silver impregnation into the skin.

The initial enthusiasm for occlusive therapy with tape (e.g., duct tape) has not been substantiated by follow-up studies. Occlusive therapy is inferior to cryotherapy, and success rates in adults are about the same as with placebo. If occlusive therapy is contemplated, a relatively impermeable tape should be used and the wart kept occluded at least 6½ and up to 7 days of the week. Fenestrated and semipermeable dressings have not been studied and may not be effective. Occlusive therapy is a good initial option for young children (<12 years) with plantar warts, in whom spontaneous resolution is high, and for others unwilling to have alternate forms of treatment. Unfortunately, in adults, the efficacy of duct tape for common warts is very low. Two months of treatment resolved common warts in only 20% of patients, and 75% of "resolved" warts recurred.

Cantharone (0.7% cantharidin) is applied to the wart, allowed to dry, and covered with occlusive tape for 24 hours or until the patient experiences burning. A blister, similar to that produced by cryotherapy, develops in 24–72 hours. These blisters may be as painful as or more painful than those following cryotherapy. Treatment is repeated every 2–3 weeks. Perhaps more than any other method, cantharidin tends to produce doughnut warts, a round wart with a central clear zone at the site of the original wart, and due to inconsistent efficacy, many do not use this modality first line. Cantharadin has the advantage that it can be applied painlessly to children.

Surgical ablation of warts can be effective treatment, but even complete destruction of a wart and the surrounding skin does not guarantee that the wart will not recur. Surgical methods should be reserved for warts that are refractory to more conservative approaches. Pulsed dye laser therapy initially appeared to have similar efficacy to cryotherapy, but low fluences were used. In recent reports, therapies with high efficacy for refractory warts (70%–90%) used fluences of 12.5–15 J/cm^2 (average 14 J/cm^2 in one study). Local anesthesia is required in the majority of patients. A short pulse duration (1.5 ms) is most effective. A 7-mm spot size is used, and treatment is extended 2 mm beyond the visible wart. The cryospray is inactivated because epidermal destruction is the goal. Immediately after treatment, the skin has a gray-black discoloration from thermal damage. The treated area becomes an eschar over 10–14 days. Treatment is repeated every 2–4 weeks, as soon as the eschar falls off, and multiple treatments may be required. In immunocompetent patients, response rates for refractory common and plantar warts are 70%–90% with this approach. The pulsed dye laser can also be used to treat warts around the nail that may have extended below the nail plate, because the laser will penetrate the nail plate. Carbon dioxide (CO_2) laser destruction requires local anesthesia, causes scarring, and may lead to nail dystrophy. Efficacy is 56%–81% in refractory warts. A potentially infectious plume is produced with the CO_2 laser. Frequency-doubled neodymium:yttrium-aluminum-garnet (Nd:YAG) laser, 532-nm potassium titanyl phosphate (KTP) laser, and PDT are options in refractory cases.

Heat treatment, either localized to the wart and delivered by radiofrequency or applied to the affected part by soaking it in a hot bath, has been reported to be effective. Treatment for 15 minutes at 43°C–50°C (107.6°F–122°F) to as short as 30 seconds at higher temperatures has been used. Extreme caution must be exercised to avoid scalding.

Immunologic Therapy. Immunotherapy with topical and intralesional agents has become a mainstay of wart therapy. The goal is not only that the wart will be eradicated, but that the immune reaction induced in the wart may also lead to widespread and permanent immunity against warts.

Oral cimetidine, 25–40 mg/kg/day, has been anecdotally reported to lead to resolution of common warts, perhaps because of its immunomodulatory effects. When used as a single agent, however, in both children and adults, the efficacy is low (30%), comparable with placebo. Cimetidine may be beneficial as an adjunct to other methods, especially for patients using immunotherapy without a brisk response to the antigen. Side effects appear to be limited.

Oral zinc seems to have benefit in patients who are zinc deficient, but efficacy was not shown in a randomized controlled trial, and therapy is limited by GI upset.

The topical agents typically used are topical DNCB, squaric acid dibutyl ester, and diphencyprone.

For the topical immunogens, patients may be initially sensitized at a distant site (usually the inner upper arm) with the topical agents, or the agents may be applied initially to the warts directly. Two treatment approaches are used, and their efficacies have not been compared. Some practitioners apply topical agents in the office in higher concentrations (2%–5%), but only about every 2 weeks. Others give their patients take-home prescriptions to use up to daily, although initially at lower concentrations (0.2%–0.5%). In most cases, the agents are dissolved in acetone. The treated wart should be kept covered for 24 hours after application. If the reaction is overly severe, the strength of the application may be reduced. Wart tenderness may indicate the need to reduce treatment concentration. Warts may begin to resolve within 1 or 2 weeks, but on average, 2–3 months or more of treatment is required. Overall cure rates for all three topical sensitizers and for intralesional antigen injection is 60%–80%. Side effects of treatment include local pruritus, local pain, and mild eczematous dermatitis. Most patients have no limitation of activities or function with topical immunotherapy.

The efficacy of imiquimod for common warts appears to be significantly less than with cryotherapy or topical immunotherapy and is considerably more expensive. The routine use of imiquimod in the treatment of common or plantar warts cannot be recommended. Unpublished placebo-controlled trials demonstrated no better response than placebo, with cure rates of about 10%.

Intralesional *Candida* antigen has become widely used with significant success rates. Injection of 0.1 mL to one to three lesions is repeated every 3–4 weeks with most benefit seen after multiple treatments. Some report up to 80% cure rate. Intralesional *Candida* injections may be associated with cytokine-mediated side effects, such as swelling, fever, shaking chills, and a flulike feeling. These begin 6–8 hours after treatment and resolve over 24–48 hours. Patients should be advised of these possible side effects. In a population previously immunized with bacille Calmette-Guérin (BCG), BCG antigen may be used.

Antiproliferative Therapy. Bleomycin has high efficacy but is reserved for recalcitrant common warts in adults. It is used at a concentration of 1 U/mL, which is injected into and immediately beneath the wart until it blanches. The multipuncture technique of Shelley—delivering the medication into the wart by multiple punctures with a needle through a drop of bleomycin—may also be used, as may an air jet injector. Even a concentration of 0.1 U/mL injected by this method can be effective. For small warts (<5 mm), 0.1 mL is used, and for larger warts, 0.2 mL. Combination use of bleomycin injections or *Candida* antigen injections with pulse dye laser may be useful in particularly refractory periungual and plantar warts. The injection of bleomycin is painful enough to require local anesthesia in some patients. Pain can occur for up to 1 week. The wart becomes black, and the black eschar separates in 2–4 weeks. Treatment may be repeated every 3 weeks, but it is unusual for common warts to require more than one or two treatments. Scarring is rare. Response rates vary by location, but average 90% with two treatments for most common, nonplantar warts, even periungual ones. Treatment of finger warts with bleomycin infrequently may be complicated by localized Raynaud phenomenon of treated fingers. Bleomycin treatment of digital warts may rarely result in digital necrosis and permanent nail dystrophy, so extreme caution should be used in treating warts around the nailfolds. Lymphangitis/cellulitis is a rare complication. In a patient receiving a total of 14 U for plantar warts, flagellate urticaria followed by characteristic bleomycin flagellate hyperpigmentation occurred.

Intralesional 5-FU and topical 5-FU have been used with variable results. Trials in which 5-FU cream was applied after cryotherapy demonstrated no additional benefit over the cryotherapy alone. Topical 5-FU is sometimes combined with salicylic acid, especially in plantar warts, with high cure rates.

Oral administration of acitretin or isotretinoin may also be used in refractory cases.

The value of quadrivalent HPV vaccination for the treatment of common warts is unknown. One study reported resolution of common and plantar warts in four young persons (three under 12 years) after HPV immunization.

Direct Antiviral Therapy. Topical cidofovir has been used in difficult situations and in immunosuppressed patients. It is compounded in a 1%–3% concentration (rarely up to 5%) and applied directly to the wart once or twice daily. The method of compounding is critical to the efficacy of topical cidofovir, so a reliable source known to compound an active gel is important. It is extremely expensive, however, and local irritation and erosion may occur. Cidofovir may also be delivered intralesionally in up to 5% concentration.

Flat Warts. Flat warts frequently undergo spontaneous remission, so therapy should be as mild as possible, and potentially scarring therapies should be avoided. If lesions are few, light cryotherapy is a reasonable consideration, although in patients with types III to VI skin, caution is advised, especially on the face due to risk of dyspigmentation. Topical salicylic acid products can also be used but not typically on the face. Treatment with topical retinoid once or twice daily, in the highest concentration tolerated (tazarotene may be most effective) to produce mild erythema of the warts without frank dermatitis, can be effective over several months. Imiquimod 5% cream used up to once daily can be effective. If the warts fail to react initially to the imiquimod, tretinoin may be used in conjunction. Should this fail, 5-FU cream 5%, applied twice daily, may be effective but in children, parents should be alerted that this is a topical chemotherapy. Anthralin, although staining, could be similarly used for its irritant effect. For refractory lesions, laser therapy in very low fluences or photodynamic therapy (PDT) might be considered before electrodesiccation because of the reduced risk of scarring. Ranitidine, 300 mg twice daily, cleared 56% of refractory flat warts in one study, with similar results using cimetidine (25–40 mg/kg). Three months of oral isotretinoin therapy at 30 mg/day was highly successful and might be considered when the previous topical approaches have failed. Immunotherapy with dinitrochlorobenzene (DNCB), squaric acid, or diphencyprone, or intralesional *Candida* or other antigens, can be used on limited areas of flat warts, with the hope that the immune response will clear distant warts. Peels have shown some benefit including those with glycolic acid and trichloracetic acid.

Genital Warts (External Genital Warts). Genital warts are the most common STD. Among sexually active young adults in the United States and Europe, infection rates as high as 50% in some cohorts have been found using sensitive PCR techniques. It is estimated that the lifetime risk for infection in sexually active young adults may be as high as 80%. The number of new U.S.

cases of genital wart infection diagnosed yearly may approach 1 million. In the about two thirds of couples in whom one has evidence of HPV infection, the partner will be found to be concordantly infected. A large portion of genital HPV infection is either subclinical or latent. Unfortunately, the infectivity of subclinical and latent infection is unknown. Subclinical and latent infection is probably responsible for most "recurrences" after treatment of genital warts. Because the methodology for determining HPV infection in men is less accurate, and women have the major complication of HPV infection, cervical cancer, virtually all data on HPV infection rates and epidemiology are derived from studies of women.

Genital HPV infection is closely linked to cancer of the cervix, glans penis, anus, vulvovaginal area, and periungual skin. Cancer occurs when there is integration of the HPV genome into the host DNA. In high-risk genital HPV types, *E6* and *E7* gene products bind to and inactivate p53 and retinoblastoma protein (pRb), respectively. This is thought to be important in their ability to cause cancer. In most persons, genital HPV infection appears to be transient, lasting about 1–2 years, and results in no sequelae. In a small proportion, about 2% of immunocompetent persons, infection persists, and in a small proportion of those with persistent HPV infection, cancer may develop (Fig. 19.48). Certain cofactors, such as the HPV type causing the infection, location of infection, cigarette smoking, uncircumcised status, and immunosuppressed status, are associated with progression to cancer. The transition zones of the cervix and anus are at highest risk for the development of cancer.

More than 30 HPV types are associated with genital warts. Patients are typically infected with multiple HPV types, although one HPV type probably causes most of the clinical lesions. Many HPV types are found in studies where the surface is sampled, but deeper in the epithelium, one type of HPV predominates, making studies that use surface sampling difficult to interpret. The HPV types producing genital infection are divided into two broad categories: those that produce benign lesions, or low-risk types, and those associated with cancer, the so-called high-risk or oncogenic types. The most common low-risk genital HPV types are HPV-6 and HPV-11, and most HPV-induced genital dysplasias are caused by HPV-16 and HPV-18. A strong correlation exists between the HPV type and the clinical appearance of HPV-induced genital lesions. Virtually all condylomata acuminata are caused by "benign" HPV-6 and HPV-11. High-risk HPV-16/18 produce flat or sessile, often hyperpigmented lesions. For this reason, biopsy and HPV typing of typical condyloma is rarely necessary. Since the advent of HPV vaccination targeting the high-risk HPV strains, the rates of HPV 6/11/16/18, as well as cervical and anogenital dysplasia, have fallen dramatically.

Genital HPV infection is strongly associated with sexual exposure. Female virgins rarely harbor HPV (about 1%). For women, insertive vaginal intercourse is strongly associated with acquiring genital HPV infection, with 50% of women testing positive for genital HPV within 5 years of the first sexual intercourse. However, sexual contact does not need to be penile-vaginal; the risk of acquiring genital HPV infection was 10% in women who had nonpenetrative sexual exposure versus 1% of women who had no such exposure. This suggests oral/digital/genital-genital exposure can transmit HPV infection to the introital skin. This infection may then be spread to other sites by self-inoculation. For this reason, women who have sex with women may have genital HPV infection and still require regular gynecologic evaluation. Condom is not fully protective for acquisition of genital HPV infection. In men, risk of genital HPV infection is associated with being uncircumcised, having had sex before age 17, having had more than six sexual partners in their lifetime, and having had sex with professional sex workers. Smokers are at increased risk of developing genital warts.

Condylomata Acuminata. Condylomata on the skin surface appear as lobulated papules that average 2–5 mm in size, but they may range from microscopic to many centimeters in diameter and height. Lesions are frequently multifocal. Numerous genital warts may appear during pregnancy. Condylomata acuminata occur in men anywhere on the penis (Fig. 19.49) or about the anus. Scrotal condylomata occur in only 1% of immunocompetent male patients with warts. Intraurethral condylomata may present with terminal hematuria, altered urinary stream, or urethral bleeding. In women, lesions appear on the mucosal surfaces of the vulva or cervix, on the perineum, or about the anus (Fig. 19.50). Cauliflower-like masses may develop in moist, occluded areas such as the perianal skin, vulva, and inguinal folds. As a result of accumulation of purulent material in the clefts, these may be malodorous. Their color is generally gray, pale yellow, or pink. When perianal lesions

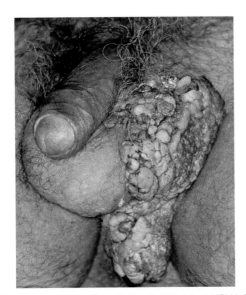

Fig. 19.48 Squamous cell carcinoma in persistent HPV infection.

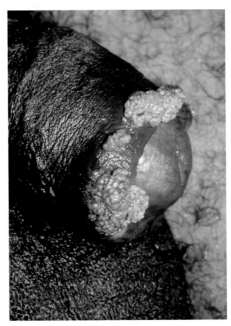

Fig. 19.49 Condylomata acuminata. (Courtesy Steven Binnick, MD.)

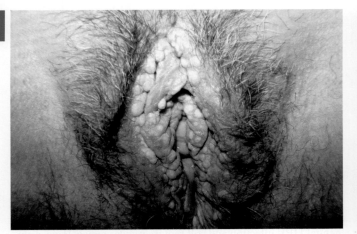

Fig. 19.50 Condylomata acuminata. (Courtesy Steven Binnick, MD.)

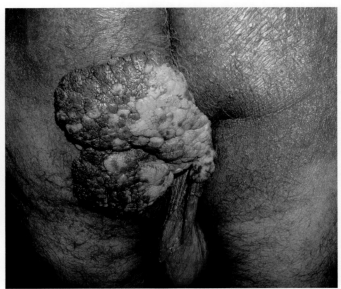

Fig. 19.52 Buschke-Lowenstein tumor. (Courtesy Shyam Verma, MBBS, DVD.)

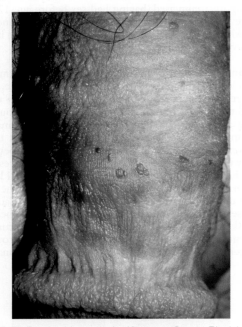

Fig. 19.51 Bowenoid papulosis. (Courtesy Steven Binnick, MD.)

occur, a prior history of receptive anal intercourse will usually predict whether intraanal warts are present and will help to determine the need for anoscopy. Immunosuppressed individuals and those with infection by known high-risk HPV types at other sites should have routine anal Papanicolaou (Pap) smears to detect malignant change.

Genital warts are sexually transmitted, and other STDs may be found in patients with genital warts. A complete history should be taken and the patient screened for other STDs as appropriate. The whole genital area should be carefully examined because external genital wart (EGW) infection is often multifocal. HIV testing is recommended. Women with EGWs should have a routine cervical cytologic screening to detect cervical dysplasia.

Bowenoid Papulosis and HPV-Induced Genital Dysplasias. Bowenoid papulosis is characterized by flat, often hyperpigmented papules a few millimeters to several centimeters in diameter. These occur singly or, more often, may be found in multiples on the penis, near the vulva, or perianally (Fig. 19.51). At times, similar lesions are seen outside the genital area in the absence of

genital bowenoid papulosis. They occur most frequently on the neck or face and are more common in men. They contain HPV-16, HPV-18, or other high-risk HPV types. In the standard terminology for lower anogenital squamous lesions, this is called HSIL (high-grade squamous intraepithelial lesion). It is usually caused by HPV-16. On the glabrous external genitalia, bowenoid papulosis usually behaves similar to other EGWs but may progress to SCC. Patients may simultaneously have bowenoid papulosis of the genitalia and SCC in situ, especially in the periungual area, both caused by the same HPV type. On the glans penis of an uncircumcised male and on the cervical, vaginal, or rectal mucosa, progression to invasive SCC is more likely. Female partners of men with bowenoid papulosis and women with bowenoid papulosis have an increased risk of cervical dysplasia. Histologically, the biopsies of SCC in situ and HSIL caused by HPV (bowenoid papulosis) are very similar. Pigmentation of the epithelium and numerous mitoses, especially in metaphase, are characteristic but not diagnostic of HPV-induced HSIL on the external genitalia.

Giant Condyloma Acuminatum (Buschke-Lowenstein Tumor). Giant condyloma acuminatum is a rare, aggressive, verrucous growth that is a verrucous carcinoma. Unlike other HPV-induced genital carcinomas, this tumor is usually caused by HPV-6. It occurs most often on the glans or prepuce of an uncircumcised male; less often, it may occur on perianal skin or the vulva (Fig. 19.52). Despite its bland histologic picture, it may invade deeply, and infrequently it may metastasize to regional lymph nodes. Treatment is by complete surgical excision. Recurrence after radiation therapy may be associated with a more aggressive course.

Diagnosis of Genital Warts. Even in women with confirmed cervical HPV infection, serologic tests are positive in only 50%, making serologic diagnosis of HPV infection of little use to the practicing clinician. HPV typing by in situ hybridization (ISH) or PCR is useful in managing HPV infection of the cervix and in some cases of prepubertal HPV infection, but not in the management of EGW. Virtually all condylomata can be diagnosed by inspection. Bright lighting and magnification should be used when examining for genital HPV infection. Flat, sessile, and pigmented lesions suggest bowenoid papulosis and may require a biopsy. Subclinical and latent infections are no longer sought or investigated because they are very common, and no management strategy is known to eradicate these forms of HPV infection. Soaking with acetic acid is not generally necessary but may be helpful to detect early lesions under the foreskin. In patients with multiple recurrences, acetic acid soaking may determine the extent of infection, helping to define the area for application of topical therapies. The procedure is performed by soaking the external genitalia in men and the vagina and cervix in women with 3%–5% acetic acid for up to 10 minutes. Genital warts turn white (acetowhitening), making them easily identifiable. Any process that alters the epidermal barrier will be acetowhite (e.g., dermatitis), however. In atypical cases, a 2-week trial is attempted with a 1% hydrocortisone preparation plus a topical anticandidal imidazole cream. If the acetowhitening persists, a biopsy is performed and histologic evidence of HPV infection sought. IP or ISH methods may aid in evaluation. PCR can aid in difficult clinical diagnosis especially in childhood cases. The high background rate of latent infection (up to 50%) makes interpretation of a positive PCR impossible. In contrast, chromogenic ISH clearing demonstrates the localization of positive nuclei within the lesion and can confirm a lesion to be HPV induced.

Treatment. Because no effective virus-specific agent exists for their treatment, genital warts frequently recur. Prevention with HPV vaccination if possible is imperative. Treatment is not proved to reduce transmission to sexual partners or to prevent progression to dysplasia or cancer. Specifically, the treatment of male sexual partners of women with genital warts does not reduce the recurrence rate of warts in these women. Therefore the goals of treatment must first be discussed with the patient and perhaps with the sexual partner. Observation represents an acceptable option for some patients with typical condylomata acuminata. Because genital warts may cause discomfort, genital pruritus, foul odor, bleeding, and substantial emotional distress, treatment is indicated if requested by the patient. Bleeding genital warts may increase the sexual transmission of HIV and hepatitis B and C. Bowenoid papulosis may be treated as discussed next when it occurs on the external genitalia. Lesions with atypical histology (high-grade squamous intraepithelial) on mucosal surfaces and periungually are special cases, and treatment must be associated with histologic confirmation of eradication in patients receiving topical treatments.

The treatment chosen is in part dictated by the size of the warts and their location. The number of EGWs at the initial evaluation is strongly predictive of wart clearance. Patients with four or fewer EGWs will be clear with three or fewer treatments, whereas only 50% of patients with 10 or more EGWs will be clear after three treatments. 20% of patients with 10 or more EGWs will still have lesions after eight treatments. A more effective or aggressive treatment approach might be considered in patients with high numbers of EGWs.

Podophyllin is more effective in treating warts on occluded or moist surfaces, such as on the mucosa or under the prepuce. It is available as a crude extract, usually in 25% concentration in tincture of benzoin. It is applied weekly by the physician and can be washed off 4–8 hours later by the patient, depending on the severity of the reaction. After six consecutive weekly treatments, approximately 40% of patients are free of warts, and 17% are free of warts at 3 months after treatment. Purified podophyllotoxin 0.5% solution or gel is applied by the patient twice daily for 3 consecutive days of each week with 4 days without therapy to allow recovery from irritation in 4- to 6-week treatment cycles. Efficacy approaches 60% for typical condylomata, and side effects are fewer than with standard, physician-applied podophyllin preparations. Therefore whenever possible, podophyllotoxin should be used instead of classic podophyllin solutions.

Imiquimod, an immune response modifier that induces IFN locally at the site of application, has efficacy similar to cryotherapy

(about 50%) and yields a low recurrence rate (22%). Imiquimod may be used to treat penile condyloma in circumcised and uncircumcised men, anal and perianal condyloma, vulvar condyloma and bowenoid papulosis. It may be used as the initial treatment or when recurrence has been frequent after attempting other forms of treatment. The 5% cream is applied daily or every other day for up to 16 weeks. The 3.75% cream is applied daily for 2 weeks, followed by a 2-week rest period, to a maximum of 8 weeks of treatment. The 3.75% cream is less effective than the 5% cream, resulting in only a 33% clearance but with fewer side effects. Imiquimod 5% cream is more effective than podophyllotoxin in treating women with EGW infection, but only equally or slightly less effective in men, especially for warts on the penile shaft. Imiquimod is less effective than cryotherapy in the treatment of EGWs. Therapeutic response to imiquimod is slow, requiring several weeks in some patients to see any effect. Treatment results in mild to moderate irritation, less than with podophyllin or cryotherapy in men, but with a similar side effect profile in women. Rare complications reported with the 5% cream include flaring of psoriasis and psoriatic arthritis, vitiligo-like hypopigmentation, induction of genital ulcers in a patient with Behçet disease, and the production of a local neuropathy. Imiquimod should be used cautiously in persons with psoriasis. Neuropathy is associated with application of excessive amounts, occlusion of the medication, and application to an eroded mucosa.

Imiquimod (and sinecatechins) has also been used as a maintenance therapy after destructive methods, the cream applied to the area for 12–16 weeks to prevent recurrence and eradicate subclinical lesions. The use of imiquimod after surgical destruction of condyloma should be considered in all immunocompetent patients, especially those with recurrence after a previous surgical procedure. Suppositories containing about 5 mg of imiquimod appear to reduce the risk of recurrence of anal condyloma in immunocompetent men after surgical ablation of extensive anal disease.

The topical application of green tea extract containing sinecatechins (Polyphenon E or Veregen) can be effective in treating EGWs. A 15% ointment applied three times daily leads to EGW clearance in 60% of women and 45% of men. Placebo cleared 35% of patients in this blinded study. The average time to complete clearance is 16 weeks. Erythema and erosions at the application site occur in 50% of patients, and 67% had moderate to severe reactions.

Bichloracetic acid or TCA 35%–85% can be applied to condylomata weekly or biweekly. TCA is safe for use in pregnant patients. Compared with cryotherapy, TCA has the same or lower efficacy and causes more ulcerations and pain. It is not generally recommended for EGWs, because other available treatments are more effective and cause less morbidity.

Cryotherapy with liquid nitrogen is more effective than podophyllin and imiquimod, approaching 70%–80% resolution during treatment and 55% at 3 months after treatment. One or two freeze-thaw cycles are applied to each wart every 1–3 weeks. A zone of 2 mm beyond the lesion is frozen. Cryotherapy is effective in dry as well as moist areas. Perianal lesions are more difficult to eradicate than other genital sites, and two freeze-thaw cycles are recommended in this location. Cryotherapy is safe to use in pregnant patients. EMLA cream with or without subsequent lidocaine infiltration may be beneficial in reducing the pain of cryotherapy. The addition of podophyllin to cryotherapy does not result in a higher cure rate but the response rate may be faster.

Electrofulguration or electrocauterization with or without snip removal of the condyloma is more effective than TCA, cryotherapy, imiquimod, or podophyllin. Wart clearance during therapy is almost 95%, and wart cure at 3 months exceeds 70%. Local anesthesia is required, and scarring may occur. Surgical removal is ideal for large, exophytic warts that might require multiple treatments with other methods. It has high acceptance in patients who have had recurrences from other methods because results are immediate and cure rates higher.

The use of CO_2 laser in the treatment of genital warts has not been shown to be more effective than simpler surgical methods. Although visible warts are eradicated by the laser, HPV DNA can still be detected at the previous site of the wart. The CO_2 laser has the advantage of being bloodless, but it is more costly and requires more technical skill. It should be reserved for treatment of extensive lesions in which more cost-effective methods have been attempted and failed. Adjunctive PDT does not prevent recurrence of EGW after CO_2 laser ablation. Compared with CO_2 laser ablation of EGWs, 5-aminolevulinic acid (ALA) with PDT demonstrated higher efficacy and fewer recurrences and was less painful. ALA-PDT response rate is about 75%. ALA-PDT should be considered before CO_2 laser ablation for the treatment of multiple small, but refractory condyloma.

Any surgical method that generates a smoke plume is potentially infectious to the surgeon. HPV DNA is detected in the plumes generated during CO_2 laser or electrocoagulation treatment of genital warts. The laser-generated plume results in longer-duration HPV aerosol contamination and wider spread of detectable HPV DNA. If these methods of wart treatment are used, an approved face mask and smoke evacuator should be used and the equipment decontaminated after the surgery.

5-Fluorouracil 5% cream applied twice daily may be effective, especially in the treatment of flat, hyperpigmented lesions, such as those in bowenoid papulosis. Care must be taken to avoid application to the scrotum, because scrotal skin is prone to painful erosions. Twice-daily instillation of 5-FU into the urethra can be used to treat intraurethral condylomata. The cone from a tube of lidocaine (Xylocaine) jelly will fit onto the thread of the 5-FU tube, or the cream may be instilled with a syringe. It is typically left in place for 1 hour before the patient voids. Care should be taken that drips of urine containing the medication do not contact the scrotum. 5-FU may also be used to treat intravaginal warts by instillation in the vagina, but this is often associated with severe irritation. Intermittent therapy (twice weekly for 10 weeks) is better tolerated than daily therapy. 5-FU is not usually recommended for the treatment of typical EGWs because other methods of treatment are available.

Immunotherapy can also be effective for refractory EGWs. This is usually delivered by injection of *Candida*, BCG, purified protein derivative (PPD), or another antigen, rather than through topical application, because of the difficulty in preventing exposure of normal skin with a topical solution. Immunotherapy may be combined with destructive methods in refractory cases. The injection of HPV-6 VLPs was found to speed the clearance of warts simultaneously treated with cryotherapy, podophyllin, or TCA.

Human Papillomavirus Vaccination. The HPV VLPs are composed of spontaneously assembling L1 molecules and have been used to develop a polyvalent vaccine against HPVs 6, 11, 16, and 18, but a newer nine-valent vaccine targets these four, as well as HPVs 31, 33, 45, 52, and 58. HPV vaccination is highly effective and is now approved in more than 100 countries for the immunization of prepubertal girls and boys. Vaccination is recommended for unvaccinated females through age 26 and males age 13–21. HIV-infected men and women should receive immunization through age 26. In older women (age 24–45) the vaccine is also effective and may be given as a "catch-up" vaccine in women with no evidence of prior genital HPV infection with HPVs 6, 11, 16, or 18. The incidence of the targeted HPVs in addition to cervical intraepithelial neoplasia have been reduced dramatically. Even condyloma in nonvaccinated women and men (who were not yet eligible for immunization) were reduced, demonstrating herd immunity. HPV-related genital HSIL was also reduced by 47% in fully vaccinated women. In countries where HPV-16/18

vaccination was widely applied, the burden of HPV disease caused by HPV-6 and HPV-11 has decreased, suggesting some benefit across HPV types.

Genital Warts in Children. Children can acquire genital warts through vertical transmission perinatally and through digital inoculation or autoinoculation, fomite or social nonsexual contact, and sexual abuse. HPV typing has demonstrated that most warts in the genital area of children are "genital" HPV types, and most children with genital warts have family members with a genital HPV infection.

Human papillomavirus typing can be performed. However, the presence of genital types of HPV does not prove abuse, and finding a nongenital HPV type does not exclude sexual abuse. In children younger than 1 year, vertical transmission is probably the most common means of acquisition. The risk for sexual abuse is highest in children older than 3 years. A careful history should be taken evaluating for any warts on the child or parent that could have been innocuously transferred to the child. When abuse is suspected, children should be referred to child protection services if the practitioner is not skilled in evaluating children for sexual abuse. Children 1–3 years old are primarily nonverbal and are difficult to evaluate but fortunately vertical transmission and not sexual abuse can be the source. Management of such patients is on a case-by-case basis. Other STDs should be screened for in children who have a genital HPV infection.

Usually, management of children with anogenital warts requires a multidisciplinary team that should include a pediatrician (Fig. 19.53). Genital warts in children often spontaneously resolve (75%), so no intervention may be a reasonable consideration. Genital warts in children usually respond quickly to topical therapy, such as podophyllotoxin, imiquimod, or light cryotherapy. In refractory cases, surgical removal or electrocautery may be used but care must be exercised not to cause undue emotional stress on the parent or child.

Recurrent Respiratory (Laryngeal) Papillomatosis

Papillomas associated with HPV may occur throughout the respiratory tract, from the nose to the lungs. Recurrent respiratory papillomatosis has a bimodal distribution: in children under age 5 years and after age 15. Affected young children are typically born to mothers with genital condylomata and present with hoarseness. The HPV types found in these lesions, HPV-6 and HPV-11, are the types seen in genital condylomata. Carcinoma

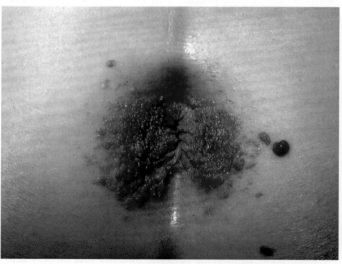

Fig. 19.53 Perianal warts in 18-month-old infant.

that is often fatal develops in 14% of patients, even in young children. The incidence of carcinoma is higher in those treated with radiation therapy. These patients often have recurrences and require numerous surgeries, usually with the CO_2 laser. Scarring can result from frequent ablations, leading to speech and breathing difficulties. Adjunctive cidofovir has been combined with surgical ablation to help reduce recurrences, with some positive preliminary results. Also, HPV vaccination has been combined with laser ablation, with preliminary results demonstrating reduced recurrences. It is hoped that HPV immunization of young women will reduce the prevalence of condyloma and thus of respiratory papillomatosis.

Heck Disease

Small, white to pinkish papules occur diffusely in the oral cavity in Heck disease, also known as focal epithelial hyperplasia. It occurs most frequently in Native Americans of North, Central, and South America; in Inuits; in Greenland Eskimos; and in descendants of Khoi-San in South Africa. In these populations, prevalence rates can be as high as 35%. It is five times more common in females. HPV-13 and HPV-32 have been classically associated with Heck disease. Clinically, the lesions may be papular or papillomatous and favor the buccal and labial mucosa and the commissures of the mouth. Lesions may spontaneously resolve. Treatment options include cryosurgery, CO_2 laser, electrosurgery, and topical, intralesional, or systemic IFN.

Epidermodysplasia Verruciformis

Epidermodysplasia verruciformis (EV) is a rare, inherited disorder characterized by widespread HPV infection and cutaneous SCCs. EV is most commonly inherited as an autosomal recessive trait, although autosomal dominant and X-linked inheritance have also been reported. About 10% of EV patients are from consanguineous marriages. HPV types associated with this syndrome include those infecting normal hosts, such as HPV-3 and HPV-10, as well as many "unique" HPV types, often β-HPVs. These HPV types are called "EV HPVs" and include HPVs 4, 5, 8, 9, 12, 14, 15, 17, 19–25, 36–38, and 47. HPV-5 and HPV-8 are found in 90% of the skin cancers in EV patients. The genetic mutations causing EV are found in two closely linked genes, *EVER1* and *EVER2*. The function of these genes and how they cause this syndrome are unknown.

The condition presents in childhood and continues throughout life. Skin lesions include flat wart–like lesions of the dorsal hands, extremities, face, and neck. They appear in childhood or young adulthood, apparently earlier in sunnier climates. The characteristic lesions are flatter than typical flat warts (Fig. 19.54) and may be quite abundant, growing to confluence. Typical flat warts may be admixed. In addition, lesions on the trunk are red, tan, or brown patches/plaques or hypopigmented, slightly scaly plaques resembling tinea versicolor. Plaques on the elbows may resemble psoriasis. Seborrheic keratosis–like lesions may also be seen on the forehead, neck, and trunk. Common warts are reported to occur infrequently in some EV cohorts.

The histologic features of an EV-specific HPV infection are very characteristic. The cells of the upper epidermis have a clear, smoky, or light-blue pale cytoplasm and a central pyknotic nucleus.

In about one third of EV patients, SCCs develop an average of 24 years after the appearance of the characteristic EV skin lesions. Most often, skin cancers appear on sun-exposed surfaces, but they can appear on any part of the body. Skin cancers are less common in African patients, suggesting a protective effect of skin pigmentation. The SCCs may appear de novo, but usually appear on the background of numerous actinic keratoses and lesions of Bowen disease (Fig. 19.55). Surgical treatment is recommended. Radiation therapy is contraindicated. If skin grafting is required,

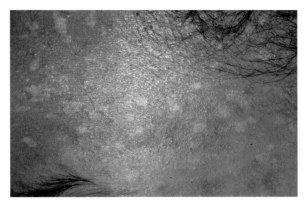

Fig. 19.54 Epidermodysplasia verruciformis in an HIV-infected patient.

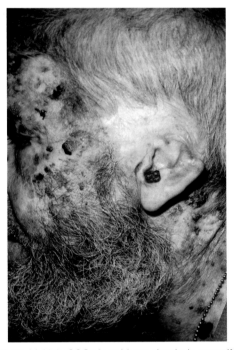

Fig. 19.55 Multiple SCCs in epidermodysplasia verruciformis.

the grafts should be taken from sun-protected skin, such as the buttocks or inner upper arm.

Aside from surgical intervention for skin cancer, treatment for EV consists largely of preventive measures. Strict sun avoidance and protection should be started as soon as the syndrome is diagnosed. An approach similar to that for children with xeroderma pigmentosa could be instituted. ALA-PDT, topical 5-FU, imiquimod, and oral retinoids may all be used to treat the lesions of patients with EV, but when treatment is discontinued, lesions usually recur.

The mechanism by which cancer occurs in patients with EV is unclear. HPV-5 proteins do not bind to p53 or pRb. The p53 mutations present in the SCCs of patients with EV are characteristic of those induced by UVB light, confirming the close association of UV exposure and the development of cancer in patients with EV. HPV DNA of EV has been reported in 35% of the general population in very low copy number, suggesting that the presence of these EV HPVs alone is not the cause of the skin cancers. Rather, the *EVER* genes apparently control important immune responses in the epidermis that control HPV replication, and in their absence, viral replication goes unchecked and can eventually lead to skin cancer in sun-damaged skin. Supporting this concept is a report of a polyomavirus-positive Merkel cell carcinoma in an EV patient. Infection with EV HPV types has been reported in immunosuppressed patients, especially those with HIV. This has been called "acquired EV." SCC has not been reported in these patients.

Other Immunodeficiencies Associated With Warts

Some patients with extensive (>100) common and plantar warts that never resolve and simply grow to confluence have been called "generalized verrucosis." These patients do not develop skin cancers and live into adulthood. Some of these patients have been identified with mutations in *GATA2* (WILD syndrome), *DOCK8*, or *CXCR4* (WHIM syndrome) or with idiopathic CD4 lymphopenia (see Chapter 5). Patients with WHIM have been treated with Plerixifor that blocks CXCL12 activation of CXCR4 and can help restore immune function. Some of these patients, unlike EV patients, are at high risk for anogenital HPV disease and its complications.

Immunosuppressed Patients

Patients with defects in cell-mediated immunity may have an increased frequency of HPV infection. Predisposing conditions include organ transplantation, immunosuppressive medications, congenital immunodeficiency diseases, lymphoma, and HIV infection.

Organ transplant recipients begin to develop warts soon after transplantation, and by 5 years, up to 90% of transplant patients have warts. Initially, these are common and plantar warts, but later, numerous flat warts appear, particularly in sun-exposed areas. Genital warts are also increased, and especially in women, genital dysplasias are more frequent. Keratotic lesions should be evaluated closely for NMSC in transplant patients. It is especially important in immunosuppressed patients to monitor the genital and anal areas regularly for changing lesions and to have a low threshold for performing a biopsy.

In HIV disease, common, plantar, flat, oral, and genital warts are all common. Warty keratoses at the angle of the mouth, often bilateral, are a characteristic manifestation of HPV infection in patients with AIDS. The warts are caused predominantly by HPVs 2, 27, and 57. HPV-7 can be found in cutaneous, oral, and perioral warts in nonbutchers with HIV infection. Genital warts are increased 15-fold among HIV-infected women. Fifty percent or more of HIV-infected MSM have evidence of anal HPV infection. Genital neoplasia associated with HPV-16 and HPV-18 occurs much more frequently in HIV-infected women and MSM. Infrequently, HIV patients develop HPV-5/8–induced EV-like lesions. With antiretroviral therapy, warts may disappear. Paradoxically, increased rates of genital and oral warts may be seen in HIV patients in the first several years of adequate control of their HIV infection, likely as part of IRIS. The likelihood of clearance of common warts in persons with HIV is related to the nadir of their Th cell count. HIV-infected persons whose Th count never falls below 200 cells are more likely to have sustained remission of their warts.

The treatment of warts in immunosuppressed hosts can be challenging. Although standard methods are used, their efficacy may be reduced. For common and plantar warts, surgically ablative methods, cryotherapy, bleomycin injections, PDT, and aggressive pulsed dye laser therapy would be expected to be more effective, because the agents designed to induce an immune response would be less effective in the immunosuppressed patient. In one study using intralesional *Candida* antigen for common warts, the response rate was less than 50% in HIV patients, and no patient showed a distant benefit for untreated warts. Imiquimod has low efficacy in these patients; only 8% had complete clearance of common

warts, and 50% had no response. For genital warts, treatment is determined by size. Any wart larger than 2 cm should be sent for consideration of surgical removal and histologic evaluation. Smaller warts can be treated with electrosurgery, cryotherapy, topical 5-FU, and ALA-PDT. Imiquimod can be attempted and is most effective for EGWs on occluded skin (intraanal, under the prepuce). Most transplant patients tolerate imiquimod well, without inducing enough systemic immune response to cause rejection of their transplanted organ. However, widespread use of imiquimod in one renal transplant patient led to acute renal failure.

Topical cidofovir (1%–5% concentration) and intralesional cidofovir (7.5 mg/mL) have been effective in refractory anogenital and common warts in immunodeficient patients. Although topical cidofovir is very expensive, is irritating, and can cause skin erosion and ulceration, it is active against the HPV and thus does not require participation of the patient's immune system to eradicate the wart. Addition of sirolimus to the immunosuppressive regimen may be associated with a decrease in the number of warts in organ transplant patients. In four pediatric transplant patients, substitution of leflunomide for mycophenolate in the immunosuppressive regimen, resulted in clearance or dramatic improvement of cutaneous warts and molluscum contagiosum. The mycophenolate was reinstituted and leflunomide stopped without recurrence of the warts. In organ transplant patients with widespread actinic damage and many precancerous lesions, PDT can be considered.

Alikhan A, et al: Use of *Candida* antigen injections for the treatment of verruca vulgaris. J Dermatolog Treat 2016; 27: 355.

Ash MM, Jolly PS: A case report of the resolution of multiple recalcitrant verrucae in a renal transplant recipient after a mycophenolate mofetil dose reduction. Transplant Proc 2017; 49: 213.

Badolato R, et al: How I treat warts, hypogammaglobulinemia, infections, and myelokathexis syndrome. Blood 2017; 130: 2491.

Bleeker MCG, et al: Penile lesions and human papillomavirus in male sexual partners of women with cervical intraepithelial neoplasia. J Am Acad Dermatol 2002; 47: 351.

Bouwes Bavinck JN, et al: Keratotic skin lesions and other risk factors are associated with skin cancer in organ-transplant recipients. J Invest Dermatol 2007; 127: 1647.

Brehm MA, et al: Case report of focal epithelial hyperplasia (Heck's disease) with polymerase chain reaction detection of human papillomavirus 13. Pediatr Dermatol 2016; 33: e224.

Broganelli P, et al: Intralesional cidofovir for the treatment of multiple and recalcitrant cutaneous viral warts. Dermatol Ther 2012; 25: 468.

Brotherton JML, Bloem PN: Population based HPV vaccination programs are safe and effective. Best Pract Res Clin Obstet Gynaecol 2017; ePub ahead of print.

Bruggink SC, et al: Cutaneous wart-associated HPV types. J Clin Virol 2012; 55: 250.

Bruggink SC, et al: HPV type in plantar warts influences natural course and treatment response. J Clin Virol 2013; 57: 227.

Bruggink SC, et al: Warts transmitted in families and schools. Pediatrics 2013; 131: 928.

Chen K, et al: Comparative study of photodynamic therapy vs CO_2 laser vaporization in treatment of condylomata acuminata, a randomized clinical trial. Br J Dermatol 2007; 156: 516.

Chow EP, et al: Ongoing decline in genital warts among young heterosexuals 7 years after the Australian human papillomavirus (HPV) vaccination programme. Sex Transm Infect 2015; 91: 214.

Cockayne S, et al: Cryotherapy versus salicylic acid for the treatment of plantar warts (verrucae). BMJ 2011; 342: d3271.

Daniel BS, Murrell DF: Complete resolution of chronic multiple verruca vulgaris treated with quadrivalent human papillomavirus vaccine. JAMA Dermatol 2013; 149: 370.

Dharancy S, et al: Conversion to sirolimus: a useful strategy for recalcitrant cutaneous viral warts in liver transplant recipients. Liver Transpl 2006; 12: 1883.

Dobson JS, Harland CC: Pulsed dye laser and intralesional bleomycin for the treatment of recalcitrant cutaneous warts. Laser Surg Med 2014; 46: 112.

Fahey LM, et al: A major role for the minor capsid protein of human papillomavirus type 16 in immune escape. J Immunol 2009; 183: 6151.

Fausch SC, et al: Human papillomavirus can escape immune recognition through Langerhans cell phosphoinositide 3-kinase activation. J Immunol 2005; 174: 7172.

Garg M, et al: Giant Buschke-Lowenstein tumour. BMJ Case Rep 2013 May 24; 2013.

Garland SM, et al: Impact and effectiveness of the quadrivalent human papillomavirus vaccine. Clin Infect Dis 2016; 63: 519.

Gibbs S: Topical immunotherapy with contact sensitizers for viral warts. Br J Dermatol 2002; 146: 705.

Gormley RH, Kovarik CL: Human papillomavirus–related genital disease in the immunocompromised host. Part I. J Am Acad Dermatol 2012; 66: 867.e1.

Gormley RH, Kovarik CL: Human papillomavirus–related genital disease in the immunocompromised host. Part II. J Am Acad Dermatol 2012; 66: 883.e1.

Grasso M, et al: Use of cidofovir in HPV patients with recurrent respiratory papillomatosis. Eur Arch Otorhinolaryngol 2014; 271: 2983.

Henrickson SE et al: Topical cidofovir for recalcitrant verrucae in individuals with severe combined immunodeficiency after hematopoietic stem cell transplantation. Pediatr Dermatol 2017; 34: e24.

Hivnor C, et al: Intravenous cidofovir for recalcitrant verruca vulgaris in the setting of HIV. Arch Dermatol 2004; 140: 13.

Imahorn E, et al: Novel TMC8 splice site mutation in epidermodysplasia verruciformis and review of HPV infections in patients with the disease. J Eur Acad Dermatol Venereol 2017; 31: 1722.

Jardine D, et al: A randomized trial of immunotherapy for persistent genital warts. Hum Vaccin Immunother 2012; 8: 623.

Kallikourdis M, et al: The *CXCR4* mutations in WHIM syndrome impair the stability of the T-cell immunologic synapse. Blood 2013; 122: 666.

Kaspari M, et al: Application of imiquimod by suppositories (anal tampons) efficiently prevents recurrences after ablation of anal canal condyloma. Br J Dermatol 2002; 147: 757.

Kimura U, et al: Long-pulsed 1064-nm neodymium:yttrium-aluminum-garnet laser treatment for refractory warts on hands and feet. J Dermatol 2014; 41: 252.

Kines RC, et al: The initial steps leading to papillomavirus infection occur on the basement membrane prior to cell surface binding. Proc Natl Acad Sci USA 2009; 106: 20458.

Kwok CS, et al: Topical treatments for cutaneous warts. Cochrane Database Syst Rev 2012; 9: CD001781.

Leiding JW, Holland SM: Warts and all: human papillomavirus in primary immunodeficiencies. J Allergy Clin Immunol 2012; 130:1030.

Li SL, et al: Identification of LCK mutation in a family with atypical epidermodysplasia verruciformis with T-cell defects and virus-induced squamous cell carcinoma. Br J Dermatol 2016; 175: 1204.

Lin JH, et al: Resolution of warts in association with subcutaneous immunoglobulin in immune deficiency. Pediatr Dermatol 2009; 26: 155.

Long FQ, et al: Vitiligo or vitiligo-like hypopigmentation associated with imiquimod treatment of condyloma acuminatum. Chin Med J 2017; 130: 503.

Mammas IN, et al: Human papilloma virus (HPV) infection in children and adolescents. Eur J Pediatr 2009; 168: 267.

Markowitz LE, et al: Prevalence of HPV after introduction of the vaccination program in the United States. Pediatrics 2016; 137: e20151968.

Martinelli C, et al: Resolution of recurrent perianal condylomata acuminata by topical cidofovir in patients with HIV infection. J Eur Acad Dermatol Venereol 2001; 15: 568.

Mavrogianni P, et al: Therapeutic combination of radiofrequency surgical dissection and oral acitretin in the management of perianal Buschke-Löwenstein tumour. Int J STD AIDS 2012; 23: 362.

M'barek LB, et al: 5% Topical imiquimod tolerance in transplant recipients. Dermatol 2007; 215: 130.

Nambudiri VE, et al: Successful treatment of perianal giant condyloma acuminatum in an immunocompromised host with systemic interleukin-2 and topical cidofovir. JAMA Dermatol 2013; 149: 1068.

Nguyen L, et al: Conversion from tacrolimus/mycophenolic acid to tacrolimus/leflunomide to treat cutaneous warts in a series of four pediatric renal allograft recipients. Transplant 2012; 94: 450.

Nofal A, et al: Treatment of recalcitrant warts with bacille Calmette-Guérin. Dermatol Ther 2013; 26: 481.

Olguin-Garcia MG, et al: A double-blind, randomized, placebo-controlled trial of oral isotretinoin in the treatment of recalcitrant facial flat warts. J Dermatolog Treat 2015; 26: 78.

Padilla Espana L, et al: Topical cidofovir for plantar warts. Dermatol Ther 2014; 27: 89.

Peterson CL, et al: Hand warts successfully treated with topical 5-aminolevulinic acid and intense pulsed light. Eur J Dermatol 2008; 18: 207.

Ruiz R, et al: Focal epithelial hyperplasia. Lancet 2014; 384: 173.

Santos-Juanes J, et al: Acute renal failure caused by imiquimod 5% cream in a renal transplant patient. Dermatology 2011; 222: 109.

Scheinfeld N: Update on the treatment of genital warts. Dermatol Online J 2013; 19: 3.

Schiller JT, Lowy DR: Understanding and learning from the success of prophylactic human papillomavirus vaccines. Nat Rev Microbiol 2012; 10: 681.

Sharma N, et al: A comparative study of liquid nitrogen cryotherapy as monotherapy versus in combination with podophyllin in the treatment of condyloma acuminata. J Clin Diagn Res 2017; 11: WC01.

Shim WH, et al: Bowenoid papulosis of the vulva and subsequent periungual Bowen's disease induced by the same mucosal HPVs. Ann Dermatol 2011; 23: 493.

Shimizu A, et al: Bowenoid papulosis successfully treated with imiquimod 5% cream. J Dermatol 2014; 41: 545.

Sparreboom EE, et al: Pulsed dye laser treatment for recalcitrant viral warts. Br J Dermatol 2014; 171: 1270.

Stefanaki C, et al: Comparison of cryotherapy to imiquimod 5% in the treatment of anogenital warts. Int J STD AIDS 2008; 19: 441.

Sterling JC, et al: British Association of Dermatologists' guidelines for the management of cutaneous warts 2014. Br J Dermatol 2014; 171: 696.

Szarewski A, et al: Efficacy of the HPV-16/18 AS04-Adjuvanted vaccine against low-risk HPV types (PATRICIA randomized trial). J Infect Dis 2013; 208: 1391.

Tripoli M, et al: Giant condylomata (Buschke-Löwenstein tumours). Eur Rev Med Pharmacol Sci 2012; 16: 747.

Vanhooteghem O, et al: Raynaud phenomenon after treatment of verruca vulgaris of the sole with intralesional injection of bleomycin. Pediatr Dermatol 2001; 18: 249.

Vicente A, et al: High-risk alpha-human papillomavirus types. J Am Acad Dermatol 2012; 68: 343.

Videla S, et al: Natural history of human papillomavirus infections involving anal, penile and oral sites among HIV-positive men. Sex Transm Dis 2013; 40: 3.

West ES, et al: Generalized verrucosis in a patient with GATA2 deficiency. Br J Dermatol 2014; 170: 1182.

Wiley DJ, et al: Smoking enhances risk for new external genital warts in men. Int J Environ Res Public Health 2009; 6: 1215.

Wong A, Crawford RI: Intralesional candida antigen for common warts in people with HIV. J Cutan Med Surg 2013; 17: 313.

Wu JK, et al: Psoriasis induced by topical imiquimod. Australas J Dermatol 2004; 45: 47.

Wu Y, et al: Aminolevulinic acid photodynamic therapy for bowenoid papulosis. Photodiagnosis and Photodynamic Therapy 2017; 17: A68.

Yew YW, Pan JY: Complete remission of recalcitrant genital warts with a combination approach of surgical debulking and oral isotretinoin in a patient with systemic lupus erythematosus. Dermatol Ther 2014; 27: 79.

Zamanian A, et al: Efficacy of intralesional injection of mumps-measles-rubella vaccine in patients with wart. Adv Biomed Res 2014; 3: 107.

Zampetti A, et al: Acquired epidermodysplasia verruciformis. Dermatol Surg 2013; 39: 974.

Trichodysplasia Spinulosa (Viral-Associated Trichodysplasia)

Immunosuppressed patients with lymphoreticular malignancies and organ transplant recipients on immunosuppressive regimens will rarely develop a characteristic eruption of erythematous, 1–3 mm fine, monomorphic facial papules. The midface, glabella, and chin are primarily affected. More widespread involvement, including the arms, has been rarely reported. Lesions are numerous, may reach confluence, and can rarely cause nasal distortion similar to that seen in rosacea and sarcoidosis (Fig. 19.56). Some papules have a central, keratotic white excrescence similar to the follicular spicules that may be seen in multiple myeloma. Alopecia of the eyebrows and eyelashes may occur, but the scalp is spared. Histology is characteristic, showing massively distended, bulbous follicles with expansion of the inner root sheath cells and containing numerous trichohyaline granules. Abrupt, inner root, sheath-type cornification is present. Abortive hair shaft–like material may be present in the affected follicles. Electron microscopy demonstrates numerous viral particles in the affected hair follicles. Immunohistochemistry may highlight select polyoma antigens. This virus has been identified as a unique polyomavirus called trichodysplasia spinulosa–associated polyomavirus. It differs from the Merkel cell polyomavirus. Treatments that may benefit patients with trichodysplasia spinulosa include reduction of the immunosuppressive regimen or topical cidofovir. Other therapies have been used in some cases, including oral valganciclovir.

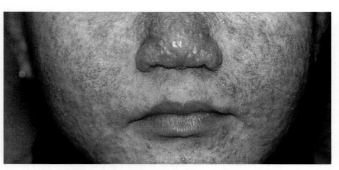

Fig. 19.56 Trichodysplasia. (Courtesy Len Sperling, MD.)

Recently one group reported on three patients, two of whom were immunosuppressed, with chronic generalized, scaly, hyperpigmented papules and plaques, with histologic findings of "tiered parakeratosis" or "peacock plumage" that demonstrated human polyomavirus 6 and 7 by PCR and cytoplasmic viral inclusions on electron microscopy. They suggest the term "HPyV6- and HPyV7-associated pruritic and dyskeratotic dermatoses."

Coogle LP, et al: Complete resolution of trichodysplasia spinulosa in a pediatric renal transplant patient. Pediatr Transplant 2017; 21.

Fischer MK, et al: Specific detection of trichodysplasia spinulosa–associated polyomavirus DNA in skin and renal allograft tissues in a patient with trichodysplasia spinulosa. Arch Dermatol 2012; 148: 726.

Kirchhof MG, et al: Trichodysplasia spinulosa. J Cutan Med Surg 2014; 18: 430.

Matthews MR, et al: Viral-associated trichodysplasia spinulosa. J Cutan Pathol 2011; 38: 420.

Nguyen KD, et al: Human polyomavirus 6 and 7 are associated with pruritic and dyskeratotic dermatoses. J Am Acad Dermatol 2017; 76: 932.

Rouanet J, et al: Trichodysplasia spinulosa. Br J Dermatol 2016; 174: 629.

Wanat KA, et al: Viral-associated trichodysplasia. Arch Dermatol 2012; 148: 219.

RETROVIRUSES

These oncoviruses are unique in that they contain RNA, which is converted by a virally coded reverse transcriptase to DNA in the host cell. The target cell population is primarily CD4+ lymphocytes (primarily helper T cells), but also, in some cases, macrophages. For this reason, the retroviruses are called human T-lymphotropic viruses (HTLVs). Transmission may be through sexual intercourse, blood products/IV drug use, and from mother to child during childbirth and breastfeeding. There is often a very long "latent" period from time of infection until presentation with clinical disease.

Human T-Lymphotropic Virus 1

Human T-lymphotropic virus 1 is endemic in Japan, the Caribbean region, South America (Brazil, Peru, Colombia), sub-Saharan Africa, and Romania; among Australian Aborigines; and in the southeastern United States. In endemic areas, infection rates may be quite high, with only a small percentage of infected patients ever developing clinical disease (estimated 3%). HTLV-1 is spread primarily by mother-to-infant transmission during breastfeeding but also can be transmitted sexually (primarily male to female) or through blood transfusion or IV drug use. HTLV-1 uses the GLUT glucose transporter to enter cells. HTLV-1 is responsible for several clinical syndromes.

About 1% of infected persons will develop adult T-cell leukemia-lymphoma (ATL), with more HTLV-1–infected persons in Japan developing ATL than in other populations. Infection in childhood through breastfeeding seems to be a risk factor for developing ATL. HTLV-1–associated myelopathy or tropical spastic paraparesis (HAM/TSP) is a less common degenerative neurologic syndrome. Patients with this have gone on to develop other autoimmune diseases, including rheumatoid arthritis, lupus, and Sjögren. There are four forms of ATL: smoldering, chronic, acute, and lymphomatous, usually progressing in that order. ATL is characterized by lymphadenopathy, hepatosplenomegaly, hypercalcemia, and skin lesions (60% of patients). Skin lesions in ATL include erythematous papules or nodules (Fig. 19.57). Prurigo may be a prodrome to the development of ATL. Histologically, the cutaneous infiltrates are pleomorphic, atypical lymphocytes with characteristic "flower cells" representing HTLV-1–infected

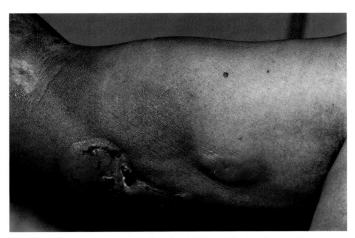

Fig. 19.57 HTLV-1–associated adult T-cell leukemia-lymphoma.

lymphocytes. Epidermotropism may be present, mimicking mycosis fungoides.

Three quarters or more of HTLV-1–infected patients will have an abnormal skin examination. The most common skin conditions are dermatophytosis (30%), seborrheic dermatitis (25%), and xerosis/acquired ichthyosis (up to 80%), and vitiligo has also been reported. In patients with HAM/TSP, chronic eczema/photosensitivity occurs in up to 20%. The disease closely resembles more common causes of eczematous dermatitis and the diagnosis can be delayed if not considered. Biopsies from the areas of chronic eczema/photosensitivity may show features of ATL in up to 25% of patients (smoldering ATL). Scabies is seen in 2% of asymptomatic HTLV-1–infected patients and in 5% of those with HAM/TSP. The scabies may be of the hyperkeratotic (crusted) type, and the presence of hyperkeratotic scabies in a person from an HTLV-1–endemic region should trigger serologic testing for the virus. The spectrum of skin disease seen in symptomatic HTLV-1–infected patients is remarkably similar to that seen in HIV-infected patients with CNS disease: xerosis/eczema, seborrheic dermatitis, and scabies.

Infective dermatitis, infective dermatitis associated with HTLV 1 infection (IDH), or HTLV-1–associated infective dermatitis (HAID) occurs in children and less frequently in adults with HTLV-1 infection. It is much rarer in Japan than other HTLV-1–endemic, more tropical countries, suggesting climate and malnutrition/socioeconomic factors may play a role. Infective dermatitis is diagnosed by major and minor criteria. Clinically, the children present at an early age (18 months onward) with a chronic eczema of the scalp, axilla, groin, external auditory canal, retroauricular area, eyelid margins, paranasal areas, and neck. Involvement of the scalp and retroauricular area is universal, followed by the body folds (neck, axillae, groin, paranasal skin, and ears). Exudation and crusting are the hallmarks of the skin lesions. Pruritus is mild. Clinically, infective dermatitis resembles a cross between infected AD and infected seborrheic dermatitis. There is a chronic nasal discharge. Cultures from the skin and nares are positive for *Staphylococcus aureus* or β-hemolytic streptococcus, and the condition responds rapidly to antibiotics and topical corticosteroids. Infective dermatitis is relapsing and recurrent. Skin biopsies show a nonspecific dermatitis; however, close examination may show atypical CD4+ cells infiltrating the epidermis, at times simulating ATL or cutaneous T-cell lymphoma. Careful neurologic examination of children with IDH will often reveal abnormal neurologic findings: weakness, lumbar pain, dysesthesias, and urinary disturbances.

De Oliveira M, et al: Infective dermatitis associated with human T-cell lymphotropic virus type 1. Clin Infect Dis 2012; 54: 1714.

Einsiedel L, et al: Clinical associations of human T-lymphotropic virus type 1 infection in an indigenous Australian population. PLoS Negl Trop Dis 2014; 8: e2643.
Hlela C, Bittencourt A: Infective dermatitis associated with HTLV-1 mimics common eczemas in children and may be a prelude to severe systemic diseases. Dermatol Clin 2014; 32: 237.
McGill NK, et al: HTLV-1-associated infective dermatitis. Exp Dermatol 2012; 21: 815.
Okajima R, et al: High prevalence of skin disorders among HTLV-1 infected individuals independent of clinical status. PLoS Negl Trop Dis 2013; 7: e2546.
Quaresma JA, et al: HTLV-1, immune response, and autoimmunity. Viruses 2015; 8: e5.
Rodriguez-Zuniga MJ, et al: Adult T-cell leukemia/lymphoma in a Peruvian hospital in human T-lymphotropic virus type 1 positive patients. Int J Dermatol 2017; 56: 503.

Human Immunodeficiency Virus

Human immunodeficiency virus (HIV) infects human helper T (Th) cells, leading to a progressive immunodeficiency disease. In its end stages, HIV infection is called *acquired immunodeficiency syndrome (AIDS)*. Patients with HIV should be screened for other STDs and often require multidisciplinary care with experienced physicians to get the most up-to-date, disease-specific care. Patients with HIV should be counseled regarding disease transmission and safe sex, and there is evidence suggesting preexposure prophylaxis with antiretroviral drugs may reduce transmission within serodiscordant couples.

Cutaneous manifestations are prominent, affecting up to 90% of HIV-infected persons. Many patients have multiple skin lesions of different types. The skin lesions or combinations of skin conditions are so unique that the diagnosis of HIV infection or AIDS can often be suspected from the skin examination alone. The skin findings can be classified into three broad categories: infections, inflammatory dermatoses, and neoplasms. The skin conditions also tend to appear at a specific stage in HIV progression, making them useful markers of the stage of HIV disease.

The natural history of HIV infection in the vast majority of patients is a gradual loss of Th cells. The rate of this decline is variable, with some patients progressing rapidly and others very slowly or not at all (long-term nonprogressors). Soon after infection, there is a seroconversion syndrome called primary HIV infection, or acute infection (group I). Patients recover from this syndrome and enter a relatively long latent period (asymptomatic infection, or group II), which averages about 10 years. During this period, patients may have persistent generalized lymphadenopathy (group III). When symptoms begin to appear, they are often nonspecific and include fever, weight loss, chronic diarrhea, and mucocutaneous disease (group IVA). Th counts in group II, III, and IVA patients usually range from 200–500 cells. The skin findings at this stage (originally called AIDS-related complex, ARC) include seborrheic dermatitis, psoriasis, Reiter syndrome, AD, herpes zoster, acne rosacea, oral hairy leukoplakia, onychomycosis, warts, *S. aureus* skin and soft tissue infections (including recurrent MRSA), and mucocutaneous candidiasis.

Once the Th count is 200 cells or less, the patient is defined as having AIDS. In this stage of HIV disease, the skin lesions are more characteristic of immunodeficiency and include characteristic opportunistic infections: chronic herpes simplex, molluscum contagiosum, bartonellosis (bacillary angiomatosis), systemic fungal infections (cryptococcosis, histoplasmosis, coccidioidomycosis, penicilliosis), and mycobacterial infection. Paradoxically, patients at this stage also have hyperreactive skin and frequently, inflammatory, often pruritic skin diseases. These skin conditions include eosinophilic folliculitis, granuloma annulare, drug reactions, enhanced reactions to insect bites, refractory seborrheic dermatitis, AD, and photodermatitis.

When the Th count falls below 50 cells, the patient is often said to have "advanced AIDS." These patients may have very unusual presentations of their opportunistic infections, including multicentric, refractory molluscum contagiosum; chronic herpes simplex; chronic cutaneous varicella-zoster infection; cutaneous CMV ulcerations, cutaneous acanthamebiasis, cutaneous atypical mycobacterial infections (including *Mycobacterium avium* complex and *Mycobacterium haemophilum*), penicilliosis, and crusted scabies. Treatment of their infections is often difficult because of the significant chronic immunosuppression.

It is now clear that HIV itself is the cause of the loss of Th cells and that effective treatment of HIV infection may halt or reverse the natural history of HIV disease. The numerous antiretroviral agents are usually used in combinations called "cocktails." This combination treatment is called highly active antiretroviral therapy (HAART). A significant percentage of HIV-infected patients respond to HAART and may show dramatic improvement of their HIV disease. HIV disappears from the blood and Th-cell counts rise. As expected, in patients who respond to HAART, opportunistic infections no longer occur, and subsequently mortality rate decreases. This is also true of cutaneous infectious conditions. HIV-associated psoriasis usually improves substantially, especially if the patient did not have psoriasis before HIV infection. Because full reconstitution of the immune system with HAART may take several years, some skin conditions may be slow to resolve (seborrheic dermatitis). Others, such as MC and KS, generally begin to improve within months.

HAART is typically associated with resolution of all forms of HIV-related cutaneous complications. However, some conditions may initially appear or be exacerbated by the sudden improvement of the immune status that occurs with eradication of HIV viremia and with increase in Th-cell counts. This complex of manifestations is called the immune reconstitution inflammatory syndrome. IRIS occurs in 15%–25% of HIV-infected persons started on HAART. Persons with an opportunistic infection (OI), specifically cryptococcosis, tuberculosis, penicilliosis, leprosy, or *Pneumocystis* pneumonia, may be at higher risk if HAART is started as the OI is being treated. This marked inflammatory syndrome can be severe, and in resource-poor countries 5% of AIDS-related deaths in treated patients can be attributed to IRIS during the first year of HAART therapy. Half of IRIS-related conditions are dermatologic. The following three forms of IRIS occur:

1. A hidden OI is unmasked as the reconstituted immune system attacks the hidden pathogen. The presentation may be atypical. The appearance of cutaneous mycobacterial infections with HAART is an example.
2. In the setting of a documented OI, when HAART is started, the patient has worsening of the infection with new findings. This is not treatment failure, but enhanced immune response to the pathogen. This typically occurs with tuberculosis or cryptococcosis.
3. The development of new disorders is seen, infectious or inflammatory, or enhanced inflammatory responses around malignancies, especially KS. Eosinophilic folliculitis, acne flares, drug eruptions, Reiter syndrome, lupus erythematosus, alopecia universalis, at times HPV infections (especially oral and genital), increased outbreaks of genital and orolabial herpes simplex, molluscum contagiosum, herpes zoster, CMV ulcerations, type I reactions in Hansen disease, cutaneous mycobacterial and fungal infections, leishmaniasis, tattoo and foreign body granulomas, and sarcoidosis can be part of IRIS in the skin.

Infection with HIV is now being effectively controlled in many patients through HAART. However, the constant struggle of the immune system to control viral replication and side effects from multiple medications has led to senescence of the immune system similar to that seen with chronologic aging. Chronic HIV disease is characterized by the same combination of immunodeficiency and inflammation that occurs with aging. This has led to increased rates and earlier onset of cardiovascular disease, metabolic disorders, osteoporosis, and some cancers in HIV disease, including KS developing in patients with normal CD4 counts due to immune senescence. Frailty, or the variability with which persons acquire health problems and the consequent inability to tolerate stressors (vulnerability), is becoming the primary consequence of HIV infection in many countries.

Primary HIV Infection (Acute Seroconversion Syndrome)

Several weeks after infection with HIV, an acute illness develops in a large proportion of individuals. The clinical syndrome is similar to primary EBV infection, with fever, sore throat, cervical adenopathy, a rash, and oral, genital, and rectal ulceration. The skin eruption can be polymorphous. Most characteristic is a papular eruption of discrete, slightly scaly, oval lesions of the upper trunk. The lesions have a superficial resemblance to pityriasis rosea, but the peripheral scale is not prominent, and there is focal hemorrhage in the lesions. A Gianotti-Crosti–like papular eruption may also occur. Purpuric lesions along the margins of the palms and soles, as seen in immune complex disease, have been reported. The mucosal erosions resemble aphthae but are larger and can affect all parts of the mouth (Fig. 19.58), pharynx, esophagus, and anal mucosa. Dysphagia may be prominent. The Th-cell count falls abruptly during seroconversion. The level of immune impairment may allow oral candidiasis or even *Pneumocystis jiroveci* (formerly *P. carinii*) pneumonia to develop. The diagnosis should be suspected in any at-risk individual with the correct constellation of symptoms. A direct measurement of HIV viral load will confirm the diagnosis, as antibody testing may be inaccurate during acute infection and seroconversion. Combination antiviral therapy is instituted immediately.

HIV-Associated Pruritus

From early in the HIV epidemic, it was clear that pruritus was a marker of HIV infection throughout the world, occurring in up to 30% of patients. Pruritus is usually not caused by HIV disease

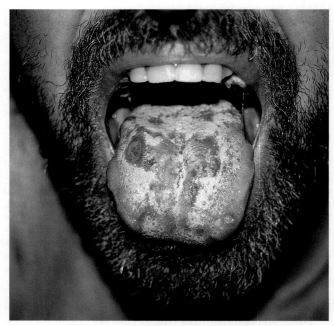

Fig. 19.58 Primary HIV infection. (Courtesy Ginat Mirowski, MD.)

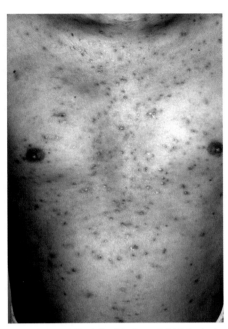

Fig. **19.59** Eosinophilic folliculitis in an HIV-infected patient.

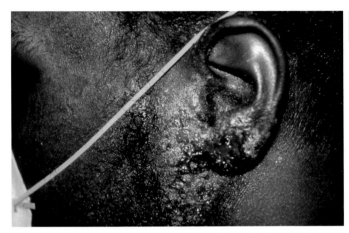

Fig. **19.60** Herpes simplex and seborrheic dermatitis in an HIV-infected patient.

itself but is related to inflammatory dermatoses associated with the disease. "Papular pruritic eruption" is not a specific disease, but rather a "wastebasket diagnosis" used to encompass patients with many forms of HIV-associated pruritus. Worldwide, it most often represents enhanced insect bite reactions. These pruritic eruptions are best subdivided into follicular and nonfollicular eruptions. The relative prevalence of these two patterns of pruritic eruptions is geographically distinct. In tropical and semitropical regions, where biting insects are prominent, nonfollicular eruptions are most common and probably represent insect bite hypersensitivity. In temperate regions, follicular pruritic eruptions are more common.

Eosinophilic folliculitis (EF) is the most common pruritic follicular eruption (Fig. 19.59). It is seen in patients with a Th count of about 200 cells. Clinically, EF presents with urticarial follicular papules on the upper trunk, face, scalp, and neck. Pustular lesions are uncommon; pustules are usually smaller than in bacterial folliculitis and represent end-stage lesions. These lesions are infrequently seen because the pruritus is so severe that the pustules are excoriated before the lesion evolves to this degree. About 90% of lesions occur above the nipple line on the anterior trunk, and lesions typically extend down the midline of the back to the lumbar spine. EF waxes and wanes in severity and may spontaneously clear, only to flare unpredictably. A peripheral eosinophilia may be present, and the serum IgE level may be elevated, suggesting this is a disorder mediated by Th2 cells. Histologically, an infiltrate of mononuclear cells and eosinophils is seen around the upper portion of the hair follicle at the level of the sebaceous gland. As lesions evolve, eosinophils and lymphocytes enter the follicular structure and the sebaceous glands. Pustules are formed late and represent aggregates of eosinophils in the uppermost part of the follicle. Rarely, there will be increased mucin within the follicular epithelium, making distinction from follicular mucinosis difficult.

Initial treatment of EF is topical corticosteroids and antihistamines. If the patient fails to respond, phototherapy (UVB or PUVA) or itraconazole, 200 mg twice daily, may be effective. In some patients, repeated applications of permethrin (every other night for up to 6 weeks) may be of benefit. Permethrin therapy is directed at *Demodex* mites, which may be the antigenic trigger

of EF. Isotretinoin is also effective, often after a few months, in a dose of about 0.5–1 mg/kg/day. HAART may lead to a flare of EF (as part of IRIS) but usually leads eventually to its resolution. Staphylococcal folliculitis, which may be severely pruritic in patients with HIV disease, and *Pityrosporum* folliculitis should be included in the differential diagnosis. These are excluded by bacterial culture and skin biopsy, respectively. *Demodex* folliculitis should also be in the differential.

The other pruritic dermatoses that are not follicular can be divided into the primarily papular eruptions and the eczematous reactions. The papular eruptions include scabies, insect bites, transient acantholytic dermatosis, granuloma annulare, and prurigo nodularis. The eczematous dermatoses include atopic-like dermatitis, seborrheic dermatitis, nummular eczema, xerotic eczema, photodermatitis, and drug eruptions. Patients may have multiple eruptions simultaneously, making differential diagnosis difficult (Fig. 19.60). A skin biopsy from a representative lesion of every morphologic type on the patient may elucidate the true diagnosis (or diagnoses). Patients on HAART who had higher VL at onset of ART may have higher rates of pruritic papular eruptions. Treatment is determined by the diagnosis and is similar to treatment in persons without HIV infection with these same dermatoses. Special considerations in AIDS patients include the use of topical therapy plus ivermectin for crusted scabies and thalidomide for prurigo nodularis and photodermatitis. Both these systemic agents are very effective if used appropriately.

HIV-Associated Neoplasia

Neoplasia is prominent in HIV infection and in some cases is highly suggestive of HIV infection. KS is an example. Other common neoplasms seen in patients with HIV infection include superficial BCCs of the trunk, SCCs in sun-exposed areas, genital HPV-induced SCC, and extranodal B-cell and T-cell lymphomas. Lipomas, angiolipomas, and dermatofibromas may occur. In the case of lipomas, their appearance is usually related to the peripheral fat loss that occurs with some HIV treatment regimens and with HIV disease itself.

Nonmelanoma skin cancers (NMSCs) are very common in HIV patients. HAART does not protect against the development of NMSC in HIV infection. BCCs usually occur as superficial multicentric lesions on the trunk in fair-skinned patients, younger than typically seen, particularly in men in their twenties to fifties. The ratio of BCC to SCC is not reversed in HIV disease as it is in organ transplant recipients, but HIV-infected patients are at higher risk than noninfected patients of developing SCC and not

BCC, and the risk correlates with lower CD4 and higher VL. BCCs behave in the same manner as they do in the immunocompetent host, and standard management is usually adequate.

Actinically induced SCCs are also quite common and present in the standard manner as nodules, keratotic papules, or ulcerations. In most cases, their behavior is relatively benign and standard management is adequate. Removal of SCCs in sun-exposed areas by curettage and desiccation in patients with HIV infection is associated with an unacceptably high recurrence rate of about 15%. Complete excision is therefore recommended. In a small subset of patients with AIDS, actinic SCCs can be very aggressive; they may double in size over weeks and may metastasize to regional lymph nodes or viscerally, leading to the death of the patient.

Genital SCCs, including cervical, vaginal, anal, penile, and periungual SCC, all occur in patients with HIV infection. These neoplasms are increased in frequency, and the progression from HPV infection to neoplasia appears to be accelerated. This is analogous to the situation in organ transplant and other immunosuppressed patients. It appears that these cancers are associated with primarily "high-risk" HPV types.

High-risk genital HPV infection in patients with HIV can produce perianal dysplasia in MSM who have a history of receptive anal intercourse. Dysplasia in this area may present as velvety white or hyperpigmented plaques involving the whole anal area and extending into the anal canal. These lesions may erode or ulcerate. Histology will demonstrate SCC in situ. The risk of progression of the lesions to anal SCC is unknown but is estimated to be at least 10 times higher than the rate of cervical cancer in women in the general population. The management of such lesions is unclear, but regular follow-up is clearly indicated, and any masses in the anal canal should be immediately referred for biopsy. At some centers, Pap smear equivalents are performed. Imiquimod has been used as an adjunct in the management of genital warts and HPV-associated genital in situ dysplasias (not genital SCC). Although it may be of benefit in patients with reconstituted immune systems receiving HAART, especially in combination with surgical ablation, the response rate is much lower than in immunocompetent patients. In the only placebo-controlled trial, done before standard HAART was available, imiquimod was no more effective than placebo in clearing genital warts (11%) in HIV infection. Small case series of patients receiving HAART suggest clearance rates of about 30%–50%. Topical cidofovir can be used to treat genital HPV infection in patients with low-risk and high-risk HPV types.

The vulvar and penile skin may develop flat, white or hyperpigmented macules from a few millimeters to several centimeters in diameter. These show SCC in situ and are analogous to bowenoid papulosis in the immunocompetent host. Lesions of the penile shaft and glabrous vulvar skin, not at a transition zone or on mucosal surfaces, have a low risk of progressing to invasive SCC. Lesions of the glans penis that are red and fixed should be biopsied. If the changes of SCC in situ are found, these should be managed aggressively as SCC in situ. Topical 5-FU and superficial radiation therapy are effective. Close clinical follow-up is indicated. Periungual SCC has also been seen in patients with HIV infection. Any persistent keratotic or hyperpigmented lesion in the periungual area must be carefully evaluated. Management is surgical excision, though digital HPV-associated SCC lesions display a high rate of recurrence, and Mohs should be considered in many cases due to the anatomic site and risk of recurrence. Some advocate for postoperative adjuvant therapy with laser, curettage, cryotherapy, or imiquimod. Perianal and vulvovaginal lesions should be managed as intraepithelial neoplasia types AIN-3 and VIN-3, respectively.

Extranodal B-cell and less often T-cell lymphomas are associated with the advanced immunosuppression of AIDS. The B-cell lymphomas and some of the T-cell lymphomas present as violaceous or plum-colored papules, nodules, or tumors. Once the diagnosis is established by biopsy, systemic chemotherapy is required. EBV is found in some cases. HAART is both protective against the development of non-Hodgkin lymphoma (NHL) and Hodgkin disease in HIV and substantially improves prognosis of HIV-infected patients with NHL. Mycosis fungoides can also be seen in patients with HIV infection, often in those who have not yet developed AIDS. It presents with pruritic patches or plaques and may progress to tumor stage. EBV is not found in these cases. CD8+ pseudolymphoma is also seen in patients with untreated HIV infection and may resolve with HAART.

Malignant melanoma (MM) is seen at increased rates in persons with HIV infection. HIV-infected melanoma patients demonstrate the same risk factors as other melanoma patients: multiple nevi, fair skin type, and prior intermittent but intense sun exposure. HIV patients with melanoma in the pre-HAART era had significantly shorter disease-free survival and reduced overall survival. Many fair-skinned patients infected with HIV complain of the new onset of atypical moles (analogous to organ transplant patients). Whether these confer an increased risk of melanoma is unknown.

AIDS and Kaposi Sarcoma

Kaposi sarcoma (KS) was, along with *Pneumocystis* pneumonia, the harbinger of the AIDS epidemic. Many MSM and bisexual men presented with this tumor in the early 1980s, with a prevalence of up to 25% in some cohorts. HHV-8, a γ-herpesvirus, has been identified in these lesions. The clinical features of KS in patients with AIDS are different than those seen in elderly men who do not have AIDS. Patients with AIDS present with symmetric widespread lesions, often numerous. Lesions begin as macules that may progress to tumors or nodules (Fig. 19.61). Any mucocutaneous surface may be involved, but areas of predilection include the hard palate, face, trunk, penis, and lower legs and soles. Visceral disease may be present and progressive. Edema may accompany lower leg lesions, and if significant, it is often associated with lymph node involvement in the inguinal area.

A diagnosis of KS is established by skin biopsy, which should be taken from the center of the most infiltrated plaque. Excessive bleeding is not usually a problem. Early macular lesions show atypical, angulated, ectatic vessels in the upper dermis associated with an inflammatory infiltrate containing plasma cells. Plaque lesions show aggregates of small vessels and endothelial cells in the upper dermis and surrounding adnexal structures. Nodules and tumors show the classic pattern of a spindle cell neoplasm with prominent extravasation of red blood cells.

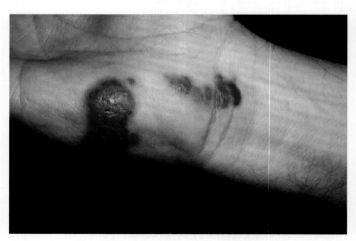

Fig. 19.61 Kaposi sarcoma in AIDS patient.

HAART has reduced the incidence of KS in HIV-infected patients by 10-fold. However, KS remains an important complication of HIV infection for the following two reasons:

1. HIV-associated KS is still common in sub-Saharan Africa. With HAART therapy, survival in Africa for HIV-infected persons for more than 1 year is almost 100%, if they do not have KS. In patients with HIV disease and KS, however, survival is only 77%. This results from the lack of effective cytotoxic therapy for KS in Africa. HIV-KS is more common in women than men in some clinics in Africa.
2. Although HAART has substantially reduced the prevalence of KS in HIV disease in the developed world, HAART has not eliminated the disease. In fact, there remains a fairly substantial proportion of primarily gay men with HIV disease who also have KS (up to 13% of some cohorts). Twenty percent or more of these AIDS-KS patients have well-controlled HIV disease with long-term undetectable viral load and CD4 counts above 300. These patients have an overall good prognosis but still may require cytotoxic or radiation therapy to control their KS. Patients with AIDS-KS and lower CD4 counts and detectable viral loads are more likely to have visceral disease. Up to one third of these AIDS-KS patients died despite HAART and chemotherapy, suggesting that AIDS-KS in the setting of poor HIV control is a poor prognostic finding.

The treatment of AIDS-associated KS depends on the extent and aggressiveness of the disease. Effective HAART after about 6 months is associated with involution of KS lesions in 50% of patients. This should be the initial management in most patients with mild to moderate disease (<50 lesions, and <10 new lesions/month) who are not receiving anti-HIV treatment. Intralesional vinblastine, can be infiltrated into lesions (as for hypertrophic scar), and lesions will involute over several weeks. Hyperpigmentation usually remains. Cryotherapy is also effective but will leave postinflammatory hypopigmentation in pigmented persons. Persistent individual lesions and lesions of the soles and penis respond well to local irradiation therapy (one single treatment of 80 Gy or fractionated treatments to 150 Gy). For patients with moderate disease (>10 lesions, or mucosal or visceral involvement), HAART alone may not be adequate in controlling KS, and liposomal doxorubicin may need to be added to the treatment. For patients with symptomatic visceral disease, aggressive skin disease, marked edema, and pulmonary disease, systemic chemotherapy is indicated. Triple therapy with vincristine, bleomycin, and etoposide has been utilized in one study of KS in Malawai.

Afonso JP, et al: Pruritic papular eruption and eosinophilic folliculitis associated with human immunodeficiency virus (HIV) infection. J Am Acad Dermatol 2012; 67: 269.

Amerson EH, Maurer TA: Immune reconstitution inflammatory syndrome and tropical dermatoses. Dermatol Clin 2011; 29: 39.

Asgari MM, et al: Association of multiple primary skin cancers with HIV infection, CD4 count, and viral load. JAMA Dermatol 2017; 153: 892.

Blaser N, et al: Impact of viral load and the duration of primary infection on HIV transmission. AIDS 2014; 28: 1021.

Brothers TD, et al: Frailty in people aging with human immunodeficiency virus (HIV) infection. J Infect Dis 2014; 210: 1170.

Brown AE, et al: Fall in new HIV diagnoses among men who have sex with men (MSM) at selected London sexual health clinics since early 2015. Euro Surveill 2017; 22: 30553.

Calabrese SK, et al: Integrating HIV preexposure prophylaxis (PrEP) into routine preventive health care to avoid exacerbating disparities. Am J Public Health 2017; 17: 1883.

Chua SL, et al: Factors associated with pruritic papular eruption of HIV infection in the antiretroviral therapy era. Br J Dermatol 2014; 170: 832.

Farsani TT, et al: Etiology and risk factors associated with a pruritic papular eruption in people living with HIV in India. J Int AIDS Soc 2013; 16: 17325.

Frater J, et al: HIV-1-specific CD4+ responses in primary HIV-1 infection predict disease progression. AIDS 2014; 28: 699.

Gormley RH, et al: Digital squamous cell carcinoma and association with diverse high-risk human papillomavirus types. J Am Acad Dermatol 2011; 64: 981.

Grinsztejn B, et al: Effects of early versus delayed initiation of antiretroviral treatment on clinical outcomes of HIV-1 infection. Lancet 2014; 14: 281.

Hausauer AK, et al: Recurrence after treatment of cutaneous basal cell and squamous cell carcinomas in patients infected with human immunodeficiency virus. JAMA Dermatol 2013; 149: 239.

Husak R, et al: Refractory human papillomavirus–associated oral warts treated topically with 1–3% cidofovir solutions in human immunodeficiency virus type 1–infected patients. Br J Dermatol 2005; 153: 382.

Khalil EA, et al: Post-Kala-Azar dermal leishmaniasis. J Trop Med 2013; 2013: 275253.

Khambaty MM, Hsu SS: Dermatology of the patient with HIV. Emerg Med Clin North Am 2010; 28: 355.

Krakower DS, et al: Infection in 2015: HIV protection with PrEP—implications for controlling other STIs. Nat Rev Urol 2016; 13: 72.

Kreuter A, et al: Clinical spectrum and virologic characteristics of anal intraepithelial neoplasia in HIV infection. J Am Acad Dermatol 2005; 52: 603.

Lehloenya R, Meintjes G: Dermatologic manifestations of the immune reconstitution inflammatory syndrome. Dermatol Clin 2006; 24: 549.

Macken M, et al: Triple therapy of vincristine, bleomycin, and etoposide for children with Kaposi sarcoma. Pediatr Blood Cancer 2018; 65.

Mani D, et al: A retrospective analysis of AIDS-associated Kaposi's sarcoma in patients with undetectable HIV viral loads and CD4 counts greater than 300 cells/mm³. J Int Assoc Physicians AIDS Care 2009; 8: 279.

Martin-Carbonero L, et al: Pegylated liposomal doxorubicin plus highly active antiretroviral therapy versus highly active antiretroviral therapy alone in HIV patients with Kaposi's sarcoma. AIDS 2004; 18: 1737.

Meyer T, et al: Human immunodeficiency virus (HIV)–associated eosinophilic folliculitis and follicular mucinosis in a black woman. Int J Dermatol 2010; 49: 1308.

Olson CM, et al: Risk of melanoma in people with HIV/AIDS in the pre- and post-HAART eras. PLoS One 2014; 9: e95096.

Özdener AE, et al: The future of pre-exposure prophylaxis (PrEP) for human immunodeficiency virus (HIV) infection. Expert Rev Anti Infect Ther 2017; 15: 467.

Picard A, et al: Human papillomavirus prevalence in HIV patients with head and neck squamous cell carcinoma. AIDS 2016; 30: 1257.

Riddel C, et al: Ungual and periungual human papillomavirus-associated squamous cell carcinoma. J Am Acad Dermatol 2011; 64: 1147.

Rodgers S, Leslie KS: Skin infections in HIV-infected individuals in the era of HAART. Curr Opin Infect Dis 2011; 2: 124.

Sabater-Marco V, et al: Eosinophilic follicular reaction induced by *Demodex folliculorum* mite. Clin Exp Dermatol 2015; 40: 413.

Seoane Reula E, et al: Role of antiretroviral therapies in mucocutaneous manifestations in HIV-infected children over a period of two decades. Br J Dermatol 2005; 153: 382.

Sherin K, et al: What is new in HIV infection? Am Fam Physician 2014; 89: 265.

Xuan L, et al: Alopecia areata and vitiligo as primary presentations in a young male with human immunodeficiency virus. Indian J Dermatol 2014; 59: 209.

Yokobayashi H, et al: Analysis of serum chemokine levels in patients with HIV-associated eosinophilic folliculitis. J Eur Acad Dermatol Venereol 2013; 27: 212.

20 Parasitic Infestations, Stings, and Bites

The major groups of animals responsible for bites, stings, and parasitic infections in humans belong to the phyla Arthropoda, Chordata, Cnidaria (formerly Coelenterata), Nemathelminthes, Platyhelminthes, Annelida, and Protozoa. This chapter reviews parasitic diseases and the major causes of bites and stings, as well as strategies for prevention.

■ PHYLUM PROTOZOA

The protozoa are one-celled organisms, divided into classes according to the nature of their locomotion. Class Sarcodina organisms move by temporary projections of cytoplasm (pseudopods); class Mastigophora by means of one or more flagella; and class Ciliata by short, hairlike projections of cytoplasm (cilia). Class Sporozoa have no special organs of locomotion.

CLASS SARCODINA

Amebiasis Cutis

Entamoeba histolytica–induced cutaneous ulcers usually result from extension of an underlying amebic abscess; the most common sites are the trunk, abdomen, buttocks, genitalia, and perineum. Those on the abdomen may result from hepatic abscesses. Penile lesions are usually sexually acquired and associated with anal intercourse. Most lesions begin as deep abscesses that rupture and form ulcerations with distinct, raised, cordlike edges, and an erythematous halo approximately 2 cm wide. The base is covered with necrotic tissue and hemopurulent pus containing amebas. These lesions are from a few centimeters to 20 cm wide. Without treatment, slow progression of the ulcer occurs in an increasingly debilitated patient until death ensues. Patients may also present with fistulas, fissures, polypoid warty lesions, or nodules. Deep lesions are more likely to be associated with visceral lesions.

The sole manifestation of early amebiasis may be chronic urticaria. An estimated 10 million invasive cases occur annually, most of them in the tropics. Infection may be asymptomatic, or bloody diarrhea and hepatic abscesses may be present. In the United States the disease occurs chiefly in institutionalized patients, world travelers, recent immigrants, migrant workers, and men who have sex with men. Penile ulcers are associated with insertive anal intercourse.

The histologic findings are those of a necrotic ulceration with many lymphocytes, neutrophils, plasma cells, and eosinophils. *E. histolytica* is found in the tissue, within blood and lymph vessels. The organism measures 50–60 μm in diameter and has basophilic cytoplasm and a single, eccentric nucleus with a central karyosome. The organism is frequently demonstrable in fresh material from the base of the ulcer by direct smear. Culture of the protozoa confirms the diagnosis. Indirect hemagglutination test results remain elevated for years after the initial onset of invasive disease, whereas the results of gel diffusion precipitation tests and counterimmunoelectrophoresis become negative at 6 months. This property can be used to test for recurrent or active disease in persons coming from endemic areas.

When the perianal or perineal areas are involved, granuloma inguinale, lymphogranuloma venereum, deep mycosis, and syphilis must be considered. In chronic urticaria, fresh stool examinations by a trained technician are necessary.

The treatment of choice is metronidazole (Flagyl), 750 mg orally three times daily for 10 days. Abscesses may require surgical drainage.

Other Amebas

Amebas of the genera *Acanthamoeba* and *Balamuthia* may also cause skin lesions in infected hosts. These organisms are ubiquitous in the environment and are found in soil, water, and air. Granulomatous amebic encephalitis is the most common manifestation of infection with these amebas. In the case of *Acanthamoeba*, invasive infections are almost always in immunocompromised individuals, including those with acquired immunodeficiency syndrome (AIDS) and organ transplant patients, although *Acanthamoeba* can also involve the cornea in those who use homemade contact lens solution. Disseminated lesions present as pink or violaceous nodules that then enlarge, suppurate, and form ulcers with a necrotic eschar (Fig. 20.1). Other findings include fever, nasal congestion or discharge, epistaxis, cough, headaches, lethargy, altered mental status, and seizures. In patients infected with *Acanthamoeba* who have disease of the central nervous system (CNS), death usually occurs within days to weeks. The organisms are visible on skin biopsy, and culture is definitive. In patients without CNS involvement, mortality rate is 75%, with successfully treated cases often managed with a combination of 5-fluorocytosine and sulfadiazine. In patients infected with *Balamuthia mandrillaris*, involvement of the central face is typical. Treatment paradigms are changing, and in vitro evidence suggests that diminazene aceturate is more active than miltefosine or pentamidine, and artemether shows promise (Fig. 20.2). Chlorhexidine topically and surgical debridement are local adjunctive measures that may prove beneficial.

Belizario V Jr, et al: Cutaneous manifestations of selected parasitic infections in western Pacific and Southeast Asian regions. Curr Infect Dis Rep 2016; 18: 30.

Deng Y, et al: Artemether exhibits amoebicidal activity against *Acanthamoeba castellanii* through inhibition of the serine biosynthesis pathway. Antimicrob Agents Chemother 2015; 59: 4680.

Eichelmann K, et al: Tropical dermatology. Semin Cutan Med Surg 2014; 33: 133.

Khan NA, et al: Targeting brain-eating amoebae infections. ACS Chem Neurosci 2017; 8: 687.

CLASS MASTIGOPHORA

Organisms belonging to this class, the mastigophorans, are also known as flagellates. Many have an undulating membrane with flagella along their crest.

Trichomoniasis

Trichomonas vulvovaginitis is a common cause of vaginal pruritus, with burning and a frothy leukorrhea. The vaginal mucosa appears bright red from inflammation and may be mottled with pseudomembranous patches. The male urethra may also harbor the organism; in the male it causes urethritis and prostatitis. Occasionally, men may develop balanoposthitis. Erosive lesions on the glans

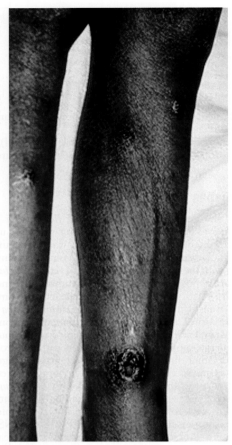

Fig. 20.1 Disseminated acanthameba in HIV disease.

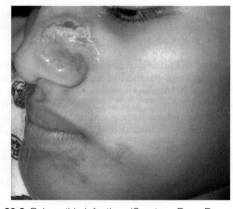

Fig. 20.2 Balamuthia infection. (Courtesy Paco Bravo, MD.)

and penis or abscesses of the median raphe may occur. Neonates may acquire the infection during passage through the birth canal, but they require treatment only if symptomatic or if colonization lasts more than 4 weeks. Because this is otherwise almost exclusively a sexually transmitted disease (STD), *Trichomonas* vulvovaginitis in a child should prompt suspicion of sexual abuse.

Trichomoniasis is caused by *Trichomonas vaginalis*, a colorless piriform flagellate 5–15 µm long. *T. vaginalis* is demonstrated in smears from affected areas. Testing by direct immunofluorescence is sensitive and specific, and polymerase chain reaction (PCR) analysis is now available.

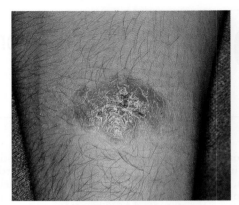

Fig. 20.3 Old World leishmaniasis.

Metronidazole, 2 g in a single oral dose, is the treatment of choice. Alternatively, 500 mg twice daily for 7 days may be given, and intravaginal metronidazole/miconazole is also effective. Patients should be warned not to drink alcohol for 24 hours after or dosing because of the disulfiram-type effects of this medication. Male sex partners should also be treated. The use of metronidazole is contraindicated in pregnant women, and clotrimazole, applied intravaginally at 100 mg a night for 2 weeks, may be used instead. Disulfiram and nithiamide show in vitro evidence of activity and could prove useful for resistant organisms.

Bouchemal K, et al: Strategies for prevention and treatment of *Trichomonas vaginalis* infections. Clin Microbiol Rev 2017; 30: 811.

de Brum Vieira P, et al: Challenges and persistent questions in the treatment of trichomoniasis. Curr Top Med Chem 2017; 17: 1249.

Leishmaniasis

All forms of leishmaniasis are caused by morphologically indistinguishable protozoa of the family Trypanosomidae, called *Leishmania* (pronounced leesh-may-nea). The clinical features of the leishmaniases differ, and in general, these diseases have different geographic distribution. The variable clinical manifestations may result from the diversity of the organism and the person's immune status and genetic ability to initiate an effective cell-mediated immune response to the specific infecting organism. It is known that the antigen-specific T-cell responses, which lead to the production of interferon (IFN) and interleukin-12 (IL-12), are important for healing of the lesions and the induction of lifelong, species-specific immunity to reinfection that results after natural infection. Both CD4+ and CD8+ lymphocytes appear to be active in the immune response. IL-10–producing natural regulatory T cells may play a role in the downregulation of infection-induced immunity.

Cutaneous Leishmaniasis

There are several types of lesion. All tend to occur on exposed parts because all are transmitted by the sandfly. Old World leishmaniasis manifests mainly in the skin and has also been called Baghdad boil, Oriental sore, leishmaniasis tropica, Biskra button, Delhi boil, Aleppo boil, Kandahar sore, and Lahore sore. Mild visceral disease may occur. Skin lesions of New World infection have been termed uta, pian bois, and bay sore or chiclero ulcer.

Clinical Features. In Old World leishmaniasis, lesions may present in two distinct types. One is the moist or rural type, a slowly growing, indurated, livid, indolent papule (Fig. 20.3), which enlarges

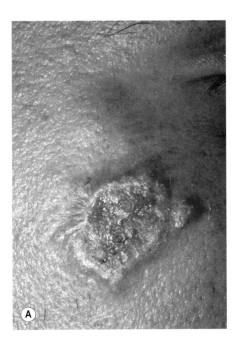

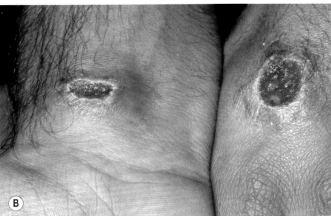

Fig. 20.4 (A and B) New World leishmaniasis.

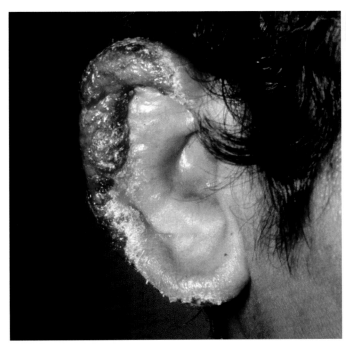

Fig. 20.5 New World leishmaniasis.

in a few months to form a nodule that may ulcerate in a few weeks to form an ulcer as large as 5 cm in diameter. Spontaneous healing usually takes place within 6 months, leaving a characteristic scar. This type is contracted from rodent reservoirs such as gerbils via the sandfly vector. The incubation period is relatively short (1–4 weeks). The dry or urban type has a longer incubation period (2–8 months or longer), develops much more slowly, and heals more slowly than the rural type. In both types, the ulcer or crust forms on a bed of edematous tissue.

Rarely, after the initial or "mother" lesion is healed, at the borders of the healed area a few soft red papules may appear that are covered with whitish scales and have the "apple jelly" characteristics of granulomatous diseases such as lupus vulgaris. These spread peripherally on a common erythematous base and are the lupoid type. This is also known as leishmaniasis recidivans and occurs most often with the urban type of disease, caused by *Leishmania tropica*. New World disease may also induce purely cutaneous lesions, of varied morphology. The primary papule may become nodular, verrucous, furuncular, or ulcerated, with an infiltrated red border (Fig. 20.4). Subcutaneous peripheral nodules, which eventually ulcerate, may signal extension of the disease. A linear or radial lymphangitic (sporotrichoid) pattern may occur

with lymphadenopathy, and the nodes may rarely yield organisms. Facial lesions may coalesce and resemble erysipelas. Recidivans lesions are unusual in the New World form of disease. In Yucatan and Guatemala, a subtype of New World disease exists: the chiclero ulcer. The most frequent site of infection is the ear (Fig. 20.5). The lesions ulcerate and occur most frequently in workers who harvest chicle for chewing gum in forests, where there is high humidity. This form is a more chronic ulcer that may persist for years, destroying the ear cartilage and leading to deformity. The etiologic agent is *Leishmania mexicana* and the sandfly vector, *Lutzomyia flaviscutellata.*

Uta is a term used by Peruvians for leishmaniasis occurring in mountainous territory at 1200–1800 m above sea level. The ulcerating lesions are found on exposed sites and mucosal lesions do not occur.

Disseminated cutaneous leishmaniasis may be seen in both New and Old World disease. Multiple nonulcerated papules and plaques, chiefly on exposed surfaces, characterize this type. The disease begins with a single ulcer, nodule, or plaque from which satellite lesions may develop and disseminate to cover the entire body. The disease is progressive, and treatment is usually ineffective. It is characterized by anergy to the organism. This type of leishmaniasis must be differentiated from lepromatous leprosy, xanthoma tuberosum, paracoccidioidal granuloma, Lobo disease, and malignant lymphoma.

Etiologic Factors

Leishmania tropica, L. major, L. aethiopica, and *L. infantum,* the cause of Mediterranean visceral leishmaniasis, may cause cutaneous leishmaniasis. Purely cutaneous leishmaniasis is also caused by several species present in the New World. *L. mexicana* does not induce mucosal disease. *Leishmania braziliensis guyanensis* produces cutaneous disease, as does *L. b. braziliensis* and *L. b. panamensis;* however, the latter two may also result in mucocutaneous disease.

Epidemiology. Cutaneous leishmaniasis is endemic in Asia Minor and to a lesser extent in many countries around the Mediterranean. Iran and Saudi Arabia have a high occurrence rate. In endemic areas, deliberate inoculation on the thigh is sometimes practiced so that scarring on the face—a frequent site for Oriental sore—may be avoided. Purely cutaneous lesions may also be found in the Americas. In the United States leishmaniasis is largely restricted to southern Texas, although rare reports of human cutaneous disease have occurred as far north as Pennsylvania, and visceral leishmaniasis in immunosuppressed humans is being recognized as an emerging infection in areas not previously thought to be endemic for the disease.

Pathogenesis. The leishmania protozoan has an alternate life in vertebrates and in insect hosts. Humans and other mammals, such as dogs and rodents, are the natural reservoir hosts. The vector hosts are *Phlebotomus* sandflies for the Old World type and *Phlebotomus perniciosus* and *Lutzomyia* sandflies for New World cutaneous leishmaniasis. After the insect has fed on blood, the flagellates (leptomonad, promastigote) develop in the gut in 8–20 days, after which migration occurs into the mouth parts; from here, transmission into humans occurs by a bite. In humans, the flagella are lost, and a leishmanial form (amastigote) is assumed.

Histopathology. An ulcer with a heavy infiltrate of histiocytes, lymphocytes, plasma cells, and polymorphonuclear leukocytes is seen. The parasitized histiocytes form tuberculoid granulomas in the dermis. Pseudoepitheliomatous hyperplasia may occur in the edges of the ulcer. Leishmanias are nonencapsulated and contain a nucleus and a paranucleus. Wright, Giemsa, and monoclonal antibody staining may be helpful in identifying the organisms within histiocytes, where they often line up at the periphery of a vacuole. PCR primers are available for a variety of species. PCR is more sensitive than microscopy but less sensitive than culture.

Diagnosis. In endemic areas, the diagnosis is not difficult. In other localities, cutaneous leishmaniasis may be confused with syphilis, yaws, lupus vulgaris, and pyogenic granulomas. The diagnosis is established by demonstration of the organism in smears. A punch biopsy specimen from the active edge of the ulcer is ideal for culture. It can be placed in Nicolle-Novy-MacNeal (NNN) medium and shipped at room temperature. Parasites can also be cultured from tissue fluid. A hypodermic needle is inserted into the normal skin and to the edge of the ulcer base. The needle is rotated to work loose some material and serum, which is then aspirated. A culture on NNN medium at 22°C–35°C (71.6°F–95°F) is recommended to demonstrate the leptomonads. PCR is now available and is the most sensitive diagnostic test for cutaneous leishmaniasis.

Treatment. Spontaneous healing of primary cutaneous lesions occurs, usually within 12–18 months, shorter for Old World disease. Reasons to treat a self-limited infection include avoiding disfiguring scars in exposed areas, avoiding secondary infection, controlling disease in the population, and failure of spontaneous healing. In the diffuse cutaneous and recidivans types, leishmaniasis may persist for 20–40 years if not treated.

In areas where localized cutaneous leishmaniasis is not complicated by recidivans or sporotrichoid forms or by mucocutaneous disease, treatment with such topical modalities as paromomycin sulfate 15% plus methylbenzethonium chloride 12%, ketoconazole cream under occlusion, cryotherapy, local heat, 5-aminolevulinic acid hydrochloride (10%) plus visible red light (633 nm), and laser ablation, or with intralesional sodium stibogluconate antimony or emetine hydrochloride may be effective and safe.

In the setting of Old World cutaneous leishmaniasis, some data suggest that intramuscular meglumine antimoniate in combination with intralesional meglumine antimoniate may be superior to intralesional therapy alone. A meta-analysis of studies of Old World cutaneous leishmaniasis concluded that pentamidine was similar in efficacy to pentavalent antimonials, and that both were

superior to the other agents studied. Since then, a Pakistani study concluded that itraconazole was more effective and more economical and had fewer side effects than meglumine antimoniate in both wet and dry types of cutaneous leishmaniasis. The number of patients studied was relatively small, and other studies have been disappointing. Oral fluconazole and zinc sulfate have been used to treat *Leishmania major* infection. A similar meta-analysis of studies of New World cutaneous leishmaniasis concluded that meglumine might be the best agent in its class. Intralesional therapy may be acceptable for small, solitary lesions in areas with a low risk of mucosal disease. Azithromycin has been used in New World disease but is inferior to antimonials. Perilesional injections of IFN-γ have also been reported to be effective but are expensive.

In immunosuppressed patients or those who acquire infection in areas where mucocutaneous disease may occur, systemic therapy is recommended. As with topical treatment, many alternatives have been reported to be effective. Sodium antimony gluconate (sodium stibogluconate) solution is given intramuscularly or intravenously, 20 mg/kg/day in two divided doses for 28 days. It can be obtained from the U.S. Centers for Disease Control and Prevention (CDC) Drug Service (Atlanta, GA 30333). Repeated courses may be given. Antimony *n*-methyl glutamine (Glucantime) is used more often in Central and South America because of its local availability.

Other systemic medications reported to be effective include fluconazole (200 mg/day for 6 weeks), ketoconazole, dapsone, rifampicin, and allopurinol. Some of these have not been subjected to controlled clinical trials, as is true of most topical treatments. The recidivans and disseminated cutaneous types may require prolonged courses or adjuvant IFN therapy. Amphotericin B may be used in antimony-resistant disease. Lipid formulations of amphotericin B are highly effective in short courses but are expensive. Liposomal amphotericin B may be especially helpful for *Leishmania braziliensis* and *L. guyanensis* infections. Intramuscular pentamidine is also used for *L. guyanensis* cutaneous leishmaniasis, because this infection is resistant to systemic antimony. Miltefosine is being used for cutaneous disease in some areas of the world and may prove to be the treatment of choice for diffuse cutaneous leishmaniasis and post–kala-azar dermal leishmaniasis. However, some studies have shown miltefosine to be ineffective in *L. major* and *L. braziliensis* infections. Posaconazole has been used in Old World disease. Control depends chiefly on the success of antifly measures taken by health authorities and personal protection with protective clothing, screening, and repellents. Vaccines are being investigated but are not available.

Mucocutaneous Leishmaniasis (Leishmaniasis Americana, Espundia)

Clinical Features. The initial leishmanial infection, which occurs at the site of the fly bite, is a cutaneous ulcer. Secondary lesions on the mucosa usually occur at some time during the next 5 years. The earliest mucosal lesion is usually hyperemia of the nasal septum with subsequent ulceration (Fig. 20.6), which progresses to invade the septum and later the paranasal fossae. Perforation of the septum eventually takes place. For some time, the nose remains unchanged externally, despite the internal destruction. At first, only a dry crust is observed, or a bright-red infiltration or vegetation on the nasal septum, with symptoms of obstruction and small hemorrhages. Despite the mutilating and destructive character of leishmaniasis, it never involves the nasal bones. When the septum is destroyed, the nasal bridge and tip of the nose collapse, giving the appearance of a parrot beak, camel nose, or tapir nose.

It is important to recall that the four great chronic infections—syphilis, tuberculosis, Hansen disease, and leishmaniasis—have a predilection for the nose. The ulcer may extend to the lips (Fig. 20.7) and continue to advance to the pharynx, attacking the soft

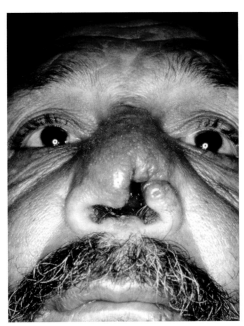

Fig. 20.6 Mucocutaneous leishmaniasis.

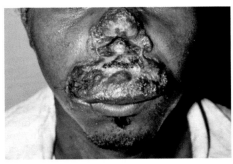

Fig. 20.7 Severe destructive mucocutaneous leishmaniasis. (Courtesy Debra Kalter, MD.)

palate, uvula, tonsils, gingiva, and tongue. The eventual mutilation is called espundia. Two perpendicular grooves at the union of the osseous palate and soft tissues, in the midst of the vegetative infiltration of the entire pharynx, are called the palate cross of espundia.

Only in exceptional cases does American leishmaniasis invade the genital or ocular mucous membranes. The frequency of mucous membrane involvement is variable. In Yucatan and Guatemala, it is an exception; in other countries, such as Brazil, it may occur in 80% of cases.

Etiologic Factors. Mucocutaneous leishmaniasis is mainly caused by *Leishmania (Viannia) braziliensis braziliensis* and *L. b. panamensis*, although some Old World organisms, including *L. infantum*, *L. major*, and *L. tropica*, can cause mucosal ulceration. Leishmania has two forms: the nonflagellated form or leishmania, which is found in the tissues of humans and animals susceptible to the inoculation of the parasite; and the flagellated form or leptomonad, which is found in the digestive tract of the vector insect (*Lutzomyia* in mucocutaneous disease) and in cultures. The typical morphology of leishmania, as found in vertebrates, is round or oval, usually with one extremity more rounded than the other, measuring 2–4 μm × 1.5–2.5 μm, with cytoplasm, nucleus, and blepharoplast or kinetoplast.

Epidemiology. Mucocutaneous leishmaniasis is predominantly a rural disease. It most often occurs in damp and forested regions. The disease can be contracted at any time of the year, but the risk is highest just after the rainy season. All ages and races and both genders are equally affected. Epidemics parallel the El Niño cycle.

Histopathology. In ulcerous leishmaniasis, marked irregular acanthosis and sometimes pseudoepitheliomatous hyperplasia can be found. The dermis shows a dense infiltration of histiocytes, lymphocytes, and plasma cells. In new lesions, some neutrophils are observed. Large Langhans giant cells or typical tubercles are occasionally seen. Numerous organisms are present (mostly in histiocytes), which are nonencapsulated and contain a nucleus and a paranucleus. Wright, Giemsa, and monoclonal antibody staining may be helpful in identifying the organisms. In patients with granulomatous infiltrates containing intracellular parasites within histiocytes, leishmaniasis is one of several diseases to be considered, including rhinoscleroma, histoplasmosis, granuloma inguinale, Chagas disease, *Penicillium marneffei* infection, and toxoplasmosis. Touch smears stained with Giemsa are helpful in many cases of cutaneous and mucocutaneous leishmaniasis.

Laboratory Findings. Leishmania is demonstrated in the cutaneous and mucous membrane lesions by direct smears or cultures. In Wright-stained biopsy material, intracellular and extracellular organisms are seen with typical morphology of two chromatic structures: nucleus and parabasal body. In later mucosal lesions, the scarcity of parasites makes identification difficult. The culture is done on NNN medium for leptomonads. PCR is now widely used, and specimens obtained from lesion scarification and blood sample–enriched leukocytes compare favorably with indirect immunofluorescence reaction and culture techniques.

Prophylaxis. Although it is impractical to eliminate the insect vector, it is still the only valid measure for the control of this prevalent disease. Effective vaccines are not available for mucocutaneous leishmaniasis.

Treatment. Treatment is the same as described for cutaneous leishmaniasis, except that antimony resistance is common in mucocutaneous disease. Combination therapy using antimonials with drugs such as rifampin or azithromycin, or adding immuno-modulators such as IFN-γ, IL-2, or imiquimod may result in cure. Amphotericin B treatment may be necessary.

Visceral Leishmaniasis (Kala-Azar, Dumdum Fever)

Clinical Features. The earliest lesion is the cutaneous nodule or leishmanioma, which occurs at the site of the initial sandfly inoculation. Kala-azar, meaning "black fever," acquired its name because of the patchy macular darkening of the skin caused by deposits of melanin that develop in the later course of the disease. These patches are most marked over the forehead and temples, periorally, and on the midabdomen.

The primary target for the parasites is the reticuloendothelial system; the spleen, liver, bone marrow, and lymph nodes are attacked. The incubation period is 1–4 months. An intermittent fever, with temperatures ranging from 39°C–40°C (102°F–104°F), ushers in the disease. Hepatosplenomegaly, agranulocytosis, anemia, and thrombocytopenia occur. Chills, fever, emaciation, weight loss, weakness, epistaxis, and purpura develop as the disease progresses. Susceptibility to secondary infection may produce pulmonary and gastrointestinal (GI) infection, ulcerations in the mouth (cancrum oris), and noma. Death occurs about 2 years from onset in untreated individuals.

Most infections are subclinical or asymptomatic. In patients with AIDS, papular and nodular skin lesions may occur.

Dermatofibroma-type or Kaposi sarcoma–like, brown to purple nodules are most frequently reported, although random biopsies of normal skin will reveal organisms. Therefore clinical correlation is necessary to attribute skin findings to *Leishmania* specifically.

Etiologic Factors. *Leishmania donovani* spp. *donovani, infantum,* and *chagasi* cause visceral leishmaniasis and are parasites of rodents, canines, and humans. They are nonflagellate oval organisms about 3 mm in diameter, known as Leishman-Donovan bodies. In the sandfly, it is a leptomonad form with flagella.

Epidemiology. *Leishmania donovani donovani* causes visceral leishmaniasis in India, with the major reservoir being humans and the vector being *Phlebotomus argentipes*. *L .donovani infantum* occurs in China, Africa, the Near East and Middle East, and the Mediterranean littoral, where the major reservoirs are dogs; *Phlebotomus perniciosus* and *P. ariasi* are the vectors of the Mediterranean type. American visceral leishmaniasis is caused by *L. donovani chagasi* and is transmitted by the sandfly *Lutzomyia longipalpis*. American visceral leishmaniasis principally affects domestic dogs, although explosive outbreaks of the human infection occur sporadically, when the number of *Lutzomyia longipalpis* builds up to a high level in the presence of infected dogs. Canine visceral infections with *Leishmania infantum* have been reported in foxhounds in various parts of the United States and Canada.

Diagnosis. Leishman-Donovan bodies may be present in the blood in individuals with kala-azar of India. Specimens for examination, in descending order of utility, include spleen pulp, sternal marrow, liver tissue, and exudate from lymph nodes. Culturing on NNN medium may also reveal the organisms.

Treatment. General supportive measures are essential. Pentavalent antimony has long been the drug of choice. In areas of drug resistance, amphotericin B is usually effective, but it is expensive and toxic, and requires intravenous administration. Miltefosine, an oral alkyl-phosphocholine analog, has proved as effective as amphotericin B in some trials. It is often used to treat visceral disease in India and Ethiopia. Mixed infections involving both *Leishmania* and *Trypanosoma cruzi* are becoming increasingly common in Central and South America because of overlapping endemic areas. Amiodarone has been used as an unconventional antiparasitic drug in this setting in addition to standard therapy.

Post–Kala-Azar Dermal Leishmaniasis

In kala-azar, the leishmanoid (amastigote) forms may be widely distributed throughout apparently normal skin. During and after recovery from the disease, a special form of dermal disease known as post–kala-azar dermal leishmaniasis appears. This condition appears during or shortly after treatment in the African form, but its appearance may be delayed up to 10 years after treatment in the Indian form. It follows the treatment of visceral leishmaniasis in 50% of Sudanese patients and 5%–10% of those seen in India. There are two constituents of the eruption: a macular, depigmented eruption found mainly on the face, arms, and upper part of the trunk and a warty, papular eruption in which amastigotes can be found. Because it may persist for up to 20 years, these patients may act as a chronic reservoir of infection. This condition closely resembles Hansen disease. High concentrations of IL-10 in the blood of visceral leishmaniasis patients predict those who will be affected by post–kala-azar dermal leishmaniasis. Miltefosine may become the drug of choice.

Viscerotropic Leishmaniasis

Twelve U.S. soldiers developed systemic infection with *Leishmania tropica* while fighting in Operation Desert Storm in Iraq and Kuwait.

None had symptoms of kala-azar, but most had fever, fatigue, malaise, cough, diarrhea, or abdominal pain, and none had cutaneous disease. Diagnostic tests yielded positive results on bone marrow aspiration; lymph node involvement was also documented. Treatment with sodium stibogluconate led to improvement.

Burza S, et al: Leishmaniasis. Lancet. 2018 Sep 15;392(10151):951-970. doi: 10.1016/S0140-6736(18)31204-2. Epub 2018 Aug 17. Review. PubMed PMID: 30126638.

Maxfield L, et al: Leishmaniasis. 2018 Oct 1. StatPearls [Internet]. Treasure Island (FL): StatPearls Publishing; 2018 Jan-. Available from http://www.ncbi.nlm.nih.gov/books/NBK531456/ PubMed PMID: 30285351.

Meireles CB, et al: Atypical presentations of cutaneous leishmaniasis. Acta Trop 2017; 172: 240.

Oryan A, et al: Worldwide risk factors in leishmaniasis. Asian Pac J Trop Med 2016; 9: 925.

Scorza BM, et al: Cutaneous manifestations of human and murine leishmaniasis. Int J Mol Sc 2017; 18.

Steverding D: The history of leishmaniasis. Parasit Vectors 2017; 10: 82.

Sundar S, et al: Recent developments and future prospects in the treatment of visceral leishmaniasis. Ther Adv Infect Dis 2016; 3: 98.

Wolf Nassif P, et al: Safety and efficacy of current alternatives in the topical treatment of cutaneous leishmaniasis. Parasitology. 2017; 144: 995.

Human Trypanosomiasis

Three species of trypanosome are pathogenic to humans: *Trypanosoma gambiense* and *T. rhodesiense* in Africa and *T. cruzi* in America. The skin manifestations are usually observed in the earlier stages of trypanosomiasis as evanescent erythema, erythema multiforme, and edema, especially angioedema.

In the early stage of African trypanosomiasis, a trypanosome chancre may occur at the site of a tsetse fly bite. Erythema with circumscribed swellings of angioedema then occurs, with enlargement of the lymph nodes, fever, malaise, headache, and joint pains. In the West African (Gambian) form, the illness is chronic, lasting several years, with progressive deterioration, whereas the East African (Rhodesian) form is an acute illness, with a stormy, fatal course of weeks to months. The Rhodesian form is more often associated with cutaneous signs. Annular or deep erythema nodosum–like lesions are frequent manifestations (Fig. 20.8). Lymphadenopathy is generalized, but frequently there is a pronounced enlargement of the posterior cervical group (Winterbottom sign).

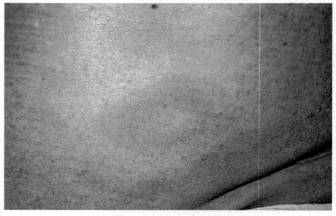

Fig. 20.8 African trypanosomiasis.

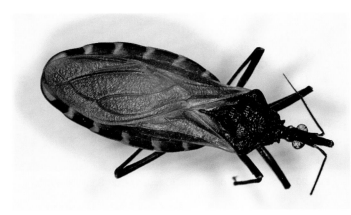

Fig. 20.9 Triatome reduviid bug.

In American trypanosomiasis (Chagas disease), similar changes take place in the skin. The reduviid bug (kissing bug, assassin bug) usually bites at night, frequently at mucocutaneous junctions, where the bug's infected feces are deposited when it feeds (Fig. 20.9). The unsuspecting sleeping person rubs the feces into the bite and becomes infected. If the bite of the infected bug occurs near the eye, Romana sign develops, consisting of unilateral conjunctivitis and edema of the eyelids, with an ulceration or chagoma in the area. The bite of a "kissing bug" becomes extremely swollen and red, whether or not trypanosomes are involved. Acute Chagas disease is usually a mild illness of fever, malaise, edema of the face and lower extremities, and generalized lymphadenopathy. Skin lesions occurring in this phase include nodules at the site of inoculation, disseminated nodules, or morbilliform and urticarial lesions. In chronic Chagas disease, which occurs in 10%–30% of infected persons years to decades later, the heart (myocarditis, arrhythmias, thromboembolism, cardiac failure) and GI system (megaesophagus, megacolon) are most often involved. During the remaining infected but asymptomatic indeterminate phase, patients may transmit the disease through transfusion. When such patients become immunosuppressed (with AIDS or organ transplantation), reactivation skin lesions may occur with a wide range of morphologies, including panniculitis.

Rhodesian trypanosomiasis is endemic among the cattle-raising tribes of East Africa, with the savannah habitat of the vectors determining its geographic distribution. Wild game and livestock are reservoir hosts, in addition to humans. The tsetse fly, *Glossina morsitans*, is the principal vector.

For Gambian trypanosomiasis, humans are the only vertebrate host, and the palpalis group of tsetse flies is the invertebrate host. These flies are found close to the water, and their fastidious biologic requirements restrict their distribution and thus that of the disease. Incidence is seasonal, with humidity and temperature being determining factors. The highest incidence is in men age 20–40 in tropical areas of West and Central Africa.

Chagas disease is prevalent in Central and South America from the United States to Argentina and Chile; the highest incidence is in Venezuela, Brazil, Uruguay, Paraguay, and Argentina. Approximately 29% of all male deaths in the 29–44 age-group in Brazil are attributed to Chagas disease.

Before CNS involvement has occurred in the Rhodesian form, suramin, a complex, non–metal-containing, organic compound, is the treatment of choice. When the CNS is involved, melarsoprol is the drug of choice. Pentamidine isethionate is the drug of choice for the Gambian disease. Eflornithine appears to be a good alternative to melarsoprol for second-stage West African trypanosomiasis. For American trypanosomiasis, treatment is of limited efficacy. The nitroaromatic compounds nifurtimox and benznidazole clear the parasitemia and reduce the severity of the acute illness,

but there is a high incidence of adverse effects. Although benznidazole reduces parasite load during the acute phase, it does not prevent chronic cardiac lesions. Ruthenium complexation improves bioavailability of benznidazole and has the potential to improve outcomes. Conservative treatment is the typical approach to the patient with congestive heart failure from Chagas myocarditis, but recent data suggest that clomipramine, a tricyclic antidepressant that inhibits *Trypanosoma cruzi*'s trypanothione reductase, improves the course of cardiac disease in animal models. GI complications may be treated surgically.

Aksoy S, et al: Human African trypanosomiasis control. PLoS Negl Trop Dis 2017; 11: e0005454.
Chatelain E: Chagas disease research and development. Comput Struct Biotechnol J 2016; 15: 98.
Cullen DR, et al: A brief review of drug discovery research for human African trypanosomiasis. Curr Med Chem 2017; 24: 701.
Duschak VG: Targets and patented drugs for chemotherapy of Chagas disease in the last 15 years-period. Recent Pat Antiinfect Drug Discov 2016; 11: 74.

CLASS SPOROZOA

Toxoplasmosis

Toxoplasmosis is a zoonosis caused by a parasitic protozoan, *Toxoplasma gondii*. Infection may be either congenital or acquired. Cerebral disease has been reported in the setting of rituximab therapy and widespread lesions can mimic melanoma metastases on positron emission tomography (PET) scans. Congenital infection occurs from placental transmission. Abortion or stillbirth may result. However, a full-term child delivered to an infected mother may have a triad of hydrocephalus, chorioretinitis, and cerebral calcification. In addition, there may be hepatosplenomegaly and jaundice. Skin changes in toxoplasmosis are rare and clinically nonspecific.

In congenital toxoplasmosis, macular and hemorrhagic eruptions predominate. Blueberry muffin lesions, reflecting dermatoerythropoiesis, may be seen. Occasionally, abnormal hair growth and exfoliative dermatitis have also been observed. The differential diagnosis of congenital toxoplasmosis is the TORCH syndrome (toxoplasmosis, other agents, rubella, cytomegalovirus, and herpes simplex). In acquired toxoplasmosis, early skin manifestations consist of cutaneous and subcutaneous nodules and macular, papular, and hemorrhagic eruptions. These may be followed by scarlatiniform desquamation, eruptions mimicking roseola, erythema multiforme, and dermatomyositis or lichen planus, as well as exfoliative dermatitis. As a rule, the exanthem is accompanied by high fever and general malaise.

Diagnosis of acquired toxoplasmosis is of special importance to three groups of adults: healthy pregnant women concerned about recent exposure; adults with lymphadenopathy, fever, and myalgia, who might have some other serious disease (e.g., lymphoma); and immunocompromised persons, such as patients with AIDS, in whom toxoplasmosis might be fatal. It is the most common cause of focal encephalitis in AIDS patients, and this may be accompanied by a widespread papular eruption.

Toxoplasma gondii is a crescent-shaped, oval, or round protozoan that can infect any mammalian or avian cell. Toxoplasmosis is often acquired through contact with animals, particularly cats. Reservoirs of infection have been reported in dogs, cats, cattle, sheep, pigs, rabbits, rats, pigeons, and chickens. The two major routes of transmission of *T. gondii* in humans are oral and congenital. Meats consumed by humans may contain tissue cysts, thus serving as a source of infection when eaten raw or undercooked. There is no evidence of direct human-to-human transmission, other than from mother to fetus.

The diagnosis cannot be made on clinical grounds alone. It may be established by isolation of *T. gondii*; demonstration of the protozoa in tissue sections, smears, or body fluids by Wright or Giemsa stain; characteristic lymph node histology; and serologic methods. In the patient with bone marrow transplantation, the organism has caused interface dermatitis, creating the potential for misdiagnosis as graft-versus-host disease.

A combination of pyrimethamine (Daraprim) and sulfadiazine acts synergistically and forms an effective treatment, but toxicity is substantial. Dosages and total treatment time vary according to the age and immunologic competence of the infected patient.

Assolini JP, et al: Nanomedicine advances in toxoplasmosis. Parasitol Res 2017; 116: 1603.

Chellan P, et al: Recent developments in drug discovery against the protozoal parasites *Cryptosporidium* and *Toxoplasma*. Bioorg Med Chem Lett 2017; 27: 1491.

■ PHYLUM CNIDARIA

The cnidarians include the jellyfish, hydroids, Portuguese men-of-war, corals, and sea anemones. These are all radial marine animals, living mostly in ocean water.

Portuguese Man-of-War Dermatitis

Stings by the Portuguese man-of-war (*Physalia physalis* in Atlantic or much smaller *Physalia utriculus* or "bluebottle" in Pacific Ocean) are characterized by linear lesions that are erythematous, urticarial, and even hemorrhagic. The forearms, sides of the trunk, thighs, and feet are common sites of involvement. The usual local manifestation is sharp, stinging, and intense pain. Internally, there may be severe dyspnea, prostration, nausea, abdominal cramps, lacrimation, and muscular pains. Death may occur if the areas stung are large in relation to the patient's size.

The fluid of the nematocysts contains toxin that is carried into the victim through barbs along the tentacle. The venom is a neurotoxic poison that can produce marked cardiac changes. Each Portuguese man-of-war is a colony of symbiotic organisms consisting of a blue to red float or pneumatophore with a gas gland, several gastrozooids measuring 1–20 mm, reproductive polyps, and the fishing tentacles bearing the nematocysts from which the barbs are ejected. The hydroid is found most frequently along the southeastern Florida coastline and in the Gulf of Mexico as well as on windward coasts throughout the mid-Pacific and South Pacific. Safe Sea, a barrier cream, has been reported as being effective at preventing jellyfish stings off the coast of Florida, but studies of barrier creams in general have been mixed.

Jellyfish Dermatitis

Jellyfish dermatitis produces lesions similar to those of the Portuguese man-of-war, except that the lesions are not so linear. Immediate allergic reactions occur infrequently as urticaria, angioedema, or anaphylaxis. Delayed and persistent lesions also rarely occur.

The Australian sea wasp, *Chironex fleckeri*, which is colorless and transparent, is the most dangerous of all jellyfish, with a sting that is often fatal (Fig. 20.10). Another sea wasp, *Carybdea marsupialis*, is much less dangerous and occurs in the Caribbean Sea. *Rhopilema nomadica*, common in the Mediterranean Sea, has been reported to cause severe delayed dermatitis.

Seabather's eruption is an acute dermatitis that begins a few hours after bathing in the waters along the Atlantic coast. It affects covered areas of the body as cnidarian larvae become entrapped under the bathing suit and the nematocyst releases its toxin because of external pressure. Thus the buttocks and waist are affected primarily, with the breast also involved in women (Fig. 20.11).

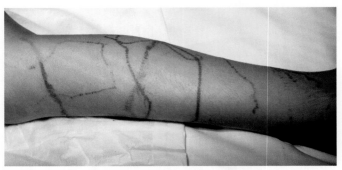

Fig. 20.10 Sea wasp dermatitis. (Courtesy Curt Samlaska, MD.)

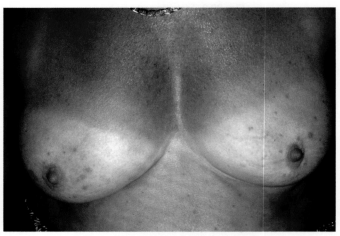

Fig. 20.11 Seabather eruption. (Courtesy Scott Norton, MD.)

Erythematous macules and papules appear and may develop into pustules or vesicles. Urticarial plaques are also present in a smaller number of patients. Crops of new lesions may occur for up to 72 hours, and the eruption persists for 10–14 days on average. It is quite pruritic.

Outbreaks in Florida are usually caused by larvae of the thimble jellyfish, *Linuche unguiculata*, which patients report as "black dots" in the water or their bathing suits. The larvae of the sea anemone *Edwardstella lineata* caused one epidemic of seabather's eruption in Long Island, New York. This organism also has nematocysts; thus the mechanism of the eruption is the same as with the jellyfish-induced eruption. It is likely that different cnidarian envenomations in different waters produce a similar clinical picture. Other reports focus on spring plants, dinoflagellates, protozoans, or crustaceans as potential causes. Because the eruption results from trapping of cnidarian larvae with their nematocysts or other toxic or irritant substances under the bathing suit, it may be limited by seabathers who remove their suit and shower soon after leaving the water.

Hydroid, Sea Anemone, and Coral Dermatitis

Patients contacting the small marine hydroid *Halecium* may develop a dermatitis. The organism grows as a 1-cm–thick coat of moss on the submerged portions of vessels or pilings. Sea anemones (Fig. 20.12) produce reactions similar to those from jellyfish and hydroids. Coral cuts are injuries caused by the exoskeleton of the corals *Milleporina*. They have a reputation for becoming inflamed and infected and for delayed healing. The combination of implantation of fragments of coral skeleton and infection (because cuts

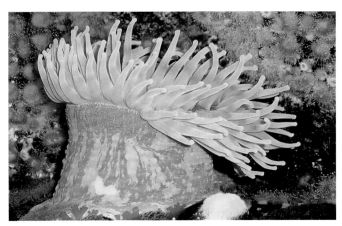

Fig. 20.12 Sea anemone.

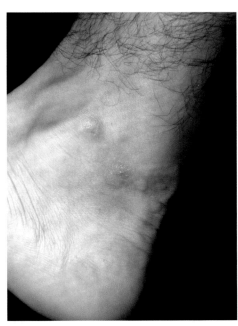

Fig. 20.13 Sea urchin granuloma. (Courtesy Steven Binnick, MD.)

occur most often on feet) probably accounts almost entirely for these symptoms. Detoxification as soon as possible after the injury is recommended for all these types of sting or cut.

Treatment of Stings and Cuts

Hot water immersion may be an effective remedy for many stings, but scald injuries must be avoided. In the case of box jellies, ice has been shown to be equally effective, but ice can worsen stings of some other jellies. Undischarged nematocytes should be removed. Fresh water, and even sea water, may cause them to discharge. Pacific *Chironex* (box jellyfish) nematocytes should always be inactivated with 5% acetic acid (vinegar) when it is available, but Pacific *Physalia* (bluebottle) nematocytes may discharge on contact with vinegar. Large, visible tentacles may be removed with forceps in a double-gloved hand. Remaining nematocysts may be removed by applying a layer of shaving cream and shaving the area gently. Meat tenderizer may cause tissue damage and has been shown to be no better than placebo in some studies.

Pressure dressings and abrasion will worsen the envenomation. Topical anesthetics or steroids may be applied after decontamination. Systemic reactions may occur through either large amounts of venom or a previously sensitizing exposure from which anaphylaxis may result, and systemic treatment with epinephrine, antihistamines, or corticosteroids may be needed. Specific antivenin is available for the box jellyfish, *Chironex fleckeri*. This should be administered intravenously to limit myonecrosis. Magnesium sulfate (MgSO₄) may also be of value in the setting of box jellyfish envenomation. Recurrent jellyfish reactions have shown partial responses to tacrolimus ointment 0.1%.

Sponges and Bristleworms

Sponges have horny spicules of silicon dioxide and calcium carbonate. Some sponges produce dermal irritants, such as halitoxin and okadaic acid, and others may be colonized by Cnidaria. Allergic or irritant reactions may result. Bristleworms may also produce stinging. All these may be treated by first using adhesive tape to remove the spicules, then applying vinegar soaks, as previously described, and lastly, topical corticosteroids.

Sea Urchin Injuries

Puncture wounds inflicted by the brittle, fragile spines of sea urchins, mainly of genus *Diadema* or *Echinothrix*, are stained blue-black by the black spines and may contain fragments of the spines. The spines consist of calcium carbonate crystals, which most frequently induce an irritant reaction with pain and inflammation of

several days' duration. Foreign body or sarcoid-like granulomas may develop (Fig. 20.13), as may a vesicular hypersensitivity reaction, 10 days after exposure. Injuries by spines of the genus *Tripneustes* have been reported to cause fatal envenomation, but this genus is not found on U.S. coasts.

Starfish also have thorny spines that can sting and burn if they are stepped on or handled. Several different types of stinging fish also produce puncture wounds. Stingrays, scorpionfish, stonefish, catfish, and weaverfish may cause such envenomations. These wounds should be immersed in nonscalding water (45°C [113°F]) for 30–90 minutes or until the pain subsides. Calcified fragments may be visible on x-ray evaluation, with fluoroscopy guiding extraction of spines, especially on the hands and feet. Sea urchin spines have been effectively removed using the erbium:yttrium-aluminum-garnet (YAG) laser. Debridement and possibly antibiotic therapy for deep puncture wounds of the hands and feet are recommended. There is a specific antivenin for stonefish stings.

Seaweed Dermatitis

Although caused by a marine alga and not by an animal, seaweed dermatitis deserves mention with other problems associated with swimming or wading. The dermatitis occurs 3–8 hours after the individual emerges from the ocean. The distribution is in parts covered by a bathing suit: scrotum, penis, perineum, and perianal area. The dermatitis is caused by a marine plant, *Lyngbya majuscula* Gomont. It has been observed only in bathers swimming off the windward shore of Oahu, Hawaii. Seabather's eruption, clam digger's itch, and swimmer's itch must be differentiated from seaweed dermatitis caused by marine algae. Prophylaxis is achieved by refraining from swimming in waters that are turbid with such algae. Swimmers should shower within 5 minutes of swimming. Active treatment in severe cases is the same as for acute burns.

Dogger Bank Itch

Dogger Bank itch is an eczematous dermatitis caused by the sea chervil *Alcyonidrium hirsutum*, a seaweed-like animal colony. These sea mosses or sea mats are found on the Dogger Bank, an immense shelflike elevation under the North Sea between Scotland and Denmark.

Isbister GK, et al: Hot water immersion v icepacks for treating the pain of *Chironex fleckeri* stings. Med J Aust 2017; 206: 258.

Jefferson J, et al: Coral contact dermatitis. Dermatol Online J 2015; 21.

Little M, et al: Successful use of heat as first aid for tropical Australian jellyfish stings. Toxicon 2016; 122: 142.

Yanagihara AA, et al: Cubozoan sting-site seawater rinse, scraping, and ice can increase venom load. Toxins (Basel) 2017; 9.

■ PHYLUM PLATYHELMINTHES

Phylum Platyhelminthes includes the flatworms, of which two classes, trematodes and cestodes, are parasitic to humans. The trematodes, or blood flukes, parasitize human skin or internal organs. The cestodes are segmented, ribbon-shaped flatworms that inhabit the intestinal tract as adults and involve the subcutaneous tissue, heart, muscle, and eye in the larval form. This is encased in a sac that eventually becomes calcified.

CLASS TREMATODA

Schistosome Cercarial Dermatitis

Cercarial dermatitis is a severely pruritic, widespread, papular dermatitis caused by cercariae of schistosomes for which humans are not hosts; the usual animal hosts are waterfowl and rodents, such as muskrats. The eggs in the excreta of these animals, when deposited in water, hatch into swimming miracidia. These enter a snail, where further development occurs. From the snail, the free-swimming cercariae emerge to invade human skin on accidental contact. The swimming, colorless, multicellular organisms are slightly less than 1 mm long. Exposure to cercariae occurs when a person swims or, more often, wades in water containing them. They attack by burrowing into the skin, where they die. The species that causes this eruption cannot enter the bloodstream or deeper tissues.

After coming out of the water, the bather begins to itch, and a transient erythematous eruption appears, but after a few hours, the eruption subsides, together with the itching. After a quiescent period of 10–15 hours, the symptoms then recur, and erythematous macules and papules develop throughout the exposed parts that were in the water (Fig. 20.14). After several days, the dermatitis heals spontaneously. There are two types: the freshwater swimmer's itch and the saltwater marine dermatitis, or clam digger's itch. Cercarial dermatitis is not communicable.

Various genera and species of organism have been reported from various locations worldwide. An outbreak of cercarial dermatitis was reported from Delaware in 1991 in which the avian schistosome *Microbilharzia variglandis* was implicated as the causative organism. *Schistosoma spindale* cercaria caused a recent epidemic in southern Thailand.

Thoroughly washing, then drying with a towel after exposure, can prevent the disease. Some advocate rubbing with alcohol as an additional preventive measure. Snail populations can be controlled, or waterfowl may be treated with medicated feed-corn to destroy the adult schistosomes and prevent outbreaks of swimmer's itch.

Visceral Schistosomiasis (Bilharziasis)

The cutaneous manifestation of schistosomiasis may begin with mild itching and a papular dermatitis of the feet and other parts after swimming in polluted streams containing cercariae. The types of schistosome causing this disease can penetrate into the bloodstream and eventually inhabit the venous system, draining the urinary bladder (*Schistosoma haematobium*) or the intestines (*Schistosoma mansoni* or *Schistosoma japonicum*). After an asymptomatic incubation period, the person may develop a sudden illness with fever and chills, pneumonitis, and eosinophilia. Petechial hemorrhages may occur.

Cutaneous schistosomal granulomas most frequently involve the genitalia, perineum, and buttocks. The eggs of *S. haematobium* or *S. mansoni* usually cause these bilharziomas (Fig. 20.15). Vegetating, soft, cauliflower-shaped masses, fistulous tracts, and extensive hard masses occur; these are riddled by sinuses that exude a seropurulent discharge with a characteristic odor. Phagedenic ulcerations and pseudoelephantiasis of the scrotum, penis, or labia are sometimes encountered. Histologically, the nodules contain bilharzial ova undergoing degeneration, with calcification and a surrounding cellular reaction of histiocytes, eosinophils, and occasional giant cells. In some cases, eventual malignant changes have been noted in chronic lesions. Animal studies have shown a moderate helper T-cell type 1 (Th1) response to parasite antigens in most tissues, but a strong Th2 response that propagates fibrogenesis within the liver. Infrequently, ectopic or extragenital lesions may occur, mainly on the trunk. This is a papular eruption tending to group in plaques and become darkly pigmented and scaly. A severe urticarial eruption known as urticarial fever or Katayama fever is frequently present along with *S. japonicum* infection; it occurs with the beginning of oviposition, 4–8 weeks after infection. This condition is seen mainly in China, Japan, and the Philippines. In addition to the urticaria, fever, malaise, abdominal cramps, arthritis, and liver/spleen involvement are seen. This is thought to be a serum sickness–like reaction.

Preventive measures include reducing infection sources, preventing contamination by human excreta of snail-bearing waters, control of snail hosts, and avoiding exposure to cercaria-infested waters. Prophylactic measures are constantly sought to control one of the world's worst parasitic diseases, but as yet, none has been found to be practical. For both *S. haematobium* and *S. mansoni*,

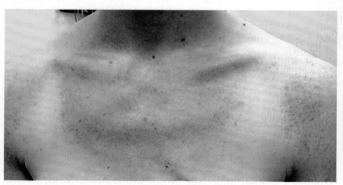

Fig. 20.14 Swimmer itch. (Courtesy Camille Introcaso, MD.)

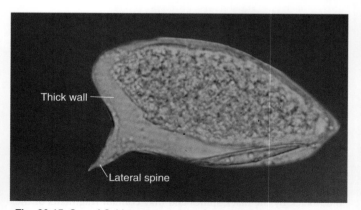

Fig. 20.15 Ova of *Schistosoma mansoni* are characterized by a thick chitinous wall and lateral spine.

praziquantel (Biltricide), 40 mg/kg orally for each of two treatments in 1 day, is the therapy of choice. *S. japonicum* treatment requires 60 mg/kg in three doses in 1 day. Schistosomicides exhibit toxicity for the host as well as for the parasite, and the risk of undesirable side effects may be enhanced by concomitant cardiac, renal, or hepatosplenic disease.

Kollipara R, et al: Emerging infectious diseases with cutaneous manifestations. J Am Acad Dermatol. 2016; 75: 19.
Patel TA, et al: Treatment of schistosomiasis in a patient allergic to praziquantel. Am J Trop Med Hyg 2016; 95: 1041.

Cysticercosis Cutis

The natural intermediate host of the pork tapeworm, *Taenia solium*, is the pig, but under some circumstances, humans act in this role. The larval stage of *T. solium* is *Cysticercus cellulosae*. Infection takes place by the ingestion of food contaminated with the eggs or by reverse peristalsis of eggs or proglottides from the intestine to the stomach. Here the eggs hatch, freeing the oncospheres. These enter the general circulation and form cysts in various parts of the body, such as striated muscles, brain, eye, heart, and lung.

In the subcutaneous tissues, the lesions are usually painless nodules that contain cysticerci. They are more or less stationary, usually numerous, and often calcified and are therefore demonstrable radiographically. Pain and ulceration may accompany the lesions. The disease is most prevalent in countries where pigs feed on human feces. It may be confused with gumma, lipoma, and epithelioma. A positive diagnosis is established solely by incision and examination of the interior of the calcified tumor, where the parasite will be found. Fine-needle aspiration has also been used to establish the diagnosis.

Albendazole or praziquantel is effective; however, the status of the CNS, spinal, and ocular involvement needs to be thoroughly assessed before treatment. The length of therapy and use of concomitant corticosteroids depend on the location of the cysts. However, none of the regimens clears the calcified parasites, which need to be surgically removed.

Sparganosis

Sparganosis is caused by the larva of the tapeworm *Spirometra*. The adult tapeworm lives in the intestines of dogs and cats. This is a rare tissue infection occurring in two forms. Application sparganosis occurs when an ulcer or infected eye is poulticed with the flesh of an infected intermediate host (such poultices are frequently used in the Orient). The larvae become encased in small nodules in the infected tissue. Ingestion sparganosis occurs when humans ingest inadequately cooked meat, such as snake or frog, or when a person drinks water that is contaminated with *Cyclops*, which is infected with plerocercoid larvae. One or two slightly pruritic or painful nodules may form in the subcutaneous tissue or on the trunk, breast, genitalia, or extremities. Cerebral disease may also occur. Diagnosis is usually made by excision of the nodule, although noninvasive imaging has also been used.

Humans are the accidental intermediate host of the sparganum, which is the alternative name for the plerocercoid larva. Treatment is surgical removal or ethanol injection of the infected nodules (Fig. 20.16). This may be difficult because of the swelling and extensive vascularity.

Echinococcosis

Echinococcosis is also known as hydatid disease. In humans, infection is produced by the ova reaching the mouth from the hands, in food, or from containers soiled by ova-contaminated feces from an infected dog. This leads to *Echinococcus granulosus* infestation of the liver and the lungs. Soft, fluctuating, semitranslucent, cystic tumors may occur

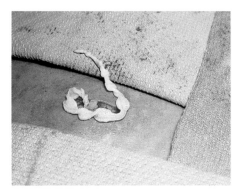

Fig. 20.16 Sparganosis.

in the skin, sometimes in the supraumbilical area as fistulas from underlying liver involvement. These tumors become fibrotic or calcified after the death of the larva. Eosinophilia, intractable urticaria and pruritus, and even acute generalized exanthematous pustulosis may be present. Such reactive findings may be present as skin manifestations of many of the helminthic infections, including other types of tapeworm. The treatment is excision, with care being taken to avoid rupturing the cyst. Albendazole combined with percutaneous drainage may also be used. *Hymenolepis nana* is a cosmopolitan dwarf tapeworm endemic in the tropics that may cause a treatment-resistant pruritic papular eruption associated with eosinophilia. Stool specimens for ova and parasites are definitive, and praziquantel is curative.

Moosazadeh M, et al: Epidemiological and clinical aspects of patients with hydatid cyst in Iran. J Parasit Dis 2017; 41: 356.

■ PHYLUM ANNELIDA

LEECHES

Leeches, of the class Hirudinea, are of marine, freshwater, or terrestrial types. After attaching to the skin or mucosa, they secrete an anticoagulant, hirudin, and then engorge themselves with blood. Local symptoms at the site of the bite may include bullae, hemorrhage, pruritus, whealing, necrosis, or ulceration. Allergic reactions, including anaphylaxis, may result. Leeches may be removed by applying salt, alcohol, or vinegar or by use of a match flame. Bleeding may then be stopped by direct pressure or by applying a styptic pencil to the site.

Leeches may be used medicinally to salvage tissue flaps that are threatened by venous congestion. However, bleeding, *Aeromonas* infection, anetoderma, and pseudolymphoma may be complications of their attachment.

Tilahun T: Vaginal leech infestation. Ethiop J Health Sci 2015; 25: 377.

■ PHYLUM NEMATHELMINTHES

Phylum Nemathelminthes includes the roundworms, both free-living and parasitic forms. Multiplication is usually outside the host. Both the larval and the adult stage may infect humans.

CLASS NEMATODA

Enterobiasis (Pinworm Infection, Seatworm Infection, Oxyuriasis)

The chief symptom of pinworm infestation, which occurs most frequently in children, is nocturnal pruritus ani. There is intense itching accompanied by excoriations of the anus, perineum, and pubic area. The vagina may become infested with the gravid pinworms. A pruritic papular dermatosis of the trunk and extremities may be observed infrequently. Restlessness, insomnia, enuresis, and irritability are a few of the many symptoms ascribed to this exceedingly common infestation. Exacerbation of mastocytosis has been described.

Oxyuriasis is caused by the roundworm *Enterobius vermicularis*, which may infest the small intestines, cecum, and large intestine of humans. The worms, especially gravid ones, migrate toward the rectum and at night emerge to the perianal and perineal regions to deposit thousands of ova; then the worm dries and dies outside the intestine. These ova are then carried back to the mouth of the host on the hands. The larvae hatch in the duodenum and migrate into the jejunum and ileum, where they reach maturity. Fertilization occurs in the cecum, thus completing the life cycle.

Humans are the only known host of the pinworm, which probably has the widest distribution of all the helminths. Infection occurs from hand-to-mouth transmission, often from handling soiled clothes, bedsheets, and other household articles. Ova under the fingernails are a common source of autoinfection. Ova may also be airborne and collect in dust that may be on furniture and the floor. Investigation may show that all members of the family of an affected person also harbor the infection. It is common in orphanages and mental institutions and among people living in communal groups.

Rarely is it feasible to identify a dead pinworm in the stool. Diagnosis is best made by demonstration of ova in smears taken from the anal region early in the morning before the patient bathes or defecates. Such smears may be obtained with a small, eye curette and placed on a glass slide with a drop of saline solution. It is also possible to use cellophane tape, looping the tape sticky-side out over a tongue depressor and then pressing it several times against the perianal region. The tape is then smoothed out on a glass slide. A drop of a solution containing iodine in xylol may be placed on the slide before the tape is applied to facilitate detection of any ova. These tests should be repeated on 3 consecutive days to rule out infection. Ova may be detected under the fingernails of the infected person.

Albendazole, 400 mg, or mebendazole, 100 mg, or pyrantel pamoate, 11 mg/kg (maximum 1 g), given once and repeated in 2 weeks, is effective. Personal hygiene and cleanliness at home are important. Fingernails should be cut short and scrubbed frequently; nails should be thoroughly cleaned on arising, before each meal, and after using the toilet. Sheets, underwear, towels, pajamas, and other clothing of the affected person should be laundered thoroughly and separately.

Hookworm Disease (Ground Itch, Uncinariasis, Ancylostomiasis, Necatoriasis)

The earliest skin lesions (ground itch) are erythematous macules and papules, which in a few hours become vesicles. These itchy lesions usually occur on the soles, toe webs, and ankles; they may be scattered or in groups. The content of the vesicles rapidly becomes purulent. These lesions are produced by invasion of the skin by the *Ancylostoma* or *Necator* larvae, and they precede the generalized symptoms of hookworm disease by 2 or 3 months. The cutaneous lesions last less than 2 weeks before the larvae continue their human life cycle. There may be as high as 40% eosinophilia about the fifth day of infection.

The onset of the constitutional disease is insidious and is accompanied by progressive iron deficiency anemia and debility. During the course of hookworm disease, urticaria often occurs. The skin ultimately becomes dry and pale or yellowish.

Hookworm is a specific communicable disease caused by *Ancylostoma duodenale* or *Necator americanus*. In the soil, under propitious circumstances, hookworms attain the stage of infective larvae in 5–7 days. When they come into accidental contact with bare feet, these tiny larvae (which can scarcely be seen with a small pocket lens) penetrate the skin and reach the capillaries. They are carried in the circulation to the lungs, where they pass through the capillary walls into the bronchi. They move up the trachea to the pharynx and, after being swallowed, eventually reach their habitat in the small intestine. Here they bury their heads in the mucosa and begin their sexual life.

Hookworm is prevalent in most tropical and subtropical countries and is often endemic in swampy and sandy localities in temperate zones. In these latter regions, the larvae are killed off each winter, but the soil is again contaminated from human sources the following summer. *N. americanus* prevails in the Western Hemisphere, Central and South Africa, South Asia, Australia, and the Pacific islands.

The defecation habits of infected individuals in endemic areas are largely responsible for its widespread distribution, as is the use of human feces for fertilization in many parts of the world. In addition, the climate is usually such that people go barefoot because of the heat or because they cannot afford shoes. Infection is thereby facilitated, especially through the toes.

Finding the eggs in the feces of a suspected individual establishes the diagnosis. The ova appear in the feces about 5 weeks after the onset of infection. The eggs may be found in direct fecal films if the infection is heavy, but in light infections, it may be necessary to resort to zinc sulfate centrifugal flotation or other concentration methods. Mixed infections frequently occur.

Albendazole, 400 mg once, or mebendazole, 100 mg twice daily for 3 days or 500 mg once, or pyrantel pamoate, 11 mg/kg (maximum 1 g) each day for 3 days, is effective. Prophylaxis is largely a community problem and depends on preventing fecal contamination of the soil. This is best attained by proper sanitary disposal of feces, protecting individuals from exposure by educating them about sanitary procedures, and mass treatment through public health methods.

Nematode Dermatitis

A patient in one report developed a persistent widespread folliculitis caused by *Ancylostoma caninum*. It was apparently acquired by lying in grass contaminated by the droppings of the patient's pet dogs and cats. A biopsy revealed hookworm larvae within the hair follicle. Oral thiabendazole was curative.

Creeping Eruption (Larva Migrans)

Creeping eruption is a term applied to twisting, winding linear skin lesions produced by the burrowing of larvae. People who go barefoot on the beach, children playing in sandboxes, carpenters and plumbers working under homes, and gardeners are often victims. The most common areas involved are the feet, buttocks, genitals, and hands.

Slight local itching and the appearance of papules at the sites of infection characterize the onset. Intermittent stinging pain occurs, and thin, red, tortuous lines are formed in the skin. The larval migrations begin 4 days after inoculation and progress at the rate of about 2 cm/day. However, they may remain quiescent for several days or even months before beginning to migrate. The linear lesions are often interrupted by papules that mark the sites of resting larvae (Fig. 20.17). As the eruption advances, the old parts tend to fade, although purulent manifestations may be caused by secondary infection in some cases; erosions and excoriations caused by scratching frequently occur. If the progress of the disease is not interrupted by treatment, the larvae usually die in 2–8 weeks, with resolution of the eruption, although rarely it has been reported to persist for up to 1 year. At times, the larvae are removed from the skin by the fingernails in scratching. Eosinophilia may be present.

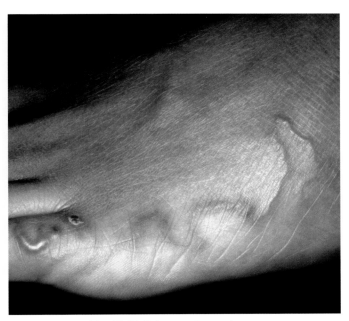

Fig. 20.17 Cutaneous larva migrans.

Loeffler syndrome, consisting of a patchy infiltrate of the lungs and eosinophilia as high as 50% in the blood and 90% in the sputum, may complicate creeping eruption.

The majority of U.S. cases of larva migrans occur along the southeast coast and are caused by penetration by the larvae of a cat and dog hookworm, *Ancylostoma braziliense*. It is acquired from body contact with damp sand or earth that has been contaminated by the excreta of dogs and cats. The larvae of *A. caninum*, which also infests the dog and the cat, rarely produce a similar dermatitis. The diagnosis is typically made clinically, although biopsy may sometimes demonstrate the organism, and even dermoscopy has been used.

Ivermectin, 200 µg/kg, generally given as a single 12-mg dose and repeated the next day, or albendazole, 400 mg/day for 3 days, is an effective treatment. Criteria for successful therapy are relief of symptoms and cessation of tract extension, which usually occurs within 1 week. Both ivermectin and metronidazole have been used topically, as has thiabendazole, compounded as a 10% suspension or a 15% cream. Another condition, not to be confused with this helminthic disease, which also is called creeping eruption (or sandworm, as it is known in South Africa, particularly in Natal and Zululand), is caused by a small mite about 300 µm long that tunnels into the superficial layers of the epidermis.

Gnathostomiasis

Migratory, intermittent, erythematous, urticarial plaques characterize human gnathostomiasis. Each episode of painless swelling lasts from 7–10 days and recurs every 2–6 weeks. Movement of the underlying parasite may be as much as 1 cm/hr. The total duration of the illness may be 10 years. Histopathologic examination of the skin swelling will demonstrate eosinophilic panniculitis. The clinical manifestation has been called larva migrans profundus.

The nematode *Gnathostoma dolorosi* or *G. spinigerum* is the cause, and most cases occur in Asia or South America. Eating raw flesh from the second intermediate host, most often freshwater fish, especially eel, in such preparations as sashimi and ceviche, allows humans to become the definitive host. Eating raw squid or snake is a less common exposure. As the larval cyst in the flesh

is digested, it becomes motile and penetrates the gastric mucosa, usually within 24–48 hours of ingestion. Symptoms then occur as migration of the parasite continues. Surgical removal is the treatment of choice, if the parasite can be located. This may be combined with albendazole, 400 mg/day or twice daily for 21 days, or ivermectin, 200 µg/kg/day for 2 days.

Creeping eruption caused by a recently recognized causative parasite of the nematode superfamily Spiruroidea has been reported in Japan. Eating raw squid was associated with the onset of long, narrow lesions that were pruritic, linear, and migratory. Surgical removal is the treatment of choice currently, as data on ivermectin are mixed.

Larva Currens

Intestinal infections with *Strongyloides stercoralis* may be associated with a perianal larva migrans syndrome called larva currens because of the rapidity of larval migration (currens means "running" or "racing"). Larva currens is an autoinfection caused by penetration of the perianal skin by infectious larvae as they are excreted in the feces. An urticarial band is the prominent primary lesion of cutaneous strongyloidiasis. Strongyloidiasis, as with the creeping eruption secondary to it, is often a chronic disease; infections may persist for more than 40 years. Approximately one third of patients infected are asymptomatic.

Signs and symptoms of systemic strongyloidiasis include abdominal pain, diarrhea, constipation, nausea, vomiting, pneumonitis, urticaria, eosinophilic folliculitis, and a peripheral eosinophilia. The skin lesions originate within 30 cm of the anus and characteristically extend as much as 10 cm/day.

Fatal cases of hyperinfection occur in immunocompromised patients; the parasite load increases dramatically and can produce a fulminant illness. Widespread petechiae and purpura are helpful diagnostic signs of disseminated infection, and chronic urticaria is a possible presenting sign. Periumbilical ecchymoses may appear as if they were caused by a thumbprint.

Administration of ivermectin, 200 µg/kg/day for 2 days, or thiabendazole, 50 mg/kg/day in two doses (maximum 3 g/day) for 2 days, is the treatment of choice. Immunosuppressed hosts may be treated with thiabendazole, 25 mg/kg twice daily for 7–10 days.

Free-living strongyloides known as *Pelodera* can also produce a creeping eruption. In one reported case, widespread follicular, erythematous, dome-shaped papules and pustules appeared on the patient within 24 hours of working under a house. This eruption persisted for 1 month before presentation. Scraping the lesions revealed live and dead larvae of the free-living soil nematode *Pelodera strongyloides*. Treatment with oral thiabendazole led to resolution.

Dracunculiasis (Guinea Worm Disease, Dracontiasis, Medina Worm)

Guinea worm disease is now limited to remote villages in several sub-Saharan African countries. It is caused by *Dracunculus medinensis* and is contracted through drinking water that has been contaminated with infected water fleas in which *Dracunculus* is parasitic. In the stomach, the larvae penetrate into the mesentery, where they mature sexually in 10 weeks. The female worm then burrows to the cutaneous surface to deposit her larvae and thus causes the specific skin manifestations. As the worm approaches the surface, it may be felt as a cordlike thickening and forms an indurated cutaneous papule. The papule may vesiculate, and a painful ulcer develops, usually on the leg. The worm is often visible. When the parasite comes in contact with water, the worm rapidly discharges its larvae, which are ingested by water fleas (*Cyclops*), contaminating the water.

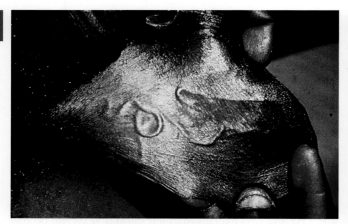

Fig. 20.18 Dracunculiasis.

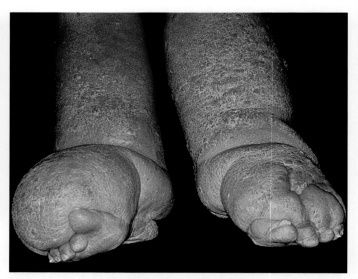

Fig. 20.19 Filarial elephantiasis.

The cutaneous lesion is usually on the lower leg, but it may occur on the genitalia, buttocks, or arms (Fig. 20.18). In addition to the ulcers on the skin, there may be urticaria, GI upset, eosinophilia, and fever.

Dracunculiasis may be prevented by boiling drinking water, providing safe drinking water through boreholes, or filtering the water through mesh fibers. Native treatment consists of gradually extracting the worm a little each day, taking care not to rupture it; otherwise, the larvae escape into the tissues and produce fulminating inflammation. Surgical removal is the treatment of choice. Metronidazole, 500 mg/day, resolves the local inflammation and permits easier removal of the worm. Immersion in warm water promotes emergence of the worm. Global eradication is within reach, and Guinea worm disease may become a historical footnote.

Filariasis

Elephantiasis Tropica (Elephantiasis Arabum)

Filariasis is a widespread tropical disorder caused by infestation with filarial worms of *Wuchereria bancrofti*, *Brugia malayi*, or *Brugia timori* species. It is characterized by lymphedema, with resulting hypertrophy of the skin and subcutaneous tissues, and by enlargement and deformity of the affected parts, usually the legs, scrotum, or labia majora. The disease occurs more frequently in young men than women.

The onset of elephantiasis is characterized by recurrent attacks of acute lymphangitis in the affected part, associated with chills and fever (elephantoid fever) that last for several days to several weeks. These episodes recur over several months to years. After each attack, the swelling subsides only partially, and as recrudescences supervene, thickening and hypertrophy become increasingly pronounced. The overlying epidermis becomes stretched, thin, and shiny, and over years, leathery, insensitive, and verrucous or papillomatous from secondary pyogenic infection. The patient may have a dozen or more attacks in a year.

In addition to involvement of the legs and scrotum, the scalp, vulva, penis, female breasts, and arms can be affected, either alone or in association with the other regions. The manifestations vary according to the part involved. When the legs are attacked, both are usually affected somewhat symmetrically, with the principal changes occurring on the posterior aspects above the ankles and on the dorsa of the feet. At first, the thickening may be slight and associated with edema that pits on pressure. Later, the parts become massive and pachydermatous, the thickened integument hanging in apposing folds, between which there is a fetid exudate (Fig. 20.19).

When the scrotum is affected, it gradually reaches an enormous size, and the penis becomes hidden in it. The skin, which at first is glazed, is later coarse and verrucous, or in far-advanced cases, ulcerated or gangrenous. Resistant urticaria may occur. Filarial orchitis and hydrocele are common. A testicle may enlarge rapidly to the size of an apple and may be extremely painful. The swelling may subside within a few days, or the enlargement may be permanent. As a result of obstruction and dilation of the thoracic duct or some of its lower abdominal tributaries into the urinary tract, chyle appears in the urine, which assumes a milky appearance. Lobulated swellings of the inguinal and axillary glands, called varicose glands, are caused by obstructive varix and dilation of the lymphatic vessels.

Filaria are transmitted person to person by the bites of a variety of mosquitoes of the *Culex*, *Aedes*, and *Anopheles* species. The adult worms are threadlike, cylindrical, and creamy white. The females are 4–10 cm long. Microfilarial embryos may be seen as coiled, each in its own membrane near the posterior tip. Fully grown, sheathed microfilariae are 130–320 μm long. The adult worms live in the lymphatic system, where they produce microfilariae. These either remain in the lymphatic vessels or enter the peripheral bloodstream. An intermediate host is necessary for the further development of the parasite.

It is important to realize that infestation by the filaria is often asymptomatic, and elephantiasis usually occurs only if hundreds of thousands of mosquito bites occur over a period of years, with episodes of intercurrent streptococcal lymphangitis. Filariasis was endemic in the considerable Samoan population of Hawaii for half a century, and only one case of elephantiasis has occurred among this group.

The microfilariae should be sought on fresh coverslip films of blood (collected at night), urine, or other body fluid and examined with a low-power objective lens. Calcified adult worms may be demonstrated on x-ray examination, and ultrasound can detect adult worms. At times, adult filariae are found in abscesses or in material taken for pathologic examination. Specific serologic tests and a simple card test for filarial antigen are available. The prognosis in regard to survival is good, but living becomes burdensome unless the condition is alleviated.

Diethylcarbamazine, in increasing doses over a 14-day period, is the treatment of choice. This regimen clears microfilariae but not adult worms. A single dose of ivermectin may also be effective. Doxycycline and rifampicin kill the intracellular symbiotic bacteria, *Wolbachia*. This leads to long-term sterility of adult female worms and both are being studied to determine their place in the treatment of both bancroftian filariasis and onchocerciasis. A worldwide effort to eliminate these diseases is underway. Surgical procedures have

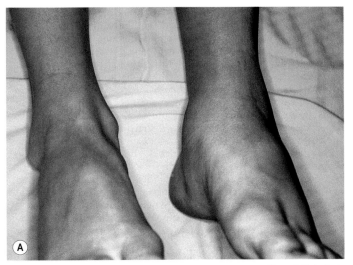

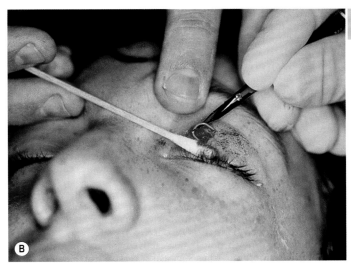

Fig. 20.20 (A and B) Loiasis. (Courtesy Curt Samlaska, MD.)

been devised to remove the edematous subcutaneous tissue from the scrotum and breast. Prophylactic measures consist of appropriate mosquito control. Diethylcarbamazine has been effective in mass prophylaxis. If a trip of over 1 month to areas with endemic *Wuchereria bancrofti* is planned and extensive exposure to mosquitoes is likely, taking diethylcarbamazine, 500 mg/day for 2 days each month, is recommended.

Loiasis (Loa Loa, Calabar Swelling, Tropical Swelling, Fugitive Swelling)

Infection with *Loa loa* is often asymptomatic. In infected persons, the parasite develops slowly, and even 3 years can elapse between infection and appearance of symptoms, although the usual interval is 1 year. The first sign is often painful, localized, subcutaneous, nonpitting edema called Calabar or fugitive swelling (Fig. 20.20A). One or more, slightly inflamed, edematous, transient swellings occur, usually about the size of a hen's egg. They typically last a few days and then subside, although recurrent swellings at the same site may eventually lead to a permanent, cystlike protuberance. These swellings may result from hypersensitivity to the adult worm or to materials elaborated by it. Eosinophilia may be as high as 90% and often is 60%–80%.

The filariae may be noticed subcutaneously in the fingers, breasts, eyelids, or submucosally under the conjunctivae. The worm may be in the anterior chamber of the eye, the myocardium, or other sites. It has a predilection for loose tissues such as the eye region, the frenum of the tongue, and the genitalia. The wanderings of the adult parasite may be noticed because of a tingling and creeping sensation. The death of the filaria in the skin may lead to the formation of fluctuant cystic lesions.

Loiasis is widely distributed in West and Central Africa, where it is transmitted by the mango fly, *Chrysops dimidia* or *Chrysops silacea*. This fly bites only in the daytime. Humans are the only important reservoir for the parasite. The observation of the worm under the conjunctiva, Calabar swellings, eosinophilia, and microfilariae in peripheral blood establish the diagnosis. Demonstration of the characteristic microfilariae in the blood during the day is possible in only about 20% of patients. Specific serologic tests are available, and luciferase immunoprecipitation systems can provide rapid diagnostic results, with improved sensitivity and specificity compared with enzyme-linked immunosorbent assay (ELISA).

Removal of the adult parasite whenever it comes to the surface of the skin is mandatory (Fig. 20.20B). This must be done quickly by seizing the worm with forceps and placing a suture under it

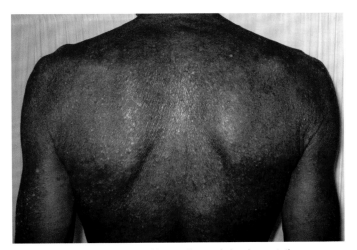

Fig. 20.21 Onchocerciasis with papules and dyspigmentation. (Courtesy Scott Norton, MD.)

before cutting down to it. Worms that are not securely and rapidly grasped may escape into the deeper tissues.

Diethylcarbamazine kills both adults and microfilariae and is given in increasing doses for 21 days. In regions where onchocerciasis and loiasis both are endemic, and where ivermectin is used in a community-based elimination strategy for onchocerciasis, simultaneously infected patients with a high *L. loa* load have a greater risk of serious side effects. If ivermectin treatment of these patients is undertaken, proper monitoring and appropriate supportive treatment should be available in anticipation of this risk. Diethylcarbamazine is an effective chemopreventive therapy, using 300 mg/week in temporary residents of regions of Africa where *L. loa* is endemic.

Onchocerciasis

The skin lesions of onchocerciasis are characterized by pruritus, dermatitis, and onchocercomas. The dermatitis is variable in appearance, probably related to chronicity of infection, age of the patient, geographic area where acquired, and relative immune responsiveness. Early in the course of the infection, an itchy papular dermatitis may occur (Fig. 20.21), and in visitors who become infected, this may be localized to one extremity. In Central America, papules may appear only on the head and neck area. This unusual localization of insect bite–appearing papules with excoriations may lead to the diagnosis in travelers returning to their home countries. In Central America, another manifestation of the acute phase of onchocerciasis is acute swelling of the face with erythema and itching, known as erisipela de la costa. In Zaire and Central America, an acute urticarial eruption is seen. The inflammation, which is accompanied by hyperpigmentation, is known as mal morado.

As time passes, the dermatitis becomes chronic and remains papular; however, thickening, lichenification, and depigmentation occur. Later, atrophy may supervene. When the depigmentation is spotted, it is known as leopard skin; when the skin is thickened, it is called elephant skin. When local edema and thickened, wrinkled, dry dermatitic changes predominate, it is sometimes called lizard skin.

In Saudi Arabia, Yemen, and East Africa, a localized type of onchocerciasis exists called sowda, Arabic for "black." It is characterized by localized, pruritic, asymmetric, usually darkly pigmented, chronic lichenified dermatitis of one leg or one body region. It is also known as the chronic hyperreactive type, and an association with antidefensin antibodies suggests a reason for this enhanced reactivity against the parasite.

After a time, firm subcutaneous nodules, pea-sized or larger, develop on various sites of the body. These nodules are onchocercomas (Fig. 20.22) containing myriad microfilariae. These occur in crops, are frequently painful, and their site varies. In parts of Africa, where natives are wholly or nearly unclothed, the lesions occur on the trunk, axillae, groin, and perineum. In Central and South America, the head, especially the scalp, is the usual site of involvement. Firm, nontender lymphadenopathy is a common finding in patients with chronically infected onchocerciasis. "Hanging groin" describes the loose, atrophic skin sack that contains these large inguinal nodes (Fig. 20.23). In about 5% of affected persons, serious eye lesions arise late in the disease, gradually leading to blindness.

Onchocerciasis is caused by *Onchocerca volvulus*, which is transmitted to humans by the bite of the black fly of the genus *Simulium*. It breeds in fast-flowing streams. When the black fly bites, it introduces larvae into the wound. The larvae reach adulthood in the subdermal connective tissue in about 1 year. Millions of the progeny then migrate back into the dermis and the aqueous humor of the eye.

Onchocerciasis occurs in Africa on the west coast, in the Sahara, Sudan, and the Victoria Nile division, where it is known as river blindness. In Central and South America, this disease can be found in Guatemala, Brazil, Venezuela, and southern Mexico.

The presence of eosinophilia, skin lesions, and onchocercomas with ocular lesions is highly suggestive in endemic areas. Frequently, the microfilariae may be found in skin shavings or dermal lymph, even when no nodules are detectable. The scapular area is the favorite site for procuring specimens for examination by means of a skin snip. This is performed in the field or office by lifting the skin with an inserted needle and then clipping off a small, superficial portion of the skin with a sharp knife or scissors. The specimen is laid in a drop of normal saline solution on a slide with a coverslip and examined under the microscope. The filariae wriggle out at the edges of the skin slice.

Specific serologic and PCR-based diagnostic tests from blood and skin biopsies are available. Other filarial parasites can be detected in similar systems. When patients with suspected onchocerciasis were given a single oral dose of 50 mg of diethylcarbamazine, a reaction consisting of edema, itching, fever, arthralgias, and exacerbation of pruritus was described as a positive Mazzotti test reaction, which supported the diagnosis of onchocerciasis.

Community-based treatment protocols have the objective of eliminating onchocerciasis from endemic areas. Severe reactions, including neurologic disease, may occur in patients simultaneously infected with *Loa loa*. Onchocercomas may be surgically excised whenever feasible. Ivermectin as a single oral dose of 150 µg/kg is the drug of choice. Skin microfilaria counts remain low at the end of 6 months' observation. Ivermectin should be repeated every 6 months to suppress the dermal and ocular microfilarial counts. More frequent dosing does not appear to reduce microfilarial counts further.

Doxycycline kills the intracellular symbiotic bacteria, *Wolbachia*, that appear to cause Mazzotti reactions and is being tested for long-term effects and determination of its place in the treatment of onchocerciasis and bancroftian filariasis. If there is eye involvement, prednisone, 1 mg/kg, should be started several days before treatment with ivermectin. Moxidectin and emodepside also appear promising as alternative drugs.

Trichinosis

Ingestion of *Trichinella spiralis* larva–containing cysts in inadequately cooked pork, bear, or walrus meat may cause trichinosis. It usually causes a puffy edema of the eyelids, redness of the conjunctivae, and sometimes urticaria or angioedema associated with hyperpyrexia, headache, erythema, GI symptoms, muscle pains, and

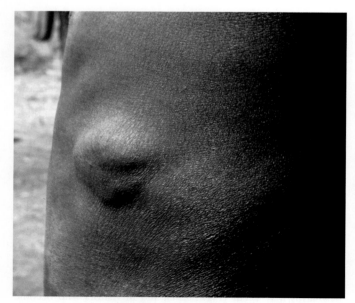

Fig. 20.22 Onchocercoma.

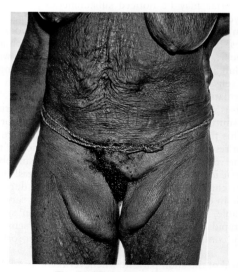

Fig. 20.23 Onchocerciasis.

neurologic signs and symptoms. Ten percent of patients develop a bilateral, asymptomatic hand swelling that is especially prominent over the digits, as well as erythema along the perimeters of the palms and volar surfaces of the digits, which progresses to desquamation. In 20% of cases, a nonspecific macular or petechial eruption occurs, and splinter hemorrhages are occasionally present. Eosinophilia is not constant but may be as high as 80%. In the average patient, eosinophilia begins about 1 week after infection and attains its height by the fourth week.

The immunofluorescence antibody test has the greatest value in establishing early diagnosis. The bentonite flocculation test, ELISA, and other serologic tests are limited by their inability to detect infection until the third or fourth week. Diagnosis is confirmed by a muscle biopsy that demonstrates larvae of *T. spiralis* in striated muscle. Unfortunately, trichinae cannot usually be demonstrated unless eosinophilic vasculitis and granulomas have been described on biopsy. A 2-mm-thick slice of the muscle biopsy may be compressed between two glass slides to demonstrate the cysts.

Trichinosis is treated with albendazole, 400 mg twice daily for 14 days. Corticosteroid agents are effective in controlling the often severe symptoms and should be given at doses of 40–60 mg/day.

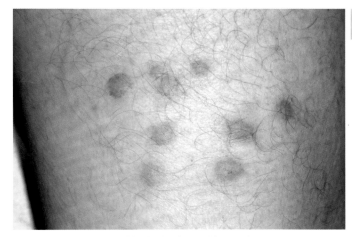

Fig. 20.24 Insect bites.

Aljayyoussi G, et al: Short-course, high-dose rifampicin achieves *Wolbachia* depletion predictive of curative outcomes in preclinical models of lymphatic filariasis and onchocerciasis. Sci Rep 2017; 7: 210.

Diaz JH: Increasing risk factors for imported and domestic gnathostomiasis in the United States. J La State Med Soc 2015; 167: 215.

Herrick JA, et al: Posttreatment reactions after single-dose diethylcarbamazine or ivermectin in subjects with *Loa loa* infection. Clin Infect Dis 2017; 64: 1017.

Hochberg NS, et al: Infections associated with exotic cuisine. Microbiol Spectr 2015; 3.

Hopkins DR, et al: Progress toward global eradication of dracunculiasis—January 2015–June 2016. MMWR Morb Mortal Wkly Rep 2016; 65: 1112.

Kaminsky RL, et al: Unsuspected Strongyloides stercoralis infection in hospital patients with comorbidity in need of proper management. BMC Infect Dis. 2016 Feb 29;16:98.

Kelly-Hope L et al: *Loa loa* vectors *Chrysops* spp. Parasit Vectors 2017; 10: 172.

Lupi O, et al: Mucocutaneous manifestations of helminth infections. J Am Acad Dermatol 2015; 73: 929.

Ng-Nguyen D, et al: A systematic review of taeniasis, cysticercosis and trichinellosis in Vietnam. Parasit Vectors 2017; 10: 150.

Rostami A, et al: Meat sources of infection for outbreaks of human trichinellosis. Food Microbiol 2017; 64: 65.

Veraldi S, et al: Treatment of hookworm-related cutaneous larva migrans with topical ivermectin. J Dermatolog Treat 2017; 28: 263.

■ PHYLUM ARTHROPODA

Phylum Arthropoda contains more species than all the other phyla combined. The classes of dermatologic significance are Myriapoda, Insecta, and Arachnida. Mosquitoes, flies, ticks, and fleas transmit diseases throughout the world. Although always prevalent, bites (Fig. 20.24) and stings increase dramatically after natural disasters such as hurricanes and flooding.

Prevention of Arthropod-Related Disease

Mosquitoes remain the most important vectors of arthropod-borne disease, and mosquito control programs are an essential component of the public health efforts of many U.S. states. Insect repellents are effective in preventing disease transmission and are especially important during travel to areas where vector-borne disease is endemic. Most are based on DEET (*N*,*N*-diethyl-3-methylbenzamide, previously called *N*,*N*-diethyl-*m*-toluamide). DEET has been tested against a wide range of arthropods, including mosquitoes, sandflies, ticks, and chiggers. The American Academy of Pediatrics recommends concentrations of 30% or less in products intended for use in children. Some evidence suggests that children do not have a higher incidence of adverse reactions than adults, but even in adults, neurotoxicity has been occasionally reported. High concentrations of DEET can produce erythema and irritation or bullous eruptions. Extended-release products reduce the need for repeated application and appear to minimize the risk of complications. Overall, DEET has a good safety record in widespread use. Picaridin is a piperidine-derived repellent ingredient that is also effective against a range of arthropods. Some studies have shown that picaridin is less irritating than DEET while providing comparable efficacy. The best studies for the evaluation of repellents are field trials that involve a range of arthropods. "Arm box" studies are still performed but must be interpreted with caution.

Citronella candles have little documented efficacy, but neem oil is an effective mosquito repellent used in many areas of the world that are endemic for malaria. Geraniol candles show some efficacy, but only in the area immediately surrounding the candles. Repellency decreases significantly at a distance of even 2 m. Candles with geraniol are twice as effective as those with linalool and five times as effective as those with citronella. IR3535 (ethyl-butyl-acetyl aminopropionate) in a variety of formulations has also demonstrated good efficacy against mosquitoes, with complete protection in field trials of 7.1–10.3 hours.

Travelers to malaria-endemic areas should follow CDC guidelines for malaria prophylaxis. They should also avoid nighttime outdoor exposure and use protective measures such as repellents and bed netting. The anopheline mosquitoes that carry malaria tend to bite at night, so bed nets and screens are important measures. Mosquitoes that carry dengue mostly bite during the day. Repellents play a greater role in protection against dengue, because it is more difficult to limit daytime outdoor activity. Mosquito control programs depend largely on drainage of stagnant water and spraying of breeding areas. In developing countries, water barrels may be stocked with fish or turtles to consume mosquito larvae. Both can soil the water, however, and the relative risks must be evaluated; some studies clearly show the risk favors stocking the barrel. Mosquito traps (e.g., Mosquito Magnet) have been effective for the control of mosquitoes in limited areas. Generally, mosquitoes fly upwind to bite and downwind to return to their resting area. Mosquito traps must be positioned between the breeding and resting areas and the area to be protected.

Mosquito traps commonly use carbon dioxide (CO_2), heat, and chemical attractants. Some *Culex* mosquitoes are repelled by octenol, and the manufacturer may provide guidelines for areas where the attractant should not be used.

Prevention of Disease From Ticks and Chiggers

Tick-borne diseases include rickettsial fevers, ehrlichiosis, Lyme disease, babesiosis, relapsing fever, and tularemia. Most require a sustained tick attachment of more than 24 hours for effective transmission, and frequent tick checks with prompt removal of ticks is an important strategy for the prevention of tick-borne illness. Unfortunately, tick inspections frequently fail to identify the tick in time for prompt removal. Some data suggest that adult ticks are found and removed only 60% of the time within 36 hours of attachment. Nymphal ticks are even more difficult to detect and may be removed in as few as 10% of patients within the first 24 hours. Because of this, repellents and acaricides remain critical for preventing tick-borne illness.

Permethrin has killing activity against a wide range of arthropods. Some North African *Hyalomma* ticks are resistant to permethrin and may exhibit a paradoxic pheromone-like attachment response when exposed to the agent, but permethrin performs very well with other species of tick, as well as mosquitoes and chiggers. It can be used to treat clothing, sleeping bags, mosquito netting, and tents. Permethrin-treated clothing, used in conjunction with a repellent, provides exceptional protection against bites in most areas of the world. Permethrin has a good record of safety, although there is a report of congenital leukemia with 11q23/*MLL* rearrangement in a preterm female infant whose mother had abused permethrin because of a pathologic fear of spiders. Permethrin can induce cleavage of the *MLL* gene in cell culture, providing a plausible link between the agent and the leukemia. It should be emphasized that permethrin in this case was not used according to the manufacturer's instructions, and the theoretic risk of carcinogenicity should be weighed against the very real risk of death from arthropod-borne disease. Cardiac glycosides have also been used topically as acaricides and have performed well in limited studies.

Ixodes scapularis is the major North American vector for Lyme disease, human granulocytic ehrlichiosis, and human babesiosis. A Lyme vaccine marketed in the United States was a commercial failure and withdrawn. Prevention of Lyme disease now centers on prevention of tick attachments and prompt tick removal. Backyards and recreational areas adjacent to wooded areas have higher rates of tick infestation. Tick numbers can be reduced by deer fencing, removal of leaf debris, application of an acaricide, and creation of border beds with wood chip mulch or gravel. Bait boxes and deer feeding stations can deliver a topical acaricide while the animal feeds. Parasitic wasps control tick numbers in nature, but wasp populations may fluctuate, and investment in wasp control may be a risky venture compared with other forms of tick control. Other natural forms of tick control have been investigated because of their potential to become self-sustaining in the environment, at least for a time; fungi and nematodes show some promise. In southern U.S. states, fire ants control tick populations by eating tick eggs.

Prevention of Flea-Borne Illness

Fleas are important vectors of plague and endemic typhus. They may also be vectors of cat-scratch disease. Lufenuron is a maturation inhibitor that prevents fleas from breeding. It is often used in oral and injectable forms for the prevention of flea infestation in cats and dogs. Fipronil is used topically for the prevention of flea and tick infestation. Other agents in use include imidacloprid, selamectin, and nitenpyram. House sprays often include pyrethroids or pyriproxyfen. Powdered boric acid may be helpful for the

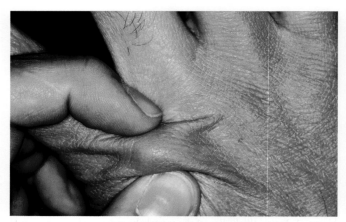

Fig. 20.25 Centipede bite.

treatment of infested carpets or floor boards. A knowledgeable veterinarian and an exterminator should be consulted.

CLASS MYRIAPODA

Morphologically and genetically, the class Myriapoda is distinct from other groups of arthropod. This group contains the centipedes and millipedes, both capable of producing significant skin manifestations.

Centipede Bites (Chilopoda)

Centipede bites are manifested by paired hemorrhagic marks that form a chevron shape caused by the large, paired mouthparts. The bite is surrounded by an erythematous swelling (Fig. 20.25) that may progress into a brawny edema or lymphangitis. Locally, there may be intense itching and pain, often associated with toxic constitutional symptoms. Most centipede bites run a benign, self-limited course, and treatment is only supportive. Children are often bitten when they try to handle centipedes. Some species of *Scolopendra* in the western United States will attain a length of 15–20 cm, and the child may describe it as a snake. Recognition of the characteristic chevron shape is important to avoid inappropriate treatment with snake antivenin. In the eastern United States, the common house centipede, *Scutigera coleoptrata*, does not bite humans. *Scolopendra subspinipes*, in Hawaii, inflicts a painful bite. As exotic species appear more often at pet stores and swap meets, envenomation by them will become more common.

In some tropical and subtropical areas, centipede bites account for about 17% of all envenomations, compared with 45% caused by snakes and 20% by scorpions. Most bites occur at home and involve an upper extremity. Local pain and edema occur in up to 96% of patients, depending on the species involved. Treatment is largely symptomatic. Rest, ice, and elevation may be sufficient, but topical or intralesional anesthetics may be required in some cases. Tetanus immunization should be considered if the patient has not been immunized within the past 10 years. Centipede bites can result in Wells syndrome, requiring topical or intralesional corticosteroids. Rarely, bites may produce more serious toxic responses, including rhabdomyolysis, myocardial ischemia, proteinuria, and acute renal failure. These have been reported after the bite of *Scolopendra heros*, the giant desert centipede. Although centipedes have sometimes been found in association with corpses, injuries from the centipede tend to be postmortem and are rarely the cause of death. Ingestion of centipedes by children is usually associated with transient, self-limited toxic manifestations.

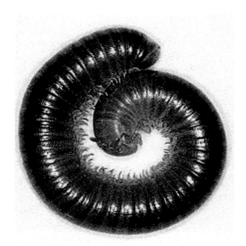

Fig. 20.26 Millipede.

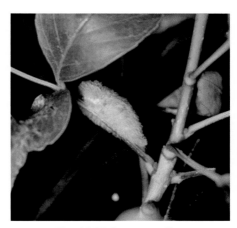

Fig. 20.27 Puss caterpillar.

Millipede Burns (Diplopoda)

Some millipedes secrete a toxic liquid that causes a brownish pigmentation or burn when it comes into contact with skin. Burns may progress to intense erythema and vesiculation. Millipedes may be found in laundry hung out to dry, and millipede burns in children have been misinterpreted as signs of child abuse. Recognition of the characteristic curved shape of the burn can be helpful in preventing misdiagnosis. Some millipedes can squirt their venom, and ocular burns are reported. Washing off the toxin as soon as possible will limit the toxic effects. Other treatment is largely symptomatic.

Diplopods have evolved a complex array of chemicals for self-defense (Fig. 20.26). Some primates take advantage of these chemicals. Two millipede compounds, 2-methyl-1,4-benzoquinone and 2-methoxy-3-methyl-1,4-benzoquinone, demonstrate a repellent effect against *Aedes aegypti* mosquitoes. Tufted and white-faced capuchin monkeys anoint themselves with the secretions to ward off mosquitoes. Effective commercial repellents are available for human use; millipede juice is not recommended.

CLASS INSECTA

Order Lepidoptera

Order Lepidoptera includes butterflies, moths, and their larval forms, caterpillars. Severe systemic reactions have resulted from ingestion of some caterpillars, and with some species, the sting alone can produce severe toxicity. *Lonomia achelous*, found in Latin America, can cause a fatal bleeding diathesis. The Spanish pine caterpillar, *Thaumetopoea pityocampa*, causes both dermatitis and anaphylactoid symptoms. Pine caterpillars are also an important cause of systemic reactions in China and Israel. The tussock moth, *Orgyia pseudotsugata*, causes respiratory symptoms in forestry workers in Oregon.

Caterpillar Dermatitis

Irritation is produced by contact of caterpillar hairs with the skin. Toxins in the hairs can produce severe pain, local pruritic erythematous macules, and wheals, depending on the species. If the hairs embed in the clothing, widespread persistent dermatitis may result. Not only the caterpillars, but also their egg covers and cocoons usually contain stinging hairs. In the United States the most common caterpillars of medical importance are the brown-tail moth caterpillar (*Nygmia phoeorrhoea*), puss caterpillar

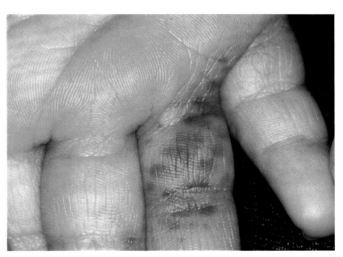

Fig. 20.28 Characteristic "railroad track" purpura of a puss caterpillar sting.

(*Megalopyge opercularis*) (Figs. 20.27 and 20.28), saddleback caterpillar (*Sibine stimulate;* Fig. 20.29), io moth caterpillar (*Automeris io*), crinkled flannel moth caterpillar (*Megalopyge crispata*), Oklahoma puss caterpillar (*Lagoa crispata*), Douglas fir tussock moth caterpillar (*Orgyia pseudotsugata*), buck moth caterpillar (*Hemileuca maia*), and flannel moth caterpillar (*Norape cretata*). The hairs of the European processionary caterpillar (*Thaumetopoea processionea*) are especially dangerous to the eyes, but ophthalmia nodosa (papular reaction to embedded hairs) can be seen with a wide variety of caterpillars and moths. Airborne processionary caterpillar hairs have caused large epidemics of caterpillar dermatitis.

Moth Dermatitis

Moth dermatitis may be initiated by the hairs of the brown-tail moth (*Euproctis chrysorrhoea*), goat moth (*Cossus cossus*), puss moth (*Dicranura vinula*), gypsy moth (*Lymantria dispar*), and Douglas fir tussock moth (*Hemenocampa pseudotsugata*). In Latin America, the moths of the genus *Hylesia* are most frequently the cause of moth dermatitis. Severe conjunctivitis and pruritus are the first signs and may persist for weeks aboard ships that have docked in ports where the moth is common. Caripito itch is named after Caripito, Venezuela, a port city where the moth is found. Korean yellow moth dermatitis is caused by *Euproctis flava* Bremer. Saturnid caterpillars (*Lonomia* sp.) are associated with a severe and often

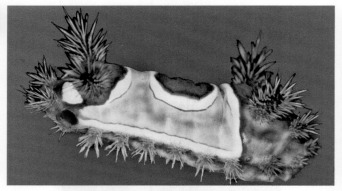

Fig. 20.29 Saddleback caterpillar.

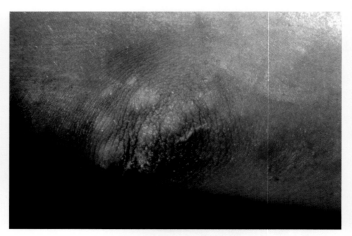

Fig. 20.31 Bedbug bites.

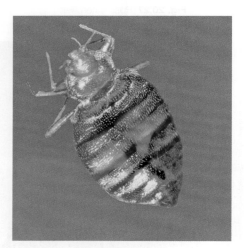

Fig. 20.30 Bedbug.

fatal hemorrhagic diathesis. In India, inhalation of tiger moth fluids, scales and hairs has been implicated as a causes of severe fever and death during the monsoon season.

Topical applications of various analgesics, antibiotics, and oral antihistamines are of little help. Topical or oral corticosteroids are sometimes helpful, as is scrubbing and tape stripping of skin. Contaminated clothing may need to be discarded if dermatitis persists after the clothing is washed.

Haddad V Jr, et al: Tropical dermatology. J Am Acad Dermatol 2012; 67: 331.e1.

Wills PJ, et al: Population explosions of tiger moth Lead to lepidopterism mimicking infectious fever outbreaks. PLoS One 2016; 11: e0152787.

Order Hemiptera

The true bugs belong to the order Hemiptera. The order includes bedbugs, water bugs, chinch bugs, stink bugs, squash bugs, and reduviid bugs (kissing bugs, assassin bugs). The latter are vectors of South American trypanosomiasis. In most true bugs, the wings are half sclerotic and half membranous and typically overlap. In bedbugs, the wings are vestigial.

Cimicosis (Bedbug Bites)

Bedbugs have flat, oval bodies and retroverted mouthparts used for taking blood meals (Fig. 20.30). *Cimex lectularius* is the most common species in temperate climates, and *Cimex hemipterus* is most common in tropical climates. Both are reddish brown and about the size of a tick. *C. hemipterus* is somewhat longer than *C. lectularius.* They breed through traumatic insemination, in which the male punctures the female and deposits sperm into her body cavity. Bedbugs hide in cracks and crevices, then descend to feed while the victim sleeps. It is common for bedbugs to inflict a series of bites in a grouping or row ("breakfast, lunch, and dinner") (Fig. 20.31). Bites may mimic urticaria, and patients with papular urticaria commonly have antibodies to bedbug antigens. Unilateral eyelid swelling has been described as a common sign of bedbug bites in children. Bullous and urticarial reactions also occur. Bedbugs have been suggested as vectors for Chagas disease, *Bartonella quintana*, and hepatitis B, although data are sparse.

Bedbugs often infest bats and birds, and these hosts may be responsible for infestation in houses. Management of the infestation may require elimination of bird nests and bat roosts. Cracks and crevices should be eliminated and the area treated with an insecticide such as dichlorvos or permethrin. Because most insecticides have poor residual effect on mud bricks, wood, and fabric, frequent retreatment may be necessary. Microencapsulation of insecticides enhances persistence. Permethrin-impregnated bednets have been shown to be effective against bedbugs in tropical climates. Ivermectin treatment is emerging as a potential ancillary measure. Bedbugs that fed once on humans 3 hours after they received 200 µg/kg of oral ivermectin had a 63% mortality rate, and survivors were unable to complete their life cycle.

Lai O, et al: Bed bugs and possible transmission of human pathogens. Arch Dermatol Res 2016; 308: 531.

Raab RW, et al: New introductions, spread of existing matrilines, and high rates of pyrethroid resistance result in chronic infestations of bed bugs (*Cimex lectularius* L.) in lower-income housing. PLoS One 2016; 11: e0117805.

Zorrilla-Vaca A: Bedbugs and vector-borne diseases. Clin Infect Dis 2014; 59: 1351.

Reduviid Bites

Triatome reduviid bugs (kissing bugs, assassin bugs, conenose bugs) descend on their victims while they sleep and feed on an exposed area of skin. The bite is typically painless, although the bugs are capable of producing a more painful defensive bite. Swelling and itching occur within hours of the bite (Fig. 20.32). Many Latin American species have a pronounced gastrocolic reflex and defecate when they feed. Romana sign is unilateral eye swelling after a nighttime encounter with a triatome bug. It resembles the "eyelid sign" associated with bedbugs. *Trypanosoma cruzi* is transmitted

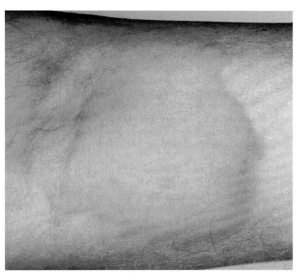

Fig. 20.32 Triatome bite.

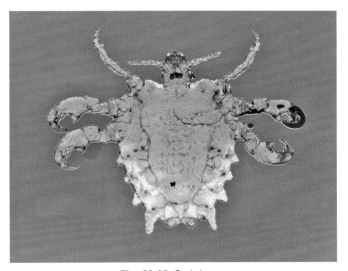

Fig. 20.33 Crab louse.

by the feces and rubbed into the bite. American trypanosomiasis can produce heart failure and megacolon. Triatome bugs infest thatch, cracks, and crevices, and infestation is associated with poor housing conditions. In nonendemic areas, bites are sporadic and often followed by a red swelling suggestive of cellulitis. Anaphylaxis has also occurred. A related arthropod, the wheel bug *Arilus cristatus*, is widely distributed and has an extremely painful defensive bite, but it is not known to carry disease.

Kapoor R, et al: What's eating you? Triatome reduviids. Cutis 2011; 87: 114.

Order Anoplura

Pediculosis

Three varieties of the flattened, wingless Anoplura insects infest humans: *Pediculus humanus* var. *capitis* (head louse), *P. humanus* var. *corporis* (body louse), and *Phthirus pubis* (pubic or crab louse) (Fig. 20.33). Rarely, zoonotic lice or louselike psocids will cause infestation.

Pediculosis Capitis. Pediculosis capitis is more common in children but also occurs in adults. Patients present with intense pruritus of the scalp and often have posterior cervical lymphadenopathy. Excoriations and small specks of louse dung are noted on the scalp, and secondary impetigo is common. Lice may be identified, especially when combing the hair. Nits may be present throughout the scalp but are most common in the retroauricular region. Generally, only those ova close to the scalp are viable, and nits noted along the distal hair shaft are empty egg cases. In extremely humid climates, however, viable ova may be present along the entire length of the hair shaft. Peripilar keratin (hair) casts are remnants of the inner root sheath that encircle hair shafts and may be mistaken for nits. Whereas nits are firmly cemented to the hair, casts move freely along the hair shaft. Head lice readily survive immersion in water but remain fixed to scalp hairs. There is no evidence that swimming pools contribute to the spread of head lice.

Effective therapeutic agents must kill or remove both lice and ova. Ulesfia (containing benzyl alcohol) is the first nonneurotoxic U.S. Food and Drug Administration (FDA)–approved treatment for lice and represents a significant advancement. Topical spinosad, 4% dimeticone liquid gel, malathion gel, and topical ivermectin are other innovations in the treatment of head lice, but permethrin remains the most widely used pediculicide in the United States, despite widespread resistance. It is available as an over-the-counter (OTC) 1% cream rinse (Nix) and a 5% prescription cream (Elimite) that is marketed for the treatment of scabies. The 1% cream rinse must be applied after shampooing and drying the hair completely. Applying to dry hair lessens dilution of the medication. Product labeling states the medication should be applied for 10 minutes, then rinsed off, but longer applications may be required. Shampooing should not take place for 24 hours afterward. Permethrin has a favorable safety profile, although congenital leukemia has been reported, as noted earlier, and the use of insecticidal shampoos is statistically associated with leukemia. Other reported side effects include acute onset of stuttering in a toddler. Pyrethrins, combined with piperonyl butoxide (RID, A-200, R+C shampoo), are other OTC products. Lindane is rarely used because of low efficacy and potential neurotoxicity. Carbaryl is used in many parts of the world, but not in the United States. Because of the potential toxicity associated with chemical pediculicides, future therapies will be asphyxiating agents, such as those containing benzyl alcohol or dimeticone. Cure rates with dimethicone are significantly higher than with permethrin in some studies, but some dimethicone products are flammable. Other agents that asphyxiate or desiccate contain isopropyl myristate 50% or Neem oil.

Nit combing is an important adjunct to treatment but is impractical as a primary method of therapy. Metal combs are more effective than plastic combs. Acidic cream rinses make the hair easier to comb but do not dissolve nit cement, which is similar in composition to amyloid. Various "natural" remedies are marketed that contain coconut oil, anise oil, and ylang ylang oil, but these agents are potential contact allergens, and data are sparse regarding their safety and efficacy. Some data support the efficacy of tea tree oil, which is more potent than lavender or lemon oil. Other studies also support combination lotions containing 5% lavender, peppermint, and eucalyptus oils, or 10% eucalyptus and peppermint oils in various combinations of water and alcohol. The addition of 10% 1-dodecanol improves efficacy.

Aliphatic alcohols show promise as pediculicides, and crotamiton (Eurax), an antiscabietic agent, has some efficacy in the treatment of pediculosis. Because no treatment is reliably ovicidal, retreatment in 1 week is reasonable for all patients.

Resistance to pediculicides is an emerging problem in many parts of the world. The emergence of resistance to an agent is related to the frequency of its use. Knockdown resistance (KDR) is a common mechanism of resistance that manifests as lack of immobilization of the lice. Responsible gene mutations (*T929I*

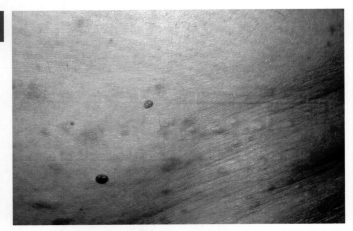

Fig. 20.34 Pediculosis corporis.

and *L932F*) have been identified and can be used to screen for KDR. Cross-resistance among pyrethroids is typical. In the United Kingdom, resistance to malathion has been reported, and multidrug-resistant lice have been identified. KDR results in slower killing of lice, but this may be overcome to some degree by longer applications. Monooxygenase-based resistance to pyrethrins may be overcome by synergism with piperonyl butoxide.

Simple public health measures are also of value when epidemics of louse infestation occur in schools. Hats, scarves, and jackets should be stored separately under each child's desk. Louse education and inspections by the school nurse facilitate targeted treatment of infested individuals.

Pediculosis Corporis. Pediculosis corporis (pediculosis vestimenti, "vagabond's disease") is caused by body lice that lay their eggs in the seams of clothing. The parasite obtains its nourishment by descending to the skin and taking a blood meal. Generalized itching is accompanied by erythematous (Fig. 20.34), blue and copper-colored macules, wheals, and lichenification. Secondary impetigo and furunculosis are common.

Body louse infestation is differentiated from scabies by the lack of involvement of the hands and feet, although infestation by both lice and scabies is common, and a given patient may have lice, scabies, and flea infestation.

Lice may live in clothing for 1 month without a blood meal. If discarding the clothing is feasible, this is best. Destruction of body lice can also be accomplished by laundering the clothing and bedding. Clothing placed in a dryer for 30 minutes at 65°C (149°F) is reliably disinfected. Pressing clothing with an iron, especially the seams, is also effective. Permethrin spray or 1% malathion powder can be used to treat clothing and reduce the risk of reinfestation.

Body lice are vectors for relapsing fever, trench fever, and epidemic typhus. These diseases are most prevalent among refugee populations. The trench fever organism is also an important cause of endocarditis among homeless persons.

Pediculosis Pubis (Crabs). Phthirus pubis, the crab louse, is found in the pubic region, as well as hairy areas of the legs, abdomen, chest, axillae, and arms. Pubic lice may also infest the eyelashes and scalp. The lice spread through close physical contact and are usually transmitted sexually. A diagnosis of pediculosis pubis should initiate a search for other STDs, including Human immunodeficiency virus (HIV) infection. Contaminated bedding is also a source of infestation. Pubic louse nits are attached to the hairs at an acute angle. Other than the presence of lice and nits in the hair, the signs and symptoms are similar to those of body louse infestation.

Occasionally, blue or slate-colored macules occur in association with pediculosis pubis. Called maculae ceruleae, these are located chiefly on the sides of the trunk and the inner aspects of the thighs and are probably caused by altered blood pigments.

Treatment of pediculosis pubis is similar to that for head lice. The affected person's sexual contacts should be treated simultaneously. For eyelash involvement, a thick coating of petrolatum can be applied twice daily for 8 days, followed by mechanical removal of any remaining nits. Fluorescein and 4% pilocarpine gel are also effective. Clothing and fomites should be washed and dried by machine, or laundered and ironed.

Arnold JD: Topical mercurials for the treatment of pediculosis. JAMA Dermatol 2017; 153: 457.
Dörge DD, et al: Flammability testing of 22 conventional European pediculicides. Parasitol Res 2017; 116: 1189.
Drugs for head lice. Med Lett Drugs Ther 2016; 58: 150.
Koch E, et al: Management of head louse infestations in the United States. Pediatr Dermatol 2016; 33: 466.
Leulmi H, et al: Assessment of oral ivermectin versus shampoo in the treatment of pediculosis (head lice infestation) in rural areas of Sine-Saloum, Senegal. Int J Antimicrob Agents 2016; 48: 627.
Semmler M, et al: Randomized, investigator-blinded, controlled clinical study with lice shampoo (Licener) versus dimethicone (Jacutin Pedicul Fluid) for the treatment of infestations with head lice. Parasitol Res 2017; 116: 1863.

Order Diptera

Order Diptera includes the two-winged biting flies and mosquitoes. Adult dipterids bite and spread disease, whereas larvae parasitize humans in the form of myiasis. Medically important families of flies include the Tabanidae (horsefly, deerfly, gadfly), which inflict extremely painful bites, and the Muscidae (housefly, stablefly, tsetse fly). Tsetse fly bites transmit African trypanosomiasis. Simulidae include the black fly (buffalo gnat, turkey gnat), the vector of onchocerciasis. These flies are dark colored and "hunchbacked." They may produce extremely painful bites that may be associated with fever, chills, and lymphadenitis. Black flies are seasonal annoyances in the northern United States and Canada.

Psychodidae sandflies (Diptera: Phlebotominae) are small, hairy-winged flies that transmit leishmaniasis, sandfly fever, and verruga peruana. Sandfly fever viruses are a problem in Africa, the Mediterranean basin, and Central Asia and are carried by *Phlebotomus* flies. *Lutzomyia* flies are common in Latin America and south Texas.

Culicidae, or mosquitoes, are vectors of many important diseases, such as filariasis, malaria, dengue, and yellow fever. Their bites may cause severe urticarial reactions. Ceratopogonidae, the biting midges or gnats, fly in swarms and produce erythematous, edematous lesions at the site of their bite.

Mosquito Bites

Moisture, warmth, CO_2, estrogens, and lactic acid in sweat attract mosquitoes. Drinking alcohol also stimulates mosquito attraction. Mosquito bites are a common cause of papular urticaria. More severe local reactions are seen in young children, individuals with immunodeficiency, and those with new exposure to indigenous mosquitoes. Immediate-type hypersensitivity can be controlled with antihistamines, and prophylactic rupatadine, 10 mg daily, has been effective in the treatment of immediate mosquito-bite allergy. Both necrotizing fasciitis and the hemophagocytic syndrome have been reported after mosquito bites, and exaggerated hypersensitivity reactions to mosquito bites are noted in a wide variety of Epstein-Barr virus (EBV)–associated lymphoproliferative disorders, especially natural killer (NK) cell proliferations.

Mosquito bites may play a key role in reactivation of latent EBV infection.

Ked Itch

The sheep ked *(Melophagus ovinus)* feeds by thrusting its sharp mouthparts into the skin and sucking blood. Occasionally, it attacks woolsorters and sheepherders, causing pruritic, often hemorrhagic papules, typically with a central punctum. Deer keds attack humans in a similar way. The papules are persistent and may last for up to 12 months. Favorite locations are the hips and abdomen.

Myiasis

Myiasis is the infestation of human tissue by fly larvae. Forms of infestation include wound myiasis, furuncular myiasis, plaque myiasis, creeping dermal myiasis, and body cavity myiasis. Wound myiasis occurs when flies lay their eggs in an open wound. Furuncular myiasis often involves a mosquito vector that carries the fly egg. Plaque myiasis typically involves many maggots and occurs after flies lay their eggs on clothing. Creeping myiasis develops when the larvae of the *Gasterophilus* fly wander intradermally. The most common species are *Gasterophilus nasalis* and *Gasterophilus intestinalis*. An itching pink papule develops, followed by a tortuous line that extends by 1–30 cm a day. Body cavity myiasis may involve the orbit, nasal cavity, GI tract, or urogenital system.

The human botfly, *Dermatobia hominis*, is a common cause of furuncular myiasis in the neotropical regions of the New World (Fig. 20.35). The female glues its eggs to the body of a mosquito, stablefly, or tick. When the unwitting vector punctures the skin by biting, the larva emerges from the egg and enters the skin through the puncture wound. Over several days, a painful furuncle develops in which the larva is present. Other larvae that frequently cause furuncular lesions in North America are the common cattle grub *(Hypoderma lineatum)*, rabbit botfly *(Cuterebra cuniculi)*, and *Wohlfahrtia vigil*. The *W. vigil* fly can penetrate infant skin, but not adult skin, so almost all reported cases have occurred in infants. The New World screw worm, *Cochliomyia hominivorax*, often involves the head and neck region. Larvae of Calliphoridae flies, especially *Phaenicia sericata*, the green blowfly, cause wound myiasis. Other blowflies, flesh flies (Sarcophagidae), and humpbacked flies (Phoridae) are less common causes of wound myiasis. In tropical Africa, the Tumbu fly *(Cordylobia anthropophaga)* deposits her eggs on the ground or on clothing. The young maggots penetrate the skin and often form a plaque with many furuncular-appearing lesions. *Cordylobia ruandae* and *Cordylobia rodhaini* are less frequent causes of plaque myiasis. *Oestrus ovis* causes ophthalmomyiasis that may be misdiagnosed as bacterial conjunctivitis.

Removal of the maggots of furuncular myiasis can be accomplished by injection of a local anesthetic into the skin, which causes the larva to bulge outward. The opening of the furuncle can also be occluded with hair gel, surgical lubricant, lard, petrolatum, or bacon, causing the larva to migrate outward. Successful treatment with ivermectin has also been reported.

Graveriau C, et al: Cutaneous myiasis. Travel Med Infect Dis 2017; 16: 70.
McGraw TA, et al: Cutaneous myiasis. J Am Acad Dermatol 2008; 58: 907.
Vasievich MP, et al: Got the travel bug? A review of common infections, infestations, bites, and stings among returning travelers. Am J Clin Dermatol 2016; 17: 451.

Order Coleoptera

Blister Beetle Dermatitis

Blister beetle dermatitis occurs after contact with several groups of beetle (Fig. 20.36). The Meloidae and Oedemeridae families produce injury to the skin by releasing a vesicating agent, cantharidin. Members of the family Staphylinidae (genus *Paederus*) contain a different vesicant, pederin. None of the beetles bites or stings; rather, they exude their blistering fluid if they are brushed against, pressed, or crushed on the skin. Many blister beetles are attracted at night by fluorescent lighting.

Slight burning and tingling of the skin occur within minutes, followed by the formation of bullae, often arranged linearly. "Kissing lesions" are observed when the blister beetle's excretion is deposited in the flexures of the elbows or other folds. Ingestion of beetles or cantharidin results in poisoning, presenting with hematuria and abdominal pain. In many tropical and subtropical habitats, rove beetles (genus *Paederus*) produce a patchy or linear, erythematous vesicular eruption (dermatitis linearis) (Fig. 20.37). In parts of South America, it is known as podo. It occurs frequently during the rainy season and appears predominantly on the neck and exposed parts. Lymphadenopathy and fever are common. In the

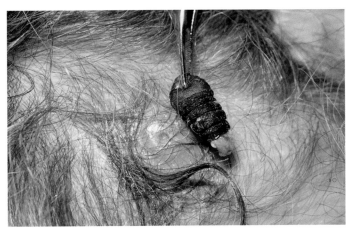

Fig. 20.35 Myiasis.

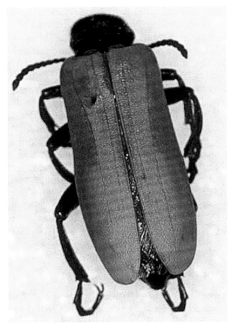

Fig. 20.36 Blister beetle.

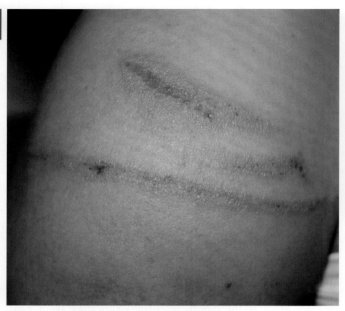

Fig. 20.37 Paederus (beetle) dermatitis. (Courtesy Shyam Verma, MBBS, DVD.)

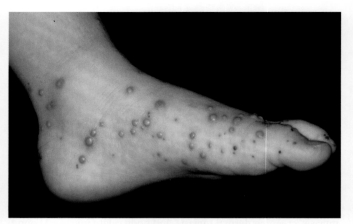

Fig. 20.38 Fire ant stings.

southwestern United States, outbreaks of rove beetle dermatitis have followed unusually rainy periods. In southeastern Australia, corneal erosions are caused by small Corylophidae beetles (*Orthoperus* spp). Blister beetle derivatives, including cantharidin, norcantharidin, cantharidimide, and norcantharimide, have significant potential as phosphoprotein phosphatase inhibitors in cancer treatment.

Treatment of blister beetle dermatitis consists of draining the bullae and applying cold wet compresses and topical antibiotic preparations. Early cleansing with acetone, ether, soap, or alcohol may be helpful to remove cantharidin.

Other Beetles

Papulovesicular and urticarial dermatitis is caused by the common carpet beetle (Dermestidae: *Anthrenus scrophulariae*). The eruption involves the chest, neck, and extremities. The larvae inhabit warm houses throughout the winter months. They are reddish brown, fusiform, about 6 mm long, and covered by hairs. A generalized pruritic eruption has been attributed to the larvae of the carpet beetle, *Anthrenus verbasci*. Bombardier beetles of the family Carabidae (subfamily Brachininae) can cause skin burns with a deep yellow-brown color. Chemicals released when these beetles are crushed include acids, phenols, hydrocarbons, and quinines. When the beetle is threatened, chemical reactions produce an explosive spray of boiling-hot benzoquinones from the tip of the abdomen. Dermestidae (skin beetles) and Cleridae (bone beetles) infest exposed human remains and are useful in estimating the postmortem interval. Rare cases of allergic angioedema have been reported after exposure to ladybugs.

Singh A, et al: Blister beetle dermatitis. Int J Prev Med 2013; 4: 241.

Order Hymenoptera

Hymenopterids include bees, wasps, hornets, and ants. Stings by any of these may manifest the characteristic clinical and histologic features of eosinophilic cellulitis (Wells syndrome), complete with flame figures.

Bees and Wasps

Yellowjackets are the principal cause of allergic reaction to insect stings, because they nest in the ground or in walls and are disturbed by outdoor activity, such as gardening or lawn mowing. Bees are generally docile and sting only when provoked, although Africanized bees display aggressive behavior. The allergens in vespid venom are phospholipase, hyaluronidase, and a protein known as antigen 5. Bee venom contains histamine, mellitin, hyaluronidase, a high-molecular-weight substance with acid phosphatase activity, and phospholipase A. The barbed ovipositor of the honeybee is torn out of the bee and remains in the skin after stinging. The bumblebee, wasp, and hornet are able to withdraw their stinger.

The reaction to these stings ranges from pain and mild local edema to exaggerated reactions that may last for days. Serum sickness, characterized by fever, urticaria, and joint pain, may occur 7–10 days after the sting. Severe anaphylactic shock and death may occur within minutes of the sting. Most hypersensitivity reactions have been shown to be mediated by specific IgE antibodies. Anaphylaxis to vespids may also be the presenting symptom of mastocytosis, with no demonstrable, specific IgE against wasp venom. Granuloma annulare and subcutaneous granulomatous reactions have been reported. Contact allergy to propolis is common among beekeepers.

Treatment of local reactions consists of immediate application of ice packs or topical anesthetics. Chronic reaction sites may be injected with triamcinolone suspension diluted to 5 mg/mL with 2% lidocaine. Oral prednisone may be required for severe local reactions.

For severe systemic reactions, 0.3 mL of epinephrine (1 : 1000 aqueous solution) is injected intramuscularly. This may need to be repeated after 10 minutes. Susceptible persons should carry a source of injectable epinephrine. Corticosteroids and epinephrine may be required for several days after severe reactions. Hyposensitization by means of venom immunotherapy can reduce the risk of anaphylaxis in people at risk. Those at risk should be evaluated by an allergist. Rush desensitization regimens exist, and ultrarush sublingual immunotherapy looks promising.

Ants

The sting of most ants is painful, but that of fire ants (*Solenopsis invicta*, *S. geminata*, or *S. richteri*) is especially painful. Fire ants are vicious and will produce many burning, painful stings within seconds if their mound is disturbed. The sting causes intense pain and whealing. Later, an intensely pruritic, sterile pustule develops at the site (Fig. 20.38). Anaphylaxis, seizures, and mononeuropathy have been reported. The sting of harvester ants and soldier ants

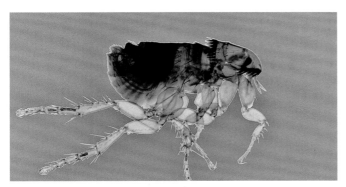

Fig. 20.39 Cat flea.

may produce similar reactions. Treatment options are similar to those for vespid stings.

Order Siphonaptera

Fleas are wingless, with highly developed legs for jumping. They are blood-sucking parasites, infesting most warm-blooded animals. Fleas are important vectors of plague, endemic typhus, brucellosis, melioidosis, and erysipeloid.

Pulicosis (Flea Bites)

The species of flea that most frequently attack humans are the cat flea (*Ctenocephalides felis*; Fig. 20.39), human flea (*Pulex irritans*), dog flea (*Ctenocephalides canis*), and oriental rat flea (*Xenopsylla cheopis*). The stick-tight flea (*Echidnophaga gallinacea*), mouse flea (*Leptopsylla segnis*), and chicken flea (*Ceratophyllus gallinae*) are sometimes implicated.

Fleas are small, brown insects about 2.5 mm long, flat from side to side, with long hind legs. They slip into clothing or jump actively when disturbed. They bite about the legs and waist and may be troublesome in houses where there are dogs or cats. The lesions are often grouped and may be arranged in zigzag lines. Hypersensitivity reactions may appear as papular urticaria (Fig. 20.40), nodules, or bullae. Camphor and menthol preparations, topical corticosteroids, and topical anesthetics can be of benefit.

Vectors of Disease

Xenopsylla cheopis and *Xenopsylla braziliensis* are vectors of plague and endemic typhus. The cat flea (*Ctenocephalides felis*) is the vector for *Rickettsia felis*, a cause of endemic typhus. Plague and tularemia are transmitted by the squirrel flea, *Diamanus montanus*. Several species of flea are intermediate hosts of the dog tapeworm and rat tapeworm, which may be an incidental parasite of humans.

Tungiasis

Tunga penetrans is also known as nigua, the chigoe, sand flea, or jigger. It is a reddish brown flea about 1 mm long. It resides in the Caribbean, equatorial Africa, Central and South America, India, and Pakistan. It was first reported in crewmen who sailed with Christopher Columbus.

The female chigoe burrows into the skin, often adjacent to a toenail, where she may be seen with the aid of dermoscopy. Once embedded, the flea becomes impregnated and ova develop (Fig. 20.41). Skin lesions are pruritic swellings the size of a small pea. These may occur on the ankles, feet, and soles, as well as the anogenital areas. The lesions become extremely painful and secondarily infected. Wearing open shoes and the presence of pigs in the area are risk factors for disease.

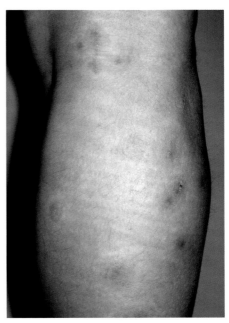

Fig. 20.40 Flea bites. (Courtesy Curt Samlaska, MD.)

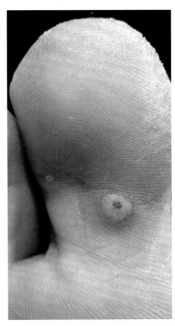

Fig. 20.41 Tungiasis. (Courtesy Catherine Quirk, MD.)

Curettage or excision may be required, but many lesions will respond to topical ivermectin, metrifonate, dimethicone, thiabendazole or oral thiabendazole, 25 mg/kg/day. Antibiotics should be used for the secondary infection and tetanus prophylaxis given. These lesions can be prevented by the wearing of shoes. Infested ground and buildings may be disinfected with insecticides and growth inhibitors.

Nordin P, et al: Treatment of tungiasis with a two-component dimeticone. Trop Med Health 2017; 45: 6.

Wafula ST, et al: Prevalence and risk factors associated with tungiasis in Mayuge district, Eastern Uganda. Pan Afr Med J 2016; 24: 77.

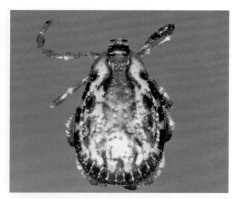

Fig. 20.42 Dermacentor variabilis.

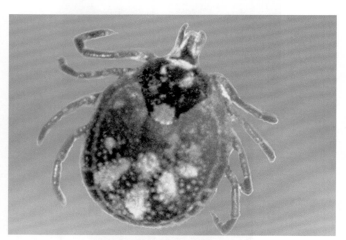

Fig. 20.43 Lone star tick.

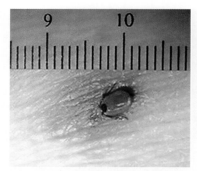

Fig. 20.44 Tick bite.

CLASS ARACHNIDA

Arachnida includes the ticks, mites, spiders, and scorpions. Adult and nymph stages of arachnids have four pairs of legs, and larval forms have six legs. Their bodies consist of cephalothorax and abdomen, in contrast to insects, which have three body segments.

Order Acarina

Tick Bite

Several varieties of the family Ixodidae (hard ticks) and Argasidae (soft ticks) will attack human skin, but only hard ticks remain attached. In the United States *Ornithodoros hermsi*, *O. turicata*, and *O. parkeri* transmit tick-borne relapsing fever. The wood tick (*Dermacentor andersoni*) is an important disease vector in western states. It carries Rocky Mountain spotted fever, tularemia, ehrlichiosis, and Colorado tick fever. The dog tick (*Dermacentor variabilis*; Fig. 20.42) is prevalent in the eastern U.S. states and is the most common vector of Rocky Mountain spotted fever. It also carries tularemia. *Dermacentor marginatus* transmits tick-borne lymphadenopathy in Spain. *Haemaphysalis longicornis* ticks are vectors for severe fever with thrombocytopenia syndrome, associated a high mortality rate in China, South Korea and Japan. The brown dog tick (*Rhipicephalus sanguineus*) is a vector of Rocky Mountain spotted fever, tularemia, and boutonneuse fever. The lone star tick (*Amblyomma americanum*; Fig. 20.43) carries Rocky Mountain spotted fever, tularemia, and human monocytic ehrlichiosis. *Ixodes ricinus* in Europe and *I. scapularis* and *I. pacificus* in the United States transmit *Borrelia burgdorferi*, the cause of Lyme disease.

Ixodes ticks also transmit human granulocytic ehrlichiosis and babesiosis. The risk of disease transmission increases with the duration of tick attachment. Unfortunately, ticks often attach in areas where they are not noticed, allowing them to engorge and transmit disease.

The female hard tick attaches itself to the skin by sticking its proboscis into the flesh to suck blood from the superficial vessels. The insertion of the hypostome is generally unnoticed by the subject. The attached tick may be mistaken by the patient for a new mole (Fig. 20.44). The parasite slowly becomes engorged and then falls off. During this time, which may last for 7–12 days, the patient may have fever, chills, headache, abdominal pain, and vomiting (tick bite pyrexia). Removal of the engorged tick causes a subsidence of the general symptoms in 12–36 hours.

The bites may be followed by small, severely pruritic, fibrous nodules (tick bite granulomas) that persist for months or by pruritic, circinate and arciform, localized erythemas that may also persist over months. Tick bite–induced alopecia has been reported, and both *Amblyomma americanum* and *Ixodes* tick bites are associated with the development of IgE antibodies to the carbohydrate galactose-α-1,3-galactose, causing delayed urticaria and anaphylaxis after consumption of red meat.

Histologically, bite reactions demonstrate wedge-shaped necrosis with a neutrophilic infiltrate and vascular thrombosis or hemorrhage. Chronic bite reactions often have atypical CD30+ lymphocytes and eosinophils. Pseudolymphomas and immunocytomas may occur.

Tick Paralysis

Tick paralysis most often affects children and carries a mortality rate of about 10%. Flaccid paralysis begins in the legs, then the arms, and finally the neck, resembling Landry-Guillain-Barré syndrome. Bulbar paralysis, dysarthria, dysphagia, and death from respiratory failure may occur. Prompt recovery occurs if the tick is found and removed before the terminal stage. *Dermacentor* ticks in North America and *Ixodes* ticks in Australia are the most important causes of tick paralysis. Because *Dermacentor* ticks typically attach to the scalp, they may go unnoticed.

Cutler SJ, et al: Diagnosing borreliosis. Vector Borne Zoonotic Dis 2017; 17: 2.
de la Fuente J, et al: Tick-pathogen interactions and vector competence. 2017; 7: 114.
Erickson TB, et al: Arthropod envenomation in North America. Emerg Med Clin North Am 2017; 35: 355.
Graves SR, et al: Tick-borne infectious diseases in Australia. Med J Aust 2017; 206: 320.
Huygelen V, et al: Effective methods for tick removal. J Evid Based Med 2017; 10: 177.
Schorderet-Weber S, et al: Blocking transmission of vector-borne diseases. Int J Parasitol Drugs Drug Resist 2017; 7: 90.

Wolver SE, et al: A peculiar cause of anaphylaxis. J Gen Intern Med 2013; 28: 322.

Zhan J, et al: Current status of severe fever with thrombocytopenia syndrome in China. Virol Sin 2017; 32: 51.

Mites

Scabies. *Sarcoptes scabiei*, the itch mite, is an oval, ventrally flattened mite with dorsal spines. The fertilized female burrows into the stratum corneum and deposits her eggs. Scabies is characterized by pruritic papular lesions, excoriations, and burrows. Sites of predilection include the finger webs (Fig. 20.45), wrists, axillae, areolae, umbilicus, lower abdomen, genitals (Fig. 20.46), and buttocks (Fig. 20.47). An imaginary circle intersecting the main sites of involvement—axillae, elbow flexures, wrists and hands, and crotch—has long been called the circle of Hebra. In adults, the scalp and face are usually spared, but in infants, lesions are usually present over the entire cutaneous surface (Fig. 20.48). The burrows appear as slightly elevated, grayish, tortuous lines in the skin. A vesicle or pustule containing the mite may be noted at the end of the burrow, especially in infants and children. To identify burrows quickly, a drop of India ink or gentian violet can be applied to the infested area, then removed with alcohol. Thin, threadlike burrows retain the ink.

The eruption varies considerably, depending on the length of infestation, previous sensitization, and prior treatment. It also varies with climate and the host's immunologic status. Lichenification, impetigo, and furunculosis may be present. Bullous lesions may contain many eosinophils, resembling bullous pemphigoid. Positive immunofluorescent findings may also be noted. Scabies has also been reported to trigger epidermolysis bullosa (EB) pruriginosa, a variant of dystrophic EB. Scabies may also resemble

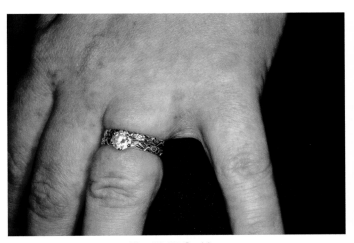

Fig. 20.45 Scabies.

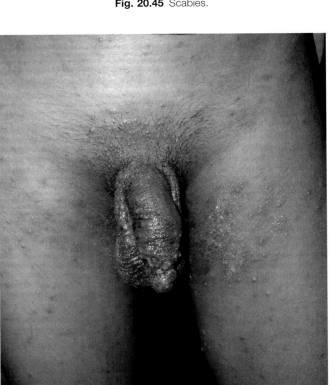

Fig. 20.46 Scabies. (Courtesy Dr. Shyam Verma.)

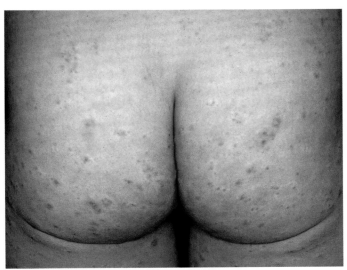

Fig. 20.47 Scabies.

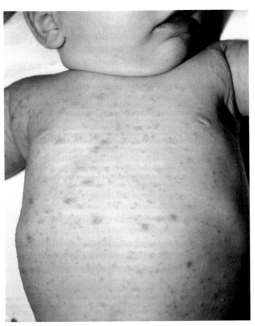

Fig. 20.48 Scabies.

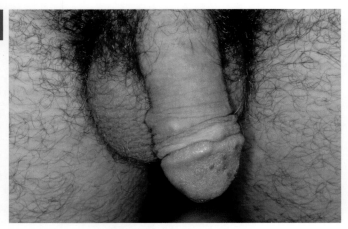

Fig. 20.49 Nodular scabies.

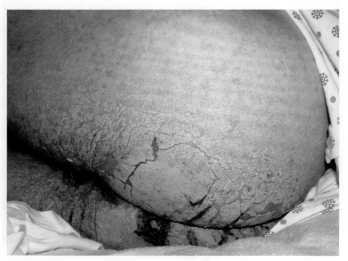

Fig. 20.50 Crusted scabies in an HIV-infected patient. (Courtesy Curt Samlaska, MD.)

Langerhans cell histiocytosis clinically and histologically. Misdiagnosis has led to systemic treatment with toxic agents.

Dull-red nodules may appear during active scabies; these are 3–5 mm in diameter, may or may not itch, and persist on the scrotum, penis (Fig. 20.49), and vulva. Intralesional steroids, tar, or excision are methods of treatment for this troublesome condition, termed nodular scabies. Histologically, the lesions may suggest lymphoma.

Crusted scabies (Norwegian or hyperkeratotic scabies) is found in immunocompromised or debilitated patients, including those with neurologic disorders, Down syndrome, organ transplants, graft-versus-host disease, adult T-cell leukemia, Hansen disease, or AIDS. In these patients, the infestation assumes a heavily scaling and crusted appearance. Crusts and scales teem with mites, and the face is involved, especially the scalp. Itching may be slight. Psoriasis-like scaling is noted around and under the nails. The tips of the fingers are swollen and crusted and the nails distorted. Severe fissuring and scaling of the genitalia and buttocks may be present (Fig. 20.50). Pressure-bearing areas are the sites of predilection for the heavy keratotic lesions, in which the mites may abound.

Scabies is usually contracted by close personal contact, although it may also be transmitted by contaminated linens and clothing. Screening for other STDs is appropriate in adults. Sensitization begins about 2–4 weeks after onset of infection. During this

time, the parasites may be on the skin and may burrow into it without causing pruritus or discomfort. Severe itching begins with sensitization of the host. In reinfections, itching begins within days, and the reaction may be clinically more intense. The itching is most intense at night, whereas during the daytime, the pruritus is tolerable but persistent. The eruption does not involve the face or scalp in adults. In women, itching of the nipples associated with a generalized pruritic papular eruption is characteristic; in men, itchy papules on the scrotum and penis are equally typical. When more than one member of the family has pruritus, scabies should be suspected. Whenever possible, however, it is advisable to identify the mite, because a diagnosis of scabies usually requires treatment of close physical contacts in addition to the patient. Because scabies cannot always be excluded by examination, treatment on presumption of scabies is sometimes necessary.

Positive diagnosis is made only by the demonstration of the mite under the microscope. A burrow is sought and position of the mite determined. A surgical blade or sterile needle is used to remove the parasite. A drop of mineral or immersion oil can be placed on a lesion and gently scraped away with the epidermis beneath it. The majority of mites are found on the hands and wrists, less frequently (in decreasing order) at the elbows, genitalia, buttocks, and axillae. Children have often gathered mites and ova under the nails when scratching. A blunt curette can be used to gather material from under the nails for examination. Noninvasive techniques include dermoscopy and digital photography.

Permethrin 5% cream, 6%–10% precipitated sulfur in petrolatum, and benzyl benzoate are the most widely used topical agents. Permethrin is a synthetic pyrethroid that has low toxicity for humans, although some concern has been raised about a possible association between topical insecticides and hematopoietic malignancy. Lindane (γ-benzene hexachloride) is rarely used as a first-line agent and is banned in some locations because of concerns about neurotoxicity. Oral ivermectin at a dose of 200 µg/kg is typically repeated in 7–10 days, but is often used in a single dose for mass infestations in resource-constrained settings. European guidelines cite permethrin, oral ivermectin and benzyl benzoate as first line agents. They list topical formulations of malathion, ivermectin and sulfur as alternatives. Japanese guidelines list topical phenothrin or oral ivermectin as first line agents and topical sulfur, crotamiton or benzyl benzoate as alternatives. German guidelines also list crotamiton as a second-line agent. Moxidectin and *Tinospora cordifolia* lotion appear promising and have the potential to replace other treatments.

Topical scabicides should be thoroughly rubbed into the skin from the neck to the feet, with particular attention given to the creases, perianal areas, umbilicus, and free nail edge and folds. They are washed off 8–10 hours later. Clothing and bed linen are changed and laundered thoroughly. Crotamiton (Eurax) has a lower cure rate than other available agents. When used, it should be applied on five successive nights and washed off 24 hours after the last use.

In the crusted type of scabies, ivermectin should be used in conjunction with a topical agent. It may need to be repeated two or three times at intervals of 1–2 weeks. Individuals in close contact with the patient should be treated. Scabies in long-term health care facilities is an increasing problem. Delays in treating close contacts may result in large numbers of persons requiring treatment. Ivermectin has no selective fetal toxicity in animal studies. Permethrin is often used in pregnancy, but because of the reported association between pyrethroids and leukemia, some prefer sulfur in this setting.

Animal Scabies. Zoonotic scabies and scab mites may affect humans who come in close contact with the animal. The reaction resembles scabies but typically runs a self-limited course. Burrows are usually absent.

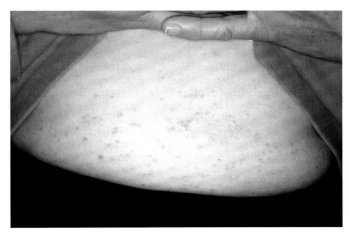

Fig. 20.51 Cheyletiella mite bites. (Courtesy Scott Norton, MD.)

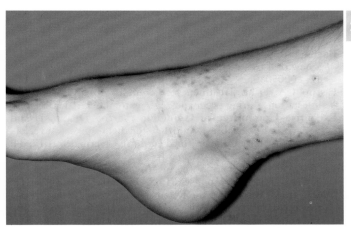

Fig. 20.52 Chigger bites.

Other Mite Diseases

Demodex Mites. *Demodex folliculorum* is a vermiform mite that inhabits the pilosebaceous units of the nose, forehead, chin, and scalp. The mite has a flattened head, four pairs of short, peglike legs, and an elongated abdomen. *Demodex brevis* is shorter and more often found on the trunk.

In dogs, the lesions of demodectic mange contain numerous mites. In humans, there are convincing reports of demodectic blepharitis, demodectic folliculitis, demodectic abscess, and demodectic alopecia that respond to eradication of the mites. Some rosacea-like lesions may also be caused by *Demodex*. Treatment of the eruptions in which *Demodex* has been implicated consists of applying permethrin, sulfur, lindane, benzyl benzoate, or benzoyl peroxide. Oral ivermectin and metronidazole have also been used.

Cheyletiella Dermatitis. *Cheyletiella yasguri, Cheyletiella blakei,* and *Cheyletiella parasitovorax* are three species of nonburrowing mite that are parasitic on dogs, cats, and rabbits, respectively, where they present as "walking dandruff." They may bite humans when there is close contact with the animals, producing an itchy dermatitis (Fig. 20.51) resembling scabies or immunobullous disease. The mites are similar in diameter to *Sarcoptes scabiei* but are elongated and have prominent anterior hooked palps. They may be found by brushing the animal's hair over a dark piece of paper. The brushings can be placed in alcohol, where the scales and hair sink while the mites float. The pet should be treated by a qualified veterinarian.

Chigger Bite. The trombiculid mites are known as chiggers, mower's mites, or red bugs. In North America, *Trombicula (Eutrombicula) alfreddugesi* attacks humans and animals. In Europe, the harvest mite, *Neotrombicula autumnalis,* is a common nuisance. Attacks occur chiefly during the summer and fall, when individuals have more frequent contact with mite-infested grass and bushes. The lesions occur chiefly on the legs (Fig. 20.52) and at the belt line and other sites where clothing causes constriction. Penile lesions are common in males. Lesions generally consist of severely pruritic, hemorrhagic puncta surrounded by red swellings. On the ankles, intensely pruritic, grouped, excoriated papules are noted. Several varieties of trombiculid mite in East Asia and the South Pacific are vectors of scrub typhus (tsutsugamushi fever).

Gamasoidosis. Gamasoidosis is caused by two genera of mites, *Ornithonyssus* and *Dermanyssus*, and occurs after contact with canaries, pigeons, and poultry. Because of the association with pigeons, the dermatitis is common among urban dwellers, and because of the small size of the mites and their tendency to leave the host after biting, the diagnosis may not be considered. In pet stores, bird mites may be transmitted to rodents with human disease related to contact with a gerbil or hamster. The mites are active at night and hide during the day. The resulting dermatosis occurs chiefly on the hands and arms as itchy macules, papules, or vesicles. Any body area may be attacked, and common additional sites are the groin, areolae, umbilicus, face, and scalp. The mites may wander from bird nests as soon as the young birds begin to fly, and they may infest terrace cushions and patio furniture. The tropical fowl mite (*Ornithonyssus bursa*) and the red chicken mite (*Dermanyssus gallina*) are the major culprits. *Dermanyssus* mites may carry *Erysipelothrix rhusiopathiae*.

Grocer's Itch. Grocer's itch is a pruritic dermatitis of the forearms, with occasional inflammatory and urticarial papules on the trunk. It results from the handling of figs, dates, and prunes, when it is caused by *Carpoglyphus passularum*, or from exposure to the cheese mite (*Glyciphagus domesticus*). This must be distinguished from grocer's eczema, which is caused by sensitization to flour, sugar, cinnamon, chocolate, and similar items.

Grain Itch. Grain itch is also known as straw itch, barley itch, mattress itch, and prairie itch. Causative mites include *Pyemotes tritici, Pyemotes ventricosus, Cheyletus malaccensis*, and *Tyrophagus putrescentiae* (copra itch mite). Those mainly affected are harvesters of wheat, hay, barley, oats, and other cereals or farm hands and packers who have contact with straw. Grain itch has a typical lesion consisting of an urticarial papule on which there is a small vesicle. There is intense pruritus, with lesions occurring predominantly on the trunk. Frequently, an initial central hemorrhagic punctum rapidly turns into an ecchymosis with hemosiderin pigmentation.

Other Mite-Related Dermatitides. *Dermatophagoides pteronyssinus* and *D. farinae* are dust mites implicated in atopic diseases. *Lepidoglyphus destructor* is the hay mite. There have been outbreaks of *Pyemotes boylei* bites in homes fumigated for termites. Although mites do not appear capable of survival when forced to share an environment with termites, they thrive in locations where there are termite carcasses. Vanillism is a dermatitis caused by *Acarus siro* and occurs in workers handling vanilla pods. Copra itch occurs on persons handling copra who are subject to *Tyrophagus longior* mite bites. Coolie itch is found on tea plantations in India and is caused by *Rhizoglyphus parasiticus;* it causes sore feet. Rat mite itch, caused by *Ornithonyssus bacoti*, the tropical rat mite, may result in an intensely pruritic dermatitis. This papulovesicular urticarial eruption is seen in workers in stores, factories, warehouses, and stockyards. The rat mite may transmit endemic typhus, rickettsialpox, equine encephalitis, tularemia, plague, and relapsing fever. Feather pillow dermatitis is a pruritic papular dermatitis traced to the Psoroptid carpet mite, *Dermatophagoides scheremetewskyi*, which may infest feather pillows. The house mouse mite, *Allodermanyssus (Liponyssoides) sanguineus*, is the vector of *Rickettsia akari*, the causative organism of rickettsialpox.

Abdel-Raheem TA, et al: Efficacy, acceptability and cost effectiveness of four therapeutic agents for treatment of scabies. J Dermatolog Treat 2016; 27: 473.

Bernigaud C, et al: Preclinical study of single-dose moxidectin, a new oral treatment for scabies. PLoS Negl Trop Dis 2016; 10: e0005030.

Elston CA, et al: Treatment of common skin infections and infestations during pregnancy. Dermatol Ther 2013; 26: 312.

Executive Committee of Guideline for the Diagnosis and Treatment of Scabies: Guideline for the diagnosis and treatment of scabies in Japan (third edition). J Dermatol 2017; 44: 991.

He R, et al: Transcriptome-microRNA analysis of *Sarcoptes scabiei* and host immune response. PLoS One 2017; 12: e0177733.

May P, et al: Protocol for the systematic review of the prevention, treatment and public health management of impetigo, scabies and fungal skin infections in resource-limited settings. Syst Rev 2016; 5: 162.

Pezzi M, et al: Gamasoidosis by the special lineage L1 of *Dermanyssus gallinae* (Acarina: Dermanyssidae). Parasitol Int 2017; 66: 666.

Reynolds HH, et al: What's eating you? Cheyletiella mites. Cutis 2017; 99: 335.

Salavastru CM, et al: European guideline for the management of scabies. J Eur Acad Dermatol Venereol 2017; 31: 1248.

Sunderkötter C, et al: S1 guidelines on the diagnosis and treatment of scabies—short version. J Dtsch Dermatol Ges 2016; 14: 1155.

Order Scorpionidae

Scorpion Sting

Scorpions are different from other arachnids in that they have an elongated abdomen ending in a stinger (Fig. 20.53). They also have a cephalothorax, four pairs of legs, pincers, and mouth pincers. Two poison glands in the back of the abdomen empty into the stinger. Scorpions are found worldwide, especially in the tropics. They are nocturnal and hide during the daytime under tabletops and in closets, shoes, and folded blankets. Ground scorpions may burrow into gravel and children's sandboxes. Buthid scorpions include the most venomous species of medical importance. Important scorpions include *Tityus serrulatus*, found in Brazil; *Buthotus tamulus*, in India; *Leiurus quinquestriatus* and *Androctonus crassicauda*, in North Africa and southwest Asia; and *Centruroides suffusus*, in Mexico. *Centruroides exilicauda* and *C. sculpturatus* are the most toxic scorpions in the United States. *Vaejovis* scorpions in the southeastern United States have been reported to cause "brown recluse–like" dermonecrotic reactions.

Scorpions sting only by accident or in self-defense. The venom causes pain, paresthesia, and variable swelling at the site. The sting of the Egyptian scorpion *(L. quinquestriatus)* has a mortality rate of 50% in children. The neurotoxic venom may produce numbness at the sting site, laryngeal edema, profuse sweating and salivation, cyanosis, nausea, and paresthesia of the tongue. There is minimal or no visible change at the sting site, and some studies have confirmed the typical absence of histologic inflammation. Death may occur from cardiac or respiratory failure, especially in children. Renal and hepatic toxicity may also occur.

Treatment depends on the species and toxic symptoms. Antiarrhythmics, antiadrenergic agents, vasodilators, and calcium channel blockers may be required. Antivenin is available for many species of scorpion and generally represents the most effective intervention.

Rodrigo C, et al: Management of scorpion envenoming. Syst Rev 2017; 6: 74.

Santos MS, et al: Clinical and epidemiological aspects of scorpionism in the world. Wilderness Environ Med 2016; 27: 504.

Order Arachnidae

Arachnidism

Spiders are prevalent throughout the world. Most are beneficial to humans, trapping many insects, but a few species are dangerous. Many spider venoms are not well characterized, and in most cases of envenomation, the responsible spider is never identified. The Brazilian armed spider *(Phoneutria nigriventer)* is well characterized. Its venom contains neurotoxins that may be fatal in children. Various reactions to spider bites have been reported, including dermonecrotic reactions, systemic toxicity, and acute generalized exanthematous pustulosis.

Latrodectism

The various species of *Latrodectus* have similar toxins and cause similar reactions in humans. The black widow spider, *Latrodectus mactans*, is of chief concern in the continental United States. It may also be found in the Caribbean region. Black widows are web-building spiders and are typically found in woodpiles and under outhouse seats. Their venom may be less potent than that of related brown widow spiders, but black widows inject more venom. *Latrodectus curacaviensis* is native to South America, and Australia and New Zealand have related red-back spiders *(Latrodectus mactans hasselti)*. *Latrodectus indistinctus* is found in Africa, and the brown widow, *Latrodectus geometricus*, is native to southern Africa and Madagascar.

The female *L. mactans* spider is 13 mm long and shiny black, with a red hourglass-shaped marking on its abdomen (Fig. 20.54). The legs are long, with a spread of up to 4 cm. The black widow

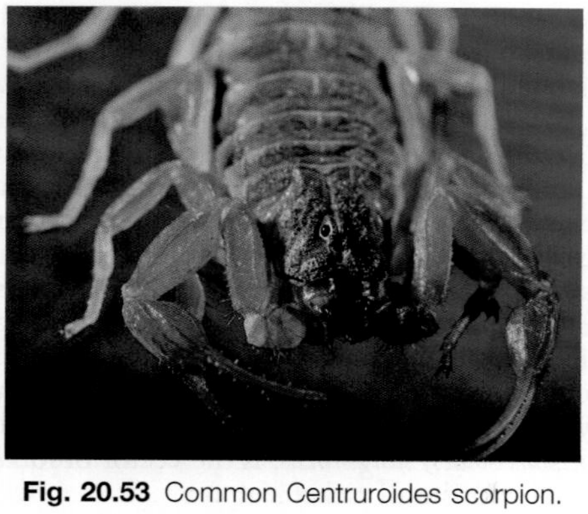

Fig. 20.53 Common Centruroides scorpion.

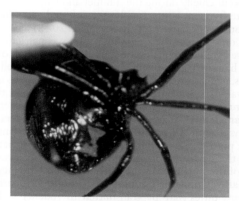

Fig. 20.54 Black widow.

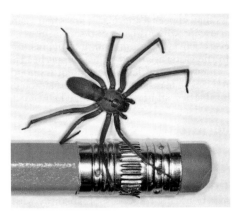

Fig. 20.55 Brown recluse spider.

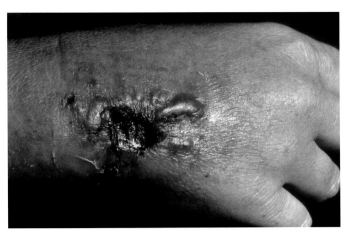

Fig. 20.56 Brown recluse spider bite. (Courtesy Steven Binnick, MD.)

spider is not aggressive and bites only when disturbed. Severe pain usually develops within a few minutes and spreads throughout the extremities and trunk. Within a few hours, the victim may have chills, vomiting, violent cramps, delirium or partial paralysis, spasms, and abdominal rigidity. The abdominal pains are frequently most severe and may be mistaken for appendicitis, colic, or food poisoning. Toxic morbilliform erythema may occur. Myocarditis has also been reported.

Antivenin is indicated for severe symptoms of envenomation. Benzodiazepines reduce the associated tetany.

Loxoscelism

The brown recluse spider *(Loxosceles reclusa)* is the major cause of necrotic arachnidism in the United States (Fig. 20.55). It is most common in the lower Midwest and Southwest. This reclusive spider may be identified by a dark, violin-shaped marking over the cephalothorax and three sets of eyes, rather than the usual four. It is light brown and about 1 cm long, with a small body and long delicate legs. It is found in storage closets, basements, and cupboards and among clothing. Outdoors it has been found in woodpiles, in grass, on rocky bluffs, and in barns. It stings in self-defense and is not an aggressive spider. The incidence of brown recluse bites is grossly overestimated. *Loxosceles rufescens*, *L. deserta*, and *L. arizonica* cause lesser degrees of skin necrosis. *Loxosceles laeta*, *L. intermedia*, *L. gaucho*, and *L. similis* are found in Latin America and produce changes similar to those of *L. reclusa*. The venom contains a phospholipase enzyme, sphingomyelinase D, which is the major toxin. Hyaluronidase contributes to a gravity-dependent spread of the necrotic lesions.

In the localized type of reaction, known as necrotic cutaneous loxoscelism, extensive local necrosis develops. A painful, severe edematous reaction occurs within the first 8 hours, with development of a bulla with surrounding zones of erythema and ischemia. In about 1 week, the central portion becomes dark, demarcated, and gangrenous (Fig. 20.56). Systemic loxoscelism is rare but may be associated with minor-appearing bite reactions. Systemic toxic symptoms are associated with disseminated intravascular coagulation.

Treatment. Treatment of loxoscelism consists of rest, ice, and elevation. Tetanus toxoid should be given if the patient has not received the immunization within 10 years. Some data suggest a trend toward better outcomes with injection of intralesional triamcinolone, with anecdotal reports of the injection site being spared necrosis but the areas above and below the site showing necrosis. Antibiotics and conservative debridement may be needed for necrotic wounds. Dapsone has been used, but some studies show that it is no better than placebo; dapsone also may be toxic,

especially in the setting of venom-induced hemolysis. Colchicine has also been disappointing in animal models, but tetracyclines show some promise and deserve further study. Hyperbaric oxygen has been used for slowly healing wounds.

Funnel Web Spiders

Funnel web spiders include *Tegenaria agrestis* (hobo spider or aggressive house spider of Pacific Northwest) and *Atrax robustus* (Sydney funnel web spider of Australia). Australian funnel web spiders are dangerous, but antivenin is available.

Tarantulas (Lycosidae: Theraphosidae)

Tarantulas are large, hairy hunting spiders. American species have urticating hairs that produce cutaneous wheal and flare reactions and embed in the cornea, causing ophthalmia nodosa.

Al Bshabshe A, et al: Black widow spider bites experience from tertiary care center in Saudi Arabia. Avicenna J Med 2017; 7: 51.

Chaves-Moreira D, et al: Highlights in the knowledge of brown spider toxins. J Venom Anim Toxins Incl Trop Dis 2017; 23: 6.

Hadanny A, et al: Nonhealing wounds caused by brown spider bites. Adv Skin Wound Care 2016; 29: 560.

Nentwig W, et al: Distribution and medical aspects of *Loxosceles rufescens*, one of the most invasive spiders of the world (Araneae: Sicariidae). Toxicon 2017; 132: 19.

Robinson JR, et al: Defining the complex phenotype of severe systemic loxoscelism using a large electronic health record cohort. PLoS One 2017; 12: e0174941.

◼ PHYLUM CHORDATA

Stingray Injury

The two stingray families, Dasyatidae and Myliobatidae, are among the most venomous fish known to humans. Attacks generally occur as a result of an unwary victim stepping on a partially buried stingray. A puncture-type wound occurs about the ankles or feet and later ulcerates. Sharp, shooting pain develops immediately, with edema and cyanosis. Symptoms of shock may occur. Histologically, granulomatous dermatitis and panniculitis with necrosis have been reported.

Persons wading in shallow, muddy waters where stingrays may be found should shuffle their feet through the mud to frighten the fish away. Successful treatment is usually attained by immersing the injured part in hot water for 30–60 minutes. The water should be as hot as can be tolerated, because the venom is detoxified by heat. Meperidine hydrochloride administered intravenously or intramuscularly may be necessary. If the ulcer remains unhealed after 8 weeks, excision is indicated.

Snakebite

Bites by venomous snakes are a serious problem in some parts of the world. In the United States the rattlesnake, water (cottonmouth) moccasin, copperhead, and coral snake are the venomous snakes most frequently encountered. Patients are usually young men, with 98% of bites on the extremities, most often the hands or arms. In Europe, 39% of envenomations from exotic pets are snakebites from rattlesnakes, cobras, mambas, or other venomous snakes. Almost 30 enzymes are found in snake venom, most of which are hydrolases. Snake venom has effects on the cardiovascular, hematologic, respiratory, and nervous systems. Severe envenomation may mimic brain death, with loss of other brainstem reflexes. Local effects at the bite site include the rapid onset of swelling, erythema, and ecchymosis. In more severe reactions, bullae and lymphangitis may appear. Fang marks are often visible and pain is common, except with Mojave rattlesnake bites. Antivenin is used in severe envenomation, and antitetanus measures are indicated. In the eastern United States, copperheads inflict most snakebites, followed by rattlesnakes and cottonmouths. Most of these children can be managed conservatively, although Crotalidae antivenin, antibiotics, and fasciotomy may be needed.

Lizard Bite

Heloderma suspectum, the Gila monster, is found chiefly in Arizona and New Mexico. Another venomous lizard is the beaded lizard of southwestern Mexico, *Heloderma horridum*. Bites from these poisonous lizards may cause paralysis, dyspnea, and convulsions. Systemic toxicity usually resolves spontaneously with supportive care within 1 or 2 days. Death is rare. There is no antivenin.

Clark AT, et al: A retrospective review of the presentation and treatment of stingray stings reported to a poison control system. Am J Ther; 24: e177.

Corbett B, et al: North American snake envenomation. Emerg Med Clin North Am 2017; 35: 339.

21   Chronic Blistering Dermatoses

In noninherited chronic blistering (vesicular or bullous) dermatoses, the cause of blistering is usually an autoimmune reaction, and the location where antibodies bind determines the clinical, histologic, and immunofluorescent pattern. A thorough understanding of the basement membrane zone (BMZ) structure and location of specific autoantigens and the target proteins of autoantibodies is critical. The desmoglein compensation hypothesis, based on the differential expression of desmoglein 1 and 3 at different amounts at different levels of the epidermis and mucosa, for instance, perfectly explains the observed differences in the phenotypes of pemphigus foliaceus and vulgaris. Autoantibodies that bind at the BMZ will often lead to tense bullae—but those that bind to proteins higher in that structure will often not scar, whereas antibodies against deeper parts of the BMZ will often lead to scarring and milia formation. High-frequency ultrasound has been anecdotally reported as a potential tool to determine blister location. Although the clinical and histologic findings are important, often it is the pattern of immunofluorescence that is critical in establishing the diagnosis. Usually, antibodies are circulating and can be found bound in perilesional and nonbullous lesional skin, whereas blistered skin often fails to demonstrate deposits. Biopsies of lower extremity skin should be avoided if possible, because it may be prone to false-negative results.

Salt-split-skin preparations are useful in determining the site of deposition of the autoantibodies. A 1-M solution of sodium chloride (NaCl) predictably splits skin at the level of the lamina lucida. Localization of immune deposits to the roof or floor of this split is diagnostically useful. On direct immunofluorescence (DIF) evaluation of nonsplit skin, the identification of n-serrated and u-serrated patterns of immunoglobulin deposition may provide the same information and may make salt-split-skin immunofluorescence unnecessary in some cases. An n-serrated pattern corresponds to a split above the basal lamina, whereas a u-serrated pattern corresponds to a sub–lamina densa split (see images on ExpertConsult). The subtle patterns are best seen in areas where the BMZ curves. Newer immunohistochemical stains such as C3d stain may also aid in the diagnosis in some cases. Immunoprecipitation, enzyme-linked immunosorbent assay (ELISA), and immunoblotting have helped to define the molecular targets of the autoantibodies and have revolutionized testing for immunobullous diseases. Data vary concerning the sensitivity and specificity of these tests, and not every test is universally available. In the setting of bullous pemphigoid, ELISA can produce apparent false-positive results at rates of 7% or higher, based on non-NC16a antibodies, as well as on anti–BP 180 antibodies that bind to the pathogenic NC16a domain but do not produce clinical disease and are not associated with positive indirect immunofluorescent findings. False-negative results also occur and are discussed later.

Transient acantholytic dermatosis (Grover disease) is an idiopathic nonimmune vesiculobullous disease that may mimic some histologic patterns of immunobullous disease, but shows no specific findings on DIF. Specific dermatoses of pregnancy are discussed under the differential diagnosis of herpes gestationis.

The outlook for immunobullous diseases has improved since the introduction of rituximab, intravenous immunoglobulins, and more targeted, autoantibody-directed therapies helping shift away from broadly toxic immunosuppressive regimens. Oral and ocular involvement often requires early aggressive therapy and a multidisciplinary approach.

PEMPHIGUS VULGARIS

Clinical Features

Pemphigus vulgaris (PV) is characterized by mucosal erosions and by thin-walled, relatively flaccid, easily ruptured bullae that appear on apparently normal skin and mucous membranes or on erythematous bases (Fig. 21.1). The fluid in the bulla is clear at first but may become hemorrhagic or even seropurulent. The bullae rupture to form erosions. The denuded areas soon become partially or totally covered with crusts that have little or no tendency to heal. When they finally heal, lesions often leave hyperpigmented patches but no scarring.

Usually, PV appears first in the mouth (60% of cases; Fig. 21.2) or at the site of a burn, radiation therapy, or other skin injury. Other common sites include the groin, scalp, face, neck, axillae, and genitals. Nikolsky sign is present (intact epidermis shearing away from underlying dermis, leaving a moist surface). The sign is elicited by slight pressure, twisting, or rubbing. The "bulla-spread phenomenon" (Asboe-Hansen sign) is elicited by pressure on an intact bulla, gently forcing the fluid to spread under the adjacent skin. The autoimmune bullous skin disorder intensity score (ABSIS), pemphigus vulgaris activity score (PVAS), and pemphigus disease activity index (PDAI) are scoring tools used in trials to track disease severity.

Short-lived bullae quickly rupture to involve most of the mucosa with painful erosions. The lesions extend onto the lips and form heavy, fissured crusts on the vermilion. Involvement of the throat produces hoarseness and difficulty in swallowing. The mouth odor is offensive. The esophagus may be involved, and sloughing of its entire lining in the form of a cast (esophagitis dissecans superficialis) may occur, even when the cutaneous disease appears to be well controlled because mucosa lacks desmoglein 1 and depends entirely on desmoglein 3. The conjunctiva, nasal mucosa, vagina, penis, and anus may also be involved. Chronic lesions may involve the face (Fig. 21.3), scalp, or flexures. Widespread cutaneous disease (Fig. 21.4) may cause death through sepsis or fluid and electrolyte imbalance.

The diagnosis is made by histology, immunofluorescence pattern of perilesional skin or plucked hairs, indirect immunofluorescence (IIF) testing of serum, or ELISA testing for anti–desmoglein 1 (Dsg1) and anti-Dsg3 autoantibodies. As in other autoimmune diseases, specific antibodies may be present in relatives of patients with pemphigus without the disease.

Epidemiology

PV occurs with equal frequency in men and women, usually in the fifth and sixth decades of life. It is rare in young persons. PV occurs more often in Jewish people and those of Mediterranean descent. Before the advent of corticosteroids, PV was frequently fatal; now, patients tend to suffer more from treatment-related complications.

Etiologic Factors

Antibodies in PV are most often directed against Dsg3. The presence of antibodies to both Dsg1 and Dsg3 correlates with

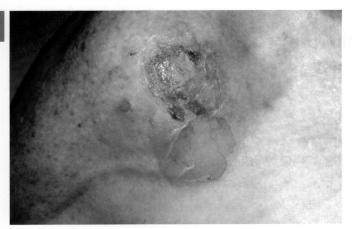

Fig. 21.1 Pemphigus vulgaris. (Courtesy Curt Samlaska, MD.)

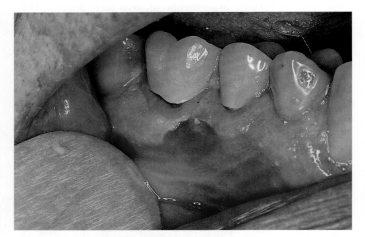

Fig. 21.2 Oral pemphigus vulgaris.

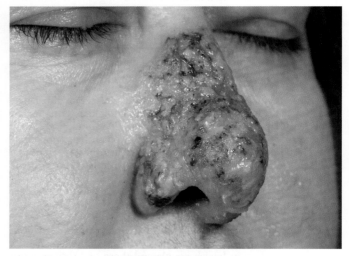

Fig. 21.3 Pemphigus vulgaris.

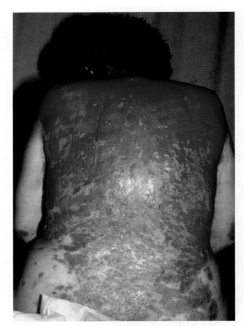

Fig. 21.4 Widespread pemphigus vulgaris.

acantholysis, without complement or inflammatory cells. Both IgG1 and IgG4 autoantibodies to Dsg3 occur in patients with pemphigus, but some data suggest that the IgG4 antibodies are pathogenic, and patients may have circulating nonpathogenic antibodies. Plasminogen activator is associated with antibody-mediated acantholysis. Involved T cells are usually CD4 cells that secrete a T-helper type 2 (Th2)–like cytokine profile, although Th1 cells may also be involved in antibody production in chronic disease. IgG is found in both involved and clinically normal skin. C3 deposits are heavier in acantholytic areas. DIF may remain positive for years after clinical remission, and conversion to negative predicts sustained remission after withdrawal of therapy. Pemphigus may be associated with myasthenia gravis and thymoma. Recent studies suggest patients with pemphigus may have an elevated rate of ulcerative colitis. PV can affect the esophagus and cause dysphagia, and patients may be misdiagnosed with steroid-side effects initially. PV-associated interstitial lung disease is reported but very rare, and some cases may have actually had paraneoplastic pemphigus.

The PV antigen (130-kD transmembrane desmosomal glycoprotein) shows homology with the cadherin family of calcium-dependent cell adhesion molecules. With IIF, circulating antibodies can be demonstrated in 80%–90% of patients. Circulating intercellular antibodies may also be present in patients with thermal or actinic burns and in patients with drug eruptions. These antibodies are not directed against Dsg3. They do not bind to the epidermis in vivo and are often directed against ABO blood-group antigens.

Drug-induced cases are uncommon, traditionally from penicillamine or angiotensin-converting enzyme (ACE) inhibitors, though recently reports of biologic-therapy associated PV have emerged. Penicillamine treatment of rheumatoid arthritis has induced pemphigus, though more often of the foliaceous type. Almost all the reported cases have had a positive DIF, and more than half have had a positive IIF. Penicillamine and captopril may induce acantholysis in organ explant cultures in the absence of autoantibody. The doses responsible for induction of disease have ranged from 250–1500 mg/day, and the drugs were taken for an average of 13 months before the onset of pemphigus. A long list of drugs, including captopril, enalapril, penicillin, thioproline, interleukin-2

mucocutaneous disease. If autoantibodies are only directed against Dsg3, mucosal lesions predominate as the mucosa lacks sufficient Dsg1 expression to compensate for the anti-Dsg3 antibody-mediated loss of keratinocyte cohesion on mucosal surfaces. Both humoral and cellular autoimmunity are important in the pathogenesis of skin lesions. Antibody alone cannot produce

(IL-2), nifedipine, piroxicam, and rifampicin, has also been reported to induce pemphigus. Many of these contain either a sulfhydryl or an amide group. Secukinumab has been reported to induce PV in one case. Only 10%–15% of patients with drug-induced pemphigus have had oral lesions. Most disease resolves when the medication is discontinued, but some cases have persisted for many months.

Many studies have indicated a genetic predisposition to pemphigus and an association with other autoimmune diseases. A strong association exists with human leukocyte antigen (HLA)–DRB1 (with variability between specific alleles in certain ethnic/racial populations), HLA-DR4, or HLA-DR6. In addition, an HLA-DQ restriction fragment has been identified in many patients with pemphigus. A non-HLA marker "suppression of tumorigenicity 18 protein" that regulates inflammation was associated with PV in Jewish and Egyptian patients but not Europeans. The incidence in Israel is among the highest in the world, with Jewish patients, particularly Ashkenazis, at three times increased risk to Arab patients, and higher rates in women than men. HLA-G is associated with pemphigus in Jewish patients. Thus there may be a genetically inherited susceptibility to the disease. Additionally, a predisposition to develop other autoimmune diseases may occur in relatives of pemphigus patients.

Histopathology

The characteristic findings of PV consist of suprabasilar acantholysis with intraepidermal blister formation. Acantholytic cells are round and show no intercellular bridges. Regeneration of the epidermis occurs and may cause the split to appear to be higher as cells regenerate beneath the cleft. At least some areas typically still demonstrate the characteristic "tombstone row" of basal keratinocytes underneath the bulla. An early intact bulla shows the most characteristic histology. Asboe-Hansen modification of the Nikolsky test may be used to extend the bulla beyond its original margin to where secondary regenerative changes have not taken place. Immunohistochemistry for IgG4 may be useful in diagnosis of PV (and PF).

In early disease, spongiosis with eosinophils may be noted in the epidermis, in the absence of acantholysis. In the setting of immunobullous disease, spongiosis with eosinophils is more likely to represent pemphigoid than pemphigus, and immunofluorescent findings readily distinguish the two. DIF demonstrates a "chicken wire" pattern of intercellular IgG in perilesional skin or plucked hairs. C3 may also be present. The staining is uniform, not granular. IIF shows a similar pattern of staining. Prozone reactions occur, so the serum should be tested at a wide range of dilutions. Positive tests may be confirmed with ELISA for the antibody.

Treatment

Pemphigus is a severe and potentially deadly disease, with patients having an increased mortality rate, and warrants aggressive immunosuppressive treatment. Large-scale, prospective, double-blinded studies are few, and the management of PV is based largely on smaller, open trials and clinical experience. A survey of 24 experienced clinicians showed that half used prednisone in doses of 1 mg/kg/day and half used higher doses. Adjuvant steroid-sparing agents were frequently employed, with almost half the respondents reporting the use of azathioprine. Because of its tolerability and simpler dosing schedule, mycophenolate mofetil (MMF) is often used in place of azathioprine. Other agents used less frequently include cyclophosphamide and methotrexate. Almost 40% of the clinicians aimed to replace prednisone with a steroid-sparing agent, whereas others were content to continue a low dose of prednisone. The survey suggests that, even among the world's experts, there is significant variation in how this difficult disease is managed. Rituximab therapy has produced dramatic responses in some

patients, and some authorities now consider rituximab appropriate first-line therapy for patients with severe disease. Intravenous immune globulin (IVIG) may also be effective, and some have combined rituximab with IVIG.

Most agents used to treat the disease are immunosuppressive, although the mechanism of action may not merely be suppression of T cells and antibody production. Methylprednisolone can directly block pemphigus antibody–induced acantholysis. It also upregulates expression of the genes encoding Dsg3 and periplakin; increases measurable levels of E-cadherin, Dsg1, and Dsg3; and interferes with phosphorylation of these adhesion molecules. Many of these effects antagonize those of pemphigus antibodies. Reversion of DIF to negative predicts sustained remission after withdrawal of medication. Plucked hairs are an alternative to skin biopsy to provide a specimen for immunofluorescence; the pilar sheath epithelium of the anagen hair typically demonstrates immunofluorescence comparable to skin.

Topical Treatment

The skin lesions are extremely painful in advanced cases. When there are extensive raw surfaces, prolonged daily baths are helpful in removing the thickened crusts and reducing the foul odor. Silver sulfadiazine (Silvadene) 1%, widely used for local therapy of burns, is an effective topical antimicrobial agent, suitable for treatment of limited disease, though broad use can lead to absorption and side effects. Silver nitrate–impregnated cotton batting, manufactured for burn units, can be used in more extensive disease. Very localized areas can be treated with silver nitrate–impregnated dressings. Painful ulcerations of the lips and mouth may benefit from topical application of a mixture of equal parts of simethicone (Maalox) and elixir of diphenhydramine hydrochloride (Benadryl) or viscous lidocaine (Xylocaine), especially before meals. The various commercial antiseptic mouthwashes are helpful in alleviating discomfort and malodor. Potent topical corticosteroids and topical tacrolimus have been successful in some patients with limited disease. The likelihood of complete remission is correlated with age of onset and initial mucosal involvement. Infection is a common complication and relates to severity of the pemphigus and the presence of diabetes mellitus.

Systemic Therapy

A common method of treatment for severe PV is to begin with doses of prednisone adequate to control the disease. High doses of prednisone (100–150 mg) are sometimes needed, but prolonged high doses are associated with significant morbidity and mortality, so adjuvant therapy should be started early. During the early phase of therapy, if prednisone at 1 mg/kg/day proves inadequate, the drug may be increased to a split dose of 1 mg/kg twice daily. As the course of corticosteroid therapy is typically longer than initially anticipated, it is good practice to begin vitamin D, calcium, weight-bearing exercise, and bisphosphonate therapy early in the course of treatment. Routine pneumocystis prophylaxis does not appear to be warranted in monotherapy, but in patients on high doses of steroids as part of combination therapy should be considered. Notably dapsone may be somewhat effective for both prophylaxis and against pemphigus. The sooner the diagnosis of PV is established and the sooner treatment is given, the more favorable the prognosis. The therapeutic effects are estimated by the number of new lesions per day and the rate of healing of new lesions. In patients with and Dsg3 antibodies, mucosal disease may still be active when cutaneous disease appears to be in remission. Pemphigus antibody titers can be performed on esophageal substrate, watching for a fall in titer. If, after 4–8 weeks of treatment, new blister formation is not suppressed, prednisone dosage may be increased to 150 mg/day. Dosage adjustments are made more frequently and aggressively in severe, progressive disease. Dividing the daily dose will usually result in greater efficacy but will also result in greater adrenal suppression. Additionally, intravenous pulse therapy with megadose corticosteroids, such as methyl-prednisolone (Solu-Medrol), at a dose of 1 g/day over 2–3 hours, repeated daily for 5 days, may be employed for patients unresponsive to oral doses. Untreated disease is often fatal, but the clinician should remember that, in treated patients, side effects of therapy are the most common cause of death. Adjuvant therapy to decrease steroid dependence has reduced the mortality rate.

Medication is continued until clinical disease is suppressed and pemphigus antibody disappears from the serum. Once the antibody is no longer present, a DIF test is repeated. A negative DIF is predictive of sustained remission after withdrawal of therapy.

MMF is usually chosen as a steroid-sparing agent, at a dose of 1–1.5 g twice daily. Gastrointestinal (GI) intolerance is the most common side effect, and blood counts must be monitored. If the disease does not respond, either plasmapheresis or IVIG may be added to the regimen. Azathioprine is less expensive than MMF and is often used as an alternative when cost is an overriding issue. Azathioprine is best dosed based on measurement of the patient's thiopurine methyltransferase (TPMT) level. Most patients metabolize the drug quickly and may be underdosed if TPMT is not measured. Patients with high levels of the enzyme may require 2.5–3 mg/kg/day of azathioprine; patients with midrange levels are treated with 1–2.5 mg/kg/day. Patients deficient in TPMT may be treated with very low doses of azathioprine or with a different agent. Allopurinol interferes with metabolism of aza-thioprine, and increased serum levels may lead to toxicity.

Rituximab is rapidly becoming a first-line option for PV, with a recent study demonstrating efficacy as initial first-line treatment. An anti-CD20 monoclonal antibody, it leads to reduction in both CD20+ B cells, and possibly T-regulatory cells, with high response rates. There is a trend toward using rituximab early in the course of treatment if patients have significant disease, though it is still used for recalcitrant cases as well. Earlier treatment with rituximab may be associated with better clinical response. Dosing regimens include either rheumatoid arthritis dosing or lymphoma dosing, though lymphoma dosing appears to have slightly better outcomes. Patients on therapy who experience relapse tend to develop relapse as CD19+ B cells return, and when either Dsg1 or Dsg3 testing returns positive; low CD4+ T-cell count was also predictive of relapse. Human anti–chimeric antibody development can limit efficacy when they develop. Rituximab is generally well tolerated, but as with other suppressive agents, infections, including progressive multifocal leukencephalopathy, have been reported.

Patients with refractory disease may be treated with rituximab, IVIG, or cyclophosphamide, either alone or with plasmapheresis. Plasmapheresis alone is followed by rebound of antibody production, but the rebounding clone of plasma cells is sensitized to the effects of cytotoxic agents. Both daily cyclophosphamide dosing and pulse dosing schedules can be used alone or in combination with dexamethasone. Pulse dosing is usually given with mesna rescue and is associated with less bladder toxicity. Both dosing schedules should be planned early in the day, with vigorous hydration to minimize the risk of bladder toxicity. Blood counts must be monitored closely. Other risks of therapy with high doses of corticosteroids and immunosuppressants include diabetes, infection, hypertension, and cardiorespiratory disease. All these risks must be monitored, and all patients must receive gentle wound care and fluid and electrolyte management. In patients who cannot tolerate cyclophosphamide, chlorambucil has been used, but it is associated with a greater risk of hematologic malignancy. Cyclosporine and infliximab have also been used. Immunoadsorp-tion represents a novel approach to therapy that could replace plasmapheresis. In addition to the use of IVIG as an adjuvant to conventional therapy, it has also been given as monotherapy. Onset of action is fairly rapid and may be seen within 1–2 weeks,

and as an immunomodulatory and not suppressive agent with a good safety profile, it may represent a good alternative in select patients.

Immunosuppressant therapy alone has been reported as a successful treatment of patients with early, stable PV. If a contraindication to the use of corticosteroids exists, or if only limited disease is present, these may be used as single agents. In general, however, combined treatment with corticosteroids is superior in gaining early control of the disease. Dexamethasone-cyclophosphamide therapy and isolated oral cyclophosphamide are very effective options, but with high rates of adverse events. Oral cyclophosphamide was successful in 17 of 20 patients who had failed therapy with prednisone and an antimetabolite. The median time to achieve complete remission was 8.5 months, and the median duration of treatment was 17 months. Plasmapheresis was used in nine patients. Hematuria developed in five patients, and infections were noted in six. One patient developed bladder cancer 15 years after therapy.

Dapsone, nicotinamide, and tetracycline can be tried in patients with milder disease. Cyclosporine, etanercept, and infliximab have been used successfully in some patients. Intramuscular or oral gold is no longer commonly used. Gold is less effective than immunosuppressive therapy, but its advantages include lack of carcinogenicity and infertility. A minimum of 6 months is required to judge the effectiveness of gold therapy. Extracorporeal photo-chemotherapy has been used in a few patients. Platelet-rich plasma was reported as beneficial in a small study of seven patients with refractory oral erosions. Cutting-edge translational research into the use of specific chimeric antigen T cells to attack the pathogenic antibody-producing cells is being explored. Other monoclonal antibodies hold promise, including ofatumumab, belimumab, and veltuzumab, but there are insufficient data to recommend their use currently.

PEMPHIGUS VEGETANS

Pemphigus vegetans may present as localized plaques in the scalp or in two classic forms, the Neumann type, which generally begins and ends as typical pemphigus, and the Hallopeau type, which usually remains localized. Both types show pseudoepitheliomatous hyperplasia, and the Hallopeau type is characterized by eosinophil microabscesses within the epidermis.

Pemphigus vegetans may begin with flaccid bullae that become erosions and form fungating vegetations or papillomatous prolifera-tions, especially in body folds or on the scalp. The tongue often shows cerebriform morphologic features early in the course of the disease. Lesions presenting as verrucous plaques on the scalp, finger, and genitalia have been reported. At times, the lesions tend to coalesce to form large patches or to arrange themselves into groups or figurate patterns.

The laboratory findings, etiologic factors, epidemiology, pathogenesis, and treatment of pemphigus vegetans are the same as those for pemphigus vulgaris. Pathogenic antibodies to desmocol-lins, specifically desmocollin-3 antibodies, have been reported in some cases and hypothesized to explain the different clinical features in vegetans versus vulgaris. Captopril-induced pemphigus vegetans has been reported.

Pemphigus vegetans must be differentiated from other condi-tions characterized by pseudoepitheliomatous hyperplasia and microabscesses, including halogenoderma, chromoblastomycosis, blastomycosis, granuloma inguinale, blastomycosis-like pyoderma, condyloma lata, and amebic granulomas. The Hallopeau type is distinguished by the presence of eosinophils, and both types by immunofluorescent findings.

Albers LN, et al: Developing biomarkers for predicting clinical relapse in pemphigus patients treated with rituximab. J Am Acad Dermatol 2017; 77: 1074.

Al-Janabi A, Greenfield S: Pemphigus vulgaris. BMJ Case Rep 2015 Oct 22; 2015.

Amber KT, et al: Determining the incidence of pneumocystis pneumonia in patients with autoimmune blistering diseases not receiving routing prophylaxis. JAMA Dermatol 2017; 153: 1137.

Atzmony L, et al: The role of adjuvant therapy in pemphigus. J Am Acad Dermatol 2015; 73: 264.

Bai YX, et al: Pemphigus vulgaris-associated interstitial lung disease. Dermatol Ther 2016; 29: 228.

Baum S, et al: Efficacy of dapsone in the treatment of pemphigus vulgaris. Dermatology 2016; 232: 578.

Baum S, et al: Epidemiological data of 290 pemphigus vulgaris patients. Eur J Dermatol 2016; 26: 382.

Cheng X, et al: High-frequency ultrasound in blistering skin diseases. J Ultrasound Med 2017; 36: 2367.

Daneshpazhooh M, et al: Immunologic prediction of relapse in patients with pemphigus vulgaris in clinical remission. J Am Acad Dermatol 2016; 74: 1160.

El-Komy MH, et al: Platelet-rich plasma for resistant oral erosions of pemphigus vulgaris. Wound Repair Regen 2015; 23: 953.

Ellebrecht CT, et al: Reengineering chimeric antigen receptor T cells for targeted therapy of autoimmune disease. Science 2016; 353: 179.

Ellebrecht CT, Payne AS: Setting the target for pemphigus vulgaris therapy. JCI Insight 2017; 2: e92021.

El-Zawahry B, et al: Rituximab treatment in pemphigus vulgaris. Arch Dermatol Res 2017; Epub ahead of print.

Glauser S, et al: Diagnostic value of immunohistochemistry on formalin-fixed, paraffin-embedded skin biopsy specimens for bullous pemphigoid. Br J Dermatol 2016; 175: 988.

Hanna S, et al: Validation studies of outcome measures in pemphigus. Int J Womens Dermatol 2016; 2: 128.

Hayashida MZ, et al: Biologic therapy-induced pemphigus. An Bras Dermatol 2017; 92: 591.

Huang A, et al: Future therapies for pemphigus vulgaris. J Am Acad Dermatol 2017; 74: 746.

Inoue-Nishimoto T, et al: IgG/IgA pemphigus representing pemphigus vegetans caused by low titres of IgG and IgA antibodies to Dsg3 and IgA antibodies to desmocollin 3. J Eur Acad Dermatol Venereol 2016; 30: 1229.

Joly P, et al: First-line rituximab combined with short-term prednisone versus prednisone alone for the treatment of pemphigus (Ritux 3). Lancet 2017; 389: 2031.

Kasperkiewicz M, et al: Pemphigus. Nat Rev Dis Primers 2017; 3: 17026.

Kridin K, et al: Ulcerative colitis associated with pemphigus. Scand J Gastroenterol 2017; 52: 1360.

Kridin K, et al: Pemphigus vulgaris and pemphigus foliaceus. Acta Derm Venereol 2017; 97: 1095.

Kridin K, et al: Remarkable differences in the epidemiology of pemphigus among two ethnic populations in the same geographic region. J Am Acad Dermatol 2016; 75: 925.

Pfaltz K, et al: C3d immunohistochemistry on formalin-fixed tissue is a valuable tool in the diagnosis of bullous pemphigoid of the skin. J Cutan Pathol 2010; 37: 654.

Ruocco V, et al: Pemphigus vegetans of the folds. Clin Dermatol 2015; 33: 471.

Saruta H, et al: Two cases of pemphigus vegetans with IgG anti-desmocollin 3 antibodies. JAMA Dermatol 2013; 149: 1209.

Sinistro A, et al: The pathogenic activity of anti-desmoglein autoantibodies parallels disease severity in rituximab treated patients with pemphigus vulgaris. Eur J Dermatol 2015; 25: 578.

Svecova D: IVIG therapy in pemphigus vulgaris has corticosteroid-sparing and immunomodulatory effects. Australas J Dermatol 2016; 57: 141.

Vinay K, et al: Pemphigus vegetans presenting as a verrucous plaque on the finger. Clin Exp Dermatol 2016; 41: 316.

Wolz MM, et al: Pemphigus vegetans variant of IgA pemphigus. Am J Dermatopathol 2013; 35: e53.

Yamaguchi Y, et al: Appearance of antidesmocollin 1 autoantibodies leading to a vegetative lesion in a patient with pemphigus vulgaris. Br J Dermatol 2018; 178: 294.

PEMPHIGUS FOLIACEUS

Pemphigus foliaceus (PF) is characterized by flaccid bullae and localized or generalized exfoliation. Antibodies target Dsg1. Lesions start as small, flaccid bullae that rupture almost as they appear, leading to crusting (Figs. 21.5 and 21.6). Below each crust is a moist surface with a tendency to bleed. Nikolsky sign may be easily elicited by rubbing the skin. After a time, the exfoliative characteristics predominate, with few bullae. Adherent scale crusts may resemble cornflakes. A variant of pemphigus that has clinical features suggestive of dermatitis herpetiformis but has immunologic features of pemphigus has been called herpetiform pemphigus. This pustular variant can be mistaken for subcorneal pustular dermatosis, IgA pemphigus, or Sneddon-Wilkinson disease. Most of these patients represent a clinical variant of PF, with the remainder being PV patients. A few have also demonstrated desmocollin antibodies. Oral lesions are rarely seen, and then only as superficial erosive stomatitis. Several patients have been described whose clinical picture shifted from PF to PV, or vice versa, with an accompanying change in antibody profile. A rare variant of a

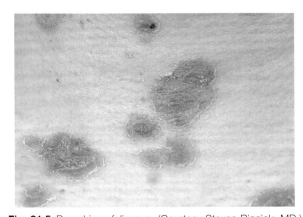

Fig. 21.5 Pemphigus foliaceus. (Courtesy Steven Binnick, MD.)

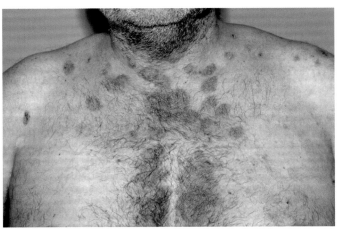

Fig. 21.6 Pemphigus foliaceus.

single fixed lesion of localized pemphigus on the face or scalp has been reported.

Most patients with PF are not severely ill. They complain of burning, pain, and pruritus. The lesions may persist for many years without affecting general health. PF occurs mostly in adults age 40–50 but has also been reported in children. The genders are affected equally. Prevalence of PF in people of Jewish heritage is much less than with PV. Endemic PF (fogo selvage) occurs in Brazil (see later discussion). The drugs listed under PV—penicillamine and ACE inhibitors, specifically captoprile—more frequently induce PF. Topical imiquimod and topical 5-fluorouracil have both been reported to induce PF in single case reports.

The principal histologic finding in PF consists of acantholysis in the upper epidermis, usually in the granular layer. The stratum corneum may be missing entirely or separated from the underlying epidermis. Individual elongated acantholytic cells are noted above the epidermis or clinging to the underside of the stratum corneum. DIF demonstrates intercellular IgG throughout the epidermis, although the deposits may be somewhat more prominent in the upper epidermis. IIF is positive in most patients, although prozone reactions occur and a wide range of dilutions should be tested. A sensitive and specific ELISA for detecting antibodies to Dsg1 is now available to confirm positive IIF results.

Patients with a distinct clinical picture of PF or PV may have a mix of antibodies. Western blot has shown Dsg1 in about 86% of PF patients and 25% of PV patients. ELISA has shown anti-Dsg1 antibodies in up to 71% of PF patients and 62% of PV patients. In one study, antibodies to Dsg3 were detected in 19 of 276 patients with PF and fogo selvagem who had only cutaneous disease. The antibody was capable of producing disease in laboratory animals, suggesting it was pathogenic in the PF patients. Therefore ELISA studies must always be interpreted in the context of clinical, histologic, and immunofluorescent findings. In PV, Dsg3 mediates mucosal disease, and cutaneous disease is associated with antibodies to Dsg1. A shift to predominantly Dsg1 antibodies has accompanied a clinical shift from PV to PF. Patients have also shifted from a pemphigus to a pemphigoid phenotype.

Dsg1, the antigen in PF, was first identified by immunoprecipitation consisting of polypeptides of molecular weight 260, 160, and 85 kilodaltons (kD). The 260-kD molecule is a complex of the 160-kD and 85-kD polypeptides. The PF antibody binds to a 160-kD glycoprotein extracted from normal epidermis. This glycoprotein is identical to Dsg1. The 85-kD glycoprotein is plakoglobulin, a desmosomal and adherens junction–associated molecule. Desmogleins are cadherin-type adhesion molecules found in desmosomes. The N-terminal extracellular domain of Dsg1 contains the dominant autoimmune epitopes in both PF and PV. Antibodies include both IgG1 and IgG4 subclasses. IgG4 antibodies appear to be pathogenic in most patients. In a subset of patients, IgG1 autoantibodies are pathogenic. E-cadherin autoantibodies often cross-react with Dsg1.

Treatment

Treatment of PF is similar to that for PVPF patients are generally less ill and may not need oral corticosteroid therapy. Dapsone and hydroxychloroquine may be useful, either alone in mild cases or to reduce the steroid dose level. Very mild disease may be treated with topical corticosteroids or topical calcineurin inhibitors. Nicotinamide and tetracycline may be more effective than in PV. Azathioprine, MMF, or cyclophosphamide may be needed, as in PV. As with PV, more reports are emerging of successful treatment with rituximab, with over 100 patients in the literature. Generally rituximab is effective though less dramatically than for PV, and patients with PF often require combination therapy or repeated treatments, and therefore have displayed slightly higher rates of infectious complications. The anti–IL6 receptor antibody tocilizumab, IVIG, and high-dose cyclophosphamide have been used

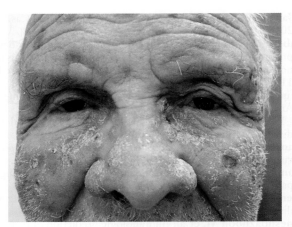

Fig. 21.7 Fogo selvagem. (Courtesy Dermatology Division, University of Campinas, Brazil.)

for refractory disease. Etanercept has been used, and immunoadsorption with tryptophan-linked polyvinyl alcohol adsorbers or adsorption with plant lectins, such as wheat germ agglutinin, has been effective and holds promise as adjuvant therapy.

Herpes simplex superinfection, or *S. aureus* impetigo, can mimic PF and should be considered in recalcitrant or flaring cases.

ENDEMIC PEMPHIGUS (FOGO SELVAGEM)

Endemic pemphigus is found in tropical regions, mostly in certain interior areas of Brazil and Colombia, but also in North Africa, including Tunisia. Fifteen percent of cases are familial. HLA-DRB1 alleles *0404, *1402, *1406, and *0102 have been identified as risk factors. The disease is common in children, adolescents, and young adults, with about one third of cases occurring before age 20 and two thirds by 40 years. The initial lesions may be flaccid bullae, but later lesions are eczematoid, psoriasiform, impetiginous, or seborrheic in appearance. The midfacial areas may be involved (Fig. 21.7). Melanoderma and verrucous vegetative lesions are not unusual, and exfoliative dermatitis may occur. The mucous membranes usually are not involved. Nikolsky sign is present. The disease is often seen in those with arthropod exposure and may be initiated by an infectious agent, possibly carried by mosquitoes, sandflies, black flies, or other vectors, with those agents carrying a molecule triggering anti-Dsg1 antibodies through molecular mimicry.

Histologically and immunohistologically, fogo selvagem is identical to PF. As with PF, antibodies to desmosomal cadherins and E-cadherin may be present. The anti-Dsg1 autoantibodies cross-react with sandfly salivary LJM11 antigen. Endemic pemphigus has also been linked to the kissing bug *Triatoma matogrossensis* and to mercury poisoning. Peripheral blood mononuclear cells from patients produce more IL-1β than those from healthy controls. A strong Th2 bias is also observed. IgM anti-Dsg1 antibodies are common in fogo selvagem, but not in other forms of pemphigus.

A distinct subset has been described in a rural area in northeastern Colombia. This subset differs from previously described forms of endemic pemphigus and shares some immunoreactivity with paraneoplastic pemphigus. It is not, however, associated with malignant tumors. Clinically, the disease resembles Senear-Usher syndrome. A systemic form may affect internal organs and has a poorer prognosis. All patients appear to have antibodies to Dsg1. In addition, many sera react with desmoplakin I, envoplakin, and periplakin. DIF is noted in the pilosebaceous unit, adjacent neurovascular bundles and meibomian glands.

A few Brazilian sera also react with plakins. None of the Colombian patients' sera reacted with Dsg3, but about half of Brazilian patients' sera reacted with Dsg3. This area of Colombia is a mining region, and the population is exposed to high environmental levels of mercuric sulfides and selenides; these compounds have been found in the skin of patients with endemic pemphigus.

PEMPHIGUS ERYTHEMATOSUS (SENEAR-USHER SYNDROME)

In Senear-Usher syndrome, the early lesions are circumscribed patches of erythema and crusting that clinically resemble lupus erythematosus and are immunopathologically positive for the lupus band in 80% of patients. The lesions are erythematous and thickly crusted, bullous, or even hyperkeratotic. These are usually localized on the nose, cheeks, and ears, sites frequently affected by lupus erythematosus. In addition, crusting and impetiginous lesions appear amid bullae on the scalp, chest, and extremities. In most patients, the disease runs an indolent course. Drug-induced cases with penicillamine, captopril, propranolol, heroin, and cefuroxime have been described.

The histopathology of pemphigus erythematosus is that of PF. DIF shows IgG and complement localized in both intercellular and BMZ sites. At the dermoepidermal junction (DEJ), the deposits are continuous and granular, as in lupus. In the epidermis, they resemble those of pemphigus. Antinuclear antibody is present in low titer in 30% of patients. Patients have demonstrated anti-Dsg1 but not anti-Dsg3 autoantibodies. Additional autoantibodies may be directed against bullous pemphigoid antigen 1 (BP230) and periplakin. Patients often respond to low doses of prednisone and may respond well to topical corticosteroids. Photoprotection is essential Immunosuppressants may be needed in severe cases. Cases have been reported in association with myasthenia and thymoma. All patients should be evaluated for features of systemic lupus.

Aoki V, et al: Update on fogo selvage, an endemic form of pemphigus foliaceus. J Dermatol 2015; 42: 18.

Atzmony L, et al: Treatment of pemphigus vulgaris and pemphigus foliaceus. Am J Clin Dermatol 2014; 15: 503.

Baroni A, et al: Cefuroxime-induced pemphigus erythematosus in a young boy. Clin Exp Dermatol 2009; 34: 708.

Callander J, Ponnambath N: Pemphigus foliaceus induced by topical 5-fluorouracil. Clin Exp Dermatol 2016; 41: 443.

Caso F, et al: Refractory pemphigus foliaceus and Behçet's disease successfully treated with tocilizumab. Immunol Res 2013; 56: 390.

de Sena Nogueira Maehara L, et al: Rituximab therapy in pemphigus foliaceus. Br J Dermatol 2015; 172: 1420.

Fernandes NC, et al: Refractory pemphigus foliaceus associated with herpesvirus infection. Rev Inst Med Trop Sao Paulo 2017; 59: e41.

Mendez-Flores S, et al: Pemphigus foliaceus with circinated plaques and neutrophil pustules. J Cutan Pathol 2016; 43: 1062.

Pritchett EN, et al: Pruritic, pink scaling plaques on the face and trunk. Pemphigus erythematosus. JAMA Dermatol 2015; 151: 1123.

Walker A, et al: Localized pemphigus foliaceus. Cutis 2017; 99: e23.

PARANEOPLASTIC PEMPHIGUS

The initial description of this entity was a group of five patients with underlying neoplasms who presented with painful mucosal ulcerations and polymorphous skin lesions, which progressed to blistering eruptions. Most patients described since then have had associated neoplasms or Castleman disease. The mucosal lesions of paraneoplastic pemphigus (PNP) may appear lichenoid or may resemble Stevens-Johnson syndrome, with severe hemorrhagic crusting of the lips (Fig. 21.8). The skin lesions may appear as erythematous macules, lichenoid lesions, erythema multiforme

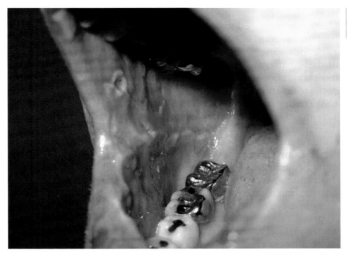

Fig. 21.8 Paraneoplastic pemphigus.

(EM)–like lesions, flaccid bullae, and erosions typical of pemphigus, or with tense, more deep-set bullae. Ocular involvement may be severe. It should be noted that all forms of pemphigus may be paraneoplastic. However, the specific disease dubbed "paraneoplastic pemphigus" has a characteristic clinical appearance as well as diagnostic immunologic findings, but it is not universally associated with a neoplasm. Many patients have devastating bronchiolitis obliterans as a manifestation of their disease.

Histologically, the lesions demonstrate epidermal acantholysis, suprabasal cleft formation, dyskeratotic keratinocytes, and vacuolar change of the basal epidermis. Biopsies that demonstrate both acantholysis and lichenoid change or individual cell necrosis should raise the suspicion of PNP. DIF reveals IgG and C3 deposition in the intercellular spaces of the epithelium. IIF shows a similar pattern in a wide range of stratified squamous epithelium and transitional epithelium (e.g., rat bladder). About 25% of cases will be negative. Immunoprecipitation is the definitive test. It reveals a complex immune response with autoantibodies directed against multiple high-molecular-weight keratinocyte proteins. Antibody targets are generally plakin family proteins at the desmosome and hemidesmosome, including desmoplakin 1 (250 kD), envoplakin (210 kD), and periplakin (190 kD), and both the major plaque protein of hemidesmosomes BPAg1 (230 kD) and plectin. Many cases also recognize an additional antigen at 170 kD. Antibodies to Dsg3, and less frequently Dsg1 and anti-α2-macroglobulin–like-1, are often present. Expanded testing has shown autoantibodies against desmocollins as well. One study suggested that antibodies to desmocollins and α2-macroglobulin–like-1 protein may be useful in making the diagnosis. Many patients have multiple antibodies. On DIF, some cases also demonstrate a linear or granular IgG and/or C3 at the BMZ. Detection of the characteristic immunologic pattern may be delayed, and tests should be repeated if the index of suspicion is high.

Whereas the dominant epitopes in PV reside in N-terminal regions of Dsg3, epitopes on Dsg3 in PNP are distributed more broadly through the extracellular domain. The N-terminal domains are still recognized more frequently than the C-terminal domains, with one study suggesting the N-terminus of envoplakin as the major epitope, particularly for patients with lichenoid inflammation and bronchiolitis obliterans. IgG subclasses in PNP are IgG1 and IgG2 dominant, contrasting with the IgG4 dominance in PV. There is a significant association in PNP with HLA-DRB1*03 allele (61.5% of those studied). In one study, eight of nine fatal PNP cases had distinctive cell surface antibodies detected in a beaded pattern by complement indirect immunofluorescence (CIIF) tests on monkey esophagus. Three long-term survivors with PNP lacked this pattern, suggesting the test may have prognostic value. One study suggested that strong cytoplasmic staining on IIF should prompt investigation for possible PNP.

A wide variety of both benign and malignant tumors are seen in these patients, and some have no identifiable neoplasm. The most common associations are hematologic malignancies, including non-Hodgkin lymphoma, chronic lymphocytic leukemia (CLL), Castleman tumor, acute myeloid leukemia (AML), and thymoma; sarcoma has also been reported. Most reported patients die of their tumor. Others have died from disease-associated bronchiolitis obliterans.

Therapy for the bullous dermatoses with prednisone and/or immunosuppressive agents should be balanced with treatment of the tumor. Severe mucosal disease, particularly ocular disease, warrants rapid, intense therapy. High dose steroids, immunoablative high-dose cyclophosphamide without stem cell rescue, cyclosporin A, plasmapheresis, immunoapheresis, and rituximab and alemtuzumab (in CLL patients), and IVIG, either alone or in combination have been successful in some cases. Occasionally the blistering disease and/or underlying disorder may be controlled, but patients may still succumb to the bronchiolitis obliterans. Even with treatment, mortality remains higher than for other immunobullous diseases.

Gong H, et al: Recurrent corneal melting in the paraneoplastic pemphigus associated with Castleman's disease. BMC Ophthalmol 2016; 16: 106.

Hirano T, et al: Rituximab monotherapy and rituximab-containing chemotherapy were effective for paraneoplastic pemphigus accompanying follicular lymphoma, but not for subsequent bronchiolitis. J Clin Exp Hematop 2015; 55: 83.

Kartan S, et al: Paraneoplastic pemphigus and autoimmune blistering diseases associated with neoplasm. Am J Clin Dermatol 2017; 18: 105.

Namba C, et al: Paraneoplastic pemphigus associated with fatal bronchiolitis obliterans and intractable mucosal erosions. J Dermatol 2016; 43: 419.

Ohzono A, et al: Clinical and immunological findings in 104 cases of paraneoplastic pemphigus. Br J Dermatol 2015; 173: 1447.

Poot AM, et al: Direct and indirect immunofluorescence staining patterns in the diagnosis of paraneoplastic pemphigus. Br J Dermatol 2016; 174: 912.

Siddiqui S, et al: Paraneoplastic pemphigus as a presentation of acute myeloid leukemia. Hematol Oncol Stem Cell Ther 2017; 10: 155.

Wang X, et al: Extremities of the N-terminus of envoplakin and C-terminus of its linker subdomain are major epitopes of paraneoplastic pemphigus. J Dermatol Sci 2016; 84: 24.

IGA PEMPHIGUS (INTRAEPIDERMAL NEUTROPHILIC IGA DERMATOSIS)

The initial description of this entity was an elderly man with chronic bullous dermatosis with unique histological and immunopathologic findings. The patient had generalized flaccid bullae, which rapidly ruptured and crusted and healed without scarring. No mucosal lesions were present. Histologically there were neutrophils linearly at the DEJ with exocytosis and some intraepidermal abscesses. DIF revealed intercellular IgA within the epidermis. No circulating antibodies were found.

Since that report, many additional patients with intraepidermal IgA deposition have been described. They have been classified as belonging to two subsets, one closely mimicking pemphigus and the second simulating subcorneal pustular dermatosis (SPD). The former starts with vesicles that become pustular within a few days, enlarge peripherally, and rupture in the center, then form a crust (Fig. 21.9). Continued peripheral vesiculation may

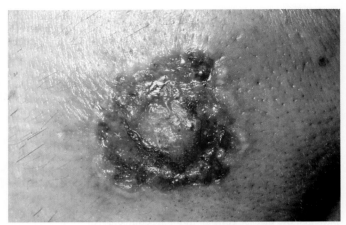

Fig. 21.9 Intraepidermal neutrophilic IgA dermatosis. (Courtesy John Stanley, MD.)

lead to a flower-like appearance. The head, neck, and trunk are frequent sites of involvement. In some patients, the condition is induced by ultraviolet (UV) A light. The second subset, SPD, presents similar to Sneddon-Wilkinson disease, with serpiginous and annular pustules. A pemphigus vegetans–like pattern has also been described. Some cases have been induced by granulocyte-macrophage colony stimulating factor (GM-CSF). Some patients have had associated malignancies, and IgA pemphigus with PNP-like clinical features has been described, showing IgA antibodies to Dsg1/3 and desmocollin 3, as well as IgG and IgA antibodies to the BMZ. Monoclonal IgA gammopathy has also been reported.

Histologically, intraepidermal bullae with neutrophils, some eosinophils, and acantholysis are seen. DIF shows intraepidermal IgA deposition, usually throughout the epidermis, and IIF may reveal circulating autoantibody that binds to the same location. There is evidence that the IgA specificity in individual cases may be directed at either Dsg1, Dsg3, or desmocollin1-3. One study suggested polymeric immunoglobulin receptor as a candidate target protein. Some patients have concurrent IgG intercellular antibodies directed at Dsg1, with a growing number of recent reports identifying IgG/IgA overlap cases. IgG/IgA pemphigus patients clinically behave more similarly to classic IgG PV patients. It should be noted that IgA antibodies to Dsg1 and Dsg3 may occur in PV, PF, and PNP. Individual patients may express both anti–desmocollin 1 and anti-Dsg1 antibodies.

Therapy with topical corticosteroids may be effective in patients with mild intraepidermal neutrophilic IgA dermatosis. Dapsone is often effective, even at doses as low as 25 mg/day in some patients. Oral corticosteroids may be necessary, and some resistant cases have required immunosuppressive agents and plasmapheresis. Colchicine, acitretin, adalimumab, MMF, Rituximab, IVIG, and isotretinoin have been effective in some patients.

Geller S, et al: The expanding spectrum of IgA pemphigus. Br J Dermatol 2014; 171: 650.

Lane N, et al: IgG/IgA pemphigus. Am J Dermatopathol 2014; 36: 1002.

Porro AM, et al: Non-classical forms of pemphigus. An Bras Dermatol 2014; 89: 96.

Toosi S, et al: Clinicopathologic features of IgG/IgA pemphigus in comparison with classic IgG and IgA pemphigus. Int J Dermatol 2016; 55: e184.

Tsuchisaka A, et al: Epidermal polymeric immunoglobulin receptor. Exp Dermatol 2015; 24: 217.

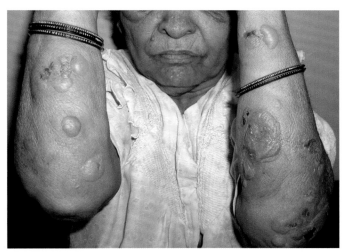

Fig. 21.10 Bullous pemphigoid. (Courtesy Shyam Verma, MBBS, DVD.)

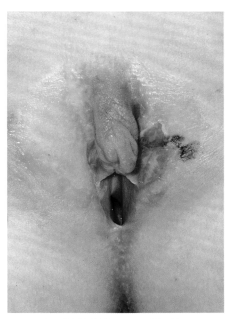

Fig. 21.12 Vulvar pemphigoid.

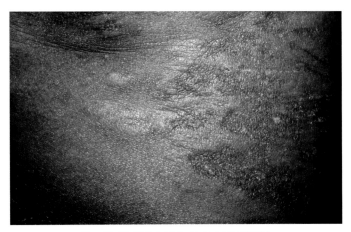

Fig. 21.11 Urticarial bullous pemphigoid.

BULLOUS PEMPHIGOID

Clinical Features

Bullous pemphigoid (BP) was described by Lever in 1953. Clinically, BP is characterized by large, tense, subepidermal bullae with a predilection for the groin, axillae, trunk, thighs, and flexor surfaces of the forearms (Fig. 21.10). Patients are frequently pruritic. Key features distinguishing BP from other immunobullous diseases include subepidermal separation at the DEJ, an inflammatory cell infiltrate that tends to be rich in eosinophils, and antibodies directed against two hemidesmosomal antigens, BP230 and BP180. Antibody detection rates vary by method, and many normal patients will have positive serologic tests but negative IIF. ELISA testing alone is not adequate for the diagnosis, and clinical examination, pathology, and immunofluorescence should be used together.

After the bullae rupture, large denuded areas are seen, but the bullae and denuded areas do not tend to increase in size as they do in PV. Instead, the denuded areas tend to heal spontaneously. In addition to the bullae, there often are erythematous patches and urticarial plaques (Fig. 21.11), with a tendency to central clearing. These patches and plaques may be present without bullae early in the course of the disease. Later, bullae often occur on an urticarial base. Sometimes, targetoid lesions are present.

BP may begin at a localized site, frequently on the thighs or shins. The disease may also be limited to areas of radiation therapy, burns, or plaques of psoriasis. BP may remain localized throughout its course or eventuate in generalized pemphigoid. Cases of the localized disease in which a vesicular eruption is limited to the palms or soles (dyshidrosiform pemphigoid) are occasionally observed. Young girls may present with localized vulvar erosions and ulcers that resemble the signs of child abuse (Fig. 21.12). These localized varieties have been shown to have circulating IgG antibody, which immunoprecipitates the 230-kD BP antigen.

Many other variants of BP have been described. A vesicular variant manifested by tense, small, occasionally grouped blisters is termed vesicular pemphigoid. Other patients, mostly women, have papules and nodules of the scalp and extremities, with sparing of the mucous membranes, in a pattern resembling prurigo nodularis (pemphigoid nodularis). Cases resembling pemphigus vegetans, but with IgG and C3 at the BMZ, are occasionally observed (pemphigoid vegetans). Erythroderma may be present (erythrodermic pemphigoid), or there may be no bullae at all (nonbullous variant). The latter type may present as generalized pruritus, pruritic eczema, or urticarial eruptions with peripheral eosinophilia. Overall, incidence of oral involvement is about 20%, but involvement of the pharynx, larynx, nasal mucosa, vulva, urethra, and eye is rare.

BP occurs most frequently in the elderly population. The age of onset averages 65–75 years. BP less commonly occurs in young children, but with clinical and pathologic findings similar to those in adults. Many of these cases begin with hand and foot bullae (Fig. 21.13). Facial involvement may be somewhat more common in children. In children, the course of disease is usually under 1 year, with most cases lasting 5 months or less.

In patients with lichen planus, a bullous eruption similar to BP may develop. This condition, called lichen planus pemphigoides, is sometimes related to the 230-kD antigen, the 180-kD antigen, or a unique 200-kD subepidermal antigen. A nonscarring eruption, with acute onset, widespread erosions, and severe mucous membrane involvement resembling toxic epidermal necrolysis or PV, has been referred to as anti-p105 pemphigoid. Linear IgG and C3 are noted at the BMZ. The 105-kD antigen is found in the lower portion of the lamina lucida.

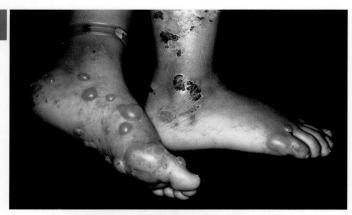

Fig. 21.13 Childhood bullous pemphigoid.

Etiologic Factors

Circulating BMZ antibodies of the IgG class are present in approximately 70% of patients with BP. In most cases, the antibodies fix complement in vitro, in contrast to pemphigus antibodies, which fail to do so. Complement is activated by both the classical and the alternate pathway. No close correlation exists between the titer of antibodies and clinical disease activity. Passive-transfer mouse models suggest that subepidermal blistering is initiated by anti-BP180 antibodies. Blister formation involves complement activation, mast cells, and neutrophils. BMZ damage is caused by proteinases and reactive oxygen species released by the infiltrating neutrophils.

The site of IgG binding has been localized to the lamina lucida, with accentuation near hemidesmosomes. BP antigen 1 (BPAg1) is synthesized by the keratinocyte and is an intracytoplasmic hemidesmosomal plaque protein of 230 kD with disulfide-linked chains. The second BP antigen (180-kD BPAg2) is a transmembrane protein with a long C-terminal collagenous domain that projects into the extracellular region below the hemidesmosome. The antibody to BPAg2 is the primary pathogenic factor. The noncollagenous (NC) 16A domain harbors the major epitopes of autoantibodies in BP. A predominance of the IgG4 subclass has been observed in several studies. In addition to this humoral response, infiltrating T-helper lymphocytes with a mixed Th1/Th2 cytokine profile may play a role in blister formation. Peripheral blood eosinophilia is present in 50% of pemphigoid patients.

Recently IgE autoantibodies to BP180 and BP230 have been reported, though widespread clinical testing is not available, and at least the anti-BP180 autoantibodies appear to be pathogenic. IgE anti-BP230 autoantibodies correlating with nodular pemphigoid have been reported. Patients with IgE levels may also have more prominent urticarial lesions in some cases.

BP has occasionally been associated with other diseases, such as psoriasis, diabetes mellitus, rheumatoid arthritis, PF, dermatomyositis, ulcerative colitis, cardiovascular disease, and thymoma. Neurologic disorders have been reported in association with BP, particularly multiple sclerosis and possibly Parkinson disease, but also stroke, dementia, amyotrophic lateral sclerosis, and epilepsy. A systematic review and meta-analysis found no association of BP with overall malignancy, though noted a possible association with hematologic malignancy; as BP is generally a disease of the elderly, age appropriate screening is warranted. Patients with BP, particularly in the acute phase, have elevated risk of venous thromboembolism.

Drug-induced cases are uncommon. Agents reported to induce BP include penicillamine, furosemide, captopril, antibiotics (penicillin, amoxicillin, quinolones), sulfasalazine, nalidixic acid, escitalopram, TNF inhibitors, ustekinumab, and enalapril. Neuroleptic and diuretic agents have been reported most commonly. Gliptins, a class of oral hypoglycemic for diabetes, appear to have high rates of drug-induced BP, particularly vildagliptin. Radiation therapy, phototherapy, and photodynamic therapy can induce BP. The new class of anticancer agents, checkpoint inhibitors, have been reported to induce BP in multiple instances, and as their use is rapidly expanding, this is expected to be a more common observation in clinical practice.

Histopathology

The histologic changes of BP are characterized by subepidermal bullae, the absence of acantholysis, and a superficial dermal infiltrate containing many eosinophils. The amount of inflammatory infiltrate varies, and individual bullae may be "infiltrate poor" or "infiltrate rich." Often, the infiltrate contains many eosinophils, although neutrophil-predominant cases exist. Spongiosis with eosinophils occurs more frequently than in pemphigus. Urticarial lesions often demonstrate eosinophils lined up along the DEJ. Immunohistochemistry is being increasingly used in the diagnosis, with C3d deposits at the DEJ a clue to the diagnosis.

Atypical presentations are fairly common. In one study of 23 new cases of BP, only 7 of 22 biopsy specimens showed subepidermal blister formation, and only 12 of these had a predominance of eosinophils in the blister cavity. In 23% of patients, the biopsy was not particularly suggestive of BP. DIF, IIF, immunoblot analysis, and ELISA are critical in establishing the diagnosis in such patients.

The DIF test is more sensitive than IIF, as in pemphigus. In a positive test, continuous linear (tubular or toothpaste pattern) immunofluorescence is seen along the BMZ. IgG and/or C3 are best found in nonbullous lesional or perilesional skin. False-negative tests are somewhat more common on the lower extremities. When using perilesional or nonbullous lesional skin of the trunk, a positive DIF test is found in a high percentage of patients, with C3 most often present and IgG present in about 80% of cases. IgA and IgM are occasionally present. About 20% of patients have negative staining for IgG on DIF, even though C3 is present. In some of these patients, IgG may be present at subthreshold levels that cannot be detected. Also, the major subclass, IgG4, shows limited reactivity with most commercial antihuman IgG conjugates. Double-sandwich antibody immunofluorescence methods have been developed that offer greater sensitivity for IgG4 antibodies.

All histologic features present in BP may also be seen in epidermolysis bullosa acquisita (EBA). Therefore immunofluorescence testing on salt-split skin is sometimes performed to differentiate EBA from BP. Salt-split skin may be replaced by assessment of u-serrated (suggests EBA) and n-serrated (suggests BP) immunoglobulin patterns in DIF specimens and by serologic testing. C3 deposition is almost always present in BP, whereas it may be absent in EBA. Type IV collagen mapping in BP localizes to the base of the blister; in EBA, it stains the roof.

Bullous scabies can also mimic both the histology and the DIF findings of BP.

Treatment

Relatively few controlled trials have been performed, and many recommendations for BP therapy are based on experience and consensus of opinion. Using Cochrane criteria, seven randomized controlled trials (RCTs) were identified through 2003, enrolling a total of 634 patients. One comparing prednisolone, 0.75 mg/kg/day, with prednisolone, 1.25 mg/kg/day, found no statistical difference between the two treatments. The same was true of a trial comparing methylprednisolone with prednisolone. Higher doses of prednisolone were associated with more severe side effects in these studies. Two trials confirmed that adjuvant therapy with azathioprine or plasma exchange could reduce the required corticosteroid dose. Another trial failed to confirm the superiority of combination treatment (with either azathioprine or plasma exchange) over corticosteroid alone, and one trial found no statistically significant difference between prednisolone and a combination of tetracycline and niacinamide. The steroid-treated group had more side effects. Another study compared ultrapotent topical corticosteroid treatment (clobetasol propionate cream, 40 g/day) with oral prednisone (0.5–1 mg/kg/day). In those with severe disease, 1-year survival was better in the topical corticosteroid group (76% vs. 58%). Disease control at 3 weeks was also better in the clobetasol than in the prednisone group (99% vs. 91%). Side effects were common in both groups, but more common in the prednisone group (29% vs. 54%). Among those with moderate disease, there were no significant differences between the two groups. One recent study randomized 132 patients to doxycycline and 121 to prednisolone, with doxycycline reducing blisters less effectively, but with half as many severe side effects. The authors concluded doxycycline is noninferior for blister control and safer long term.

Even in those with fairly extensive disease, topical corticosteroid treatment should be attempted. Prednisone has long been the standard approach to oral therapy, but the complication rate must be weighed carefully, especially in those with severe disease. Oral therapy with tetracycline, 500 mg four times daily, combined with niacinamide, 500 mg three times daily, is effective in some patients. Occasionally, patients with BP may respond to tetracycline or nicotinamide alone. Rituximab has proved effective in adults and has been used in infancy. Dapsone is also effective in some patients. Immunosuppressive therapy may still be necessary in resistant cases, either in combination with systemic or topical corticosteroids or as sole therapy. Azathioprine and MMF demonstrate similar efficacy when used as steroid-sparing agents, and cumulative corticosteroid doses are similar. MMF is more expensive but is easier to dose and associated with less toxicity. Methotrexate, cyclophosphamide, chlorambucil, IVIG, and cyclosporine have also proved effective in some patients, and some data suggest that outcomes are better with methotrexate than with prednisone. Low-dose oral methotrexate has been shown to induce apoptosis of tissue eosinophils in patients with BP. IVIG alone was effective in one study of 56 patients recalcitrant to steroids. The effectiveness of IVIG is often improved by the addition of an immunosuppressive agent. In exceptionally severe cases, pulse therapy with methylprednisolone can be rapidly effective. Again, some patients may also respond to dapsone, as well as sulfapyridine; these agents tend to be more effective in neutrophil-rich BP. Oral erythromycin and topical macrolactams have proved effective in some patients.

Double-filtration plasmapheresis (DFPP) may be more effective than conventional plasma exchange, possibly because it removes pathogenic cytokines. DFPP reduces a variety of cytokines, including IL-8, tumor necrosis factor (TNF)–α, and IL-2. IVIG produces faster clearance of antibody titers and may be helpful in inducing and maintaining remission. Some data suggest that single-chain variable fragments of anti–collagen XVII antibodies can interfere with pathogenic binding of autoantibodies, suggesting that interference with antibody binding may represent an alternative treatment approach to BP.

Rituximab is used less frequently for BP than for PV, but remains a highly effective option. One series of 12 patients treated with rituximab and IVIG achieved sustained remission in all cases, though 2 patients required redosing of rituximab. One single-center study of 19 patients treated with rituximab with steroids together as first-line treatment demonstrated good response rates, with a 20% rate of infection or serious adverse event. Omalizumab, a humanized monoclonal anti-IgE antibody, has been used in increasing numbers of reports recently, particularly in light of emerging studies highlighting the importance of IgE autoantibodies in the pathogenesis of BP in some patients.

A consensus statement from the European Academy of Dermatology and Venereology in 2015 provides expert opinion guidance for initial therapy. For limited disease, the Academy suggests that first-line treatment is high-potency topical steroids, with second-line options being oral steroids, tetracycline, or dapsone; for generalized disease, either ultrapotent topical or oral steroids, with second-line options azathioprine, mycophenolate, tetracycline, methotrexate, or chlorambucil. Rituximab, IVIG, cyclophosphamide, immunoadsorption, and plasma exchange are available as third-line options or for severe/recalcitrant cases.

Course and Prognosis

BP is usually self-limited over 5–6 years. This period is generally a year or less in children. Relapse occurs in 10%–15% of patients once therapy is discontinued. The presence of circulating anti-BP180 antibodies, but not anti-BP230, is associated with a statistically increased mortality risk in the first year after diagnosis. Other risk factors for death during the first year include older age, higher daily steroid dosage at discharge, low serum albumin, and erythrocyte sedimentation rate greater than 30 mm/hr. Much of the morbidity and mortality now relate to infection and side effects of drug therapy, but with improvements in treatment, pemphigoid patients have similar mortality to age-matched controls. Although IIF titers do not always correlate with disease activity, ELISA measurements of BP180NC16a show better correlation. The presence of IgE autoantibodies to BP180 correlate with a more severe course.

Ahmed AR, et al: Treatment of recalcitrant bullous pemphigoid with a novel protocol. J Am Acad Dermatol 2016; 74: 700.

Akasaka E, et al: Elevated levels of circulating immunoglobulin E autoantibodies against BP180 and BP230 in an intractable case of bullous pemphigoid. J Dermatol Sci 2016; 84: 110.

Al-Shenawy HA: Can immunohistochemistry replace immunofluorescence in diagnosis of skin bullous diseases? APMIS 2017; 125: 114.

Amagai M, et al: A randomized double-blind trial of intravenous immunoglobulin for bullous pemphigoid. J Dermatol Sci 2017; 85: 77.

Bakker CV, et al: Bullous pemphigoid as pruritus in the elderly. JAMA Dermatol 2013; 149: 950.

Bardazzi F, et al: Autoantibody serum levels and intensity of pruritus in bullous pemphigoid. Eur J Dermatol 2016; 26: 390.

Béné J, et al: Bullous pemphigoid and dipeptidyl peptidase IV inhibitors. Br J Dermatol 2016; 175: 296.

Caccavale S, et al: Bullous pemphigoid induced by escitalopram in a patient with depression. G Ital Dermatol Venereol 2016; 151: 122.

Chalmers JR, et al: A randomized controlled trial to compare the safety, effectiveness, and cost-effectiveness of doxycycline with that of oral prednisone for initial treatment of bullous pemphigoid. Health Technol Assess 2017; 21: 1.

Cho YT, et al: High serum anti-BP180 IgE levels correlate to prominent urticarial lesions in patients with bullous pemphigoid. J Dermatol Sci 2016; 83: 78.

Cho YT, et al: First-line combination therapy with rituximab and corticosteroids provides a high complete remission rate in moderate-to-severe bullous pemphigoid. Br J Dermatol 2015; 173: 302.

Cozzani E, et al: Ciprofloxacin as a trigger for bullous pemphigoid. Am J Ther 2016; 23: 1202.

Cugno M, et al: Increased risk of venous thromboembolism in patients with bullous pemphigoid. Thromb Haemost 2016; 115: 193.

Feliciani C, et al: Management of bullous pemphigoid. Br J Dermatol 2015; 172: 867.

Glauser S, et al: Diagnostic value of immunohistochemistry on formalin-fixed, paraffin-embedded skin biopsy specimens for bullous pemphigoid. Br J Dermatol 2016; 175: 988.

Hammers CM, Payne AS: Clinical significance of immunoglobulin E in bullous pemphigoid. Br J Dermatol 2017; 177: 13.

Hashimoto T, et al: Detection of IgE autoantibodies to BP180 and BP230 and their relationship to clinical features in bullous pemphigoid. Br J Dermatol 2017; 177: 141.

Keller JJ, et al: Evaluation of ELISA testing for BP180 and BP230 as a diagnostic modality for bullous pemphigoid. Arch Dermatol Res 2016; 308: 269.

Kibsgaard L, et al: Increased frequency of multiple sclerosis among patients with bullous pemphigoid. Br J Dermatol 2017; 176: 1486.

Kluger N, et al: Photodynamic therapy-triggered BP. Int J Dermatol 2017; 56: e41.

Kridin K, et al: Association between bullous pemphigoid and psoriasis. J Am Acad Dermatol 2017; 77: 370.

Lai YC, et al: Bullous pemphigoid and its association with neurological diseases. J Eur Acad Dermatol Venereol 2016; 30: 2007.

Meijer JM, et al: Current practice in treatment approach for bullous pemphigoid. Clin Exp Dermatol 2016; 41: 506.

Nakane S, et al: A potential link between amyotrophic lateral sclerosis and bullous pemphigoid. Intern Med 2016; 55: 1985.

Onsun N, et al: Bullous pemphigoid during ustekinumab therapy in a psoriatic patient. Eur J Dermatol 2017; 27: 81.

Patsatsi A, et al: Multiple sclerosis is the neurological disorder most highly associated with bullous pemphigoid. Br J Dermatol 2017; 176: 1428.

Rofe O, et al: Severe bullous pemphigoid associated with pembrolizumab therapy for metastatic melanoma with complete regression. Clin Exp Dermatol 2017; 42: 309.

Shetty S, et al: Treatment of bullous pemphigoid with rituximab. J Drugs Dermatol 2013; 12: 672.

Tan CW, et al: The association between drugs and bullous pemphigoid. Br J Dermatol 2017; 176: 549.

Terra JB, et al: The n- vs. u-serration is a learnable criterion to differentiate pemphigoid from epidermolysis bullosa acquisita in direct immunofluorescence serration pattern analysis. Br J Dermatol 2013; 169: 100.

PEMPHIGOID GESTATIONIS (HERPES GESTATIONIS)

Clinical Features

Pemphigoid gestationis (PG) is an autoimmune, inflammatory, bullous disease with onset during pregnancy or during the postpartum period. It occurs in approximately 1 in 20,000 to 1 in 50,000 pregnancies. The onset is usually during the second trimester, though multigravida patients develop the disease earlier (21 weeks) than primigravid patients (31 weeks). Clinically urticarial plaques and papules developing around the umbilicus and extremities. Targetoid lesions may be present (Fig. 21.14). As the disease progresses, lesions may spread over the abdomen, back, chest, and extremities, including the palms and soles. The face, scalp, and oral mucosa are usually spared. Within the infiltrated erythematous plaques, tense vesicles and bullae erupt, often in an annular or polycyclic configuration. Pruritus is severe and universally present, and may be paroxysmal. The disease will often flare shortly after delivery and then remit spontaneously, usually within 3–6 months of delivery. There is no scarring, except that caused by excoriations or secondary infections. Recurrences with subsequent pregnancies are common, and the disease may be provoked by subsequent menstrual periods or oral contraceptives (OCs). A number of cases of persistent disease have been reported.

Most study data suggest that fetal loss is not statistically increased, although infants are often born prematurely and are

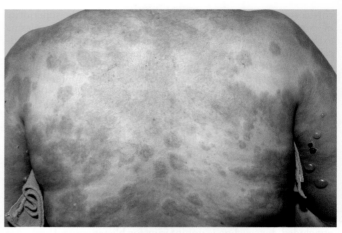

Fig. 21.14 Pemphigoid gestationis.

small for gestational age. In fewer than 5% of cases, infants manifest the disease in the form of urticarial lesions or bullae. The lesions are usually limited, and clear spontaneously without the need for therapy. Neonatal convulsions have been reported.

Etiologic Factors

PG is an autoimmune, antibody-mediated disease, primarily caused by antibodies against the NC16-a domain of BP180. A complement-fixing IgG antibody is present in the serum and is deposited in the lamina lucida. The antigen, transmembrane collagen XVII, is a component of fetal membranes and promotes migration of placental cytotrophoblastic cells. The antigenic epitopes are usually restricted to the N-terminal portion of the extracellular domain of BP180 (BPAg2). The antigenic N-terminal portion of MCW-1 is located in the noncollagenous domain (NC16A) of BP180. Other antigens are located nearby, and four major PG epitopes are clustered within a 22–amino acid region of the BP180 ectodomain. ELISA-based assays correlate antibody levels to disease activity. Both IgG1 and IgG3 subtypes have been noted, but a more recent study found IgG4 to be the predominant subtype, as in BP.

Studies have documented an increased frequency of HLA-DR3, HLA-DR4, and HLA-C4 null alleles in patients with PG. A woman may have antibodies directed against her husband's HLA antigens. Black women rarely manifest PG, possibly related to the low incidence of HLA-DR4 in American black persons. From 10%–11% of patients develop Graves disease.

Pathogenesis

Pathogenesis is similar to that of BP. However, hormonal factors influence the disease manifestation. In addition to being seen in pregnant patients, menstruating women, and those taking OCs, the disease may occur in association with hydatidiform mole and choriocarcinoma. The IgG antibodies bind to the lamina lucida and fix complement. Activated eosinophils, neutrophils, and T cells with a predominant Th2 phenotype are involved in blister formation. Evidence of fetal microchimerism is lacking. Estrogen and progesterone may play a role given the diseases may flare immediately postpartum, during menstruation, and with OC use.

Patients with chronic PG tend to be older and multigravid, with a history of PG during previous pregnancies. They often have widespread cutaneous and mucosal involvement. The IgG1 subclass is often present. Antibodies to a C-terminal portion of BP180 have been noted in a patient with chronic PG. This same region is targeted in patients with cicatricial pemphigoid and some with BP.

Histopathology

A subepidermal bulla with eosinophils and some neutrophils is usually present in PG. In the urticarial stage, eosinophils may line up along the DEJ, as in urticarial BP. Civatte bodies may be present. On DIF, all patients have C3 deposited in a linear pattern at the DEJ; 25%–40% also have detectable IgG. On conventional IIF testing, approximately 25% of patients have a circulating IgG anti-BMZ antibody, but in almost 75%, the PG factor, a complement-fixing IgG antibody, can be demonstrated by complement-enhanced immunofluorescence. Immunoelectron microscopy has demonstrated that the blister occurs at the level of the lamina lucida, with deposition of C3 and IgG at this site, exactly as in BP.

Differential Diagnosis

The main diagnosis to be considered is pruritic urticarial papules and plaques of pregnancy (PUPPP). The differential diagnosis of PG also includes EM, drug reactions, and bullous scabies. Acrodermatitis enteropathica has also been reported to flare as a bullous eruption with each pregnancy. Biopsy, immunofluorescence findings, and clinical course establish the diagnosis.

Treatment

The use of potent topical steroids may be adequate in some patients with milder PG. Prednisone, about 40 mg/day orally, is usually effective in the remaining women. The dose is tapered to the lowest effective amount given on alternate days. Pyridoxine has been reported to be effective in some patients. Persistent PG after delivery has been treated with various tetracyclines, together with nicotinamide. A few women with severe PG have required treatment with rituximab, cyclophosphamide, dapsone, methotrexate, IVIG, or plasmapheresis.

OTHER PREGNANCY-RELATED DERMATOSES

Intrahepatic Cholestasis of Pregnancy (Prurigo Gravidarum)

This rare condition has wide geographic variability in reported frequency, with 4% of pregnancies in Chile versus 0.7% in the United Kingdom, though these numbers may overestimate the true rate. There may be a genetic predisposition, though seasonality, dietary factors, and hormones may confer additional risk. Women with prurigo gravidarum have no primary skin lesions and usually manifest only severe, generalized pruritus. Secondary excoriations may be present. The disease is caused by cholestasis with elevated serum bile salts and often other signs of liver dysfunction; serum bilirubin is elevated in 10%, and those patients develop jaundice. It occurs late in pregnancy, resolves after delivery, and recurs with subsequent pregnancies. There is an increased incidence of fetal complications. There may be an increased risk of preeclampsia. Both ursodeoxycholic acid and *S*-adenosylmethionine improve pruritus, but the former is more effective in improving liver function. Rifampicin has been used in severe cases in combination with ursodeoxycholic acid. Mentholated topical emollients may relieve the pruritus. Delivery closer to 37 weeks of gestation may be associated with better outcomes.

Polymorphic Eruption of Pregnancy

Some investigators have proposed grouping all the pruritic inflammatory dermatoses of pregnancy into the designation "polymorphic eruption of pregnancy." This argument has some merit, because many of the pruritic eruptions of pregnancy are nonspecific or variable manifestations of PUPPP, and there are no consistent

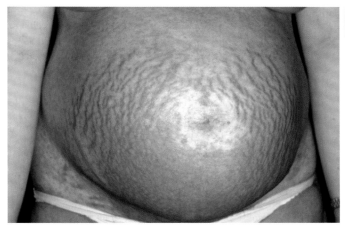

Fig. 21.15 Pruritic urticarial papules and plaques of pregnancy.

hormonal or immunopathogenetic factors that reliably separate them. These eruptions occur in approximately 1 in 120 to 1 in 240 pregnancies. They are more common with male fetuses and multiple-gestation pregnancies.

Pruritic Urticarial Papules and Plaques of Pregnancy

This eruption was first reported in 7 patients under the name pruritic urticarial papules and plaques of pregnancy in 1979. PUPPP is characterized by erythematous papules and plaques that begin as 1- or 2-mm lesions within the abdominal striae (Fig. 21.15). These then spread over a few days to involve the abdomen, buttocks, thighs, and in some cases the arms and legs. The upper chest, face, and mucous membranes are generally spared. The lesions coalesce to form urticarial plaques, sometimes in figurate patterns, and occasionally spongiotic vesicles are present. Intense pruritus is characteristic. In contrast to PG, postpartum onset or exacerbation is uncommon. Fetal and maternal outcomes are not affected by this eruption, and only rarely do newborns manifest transient lesions of PUPPP.

This eruption occurs in primigravidas 75% of the time and rarely recurs with subsequent pregnancies. It begins late in the third trimester and resolves with delivery. Many studies have investigated the relationship of maternal weight gain to the development of this dermatosis. Patients with PUPPP average more weight gain and greater abdominal distention than those without the disease. It is more common in primigravid women and those carrying twins or triplets.

Histologic findings consist of a perivascular lymphohistiocytic infiltrate in the upper and middle dermis, with a variable number of eosinophils and dermal edema. The epidermis is usually normal, although focal spongiosis, parakeratosis, or scales or crust may be present. The results of a DIF test are negative or nonspecific.

Usually, potent topical corticosteroids are required to control the eruption. Even short-duration use of strong steroids can lead to maternal absorption and fetal effects, and patients should be counseled and the use discussed with the obstetrician. A few patients require prednisone. PUPPP remits after delivery.

Papular Dermatitis of Pregnancy

Papular dermatitis of pregnancy is a controversial entity. It is defined as a pruritic, generalized eruption of 3–5 mm, erythematous papules, each surmounted by a small, firm, central crust. The lesions may erupt at any time during pregnancy and usually resolve with delivery. Marked elevation of the 24-hour urinary chorionic gonadotropin has been cited as a marker for the condition.

Administration of systemic corticosteroids is reportedly effective in controlling the eruption. Papular dermatitis may recur in subsequent pregnancies. The high incidence of fetal deaths reported by Spangler is now thought to have been overstated.

Prurigo Gestationis (Besnier)

Prurigo gestationis consists of pruritic, excoriated papules of the proximal limbs and upper trunk, occurring most often between the 20th and 34th weeks of gestation. It clears in the postpartum period and usually does not recur. Therapy with potent topical corticosteroids is recommended. No adverse effects on maternal or fetal health are seen. This eruption may simply be an expression of atopic dermatitis in pregnancy.

Pruritic Folliculitis of Pregnancy. Several authors have reported on pruritic folliculitis in gravid women, with small follicular pustules scattered widely over the trunk appearing during the second or third trimester and resolving by 2 or 3 weeks after delivery. Acute folliculitis and focal spongiosis with exocytosis of polymorphonuclear leukocytes are present on biopsy, and DIF results are negative. This condition may be a type of hormonally induced acne.

Linear IgM Dermatosis of Pregnancy

This entity was reported in a woman who developed small, red, follicular papules and pustules that, on immunofluorescence testing, showed linear deposits of IgM. This finding is common in a wide variety of dermatoses and is nonspecific.

Impetigo Herpetiformis

Impetigo herpetiformis is a form of severe pustular psoriasis occurring in pregnancy. It consists of an acute, usually febrile onset of grouped pustules on an erythematous base, which begins in the groin, axillae, and neck. There is a high peripheral white blood cell count, and hypocalcemia may be present. The histopathology is that of pustular psoriasis. The condition resolves with delivery, but recurrences with subsequent pregnancies may be expected. Fetal death can occur and results from placental insufficiency. Initial treatment is with systemic corticosteroids, in the range of 40–60 mg/day of oral prednisone. Impetigo herpetiformis is discussed in more detail in Chapter 10.

Al-Saif F, et al: Retrospective analysis of pemphigoid gestationis in 32 Saudi patients. J Reprod Immunol 2016; 116: 42.

Brandao P, et al: Polymorphic eruption of pregnancy. J Obstet Gynaecol 2017; 37: 137.

Kanwar AJ: Pemphigoid gestationis. Br J Dermatol 2015; 172: 6.

Ovadia C, et al: Intrahepatic cholestasis of pregnancy. Clin Dermatol 2016; 34: 327.

Sadik CD, et al: Pemphigoid gestationis. Clin Dermatol 2016; 34: 378.

Seidel R, et al: Pemphigoid gestationis. J Drugs Dermatol 2015; 14: 904.

Tani N, et al: Clinical and immunological profiles of 25 patients with pemphigoid gestationis. Br J Dermatol 2015; 172: 120.

Taylor D, et al: Polymorphic eruption of pregnancy. Clin Dermatol 2016; 34: 383.

CICATRICIAL PEMPHIGOID (MUCOUS MEMBRANE PEMPHIGOID)

In 1953 Lever suggested the designation "benign mucosal pemphigoid" for what had previously been called ocular pemphigus, cicatricial pemphigoid, or essential shrinkage of the conjunctiva.

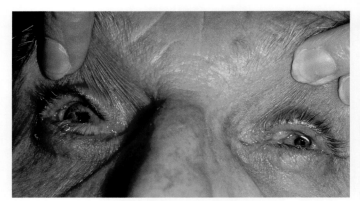

Fig. 21.16 Cicatricial pemphigoid.

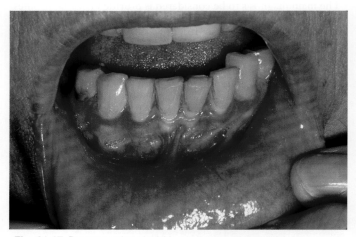

Fig. 21.17 Desquamative gingivitis secondary to cicatricial pemphigoid.

Because of its scarring nature, the designation cicatricial pemphigoid (CP) has gained predominance, as "benign" is a misnomer. The term encompasses a group of immunologically distinct immunobullous diseases with scarring.

Clinical Features

CP usually occurs in older women, with a female/male ratio of approximately 2 : 1. CP is characterized by evanescent vesicles that rupture quickly, leaving behind erosions and ulcers. In most patients, the vesicles primarily occur on the mucous membranes, especially the conjunctiva (Fig. 21.16) and oral mucosa. Oral lesions occur in approximately 90% of patients and conjunctival lesions in 66%. The oral mucosa may be the only affected site for years. Desquamative gingivitis, diffuse erythema of the marginal and attached mucosa associated with mucosal desquamation and pain, is often the presenting sign (Fig. 21.17). The mucosa readily peels away in response to pressure from a cotton-tipped applicator or stream of air from a dental air hose. The gingivae are almost always involved, and the lingual surfaces less regularly. The palate, tongue, and tonsillar pillars may be involved. Patients may be misdiagnosed initially with mucosal lichen planus.

In contrast to BP, CP shows little tendency for remission. Although the disease is chronic and produces significant morbidity, the patient's general health is usually not jeopardized. In ocular cases, CP leads to scarring and progressive shrinkage of the ocular mucous membranes. Blindness may quickly result. It is usually bilateral and associated with redness and flaccid vesicles on the conjunctiva, xerosis, and fibrous adhesions (symblepharon).

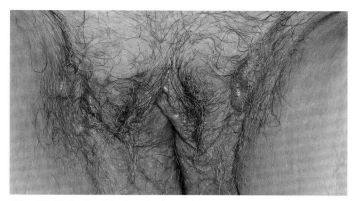

Fig. 21.18 Antilaminin cicatricial pemphigoid with inguinal involvement. Blisters began at the same time colonic cancer was diagnosed.

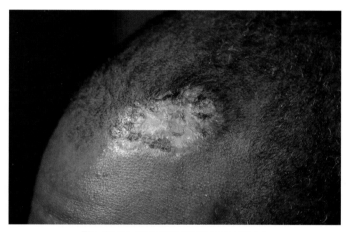

Fig. 21.19 Brunsting-Perry pemphigoid.

Entropion, trichiasis, and corneal opacities develop, and ultimately, the adhesions attach both lids to the eyeball and narrow the palpebral fissure. Scarring may also develop in the pharynx, esophagus, larynx, and anogenital mucosa. Esophageal stricture may occur, and deafness has been reported.

Cutaneous lesions are seen in approximately 25% of CP patients. These begin as tense bullae, similar to those in BP. The bullae may occur on the face, scalp, neck, inguinal region (Fig. 21.18), or extremities. Generalized lesions may also occur. Some of these patients will have circulating antibodies targeted against the classic BP antigens and should be classified as mucosal-predominant BP. Some have secondary antibodies against other antigens. Some patients have EBA, as their IgG autoantibody targets type VII collagen. Vegetating intertriginous lesions have been dubbed CP vegetans. Some patients have developed esophageal involvement, which can lead to strictures and other complications.

In Brunsting-Perry pemphigoid, there are no mucosal lesions, but one or several circumscribed erythematous patches develop, on which recurrent crops of blisters appear. Ultimately, atrophic scarring results (Fig. 21.19). Generally, the areas of involvement are confined to the head and neck. The average age at onset is 58, with a 2:1 male/female ratio.

Etiologic Factors

Although patients share a similar phenotype, CP is a heterogeneous group of autoimmune subepidermal blistering diseases. Circulating autoantibodies target the hemidesmosomal protein BP180, but the target epitopes differ from those usually targeted in BP. Whereas

most BP patients react with the noncollagenous domain (NC16a) on the extracellular N-terminal portion of BP180, most CP antibodies target C-terminal domains. Fluorescence typically is found on the epidermal side of 1-M NaCl-split skin. The deeper location within the BMZ of the target autoantigen in this entity helps explain the observed scarring phenotype.

Whereas most patients' autoantibodies target BP180, others target laminin 5 (also called laminin 3-3-2), termed *antiepiligrin* or *antilaminin cicatricial pemphigoid*, or the β4 subunit of α6 β4 integrin. Integrin β4 appears to be the major autoantigen for pure ocular mucous membrane pemphigoid (MMP). Some patients with a CP phenotype have antibodies to multiple epitopes, including the β4 subunit, BP180, and BP230. Other subsets of patients targeting unique BMZ antigens will likely be identified.

A sensitive ELISA test for laminin 5 antibodies has made it easier to identify this subset of patients. Among those whose antibodies target laminin 5 (antiepiligrin CP), most exhibit antibodies to the α subunit, especially the G domains of the α3 subunit. Antibodies may also target the β3 and γ2 subunits. Other patients have been found to have autoantibodies that react with both laminin 6 and laminin 5, prompting the proposed designation of antilaminin cicatricial pemphigoid. In antilaminin cicatricial pemphigoid, IgG anti-BMZ autoantibodies bind to the dermal side of 1-M NaCl-split skin. As with other forms of CP, the disease rarely remits spontaneously. Some data suggest an increased relative risk for solid cancers (mostly adenocarcinomas) in these patients. Tumors are usually found during the first year of the disease. Other data suggest that antilaminin 332 autoantibodies are associated with severe MMP but not malignancy. These patients also have higher rates of oropharyngeal involvement. In contrast to the possible increased tumor risk in antilaminin 5 CP, some data suggest that patients with antibodies to the β4 integrin subunit have a decreased risk of cancer.

Histopathology

The histologic findings of CP are identical to those of BP, except that fibrosis and scarring may be present in the upper dermis. Basement membrane separation occurs in the lamina lucida or below the lamina densa, depending on the targeted antibody. The inflammatory infiltrate is variable. DIF testing of perilesional skin or mucosa reveals C3 and IgG at the lamina lucida in 80%–95% of patients. The BMZ of mucosal glands stains as well. IgA may be found occasionally. False-negative studies are not uncommon, and repeated biopsies increase the sensitivity for DIF to detect the disease. A circulating antibody to the BMZ is found by IIF in about 20% of CP patients. Immunoelectron microscopy shows that lamina lucida antibodies bind at a deeper level than with BP. Most IIF-positive cases show IgG binding to the epidermal side of salt-split skin, although combined staining and dermal staining may be present in different subtypes, as previously noted. Laser scanning confocal microscopy using fluorescein isothiocyanate–conjugated antihuman IgG antibody has been employed to determine the localization of IgG at the BMZ, and may be of value in patients with negative IIF. "Knockout" skin substrates and fluorescent overlay antigen mapping have also been used to differentiate between antiepiligrin CP and EBA.

Treatment

Because patients can rapidly develop blindness, early, aggressive treatment is indicated. Cyclophosphamide or rituximab-containing regimens are generally advised. A review of studies using the Cochrane criteria found two small RCTs, both in patients with severe eye involvement. In one, 6 months of cyclophosphamide was superior to prednisone. In the second RCT, 20 of 20 patients responded well to 3 months of cyclophosphamide, but only 14 of 20 responded to dapsone. Based on these limited data and other, uncontrolled trials, the reviewers concluded that patients with severe ocular CP respond best to cyclophosphamide combined with corticosteroids, and that those with mild to moderate disease may respond to dapsone. MMF, methotrexate, and azathioprine have also been used effectively in some cases and are more effective than dapsone. Rituximab has emerged as an excellent additional option, with multiple studies indicating patients with rituximab added to their regimen demonstrating improved outcomes. One retrospective study showed 24 patients treated with rituxan with 100% achieving disease control, versus 25 patients treated with conventional immunosuppression. IVIG has been used in recalcitrant cases. TNF inhibitors have been reported to help some patients with severe, refractory disease (etanercept, infliximab, and also pentoxifylline).

In patients with mild CP, oral hygiene, topical corticosteroids, intralesional or perilesional triamcinolone, topical calcineurin inhibitors, or topical steroids occluded under vinyl inserts may be effective for desquamative gingivitis and other oral, genital, or cutaneous disease. Cream and gel formulations may be used, or the steroid may be compounded in Orabase. Topical sucralfate suspension may decrease the pain and healing time of the oral and genital ulcers. There have been reports of efficacy of thalidomide, tetracycline combined with niacinamide, dapsone, IVIG, etanercept, systemic corticosteroids, and immunosuppressive drugs.

Amber KT, et al: A systematic review with pooled analysis of clinical presentation and immunodiagnostic testing in mucous membrane pemphigoid. J Eur Acad Dermatol Venereol 2016; 30: 72.

Broussard KC, et al: Autoimmune bullous diseases with skin and eye involvement. Clin Dermatol 2016; 34: 205.

Fukuda A, et al: Four cases of mucous membrane pemphigoid with clinical features of oral lichen planus. Int J Dermatol 2016; 55: 657.

Kalinska-Bienias A, et al: Efficacy and safety of perilesional/intralesional triamcinolone injections in oral mucous membrane pemphigoid. Br J Dermatol 2016; 174: 436.

Li X, et al: Integrin β4 is a major target antigen in pure ocular mucous membrane pemphigoid. Eur J Dermatol 2016; 26: 247.

Maley A, et al: Rituximab combined with conventional therapy versus conventional therapy alone for the treatment of mucous membrane pemphigoid. J Am Acad Dermatol 2016; 74: 835.

Nottage JM, et al: Treatment of mucous membrane pemphigoid with mycophenolate mofetil. Cornea 2013; 32: 810.

Queisi MM, et al: Update on ocular cicatricial pemphigoid and emerging treatments. Surv Ophthalmol 2016; 61: 314.

Rubsam A, et al: Rituximab preserves vision in ocular mucous membrane pemphigoid. Expert Opin Biol Ther 2015; 15: 927.

Shetty S, et al: Critical analysis of the use of rituximab in mucous membrane pemphigoid. J Am Acad Dermatol 2013; 68: 499.

Shimanovich I, et al: Multiple and repeated sampling increases the sensitivity of direct immunofluorescence testing for the diagnosis of mucous membrane pemphigoid. J Am Acad Dermatol 2017; 77: 700.

You C, et al: Rituximab in the treatment of ocular cicatricial pemphigoid. Graefes Arch Clin Exp Ophthalmol 2017; 255: 1221.

Yuan H, et al: Endoscopic characteristics of oesophagus involvement in mucous membrane pemphigoid. Br J Dermatol 2017; 177: 902.

EPIDERMOLYSIS BULLOSA ACQUISITA

Initial proposed criteria for EBA included the following:

1. Clinical lesions of dystrophic epidermolysis bullosa, including increased skin fragility, trauma-induced blistering with erosions

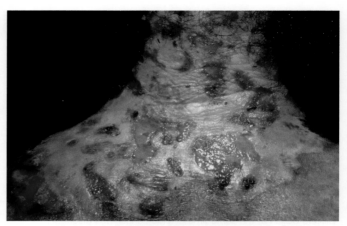

Fig. 21.20 Epidermolysis bullosa acquisita.

(Fig. 21.20), atrophic scarring, milia over extensor surfaces, and nail dystrophy
2. Adult onset
3. Lack of a family history of epidermolysis bullosa
4. Exclusion of all other bullous diseases, such as porphyria cutanea tarda, pemphigoid, pemphigus, dermatitis herpetiformis, and bullous drug eruption

In 1981 Roenigk et al. extended these criteria to include the following:

5. IgG at the basement membrane zone by DIF
6. Demonstration of blister formation beneath the basal lamina
7. Deposition of IgG beneath the basal lamina

Patients may also have mucosal involvement. The antibodies have been found to target type VII collagen, a major component of anchoring fibrils. The target is the same as that in bullous lupus erythematosus. In some patients, it has been shown that autoantibodies bind to the NC-1 domain of collagen VII within the lamina densa. IIF studies reveal circulating anti-BMZ antibodies in approximately half of cases. B cells, dendritic cells, and macrophages are required to induce the CD4 helper T-cell response that results in the formation of pathogenic antibodies. Neutrophil activation and recruitment appear to play an important role. Type VII collagen ELISA using the NC1 and NC2 domains is useful for diagnosis, and antibody levels have been shown to correlate with disease severity.

The noninflammatory clinical presentation of EBA is the most frequently recognized type. A rare erythrodermic presentation has been reported. The association of EBA with many systemic diseases, such as myeloma, inflammatory bowel disease (especially Crohn disease), diabetes, lymphoma, leukemia, amyloidosis, hepatitis C infection, and carcinoma, is well established. EBA is associated with HLA-DR2, and in patients of African descent, HLA-DRB1*15:03.

Cases were reported describing patients with generalized inflammatory bullous disease that resembled BP clinically but with immunologic and ultrastructural features of EBA. Many of these patients have associated diabetes mellitus, are HLA-DR2 positive, and progress to the trauma-induced scarring type of EBA in the long term. Approximately 5%–10% of patients referred to medical centers as having BP may actually have EBA. Rare patients have been reported who meet criteria for both BP and EBA and appear to have both diseases.

Patients with EBA usually have a predominance of neutrophils over eosinophils, although this is variable. On IIF, EBA patients are more likely to have linear IgG without concomitant C3

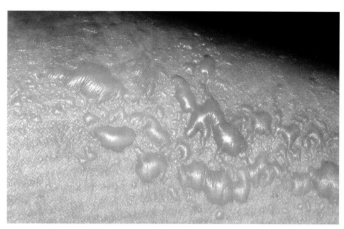

Fig. 21.21 Inflammatory epidermolysis bullosa acquisita.

deposition than are patients with BP. Immunofluorescence on salt-split skin allows differentiation of the majority of cases without the need to resort to immunoblot techniques or immunoelectron microscopy. By DIF testing of the patient's salt-split-skin biopsy, EBA will manifest IgG deposition only on the dermal side of the split, whereas the majority of BP patients will have IgG bound only to the epidermal side or to both sides. The finding of a u-serrated pattern on DIF may make the salt-split-skin assay unnecessary. As noted earlier, some patients with BP have antibodies that target sub–lamina densa antigen. Absolute differentiation of these diseases is obtained by immunoelectron microscopy or immunoblot findings. In EBA, immunoblotting identifies 290-kD and 145-kD proteins, corresponding to type VII collagen. Blistering appears to be T-cell dependent.

Bullous systemic lupus erythematosus (SLE) and EBA demonstrate clinical and histologic overlap, but the following features favor EBA: skin fragility, predilection for traumatized areas, and healing with scars and milia. In bullous SLE, sun-exposed skin is involved by preference, and the patient has a diagnosis of SLE established by American College of Rheumatology criteria; bullous SLE patients usually have a dramatic response to dapsone. In addition to the cases of bullous SLE that show linear IgG staining below the lamina densa with circulating IgG autoantibodies to the 290-kD and 145-kD antigens, some patients will show granular staining of IgG at the BMZ without circulating IgG. EBA-like eruptions are rarely seen as a result of penicillamine therapy.

Purely IgA-mediated EBA has been described. The patients resemble linear IgA dermatosis or inflammatory IgG-mediated EBA. Only a minority demonstrate milia or scarring. Immunoblotting or fluorescence overlay antigen mapping using laser scanning confocal microscopy can distinguish the two diseases. IgM-type EBA has also been reported, with a milder phenotypes and predominantly mechanically induced bullae at sites of pressure.

Treatment

A review of the literature using Cochrane criteria failed to identify any RCTs. EBA is often resistant to therapy, but good responses have been reported in some patients treated with systemic corticosteroids alone or in combination with azathioprine or dapsone. Rituximab and IVIG together have helped patients resistant to standard therapy. Other agents reported to be effective include rituximab, MMF, IVIG, cyclosporine, colchicine, plasmapheresis, photophoresis, infliximab, minocycline, and daclizumab. Given the role of neutrophils, some have suggested further examination of treatments blocking neutrophil chemokines and cytokines. PDE-4 inhibitors were effective in an in vitro model.

Supportive therapy, including control of infection, careful wound management, and maintenance of good nutrition, should be emphasized.

Adachi A, et al: Oral colchicine monotherapy for epidermolysis bullosa acquisita. J Dermatol 2016; 43: 1389.
Hafliger S, et al: Erythrodermic epidermolysis bullosa acquisita. JAMA Dermatol 2015; 151: 1566.
Hashimoto T, et al: Clinical and immunological studies for 105 Japanese seropositive patients of epidermolysis bullosa acquisita examined at Kurume University. Expert Rev Clin Immunol 2016; 12: 895.
Iranzo P, et al: Epidermolysis bullosa acquisita. Br J Dermatol 2014; 171: 1022.
Kasperkiewicz M, et al: Epidermolysis bullosa acquisita. J Invest Dermatol 2016; 136: 24.
Kim JH, et al: Serum levels of anti-type VII collagen antibodies detected by enzyme-linked immunosorbent assay in patients with epidermolysis bullosa acquisita are correlated with the severity of skin lesions. J Eur Acad Dermatol Venereol 2013; 27: e224.
Kim JH, et al: Successful treatment of epidermolysis bullosa acquisita with rituximab therapy. J Dermatol 2012; 39: 477.
Koga H, et al: PDE4 inhibition as potential treatment of epidermolysis bullosa acquisita. J Invest Dermatol 2016; 136: 2211.
Ludwig RJ: Clinical presentation, pathogenesis, diagnosis, and treatment of epidermolysis bullosa acquisita. ISRN Dermatol 2013; 2013: 812029.
Oktem A, et al: Long-term results of rituximab-intravenous immunoglobulin combination therapy in patients with epidermolysis bullosa acquisita resistant to conventional therapy. J Dermatolog Treat 2017; 28: 50.
Omland SH, et al: IgM-type epidermolysis bullosa acquisita. Br J Dermatol 2015; 173: 1566.
Reddy H, et al: Epidermolysis bullosa acquisita and inflammatory bowel disease. Clin Exp Dermatol 2013; 38: 225.
Vorobyey A, et al: Clinical features and diagnosis of epidermolysis bullosa acquisita. Expert Rev Clin Immunol 2017; 13: 157.
Yamase A, et al: An autoimmune bullous dermatosis with clinical, histopathological, and immunological features of bullous pemphigoid and epidermolysis bullosa acquisita in an adult. Br J Dermatol 2016; 175: 790.

DERMATITIS HERPETIFORMIS (DUHRING DISEASE)

Clinical Features

Dermatitis herpetiformis (DH) is a chronic, relapsing, severely pruritic disease characterized by grouped, symmetric lesions on extensor surfaces, the scalp, nuchal area, and buttocks. The lesions are severely pruritic and thus generally present as excoriations rather than vesicles or bullae. The eruption usually occurs on an erythematous base and may be papular, papulovesicular, vesiculobullous (Fig. 21.22), bullous, or urticarial. Linear petechial lesions may be noted on the volar surfaces of the fingers, as well as the palms. Pigmented spots alone over the lumbosacral region should arouse suspicion of DH. The mucous membranes are involved in rare cases, mostly when bullae are numerous. Laryngeal lesions may manifest as hoarseness. Itching is usually intense, but spontaneous remissions lasting as long as 1 week and terminating abruptly with a new crop of lesions are a characteristic feature of the disease. Perimenstrual flares may rarely occur.

Between 77% and 90% of patients with DH and IgA deposits in the skin are HLA-B8 positive, a similar frequency to that observed in gluten-sensitive enteropathy (GSE). HLA antigens DR3 and DQw2 are also increased in frequency. Black and Asian patients are uncommon, possibly because of HLA differences. These HLA markers are associated with other autoimmune diseases

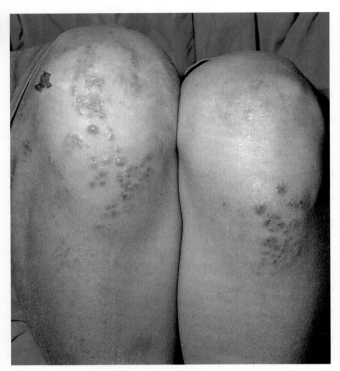

Fig. 21.22 Dermatitis herpetiformis.

and indicate patients who appear to have an overactive immune response to common antigens and who may clear immune complexes slowly. DH is more common in those with affected family members.

In childhood DH is usually similar to the adult type, has identical histologic and immunofluorescent findings, and has a high incidence of HLA-B8 and HLA-DR3 and abnormal jejunal biopsies. Palmar blisters and brown, hemorrhagic, purpuric macules may be more common than in adults. Treatment with sulfones results in prompt response in children, as in adults.

Gluten, a protein found in cereals, except for rice and corn, provokes flares of the disease. Villous atrophy of the jejunum and inflammation of the small bowel occur. IgA is bound to the skin, and this apparently activates complement, primarily through the alternate pathway. Oral iodides will cause a flare of the disease. Patch tests with 50% potassium iodide in petrolatum produce a bulla in uncontrolled DH, but only exceptionally in patients controlled by a gluten-free diet or by sulfone therapy.

Associated Disease

Thyroid disorders are increased in incidence in patients with DH. Neurologic disease, including ataxia, may occur. An increased incidence of malignancy, especially small bowel lymphoma, has also been noted in some studies, although others have reported this increase with celiac disease but not DH. In fact, the incidence of breast cancer may be lower in those with DH than in the general population. A high prevalence of cryofibrinogenemia was reported in one study.

Enteropathy

Between 70% and 100% of patients with DH have abnormalities in the jejunal mucosa, but most are asymptomatic. If given a high-gluten diet, virtually all patients with DH develop findings indistinguishable from celiac disease, and DH affects approximately 25% of patients presenting with celiac disease.

The dapsone requirement in DH is usually decreased after 3–6 months of a gluten-free diet. The majority of patients who adhere to a strict gluten-free diet can eventually stop their medication or significantly reduce the dosage. A gluten-free diet is not easy to follow but may decrease the incidence of intestinal lymphoma.

Diagnosis

The distinction of DH from linear IgA bullous dermatosis is often clinically impossible. Other conditions considered in the differential diagnosis at times are BP, bullous EM, scabies, contact dermatitis, atopic dermatitis, nummular eczema, neurotic excoriations, insect bites, and chronic bullous disease of childhood. The finding of IgA in a granular pattern at the DEJ with accentuation in the dermal papillae is specific for DH.

Autoantibodies

Circulating IgA antibodies against the smooth muscle cell endomysium (antiendomysial antibodies) are present in 70% of DH patients, in almost all patients with active celiac disease, and almost never in other conditions. Tissue transglutaminase (TTG) is the major autoantigen in GSE. IgA antibodies directed at TTG2 are common in patients with DH or celiac disease, but epidermal transglutaminase (TTG3) appears to be the most important antigen. Dietary exposure to gliadin proteins in wheat and related proteins from barley and rye induce flares of the disease. These proteins are high-affinity substrates for TTG. The two are often tightly bound, which may explain why an antibody response is generated against both gliadin and TTG. Gliadins can also be found in rice, corn, and oats, but these proteins are poor substrates for TTG.

Epidemiology

This disease has an equal male-to-female incidence. The average age of onset is 20–40 years. DH does occur with some frequency in children. Black and Asian persons are rarely affected.

Histopathology

The initial changes of DH are noted at the tips of the dermal papillae, where edema, focal fibrin, and neutrophilic microabscesses are seen. The cellular infiltrate contains many neutrophils but may also include a few eosinophils. A subepidermal separation is noted histologically. Ultrastructurally, the split may begin in the lamina lucida. In a study of 24 patients with confirmed DH, 37.5% had nonspecific findings on hematoxylin and eosin (H&E) staining, including a lymphocytic infiltrate, ectatic capillaries, and fibrosis in the dermal papillae. Because of the potential for nonspecific biopsy findings, DIF studies are essential. Histologic differentiation of linear IgA bullous dermatosis from DH is extremely difficult unless DIF is performed. DIF of noninvolved perilesional skin reveals deposits of IgA alone or together with C3 arranged in a granular pattern at the DEJ. The deposits are typically accentuated in the dermal papillae. IgM and IgG deposits are occasionally observed in association with IgA. Deposits may be focal, so multiple biopsies may be needed, and the deposits of antibody are more often seen in previously involved skin or normal-appearing skin adjacent to involved skin. IgA is observed by immunoelectron microscopy, either alone or in conjunction with C3, IgG, or IgM, as clumps in the upper dermis. A vertically oriented fibrillar staining pattern exists in a subset of patients, with immune deposits along dermal microfibrils, creating a "picket fence" pattern of immunofluorescence. The fibrillar pattern is present in a third of Japanese patients, and this group lacks the typical distribution of skin lesions and has a low association with celiac disease. A few patients will have negative DIF despite typical clinical findings and evidence of antiendomysial antibodies. IIF is rarely positive.

Treatment

Adherence to a gluten-free diet is important, because it reduces the risk of intestinal disease. Compliance can often reduce the need for or dose of treatment. The drugs chiefly used for DH are dapsone and sulfapyridine. The most effective sulfone is diaminodiphenylsulfone (dapsone). The dose usually ranges from 50 mg/d to 150mg/d, with rare cases requiring up to 300mg/day. Doses are increased gradually to an effective level or until side effects occur. Once a favorable response is attained, the dosage is decreased to the minimum that does not permit recurrence of signs and symptoms. When dapsone is discontinued abruptly, large bullae similar to those seen in BP frequently occur. Hemolytic anemia, leukopenia, methemoglobinemia, agranulocytosis, or peripheral neuropathy may occur with dapsone. Acute hemolytic anemia (which may be severe) occurs in patients with glucose-6-phosphate dehydrogenase (G6PD) deficiency; therefore G6PD level should be measured before therapy. In those whose ethnic background makes G6PD deficiency unlikely, some authorities begin dapsone at a low starting dose (25 mg/day) and watch the patient closely for dark urine. The patient should be warned to report by telephone any incident of red or brown urine or blue nail beds or lips. A blood count should be done weekly for 4 weeks, bimonthly for the next 3 months, and every 2–6 months thereafter. Liver function tests should be monitored bimonthly for the first 4 months, then checked with the hematologic studies every 4–6 months.

Agranulocytosis is rare. It typically occurs 1–3 months after initiation of drug therapy and presents with sore throat, aphthae, or evidence of infection. The risk of agranulocytosis is higher in older patients (>60 years) and nonwhite persons. The incidence varies with the disease. It is rarely seen in patients with Hansen disease, but patients with DH have a 25-fold to 33-fold increased risk.

Sulfapyridine can also be used to treat the disease. After a test dose of 0.5 g of sulfapyridine, 1 tablet (0.5 g) is given four times daily. The dose is then increased if necessary, or reduced if possible. Usually 1–4 g/day is required for good control. The drug is less water soluble than dapsone, and patients should remain hydrated. Sulfasalazine, 500 mg three times daily, increased to 1.5 g three times daily as tolerated, may also be used, because sulfapyridine is a metabolic product. GI intolerance may limit the dosage.

In rare patients, it is necessary to find alternatives to the sulfone drugs. Tetracycline/nicotinamide and colchicine have controlled individual patients. Topical dapsone 5% gel may be effective. Rituximab has been used in one case of recalcitrant DH. Heparin has been used in the past but is generally unnecessary with newer options.

Gluten-Free Diet

Patients must strictly avoid wheat, barley, and rye. Moderate amounts of oats may be tolerated. In Canada, standards for growing, processing, testing, and labeling of pure, uncontaminated oats have allowed adults to consume up to 70 g (about one half to three quarters cup) of oats and children to consume up to 25 g (one quarter cup) daily without flares of disease. Corn and rice are generally well tolerated, corresponding to the poor binding of their gliadin proteins to TTG, but exacerbation of disease related to cornstarch has been reported. If a gluten-free diet is followed strictly, the patient will almost certainly be able to take less medication or stop it altogether. Some evidence suggests that this may decrease the incidence of associated malignancy; however, it is a very difficult diet to follow.

Once a prolonged remission has been obtained, some gluten may be tolerated in a subset of patients. In one study, 38 patients who had followed a gluten-free diet for a mean of 8 years reintroduced gluten to their diets. Thirty-one experienced recurrence within an average of 2 months, but seven remained in remission for a mean follow-up of 12 years. IgA deposits did not recur in their skin. This report suggests that clinical and histologic remission can be maintained in some patients with DH despite the reintroduction of dietary gluten.

For most patients, however, a gluten-free diet remains an important aspect of disease management. Fortunately, many grocery stores now have a section devoted to gluten-free products. Support may be obtained from the American Celiac Society/Dietary Support Coalition (www.americanceliacsociety.org/diet.html) or from celiac societies (www.nowheat.com/grfx/nowheat/primer/celisoc.htm or www.enabling.org/ia/celiac/groups/groupsus.html). A commercial website with a search engine can be found at www.celiac.com. Another commercial source for products can be found at www.glutenfreemall.com. An Internet search using the terms "celiac society" or "gluten-free diet" is a good starting point for patients with the disease who want more information about the diet and commercially available products.

Albers LN, et al: Rituximab treatment for recalcitrant dermatitis herpetiformis. JAMA Dermatol 2017; 153: 315.

Antiga E, et al: Clinical and immunopathological features of 159 patients with dermatitis herpetiformis. G Ital Dermatol Venereol 2013; 148: 163.

Bognar P, et al: High prevalence of cryofibrinogenaemia in dermatitis herpetiformis. J Eur Acad Dermatol Venereol 2016; 30: 517.

Burbidge T, et al: Topical dapsone 5% gel as an effective therapy in dermatitis herpetiformis. J Cutan Med Surg 2016; 20: 600.

Clarindo MV, et al: Dermatitis herpetiformis. An Bras Dermatol 2014; 89: 865.

Fabbri P, et al: Novel advances in dermatitis herpetiformis. Clin Dev Immunol 2012; 2012: 450109.

Fasano A: Novel therapeutic/integrative approaches for celiac disease and dermatitis herpetiformis. Clin Dev Immunol 2012; 2012: 959061.

Hervonen K, et al: Dermatitis herpetiformis refractory to gluten-free dietary treatment. Acta Derm Venereol 2016; 96: 82.

Huber C, et al: Negative direct immunofluorescence and non-specific histology do not exclude the diagnosis of dermatitis herpetiformis Duhring. Int J Dermatol 2013; 52: 248.

Jakes AD, et al: Dermatitis herpetiformis. BMJ 2014; 348: g2557.

Zaghi D, et al: Petechial eruption on fingers. JAMA Dermatol 2014; 150: 1353.

LINEAR IGA BULLOUS DERMATOSIS

Linear IgA bullous dermatosis (LAD) is characterized by subepidermal blisters, a neutrophilic infiltrate, and a circulating IgA anti-BMZ antibody with linear BMZ deposits on DIF. As with CP, LAD is really a group of diseases with a similar immunofluorescent pattern.

Adult Linear IgA Disease

Adult patients with LAD may present with a clinical pattern of vesicles indistinguishable from DH or with vesicles and bullae having a BP-like appearance, with severe cases mimicking Stevens-Johnson syndrome. They may have urticarial lesions, and bullae may occur on an urticarial base, as in BP (Fig. 21.23). Unusual variants include morbilliform, prurigo-like, and eczematous presentation. Mucous membrane involvement may occur in up to 50% of patients. In some, oral and conjunctival lesions dominate the presentation, and scarring may occur, as in CP. Younger patients

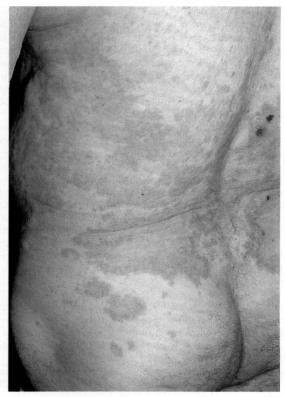

Fig. 21.23 Adult linear IgA disease.

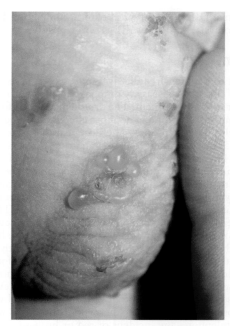

Fig. 21.24 Childhood linear IgA disease.

and those with mucosal disease appear to be at risk for chronic disease and less likely to achieve remission. In the majority of patients, there is no association with enteropathy or with HLA-B8. The disease remits after several years in approximately 60% of patients. IgA is typically directed against a 97-kD antigen in the lamina lucida. Some patients demonstrate both IgA and IgG antibodies to BP180, and IgA to LAD285. IgA and IgG reactivity has been found to all three portions of the BP180 ectodomain. In some patients, the strongest reactivity is to the C-terminal portion of BP180 (major antigenic area in CP). This may explain cases of clinical overlap with CP. Type VII collagen has been reported as the major autoantigen for LAD targeting the sublamina densa, possibly explaining the overlap with bullous SLE and EBA. Antigenic targets for LAD are expressed by both keratinocytes and fibroblasts. Recent cases have demonstrated LAD to laminin-332.

Linear IgA dermatosis frequently occurs as a drug-induced disease. In drug-induced LAD the eruption is self-limited, there is less mucosal involvement, and usually there is no detectable circulating autoantibody. The IgA may be deposited in the sub–basal lamina area. Vancomycin is the most frequently implicated culprit. Other causes of drug-induced disease include lithium, amiodarone, carbamazepine, captopril, penicillin, amoxicillin, trimethoprim/sulfamethoxazole, piperacillin-tazobactam, moxifloxacin, UV light, furosemide, oxaprozin, IL-2, interferon-α, phenytoin, ketoprofen, diclofenac, statins, tea tree oil, angiotensin receptor antagonists, sulfasalazine, buprenorphine, ustekinumab, infliximab, and gliben-clamide. The lymphocyte stimulation test has been reported as a possible method to assess drug causality with improved specificity.

Some cases have been associated with internal malignancy, paraproteinemia, or infection. Sporadic reports have linked single cases with dermatomyositis, rheumatoid arthritis, acquired hemophilia, and multiple sclerosis, although these may be fortuitous associations.

Biopsies typically demonstrate papillary dermal microabscess with neutrophils. As in DH, eosinophils may be present. On DIF, a homogeneous linear (tubular or toothpaste) pattern of IgA is present at the BMZ. Some patients will have both linear IgA and IgG in combination at the BMZ. A lack of C3 may be a clue that both immunoglobulins recognize the 97-kD antigen.

By IIF, only a minority of LAD patients will have circulating IgA autoantibody with anti-BMZ specificity, and this is usually present in low titer. On salt-split skin, deposition may occur on the roof or base, or a combination of the two.

In drug-induced disease, the drug must be stopped. Many cases resolve quickly, but some patients require drug therapy with corticosteroids or dapsone. Idiopathic disease generally responds to dapsone in doses similar to that described for DH; sulfapyridine may also be used. Other patients require topical or systemic corticosteroids in addition, or as sole treatment. A combination of tetracycline, 2 g/day, and nicotinamide, 1.5 g/day, may be effective. Other patients have responded to MMF, IVIG, colchicine, trimethoprim-sulfamethoxazole, or erythromycin. The rare patients with associated GSE may respond to a gluten-free diet.

Childhood Linear IgA Disease (Chronic Bullous Disease of Childhood)

Chronic bullous disease of childhood (CBDC) is an acquired, self-limited bullous disease that may begin by the time the patient is 2 or 3 years old and usually remits by age 13. The average age of onset is 5 years. Bullae develop on either erythematous or normal-appearing skin, preferentially involving the lower trunk, buttocks, genitalia, and thighs (Fig. 21.24). Perioral and scalp lesions are common, and oral mucous membrane lesions may occur in up to 75% of patients. Bullae are often arranged in rosettes or an annular array, the so-called string of pearls configuration (Fig. 21.25). Tense individual bullae similar to those in BP are also seen. Pruritus is often severe.

The prime histologic finding is the presence of a subepidermal bulla filled with neutrophils. Eosinophils may be present, and in some cases they predominate. DIF reveals a linear deposition of IgA at the BMZ identical to that seen in the adult forms of the disease. IIF is positive for circulating IgA anti-BMZ antibodies

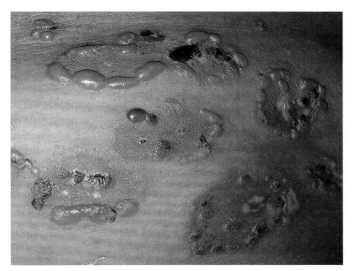

Fig. 21.25 Childhood linear IgA disease. (Courtesy Debabrata Bandyopadhyay, MD.)

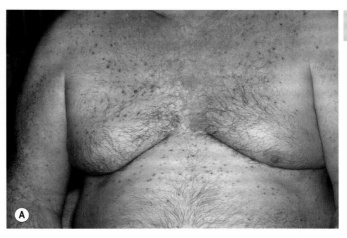

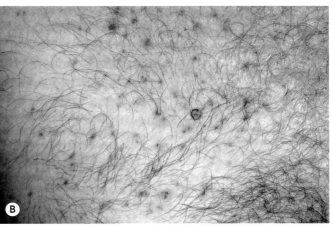

Fig. 21.26 (A and B) Transient acantholytic dermatosis. (Courtesy Steven Binnick, MD.)

in approximately 50% of patients, usually in low titer. In contrast to adults with LAD, children demonstrate an increased frequency of B8, DR3, and DQ2 and may be homozygous for these antigens. As in the adult disease, immunoelectron microscopy and immunomapping studies may demonstrate immune deposits within the lamina lucida, below the lamina densa, or both. Also as in adult disease, some children have both IgG and IgA deposits. GSE is rare, but IgA nephropathy may occur. Childhood linear IgA disease has occurred in conjunction with Crohn disease.

Many patients' antibodies target the 97-kD peptide. Some children with sub–basal lamina deposits target type VII collagen and have EBA. Patients with only IgA or with both IgG and IgA circulating autoantibodies may target BP230 or BP180. Individual patients may have a combination of IgA against the 97-kD peptide, and IgG against BP230 and BP180. Collagen XVII/BP180 is a transmembrane protein with a soluble 120-kD ectodomain. In linear IgA dermatosis and CBDC, IgA targets the soluble ectodomain more efficiently than the full-length protein. Some sera target the Col15 domain.

The untreated disease runs a variable course, typically with eventual spontaneous resolution by adolescence. Treatment with either dapsone or sulfapyridine is usually successful. Occasional cases respond to topical corticosteroids alone, and systemic corticosteroids are sometimes necessary. Other patients have responded to MMF, colchicine, topical calcineurin inhibitors, or dicloxacillin.

Adler NR, et al: Piperacillin-tazobactam-induced linear IgA bullous dermatosis presenting as Stevens-Johnson syndrome/toxic epidermal necrolysis overlap. Clin Exp Dermatol 2017; 42: 299.

Concha-Garzon MJ, et al: Ketoprofen-induced lamina lucida-type linear IgA bullous dermatosis. J Eur Acad Dermatol Venereol 2016; 30: 350.

Gottlieb J, et al: Idiopathic linear IgA bullous dermatosis. Br J Dermatol 2017; 177: 212.

Hoffmann J, et al: Linear IgA bullous dermatosis secondary to infliximab therapy in a patient with ulcerative colitis. Dermatology 2015; 231: 112.

Ishii N: Prognostic factors of patients with linear IgA bullous dermatosis. Br J Dermatol 2017; 177: 16.

Lings K, et al: Linear IgA bullous dermatosis. Acta Derm Venereol 2015; 95: 466.

Tomida E, et al: Causative drug detection by drug-induced lymphocyte stimulation test in drug-induced linear IgA bullous dermatosis. Br J Dermatol 2016; 175: 1106.

Tsuchisaka A, et al: Type VII collagen is the major autoantigen for sublamina densa-type linear IgA bullous dermatosis. J Invest Dermatol 2015; 135: 626.

Wozniak K, et al: UV-induced linear IgA bullous dermatosis. Br J Dermatol 2014; 171: 1578.

Zenke Y, et al: A case of vancomycin-associated linear IgA bullous dermatosis and IgA antibodies to the a3 subunit of laminin-332. Br J Dermatol 2014; 170: 965.

TRANSIENT ACANTHOLYTIC DERMATOSIS (GROVER DISEASE)

In 1970 Grover described a new dermatosis that occurred predominantly in persons over 50 years of age and consisted of a sparse eruption of limited duration. The lesions were fragile vesicles that rapidly turned into crusted and keratotic erosions. He termed the condition *transient acantholytic dermatosis* (TAD). Since then, the majority of cases have been found to persist or recur, and the term *persistent and recurrent acantholytic dermatosis* may be a more accurate description of the disorder. The distribution is predominantly limited to the chest or shoulder girdle area and upper abdomen, and there is a strong male predominance (Fig. 21.26). The condition often appears or flares during periods of heat, sweating, or hospitalization. Many patients are asymptomatic, and the condition may be an incidental finding on examination. Other patients complain of pruritus. Asteatotic eczema occurs five times as often among patients with TAD as in controls. The disorder has been described in the setting of a variety of malignancies, but it may be associated with the hospitalization or type B symptoms rather than the malignancy itself. TAD has been reported with cetuximab. This pattern may also occur rarely as a side effect from chemotherapy. Patients on strict bed rest appear to have a higher incidence of the disease. The clinical differential diagnosis includes Galli-Galli disease, an acantholytic variant of Dowling-Degos disease that may resemble TAD clinically.

There are five histologic types, resembling Darier disease, PV, PF, benign familial pemphigus, or spongiotic dermatitis. The Darier type predominates. Often, two or more types can be found in a single biopsy specimen. DIF studies yield negative or nonspecific results. Although heat and sweating are significant risk factors, only a minority of cases are associated with acrosyringia histologically. Impairment of keratinocytic cholinergic receptors has been suggested as a pathogenic mechanism.

About 50% of patients respond to topical corticosteroids. Control of fever, hospital discharge, and avoidance of sun and sweating often result in improvement. Sustained remission has been described after a course of systemic corticosteroids. Topical antibiotics, topical calcipotriol, isotretinoin, and dapsone have been successful in some patients. Psoralen plus UVA (PUVA) has been reported to result in an initial flare followed by slow clearance, and UVB therapy may produce clearing in some patients. Photodynamic therapy with red light and 5-aminolevulinic acid has been reported as successful, and rituximab has produced clearing of TAD in patients being treated for lymphoma.

Arbache ST, et al: Immunofluorescence testing in the diagnosis of autoimmune blistering diseases. An Bras Dermatol 2014; 89: 885.

Braunstein I, et al: Treatment of dermatologic connective tissue disease and autoimmune blistering disorders in pregnancy. Dermatol Ther 2013; 26: 354.

Fine JD: Prevalence of autoantibodies to bullous pemphigoid antigens within the normal population. Arch Dermatol 2010; 146: 74.

Liu S, et al: Successful novel treatment of recalcitrant transient acantholytic dermatosis (Grover disease) using red light 5-aminolevulinic acid photodynamic therapy. Dermatol Surg 2013; 39: 960.

Paslin D: Grover disease may result from the impairment of keratinocytic cholinergic receptors. J Am Acad Dermatol 2012; 66: 332.

Phillips C, et al: Is Grover's disease an autoimmune dermatosis? Exp Dermatol 2013; 22: 781.

Segura S, et al: High-dose intravenous immunoglobulins for the treatment of autoimmune mucocutaneous blistering diseases. J Am Acad Dermatol 2007; 56: 960.

22 Nutritional Diseases

A nutritional disease is caused either by insufficiency or, less often, by excess of one or more dietary essentials. Nutritional deficiencies are particularly common in developing countries but can also occur due to fad diets or restrictive eating practices in patients with behavioral or autism spectrum disorders. Infants and children are particularly at risk for deficiency states, especially malnutrition. Infants diagnosed with multiple food allergies who substitute other nutrition such as rice milk for breast milk or standard baby formulas are at particular risk. Frequently, patients have features of several nutrient deficiencies if their diet has generally been restricted. An intertriginous or acral eruption, a seborrheic dermatitis–like facial eruption, atrophic glossitis, and alopecia are common features of many nutritional deficiencies. This occurs because these nutrients are essential to overlapping metabolic pathways of fatty acid metabolism, resulting in abnormal differentiation of the epidermis and defective barrier function. The histologic findings in many types of nutritional dermatosis are also similar.

In developed countries, alcoholism is the main cause of nutritional diseases in adults. Nutritional diseases should also be suspected in postoperative patients; psychiatric patients, including those with anorexia nervosa and bulimia; patients on the autism spectrum who have textural issues with certain foods; patients on restrictive diets; patients with surgical or inflammatory bowel dysfunction, especially Crohn disease; patients who have had bowel bypass surgery; cystic fibrosis patients; and patients with severe oral erosive disease (e.g., pemphigus) that prevents eating. In the pediatric setting, nutritional deficiency may also occur because of parental ignorance of the nutritional requirements or restriction due to concern for perceived or actual food allergies.

The diagnosis of nutritional deficiency is often missed because physicians fail to take an adequate dietary history. When children have protein malnutrition, their albumin is low and thus cannot serve its role as an osmotic agent to hold serum in the vessels. Therefore children will gain weight, which clinically masks their severe deficiency in protein. The dermatitis produced by elevated glucagon levels from islet cell tumors of the pancreas (necrolytic migratory erythema) and a similar dermatosis seen in hepatitis C infection and other forms of hepatic insufficiency (necrolytic acral erythema, pseudoglucagonoma) probably also represent nutritional deficiency dermatoses. Deficiency states caused by inborn errors of metabolism are discussed in Chapter 26. In many cases, the clinical findings and socioeconomic scenario are adequate to lead to suspicion of a specific deficiency state, and replacement therapy can confirm the diagnosis. Laboratory testing may be costly and inaccurate in some deficiency states, and patients with poor nutrition are often deficient in many nutrients simultaneously. Testing is indicated to confirm the diagnosis of zinc deficiency, as well as the inborn errors of metabolism that can mimic zinc deficiency, such as propionyl-CoA carboxylase deficiency, methylmelnonic acidemia, isoleucine deficiency, holocarboxylase synthetase deficiency, and biotinidase deficiency; to assess essential fatty acid (EFA) deficiency; and to evaluate for possible glucagonoma syndrome in a child.

VITAMIN A

Hypovitaminosis A (Phrynoderma)

Vitamin A is a fat-soluble vitamin found as retinyl esters in milk, fish oil, liver, and eggs and as carotenoids in plants. Vitamin A deficiency is common in children in the developing world. It is rare in developed countries, where it is most often associated with diseases of fat malabsorption, such as bowel bypass surgery for obesity, pancreatic insufficiency, Crohn disease, inflammatory bowel disease (IBD), celiac disease, cystic fibrosis, and liver disease. Vitamin A is required for the normal keratinization of many mucosal surfaces. When it is deficient, the resultant abnormal keratinization leads to increased mortality risk from inflammatory disease of the gut and lung—diarrhea and pneumonia (especially in measles). Vitamin A supplementation of 200,000 IU/day for 2 days is recommended for children with measles; this may also prevent the risk of blindness.

Although phrynoderma had classically been ascribed to, and thought to be specific for, vitamin A deficiency, this clinical sign is in fact most frequently found as a disorder of multiple deficiencies, including vitamins A, B, C, and E and EFAs. Replacing all these deficiencies leads to rapid improvement. This explains patients in whom the cutaneous findings of phrynoderma were found without the classic eye findings of vitamin A deficiency. The skin eruption, termed *follicular hyperkeratosis* or *phrynoderma* ("toadskin"), resembles keratosis pilaris and the genodermatosis keratosis follicularis spinuloas decalvans. It consists of keratotic papules of various sizes distributed symmetrically over the extremities and shoulders, surrounding and arising from the pilosebaceous follicles (Fig. 22.1). Individual lesions are usually asymptomatic firm, pigmented papules containing a central, intrafollicular keratotic plug that projects from the follicle as a horny spine and leaves a pit when expressed. Lesions are of two sizes: 1–2 mm papules closely resembling keratosis pilaris and the more diagnostic, large, 2–6 mm, crateriform papules filled with a central keratotic plug. These latter lesions may simulate a perforating disorder. The eruption of small lesions usually begins on the anterolateral aspect of the thighs or the posterolateral aspect of the upper arms, although one study showed that the elbows were the most common initial site in 84%. It then spreads to the extensor surfaces of both the upper and the lower extremities, the shoulders, abdomen, back, and buttocks and finally reaches the face and posterior aspect of the neck. The hands and feet are not involved, and lesions occur only occasionally on the midline of the trunk or in the axillary and anogenital areas. On the face, the eruption resembles acne because of the presence of many large comedones, but it differs from acne in regard to dryness of the skin. The large, dome-shaped nodules are on the elbows and knees and have a surrounding red or brown rim. There is generalized dryness, fine scaling, and hyperpigmentation. Hair casts may also be seen.

Vitamin A deficiency may mimic vitamin C deficiency (scurvy) because both conditions cause follicular hyperkeratosis, although the characteristic follicular hemorrhage is more prominent in vitamin C deficiency. Bleeding and gingival disease can be a feature of vitamin A deficiency as well as scurvy. The histologic findings of "deficiency dermatitis," which are common to many deficiency states (zinc, EFAs, amino acids, glucagonoma, cystic

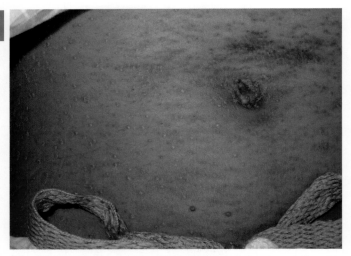

Fig. 22.1 Phrynoderma in a patient with inflammatory bowel disease.

fibrosis), are not features of either vitamin A or vitamin C deficiency.

In vitamin A deficiency, eye findings are prominent and often pathognomonic. These include night blindness, an inability to see bright light, xerophthalmia, xerosis corneae, and keratomalacia. The earliest finding is delayed adaptation to the dark (nyctalopia). Some patients have circumscribed areas of xerosis of the conjunctiva lateral to the cornea, occasionally forming well-defined white spots (Bitot spots); these are triangular, with the apex toward the canthus. Vitamin A deficiency is a major cause of blindness in children in developing countries.

The histologic findings of vitamin A deficiency are hyperkeratosis, horny plugs in the upper portion of the hair follicle, coiled hairs in the upper part of the follicle, severe atrophy of the sebaceous glands, and squamous metaplasia of the secretory cells of the eccrine sweat glands. If the follicles rupture, perifollicular granulomatous inflammation is found.

The diagnosis of vitamin A deficiency is confirmed by determination of the serum retinol level. The treatment is oral vitamin A, 100,000 IU/day for 2–3 days, followed by the recommended dietary requirement. Serum retinol levels are monitored to determine adequacy of supplementation and to avoid vitamin A toxicity.

HYPERVITAMINOSIS A

The skin findings of hypervitaminosis A are similar to the side effects of synthetic retinoid therapy (such as isotretinoin). Children are at greater risk for toxicity than adults. Excess megavitamin ingestion may be the cause. In adults, doses as small as 25,000 IU/day may lead to toxicity, especially in persons with hepatic compromise from alcoholic, viral, or medication-induced hepatitis. Patients on dialysis also are at increased risk, because vitamin A is not removed by dialysis. Standard hyperalimentation solutions contain significant amounts of vitamin A, and in burn victims with renal compromise, vitamin A toxicity can occur. If the patient is taking a synthetic retinoid, all vitamin A supplementation should be stopped.

Most cases of chronic hypervitaminosis A have been reported in children. There is loss of hair and coarseness of the remaining hair, loss of the eyebrows, exfoliative cheilitis, generalized exfoliation and pigmentation of the skin, and clubbing of the fingers. Moderate widespread itching may occur. Hepatomegaly, splenomegaly, hypochromic anemia, depressed serum proteins, and elevated liver function tests may be found. Bone growth may be impaired by premature closure of the epiphyses in children. Pseudotumor cerebri with papilledema may occur early, before any other signs appear. In infants, this may present as a bulging fontanelle.

In adults, the early signs are dryness of the lips and anorexia. These symptoms may be followed by joint and bone pains, follicular hyperkeratosis, branny desquamation of the skin, fissuring of the corners of the mouth and nostrils, dryness and loss of scalp hair and eyebrows, and dystrophy of the nails. Fatigue, myalgia, depression, anorexia, headache (from pseudotumor cerebri), strabismus, and weight loss frequently occur. Liver disease may be progressive and may lead to cirrhosis with chronic toxicity. Hypercalcemia often occurs in dialysis patients and be worsened by the hypervitaminosis A. Retinoids are teratogens, and birth defects may occur with excess vitamin A supplementation during pregnancy.

Bello S, et al: Routine vitamin A supplementation for the prevention of blindness due to measles infection in children. Cochrane Database Syst Rev 2016; 8: CD007719.

Bremner NA, et al: Vitamin A toxicity in burns patients on long-term enteral feed. Burns 2007; 22: 266.

Brown CA, et al: Medical complications of self-induced vomiting. Eat Disord 2013; 21: 287.

Cheruvattath R, et al: Vitamin A toxicity. Liver Transpl 2006; 12: 1888.

Duignan E, et al: Ophthalmic manifestations of vitamin A and D deficiency in two autistic teenagers. Case reports in ophthalmology 2015; 24.

Galimberti F, Mesinkovska NA: Phrynoderma. J Am Acad Dermatol 2017; 76: AB197.

Grauel E, et al: Necrolytic acral erythema. J Drugs Dermatol 2012; 11: 1370.

Halawi A, et al: Bariatric surgery and its effects on the skin and skin diseases. Obes Surg 2013; 23: 408.

Jen M, et al: Syndromes associated with nutritional deficiency and excess. Clin Dermatol 2010; 28: 669.

Monshi B, et al: Phrynoderma and acquired acrodermatitis enteropathica in breastfeeding women after bariatric surgery. J Dtsch Dermatol Ges 2015; 13: 1147.

Ragunatha S, et al: A clinical study of 125 patients with phrynoderma. Indian J Dermatol 2011; 56: 389.

Raphael BA, et al: Low prevalence of necrolytic acral erythema in patients with chronic hepatitis C virus infection. J Am Acad Dermatol 2012; 67: 962.

Romano ME, et al: Dermatologic findings in the evaluation of adolescents with suspected eating disorders. Adolesc Med State Art Rev 2011; 22: 11.

Shmaya Y, et al: Nutritional deficiencies and overweight prevalence among children with autism spectrum disorder. Res Dev Disabil 2015; 38: 1.

Tiang S, et al: Nyctalopia. BMJ Case Reports 2010 Aug 26; 2010.

VITAMIN D

Although active vitamin D is produced in the skin, deficiency of vitamin D has no primary skin manifestations, except for alopecia. Low vitamin D levels correspond in some children with atopic dermatitis (AD) severity, but studies are conflicting. Some studies have found genetic polymorphisms associated with vitamin D not to be more prevalent in atopic patients, but more recently patients with polymorphisms in the CYp24a1 vitamin D–inactivating enzyme were found to have more severe AD. Some patients with AD may improve and manifest fewer infections with vitamin D supplementation. Elderly persons have decreased vitamin D cutaneous photosynthesis because of decreased sun exposure and poor intake of vitamin D, both of which predispose them to osteomalacia. Aggressive photoprotection may also reduce vitamin D levels. Patients with cutaneous lupus and other photosensitive diseases who are counseled to avoid the sun and use high sun protection factor (SPF) sunscreens are at particular risk. Other patients at risk include those who are debilitated with limited sun exposure; those taking anticonvulsants; those with fat malabsorption; and patients with human immunodeficiency virus (HIV) infection, especially dark-skinned patients living in northern climes. Vitamin D_3 supplementation of 600 IU/day should be recommended in all these groups of patients for those up to age 70, and 800 IU for older patients; pediatric dosing is lower and based on age. Dermatologists who have patients at risk should also consider measuring vitamin 25 OH vitamin D levels.

Camargo CA Jr, et al: Randomized trial of vitamin D supplementation for winter-related atopic dermatitis in children. J Allergy Clin Immunol 2014; 134: 831.

Hallau J, et al: A promoter polymorphism of the vitamin D metabolism gene CYP24A1 is associated with severe atopic dermatitis in adults. Acta Derm Venereol 2016; 96: 169.

Malloy PJ, et al: The role of vitamin D receptor mutations in the development of alopecia. Mol Cell Endocrinol 2011; 347: 90.

Manousaki D, et al: Vitamin D levels and susceptibility to asthma, elevated immunoglobulin E levels, and atopic dermatitis. PLoS Med 2017; 14: e1002294.

Pinzone MR, et al: Vitamin D deficiency in HIV infection. Eur Rev Med Pharmacol Sci 2013; 17: 1218.

Vanchinathan V, et al: A dermatologist's perspective on vitamin D. Mayo Clin Proc 2012; 87: 372.

Wang SS, et al: Vitamin D deficiency is associated with diagnosis and severity of childhood atopic dermatitis. Pediatr Allergy Immunol 2014; 24: 30.

VITAMIN K DEFICIENCY

Dietary deficiency of vitamin K, a fat-soluble vitamin, usually does not occur in adults because it is synthesized by bacteria in the large intestine. However, deficiency may occur in adults because of malabsorption caused by biliary disease, malabsorption syndromes, cystic fibrosis, or anorexia nervosa. Drugs such as coumarin, salicylates, cholestyramine, and antibiotics such as trimethoprim-sulfamethoxazole and the cephalosporins may induce a deficiency state. Newborns of mothers taking coumarin or phenytoin and premature infants with an uncolonized intestine can be vitamin K deficient. Standard practice is to administer intramuscular (IM) vitamin K at birth; however, some parents decline this, and those children are at 81 times greater risk of developing vitamin K bleeding than those who do receive it. Additionally, a rare condition exists that predisposes to bleeding, called hereditary combined deficiency of the vitamin K–dependent clotting factors. The liver synthesizes vitamin K–dependent clotting factors II, VII, IX, and X, and requires vitamin K as a cofactor. The result of vitamin K deficiency or severe liver disease is a decrease in the vitamin K–dependent clotting factors. The resulting cutaneous manifestations are purpura, hemorrhage, and ecchymosis and are similar to those seen with coumarin skin necrosis given the shared pathophysiology. Treatment is IM vitamin K for several days. In acute crises, fresh frozen plasma is used because it contains the clotting factors.

Burke CW: Vitamin K deficiency bleeding. J Pediatr Health Care 2013; 27: 215.

Centers for Disease Control and Prevention (CDC): Notes from the field: late vitamin K deficiency bleeding in infants whose parents declined vitamin K prophylaxis—Tennessee, 2013. MMWR Morb Mortal Wkly Rep 2013; 62: 901.

Fotouhie A, et al: Gastrointestinal bleeding secondary to trimethoprim-sulfamethoxazole-induced vitamin K deficiency. BMJ Case Rep 2016 Jun 6; 2016.

Lapecorella M, et al: Effective hemostasis during minor surgery in a case of hereditary combined deficiency of vitamin K–dependent clotting factors. Clin Appl Thromb Hemost 2010; 16: 221.

Napolitano M, et al: Hereditary combined deficiency of the vitamin K–dependent clotting factors. Orphanet J Rare Dis 2010; 5: 21.

Tie JK, et al: Characterization of vitamin K–dependent carboxylase mutations that cause bleeding and nonbleeding disorders. Blood 2016; 127: 1847.

VITAMIN B₁ DEFICIENCY

Vitamin B_1 (thiamine) deficiency results in beriberi. The skin manifestations are limited to edema and red, burning tongue. Peripheral neuropathy is common, and congestive heart failure may develop. In addition to alcoholism and lack of dietary intake, deficiency in vitamin B_1 can occur from bariatric surgery and in intensive care settings without proper nutrition.

Lee LW, et al: Skin manifestations of nutritional deficiency disease in children. Int J Dermatol 2012; 51: 1407.

Leite HP, de Lima LFP: Thiamine (vitamin B_1) deficiency in intensive care: physiology, risk factors, diagnosis, and treatment. In R Rajendram, VR Preedy, VB Patel (Eds.), *Diet and Nutrition in Critical Care* (pp 959-972). New York: 2015, Springer.

Tack J, Deloose E: Complications of bariatric surgery. Best Pract Res Clin Gastroenterol 2014; 28: 741.

VITAMIN B₂ DEFICIENCY

Vitamin B_2 (riboflavin) deficiency is seen most often in alcoholic patients; however, phototherapy for neonatal icterus, acute boric acid ingestion, hypothyroidism, and chlorpromazine therapy have also been reported as causes. The classic findings are the oral-ocular-genital syndrome. The lips are prominently affected with angular cheilitis (perlèche) and cheilosis. The tongue is atrophic and magenta in color (Fig. 22.2). A seborrheic-like dermatitis with follicular keratosis around the nares primarily affects the face. Genital dermatitis is worse in men than in women who have riboflavin deficiency. There is a confluent dermatitis of the scrotum, sparing the midline, with extension onto the thighs. In its mildest form, the dermatitis is slightly "irritating" and pruritic, especially when sweating. As the deficiency progresses, the scrotum goes through a mild, acute dry phase with erythema and slight scale to a severe, chronic dry phase with confluent red papules that spread to involve the perianal area and inner thighs, accompanied by fissuring and pain. Balanitis and phimosis may occur, requiring circumcision. In severe deficiency, the entire scrotum becomes wet, with increasing pain and fissuring. The final stage is accompanied by massive swelling, and the scrotum may reach the size

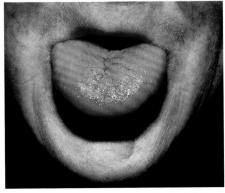

Fig. 22.2 Magenta tongue in riboflavin deficiency.

of a football. Photophobia and blepharitis angularis occur. The response to repletion is dramatic.

Roe DA: Riboflavin deficiency. Semin Dermatol 1991; 10: 293.
Tolkachjov SN, Bruce AJ: Oral manifestations of nutritional disorders. Clin Dermatol 2017; 35: 441.

VITAMIN B$_6$

Pyridoxine Deficiency

Pyridoxine (vitamin B$_6$) deficiency may occur in patients with uremia and cirrhosis, as well as with the use of certain pharmacologic agents. Skin changes include a seborrheic dermatitis–like eruption, atrophic glossitis with ulceration, angular cheilitis, conjunctivitis, and intertrigo. Occasionally, a pellagra-like eruption may occur. Neurologic symptoms include somnolence, confusion, and neuropathy. Pyrodoxine has been used to prevent or treat chemotherapy-induced hand-foot syndrome but has not been consistently successful.

Pyridoxine Excess

A patient who ingested large doses of pyridoxine developed a subepidermal vesicular dermatosis and sensory peripheral neuropathy. The bullous dermatosis resembled epidermolysis bullosa acquisita. Exacerbation of rosacea was also reported in a patient taking isoniazide and pyridoxine.

Friedman MA, et al: Subepidermal vesicular dermatosis and sensory peripheral neuropathy caused by pyridoxine abuse. J Am Acad Dermatol 1986; 14: 915.
Macedo LT, et al: Prevention strategies for chemotherapy-induced hand-foot syndrome. Support Care Cancer 2014; 22: 1585.
Rezaković S, et al: Pyridoxine induced rosacea-like dermatitis. Acta Clin Croat 2015; 54: 99.

VITAMIN B$_{12}$ DEFICIENCY

Vitamin B$_{12}$ (cyanocobalamin) is absorbed through the distal ileum after binding to gastric intrinsic factor in an acid pH. Deficiency is caused mainly by gastrointestinal (GI) abnormalities, such as a deficiency of intrinsic factor, achlorhydria (including that induced by medications), ileal diseases, and malabsorption syndromes resulting from pancreatic disease or sprue. Aggressive treatment for the eradication of *Helicobacter pylori* may cause B$_{12}$ deficiency, as can metformin administration and long-term antacid ingestion. In food-cobalamin malabsorption syndrome, the body is unable to release vitamin B$_{12}$ from food or intestinal transport proteins, especially with accompanying achlorhydria. These patients have adequate dietary vitamin B$_{12}$ but often have atrophic gastritis. A Schilling test will be normal. Congenital lack of transcobalamin II can also produce B$_{12}$ deficiency. Because of the large body stores of B$_{12}$ in adults, deficiency occurs 3–6 years after GI abnormalities.

Glossitis, hyperpigmentation, and canities are the main dermatologic manifestations of vitamin B$_{12}$ deficiency. The tongue is bright red, sore, and atrophic. Linear atrophic lesions may be an early sign. The hyperpigmentation is generalized, but more often it is accentuated in exposed areas, such as the face and hands, and in the palmar creases and flexures, resembling Addison disease. The nails may be pigmented. Premature gray hair may occur paradoxically. Megaloblastic anemia is often present. Weakness, paresthesias, numbness, ataxia, and other neurologic findings occur. Repletion of vitamin B$_{12}$ can aid in chronic aphthous stomatitis in some patients.

Parenteral replacement with IM injections of B$_{12}$, 1, leads to a reversal of the pigmentary changes in the skin, nails, mucous membranes, and hair. Megadose oral replacement of 1–2 mg/day may replace body stores by simple diffusion, independent of intrinsic factor. Neurologic defects may or may not improve with vitamin B$_{12}$ replacement.

FOLIC ACID DEFICIENCY

Diffuse hyperpigmentation, glossitis, cheilitis, and megaloblastic anemia, identical to vitamin B$_{12}$ deficiency, occur in folic acid deficiency. Low folic acid is associated with neural tube defects, which are more common in light-skinned people, suggesting an association between ultraviolet (UV) light exposure and reduction in folic acid. Folic acid supplementation leads to fewer GI and liver side effects in patients on methotrexate.

Andrès E, et al: Oral manifestations of vitamin B$_{12}$ and B$_9$ deficiencies. J Oral Pathol Med 2016; 45: 154
Cui RZ, et al: Recurrent aphthous stomatitis. Clin Dermatol 2016; 34: 475.
De Giuseppe R, et al: Burning mouth syndrome and vitamin B$_{12}$ deficiency. J Eur Acad Dermatol Venereol 2011; 25: 868.
Downham TF, et al: Hyperpigmentation and folate deficiency. Arch Dermatol 1976; 112: 562.
Graells J, et al: Glossitis with linear lesions. J Am Acad Dermatol 2009; 60: 498.
Shea B, et al: Folic acid and folinic acid for reducing side effects in patients receiving methotrexate for rheumatoid arthritis. J Rheumatol 2014; 41: 1049.
Stabler SP: Vitamin B$_{12}$ deficiency. N Engl J Med 2013; 368: 149.
Stoopler ET, et al: Glossitis secondary to vitamin B$_{12}$ deficiency anemia. CMAJ 2013; 185: E582.

VITAMIN C DEFICIENCY (SCURVY)

Scurvy, or vitamin C deficiency, is often diagnosed by dermatologists, because cutaneous manifestations are early and prominent. Elderly male alcoholics and patients with behavioral health and autism spectrum disorders on restrictive diets are most frequently affected. Iron overload due to multiple transfusions, neurologic disorders, smoking, and history of chemotherapy and dialysis patients are also risk factors. One patient with scurvy related to nilotinib has been reported.

The "four Hs" are characteristic of scurvy: hemorrhagic signs, hyperkeratosis of the hair follicles, hypochondriasis, and hematologic abnormalities. Perifollicular petechiae are the characteristic cutaneous finding (Fig. 22.3). In addition, ecchymoses of various sizes, especially on the lower extremities, are common. These may

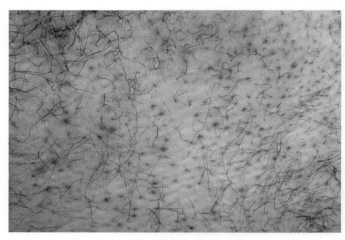

Fig. 22.3 Scurvy.

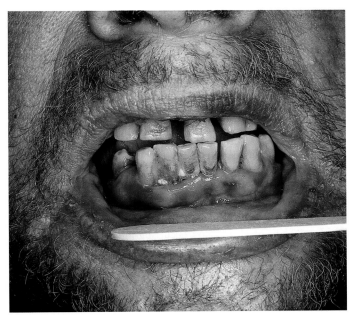

Fig. 22.4 Scurvy, gingivitis.

be associated with tender nodules (subcutaneous and intramuscular hemorrhage) and subperiosteal hemorrhage, leading to bone pain and possible pseudoparalysis in children. Woody edema may be present, simulating cellulitis. Subungual, subconjunctival, intramuscular, periosteal, and intraarticular hemorrhage may also occur. The referring diagnosis is often vasculitis due to the perifollicular hemorrhage with bone pain a prominent feature in advanced disease; Henoch-Schönlein purpura can easily be confused with scurvy. Another characteristic finding is keratotic plugging of the hair follicles, chiefly on the anterior forearms, abdomen, and posterior thighs. The hair shafts are curled in follicles capped by keratotic plugs, a distinctive finding called "corkscrew hairs." Hemorrhagic gingivitis occurs adjacent to teeth and presents as swelling and bleeding of the gums (Fig. 22.4). The teeth can be loose and the breath may be foul. Gingival hyperplasia and bleeding may be absent or may be the sole sign of scurvy. Edentulous areas do not develop gingivitis, and those with good oral hygiene have less prominent gingival involvement. Epistaxis, delayed wound healing, and depression may also occur. Frequently, anemia is present and may be the result of blood loss or associated deficiencies of other nutrients, such as folate.

The diagnosis of scurvy is usually made on clinical grounds and confirmed by a positive response to vitamin C supplementation or a low vitamin C level. Because vitamin C levels normalize very quickly, if needed, the blood test must be checked before any diet change. A biopsy will exclude vasculitis and demonstrate follicular hyperkeratosis, coiled hairs, and perifollicular hemorrhage in the absence of inflammation. Treatment is with ascorbic acid, 1000 mg/day for a few days to 1 week, and a maintenance dose of 100 mg/day should be considered.

Arron ST, et al: Scurvy. J Am Acad Dermatol 2007; 57: S8.

Bacci C, et al: A rare case of scurvy in an otherwise healthy child. Pediatr Dent 2010; 32: 536.

Chisolm C, et al: Lower extremity purpura in a woman with psychosis. Arch Dermatol 2010; 146: 1167.

Daff M, et al: Vitamin C deficiency in psychiatric illness. Asian J Psychiatr 2017; 28: 97.

Duggan CP, et al: Case 23-2007: a 9-year-old boy with bone pain, rash, and gingival hypertrophy. N Engl J Med 2009; 357: 392.

Fossitt DD, et al: Classic skin findings of scurvy. Mayo Clin Proc 2014; 89: e61.

Golriz F, et al: Modern American scurvy—experience with vitamin C deficiency at a large children's hospital. Pediatr Radiol 2017; 47: 214.

Krutzman D, et al: Fatigue and lower extremity ecchymosis in a 36-year-old woman. Arch Dermatol 2012; 148: 1073.

Li R, et al: Gingival hypertrophy. Am J Otolaryngol 2008; 29: 426.

Maltos AL, et al: Scurvy in a patient with AIDS. Rev Soc Bras Med Trop 2011; 44: 122.

Oak AS, et al: A case of scurvy associated with nilotinib. J Cutan Pathol 2016; 43: 725.

Pullar JM, et al: The roles of vitamin C in skin health. Nutrients 2017; 9: 866.

Seya M, et al: Scurvy. J Pediatr 2016; 177: 331.

Singer R, et al: High prevalence of ascorbate deficiency in an Australian peritoneal dialysis population. Nephrology 2008; 13: 17.

Swanson AM, et al: Acute inpatient presentation of scurvy. Cutis 2010; 86: 205.

Woodier N, et al: Scurvy. Emerg Med J 2012; 29: 103.

NIACIN DEFICIENCY (PELLAGRA)

Pellagra usually results from a deficiency of nicotinic acid (niacin, vitamin B₃) or its precursor amino acid, tryptophan. It is associated classically with a diet almost entirely composed of corn, millet, or sorghum. Pellagra can occur within 60 days of dietary niacin deficiency. Malnutrition or other vitamin deficiencies, especially pyridoxine, which interfere with the conversion of tryptophan to niacin, often coexist. In developed countries, most cases of pellagra occur in alcoholics. Other possible causes of pellagra are as follows:

- Carcinoid tumors, which divert tryptophan to serotonin
- Hartnup disease (impaired absorption of tryptophan)
- Gastrointestinal disorders (e.g., Crohn disease, GI surgery)
- Prolonged intravenous (IV) supplementation
- Psychiatric disease, including anorexia nervosa
- Restrictive diets in adult patients with atopic dermatitis concerned about "food allergy"

Pellagra can also be induced by medications, most often isoniazid, azathioprine (and its metabolite 6-mercaptopurine), 5-fluorouracil, ethionamide, protionamide, and pyrazinamide. These medications may induce pellagra by interfering with niacin biosynthesis. The anticonvulsants, including hydantoins, phenobarbital, and carbamazepine, may rarely produce pellagra in a dose-dependent manner.

Clinical Features

Pellagra is a chronic disease affecting the GI tract, nervous system, and skin; thus the mnemonic of the "three Ds"—diarrhea, dementia, and dermatitis.

The most characteristic cutaneous finding is the photosensitive eruption, which worsens in the spring and summer. It occurs symmetrically on the face, neck, and upper chest (Casal necklace; Fig. 22.5); extensor arms; and backs of the hands. Initially, there is erythema and swelling after sun exposure, accompanied by itching and burning or pain. In severe cases, the eruption may be vesicular or bullous (wet pellagra). Compared with normal sunburn, the pellagrous skin takes about four times longer to recover from the acute phototoxic injury. After several phototoxic events, thickening, scaling, and hyperpigmentation of the affected skin occur. The skin has a copper or mahogany hue. In protracted cases, the skin ultimately becomes dry, smooth, paper-thin, and glassy with a parchment-like consistency. Scarring rarely occurs.

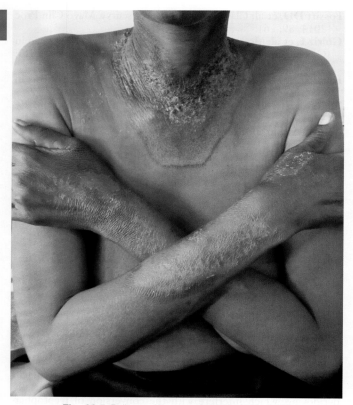

Fig. 22.5 Pellagra. (Courtesy Michelle Weir, MD.)

The nose is fairly characteristic. There is dull erythema of the bridge of the nose, with fine, yellow, powdery scales over the follicular orifices (sulfur flakes). The eruption resembles seborrheic dermatitis, except for its location. Plugs of inspissated sebum may project from dilated orifices on the nose, giving it a rough appearance.

At the onset, the patient has weakness, loss of appetite, abdominal pain, diarrhea, mental depression, and photosensitivity. Skin lesions may be the earliest sign, with phototoxicity the presenting symptom in some cases. Neurologic and GI symptoms can occur without skin changes. Delusions of parasitosis have been reported in pellagra. In the later stages, the neurologic symptoms may predominate. Apathy, depression, muscle weakness, paresthesias, headaches, and attacks of dizziness or falling are typical findings. Hallucinations, psychosis, seizures, dementia, neurologic degeneration, and coma may develop. Pellagra is progressive and can be fatal if untreated.

Histopathology

Histologically, the findings in the skin vary according to the stage of the disease. The most characteristic finding is pallor and vacuolar changes of the keratinocytes in a band in the upper layers of the stratum malpighii, just below the granular cell layer, which may be attenuated. If marked, a cleft may form in the upper epidermis, correlating with the blistering seen in wet pellagra. Langerhans cells were shown to be depleted in the skin of patients with pellagra.

Diagnosis and Treatment

If the characteristic skin findings are present, the diagnosis of pellagra is not difficult clinically. Dietary treatment to correct the malnutrition is essential. Animal proteins, eggs, milk, and vegetables are beneficial. Supplementation with nicotinamide, 100 mg three times daily for several weeks, should be given. Fluid and electrolyte loss from diarrhea should be replaced, and in patients with GI symptoms possibly interfering with absorption, initial IV supplementation should be considered. Within 24 hours of niacin therapy initiation, the skin lesions begin to resolve, confirming the diagnosis. Alcoholism must be treated if present, and the factors that may have led to pellagra must be corrected.

Bell HK, et al: Cutaneous manifestations of the malignant carcinoid syndrome. Br J Dermatol 2005; 152: 71.

Bilgili SG, et al: Isoniazid-induced pellagra. Cutan Ocul Toxicol 2011; 30: 317.

Desai NK, et al: Dermatitis as one of the 3 Ds of pellagra. Mayo Clin Proc 2012; 87: e113.

Frank GP, et al: Pellagra. Trop Doct 2012; 42: 182.

Kleyn CE: Cutaneous manifestations of the malignant carcinoid syndrome. J Am Acad Dermatol 2004; 50: P437.

Ladoyanni E, et al: Pellagra occurring in a patient with atopic dermatitis and food allergy. J Eur Acad Dermatol Venereol 2006; 21: 394.

Li R, et al: Pellagra secondary to medication and alcoholism. Nutr Clin Pract 2016; 31: 785.

Oliveira A, et al: Azathioprine-induced pellagra. J Dermatol 2011; 38: 1035.

Savvidou S: Pellagra. Clin Pract 2014; 4: 637.

Yamaguchi S, et al: Depletion of epidermal Langerhans cells in the skin lesions of pellagra patients. Am J Dermatopathol 2017; 39: 428.

Wan P, et al: Pellagra. Br J Dermatol 2011; 164: 1188.

DISORDERS THAT PRESENT WITH ACRODERMATITIS-LIKE SKIN CHANGES

Biotin Deficiency

Biotin is universally available and is produced by intestinal bacteria. Therefore deficiency is rare but can occur in patients with a short gut or malabsorption. Sometimes biotin deficiency occurs in patients taking antibiotics or receiving parenteral nutrition. Avidin, found in raw egg white, may bind biotin, leading to deficiency. The three autosomal recessive syndromes of holocarboxylase synthetase deficiency (multiple carboxylase deficiency), biotinidase deficiency, and the rare syndrome of inability to transport biotin into cells all have similar clinical features, referred to as "multiple carboxylase deficiency." The holocarboxylase deficiency presents earlier and is termed the *neonatal* form, whereas the biotinidase deficiency may present later and is termed the *juvenile* form. Clinical presentation is variable, with some patients manifesting only certain features. Biotin deficiency may increase the inflammatory response from dendritic cells leading to excess inflammation.

The skin and nervous system are primarily affected. Dermatitis similar to that found in patients with zinc deficiency and EFA deficiency is seen. This periorificial dermatitis is characterized by patchy, red, eroded lesions on the face and groin (Fig. 22.6). *Candida* is regularly present on the lesions. Alopecia, in some cases total, including loss of the eyebrows and eyelashes, can occur. Congenital trichorrhexis nodosa may be present, and conjunctivitis may occur. Neurologic findings are prominent; in adults these include depression, lethargy, hallucinations, and limb paresthesias, and in infants, hypotonia, lethargy, a withdrawn behavior, ataxia, seizures, deafness, and developmental delay.

The diagnosis of the inherited forms is made by detecting organic aminoaciduria of 3-hydroxyisovaleric acid. Measurement of serum biotinidase can distinguish biotinidase deficiency from holocarboxylase deficiency.

Treatment consists of 10 mg/day of biotin, but depending on the severity of the enzyme mutation, higher doses may be required.

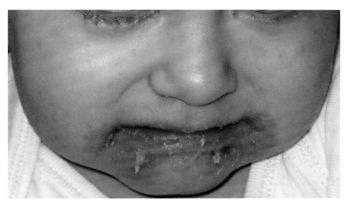
Fig. 22.6 Multiple carboxylase deficiency.

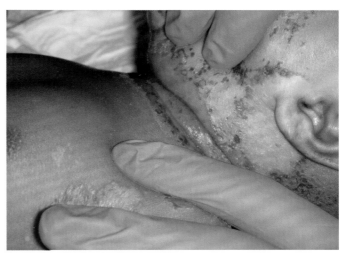
Fig. 22.7 Acrodermatitis enteropathica.

Skin lesions resolve rapidly, but the neurologic damage may be permanent; thus early diagnosis is important. Valproic acid treatment in children, may lead to partial biotinidase deficiency, and that the skin lesions (seborrheic dermatitis–like rash and alopecia) improved with biotin supplementation.

Agrawal S, et al: Biotin deficiency enhances the inflammatory response of human dendritic cells. Am J Physiol Cell Physiol 2016; 311: C386.

Bassi A, et al: A 2-month-old boy with desquamative skin fold dermatitis. J Pediatr 2014; 164: 211.

Esparza EM, et al: What syndrome is this? Infantile periorificial and intertriginous dermatitis preceding sepsis-like respiratory failure. Pediatr Dermatol 2011; 28: 333.

Fleischman MH, et al: Case report and review of congenital biotinidase deficiency. J Am Acad Dermatol 2004; 50: P513.

Hove JLK, et al: Management of a patient with holocarboxylase synthetase deficiency. Mol Genet Metab 2008; 95: 201.

Lunnemann L, et al: Hair-shaft abnormality in a 7-year-old girl. JAMA Dermatol 2013; 149: 357.

Rathi N, Rathi M: Biotinidase deficiency with hypertonia as unusual feature. Indian Pediatr 2009; 46: 65.

Tammachote R, et al: Holocarboxylase synthetase deficiency. Clin Genet 2010; 78: 88.

ZINC DEFICIENCY

Zinc deficiency may be an inherited abnormality, acrodermatitis enteropathica, or it may be acquired. Acrodermatitis enteropathica is an autosomal recessive disorder caused by mutations in the *SLC39A4* gene, which encodes the zinc transporter ZIP4. ZNT Acquired cases are termed *acquired acrodermatitis enteropathica* or *acrodermatitis enteropathica–like syndrome*. Premature infants are at particular risk because of inadequate body zinc stores, suboptimal absorption, and high zinc requirements. Normally, human breast milk has adequate zinc, and weaning classically precipitates clinical zinc deficiency in premature infants and in infants with acrodermatitis enteropathica. Zinc-binding proteins in cow's milk may also inhibit the bioavailability of zinc. However, clinical zinc deficiency may occur in full-term and premature infants still breastfeeding. This results from either low maternal breast milk zinc levels or a higher zinc requirement by the infant than the breast milk can provide (even though zinc level in breast milk is normal). A rare syndrome of congenital myopathy, recurrent diarrhea, microcephaly, and deafness has been associated with a neonatal bullous eruption characteristic of nutritional deficiency. These children have required very high doses of zinc supplementation.

Parenteral nutrition without adequate zinc content may lead to zinc deficiency. Acquired zinc deficiency also occurs in alcoholics as a result of poor nutritional intake and increased urinary excretion; as a complication of malabsorption, IBD, chronic granulomatous disorder, or GI surgery; and occasionally in patients with anorexia nervosa or acquired immunodeficiency syndrome (AIDS). Patients with severe erosive oral disease, such as pemphigus or graft-versus-host disease, may develop zinc deficiency from malnutrition. Zinc requirements increase during metabolic stress, so symptomatic deficiency may present during infections, after trauma or surgery, with malignancy, during pregnancy, and with renal disease. Diets containing mainly cereal grains are high in phytate, which binds zinc, and has caused endemic zinc deficiency in certain areas of the Middle East and North Africa.

The dermatitis found in all forms of zinc deficiency is pustular and bullous, but the lesions are often flaccid leading to the clinical appearance of crusting. There is an acral and a periorificial distribution. On the face, in the groin, and in other flexors there is a patchy, red, dry scaling with exudation and crusting (Fig. 22.7). Angular cheilitis and stomatitis may be present. The periungual areas are erythematous and scaling and may have superficial, flaccid pustules. Nail dystrophy may result, with thinning of the nails and accentuated longitudinal ridges. Low zinc levels have been found in patients with burning mouth syndrome, and zinc supplementation may alleviate the symptoms. Chronic lesions may be more psoriasiform. Generalized alopecia may occur. Inborn errors of metabolism, such as methylmelonic academia, biotinidase deficiency, propionic acidemia, and multiple carboxylase deficiency, as well as isoleucine deficiency during treatment of maple syrup urine disease, can all manifest with the scaling, intertriginous clinical appearance of acrodermatitis enteropathica.

Diarrhea is present in most cases. Growth retardation, ophthalmic findings, impaired wound healing, and central nervous system manifestations occur. Patients are particularly irritable and emotionally labile.

The histopathology of acquired and hereditary zinc deficiency is identical. There is vacuolation of the keratinocytes of the upper stratum malpighii. These areas of vacuolation may become confluent, forming a subcorneal bulla. In larger lesions, there may be total epidermal necrosis with subepidermal blister formation. Neutrophils are typically present. In the late stages of acrodermatitis enteropathica, this characteristic upper epidermal pallor is frequently absent, and the biopsy demonstrates only a psoriasiform dermatitis.

The diagnosis of zinc deficiency should be suspected in at-risk individuals with acral or periorificial dermatitis. In particular,

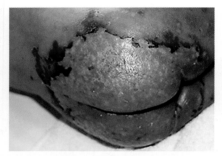

Fig. 22.8 Acrodermatitis enteropathica. (Courtesy Carrie Kovarik, MD.)

chronic diaper rash with diarrhea in an infant should lead to evaluation for zinc deficiency (Fig. 22.8). The diagnosis can be confirmed by low serum zinc levels. A low level of serum alkaline phosphatase, a zinc-dependent enzyme, may be a valuable (and more quickly reported) adjunctive test in which the serum zinc level is normal or near-normal. In some patients, even if the zinc level is in the normal range, a trial of zinc supplementation should be considered if the skin lesions are characteristic. Replacement is with zinc sulfate, 1–2 mg/kg/day (50 mg of elemental zinc per 220 mg zinc sulfate tablet).

In acquired cases, transient treatment and addressing the underlying condition are adequate. In patients with genetic causes of acrodermatitis enteropathica, zinc supplementation is 3 mg/kg/day and should be lifelong, whereas patients with inappropriate intake can be supplemented and, with appropriate changes in diet, stop the supplementation once replete. Overzealous zinc supplementation should be avoided, because it may lead to low serum copper levels.

Afrin LB: Fatal copper deficiency from excessive use of zinc-based denture adhesive. Am J Med Sci 2010; 340: 164.

Alhaj E, et al: Diffuse alopecia in a child due to dietary zinc deficiency. Skinmed 2007; 6: 199.

Bock DE, et al: Picture of the month—diagnosis. Arch Pediatr Adolesc Med 2009; 163: 763.

Centers for Disease Control and Prevention (CDC): Zinc deficiency dermatitis in cholestatic extremely premature infants after a nationwide shortage of injectable zinc. MMWR Morb Mortal Wkly Rep 2013; 62: 136.

Cho GS, et al: Zinc deficiency may be a cause of burning mouth syndrome as zinc replacement therapy has therapeutic effects. J Oral Pathol Med 2010; 39: 722.

Chue CD, et al: An acrodermatitis enteropathica–like eruption secondary to acquired zinc deficiency in an exclusively breast-fed premature infant. Int J Dermatol 2008; 46: 372.

Corbo MD, et al: Zinc deficiency and its management in the pediatric population. J Am Acad Dermatol 2013; 69: 616.

Cunha SF, et al: Acrodermatitis due to zinc deficiency after combined vertical gastroplasty with jejunoileal bypass. São Paulo Med J 2012; 130: 330.

Inzinger M, et al: Acquired zinc deficiency due to long-term tube feeding. Eur J Dermatol 2011; 21: 633.

Iyengar S, et al: Bullous acrodermatitis enteropathica. Dermatol Online J 2015; 21.

Jensen SL, et al: Bullous lesions in acrodermatitis enteropathica delaying diagnosis of zinc deficiency. J Cutan Pathol 2008; 35: 1.

Karashima T, et al: Oral zinc therapy for zinc deficiency–related telogen effluvium. Dermatol Ther 2012; 25: 210.

Kobayashi K, et al: Severe acquired acrodermatitis enteropathica caused by anorexia nervosa. J Dermatol 2016; 43: 456.

Ladinsky HT, et al: Chronic granulomatous disease associated colitis leading to profound zinc deficiency. J Allergy Clin Immunol Pract 2014; 2: 217.

Macdonald JB, et al: Think zinc deficiency: acquired acrodermatitis enteropathica due to poor diet and common medications. Arch Dermatol 2012; 148: 961.

Mankaney GN, et al: Images in clinical medicine. N Engl J Med 2014; 371: 67.

Maskarinec SA, et al: Persistent rash in a patient receiving total parenteral nutrition. JAMA 2016; 315: 2223.

Maverakis E, et al: Acrodermatitis enteropathica and an overview of zinc metabolism. J Am Acad Dermatol 2007; 56: 116.

Salle A, et al: Zinc deficiency. Obes Surg 2010; 20: 1660.

ESSENTIAL FATTY ACID DEFICIENCY

Essential fatty acids (EFAs) are those that cannot be synthesized by the body. EFA deficiency may develop in multiple settings, including low-birth-weight infants, cystic fibrosis, GI abnormalities with diarrhea (e.g., IBD, intestinal surgery), and prolonged parenteral nutrition without EFA supplementation. The resulting dermatitis is similar to that seen in zinc and biotin deficiency, although characteristically more widespread, and with less prominent periorificial, mucous membrane, and nail involvement. There is a generalized xerosis because EFAs constitute up to one quarter of the fatty acids of the stratum corneum and are required for normal epidermal barrier function. Widespread erythema and an intertriginous weeping eruption are seen. The hair becomes lighter in color, and diffuse alopecia is present. Poor wound healing, growth failure, and increased risk of infection may occur. There is a decrease in linoleic acid and an increase in palmitoleic and oleic acids. A ratio of eicosatrienoic acid to arachidonic acid of more than 0.4 is diagnostic of EFA deficiency. IV lipid therapy reverses the process. In patients who develop pancreatitis from the fat emulsion infusion, topical safflower oil emulsion or soybean oil applications may be considered as a stopgap measure, waiting for the pancreatitis to improve. Topical treatment does not maintain liver and tissue stores.

The nutrient deficiency eruption seen in children with cystic fibrosis has been called "cystic fibrosis nutrient deficiency dermatitis" (CFNDD). It shares features of acrodermatitis enteropathica, kwashiorkor, and EFA deficiency. It presents at 2 weeks to 6 months of age with erythematous papules that may be annular. The diaper area and perioral/periorbital regions are initially affected. It spreads to the extremities and progresses to widespread plaques. The hair may turn gray, then repigment on supplementation. Laboratory abnormalities include anemia, hypoalbuminemia, elevated liver function tests (e.g., alkaline phosphatase), low or normal zinc, low vitamin E, and at times EFA deficiency. Biopsy shows psoriasiform dermatitis, but the upper dermal pallor may be absent. Treatment of CFNDD is general enhancement of the child's nutrition, addressing zinc, protein, and EFA deficiencies, as well as other nutritional deficits. Zinc therapy alone does not improve CFNDD.

Bernstein ML, et al: Cutaneous manifestations of cystic fibrosis. Pediatr Dermatol 2008; 25: 150.

Dalgic B, et al: Gray hair and acrodermatitis enteropathica–like dermatitis. Eur J Pediatr 2011; 170: 1305.

Lakdawala N, et al: Acrodermatitis caused by nutritional deficiency and metabolic disorders. Clin Dermatol 2017; 35: 64.

Marcason W: Can cutaneous application of vegetable oil prevent an essential fatty acid deficiency? J Am Diet Assoc 2007; 107: 1262.

Peroni DG, et al: Severe refractory dermatitis and cystic fibrosis. Arch Dis Child 2012; 97: 205.

Roongpisuthipong W, et al: Essential fatty acid deficiency while a patient receiving fat regimen total parenteral nutrition. BMJ Case Rep 2012 Jun 14; 2012.

Wenk KS, et al: Cystic fibrosis presenting with dermatitis. Arch Dermatol 2010; 146: 171.

IRON DEFICIENCY

Iron deficiency is common, especially among actively menstruating women, and particularly if they have minimal red meat in their diets and have not compensated with other foods. Iron deficiency has recently been reported in patients treated with extracorporeal photopheresis. Mucocutaneous findings include koilonychia, glossitis, angular cheilitis, pruritus, and telogen effluvium. Plummer-Vinson syndrome is the combination of microcytic anemia, dysphagia, and glossitis, seen almost entirely in middle-aged women. The lips are thin and the opening of the mouth is small and inelastic, creating a rather characteristic appearance. Smooth atrophy of the tongue is pronounced. Koilonychia is present in 40%–50% of patients, and alopecia may be present. An esophageal web in the postcricoid area may occur, presenting as difficulty swallowing, or the feeling that food is stuck in the throat. The diagnosis is confirmed by measuring the serum iron level. Treatment consists of iron sulfate supplementation.

Anderson J, et al: Iron deficiency anemia in patients undergoing extracorporeal photopheresis for cutaneous T-cell lymphoma. J Clin Apher 2015; 30: 69.
Reveiz L, et al: Treatments for iron-deficiency anaemia in pregnancy. Cochrane Database Syst Rev 2011; 10: CD003094.
St Pierre SA, et al: Iron deficiency and diffuse nonscarring scalp alopecia in women. J Am Acad Dermatol 2010; 63: 1070.

SELENIUM DEFICIENCY

Selenium deficiency occurs in patients receiving parenteral nutrition, in areas where soil selenium content is poor, in cirrhosis patients with ineffective metabolism of selenomethionine, and in low-birth-weight infants. Manifestations in children include hypopigmentation of the skin and hair (pseudoalbinism). Leukonychia and Terry-like nails have been reported. Cardiomyopathy, muscle pain, and weakness with elevated levels of muscle enzymes are the major features. Autoimmune thyroid disease has also been reported in patients with selenium deficiency. Treatment of deficiency consists of 3 μg/kg/day of selenium.

Burk RF, et al: Selenium deficiency occurs in some patients with moderate-to-severe cirrhosis and can be corrected by administration of selenate but not selenomethionine. Am J Clin Nutr 2015; 102: 1126.
Vinton NE, et al: Macrocytosis and pseudoalbinism. J Pediatr 1987; 111: 711.
Wichman J, et al: Selenium supplementation significantly reduces thyroid autoantibody levels in patients with chronic autoimmune thyroiditis. Thyroid 2016; 26: 1681.

PROTEIN-ENERGY MALNUTRITION

Protein-energy malnutrition is a spectrum of related diseases, including marasmus, kwashiorkor, and marasmic kwashiorkor. These conditions are more common in parts of the developing world. Marasmus represents prolonged deficiency of protein and calories and is diagnosed in children who are below 60% of their ideal body weight without edema or hypoproteinemia. Kwashiorkor occurs with protein deficiency but a relatively adequate caloric intake and is diagnosed in children at 60%–80% of their ideal body weight with edema or hypoproteinemia. Marasmic kwashiorkor shows features of both conditions and is diagnosed in children who are less than 60% of their ideal body weight with features of edema or hypoproteinemia.

These conditions are rare in developed countries, but occasionally kwashiorkor may occur as a result of severe dietary restrictions. In the United States this may occur in infants because they garner most of their protein from breast milk or formula. When rice beverages or other low-protein beverage are substituted for breast milk, baby formula, or cow's milk (in older children) due to food allergies, they can become deficient in multiple nutrients, including protein. Therefore patients with food protein–induced enterocolitis or extensive food allergies should be counseled on proper nutrition while avoiding their allergens.

Marasmus

In cases of marasmus, the skin is dry, wrinkled, and loose because of marked loss of subcutaneous fat. The loss of the buccal fat pad is characteristic. In contrast to kwashiorkor, there is no edema or dermatosis.

Kwashiorkor

Kwashiorkor produces hair and skin changes, edema, impaired growth, and the characteristic potbelly. U.S. cases are caused by dietary restriction often seen in patients with eating disorders, autism spectrum disorders, or restrictive diets due to avoidance of food allergies. Altered gut microbiome may put certain infants at risk for kwashiorkor. Infants with atopy and multiple food allergies are at especially high risk if breastfeeding is stopped and properly fortified infant formula is not substituted. The resultant scaling can be confused for worsening atopic dermatitis. Patients with kwashiorkor have edema that can mask true growth failure due to the weight of the edema, delaying the diagnosis of malnutrition. The hair and skin changes are usually striking. The hair is hypopigmented, varying in color from a reddish yellow to gray or even white. The hair is dry and lusterless; curly hair becomes soft and straight; and marked scaling (crackled hair) is seen. Especially striking is the "flag sign," affecting long, normally dark hair. The hair grown during periods of poor nutrition is pale, so that alternating bands of pale and dark hair can be seen along a single strand, indicating alternating periods of good and poor nutrition. The nails are soft and thin.

The skin lesions are hypopigmented on dark skin and erythematous or purple on lighter skin (Fig. 22.9). Lesions first appear in areas of friction or pressure: the flexures, groin, buttocks, and elbows (Fig. 22.10). Hyperpigmented patches occur with slightly raised edges. As they progress, lesions resemble old, dark, deteriorating enamel paint with peeling or desquamation (Fig. 22.11). This has been described variously as "crazy pavement," crackled skin, mosaic skin, enamel paint, and flaky paint. In severe cases, the peeling leaves pale, ulcerated, hypopigmented areas with hyperpigmented borders. There may be concomitant zinc deficiency

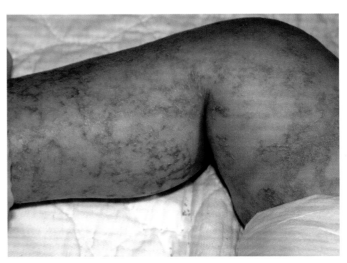

Fig. 22.9 Kwashiorkor.

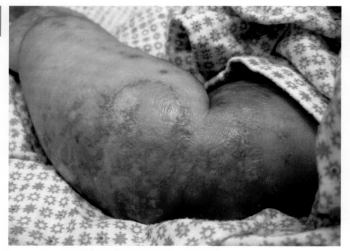

Fig. 22.10 Kwashiorkor. (Courtesy Campbell Stewart, MD.)

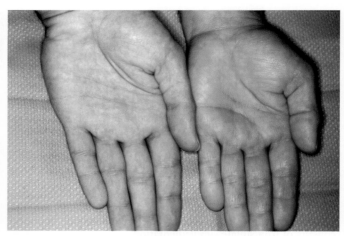

Fig. 22.12 Carotenemia.

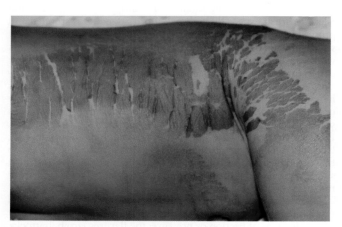

Fig. 22.11 Flaky paint appearance in Kwashiorkor. (Courtesy Shyam Verma, MBBS, DVD.)

leading to the superimposed appearance of acrodermatitis enteropathica.

Buno IJ, et al: The enamel paint sign in the dermatologic diagnosis of early-onset kwashiorkor. Arch Dermatol 1998; 134: 107.

Cox JA, et al: Flaky paint dermatosis. JAMA Dermatol 2014; 150: 85.

Diamanti A, et al: Iatrogenic kwashiorkor in three infants on a diet of rice beverages. Pediatr Allergy Immunol 2011; 22: 878.

Grover Z, et al: Protein energy malnutrition. Pediatr Clin North Am 2009; 56: 1055.

Heath ML, Sidbury R: Cutaneous manifestations of nutritional deficiency. Curr Opin Pediatr 2006; 18:417.

Henrique DS, et al: A child with kwashiorkor misdiagnosed as atopic dermatitis. Dermatol Online J 2017; 23.

Mann D, et al: Cutaneous manifestations of kwashiorkor. An Bras Dermatol 2011; 86: 1174.

Palm CV, et al: Kwashiorkor. BMJ Case Rep 2016 Nov 15; 2016.

Smith MI, et al: Gut microbiomes of Malawian twin pairs discordant for kwashiorkor. Science 2013; 339: 548.

CAROTENEMIA AND LYCOPENEMIA

Excessive ingestion of fruits and vegetables containing large amounts of β-carotene and lycopene can result in a yellow-orangish discoloration of the skin, which is especially prominent on the palms (Fig. 22.12), soles, and central face (areas of high sweat gland density). The sclerae are spared. Infants are most frequently affected, perhaps because pureeing fruits and vegetables makes these pigments more available for absorption. Carotenemia may also result from excess ingestion of β-carotene nutritional supplements and can be seen in hypothyroidism, patients with food allergies, and anorexia nervosa. Hypothyroidism can lead to carotenemia because thyroid hormone helps the conversion of beta carotene into retinol. In addition a familial form can be due to a deficiency in carotenoid 15,15′-monooxygenase, which is responsible for breaking β-carotene into vitamin A.

Gangakhedkar A, et al: Carotenemia and hepatomegaly in an atopic child on an exclusion diet for a food allergy. Australas J Dermatol 2017; 58: 42.

Kaimal S, et al: Diet in dermatology. Indian J Dermatol Venereol Leprol 2010; 76: 103.

Lee LW, et al: Skin manifestations of nutritional deficiency disease in children. Int J Dermatol 2012; 51: 1407.

Lindqvist A, et al: Loss-of-function mutation in carotenoid 15,15-prime-monooxygenase identified in a patient with hypercarotenemia and hypovitaminosis A. J Nutr 2007; 137: 2346.

Nagao A, et al: Inhibition of beta-carotene-15,15′-dioxygenase activity by dietary flavonoids. J Nutr Biochem 2000; 11: 348.

Sivaramakrishnan VK, et al: Carotenemia in infancy and its association with prevalent feeding practices. Pediatr Dermatol 2006; 23: 571.

Yuko T, et al: A case of carotenemia associated with ingestion of nutrient supplements. J Dermatol 2006; 2: 132.

23 Diseases of Subcutaneous Fat

An inflammatory disorder that is primarily localized in the sub-cutaneous fat is termed a *panniculitis*. This group of disorders may be challenging for both the clinician and the dermatopathologist. Clinically, in all forms of panniculitis, lesions present as subcutaneous nodules. Histopathologically, the subcutaneous fat is a rather homogeneous tissue, and inflammatory processes may show considerable overlap. One way of classifying panniculitis is to separate them into those that involve the septae between fat lobules (septal panniculitides) from those processes that primarily involve the fat lobules (lobular panniculitides). The prototypical septal panniculitis is erythema nodosum. Some lobular panniculitides are caused by vasculitis (e.g., polyarteritis nodosa) and are discussed in other chapters. The remaining lobular panniculitides are categorized by their pathogenesis. Weber-Christian disease, Rothmann-Makai disease, lipomembranous or membranocystic panniculitis, and eosinophilic panniculitis are reaction patterns and are not specific entities. Neutrophilic panniculitis may be infectious or may represent a variant of Sweet syndrome with primary involvement of the panniculus.

Given the depth of lesions in the panniculus, the choice of biopsy is critical in establishing the diagnosis. An incisional or excisional biopsy, narrow at the skin surface and wider in the panniculus, is the optimal procedure. An alternative double-punch method, using a 6–8 mm punch first, followed by a 4–6 mm punch at the depth of the first punch, may be considered, but it is less ideal. Depending on the amount of fat in the particular body location that is being biopsied and the age of the patient, the fat can be adequately sampled with the initial punch. Panniculitis is an area of dermatopathology where the skill of the dermatopathologist is critical in establishing good clinicopathologic correlation. If the biopsy report from an adequate specimen does not match the clinical findings, the clinician should repeat the biopsy or ask for a second opinion on the original specimen.

Requena L: Normal subcutaneous fat, necrosis of adipocytes and classification of the panniculitides. Semin Cutan Med Surg 2007; 26: 66.

Zelger B: Panniculitides, an algorithmic approach. G Ital Dermatol Venereol 2013; 148: 351.

SEPTAL PANNICULITIS (ACUTE AND CHRONIC ERYTHEMA NODOSUM)

Erythema nodosum (EN) is the most common inflammatory panniculitis. It occurs in two forms: acute, which is more common, and chronic, which is rare. Acute EN may occur at any age and in both genders, but most cases occur in young adult women (female/male ratio, 3 : 1–6 : 1). The eruption consists of bilateral, symmetric, deep, tender nodules and plaques 1–10 cm in diameter. Usually, there are up to 10 lesions, but in severe cases many more may be found. Initially, the skin over the nodules is red, smooth, slightly elevated, and shiny (Fig. 23.1). The most common location is the pretibial area and lateral shins.

In general, the lesions should be primarily anterior rather than posterior calf. Lesions may also be seen on the upper legs, extensor arms, neck, and rarely the face. The onset is acute and is frequently preceded by malaise and leg edema. Arthritis or arthralgia, usually of the ankles, knees, or wrists, can occur. Fever, headache, episcleritis, conjunctivitis, and various gastrointestinal (GI) complaints may also be present. EN is a panniculitis that is a reactive response to another disease, therefore some of these symptoms may be related to the associated disease. Over a few days, the lesions flatten, leaving a purple or blue-green color resembling a deep bruise (erythema contusiforme). Ulceration does not occur, and the lesions resolve without atrophy or scarring. The natural history is for the nodules to last a few days or weeks, appearing in crops, and then slowly involute. EN in children affects boys and girls equally.

EN is a reactive process although approximately half of cases are idiopathic. It is frequently associated with a streptococcal infection (especially in children). Tuberculosis (TB) remains an important cause in areas where TB is endemic. Intestinal infection with *Yersinia, Salmonella,* or *Shigella* may precipitate EN. Other infectious causes include systemic fungal infections (coccidioidomycosis, histoplasmosis, sporotrichosis, blastomycosis) and toxoplasmosis. EN-like lesions have been described in other infectious diseases such as *Helicobacter* septicemia, brucellosis, psittacosis, and cat-scratch fever. Because these organisms are fastidious, it has not always been possible to exclude the possibility that the EN-like lesions seen in these diseases actually represent septic foci in the fat.

Sarcoidosis may present with fever, cough, joint pains, hilar adenopathy, and EN. This symptom complex, known as Löfgren syndrome, is especially common in Scandinavian, Irish, and Puerto Rican women. Sarcoidosis associated EN has been linked to a tumor necrosis factor–α (TNF-α) polymorphism. It generally responds well to therapy and runs a self-limited course. EN is frequently seen in patients with inflammatory bowel disease (IBD), more often Crohn disease than ulcerative colitis, and has been linked to mutations in genes controlling immune signaling, including *PTGER4, ITGAL,* and *IKZF1*. In IBD patients, EN is not associated with overall disease severity but is strongly associated with female gender, eye and joint involvement, and isolated colonic involvement. Fecal calprotectin is a marker of inflammation in the GI tract and can be a sensitive marker for active IBD and thus a useful screening test. EN has been rarely reported in association with various hematologic malignancies, but Sweet syndrome and pyoderma gangrenosum are more commonly neutrophilic dermatoses associated with hematologic malignancy. EN has also been associated with idiopathic granulomatous mastitis, which is usually unilateral and mimics infection and breast carcinoma.

Drugs may also induce EN. The bromides and iodides were once the most frequent causative agents. Currently, oral contraceptives, hormone replacement therapy, sulfonamides, and penicillins are the most common medications inducing EN. Azathioprine has also been implicated in causing neutrophilic dermatoses including EN. Other newer associated medications include lenalidomide, methimazole, and Echinacea. The association with hormonal-based therapy, predominantly in young women, and the occurrence of EN in pregnancy suggest that estrogens may predispose to the development of EN. BRAF targeting therapy with vemurafenib, dabrafenib, or trametinib may also induce EN. Although infliximab has been used to treat EN associated with Crohn disease, it has also produced EN on multiple challenges in the setting of ankylosing spondylitis.

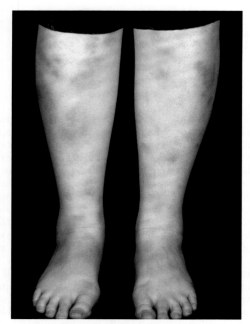

Fig. 23.1 Erythema nodosum.

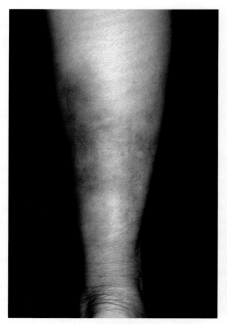

Fig. 23.2 Chronic erythema nodosum.

Erythema nodosum–like lesions have been described in Behçet syndrome and Sweet syndrome and probably represent these inflammatory processes occurring in the fat, rather than the coexistence of two disorders. Histologically, the subcutaneous lesions of Behçet syndrome show features different from EN: a lobular or mixed lobular and septal pattern and, most important, a vasculitis that may be lymphocytic or leukocytoclastic or that may involve a small arteriole. This vasculitis is proposed to be the primary event producing the subcutaneous lesions in Behçet syndrome.

A more chronic variant of EN, called chronic EN, erythema nodosum migrans, or subacute migratory panniculitis of Vilanova and Piñol, is well described. This form of septal panniculitis is much less common than acute EN. It is distinguished from acute EN because it is unilateral, or asymmetric if bilateral (Fig. 23.2); it tends to occur in older women; and it is not associated with associated systemic symptoms except arthralgias. Additionally, the lesions in chronic EN begin as a single red nodule that tends to resolve but migrates centrifugally, forming annular plaques of subcutaneous nodules with central clearing. The lesions are painless or less tender than acute EN, and they have a prolonged course of months to years. TNF-α antagonists seem to be helpful in some cases.

In the differential diagnosis of EN, other forms of panniculitis must be considered. Erythema induratum is a reactive process due to *Mycobacterium tuberculosis.* It usually affects primarily the posterior calves alone and runs a more chronic course, with the possibility of ulceration and scarring. Syphilitic gummas, as well as the nodules of sporotrichosis, are generally unilateral. Subcutaneous fat necrosis associated with pancreatitis and nodular vasculitis may also occur on the shins, but associated clinicohistologic features allow the differentiation from EN. Subacute infectious processes, such as *Helicobacter* cellulitis and primary atypical mycobacterial infection, may closely mimic EN. In most cases, the classic picture of the acute onset of symmetric, red, tender nodules on the anterior shins of a young woman readily leads to the diagnosis of EN without a biopsy. However, if the case is atypical or does not evolve typically, a biopsy should be performed. When the diagnosis of EN has been made in error, either the clinical features were atypical and a biopsy was not performed or was inadequate (punch biopsy), or the biopsy was misinterpreted by the pathologist.

The histopathology of EN is a septal panniculitis; the inflammatory infiltrate principally involves the connective tissue septa between fat lobules throughout the evolution of the lesion. The infiltrate may be composed of either neutrophils (early) or lymphocytes and other mononuclear cells (later), or a mixture, depending on the stage at which the lesion is biopsied. In older lesions, histiocytes and multinucleate giant cells may predominate. Fat lobules are only secondarily affected by the inflammation, but some foamy histiocytes may be seen in the evolution of the lesions. Meischer radial granulomas, which are aggregates of histiocytes around stellate clefts, are characteristic but not diagnostic of EN. Leukocytoclastic vasculitis is not a histologic feature of EN. In chronic EN, septal fibrosis and septal granulomas composed of epithelioid histiocytes are seen.

The management of EN involves three components: identifying the trigger, rest and elevation of the affected extremities, and antiinflammatory medications. Because streptococcus is a common trigger, throat culture (or perianal culture in young children) and antistreptolysin O (ASO) titer are indicated, especially in children. Some basic laboratory testing is done to rule out pregnancy in women, and stool calprotectin level is determined to evaluate for IBD. A complete history of any preceding illness will often lead to clues; for example, previous diarrhea might suggest *Yersinia* infection and a stool culture can be helpful if warranted based on symptoms. A travel and exposure history is especially important when considering endemic fungal infections. Because 4% of patients with histoplasmosis present with EN, this cause should be excluded in endemic areas, and TB should be excluded in patients who may have had exposure.

Early treatment of the infectious cause does not appear to shorten the duration of the EN, although EN triggered by infections tends to last longer with a more chronic infection, and streptococcal-induced EN tends to be shorter than TB-triggered EN. Bed rest is of great value and may be all that is required in mild cases, especially in children. Gentle support hose are also helpful. Curtailing vigorous exercise during the acute attacks will shorten the course, and restriction of physical activities might prevent exacerbations and recurrences. Aspirin and nonsteroidal antiinflammatory drugs (NSAIDs) such as indomethacin are often helpful. Potassium iodide is a safe and effective treatment for both acute and chronic EN. As a supersaturated solution, 5 drops three times a day, increased by 1 drop per dose per day up to 30 drops three times a day, is one easy-to-remember dose schedule. As a tablet, the dose is one 300-mg tablet three times daily. Induction of hypothyroidism by prolonged iodide therapy may occur and should be monitored for. Once controlled, the therapy is gradually reduced over 2–3 weeks. Intralesional corticosteroid injections will control persistent lesions. Systemic corticosteroids will result in rapid resolution of lesions, if not contraindicated by the underlying precipitating cause. In acute lesions, colchicine is often rapidly effective at a dose of 0.6 mg twice daily. In refractory cases, antimalarials such as hydroxycholoroquine may be tried. TNF-α medications may also be effective, but a paradoxic reaction in which adalimumab may have caused EN has been reported.

The prognosis in patients with acute EN is typically good, with the attack running its course in 3–6 weeks. Recurrences do occur, especially if the underlying condition or infection is still present, or if physical activity is resumed too quickly. Chronic or atypical lesions should suggest an alternative diagnosis and require a biopsy.

Acosta KA, et al: Etiology and therapeutic management of erythema nodosum during pregnancy. Am J Clin Dermatol 2013; 14: 215.

Blake T, et al: Erythema nodosum–a review of an uncommon panniculitis. Dermatol Online J 2014; 20.

Dengen A, et al: Erythema nodosum in a patient undergoing vemurafenib therapy for metastatic melanoma. Eur J Dermatol 2013; 23: 118.

Emre S, et al: A case of severe erythema nodosum induced by methimazole. Saudi Pharm J 2017; 25: 813.

Fruchter R, et al: Erythema nodosum in association with idiopathic granulomatous mastitis. J Eur Acad Dermatol Venereol 2017; 31: e391.

Ilhanli I, et al: Erythema nodosum during adalimumab therapy. Am J Internal Med 2015; 3: 210.

Kisacik B, et al: Multiclinical experiences in erythema nodosum. Rheumatol Int 2013; 33: 315.

Labunski S, et al: Tumour necrosis factor-alpha promoter polymorphism in erythema nodosum. Acta Derm Venereol 2001; 81: 18.

Mössner R, et al: Erythema nodosum-like lesions during BRAF inhibitor therapy. J Eur Acad Dermatol Venereol 2015; 29: 1797.

Passarini B, et al: Erythema nodosum. G Ital Dermatol Venereol 2013; 148: 413.

Uceda J et al: A6.15 refractory chronic erythema nodosum and treatment with anti TNF. Annals of the Rheumatic Diseases 2013; 72: A47.

Vargas-Hitos JA, et al: Erythema nodosum as azathioprine hypersensitivity reaction in a patient with bullous pemphigoid. Indian J Dermatol 2014; 58: 406.

Weizman A, et al: Clinical, serologic, and genetic factors associated with pyoderma gangrenosum and erythema nodosum in inflammatory bowel disease patients. Inflamm Bowel Dis 2014; 20: 525.

■ LOBULAR PANNICULITIS

Vessel-Based Lobular Panniculitis

Inflammation or thrombosis of blood vessels may lead to fat necrosis caused by ischemia. This can occur in primary forms of vasculitis, such as polyarteritis nodosa and Churg-Strauss syndrome, in metabolic disorders such as oxalosis and calciphylaxis, with atheromatous emboli, with heparin and coumarin necrosis, and with various coagulopathies. These entities are discussed in other chapters.

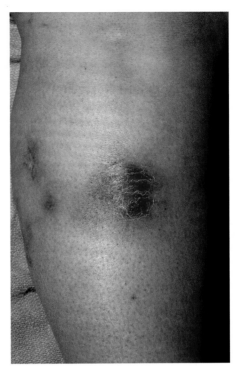

Fig. 23.3 Nodular vasculitis.

Nodular Vasculitis and Erythema Induratum

Clinically and histologically, nodular vasculitis is identical to erythema induratum (EI). The two differ only by the presence of TB as a precipitating factor in EI. Nodular vasculitis presents as tender, subcutaneous nodules on the calves of middle-aged women (Fig. 23.3). Venous insufficiency may be present. Lesions are bilateral and less red and tender than EN; they often ulcerate, drain oily liquid, and recur over years.

The early lesions may show a suppurative vasculopathy, proposed by various authors to be an arteritis, a venulitis, or both. In some cases, no vasculitis is found, and despite its name, the presence of a vasculitis is not required to establish the diagnosis. Nodular vasculitis results in substantial lobular necrosis of adipocytes with suppuration. Necrosis of the lobule results in loss of the lipocyte membrane and pooling of lipid into variably sized round aggregates. As lesions evolve, the fat becomes increasingly necrotic, forming microcysts, and the disease progresses to the point where it may perforate through the epidermis, forming ulceration. Granulomatous inflammation appears adjacent to areas of fat necrosis, and eventually lesions resolve with fibrosis.

Nontuberculous nodular vasculitis must be distinguished from EI. Nodular vasculitis has many reported causes, including *Chlamydia* infections, Crohn disease, Takayasu arteritis, BCG vaccination, TNF-α antagonist therapy, and non-TB mycobacterial infections. Because clinicopathologic features are identical in EI and nodular vasculitis, the differentiation is made by evaluating for tuberculous infection in the patient. A Quantiferon gold or tuberculin skin test can be administered. If this is positive, the appropriate diagnosis is EI. Polymerase chain reaction (PCR) of the affected tissue may reveal the DNA of *M. tuberculosis* in 50%–70% of cases of EI. As a tuberculid (inflammatory response to tuberculosis), EI is a manifestation of cellular immunity to TB, and the purified protein derivative (PPD) test will always be positive. PCR of the tissue is not recommended in patients who are tuberculin skin test negative. It should be noted that even in areas where TB is prevalent, EI is rare, representing only 1% of cutaneous manifestations of TB in one study. When present, EI may signal serious genitourinary involvement, including tuberculous epididymo-orchitis.

EI requires antibiotic therapy for the underlying TB. Treatment of nodular vasculitis is usually supersaturated solution of potassium iodide (SSKI) supersaturated solution of potassium iodide, as outlined for EN, and is effective in about half of patients. In the others, trials of colchicine, antimalarials, NSAIDs, mycophenolate mofetil, and systemic corticosteroids have been helpful. Support stockings, elevation, and treatment of associated venous insufficiency may also improve nodular vasculitis.

Chen S, et al: *Mycobacterium tuberculosis* infection is associated with the development of erythema nodosum and nodular vasculitis. PLoS One 2013; 8: e62653.

Gilchrist H, et al: Erythema nodosum and erythema induratum (nodular vasculitis). Dermatol Ther 2010; 23: 320.

Kabuto M, et al: Erythema induratum (nodular vasculitis) associated with Takayasu arteritis. Eur J Dermatol 2017; 27: 410.

Misago N, et al: Erythema induratum (nodular vasculitis) associated with Crohn's disease. Am J Dermatopathol 2012; 34: 325.

Papathemeli D, et al: Explosive generalization of nodular vasculitis–*Mycobacterium marinum* challenges the paradigm. J Eur Acad Dermatol Venereol 2016; 30: e189.

Park SB, et al: Nodular vasculitis that developed during etanercept (Enbrel) treatment in a patient with psoriasis. Ann Dermatol 2015; 27: 605.

Sekiguchi A, et al: Erythema induratum of Bazin associated with bacillus Calmette–Guérin vaccination. J Dermatol 2016; 43: 111.

Taverna JA, et al: Case reports: nodular vasculitis responsive to mycophenolate mofetil. J Drugs Dermatol 2006; 5: 992.

Wee E, Kelly RI: Treatment of nodular vasculitis with colchicine. Australas J Dermatol 2017; 58: e79.

Lipodermatosclerosis

Lipodermatosclerosis, or sclerosing panniculitis, occurs primarily on the medial lower third of the lower legs of women older than 40 (Fig. 23.4), with an above-average body mass index (BMI). It

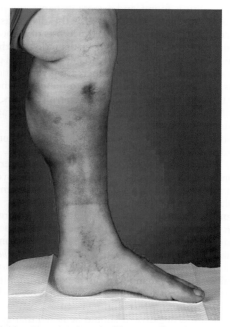

Fig. 23.4 Lipodermatosclerosis. (Courtesy Douglas Pugliese, MD.)

is often bilateral. In the acute phase, red to purple, poorly demarcated, indurated plaques are present on the lower legs. The lesions are painful and the differential diagnosis includes cellulitis, phlebitis, EN, or inflammatory morphea. In the chronic phase there is marked woody induration in a stocking distribution, resulting in calves that resemble inverted champagne bottles. This thick, tight, hyperpigmented skin results from fibrosis in the subcutaneous fat, which may occur without the primary inflammatory panniculitis ever being clinically observed. Fibrosis occurs multifocally and microscopically throughout the affected area.

The etiology of lipodermatosclerosis is venous insufficiency. These patients may have venous varicosities, superficial thrombophlebitis, deep venous thrombosis, or several of these conditions. Even when venous disease is not clinically evident, evaluation of the venous system of the lower leg will frequently reveal insufficiency. Laboratory evaluation is rarely done but may reveal a genetic mutation in the fibrinolytic system resulting in increased thrombosis in these patients. Venous insufficiency results in hypoxia, necrosis of fat, inflammation, and eventual fibrosis. If hypoxemia is present from other causes, such as pulmonary disease, sclerosing panniculitis may be more severe. Angiosarcoma has been reported as a rare complication in the setting of postphlebitic lipodermatosclerosis.

The histologic features of sclerosing panniculitis are characteristic, but not all features may be seen on every biopsy, because the histologic features change over time within the lesion. The overlying dermis frequently shows changes of stasis with nodular proliferation of thick-walled vessels, hemosiderin deposition, fibrosis, and atrophy. In early lesions, there is ischemic necrosis in the center of the fat lobules manifested as "ghost cells"—pale cell walls with no nuclei along with thickened septae. Pseudomembranous changes in the dermis may also be a clue to early disease. There is a sparse lymphocytic infiltrate in the fat septa. As the lesions evolve, the septa are thickened and fibrosed, and there is a mixed inflammatory infiltrate of lymphocytes, plasma cells, and macrophages. Foamy histiocytes are present around the areas of fat necrosis. Fat microcysts are characteristic (but not diagnostic) and appear as small cysts with feathery eosinophilic remnants of adipocytes lining the cyst cavity and resembling frost on a window, so-called lipomembranous fat necrosis. In lesions later, these microcysts collapse and are replaced by fibrosis. Despite these characteristic features, biopsy should be avoided in these patients. Biopsies heal poorly and may lead to chronic leg ulcers. The diagnosis can usually be made clinically. Noninvasive techniques such as magnetic resonance imaging (MRI) have been used to avoid poorly healing wounds related to a biopsy. If a biopsy must be performed, it should be from the most proximal edge of involvement.

This diagnosis can be clinically confirmed if a careful vascular evaluation is performed. The location on the lower medial calf is unusual for EN. Most other panniculitides favor the posterior midcalf. The gradual progression from the ankles proximally is characteristic of sclerosing panniculitis and not other forms of lobular panniculitis.

The treatment of lipodermatosclerosis may be difficult. The fibrosis may be irreversible. Graded compression stockings with elevation and standard treatments for venous insufficiency are most effective in this condition. Application of pressure dressings, such as an Unna boot, can produce dramatic, if temporary, improvement. Greater compression—Unna boot with Coban and a foam buttress (bolster material to apply extra pressure to the red inflamed area) or the Profore boot—can be beneficial. Unfortunately, some patients cannot tolerate compression because of the pain of the lesions. Intralesional triamcinolone and ultrasound therapy have been used, but this is most effective when used in conjunction with compression. Pentoxiphylline, may be useful, especially in patients not responding to compression and elevation alone, or in patients who are initially intolerant of compression dressings. The addition of hydroxychloroquine to pentoxiphylline may provide additional improvement. Apparently, by enhancing the fibrinolytic capacity of affected patients, stanozolol, or oxandrolone, may benefit some patients. This is rarely required, however, if appropriate pressure dressings are applied and the patient is able to take full doses of pentoxiphylline. Stanozolol and oxandrolone may be virilizing for women and should be avoided in women of childbearing age. Stanozolol may induce hepatitis. Surgical treatment of varicosities and incompetent perforators may result in dramatic improvement in some patients.

Ayele A, et al: Pseudomembranous changes in the dermis. J Cutan Pathol 2017; 44: 1070.
Balasubramanyam S, et al: Venous treatment of lipodermatosclerosis to improve ambulatory function. Dermatolog Surg 2017 Aug 29; ePub ahead of print.
Chan CC, et al: Magnetic resonance imaging as a diagnostic tool for extensive lipodermatosclerosis. J Am Acad Dermatol 2008; 58: 525.
Choonhakarn C, Chaowattanapanit S: Lipodermatosclerosis. J Am Acad Dermatol 2012; 66: 1013.
Choonhakarn C, et al: Lipodermatosclerosis. Int J Dermatol 2016; 55: 303.
Damian DL, et al: Ultrasound therapy for lipodermatosclerosis. Arch Dermatol 2009; 145: 330.
Jeong, KH, et al: Refractory lipodermatosclerosis treated with intralesional platelet-rich plasma. J Am Acad Dermatol 2011; 65: e157.
Jowett AJ, et al: Angiosarcoma in an area of lipodermatosclerosis. Ann R Coll Surg 2008; 90: W15.
Segura S, et al: Lipomembranous fat necrosis of the subcutaneous tissue. Dermatol Clin 2008; 26: 509.
Vesić S, et al: Acute lipodermatosclerosis. Dermatol Online J 2008; 14: 1.
Walsh SN, et al: Lipodermatosclerosis. J Am Acad Dermatol 2010; 62: 1005.

PHYSICAL PANNICULITIS

The category of panniculitis includes processes in the fat that occur from physical factors. Some are characterized by the presence of needle-like clefts: sclerema neonatorum, subcutaneous fat necrosis, and poststeroid panniculitis. Infants and children are most frequently affected likely in part due the higher amount of brown fat in children. Fat is typically in a liquid form in lobules. Brown fat freezes into a solid at higher temperatures than regular fat in adults, so slight cooling can lead to solidification and necrosis.

Sclerema Neonatorum

Sclerema neonatorum is the most severe and rarest disorder of the physical panniculitides. It affects premature neonates who are critically ill for other reasons or have experienced profound hypothermia. With more adequate neonatal intensive care, this disorder has become extremely rare. Neonates affected with sclerema neonatorum usually die, unless the underlying diseases can be reversed. In the first few days of life, the skin begins to harden, usually initially on the buttocks or lower extremities, then rapidly spreads to involve the whole body. The skin on the palms, soles, and genitalia is spared. The skin becomes dry, livid, cold, rigid, and boardlike, limiting the mobility of the parts. The skin in the involved areas cannot be picked up. The skin of the entire body may appear half-frozen and is yellowish white. Visceral fat may also be involved. Therapy is mostly supportive, but some data suggest exchange transfusion may improve survival.

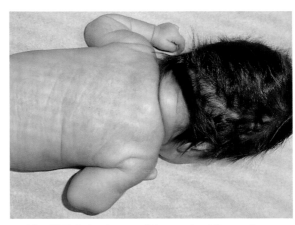

Fig. 23.5 Subcutaneous fat necrosis of the newborn.

Histologically, adipocytes are enlarged and filled with needle-like clefts in a radial array Recently, this unusual histologic finding was documented in a reaction to gemcitabine. Affected fat cells undergo necrosis. There is sparse inflammation, and histiocytes containing needle-like clefts are rare, possibly because most children die before granulomas can form.

Subcutaneous Fat Necrosis of the Newborn

Subcutaneous fat necrosis of the newborn (SCFN) occurs during the first 4 weeks of life (half in the first week) in term or postterm infants. There is often a history of fetal distress such as birth asphyxia, maternal-fetal disproportion, or meconium aspiration. More recently, intensive care unit protocols for neonates with neural depression may initiate hypothermia, which can lead to widespread SCFN that can even involve the viscera. Septicemia, severe neonatal anemia, thrombocytopenia, and maternal cocaine use have also been associated with SCFN.

SCFN is characterized by painful, firm to rubbery, erythematous nodules usually on areas that have significant subcutaneous tissue and are susceptible to crush injury during birth such as the upper back, buttocks, cheeks, or proximal extremities (Fig. 23.5). The arms, shoulders, and back were most common in a recent larger series. Lesions may fuse to form plaques. They heal spontaneously within 3 months with no scarring unless there is ulceration. In general, the infants remain well; however, hypoglycemia, thrombocytopenia, hypertriglyceridemia, lactic acidosis, and potentially life-threatening hypercalcemia may rarely occur. Some degree of hypercalcemia occurred in more than 50% of recently reported cases. The hypercalcemia may appear weeks to months after the appearance and resolution of the skin lesions. Periodic measuring of serum calcium for the first 3–6 months of life or until the lesions resolve has been recommended as the calcium can increase even as the lesions are resolving. Hypercalcemia may result in failure to thrive, irritability, lethargy, hypotonia, seizures, and renal failure. Rarely nephrocalcinosis and calcinosis of the gallbladder were reported. Significant hypercalcemia is treated with hyperhydration, calcium-wasting diuretics (furosemide), and formulas low in calcium and vitamin D. Systemic corticosteroids, calcitonin, and bisphosphonates may also be effective when other methods fail to reduce the hypercalcemia.

Histologically, SCFN is a lobular panniculitis with granular necrosis of adipocytes. Needle-shaped clefts are arranged radially within histiocytes, and multinucleate foamy histiocytes are present. Degranulating eosinophils may also be present. Lesions may resolve with calcification and fibrosis. Fine-needle aspiration and touch preparations can confirm this diagnosis, and a biopsy is diagnostic. Characteristic ultrasound and MRI findings have been reported.

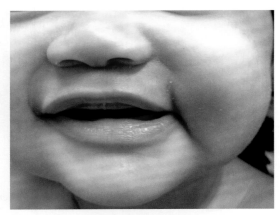

Fig. 23.6 Cold panniculitis.

Cold Panniculitis

Infants and young children are particularly predisposed to cold panniculitis. It has been described in children who suck on ice, use frozen teething rings, or popsicles (popsicle panniculitis); in the scrotum of prepubertal males (Fig. 23.6); and in infants treated for supraventricular tachycardia with the application of cold packs to the face. Lesions occur within a few days of the cold application and appear as slightly erythematous, nontender, firm subcutaneous nodules. Equestrian panniculitis on the upper outer thighs (although it can be medial) of people riding horses in the cold more closely resembles a form of perniosis rather than true panniculitis (see Chapter 3). Overlapping histology may occur in adults using ice packs for pain relief.

The typical patient with fat necrosis of the scrotum is a prepubertal (age 9–14) boy, who is heavyset or even obese, with scrotal swelling, usually bilateral, associated with mild to moderate pain. There is a lack of systemic complaints and no symptoms related to voiding. The scrotal masses are bilateral and symmetric in most cases. However, the lesions may be unilateral, and there may be more than two. The masses are firm and tender and do not transmit light. The overlying scrotal skin is normal or red. The most common location of the lesions is near the perineum, consistent with the area of greatest concentration of scrotal fat in children. The adult scrotum lacks this fatty tissue. Without treatment, lesions resolve over several days to weeks.

Histologically, there is necrosis of adipocytes within lobules of the upper subcutaneous fat adjacent to the lower dermis. A mixed inflammatory infiltrate of lymphocytes, neutrophils, and foam cells is present, and microcysts sometimes occur. This histology is not specific, and the diagnosis of cold panniculitis relies largely on obtaining a history of cold exposure.

Akcay A, et al: Hypercalcemia due to subcutaneous fat necrosis in a newborn after total body cooling. Pediatr Dermatol 2013; 30: 120.

Bolotin D, et al: Cold panniculitis following ice therapy for cardiac arrhythmia. Pediatr Dermatol 2011; 28: 192.

Del Pozzo-Magaña BR, Ho N: Subcutaneous fat necrosis of the newborn. Pediatr Dermatol 2016; 33: e353.

Ferrara G, et al: Cold-associated perniosis of the thighs ("equestrian-type" chilblain). Am J Dermatopathol 2016; 38: 726.

Khedr S, et al: Occult massive visceral fat necrosis following therapeutic hypothermia for neonatal encephalopathy. Pediatr Dev Pathol 2017; Epub ahead of print.

Lopez V, et al: Usefulness of fine-needle aspiration in subcutaneous fat necrosis of the newborn diagnosis. Pediatr Dermatol 2010; 27: 317.

Mahé E, et al: Subcutaneous fat necrosis of the newborn. Br J Dermatol 2007; 156: 709.

Patel AR, et al: Circular erythematous patch in a febrile infant. Pediatr Dermatol 2012; 29: 659.

Saenz Ibarra B, et al: Cold-induced dermatoses. Am J Dermatopathol 2017 Sept 27; ePub ahead of print.

Samedi VM, et al: Neonatal hypercalcemia secondary to subcutaneous fat necrosis successfully treated with pamidronate. AJP Rep 2014; 4: e93.

Schubert PT, et al: Fine-needle aspiration cytology of subcutaneous fat necrosis of the newborn. Diagn Cytopathol 2012; 40: 245.

Stewart CL, et al: Equestrian perniosis. Am J Dermatopathol 2013; 35: 237.

Zeb A, et al: Sclerema neonatorum. J Perinatol 2008; 28: 453.

Poststeroid Panniculitis

This rare form of panniculitis occurs predominantly in children treated acutely with high doses of systemic corticosteroids during rapid corticosteroid withdrawal. Substantial weight gain has usually occurred during the corticosteroid therapy. Firm subcutaneous nodules begin to appear within 1 month of tapering the corticosteroids. Areas of abundant subcutaneous fat are favored: the cheeks, trunk, and proximal extremities. Most cases resolve spontaneously within weeks, but if severe, the corticosteroids must be reinstituted and tapered more slowly.

Histologically, the changes are identical to those seen in subcutaneous fat necrosis of the newborn. There is a lobular panniculitis with necrosis of adipocytes and needle-shaped clefts in both adipocytes and histiocytes. Foamy histiocytes are also present.

Sacchidanand SA, et al: Post-steroid panniculitis. Indian Dermatol Online J 2013; 4: 318.

Traumatic Panniculitis

Accidental trauma to the skin may induce necrosis of the fat. The prior history of trauma is frequently not recalled. There may be erythema that develops over top of the area of panniculitis. Lesions present similar to a lipoma, as a firm, mobile subcutaneous mass (formerly reported as mobile encapsulated lipoma). The term *myospherulosis* (spherulocytosis) has been used to describe subcutaneous cystic lesions induced by trauma with hemorrhage into areas of high lipid content. Many cases are caused by exogenous lipids from postoperative packing, often in parasinus tissues or subcutaneous fat. The structures resemble the sporangia of rhinosporidiosis but represent degenerated red blood cells rather than true fungal organisms. Accidental trauma to the upper anterolateral thigh from a desk or chair may result in semicircular bands of atrophy of fat called lipoatrophia semicircularis. Airbag injury may induce fat necrosis.

Histologically, there is a granulomatous lobular panniculitis with foamy histiocytes, membranous fat necrosis, and microcysts. Lesions heal with fibrosis of the septa. In myospherulosis, large round structures containing many smaller round eosinophilic bodies are noted. These represent degenerated erythrocytes.

Boyd AS, et al: Revision: cutaneous Munchausen syndrome. J Cutan Pathol 2014; 41: 33.

Grassi S, et al: Post-surgical lipophagic panniculitis. G Ital Dermatol Venereol 2013; 148: 435.

Lee DJ, et al: Traumatic panniculitis with hypertrichosis. Eur J Dermatol 2011; 21: 258.

Sacchidanand SA, et al: Post-steroid panniculitis. Indian Dermatol Online J 2013; 4: 318.

Factitial Panniculitis

Self-induced panniculitis is rarely reported, but it does occur. It may be induced by the injection of organic materials, povidone, feces, saliva, vaginal fluid, and oils. In many cases, ulceration will occur. Cupping and other trauma may also induce a panniculitis. Some patients have a medical background because they have ready access to syringes and needles. Pointed, detailed questioning of the patient may identify inconsistencies in the history or the underlying cause for the behavior (e.g., attention seeking, revenge, malingering).

The clinician must have a high index of suspicion with patients in whom the clinical pattern is not characteristic of a known form of panniculitis. Inspection of early lesions for telltale healing injection sites may help confirm the diagnosis. A biopsy is often required. Culture may demonstrate many different microbes representative of fecal, oral, or vaginal flora. Biopsy demonstrates an acute lobular panniculitis with fat necrosis and a neutrophilic infiltrate. Careful evaluation of the biopsy material with polarization may identify foreign material. When the suspicion is high and no foreign material can be seen in the tissue, special evaluation by incineration and mass spectroscopy may identify the injected substance. Electron microscopy with x-ray emission spectrography can identify inorganic substances. Radiographs may demonstrate fractured needles or foreign bodies.

Kim TH, et al: Adverse events related to cupping therapy in studies conducted in Korea. Eur J Integr Med 2014; 6: 434.
Sanmartín O, et al: Factitial panniculitis. Dermatol Clin 2008; 26: 519.

Sclerosing Lipogranuloma

Sclerosing lipogranuloma describes the granulomatous and fibrotic reaction that occurs in the panniculus from the injection of silicone or mineral oils. In most cases, the injections are intentional and cosmetic. The time from injection to onset of symptoms may be months to more than 10 years. Topical application of an antibacterial ointment to an open wound can rarely result in the formation of lipogranuloma. Exenatide injections for type 2 diabetes may induce such changes as well.

Lesions are usually localized to the penis, scrotum, breasts, nose, and buttocks, often after an attempt to augment the area by injection. The overlying skin is hyperpigmented and erythematous. Lesions are frequently diagnosed initially as cellulitis. On palpation, the skin is indurated and cannot be picked up between the fingers. The subcutaneous tissue is indurated, thickened, and lumpy. Some patients will have focal ulceration. MRI can be helpful in establishing the location and extent of the material, ruling out malignancy, and ensuring normal anatomy underneath. The injected material will frequently migrate locally, extending beyond the sites of implantation. In some cases, it is carried to other tissues, specifically the lymphoreticular system and lungs. Hepatosplenomegaly and pulmonary fibrosis may occur.

Histologically, the panniculus is replaced by the injected material, which is in various-sized vacuoles, giving the affected tissue a "Swiss cheese" appearance. Because the material is usually washed out during the tissue processing, the material itself is not seen, only the spaces it occupied in the tissue in vivo. The vacuoles are surrounded by histiocytes, many of which have ingested the material, giving their cytoplasm a vacuolated appearance. Fibrosis may be prominent. Frozen section can be used to demonstrate the lipid.

Eun YS, et al: A woman with a nose like an "elephant's trunk." J Cosmet Laser Ther 2014; 16: 153.
Foxton G, et al: Sclerosing lipogranuloma of the penis. Australas J Dermatol 2011; 52: e12.

Nyirády P, et al: Treatment and outcome of Vaseline-induced sclerosing lipogranuloma of the penis. Urology 2008; 71: 1132.
Shan SJ, et al: Exenatide-induced eosinophilic sclerosing lipogranuloma at the injection site. Am J Dermatopathol 2014; 36: 510.
Tirico MC, et al: Sclerosing lipogranuloma with multiple skin lesions and pulmonary involvement, secondary to a factitious disorder. Acta Derm Venereol 2016; 96: 268.
Tsili AC, et al: Silicone-induced penile sclerosing lipogranuloma. J Clin Imaging Sci 2016; 6: 3.

■ ENZYME-RELATED PANNICULITIS

The enzyme-related category includes panniculitis induced by enzymes that damage fat (pancreatic panniculitis) and panniculitis caused by the absence of an enzyme critical in preventing tissue inflammation after injury (α_1-antitrypsin).

PANCREATIC PANNICULITIS (SUBCUTANEOUS FAT NECROSIS)

Subcutaneous fat necrosis is most often associated with pancreatitis or pancreatic carcinoma, and rarely with anatomic pancreatic abnormalities, pseudocysts, hypertriglyceridemia in association with nephrotic syndrome, pancreatic portal fistule, endoscopic retrograde cholangiopancreatography, or drug-induced pancreatitis. Men outnumber women 2:1 in cases of pancreatitis and 7:1 in cases of pancreatic carcinoma. In cases associated with pancreatic carcinoma, acinar cell carcinoma is most common. Even metastatic pancreatic carcinoma with no residual tumor in the pancreas may induce the syndrome. In 40% of patients, the skin lesions are the first symptom of the underlying pancreatic pathology and therefore represent an important clue to the diagnosis.

Skin lesions appear as tender or painless, erythematous subcutaneous nodules 1–5 cm in diameter (Fig. 23.7). The lower leg is the most common location and is affected in more than 90% of cases. Subcutaneous fat elsewhere may also be affected, except rarely on the head and neck. The number of lesions is usually fewer than 10 but may reach the hundreds. In most patients, the lesions involute, leaving an atrophic scar. If the fat necrosis is severe, however, the lesion develops into a sterile abscess that may break down, draining a thick, brown, oily material.

Pancreatic panniculitis is frequently accompanied by a constellation of findings related to fat necrosis in other organs. Importantly, abdominal symptoms may be completely absent. Arthritis is found in 54%–88% of patients and may be monoarticular, oligoarticular, and rarely polyarticular. This has been labeled PPP (pancreatitis, panniculitis, and polyarthritis) syndrome. The arthritis may be intermittent, migratory, or persistent and is usually in joints adjacent

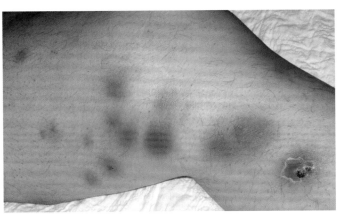

Fig. 23.7 Pancreatic panniculitis.

to the lesions of panniculitis. Examination of the joint fluid reveals the presence of free fatty acids, suggesting it is caused by fat necrosis adjacent to the joint space. Other findings are medullary fat necrosis of bone, polyserositis, and pulmonary infiltrates or embolism.

Laboratory evaluation is useful in establishing the diagnosis. In most patients the amylase or lipase (or both) is elevated. In many cases, however, one of the tests may be normal and the other abnormal, so both tests must be performed. About 60% of patients with pancreatic carcinoma and panniculitis will have a peripheral eosinophilia.

The histologic features of pancreatic panniculitis are diagnostic. These include focal areas of fat necrosis with anucleate "ghost cells"; finely stippled basophilic material, representing calcium, within the residual rim of the necrotic cells and at the periphery of the affected foci; and a dense, inflammatory polymorphous infiltrate at the periphery of the affected fat. The affected necrotic areas are relatively acellular. Several reports have suggested that the early features are those of a septal panniculitis, resembling EN. This may have represented sampling error but does indicate that if the initial sample is not diagnostic, another, perhaps more adequate, sample of a more advanced lesion should be considered. Panniculitis caused by interferon-beta injections can have a histologic appearance similar to pancreatic panniculitis.

The necrosis of fat at all affected sites is at least partly caused by the release of fat-digesting enzymes, lipases, from the affected pancreatic tissue. These lipases spread hematogenously to the affected sites.

EN represents the primary differential consideration, because pancreatic panniculitis may not have abdominal symptoms, also favors the lower legs, and may be accompanied by joint symptoms. The distinction can be made by skin biopsy, serum amylase, and lipase determinations, and especially if eosinophilia is present, a search for a pancreatic neoplasm.

Treatment mainly involves treating the cause of the pancreatitis. Obstruction or stenosis of ducts should be repaired, pseudocysts drained, and in the case of pancreatic carcinoma, surgery or other interventions as indicated.

Ball, NJ, et al: Lobular panniculitis at the site of subcutaneous interferon beta injections for the treatment of multiple sclerosis can histologically mimic pancreatic panniculitis. J Cutan Pathol 2009; 36: 331.
Evans AC, et al: An unexpected etiology of pancreatic panniculitis. J Pancreat Cancer 2017; 3: 1.
Manawish K, et al: Pancreatic panniculitis. BMJ Case Rep 2014 Aug 22; 2014.
Zundler S, et al: Pancreatic panniculitis and polyarthritis. Curr Rheum Rep 2017; 19: 62.

α₁-ANTITRYPSIN DEFICIENCY PANNICULITIS

α_1-Antitrypsin is the most abundant antiprotease in circulation and a potent and irreversible inactivator of neutrophil elastase. Heterozygous deficiency of this enzyme occurs in 1 in 50 persons and homozygous deficiency in 1 in 2500 persons of European descent. Emphysema and liver disease are the most common manifestations of antitrypsin deficiency. A small percentage of patients with homozygous deficiency and the PiZZ or PiSZ phenotypes will develop panniculitis. It is caused by a mutation in SERPINA1 gene.

The panniculitis usually appears between ages 20 and 40 but can occur in childhood. Both genders are equally affected. Lesions appear after relatively minor trauma and present as painful nodules on the extremities or trunk. They may spontaneously drain an oily, brown liquid. Multiple draining sinus tracts can occur, with lesions coalescing into large, draining plaques.

The histologic findings in this form of panniculitis depend on the stage of the lesion. Early lesions show neutrophils splaying the collagen of the reticular dermis and subcutaneous septa. More fully evolved lesions show dissolution of the septa, with islands of normal fat "floating" in the spaces that represented the destroyed septa. This later finding is considered diagnostic by some. Elastic tissue stains may reveal decreased elastic tissue in the affected areas.

The clinical and histologic differential diagnosis is factitial panniculitis. This is not surprising because trauma produces both lesions, and in the case of α_1-antitrypsin deficiency, the inflammation-produced enzymes are simply not inactivated, leading to more pronounced lesions than would be expected from that degree of trauma.

Replacement of the deficient antitrypsin will lead to resolution of the skin lesions, but is costly. Dapsone, colchicine, and doxycycline can also be effective. These agents can reduce the requirement for enzyme replacement and should be considered as maintenance treatment in affected patients. Systemic corticosteroids may exacerbate the panniculitis. Liver transplantation leads to normal levels of α_1-antitrypsin and resolution of the panniculitis. Gene therapy and stem cell therapy appear promising.

Blanco I, et al: Neutrophilic panniculitis associated with alpha-1-antitrypsin deficiency. Br J Dermatol 2016; 174: 753.
Laureano A, et al: Alpha-1-antitrypsin deficiency–associated panniculitis. Dermatol Online J 2014; 20: 21245.

CYTOPHAGIC HISTIOCYTIC PANNICULITIS

Cytophagic histiocytic panniculitis (CHP) is a multisystem disease characterized by widespread erythematous, painful, subcutaneous nodules that may occasionally become ecchymotic or break down and form crusted ulcerations. There is a progressive febrile illness, with hepatosplenomegaly, pancytopenia, hypertriglyceridemia, and liver dysfunction. These result from the proliferation of benign-appearing histiocytes, which have a marked phagocytic capacity and extensively involve the reticuloendothelial system. Some patients progress to a terminal phase characterized by profound cytopenia, liver failure, and a terminal hemorrhagic diathesis. CHP represents a spectrum of disease that occurs in children and adults. Some cases are triggered by viral infections, such as Epstein-Barr virus (EBV) or human immunodeficiency virus (HIV), or viral vaccines, and others represent subcutaneous B-cell or T-cell lymphomas. CHP can also occur in hemophagocytic lymphohistiocytosis and has been associated with *STX 11* gene mutation. The benign cases are EBV negative and the lymphoma-associated cases are EBV positive.

Histologically, there is infiltration of the lobules of subcutaneous fat by histiocytes and inflammatory cells, primarily helper T cells, with fat necrosis and hemorrhage. The characteristic cell is a "beanbag" cell: a histiocyte stuffed with phagocytized red blood cells, lymphocytes, neutrophils, platelets, or fragments of these cells. These beanbag cells are not diagnostic of CHP and can be seen infrequently in other panniculitides, especially lupus profundus. The presence of atypical lymphocytes or the detection of a clonal B-cell or T-cell proliferation supports the diagnosis of subcutaneous lymphoma in patients with CHP.

The treatment of CHP is difficult. If malignancy cannot be detected, cyclosporine has been effective in many patients, and combination treatment with high-dose corticosteroids, cyclosporine, and anakinra has been reported. Tacrolimus is another option that has improved some patients. If malignancy is detected, aggressive chemotherapy and perhaps bone marrow transplantation may be considered.

Bader-Meunier B, et al: Clonal cytophagic histiocytic panniculitis in children may be cured by cyclosporine A. Pediatrics 2013; 132: e545.

Krilis M, et al: Cytophagic histiocytic panniculitis with haemophagocytosis in a patient with familial multiple lipomatosis and review of the literature. Mod Rheumatol 2012; 22: 158.

Miyabe Y, et al: Successful treatment of cyclosporine-A–resistant cytophagic histiocytic panniculitis with tacrolimus. Mod Rheumatol 2011; 21: 553.

Pasqualini C, et al: Cytophagic histiocytic panniculitis, hemophagocytic lymphohistiocytosis and undetermined autoimmune disorder. Ital J Pediatr 2014; 40: 17.

■ MISCELLANEOUS FORMS OF PANNICULITIS

GOUTY PANNICULITIS

Uric acid crystals may deposit initially in the subcutaneous fat of patients with gouty panniculitis, leading to lesions resembling other forms of panniculitis. Histologically, there is a lobular panniculitis with necrosis of adipocytes and infiltration of polymorphonuclear leukocytes. Feathery, needle-like crystals in sheaves are present.

Martin D, et al: An unusual location of gouty panniculitis. Medicine (Baltimore) 2017; 96: e6733.

Pattanaprichakul P, et al: Disseminated gouty panniculitis. Dermatol Pract Concept 2014; 4: 33.

■ LIPODYSTROPHY (LIPOATROPHY)

The lipodystrophies are conditions characterized by a marked reduction in subcutaneous fat. Lipodystrophies can be generalized (total), partial, or localized and may be congenital or acquired. In the congenital types, females are more frequently and more severely affected. Hypertriglyceridemia and diabetes mellitus (DM) with insulin resistance occur in many of the congenital and acquired forms of lipodystrophy. These syndromes were quite rare until the 1990s. With the advent of combination antiviral therapy for HIV infection (highly active antiretroviral therapy [HAART]), acquired lipodystrophy has become common in geographic regions where HIV infection is prevalent. In addition, localized fat loss can be a consequence of therapeutic injections into the fat.

CONGENITAL LIPODYSTROPHIES

Congenital Generalized Lipodystrophy

Congenital generalized (total) lipodystrophy, also known as Berardinelli-Seip syndrome, is a rare autosomal recessive condition that is often due to parental consanguinity. At birth or soon after, there is noted an extreme paucity of fat in the subcutaneous tissue and other adipose tissues, giving affected persons a generalized muscular appearance. The mechanical fat of the palms, soles, joints, orbits, and scalp is often not affected. The children have a voracious appetite. They have increased height and height velocity, advanced bone age, muscular hypertrophy, and a masculine habitus. This habitus plus enlargement of the genitalia in infancy (clitoromegaly) can lead to the misdiagnosis of precocious puberty. Scalp hair is abundant and curly, and there is generalized hypertrichosis and hyperhidrosis. The abdomen is protuberant, and the liver and spleen are enlarged. The overall appearance is acromegalic (Fig. 23.8) from enlargement of the mandible, hands, and feet. Acanthosis nigricans is invariably present and often generalized. Hyperinsulinemia, insulin resistance, and DM appear often at about puberty. Women often have menstrual irregularity. The DM resists insulin and oral hypoglycemic therapy, but ketoacidosis does not occur. Hypertriglyceridemia occurs and can produce eruptive xanthomas, pancreatitis, and fatty liver, which may eventuate in cirrhosis. Hypertrophic cardiomyopathy and mild mental retardation may occur. Life span is shortened, with patients frequently dying in

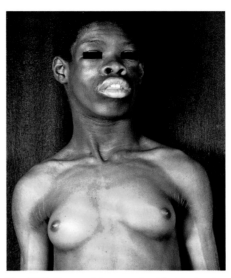

Fig. 23.8 Congenital generalized lipodystrophy.

young adulthood from complications of diabetes or from liver or heart disease.

Mutations in four genes, encoding for 1-acylglycerol 3-phosphate-*O*-acyltransferase 2 (*AGPAT2*), seipin, caveolin-1 (*CAV1*), and cavin-1, cause different subtypes of congenital generalized lipodystrophy. Type B mandibuloacral dysplasia from *ZMPSTE24* mutations, proteasome-associated autoinflammatory syndromes caused by beta subunit type 8 mutations (e.g., seemingly acquired lipodystrophies seen in Candle syndrome, and three other subtypes), glycosylation disorders, *FBNI* mutations, and *c-Fos* and *BANF1* mutations are other causes of generalized lipodystrophies that are inherited. A novel subtype with preservation of bone marrow fat, congenital muscular weakness, and cervical spine instability has also been described. Serum leptin and adiponectin levels are extremely low in various types. If leptin levels are low, leptin replacement decreases serum triglycerides and improves hyperglycemia. Metreleptin was approved in 2014 for replacement. Some patients with congenital generalized lipodystrophy do not have mutations in these genes, suggesting that there are other genetic causes.

Familial Partial Lipodystrophy

Familial partial lipodystrophy is a heterogeneous autosomal dominant group of disorders with distinct phenotypes. The most common variant is the Dunnigan type. Patients are normal at birth, but at about puberty, subcutaneous tissue is gradually lost from the arms and legs and variably from the chest and anterior abdomen. Fat gain occurs in the face, neck, and intraabdominally, resulting in a cushingoid appearance. Increased levels of dipeptidyl peptidase-4 involved in glucose metabolism have been found. DM, hypertriglyceridemia, and atherosclerosis occur more frequently in female patients. The hypertriglyceridemia may result in pancreatitis and fatty liver, but cirrhosis has not been reported. The genetic defect in the Dunnigan variant of partial lipodystrophy is in the gene encoding lamins A and C (*LMNA*). Lamins are intermediate filaments integral to the nuclear envelope. The site of the mutation determines the phenotype expressed. Myopathy, muscular dystrophy, cardiomyopathy, and conducting system disturbances can occur in a minority of patients.

A second characterized form of familial partial lipodystrophy is related to mutations in the *PPAR*-γ gene. This rare syndrome is associated with marked loss of subcutaneous tissue of the forearms and calves, and less prominently on the upper arms and thighs.

The trunk is spared, and there is no excess fat on the neck. DM, hypertriglyceridemia, hypertension, and hirsutism also occur. Other forms of familial partial lipodystrophy not associated with the previous two mutations have been described, suggesting additional genetic causes of this syndrome.

Mandibuloacral dysplasia is an extremely rare autosomal recessive condition with hypoplasia of the mandible and clavicle, acro-osteolysis, joint contractures, mottled cutaneous pigmentation, skin atrophy, alopecia, a birdlike facies, and dental anomalies. Two distinct patterns of lipodystrophy occur. Type A is characterized by loss of subcutaneous fat from the arms and legs, but normal to excess fat of the face and neck. Hyperinsulinemia, insulin resistance, DM, and hyperlipidemia occur in some patients. Mutations in the *LMNA* gene have been reported in type A patients. Mutations in the zinc metalloproteinase *(ZMPSTE24)*, which is involved in the processing of prelamin A, have also been responsible for mandibuloacral dysplasia. Other gene mutations responsible for rarer types include those of *AKT2*, *CIDEC*, and perilipin. Autosomal recessive neonatal progeroid syndrome is characterized by near-total absence of fat from birth, with sparing of the sacral and gluteal areas.

ACQUIRED LIPODYSTROPHY

Most cases of acquired lipodystrophy are related to antiretroviral therapy, and the severity may be related to genetic variations in resistin. Lipodystrophy occurs in up to 80% of HIV-infected patients, most of whom are being treated with combination anti-HIV therapy (HAART). The fat of the face (especially buccal fat pads), buttocks, and limbs is lost. There is increased fat deposition in other areas, especially the neck, upper back (buffalo hump), and intraabdominally. It is related to nonnucleoside reverse transcriptase inhibitors, which also inhibit the γ-DNA polymerase of mitochondria, leading to adipocyte apoptosis. There are elevated levels of FGF21 in HIV patients with lipodystrophy, but it is more elevated in those treated with HAART and this may explain the metabolic abnormalities. As with the other acquired and inherited forms of lipodystrophy, patients may have hypertriglyceridemia, hypercholesterolemia, and insulin resistance, especially if a protease inhibitor is a part of their treatment. Metformin or thiazolidinediones combined with exercise can reduce insulin resistance and waist circumference. Antiretroviral-associated lipoatrophy slowly improves with prolonged rosiglitazone. Growth hormone reduces visceral fat, but the effects are short lived, unlike with the growth hormone–releasing factor analog tesamorelin, which has long-term benefit. Various injectable agents may provide cosmetic improvement.

Acquired lipodystrophy has several idiopathic forms, and it can be partial or generalized. In addition, hyperinsulinemia, hyperlipidemia, and DM may occur in patients with acquired lipodystrophy. Management involves controlling the hyperinsulinemia and its complications.

Acquired Partial Lipodystrophy (Barraquer-Simons Syndrome)

Until HAART-associated lipodystrophy appeared, the acquired partial type was the most common form of lipodystrophy. Affected females outnumber males 4:1. The syndrome presents in the first and second decades of life. This progressive fat disorder is characterized by a diffuse and progressive loss of the subcutaneous fat that usually begins in the face and scalp, progressing downward as far as the iliac crests but sparing the lower extremities. The upper half of the body looks emaciated, and the patient has sunken cheeks (Fig. 23.9A). There is an apparent, and sometimes real, adiposity of the buttocks, thighs, and legs, especially in affected women (Fig. 23.9B). The onset is insidious, with no discomfort or inflammation in the areas of fat loss. A few patients have developed other autoimmune diseases, including systemic lupus erythematosus and juvenile dermatomyositis.

Histologically, the skin is normal except for the absence of fat. Most patients with acquired partial lipodystrophy have reduced levels of C3 resulting from a circulating polyclonal IgG called "C3 nephritic factor." Proteinuria caused by membranoproliferative glomerulonephritis occurs in about 20% of patients, appearing about 8 years after the onset of the lipodystrophy. C3 nephritic

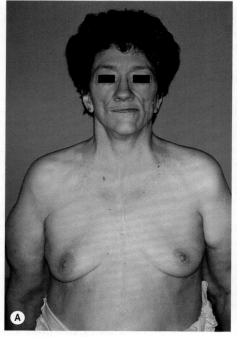
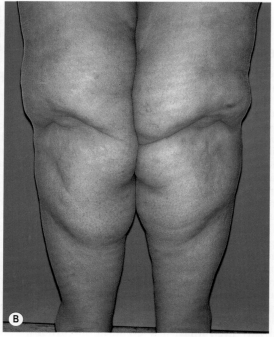

Fig. 23.9 Partial lipodystrophy, acquired. (A) Face. (B) Hypertrophy of subcutaneous fat on lower half of the body.

factor stabilizes C3b,Bb (C3 convertase), leading to unopposed activation of the alternative complement system and excessive consumption of C3.

Acquired Generalized Lipodystrophy

This rare form of lipodystrophy appears during childhood or adolescence. Females with acquired generalized lipodystrophy outnumber males 3 : 1. The fat loss affects large areas of the body, particularly the face, arms, and legs. Mechanical fat of the palms and soles may be lost, but ocular and bone marrow fat are spared. Acanthosis nigricans is present. Hepatic steatosis and voracious appetite may be present. Cirrhosis occurs in about 20% of patients due to hepatitic steatosis or autoimmune hepatitis. DM and hypertriglyceridemia may occur.

About 25% of patients will have a preceding inflammatory panniculitis at the onset of the syndrome. These patients tend to have less severe manifestations. Another 25% of patients with acquired generalized lipodystrophy have an associated connective tissue disease, especially juvenile dermatomyositis. Half the patients give no history of panniculitis and have no connective tissue disease. Other associations include graft-versus-host disease, lymphoma, and glucocorticoid administration.

CENTRIFUGAL ABDOMINAL LIPODYSTROPHY

Most cases of "lipodystrophia centrifugalis abdominalis infantilis," as described by Imamura et al., have been reported nearly exclusively from a single region of Japan. The cause is unknown. It is almost invariably a disease of childhood; 90% of cases begin at age 3. Girls outnumber boys 2 : 1. It is characterized by depression of the skin caused by loss of fat in the groin (80% of patients) or axilla (20%). The atrophic area slowly enlarges centrifugally for 3–8 years in most patients, often stopping with the onset of puberty. In 80% the depressed area was surrounded by a discrete, erythematous border with scale. One third of patients have multiple lesions, and regional lymph nodes are enlarged in 65%. The affected children are otherwise well. When the lesion stops expanding, the erythematous rim and lymphadenopathy disappear. After the progression stops, the skin returns to normal within 1 or 2 years.

LIPOATROPHIA ANNULARIS (FERREIRA-MARQUES SYNDROME)

Lipoatrophia annularis primarily affects women and usually involves the upper extremity. The lipoatrophy may be preceded by erythema, a bracelet-shaped swelling, and tenderness of the entire extremity. This is followed by loss of subcutaneous fat, with the arm divided into two parts by a depressed, atrophic, bracelet-like constriction. The depressed band is usually about 1 cm wide and up to 2 cm in depth. Arthralgias and pain of the affected extremity precede and accompany the process. The band persists for up to 20 years. The histology shows atrophy of the subcutaneous fat. The cause is unknown.

LOCALIZED LIPODYSTROPHY

A few months after subcutaneous injections, localized atrophy of fat may develop. Many different medications have been implicated, including insulin (more commonly nonhumanized), antibiotics, and vaccinations, and the reports are more frequent in children and women than in men. Acupuncture has also been associated. Localized lipodystrophy may also be a manifestation of connective tissue disease. Pegvisomant and insulin have also been associated with lipohypertrophy.

Benedini S, et al: Lipodystrophy HIV-related and FGF21. J Transl Int Med 2016; 4: 150.

Brown RJ, et al: Lymphoma in acquired generalized lipodystrophy. Leuk Lymphoma 2016; 57: 45.

Chan JL, et al: Clinical classification and treatment of congenital and acquired lipodystrophy. Endocr Pract 2010; 16: 310.

De Waal R, et al: Systematic review of antiretroviral-associated lipodystrophy. PLoS One 2013; 8: e63623.

Eren E, et al: Acquired generalized lipodystrophy associated with autoimmune hepatitis and low serum C4 level. J Clin Res Pediatr Endocrinol 2010; 2: 39.

Florenza CG, et al: Lipodystrophy. Nat Rev 2011; 7: 137.

Hussain I, Garg A: Lipodystrophy syndromes. Endocrinol Metab Clin North Am 2016; 45: 783.

Imamura S, et al: Lipodystrophia centrifugalis abdominalis infantilis. Archives of dermatology 1971; 104(3):29–18.

Kerns MJ, et al: Annular lipoatrophy of the ankles. Pediatr Derm 2011; 28: 142.

Oliveira J, et al: Barraquer-Simons syndrome. BMC Res Notes 2016; 9: 175.

Park SM, et al: Adverse events associated with acupuncture. Int J Dermatol 2016; 55: 757.

Rahul SK: Localized lipoatrophy following DPT injection. JCR 2016; 6: 132.

Sarpa HG, et al: Lipodystrophia centrifugalis abdominalis infantilis in a Caucasian girl. J Cutan Pathol 2008; 35: 971.

Shuck J, et al: Autologous fat grafting and injectable dermal fillers for human immunodeficiency virus–associated facial lipodystrophy. Plast Reconstr Surg 2013; 131: 499.

Tsoukas MA, et al: Leptin in congenital and HIV-associated lipodystrophy. Metabolism 2015; 64: 47.

Valerio CM, et al: Dipeptidyl peptidase-4 levels are increased and partially related to body fat distribution in patients with familial partial lipodystrophy type 2. Diabetol Metab Syndr 2017; 9: 26.

Vantyghem MC, et al: How to diagnose a lipodystrophy syndrome. Ann Endocrinol (Paris) 2012; 73: 170.

Vázquez-Osorio I, et al: Localized lipoatrophy in a boy after an intramuscular injection of penicillin. Actas Dermosifiliogr 2016; 107: 620.

The skin interacts with the endocrine system in many ways. Some of these are discussed in this chapter.

Leventhal JS, et al: Skin manifestations of endocrine and neuroendocrine tumors. Semin Oncol 2016; 43: 335.
Quatrano NA, et al: Dermatologic manifestations of endocrine disorders. Curr Opin Pediatr 2012; 24: 487.

ACROMEGALY

Excess growth hormone (GH) in prepubertal children leads to gigantism, whereas once the epiphyseal growth plates close, such excess leads to acromegaly. In acromegaly, changes in the soft tissues and bones form a characteristic syndrome. In association with the well-known changes in the facial features caused by gigantic hypertrophy of the chin, nose, and supraorbital ridges, there is thickening, reddening, and wrinkling of the forehead and exaggeration of the nasolabial grooves. The lips and tongue are thick. Cutis verticis gyrata is present in approximately 30% of patients. The hands and feet enlarge (Fig. 24.1), and there is gradual growth of the fingertips until they resemble drumsticks. There is diffuse hypertrophy of the skin, which is at least partly caused by deposition of colloidal iron-positive material in the papillae and reticular dermis. This increased skin thickness can be demonstrated in lateral radiographs of the heel, with reversal toward normal after treatment. Skin thickness does not correlate well with GH levels at the time of diagnosis. Skin tags are often present and the skin has an oily feel. Hypertrichosis, hyperpigmentation, and hyperhidrosis occur in many patients. The viscera also enlarge and patients may develop a variety of rheumatologic, cardiovascular, metabolic, and respiratory complications.

The clinical changes may suggest the leonine facies of Hansen disease, as well as Paget disease, myxedema, and pachydermoperiostosis. Acromegaloid facial appearance syndrome is an inherited condition in which only the facial changes are present, and no abnormality of GH exists. Pseudoacromegaly is an acquired condition that may be seen in patients with severe insulin-resistant diabetes, which appears to be a fibroblast defect, in patients receiving long-term minoxidil.

The cause of 98% of acromegaly is hypersecretion of GH by a pituitary adenoma. Rare cases of ectopic GH-releasing hormone (GHRH) producing tumors of the lung and pancreas have been reported. The peak age of diagnosis is in the forties. Measurement of serum insulin-like growth factor (IGF, somatomedin C), measurement of serum GH after a glucose load, and magnetic resonance imaging (MRI) of the pituitary are diagnostic tests. It may occur as one of the manifestations of Carney complex, McCune-Albright syndrome, or multiple endocrine neoplasia (MEN) type I.

The currently preferred treatment is a transsphenoidal microsurgical excision of the tumor. Medical therapy may be used as a primary treatment for those unsuitable for surgery, as a preoperative treatment, or as secondary therapy after failed surgery. Octreotide and lanreotide are potent, long-acting inhibitors of GH (somatostatin analogs) that are given as once-monthly or biweekly intramuscular (IM) depot injections. Fatigue, paresthesias, and headaches improve rapidly. With continuous treatment, soft tissue swelling and facial coarsening improve as GH levels decline in almost all patients. After 18–24 months of therapy, 50% of patients will completely normalize, with the exception of hyperhidrosis, which persists in most patients. The dopamine agonists bromocriptine and cabergoline suppress GH secretion and are used as an adjuvant medical therapy in some cases. The GH receptor antagonist pegvisomant is another medical option to normalize GH secretion. Radiation is generally reserved for recalcitrant cases.

Akoglu G, et al: Cutaneous findings in patients with acromegaly. Acta Dermatovenereol Croat 2013; 21: 224.
Borson-Chazot F, et al: Acromegaly induced by ectopic secretion of GHRH. Ann Endocrinol 2012; 73: 497.
Chakraborty PP, et al: Pseudoacromegaly in congenital generalized lipodystrophy (Berardinelli-Seip syndrome). BMJ Case Rep 2016 Apr 11; 2016.
Davidovici BB, et al: Cutaneous manifestations of pituitary gland diseases. Clin Dermatol 2008; 26: 288.
Ghazi A, et al: Acromegaloid facial appearance. Case Rep Endocrinol 2013; 2013: 970396.
Jallad RS, et al: The place of medical treatment of acromegaly. Expert Opin Pharmacother 2013; 14: 1001.
Ribeiro-Oliveira A, et al: The changing face of acromegaly: advances in diagnosis and treatment. Nat Rev 2012; 8: 605.

CUSHING SYNDROME

Chronic excess of glucocorticoids leads to a wide variety of signs and symptoms. The most prominent features of Cushing syndrome include central obesity, affecting the face, neck, trunk, and especially the abdomen, but sparing the limbs. There is classically deposition of fat over the upper back, referred to as a buffalo hump. This may be treated with liposuction. The face becomes moon shaped, being wide and round. The peak age of onset is in the twenties and thirties.

The striking and distressing skin changes include hypertrichosis, dryness, acne, susceptibility to superficial dermatophyte and *Pityrosporon* infections, a plethora over the cheeks, anterior neck, and V of the chest, and the characteristic purplish, atrophic striae that may involve the abdomen (Fig. 24.2), buttocks, back, breasts, upper arms, and thighs. Skin fragility and thinning occur such that easy bruising and a cigarette paper–type wrinkling are present. The skin may easily pull off when adhesive tape is removed (Liddle sign). The thinning of the skin can be demonstrated and measured in lateral radiographs of the heels. There is reversal with treatment. Women, who are affected four times more frequently than men in noniatrogenic cases, develop facial lanugo hypertrichosis, with thinning of the scalp hair. Occasionally, there may be livedo reticularis, purpura, ecchymosis, or brownish pigmentation. Poikiloderma-like changes have been observed. Opportunistic fungal infections occur, either with organisms that are not normally pathogenic or as uncommon presentations of common infections.

Patients with Cushing syndrome usually have hypertension and marked generalized arteriosclerosis, with progressive weakness, prostration, and pains in the back, limbs, and abdomen; kyphosis of the dorsal spine also occurs, accentuating the buffalo hump appearance. Osteoporosis occurs, and there is generally a loss of libido. In 20% of patients, a disturbance in carbohydrate metabolism develops, with hyperglycemia, glycosuria, and diabetes mellitus.

These varied symptoms indicate a marked and widespread disturbance caused by the hyperactive adrenal cortex. When microadenomas of the pituitary gland produce these clinical findings, it is referred to as Cushing disease; this accounts for only 10% of patients. Between 40% and 60% of additional cases are caused by increased adrenocorticotropic hormone (ACTH, corticotropin) production by the pituitary, but no adenoma is identified. Adrenal adenomas and carcinomas, with ectopic production of ACTH by other tumors, account for the remainder of cases of noniatrogenic Cushing syndrome. Iatrogenic Cushing syndrome is usually secondary to systemic administration of corticosteroids; however, absorption from topical corticosteroids to the skin, nasal mucosa, the conjunctiva, or the gingiva may occur, especially in children. Primary pigmented nodular adrenocortical disease leading to Cushing syndrome occurs in 30% of patients with Carney complex. It is a rare feature of McCune-Albright and MEN type I syndrome. With alcohol abuse, the clinical findings of Cushing syndrome may be mimicked, producing the pseudo–Cushing syndrome.

A rapid screening test for Cushing syndrome consists of oral administration of 1 mg of dexamethasone at 11 PM, followed at 8 AM by a fluorometric determination of plasma cortisol. A cortisol level below 50 nmol/L essentially rules out Cushing syndrome, except for the iatrogenic variety, in which there is adrenocortical hypoplasia, and the serum cortisol level is very low, even without dexamethasone suppression. If this test is positive, it must be confirmed by doing a 24-hour urinary free cortisol test. A value of at least three times the upper limit of normal is 95%–100% sensitive and specific. A serum ACTH is then obtained to determine whether the source is the adrenal glands or whether it is a pituitary tumor or an ectopic tumor (low, normal or high, and very high, respectively). Treatment is primarily surgical removal of the tumor; however, radiation, chemotherapy, or medication that blocks steroid synthesis is occasionally used.

Al Ojaimi EH: Cushing's syndrome due to an ACTH-producing primary ovarian carcinoma. Hormones (Athens) 2014; 13: 140.
Brown RJ, et al: Cushing syndrome in the McCune-Albright syndrome. J Clin Endocrinol Metab 2010; 95: 1508.
Ceccato F, Boscaro M: Cushing's syndrome. High Blood Press Cardiovasc Prev 2016; 23: 209.
Davidovici BB, et al: Cutaneous manifestations of pituitary gland diseases. Clin Dermatol 2008; 26: 288.
Fukuhara D, et al: Iatrogenic Cushing's syndrome due to topical ocular glucocorticoid treatment. Pediatric 2017; 139: e20161233.
Pichardo-Lowden A, et al: Cushing syndrome related to gingival application of a dexamethasone-containing preparation. Endocr Pract 2010; 16: 336.
Pluta RM, et al: Cushing syndrome and Cushing disease. JAMA 2011; 306: 2742.
Sattar H, et al: Iatrogenic Cushing's syndrome in children presenting at Children's Hospital Lahore using nappy rash ointments. J Pak Med Assoc 2015; 65: 463.
Sikorska D, et al: Bilateral primary pigmented nodular adrenal disease as a component of Carney syndrome—case report. Endokrynol Pol 2017; 68: 70.

ADDISON DISEASE

Adrenal insufficiency is manifested in the skin primarily by hyperpigmentation (Fig. 24.3). It is diffuse but most prominently observed in sun-exposed areas and sites exposed to recurrent trauma or pressure. The axillae, perineum, and nipples are also affected. Palmar crease darkening in patients of lighter skin type, scar hyperpigmentation, and darkening of nevi, mucous membranes, hair, and nails may all be seen. Multifocal oral melanoacanthoma, a reactive mucosal hyperpigmentation, may occur. An eruptive onset of multiple new nevi may be an early sign of Addison disease. Occasionally, pigmentation may not occur; this is referred to as white Addison disease. Decreased axillary and pubic hair is seen in women, because their androgen production primarily occurs

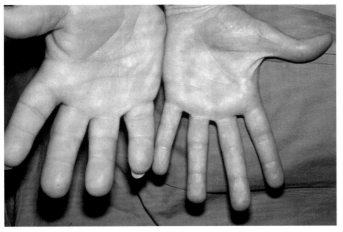

Fig. 24.1 Acromegalic hand compared with normal.

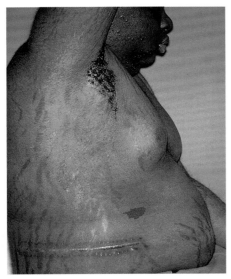

Fig. 24.2 Cushing syndrome.

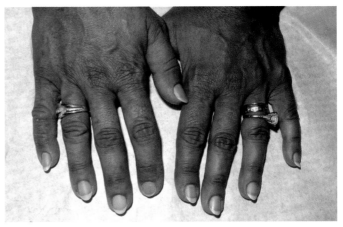

Fig. 24.3 Hyperpigmentation in Addison disease. (Courtesy Steven Binnick, MD.)

in the adrenals. Fibrosis and calcification of the pinnae of the ears are rare complications.

Systemic signs such as weight loss, nausea, vomiting, diarrhea, weakness, fatigue, and hypotension add specificity to the cutaneous abnormalities. Addison disease is usually the result of autoantibody destruction of adrenocortical tissue; however, infection, hemorrhage, or infiltration may be the cause of adrenal insufficiency. In young boys suspected of having Addison disease, adrenoleukodystrophy, a peroxisomal disease, must be considered. Hyperpigmentation associated with adrenocortical insufficiency usually occurs in childhood, and precedes the adult onset of neurologic signs, so very-long-chain fatty acid levels should be determined and analysis for a mutation of the *ABCD1* gene done. Addison disease may be part of polyglandular autoimmune syndrome types I, II, and IV, in which various combinations of hypoparathyroidism, chronic candidiasis, vitiligo or autoimmune thyroiditis, and diabetes may occur.

Diagnosis of Addison disease is made by obtaining a paired serum cortisol and plasma ACTH, followed by stimulation with cosyntropin. Failure to see an elevation above 550 nmol/L in 1 hour is diagnostic. Plasma ACTH is elevated in primary insufficiency but normal to low in patients with secondary adrenal insufficiency, in whom the damage is in the hypothalamic-pituitary axis. The adrenals should be imaged with computed tomography (CT) to exclude infiltration or infection.

Treatment of Addison disease is replacement of the glucocorticoids and mineralocorticoids.

Cutolo M: Autoimmune polyendocrine syndromes. Autoimmun Rev 2014; 13: 85.

Dantas TS, et al: Multifocal oral melanoacanthoma associated with Addison's disease and hyperthyroidism. Arch Endocrinol Metab 2017; 61: 403.

Engelen M, et al: X-linked adrenoleukodystrophy. Curr Neurol Neurosci Rep 2014; 14: 486.

Husebye ES, et al: Consensus statement on the diagnosis, treatment and follow-up of patients with primary adrenal insufficiency. J Intern Med 2014; 275: 104.

Koelemji I, et al: Eruptive melanocytic naevi as a sign of primary adrenocortical insufficiency. Clin Exp Dermatol 2013; 38: 927.

Prat C, et al: Longitudinal melanonychia as the first sign of Addison's disease. J Am Acad Dermatol 2008; 58: 522.

COMBINED PITUITARY HORMONE DEFICIENCY AND GROWTH HORMONE DEFICIENCY

Pituitary failure results in many changes in the skin, hair, and nails because of the absence of pituitary hormone action on these sites. Pale, thin, dry skin is seen. Hypohidrosis is present. Diffuse loss of body hair occurs, with axillary, pubic, and head hair being especially thin. The nails are thin, fragile, and opaque and grow slowly. Compromise of the pituitary gland is usually caused by a pituitary tumor, although infiltration, autoimmunity and other inflammatory processes, infection, genetic mutations, trauma, radiation, hemorrhage, or hypothalamic tumors may be the etiology. Isolated GH deficiency is the most common sporadic form of hypopituitarism; however, thyroid hormone, glucocorticoids, and sex steroids may be low and require replacement in combined pituitary hormone deficiency (or panhypopituitarism). A pituitary MRI will screen for tumors or infiltrative processes. Mutations in a large number of genes encoding transcription factors and specific autoantibodies such as anti-pit-1 may also be responsible.

Castinetti F, et al: Combined pituitary hormone deficiency. J Endocrinol Invest 2015; 38: 1.

Davidovici BB, et al: Cutaneous manifestations of pituitary gland diseases. Clin Dermatol 2008; 26: 288.

Di Iorgi N, et al: Classical and non-classical causes of GH deficiency in the paediatric age. Best Pract Res Clin Endocrinol Metab 2016; 30: 705.

ANDROGEN-DEPENDENT SYNDROMES

The androgen-dependent syndromes are caused by the excessive production of adrenal or gonadal androgens by adrenal adenomas, carcinoma, or hyperplasia, Leydig cell tumors in men, and arrhenoblastomas and polycystic ovarian syndrome (PCOS) in women.

PCOS is defined as the association of polycystic ovaries with biochemical (the best screening laboratory test is free testosterone) or clinical signs of hyperandrogenism and chronic anovulation (less than nine periods per year), without specific underlying disease of the adrenal or pituitary glands. The cutaneous signs of excessive androgen in women include acne, hirsutism, and androgen-induced patterned scalp hair loss. Hyperpigmentation of the skin, areolae, genitalia, palmar creases, and buccal mucosa develops in some patients. Acanthosis nigricans is common in PCOS, reflecting insulin resistance. Women who meet the criteria of PCOS have more severe truncal hirsutism and axillary acanthosis nigricans. Diabetes mellitus, cardiovascular complications, and sleep apnea are associated comorbidities of PCOS. In patients who are obese, weight loss is a prime target of therapy to prevent morbidity and mortality from the associated metabolic syndrome. An association of endometrial cancer is suggested but remains unproven.

In the congenital adrenogenital syndrome (Fig. 24.4), excess androgen is produced by an inherited defect in any of the five enzymatic steps required to convert cholesterol to cortisol. The formation of inadequate amounts of cortisol stimulates the pituitary to secrete excessive ACTH, which leads to excess androgen production. In boys, precocious puberty results. In girls, masculinization occurs, with the prominent cutaneous signs of excess androgen production. These signs may include acne. Acne with onset between ages 1 and 7 with physical findings suggestive of a hormonal disorder, such as sexual precocity, virilization, and growth abnormalities, should be referred to a pediatric endocrinologist. Acne that begins from ages 7 to 12 often manifests primarily as comedonal lesions in the central face. Unless there are other signs of androgen excess, these patients do not need a workup. Accelerated bone growth with early closure of the epiphyseal plates results in short stature. Early appearance of pubic and axillary hair is also seen.

Testing includes serum total testosterone and dehydroepiandrosterone sulfate (DHEA-S) levels. If the total testosterone concentration is greater than 200 ng/dL, ovarian imaging is indicated to assess for an ovarian tumor. If the DHEA-S level is

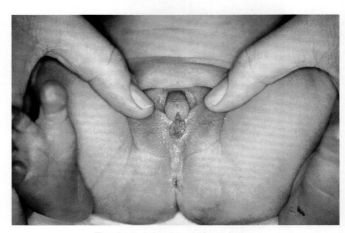

Fig. 24.4 Adrenogenital syndrome.

two to three times the upper limit, an adrenal mass should be suspected, and CT scan of the adrenals is required. Tumors causing such elevations in serum androgens often cause more dramatic masculinization with clinical findings such as a deepening voice, increased muscle mass, enlargement of the clitoris, decreased breast size, galactorrhea, and absent periods. In congenital adrenal hyperplasia, testing should include levels of cortisol, aldosterone, and precursor hormones, and in some patients, cosyntropin (Cortrosyn) stimulation tests. Nonclassic adrenal hyperplasia is most often related to 21-hydroxylase deficiency and may present as PCOS. It is best diagnosed by a corticotropin-stimulated 17-hydroxyprogesterone (17-HP) level greater than 10 ng/mL (30.3 nmol/L). The diagnosis can be confirmed by genotyping of the *CYP21* gene. The question remains whether treatment with corticosteroid replacement results in better outcomes than empiric antiandrogen therapy.

Treatment of the cutaneous signs of androgen excess is successful with an oral contraceptive and often also an androgen-blocking agent such as cyproterone acetate, flutamide, or finasteride. Spironolactone, which competes for the androgen cytosol receptors, has proved useful as a systemic antiandrogen in the treatment of hirsutism and acne. Laser hair removal and standard acne therapy are also effective. Adrenal-androgenic female pattern alopecia may improve with topical minoxidil or spironolactone. Metformin is frequently used to improve insulin responsiveness. Chorionic villous biopsy may identify homozygous adrenogenital female fetuses and allow for dexamethasone therapy to prevent intrauterine virilization of the external genitalia.

Auchus RJ, et al: Approach to the patient: the adult with congenital adrenal hyperplasia. J Clin Endocrinol Metab 2013; 98: 2645.

Goodman NF, et al: Guide to the best practice in the evaluation and treatment of polycystic ovary syndrome—part 1. Endocr Pract 2015; 21: 1291.

Goodman NF, et al: Guide to the best practice in the evaluation and treatment of polycystic ovary syndrome—part 2. Endocr Pract 2015; 21: 1415.

Heidelbaugh JJ: Endocrinology update: hirsutism. FP Essent 2016; 451: 17.

Housman E, Reynolds RV: Polycystic ovary syndrome. J Am Acad Dermatol 2014; 71: 847.e1.

Schmidt TH, et al: Cutaneous findings and systemic associations in women with polycystic ovary syndrome. JAMA Dermatol 2016; 152: 391.

Schmidt TH, et al: Rotterdam criteria-based diagnostic subtype is not a strong predictor of cutaneous phenotype in patients with polycystic ovary syndrome. J Am Acad Dermatol 2017; 77: 174.

Setji TL, et al: Polycystic ovary syndrome. Am J Med 2014; 127: 912.

Voutilainen R, Jääskeläinen J: Premature adrenarche. J Steroid Biochem Mol Biol 2015, 145: 226.

HYPOTHYROIDISM

Hypothyroidism is a deficiency of circulating thyroid hormone, or rarely, peripheral resistance to hormonal action. Deficiency may be caused by iodine deficiency, late-stage Hashimoto autoimmune thyroiditis, or pituitary or hypothalamic disease causing central hypothyroidism, or it may be iatrogenic secondary to surgery, radioactive iodine treatment, or drug therapy with lithium, interferon, multikinase inhibitors, ipilimumab alone or particularly if given in combination with nivolumab, valproic acid, or bexarotene. It may also complicate anticonvulsant and minocycline hypersensitivity syndromes, appearing approximately 2 months after the eruption has resolved. The endothelium in infantile hemangiomas may produce elevated type 3 iodothyronine deiodinase, leading to consumptive hypothyroidism. Hypothyroidism produces various clinical manifestations, depending on the age when it occurs and on its severity. Middle-aged women are the adults most often affected. Patients with Turner and Down syndrome are predisposed to hypothyroidism and the production of thyroid autoantibodies. A wide array of immunologic conditions are associated with Hashimoto thyroiditis, including polyglandular autoimmune syndrome types II and III, vitiligo, connective tissue disease, and autoimmune urticaria.

An autosomal recessive variant of ectodermal dysplasia has been described as ANOTHER syndrome: alopecia, nail dystrophy, ophthalmic complications, thyroid dysfunction, hypohidrosis, ephelides and enteropathy, and respiratory tract infections. Other associations with hypothyroidism include lichen planopilaris and cutaneous sarcoidosis.

Congenital Hypothyroidism

Thyroid deficiency in fetal life produces the characteristic picture of cretinism at birth and in the next few months of life. Various mutations in the thyroglobulin gene, the thyroid peroxidase gene, and the thyroid-stimulating hormone (TSH) receptor may be causative. True absence of the gland may occur, as was documented in a patient with PHACE syndrome. Depending on the degree of thyroid deficiency, a wide variety of signs and symptoms may be evident. The main consequence of extreme thyroid deficiency is cretinism and its attendant mental retardation, but much more prevalent are lesser degrees of intellectual and neurologic deficits seen in areas of the world where iodized salt is still not routinely available.

The person with cretinism has cool, dry, pasty-white to yellowish skin. Disturbances in the amount, texture, and distribution of the hair with patchy alopecia are common. Pigmentation is less than normal after exposure to sunlight. Sweating is greatly diminished. The lips are pale, thick, and protuberant. The tongue is usually enlarged, and there is delayed dentition. Wide-set eyes, a broad, flat nose, and periorbital puffiness characterize the face. A protuberant abdomen with umbilical hernia; acral swelling; coarse, dry, brittle nails; a clavicular fat pad; and hypothermia with cutis marmorata are also seen. Mandatory screening programs for congenital hypothyroidism (as in the United States) has led to dramatically improved cognitive outcomes.

Myxedema

When lack of secretion of thyroid hormone is severe, myxedema is produced. The skin becomes rough and dry, and in severe cases of primary myxedema, ichthyosis vulgaris may be simulated. The facial skin is puffy; the expression is often dull and flat; macroglossia, swollen lips, and a broad nose are present; and chronic periorbital infiltration secondary to deposits of mucopolysaccharides frequently develops (Fig. 24.5A). Such infiltrate can lead to a cutis verticis gyrata appearance of the scalp. Carotenemia may cause a yellow tint in the skin that is especially prominent on the palms and soles. Diffuse hair loss is common, and the outer third of the eyebrows is shed (Fig. 24.5B). The hair becomes coarse and brittle. The free edges of the nails break easily, and onycholysis may occur.

Mild Hypothyroidism

Lesser degrees of thyroid deficiency are common and much less easily diagnosed. Coldness of hands and feet in the absence of vascular disease, sensitivity to cool weather, lack of sweating, tendency to put on weight, need for extra sleep, drowsiness in the daytime, and constipation all suggest possible hypothyroidism and the need for appropriate tests. Palmoplantar keratoderma may be a sign of hypothyroidism and will resolve after thyroid hormone replacement is given.

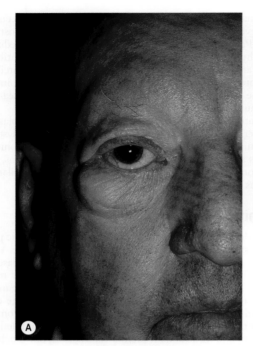
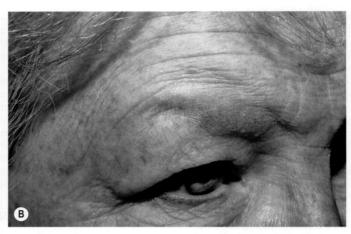

Fig. 24.5 (A) Periorbital infiltration with mucopolysaccharides. (B) Loss of lateral eyebrow.

Diagnosis and Treatment

An elevated TSH is the best diagnostic test for primary hypothyroidism. Triiodothyronine (T₃) and thyroxine (T₄) are low. In Hashimoto thyroiditis, the most common cause of hypothyroidism in the United States, thyroid peroxidase antibodies are present in 95% of patients and antithyroglobulin antibodies in 65%. In those with positive antibodies but normal thyroid function, hypothyroidism will develop at a rate of 5% per year. Thyroid hormone replacement will reverse the skin findings of hypothyroidism.

Abduljabbar MA, et al: Congenital hypothyroidism. J Pediatr Endocrinol Metab 2012; 25: 13.

Almandoz JP, et al: Hypothyroidism. Med Clin North Am 2012; 96: 203.

Anolik RB, et al: Thyroid dysfunction and cutaneous sarcoidosis. J Am Acad Dermatol 2012; 66: 167.

Bouras M, et al: Palmoplantar keratoderma. Ann Dermatol Venereol 2014; 141: 39.

Brown RJ, et al: Minocycline-induced drug hypersensitivity syndrome followed by multiple autoimmune sequelae. Arch Dermatol 2009; 145: 63.

Funakoshi T, et al: Risk of hypothyroidism in patients with cancer treated with sunitinib. Acta Oncol 2013; 52: 691.

Mamlouk MD, et al: PHACE syndrome and congenitally absent thyroid gland at MR imaging. Clin Imaging 2016; 40: 237.

Mesinkovska NA, et al: Association of lichen planopilaris with thyroid disease. A retrospective case-control study J Am Acad Dermatol. 2014; 70: 889.

Persani L, et al: Clinical review: central hypothyroidism. J Clin Endocrinol Metab 2012; 97: 3068.

Ryder M, et al: Endocrine-related adverse events following ipilimumab in patients with advanced melanoma. Endocr Relat Cancer 2014; 21: 371.

Van Vliet G, Deladoëy J: Diagnosis, treatment and outcome of congenital hypothyroidism. Endocr Dev 2014; 26: 50.

HYPERTHYROIDISM

Excessive quantities of circulating thyroid hormone may be caused by Graves thyroiditis (diffuse toxic goiter), a multinodular toxic goiter (Plummer disease), or a single, toxic thyroid nodule, early Hashimoto autoimmune thyroiditis, a TSH-secreting pituitary adenoma, pituitary resistance to thyroid hormone, metastatic thyroid cancer, or excessive human chorionic gonadotropin. The most common etiology is Graves disease, which accounts for about 55% of cases; it is mediated by thyroid-stimulating antibodies that bind to the TSH receptor, mimic the effects of TSH, and induce hyperthyroidism. Many skin changes are common to all forms of hyperthyroidism. The cutaneous surface is warm, moist, and smooth. Palmar erythema or facial flushing may be seen. The hair is thin and has a downy texture, and nonscarring diffuse alopecia may be observed. The skin may darken to produce a bronzed appearance or melanoderma; melasma of the cheeks is seen is some cases. Nail changes are present in approximately 5% of patients with Plummer nails, a concave contour of the plate with characteristic distal onycholysis. Hyperhidrosis may be noted.

Graves disease has a female/male ratio of 7:1, and the peak age of onset is 20–30 years. Ophthalmopathy, pretibial myxedema, and thyroid acropachy are findings almost always limited to patients with Graves disease (Fig. 24.6). Thyroid acropachy, seen in approximately 0.1%–1% of patients with Graves disease, is characterized by digital clubbing, soft tissue swelling of the hands and feet, and diaphyseal proliferation of the periosteum in acral and distal long bones (tibia, fibula, ulna, radius). It usually occurs after treatment of hyperthyroidism and is frequently associated with exophthalmos and pretibial myxedema. It may, however, occasionally precede the thyrotoxicosis and has been recognized in euthyroid and hypothyroid patients. It can be confused clinically with acromegaly, pachydermoperiostosis, pulmonary osteoarthropathy, or osteoperiostitis, but the radiologic findings are pathognomonic.

Pretibial myxedema, consisting of bilateral, localized, cutaneous accumulations of glycosaminoglycans, occurs in 4% of patients who have or have had Graves disease. The morphology may vary from a nonpitting infiltration to nodules, plaques, and even an

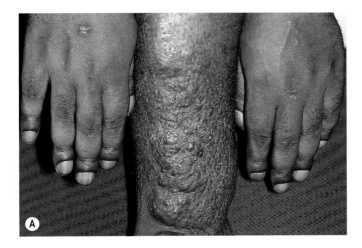

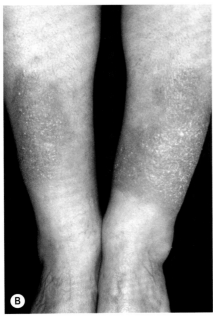

Fig. 24.6 (A) Thyroid acropachy and pretibial myxedema. (B) Pretibial myxedema.

Vitiligo is present in 7% of patients with Graves disease and occurs with an increased frequency in Hashimoto thyroiditis. Urticaria may be seen in patients with thyroid autoantibodies and may clear with the administration of thyroid hormone, even in euthyroid patients. A wide range of other autoimmune disorders may be seen in patients with Graves disease or Hashimoto autoimmune thyroiditis.

The TSH level is low in all patients except those with a TSH-secreting pituitary adenoma. Free T_3 and T_4 are elevated. Anti-TSH antibodies are present in almost all patients with Graves disease. A 24-hour radioiodine scan will also help define the etiology. Treatment is with radioactive iodine or antithyroid drugs such as methimazole or propylthiouracil.

Guerrero C, Pittelkow MR: Thyroid ophthalmopathy, dermopathy, and acropachy. N Engl J Med 2016; 21: 375.

Heymann W (ed): Thyroid Disorders with Cutaneous Manifestations. Heidelberg: Springer, 2008.

Ramos LO, et al: Pre-tibial myxedema. An Bras Dermatol 2015; 90: 143.

Shirai K, et al: Dramatic effect of low-dose oral steroid on elephantiasic pretibial myxedema. J Dermatol 2014; 41: 941.

Takasu N, et al: Treatment of pretibial myxedema (PTM) with topical steroid ointment application with sealing cover (steroid occlusive dressing technique). Intern Med 2010; 49: 665.

Yu H, et al: Elephantiasic pretibial myxedema in a patient with Graves disease that resolved after 131I treatment. Clin Nucl Med 2014; 39: 758.

HYPOPARATHYROIDISM

Varied changes in the skin and its appendages may be evident in parathyroid hormone (PTH, parathormone) deficiency. Most pronounced is faulty dentition when hypoparathyroidism is present during development of the permanent teeth. The skin is dry and scaly. A diffuse scantiness of the hair and complete absence of axillary and pubic hair may be found. The nails are brittle and malformed. Onycholysis with fungal infection may be present. Of patients with idiopathic hypoparathyroidism, 15% develop mucocutaneous candidiasis. Hypoparathyroidism is the most frequent endocrine abnormality present in patients with the APECED (autoimmune polyendocrinopathy, candidiasis, ectodermal dystrophy) syndrome. In this syndrome caused by mutations in the autoimmune regulator (*AIRE*) gene, hypoparathyroidism is present in association with Addison disease and chronic candidiasis. Hypoparathyroidism may also occur in DiGeorge syndrome, or with parathyroid infiltration or their inadvertent surgical removal during thyroid surgery. The causative genetic defects and specific autoantibodies responsible for PTH deficiency and pseudohypoparathyroidism are well defined. Hypoparathyroidism with resultant hypocalcemia may trigger bouts of impetigo herpetiformis or pustular psoriasis.

Pseudohypoparathyroidism (PH) is an autosomal dominant or X-linked inherited disorder characterized by end-organ unresponsiveness to PTH. The PTH and phosphorus levels are high, whereas the serum calcium is low. The typical clinical findings include short stature; obesity; round face; prominent forehead; low nasal bridge; attached earlobes; short neck; short, wide nails; delayed dentition; mental deficiency; amenorrhea; blue sclerae; and cataracts. Brachycephaly, microcephaly, and shortened metacarpals or metatarsals, especially of the fourth and fifth digits (Fig. 24.7), occur because of premature epiphyseal closure. This results in short, stubby fingers and toes, with dimpling over the metacarpophalangeal joints (Albright sign). Subcutaneous calcification and ossification occur frequently in PH, as they may in pseudopseudohypoparathyroidism (PPH), which has the same phenotype, but patients have normal serum and calcium levels. Mutations or epigenetic changes in the complex GNAS locus in the mother

elephantiasic form where the skin is thickened, firm, and hyperpigmented from just below the knees to the feet. It may also occur infrequently during the course of Hashimoto thyroiditis and primary hypothyroidism. Patients with pretibial myxedema regularly have associated ophthalmopathy and occasionally thyroid acropachy. Although usually not clinically apparent, approximately half of patients with Graves disease have mucopolysaccharide deposition in the preradial area of the extensor aspects of the forearms. Lesions of the shoulder, hands, thigh, and scalp have been reported.

Improvement in the plaques of pretibial myxedema has resulted from intralesional injections of triamcinolone acetonide and with high-potency topical corticosteroids under occlusion. Systemic corticosteroids may also be helpful. Compression stockings or complete decongestive physiotherapy, and a combination of manual lymphatic drainage, bandaging, and exercise, are useful and safe. With intravenous immune globulin (IVIG) administration, improvement of the skin, eye, and immunologic parameters has been reported in small series of patients. Pentoxifylline, octreotide, plasmapheresis, and cytotoxic drugs have all been reported to help in small numbers of patients, but negative reports also exist.

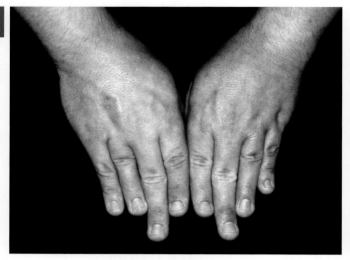

Fig. 24.7 Pseudohypoparathyroidism.

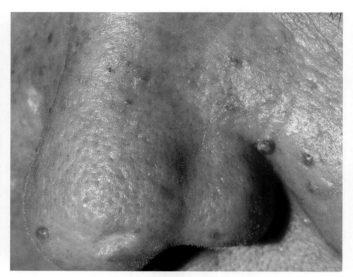

Fig. 24.8 Multiple endocrine neoplasia type 1 angiofibromas. (Courtesy Thomas Darling, MD, PhD.)

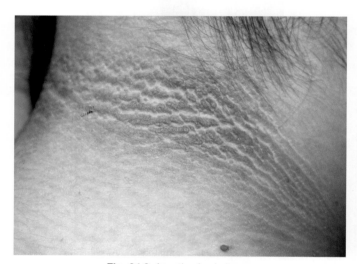

Fig. 24.9 Acanthosis nigricans.

result in PH, whereas if present in the father PPH results. PH and PPH are two types of Albright hereditary osteodystrophy.

Abate EG, Clarke BL: Review of hypoparathyroidism. Front Endocrinol (Lausanne) 2017; 7: 172.

De Martino L, et al: Novel findings into AIRE genetics and functioning. Front Pediatr 2016; 4: 86.

Tafaj O, Jüppner H: Pseudohypoparathyroidism. J Endocrinol Invest 2017; 40: 347.

HYPERPARATHYROIDISM

Whereas PTH regulates calcium levels, calcinosis cutis may develop from excess PTH. This can occur when the serum calcium/phosphorus product is greater than 65 mg/dL. This may manifest as large, subcutaneous nodules or white, often linearly arranged papules centered around joints. Additionally, calciphylaxis, although most common in the patient with secondary hyperparathyroidism and renal failure, may be seen occasionally in primary hyperparathyroidism.

Multiple endocrine neoplasia type I (MEN-1) is characterized by tumors of the parathyroid glands, endocrine pancreas, anterior pituitary, thyroid, and adrenal glands. The most frequently observed abnormality is hypercalcemia from hypersecreting tumors of the parathyroid glands. This autosomal dominant inherited disease usually presents in the fourth decade of life with clinical symptoms related to hypersecretion of hormones specific for the type of tumor present. Skin findings in MEN-1 include multiple angiofibromas (Fig. 24.8), collagenomas, café au lait macules, lipomas, confetti-like hypopigmentation, and gingival macules. The angiofibromas are smaller and less numerous than those present in tuberous sclerosis. MEN-1 is caused by *MENIN* mutations. MEN types 2A and 4 also may manifest parathyroid tumors. The latter is caused by mutations of *CDNK1B*.

Li Y, Simonds WF: Endocrine neoplasms in familial syndromes of hyperparathyroidism. Endocr Relat Cancer 2015; 23: R229.

Vidal A, et al: Cutaneous lesions associated to multiple endocrine neoplasia syndrome type 1. J Eur Acad Dermatol Venereol 2008; 22: 835.

ACANTHOSIS NIGRICANS

Acanthosis nigricans (AN) is characterized by hyperpigmentation and velvet-textured plaques, which are symmetrically distributed. The regions affected may be the face, neck (Fig. 24.9), axillae, external genitals, groin, inner aspects of the thighs, flexor and extensor surface of the elbows and knees, dorsal joints of the hands, umbilicus, nasal crease, and anus. With extensive involvement, lesions can be found on the areolae, conjunctivae, lips, and buccal mucosa, and around the umbilicus. Rarely, the involvement may be almost universal. The color of the patches is grayish, brownish, or black. The palms or soles may show thickening of the palmar or plantar skin with exaggeration of the dermatoglyphs. In severe cases, a rugose hypertrophy occurs and can be a sign of malignancy. Small, papillomatous, nonpigmented lesions and pigmented macules may occasionally be found in the mucous membranes of the mouth, pharynx, and vagina. Acrochordons are a frequent accompaniment in the axillae and groin. There is a clear predisposition for certain racial groups, independent of obesity, to manifest AN, with Native Americans most often affected, followed by African Americans and Hispanics, all above the rates in Caucasians.

Acanthosis nigricans can best be understood by grouping the associations in the following manner.

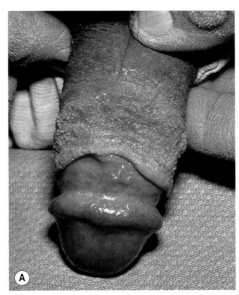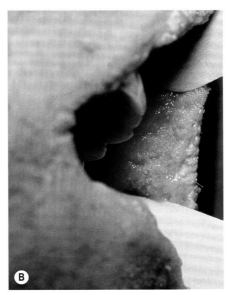

Fig. 24.10 (A and B) Extensive acanthosis nigricans in patient with stomach cancer.

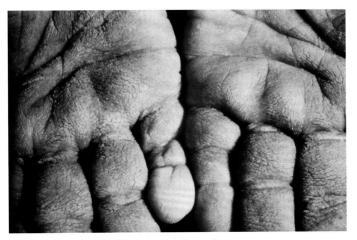

Fig. 24.11 Tripe palms.

Acanthosis Nigricans Associated With Malignancy

The rare type I AN may either precede (18%), accompany (60%), or follow (22%) the onset of the internal cancer. It is generally the most striking type clinically, from both the extent of involvement and the pronounced nature of the lesions (Fig. 24.10). Most cases are associated with adenocarcinoma, especially of the gastrointestinal tract (60% stomach), lung, and breast, or less often the gallbladder, pancreas, esophagus, liver, prostate, kidney, colon, rectum, uterus, and ovaries. Other types of cancer and lymphoma may be seen as well. A few cases have been observed in childhood, but most begin after puberty or in adulthood. Type I AN should be highly suspected if widespread lesions develop in a nonobese man over age 40.

Tripe palms (acanthosis palmaris) are characterized by thickened, velvety palms with pronounced dermatoglyphics; 95% occur in patients with cancer, and 77% are seen with AN (Fig. 24.11). In 40% of these patients, tripe palms are the presenting sign of an undiagnosed malignancy. If only the palms are involved, lung cancer is most common, whereas in tripe palms associated with AN, gastric cancer is most frequent.

Familial Acanthosis Nigricans and *Fgfr* Gene Mutation Syndromes

The exceedingly rare type II AN is present at birth or may develop during childhood. It is commonly accentuated at puberty. It is not associated with an internal cancer and is inherited in an autosomal dominant manner. Some patients will have a mutation in a fibroblast growth factor receptor gene, as also occurs in Cruzon and other syndromes with associated AN such as Beare-Stevenson cutis gyrata syndrome, severe achondroplasia with developmental delay and AN (SADDAN), and thanatophoric dysplasia.

Acanthosis Nigricans Associated With Insulin-Resistant States and Syndromes

This is the most common variety of AN. It presents as a grayish, velvety thickening of the skin of the sides of the neck, axillae, and groins. It occurs in obese persons with or without endocrine disorders. When AN accompanies obesity there is more severe hyperinsulinemia and hyperuricemia and lower serum testosterone in men than in obese patients without AN.

It also occurs in acromegaly and gigantism, pseudoacromegaly, PCOS, Cushing syndrome, diabetes mellitus, MORFAN syndrome (mental retardation, overgrowth, remarkable face, and AN), Addison disease, Prader-Willi syndrome, Alström syndrome, ataxia-telangiectasia, hyperandrogenic states, hypogonadal syndromes, and the various well-recognized insulin-resistant states. These states include lipoatrophic diabetes, leprechaunism, Rabson-Mendenhall syndrome, pineal hypertropic syndrome, and acral hypertrophy syndrome, as well as type A syndrome, with a defect in the *INSR* (insulin receptor) gene and postreceptor pathways, or a lamin A mutation, and type B syndrome, with the presence of autoantibodies to the insulin receptor. Whereas both type A and type B syndromes occur most often in black females, type A predominates in young children with hyperandrogenic manifestations. Many of the conditions associated with insulin resistance and AN manifest as hyperandrogenism and have been called the HAIR-AN syndrome. In one group of women with hirsutism, obesity, and hyperandrogenism, vulvar AN was present in all patients, with other sites less frequently involved. Type B syndrome is seen in middle-aged patients with autoimmune disease (Fig. 24.12). Most, if not all, patients with this type of AN may

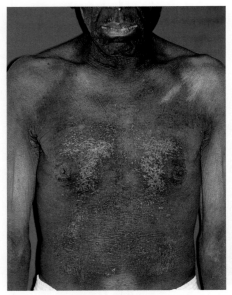

Fig. 24.12 Diffuse acanthosis nigricans in type B syndrome.

have either clinical or subclinical insulin resistance, and patients should have a glucose and insulin level drawn simultaneously. In adults a glucose-to-insulin ratio of less than 4.5 is abnormal, and in prepubertal children less than 7 is abnormal. Fasting glucose and lipoprotein profile, hemoglobin A1c, body weight, blood pressure, and an alanine transaminase (ALT) test for evaluation for fatty liver are other investigations that are useful in assessing patients with suspected insulin-resistant states.

Drug-Induced Acanthosis Nigricans

Drugs known to induce AN include nicotinic acid, niacinamide, somatotrophin, testosterone, triazinate, diethylstilbestrol, oral contraceptives, insulin, protease inhibitors, and glucocorticoids.

Miscellaneous Associations

Other syndromes and conditions not mentioned previously that may manifest AN include Bloom syndrome, Costello syndrome, Wilson disease, benign encephalopathy, Hirschowitz syndrome, Capozucca syndrome, Down syndrome, Hermansky-Pudlack syndrome, Kabuki syndrome, hypothyroidism, Rud syndrome, Lelis syndrome, and primary biliary cirrhosis. Approximately 10% of renal transplant patients have AN.

Diagnosis and Treatment

The histopathology of AN shows papillomatosis without thickening of the malpighian layer. "Acanthosis" was applied here to indicate the clinical bristly thickening of the skin and not as a histologic term. Hyperkeratosis and slight hyperpigmentation of the basal layer is present in most cases; it appears, however, that the clinically

observed hyperpigmentation is caused by hyperkeratosis and clinical thickening rather than by melanin.

The differential diagnosis includes intertriginous granular parakeratosis and several disorders of reticulated hyperpigmentation, including confluent and reticulated papillomatosis (Gougerot-Carteaud syndrome), Dowling-Degos disease, Haber syndrome, and acropigmentation reticularis of Kitamura. Granular parakeratosis presents as erythematous to brownish hyperkeratotic papules and plaques of the intertriginous regions. It is most often seen in middle-aged women in the axillae; however, the inguinal folds and submammary areas may be involved. Histology reveals a thickened stratum corneum, severe compact parakeratosis with retention of keratohyalin granules, and vascular proliferation and ectasia. The cause is likely to be an irritant response to rubbing or to antiperspirants or deodorants. Dowling-Degos disease is a familial nevoid anomaly with delayed onset in adult life. There is progressive, brown-black hyperpigmentation of flexures with associated soft fibromas and follicular hyperkeratoses. Pitted acneiform scars occur periorally.

Treatment of type I AN, associated with malignancy, consists of finding and removing the causal tumor. Early recognition and treatment may be lifesaving. AN occurring with obesity (type III) usually improves with weight loss. If there is associated endocrinopathy, it must be treated as well. One patient with lipodystrophic diabetes improved during dietary supplementation with fish oil. Etretinate, metformin, or other medications to control insulin resistance, as well as tretinoin, calcipotriol, urea, salicylic acid, glycolic acid peels, CO_2 laser ablation, and long-pulsed alexandrite laser therapy, have been reported as successful treatments in individual cases.

Bustan RS, et al: Specific skin signs as a cutaneous marker of diabetes mellitus and the prediabetic state—a systematic review. Dan Med J 2017; 64: A5316.

Chakraborty PP, et al: Tripe palm. BMJ Case Rep 2014 Oct 16; 2014.

Huang Y, et al: The clinical characteristics of obese patients with acanthosis nigricans and its independent risk factors. Exp Clin Endocrinol Diabetes 2017; 125: 191.

Ichiyama S, et al: Effective treatment by glycolic acid peeling for cutaneous manifestation of familial generalized acanthosis nigricans caused by FGFR3 mutation. J Eur Acad Dermatol Venereol 2016; 30: 442.

Jagwani AV, et al: Resolution of acanthosis nigricans following curative gastric carcinoma resection. Clin Ter 2016; 167: 99.

Malek R, et al: Treatment of type B insulin resistance. J Clin Endocrinol Metab 2010; 95: 3641.

Mir A, et al: Cutaneous features of Crouzon syndrome with acanthosis nigricans. JAMA Dermatol 2013; 149: 737.

Rafalson L, et al: The association between acanthosis nigricans and dysglycemia in an ethnically diverse group of eighth grade students. Obesity 2013; 21: E328.

Schmidt TH, et al: Cutaneous findings and systemic associations in women with polycystic ovary syndrome. JAMA Dermatol 2016; 152: 391.

Sinha S, et al: Juvenile acanthosis nigricans. J Am Acad Dermatol 2007; 57: 502.

25   Abnormalities of Dermal Fibrous and Elastic Tissue

COLLAGEN

Many types of collagen have been identified in tissues of vertebrates (Table 25.1). Collagens help form the support structure and scaffolding for many parts of the body, including tissues, blood vessels, and bones. Fibrillar collagens (types I, II, III, V, and XI) form fibrils that are among the most abundant proteins in the body. Type I collagen accounts for 60%–90% of the dry weight of skin, ligaments, and demineralized bone. Type III collagen is abundant in fetal skin and blood vessels. It comprises 35% of the collagen in normal adult skin, but up to 40% in inflamed skin in the setting of contact dermatitis. Basement membrane–associated collagen is made up of types IV and VII. Fiber-associated collagens (types VIII, IX, and XIV) are found on the surface of type I and II collagens and are believed to serve as flexible spacers among fibrils. Fibril-associated collagens with interrupted triple helices (FACITs) do not form fibrils themselves but are found attached to the surfaces of preexisting fibrils of the fibril-forming collagens. FACITs are composed of types IX, XII, XIV, XVI, XIX, XX, and XXI. Network-forming collagens are sheets formed from types VIII and X. Studies on types XV, XVII, and XIX demonstrate their widespread presence in basement membranes, particularly vascular endothelium, which may represent a new subgroup of collagens associated with angiogenic and pathologic processes. Type XVII collagen is also known as BP180, and contains the target antigens for several immunobullous diseases. Type VII collagen contains the target antigens for bullous lupus and epidermolysis bullosa acquisita. Type II collagen contains the target antigens for relapsing polychondritis. Genetic mutations leading to defects in or absence of various collagens (VII and XVII) can lead to epidermolysis bullosa.

The regulation of collagen synthesis and degradation is complex. Dermal fibrosis is largely related to increases in type I collagen mediated by proα1 and proα2 collagen genes. Transforming growth factor–beta (TGF-β) results in increased type I procollagen synthesis. Angiotensin II type 1 receptor stimulation increases collagen production and inhibits collagen degradation, whereas type 2 receptor stimulation exerts the reverse effects. Mutations in collagens or disruption of their function due to autoimmunity or medications can lead to disease.

Czarny-Ratajczak M, et al: Collagens, the basic proteins of the human body. J Appl Genet 2000; 41: 317.

ELASTOSIS PERFORANS SERPIGINOSA

In 1953 Lutz described a chronic papular keratotic eruption in an arciform shape located on the sides of the nape of the neck. The papules range from 2–5 mm in diameter and are grouped in a serpiginous or horseshoe-shaped arrangement (Fig. 25.1). The papules have a keratotic top that extrudes elastic fibers likely by binding to an elastin receptor on keratinocytes. Although the lesions typically occur on the neck, other sites may be involved, such as the upper arms, face, lower extremities, and rarely the trunk. Disseminated lesions may occur in Down syndrome. The disease runs a variable course, with spontaneous resolution often occurring from 6 months to 5 years after onset. Often, atrophic scarring remains. Progressive vasoocclusive disease with stroke has been reported.

Elastosis perforans serpiginosa (EPS) is most common in young adults. Men outnumber women 4 : 1. Approximately one third of EPS cases occur in patients with associated diseases; the most common concomitant disorder is Down syndrome. Approximately 1% of patients with Down syndrome have EPS, and the lesions are likely to be more extensive and persistent than in other patients. EPS has also been reported in Ehlers-Danlos syndrome, osteogenesis imperfecta, Marfan syndrome, Rothmund-Thomson syndrome, acrogeria, systemic sclerosis, morphea, XYY syndrome, and renal disease. Reports of EPS associated with pseudoxanthoma elasticum have occurred with penicillamine administration. EPS can also be idiopathic. Evaluation for associated disease should be driven by associated signs and symptoms.

The distinctive histopathologic changes of EPS consist of elongated, tortuous channels in the epidermis into which eosinophilic elastic fibers perforate. The fibers are extruded from the dermis. There is degeneration and alteration of the elastic tissue in the adjacent papillary dermis with an accompanying inflammatory response. In penicillamine-associated disease, the fibers may have an irregular (bramble bush) contour when examined with electron microscopy.

Treatment of EPS is difficult, but individual lesions may resolve after liquid nitrogen cryotherapy. Some cases have responded to carbon dioxide (CO$_2$) (fractional in some reports), erbium:yttrium-aluminum-garnet (Er:YAG), or pulsed dye laser therapy. Topical retinoids and imiquimod have been reported to be of benefit.

Kelati A, et al: Treatment of elastosis perforans serpiginosa using a fractional carbon dioxide laser. JAMA Dermatol 2017; 153: 1063.
Kim SW, et al: A clinicopathologic study of thirty cases of acquired perforating dermatosis in Korea. Ann Dermatol 2014; 26: 162.
Lee SH, et al: Elastosis perforans serpiginosa. Ann Dermatol 2014; 26: 103.
Nasca MR, et al: Perforating pseudoxanthoma elasticum with secondary elastosis perforans serpiginosa-like changes. J Cutan Pathol 2016; 43: 1021.
Polańska A, et al: Elastosis perforans serpiginosa. Postepy Dermatol Alergol 2016; 33: 392.
Vearrier D, et al: What is standard of care in the evaluation of elastosis perforans serpiginosa? A survey of pediatric dermatologists. Pediatr Dermatol 2006; 23: 219.
Yang JH, et al: Treatment of elastosis perforans serpiginosa with the pinhole method using a carbon dioxide laser. Dermatol Surg 2011; 37: 524.

REACTIVE PERFORATING COLLAGENOSIS

In 1967 Mehregan reported a rare, familial, nonpruritic skin disorder characterized by papules that grow to a diameter of 4–6 mm and develop a central area of umbilication in which keratinous material is lodged. The discrete papules may be numerous (Fig. 25.2) and involve sites of frequent trauma, such as the backs of the hands, the forearms, elbows, and knees. The lesion reaches a maximum size of about 6 mm in 4 weeks and then regresses spontaneously in 6–8 weeks. The lesions are broader than those of EPS, and a broad crust containing collagen fibers is extruded centrally. Koebnerization is often observed. Young children are most frequently affected. Most reports support an autosomal recessive mode of inheritance, although apparent autosomal dominant inheritance was reported in one family but

TABLE 25.1 Collagen Types

Collagen Type	Gene*	Chromosome	Tissue Distribution
I	COL1A1–2	17q21.3–q22	Skin, bone, tendon
I-trimer			Tumors, cell cultures, skin, liver
II	COL2A1	7q21.3–q22	Cartilage, vitreous
III	COL3A1	12q13–q14	Fetal skin, blood vessels, intestines
IV	COL4A1–6	13q34, 2q35–q37, Xq22	Basement membranes
V	COL5A1–3	9q34.2–q34.3	Ubiquitous
VI	COL6A1–3	21q22.3, 2q37	Aortic intima, placenta
VII	COL7A1	3p21	Amnion, anchoring fibrils
VIII	COL8A1–2	3q12–q13.1, 1p32.3–p34.3	Endothelial cell cultures
IX	COL9A1–3	6q12–q14, 1p32	Cartilage, type II collagen tissue
X	COL10A1	6q12–q22	Cartilage
XI	COL11A1–2, COL2A1	1p21	Cartilage, skin
XII	COL12A1	6	Skin, cartilage, cornea, limbal
XIII	COL13A1	10q22	Ubiquitous
XIV	COL14A1	8q23	Ubiquitous, fetal hair follicles, basement membranes
XV	COL15A1	9q21–22	Skin hemidesmosomes, kidney, liver, spleen
XVI	COL16A1	1p34–35	Ubiquitous
XVII	COL17A1	10q24.3	Skin hemidesmosomes (BP180)
XVIII	COL18A1	21q22.3	Ubiquitous, basement membranes
XIX	COL19A1	6q12–q14	Ubiquitous, basement membranes
XX	COL20A1		Corneal epithelium, embryonic skin, sternal cartilage, tendon
XXI	COL21A1	6p11.2–12.3	Blood vessel walls
XXII	COL22A1	8q24.2	Tissue junctions such as basement membrane zone of anagen hair follicle
XXIII			Rat prostate carcinoma cells
XXIV			Fetal cornea and bone
XXV			Precursor to Alzheimer amyloid plaque component
XXVI			Testis, ovary
XXVII			Chondrocytes; developing tissues, including stomach, lung, gonad, skin, cochlea, teeth

*A dash denotes a series of genes; e.g., COL14A1–2 indicates both the COL14A1 and the COL14A2 gene.

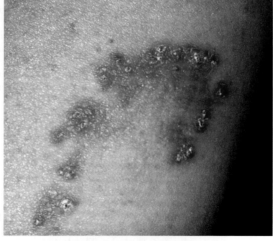

Fig. 25.1 Elastosis perforans serpiginosa.

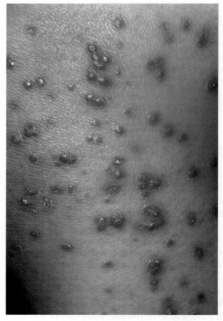

Fig. 25.2 Reactive perforating collagenosis. (Courtesy Steven Binnick, MD.)

the genetics have not been elucidated. Acquired reactive perforating collagenosis is discussed further in Chapter 33.

No specific treatment is typically indicated for reactive perforating collagenosis because the lesions involute spontaneously. Topical retinoids may be helpful in patients who require treatment.

Ramesh V, et al: Familial reactive perforating collagenosis. J Eur Acad Dermatol Venereol 2007; 21: 766.

Tiwary AK, et al: A rare case of familial reactive perforating collagenosis. Indian J Dermatol 2017; 18: 230.

PSEUDOXANTHOMA ELASTICUM

Pseudoxanthoma elasticum (PXE) is an inherited disorder involving the connective tissue of the skin, eye, and cardiovascular system. Many cases are sporadic. In familial cases, both a recessive and a dominant inheritance pattern have been reported, with the recessive form apparently more common. The skin changes generally present as small, circumscribed, yellow to cream-colored papules on the sides of the neck and flexures, giving the skin a "plucked chicken skin" appearance (Fig. 25.3). Lax, redundant folds of skin may be present (Fig. 25.4). Nuchal comedones and milia en plaque may also be seen. Characteristic exaggerated nasolabial folds and mental creases are common. Mental creases (horizontal creases across the chin) appearing in patients under age 30 are highly suggestive of PXE. In addition, the inguinal, periumbilical, and periauricular skin, as well as the mucosa of the soft palate, inner lip, tonsils, stomach, rectum, and vagina, may be involved.

The characteristic retinal change is the angioid streak, which is the result of breaks in Bruch's elastic membrane. PXE can be demonstrated in more than half of patients with angioid streaks, and 85% of PXE patients will have retinal findings. The angioid streaks appear earlier than the skin changes, so most cases are discovered by ophthalmologists. Angioid streaks may be the only sign of the disease for years. Biopsies of the midportions of old scars may be diagnostic of PXE. Angioid streaks may also be seen in Ehlers-Danlos syndrome, Paget disease of bone, diabetes, hemochromatosis, hemolytic anemia, hypercalcinosis, solar elastosis, neurofibromatosis, Sturge-Weber syndrome, tuberous sclerosis, myopia, sickle cell anemia, trauma, lead poisoning, hyperphosphatemia, pituitary disorders, and intracranial disorders. PXE, Paget disease of the bone, and sickle cell disease account for the vast majority of patients with angioid streaks.

On funduscopic examination, a reddish brown band is evident around the optic disk, from which glistening streaks extend. In addition, there may be hemorrhages and exudates. Progressive loss of vision often starts after minor trauma to the eye. Drusen-like spots are often present and show increased autofluorescence, unlike age-related drusen.

Vascular involvement frequently leads to hemorrhage. These vascular events are caused by the degeneration of the elastic fibers in the vascular media. Gastric hemorrhage occurs in 10% of patients, and on gastroscopy, diffuse bleeding is common. Epistaxis occurs frequently, but hematuria is rare. PXE affects the elastic tissue of the cardiac valves, myocardium, and pericardium. In one study, mitral valve prolapse was found in 71% of 14 patients examined. Hypertension occurs in many patients older than age 30. Any patient with hypertension at a young age should be examined for stigmata of PXE. Leg cramps and intermittent claudication occur prematurely, and peripheral pulses are diminished or absent. Calcification of peripheral arteries is seen in many patients over age 30 and may be detected by radiography. Accelerated coronary artery disease (CAD) can occur, especially in association with hypertension. Extensive cutaneous calcification and renal and testicular stones may occur.

Mutations in the adenosine triphosphate (ATP)–binding cassette transporter protein subfamily C member 6 gene (*ABCC6*) have been implicated in the pathogenesis of PXE in a majority of patients, who also have a higher incidence of CAD. Defective release of ATP leads to less inorganic pyrophosphate (PPi), which is important

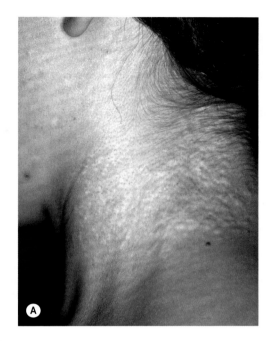

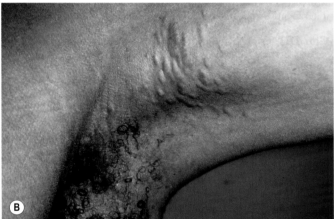

Fig. 25.3 (A and B) Pseudoxanthoma elasticum.

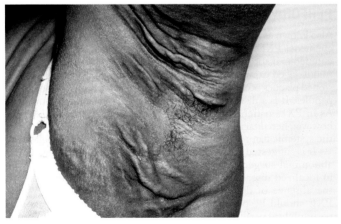

Fig. 25.4 Pseudoxanthoma elasticum.

in inhibiting mineralization; thus the mineralization goes unchecked. Although the most prominent manifestations of the disease are in the skin, eye, gut, and heart, mineralization of elastic fibers can be found in many organs.

Histologically, elastic fibers are fragmented and mineralized with calcium. The fibers stain gray-blue with hematoxylin and eosin (H&E) and are twisted, curled, and broken, suggesting "raveled wool." Blind biopsies of scars or axillary skin in patients with a family history of PXE or with angioid streaks may show early changes of PXE. Calcium stains are helpful in identifying early disease.

The differential diagnosis includes PXE-like papillary dermal elastolysis, perforating calcific elastosis, connective tissue nevus with elastorrhexis, and cutis laxa. Patients with PXE-like papillary dermal elastolysis may have cobblestoned, yellow papules on the neck, similar to PXE, but lack any retinal or vascular alterations and the typical fragmentation of elastic fibers with calcium deposition on histology. Patients described with connective tissue nevus with elastorrhexis have tiny white papules coalescing into a plaque on the upper chest and lower neck that are not associated with any internal findings. Penicillamine may induce similar clinicohistologic features in patients with Wilson disease or homocystinuria.

No definitive therapy is available to treat the skin disease. Some data suggest that PXE patients benefit from limiting dietary calcium and phosphorus to the minimal daily requirement. Intravitreal bevacizumab has been used to treat choroidal neovascularization. Atorvastatin treatment appears promising in a mouse model. Therapeutic trials of magnesium and a bisphosphonate are ongoing.

Chu DH, et al: A new variant of connective tissue nevus with elastorrhexis and predilection for the upper chest. Pediatr Dermatol 2015; 32: 518.

Decani S, et al: Pseudoxanthoma elasticum of the palate. Oral Surg Oral Med Oral Pathol Oral Radiol 2016; 121: e6.

Finger RP, et al: Intravitreal bevacizumab for choroidal neovascularisation associated with pseudoxanthoma elasticum. Br J Ophthalmol 2008; 92: 483.

Guo H, et al: Atorvastatin counteracts aberrant soft tissue mineralization in a mouse model of pseudoxanthoma elasticum (Abcc6−/−). J Mol Med (Berl) 2013; 91: 1177.

Hendig D, et al: New insights into the pathogenesis of pseudoxanthoma elasticum and related soft tissue calcification disorders by identifying genetic interactions and modifiers. Front Genet 2013; 4: 114.

Plomp AS, et al: Proposal for updating the pseudoxanthoma elasticum classification system and a review of the clinical findings. Am J Med Genet 2010; 152A: 1049.

Uitto J, et al: Insights into pathomechanisms and treatment development in heritable ectopic mineralization disorders. J Invest Dermatol 2017; 137: 790.

PERFORATING CALCIFIC ELASTOSIS

Also known as periumbilical perforating PXE and localized acquired cutaneous PXE, perforating calcific elastosis is an acquired, localized cutaneous disorder most frequently found in obese, multiparous, middle-aged women. Lax, well-circumscribed, reticulated, or cobblestoned plaques occur in the periumbilical region with keratotic surface papules. It is a distinct disorder that shares some features of PXE. As in PXE, patients may have calcific elastosis in the middermis; however, hereditary PXE rarely causes perforating channels. None of the systemic features of PXE occurs in perforating calcific elastosis.

It is suggested that repeated trauma of pregnancy, obesity, and abdominal surgery promote elastic fiber degeneration, resulting in localized disease. PXE can cause periumbilical lesions, and in the absence of documented perforation, evaluations to exclude PXE should be performed as patients with angioid streaks and periumbilical perforating PXE clinical findings have been reported. There is no effective therapy for perforating calcific elastosis.

Kumar P, et al: Periumbilical perforating pseudoxanthoma elasticum. Dermatol Online J 2016; 22.

EHLERS-DANLOS SYNDROMES

Ehlers-Danlos syndromes (EDSs) are a group of genetically distinct connective tissue disorders characterized by excessive stretchability and fragility of the skin (Fig. 25.5), with hyperextensibility of the joints (Fig. 25.6) and a tendency toward easy scar formation and formation of fibrous or calcified pseudotumors. The dermatologist's role is to help identify people who may have EDS and guide them to workup by a geneticist and if necessary other specialties including cardiology.

Recently EDS was reclassified into 13 subtypes. Type IX EDS, an allelic variant of Menkes disease, is now reclassified as the occipital horn syndrome and is identical to X-linked cutis laxa. It is related to mutations in an X-linked gene, *ATP7A*. The most clinically relevant features of EDS (for a dermatologist) are reviewed in Table 25.2. For a full review of the symptoms the reader is referred to the Malfait et al. review.

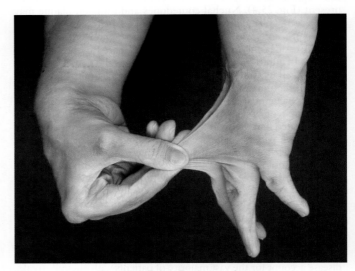

Fig. 25.5 Ehlers-Danlos syndrome.

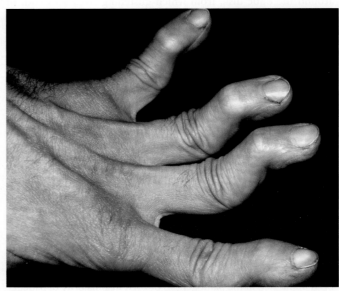

Fig. 25.6 Ehlers-Danlos syndrome, hyperextensible joints. (Courtesy Steven Binnick, MD.)

TABLE 25.2 Features of Ehlers-Danlos Syndromes Based on 2017 Classification

Ehlers-Danlos Type and Clinical Name	Gene (Protein) and Inheritance	Selected Clinical Features[a]	
		Major Criteria	*Minor Criteria*
1 Classical	COL5A1 (type 5 collagen) AD COL1A1 (type I collagen) AD	Skin hyperextensibility Joint hypermobility Atrophic scars	Easy bruising Soft doughy skin Molluscoid pseudotumors Epicanthal folds
2 Classical-like	TNXB (tenascin XB) AR	Skin hyperextensibility Velvety skin but no atrophic scars Joint hypermobility Easy bruising	Broad forefoot Pes planus Polyneuropathy Edema Vaginal/rectal prolapse
3 Cardiac Valvular	Col1A2 (type I collagen) AR	Aortic and mitral valve disease Skin hyperextensibility Atrophic scars Joint hypermobility Easy bruising	Inguinal hernia Pectus excavatum Joint dislocations
4 Vascular	COL3A1 (type III collagen) Col1A1 (type I collagen) AD	Arterial rupture Colon perforation Uterine rupture	Easy bruising Thin translucent skin Congenital hip dislocation
5 Hypermobile	Unknown AD	Joint hypermobility Velvety skin Hyperextensiblity Striae Piezogenic papules Abdominal hernia	Joint dislocations or laxity Musculoskeletal pain
6 Arthrochalasia	Col1A1–2 (type I collagen) AD	Congenital hip dislocation (bilateral) Severe joint hypermobility Skin Hyperextensibility	Hypotonia Easy bruising
7 Dermatosparaxis	ADAMTS2 (ADAMTS-2) AD	Fragile skin with tears Skin laxity Easy bruising Short limbs, hands, and feet	Doughy skin Skin hyperextensibility Atrophic scars Joint hypermobility Bladder rupture/diaphragm rupture
8 Kyphoscoliosis	PLOD1 (LH1) FKBP14 (FKBP22) AR	Congenital hypotonia Kyphoscoliosis Joint hypermobility	Skin hyperextensibility Easy bruising Rupture of arteries Blue sclerae Marphanoid Pectus deformity PLOD1 (skin more fragile, scleral rupture, microcornea) FKBP14 (hearing impairment, follicular hyperkeratosis, muscle atropy)
9 Brittle Cornea Syndrome	ZNF469 (ZNF469) PRDM5 (PRDM5) AR	Thin cornea Keratoconus Blue sclerae	Hypotonia Hypermobile joints Finger contractures Velvety translucent skin
10 Spondylodysplastic	B4GALT7 (B4GalT7) B3GALT6 (B3GalT6) SLC39a13 (ZIP13) AR	Short stature Muscle hypotonia Bowing limbs	Skin hyperextensibility Cognitive impairment B4GALT7 (elbow contractures, clouded cornea) B3GALT6 (joint contractures and hypermobility, tooth discoloration) SLC39a13 (protuberant eyes, blue sclerae, atrophy of thenar eminences and wrinkled palms)
11 Musculocontractural	CHST14 (D4ST1) DSE (DSE) AR	Congenital contractures, skin hyperextensibility Easy bruising Fragile skin	Dislocations Finger anomalies Spinal deformities Pneumothorax nephrolithiasis
12 Myopathic	COL12A1 (type XII collagen) AD or AR	Congenital hypotonia Proximal contractures Hypermobility of joints	Doughy skin Atrophis scars
13 Periodontal	C1R (C1r) C1S (C1s) AD	Severe periodontitis Pretibial plaques Lack of attached gingiva	Easy bruising Joint hypermobility Skin hyperextensibility

AD, Autosomal dominant; *AR,* autosomal recessive.
[a]Not all criteria listed; see full classification from Malfait et al.

Joint hypermobility, skin hyperextensibility, and tissue fragility are the hallmark cutaneous findings of EDS. There are multiple clinical tests to help evaluate for these. Remvig et al. described that if the skin can be pinched and stretched over 1.5 cm on the dorsal hand or volar forearm or over 3 cm at the neck, this is defined as hyperextensible. In hyperextensible skin the integument may be stretched like a rubber band and snaps back with equal resilience. This rubbery skin is most pronounced on the elbows, neck, and sides of the abdomen. The skin may be velvety in appearance and feel like wet chamois cloth.

The Beighton score grades joint hypermobility; a point is given for each side of the body that can do the following: if the fifth digit can be pulled back more than 90 degrees with the palm on a flat surface, with the arm stretched out and the palm pronated if the thumb can be pulled to touch the forearm, if the elbows can bend more than 10 degrees with the arms outstretched and hands supinated, if the knees extend more than 10 degrees while standing with knees locked, with knees locked if the patient can lean over and put the palms flush on the floor. A score of 5 to 9 is positive.

Other prominent features in many forms of EDS include easy bruising and scarring. Minor trauma may produce a gaping "fish-mouth" wound with large hematomas underneath. Two types of nodules occur in patients with EDS. Molluscoid pseudotumors are soft, fleshy nodules seen in easily traumatized areas such as the ulnar forearms and shins. From 2–8 mm oval subcutaneous calcifications can occur, mostly on the legs, and probably result from fat necrosis. Trauma over the shins, knees, hands, and elbows produces cigarette paper–thin scars. Atrophic scarring on the distal fingers and wide atrophic "fish-mouth" scars are typical. Patients demonstrate reduced thickness of the dermis. The reduction in thickness is most marked on the chest and distal lower leg. Approximately 50% of these patients can touch the tip of the nose with their tongue (Gorlin sign), compared with 10% of persons without the disorder. Aortic root dilation is seen in up to 20% of patients with EDS and patients should be referred to cardiology to consider an echocardiogram.

Patients must be counseled to avoid trauma and may need physical therapy. Unfortunately, invasive cardiovascular procedures have generally not improved outcomes for patients with severe disease, but echocardiograms are generally recommended. Matrix metalloproteinase (MMP) inhibitors produce changes in connective tissue and are being evaluated as possible therapeutic agents.

Beighton P, et al: Articular mobility in an African population. Ann Rheum Dis 1973; 13: 413.

Bergqvist D, et al: Treatment of vascular Ehlers-Danlos syndrome. Ann Surg 2013; 258: 257.

Bloom L, et al: The international consortium on the Ehlers-Danlos syndromes. Am J Med Genet C Semin Med Genet 2017; 175: 5.

Callewaert B, et al: Ehlers-Danlos syndromes and Marfan syndrome. Best Pract Res Clin Rheumatol 2008; 22: 165.

Malfait F, et al: The 2017 international classification of the Ehlers-Danlos syndromes. Am J Med Genet C Semin Med Genet 2017; 175: 8.

Müller T, et al: Loss of dermatan sulfate epimerase (DSE) function results in musculocontractural Ehlers-Danlos syndrome. Hum Mol Genet 2013; 22: 3761.

Petersen JW, et al: Tenascin-X, collagen, and Ehlers-Danlos syndrome. Med Hypotheses 2013; 81: 443.

Remvig L, et al: Are diagnostic criteria for general joint hypermobility and benign joint hypermobility syndrome based on reproducible and valid tests? J Rheumatol 2007; 34: 798.

Wiesmann T, et al: Recommendations for anesthesia and perioperative management in patients with Ehlers-Danlos syndrome(s). Orphanet J Rare Dis 2014; 9: 109.

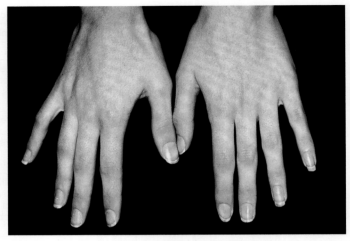

Fig. 25.7 Marfan syndrome.

MARFAN SYNDROME

Marfan syndrome is an autosomal dominant disorder of connective tissue caused by mutations in the gene encoding fibrillin-1. It is one of the more common inherited diseases, with estimated incidence rates of 1 in 10,000 in the United States. Important clinical findings include tall stature, loose-jointedness, a dolichocephalic skull, high-arched palate, arachnodactyly (Fig. 25.7), pigeon breast, pes planus, poor muscle tone, and large, deformed ears. The aorta, chordae tendineae, and aortic and mitral valves are often involved. Ascending aortic aneurysm and mitral valve prolapse are frequently seen. Ectopia lentis (typically upwardly displaced), extensive striae over the hips and shoulders, dental anomalies, and rarely EPS have been reported. Several cases document the occasional occurrence of spontaneous pneumothorax and congenital lung abnormalities.

Marfan syndrome is caused by a gene defect in fibrillin-1 (aorta adventitia, suspending ligaments of lens and skin). Fibrillin-2 mutations are associated with congenital contractural arachnodactyly (arachnodactyly, camptodactyly and contractures, crumpled-appearing ears, and pectus carinatum).

In Marfan syndrome, echocardiography is helpful for early detection of cardiovascular involvement. Surgical intervention may be required for aneurysms of the aortic root or for aortic dissection. Death may result from aortic root aneurysm rupture or dissection. Long-term administration of propranolol may significantly reduce the rate of aortic dilation, as does angiotensin II blockade with losartan. Long-term doxycycline may be helpful to inhibit MMPs. Some evidence suggests that doxycycline may be more effective than atenolol in preventing progression of thoracic aortic aneurysms. Antisense ribozymes are promising for gene therapy.

LOEYS DIETZ SYNDROME

Loeys Dietz is a syndrome caused by mutations in the TGF-β pathway that clinically resembles Marfan syndrome without the tall stature. Affected individuals have pectus abnormalities, flat feet, and arachnodactyly, along with arterial tortuosity and risk of aortic dissection. Their skin is translucent, with easy bruising, and they get striae and atrophic scars with impaired wound healing. They have a higher rate of atopic disease and they have joint hypermobility and hypotonia.

Brooke BS, et al: Angiotensin II blockade and aortic-root dilation in Marfan's syndrome. N Engl J Med 2008; 358: 2787.

Cui JZ, et al: Evaluation of the protective effects of long-term doxycycline treatment on progression of Marfan-associated aortic aneurysm by high-resolution ultrasound imaging. Circulation 2015; 132: A14680.

Groenink M, et al: Losartan reduces aortic dilatation rate in adults with Marfan syndrome. Eur Heart J 2013; 34: 3491.

MacCarrick G, et al: Loeys-Dietz syndrome. Genet Med 2014; 16: 576.

Mehar V, et al: Congenital contractural arachnodactyly due to a novel splice site mutation in the FBN2 gene. J Pediatr Genet 2014; 3: 163.

HOMOCYSTINURIA

Homocystinuria, an inborn error in the metabolism of methionine, is characterized by the presence of homocysteine in the urine and deficiency of the enzyme cystathionine synthetase or methylene-tetrahydrofolate reductase. Cystathionine β-synthase is a heme-containing enzyme that catalyzes pyridoxal 5′-phosphate–dependent conversion of serine and homocysteine to cystathionine. The defect results in increased levels of homocysteine and methionine and decreased levels of cysteine. The incidence of the disorder varies from 1 in 344,000 worldwide to 1 in 65,000 in Ireland, where homocystinuria is more common.

Signs of homocystinuria include ectopia lentis, genu valgum, kyphoscoliosis, pigeon breast deformity, and frequent fractures. The facial skin has a characteristic flush, especially on the malar areas, and the color tends to become violaceous when the patient is reclining. Elsewhere, the skin is blotchy red, suggestive of livedo reticularis. The hair is typically fine, sparse, and blond, and the teeth are irregularly aligned. Generalized osteoporosis, arterial and venous thrombosis, and mental retardation are features of homocystinuria not found in Marfan syndrome. Half of all patients will have a serious vascular event before age 30, and 25% experience a serious event before age 16. Downward dislocation of the lens, unlike the upward displacement seen in Marfan syndrome, is a prominent feature.

Treatment with pyridoxine, folic acid, and vitamin B_{12} produces variable results in homocystinuric patients. A methionine-restricted, cysteine-supplemented diet is generally recommended. Betaine supplementation has been shown to be effective. Some recommend that methionine-free formulas be supplemented with 150 mg/dL of betaine. Alfalfa and bean sprouts contain ample homocysteine, and excessive amounts should be avoided. Other vegetables do not contain large amounts of homocysteine. Vitamin C ameliorates endothelial dysfunction, and the effect appears to be independent of homocysteine concentration. Some of the beneficial effects of folate are also independent of homocysteine reduction. In an animal model of homocystinuria, 5-methyltetrahydrofolate decreased mortality rate, but folic acid did not.

Li D, et al: Mefolinate (5-methyltetrahydrofolate), but not folic acid, decreases mortality in an animal model of severe methyl-enetetrahydrofolate reductase deficiency. J Inherit Metab Dis 2008; 31: 403.

Walter JH, et al: Newborn screening for homocystinuria. Cochrane Database Syst Rev 2013; 8: CD008840.

CUTIS LAXA (GENERALIZED ELASTOLYSIS)

Cutis laxa is characterized by inelastic, loose, redundant skin. Around the eyelids, cheeks, and neck, the drooping skin produces a "bloodhound-like" facies. Usually, the entire integument is involved. The shoulder girdle skin may resemble that of a St. Bernard dog. The abdomen is frequently the site of large, pendulous folds. There are two well-described genetic forms of cutis laxa, the autosomal dominant and autosomal recessive types, and there is also acquired cutis laxa as described later. The dominant form is primarily a cutaneous, cosmetic form, with a good prognosis. The recessive form is more common and associated with significant

internal involvement, including hernias, diverticula, pulmonary emphysema, cor pulmonale, aortic aneurysm, dental caries, large fontanelles, and osteoporosis. Pulmonary emphysema, cor pulmonale, and right-sided heart failure are often seen already in infancy. Frameshift and splicing mutations in the elastin gene have been reported in autosomal dominant disease. Both homozygous and heterozygous missense mutations in the gene for fibulin 5 have been reported in some patients with the disease, especially in families with the recessive form. Gene mutations in fibulin 4 may cause autosomal recessive cutis laxa associated with emphysema, vascular tortuosity, ascending aortic aneurysm, inguinal and diaphragmatic hernia, joint laxity, and pectus excavatum. X-linked recessive cutis laxa is now known as the occipital horn syndrome (formerly type IX EDS). It is caused by a mutation in the copper-binding ion-transporting ATPase, *ATP7A*, and is allelic to another X-linked disorder, Menkes disease.

Acquired cases have been associated with urticaria, Sweet syndrome (Marshall syndrome), lupus erythematosus, glomerulonephritis, plasma cell dyscrasias, and systemic amyloidosis. These acquired cases may have a preceding inflammatory phase with large numbers of interstitial neutrophils, eosinophils, or macrophages engulfing elastic fibers. Isolated acral disease has been associated with myeloma and rheumatoid arthritis. Middermal elastolysis is an acquired, noninherited condition that usually affects young women. Wide areas of skin demonstrate atrophic wrinkling. Histologically, elastic tissue is absent from the middle dermis. Many cases appear to be induced or aggravated by ultraviolet light exposure.

There are a few genetic disorders that have cutis laxa as a component. Costello syndrome is characterized by increased prenatal growth, postnatal growth retardation, coarse facies, loose skin that resembles cutis laxa, cardiomyopathy, and gregarious personality. Patients are predisposed to abdominal and pelvic rhabdomyosarcoma in childhood. The disorder appears to be inherited as an autosomal dominant trait. De Barsy syndrome is associated with severe cutis laxa, mental and growth retardation, joint laxity, ocular abnormalities, and skeletal disease.

Bangaru H, et al: Sweet's syndrome leading to acquired cutis laxa in a child (Marshall's syndrome). Indian J Paediatr Dermatol 2016; 17: 135.

Callewaert B, et al: Comprehensive clinical and molecular analysis of 12 families with type 1 recessive cutis laxa. Hum Mutat 2013; 34: 111.

Duz MB, et al: A novel case of autosomal dominant cutis laxa in a consanguineous family. Clin Dysmorphol 2017; 26: 142.

Mohamed M, et al: Cutis laxa. Adv Exp Med Biol 2014; 802: 161.

Tas A, et al: Oculoplastic approach to congenital cutis laxa syndrome. Aesthetic Plast Surg 2013; 37: 417.

BLEPHAROCHALASIS

In blepharochalasis, the eyelid skin becomes lax and falls in redundant folds over the lid margins. The condition may affect young adults, in whom a preceding inflammatory phase presents with episodes of lid swelling, such as from allergies or bee stings, that lead to disruption of elastin. Most cases are bilateral, but unilateral involvement may occur. Rarely, elastolysis of the earlobes may accompany blepharochalasis. It is generally sporadic, but a dominantly inherited form has been described. Biopsy shows lack of elastic fibers, and abundant IgA deposits have been demonstrated in some cases, possibly binding to fibulin and fibronectin. Sequelae include excess thin skin, fat herniation, lacrimal gland prolapse, ptosis, blepharophimosis, pseudoepicanthic fold, proptosis, conjunctival injection and cysts, entropion, and ectropion.

Ascher syndrome consists of progressive enlargement of the upper lip and blepharochalasis (Fig. 25.8). The minor salivary

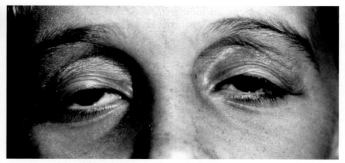

Fig. 25.8 Blepharochalasis in Ascher syndrome. (Courtesy Ken Greer, MD.)

Fig. 25.9 Anetoderma.

glands of the affected areas are inflamed, resulting in superfluous folds of mucosa, giving the appearance of a double lip. There is a superficial resemblance to angioedema.

Treatment is generally by surgical correction, although successful medical treatment has been reported with systemic acetazolamide in combination with topical hydrocortisone cream. Doxycycline has also been reported as effective, presumably through MMP inhibition.

Browning RJ, et al: Blepharochalasis. J Cutan Pathol 2017; 44: 279.

Drummond SR, et al: Successful medical treatment of blepharochalasis. Orbit 2009; 28: 313.

Karaconji T, et al: Doxycycline for treatment of blepharochalasis via inhibition of matrix metalloproteinases. Ophthal Plast Reconstr Surg 2012; 28: e76.

Sacchidanand SA, et al: Transcutaneous blepharoplasty in blepharochalasis. J Cutan Aesthet Surg 2012; 5: 284.

ANETODERMA (MACULAR ATROPHY)

Anetoderma is characterized by localized loss of elastic tissue resulting in herniation of subcutaneous tissue. The lesions protrude from the skin (Fig. 25.9) and on palpation have less resistance than the surrounding skin, producing the "buttonhole" sign identical to a neurofibroma. The surface skin may be slightly shiny, white, and crinkly. The usual locations are the trunk, especially on the shoulders, the upper arms, and thighs. The intervening skin is normal.

Up to half of patients with anetoderma have an accompanying abnormality, such as lupus, antiphospholipid antibodies, Graves disease, scleroderma, hypocomplementemia, hypergammaglobulinemia, autoimmune hemolysis, or human immunodeficiency virus

(HIV) infection. Screening for antiphospholipid antibodies is of particular importance because these may produce a prothrombotic state, and some patients fulfill criteria for the antiphospholipid syndrome. The antibodies may be detected as anticardiolipin antibodies, anti-β_2-glycoprotein-I antibodies, or a lupus anticoagulant. Patients may experience recurrent fetal loss, recurrent strokes, or recurrent deep vein thrombosis. Thrombosis-associated anetoderma with ulceration has been related to antithrombin III deficiency. Some cases of anetoderma may be related to borreliosis. Rare familial cases have been noted. Secondary anetoderma may be associated with previous lesions of acne, secondary syphilis, measles, lupus erythematosus, Hansen disease, sarcoidosis, tuberous xanthoma, varicella, granuloma annulare, mastocytosis, and lymphoreticular malignancy.

Anetoderma of prematurity (congenital anetoderma) occurs in premature infants who have immature epidermis. This is almost always caused by direct damage to the epidermis from the lifesaving care necessary to keep these infants alive; much more rarely, intrauterine borreliosis has also been implicated. Application of adhesives to keep indwelling lines and catheters in place, aggressive epidermal cleansing in preparation for procedures, or pressure from medical equipment can lead to areas of anetoderma. Typical locations include periumbilical due to fastening of umbilical artery lines and on extremities around locations of intravenous access. Recommendations to avoid this include using silicone-based tapes, avoiding stronger adhesives, washing with cleansers that are pH neutral, and avoiding baby wipes in infants under 28 weeks. Chlorhexadine cleansers typically come in 70% isopropyl alcohol and may be an irritant as well and should never be allowed to collect in skinfolds. Some advocate for using 10% povidone-iodine solution preparation for medical procedures for the first 2 weeks of life in infants born before 26 weeks.

Histologically, loss of elastic tissue is noted with special stains. In the late stage, the skin looks normal in H&E sections. In the acute stage, a neutrophilic, lymphoid, or granulomatous response may be noted. Ablative laser treatment has been reported as helpful in some adult patients with anetoderma but treatment is general unsatisfactory.

Clark ER, et al: Thrombosis-induced ulcerations of the lower legs with coexistent anetoderma due to anti-thrombin III deficiency. J Am Acad Dermatol 2011; 65: 880.

Emer J, et al: Generalized anetoderma after intravenous penicillin therapy for secondary syphilis in an HIV patient. J Clin Aesthet Dermatol 2013; 6: 23.

Haider M, et al: Lupus erythematosus–associated primary and secondary anetoderma. J Cutan Med Surg 2012; 16: 64.

Hodak E, et al: Primary anetoderma and antiphospholipid antibodies. Clin Rev Allergy Immunol 2007; 32: 162.

Johnson DE: Extremely preterm infant skin care. Adv Neonatal Care 2016; 16: S26.

STRIAE DISTENSAE (STRETCH MARKS)

Striae distensae are depressed lines or bands of thin, reddened skin (Fig. 25.10), which later become white, smooth, shiny, and depressed. Elastotic striae have a yellow-gold iridescent appearance. Striae occur in response to changes in weight or muscle mass and skin tension, such as that induced by weightlifting. They are common on the abdomen during and after pregnancy (striae gravidarum) and breasts due to pregnancy as well. They also occur on the buttocks and thighs, the inguinal areas, and more rarely over the knees and elbows in children during the growth spurt of puberty. Horizontal striae on the midback are common in adolescent males and although the cause is unknown, they are typically not associated with any systemic disease and in various studies have been seen in approximately 25%–50% of young adult males. People with Cushing syndrome have much more purple and

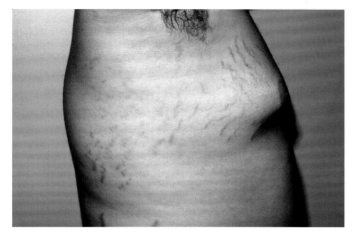

Fig. 25.10 Striae distensae.

Fig. 25.11 Elastotic striae.

wide (greater than 1 cm) striae. They will also often have other signs of Cushing syndrome, including "cigarette paper" skin on the elbows and knees that tears easily, acanthosis nigricans, and decreased linear but increased weight growth. An important cause of striae is either endogenous or induced by systemic corticosteroid treatment. They may occur after application of potent topical corticosteroid preparations, especially under occlusion or in skinfolds. Striae are common in patients with Marfan syndrome.

The histologic findings are variable and depend on the stage of development. In some early lesions, perivascular and interstitial infiltration of lymphocytes and sometimes eosinophils is noted. In older lesions, the primary changes are in the connective tissue. The collagen of the upper dermis is decreased, and thin collagen bundles lie parallel to the overlying epidermis, as in a scar. Elastic tissue often appears increased, but this may result from a loss of collagen in many cases. Dilated upper dermal vessels may be prominent.

A Cochrane review found no high-quality evidence to support the use of any topical preparation for the prevention of stretch marks during pregnancy. Over time, striae become less noticeable without treatment. Both silicone gel and placebo have demonstrated some positive effects in clinical studies, complicating interpretation of results. Topical tretinoin and vascular lasers may produce some improvement in appearance, although the benefits are more marked in the early erythematous phase and tretinoin should be avoided during pregnancy. Pulsed dye lasers (585 nm) result in a moderate decrease in erythema in striae rubra. Although the total collagen per gram of dry weight increases in striae treated with pulsed dye laser, this change may not result in a clinically evident change in striae alba. Pulsed dye laser has also been used in conjunction with a radiofrequency device. Intense pulsed light has also demonstrated potential for improvement in the appearance of some striae, although with greater risk and lower efficacy in darker skin types. Some data suggest that 590-nm light is more effective than 650-nm light. Fractional photothermolysis has been used in a variety of skin types for both rubra and alba types of striae.

LINEAR FOCAL ELASTOSIS (ELASTOTIC STRIAE)

This elastosis variant presents with asymptomatic, palpable, or atrophic, yellow lines of the middle and lower back, thighs, arms, and breasts (Fig. 25.11). Linear focal elastosis can be differentiated from striae because they are more yellow and raised but may just be the end stage of striae. They are often reported after a sudden increase in exercise. Linear focal elastosis is more common in males. Histologically, increased elastic fibers are seen, characterized by thin, wavy, and elongated as well as fragmented bundles. Electron

microscopy reveals thin, elongated, irregularly shaped, swollen elastic fibers with degenerative changes.

Chantes A, et al: Clinical improvement of striae distensae in Korean patients using a combination of fractionated microneedle radiofrequency and fractional carbon dioxide laser. Dermatol Surg 2014; 40: 699.

Florell AJ, et al: Linear focal elastosis associated with exercise. JAAD Case Rep 2017; 3: 39.

Kim BJ, et al: Fractional photothermolysis for the treatment of striae distensae in Asian skin. Am J Clin Dermatol 2008; 9: 33.

Lause M, et al: Dermatologic manifestations of endocrine disorders. Transl Pediatr 2017; 6: 300.

Leung AK, et al: Physiological striae atrophicae of adolescence with involvement of the upper back. Case Rep Pediatr 2013; 2013: 386094.

Naeini FF, et al: Comparison of the fractional CO_2 laser and the combined use of a pulsed dye laser with fractional CO_2 laser in striae alba treatment. Adv Biomed Res 2014; 3: 184.

Ud-Din S, et al: A double-blind controlled clinical trial assessing the effect of topical gels on striae distensae (stretch marks). Arch Dermatol Res 2013; 305: 603.

ACRODERMATITIS CHRONICA ATROPHICANS

Patients with acrodermatitis chronica atrophicans present with diffuse thinning of the skin on the extremities, sometimes associated with fibrous bands. This condition is reviewed with bacterial infections in Chapter 14, because it results from *Borrelia* infection.

OSTEOGENESIS IMPERFECTA

Osteogenesis imperfecta (OI), also known as Lobstein syndrome, affects the bones, joints, eyes, ears, and skin. It is estimated to affect approximately 10,000 persons in the United States (4–5 in 100,000 population). There are seven recognized forms based on differences in clinical presentation and bone architecture. Types I and IV have only an autosomal dominant inheritance, whereas types II and III have both autosomal dominant and autosomal recessive forms. Fifty percent of OI patients have the type I form. The type II form is lethal, and deaths usually occur within the first week of life.

The brittle bones result from a defect in the collagenous matrix. Fractures occur early in life, sometimes in utero. Children with unexplained fractures are often referred to rule out child abuse and therefore it is vital to recognize OI to avoid emotionally

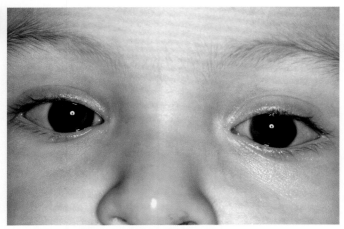

Fig. 25.12 Osteogenesis imperfecta with blue sclera. (Courtesy Scott Norton, MD.)

traumatic workups for parents. Loose-jointedness may be striking, and dislocation of joints can be a problem. Blue sclerae, when present, are a valuable diagnostic clue (Fig. 25.12). Scoliosis and defective teeth may be present. Deafness develops in many patients by the second decade of life and is audiologically indistinguishable from otosclerosis. The skin is thin and translucent, and healing wounds result in spreading atrophic scars. EPS may occur. Some patients experience unusual bruisability, probably from a structural defect in either the blood vessel wall or the supporting dermal connective tissue.

The basic defect is abnormal collagen synthesis, resulting in type I collagen of abnormal structure. Most forms of OI result from mutations in the genes for the proα1 or proα2 chains of type I collagen. Types V, VI, and VII are not associated with type I collagen gene defects. In type I (blue scleral dominant) there is diminished type I collagen with a mutation of *COL1A1* gene; in type II (perinatal lethal) there is diminished type I collagen synthesis and decreased integrity of the helical domain of the α1(I) gene; in type III (progressive deforming) there is delayed secretion of type I collagen with altered mannosylation; and in type IV (white sclerae dominant) there is a defective proα1(I) gene. A distinct subset of type IV with clinical improvement over time has been mapped to chromosome 11q.

The major causes of death attributed to OI are respiratory failure secondary to severe kyphoscoliosis and head trauma, mostly observed in type III disease. Aortic dissection has also been described. Patients with type I and type IV disease have a normal life span. Brack syndrome is a combination of OI and arthrogryposis multiplex.

Treatment includes surgical intervention, such as intramedullary stabilization. Bisphosphonates and calcitriol are the most effective pharmacologic agents. Specifically, cyclic pamidronate therapy has been shown to suppress bone turnover, reduce bone pain and fracture incidence, and increase bone density and level of ambulation. Gene therapy is promising but is complicated by the genetic heterogeneity of the disease.

Alcausin MB, et al: Intravenous pamidronate treatment in children with moderate-to-severe osteogenesis imperfecta started under three years of age. Horm Res Paediatr 2013; 79: 333.

Ben Amor M, et al: Osteogenesis imperfecta. Pediatr Endocrinol Rev 2013; 10: 397.

Zhang Z, et al: Phenotype and genotype analysis of Chinese patients with osteogenesis imperfecta type V. PLoS One 2013; 8: e72337.

26   Errors in Metabolism

AMYLOIDOSIS

Amyloid is a material deposited in the skin and other organs that is eosinophilic, homogeneous, and hyaline in appearance. It represents beta-pleated sheet forms of various host-synthesized molecules processed into this configuration by host cells.

Amyloidosis can be classified as systemic, localized, and heredofamilial types. The systemic types can deposit amyloid in multiple organs due to an overproduction of a host protein that cannot be adequately excreted or metabolized by the host. The excess protein is metabolized into amyloid precursors that interact with tissue proteoglycans/glycosaminoglycans, forming soluble amyloid oligomers. These oligomers complex with serum amyloid P (SAP), forming amyloid deposits in the affected organ. Over 30 proteins have been associated with amyloidosis, including immunoglobulin light chains (myeloma associated amyloid), tranthyretin (senile amyloid), beta-2 microglobulin (diabetic amyloid), and alpha natriuretic protein. In all forms of amyloid, the pattern of deposition is characteristic, although there can be overlap between various forms. The diagnosis of a specific type of amyloid should only be made if the clinical features are characteristic and if the deposited protein is identified histochemically. Primary localized amyloidosis (also called primary cutaneous amyloidosis when the skin is affected) is very common. Rare familial syndromes may be complicated by secondary systemic amyloidosis or may have genetic defects that lead to amyloid deposition (heredofamilial amyloidosis). Classification of cutaneous amyloidoses is as follows:

I. Systemic amyloidosis
   A. Primary (myeloma-associated) systemic amyloidosis
   B. Secondary systemic amyloidosis
   C. Dialysis-related amyloidosis
   D. Senile systemic amyloidosis
II. Cutaneous amyloidosis
   A. Macular amyloidosis
   B. Lichen amyloidosis
   C. Nodular amyloidosis
   D. Secondary (tumor-associated) cutaneous amyloidosis
   E. Familial primary cutaneous amyloidosis
   F. Pharmaceutical amyloidosis
III. Heredofamilial amyloidosis

All forms of amyloid have relatively identical histologic and electron microscopic findings. The amyloid in all forms is made up of three distinct components: protein-derived amyloid fibers, amyloid P component (about 15% of amyloid), and ground substance. The protein-derived amyloid fibers are those that differ among the various forms of amyloid.

Amyloid is weakly periodic acid–Schiff (PAS) positive and diastase resistant, Congo red positive, purple with crystal violet, and positive with thioflavin T. Amyloid stained with Congo red exhibits apple-green birefringence under polarized light. Secondary systemic amyloid (AA amyloid) loses its birefringence after treatment with potassium permanganate, whereas primary and localized cutaneous forms do not.

Amyloid stains an intense, bright orange with cotton dyes such as Dylon, Pagoda red, RIT Scarlet No. 5, or RIT Cardinal Red

No. 9. Ultrastructurally, amyloid has a characteristic fibrillar structure that consists of straight, nonbranching, nonanastomosing, often irregularly arranged filaments 60–100 nm in diameter. In most cases, specific antibodies against the protein component should be used to confirm the type of amyloidosis. Because amyloid substance P is present in all forms of amyloid, immunoperoxidase staining against this component will stain all forms of amyloid. In addition, because SAP is avidly bound to amyloid, radiolabeled, highly purified SAP can be used to localize amyloidosis, determine the extent of organ infiltration, study progression of disease, and determine whether therapy reduces the amount of amyloid in various organs. Radiolabeled SAP scintigraphy and identification of specific amyloid proteins immunohistochemically can be done at some specialized centers, although the amount of deposition is not directly correlated with organ dysfunction.

SYSTEMIC AMYLOIDOSES

Primary Systemic Amyloidosis (AL Amyloidosis)

Primary systemic amyloidosis typically involves the kidneys, liver, heart, gastrointestinal (GI) tract, peripheral nerve tissue, and skin. Myeloma-associated amyloidosis is included in this category. The amyloid fibril proteins in primary systemic amyloidosis are composed of the protein AL amyloid, a portion of the immunoglobulin (Ig) light chain. It is usually of the lambda (λ) subtype, and certain germline Ig light-chain V chains (6aVλVI and 3rVλIII) are responsible for AL amyloidosis in 40% of patients.

Cutaneous manifestations occur in approximately 40% of patients with primary systemic amyloidosis. The cutaneous eruption usually begins as shiny, smooth, firm, flat-topped, or spherical papules of waxy color that have the appearance of translucent vesicles. These lesions coalesce to form nodules and plaques of various sizes and, in some cases, bandlike lesions. The regions around the eyes, nose, mouth, and mucocutaneous junctions are frequently involved (Fig. 26.1). Vulvar lesions may resemble giant condylomata. Lesions may also be uniform small papules resembling milia or even microcystic lymphatic malformations. Follicular plugging may occur, resulting in milia.

Purpuric lesions and ecchymoses occur in about 15% of patients and are the most common cutaneous manifestation of primary systemic amyloidosis. There are several mechanisms by which AL amyloid leads to purpura. Amyloid may infiltrate blood vessels, making them fragile. AL amyloid may also bind factor X, inhibiting its function and thus leading to pupura. Last, amyloid infiltration of the liver may lead to reduced production of fibrinogen and factor X, adversely affecting clotting. Purpura chiefly involves the eyelids, limbs, and oral cavity. It typically occurs after trauma (pinch purpura) and can be reproduced by the physician by rubbing a pen or dull instrument over the skin, analogous to trying to demonstrate dermatographism. Purpuric lesions also classically appear after actions or procedures that result in increased pressure in the vessels of the face, such as after vomiting, coughing, proctoscopic examination, or pulmonary function testing.

Glossitis, with macroglossia, occurs in at least 20% of patients, may be an early symptom, and can lead to dysphagia. The tongue becomes greatly enlarged, and furrows develop. The lateral aspects show indentations from the teeth. Papules or nodules, sometimes with hemorrhage, occur on the tongue (Fig. 26.2).

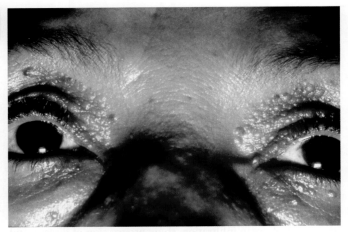

Fig. 26.1 Amyloidosis.

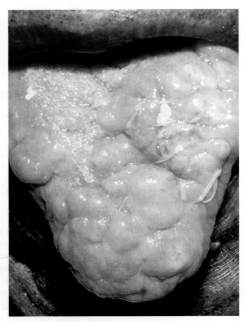

Fig. 26.2 Amyloidosis of the tongue.

Bullous amyloidosis is a rare but important clinical manifestation of amyloidosis. Skin fragility and tense, hemorrhagic or clear, noninflammatory bullae appear at areas of trauma, usually the hands, forearms, and feet. Lesions heal with scarring and milia. The esophagus and oropharyngeal mucosae may also be involved. Histologically, the lesions are subepidermal and pauci-inflammatory. Epidermolysis bullosa acquisita and porphyria cutanea tarda are in the differential diagnoses because they both cause blisters that heal with milia. Amyloid staining may yield negative results, and direct immunofluorescence (DIF) may be falsely positive because of AL protein deposition at the dermoepidermal junction (DEJ). The diagnosis is confirmed by evaluation of the patient's serum and urine for Ig fragments and by amyloid stains or electron microscopy of the skin biopsies.

A diffuse or patchy alopecia, cutis verticis gyrata, and a scleroderma-like, scleromyxedema-like, or a cutis laxa–like appearance have also rarely been described. Cutis laxa–like findings may be generalized or localized to the acral parts. Lesions in the flexors and lateral neck may resemble pseudoxanthoma elasticum (PXE). At times, lesions with cutis laxa–like or PXE-like appearance may

show amyloid bound to elastic fibers. The nail matrix may be infiltrated, resulting in atrophy of the nail plate, presenting as longitudinal striae, partial anonychia, splitting, and crumbling of the nail plate. Cordlike thickening along blood vessels can also occur. Bilateral stenosis of the external auditory canals has been reported. Patients with systemic amyloidosis are at increased risk for skin cancer.

Patients may present with or develop a plethora of systemic findings. Most characteristically, they develop carpal tunnel syndrome, other peripheral neuropathies, a rheumatoid arthritis (RA)–like arthropathy of the small joints, orthostatic hypotension, GI bleeding, nephrotic syndrome, and cardiac disease.

About 90% of patients will have the Ig fragment detectable in the serum or urine; in the other 10%, the serum free light-chain assay will detect a clear excess of one of the light chains (κ or λ), confirming the diagnosis. Also, reduction of the urine free light chains by more than 50% correlates with substantial benefit from treatment. Cardiac troponins are elevated and are powerful prognostic determinants in AL amyloidosis. Elevated troponins are associated with a 6-month survival. AL patients may appear to have prominent deltoid muscles as a result of deposition of amyloid in the muscles (shoulder pad sign). Cardiac arrhythmias and right-sided congestive heart failure are common causes of death.

The prognosis for patients with primary systemic amyloidosis is poor, and therapy is targeted toward decreasing the production of the initial protein that makes the amyloid. Those presenting with neurologic findings survive longer than patients presenting with cardiac disease. Approximately 15% of patients with AL amyloidosis will have myeloma, and 15% of patients with myeloma will have AL amyloidosis.

Secondary Systemic Amyloidosis (AA Amyloidosis)

Secondary systemic amyloidosis is caused by a chronic infectious or inflammatory process. In these conditions, the precursor protein, serum amyloid A (SAA), an acute-phase reactant, is chronically elevated and cannot be adequately cleared from the body. It is processed to AA amyloid in affected tissues. With more effective treatment for chronic infections (especially tuberculosis, schistosomiasis, osteomyelitis, bronchiectasis, pyelonephritis, and decubitus ulcer), infection-related AA amyloid is much less common. Most cases are now related to chronic inflammatory conditions, especially RA, juvenile idiopathic arthritis, ankylosing spondylitis, adult Still disease, inflammatory bowel disease, and Behçet disease. Amyloidosis has also been reported in alkaptonuria. The newer and more aggressive management strategies for these inflammatory conditions have led to reduced numbers or delayed onset of AA amyloidosis in these patients. Maintaining SAA below 4 mg/L is associated with a good outcome in AA amyloidosis. The organs involved most commonly by AA amyloidosis are the kidneys, adrenals, liver, and spleen. The skin is not involved, but biopsy of skin in patients with AA amyloidosis will detect amyloid deposits in the dermis perivascularly. Certain skin conditions, such as hidradenitis suppurativa, stasis ulcers, psoriatic arthritis, and dystrophic epidermolysis bullosa, may be complicated by AA amyloidosis. Many inherited conditions associated with elevated SAA may be complicated by AA amyloidosis as well. These include familial Mediterranean fever, cryopyrin-associated periodic syndromes, and tumor necrosis factor (TNF) receptor–associated periodic syndrome (TRAPS).

Dialysis-Associated Amyloidosis (β_2-Microglobulin Amyloidosis)

β_2-Microglobulin is excreted primarily by the kidneys. In patients with severe renal failure on dialysis or predialysis, the excess β_2-microglobulin may be processed to amyloid in certain tissues.

Almost 100% of patients receiving dialysis for 15 years or more will develop this form of amyloidosis. It primarily affects the synovium, causing musculoskeletal symptoms, carpal tunnel syndrome, and, less often, triggers finger, bone cysts, and spondyloarthropathy. Rarely subcutaneous tumors can arise often of the buttocks overlying the sacrum. Pedunculated sacral masses, lichenoid papules, and localized hyperpigmentation can also be seen. The diagnosis is confirmed by biopsy, which demonstrates that the amyloid material is β_2-microglobulin on immunohistochemical stains. The treatment is high-flux dialysis or kidney transplantation.

Senile Systemic Amyloidosis

Senile systemic amyloidosis is increasingly recognized as an important cause of cardiac disease in the elderly population (>70 years). Carpal tunnel syndrome can also occur. Senile systemic amyloidosis is caused by deposition of normal transthyretin, a transporter protein, in tissue. Skin lesions have not been reported, but vascular deposition has led to tongue necrosis. The diagnosis can be confirmed in about three quarters of patients with a deep abdominal fat biopsy.

CUTANEOUS AMYLOIDOSIS

Primary Localized Cutaneous Amyloidosis

The primary localized cutaneous amyloidoses have been divided into four forms: macular, lichen, nodular, and familial. Macular and lichen forms of amyloidosis are also called "keratinocyte-derived" amyloidosis, frictional amyloidosis, and frictional melanosis. Some cases of these two forms of cutaneous amyloidosis are familial, but the relationship between these and cases of familial primary localized cutaneous amyloidosis is unclear. Patients with macular and lichen amyloidosis often have coexistent atopic dermatitis and the scratching is likely the cause of the amyloid. Nodular and familial cases of cutaneous amyloidosis are rare and have a unique pathogenesis.

Nonfamilial macular and lichen amyloidosis have the same pathogenic basis (rubbing and friction), and overlap cases (biphasic cutaneous amyloidosis) can be seen. Individuals of Asian, Hispanic, or Middle Eastern ancestry seem to be predisposed and use of abrasive devices during bathing is a precipitant. In cases of acquired macular and lichen amyloidosis, the deposited amyloid material contains keratin (primarily keratin 5) as its protein component, strongly suggesting that traumatic damage to basal keratinocytes results in the deposits. A rare form localized to the conchae has been described. Many pruritic skin conditions such as primary biliary cirrhosis and chronic renal failure have been associated.

The histologic picture of acquired macular and lichen amyloidosis is similar; the only difference is the size of the amyloid deposits and the extent of the overlying epidermal changes. The overlying epidermis is frequently hyperkeratotic and focally acanthotic, as a result of the chronic rubbing. Focal necrotic keratinocytes may be observed in the basal cell layer. Microscopic and rarely macroscopic bullae (analogous to those in lichen planus) may be seen. Dermal papillae are expanded by amorphous deposits of amyloid that abut immediately below the epidermis. Melanin deposits are classically present in the amyloid. In cases of postinflammatory hyperpigmentation with incontinence of pigment, the architecture of the areas of dermal melanosis should be examined carefully to exclude amyloidosis. Systemic amyloidosis is excluded by the absence of amyloid deposits around blood vessels. Special stains may be used to confirm the diagnosis, but this is rarely required if the classic histology is found. In difficult cases, immunoperoxidase for keratin will stain the amyloid deposits and confirm the diagnosis of primary cutaneous amyloidosis. DIF may demonstrate immunoglobulin (usually IgM) in a globular pattern in the keratin-derived cutaneous

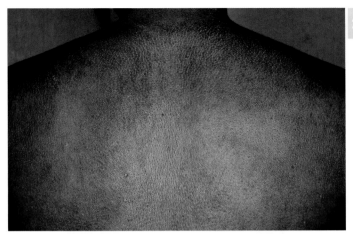

Fig. 26.3 Macular amyloid. (Courtesy Dr. Debabrata Bandyopadhyay.)

amyloidoses, but this is caused by passive absorption rather than specific deposition. This phenomenon is seen in all disorders with prominent apoptosis of keratinocytes.

Macular Amyloidosis

Typically, patients with macular amyloidosis exhibit moderately pruritic, brown, rippled macules characteristically located in the interscapular region of the back (Fig. 26.3). Women outnumber men by 5 : 1 and the disease is chronic. Pigmentation is generally not uniform, giving the lesions a "salt and pepper" or rippled appearance. Many cases of macular amyloid between the scapulae probably result from rubbing dysesthetic areas of notalgia paresthetica. Occasionally, the thighs, shins, arms, breasts, and buttocks may be involved, and these more diffuse cases are usually associated with diffuse pruritus.

Lichen Amyloidosis

Lichen amyloidosis is characterized by the appearance of paroxysmally itchy lichenoid papules, virtually always appearing bilaterally on the shins (Fig. 26.4). Some patients may deny itching but there is still chronic rubbing. Men outnumber women 2 : 1. Lichen amyloidosis may be found in approximately one third of patients with multiple endocrine neoplasia type IIA (see later discussion). The primary lesions are small, brown, discrete, slightly scaly papules that group to form large, infiltrated plaques. Less frequently, these may occur on the thighs, forearms, face, and even the upper back.

Treatment

Treatment of lichen and macular cutaneous amyloidosis is frequently unsatisfactory. Reducing friction is critical. Identifying the cause of the rubbing, and whether it is habit, pruritus, or neuropathy (as in notalgia paresthetica), directs treatment. Occlusion of therapy is helpful because it both enhances topical treatments and provides a physical block to prevent trauma to the skin. High-potency topical corticosteroids can be beneficial, as can intralesional corticosteroid therapy when small areas are involved. Topical tacrolimus 0.1% ointment, psoralen plus ultraviolet A light (PUVA) and with retinoids (Re-PUVA), ultraviolet B (UVB) light, tar, and calcipotriol benefit individual patients. Amitriptyline (for itching), oral retinoids, thalidomide, and systemic immunosuppressants, including corticosteroids, may be used in refractory cases. The pigmentation of macular amyloidosis reportedly has been improved by laser therapy, especially the 532-nm Q-switched neodymium-doped yttrium-aluminum-garnet (Nd:YAG) laser.

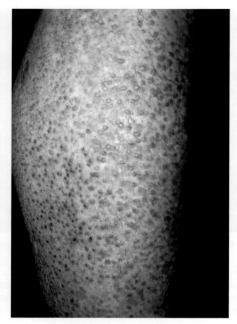

Fig. 26.4 Lichen amyloidosis.

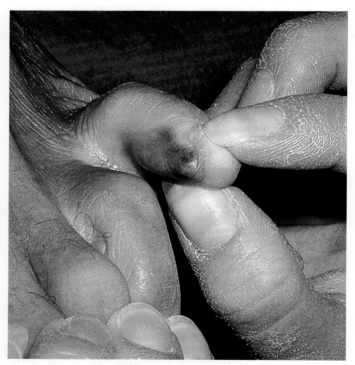

Fig. 26.5 Nodular amyloidosis.

Nodular Amyloidosis

Nodular amyloidosis is a rare form of primary localized cutaneous amyloidosis in which single or, less often, multiple nodules or tumefactions preferentially involve the acral areas (Fig. 26.5). However, trunk, genital, or facial lesions may be seen as well. The lesions are asymptomatic, vary in size from several millimeters to several centimeters, and may grow slowly after their initial appearance. The overlying epidermis may appear atrophic, and lesions may resemble large bullae. Numerous conditions have been

associated with nodular primary localized cutaneous amyloidosis (NPLCA), especially Sjögren syndrome, but also systemic sclerosis (including CREST) and RA. In Sjögren syndrome the nodular amyloidosis typically appears around age 60, more frequently in females, and may precede the diagnosis of Sjögren syndrome by many years. The dermis and subcutis may be diffusely infiltrated with amyloid. The lesions may contain numerous plasma cells and may be early MALT lymphomas. The amyloid in these patients is Ig-derived AL, as is seen in primary systemic amyloidosis, and is unrelated to keratinocyte-related amyloid or to AA amyloid. Progression to systemic amyloidosis may occur in about 7% of cases, so they should be regularly evaluated for progression. Treatment is physical removal or destruction of the lesion with shave removal and destruction of the base.

Secondary Cutaneous Amyloidosis

After PUVA therapy and in benign and malignant cutaneous neoplasms, deposits of amyloid may be found. Most frequently, the associated neoplasms are nonmelanoma skin cancers or seborrheic keratoses. Discoid lupus, dermatomyositis (DM), and graft-versus-host disease (GVHD), as interface dermatoses with apoptosis of keratinocytes, can occasionally demonstrate amyloid in the upper dermis. In all cases, this is keratin-derived amyloid.

Hereditary Cutaneous Amyloidosis Syndromes

Familial primary localized cutaneous amyloidosis (FPLCA) is an autosomal dominant syndrome associated with chronic itching (although some deny it) and cutaneous lesions resembling macular and lichen amyloidosis. It is seen most often in Japan, Brazil, China. The age of onset is 5–18 years. In some families, sun exposure may be an exacerbating factor. Lesions are often widespread on the limbs, chest, and upper and lower back. The buttocks, conchae, and dorsal feet and hands may also be involved. Mutations in the *OSMRβ* or interleukin-31 receptor A *(IL-31RA)* genes that code for proteins that form the two subunits of the transmembrane receptor for IL-31. IL-31 induces the secretion of monocyte chemotactic protein 1 (MCP-1), and levels of MCP-1 expression are very low in FPLCA. MCP-1 recruits monocytes to clear the cellular debris resulting from keratinocyte damage. In the absence of this signal, cellular debris accumulates, and the keratin is processed to amyloid. There is hypersensitivity of small nerve fibers leading to itching. Rare cases of macular amyloidosis in a blaschkoid distribution suggest that mosaicism for FPLCA can be seen, giving this unusual cutaneous distribution. Some FPLCA cases demonstrate extensive poikilodermatous lesions, and less frequently a patient may have multiple morphologies of lichen amyloid, poikiloderma, and dyschromica and even small bullous lesions.

Amyloidosis cutis dyschromica is a distinct type of FPLCA with onset in childhood, no pruritus, a dotted reticular hyperpigmentation with hypopigmented spots without papulation covering almost all the body, and small foci of amyloid just below the epidermis. The nature of the amyloid is unclear. Most affected families are from Japan, and India. UVB hypersensitivity is often reported by these patients.

Multiple endocrine neoplasia type IIA (MEN-2A) syndrome and familial medullary thyroid carcinoma (FMTC) are both caused by mutations in the *RET* proto-oncogene. Cutaneous amyloidosis, most often keratin-derived macular amyloidosis, may be seen in these patients. The macular amyloid may be restricted to the upper back and also unilateral (associated with notalgia paresthetica), or it may be bilateral and more extensive. Age of onset is usually before 20. Thirty of 31 patients with MEN-2A had cutaneous amyloidosis before the diagnosis of MEN-2A was made. In a patient with macular amyloidosis of early onset (before age 20), a careful family history should be taken for endocrine neoplasias, the skin and mucosa examined for neuromas, the blood pressure taken (checking for pheochromocytoma), and the thyroid palpated. A serum calcitonin level should be ordered and, if elevated, a thyroid ultrasound performed.

Pharmaceutical Amyloidosis

When injected into the skin, insulin can create deposits of amyloid composed of the A and B subunits of insulin. This is termed *AIns*. Lesions present as deep subcutaneous nodules, usually on the lower abdomen. If patients inject into these sites, their glucose control may be impaired as their insulin is less effective. Injecting into new areas or surgically removing the nodules improves glucose control. Enfuvirtide, a human immunodeficiency virus (HIV) fusion–inhibiting peptide administered subcutaneously, can produce similar lesions.

FAMILIAL SYNDROMES ASSOCIATED WITH AMYLOIDOSIS (HEREDOFAMILIAL AMYLOIDOSIS)

Most forms of familial amyloidosis are caused by abnormal host proteins that cannot be adequately processed, resulting in their deposition in various tissues in the form of amyloid. Only 50% of patients with hereditary amyloidosis will have a positive family history. Liver, kidney, heart, eye, and nervous system may be involved. Several types of hereditary amyloidosis have been identified; some forms are caused by genetic defects in transthyretin. These are autosomal dominant syndromes, and most affected patients are heterozygotes. Others are caused by a genetic defect in apolipoprotein A-I or A-II, by a defect in gelsolin, fibrinogen A-α, cystatin C, or lysozyme. These syndromes must often be diagnosed by genetic testing or immunohistochemical identification of the deposited pathogenic protein.

Alvarez-Ruiz SB, et al: Unusual clinical presentation of amyloidosis. Int J Dermatol 2007; 46: 503.

An Q, et al: Thalidomide improves clinical symptoms of primary cutaneous amyloidosis. Dermatol Ther 2013; 26: 263.

Andoh T, et al: Increase in sensory sensitivity around, but not in the central part of, the hyperkeratotic papule in lichen amyloidosis. Br J Dermatol 2017; ePub ahead of print.

Arnold SJ, Bowling JC: "Shiny white streaks" in lichen amyloidosis. Australas J Dermatol 2012; 53: 272.

Barja J, et al: Systemic amyloidosis with an exceptional cutaneous presentation. Dermatol Online J 2013; 19: 11.

Chandran NS, et al: Case of primary localized cutaneous amyloidosis with protean clinical manifestations. J Dermatol 2011; 38: 1066.

Chu H, et al: Successful treatment of lichen amyloidosis accompanied by atopic dermatitis by fractional CO_2 laser. J Cosmet Laser Ther 2017; 19: 345.

Clos AL, et al: Role of oligomers in the amyloidogenesis of primary cutaneous amyloidosis. J Am Acad Dermatol 2011; 65: 1023.

De Sousa SM, McCormack AI: Cutaneous lichen amyloidosis in multiple endocrine neoplasia. Intern Med J 2016; 46: 116.

D'Souza A, et al: Pharmaceutical amyloidosis associated with subcutaneous insulin and enfuvirtide administration. Amyloid 2014; 21: 71.

Garg T, et al: Amyloidosis cutis dyschromica. J Cutan Pathol 2011; 38: 823.

Grimmer J, et al: Successful treatment of lichen amyloidosis with combined bath PUVA photochemotherapy and oral acitretin. Clin Exp Dermatol 2007; 32: 39.

Haemel A, et al: Keratinocyte-derived amyloidosis as a manifestation of chronic graft-versus-host disease. J Cutan Pathol 2013; 40: 291.

Hanami Y, Yamamoto T: Secondary amyloid deposition in a melanocytic nevus. Int J Dermatol 2013; 52: 1031.

Hemminki K, et al: Cancer risk in amyloidosis patients in Sweden with novel findings on non-Hodgkin lymphoma and skin cancer. Ann Oncol 2014; 25: 511.

Kalkan G, et al: An alternative treatment model: the combination therapy of narrow band ultraviolet B phototherapy and tacrolimus ointment 0.1% in biphasic amyloidosis. J Pak Med Assoc 2014; 64: 579.

Kandhari R, et al: Asymptomatic conchal papules. Indian J Dermatol Venereol Leprol 2013; 79: 445.

Koh M, et al: A rare case of primary cutaneous nodular amyloidosis of the face. J Eur Acad Dermatol Venereol 2008; 22: 1011.

Konopinski JC, et al: A case of nodular cutaneous amyloidosis and review of the literature. Dermatol Online J 2013; 19: 10.

Kumar S, et al: Skin involvement in primary systemic amyloidosis. Mediterr J Hematol Infect Dis 2013; 5: e2013005.

Kurian SS, et al: Amyloidosis cutis dyschromica. Indian Dermatol Online J 2013; 4: 344.

Kuseyri, O et al: Amyloidosis cutis dyschromica, a rare cause of hyperpigmentation. Pediatrics 2017; 139: e20160170.

LaChance A, et al: Nodular localized primary cutaneous amyloidosis. Clin Exp Dermatol 2014; 39: 344.

Lin JR, et al: Tongue necrosis and systemic vascular amyloidosis. Human Pathol 2011; 42: 734.

Love WE, et al: The spectrum of primary cutaneous nodular amyloidosis. J Am Acad Dermatol 2008; 58: S33.

Meijer JM, et al: Sjögren's syndrome and localized nodular cutaneous amyloidosis. Arthritis Rheum 2008; 58: 1992.

Merchand A, et al: Cutaneous amyloid elastosis revealing multiple myeloma with systemic amyloidosis. Acta Derm Venereol 2013; 93: 204.

Millucci L, et al: Diagnosis of secondary amyloidosis in alkaptonuria. Diagn Pathol 2014; 9: 185.

Mohty D, et al: Cardiac amyloidosis. Arch Cardiovasc Dis 2013; 106: 528.

Nagaste T, et al: Insulin-derived amyloidosis and poor glycemic control Am J Med 2014; 127: 450.

Ostovari N, et al: 532-nm and 1064-nm Q-switched Nd:YAG laser therapy for reduction of pigmentation in macular amyloidosis patches. J Eur Acad Dermatol Venereol 2008; 22: 442.

Pardo Arranz L, et al: Familial poikylodermic cutaneous amyloidosis. Eur J Dermatol 2008; 18: 289.

Park MY, Kim YC: Macular amyloidosis with an incontinentia pigmenti–like distribution. Eur J Dermatol 2008; 18: 477.

Renker T, et al: Systemic light-chain amyloidosis revealed by progressive nail involvement, diffuse alopecia and sicca syndrome. Dermatology 2014; 228: 97.

Ritchie SA, et al: Primary localized cutaneous nodular amyloidosis of the feet. Cutis 2014; 93: 89.

Rothberg AE, et al: Familial medullary thyroid carcinoma associated with cutaneous lichen amyloidosis. Thyroid 2009; 19: 651.

Sakuma TH, et al: Familial primary localized cutaneous amyloidosis in Brazil. Arch Dermatol 2009; 145: 695.

Salim T, et al: Lichen amyloidosis. Indian J Dermatol Venereol Leprol 2005; 71: 166.

Shiao YM, et al: MCP-1 as an effector of IL-31 signaling in familial primary cutaneous amyloidosis. J Invest Dermatol 2013; 133: 1375.

Susantitaphong P, Dember LM, Jaber BL: Dialysis-associated amyloidosis. In: Picken M, Herrera G, Dogan A (Eds.), *Current Clinical Pathology: Amyloid and Related Disorders* (pp. 81-94). New York: 2015, Humana Press.

Taniquchi Y, et al: Cutaneous amyloidosis associated with amyopathic dermatomyositis. J Rheumatol 2009; 36: 1088.

Tey HL, et al: Pathophysiology of pruritus in primary localized cutaneous amyloidosis. Br J Dermatol 2016; 174: 1345.

Tong PL, et al: Primary localized cutaneous nodular amyloidosis successfully treated with cyclophosphamide. Australas J Dermatol 2013; 54: e12.

Walsh N, et al: Sjogren's syndrome and localized nodular cutaneous amyloidosis. Lupus Sci Med 2017; 4.

Wang WH, et al: A new c.1845A→T of oncostatin M receptor-β mutation and slightly enhanced oncostatin M receptor-β expression in a Chinese family with primary localized cutaneous amyloidosis. Eur J Dermatol 2012; 22: 29.

Wat H, et al: Primary systemic (amyloid light-chain) amyloidosis masquerading as pseudoxanthoma elasticum. JAMA Dermatol 2014; 150: 1091.

Wechalekar AD, et al: Systemic amyloidosis. Lancet 2016; 387: 2641.

Weidner T, et al: Primary localized cutaneous amyloidosis. Am J Clin Dermatol 2017; 18: 629.

Yang W, et al: Amyloidosis cutis dyschromica in two female siblings. BMC Dermatol 2011; 11: 4.

Yasuyuki F, et al: Nail dystrophy and blisters as sole manifestations in myeloma-associated amyloidosis. J Am Acad Dermatol 2006; 54: 712.

Yew YW, Tey HL: Itch in familial lichen amyloidosis. Dermatol Ther 2014; 27: 12.

Zhao JY, et al: A case of systemic amyloidosis beginning with purpura. Chin Med J 2012; 125: 555.

■ PORPHYRIAS

Porphyrinogens are the building blocks of all the hemoproteins, including hemoglobin and the cytochrome enzymes, and are produced primarily in the liver and bone marrow. Each form of porphyria has now been associated with a deficiency in an enzyme in the metabolic pathway of heme synthesis. These enzyme deficiencies lead to accumulation of the precursor molecules before the mutation. The precursors are porphyrins, and the diseases are called porphyrias. Many of the porphyrins lead to severe photosensitivity that accounts for most of the cutaneous findings.

Understanding the biosynthetic pathway of heme has clarified the biochemical basis of the porphyrias. Delta-aminolevulinic acid (dALA) is synthesized in the mitochondria by dALA synthetase. From it are formed, successively, porphobilinogen (PBG), uroporphyrin III, coproporphyrin III, and protoporphyrin IX. Protopoyphyrin IX reenters the mitochondrion, to be acted on by ferrochelatase to produce heme. Each step in this process is catalyzed by a specific enzyme. The final product, heme, by negative feedback, represses the production, or activity, of dALA synthetase. If the amount of heme produced is inadequate due to a missing enzyme, dALA synthetase activity may be increased, leading to the production of more porphyrins. Because this enzyme system is inducible, medications that increase the cytochrome drug-metabolizing system in the liver can lead to exacerbation of the porphyrias by increasing the production of the porphyrin intermediates.

The current grouping of the porphyrias is based on the primary site of increased porphyrin production, either liver or bone marrow—the hepatic or erythropoietic porphyrias, respectively. Some include a hepatoerythropoietic category. Congenital erythropoietic porphyria (CEP), X-linked dominant protoporphyria (XLDPP), and erythropoietic protoporphyria (EPP) are the erythropoietic forms. Acute intermittent porphyria (AIP), ALA dehydratase deficiency (ADP), hereditary coproporphyria (HCP), variegate porphyria (VP), and porphyria cutanea tarda (PCT) are the hepatic forms. Hepatoerythrocytic porphyria (HEP) has been classified as either a hepatic or a hepatoerythropoietic type.

Another way to classify the porphyrias is by their symptomatology. This system divides those diseases that have acute episodes, called the acute porphyrias, and those that have skin findings, called the cutaneous porphyrias. Some conditions have both skin disease and acute episodes. The acute porphyrias are ADP, AIP, HCP, and VP. The cutaneous porphyrias are PCT, CEP, XLDPP, and EPP. VP and HCP can have both acute attacks and skin lesions. The acute attacks are induced by conditions that activate the heme biosynthesis pathway. Due to the enzymatic "blocks" as the pathway is activated, large amounts of the heme precursors (specifically, dALA and PBG) are produced by the liver and dumped into the bloodstream. These substances are neurotoxic and affect primarily the autonomic and peripheral nerves. In the cutaneous porphyrias, photosensitivity is observed. The photosensitivity is caused by the absorption of UV radiation in the Soret band (400–410 nm) by the porphyrins, primarily in the blood vessels of the upper dermis. These activated porphyrins are unstable, and as they return to a ground state, they transfer energy to oxygen, creating reactive oxygen species. These unstable oxygen species interact with biologic systems, primarily plasma and lysosomal membranes, causing tissue damage. Mediators released from mast cells and polymorphonuclear leukocytes, acting through complement and metalloproteinase, eicosanoids, or factor XII pathways, may augment tissue effects. The skin lesions are determined by the biochemical nature of the excess porphyrin. Hydrophobic protoporphyrin has more affinity to lipid membranes, specifically endothelial cells. This correlates with acute burning and purpura exhibited in EPP, as well as the prominent reduplication of the basement membranes (seen as perivascular hyaline deposits) of the upper dermal vessels from constant repair of the phototoxic damage to the endothelial cells. The more water-soluble porphyrins (uroporphyrin and coproporphyrins) diffuse into and accumulate in the dermis and along the DEJ. The resulting skin lesions, subepidermal blisters, are caused by the phototoxic damage in this region.

The porphyrias have classically been diagnosed by identifying characteristic clinical and biochemical abnormalities, typically elevated levels of porphyrins in the urine, serum, red blood cells (RBCs), or stool. Because there is some clinical overlap, biochemical testing should be performed to confirm any diagnosis of porphyria. In the acute porphyrias, patients are often asymptomatic between attacks. During attacks, porphyrin assays will be abnormal in all forms of porphyria. Between attacks, some patients with AIP may have normal porphyrin assays so genetic testing is necessary to make the diagnosis. The genetic defect and the points of the most common mutations for each gene are now known for most forms of the porphyrias. Genetic testing is now recommended in most porphyrias, except PCT and EPP. There is considerable clinical overlap in these rarer porphyrias; dual porphyrias exist, with mutations in two different heme synthesis genes; and low-level mutations causing atypical presentations are now well described. Accurate diagnosis in such cases requires genetic testing and allows for genetic counseling and prenatal diagnosis.

PORPHYRIA CUTANEA TARDA

Porphyria cutanea tarda (PCT) is the most common type of porphyria. Patients with PCT present most often in midlife, averaging 45 years of age at disease onset. The disease is characterized by photosensitivity resulting in skin fragility and bullae, especially on sun-exposed parts. The dorsal hands and forearms, ears, and face are primarily affected. The bullae are noninflammatory and rupture easily to form erosions or shallow ulcers (Fig. 26.6). These heal with scarring, milia, and dyspigmentation. Lesions on the legs, especially the shins and dorsal feet, occur primarily in women. There is hyperpigmentation of the skin, especially of the face, neck, and hands. Hypertrichosis of the face, especially over the cheeks and temples. The face and neck, especially in the periorbital area, may show a pink to violaceous tint. Sclerodermatous thickenings may develop on the back of the neck, in the preauricular areas, or on the thorax (Fig. 26.7), fingers, and the scalp, with associated alopecia. There is a direct relationship between the levels of uroporphyrins in the urine and sclerodermatous changes.

Liver disease is frequently present in patients with PCT. A history of alcoholism is common. PCT is a well-recognized cutaneous complication of hepatitis C virus (HCV) infection. All

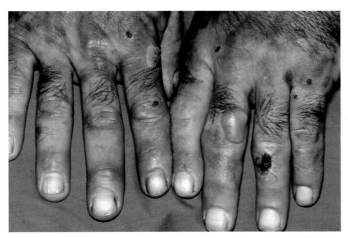

Fig. 26.6 Porphyria cutanea tarda. (Courtesy Steven Binnick, MD.)

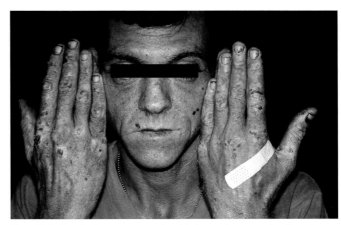

Fig. 26.8 Porphyria cutanea tarda with hemochromatosis. (Courtesy Curt Samlaska, MD.)

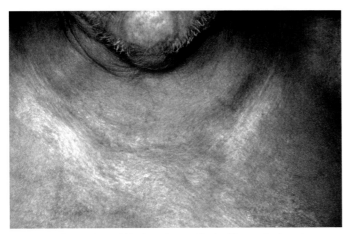

Fig. 26.7 Sclerodermoid lesions in a patient with porphyria cutanea tarda.

PCT patients should be screened for HCV infection especially with new therapeutics so effective for HCV. A recent report documented clearance of PCT with cure of the Hep C. Iron overload in the liver is frequently found in patients with PCT as a result of chemical or viral liver damage, or because a significant number of patients with PCT have a *C282Y* mutation (and a few with *H63D* mutation), the genetic cause of hemochromatosis (Fig. 26.8). The net result of all these liver and iron metabolism abnormalities is an increase in ferritin, with hepatic iron overload. Hepatocellular carcinoma may rarely present with PCT, and PCT patients are at 3.5 times the risk of developing hepatocellular carcinoma.

PCT has been frequently associated with other diseases. It is estimated that adult-onset (type 2) diabetes mellitus occurs in 15%–20% of patients with PCT usually about a decade after the PCT diagnosis. Type 2 diabetes and the metabolic syndrome are associated with hyperferritinemia. It has been proposed that in some patients, nonalcoholic steatohepatitis (NASH) of diabetes may contribute to the development of PCT. In one patient, weight reduction led to improvement of PCT and antimalarial treatment of PCT has lead to enhanced glucose control. Moderate smoking (>10 cigarettes/day) may lead to earlier presentation of PCT by almost a decade. Numerous cases of lupus erythematosus (systemic of purely cutaneous) concomitant with PCT have been reported.

PCT can occur in patients with HIV infection. This is not only accounted for by coexistent HCV infection, which is increased in some risk groups of HIV-infected persons. Subtle porphyrin abnormalities (typically below concentrations capable of inducing disease) are found in HIV disease due to interference with normal porphyrin metabolism. Other risk factors, such as alcoholism, should be evaluated, and the existence of PCT should not be attributed to the HIV disease alone. However, effective anti-HIV therapy has led to improvement of PCT in one HIV/HCV-infected patient.

Estrogen treatment is associated with the appearance of PCT by an unknown mechanism. Before oral contraceptives were introduced, PCT cases occurred predominantly among men, but in most recent series, 60% of cases occurred in men and 40% in women. Men treated with estrogens for prostate cancer may develop PCT.

PCT is caused by a deficiency in the enzyme uroporphyrinogen decarboxylase (UROD). Several types have been described. The most common is the sporadic, nonfamilial form, which represents about 75%–80% of cases. Enzymatic activity of UROD is abnormal in the liver but normal in other tissues. This is the form associated with the cofactors previously listed. The enzyme deficiency is related to loss of enzyme activity caused by the liver damage or estrogens triggering the PCT. The enzyme UROD is inhibited by iron, so conditions that lead to iron overload in the liver (cirrhosis, alcoholism, HCV infection, type 2 diabetes, hemochromatosis) can all induce the clinical signs and symptoms of PCT. Removal of this iron in the liver may result in improvement in PCT. With remission, the enzyme activity in the liver may return to normal.

The second, or familial, type of PCT is an autosomal dominant inherited deficiency of UROD in the liver and RBCs of patients and of clinically unaffected family members. Both the activity and the concentration of the enzyme decrease by about 50%. Multiple genetic defects have been reported that produce the same phenotype. Familial PCT tends to present at an earlier age because it does not require a second insult to the liver to decrease enzyme activity further, and development of PCT before age 20 strongly suggests familial PCT.

A third form, acquired toxic PCT, is associated with acute or chronic exposure to hepatotoxins, specifically, polyhalogenated hydrocarbons such as hexachlorobenzene and dioxin. These patients have biochemical and clinical features identical to those of patients with sporadic and familial PCT.

A diagnosis of PCT can be strongly suspected on clinical grounds. A useful confirmatory test that can be performed in the office is the characteristic pink or coral-red fluorescence of a random urine specimen under Wood's light. A 24-hour urine specimen usually contains less than 100 µg of porphyrins in a normal individual, whereas in the PCT patient it may range from 300 μg to several thousand. The ratio of uroporphyrins to coproporphyrins in PCT is typically 3:1 to 5:1, distinguishing PCT from variegate porphyria. Plasma porphyrins will also be abnormal and may be detected by peak plasma fluorescence at less than 623 nm. The diagnosis of hereditary PCT is made by demonstrating reduced UROD activity in erythrocytes. There are a few reference laboratories in the United States that have special expertise in evaluation of porphyrins and they often recommend shielding the sample from light after it is collected.

Biopsy of a blister reveals a noninflammatory subepidermal bulla with an undulating, festooned base. PAS-positive thickening of blood vessel walls in the upper and middle dermis is present. A useful and highly characteristic, but not diagnostic, feature is the presence of the so-called caterpillar bodies. These eosinophilic, elongated, wavy structures are present in the lower and middle epidermis and lie parallel to the basement membrane zone (BMZ). They stain positively with PAS and are positive for type IV collagen and laminin, suggesting they represent BMZ material present in the epidermis. DIF of involved skin shows IgG and C3 at the DEJ and in the vessel walls in a granular-linear pattern.

Initial treatment of PCT involves removal of all precipitating factors, such as alcohol, medications, and therapy for HCV and metabolic syndrome if present. This may lead to sufficient improvement so that further therapy is not required. Chemical sunscreens are of little value because they do not typically absorb radiation in the near-visible UVA range. Barrier sunscreens such as titanium dioxide and zinc oxide with nonionized zinc oxide being superior. Physical barriers such as hats and gloves should be used.

Phlebotomy is a highly effective treatment for PCT. UROD is inhibited by iron, and removal of hepatic iron may therefore lead to recovery of enzyme activity. Typically, phlebotomy of 500 mL at 2-week intervals is performed until the hemoglobin reaches 10 g/dL or the serum iron 50–60 μg/dL. Ideally, serum ferritin will become normal as well. Urinary porphyrin excretion initially increases, but gradually, 24-hour uroporphyrin levels are greatly reduced, with most patients able to achieve normal levels. This process takes several months, usually requiring a total of 6–10 phlebotomies. As the porphyrins fall, the skin lesions also involute. Initially, blistering improves, then skin fragility decreases, and finally the cutaneous sclerosis and hypertrichosis can eventually reverse. A common error in management is coadministration of oral iron supplementation during the phlebotomies to treat the anemia.

Antimalarial therapy is an alternative to phlebotomy and may be combined with phlebotomy in difficult cases. Antimalarials complex the excess porphyrins, enhancing their excretion. Full doses of antimalarials may produce a severe hepatotoxic reaction. The initial dose is 125 mg of chloroquine or 100–200 mg of hydroxychloroquine twice weekly. Improvement is gradual and parallels the reduction in porphyrins.

The duration of treatment to reach a biochemical remission is the same for phlebotomy and antimalarial therapy, about 6–7 months. This remission may last many years. If the patient relapses, these treatments can be repeated. Alternative treatments, which are rarely required, include desferrioxamine or deferasirox (iron chelation) and erythropoietin treatment. Erythropoietin may be combined with phlebotomy. PCT in renal failure may respond to erythropoietin and low-volume phlebotomy, desferrioxamine given at the end of dialysis, or renal transplantation. If HCV infection coexists, interferon alfa treatment of the HCV infection may lead to improvement of the PCT. The management of PCT associated with hemodialysis is much more difficult. High-flux, high-efficiency hemodialysis should be instituted. N-acetylcysteine, 400 mg of powder dissolved in orange juice twice daily, can be added to augment dialysis. Erythropoietin, at times at very high dose, in combination with miniphlebotomy can be used in anuric patients with PCT not controlled by other methods.

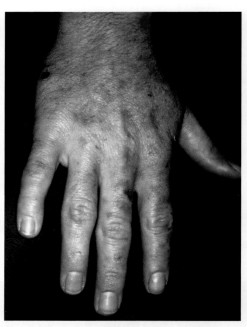

Fig. 26.9 Pseudoporphyria cutanea tarda in a 16-year-old girl who was taking tetracycline for acne.

PSEUDOPORPHYRIA

In certain settings, patients develop blistering and skin fragility identical to PCT, with the histologic features of PCT but with normal urine and serum porphyrins. Hypertrichosis, dyspigmentation, and cutaneous sclerosis do not occur. This pseudoporphyria is most often caused by medications, typically a nonsteroidal antiinflammatory drug (NSAID), usually naproxen. Other NSAIDs, such as nabumetone, diclofenac, and rofecoxib, as well as voriconazole, tetracycline (Fig. 26.9), tolterodine, imatinib mesylate and sunitinib, metformin, finasteride, estrogen, chlorophyll, and multiple other medications, can cause a similar clinical picture. Tanning bed use can also produce pseudo-PCT. Some patients on hemodialysis develop a similar PCT-like picture. Less frequently, dialysis patients develop true PCT. In the anuric dialysis patient, true PCT and pseudo-PCT are distinguished by analysis of serum porphyrins in a laboratory knowledgeable in the normal porphyrin levels in patients undergoing hemodialysis. The treatment of pseudoporphyria is physical sun protection and discontinuance of any inciting medication. Ibuprofen is a safer alternative NSAID that usually does not cause pseudoporphyria. In medication-induced PCT, blistering resolves over several months once the medication is stopped. Skin fragility may persist for much longer. N-acetylcysteine and glutamine have been reported to improved dialysis-associated pseudo-PCT.

HEPATOERYTHROPOIETIC PORPHYRIA

Hepatoerythropoietic porphyria (HEP) is the homozygous form of PCT. It is caused by a homozygous or compound heterozygous deficiency of UROD, which is about 10% of normal in both the liver and the erythrocytes. The biochemical abnormalities are similar to but more marked than those in PCT, although the clinical features are similar to CEP. Dark urine is usually present from birth. In infancy, vesicles occur in sun-exposed skin, followed by sclerodermoid scarring, hypertrichosis, pigmentation, red fluorescence of the teeth under Wood's light, and nail damage. Neurologic disease has been reported. The diagnosis of HEP is confirmed by abnormal urinary uroporphyrins (as seen in PCT), elevated erythrocyte protoporphyrins, and increased coproporphyrins in the feces. In CEP uroporphyrins are elevated in the erythrocytes, allowing differentiation from HEP. Sun protection is necessary, but often inadequate. Bone marrow transplantation, as in CEP, may be required for HEP patients.

VARIEGATE PORPHYRIA

Variegate porphyria (VP) is also known as mixed porphyria, South African genetic porphyria, and mixed hepatic porphyria. VP has an autosomal dominant inheritance with a high penetrance. It results from a decrease in activity of protoporphyrinogen oxidase (PPOX). Between 40% and 70% of patients with VP have skin symptoms, 27% have acute attacks, and only 14% have both acute attacks and skin symptoms. Many affected relatives have silent VP, in which there is reduced enzyme activity but no clinical lesions. Such persons should be identified and evaluated.

VP is characterized by the combination of the skin lesions of PCT and the acute GI and neurologic disease of AIP. In 50% of VP patients, skin lesions are the presenting finding. Vesicles and bullae with erosions, especially on sun-exposed areas, are the chief manifestations. In addition, hypertrichosis is seen in the temporal area, especially in women. Hyperpigmentation of sun-exposed areas is also a feature. Facial scarring and thickening of the skin may give the patient a prematurely aged appearance. The visceral attacks include hypertension, fever and paralysis of the respiratory system.

The presence of VP should be suspected in a patient when findings indicate both PCT and AIP, especially if the patient is of South African ancestry. Fecal coproporphyrins and protoporphyrins are always elevated, and during attacks, urine PBG and ALA are elevated. Normal levels of fecal protoporphyrin in adulthood predicts lack of both skin symptoms and acute attacks. Urinary coproporphyrins are increased over uroporphyrins, distinguishing VP from PCT. Urinary coproporphyrin level greater than 1000 nmol/day predicts increased risk for acute attacks and skin symptoms and indicates the need for preventive treatment to reduce porphyrins. A finding in the plasma of a unique fluorescence at 626 nm is characteristic of VP and distinguishes it from all other forms of porphyria. Lymphocyte PPOX can be measured, but because of the profound founder effect in this condition, genetic testing should be used to confirm the diagnosis.

Treatment of the skin lesions is symptomatic, because antimalarials and phlebotomy are not effective in modifying cutaneous disease in VP. Gonadotropin-releasing hormone (GnRH) analogs may prevent premenstrual attacks, and "hemin" and glucose loading can be used for acute attacks. VP patients, as well as those with other acute porphyrias (HCP and AIP), are at increased risk for hepatocellular carcinoma, and regular liver imaging should be performed after age 50. Education of patients and unaffected PPOX-deficient relatives is essential to avoid triggering medications.

Homozygous VP is a very rare autosomal recessive condition that presents in childhood with PCT-like acral blistering, vermiculate scarring of the cheeks, finger shortening, and developmental delay. Brain myelin is completely absent.

HEREDITARY COPROPORPHYRIA

Hereditary coproporphyria (HCP) is a rare, autosomal dominant porphyria resulting from a deficiency of coproporphyrinogen oxidase (CPO). About one third of patients are photosensitive, with blistering similar to but less severe than in VP. About 35% have acute attacks with GI and neurologic symptoms similar to those seen in AIP and VP. Fecal coproporphyrin III is always increased; urinary coproporphyrin, ALA, and PBG are increased only during attacks. Plasma fluorescence at 619 nm is seen. Mutation screening can be used to confirm the diagnosis and identify unaffected but CPO-deficient relatives. Homozygous hereditary

coproporphyria, or harderoporphyria, is caused by a homozygous defect of CPO, with patients having 10% or less of normal activity. Harderoporphyrin is the natural intermediate between coproporphyrinogen and protoporphyrinogen. There is a report of HCP induced by efavirenz and liver failure in a patient who used "hydroxycut" over-the-counter weight loss therapy. Children present with photosensitivity, hypertrichosis, and hemolytic anemia, and a neonatal form was recently described. The biochemical findings in plasma, feces, and urine are identical to HCP, but more marked.

ERYTHROPOIETIC PROTOPORPHYRIA

Erythropoietic protoporphyria (EPP) is caused by decreased ferrochelatase (FECH) activity. There is a wild-type allele that has low function (hypomorphic) and when this is combined with a mutated allele leading to dysfunction. Therefore it is usually inherited in an autosomal dominant pattern with only one gene being truly mutated (pseudodominant). Autosomal recessive EPP from inheritance of 2 loss of function mutations is much more severe and typically requires bone marrow transplantation. FECH activity below 35% will lead to disease and most affected patients have 10%–25% of normal function. In Europe, up to 10%–15% of the population carries the low-expression (hypomorphic) allele that is only 50% as active as the wild-type enzyme.

Typically, EPP presents early in childhood (3 months to 2 years), although presentation late in adulthood can occur. The diagnosis of EPP in children is frequently delayed because of its rarity. Older children at times are referred to psychiatrists until the diagnosis is suspected.

Unique among the more common forms of porphyria is an immediate burning of the skin on sun exposure. Because the elevated protoporphyrin IX absorbs both in the Soret band and at 500–600 nm, visible light through window glass, in the operating room, or during neonatal exposure to a bili-light (Fig. 26.10) may precipitate symptoms. Infants cry when exposed to sunlight. Erythema, plaquelike edema, and wheals such as those seen in solar urticaria can be seen. These lesions appear solely on sun-exposed areas. In severe cases, purpura is seen in the sun-exposed areas.

With repeated exposure, the skin develops a weather-beaten appearance. Shallow linear or elliptical scars, waxy thickening and pebbling of the skin on the nose and cheeks and over metacarpophalangeal joints, and atrophy of the rims of the ears have been described. Perioral furrow-like scars are characteristic. The dorsal

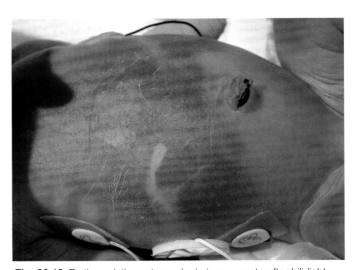

Fig. 26.10 Erythropoietic protoporphyria in a neonate after bili-light exposure.

hands and face of EPP patients appear much older than their chronologic age.

About 2.5% of patients with EPP have a seasonal palmar keratoderma. It is worse in the summer and resolves in winter or with occlusion of the palm by a plaster cast. The keratoderma is waxy and may cover the whole palm or may be localized to the first web space. It is sharply demarcated at the wrist and has no red border. The thickening is moderate in severity. The nails are usually unaffected but may show minimal onycholysis. Patients with nail changes all have true autosomal recessive EPP, with lower levels of erythrocyte protoporphyrin but increased levels of fecal total porphyrin compared with pseudodominant EPP patients. In fact, their erythrocyte protoporphyrin may be near normal. About 45% of patients with autosomal recessive EPP have this keratoderma.

Between 20% and 30% of EPP patients have liver complications because of excessive porphyrin deposits in hepatocytes. This can occur anywhere along the spectrum, from mild elevation of liver function tests to cirrhosis. Only 5% of patients with EPP and liver disease develop hepatic failure, or 0.5%–1% of all EPP patients. Liver transplantation may be required. It is extremely important during liver transplantation to use filters on the operating room lights. A yellow filter that only emits below 470 nm has been reported to be safe. Autosomal recessive inheritance of EPP may be a risk factor for the development of liver failure. There is currently no marker for progressive liver disease (not laboratory porphyrins or genetic defect), so all patients must be monitored. Ten percent of patients develop gallstones, often in childhood. A mild microcytic anemia is present in 25% of patients with EPP, but therapy with iron should be used only if iron deficiency is detected, because it may exacerbate symptoms. Because of sun avoidance, vitamin D deficiency can occur.

The rare syndrome of EPP appearing de novo in adults has been reported multiple times. These cases are associated with a myeloproliferative disorder or myelodysplastic syndrome. The malignant cells in the bone marrow, caused by a translocation, lose the *FECH* gene on chromosome 18, and the patient "acquires" a FECH deficiency. Bone marrow transplantation is associated with resolution of this form of EPP.

Histologically, there is prominent ground-glass, PAS-positive material in the upper dermis, mostly perivascularly. This material is type IV collagen. On DIF, IgG and C3 may be found perivascularly. If an acute purpuric lesion is biopsied, the features of a leukocytoclastic vasculitis may be seen.

A diagnosis of EPP can usually be suspected on clinical grounds, especially if both the acute symptoms and the chronic skin changes are found. Because protoporphyrin IX is not water soluble, urine porphyrin levels are normal. Erythrocyte protoporphyrin is elevated and can be detected by RBC fluorescence. Erythrocyte, plasma, and fecal protoporphyrin can also be assayed to confirm the diagnosis. Erythrocyte protoporphyrin levels in affected persons may range from several hundred to several thousand micrograms per 100 mL of packed RBCs (normal values, <35 μg/100 mL of packed RBCs). Plasma fluorescence shows a peak at 634 nm.

The differential diagnosis of EPP includes hydroa vacciniforme, pseudoporphyria, xeroderma pigmentosa, and solar urticaria. In infancy, before the appearance of the chronic skin changes, erythrocyte porphyrins may need to be screened to confirm the diagnosis. Once chronic changes are present, a skin biopsy will confirm the diagnosis.

The treatment of EPP patients consists of protection from exposure to sunlight with clothing and barrier sunscreens containing titanium dioxide or zinc oxide. Beta carotene, 60–180 mg/day in adults and 30–90 mg/day for children, to maintain a serum level of 600 μg/100 mL, provides some modest protection. As the child grows, the dose must be increased to maintain adequate tissue levels. Early-spring hardening with narrow-band UVB or PUVA (wavelengths below the action spectrum of the incriminated

porphyrins) is being increasingly used. Preliminary trials of colestipol, 2 g daily, and oral zinc sulfate, 600 mg daily, have led to substantial increases in light tolerance in EPP patients. Alpha melanocyte stimulating hormone analogs (alfamelanotide) can help increase photoprotection by inducing melanin production. Alfamelanotide has been demonstrated to increase light tolerance in patients with EPP, in a 20-mg sustained-release form implanted every 2 months. There are reports of increased pigmentation and number of nevi.

X-LINKED DOMINANT PROTOPORPHYRIA

X-linked dominant protoporphyria (XLDPP) is caused by deletions in the dALA synthetase 2 (*ALAS2*) gene. These mutations result in gain of function of the *ALAS2* gene, with increased production of protoporphyrin. Erythrocyte protoporphyrins are elevated from this overproduction of protoporphyrin, which exceeds the capacity of the ferrochelatase to incorporate the protoporphyrin into heme, resulting in excess protoporphyrin. Patients present with symptoms identical to EPP. About 10% of patients in North America with "EPP" actually have XLDPP. More severe photosensitivity and more frequent liver disease (15%) occur in XLDPP due to higher levels of protoporphyrins, about two times higher than in EPP patients. One case of late-onset XLDPP associated with myelodysplasia has been reported. Intravenous iron therapy has improved skin symptoms.

CONGENITAL ERYTHROPOIETIC PORPHYRIA

Congenital erythropoietic porphyria (CEP) is a very rare form of porphyria that is inherited as an autosomal recessive trait. It is caused by a homozygous defect of the enzyme uroporphyrinogen III synthase (UROS). The coinheritance of a gain-of-function mutation in *ALAS2* can lead to a more severe phenotype. One family with a *GATA1* mutation also developed CEP.

CEP presents soon after birth with the appearance of red urine (noticeable on diapers). Severe photosensitivity occurs and may result in immediate pain and burning, so that the affected child screams when exposed to the sun. The laser used in pulse oximeters may lead to skin lesions of the nail bed. Redness, swelling, and blistering occur and result in scarring of the face (Fig. 26.11), dorsal hands, and scalp (with subsequent alopecia). Ectropion can occur, with subsequent corneal damage and loss of vision. Erythrodontia of both deciduous and permanent teeth is also characteristic

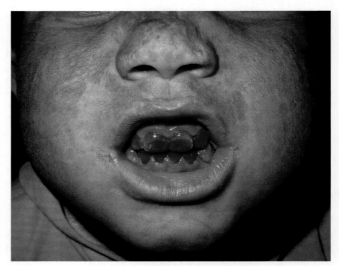

Fig. 26.11 Congenital erythropoietic porphyria. (Courtesy Dr. Debabrata Bandyopadhyay.)

(see Fig. 26.11). This phenomenon is demonstrated by the coral-red fluorescence of the teeth when exposed to Wood's light. Mutilating scars, especially on the face, and hypertrichosis of the cheeks, with profuse eyebrows and long eyelashes, occur. Other features seen in CEP include growth retardation, hemolytic anemia, thrombocytopenia, porphyrin gallstones, osteopenia, and increased fracturing of bones.

A diagnosis of CEP can be easily suspected when an infant has dark urine and is severely photosensitive. There is a direct correlation among the severity of the disease, the levels of plasma porphyrins, and the residual activity of UROS. Abnormally high amounts of uroporphyrin I and coproporphyrin I are found in urine, stool, and RBCs. There is stable red fluorescence of erythrocytes. On biopsy, a subepidermal bulla is seen, identical to that in PCT.

Treatment of CEP patients is strict avoidance of sunlight and, in some cases, splenectomy for the hemolytic anemia. Oral activated charcoal is efficacious, presumably impairing the absorption of endogenous porphyrins. Repeated transfusions of packed RBCs are given at volumes sufficient to maintain the hematocrit level at 33%, turn off the demand for heme, and reduce porphyrin production. A report of using deferasirox to induce iron deficiency also reduced symptoms. Bone marrow transplantation should be considered in severely affected children, typically those with transfusion requiring anemia or thrombocytopenia, but also those with progressive photomutilation and genotypes associated with poor outcome. Proteosome inhibitors and induced pluripotent stem cells are newer treatment opportunities.

Adult-onset CEP is extremely rare, presenting as a mild, photosensitive blistering disease resembling PCT. Usually, patients with CEP live into adulthood. Preauricular fibrosis with loss of earlobes occurs. A corticobasal syndrome resembling Parkinson disease can also occur.

ACUTE INTERMITTENT PORPHYRIA

Acute intermittent porphyria (AIP), the second most common form of porphyria after PCT, is characterized by periodic attacks of abdominal pain (up to 95% of patients), GI disturbances (up to 90% of patients), pain and paresis (50%–70%), seizures (10%–20%), and mental symptoms (40%–60%), including agitation, hallucinations, and depression. Skin lesions do not occur because the elevated porphyrin precursors are not photosensitizers. AIP is inherited as an autosomal dominant trait and is caused by a deficiency in PBG deaminase, which has 50% activity in affected persons. Only 10% of those with the genetic defect develop disease, but all may be at risk for primary liver cancer. AIP is particularly common in Scandinavia, especially Lapland. AIP usually presents after puberty in young adulthood, and women outnumber men 1.5:1 to 2:1.

Severe abdominal colic is most often the initial symptom of AIP. Patients usually have no abdominal wall rigidity, although tenderness and distention are present. Nausea, vomiting, and diarrhea or constipation accompany the abdominal pain. Peripheral neuropathy, mostly motor, is present. Severe pain in the extremities occurs. Optic atrophy, diaphragmatic weakness, respiratory paralysis, flaccid quadriplegia, facial palsy, and dysphagia are some of the many neurologic signs.

Attacks of AIP are triggered by certain medications and other conditions. These triggers frequently require increased hepatic heme synthesis (e.g., to make the cytochrome P450 enzymes required for metabolism of medications). Progesterone is one trigger, explaining the increased prevalence of AIP in women and the relationship to menses. Anticonvulsants, griseofulvin, rifampin, and sulfonamides are common drugs implicated in triggering AIP. The implicated medication list is constantly being modified as new drugs enter the market. The website of the European Porphyria Initiative is the best source for an up-to-date list of both patients and health care providers (www.porphyria-europe.com). Crash dieting, cigarette smoking, infections, and surgery are additional triggers.

A diagnosis of AIP is established by finding elevated levels of urinary PBG and increased dALA in the plasma and urine during attacks. During remissions, the diagnosis can be confirmed in 88% of patients by detecting elevated urinary PBG. A normal test between attacks suggests less likelihood of subsequent attacks. Erythrocyte and fecal porphyrin levels are normal. AIP must be distinguished from VP, CP, and ALA dehydratase deficiency porphyria (ALAD), an autosomal recessive condition presenting in an almost identical manner to AIP. Increased dALA in the urine is found in ALAD patients and those with lead poisoning.

No specific treatment is available for AIP. It is important for the patient to avoid such precipitating factors as a wide variety of medications, including sex steroid hormones, and to maintain adequate nutrition. Glucose loading has been used extensively and appears to be beneficial in many cases. Hematin infusions, in the form of heme arginate, result in clinical improvement and a marked decrease in ALA and PBG excretion. Early treatment may ameliorate attacks. The phenothiazines (e.g., chlorpromazine) may be helpful for pain; opiates and propoxyphene are also useful for analgesia. Because 10% of patients with AIP die of hepatoma (without the development of cirrhosis), yearly ultrasound and alpha-fetoprotein determination should be undertaken in all AIP patients over age 50.

TRANSIENT ERYTHROPORPHYRIA OF INFANCY (PURPURIC PHOTOTHERAPY-INDUCED ERUPTION)

Paller et al. reported seven infants exposed to 380–700 nm blue lights for the treatment of indirect hyperbilirubinemia who developed marked purpura in skin exposed to UV light. Extensive blistering and erosions occurred in one patient. Biopsies of the skin showed hemorrhage without epidermal changes in the cases associated with purpura, and a pauci-inflammatory, subepidermal bulla in the patient with blistering. The infants had all received transfusions. Elevated plasma coproporphyrins and protoporphyrins were found in the four infants examined. The pathogenesis is unknown.

Allo G, et al: Bone mineral density and vitamin D levels in erythropoietic protoporphyria. Endocrine 2013; 44: 803.

Azak A, et al: Pseudoporphyria in a hemodialysis patient successfully treated with oral glutamine. Hemodial Int 2013; 17: 466.

Badadams EL, et al: Cascade testing of primary care blood samples with hyperferritinaemia identifies subjects with iron overload and porphyria cutanea tarda. Ann Clin Biochem 2014; 51: 499.

Balwani M, et al; Porphyrias Consortium of the NIH-Sponsored Rare Diseases Clinical Research Network. Erythropoietic protoporphyria, autosomal recessive. 2012 Sep 27 [Updated 2017 Sep 7]. In: Adam MP, Ardinger HH, Pagon RA, et al., editors. GeneReviews [Internet]. Seattle: University of Washington, Seattle.

Balwani M, et al: Loss-of-function ferrochelatase and gain-of-function erythroid-specific 5-aminolevulinate synthase mutations causing erythropoietic protoporphyria and X-linked protoporphyria in North American patients reveal novel mutations and a high prevalence of X-linked protoporphyria. Mol Med 2013; 19: 26.

Beer K, et al: Pseudoporphyria. J Drugs Dermatol 2014; 13: 990.

Bentley DP, Meek EM: Clinical and biochemical improvement following low-dose intravenous iron therapy in a patient with erythropoietic protoporphyria. Br J Haematol 2013; 163: 277.

Berghoff AT, English JC: Imatinib mesylate–induced pseudoporphyria. J Am Acad Dermatol 2011; 63: e14.

Bishop DF, et al: Molecular expression and characterization of erythroid-specific 5-aminolevulinate synthase gain-of-function mutations causing X-linked protoporphyria. Mol Med 2013; 19: 18.

Blouin JM, et al: Therapeutic potential of proteasome inhibitors in congenital erythropoietic porphyria. Proc Natl Acad Sci USA 2013; 110: 18238.

Crawford RI, et al: Transient erythroporphyria of infancy. J Am Acad Dermatol 1996; 35: 833.

Ergen EN, et al: Is non-alcoholic steatohepatitis a predisposing factor to porphyria cutanea tarda? Photodermatol Photoimmunol Photomed 2013; 29: 106.

Erwin A, et al; Porphyrias Consortium of the NIH-Sponsored Rare Diseases Clinical Research Network. Congenital erythropoietic porphyria. 2013 Sep 12 [Updated 2016 Apr 7]. In: Adam MP, Ardinger HH, Pagon RA, et al., editors. GeneReviews [Internet]. Seattle: University of Washington, Seattle.

Frank J, et al: Photosensitivity in the elderly—think of late-onset protoporphyria. J Invest Dermatol 2013; 133: 1467.

García-Martín P, et al: Phototolerance induced by narrow-band UVB phototherapy in severe erythropoietic protoporphyria. Photodermatol Photoimmunol Photomed 2012; 28: 261.

Gibson GE, et al: Coexistence of lupus erythematosus and porphyria cutanea tarda in 15 patients. J Am Acad Dermatol 1998; 38: 569.

Gonzalez-Estrada A, et al: Sporadic porphyria cutanea tarda: treatment with chloroquine decreases hyperglycemia and reduces development of metabolic syndrome. Eur J Intern Med 2014; 25: e76.

Grimes R, et al: A case of hereditary coproporphyria precipitated by efavirenz. AIDS 2016; 30: 2142.

Haimowitz S, et al: Liver failure after Hydroxycut use in a patient with undiagnosed hereditary coproporphyria. J Gen Intern Med 2015; 30: 856.

Hasegawa K, et al: Neonatal-onset hereditary coproporphyria. JIMD Rep 2017; 37: 99.

Hatch MM, et al: Can curative antivirals benefit porphyria cutanea tarda in hepatitis C patients? J Eur Acad Dermatol Venereol 2017; 31: e194.

Hivnor C, et al: Cyclosporine-induced pseudoporphyria. Arch Dermatol 2003; 139: 1373.

Holme SA, et al: Seasonal palmar keratoderma in erythropoietic protoporphyria indicates autosomal recessive inheritance. J Invest Dermatol 2009; 129: 599.

Horner ME, et al: Cutaneous porphyrias part I. Int J Dermatol 2013; 52: 1464.

Jenkins SM, et al: Rash associated with phototherapy in a 2-day-old preterm male infant. NeoReviews 2016; 17: e55.

Katoulis AC, et al: Pseudoporphyria associated with non-hemodialyzed renal insufficiency, successfully treated with oral *N*-acetylcysteine. Case Rep Dermatol Med 2013; 2013: 271873.

Katugampola RP, et al: A management algorithm for congenital erythropoietic porphyria derived from a study of 29 cases. Br J Dermatol 2012; 167: 888.

Katugampola RP, et al: Congenital erythropoietic porphyria. Br J Dermatol 2012; 167: 901.

LaRusso J, et al: Phototherapy-induced purpuric eruption in a neonate. J Clin Aesthet Dermatol 2015; 8: 46.

Lenfestey A, et al: Metformin-induced pseudoporphyria. J Drugs Dermatol 2012; 11: 1272.

Liu LU, et al; Porphyrias Consortium of the NIH-Sponsored Rare Diseases Clinical Research Network. Familial porphyria cutanea tarda. 2013 Jun 6[Updated 2016 Sep 8]. In: Adam MP, Ardinger HH, Pagon RA, et al., editors. GeneReviews [Internet]. Seattle: University of Washington, Seattle.

Livideanu CB, et al: Late-onset X-linked dominant protoporphyria: an etiology of photosensitivity in the elderly. J Invest Dermatol 2013; 133: 1688.

Mungo N, et al: An unusual case of voriconazole induced pseudoporphyria. Ann Allergy Asthma Immunol 2017; 119: S24.

Oshikawa Y, et al: Photosensitivity and acute liver insufficiency in late-onset erythropoietic protoporphyria with a chromosome 18q abnormality. Case Rep Dermatol 2012; 4: 144.

Paller AS, et al: Purpuric phototherapy-induced eruption in transfused neonates. Pediatrics 1997; 100: 360.

Panton NA, et al: Iron homeostasis in porphyria cutanea tarda. J Clin Pathol 2013; 66: 160.

Pérez NO, et al: Pseudoporphyria induced by imatinib mesylate. Int J Dermatol 2014; 43: e143.

Petersen AB, et al: Zinc sulphate: a new concept of treatment of erythropoietic protoporphyria. Br J Dermatol 2012; 166: 1121.

Pham HP, et al: Therapeutic plasma exchange in a patient with erythropoietic protoporphyria status post orthotropic liver transplantation as a bridge to hematopoietic stem cell transplantation. J Clin Apher 2014; 29: 341.

Pinder VA, et al: Homozygous variegate porphyria presenting with developmental and language delay in childhood. Clin Exp Dermatol 2013; 38: 737.

Santo Domingo D, et al: Finasteride-induced pseudoporphyria. Arch Dermatol 2011; 147: 747.

Sarkany RP, et al: Acquired erythropoietic protoporphyria as a result of myelodysplasia causing loss of chromosome 18. Br J Dermatol 2006; 155: 464.

Schneider-Yin X, et al: Hepatocellular carcinoma in a variegate porphyria. Acta Derm Venereol 2010; 90: 512.

Seager MJ, et al: X-linked dominant protoporphyria. Clin Exp Dermatol 2014; 39: 35.

Sidorsky TI, et al: Development of corticobasal syndrome in a patient with congenital erythropoietic porphyria. Parkinsonism Relat Disord 2014; 20: 349.

Singal AK, Anderson KE: Variegate porphyria. 2013 Feb 14. In: Adam MP, Ardinger HH, Pagon RA, et al., editors. GeneReviews [Internet]. Seattle: University of Washington, Seattle.

Singal AK, et al: Liver transplantation in the management of porphyria. Hepatology 2014; 60: 1082.

Sivaramakrishnan M, et al: Narrowband ultraviolet B phototherapy in erythropoietic protoporphyria. Br J Dermatol 2014; 170: 987.

Spelt JM, et al: Vitamin D deficiency in patients with erythropoietic protoporphyria. J Inherit Metab Dis 2010; 33: S1.

Tewari A, et al: A case of extensive hyaline deposition in facial skin caused by erythropoietic protoporphyria. Br J Dermatol 2014; 171: 412.

Thom G, et al: Leukocytoclastic vasculitis masking chronic vascular changes in previously undiagnosed erythropoietic protoporphyria. J Cutan Pathol 2013; 40: 966.

Tintle S, et al: Cutaneous porphyrias part II. Int J Dermatol 2014; 53: 3.

Tishler PV, Rosner B: Treatment of erythropoietic protoporphyria with the oral sorbent colestipol. J Am Acad Dermatol 2013; 70: 391.

Turnbull N, et al: Diclofenac-induced pseudoporphyria. Clin Exper Dermatol 2014; 39: 348.

Van Tuyll van Serooskerken AM, et al: Digenic inheritance of mutations in the coproporphyrinogen oxidase and protoporphyrinogen oxidase genes in a unique type of porphyria. J Invest Dermatol 2011; 131: 2249.

Vasconcelos P, et al: Desferrioxamine treatment of porphyria cutanea tarda in a patient with HIV and chronic renal failure. Dermatol Ther 2014; 27: 16.

Verma A, et al: Congenital erythropoietic porphyria. Br J Dermatol 2014; 171: 422.

Wahlin S, et al: Protection from phototoxic injury during surgery and endoscopy in erythropoietic protoporphyria. Liver Transpl 2008; 14: 1340.

Whatley SD, Badminton MN: Role of genetic testing in the management of patients with inherited porphyria and their families. Ann Clin Biochem 2013; 50: 204.

Willis ZI, et al: Phototoxicity, pseudoporphyria, and photo-onycholysis due to voriconazole in a pediatric patient with leukemia and invasive aspergillosis. J Pediatric Infect Dis Soc 2014; 4: e22.

Zhao CY et al: A case series of chlorophyll-induced pseudoporphyria and proposed pathogenesis. J Am Acad Dermatol 2015; 72: AB213.

CALCINOSIS CUTIS

Cutaneous calcification results from deposits of calcium and phosphorus in the skin. Calcinosis cutis is divided into five forms. Dystrophic calcinosis includes conditions in which calcification occurs in damaged tissue, usually collagen or elastic tissue. Serum calcium and phosphorus levels are normal. DM is a classic example of a disease in which the inflamed skin can have dystrophic calcinosis. Metastatic calcification refers to deposition of calcium resulting from elevated serum levels of calcium or phosphorus. Hyperparathyroidism can cause this form of calcification. Iatrogenic and traumatic calcinosis is associated with medical procedures or occupational exposures that may involve both tissue damage and local elevated calcium concentrations. Idiopathic calcinosis cutis refers to the forms of cutaneous calcification of unknown cause with normal serum calcium. In osteoma cutis, true bone is formed in the skin. Calciphylaxis is discussed in Chapter 35.

DYSTROPHIC CALCINOSIS CUTIS

The dystrophic type occurs in a preexisting lesion or inflammatory process. Systemic calcium metabolism is normal, and lesions affect the skin only. Dystrophic calcinosis cutis presents as small deposits of chalky granular material around the fingers and on the elbows, at areas of trauma. The deposits may spontaneously extrude from the skin. The dystrophic form often occurs in limited scleroderma (the CREST syndrome: calcinosis cutis, Raynaud phenomenon, esophageal disorders, sclerodactyly, and telangiectasia) (Fig. 26.12), as well as polymyositis systemic sclerosis overlap. Pancreatic and lupus panniculitis typically demonstrate dystrophic calcification, but the process tends to remain microscopic. Dystrophic calcification of facial lesions of systemic lupus erythematosus and GVHD have also been reported. Patients with Werner syndrome and PCT may also develop calcifications within the scleroderma-like lesions.

Calcinosis cutis occurs in about 10% of patients with DM, especially juvenile cases. Fingertip ulcers and disease duration are associated with calcinosis cutis. Autoantibodies to NXP-2 increase the risk for cutaneous calcinosis in DM by 15-fold. MDA-5 antibodies are associated with fingertip ulcers but don't seem to be independently associated with calcification. Calcification in DM can occur in multiple forms, including hard nodules or plaques in the subcutaneous or periarticular areas; large tumors; deposits in the intermuscular fascia leading to decreased mobility; and as an exoskeleton.

Various benign and malignant neoplasms may develop calcification or ossification, with pilomatrixomas and pilar cysts most frequently reported. Nephrogenic systemic fibrosis, Hutchinson-Gilford progeria, and poikiloderma with neutropenia (Clericuzio type) may all be complicated by calcinosis cutis.

The treatment of dystrophic calcification is determined by the location, size/extent, and underlying condition. Limited surgical

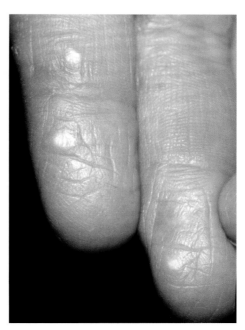

Fig. 26.12 Dystrophic calcinosis cutis.

removal, as needed to control discomfort, can be very beneficial. Curetting out the calcium deposits around the fingers can bring dramatic relief to the patients with CREST and DM. Systemic therapies have not been consistently beneficial, with some patients having dramatic response, and the same treatment for the same disease having no effect in other patients. Bisphosphonates (alendronate, etidronate, pamidronate), diltiazem (30–180 mg/day), warfarin, antiinflammatory agents, TNF inhibitors, intravenous immune globulin (IVIG), thalidomide, and colchicine have all been used as single agents or in combination. Sodium thiosulfate, 10%–25% by topical application and 12.5 mg/50 mL by injection, has reduced dystrophic calcifications in various areas. Eight patients with dystrophic calcification treated with lithotripsy had a decrease in size of the calcium deposits and a dramatic reduction in pain.

METASTATIC CALCINOSIS CUTIS

Metastatic calcinosis cutis is a rare entity characterized by calcifications in the skin due to elevated serum calcium, and sometimes hyperphosphatemia. It is often associated with bone loss or destruction, with the bone providing the source of the elevated serum calcium. Conditions associated with metastatic calcinosis include parathyroid neoplasms, primary hyperparathyroidism, chronic renal failure, hypervitaminosis D, sarcoidosis, and excessive intake of milk and alkali. Destruction of bone by osteomyelitis, leukemia, Paget disease of the bone, myeloma, and metastatic carcinoma may lead to elevated serum calcium and metastatic calcification. In calcinosis cutis with hyperparathyroidism, many skin manifestations are seen, with small, firm, white papules, about 1–4 mm in diameter, occurring symmetrically in the popliteal fossae, over the iliac crests, and in the posterior axillary lines. At times, metastatic calcinosis cutis localizes to areas of damaged elastic tissue (e.g., striae, solar elastosis).

The most common metabolic condition associated with metastatic calcification is renal failure. Usually, there is an elevated phosphorus level and secondary hyperparathyroidism, resulting in high calcium and phosphorus production and deposition of calcium phosphate in tissues. Less often, cutaneous calcification in renal disease can occur with normal serum calcium and phosphorus levels. Three forms of cutaneous calcification in renal disease have been described: tumoral calcinosis, calcifying panniculitis, and calciphylaxis. Tumoral calcinosis is a rare complication of renal disease. Managing the metabolic abnormalities may lead to resolution of the large deposits of calcium.

Often, calcifying panniculitis and calciphylaxis occur in the same patient at the same time, suggesting a common pathogenesis. Isolated, firm, indurated nodules, usually on the legs or thighs in the subcutaneous fat, have been called calcifying panniculitis. Usually these are seen with the most severe complication of the abnormal calcium and phosphorus metabolism of renal disease, calciphylaxis. This life-threatening condition leads to livedo reticularis and ischemic tissue necrosis (see Chapter 35).

IATROGENIC AND TRAUMATIC CALCINOSIS CUTIS

Medical procedures that may inadvertently introduce calcium into tissue, in association with tissue trauma, may lead to cutaneous calcification. This has been reported after extravasation of calcium chloride or calcium gluconate infusion and after electroencephalography or electromyography. Electrode paste is high in calcium, and the skin is traumatized during the procedure, leading to calcifications at the sites of electrode insertion. The most common setting is on the scalp of children. Performing frequent heel sticks in neonates has led to similar lesions that are characteristically on the side of the heel. Injections of low-molecular-weight calcium–containing heparins in patients with renal failure may result in calcification at the sites of injection. Frequent subcutaneous injection of interferon beta in the abdomen has resulted in localized calcification in the fat. Lesions spontaneously resolve over months. Topical thiosulfate has also been reported to help speed resolution.

During liver transplantation, hypocalcemia can result from calcium chelation by the citrate in transfused blood products. Intravenous calcium infusions are regularly given. Calcifications on the upper extremities have been reported, occurring 1–3 weeks after transplantation and resolving over 6 months.

Traumatic calcinosis may occur as a result of occupational exposure to calcium-containing materials, as in the cases reported in oil-field workers and coal miners. Exposure of the skin to cloth sacks of calcium chloride, limewater compresses, and refrigerant calcium chloride can all cause calcinosis cutis.

IDIOPATHIC CALCINOSIS CUTIS

Idiopathic Scrotal Calcinosis

Idiopathic scrotal calcinosis is the most common form of idiopathic calcinosis cutis. Lesions present in young to middle-aged adult men as multiple, asymptomatic, firm, round, yellow papules from several millimeters up to 1 cm in diameter (Fig. 26.13). The papules resemble infundibular follicular cysts. Similar lesions, usually 1 mm to several millimeters in size, may be seen rarely in girls or women on the labia majora. In men with scrotal lesions, similar lesions rarely will be found on the shaft of the penis, termed idiopathic calcinosis cutis of the penis. Calcinosis of the areola can have a similar appearance and is extremely rare. Histologically, localized deposits of calcium are surrounded by a foreign body reaction. At least some are calcified scrotal infundibular cysts. Why they have such a high proclivity to calcification at this anatomic location is unclear. Treatment is not required, but surgical removal cures individual lesions.

Subepidermal Calcified Nodule and Milia-Like Idiopathic Calcinosis Cutis

These two similar conditions are uncommon but distinct types of idiopathic calcinosis. Subepidermal calcified nodule occurs most frequently as one or a few lesions on the eyelid, scalp, or face of

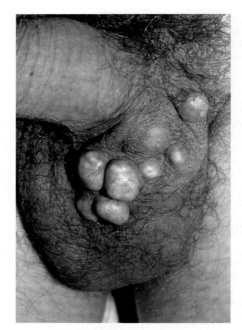

Fig. 26.13 Scrotal calcinosis.

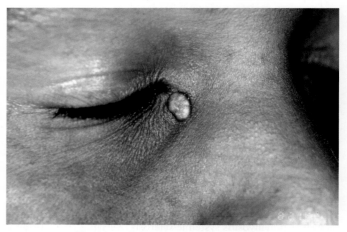

Fig. 26.14 Subepidermal calcified nodule.

children (Fig. 26.14) and occasionally adults. Males outnumber females by almost 2:1, and the average age at onset is 7 years. Lesions present as fixed, noninflamed papules that closely resemble those of molluscum contagiosum with a central umbilication. The affected children usually do not have an underlying medical condition. The differential diagnosis includes pilomatrixomas, which also commonly occur on the head and neck, including the eyelids.

A similar condition, milia-like idiopathic calcinosis cutis, has a wider distribution; eyelids, hands, feet, elbows, and knees are common sites. Two thirds of patients have Down syndrome. Treatment is not required, but surgical removal will cure any individual lesion.

Tumoral Calcinosis

Investigation of the rare cases of tumoral calcinosis, discovery of the causal genes, and development of animal models have led to improved understanding of the mechanisms of ectopic mineralization. Familial tumoral calcinosis has two genetic causes.

Normophosphatemic familial tumoral calcinosis (NFTC) is seen in young adults, primarily of African descent. Lesions are associated with antecedent trauma. The genetic cause is mutation in *SAMD9*. Hyperphosphatemic familial tumoral calcinosis (HFTC) is characterized by periarticular calcifications. Mutations in three genes have been described as causing this syndrome: fibroblast growth factor 23 (*FGF23*), *GALNT3*, and *KLOTHO*. Most patients present before the second decade of life. Three quarters of these individuals have affected siblings. Multiple lesions predominate, and there is no preceding history of trauma. The serum calcium level is normal, but serum phosphorus and calcitriol levels are elevated.

Lesions in both types present as large subcutaneous masses of calcium overlying pressure areas and large joints, usually the hips, elbows, shoulders, or knees. Skin involvement, apart from the tumoral masses, is extremely rare but may occur as localized calcinosis cutis. The internal organs are not involved, and serum calcium levels are generally normal. Surgical excision has been the mainstay of therapy; however, recurrences are frequent after incomplete removal. Various dietary restrictions to lower calcium and phosphorus intake have shown some success. The combination of a phosphate binder and a carbonic anhydrase inhibitor (acetozolamide), along with a low-phosphorus diet, has been reported to lead to significant improvement.

OSTEOMA CUTIS

Bone formation within the skin may be primary, occurring in cases with no preceding lesion; metastatic, in cases associated with abnormalities of parathyroid metabolism; or dystrophic, in which ossification occurs in a preexisting lesion or inflammatory process.

Primary osteoma cutis occurs in several clinically distinct disorders: Albright's hereditary osteodystrophy (AHO), pseudohypoparathyroidism (PHP), progressive osseous heteroplasia (POH), and widespread or single, platelike osteoma cutis (PLOC). Mutations in all four of these conditions occur in the *GNAS* gene.

Progressive osseous heteroplasia is a rare form of cutaneous ossification initially seen between birth and 6 months of age, often in the first month of life. Females are preferentially affected. Lesions begin as small papules that can coalesce to large plaques. Sometimes these plaques will have small, firm, calcified papules overlying them. Lesions are randomly distributed and may be unilateral or may involve only one anatomic area. There is no preceding trauma or inflammatory phase. Serum calcium, phosphorus, parathyroid hormone (PTH), and calcitriol are normal, but alkaline phosphatase (ALP), lactate dehydrogenase (LDH), and creatine phosphokinase (CPK) may be elevated, indicating increased bone formation (ALP) or muscle destruction (CPK and LDH). Histologically, the lesions reveal intramembranous bone formation and can affect the soft tissues as well as skin. Only calcification without ossification may be found in superficial dermal biopsies, so a deep biopsy, including subcutaneous fat, may be required to confirm the diagnosis. The condition is progressive and can lead to serious sequelae, including ulceration, infection, and severe pain. Plate-like osteoma cutis occurs in newborns or young children, but also in adults. It is not associated with dysmorphic features or abnormalities of calcium or phosphorus metabolism, but shows intramembranous bone formation histologically. These disorders are most likely polar ends of a spectrum of disease; one family has been described with members having either condition. AHO is characterized by childhood development of intramembranous bone formation in the dermis and subcutaneous tissue (see Chapter 24). The cutaneous ossifications may be noted soon after birth and are usually multiple, small, superficial plaques that favor the scalp, hands, feet, periarticular regions, abdomen, and chest wall. Small lesions are of little consequence, but large subcutaneous masses may disrupt underlying structures. The patient may have characteristic dysmorphic features and pseudohypoparathyroidism or pseudopseudohypoparathyroidism. AHO also is associated with mutations of the *GNAS1* gene.

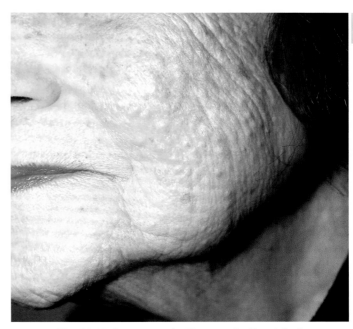

Fig. 26.15 Osteoma cutis. (Courtesy Dr. Don Adler.)

Multiple miliary osteomas of the face are clinically the most common form of osteoma cutis. These are usually seen in women (Fig. 26.15). The osteomas probably represent dystrophic ossification because they occur in patients with acne, are localized to the face, and are associated with acne scars. If oral tetracycline or minocycline is taken to treat the acne, the cutaneous osteomas may be pigmented or may fluoresce under Wood's light. Improvement with topical tretinoin, erbium:YAG laser, or incision, curettage, and primary closure has been reported.

AlWadani S, et al: Subepidermal calcified nodules of the eyelid differ in children and adults. Ophthal Plast Reconstr Surg 2017; 33: 304.

Bair B, Fivenson D: A novel treatment for ulcerative calcinosis cutis. J Drugs Dermatol 2011; 10: 1042.

Balin SJ, et al: Calcinosis cutis occurring in association with autoimmune connective tissue disease. Arch Dermatol 2012; 148: 455.

Caravaglio JV, et al: Multiple miliary osteoma cutis of the face associated with Albright hereditary osteodystrophy in the setting of acne vulgaris. Dermatol Online J 2016; 23.

Chabra IS, Obagi S: Evaluation and management of multiple miliary osteoma cutis. Dermatol Surg 2014; 40: 66.

Chantorn R, Shwayder T: Poikiloderma with neutropenia: report of three cases including one with calcinosis cutis. Pediatr Dermatol 2012; 29: 463.

Cheng PS, Lai FJ: Sporotrichoid-like calcinosis cutis and calcifications in vessel walls and eccrine sweat glands following intravenous infusion and calcium gluconate. Br J Dermatol 2012; 166: 892.

Cho E, et al: Subcorneal milia-like idiopathic calcinosis cutis. Ann Dermatol 2013; 25: 249.

Chung EH, et al: Iatrogenic calcinosis cutis of the upper limb arising from the extravasation of intravenous anticancer drugs in a patient with acute lymphoblastic leukemia. Arch Plast Surg 2016; 43: 214.

Cohen PR, Tschen JA: Idiopathic calcinosis cutis of the penis. J Clin Aesthet Dermatol 2012; 5: 23.

Elli FM, et al: Screening for *GNAS* genetic and epigenetic alterations in progressive osseous heteroplasia. Bone 2013; 56: 276.

Fabreguet I, et al: Calcinosis cutis associated with connective tissue diseases. Rev Med Suisse 2015; 11: 668.

Finer G, et al: Hyperphosphatemic familial tumoral calcinosis. Am J Med Genet A 2014; 164A: 1545.

Fox GN, et al: Acral milia-like idiopathic calcinosis cutis in a child with Down syndrome. Pediatr Dermatol 2013; 30: 263.

Hershkovitz D, et al: Functional characterization of SAMD9, a protein deficient in normophosphatemic familial tumoral calcinosis. J Invest Dermatol 2011; 131: 662.

Huh JY, et al: Novel nonsense *GNAS* mutation in a 14-month-old boy with plate-like osteoma cutis and medulloblastoma. J Dermatol 2014; 41: 319.

Jaeger VA, et al: Metastatic calcinosis cutis in end-stage renal disease. Proc (Bayl Univ Med Cent) 2017; 30: 368.

Killedar MM, et al: Idiopathic scrotal calcinosis. Indian J Surg 2016; 78: 329.

Kucukemre Aydin B, et al: Osteoma cutis. Pediatr Int 2013; 55: 257.

Li Q, Uitto J: Mineralization/anti-mineralization networks in the skin and vascular connective tissues. Am J Pathol 2013; 183: 10.

Lopez AT, et al: Facial calcinosis cutis in a patient with systemic lupus erythematosus. JAAD Case Rep 2017; 3: 460.

Lykoudis EG, et al: Huge recurrent tumoral calcinosis needing extensive excision and reconstruction. Aesth Plast Surg 2012; 36: 1194.

Macbeth AE, et al: Calcified subcutaneous nodules. Br J Dermatol 2007; 157: 624.

Myllylä RM, et al: Multiple miliary osteoma cutis is a distinct disease entity. Br J Dermatol 2011; 164: 544.

Nagai Y, et al: Nephrogenic systemic fibrosis with multiple calcification and osseous metaplasia. Acta Derm Venereol 2008; 88: 597.

Nakamura S, et al: Hutchinson-Gilford progeria syndrome with severe skin calcinosis. Clin Exp Dermatol 2007; 32: 525.

Nguyen Y, et al: Cutaneous nodules in the genital area in a patient With chronic graft-vs-host disease. JAMA Dermatol 2017; 153: 465.

Ozuguz P, et al: Multiple sub-epidermal calcified nodule mimicking eruptive xanthoma. Indian J Dermatol 2013; 58: 406.

Piombino L, et al: A novel surgical approach to calcinosis cutis using a collagen-elastin matrix. J Wound Care 2013; 22: 22.

Reiter N, et al: Calcinosis cutis. Part I. J Am Acad Dermatol 2011; 65: 1.

Reiter N, et al: Calcinosis cutis. Part II. J Am Acad Dermatol 2011; 65: 15.

Riahi RR, Cohen PR: Multiple miliary osteoma cutis of the face after initiation of alendronate therapy for osteoporosis. Skinmed 2011; 9: 258.

Shah V, Shet T: Scrotal calcinosis results from calcification of cysts derived from hair follicles. Am J Dermatopathol 2007; 29: 172.

Shinjo SK, Souza FH: Update on the treatment of calcinosis in dermatomyositis. Rev Bras Reumatol 2013; 53: 211.

Slavin RE, et al: Tumoral calcinosis—a pathogenetic overview. Int J Surg Pathol 2012; 20: 462.

Smith GP: Intradermal sodium thiosulfate for exophytic calcinosis cutis of connective tissue disease. J Am Acad Dermatol 2013; 69: e146.

Smith S, Henson J: Extensive dystrophic calcinosis cutis. J Clin Rheumatol 2017; 23: 445.

Valenzuela A, et al: Identification of clinical features and auto-antibodies associated with calcinosis in dermatomyositis. JAMA Dermatol 2014; 150: 724.

Ward S, et al: Three cases of osteoma cutis occurring in infancy. Australas J Dermatol 2011; 52: 127.

Yong AS, et al: Vitamin D deficiency–associated calcinosis cutis, with secondary granulomatous changes. Clin Exp Dermatol 2013; 38: 814.

■ LIPID DISTURBANCES

XANTHOMAS

Xanthomas are deposits of lipids in tissue. For the dermatologist, the important areas to look for lipid deposits are on the skin, tendon, and eyes. Xanthomas appear when abnormalities of lipid amount or processing occur in the body and thus are important markers of underlying dyslipidemia and potentially increased cardiovascular risk. The histologic features in all varieties of xanthoma are similar, characterized by the presence of numerous large, xanthoma or foam cells, that are phagocytes (fat-laden histiocytes). The cells may be multinucleated. In addition to the foam cells, touton giant cells can occur. Clefts representing cholesterol and fatty acids dissolved by processing agents may be noted. Generally, a connective tissue reaction occurs around the nests of foam cells, and in old lesions, most of the foam cells are replaced with fibrosis. CD68 and adipophilin immunoperoxidase may aid in identifying foam cells.

In addition to inherited genetic defects of molecules involved in lipid homeostasis, systemic diseases (e.g., diabetes mellitus) and medications (e.g., systemic retinoids) can also cause hyperlipidemias and result in xanthomas especially in people who have some genetic predisposition. The names of the various forms of cutaneous xanthomas are based on clinical morphology. Numerous genetic mutations that result in hyperlipidemias have been identified. Several different genetic diseases may present with similar cutaneous xanthoma patterns, so referral to a "lipid" clinic is recommended for xanthoma patients with familial patterns of hyperlipidemia, as well as for those without an obvious medical cause for their dyslipidemia. The morphologies are relatively specific for the associated elevated lipid, or triglycerides. The clinical phenotype of the lesions will be discussed first and then the syndromes associated with each type of xanthoma are reviewed.

Lipids can either be endogenous or exogenous (ingested). Exogenous lipids in the diet are absorbed and incorporated into triglyceride-rich chylomicrons. These are hydrolyzed by the action of lipoprotein lipase and certain cofactors, including apoprotein CII. The resulting remnants are taken up by the liver. Endogenously produced very-low-density lipoproteins (VLDLs) are synthesized in the liver and, again through the action of lipoprotein lipase. They are converted to cholesterol-rich IDLs and eventually into low-density lipoproteins (LDLs). These are then available for uptake by peripheral tissues, as well as by the liver. Specific receptors in different tissues guide uptake of LDL, IDL, and chylomicron remnants. Abnormalities of lipoprotein lipase, the apolipoproteins, cofactors, receptors, or stimulators or retarders of endogenous production or catabolism, whether on a genetic or a sporadic basis, may accelerate or block the pathway in different areas. If blockade occurs early and results in elevation of triglyceride-rich particles, eruptive xanthoma may result. If a defect occurs later in the pathway and cholesterol-rich particles accumulate, xanthelasma, tuberous xanthomas, and tendinous xanthomas should be expected, along with premature atherosclerotic cardiovascular disease.

Xanthoma Tuberosum

Tuberous xanthomas are variously found as flat or elevated and rounded, grouped, yellowish or orange nodules located over the joints, particularly on the elbows and knees (Fig. 26.16). The lesions are indurated and tend to coalesce. They may also occur over the face, knuckles, toe joints, axillary and inguinal folds, and buttocks. Solitary lesions may be found. Early lesions are usually

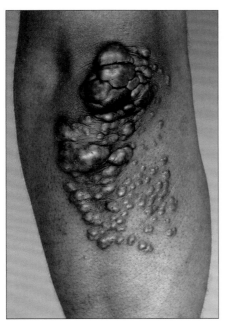

Fig. 26.16 Tuberous xanthomas.

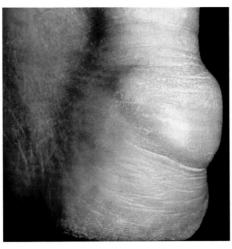

Fig. 26.17 Tendinous xanthomas.

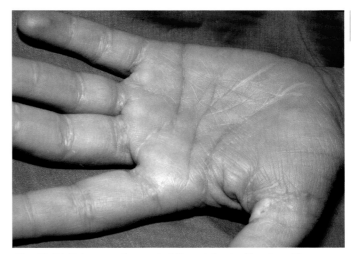

Fig. 26.18 Palmar xanthomas in biliary cirrhosis. (Courtesy Steven Binnick, MD.)

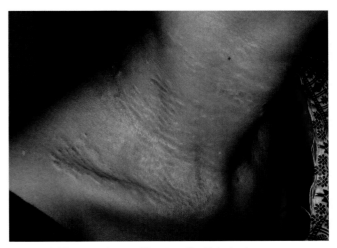

Fig. 26.19 Plane xanthoma. (Courtesy Dr. Debabrata Bandyopadhyay.)

bright yellow or erythematous; older lesions tend to become fibrotic and lose their color. Pedunculated, fissured, and suppurative nodules may also be seen.

Xanthoma Tendinosum

Papules or nodules 5–25 mm in diameter are found in the tendons, especially in extensor tendons on the backs of the hands and dorsa of the feet and in the Achilles tendons (Fig. 26.17). These predominate in conditions with elevated LDL cholesterol (see later discussion) and can be seen in association with tuberous xanthomas and xanthelasma. The lesions also occur in obstructive liver disease, diabetes, myxedema, cerebrotendinous xanthomatosis, and phytosterolemia.

Palmar Xanthomas

Palmar xanthomas consist of nodules and irregular yellowish plaques involving the palms and flexural surfaces of the fingers. Striated

xanthomas appear as yellowish streaks that follow the distribution of creases of the palms and soles (Fig. 26.18). These lesions are seen in familial dysbetalipoproteinemia, multiple myeloma, and primary biliary cirrhosis. In patients with primary hyperlipoproteinemias, palmar xanthomas have been proposed to be pathognomonic of familial dysbetalipoproteinemia.

Xanthoma Planum (Plane Xanthoma)

Plane xanthomas appear as flat macules or slightly elevated plaques with a yellowish tan or orange coloration of the skin spread diffusely over large areas. Characteristically, plane xanthomas may occur around the eyelids, neck, trunk, shoulders, or axillae (Fig. 26.19). These well-defined macular patches may be situated on the inner surface of the thighs and antecubital and popliteal spaces. Although these can be seen as a complication of elevated lipid levels, as in primary biliary cirrhosis, they are the one form of xanthoma that may not be associated with increased lipids. Normolipemic plane xanthomas are most frequently seen in patients with myeloma or a monoclonal gammopathy and less often in other myelodysplasias, such as mycosis fungoides, lymphoma, leukemia, and adult T-cell lymphoma/leukemia caused by human lymphotropic virus type 1 (HTLV-1). In myeloma and monoclonal gammopathy,

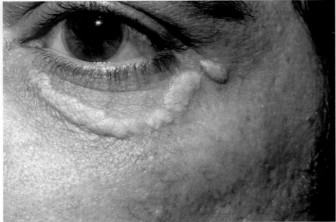

Fig. 26.20 Xanthelasma.

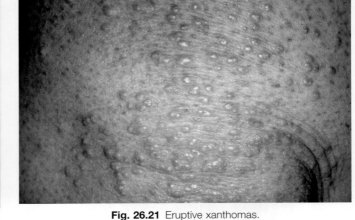

Fig. 26.21 Eruptive xanthomas.

the paraprotein complexes with LDL, and these complexes are phagocytosed by histiocytes in tissue, forming the plane xanthomas. In patients with monoclonal gammopathy–associated xanthoma, a reduced CH50 and reduced C4 (both in 80% of patients) are also usually detected, as well as a decreased C1 inhibitor level (50%) and the presence of a cryoglobulin (30%). Treatment of the underlying myelodysplasia may lead to resolution of the xanthomas.

A rare form of normolipemic xanthomatosis can occur in childhood termed *normolipemic papuloeruptive xanthomatosis*. Yellowish papules 2–5 mm in diameter occur on the face. They can coalesce to form large confluent plaques, especially on the face, nape of the neck, and axillae. Spontaneous involution occurs. It is unclear whether this is a rare disease in its own right or a variant of benign cephalic histiocytosis or papular xanthoma of childhood.

Xanthelasma Palpebrarum (Xanthelasma)

Xanthelasma is the most common type of xanthoma. It occurs on the eyelids and is characterized by soft, chamois-colored or yellowish orange oblong plaques, usually near the inner canthi (Fig. 26.20). They usually appear between ages 40 and 60. The xanthelasmas vary from 2–30 mm in length and are usually symmetric. Xanthelasmas are typically seen without other forms of xanthomas and often with "normal" lipids. In 60% of xanthelasma patients, however, dyslipidemia is detected. New patients with xanthelasma should be evaluated with a full lipoprotein profile, as well as a careful history and physical examination. Consultation with a lipid clinic may be appropriate. Early (childhood) onset of xanthelasma should suggest a hereditary lipid abnormality, especially familial hypercholesterolemia. Xanthelasma has been reported after injection of hyaluronic acid and polymethacrylate collagen fillers.

Treatment of xanthelasma is discussed here because of its uniqueness among the xanthomas, in that surgical therapy is often successful. The best method is surgical excision. The anesthetized lesion is grasped with mouse-tooth forceps and clipped off with scissors, and the skin edges are undermined and sutured. Excellent cosmetic results are obtained, even if the wound is not closed. Fulguration, trichloroacetic acid cauterization, and carbon dioxide (CO$_2$), erbium:YAG, or Nd:YAG laser therapy are other methods. Complete removal of the lesions does not preclude the possibility that other new lesions will develop.

Eruptive Xanthoma

Xanthoma eruptivum consists of small, yellowish orange to reddish brown papules that appear in crops over the entire body (Fig. 26.21). The papules may be surrounded by an erythematous halo and may be grouped in various favored locations, such as the buttocks, extensor surfaces of the arms and thighs, knees, inguinal and axillary folds, and oral mucosa. Koebnerization may occur. Pruritus is variable. Eruptive xanthomas strongly suggest the presence of elevated triglyceride levels. Eruptive xanthomas are seen most often in poorly controlled type 2 diabetes mellitus but can also be seen in chronic renal failure, hypothyroidism, and treatment with estrogens, corticosteroids, or systemic retinoids.

PRIMARY HYPERLIPOPROTEINEMIAS

Lipoproteins are responsible for carrying fat molecules in the blood, and the β-lipoproteins (VLDL, LDL, IDL, and chylomicron) have ApoB on their surface so they can invade into the intima of blood vessels and lead to artherosclerotic plaques. α-Lipoproteins (HDL) are antiartherogenic. Frederickson classified hyperlipoproteinemias into six types on the basis of electrophoretic patterns, now called the World Health Organization International Classification of Diseases (WHO ICD) hyperlipoprotein (HLP) phenotypes, as follows.

- HLP1/type I (chylomicronemia): excess chylomicrons (triglycerides).
  - Clinical: There are monogenic as well as polygenic forms. The monogenic familial forms present in childhood and the polygenic forms typically require a secondary illness such as diabetes to unmask the predisposition toward hypertriglyceridemia. Familial monogenic chylomicronemia (hypertriglycerideamia) is caused by many different gene mutations including lipoprotein lipase deficiency. With levels of triglycerides above 1000 mg/dL, a high risk of pancreatitis and eruptive xanthomas exists (Fig. 26.22). This monogenic familial version often manifests in early childhood with xanthomas, pancreatitis, lipema retinalis, abdominal pain and failure to thrive. Alipogene tiparvovec is a gene therapy available to treatment.
- HLP2A/type IIa (familial hypercholesterolemia): excess β-lipoprotein (LDL predominantly).
  - Familial hypercholesterolemia (FH) has an HLP2A (Frederickson type IIa) lipid profile. It is caused by mutations in multiple genes, most often the LDL receptor. One in 500 persons carry a mutation in this gene, and these heterozygotes present with planar, tendon, or tuberous xanthomas from age 30–60. Their LDL cholesterol is two to three times normal, and they have a twofold to threefold increase in cardiovascular disease. People with homozygous recessive

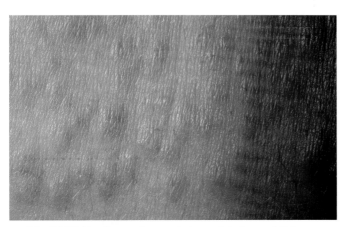

Fig. 26.22 Eruptive xanthomas in lipoprotein lipase deficiency.

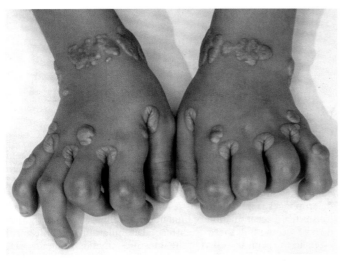

Fig. 26.23 Homozygous hypercholesterolemia with intertriginous xanthomas.

defects in LDL receptor gene will present in childhood (teens or early twenties) with xanthomas, LDL cholesterol four to six times normal, and cardiovascular disease with aortic stenosis. Homozygous FH patients may have large xanthelasmas (xanthomatous pseudospectacles) and xanthomas of the interdigital web spaces and the gluteal cleft (Fig. 26.23). Statin medications have less effect due to the lack of LDL receptor, but a medication (evinacumab) that targets angiopoietin-like 3 (a liver-secreted protein that increases LDL and VLDL in blood) was effective in a small series.

- HLP2B/type IIb (familial combined hyperlipidemia): excess β-lipoprotein (VLDL and LDL).
  - Clinical: similar to the polygenic HLP1 there is typically a secondary event such as diabetes or metabolic syndrome that leads to artherosclerosis but xanthomas are less common.
- HLP3/type III (familial dysbetalipidemia): increased IDL and chylomicron remnants.
  - Clinical: eruptive or tuberous xanthomas. Planar and palmar crease xanthomas also noted and the latter have been deemed pathognemonic for HLP3
- HLP4/type IV: increased pre–β-lipoprotein (VLDL).
  - Clinical: increased cardiovascular risk along with hypertension and hyperuricemia.

- HLP5/type V (mixed dyslipidemia): increased pre–β-lipoproteins (VLDL) and chylomicrons.
  - Clinical: Presentation typically in adults. Risk for pancreatitis due to eruptive xanthoma, hepatosplenomegaly, or lipema retinalis.

Familial Apoprotein CII Deficiency

Patients with the rare familial apoprotein CII deficiency lack lipoprotein lipase activator and have very high triglyceride levels, up to 10,000 mg/dL. They are at risk for pancreatitis and eruptive xanthomas.

SECONDARY HYPERLIPOPROTEINEMIA

Obstructive Liver Disease (Xanthomatous Biliary Cirrhosis)

Lipoprotein X is an aberrant protein formed when there is biliary obstruction of multiple different etiologies including primary biliary cirrhosis and Alagille syndrome. Lipoprotein X has the ability to carry large quantities of free cholesterol and phospholipids, but when oxidized in the periphery and taken up by macrophages it leads to foamy macrophages that can be detected in xanthomas. The xanthomatous lesions are plane xanthomas, with lesions on the face, flexor surfaces of the extremities, and trunk. Striate palmar and plantar lesions and xanthelasmas can also be seen. Tuberous xanthomas may occur. Pruritus is extremely severe. Hepatomegaly and jaundice are present. Cholestyramine can help in allaying pruritus. The triglycerides are not elevated, and the plasma is clear, showing no chylomicrons, giving a type II lipoprotein pattern.

Alagille syndrome is a congenital disorder characterized by intrahepatic bile ductular atresia, patent extrahepatic bile ducts, a characteristic facies (prominent forehead, deep-set eyes, straight nose, and small, pointed chin), cardiac murmur, vertebral and ocular abnormalities, low intelligence, and hypogonadism. It is an autosomal dominant inherited condition. There is persistent cholestasis early in life, with pruritus and hyperbilirubinemia. Lipid levels increase by age 2 years, and planar or papular xanthomas may occur. Alagille syndrome is treatable with cholestyramine and fat-soluble vitamins leading to long-term improvement.

Pancreatitis

Hyperlipidemia in the hyperchylomicronemic syndromes (HLP types I and V) may cause pancreatitis; it may be recurrent, and pancreatic necrosis and death may occur. Alternatively, pancreatitis may cause type I or V hyperlipoproteinemia by inducing insulin deficiency and a relative lack of lipoprotein lipase activity. A triglyceride level of 1000 mg/dL is required for pancreatitis to occur in the setting of hypertriglyceridemia. The amylase may be normal, but the lipase will be elevated.

Medication-Induced Hyperlipoproteinemia

Estrogens, by decreasing lipoprotein lipase activity and increasing VLDL synthesis, may cause HLP1 or HLP5 patterns. Eruptive xanthomas may occur. Oral prednisone may induce insulin resistance and cause HLP4 or HLP5 patterns to develop. Oral retinoids, indomethacin, protease inhibitors for HIV, and olanzapine may also cause eruptive xanthomas through hypertriglyceridemia.

Cerebrotendinous Xanthomatosis

Cerebrotendinous xanthomatosis is a rare autosomal recessive disease caused by an accumulation of cholestanol in plasma lipoproteins, brain, and xanthomatous tissue. The underlying abnormality is a mutation in the sterol 27-hydroxylase gene

(*CYP27A1*) in the mitochondria, leading to incomplete oxidation of cholesterol to bile acids. As a result, cholestanol, an intermediate, accumulates in tendons, brain, heart, lungs, and the lens of the eye. The disorder is characterized by prominent tendinous xanthomas, especially of the Achilles tendons (not present in all patients), macroglossia, progressive neurologic dysfunction in many forms, infantile diarrhea, developmental cataracts, and atherosclerotic coronary artery disease. Plasma cholestanol is elevated and can exceed more than 10 times normal levels. Patients with cerebrotendinous xanthomatosis are treated with chenodeoxycholic acid, and early treatment can prevent the progressive neurologic impairment.

Sitosterolemia (Phytosterolemia)

In sitosterolemia, a rare autosomal recessive disorder, plasma plant sterols are extremely elevated (>30 times normal). This disorder is caused by mutations in the genes encoding the ABCG5 and ABCG8 transporters, which are expressed only in the intestine and liver. In the intestine, they pump plant sterols and cholesterol out of intestinal cells back into the lumen of the gut, limiting sterol and cholesterol absorption. In the liver, they pump plant sterols into the bile, aiding in their excretion. Absence of either of these genes results in increased absorption and decreased excretion of plant sterols, leading to their accumulation in the body. There is also excess absorption of cholesterol leading to somewhat elevated LDL levels. Patients develop tendinous xanthomas, xanthelasma, and tuberous, intertriginous, and palmar xanthomas (similar to HLP IIa familial hypercholesterolemia). The diagnosis of sitosterolemia should be considered in any child or adolescent with xanthomas and an LDL less than 130–400 (thus lower than would be expected with homozygous LDL receptor mutation). It can also present as dietary-responsive hypercholesterolemia in infancy. Phytosterolemia can also mimic FH in the adult because most patients also have type IIa hyperlipoproteinemia and accelerated atherosclerosis due to the enhanced absorption of cholesterol. Treatment is dietary restriction of plant sterols, cholesterol, and some shellfish (clam, oysters, scallops) whose sterols are also hyperabsorbed. In addition, bile sequestrants (chenodeoxycholic acid) can be used. Ezetimibe, an inhibitor of NPC1L1 (Niemann-Pick C1-like 1), inhibits absorption of plant sterols and can be effective in reducing plasma sterol levels.

Verruciform Xanthoma

Verruciform xanthoma (VX) is an uncommon lesion that occurs as a reddish or light orange hyperkeratotic plaque or papillomatous growth with a pebbly or verrucous surface. The most common site is the oral mucosa. VX has also been reported on other mucosal surfaces, genitalia (Fig. 26.24), lower extremities, and elsewhere. On the external genitalia in men, the lesions frequently resemble condylomata acuminata and are not associated with any other condition. Disorders with damage of the papillary dermis have been associated with VX, including recessive dystrophic epidermolysis bullosa, lymphedema, and GVHD. Similarly, vulvar VX have been associated with lichen sclerosus, lichen planus, Paget disease, and radiodermatitis. Additionally, VX has been reported in a patient with psoriatic lesions undergoing PUVA therapy and in psoriasiform skin lesions in an HIV-positive patient. Histologically, there is acanthosis without atypia, parakeratosis, and xanthoma cells in the papillary dermis. In CHILD syndrome (congenital hemidysplasia with ichthyosiform erythroderma and limb defects) the blaschkoid epidermal lesions have histologic characteristics of VX. In a small percentage of VX patients, a mutation in the *NSDHL* gene (3β-hydroxysteroid dehydrogenase) has been found. This gene is also mutated in CHILD syndrome, explaining why it and VX share the same histology. In one child, a genital VX responded to topical imiquimod treatment.

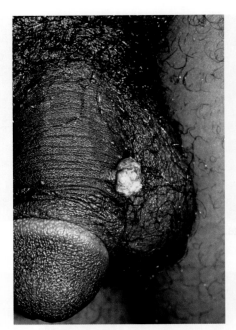

Fig. 26.24 Verruciform xanthoma.

Familial α-Lipoprotein Deficiency (Hypoalphalipoproteinemia, Tangier Disease)

Tangier disease is caused by mutations in the cell membrane protein ABCA1, which mediates the secretion of excess cholesterol from cells into the HDL metabolic pathway. This results in a profound deficiency of HDL and accumulation of cholesterol in tissue macrophages. The characteristic clinical finding is enlarged yellow tonsils from accumulation of lipid in this localized area. Xanthomas do not occur, but there is diffuse accumulation of cholesterol esters in the skin, as well as in the intestines, thymus, bone marrow, lymph nodes, and spleen. Peripheral neuropathy, splenomegaly (with thrombocytopenia), and premature coronary artery disease are other features of Tangier disease.

Björkhem I: Cerebrotendinous xanthomatosis. Curr Opin Lipidol 2013; 24: 283.

Blankenship DW, et al: Verruciform xanthoma of the upper extremity in the absence of chronic skin disease or syndrome. J Cutan Pathol 2013; 40: 745.

Boyd AS, Roffwarg D: Cutaneous verrucous xanthoma in a bone marrow transplant recipient with recessive dystrophic epidermolysis bullosa. Pediatr Dermatol 2013; 30: 480.

Brahm A, et al: Hypertriglyceridemia. Nutrients 2013; 5: 981.

Broeshart JH, et al: Normolipemic plane xanthoma associated with adenocarcinoma and severe itch. J Am Acad Dermatol 2003; 49: 119.

Brown CA, et al: Tuberous and tendinous xanthomata secondary to ritonavir-associated hyperlipidemia. J Am Acad Dermatol 2005; 52: S86.

Chung HG, et al: CD 30 (Ki-1)–positive large-cell cutaneous T-cell lymphoma with secondary xanthomatous changes after radiation therapy. J Am Acad Dermatol 2003; 48: S28.

Curtis JA, et al: Xanthelasma palpebrarum after artecoll (polymethylmethacrylate collagen) injections to the bilateral tear troughs. Am J Dermatopathol 2017; 39: 553.

D'Acunto C, et al: Xanthelasma palpebrarum. Br J Dermatol 2013; 168: 437.

Dey A, et al: Cardiovascular profile of xanthelasma palpebrarum. Biomed Res Int 2013; 2013: 932863.

Duzayak S, et al: Acute pancreatitis with eruptive xanthoma. BMJ Case Rep 2017 Oct 9;2017.

Fite C, et al: Vulvar verruciform xanthoma. Arch Dermatol 2011; 147: 1087.

Fujimoto N, et al: Verruciform xanthoma results from epidermal apoptosis with galectin-7 overexpression. J Eur Acad Dermatol Venereol 2013; 27: 922.

Fujimoto N, et al: Ultraviolet irradiation may generate plane xanthomas on mycosis fungoides. Br J Dermatol 2013; 168: 213.

Gaudet D, et al: ANGPTL3 inhibition in homozygous familial hypercholesterolemia. N Engl J Med 2017; 377: 296.

Gaudet D, et al: Long-term retrospective analysis of gene therapy with alipogene tiparvovec and its effect on lipoprotein lipase deficiency-induced pancreatitis. Hum Gene Ther; 27: 916.

Gregorious S, et al: Treatment of mycosis fungoides with bexarotene results in remission of diffuse plane xanthomas. J Cutan Med Surg 2013; 17: 52.

Guo Y, et al: Successful treatment of verruciform xanthomas with imiquimod. J Am Acad Dermatol 2013; 69: e184.

Helm TN, et al: Verruciform xanthomas with porokeratosis-like features but no clinically apparent lymphedema. J Cutan Pathol 2012; 39: 887.

Heng JK, et al: Treatment of xanthelasma palpebrarum with a 1064-nm, Q-switched Nd:YAG laser. J Am Acad Dermatol 2017; 77: 728.

Huang HY, et al: Normolipemic papuloeruptive xanthomatosis in a child. Pediatr Dermatol 2009; 26: 360.

Johansen CT, Hegele RA: Genetic bases of hypertriglyceridemic phenotypes. Curr Opin Lipidol 2011; 22: 247.

Kashif M, et al: An unusual presentation of eruptive xanthoma. Medicine (Baltimore) 2016; 95: e4866.

Kose R: Treatment of large xanthelasma palpebrarums with full-thickness skin grafts obtained by blepharoplasty. J Cutan Med Surg 2013; 17: 197.

Kwiterovich PO: Diagnosis and management of familial dyslipoproteinemias. Curr Cardiol Rep 2013; 15: 371.

Lee HY, et al: Outcomes of surgical management of xanthelasma palpebrarum. Arch Plast Surg 2013; 40: 380.

Mehra S, et al: A novel somatic mutation of the 3β-hydroxysteroid dehydrogenase gene in sporadic cutaneous verruciform xanthoma. Arch Dermatol 2005; 141: 1263.

Mignarri A, et al: A suspicion index for early diagnosis and treatment of cerebrotendinous xanthomatosis. J Inherit Metab Dis 2014; 37: 421.

Park JH, et al: Sitosterolemia presenting with severe hypercholesterolemia and intertriginous xanthomas in a breastfed infant. J Clin Endocrinol Metab 2014; 99: 1512.

Park JS, et al: Hepatic ABC transporters and triglyceride metabolism. Curr Opin Lipidol 2012; 23: 196.

Rosmaninho A, et al: Diffuse plane xanthomatosis associated with monoclonal gammopathy. An Bras Dermatol 2011; 86: S50.

Rothschild M, et al: Pathognomonic palmar crease xanthomas of apolipoprotein E2 homozygosity-familial dysbetalipoproteinemia. JAMA Dermatol 2016; 152: 1275.

Ryu DJ, et al: Verruciform xanthoma of the palatal gingiva. J Korean Assoc Oral Maxillofac Surg 2013; 39: 292.

Shirdel A, et al: Diffuse normolipaemic plane xanthomatosis associated with adult T-cell lymphoma/leukaemia. J Eur Acad Dermatol Venereol 2008; 22: 1252.

Sorrell J, et al: Eruptive xanthomas masquerading as molluscum contagiosum. Pediatrics 2014; 134: e257.

Suzuki L, et al: Lipoprotein-X in cholestatic patients causes xanthomas and promotes foam cell formation in human macrophages. J Clin Lipidol 2017; 11: 110.

Szalat R, et al: Pathogenesis and treatment of xanthomatosis associated with monoclonal gammopathy. Blood 2011; 118: 3777.

Teixeira V, et al: Verruciform xanthomas. Dermatol Online J 2012; 18: 10.

Tsubakio-Yamamoto K, et al: Current therapy for patients with sitosterolemia. J Atheroscler Thromb 2010; 17: 891.

Wolska A, et al: Apolipoprotein C-II. Atherosclerosis 2017; 267: 49.

Yamamoto T, et al: Numerous intertriginous xanthomas in infant. J Dermatol 2016; 43: 1340.

Yoo EG: Sitosterolemia. Ann Pediatr Endocrinol Metab 2016; 21: 7.

Zhao Y, et al: 1064-nm Q-switched Nd:YAG laser in an effective and safe approach to treat xanthelasma palpebrarum in Asian population. J Eur Acad Dermatol Venereol 2015; 29: 2263.

NIEMANN-PICK DISEASE

Niemann-Pick disease is a rare autosomal recessive condition originally described in people of Ashkenazi Jewish descent that has three recognized subtypes. Type A and type B are both caused by mutations in the acid sphingomyelinase gene (*SMPD1*). There can be hyperlipidemia with rarely associated xanthomatous lesions, including xanthomas and xanthogranulomas, in addition to waxy yellow-brown skin. Type A is more severe, presents in infancy with neurovisceral disease, and is often fatal, and skin manifestations may arise. Type B is purely visceral (nonneurologic), and survival into adulthood is characteristic and lichen nitidus has been reported. Histologically, foamy histiocytes are found, which on electron microscopy have characteristic cytoplasmic inclusions. Niemann-Pick disease type C is caused by mutations in the *NPC1* and *NPC2* genes, which are involved in endosomal-lysosomal cholesterol trafficking. Type C is a neurovisceral disease with a variable age of onset and neurodegenerative course. Patients may present from the perinatal period to adulthood. Cholestatic jaundice is characteristic.

Grasko Y, et al: A novel missense SMPD I gene mutation, *T460P*, and clinical findings in a patient with Niemann-Pick disease type B presenting to a lipid disorders clinic. Ann Clin Biochem 2014; 51: 615.

Stern G, et al: Niemann-Pick's and Gaucher's diseases. Parkinsonism Relat Disord 2014; 2051: S143.

Texeira VB, et al: Generalized lichen nitidus in a boy with Niemann-Pick disease type B. An Bras Dermatol 2013; 88: 977.

Toussaint M, et al: Specific skin lesions in a patient with Niemann-Pick disease. Br J Dermatol 1994; 131: 895.

GAUCHER DISEASE

Although rare, Gaucher disease is the most common lysosomal storage disease and occurs most frequently among people of Ashkenazi Jewish descent. It is an autosomal recessive disorder caused by insufficient activity of the lysosomal enzyme acid β-glucosidase (glucocerebrosidase, GBA, glucosylceramidase). Lysosomal accumulation of glucosylceramide, the substrate of GBA in macrophages, causes the disease manifestations. In rare cases, Gaucher disease is caused by mutations in the prosaposin gene, which encodes the saposin C activator protein that is necessary for optimal activity of β-glucosidase. Gaucher cells are identified histologically as large macrophages, 20–100 μm in diameter, with one nucleus or a few small nuclei, and pale cytoplasm that stains faintly for fat but is PAS positive.

Gaucher disease occurs at any age, but three types are recognized: type 1 (adult form), without neurologic involvement; type 2, the infantile form, with acute early neurologic manifestations;

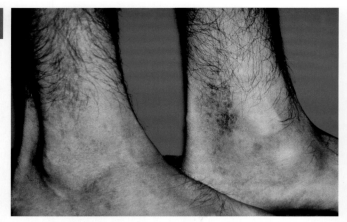

Fig. 26.25 Pigmentation of the lower leg in Gaucher disease.

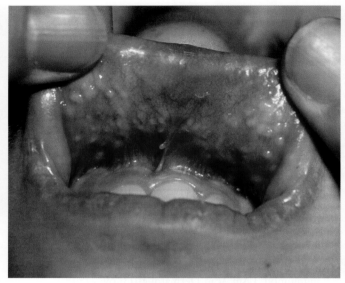

Fig. 26.26 Lipoid proteinosis.

and type 3, the juvenile chronic neuropathic form. The diagnosis is confirmed by genetic testing. Some type 2 patients are born with a collodion membrane, and there is one report of blueberry muffin lesions. The collodion can transition into and ichthyosis that precedes neurologic manifestations thus can be helpful in diagnosis. Epidermal ultrastructural and biochemical abnormalities occur in all type 2 patients. Hepatosplenomegaly, osteopenia/osteoporosis of the long bones, pingueculae of the sclera, and a distinctive bronze coloration of the skin from melanin characterize the adult type. A deeper pigmentation may extend from the knees to the feet (Fig. 26.25). This is often caused by hemosiderin and may be accompanied by thrombocytopenia and splenomegaly.

Therapy for Gaucher disease types 1 and 3 now consists of enzyme replacement therapy (ERT) with intravenous mannose-terminated glucocerebrosidase; ERT does not benefit type 2 patients. ERT is successful in treating some of the manifestations of the adult form (Gaucher disease type 1). Substrate reduction therapy using the glycolipid synthesis inhibitor *N*-butyldeoxynojirimycin (miglustat) is also available.

Adult patients with Gaucher disease can develop monoclonal gammopathy, myelodysplasia (myeloma or lymphoma). Heterozygous carriers of GBA mutations are frequently found in patients with Parkinson disease. Parkinson disease is associated with certain "pathogenic" variant GBA mutations.

Carr PC, et al: Gaucher disease type 2 presenting with collodion membrane and blueberry muffin lesions. Pediatr Dermatol 2016; 33.

Hughes DA: Enzyme, substrate, and myeloma in Gaucher disease. Am J Hematol 2009; 84: 199.

Mignot C, et al: Gaucher disease. Handb Clin Neurol 2013; 113: 1709.

LIPOID PROTEINOSIS

Also known as Urbach-Wiethe disease and hyalinosis cutis et mucosae, lipoid proteinosis is a rare autosomal recessive condition that usually presents in infancy with a hoarse cry or voice (99%). Mucosal lesions include yellowish white infiltrative deposits on the inner surface of the lips (Fig. 26.26), undersurface of the tongue, buccal mucosa, fauces, and uvula. Inability to protrude the "woody" tongue because of frenulum shortening is characteristic. Xerostomia may occur. In childhood, beaded eyelid papules are seen in over 90% (Fig. 26.27). Uveitis and hyaline deposits on and in the eye may develop. Waxy, yellow papules and nodules with generalized skin thickening occur. Mechanical friction leads to hyperkeratosis of the hands, elbows, knees, buttocks, and axillae. Acral hyperkeratotic papules occur in about 20% of patients and

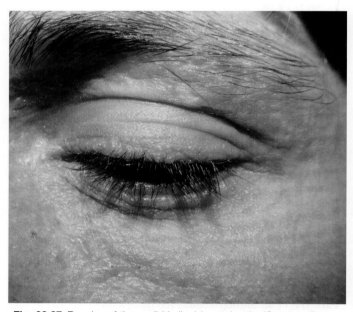

Fig. 26.27 Papules of the eyelid in lipoid proteinosis. (Courtesy Dr. Eric Krause.)

have been described as "verrucous." In fact, in some patients these lesions are induced by human papillomavirus (HPV). In one patient with lipoid proteinosis, epidermodysplasia verruciformis was diagnosed. Minor trauma leads to bullae that heal with pocklike or acnelike scars, especially on the face. This may be related to the increased risk for bacterial skin infections in these patients. Scalp involvement may lead to mild loss of hair. Neurologic sequelae include epilepsy, dystonia, and cognitive impairments.

Distinctive histologic features include extreme dilation of the blood vessels, thickening of the vessel walls, progressive hyalinization of sweat glands, and infiltration of the dermis and subcutaneous tissue with extracellular hyaline deposits. Normal skin and mucous membranes also show changes of endothelial proliferation of the subpapillary vessels and a homogeneous thickening of the walls of the deeper vessels. Type IV collagen and laminin are increased around blood vessels.

Lipoid proteinosis is caused by mutations in the extracellular matrix protein 1. This protein binds to heparin sulfate proteoglycans, which are also the binding substances for HPV, perhaps explaining the frequency of HPV infection. Differentiation from erythropoietic protoporphyria may be difficult, especially histologically.

Numerous patients with lipoid proteinosis have been treated with systemic retinoids with positive results. A dose of about 0.5 mg/kg of acitretin is well tolerated and effective. Hoarseness improves in most patients, palmar and plantar hyperkeratosis is reduced, and patients may note reduction in skin blisters. Oral ulcerations improve. Earlier treatment (before age 11) was associated with a better response. Histologically, the epidermis is less thick, but the hyaline deposition is unchanged. Although death from respiratory obstruction occasionally occurs in infancy, the disease is otherwise compatible with a normal life span.

Bakry OA, et al: Two Egyptian cases of lipoid proteinosis successfully treated with acitretin. J Dermatol Case Rep 2014; 1: 29.

Dertlioğlu SB, et al: Demographic, clinical, and radiologic signs and treatment responses of lipoid proteinosis patients. Int J Dermatol 2014; 53: 516.

Frenkel B, et al: Lipoid proteinosis unveiled by oral mucosal lesions. Clin Oral Investig 2017; 21: 2245.

Luo XY, et al: Treatment of lipoid proteinosis with acitretin in two patients from two unrelated Chinese families with novel nonsense mutations of the ECM1 gene. J Dermatol 2016; 43: 804.

O'Blenes C, et al: Epidermodysplasia verruciformis in lipoid proteinosis. Pediatr Dermatol 2015; 32: 118.

ANGIOKERATOMA CORPORIS DIFFUSUM (FABRY DISEASE)

Fabry disease (FD) is a rare X-linked lysosomal storage disease. It is caused by mutations in the α-galactosidase A gene (*GLA*), leading to a deficiency in α-galactosidase A. This results in the inability to catabolize glycosphingolipids, and globotriaosylceramide accumulates in lysosomes in many tissues, including endothelial cells, erector pili muscles, dorsal root ganglion nerves, and visceral organs. Males are affected more severely and earlier. Female heterozygotes (carriers of the defective gene) can have a broad spectrum of disease, from asymptomatic to disease as severe as males, depending on patterns of lyonization. This can make confirming the diagnosis of FD in a female with limited cutaneous and visceral disease quite difficult.

Skin lesions are common, and in about one quarter of male patients a dermatologist makes the diagnosis. The most characteristic skin lesions are widespread punctate telangiectatic vascular papules that on first inspection suggest purpura, but are actually angiokeratomas. Some show hyperkeratotic tops, but these are less prominent than in other forms of angiokeratoma. Angiokeratomas occur in 66% of male and 36% of female patients with FD. The average age of onset in males is about age 20 and in females, about 10 years later. Lesions can be present as early as age 1 year. Lesions tend to occur in the "bathing trunk" area, from the umbilicus to the genitalia, where they may be present in large numbers (Fig. 26.28). Smaller "macular angiomas" are seen, especially on the proximal limbs, palms, and soles, around the nailfolds of the digits, and on the vermilion border of the lips. Telangiectasias occur in about 25% of men presenting about age 25 and in women about age 40. Vascular tortuosities of the upper eyelid are seen in 95% of FD patients, with 40% showing microaneurysms. The ophthalmologist should examine for these lesions when screening for the characteristic corneal opacities.

Other skin manifestations of FD include lower limb edema and lymphedema. Leg ulceration can occur. Hair growth is scanty. Lack of sweating can lead to overheating. Hypohidrosis is reported

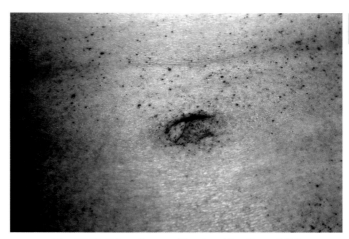

Fig. 26.28 Fabry disease. (Courtesy Ken Greer, MD.)

by 50% or more of male and about one third of female patients, starting in their twenties. Anhidrosis occurs in 25% of male patients. About 12% of female and 6% of male patients complain of hyperhidrosis.

Visceral disease is common, especially of the kidneys, cardiovascular system, nervous system, and GI tract, although only one organ may be involved. Abdominal pain, nausea, vomiting and diarrhea can all occur. Proteinuria followed by renal failure may begin as early as the second decade and typically presents around age 40. Cardiovascular events (myocardial infarction, arrhythmia, angina, congestive heart failure) typically appear around age 40, contributing to premature death. About 5% of men and women have a cerebrovascular accident (stroke) around age 40 that is often "cryptogenic."

Neuropathic pain is the most common initial presentation, affecting about two thirds of FD patients. It may begin in childhood, but its nonspecific nature and the lack of physical findings delay the diagnosis, usually by more than a decade, until other stigmata appear. Thermohypesthesia is often present. The acroparesthesia or burning pain affects primarily the longest nerves and is severest on the hands and feet. This is similar in distribution to erythromelalgia. The pain in fabrys may be transient or may last for hours. Treatment is as for neuropathy, with tricyclics, gabapentin, capsaicin, and anticonvulsants. About 25% of FD patients develop carpal tunnel syndrome. Cramps and fasciculation may be the presenting neurologic symptoms. Female patients may be misdiagnosed as having multiple sclerosis.

Distinctive whorl-like opacities of the cornea occur in 90% of patients, and 50% develop characteristic spokelike cataracts in the posterior capsular location. Telangiectasias may be present on the conjunctiva and in the eye.

The diagnosis of FD may be confirmed by finding diminished levels of α-galactosidase A in leukocytes, serum, fibroblasts, or amniotic fluid cells. Less than 10% enzyme activity is usually detected in affected males. In females, the diagnosis requires the identification of a genetic mutation in the *GLA* gene. This can be quite difficult if an affected male relative is not identified, because hundreds of *GLA* mutations have thus far been described that cause FD.

Histologically, there is dilation of capillaries in the papillary dermis, resulting in endothelium-lined lacunae filled with blood and surrounded by acanthotic and hyperkeratotic epidermis. Electron microscopy reveals characteristic electron-dense bodies in endothelial cells, pericytes, erector pili muscles, and fibroblasts. They are also present in normal skin of affected adults and children.

Enzyme replacement therapy is safe and can reverse substrate storage in the lysozyme. ERT leads to a reduction in neuropathic pain, relief of GI symptoms, and stabilization of cardiomyopathy; left ventricular mass decreases. Stroke and vascular coronary disease still occur, but perhaps at a lower rate. Early treatment may be more effective in preventing progression of FD.

Although widespread angiokeratomas are typical of FD, patients with other rare autosomal recessive lysosomal storage diseases, such as galactosialidosis, aspartylglycosaminuria, GM1 gangliosidosis (β-galactosidase deficiency, which may also manifest extensive dermal melanocytosis), and α-N-acetylgalactosaminidase deficiency (Kanzaki disease), have been reported to have Fabry-like angiokeratomas. Also, several patients with no detectable enzyme deficiency have been reported, including a family with autosomal dominant inherited Fabry-like angiokeratomas associated with arteriovenous malformations. It should be emphasized that there are many normal patients who have widespread small, petechia-like lesions that erupt in adulthood, a variant of cherry angiomas.

FUCOSIDOSIS

Angiokeratomas identical to those of FD occur in types II and III of this rare lysosomal storage disease. Fucosidosis can be distinguished clinically by the frequent presence of facial dysmorphism, severe mental retardation, weakness, spasticity, and seizures. The most severely affected patients die in childhood (type I), without the development of typical angiokeratomas. Patients with type II disease have severe spondyloepiphyseal dysplasia and normal intelligence. The adolescent type III patient can also have angiokeratomas. Fucosidosis is autosomal recessive and is caused by a deficiency in α-L-fucosidase, usually detected in leukocytes.

SIALIDOSIS

Sialidosis (mucolipidosis type I) is an autosomal recessive lysosomal storage disease caused by mutations in the sialidase gene *NEU1*. Two types are described, the severest of which is the infantile form (type II), in which the children die within the first 2 years of life. Type I sialidosis is less severe and is characterized by mental retardation, myoclonus, cerebellar ataxia, hypotonia, skeletal abnormalities, and facial dysmorphism. Angiokeratoma can occur.

β-MANNOSIDASE DEFICIENCY

This rare autosomal recessive lysosomal storage disease of glycoprotein metabolism is caused by a deficiency of β-mannosidase that results in the accumulation of a characteristic disaccharide in the lysosomes, which may also be found in the urine. In addition to the Fabry-like angiokeratomas, mental retardation, hearing loss, aggressive behavior, peripheral neuropathy, recurrent infections, epilepsy, coarse facies, and skeletal abnormalities are often present.

Böttcher T, et al: Fabry disease. PLoS One 2013; 8: e71894.
Canafoglia L, et al: Expanding sialidosis spectrum by genome-wide screening. J Am Acad Neurol 2014; 82: 2003.
Ferraz MJ, et al: Gaucher disease and Fabry disease. Biochem Biophys Acta 2014; 1841: 811.
Juan P, et al: Fabry disease. JIMD Rep 2014; 16: 7.
Kanitakis J, et al: Fucosidosis with angiokeratoma. J Cutan Pathol 2005; 32: 506.
Mahmud HM: Fabry's disease. J Pak Med Assoc 2014; 64: 189.
Michaud L: Vascular tortuosities of the upper eyelid. J Ophthamol 2013; 2013: 207573.
Molho-Pessach V, et al: Angiokeratoma corporis diffusum in human beta-mannosidosis. J Am Acad Dermatol 2007; 57: 407.
Nance CS, et al: Later-onset Fabry disease. Arch Neurol 2006; 63: 453.
Rombach SM, et al: Natural course of Fabry disease and the effectiveness of enzyme replacement therapy. J Inherit Metab Dis 2014; 37: 341.
Schiffmann R, et al: Screening, diagnosis, and management of patients with Fabry disease. Kidney Int 2017; 91: 284.
Toyooka K: Fabry disease. Handb Clin Neurol 2013; 113: 1437.
Van der Tol L, et al: A systematic review on screening for Fabry disease. J Med Genet 2014; 51: 1.

■ SKIN DISORDERS IN DIABETES MELLITUS

Skin lesions are common in diabetic patients, with two thirds or more having at least one skin finding. Xerosis appears to be particularly common, affecting 50% of those with type 1 diabetes. Keratosis pilaris is also common. Other specific cutaneous findings of diabetes are discussed next.

NECROBIOSIS LIPOIDICA/NECROBIOSIS LIPOIDICA DIABETICORUM

Necrobiosis lipoidica (NL) is characterized by well-circumscribed, firm, depressed, waxy, yellow-brown plaques, usually of the anterior shin. Although NL can occur in persons without diabetes mellitus, 60% of cases of NL occur in insulin-dependent (type 1) diabetic patients, and 20% occur in persons at risk for the development of diabetes (who have glucose intolerance or a family history of diabetes). If NL occurs in the setting of diabetes, it is called necrobiosis lipoidica diabeticorum (NLD). In diabetics who have NL they tend to have worse hyperglycemia but also more associated autoimmune disease such as celiac. Women are affected three times more often than men; the condition usually appears between ages 20 and 40 but may occur in children or elderly people as well. The average age of onset is 34 for all diabetic patients, but 22 years, on average, in insulin-dependent patients, and 49 in non–insulin-dependent patients. Although NL is reported to affect only 0.3% of diabetic patients, the prevalence was much higher (>2%) in series of patients with type 1 diabetes. In 15%, NL precedes the onset of frank diabetes by an average of 2 years. Control of the diabetes does not influence the course of the NL.

The earliest changes are small, sharply bordered, red papules that may be capped by a slight scale and that do not disappear under diascopic pressure. Later, the lesions develop into irregularly round or oval lesions with well-defined borders and a smooth, glistening (glazed) surface. The center becomes depressed and sulfur yellow, so that a firm yellowish lesion forms, surrounded at times by a violet-red or pink border. In the yellow portion, numerous telangiectases and ectatic veins are evident. Ulceration occurs in one third of NLD patients. In an unusual case, the plaques were studded with exophytic nodules resembling tuberous xanthomas. This patient had marked hyperlipidemia, perhaps contributing to the morphology. Rarely, squamous cell carcinoma may occur in chronic ulcers.

The most common location of the lesions is the shins (Fig. 26.29). Much less often, lesions will appear on the forearms, and rarely, lesions have been reported on the trunk, face, scalp, palms, and soles.

Histologically, well-developed lesions of NL demonstrate a superficial, deep, and interstitial inflammatory process that involves the whole reticular dermis and often the panniculus. Because the dermis is firm, punch biopsy specimens appear rectangular rather than tapered. The inflammatory cells include lymphocytes, histiocytes, multinucleate giant cells, and plasma cells. At low magnification, there are layered palisaded granulomas with pale-pink degenerated collagen alternating with amphophilic-staining histiocytes. In contrast to granuloma annulare, mucin is not increased in the centers of the granulomas, and there is no normal dermis in NL lesions. Between granulomas in granuloma annulare, the collagen pattern is relatively normal, although inflammatory cells may be present. In NL, the overlying epidermis tends to be thinned, with loss of the normal rete ridge pattern.

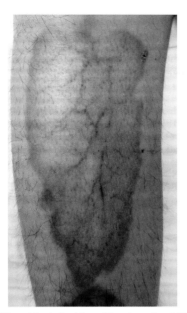

Fig. 26.29 Necrobiosis lipoidica. (Courtesy Scott Norton, MD.)

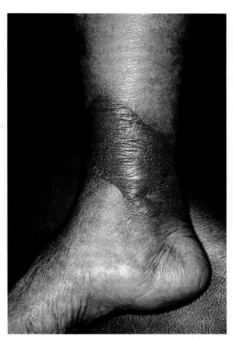

Fig. 26.30 Bullous eruption of diabetes.

Treatment of NLD, after control of the diabetes is achieved, is not completely satisfactory. Initial therapy is superpotent topical corticosteroids with occlusion. Topical calcineurin inhibitors can also be effective. Intralesional injections of triamcinolone suspension into the inflammatory papules and active advancing edges can be quite effective. Injection into the yellow center is of little benefit and may result in ulceration. It had been proposed that NLD is caused by the microangiopathy of diabetes. For this reason, agents designed to improve circulation have been used, at times with success. These include low-dose aspirin, nicotinamide, pentoxifylline, and dipyridamole. The blood flow in lesions of NLD is normal, however, suggesting that this is better considered as an inflammatory dermatosis. Phototherapy, including PUVA and UVA1, has been effective in select patients. Oral immunomodulatory therapy should be considered in patients unresponsive to topical treatment. Antimalarial treatment and thalidomide are nonimmunosuppressive options that would not alter blood sugar control. Systemic antiinflammatories reported to be effective in select cases include systemic corticosteroids, mycophenolate mofetil (MMF), and cyclosporin A. TNF inhibitors (specifically infliximab and etanercept) have been effective in refractory cases, either systemically or by intralesional injection. However, patients being treated with TNF inhibitors for other conditions have developed NLD, similar to the paradox of patients who take TNF inhibitors developing psoriasis. Hyperbaric oxygen may be used for patients with chronic ulceration. Intense pulse light has also been reported to be effective. In severe cases with persistent ulceration, excision and skin grafting have been effective, although the NLD may recur in or at the edges of the grafts. Despite initial reports of success, photodynamic therapy only improves about one third of treated patients. Pioglitazone treatment may be beneficial. Pancreas-kidney transplantation led to resolution in one case, but the patient also received MMF, prednisone, and tacrolimus orally.

Diabetic Dermopathy (Shin Spots)

Dull-red papules that progress to small, well-circumscribed, round, atrophic, hyperpigmented lesions on the shins are a common cutaneous sign of diabetes, occurring in up to 40% of diabetic patients. Lesions begin on the lower extremities as crops of four or five dull-red macules 0.5–1 cm in diameter. As the lesions resolve, they become shallow, depressed, and hyperpigmented scars. The lesions are twice as common in men; 70% of diabetic men over age 60 have diabetic dermopathy. Although shin spots occur individually in people who do not have diabetes, if four or more are present, the specificity is high for diabetes. Patients with diabetic dermopathy have a higher risk of nephropathy and retinopathy.

Diabetic Bullae

Noninflammatory, spontaneous, painless blistering, most often in acral locations, is characteristic of diabetic bullae (Fig. 26.30). Lesions tend to involve the lower legs and to be 10 cm or more in diameter. The incidence is 0.16% per year. In many cases, lesions heal spontaneously in 4–5 weeks, usually without scarring. However, lesions may be complicated at times by chronic ulceration. Aggressive and cautious management with dressings and diabetic foot care is required. Lesions appear after periods of relative hypoglycemia, perhaps explaining the clinical resemblance of diabetic bullae to pressure bullae.

The blisters are subepidermal. Electron microscropic studies show separation at the lamina lucida level. DIF is negative. Treatment is diabetic control, aspiration of the bulla to prevent expansion by hydrostatic pressure, and aggressive wound management to optimize healing and prevent infection.

Carotenosis

Carotenosis is a yellowish discoloration of the skin, especially of the palms and soles (Fig. 26.31), which is sometimes seen in diabetic patients and patients with trisomy 21.

Limited Joint Mobility and Waxy Skin

Limited joint mobility and waxy skin are important not only because of the 30%–50% prevalence of these conditions in diabetic patients with long-standing disease, but also because they are associated with microvascular complications, such as nephropathy and retinopathy. Joint symptoms begin with limitation of joint mobility in the fifth finger at the metacarpophalangeal and proximal joints and progress radially to the other fingers. The condition is bilateral,

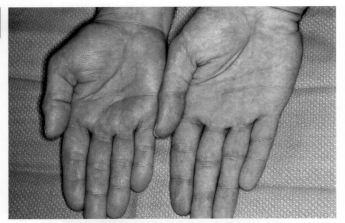

Fig. 26.31 Carotenemia, yellow palm shown next to normal palm.

symmetric, and painless. Dupuytren contractures and palmar fibrosis may occur. Involvement of the feet also occurs and is thought to contribute to the development of chronic ulcerations. Such open sores on the neuropathic, microvascularly compromised, infection-prone diabetic foot pose a constant threat to life and limb.

Other Associated Conditions in Patients With Diabetes

Various abnormalities associated with diabetes are erysipelas-like erythema of the legs or feet; sweating disturbances; paresthesias of the legs; mal perforans ulcerations; a predisposition to certain infections such as mucormycosis, group B streptococcal infections, nonclostridial gas gangrene, and malignant external otitis resulting from *Pseudomonas;* disseminated granuloma annulare; eruptive xanthomas; clear cell syringomas; rubeosis of the face; lipoatrophy or lipohypertrophy at sites of insulin injection; acquired perforating disorders; acanthosis nigricans; skin tags; and finger pebbling. Pruritus is common in adult diabetic patients, typically of the central trunk. It is associated with evidence of diabetic neuropathy and probably represents a form of neuropathic pruritus. Treatment is similar to that for neuropathy, starting with gabapentin.

Basoulis D, et al: Anti-TNFα treatment for recalcitrant ulcerative necrobiosis lipoidica diabeticorum. Metabolism 2016; 65: 569.
Bouhanick B, et al: Necrobiosis lipoidica. Diabetes Metab 1998; 24: 156.
Chatterjee N, et al: An observational study of cutaneous manifestations in diabetes mellitus in a tertiary care hospital of eastern India. Indian J Endocrinol Metab 2014; 18: 217.
da Cunha MG, et al: Necrobiosis lipoidica treated with intense pulsed light. J Surg Dermatol 2017; 2: 39.
Fehlman JA, et al: Ulcerative necrobiosis lipoidica in the setting of anti–tumor necrosis factor-α and hydroxychloroquine treatment for rheumatoid arthritis. JAAD Case Rep 2017; 3: 127.
Hammer E, et al: Risk factors for necrobiosis lipoidica in type 1 diabetes mellitus. Diabet Med 2017; 34: 86.
Kato M, et al: Necrobiosis lipoidica with infiltration of Th17 cells into vascular lesions. J Dermatol 2014; 41: 459.
Lopez PR, et al: Bullosis diabeticorum associated with a prediabetic state. South Med J 2009; 102: 643
Mahmood T, et al: Cutaneous manifestations of diabetes mellitus. JPAD 2016; 15: 227.
Mirhoseini M, et al: A study on the association of diabetic dermopathy with nephropathy and retinopathy in patients with type 2 diabetes mellitus. J Nephropathol 2016; 5: 139.
Mitre, V et al: Necrobiosis lipoidica. J Pediatr 2016; 179: 272.
Murao K: Photodynamic therapy for necrobiosis lipoidica is an unpredictable option. Int J Dermatol 2013; 52: 1567.
Murphy-Chutorian B, et al: Dermatologic manifestations of diabetes mellitus. Endocrinol Metab Clin North Am 2013; 42: 869.
Quondamatteo F: Skin and diabetes mellitus. Cell Tissue Res 2014; 355: 1.
Reid SD, et al: Update on necrobiosis lipoidica. J Am Acad Dermatol 2013; 69: 783.
Schilling WH, et al: Cutaneous stigmata associated with insulin resistance and increased cardiovascular risk. Int J Dermatol 2014; 53: 1062.
Shenavandeh S, et al: Diabetic muscle infarction and diabetic dermopathy two manifestations of uncontrolled prolong diabetes mellitus presenting with severe leg pain and leg skin lesions. J Diabetes Metab Disord 2014; 13: 38.
Silverberg NB, Lee-Wong M: Generalized yellow discoloration of the skin. The diagnosis: carotenemia. Cutis 2014; 93: E11.
Wee E, Kelly R: Pentoxifylline: an effective therapy for necrobiosis lipoidica. Australas J Dermatol 2017; 58: 65.

■ OTHER METABOLIC DISORDERS

CITRULLINEMIA

Citrullinemia occurs in two forms. Type I is caused by a deficiency of the enzyme argininosuccinic acid synthetase (*ASS1* gene). This enzyme converts citrulline and aspartic acid to arginino-succinic acid, as a part of the urea cycle. Low plasma arginine levels result, and the hypothesis is that, because keratin is 16% arginine, dermatitis may occur. Neonates who present with severe deficiencies and hyperammonemic crises may develop erosive, erythematous, scaling patches and plaques prominent in the perioral, lower abdominal, diaper, and buttock regions or erythroderma similar to psoriasis. Short, sparse hair may also be present. This eruption clears with arginine supplementation. Citrullinemia type II is caused by a defect in the *SCL25A13* gene and is seen primarily in East Asia, usually presenting in adolescence or adulthood.

In carbamoyl phosphate synthetase deficiency, low plasma arginine levels may also occur, and similar cutaneous findings have been reported in this second metabolic defect of the urea cycle.

Diets high in arginine will heal the skin lesions.

Diez-Fernandez C, et al: Mutations in the human argininosuc-cinate synthetase (ASS1) gene, impact on patients, common changes, and structural considerations. Hum Mut 2017; 38: 471.
Fiermonte G, et al: An adult with type 2 citrullinemia presenting in Europe. N Engl J Med 2008; 358: 1408.
Kumar P, et al: Infantile erythrodermic psoriasis. Indian J Paediatr Dermatol 2017; 18: 248.

HARTNUP DISEASE

Hartnup disease is an inborn error of tryptophan excretion named after the Hartnup family, in whom it was first noted. It is the second most common inherited aminoaciduria after phenylketon-uria. The characteristic findings are a pellagra-like dermatitis following exposure to sunlight, intermittent cerebellar ataxia, psychosis, and constant aminoaciduria.

The dermatitis occurs on exposed parts of the skin, chiefly the face, neck, hands, and legs. The erythematous scaly patches flare up into a hot, red, exudative state after exposure to sunlight, followed by hyperpigmentation. Stomatitis and vulvitis also occur. The disease becomes milder with increasing age. Rarely, an acrodermatitis enteropathica–like eruption with normal zinc levels may occur in patients with Hartnup disease.

Hartnup disease is an autosomal recessive trait caused by mutations in the *SLC6A19* gene coding an enzyme that transports neutral amino acids across the apical membrane of epithelial cells in the gut and kidneys. Large amounts of neutral amino acids, including tryptophan, are present in the urine, establishing the diagnosis. The skin lesions respond to niacinamide, but the neurologic disease may not improve.

Ciecierega T, et al: Severe persistent unremitting dermatitis, chronic diarrhea and hypoalbuminemia in a child; Hartnup disease in setting of celiac disease. BMC Pediatr 2014; 14: 311.
Orbak Z, et al: Hartnup disease masked by kwashiorkor. J Health Popul Nutr 2010; 28: 413.

PROLIDASE DEFICIENCY

Prolidase deficiency (PD) is an autosomal recessive inherited inborn error of metabolism caused by mutations in the *PEPD* gene. Prolidase cleaves dipeptides containing C-terminal proline or hydroxyproline. When this enzyme is deficient, the normal recycling of proline residues obtained from collagen degradation is impaired. A buildup of iminodipeptides results, with disturbances in connective tissue metabolism and excretion of large amounts of iminodipeptides in the urine. Clinically, 85% of patients have some dermatologic manifestations. The most important cutaneous signs, which almost always appear before the affected person is 12 years old, are skin fragility; ulceration and scarring of the lower extremities; photosensitivity and telangiectasia; poliosis; scaly, erythematous, maculopapular, and purpuric lesions; and thickening of the skin with lymphedema of the legs. Systemic signs and symptoms include mental deficiency, splenomegaly, recurrent infections and facial dysmorphism with low hairline, frontal bossing, and saddle nose. About 10% of patients with PD meet American Rheumatology Association (ARA) criteria for the diagnosis of systemic lupus erythematosus. Antinuclear antibodies, extractable nuclear antigen, and anti-dsDNA may be positive; C3 and C4 are low; and cytopenias are present. Because C1q has a high proline content, a relative deficiency of functional C1q may explain the high frequency of lupus erythematosus in these patients.

PD is confirmed by determining prolidase activity in erythrocytes, leukocytes, or fibroblasts in culture or by sequence analysis of the *PEPD* gene. In long-standing ulcerations, squamous cell carcinomas may occur.

Bertolini F: Leg ulcers caused by genetic disease 'prolidase deficiency'. J Eur Acad Dermatol Venereol 2017; 31: e377.
Butbaul Aviel Y, et al: Prolidase deficiency associated with systemic lupus erythematosus (SLE). Pediatr Rheumatol 2012; 10: 18.

PHENYLKETONURIA

Phenylketonuria (PKU) is an autosomal recessive disorder of phenylalanine metabolism caused by a deficiency in the enzyme phenylalanine hydroxylase. Phenylalanine is not metabolized to tyrosine. PKU is the most common form of inherited aminoaciduria, affecting 1 in 15,000 live births in the United States. It is characterized by mental deficiency; epileptic seizures; pigmentary dilution of skin, hair, and eyes; pseudoscleroderma; and dermatitis (Fig. 26.32). It is most common in white persons.

Affected children are blue-eyed, with blond hair and fair skin. They are usually extremely sensitive to light, and about 50% have an eczematous dermatitis. It is clinically similar to atopic dermatitis, with a predilection for the flexures. The dermatitis is worst in the youngest patients, may improve with dietary treatment, and has been exacerbated by phenylalanine challenge in a carrier of the recessive gene. Indurations of the thighs and buttocks are present early in infancy and increase with time. After many years, the lesions soften and become atrophic.

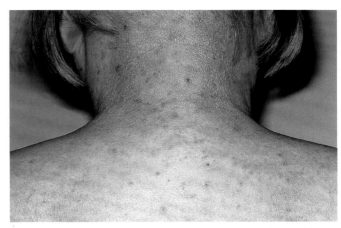

Fig. 26.32 Light-skinned, light-haired phenylketonuria patient with dermatitis. (Courtesy Dr. Jeff Miller.)

Blood levels of phenylalanine are high. The presence of phenylpyruvic acid in the urine is demonstrated by a characteristic deep-green color when a few drops of ferric chloride solution are added. Green diapers occur in histidinemia as well as in PKU.

In developed countries, universal screening for PKU is practiced, so dietary therapy with phenylalanine restriction is instituted. Sapropterin dihydrochloride may also be given. This prevents the manifestations of the disease. If compliance is poor, the manifestations, including eczema, may develop at any age, followed by improvement of the skin with reinstitution of the diet.

Al-Mayouf SM, Al-Owain MA: Progressive sclerodermatous skin changes in a child with phenylketonuria. Pediatr Dermatol 2006; 23: 136.
Eichenfield LF, Stein Gold LF: Practical strategies for the diagnosis and assessment of atopic dermatitis. Semin Cutan Med Surg 2017; 36: S36.
Longo N, et al: Single-dose, subcutaneous recombinant phenylalanine ammonia lyase conjugated with polyethylene glycol in adult patients with phenylketonuria. Lancet 2014; 384: 37.
Somaraju UR, Merrin M: Sapropterin dihydrochloride for phenylketonuria. Cochrane Database Syst Rev 2012; 12: CD008005.

ALKAPTONURIA AND OCHRONOSIS

Alkaptonuria (endogenous ochronosis), inherited as an autosomal recessive trait, is caused by the lack of renal and hepatic homogentisic acid oxidase, the enzyme necessary for the catabolism of homogentisic acid (HGA), a product of tyrosine and phenylalanine metabolism. Excess HGA is excreted in the urine and deposited in connective tissues throughout the body, especially the cartilage leading to a dark color. The urine is dark and becomes black on standing. Men with alkaptonuria outnumber women by 2:1.

For many years, the dark urine may be the only indication of the presence of alkaptonuria. In the meantime, large amounts of HGA accumulate in the body tissues. By the third decade of life, the deposition of pigment becomes apparent. The early sign is the pigmentation of the sclera (Osler sign; Fig. 26.33) and the cartilage of the ears (Fig. 26.34). Later, the cartilage of the nose and tendons, especially those on the hands, becomes discolored.

Blue or mottled brown macules appear on the skin. The bluish macules have a predilection for the fingers, ears, nose, genital regions, apices of the axillae, and buccal and vaginal mucosae. Palmoplantar pigmentation may occur and may be accentuated along the thenar and hypothenar eminences as pigmented pitted areas some with hyperkeratosis. The transgradience of the index

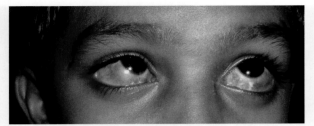

Fig. 26.33 Osler sign.

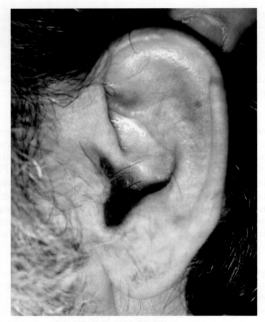

Fig. 26.34 Alkaptonuria.

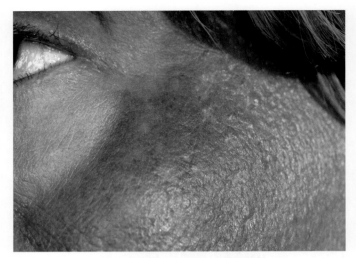

Fig. 26.35 Exogenous ochronosis.

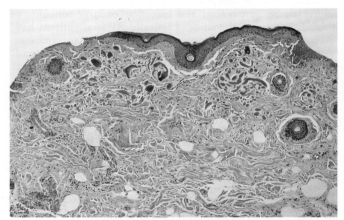

Fig. 26.36 Exogenous ochronosis.

fingers is also affected, closely resembling degenerative collagenous plaques the hand and acrokeratoelastoidosis. The apocrine sweat glands are rich in ochronotic pigment granules, and the intradermal injection of epinephrine into the skin of the axillary vault will yield brown-black sweat droplets in the follicular orifices. The cerumen is often black. Histologically, there are large, irregular ochre bodies within the reticular dermis. These represent degenerated elastic fibers with deposition of ochronotic pigment and stain black with crystal violet or methylene blue.

Ochronotic arthropathy first involves the axial spine joints, followed by the knees, shoulders, and hips. Radiographs show a characteristic appearance of early calcification of the intervertebral disk and later narrowing of the intervertebral spaces with eventual disk collapse. Tendon rupture may occur. Heart disease results from HGA deposition in the aortic and mitral valves. Renal disease is caused by HGA stones in the urinary system and can progress to renal failure.

There is no effective treatment for alkaptonuria. Dietary restriction of tyrosine and phenylalanine is recommended but may not prevent progression of disease. Joint and cardiac valve replacement may be necessary. Nitisinone can greatly reduce HGA excretion but does not appear to be effective once joint disease is present. Tyrosine keratopathy can result from nitisinone treatment. Life span is generally unaffected.

Exogenous Ochronosis

Topically applied phenolic intermediates, such as hydroquinone, carbolic acid (phenol), picric acid, and resorcinol, may produce exogenous ochronosis. Even 2% over-the-counter hydroquinone can produce ochronosis if used regularly for a long period. Hydroquinone specifically inhibits the enzyme HGA oxidase locally instead of the systemic inhibition of alkaptonuria. This results in accumulation of the blue discoloration on the collagen fibers where hydroquinone is applied. All skin types can be affected, but ethnic groups with the highest prevalence of melasma and hydroquinone use are primarily reported: African Americans, Africans, and Asians. Because most patients use the hydroquinone to treat melasma, findings of melasma may overlay the skin findings of exogenous ochronosis. The typical findings are gray-brown or blue-black macules, usually over the zygomatic regions (Fig. 26.35). Hyperchromic pinpoint papules may occur, that on dermoscopy can be seen associated with follicular openings. Confetti-like depigmentation (from the hydroquinone) may be admixed with the hyperpigmentation. Histologically, exogenous ochronosis and alkaptonuria show identical changes (Fig. 26.36). Treatment is challenging but stopping the application of hydroquinone may lead to improvement. Q-switched lasers and IPL have shown some inconsistent improvement.

Chandrakala C, et al: A case of alkaptonuria with degenerative collagenous plaques and foot drop. Indian J Dermatol 2016; 61: 678.

Khaled A, et al: Endogenous ochronosis. Int J Dermatol 2011; 50: 262.

Liu WC, et al: Exogenous ochronosis in a Chinese patient. Singapore Med J 2014; 55: e1.

Moche MJ, et al: Cutaneous annular sarcoidosis developing on a background of exogenous ochronosis. Clin Exp Dermatol 2009; 35: 399.

Ranganath LR, et al: Recent advances in management of alkaptonuria. J Clin Pathol 2013; 66: 367.

Ranganath LR, et al: Suitability of nitisinone in alkaptonuria 1 (SONIA 1). Ann Rheum Dis 2016; 75: 362.

Simmons BJ, et al: Exogenous ochronosis. Am J Clin Dermatol 2015; 16: 205.

Thomas M, et al: Acral pigmentation in alkaptonuria resembling degenerative collagenous plaques of the hands. J Am Acad Dermatol 2010; 65: e45.

WILSON DISEASE (HEPATOLENTICULAR DEGENERATION)

Wilson disease is an autosomal recessive derangement of copper transport. The disease is caused by dysfunction of a copper-transporting enzyme, P-type adenosine triphosphatase (ATP7B), which is required to excrete copper into the bile. This leads to accumulation of copper in the liver, brain, cornea, and kidney. Affected persons develop hepatomegaly, splenomegaly, and neuropsychiatric changes. Slurred speech, a squeaky voice, salivation, dysphagia, tremors, incoordination, and spasticity may all occur. There is progressive, fatal, hepatic and central nervous system degeneration.

Azure lunulae ("sky-blue moons") of the nails occur in 10% of patients, and the smoky, greenish brown Kayser-Fleischer rings develop at the edges of the corneas. Hyperpigmentation develops on the lower extremities in most patients. A vague greenish discoloration of the skin on the face, neck, and genitalia may also be present. An idiopathic blistering eruption that ceased with treatment of Wilson disease has been reported. Lipomas can occur in approximately 25% of patient with Wilson disease. Skin changes of cirrhosis (vascular spiders and palmar erythema) may occur. Low ceruloplasmin level in the serum leads to the suspected diagnosis, along with elevated 24-hour urinary copper excretion and elevated free serum copper. Ten percent of carriers for Wilson disease have a low ceruloplasmin level, so additional tests should be performed to confirm the diagnosis.

The treatment is a low-copper diet, often with agents that bind copper and enhance its excretion from the body. D-Penicillamine, 1 or 2 g/day orally, removes copper by chelating it. Potential side effects include pemphigus, cutis laxa, and elastosis perforans serpiginosa, which has been reported repeatedly in Wilson patients receiving penicillamine. Trientine, another copper chelator, enhances copper excretion. It has less toxicity, but is somewhat less effective than D-penicillamine. Zinc supplementation leads to increased metallothionein in the gut and liver. This leads to more copper excretion in the stool. Zinc can be given at the same time as D-penicillamine. Treatment must be continued for life.

Harada M: Pathogenesis and management of Wilson disease. Hepatol Res 2014; 44: 395.

Neri I, et al: Detection of D-penicillamine in skin lesions in a case of dermal elastosis after a previous long-term treatment for Wilson's disease. J Eur Acad Dermatol Venereol 2015; 29: 383.

Schaefer M, et al: Increased prevalence of subcutaneous lipomas in patients with Wilson disease. J Clin Gastroenterol 2015; 49: e61.

TYROSINEMIA II (RICHNER-HANHART SYNDROME)

Tyrosinemia is an autosomal recessive syndrome resulting from a deficiency of hepatic tyrosine aminotransferase, an important enzyme in the degradation of tyrosine and phenylalanine caused by mutations in the *TAT* gene. Clinical features are mild to severe keratitis and painful hyperkeratotic, erosive lesions of palms and soles, often with mild mental retardation. Photophobia and tearing usually occur as the keratitis begins, and ultimately, neovascularization is seen; occasionally only the eye findings are present or they are totally absent. Painful palmar and plantar hyperkeratosis are usually on weight-bearing areas and the keratosis can track along dermatoglyphs. Bullae can also be present. The skin manifestations, although usually present in the first year, can first present in the second decade. Initially, only the soles may be affected, with hyperkeratosis mainly over the tips of the digits and on weight-bearing surfaces. The fingertips and the hypothenar and thenar eminences are primarily affected on the palms. In any child presenting with palmoplantar keratoderma, the diagnosis of tyrosinemia type II must be considered, especially if there is tearing and photophobia (which is usually present by age 1). The diagnosis is confirmed by identifying elevated levels of serum tyrosine. A low-tyrosine, low-phenylalanine diet may improve or prevent the eye and skin lesions, but it may or may not benefit established mental retardation.

Peña-Quintana L, et al: Tyrosinemia type II. Clin Genet 2017; 92: 306.

HURLER SYNDROME (MUCOPOLYSACCHARIDOSIS I)

Hurler syndrome is an autosomal recessive lysosomal storage disease of mucopolysaccharide metabolism caused by a deficiency of α-iduronidase. This enzyme is responsible for the breakdown of heparan sulfate and dermatan sulfate. All patients have undetectable enzyme activity, yet there is significant polymorphism in the severity and age of onset. In general, cases are divided into severe mucopolysaccharidosis (MPS-I, Hurler syndrome) and attenuated MPS-I (Hurler-Scheie syndrome, Scheie syndrome).

Hurler syndrome is characterized by mental retardation, hepatosplenomegaly, umbilical and inguinal hernia, genital infantilism, corneal opacities, and skin abnormalities. Patients with Hurler syndrome have facial dysmorphism, with a broad saddle nose, thick lips, and a large tongue. The skin is thickened, with ridges and grooves, especially on the upper half of the body. Fine lanugo hair is profusely distributed all over the body. Large, coarse hair is prominent, especially on the extremities. Dermal melanocytosis (Mongolian spots), characterized by extensive blue pigmentation with both a dorsal and a ventral distribution, indistinct borders, and a persistent or progressive course, occurs in approximately 15% of patients with lysosomal storage disease, including patients with Hurler syndrome, Hunter syndrome, and GM1–gangliosidosis type 1. Because the dermal melanocytosis is prominent in infancy, this may be the initial clinical manifestation. The skeletal system is deformed, with hydrocephalus, kyphosis, and gibbus (cat-back shape). The hands are broad and have clawlike fingers.

The diagnosis of MPS-I is made by demonstrating elevated urinary glycosaminoglycan levels and deficient enzyme activity in fibroblasts, leukocytes, serum, or blood spots. Prenatal diagnosis is possible. Hematopoietic stem cell transplantation (HSCT) is the most effective treatment for Hurler syndrome. It can prevent mental deterioration if performed early enough (before age 2 and before developmental quotients fall below 70). ERT with recombinant human α-iduronidase (Aldurazyme) is an option in patients who are not candidates for HSCT.

Kiely BT et al: Early disease progression of Hurler syndrome. Orphanet Journal of Rare Diseases 2017 Feb 14; 12(1): 32.

HUNTER SYNDROME (MUCOPOLYSACCHARIDOSIS II)

Hunter syndrome is X-linked recessive lysosomal storage disease caused by deficiency of the enzyme iduronate-2-sulfatase. The initial

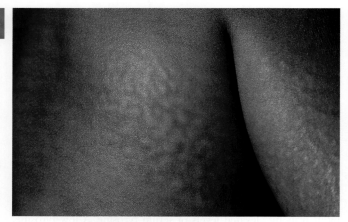

Fig. 26.37 Hunter syndrome papules.

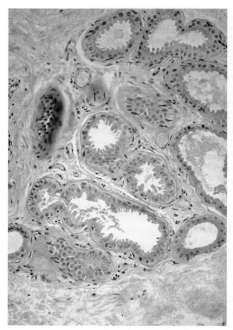

Fig. 26.38 PAS-stained inclusions in Lafora disease.

presentation of Hunter syndrome may be to the dermatologist due to the extensive dermal melanocytosis (Mongolian spots) that are large and located in atypical locations (not just along the back and buttocks) seen in infancy. Often these children are otherwise asymptomatic. The pebbly lesions of MPS-II in the skin of the upper back, neck, chest, proximal arms, or thighs occur in approximately 10% of patients. The lesions are firm, flesh-colored to white papules and nodules that coalesce into a cobblestone or reticular pattern as a connective tissue nevus (Fig. 26.37). At time of these skin lesions (around age 10), patients will typically have large head circumference, high body mass index, and short stature. Histologically, the lesions demonstrate increased dermal mucin and metachromatic granules in the cytoplasm of dermal fibroblasts and at times in eccrine sweat glands and epidermal keratinocytes.

Dermatan sulfate and heparan sulfate are excreted in the urine in large amounts, and the diagnosis of Hunter syndrome can be confirmed by absent iduronate-2-sulfatase in leukocytes. HSCT and ERT can be useful in appropriately evaluated patients.

Amartino H, et al: Aberrant mongolian spots as a clue to early diagnosis of Hunter syndrome. Mol Genet Metab 2016; 117: S19.

Parini R, et al: The natural history of growth in patients with Hunter syndrome. Mol Genet Metab 2016; 117: 438.

Sakata S, et al: Skin rash with the histological absence of metachromatic granules as the presenting feature of Hunter syndrome in a 6-year-old boy. Br J Dermatol 2008; 159: 249.

Schwartz IV, et al: A clinical study of 77 patients with mucopolysaccharidosis type II. Acta Paediatr 2007; 96: 63.

Tanjuakio J et al: Activities of daily living in patients with Hunter syndrome. Mol Genet Metab 2015; 114: 161.

You HS, et al: Hunter syndrome with extensive mongolian spots. Ann Dermatol 2017; 29: 381.

LAFORA DISEASE

Lafora disease is an autosomal recessive form of progressive myoclonic and tonic-clonic epilepsy beginning at puberty that is caused by a mutation in EPM2A or NHLRC1. The products of these two genes form a complex critical to the regulation of neuronal function. It is characterized by myoclonic jerks followed by progressive ataxia, dysphagia, dysarthria, dementia, and death in early adulthood. Diagnosis is established in the proper clinical setting by demonstration of characteristic PAS-positive cytoplasmic inclusion bodies in the eccrine ducts, axillary apocrine myoepithelial cells (Fig. 26.38), and peripheral nerves. The best site to biopsy is the axilla. Other conditions in which similar polyglucosan inclusions can be seen include normal aging (amyloid bodies),

double-athetosis syndrome, amyotrophic lateral sclerosis, and glycogen storage disease type IV.

Cutaneous manifestations are rare in Lafora disease. Papulonodular lesions on the ears and indurated, thickened plaques on the arms have been reported. Large amounts of acid mucopolysaccharides were demonstrated histologically in these lesions.

Casciato S, et al: Severe and rapidly-progressive Lafora disease associated with *NHLRC1* mutation. Int J Neurosci 2017; 127: 1150.

Karimipour D, et al: Lafora's disease. J Am Acad Dermatol 1999; 41: 790.

Yildiz EP, et al: A novel *EPM2A* mutation in a patient with Lafora disease presenting with early parkinsonism symptoms in childhood. Seizure 2017; 51: 77.

CADASIL SYNDROME

Cerebral autosomal dominant arteriopathy with subcortical infarcts and leukoencephalopathy (CADASIL) is a neurovascular disease of young and middle-aged people caused by mutations in NOTCH3. It is the most common heritable cause of stroke and vascular dementia in adults, but, due to the characteristic skin findings on histology, skin biopsies can aid in diagnosis. Children have cognitive impairment; young adults have depression and migraine with aura; and patients in their forties and fifties experience apathy, executive dysfunction, mood disturbances, and motor disability followed by dementia. The diagnosis should be confirmed by genetic testing, which will identify most but not all patients with CADASIL. When genetic testing is negative, a skin biopsy can be done showing deposition of a granular osmophilic material in the media of arterial walls with an electron-lucent halo on electron microscopy or demonstrated by a specific immunostain.

Lee YC, et al: The remarkably variable expressivity of CADASIL. J Neurol 2009; 256: 1026.

Lorenzi T, et al: CADASIL. Brain Behav 2017; 7: e00624.

Moreton FC, et al: Changing clinical patterns and increasing prevalence in CADASIL. Acta Neurol Scand 2014; 130: 197.

Ratzinger G, et al: CADASIL. Br J Dermatol 2005; 152: 246.

FARBER DISEASE

Also known as Farber lipogranulomatosis, Farber disease is characterized by periarticular nodules; joint swelling and deformation (usually the initial presentation); a weak, hoarse cry (from laryngeal involvement); pulmonary failure; and motor and mental retardation. It is caused by deficiency of lysosomal acid ceramidase resulting from mutations in the *ASAH1* gene. Progressive accumulation of ceramide in affected tissues results in the complications. Testing for C26-ceramide is the most sensitive.

The rubbery subcutaneous nodules have a distinct yellowish hue and are 1–2 cm in diameter. They are usually located over the joints, lumbar spine, scalp, and weight-bearing areas. Histologically, these are granulomas. Farber disease presents with a highly variable spectrum, with the most severely affected children dying by age 2 years and mildly affected children reaching their teens. There is no correlation between the genotype or the residual ceramidase level and the phenotype. In more mildly affected cases that have not been diagnosed in infancy, the periarticular swellings and predominant joint disease, in about one third of patients, leads to the incorrect diagnosis of juvenile idiopathic arthritis. An animal model has allowed treatment strategies to be tested.

Cozma C, et al: C26-ceramide as highly sensitive biomarker for the diagnosis of Farber Disease. Sci Rep 2017; 7: 6149.

Sands MS, et al: Farber disease. EMBO Mol Med 2013; 5: 799.

Schuchman E: Farber disease explains subset of juvenile idiopathic arthritis. Arthritis Rheum 2014; 66: S173.

Solyom A, et al: Farber disease (acid ceramidase deficiency) epidemiology. Mol Genet Metab 2017; 120: S124.

ADRENOLEUKODYSTROPHY (SCHILDER DISEASE)

Adrenoleukodystrophy (X-ALD) is an X-linked disorder in which cerebral white matter becomes progressively demyelinated and serious adrenocortical insufficiency usually occurs. X-ALD is caused by mutations in the *ABCD1* gene. The gene defect results in impaired degradation of very-long-chain fatty acids (>22 carbons). Skin hyperpigmentation including the buccal mucosa and palmar creases often calls attention to the adrenal disease (Addison disease), and mental deterioration indicates the even graver diagnosis of X-ALD. A mild ichthyotic appearance to the skin of the trunk and legs and sparse hair with trichorrhexis nodosa–like features may occur. Although males are most severely affected, female heterozygote carriers can, in adulthood, develop Addison disease and chronic myelopathy and peripheral neuropathy, often with fecal incontinence. Skin biopsies may show characteristic vacuolization of eccrine secretory coils (duct cells being spared), and biopsies of the skin and conjunctiva may show diagnostic clefts in Schwann cells surrounding myelinated axons. Lorenzo's oil and pioglitazone are potential therapies. Bone marrow transplantation may benefit X-ALD patients, but gene therapy trials are in progress and show promise.

Chen X, et al: Adult cerebral adrenoleukodystrophy and Addison's disease in a female carrier. Gene 2014; 544: 248.

Eichler F, et al: Hematopoietic stem-cell gene therapy for cerebral adrenoleukodystrophy. N Engl J Med 2017; 377: 1630.

Engelen M, et al: X-linked adrenoleukodystrophy in women. Brain 2014; 137: 693.

Pujol A: Novel therapeutic targets and drug candidates for modifying disease progression in adrenoleukodystrophy. Endocr Dev 2016; 30: 147.

Suryawanshi A, et al: An unusual presentation of X-linked adrenoleukodystrophy. Endocrinol Diabetes Metab Case Rep 2015; 2015: 150098.

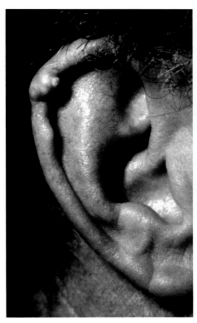

Fig. 26.39 Gout.

GOUT

Classic gout presents as an acute monoarthritis, usually of the great toe or knee, in a middle-aged to elderly man with hyperuricemia. In such patients with chronic disease, usually present for more than 10 years, monosodium urate monohydrate may be deposited in the dermal or subcutaneous tissues, forming papules or nodules called tophi. Rarely, tophi may be the initial presentation of gout, even with normal serum uric acid levels. Gouty tophi vary from pinhead to pea sized or rarely even baseball sized. Tophi are typically found on the pinna (Fig. 26.39) or outer helix of the ears and over the distal interphalangeal articulations. Tophi are of a yellow or cream color. Over time, tophi tend to break down and discharge sodium urate crystals, afterward healing and perhaps breaking down again. Atypical locations for gout include nasal bridge tophi, gouty panniculitis (inflammatory subcutaneous nodules mimicking other forms of panniculitis, possibly with normal serum uric acid), disseminated gout not associated with joints and finger pad tophi. When urate crystal deposition occurs in the dermis, the lesions have been described as "pustular" or "intradermal" tophi.

The diagnosis of gout is verified histologically by finding the characteristic long, needle-shaped crystals of monosodium urate. Because routine processing dissolves these deposits, fixation in absolute ethanol or freezing is optimal for their demonstration, but this is rarely done because most specimens are submitted in formalin. Rather, 10-µm unstained sections from formalin-fixed specimens can demonstrate characteristic crystals under polarized light. Atypical gout occurs as a polyarticular chronic arthritis, often of the hands. It occurs equally in women and men, and there may be tophi, frequently overlying Heberden nodes, at presentation. Another risk group is organ transplant patients, 10% of whom develop gout. Treatment with certain medications has been associated with the appearance of tophi. These include diuretics, methotrexate, cyclosporine, and etanercept. Treatment with allopurinol can result in disappearance of the tophi.

LESCH-NYHAN SYNDROME

Also known as juvenile gout, Lesch-Nyhan syndrome is a rare X-linked recessive inherited disorder characterized by childhood

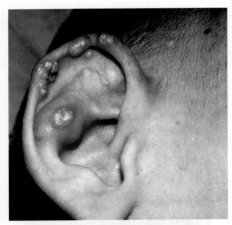

Fig. 26.40 Lesch-Nyhan syndrome.

hyperuricemia, gout, tophi (Fig. 26.40), choreoathetosis, progressive mental retardation, and self-mutilation. The cutaneous lesions are distinctive. Massive self-mutilation of lips with the teeth occurs. The fingers are also severely chewed. The ears and nose are occasionally mutilated. An early diagnostic clue is orange crystals in the diaper. The blood uric acid is increased, and allopurinol, 200–400 mg/day, is given. There is a marked deficiency in an enzyme of purine metabolism, hypoxanthine guanine phosphoribosyltransferase.

Forbess LJ, Fields TR: The broad spectrum of urate crystal deposition: unusual presentations of gouty tophi. Semin Arthritis Rheum 2012; 42: 146.

Jung HY, et al: Disseminated cutaneous gout. Indian J Dermatol Venereol Leprol 2016; 82: 204.

Uy JL, et al: Oral hemorrhage in a 3-year-old boy caused by self-mutilating behavior. Pak J Med Sci 2016; 32: 1583.

Weaver J, et al: Simple non-staining method to demonstrate urate crystals in formalin-fixed, paraffin-embedded skin biopsies. J Cutan Pathol 2009; 36:5 60.

27 Genodermatoses and Congenital Anomalies

The genetic basis for common diseases such as atopic dermatitis and psoriasis, in addition to rare diseases, has been partially elucidated. Some genetic disorders are explained by mutations in a specific gene or genes that lead to a specific clinical phenotype that can be recognized based in part on the skin manifestations. These are termed *genodermatoses*, and recognizing the skin features can lead to earlier diagnosis and management, potentially preventing disease. Genetic disorders are often grouped into three categories: chromosomal, single gene, and polygenic. The advancement of genetic testing has allowed the discovery of postzygotic mutations that only affect a small area of the body. Many segmental patterns of congenital lesions are due to postzygotic mutations. These postzygotic mutations leading to congenital lesions of the vascular system and epidermal nevi are discussed in their respective chapters. Chromosomal disorders can be numeric, such as trisomy and monosomy, or structural, resulting from translocations or deletions. Most genodermatoses show single-gene or mendelian inheritance (autosomal dominant, autosomal recessive, or X-linked recessive genes). Polygenetic syndromes often involve complex interactions of genes. Occasionally a second genetic hit is required to manifest skin findings.

Autosomal dominant conditions require only a single gene to produce a given phenotype. Usually the patient has one affected parent or is affected by a new mutation. The disease is transmitted from generation to generation. Autosomal recessive traits require a homozygous state to produce the abnormality. The pedigree may reveal parental consanguinity. Parents will be clinically unaffected or have mild manifestations but often have affected relatives. X-linked conditions occur when the mutated gene is carried on the X chromosome. If a disease is X-linked recessive, the loss is evident in males (XY), who do not have a second X chromosome to express the normal allele. Therefore X-linked recessive traits occur almost exclusively in males. They cannot transmit the disease to sons (who inherit their Y chromosome), but all their daughters will be carriers. Carrier females who are heterozygous (having one normal and one abnormal X chromosome) occasionally show some evidence of the disease. This occurs as a result of lyonization, the physiologic inactivation of one of the X chromosomes. X-linked dominant disease states are usually lethal in males. Survival is possible in females who retain a normal allele. Because the mutation is lethal in many affected cell lines, females typically demonstrate loss of normal tissue in the affected segments (narrow Blaschko segments, loss of digits, microphthalmia, loss of teeth). X-linked dominant traits result in pedigrees in which more than one female is affected but no males express the disease. Rarely, males may survive, especially if they have Klinefelter syndrome (XXY) or a postzygotic mutation leading to mosaicism such that only some cells are affected.

Mosaicism is the presence of two or more genetically distinct cell lines in a single individual. It may occur as a result of physiologic inactivation of one X chromosome (lyonization) or as the result of a postzygotic somatic mutation. Mosaicism often presents in a linear and whorled pattern along the lines of Blaschko. In mosaic states, genes that are detrimental to a cell population during fetal development (e.g., incontinentia pigmenti) typically result in thin segments because they are overgrown by the adjacent normal tissue. Conversely, genes that confer a growth advantage during fetal development (e.g., mutated tumor suppressor gene in segmental neurofibromatosis) may result in broad, plaque-type lesions that have grown beyond the boundaries of a typical Blaschko segment.

In autosomal dominant conditions, a normal allele remains but is not enough to prevent disease. Loss of heterozygosity (LOH) is a second genetic mutation leading to a defect in the remaining normal allele that explains why a lesion is only in a limited part of the skin. LOH may give rise to segments of the body with an exaggerated presentation of the syndrome. The affected area corresponds to a Blaschko segment or plaque. The forehead plaque of tuberous sclerosis is related to a mutation in a tumor suppressor gene. The loss of the tumor suppressor gene imparts a growth advantage, and LOH leaves no suppressor gene product in the segment. As a result, the affected segment grows beyond its Blaschko boundaries, forming a broad plaque.

When a patient presents with segmental distribution of a disorder, it is critical to determine whether the disorder is a result of mosaicism or LOH. In LOH, the abnormal allele is present throughout the body, including gonadal tissue. In a patient who presents with segmental neurofibromatosis but has Lisch nodules or axillary freckling, LOH rather than mosaicism is likely to account for the segmental presentation. The risk of passing the gene to a child is about 50/50. A genetic counselor should be involved to discuss risk of transmission to offspring because the mechanisms may be complex. Patients with mosaicism based on postzygotic somatic gene mutation may have gonadal mosaicism and may be capable of passing on the gene. Gonadal mosaicism is more likely when more than one segment is present on different regions of the body. Before gastrulation, when a cavity forms in the embryo, every cell is pluripotent and can give rise to an entire organism, or it can contribute to multiple sites of the body. At gastrulation, cells become dedicated to produce specific segments of the body. Blaschko segments in different regions suggest a mutation that occurred before gastrulation, when the involved cell lines could contribute to different parts of the body, including the gonads. Polygenetic disorders, such as psoriasis, may also present with limited and linear forms that may relate to segmental LOH or postzygotic mutation.

Online Mendelian Inheritance in Man (OMIM.org) contains a comprehensive database of known genetic disorders and has a search function that allows the clinician to match clinical manifestations with possible diagnoses. When a patient has more than one very unusual finding OMIM can help determine whether the patient may have a genetic disorder linking the findings. PubMed's clinical query function can also be used to match manifestations with syndromes, and Genetest.org lists sources for genetic testing.

Happle R: Superimposed segmental manifestation of polygenic skin disorders. J Am Acad Dermatol 2007; 57: 690.

■ X-LINKED, MOSAIC AND RELATED DISRODERS WITH ABNORMAL PIGMENT

INCONTINENTIA PIGMENTI

Also known as Bloch-Sulzberger disease, incontinentia pigmenti is an X-linked dominant condition characterized by whorled pigmentation on the trunk, preceded by vesicular and verrucous changes. It appears in girls during the first weeks after birth (Fig.

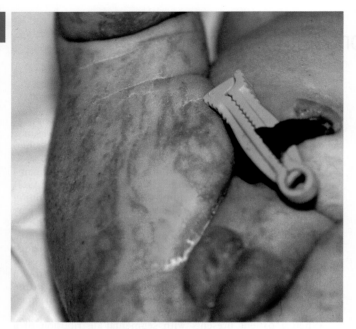

Fig. 27.1 Incontinentia pigmenti, early inflammatory phase.

27.1). Most lesions are evident by the time the infant is 4–6 weeks old. A vesicular phase is present in nearly all cases. This first stage begins in most individuals before 6 weeks of age and is replaced by verrucous lesions after several weeks to months in two thirds of patients. Although these usually resolve by 1 year of age, lesions may persist or recurr for many years. In the third, or pigmentary, phase, pigmented macules in streaks, sprays, splatters, and whorls follow the lines of Blaschko. The pigmentary stage may last for many years and then fade away, leaving no sequelae. The stages are not mutually exclusive. Therefore it is not uncommon for a young child to have some areas still in a verrucous stage while others are hyperpigmented. A fourth stage may be seen in some adult women, manifesting subtle, faint, hypochromic or atrophic linear lesions, most often on the extremities.

Histologically, the vesicular stage is characterized by spongiosis with eosinophils. As the lesions mature, clusters of dyskeratotic cells appear within the epidermis. Dyskeratotic cells predominate in the verrucous stage, and pigment incontinence (dermal melanophages) predominates in hyperpigmented lesions.

Other cutaneous changes include patchy alopecia at the vertex of the scalp, atrophic changes simulating acrodermatitis chronica atrophicans on the hands, onychodystrophy, late subungual tumors that resemble subungual keratoacanthoma and may have underlying lytic bone lesions, and palmoplantar hyperhidrosis. Extracutaneous manifestations occur in 70%–90% of patients. Most frequently involved are the teeth (up to 90%), bones (40%), central nervous system (CNS; 33%), and eyes (35%). Immune dysfunction with defective neutrophil chemotaxis and elevated immunoglobulin E (IgE) has been reported. Eosinophilia is common. Incontinentia pigmenti is an important cause of neonatal seizures and encephalopathy.

Dental abnormalities usually manifest by the time the individual is 2 years old. Dental defects may be the only stigmata still present in the mother and thus can be helpful in the diagnosis of an affected child. Dental defects include delayed eruption, partial anodontia (43%), microdontia, and cone- or peg-shaped teeth (30%). The most common CNS findings are seizures in approximately 10% followed by mental retardation, spastic paralysis, microcephaly, destructive encephalopathy, and motor impairment.

The eye changes include strabismus, cataracts, retinal detachments, optic atrophy, vitreous hemorrhage, blue sclerae, and exudative chorioretinitis. Skeletal abnormalities include syndactyly, skull deformities, dwarfism, spina bifida, clubfoot (talipes), supernumerary ribs, hemiatrophy, and shortening of the legs and arms. Rarely, tricuspid insufficiency, right ventricular hypertrophy, and pulmonary hypertension have been described.

Incontinentia pigmenti is caused by a mutation in the nuclear factor-κB (*NEMO*) gene on the X chromosome, localized to Xq28. Therefore it is typically passed from mother to daughter although there are reports of germline mosaic males giving birth to affected daughters. The gene is generally lethal in male fetuses, although males with Klinefelter syndrome (47,XXY) may survive. Mosaicism may also account for some cases in males. *NEMO* mutations also cause X-linked ectodermal dysplasia with immunodeficiency, characterized by alopecia, hypohidrosis, dental anomalies, and defects in humoral immunity. Osteopetrosis and lymphedema may be present.

Incontinentia pigmenti achromians is a term that has been replaced with the term *pigmentary mosaicism* (see section on pigmentary mosaicism). Mendelian susceptibility to mycobacterial disease is a rare syndrome predisposing to infection with weakly virulent mycobacteria, such as *Mycobacterium avium* complex, *Mycobacterium bovis*, bacille Calmette-Guérin (BCG), and environmental nontuberculous mycobacteria. The causative mutations in *NEMO* selectively affect the CD40-dependent induction of interleukin-12 (IL-12) in mononuclear cells. These patients typically clinically manifest with hypohidrotic ectodermal dysplasia or rarely incontinentia pigmenti.

Use of ruby lasers to treat pigmented lesions in infants and young children may worsen the condition. Usually, the end stage of streaks of incontinentia pigmenti start to fade at age 2 years, and by adulthood, there may be minimal residual pigmentation.

NAEGELI-FRANCESCHETTI-JADASSOHN SYNDROME

Naegeli-Franceschetti-Jadassohn syndrome differs from incontinentia pigmenti in that the pigmentation is reticular, with no preceding inflammatory changes, vesiculation, or verrucous lesions. Vasomotor changes and hypohidrosis are present. There is reticulate pigmentation involving the neck, flexural skin, and perioral and periorbital areas. Diffuse keratoderma and punctiform accentuation of the palms and soles may occur. Dermatoglyphics are abnormal, producing atrophic or absent ridges on fingerprints. Congenital malalignment of the great toenails may be found. Dental abnormalities are common, and many patients are edentulous. Both genders are equally affected, and the syndrome appears to be transmitted as an autosomal dominant trait related to mutations in keratin 14, causing increased susceptibility to tumor necrosis factor (TNF)-α–induced apoptosis. The syndrome is allelic to dermatopathia pigmentosa reticularis (DPR), which manifests with similar cutaneous findings but DPR patients have absent dermatoglyphs.

Bustamante J, et al: Genetic lessons learned from X-linked mendelian susceptibility to mycobacterial diseases. Ann NY Acad Sci 2011; 1246: 92.

Fusco F, et al: Incontinentia pigmenti. Orphanet J Rare Dis 2014; 9: 93.

Fusco F, et al: Unusual father-to-daughter transmission of incontinentia pigmenti due to mosaicism in IP males. Pediatrics 2017; 140: e20162950.

Itin PH, et al: Spontaneous fading of reticular pigmentation in Naegeli-Franceschetti-Jadassohn syndrome. Dermatology 2010; 221: 135.

Mahmoud BH, et al: Controversies over subungual tumors in incontinentia pigmenti. Dermatol Surg 2014; 40: 1157.

Marques GF, et al: Incontinentia pigmenti or Bloch-Sulzberger syndrome. An Bras Dermatol 2014; 89: 486.
Minić S, et al: Systematic review of central nervous system anomalies in incontinentia pigmenti. Orphanet J Rare Dis 2013; 8: 25.
Okita M, et al: *NEMO* gene rearrangement (exon 4-10 deletion) and genotype-phenotype relationship in Japanese patients with incontinentia pigmenti and review of published work in Japanese patients. J Dermatol 2013; 40: 272.
Poziomczyk CS, et al: Incontinentia pigmenti. An Bras Dermatol 2014; 89: 26.
Zhang Y, et al: Incontinentia pigmenti (Bloch-Siemens syndrome). Eur J Pediatr 2013; 172: 1137.

PIGMENTARY MOSAICISM

Pigmentary mosaicism is a term that encompasses congenital hypopigmentation and hyperpigmentation in multiple patterns that is due to alterations in genetic pathways responsible for pigmentation. Pigmentation changes can be either hypopigmentation or hyperpigmentation and are often manifested along lines of Blaschko. Some of the affected genes are also important in other tissues and thus markers of systemic disease. For example, if there are defects in neural crest cells that are programmed to form both the skin and the CNS or eye there can be manifestations in all of the tissues. Genetic mutations that occur in earlier in development lead to a more widespread pattern of pigmentation changes and likely a greater chance that some of those cells with mutations were the progenitors for other tissues, thus increasing the risk for systemic disease associations. Many patients with localized pigmentary mosaicism especially when unilateral and blocklike have no associated systemic findings (segmental pigmentary disorder). There are many historical descriptive terms for different types of pigment but because the pathophysiology is the same, the term *pigmentary mosaicism* is more correct. Pigmentary mosaicism can result from chromosomal abnormalities, with most demonstrating mosaicism for aneuploidy or unbalanced translocations. There is no treatment for pigmentary mosaicism although the pigment may normalize over time in some.

PIGMENTARY MOSAICISM WITH HYPOPIGMENTATION

Incontinentia pigmenti achromians (IPA) and *hypomelanosis of Ito* (HI) are terms that have historically been used, but because most people with HI have been described as having seizures and/or developmental delay whereas many people with blaschkoid hypopigmentation do not have these manifestations, it is favored to use the term *pigmentary mosaicism* to avoid the assumption that children with hypopigmentation will have poor prognosis. The hypopigmentation typically follows the lines of Blaschko (Fig. 27.2). If there are system findings, which may be more likely in children with more diffuse cutaneous involvement, affected individuals can have associated anomalies of the CNS, eyes, hair, teeth, skin, nails, musculoskeletal system, or internal organs, including polycystic kidney disease. Patients may manifest psychomotor or mental impairment, autism, microcephaly, coarse facies, and dysmorphic ears.

Because there are many different types of mutations that can lead to hypopigmentation, these patients should not be considered to have one syndrome but instead multiple rare syndromes many of which have not been named. Some patients have had associated Sturge-Weber syndrome–like leptomeningeal angiomatosis. A recent group of patients was described mammalian target of rapamycin (mTOR) with pigmentary mosaicism of the hypopigmented type with megalencephaly and focal cortical dysplasia due to mosaic mTOR mutations. Several patients have demonstrated trisomy 13 with hypopigmented mosaicism.

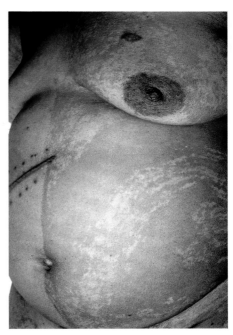

Fig. 27.2 Incontinentia pigmentary mosaicism.

Baxter LL, et al: The etiology and molecular genetics of human pigmentation disorders. Wiley Interdiscip Rev Dev Biol 2013; 2: 379.
Hogeling MI, Frieden IJ: Segmental pigmentation disorder. Br J Dermatol 2010; 162: 1337.

PIGMENTARY MOSAICISM WITH HYPERPIGMENTATION

Linear and whorled nevoid hypermelanosis is the term historically used to describe blaschkoid distribution of hyperpigmented streaks without preceding bullae or verrucous lesions. Sparing of mucous membranes, eyes, palms, and soles is noted. Congenital anomalies, such as mental retardation, cerebral palsy, atrial septal defects, dextrocardia, auricular atresia, hemiatrophy, and patent ductus arteriosus, may be present but seem to be less prevalent with hyperpigmentation than with hypopigmented mosaicism. Bilateral giant cerebral aneurysms have been reported. Biopsy of pigmented areas demonstrates increased pigmentation of the basal layer and prominence of melanocytes without incontinence of pigment. Again, patients who have localized pigmentation especially in blocklike unilateral patterns seem to be less likely to have systemic manifestations. Most cases appear to be sporadic, although familial cases have been reported. The differential diagnosis includes other causes of blaschkoid hyperpigmentation such as incontinentia pigmenti, verrucous epidermal nevi that have not proliferated yet, and McCune-Albright syndrome.

Cohen J 3rd, et al: Analysis of 36 cases of Blaschkoid dyspigmentation. Pediatr Dermatol 2014; 31: 471.
Mehta V, et al: Linear and whorled nevoid hypermelanosis. Int J Dermatol 2011; 50: 491.
Metta AK, et al: Linear and whorled nevoid hypermelanosis in three successive generations. Indian J Dermatol Venereol Leprol 2011; 77: 403.

DISORDERS DUE TO SEX CHROMOSOMES

X-Linked Reticulate Pigmentation Disorder

X-linked reticulate pigmentation disorder with systemic manifestations that presents with reticulate hyperpigmentation due a mutation that leads to amyloid buildup. In males, cutaneous involvement is characterized by reticulate hyperpigmentation of the skin, characteristic facies, and severe systemic involvement. In the carrier females, manifestations are limited to the skin.

Anderson RC, et al: X-linked reticulate pigmentary disorder with systemic manifestations. Pediatr Dermatol 2005; 22: 122.

Klinefelter Syndrome

Klinefelter syndrome, the most common sex chromosome disorder, consists of hypogonadism, gynecomastia, eunuchoidism, small or absent testicles, and elevated gonadotropins. The patient may have a low frontal hairline, sparse body hair with only a few hairs in the axillary and pubic areas, scanty or absent facial hair in men, and shortening of the fifth digit of both hands.

Thrombophlebitis and recurrent or chronic leg ulcerations may be a presenting manifestation; these may be more common than previously reported. The cause of the hypercoagulable state is believed to be an increase in plasminogen activator inhibitor 1 levels. Patients are at an increased risk of lupus erythematosus and a variety of cancers, especially male breast cancer, hematologic malignancies, and sarcomas (retinoblastoma and rhabdomyosarcoma).

Many of these patients are tall; some are obese. Psychiatric disorders occur in about one third of patients and patients can have decreased mental capacity. Klinefelter syndrome is most frequently associated with an XXY sex chromosome pattern, although other variations occur as the number of X chromosomes increases. Androgen therapy may result in improvements in appearance and function.

XXYY Genotype

The XXYY genotype is considered to be a variant of Klinefelter syndrome. In addition to the changes seen in Klinefelter, vascular changes occur in XXYY patients, such as cutaneous angiomas, acrocyanosis, and peripheral vascular disease leading to stasis dermatitis. Hypertelorism, clinodactyly, pes planus, and dental abnormalities are common. Systemic manifestations include asthma, cardiac defects, radioulnar synostosis, inguinal hernia, cryptorchidism, CNS defects, attention-deficit disorder, autism, and seizures.

XYY Genotype

Patients with an XYY karyotype can have very severe acne with onset in childhood and be more aggressive and have cognitive delays, although these studies were performed on prisoners so there may be a selection bias.

Turner Syndrome

Turner syndrome, also known as gonadal dysgenesis, is characterized by a webbed neck, low posterior hairline margin, increased carrying angle at the elbow (cubitus valgus), congenital lymphedema, and a triangular mouth. Patients may demonstrate alopecia of the frontal area on the scalp, koilonychia, cutis laxa, cutis hyperelastica, mental retardation, short stature, infantilism, impaired sexual development, primary amenorrhea, numerous melanocytic nevi, angiokeratomas, and an increased risk of melanoma, pilomatricoma, and thyroid disease. Coarctation of the aorta is frequently found. There may be an increased incidence of alopecia areata and halo nevi in these patients.

Patients with Turner syndrome are females who have only one X chromosome. Mosaic Turner syndrome exists in which only some cells are missing the other X. Loss of long-arm material (Xq) can result in short stature and ovarian failure, but deletions distal to Xq21 do not appear to affect stature. Loss of the short arm (Xp) produces the full phenotype. Patients with very distal Xp deletions usually have normal ovarian function.

No specific treatment is available for Turner syndrome. Human growth hormone (hGH) has been used to treat the short stature. A review of the Cochrane Central Register of Controlled Trials determined that hGH increases short-term growth, but few data exist regarding its effects on final height.

Multiple pterygium syndrome (Escobar syndrome) is a rare autosomal recessive disorder characterized by multiple congenital joint contractures and multiple skin webs that may mimic Turner syndrome.

Balsera AM, et al: Distinct mechanism of formation of the 48, XXYY karyotype. Mol Cytogenet 2013; 6: 25.
Castelo-Branco C: Management of Turner syndrome in adult life and beyond. Maturitas 2014; 79: 471.
Dillon S, et al: Klinefelter's syndrome (47,XXY) among men with systemic lupus erythematosus. Acta Paediatr 2011; 100: 819.
Güven A, et al: Multiple pterygium syndrome. J Pediatr Endocrinol Metab 2011; 24: 1089.
Kasparis C et al: Childhood acne in a boy with XYY syndrome. BMJ Case Rep 2014 Jan 6; 2014.
Rogol AD, et al: Considerations for androgen therapy in children and adolescents with Klinefelter syndrome (47, XXY). Pediatr Endocrinol Rev 2010; 8: 145.

RASOPATHIES

The Ras-Map kinase pathway (including Raf, ERK, and MEK) is critical for cellular growth. Many different genetic disorders involving mutations in the genes controlling various parts of this pathway present with similar features. Historically as these diseases were described they had significant clinical overlap and this is due to the defects involving the same pathway. These disorders are now grouped under the category of RASopathies.

Neurofibromatosis Type 1

The four types of neurofibromatosis are neurocutaneous syndromes that are manifested by developmental changes in the nervous system, bones, and skin.

Patients with neurofibromatosis type I (NF-1, von Recklinghausen disease), which accounts for more than 85% of cases, typically present in infancy. NF-1 is either inherited autosomal dominantly or occurs due to de novo mutations. The most common initial manifestations are a large head circumference along with six or more café au lait macules. The typical café au lait macules of NF-1 should have a smooth margin and are oval or round and typically very clinically apparent (Fig. 27.3). Most often, these macules are present at birth and almost always present by 1 year of age. The finding of six or more of these lesions measuring at least 1.5 cm in diameter is diagnostic, usually indicating NF-1. In children, the minimum diameter for a significant lesion is 0.5 cm. There are many children who have brown patches with jagged margins that appear splattered onto the skin or arranged in blaschkoid pattern and these are not typical for NF-1. Histologically, basilar hyperpigmentation is noted, and giant melanosomes may be seen. Axillary freckling (Fig. 27.4) and/or inguinal freckling (Crowe sign) may also be present at birth and can extend to the neck and involve the inguinal, genital, and perineal areas.

Neurofibromas (Fig. 27.5) develop later in childhood and continue to develop into adulthood but are rarely present in infants unless there is a plexiform neurofibroma. Neurofibromas of the areolae

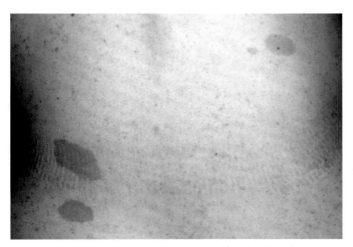
Fig. 27.3 Neurofibromatosis with café au lait macule.

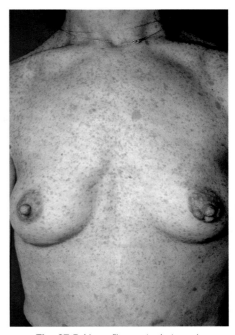
Fig. 27.5 Neurofibromatosis type 1.

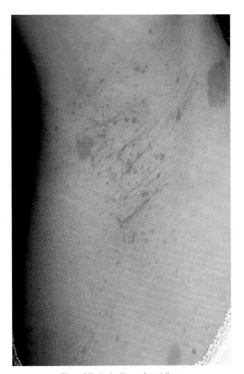
Fig. 27.4 Axillary freckling.

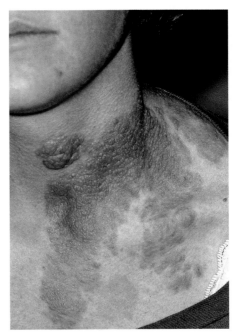
Fig. 27.6 Plexiform neurofibroma.

occur in more than 90% of women with NF-1. Neurofibromas are soft tumors that can be pushed down into the panniculus by light pressure with the finger ("buttonholing") and spring back when released. Histologically, these are well-circumscribed, but rarely encapsulated, spindle cell proliferations with an amphophilic myxoid stroma and many mast cells. The spindle cells have a wavy appearance. Neurofibromas result from proliferation of all supporting elements of the nerve fibers, including Schwann, perineurial, endoneurial, and mast cells and blood vessels. Axon stains demonstrate individual axons spread randomly throughout the tumor, in contrast to a schwannoma, where a nerve trunk is compressed at one edge of the tumor, but no axons are present within its bulk.

Subcutaneous plexiform neurofibromas are virtually pathognomonic of NF-1 and are often a manifestation of LOH. On palpation, these resemble a "bag of worms." The overlying skin is usually hyperpigmented and may resemble a giant café au lait macule (Fig. 27.6). Because the plexiform neurofibromas can take time to grow and manifest the larger café au lait may be the only marker of its presence in infancy. Plexiform neurofibromas within the spine can cause paralysis. Histologically, plexiform neurofibromas demonstrate numerous elongated encapsulated neurofibromas, often embedded in diffuse neurofibroma that involves the dermis and subcutaneous fat.

Many organ systems may be involved. Optic gliomas can be present in infancy and patients should be referred to an ophthalmologist immediately. Lisch nodules are found in the irides of about one quarter of patients under 6 years of age and in 94% of adult patients. Acromegaly, cretinism, hyperparathyroidism, myxedema, pheochromocytoma (<1%), or precocious puberty may be present. Patients with NF-1 can present with hypertension either due to renal artery stenosis or aortic coarctation (early in life) or a pheochromocytoma usually manifested later, and thus all patients with NF-1 should have their blood pressure closely monitored. Bone changes (usually erosive) may produce lordosis, kyphosis, and pseudoarthrosis, as well as spina bifida, dislocations, and atraumatic fractures. The pseudoarthrosis (pseudojoints) can be seen on imaging of long bones in childhood in some patients.

Patients with NF-1 are four times more likely to develop malignancies than the general population. Cutaneous neurofibromas rarely develop into malignant, peripheral nerve sheath tumors. A painful, growing or hardening lesion is an indication for biopsy. An increased incidence of breast carcinoma, Wilms tumor, rhabdomyosarcomas, gastrointestinal (GI) malignancies, and chronic myelogenous leukemia (CML) has also been reported. Children with NF-1 are 200–500 times more likely to develop malignant myeloid disorders than age-matched controls, and the risk for juvenile chronic myelomonocytic leukemia (JCMML) may be higher for those with juvenile xanthogranulomas (JXGs). Therefore some experts advocate for regular complete blood counts for the first few years in patients with NF-1 who have JXG.

Mental retardation, dementia, epilepsy, and a variety of intracranial malignancies may occur. Hypertelorism heralds a severe expression of neurofibromatosis with brain involvement. Diffuse interstitial lung disease occurs in 7% of patients.

Approximately 50% of cases of NF-1 represent new mutations. The gene for NF-1 codes for neurofibromin, a protein that negatively regulates signals transduced by Ras proteins. There is a high rate of spontaneous postzygotic mutation of this gene. Both alleles must be affected for the individual to grow a neurofibroma. In patients with the syndrome, there is germline loss of one allele, and each neurofibroma that develops represents a late spontaneous mutation knocking out the remaining allele.

Segmental neurofibromatosis (also called mosaic neurofibromatosis) arises from postzygotic somatic mutation (Fig. 27.7). Early postzygotic mutation affecting the second allele in fetal life results in LOH affecting an entire Blaschko segment. Within this affected lesion any of the other features of NF-1 could occur, but in one series 29% of the patients were found to have features of NF-1 affecting other tissues and thus patients with segmental NF-1 should be monitored similarly to patients with nonsegmental NF-1. Diagnosis is by biopsying affected tissues for genetic testing because the peripheral blood may be negative.

Diagnosis

The diagnosis of NF-1 requires two or more of the following criteria to be fulfilled:

1. Six or more café au lait macules with a greatest diameter of more than 5 mm in prepubertal individuals, and a greatest diameter of more than 15 mm in postpubertal individuals
2. Two or more neurofibromas of any type or one plexiform neurofibroma
3. Freckling in the axillary or inguinal regions
4. Optic gliomas
5. Two or more Lisch nodules
6. Distinctive osseous lesion, such as a sphenoid dysplasia or thinning of the long-bone cortex with or without pseudarthrosis
7. First-degree relative (parent, sibling, or offspring) with the disease

A diagnosis of NF-2 requires either of the following:

1. Bilateral eighth cranial nerve masses, as demonstrated on computed tomography (CT) or magnetic resonance imaging (MRI)

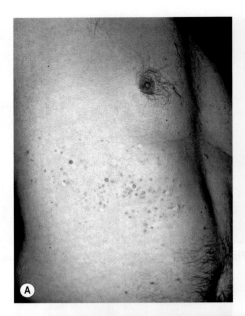

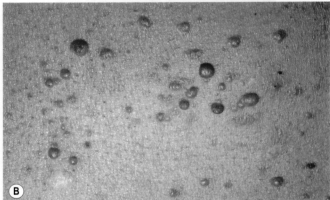

Fig. 27.7 (A and B) Segmental neurofibromatosis.

2. First-degree relative with NF-2 and either unilateral eighth nerve mass or two of the following: a neurofibroma, meningioma, glioma, schwannoma, and juvenile posterior subcapsular lenticular opacity

Although not listed in the previous criteria, the presence of nevus anemicus, xanthogranuloma, and glomus tumors is strongly associated with a diagnosis of NF-1, and the prevalence is high during the first 2 years of life, when other diagnostic criteria may be absent so they are vital to recognize. Nevus anemicus is usually found on the neck and upper chest, whereas the xanthogranulomas tend to be cephalic or genital.

Screening and Monitoring for Complications

In one study of 93 asymptomatic patients with NF-1 who underwent cerebral imaging, 12 optic gliomas were detected, suggesting that screening MRI or CT may be of value. Positron emission tomography (PET) scanning has shown some value in discriminating between benign and malignant tumors. The National Institutes of Health (NIH) consensus panel concluded that studies should be dictated by findings on clinical evaluation. It concluded that laboratory tests in asymptomatic patients are unlikely to be of value. In the majority of patients with NF-1, imaging studies should only be performed as indicated by signs or symptoms.

Therapy for individual symptomatic lesions is with surgical removal, but sirolimus has shown some efficacy for plexiform neurofibromas that are causing morbidity. Trials of targeted therapy to reduce the growth of cutaneous neurofibromas are ongoing and are likely to result in better treatment options for severely affected patients.

Type 2 neurofibromatosis (NF-2), central or acoustic neurofibromatosis, is distinguished by bilateral acoustic neuromas, usually in the absence of cutaneous lesions, although neurofibromas and schwannomas may occur. The gene for NF-2 encodes for merlin (schwannomin), a protein that links the actin cytoskeleton to cell surface glycoproteins and functions as a negative growth regulator. NF-2 patients, in contrast, often require imaging studies. Screening studies should include an audiogram and brainstem auditory evoked responses. MRI is the best imaging procedure for patients with evidence of hearing impairments or abnormal evoked responses. Tests of vestibular function may be useful, because eighth cranial nerve tumors develop on the vestibular division. A screening MRI should be performed by puberty. Other tests should be performed as dictated by signs and symptoms. Pediatric patients with NF-2 have a worse prognosis, with 75% demonstrating hearing loss, 83% visual impairment, and 25% abnormal ambulation. Type 3 (mixed) and type 4 (variant) forms resemble type 2 but have cutaneous neurofibromas. Patients with these types are at greater risk for developing optic gliomas, neurilemmomas, and meningiomas. These forms are inherited as autosomal dominant traits.

SPRED1 (Legius Syndrome)

Germline loss-of-function mutations in the *SPRED1* gene have been associated with an NF-1–like phenotype with café au lait macules and axillary or inguinal freckling but no neurofibromas or lisch nodules (Legius syndrome). Patients present with similar café au laits and increased head circumference to NF-1, and most laboratories that do genetic testing for NF-1 will do *SPRED1* reflexively if NF-1 testing is negative because the diseases match each other so closely. Developmental delay in patients with mosaic *SPRED1* has now been reported as well.

Noonan Syndrome

Noonan syndrome is an autosomal dominant RASopathy associated with a webbed neck that mimics Turner syndrome but affects males and females equally. The other major features are a characteristic facies with hypertelorism, prominent ears, short stature, undescended testicles, low posterior neck hairline, cardiovascular abnormalities (e.g., pulmonary stenosis), and cubitus valgus. From 25%–40% of patients have dermatologic findings: lymphedema, short curly hair, dystrophic nails, tendency toward keloid formation, soft elastic skin, keratosis pilaris atrophicans (ulerythema of eyebrows), multiple granular cell tumors, and abnormal dermatoglyphics. Growth hormone can help patients achieve more normal stature.

Genetic changes in Noonan affect the RAS/MAPK pathway. The majority of Noonan cases are caused by defects in *PTPN11*. Patients with *PTPN11* have more café au lait macules. Patients with Noonan syndrome may have *SOS1* mutations associated with normal cognition and stature along with keratosis pilaris, *RAF1* mutations entailing a high risk of hypertrophic cardiomyopathy. *PTPN11* mutations predispose to juvenile myelomonocytic leukemia. When differentiating RAsopathies, feeding difficulties and developmental motor delay are the most common features with the cardiofaciocutaneous syndrome and Costello syndrome. Noonan-associated RASopathies appear to have an increased risk of lupus erythematosus.

Noonan Syndrome–Like Disorder With Loose Anagen Hair (NSLAH)

Recently a group of patients with Noonan-like features (short stature, typical facies, and pectus excavatum) along with loose anagen have been documented. They also have more hyperactive behavior, a hoarse voice, and more severe developmental delay. This is caused by a *SHOC2* mutation (or more recently described with *PPP1CB*). The hair demonstrates an anagen hair bulb (hockey stick or tube sock at the end) on dermoscopy, but recently trichorrhexis nodosa and trichoptilosis along with darkened or hairless skin have been described.

Noonan Syndrome With Lentigines (LEOPARD)

The LEOPARD syndrome—multiple lentigines, electrocardiographic conduction abnormalities, ocular hypertelorism, pulmonary stenosis, abnormal genitalia, retardation of growth, and sensorineural deafness—also known as multiple lentigines syndrome, cardiocutaneous syndrome, lentiginosis profusa syndrome, or progressive cardiomyopathic lentiginosis has been renamed Noonan syndrome with lentigines. The lentigines occur in nearly all patients and are small, dark-brown, polygonal, and irregularly shaped macules, usually measuring 2–5 mm in diameter that start around age 5 and increase dramatically over time. There are none in the mucosa. Individual lesions may be larger, even up to 1–1.5 cm. Melanoma has been described in these patients, so atypical lesions should be biopsied.

The LEOPARD syndrome shares many clinical features with Noonan syndrome. These are allelic disorders; patients with both syndromes (Fig. 27.8) demonstrate mutations in the Noonan syndrome gene, *PTPN11*, although patients with *BRAF*, *RAF1*, and *MAP2K1* mutations are described. Although the "R" in LEOPARD indicates growth retardation, some patients with the syndrome also exhibit mild mental retardation or speech difficulties. Many cases appear sporadically; however, inheritance as an autosomal dominant genetic trait has also been reported. Patients should be referred for cardiovascular and hearing evaluation and screened for cryptorchidism.

Costello Syndrome

Costello syndrome is characterized by growth retardation; failure to thrive in infancy; coarse facies; redundant velvety skin on the neck, palms, soles, and fingers; acanthosis nigricans; and nasal papillomata caused by HRAS mutations. Ventricular dilation

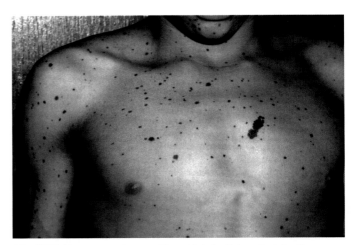

Fig. 27.8 Noonan syndrome with multiple lentigines (previously LEOPARD syndrome). (Courtesy Paul Honig, MD.)

is observed in more than 40% of cases. Hydrocephalus, brain atrophy, Chiari malformation, and syringomyelia may occur. Mild to moderate mental deficiency is frequently discovered, and most patients exhibit a characteristic sociable and friendly personality.

CARDIOFACIOCUTANEOUS SYNDROME

Cardiofaciocutaneous (CFC) syndrome is characterized by a distinctive facial appearance, heart defects, and mental retardation. Facial characteristics include high forehead with bitemporal constriction, downslanting palpebral fissures, hypoplastic supraorbital ridges, a depressed nasal bridge, and posteriorly angulated ears with prominent helices. The heart defects include pulmonic stenosis, atrial septal defect, and hypertrophic cardiomyopathy. Patients may have ectodermal abnormalities. The most frequent dermatologic findings in CFC patients involve the hair, which may be sparse, curly, fine or thick, or woolly or brittle. In the majority reported cases, the patient had dry, scaly, ichthyotic skin with follicular hyperkeratosis (keratosis pilaris, or keratosis pilaris atrophicans faciei). Other cutaneous findings include sparse or absent eyebrows and eyelashes, low posterior hairline, patchy alopecia, scant body hair, seborrheic dermatitis, eczema, lymphedema, hemangiomas, café au lait spots, pigmented nevi, hyperpigmented macules or stripes, cutis marmorata, and sacral dimples. Nail dystrophy, koilonychia, and dysplastic teeth have also been reported.

Most cases occur sporadically, but autosomal dominant transmission has been reported. Various subtypes relate to different genes in the RAS/MAPK pathway, including *KRAS*, *BRAF*, and *MEK1* or *MEK2* mutations.

Aoki Y, et al: Ras/MAPK syndromes and childhood hemato-oncological diseases. Int J Hematol 2013; 97: 30.

Bader-Meunier B, et al: Are RASopathies new monogenic predisposing conditions to the development of systemic lupus erythematosus? Semin Arthritis Rheum 2013; 43: 217.

Blakeley J: Development of drug treatments for neurofibromatosis type 2–associated vestibular schwannoma. Curr Opin Otolaryngol Head Neck Surg 2012; 20: 372.

Duan L, et al: Renal artery stenosis due to neurofibromatosis type 1. Eur J Med Res 2014; 19: 17.

Ferner RE, et al: Neurofibromatosis type 1 (NF1). Handb Clin Neurol 2013; 115: 939.

Ferrari F, et al: Juvenile xanthogranuloma and nevus anemicus in the diagnosis of neurofibromatosis type I. JAMA Dermatol 2014; 150: 42.

García-Romero MT, et al: Mosaic neurofibromatosis type 1. Pediatr Dermatol 2016; 33: 9.

Gelb, BD, Tartaglia M: Noonan syndrome with multiple lentigines. 2007 Nov 30 [Updated 2015 May 14]. I: Adam MP, Ardinger HH, Pagon RA, et al [Eds.] GeneReviews® [Internet]. Seattle (WA): University of Washington, Seattle.

Gripp KW, et al: A novel rasopathy caused by recurrent de novo missense mutations in PPP1CB closely resembles Noonan syndrome with loose anagen hair. Am J Med Genet A 2016; 170: 2237.

Gutmann DH, et al: Optimizing biologically targeted clinical trials for neurofibromatosis. Expert Opin Investig Drugs 2013; 22: 443.

Harrison B, Sammer D: Glomus tumors and neurofibromatosis. Plast Reconstr Surg Glob Open 2014; 2: e214.

Jobling RK, et al: Mosaicism for a SPRED1 deletion revealed in a patient with clinically suspected mosaic neurofibromatosis. Br J Dermatol 2017; 176: 1077.

Kane J, et al: Noonan syndrome with loose anagen hair associated with trichorrhexis nodosa and trichoptilosis. Clin Case Rep 2017; 5: 1152.

Madanikia SA, et al: Increased risk of breast cancer in women with NF1. Am J Med Genet 2012; 158A: 3056.

Martínez-Quintana E, et al: LEOPARD syndrome. Mol Syndromol 2012; 3: 145.

Morice-Picard F, et al: Cutaneous manifestations in Costello and cardiofaciocutaneous syndrome. Pediatr Dermatol 2013; 30: 665.

Myers A, et al: Perinatal features of the RASopathies. Am J Med Genet A 2014; 164: 2814.

Niemeyer CM: RAS diseases in children. Haematologica 2014; 99: 1653.

Pasmant E, et al: Neurofibromatosis type 1. J Med Genet 2012; 49: 483.

Pečina-Šlaus N: Merlin, the NF2 gene product. Pathol Oncol Res 2013; 19: 365.

Rauen KA: The RASopathies. Annu Rev Genomics Hum Genet 2013; 14: 355.

Treglia G, et al: Usefulness of whole-body fluorine-18-fluorodeoxyglucose positron emission tomography in patients with neurofibromatosis type 1. Radiol Res Pract 2012; 2012: 431029.

Tumurkhuu M, et al: A novel *SOS1* mutation in Costello/CFC syndrome affects signaling in both RAS and PI3K pathways. J Recept Signal Transduct Res 2013; 33: 124.

Vranceanu AM, et al: Quality of life among adult patients with neurofibromatosis 1, neurofibromatosis 2 and schwannomatosis. J Neurooncol 2013; 114: 257.

Weiss B, et al: Sirolimus for progressive neurofibromatosis type 1–associated plexiform neurofibromas. Neuro Oncol 2015; 17: 596.

EPIDERMAL NEVUS SYNDROMES

Epidermal nevi are overgrowths of specific epidermal structures and can be isolated to skin findings or if more widespread or extensive can be a marker for a syndrome. Important clues to the diagnosis of specific epidermal nevus (EN) syndromes include linear lesions following blaschkoid lines because the lesions and syndromes are caused by postzygotic mutations leading to mosaicism. Many of the following syndromes are reviewed in other chapters: linear nevus sebaceous (NS) in Schimmelpenning syndrome, NS and papular nevus spilus in phacomatosis pigmentokeratotica, soft white hair in angora hair nevus syndrome (Schauder syndrome), breast hypoplasia in Becker nevus syndrome, mosaic R248 C mutation in fibroblast growth factor receptor 3 EN syndrome (characterized by soft velvety EN and CNS abnormalities), and acral strawberry papillomatous lesions on tips of fingers or toes in CHILD syndrome (see Congenital Hemidysplasia with Ichthyosiform Erythroderma and Limb Defects [CHILD] Syndrome, later in this chapter). Other EN syndromes include nevus trichilemmocysticus (cysts in blaschkoid distribution), didymosis aplasticosebacea (NS with aplasia cutis congenita), SCALP syndrome (NS, CNS malformations, aplasia cutis, limbal dermoid, and pigmented nevus), Gorbello syndrome (systematized linear velvety EN with bone defects), NEVADA syndrome (nevus epidermicus verrucosus with angiodysplasia and aneurysms), and CLOVE syndrome (congenital lipomatous overgrowth [see Chapter 28], vascular malformations, and EN with nonprogressive proportionate overgrowth).

Cirstea IC, et al: Diverging gain-of-function mechanisms of two novel *KRAS* mutations associated with Noonan and cardio-facio-cutaneous syndromes. Hum Mol Genet 2013; 22: 262.

Hafner C, et al: Keratinocytic epidermal nevi are associated with mosaic *RAS* mutations. J Med Genet 2012; 49: 249.

Hafner C, et al: Mosaic RASopathies. Cell Cycle 2013; 12: 43.

Laura FS: Epidermal nevus syndrome. Handb Clin Neurol 2013; 111: 349.

Proteus Syndrome

Proteus syndrome is an overgrowth syndrome caused by an *AKT1* mutation. The mutation appears to be mosaic and activating leading to overgrowth. Proteus shares many features with other syndromes such as PTEN hamartoma syndrome and CLOVE syndrome (see Chapter 28) because they are within a common cellular pathway. Proteus syndrome is named after the Greek god Proteus. The syndrome has protean manifestations that include disproportionate, asymmetric, and distorting segmental overgrowth; cerebriform plantar hyperplasia (Fig. 27.13); epidermal nevi; patchy dermal hypoplasia; macrocephaly; hyperostosis; muscular hypoplasia; hypertrophy of long bones; vascular malformations of the capillary, venous, or lymphatic types; lipomas, lipohypoplasia; fatty overgrowth; bullous lung alterations; intellectual disability; seizures; brain malformations; and deep vein thrombosis. The cerebriform hyperplasia is histopathologically a connective tissue nevus made of collagen and can occur most commonly on the plantar foot but also the palm, abdomen, and nose and is a major diagnostic criterion of Proteus syndrome and very suggestive if present. The vascular lesions are capillary malformations and tend to be darker purple and geometric. Patients with a greater number of cutaneous lesions also have the most extracutaneous abnormalities. There is a high risk of deep vein thrombosis. The vascular stains and epidermal nevi may be the first manifestations because the overgrowth can take time to present (different from CLOVE syndrome) that has similar features. There is progressive severe bony overgrowth in Proteus syndrome that can be extremely distorting.

Cohen MM Jr: Proteus syndrome review. Clin Genet 2014; 85: 111.

Lindhurst MJ, et al: *AKT1* gene mutation levels are correlated with the type of dermatologic lesions in patients with Proteus syndrome. J Invest Dermatol 2014; 134: 543.

Rozas-Muñoz E, et al: Vascular stains: proposal for a clinical classification to improve diagnosis and management. Pediatr Dermatol 2016; 33: 570.

■ PHAKOMATOSES

The phakomatoses are the various inherited disorders of the CNS associated with cutaneous and often ocular involvement. The term was more helpful in organizing genodermatoses before the current genetic pathophysiologic classifications. Phakomatoses include tuberous sclerosis, neurofibromatosis, von Hippel–Lindau disease, ataxia-telangiectasia, nevoid basal cell carcinoma syndrome, nevus sebaceous, and Sturge-Weber syndrome. Many of these disorders have been grouped into more specific groups in this book due to more specific understanding of the pathogenisis of each syndrome.

TUBEROUS SCLEROSIS

Tuberous sclerosis was first described by Desiree-Magloire Bourneville in 1880. The classic triad of adenoma sebaceum (Fig. 27.9), mental deficiency, and epilepsy, however, is present in only a minority of patients. Other associated features include periungual fibromas, shagreen plaques (collagenoma), oral papillomatosis, gingival hyperplasia, ash-leaf hypomelanotic macules, skin fibromas, and café au lait spots.

The first cutaneous lesions are typically the white patches that are oval and shaped like an "ash leaf" (Fig. 27.10). These congenital white, leaf-shaped macules, also called hypomelanotic macules, are found in 85% of patients with tuberous sclerosis and range in number from 1 to 100, although 3 lesions greater than 5 mm must be present to satisfy the criteria. Occasional patients may not develop the macules until 6–8 years of age. These may be

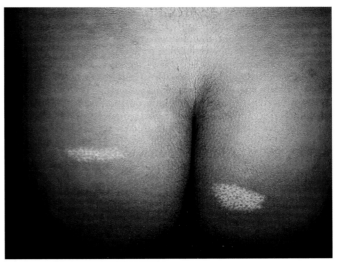

Fig. 27.10 Ash-leaf macules.

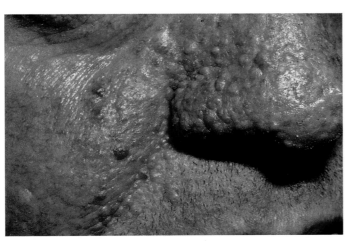

Fig. 27.9 Angiofibromas (adenoma sebaceum).

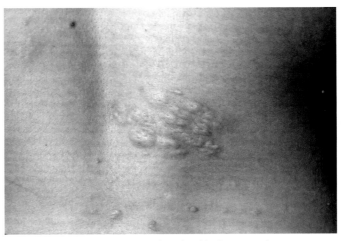

Fig. 27.11 Tuberous sclerosis with shagreen plaque.

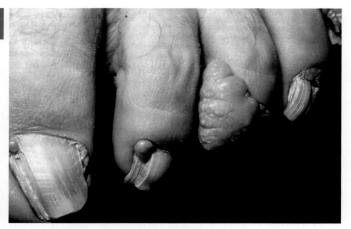

Fig. 27.12 Tuberous sclerosis with periungual fibromas.

shaped like an ash leaf, but linear and confetti-type white macules may also be present. Wood's light examination will highlight these lesions because they can be subtle. Focal poliosis (localized tufts of white hair) may be present at birth. Solitary ash-leaf macules can occur in the general population and may be difficult to distinguish from pigmentary mosaicism and nevus depigmentosus.

Adenoma sebaceum lesions (angiofibromas) are 1–3 mm, yellowish red, translucent, discrete, waxy papules that are distributed symmetrically, principally over the cheeks, nose, and forehead. These lesions are present in 90% of patients older than 4 years, persist indefinitely, and may increase in number. A fibrous forehead plaque (newly named "fibrous cephalic plaque" because they can be anywhere on the head) is usually on the forehead and histopathologically appears to be an angiofibroma. Angiofibromas have also been reported in patients with multiple endocrine neoplasia (MEN-1) and the Birt-Hogg-Dube syndrome.

Shagreen plaque is named after a type of leather tanned to produce knobs on the surface, resembling shark skin. Patches of this type of "knobby" skin, varying from 1–8 cm in diameter, are found on the trunk, most often on the lumbosacral area (Fig. 27.11). These are connective tissue nevi composed almost exclusively of collagen, occur in 40% of patients, and develop in the first decade of life.

Koenen tumors (periungual angiofibromas) occur in 50% of patients (Fig. 27.12). The tumors are small, digitate, protruding, asymptomatic, and periungual/subungual. They appear at puberty. Similar lesions may occur on the gingiva. Nails may also demonstrate longitudinal grooves, long leukonychia, and short red streaks.

Gingival fibromas in the mouth can occur on the buccal mucosa, the labial mucosa, and the tongue.

Mental deficiency, usually appreciated early in life, is present in 40%–60% of patients, varying widely in its manifestations. Epilepsy also occurs, is variable in its severity, and usually also presents early in life. Between 80% and 90% of patients have seizures or nonspecific electroencephalographic abnormalities. Hamartomatous proliferations of glial and neuronal tissue produce potato-like nodules in the cortex. X-ray evaluation will reveal these once calcified, but CT, cranial ultrasonography, and MRI may define these lesions as early as 6 weeks of age and thus are useful in making an early diagnosis. These brain tumors may progress to gliomas. Subependymal nodules ("candle drippings") are similar lesions in the ventricular walls. Astrocytomas may also occur. Forehead plaques may be a marker for more serious intracranial involvement.

Retinal tumors (phakomas) are optic nerve or retinal nerve hamartomas. Various ophthalmologic findings, such as pigmentary changes, nystagmus, and angioid streaks, occur in 50% of patients. Renal hamartomas (angiomyolipomas, cystic disease,

fibroadenomas, or mixed tumors) and cardiac tumors (rhabdomyomas in 43%) may also occur. Renal angiomyolipomas are bilateral and cause renal failure. The cardiac rhabdomyomas may only be seen prenatally and regress after birth but are highly specific for tuberous sclerosis (TS). Pulmonary lymphangioleiomyomatosis is more common in women, especially in their thirties and forties, and can lead to progressive respiratory failure or spontaneous pneumothorax. The condition is characterized by diffuse proliferation of smooth muscle cells and cystic degeneration of the pulmonary parenchyma, associated with the perivascular epithelioid cells ("PEC" cells) implicated in various PEComas. Almost half of patients with TS have bony abnormalities such as bone cysts and sclerosis, which can be seen on x-ray evaluation. Five or more pits in the enamel of permanent teeth are a marker for this disease.

Tuberous sclerosis is a common inherited autosomal dominant disease with highly variable penetrance. Prevalence estimates range from 1 in 5800 to 1 in 15,000. Up to 50% of cases may result from spontaneous mutations. There are two genes, the mutations of which produce indistinguishable phenotypes *TSC1* and *TSC2*. These are tumor suppressor genes. *TSC2* encodes for tuberin, a putative guanosine triphosphatase (GTPase)–activating protein for rap1 and rab5. *TSC1* encodes for hamartin, a novel protein with no significant homology to tuberin or any other vertebrate protein. Hamartin and tuberin associate physically in vivo, suggesting that they function in the same complex rather than in separate pathways. This interaction of tuberin and hamartin explains the indistinguishable phenotypes caused by mutations in either gene. Hamartomas frequently demonstrate loss of the remaining normal allele (loss of heterozygosity).

Diagnosis

The major criteria for TS are three or more hypomelanotic macules, three or more angiofibromas or a fibrous cephalic plaque, two or more periungual fibromas, shagreen patch, retinal hamartomas, cortical dysplasia, subependymal nodules, subependymal giant cell astrocytoma, cardiac rhabdomyoma, lymphangioleiomyomatosis, and angiomyolipomas.

The minor criteria are confetti-like macules, three or more dental enamel pits, two more intraoral fibromas, retinal achromic patch, multiple renal cysts, and nonrenal hamartomas.

A diagnosis of TS is made either with positive TSC 1 or 2 testing or with two major or one major and two or more minor criteria. A possible diagnosis is with one major or two or more minor criteria.

Workup should include a full skin examination for cutaneous features including a Wood's light examination. If x-ray examination fails to show calcified intracranial nodules, ultrasonography, CT, or MRI should be performed. Funduscopic examination, hand and foot x-ray evaluation, and renal ultrasonography are often revealing in a patient with few clinical findings; up to 31% of asymptomatic parents have been identified using these tests.

Treatment

Adenoma sebaceum can be treated by shaving, dermabrasion, or laser therapy, but topical rapamycin ranging from 0.1%–1% applied to the lesions can eradicate them noninvasively. Lesions are likely to recur, requiring maintenance treatment. Everolimus was the first mTOR inhibitor approved in the United States and Europe as a treatment for subependymal giant cell astrocytomas. Clinical evidence also supports the use of mTOR inhibitors, including sirolimus, in a variety of tuberous sclerosis complex–associated disease manifestations, including facial angiofibromas, renal angiomyolipoma, and epilepsy. Cranial irradiation of astrocytomas should be avoided because this may result in the subsequent development of glioblastomas.

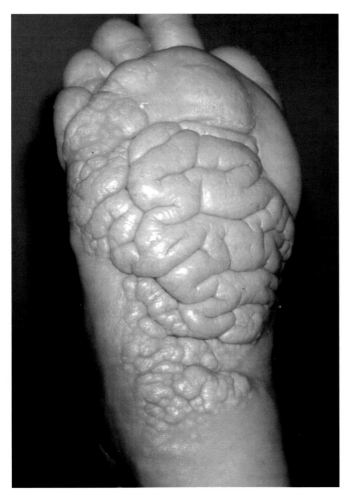

Fig. 27.13 Proteus syndrome with connective tissue nevus.

Cudzilo CJ, et al: Lymphangioleiomyomatosis screening in women with tuberous sclerosis. Chest 2013; 144: 578.

Curatolo P, et al: mTOR inhibitors in tuberous sclerosis complex. Curr Neuropharmacol 2012; 10: 404.

Ebrahimi-Fakhari D, et al: Topical rapamycin for facial angiofibromas in a child with tuberous sclerosis complex (TSC). Dermatol Ther (Heidelb) 2017; 7: 175.

Liebman JJ, et al: Koenen tumors in tuberous sclerosis. Ann Plast Surg 2014; 73: 721.

Northrup H, et al: Tuberous sclerosis complex diagnostic criteria update. Pediatr Neurol 2013; 49: 243.

Teng JM, et al: Dermatologic and dental aspects of the 2012 International Tuberous Sclerosis Complex Consensus Statements. JAMA Dermatol 2014; 150: 1095.

Tu J, et al: Topical rapamycin for angiofibromas in paediatric patients with tuberous sclerosis. Australas J Dermatol 2014; 55: 63.

VON HIPPEL–LINDAU SYNDROME

Von Hippel–Lindau syndrome is an autosomal dominant disorder consisting of retinal angiomas, cerebellar medullary angioblastic tumors, pancreatic cysts, and renal tumors and cysts. Ocular lesions may lead to retinal detachment. Pheochromocytoma has been associated in several kindreds with von Hippel–Lindau disease. Usually, the skin is not involved, although capillary malformations on the head and neck and café au lait macules have been described.

Patiroglu T, et al: Cerebellar hemangioblastoma associated with diffuse neonatal hemangiomatosis in an infant. Childs Nerv Syst 2012; 28: 1801.

ATAXIA-TELANGIECTASIA

Also known as Louis-Bar syndrome, ataxia-telangiectasia (AT) consists of cerebellar ataxia, oculocutaneous telangiectasia, and sinopulmonary infections. Patients may have a marked IgA deficiency, with decreased lymphocytes and a small to absent thymus. In 80% of cases, IgA is absent or deficient; in 75%, absent or deficient IgE is seen; and in 50%, IgG is very low. There also can be T-cell lymphopenia. AT is caused by a mutation in the ATM gene. It is usually first noted when the child begins to walk. There is awkwardness and a swaying gait, which results in the child needing to use a wheelchair by about 10 years of age. Choreic and athetoid movements and pseudopalsy of the eyes are other features. Fine telangiectases appear on the exposed surfaces of the conjunctiva at about age 3. Telangiectases also appear later on the butterfly area of the face, inside the helix and over the backs of the ears, in the roof of the mouth, in the necklace area, in the flexures, and over the dorsa of the hands and feet. The skin tends to be dry and coarse and over time becomes tight and inelastic, as in scleroderma. Atrophic, granulomatous, scarring plaques may occur. Granulomatous plaques occur in various immunodeficiency syndromes including cartilage hair hypoplasia, combined variable immunodeficiency and DNA ligase deficiency. Rubella virus has been documented by PCR in the granulomatous lesions and likely is a result of the immune system not being able to handle the killed virus that is introduced during vaccination that occurs with the live vaccine at age 1 before knowing the child has immunodeficiency.

Other cutaneous stigmata are café au lait patches, hypopigmented macules, melanocytic nevi, hypertrichosis, seborrheic dermatitis, premature graying and sparsity of the hair, and progeroid features. The most common types of malignancy are lymphomas, usually of the B-cell type, and leukemias. It has been shown that homozygous patients also have a higher risk of breast cancer—100 times higher than age-matched controls. Heterozygous carriers share the defective repair of radiation-induced damage, and there is a threefold to fivefold higher risk for development of neoplasms, especially breast cancer, in heterozygotes under age 45. The ovaries and testicles do not develop normally. There is deficient thymus development, with absence of Hassall's corpuscles and a lack of T-helper cells. Suppressor T cells are normal.

Early death from bronchiectasis occurs in more than half these patients, most of whom have recurrent sinus and lung infections that begin between 3 and 8 years of age.

Ataxia-telangiectasia is transmitted as an autosomal recessive trait, and heterozygotes, although they lack clinical findings, are cancer prone. The ATM gene is involved in cell cycle control, meiotic recombination, telomere length monitoring, and DNA damage response. Affected cells are hypersensitive to ionizing radiation.

Early diagnosis can be difficult and the most frequent misdiagnosis is cerebral palsy. The ataxia, along with telangiectasias, persistently elevated levels of α-fetoprotein, and carcinoembryonic antigen, along with the immunodeficiency, are useful in early diagnosis. Genetic testing is diagnostic.

Greenberger S, et al: Dermatologic manifestations of ataxia-telangiectasia syndrome. J Am Acad Dermatol 2013; 68: 932.

Knoch J, et al: Rare hereditary diseases with defects in DNA-repair. Eur J Dermatol 2012; 22: 443.

Rothblum-Oviatt C et al: Ataxia telangiectasia. Orphanet J Rare Dis 2016; 11: 159.

Zakko L, et al: Von Hippel–Lindau syndrome. In Wu G, Selsky N, Grant-Kels J [Eds.] *Atlas of Dermatological Manifestations of Gastrointestinal Disease.* New York, NY: Springer, 2013.

EPIDERMOSYSIS BULLOSA

Epidermolysis bullosa (EB) is a group of rare genetic disorders characterized by skin fragility with formation of blisters from minor physical injury. EB occurs due to congenital absence of proteins involved in keeping the epidermis together or connected to the dermis. Autoimmune blistering diseases often target similar proteins but are acquired. EB has been reclassified based on where the splitting of the skin occurs. The severity of EB subtypes is associated with the location of blistering, extent of loss of the skin, and other abnormalities associated with the protein that is defective or absent. The split in EB simplex (EBS) is within the epidermis (and is further divided into suprabasal and basal), junctional EB (JEB) splits within the basement membrane, and dystrophic EB (DEB) splits below the basement membrane. There are mixed pattern as well (Kindler). The inherited types of EB are classified as listed in Box 27.1.

Some of the mutations leading to EB are in genes that expressed in other tissues and therefore have extracutaneous manifestations. Esophageal and laryngeal complications are seen primarily in recessive dystrophic EB but may be present in JEB (Herlitz). Pyloric atresia can occur in JEB. Ocular lesions may be severe in dystrophic EB, and mild lesions have been reported in simplex and junctional disease. Congenital absence of the leg skin (Bart syndrome) presents with geometric loss of large areas of skin often on the medial legs extending to the calves possibly from one leg rubbing on the other in utero. This phenotype can be seen in multiple different forms of EB although it is most commonly reported with dystrophic EB.

Clinical findings and routine histologic features overlap in EB. Electron microscopy (EM) studies and immunofluorescent mapping can be used to determine the location of the split and the presence or absence of certain proteins. Immunofluorescent mapping may define the level of the split without resorting to EM. By staining biopsy specimens for normal components of the basement membrane zone (BMZ), such as bullous pemphigoid antigen, laminin, type IV collagen, or LDA-1 antigen, the level of the split may be determined by whether the antigen localizes at the roof or base of the blister. Biopsy should be done by inducing a new blister (usually with a pencil eraser) in clinically normal skin and sending to a specialized laboratory. EM and immunofluorescence do not always fully differentiate between various phenotypes that can be caused by mutations in the same genes, and genetic testing can be done to confirm a diagnosis. Now that genetic panels are available that include nearly all described EB mutations and are less expensive and faster than previously, it is reasonable to start with genetic testing because it will avoid a procedure and give a more definitive diagnosis. However, caution is advised predicting severity from genetic testing because not all patients with the same mutation will have the same clinical symptoms.

Intraepidermal Forms (Epidermolysis Bullosa Simplex)

Suprabasal Epidermolysis Bullosa Simplex

Suprabasal forms of EBS are caused by defects in transglutaminase 5, plakophilin, desmoplakin, and plakoglobin. They present with skin fragility and peeling.

Acral peeling skin syndrome is caused by transglutaminase 5 mutations and leads to superficial peeling, especially on the palms and soles, and heals without scarring.

EBS superficialis presents with superficial blisters and has no causal known mutation.

Skin fragility syndromes include EBS desmoplakin skin fragility and woolly hair syndrome, skin fragility–ectodermal dysplasia syndrome, and skin fragility–plakoglobin deficiency. Mutations in

---

BOX 27.1 Inherited Types of Epidermolysis Bullosa

INTRAEPIDERMAL

- Epidermolysis bullosa (EB) simplex, generalized intermediate, *KRT5* or *KRT14* mutation
- EB simplex, localized, *KRT5* or *KRT14* mutation
- EB, generalized severe, *KRT5* or *KRT14* mutation
- EBS with muscular dystrophy, pyloric atresia and Ogna are caused by Plectin mutations
- EB simplex-migratory circinate is caused by keratin 5 mutations
- EB simplex with mottled pigmentation, *KRT5* mutation
- EBS with muscular dystrophy, pyloric atresia and Ogna (above) are caused by Plectin mutations)
- EB superficialis
- Acantholytic EB simplex, *DSP* or *JUP* mutations
- Acral peeling skin syndrome is caused by TGM5 mutation
- Skin fragility syndromes
  - **Skin fragility–wooly hair syndrome (desmoplakin mutation)**
  - **Skin fragility (plakoglobin mutation)**
  - **Skin fragility–ectodermal dysplasia syndrome (plakophilin mutation)**
- EB simplex autosomal recessive–BP230 mutation
- EB simplex autosomal recessive–exophilin 5 mutation
- EB simplex autosomal recessive–K14 mutation

JUNCTIONAL (INTRALAMINA LUCIDA)

- Junctional epidermolysis bullosa (JEB), generalized severe, *LAMA3*, *LAMB3*, or *LAMC2* mutations
- JEB, generalized intermediate, *LAMA3*, *LAMB3*, *LAMC2*, or *COL17A1* mutations
- JEB localized
- JEB with pyloric atresia (α6β4-integrin)
- JEB, late onset (Collagen XVII mutation)
- JEB with respiratory and renal involvement (α3-integrin subunit)
- JEB inversa

DERMOLYTIC OR DYSTROPHIC (SUBLAMINA DENSA)

Dominant Forms

- Dystrophic EB, generalized, *COL7A1* mutation
- EB pruriginosa
- Pretibial EB
- Bullous dermolysis of the newborn

Recessive Forms

- Generalized severe, collagen VII absent, *COL7A1* mutations
- Generalized intermediate, *COL7A1* mutations
- Bullous dermolysis of the newborn, *COL7A1* mutations
- Localized (various types, including EB pruriginosa and pretibial EB)

---

the genes that encode the plakin family (desmoplakin, plakoglobin, and plakophilin) can present with widely variable phenotypes, including with systemic findings.

Skin Fragility (Plakoglobin Mutation)

Plakoglobin mutations can affect skin, hair and heart. Different mutations can lead to isolated skin findings of fragility or isolated cardiac findings. The phenotype of wooly hair, palmoplantar keratoderma and cardiomyopathy is called Naxos disease.

Skin Fragility and Woolly Hair Syndrome (Desmoplakin Mutation)

Mutations in desmoplakin can lead to multiple different phenotypes depending in part on the specific mutation because desmoplakin is expressed in skin, hair, nails, and cardiac tissue. Skin fragility with wooly hair is isolated to the skin. Desmoplakin mutations can also cause a striate PPK in isolation, a striate PPK with wooly hair and cardiomyopathy (Carvajal syndrome), cardiac disease in isolation, or a lethal acantholytic EB with complete alopecia.

Skin Fragility–Ectodermal Dysplasia Syndrome (Plakophilin Mutation)

This syndrome is characterized by inflammation around the mouth with fissuring, nail dystrophy, trauma-induced skin fragility, and defects of the hair, nails, and sweat glands. Trauma-induced blisters are generalized with skin tearing noted on the pressure points, especially after prolonged standing or walking. Plakophilins are not expressed in cardiac tissue so there are no cardiac findings thus far reported.

Epidermolysis Bullosa Simplex, Basalar

There are multiple forms of EBS caused by mutations in the genes encoding keratins 5 or 14, and the severity and pattern depend on the how much the mutation disrupts function. Basal EBS mutations in Krt5 or Krt14 can cause EBS localized, EBS generalized-severe, or EBS generalized-intermediate. Mutations in Krt5 cause EBS with mottled pigmentation and EBS migratory circinate.

Mutations in K14 can cause an autosomal recessive EBS (EBS autosomal recessive-K14). EBS with muscular dystrophy, pyloric atresia, and Ogna are caused by plectin mutations. Two other types of autosomal recessive EBS are caused by BPAG-1 or exophillin 5 mutations.

Epidermolysis Bullosa Simplex, Localized

Recurrent bullous eruption of the hands and feet is autosomal dominantly determined and appears in a chronic form in early childhood with exacerbations as an adult based on activities that increase friction. The Weber-Cockayne designation has been dropped in recent classification schemes. The lesions worsen during hot weather and when the patient is subjected to prolonged walking or marching, as in military service. Hyperhidrosis may be an associated finding. In localized EBS, the bullae are intraepidermal and suprabasal, and healing occurs without scarring.

Application of aluminum chloride hexahydrate in anhydrous ethanol (Drysol) on the normal skin of hands and feet twice a day has been shown to reduce blistering in this form of EBS. After 2 weeks of daily therapy, the patient can be switched to weekly or twice-weekly applications.

Epidermolysis Bullosa Simplex, Generalized Intermediate

The generalized type of EBS, dominantly inherited with complete penetrance, occurs in 1 in 500,000 births. It is characterized by the development of vesicles, bullae, and sometimes milia over the joints of the hands, elbows, knees, and feet, as well as other sites subject to repeated trauma. The child is affected at birth or shortly thereafter, with improvement within the first few months, but there are more blisters when the child begins crawling. The blistering is worse during the summer and improves during the winter. The lesions are sparse and do not lead to severe atrophy.

Usually, the mucous membranes and nails are not involved. EBS is usually milder than other forms of EB.

Inherited as an autosomal dominant trait, EBS is a disease in which keratin gene mutations cause the production of defective intermediate filaments, that lead to epidermal basal cell fragility and subsequent blistering. The genes encoding keratins 5 or 14 (expressed in the basal layer) are mutated. Patients heterozygous for abnormal keratin 14 have blistering limited to the hands and feet, but homozygotes have more severe and widespread blistering of the skin and mucous membranes. Separation occurs through the basal cell layer.

Epidermolysis Bullosa Simplex, Generalized Severe

In this autosomal dominant variant of EBS, active blisters (Fig. 27.14) with circinate configuration occur in infancy. Milia may develop, but there is no scarring. The oral mucosa is involved. Nails are shed but may regrow, sometimes with dystrophy. Blistering lessens with age. Hyperkeratosis of the palms and soles may occur. Histologically, the split is through the basal layer, and tonofilaments are clumped on EM. Point mutations have been shown in keratin 5 and 14 genes.

Epidermolysis Bullosa Simplex With Mottled Pigmentation

Patients have been reported with autosomal dominant EBS with congenital scattered hyperpigmented and hypopigmented macules that fade slowly after birth. The remaining features are similar to those of generalized EBS. Ultrastructural studies show vacuolization of the basal cell layer.

Epidermolysis Bullosa Simplex Migratory Circinate

Affected individuals present with slowly advancing erythema with blisters, and the lesions resolve with pigmentation. The mutation in EBS migratory circinate is the same as mottled pigmentation, so they are likely on a spectrum with some cases showing more erythema in early life and mottled pigmentation later.

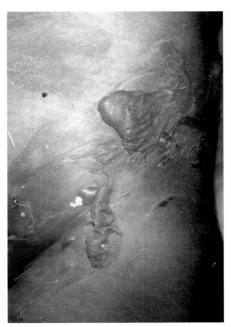

Fig. 27.14 Epidermolysis bullosa simplex, generalized.

Epidermolysis Bullosa Simplex With Muscular Dystrophy

A form of EBS is associated with late-onset neuromuscular disease and is caused by plectin mutation. Widespread blistering at birth is associated with scarring, milia, atrophy, nail dystrophy, dental anomalies, laryngeal webs, and urethral strictures. Progressive muscular dystrophy with weakness and wasting begins in childhood or later so patients should be followed over time.

Epidermolysis Bullosa Simplex With Pyloric Atresia

EBS with pyloric atresia is also caused by plectin mutation as well as integrin beta-4 and alpha-6 because integrin beta-4 binds plectin in the hemidesmosome. Late urologic complications have been described in patients with EBS with pyloric atresia.

Epidermolysis Bullosa Simplex (Ogna)

Generalized bruising and hemorrhagic blisters occur. EBS is transmitted as an autosomal dominant trait. At birth there are small, acral, traumatic sanguineous blisters. The basal keratinocytes in this syndrome do not stain with antiplectin antibodies.

Junctional Forms

Junctional epidermolysis bullosa (JEB) presents with severe generalized blistering usually at birth (Fig. 27.15), and in most forms extensive denudation may prove fatal. JEB is caused by mutations in three genes: *LAMA3*, *LAMB3*, or *LAMC2*, that code for polypeptide subunits of laminin 332 (also referred to as laminin 5), COL XVII, and integrins alpha-3 or -6 or beta-4.

Junctional Epidermolysis Bullosa

JEB can classified as localized, generalized, or generalized severe. The more severe phenotypes are characterized by more blisters, scarring, and intraoral involvement. There is little to no GI, ocular genitourinary, or respiratory involvement in the less severe forms. JEB is characteristic perioral and perinasal hypertrophic granulation tissue. Eventually, the lesions heal without scarring or milia formation, but erosions may persist for years. Dysplastic teeth are common. Laryngeal and bronchial lesions may cause respiratory

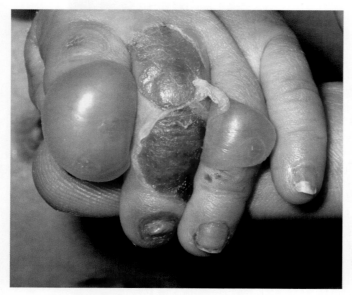

Fig. 27.15 Junctional epidermolysis bullosa.

distress and death in more severe forms. Additional systemic complications include GI tract, gallbladder, corneal, and vaginal disease. Patients who survive infancy have growth retardation and, often, moderate to severe refractory anemia.

In addition to good wound care and control of infection, epidermal autographs of cultured keratinocytes, isolated from clinically uninvolved skin and grown on collagen sponges, may be useful for chronic facial erosions.

Junctional Epidermolysis Bullosa With Pyloric Atresia

This rare autosomal recessive inherited form of JEB presents at birth with severe mucocutaneous fragility and gastric outlet obstruction. Often the ears are crumpled and misshapen. Even if the pyloric atresia is repaired, the neonates may die of the severity of their skin disease. If they survive the neonatal period, the blistering diminishes. Persistent scarring of the urinary tract may occur, however, with stenosis of the ureteral-vesicular junction, requiring numerous urologic procedures. This syndrome is usually caused by a genetic mutation in either the α6- or β4-integrin genes (*ITGA6* and *ITGB4*). This α6β4-integrin complex is uniquely expressed on epithelial surfaces.

Other Forms of Junctional Epidermolysis Bullosa

JEB with late onset is caused by collagen XVII mutations and is generally more mild than typical JEB. JEB with respiratory or renal involvement is caused by mutations in integrin alpha-3.

Dermolytic or Dystrophic Forms of Epidermolysis Bullosa

The cause of dystrophic EB in both autosomal dominant and autosomal recessive inherited forms is mutation in the *COL7A1* gene encoding for type VII collagen. The anchoring fibrils in these patients are defective or deficient. Presumably, because of antigen exposure, anti–type VII collagen, anti-BP180, and anti-BP230 autoantibodies may be detected.

Dominant Dystrophic Epidermolysis Bullosa

Dominant dystrophic EB (DDEB) typically presents at or soon after birth with blisters but the overall course of it is favorable. The blisters are most pronounced over the joints, especially over the toes, fingers, knuckles, ankles, and elbows (Figs. 27.16 and Fig. 27.17). Spontaneous, flesh-colored, scarlike (albopapuloid) lesions may appear on the trunk, often in adolescence, with no previous trauma and may be associated with more severe disease. The nails may be thickened. Usually, Nikolsky sign is present, and frequently the accumulated fluid in a bulla can be moved under the skin several centimeters away from the original site. Healing usually occurs with scarring and atrophy. Milia are often present on the rims of the ears, dorsal surfaces of the hands, and extensor surfaces of the arms and legs.

The mucous membranes are frequently involved. Bullae, vesicles, and erosions are encountered on the buccal mucosa, tongue, palate, esophagus, pharynx, and larynx. The latter involvement is manifested by persistent hoarseness in some of these patients. There may be angular contractures at the gingivolabial sulcus and dysphagia from pharyngeal scarring. Scarring on the tip of the tongue can happen. The teeth are normal. Usually, the conjunctiva is not involved.

EB pruriginosa is a form for DDEB is characterized by extreme pruritus, lichenified plaques, prurigo-like lesions, and violaceous linear scarring often worst on the pretibial area. Nail dystrophy is common.

Bullous dermolysis of the newborn (BDN), also called transient BDN, is a mild form of DDEB in which the blisters dissipate or

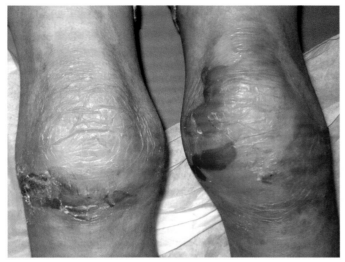

Fig. 27.16 Dominant dystrophic epidermolysis bullosa.

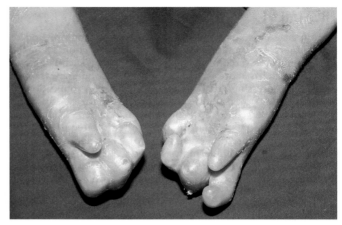

Fig. 27.18 Epidermolysis bullosa, recessive dystrophic type.

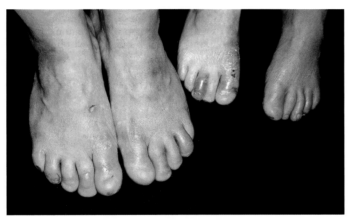

Fig. 27.17 Epidermolysis bullosa, dominant dystrophia.

stop forming all together after infancy. The presence of intracytoplasmic collagen VII retention seen on immunofluorescence or stellate bodies on EM has been proposed as a way of distinguishing BDN from DDEB. The mechanism for the transient nature of reduced amounts of type VII collagen along the dermoepidermal junction remains to be defined.

Histologically, in DDEB a noninflammatory subepidermal bulla is generally present. On electron microscopy, cleavage occurs beneath the basal lamina, and anchoring fibrils are rudimentary and reduced in number. In blistered areas, these are not demonstrable.

Recessive Dystrophic Epidermolysis Bullosa, Generalized Severe

All forms of recessive dystrophic EB result from mutations in the gene encoding type VII collagen, *COL7A1*. Generalized recessive dystrophic EB in its mildest form has blisters limited primarily to the hands, feet, elbows, and knees, and limited complications. The more severe variety characteristically begins at birth with generalized cutaneous and mucosal blistering. Digital fusion with encasement of the fingers and toes in scar tissues, forming a "mitten-like" deformity (Fig. 27.18), is characteristic of the severe form of recessive dystrophic EB, occurring in up to 90% of patients by

age 25. Dental complications may be severe, including extensive dental caries and microstomia. Esophageal stricture may be present. Anemia and growth retardation are frequently seen in the most severe cases, and progressive nutritional deficiency can result in fatal cardiomyopathy. Monitoring for anemia, hypoproteinemia, zinc deficiency, selenium levels, and carnatine levels is recommended. Fatal systemic amyloidosis (AA type) has also been reported. There is a high risk of developing cutaneous squamous cell carcinomas (SCCs), with up to 50% of patients affected by age 35. These SCCs may be multiple and can metastasize and cause death.

Although gene therapy is promising, treatment remains primarily palliative. Gentle wound care and proper nutrition are critical. Debilitating oral lesions produce pain, scarring, and microstomia. Aggressive dental intervention is recommended. Nutritional support is of critical importance. Autologous meshed split-thickness skin grafts and allogeneic cultured keratinocytes have been useful in treating nonhealing cutaneous defects, or may be used for closure after removal of large cutaneous malignancies. A single injection of allogeneic fibroblasts at the margins can accelerate early healing of chronic recessive dystrophic EB erosions. Family education and referral to DEBRA (Dystrophic Epidermolysis Bullosa Research Association of America, 5 West 36th Street, Room 404, New York, NY 10018, www.debra.org) are strongly recommended.

Kindler Syndrome (Acrokeratotic Poikiloderma, Weary-Kindler Syndrome)

In 1954 Kindler reported a combination of poikiloderma congenitale and traumatic blistering of the feet from minor trauma. The disorder shares some clinical features with dominant dystrophic EB, but in the largest reported familial cluster, inheritance followed an autosomal recessive pattern. Characteristic features include skin fragility with blistering, congenital acral bullae, generalized poikiloderma with prominent atrophy, photosensitivity, acral keratoses, severe periodontal disease, and phimosis. Some patients develop intestinal dysfunction or ulcerative colitis. Pseudoainhum and sclerotic bands were reported in one case. The principal histologic change is absence of elastic fibers in the papillary dermis and fragmented fibers in the middermis. Ultrastructural studies have shown replication of the lamina densa. Acrokeratotic poikiloderma is caused by loss-of-function mutations in fermitin family homolog 1, an actin cytoskeleton-associated protein encoded by the gene *FERMT1*, which plays a role in keratinocyte adhesion, migration, and proliferation. The protein is mainly expressed in basal keratinocytes. It binds to fermitin family homolog 2, as well as beta-1 and beta-3 integrins.

TREATMENT

Treatment consists of prevention of trauma, decompression of large blisters, and monitoring for and treating infection. Denuded areas should be covered with nonadherent dressings such as silicone or petrolatum based dressings as a contact layer and then wrapped with elastic dressings that do not require tape. Application of prophylactic antibiotics may lead to resistance, so topical antibiotics are typically reserved for acute infections and the type of antibiotic (mupirocin, bacitracin, retapamulin) is often rotated to decrease the risk of resistance. In severe forms of EB including JEB and recessive dystrophic epidermolysis bullosa (RDEB), patients are often colonized with *Staphylococcus aureus* or other bacteria, including *Pseudomonas aeruginosa*. Infection with candida species or even herpes simplex can be difficult to differentiate in chronic wounds and blistered areas so there should be a low threshold for culture.

Autologous meshed split-thickness skin grafts and allogeneic cultured keratinocytes may be used in treating nonhealing skin defects. Bone marrow or cord blood transplantation for more severe forms of EB has been tried but the benefits may be transient and there is significant risk related to the transplantation itself. Recently a JEB patient's entire epidermis was regenerated with autologous keratinocytes grown in culture.

Abdul-Wahab A, et al: Gene therapies for inherited skin disorders. Semin Cutan Med Surg 2014; 33: 83.

Chu MB, et al: Speedy simple technique for subungual blister evacuation in epidermolysis bullosa. J Am Acad Dermatol 2013; 69: e7.

Fine JD, et al: Inherited epidermolysis bullosa. J Am Acad Dermatol 2014; 70: 1103.

Fortuna G, et al: The largest family of the Americas with dominant dystrophic epidermolysis bullosa pruriginosa. J Dermatol Sci 2013; 71: 217.

Gonzalez ME: Evaluation and treatment of the newborn with epidermolysis bullosa. Semin Perinatol 2013; 37: 32.

Has C, et al: The genetics of skin fragility. Annu Rev Genomics Hum Genet 2014; 15: 245.

Heinecke G, et al: Intraepidermal type VII collagen by immunofluorescence mapping. Pediatr Dermatol 2017; 34: 308.

Hirsch T, et al: Regeneration of the entire human epidermis using transgenic stem cells. Nature 2017; 551: 327.

Hook K, et al: Bone marrow/cord blood transplantation (BMCBT) ameliorates symptoms in some, but not all, subtypes of severe generalized junctional epidermolysis bullosa (JEB). J Investig Dermatol 2017; 137: S52.

Kindler T, et al: Congenital poikiloderma with traumatic bulla formation and progressive cutaneous atrophy. Br J Dermatol 1954; 66 (3): 104–11. PMID 13149722.

Kroeger JK, et al: Amino acid duplication in the coiled-coil structure of collagen XVII alters its maturation and trimerization causing mild junctional epidermolysis bullosa. Hum Mol Gen 2016; 26: 479.

Kumagai Y, et al: Distinct phenotype of epidermolysis bullosa simplex with infantile migratory circinate erythema due to frameshift mutations in the V2 domain of KRT5. J Eur Acad Dermatol Venereol 2017; 31: e241.

Mahto A, et al: Late-onset pretibial recessive dystrophic epidermolysis bullosa. Clin Exp Dermatol 2013; 38: 630.

Murrell DF: The pitfalls of skin biopsies to diagnose epidermolysis bullosa. Pediatr Dermatol 2013; 30: 273.

Petrof G, et al: Desmosomal genodermatoses. Br J Dermatol 2012; 166: 36.

Pigors M, et al: Lack of plakoglobin leads to lethal congenital epidermolysis bullosa. Hum Mol Gen 2011; 20: 1811.

Velden JJ, et al: Novel TGM5 mutations in acral peeling skin syndrome. Exp Dermatol 2015; 24: 285.

Villa CR, et al: Left ventricular non-compaction cardiomyopathy associated with epidermolysis bullosa simplex with muscular dystrophy and PLEC1 mutation. Neuromuscul Disord 2015; 25: 165.

Yang CS, et al: An incompletely penetrant novel mutation in *COL7A1* causes epidermolysis bullosa pruriginosa and dominant dystrophic epidermolysis bullosa phenotypes in an extended kindred. Pediatr Dermatol 2012; 29: 725.

OTHER GENETIC BLISTERING DISEASES

Familial Benign Chronic Pemphigus (Hailey-Hailey Disease)

In 1939 Hailey and Hailey described a familial disease characterized by persistently recurrent bullous and vesicular dermatitis of the sides of the neck, axillae, and flexures. The eruption may remain localized or may become widespread. Usually, intact blisters are not evident. Instead, the lesions appear as macerated plaques with a linear or reticulated pattern of fissuring (Fig. 27.19). Lesions may become thickly crusted producing circinate and figurate patterns that resemble impetigo. The onset is usually in the late teens or early twenties. The condition is typically worse during the summer. Lesions tend to recur at sites of prior involvement. There may be tenderness and enlargement of the regional lymph glands caused by secondary bacterial infection. Longitudinal

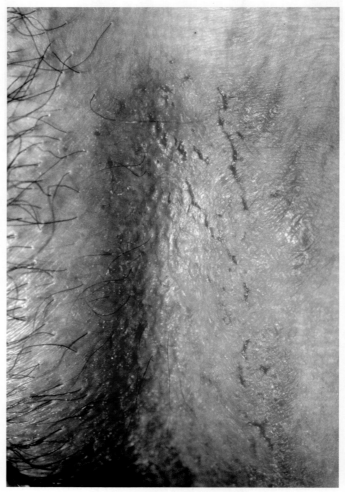

Fig. 27.19 Hailey-Hailey disease.

leukonychia may occur. Involvement of the esophagus, mouth, and labia majora is rare.

In predisposed persons with Hailey-Hailey disease, skin trauma, sunburn, bacterial or fungal infection, and dermatoses may trigger lesions. Widespread bullous lesions may occur in response to drug eruptions and may be misdiagnosed as toxic epidermal necrolysis. Histopathologically, there is acanthosis and full-thickness acantholysis resembling a dilapidated brick wall. A red band of dyskeratosis is present surrounding the nucleus, with no evidence of the blue or clear bands that occur in Darier disease. Hailey-Hailey disease is caused by a genetic defect in a calcium adenosine triphosphatase *(ATP2C1)*,inherited in an autosomal dominant manner, and 30% of patients express new mutations.

The treatment of Hailey-Hailey disease is difficult. Many patients improve with the use of systemic antibiotics against *S. Aureus*. Topical ckindamycin and mupirocin as well as antifungal agents can be helpful. Corticosteroids, administered topically, systemically, or both, have shown benefit. Cyclosporine, methotrexate, oral retinoids, topical calcineurin inhibitors, topical calcitriol, tacalcitol, botulinum toxin, photodynamic therapy (PDT), narrowband ultraviolet B therapy (NB-UVB), terbinafine, minocycline/niacinamide, and dapsone have been used in severe cases. Low-dose naltrexone was recently reported for pruritus relief. Dermabrasion and carbon dioxide (CO_2) laser vaporization have been effective in refractory disease, as the epidermis heals from uninvolved adnexal structures. Grafting and electron beam therapy have been helpful in the most severe forms of Hailey-Hailey disease.

Campbell V, et al: Low dose naltrexone: a novel treatment for Hailey-Hailey disease. Br J Dermatol 2017 Oct 9; ePub ahead of print.

D'Errico A, et al: Hailey-Hailey disease treated with methotrexate. J Dermatol Case Rep 2012; 6: 49.

Hailey and Hailey, et al: Familial benign chronic pemphigus. Arch Dermatol 1982; 118(10): 774–83. PMID 13149722.

Hamada T, et al: Successful therapeutic use of targeted narrowband ultraviolet B therapy for refractory Hailey-Hailey disease. Acta Derm Venereol 2013; 93: 110.

Vanderbeck KA, et al: Combined therapeutic use of oral alitretinoin and narrowband ultraviolet-B therapy in the treatment of Hailey-Hailey disease. Dermatol Reports 2014; 6: 5604.

Varada S, et al: Remission of refractory benign familial chronic pemphigus (Hailey-Hailey disease) with the addition of systemic cyclosporine. J Cutan Med Surg 2014; 18: 1.

DISORDERS OF CORNIFICATION (ICHTHYOSES AND ICHTHYOSIFORM SYNDROMES

Ichthyoses are a group of diseases in which the homeostatic mechanism of epidermal cell kinetics or differentiation is altered, resulting in the clinical appearance of scale. The stratum corneum is made of many different proteins, ceramides, and cholesterols, along with keratinocytes, and helps with epidermal barrier function. Disorders that affect cornification and the proper shedding of the cornified layer lead to symptoms of itching, overheating, and increased epidermal infection. Because these disorders manifest as abnormal differentiation of the epidermis, the term *disorders of cornification* is also used. Ichthyoses can be isolated or part of a systemic syndrome. Some ichthyoses start with collodion membranes.

Isolated Ichthyoses

Ichthyosis Vulgaris

Ichthyosis vulgaris is an autosomal dominant ichthyosis caused by mutations in filaggrin. It is characterized by onset in early childhood, usually between 3 and 12 months, with fine scales that appear "pasted on" over the entire body. Varying degrees of dryness of the skin may be evident. The scales are more coarse on the lower extremities than on the trunk and are especially apparent along the shins. The axillary and gluteal folds are usually not affected. Although the antecubital and popliteal fossae are usually spared by ichthyosis vulgaris, atopic changes may be present, because these disorders are frequently associated. Accentuated skin markings, hyperkeratosis of the palms, and keratosis pilaris are frequently associated. The scalp is involved, with only slight scaling. Keratotic lesions may be found on the palmar creases (keratosis punctata). Atopy manifested as seasonal allergies, atopic dermatitis, and asthma are often present. The course is favorable, with limited findings by the time the patient is an adult.

Histologically, there is compact eosinophilic orthokeratosis. The granular layer is reduced or absent, and keratohyalin granules may appear spongy or fragmented on EM. The spinous layer is of normal thickness. Filaggrin is reduced in involved epidermis, and profilaggrin messenger RNA is unstable in keratinocytes. This is a retention hyperkeratosis, with a normal rate of epidermal turnover. Therapy is similar to that for atopic dermatitis with thick emollients and gentle cleansers. Bathing more frequently can help desquamate the extra scaling. The differential diagnosis includes severe xerosis, X-linked ichthyosis, and acquired ichthyosis.

X-Linked Ichthyosis

X-linked ichthyosis is transmitted only to males by heterozygous mothers as an X-linked recessive trait. This condition results from a deficiency of steroid sulfatase (arylsulfatase C) and occurs in 1 : 2000 to 1 : 5000 male births. Onset is usually before age 3 months. Cesarean birth is typical, with failure in progression of labor because of a placental sulfatase deficiency. Scales are dark, large, and prominent on the anterior neck, extensor surfaces of the extremities (Fig. 27.20), and the trunk. The sides of the neck are invariably involved, giving the child an unwashed look. The elbow and knee flexures are relatively spared, as are the face and scalp; the palms and soles are almost always spared.

The condition may be confused with ichthyosis vulgaris but typically has darker scales and demonstrates dramatic clearing during the summer months. A diagnosis of X-linked ichthyosis is likely if the abdomen is more involved than the back, and if the ichthyosis extends down the entire dorsum of the leg. Keratosis pilaris is not present, and the incidence of atopy is not increased.

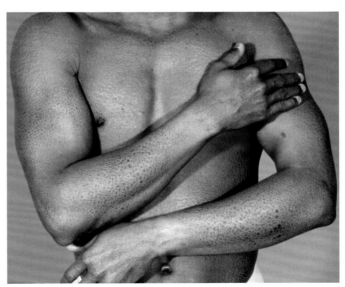

Fig. 27.20 X-linked ichthyosis.

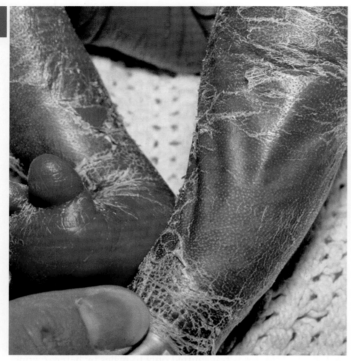

Fig. 27.21 Collodion baby.

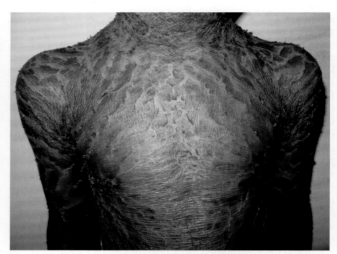

Fig. 27.22 Lamellar ichthyosis. (Courtesy Dr. Debabrata Bandyopadhyay.)

Corneal opacities (which do not affect vision) are seen by slit-lamp examination on the posterior capsule or Descemet membrane in about 50% of affected males and female carriers. Another extracutaneous feature is a 12%–15% incidence of cryptorchidism (undescended testicle) and an independently increased risk of testicular cancer. Unlike ichthyosis vulgaris, X-linked ichthyosis does not improve with age, but gradually worsens in both extent and severity.

There is usually a deletion at Xp22.3, and steroid sulfatase is lacking in fibroblasts, leukocytes, and keratinocytes. The diagnosis can be confirmed by genetic testing or lipoprotein electrophoresis, because the increase in cholesterol sulfate makes the low-density lipoproteins (LDLs) migrate much more rapidly, and cholesterol sulfate is elevated in serum, erythrocyte membranes, and keratin. The reduced enzyme activity can be assessed in fibroblasts, keratinocytes, leukocytes, and prenatally in amniocytes.

Autosomal Recessive Congenital Ichthyosis

Biochemical and genetic studies have helped to define the specific ichthyotic subtypes. Clinical features often overlap, and in the past, the severity of the disease determined the classification. Identification of specific defects is the basis for classification of ichthyotic disorders. These disorders typically present with a collodion membrane that is a thin layer that looks like plastic wrap and depending on the severity can be associated with ectropion and eclabium.

Lamellar Ichthyosis

Lamellar ichthyosis usually presents with a collodion membrane with ectropion that then desquamates over the first 2–3 weeks of life (Fig. 27.21). The ensuing ichthyosis is characterized by large (5–15 mm), grayish brown scales, which are strikingly quadrilateral, free at the edges, and adherent in the center (Fig. 27.22). In severe cases, the scales may be so thick that they are like armor plate. Moderate hyperkeratosis of the palms and soles is frequently present. The follicles in most cases have a crateriform appearance.

Lamellar ichthyosis is inherited as an autosomal recessive trait. About half the patients have decreased or absent TGM1 activity. An acral presentation of lamellar ichthyosis was recently described. Patients with no collodion but a lamellar phenotype with erythroderma of the hands and feet is caused by CYP4F22.

Patients should be kept in high humidity isolettes at first with gradual weaning to decrease insensible water losses. In addition to the topical agents recommended for the treatment of other ichthyoses, tazarotene and oral retinoids can improve symptoms. Topical 10% N-acetylcysteine in 5% urea has also been used with excellent success (although it smells of rotten eggs, so rosemary oil is often added). The adverse effects of prolonged oral retinoid therapy make their use for long-term maintenance therapy difficult.

Bathing Suit Ichthyosis

Bathing suit ichthyosis is an ichthyosis caused by a temperature-sensitive mutation in TGM1 that worsens in hot temperature (opposite of most ichthyoses). Therefore the scaling is worse in the bathing suit distribution and the summertime.

Congenital Ichthyosiform Erythroderma

Most infants with congenital ichthyosiform erythroderma (CIE; formerly nonbullous CIE) are born with a collodion membrane often with ectropion. Because the clinical phenotype at birth is similar to lamellar ichthyosis the two cannot be reliably differentiated at birth. Within 24 hours of birth, fissuring and peeling begin, and large, keratinous lamellae are cast off in 10–14 days, coincident with rapid improvement. As the membrane is shed, underlying redness and scaling are apparent (Fig. 27.23). Generalized involvement is the rule, including the face, palms, soles, and flexures. Cicatricial alopecia can occur, and nail dystrophy and some ectropion are common. Scales are more fine on the trunk, face, and scalp.

Histologically, parakeratosis and inflammation are seen more frequently in CIE than in lamellar ichthyoses. The stratum corneum is usually thicker in lamellar ichthyoses and is usually not parakeratotic. Mutations in *ALOXE3*, *ALOX12B*, and ichthyin (NIPAL4) can lead to either CIE or lamellar ichthyoses; the entities are separated largely on the basis of the clinical phenotype.

Harlequin Ichthyosis

Harlequin ichthyosis (HI) is the most severe type of autosomal recessive congenital ichthyosis (ARCI) caused by ABAC12

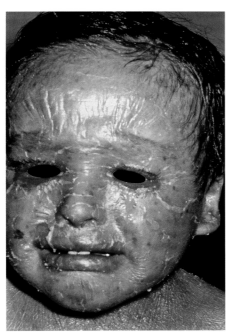

Fig. 27.23 Nonbullous congenital ichthyosiform erythroderma.

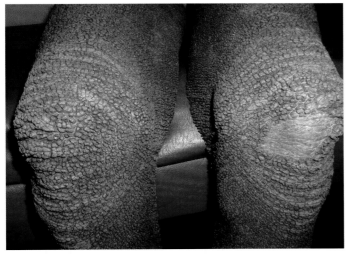

Fig. 27.24 Epidermolytic hyperkeratosis. (Courtesy Dr. Shyam Verma.)

mutations. HI presents with a thick collodion, with thick, horny, armor-like plates covering the entire surface with very severe ectropion and eclabium. The ears are rudimentary or absent. The mortality rate is high but, with aggressive management with emoliation and systemic retinoids, there have been many long-term survivors. Acitretin and isotretinoin have been used with success in infancy. Patients who survive develop features of CIE or lamellar ichthyosis. Absent or abnormal lamellar granules, a lack of extracellular lipid lamellae, and lipid droplets in the stratum corneum have been reported.

Epidermolytic Ichthyosis

Epidermolytic ichthyosis (EI) comprises what used to be called nonbullous congenital ichthyosiform erythroderma, epidermolytic hyperkeratosis (EHK), and ichthyosis bullosa of siemens. EI is usually manifested by blisters at or shortly after birth. Superficial

EI (formerly ichthyosis bullosa of siemens) is less severe and typically lacks blisters at birth. In EI, thickened, horny, warty, or spinelike ridged scales predominate (Fig. 27.24). They are particularly prominent at the flexures. There is remarkable heterogeneity, particularly in regard to the degree of hyperkeratosis, extent of body surface involvement, presence or absence of erythroderma, and palm and sole involvement. An association with hypocalcemic vitamin D–resistant rickets has been reported. Keratinocytic epidermal nevi with epidermolysis type are mosaic expressions of epidermolytic ichthyosis. There are reports of people with epidermal nevi that have epidermolysis having offspring with EI. Superficial EI is characterized by a lack of erythema, relatively mild hyperkeratosis usually limited to the flexures, and superficial molting or peeling of the skin (the "mauserung" phenomenon).

Epidermolytic ichthyosis is caused by mutations in the genes for K1 and K10 (or K2e in the case of ichthyosis bullosa of Siemens). Keratin distribution patterns in keratinocytes are abnormal, suggesting an altered assembly process of cornified cell envelopes. A recessive form related to K10 mutation has been described.

Histologically, the lesional skin demonstrates compact hyperkeratosis. The granular layer is greatly thickened and contains coarse, blue and red, keratohyaline granules. Epidermal cells detach in the granular cell layer and may appear vacuolated. EM reveals the formation of perinuclear halos. Epidermolysis has been described as an incidental finding in normal skin, skin adjacent to benign and malignant epidermal tumors, and normal oral mucosa.

Thick emollients are the mainstay of therapy but topical and systemic retinoids can be tried. Pyogenic infection is a common problem, and appropriate antibiotics should be administered. A water solution of 10% glycerin and 3% lactic acid applied to wet skin can result in clinical improvement. The disease tends to become less severe with age.

Acquired Ichthyosis

Ichthyosis clinically similar to ichthyosis vulgaris may develop in patients with several systemic diseases. Acquired ichthyosis has been reported with Hodgkin disease and may be a presenting symptom. It has also occurred in non-Hodgkin lymphoma, mycosis fungoides, multiple myeloma, and carcinomatosis. In hypothyroidism, patients may develop fine scaling of the trunk and extremities, as well as carotenemia and diffuse alopecia. Characteristic ichthyosiform lesions may develop in patients with sarcoidosis, particularly over the lower extremities. Biopsy of the lesion will often show granulomas. Ichthyosiform changes have also been reported in patients with Hansen disease, nutritional deficiency, acquired immunodeficiency syndrome (AIDS), human T-cell lymphotropic virus infection, lupus erythematosus, and dermatomyositis. Drug-induced ichthyosis may occur with nicotinic acid, statins, triparanol, and butyrophenones.

Treatment

Topical keratolytics and retinoids can be used for ichthyosis, but caution is advised in young children because systemic absorption can be assumed given the large body surface area that needs to be covered along with the defective skin barrier. Widespread use of topical salicylic acid in children may lead to salicylism, and lactic acid can lead to lactic acidemia. Symptomatic treatment with α-hydroxy acids, such as lactic acid or 12% ammonium lactate lotion, is helpful, but patients with atopic dermatitis and ichthyosis vulgaris may find that these products sting. Other compounds with hydrating and keratolytic properties are also beneficial. Creams containing 5%–10% urea are effective humectants. Response to topical retinoids has been variable but can be very effective for the face and ectropion in more severe ARCI. Baths may help by hydrating the horny layer, but immediate application of a thick emollient such as white petrolatum is vital. Topical calcipotriene ointment has proved effective in a variety of ichthyoses, and topical maxacalcitol, a vitamin D_3 analog, has been used successfully in mosaic-type bullous congenital ichthyosiform erythroderma. Application of a 40%–60% solution of propylene glycol in water under an occlusive suit removes the scales, especially on the palms and soles. Propylene glycol can produce renal failure and cardiac toxicity when given systemically, but few reports of adverse effects have been noted with topical use. Many patients benefit from the use of a sauna suit (unless they have bathing suit ichthyosis).

Abdul-Wahab A, et al: Gene therapies for inherited skin disorders. Semin Cutan Med Surg 2014; 33: 83.

Chang LM, et al: A case of harlequin ichthyosis treated with isotretinoin. Dermatol Online J 2014; 20.

Davila-Seijo P, et al: Topical N-acetylcysteine for the treatment of lamellar ichthyosis. Pediatr Dermatol 2014; 31: 395.

de Almeida H Jr, et al: Acral lamellar ichthyosis—expanding the phenotype of temperature-sensitive keratinization disorders. J Eur Acad Dermatol Venereol 2017 Dec 1; ePub ahead of print.

Digiovanna JJ, et al: Systemic retinoids in the management of ichthyoses and related skin types. Dermatol Ther 2013; 26: 26.

Dufresne H, et al: Importance of therapeutic patient education in ichthyosis. Orphanet J Rare Dis 2013; 8: 113.

Dyer JA, et al: Care of the newborn with ichthyosis. Dermatol Ther 2013; 26: 1.

Fleckman P, et al: Topical treatment of ichthyoses. Dermatol Ther 2013; 26: 16.

Gruber R, et al: Morphological alterations in two siblings with autosomal recessive congenital ichthyosis associated with CYP4F22 mutations. Br J Dermatol 2017; 176: 1068.

Hanson B, et al: Ectropion improvement with topical tazarotene in children with lamellar ichthyosis. Pediatr Dermatol 2017; 34: 584.

Hernández-Martin A, et al: A systematic review of clinical trials of treatments for the congenital ichthyoses, excluding ichthyosis vulgaris. J Am Acad Dermatol 2013; 69: 544.

Lai-Cheong JE, et al: Pathogenesis-based therapies in ichthyoses. Dermatol Ther 2013; 26: 46.

Madan RK, Levitt J: A review of toxicity from topical salicylic acid preparations. J Am Acad Dermatol 2014; 70: 788.

Marukian NV, et al: Expanding the genotypic spectrum of bathing suit ichthyosis. JAMA Dermatol 2017; 153: 537.

McLean WH: Filaggrin failure—from ichthyosis vulgaris to atopic eczema and beyond. Br J Dermatol 2016; 175: 4.

Prado R, et al: Collodion baby. J Am Acad Dermatol 2012; 67: 1362.

Richard G, et al: Management of ichthyosis and related conditions, gene-based diagnosis and emerging gene-based therapy. Dermatol Ther 2013; 26: 55.

CONGENITAL SYNDROMES WITH ICHTHYOSIS

Chondrodysplasia Punctata

There are four forms of chondrodysplasia punctata, classified by their inheritance patterns and clinical feature of punctiform bone calcification (stippled epiphyses). Chondrodysplasia punctata is characterized by ichthyosis of the skin similar to that of the collodion baby, followed by a blaschkoid pattern of hyperkeratosis on erythematous skin (Fig. 27.25). In addition to reddening, the waxy, shiny skin has hyperkeratotic scales of a peculiar, crushed-eggshell configuration. As the child grows, follicular atrophoderma and pseudopelade develop. Usually, the ichthyosis clears within the first year of life but may leave behind blaschkoid hyperpigmentation similar to that seen in incontinentia pigmenti. Additional features are nail findings such as platonychia and onychoschizia.

The Conradi-Hünermann type is caused by autosomal dominantly inherited EBP mutation. Affected individuals present with

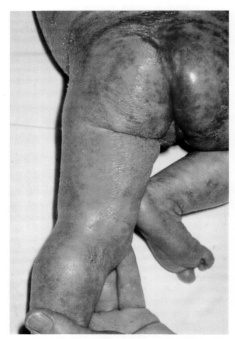

Fig. 27.25 Chondrodysplasia punctata.

facial dysmorphia with a low nasal bridge, short stature, mild disease, cataracts, and few skin lesions. The rhizomelic (rhizomelia here means shortening of the long bones of the upper arms and legs) form (caused by PEX7 mutation) has autosomal recessive inheritance, marked shortening of the extremities, cataracts, ichthyosis, and nasal hypoplasia. Patients typically do not survive infancy. The X-linked recessive type has been described as part of contiguous gene deletion syndromes, with short stature, telebrachydactyly, and nasal hypoplasia. The X-linked dominant form (Happle syndrome, Conradi-Hünermann-Happle syndrome, or CDPX2) is lethal in males. Happle syndrome (X-linked dominant chondrodysplasia punctata) has ichthyosiform erythroderma along the lines of Blaschko, cataracts, asymmetric limb shortening, and calcified stippling of the epiphyses of long bones. CDPX2 is caused by a defect in the EBP gene, leading to increase of sterols.

The skeletal defects revealed on radiographic evaluation include irregular calcified stippling of the cartilaginous epiphyses in the long bones, costal cartilages, and vertebral diaphysis. The stippling occurs in the fetus and persists until age 3 or 4 years. The humeri and femurs may be shortened, and joint dysplasia may occur. Histologic evaluation of the ichthyotic lesions reveals a thinned, granular cell layer, calcification of keratotic follicular plugs, and focal hyperpigmentation of basal keratinocytes. The keratotic follicular plugs and calcium deposits are characteristic of chondrodysplasia punctata and helpful in establishing the diagnosis in newborns. Various types are related to defects in peroxisomal metabolism, plasmalogen, and cholesterol biosynthesis. X-linked recessive chondrodysplasia punctata (CDPX1) is caused by a defect in arylsulfatase E, located on Xp22.3. There may be an association between the rhizomelic variety and maternal autoimmunity and connective tissue disease. A contiguous gene deletion syndrome can affect arylsulfatase E and *KAL1* (the gene defect responsible for Kallman syndrome), leading to anosmia and hypogonadism.

Aubourg P, et al: Peroxisomal disorders. Handb Clin Neurol 2013; 113: 1593.

Kanungo S, et al: Sterol metabolism disorders and neurodevelopment. Dev Disabil Res Rev 2013; 17: 197.

Lambrecht C, et al: Conradi-Hünermann-Happle syndrome. Pediatr Dermatol 2014; 31: 493.

Netherton Syndrome

Netherton syndrome is an inherited autosomal recessive disorder of cornification. It may first appear as severe congenital generalized exfoliative erythroderma in infancy. Then children develop migratory annular and polycyclic patches of ichthyosis linearis circumflexa (Fig. 27.26). Lesions predominate on the trunk and extremities, and appear as a polycyclic serpiginous eruption characterized by constantly changing patterns. Individual lesions grow over about a week and then attain their maximum diameter and involute, leaving no atrophy, scarring, or pigmentation. The lesions may clear almost completely during the summer. Most patients are found to have bamboo hair (trichorrhexis invaginata). The association of ichthyosiform dermatitis, hair abnormality, and atopic diathesis is called Netherton syndrome. Because of coexistent atopic dermatitis, the scalp, face, and eyebrow regions are erythematous and scaly. Hairs may fracture below the surface of the scalp, so that the patient appears bald. Mutations in *SPINK5*, which encodes the serine protease inhibitor Kazal-type 5 protein, have been identified in Netherton syndrome and result in unopposed kallikrein-related peptidase 5 (KLK5) and KLK7 activities and overactivity of elastase 2 (ELA2).

Histologic examination shows hyperkeratosis, parakeratosis, and acanthosis. The granular layer is typically absent.

Acitretin has been effective in some patients but should be avoided in erythrodermic neonates; long-term use is limited by toxicity. Topical tacrolimus has also been reported as effective, but in one report, three patients treated twice with 0.1% tacrolimus ointment were found to have significant tacrolimus blood levels. Although none of these patients developed signs or symptoms of toxic effects, monitoring of blood levels is advised if tacrolimus is used in this setting. NB-UVB has been reported as effective. There is IL-17 activation and thus IL-17 blockade with ustekinumab may be helpful.

Hovnanian A: Netherton syndrome. Cell Tissue Res 2013; 351: 289.

Maatouk I, et al: Narrowband ultraviolet B phototherapy associated with improvement in Netherton syndrome. Clin Exp Dermatol 2012; 37: 364.

Paller AS, et al: An IL-17–dominant immune profile is shared across the major orphan forms of ichthyosis. J Allergy Clin Immunol 2017; 139: 152.

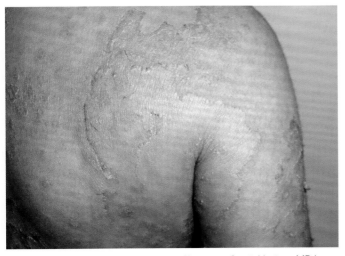

Fig. 27.26 Netherton syndrome. (Courtesy Scott Norton, MD.)

Neutral Lipid Storage Disease

Neutral lipid storage disease (Dorfman-Chanarin syndrome) is a rare autosomal recessive disorder characterized by an ichthyosiform erythroderma, myopathy, and vacuolated leukocytes. Affected infants can be born with a collodion membrane. Associated cutaneous disorders include poikiloderma atrophicans vasculare. The ichthyosis is more severe in warmer weather. Lipid vacuoles are present in all circulating granulocytes and monocytes, as well as in dermal fibroblasts, Schwann cells, smooth muscle cells, and sweat gland cells. Other organ systems, such as the CNS, liver, muscles, ears, and eyes, may also have deposits. Neutral lipid storage disease is caused by a regulatory defect that alters the rates of synthesis and degradation of the major cellular phospholipids, particularly triacylglycerol-derived diacylglycerol. EM findings show electron-lucent globular inclusions in lamellar structures. Dietary intervention, with modulation of dietary fats, along with fibrates have been shown to aid in controlling the disease. Recently a report of application of menthol for "cold-sensing" significantly improved the ichthyosis.

Nakajima K, et al: 137 Cold-sensing ameliorated ichthyosis in a patient with Dorfman-Chanarin syndrome likely through reversed lypolysis under thermo-regulation in keratinocytes. J Investig Dermatol 2017; 137: S216.

Nur BG, et al: Chanarin-Dorfman syndrome. Eur J Med Genet 2015; 58: 238.

Van de Weijer T, et al: Effects of bezafibrate treatment in a patient and a carrier with mutations in the *PNPLA2* gene, causing neutral lipid storage disease with myopathy. Circ Res 2013; 112: e51.

Sjögren-Larsson Syndrome

Sjögren-Larsson syndrome is characterized by ichthyosis, spastic paralysis, oligophrenia, mental retardation, and a degenerative retinitis. The ichthyosis is usually generalized, with minimal or no involvement of the scalp, hair, or nails and rarely infants present with a collodion membrane. There is flexural and lower abdominal accentuation. The central face is spared, ectropion is unusual, and palms and soles are involved. Beginning by age 2 or 3 years, there is spastic paralysis consisting of a stiff, awkward movement of the extremities. EM reveals prominent Golgi apparatus and increased numbers of mitochondria in keratinocytes. Usually, a severe mental deficiency with seizures is present. This syndrome is caused by a mutation in fatty aldehyde dehydrogenase (FALDH).

Dutra LA, et al: Sjogren-Larsson syndrome. Adv Exp Med Biol 2012; 724: 344.

Srinivas SM, et al: Sjögren-Larsson syndrome. Indian Dermatol Online J 2014; 5: 185.

Refsum Syndrome

Refsum syndrome (heredopathia atactica polyneuritiformis) is an autosomal recessive inherited ichthyosis with atypical retinitis pigmentosa, hypertrophic peripheral neuropathy, cerebellar ataxia, nerve deafness, and cardiomyopathy. The ichthyosis resembles ichthyosis vulgaris and presents later in childhood. It may be generalized or localized to the palms and soles. There are lipid vacuoles in the epidermal basal layer with decreased granular cell layer. Biochemically, the disease is a peroxisomal disorder characterized by excessive accumulation of phytanic acid, pristanic acid, and picolinic acid in fatty tissues, myelin sheaths, heart, kidneys, and retinal tissues.

Refsum syndrome is caused by a deficiency of phytanolyl/pristanoyl-CoA-hydroxilase. *PHYH* mutations account for the majority but some patients with mutations in *PEX*7 (a gene also associated with rhizomelic chondrodysplasia punctata type 1) have been identified. Dietary restriction of phytanic acid–containing vegetables can lead to an improvement of neurologic symptoms but does not affect retinal changes. Unfortunately, in many patients, dietary restriction is not sufficient to prevent acute attacks or stabilize the progressive course. The acids are localized within very-low-density lipoprotein (VLDL), LDL, and high-density lipoprotein (HDL) particles and may be removed by extracorporeal LDL apheresis.

Braverman NE, et al: Peroxisome biogenesis disorders. Dev Disabil Res Rev 2013; 17: 187.
Wanders RJ, Waterham HR, Leroy BP: Refsum disease. 2006 Mar 20 [Updated 2015 Jun 11]. In: Adam MP, Ardinger HH, Pagon RA, et al [Eds.] GeneReviews® [Internet]. Seattle, WA: University of Washington, Seattle, 2015.
Yoneda K: Inherited ichthyosis. J Dermatol 2016; 43: 252.

Rud Syndrome

Rud syndrome is characterized by ichthyosis, hypogonadism, small stature, mental retardation, acanthosis nigricans, epilepsy, macrocytic anemia, and, rarely, retinitis pigmentosa. Most kindreds have shown autosomal recessive inheritance and may be atypical variants of well-described disorders, such as Sjögren-Larsson syndrome or Refsum syndrome, rather than representing a distinct inherited disorder. Some patients have X-linked steroid sulfatase deficiency.

Happle R: Rud syndrome does not exist. Eur J Dermatol 2012; 22: 7.

Keratitis-Ichthyosis-Deafness Syndrome

The keratitis-ichthyosis-deafness (KID or Senter) syndrome is characterized by vascularization of the cornea, an extensive congenital ichthyosiform eruption, neurosensory deafness, reticulated hyperkeratosis of the palms and soles, hypotrichosis, partial anhidrosis, nail dystrophy, and tight heel cords. Distinctive leathery, verrucoid plaques involve the central portion of the face (Fig. 27.27) and ears. These changes, with absent eyebrows and eyelashes and furrows about the mouth and chin, give the children a unique facies. Occasionally, hairs may demonstrate bright and dark bands on polarized microscopy, as seen in trichothiodystrophy. Chronic mucocutaneous candidiasis and superinfection of skin lesions is common. Benign trichilemmal tumors and SCC occur in approximately 15% of patients. The candidal lesions can appear heaped up and mimic SCC, so there should be a low threshold for biopsy.

Some kindreds lack deafness. The disorder is related to missense mutations in the *GJB2* gene that encodes connexin 26 (Cx26). Most cases are sporadic.

Initial therapy with topical retinoids or keratolytics may help some. Isotretinoin treatment may exacerbate and promote corneal vascularization. Treatment with acitretin has been reported to clear the hyperkeratotic ichthyotic lesions with minimal effect on the cornea or hearing. Cyclosporin A eyedrops have been used to treat corneal neovascularization.

Porokeratotic Eccrine Ostial and Dermal Duct Nevus

Porokeratotic eccrine ostial and dermal duct nevus (PEODDN) is a keratotic condition that affects the eccrine ostia keratosis resembling music box spines and typically presents on the palms (Fig. 27.28) or soles. It is caused by a mosaic *GJB2* mutation and PEODDN has been seen in KID syndrome (also caused by *GJB2* mutations), thus PEODDN can be considered a mosaic limited form of KID syndrome.

Coggshall K, et al: Keratitis, ichthyosis, and deafness syndrome. J Am Acad Dermatol 2013; 69: 127.
Levinsohn JL, et al: A somatic p. G45E GJB2 mutation causing porokeratotic eccrine ostial and dermal duct nevus. JAMA Dermatol 2015; 151: 638.
Patel V, et al: Treatment of keratitis-ichthyosis-deafness (KID) syndrome in children. Dermatol Ther 2015; 28: 89.
Sakabe J, et al: Connexin 26 *(GJB2)* mutations in keratitis-ichthyosis-deafness syndrome presenting with squamous cell carcinoma. J Dermatol 2012; 39: 814.

Congenital Hemidysplasia With Ichthyosiform Erythroderma and Limb Defects (CHILD) Syndrome

Present at birth, congenital hemidysplasia with ichthyosiform erythroderma and limb defects (CHILD) syndrome is characterized by unilateral inflammatory epidermal nevi and ipsilateral limb hypoplasia or limb defects (Fig. 27.29). Features may vary widely, from complete absence of an extremity to defects of internal organs involving the musculoskeletal system, cardiovascular system, or CNS. The condition is X-linked dominant caused by a mutation in the *NSDHL* gene that is involved in cholesterol metabolism. CHILD is lethal in hemizygous males. Survival in males has been reported as a result of mosaicism. In females, lyonization may produce cutaneous patterns following the lines of Blaschko. When unilateral epidermal nevi show features of verruciform xanthoma,

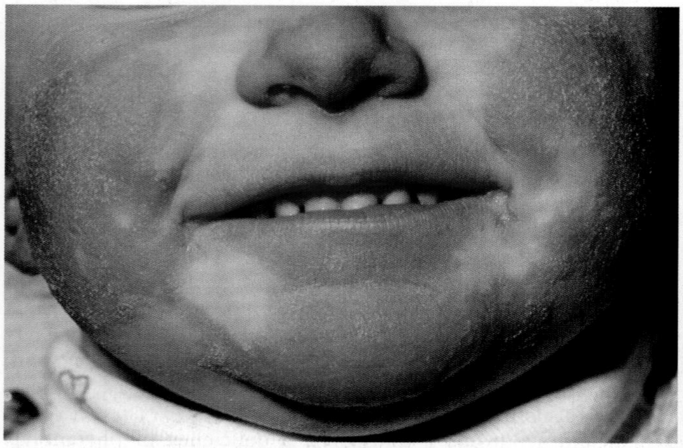

Fig. 27.27 Keratosis ichthyosis deafness syndrome. (Courtesy Paul Honig, MD.)

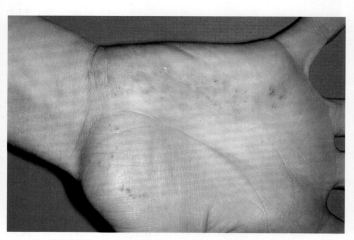

Fig. 27.28 Porokeratotic eccrine ostial and dermal duct nevus.

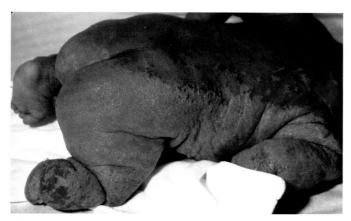

Fig. 27.29 Congenital hemidysplasia with ichthyosiform erythroderma and limb defects (child) syndrome. (Courtesy Paul Honig, MD.)

CHILD syndrome should be suspected. The CHILD nevus is distinguished by ptychotropism (flexural involvement), waxy yellowish scaling, lateralization showing both diffuse and linear involvement, and the presence of foamy macrophages in the dermal papillae.

Therapy with a topical formulation of 2% lovastatin/2% cholesterol that bypasses hepatic first-pass metabolism to deliver cholesterol directly to the skin is extremely effective for the cutaneous features.

Paller AS, et al: Pathogenesis-based therapy reverses cutaneous abnormalities in an inherited disorder of distal cholesterol metabolism. J Investig Dermatol 2011; 131: 2242.

Raychaudhury T, et al: A novel X-chromosomal microdeletion encompassing congenital hemidysplasia with ichthyosiform erythroderma and limb defects. Pediatr Dermatol 2013; 30: 250.

Multiple Sulfatase Deficiency

Patients with multiple sulfatase deficiency display an overlap of steroid sulfatase deficiency, mucopolysaccharidosis, and metachromatic leukodystrophy. The scaling is sometimes milder than X-linked recessive ichthyosis. Patients present around age 3 with regressed development, ataxia, hypotonia and the ichthyosis. Histologic examination shows hyperkeratosis with a normal granular cell layer. This autosomal recessive disorder is caused by a lack of or deficiency in all known sulfatases.

Sreekantam S, et al: Clinical features and outcomes in multiple sulfatase deficiency. Mol Genet Metab 2016; 117: S108.

Erythrokeratodermias

The erythrokeratodermias are closely related and have significant clinical overlap but are genotypically distinct. Erythrokeratodermia variabilis (EKV), also called erythrokeratodermia figurata variabilis, is characterized by erythematous patches and hyperkeratotic plaques of sparse but generalized distribution. Progressive symmetric erythrokeratodermia (erythrokeratodermia progressiva symmetrica) manifests soon after birth with erythematous, hyperkeratotic plaques that are symmetrically distributed on the extremities, buttocks, and face, sparing the trunk and palmoplantar keratoderma (often striate). The lesions may regress at puberty. Occipital alopecia, oligodontia, and severe caries have been reported. *Erythrokeratodermia variabilis et progressiva* (EKVP) has been proposed as a term that encompasses the full spectrum of either localized hyperkeratotic plaques to more widespread disease.

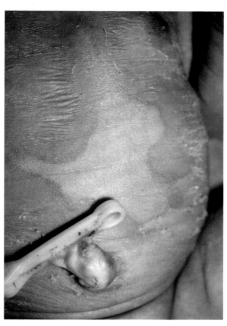

Fig. 27.30 Erythrokeratoderma variabilis. (Courtesy Ken Greer, MD.)

The erythematous patches of EKV may assume bizarre geographic configurations that are sharply demarcated (Fig. 27.30). Over time, they change shape or size or involute completely. The keratotic plaques are reddish brown, often polycyclic, and fixed in location. The extensor surfaces of the limbs, buttocks, axillae, groins, and face are most often involved. Approximately 50% of patients display a palmoplantar keratoderma associated with peeling. Hair, nails, and mucous membranes are spared. The onset of EKV is shortly after birth, or rarely at birth, or in early adult life. There may be some improvement with age, particularly after menopause. Exacerbations have been seen during pregnancy. The figurate erythematous component may be accentuated by exposure to heat, cold, or wind. Emotional upsets may also be a factor. Histologically, there is hyperkeratosis and parakeratosis and a diminished granular layer. Acanthosis may occur. Ultrastructurally, epidermal keratinosomes are diminished.

Mutations in *GJB3*, *GJB4*, and *GJA1* have all been associated with EKVP. Recently a mutation in keratin 83 has been shown to cause progressive symmetric erythrokeratodermia. Interestingly, *GJA1* mutations were recently found in inflammatory linear verrucous epidermal nevus (ILVEN), therefore ILVEN may represent mosaic EKV.

Systemic retinoids such as acitretin or isotretinoin alone or combined with psoralens and ultraviolet A (UVA) therapy can restore the deficient keratinosomes and partially clear the hyperkeratotic plaques for severe widespread disease. EKV often relapses when therapy is discontinued. Urea, salicylic acid, and lactic acid have proved useful for the hyperkeratotic plaques.

Boyden LM, et al: Dominant de novo mutations in *GJA1* cause erythrokeratodermia variabilis et progressiva, without features of oculodentodigital dysplasia. J Investig Dermatol 2015; 135: 1540.

Umegaki-Arao N, et al: Inflammatory linear verrucous epidermal nevus with a postzygotic *GJA1* mutation is a mosaic erythrokeratodermia variabilis et progressiva. J Investig Dermatol 2017; 137: 967.

Wei S, et al: Evidence for the absence of mutations at *GJB3*, *GJB4* and *LOR* in progressive symmetrical erythrokeratodermia. Clin Exp Dermatol 2011; 36: 399.

Yüksek J, et al: Erythrokeratodermia variabilis. J Dermatol 2011; 38: 725.

Colobomas of the Eye, Heart Defects, Ichthyosiform Dermatosis, Mental Retardation, and Ear Defects (CHIME)

Colobomas of the eye, heart defects, ichthyosiform dermatosis, mental retardation, and ear defects (CHIME) syndrome is a neuroectodermal disorder. The ichthyosis is usually congenital and migratory and is most pronounced in the flexural surfaces. Other features may include facial anomalies, epidermal nevi, developmental delay, infantile macrostomia, recurrent infections, acute lymphoblastic leukemia, and duplicated renal collecting system. The inheritance is believed to be autosomal recessive, related to mutations in the glycosylphosphatidylinositol gene *PIGL*.

Richner-Hanhart Syndrome

Richner-Hanhart syndrome (tyrosinemia type 2) is characterized by corneal opacities and keratosis palmoplantaris. The skin manifestations of painful keratotic plaques on the palms and soles usually develop after the first year of life and relate to defects in tyrosine aminotransferase. Newborn screening can allow early intervention with dietary restriction with a low-protein diet that may help the skin as well by lowering tyrosine levels.

Knight Johnson A, et al: Alu-mediated deletion of *PIGL* in a patient with CHIME syndrome. Am J Med Genet A 2017; 173: 1378.

Sidbury R, et al: What syndrome is this? CHIME syndrome. Pediatr Dermatol 2001; 18: 252.

PITYRIASIS ROTUNDA

Pityriasis rotunda (pityriasis circinata) manifests as perfectly circular scaly patches on the torso and proximal portions of the extremities (Fig. 27.31). The scale is adherent and resembles that of ichthyosis vulgaris. There is a strong ethnic predisposition, with a preponderance of reports in black persons, Japanese, Koreans, and Italians suggesting it may have a genetic cause. Two forms of pityriasis rotunda occur. Type I is found in black or Asian persons, usually has fewer than 30 hyperpigmented lesions, is nonfamilial, and

may be associated with systemic disease. Type II disease occurs in white persons, has larger numbers of hypopigmented lesions, is often familial, and usually is not associated with internal disease. Some cases are associated with systemic illnesses, especially in darker-skinned patients. Associated illnesses include tuberculosis, other pulmonary disorders, liver disease, malnutrition, leukemia, lymphoma, and carcinoma of the esophagus or stomach. Familial cases with autosomal dominant transmission have also been described.

The differential diagnosis includes tinea versicolor, tinea corporis, erythrasma, Hansen disease, fixed drug eruptions, and pityriasis alba. Some patients note a seasonal improvement during the summer, and some respond to emollients during the winter months. Low levels of steroid sulfatase have been identified, the profilaggrin N-terminal domain is absent in some patients, and filaggrin-2 expression has also been reported to be diminished in some. Topical and systemic retinoids have been used successfully, but pityriasis rotunda often is unresponsive unless the patient has an underlying systemic illness that can be treated.

Makino T, et al: Decreased filaggrin-2 expression in the epidermis in a case of pityriasis rotunda. Clin Exp Dermatol 2016; 41: 215.

Yoneda K, et al: The profilaggrin N-terminal domain is absent in pityriasis rotunda. Br J Dermatol 2012; 166: 227.

Zur RL, et al: Pityriasis rotunda diagnosed in Canada. J Cutan Med Surg 2013; 17: 1.

POROKERATOSIS

Porokeratosis comprises a heterogeneous group of disorders that can be inherited in an autosomal dominant fashion. Except for the punctate type, they are characterized by distinct clinical findings of a keratotic ridge with a central groove that corresponds to the cornoid lamella on histology (Fig. 27.32). The groove may be accentuated by the application of gentian violet, followed by removal with alcohol. The dye remains in the groove. Povidone-iodine has been similarly used. Immunosuppression, UV exposure, and radiation therapy may exacerbate porokeratosis and promote the development of skin cancers within the lesions. The linear type has the greatest risk of malignant transformation. Segmental forms have been reported in a blaschkoid distribution and after radiation therapy.

Topical 5-fluorouracil (5-FU) can be effective in destroying individual lesions; it may need to be applied under occlusion but may result in scarring. In disseminated superficial actinic porokeratosis

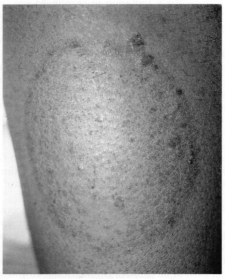

Fig. 27.31 Pityriasis rotunda.

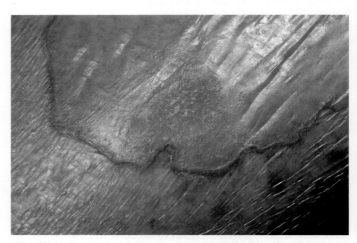

Fig. 27.32 Porokeratosis with keratotic ridge. (Courtesy Dr. Curt Samlaska.)

(DSAP), where the risk of malignant transformation is very low, the risks of treatment with 5-FU must be weighed against the generally indolent course of the lesions. PDT has been used with incubation under a heating pad to promote porphyrin conversion. Sun protection, emollients, and observation for signs of malignant degeneration may be the most suitable course of action for many patients with DSAP. Other agents that have been shown to be effective for some patients with DSAP include topical imiquimod, vitamin D_3 analogs, diclofenac gel, and topical retinoids, including tazarotene. Salicylic acid and α-hydroxyl acids may make the lesions less noticeable. Oral retinoids have shown efficacy, but the lesions frequently recur after treatment, and long-term treatment with these agents is impractical. Combinations of oral retinoids and topical 5-FU have been effective for refractory DSAP and porokeratosis plantaris, palmaris, et disseminata, but the side effects of treatment may be considerable. Destructive modalities must extend into the dermis and produce scarring to prevent recurrence. Destructive modalities employed include cryotherapy, electrodesiccation and curettage, CO_2 laser ablation, Q-switched ruby laser, fractional photothermolysis, flashlamp-pumped pulsed dye laser, frequency-doubled neodymium-doped yttrium-aluminum-garnet (Nd:YAG) laser, dermabrasion, and grenz ray radiotherapy.

Plaque-Type Porokeratosis (Mibelli)

Plaque-type porokeratosis is a chronic, progressive disease characterized by the formation of slightly atrophic patches surrounded by an elevated, warty border. The lesion begins as a small keratotic papule, which spreads peripherally and becomes depressed centrally. Eventually, it becomes a circinate or serpiginous, well-defined plaque surrounded by a keratotic wall or collar. This wall is grayish or brownish and frequently is surmounted by a tiny groove or linear ridge running along its summit. The enclosed central portion of the plaque consists of dry, smooth, atrophic skin; the lanugo hairs generally are absent when the patches occur in hairy areas. Linear or zosteriform distribution of the lesions may also occur. If the nail matrix is involved, nail dystrophy may develop. Lesions may appear during chemotherapy for malignancy, after renal transplantation, while on psoralen plus UVA (PUVA) treatment, and in areas of chronic sun damage or chemical exposure, such as benzylhydrochlorothiazide.

Sites of predilection are the surfaces of the hands and fingers, as well as the feet and ankles. The disease also occurs on the face and scalp (where it produces bald patches), on the buccal mucosa (where the ridge becomes macerated by moisture and appears as a milky white, raised cord), and on the glans penis (where it causes erosive balanitis).

Histologically, the principal diagnostic changes are in the area of the cornoid lamella. This area demonstrates a column of parakeratotic keratin extending at about a 45-degree angle from a focus of dyskeratotic cells in the malpighian layer. The column trails behind the focus of dyskeratosis as the focus expands peripherally. The granular cell layer is absent beneath the parakeratotic column. The central portion of the lesion may demonstrate atrophy with loss of the rete ridge pattern, lichenoid dermatitis, or psoriasiform hyperplasia.

Disseminated Superficial Actinic Porokeratosis

Disseminated superficial actinic porokeratosis (DSAP) is characterized by numerous superficial, circinate, keratotic, brownish red macules found on sun-exposed skin (Fig. 27.33). It is more common in women. The distribution of the lesions on the sun-exposed areas indicates that actinic radiation is an important factor in the pathogenesis, and new lesions have been induced by exposure at commercial tanning salons. Exacerbations occur in up to two thirds of patients during summer. Immunosuppression is also well documented as exacerbating the disease. DSAP has been seen in patients

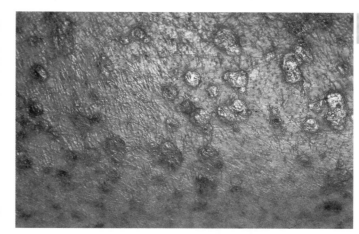

Fig. 27.33 Disseminated superficial actinic porokeratosis.

with AIDS, cirrhosis, and Crohn disease. Organ transplant patients may develop DSAP. Improvement of the immunosuppression may lead to resolution of the lesions. Gene loci have been localized to chromosomes 12q23.2–24.1 and 15q25.1–26.1, suggesting that DSAP is a genetically heterogeneous disorder. An eruptive form of porokeratosis has been named eruptive disseminated porokeratosis and this may be paraneoplastic (GI, lymphoma, or ovarian), or from an autoimmune or inflammatory disorder or idiopathic.

Linear Porokeratosis

Linear porokeratosis may be segmental or generalized. It may be identified during the newborn period, and when found in the segmental pattern, may follow the lines of Blaschko. Ulcerations and erosions involving the face or extremities may delay the correct diagnosis, and linear porokeratosis should be included in the differential diagnosis of ulcerative lesions in the neonatal period. This form of porokeratosis has the highest risk of developing cutaneous malignancies, including SCC (Fig. 27.34), Bowen disease, and basal cell carcinoma.

Porokeratosis Palmaris, Plantaris, et Disseminata

In this distinctive form of porokeratosis, lesions first appear on the palms or soles, or more often both. Onset is frequently noted when patients are in their twenties. Slowly, the lesions may extend over the entire body. In porokeratosis eccrine ostial and dermal duct nevus, the presentation clinically appears as a nevus comedonicus of the palm or sole (see Fig. 27.28), but histologic analysis reveals multiple coronoid, lamella-like, parakeratotic columns. In porokeratosis punctata, palmaris, et plantaris or punctate porokeratosis, lesions are limited to the hands and feet.

Aird GA, et al: Light and laser treatment modalities for disseminated superficial actinic porokeratosis. Lasers Med Sci 2017; 32: 945.

Anderson I, et al: Disseminated superficial actinic porokeratosis treated with ingenol mebutate gel 0.05. Cutis 2017; 99: E36.

Ferreira FR, et al: Porokeratosis of Mibelli—literature review and a case report. An Bras Dermatol 2013; 88: 179.

Friedman B, et al: Linear porokeratosis associated with multiple squamous cell carcinomas. Cutis 2017; 100: E11.

Lorenz GE, et al: Linear porokeratosis. Cutis 2008; 81: 479.

Moon SH, et al: A case of linear porokeratosis superimposed on disseminated superficial actinic porokeratosis. Korean J Dermatol 2016; 54: 819.

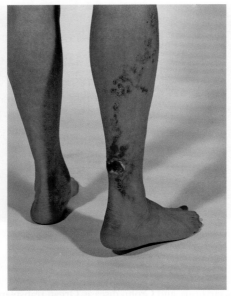

Fig. 27.34 Linear porokeratosis with squamous cell carcinoma.

Shoimer I, et al: Eruptive disseminated porokeratosis. J Am Acad Dermatol 2014; 71: 398.

Weidner T, et al: Treatment of porokeratosis. Am J Clin Dermatol 2017; 18: 435.

Zhang SQ, et al: Exome sequencing identifies *MVK* mutations in disseminated superficial actinic porokeratosis. Nat Genet 2012; 44: 1156.

DARIER DISEASE (KERATOSIS FOLLICULARIS, DARIER-WHITE DISEASE)

Darier disease is an autosomal dominant inherited skin disorder characterized by brown keratotic papules that tend to coalesce into patches in a seborrheic distribution. Early lesions are small, firm papules, almost the color of normal skin. Each papule becomes covered with a greasy, gray-brown crust that fits into a small concavity in the summit of the papule. As the lesions age, their color darkens. Over years, the papules grow and may fuse to form malodorous, papillomatous, vegetating growths.

The neck, shoulders, face, extremities, front of the chest (Fig. 27.35), and midline of the back are sites of predilection for the disease. A frequent site for the earliest lesions is behind the ears. As the eruption spreads, the entire trunk, buttocks, genitals, and other parts of the skin may be involved. Usually, the eruption is symmetric and widespread, but unilateral or segmental involvement may also occur probably representing postzygotic mutations.

Vegetations appear chiefly in the axillae, gluteal crease, and groin and behind the ears. The scalp is generally covered with greasy crusts. Lesions on the face are often prominent about the nose. The lips may be crusted, fissured, swollen, and superficially ulcerated, and there may be a patchy keratosis with superficial erosions on the dorsum of the tongue. Small white papules or pebbling may be present on the gingiva and palate. Involvement of the oropharynx, esophagus, hypopharynx, larynx, and anorectal mucosa has been reported. Punctate keratoses are frequently noted on the palms and soles. A general horny thickening of the palms and soles may be present because of innumerable, closely set, small papules. On the dorsa of the hands and on the shins, the flat verrucous papules may resemble verrucae planae. The nails show subungual hyperkeratosis, fragility, and splintering, with longitudinal alternating white and red streaks, and triangular nicking of the free edges (Fig. 27.36). Cutaneous herpes simplex may be

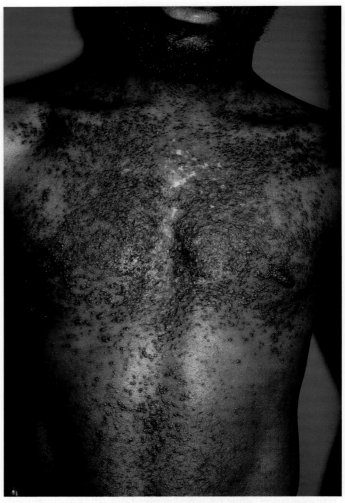

Fig. 27.35 Darier disease. (Courtesy Dr. Lawrence Lieblich.)

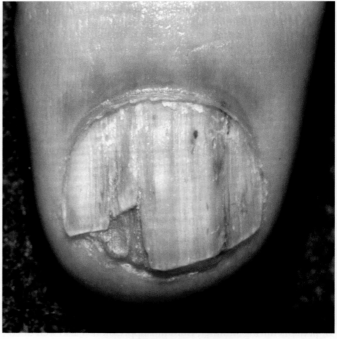

Fig. 27.36 Darier disease.

a complication of the disease. Esophageal involvement, renal anomalies (including agenesis), and gonal hypoplasia have been described. Recently an association with hidradenitis in two patients was proposed.

Darier disease is usually worse in the summer. It may begin after severe sunburn, and in some patients the lesions may be reproduced with suberythema doses of UVB light. Lithium carbonate has been shown to induce Darier disease in some individuals.

Abnormal dissolution of desmosomal plaque proteins is seen, specifically desmoplakin I and II, plakoglobin, and desmoglein. Calcium ion (Ca^{2+})–dependent cell-cell adhesion molecules (epithelial cadherins) are greatly reduced on the acantholytic cells of patients with Darier's disease. The Darier gene *(ATP2A2)* codes for the second isoform of a calcium ATPase of the sarcoplasmic/endoplasmic reticulum (SERCA2) pump, which transports Ca^{2+} from the cytosol into the endoplasmic reticulum. Inhibition of SERCA impairs trafficking of desmoplakin to the cell surface, contributing to acantholysis.

Histology

Darier disease is characterized by acantholytic dyskeratosis with overlying hyperkeratosis. Round, acantholytic dyskeratotic cells (corps ronds) typically demonstrate a pale or blue halo surrounding the nucleus. Grains are flat, deeply basophilic, dyskeratotic cells, seen most frequently in the stratum granulosum and stratum corneum. Formation of a suprabasal cleft (lacuna) is noted and may involve hair follicles as well as the surface epidermis. Dermal papillae covered by a single layer of basal cells project as villi into the acantholytic space.

Treatment

During flares, topical antibacterial agents, oral antibiotics, and short-term application of a corticosteroid may be of benefit. For localized disease, topical retinoids may be effective, but papules often occur at the periphery of the treated region. Topical diclofenac sodium has also been used. Oral retinoids are the drugs of choice for most severe cases. Cyclosporine may control severe flares, and topical sunscreens and ascorbic acid can prevent disease flares in some patients. For hypertrophic lesions, dermabrasion, laser vaporization, or excision and grafting can be considered. PDT using topical 5-aminolevulinic acid produces an initial inflammatory response that lasts 2–3 weeks. In some patients with Darier disease, this is followed by sustained improvement. Because of the initial inflammatory response, it is only appropriate for patients who have failed most other options.

Anuset D, et al: Efficacy of oral alitretinoin for the treatment of Darier disease. J Am Acad Dermatol 2014; 71: e46.

Letulé V, et al: Treatment of Darier disease with oral alitretinoin. Clin Exp Dermatol 2013; 38: 523.

Matsuoka LY, et al: Renal involvement in Darier disease. J Am Acad Dermatol 2016; 75: e235.

Millán-Parrilla F, et al: Improvement of Darier disease with diclofenac sodium 3% gel. J Am Acad Dermatol 2014; 70: e89.

Ornelas J, et al: A report of two patients with Darier disease and hidradenitis suppurativa. Pediatr Dermatol 2016; 33: e265.

Stewart LC, et al: Vulval Darier's disease treated successfully with ciclosporin. J Obstet Gynaecol 2008; 28: 108.

ACROKERATOSIS VERRUCIFORMIS

This rare autosomal dominant genodermatosis is characterized by numerous flat verrucous papules occurring on the backs of the hands, insteps, knees, and elbows. The papules are closely grouped and resemble warts, except that they are flatter and more localized. The verrucous lesions are identical to those in Darier disease, and

some, but not all, cases of acrokeratosis verruciformis of Hopf are caused by mutations in the *ATP2A2* gene.

Histologically, hyperkeratosis, thickening of the granular layer, acanthosis, and church spire papillomatosis characterize the disease. Available treatments are liquid nitrogen therapy, shave excision, and CO_2 laser ablation. Recurrence is common. Acitretin has been used successfully.

DeFelice T, et al: Acrokeratosis verruciformis. Dermatol Online J 2012; 18: 12.

Serarslan G, et al: Acitretin treatment in acrokeratosis verruciformis of Hopf. J Dermatolog Treat 2007; 18: 123.

PACHYONYCHIA CONGENITA

In 1906 Jadassohn and Lewandowsky described a rare, often familial, anomaly of the nails that they named pachyonychia congenita. It is characterized by thickened nail beds of all fingers and toes, painful palmar and plantar hyperkeratosis, blistering under the callosities, palmar and plantar hyperhidrosis, spiny follicular keratoses, and benign leukokeratosis of the mucous membranes. The nail plates are extremely hard and are firmly attached to the nail beds. The nail bed is filled with yellow, horny, keratotic debris, which may cause the nail to project upward at the free edge (Fig. 27.37). Paronychial inflammation is frequently present. Delayed onset of pachyonychia in young adulthood has been described, as has acro-osteolysis.

On the extensor surfaces of the extremities, buttocks, and lumbar regions, spinelike follicular keratotic papules are found. Removal of these central cores leaves a slightly bleeding cavity. The eruption on the outer aspects of the upper and lower extremities is also follicular, resembling keratosis pilaris. This latter condition is not constant and disappears at times.

Painful friction blisters may develop on the plantar aspects of the toes or heels or along the edges of the feet, and cases have been misdiagnosed as epidermolysis bullosa. In a study of 254 patients, the triad of toenail thickening, plantar keratoderma, and plantar pain was reported by 97% of patients by age 10. Leukokeratosis of the tongue and oral mucosa, as well as occasional laryngeal involvement with hoarseness, may occur. This oral leukokeratosis resembles an oral white sponge nevus histologically and is not predisposed to the development of malignancy.

Pachyonychia congenita was formerly divided into four types but, with more exact genetic diagnosis, patients are now divided based on keratin (KRT6A, KRT6B, KRT6C, KRT16, or KRT17;

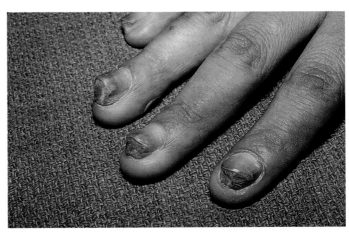

Fig. 27.37 Pachyonychia congenita.

e.g., PC-6A). There is overlap in clinical findings even with different genetic mutations so a panel of testing including each gene is usually ordered. There is a higher likelihood of oral leukokeratosis with *KRT6A* mutations, and natal teeth and cysts are strongly associated with *KRT17* mutation. Focal nonepidermolytic PPK is more associated with *KRT6c* and *16*. Homozygous dominant missense mutation in *K17* has been associated with severe pachyonychia congenita and alopecia.

Avulsion of the nails brings about only temporary relief. Vigorous curettage of the matrix and nail bed is the simplest and most effective therapy. Destruction of the nail matrix with phenol may be partially effective, but recurrence of nail bed hyperkeratosis is common. The keratoderma is difficult to treat, but topical lactic acid, ammonium lactate, salicylic acid, or urea may be of some benefit. Isotretinoin has been reported to clear the keratotic papules and the oral leukokeratosis, but not the palms or soles. Acitretin has been shown to be effective in treating the late-onset form.

Eliason MJ, et al: A review of the clinical phenotype of 254 patients with genetically confirmed pachyonychia congenita. J Am Acad Dermatol 2012; 67: 680.

Irvine AD: Double trouble: homozygous dominant mutations and hair loss in pachyonychia congenita. J Invest Dermatol 2012; 132: 1757.

Jadassohn J, et al: Jacob's Ikonographia Dermatologica. 1st ed. Berlin: Urban und Schwarzenberg; 1906. Pachyonychia congenita. Keratosis disseminata circumscripta (follicularis). Tylomata. Leukokeratosis linguae; pp. 29–31.

McLean WI, et al: The phenotypic and molecular genetic features of pachyonychia congenita. J Investig Dermatol 2011; 131: 1015.

O'Toole EA, et al: Pachyonychia congenita cornered. Br J Dermatol 2014; 171: 974.

Smith FJD, Hansen CD, Hull PR, et al: Pachyonychia congenita. 2006 Jan 27 [Updated 2017 Nov 30]. In: Adam MP, Ardinger HH, Pagon RA, et al. [Eds.] GeneReviews® [Internet]. Seattle (WA): University of Washington, Seattle.

Wilson NJ, et al: Homozygous dominant missense mutation in keratin 17 leads to alopecia in addition to severe pachyonychia congenita. J Invest Dermatol 2012; 132: 1921.

DYSKERATOSIS CONGENITA (ZINSSER-COLE-ENGMAN SYNDROME)

Dyskeratosis congenita is a rare congenital syndrome characterized by cutaneous poikiloderma, nail dystrophy, premalignant leukoplakia, and bone marrow failure in some. Atrophy and telangiectasia are accompanied by tan-gray, mottled, hyperpigmented and hypopigmented macules or reticulated patches (Fig. 27.38). Commonly affected areas are on the upper torso, neck, and face, although the extremities may also be involved.

The nails may be thin and dystrophic, although only ridging and longitudinal fissuring may be seen in mild cases. This is the first component of the syndrome to appear, becoming apparent between ages 5 and 15. The other cutaneous lesions generally follow within 3–5 years. Leukoplakia occurs mostly on the buccal mucosa, where extensive involvement with verrucous thickening may be present. The anus, vagina, conjunctiva, and urethral meatus can be involved. Malignant neoplasms of the skin, mouth, nasopharynx, esophagus, rectum, and cervix may occur in sites of leukoplakia. Other manifestations of dyskeratosis congenita include hyperhidrosis of the palms and soles, bullous conjunctivitis, gingival disorders, dental caries, hypodontia, thin tooth enamel, periodontitis, dysphagia resulting from esophageal strictures and diverticula, skeletal abnormalities, aplastic anemia, mental deficiency, and hypersplenism. In many cases, a Fanconi type of anemia develops, beginning with leukopenia and thrombocytopenia, and progressing to severe pancytopenia (bone marrow failure). Pulmonary

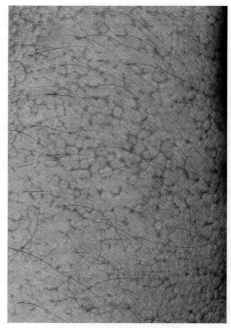

Fig. 27.38 Dyskeratosis congenita. (Courtesy Dr. Lawrence Lieblich.)

complications include interstitial fibrosis and *Pneumocystis jiroveci* (formerly *P. carinii*) pneumonia.

Patients with dyskeratosis congenita have short telomeres, related to mutations in genes that encode components of the telomerase complex. These include dyskerin, *TERC*, *TERT*, *NHP2*, and *NOP10*. The genetic defect for the X-linked form is caused by a mutation in the *DKC1* gene for dyskerin, a protein implicated in both telomerase function and ribosomal RNA processing. The presence of short leukocyte telomeres can be helpful diagnostically. Autosomal dominant inheritance is often associated with mutations in hTR (*hTERC*), involved in the RNA component of telomerase. Some autosomal dominant cases have anemia and reticulated pigmentation following the lines of Blaschko. Of interest, some patients with idiopathic aplastic anemia or myelodysplastic syndrome without skin findings demonstrate *hTERC* mutations.

Granulocyte colony-stimulating factor and erythropoietin may provide short-term benefits in treating bone marrow failure. Bone marrow transplantation or hematopoietic stem cell transplantation with nonmyeloablative conditioning affords the best outcomes.

Hoyeraal-Hreidarsson syndrome is a severe variant of dyskeratosis congenita characterized by intrauterine onset with growth retardation, cerebellar hypoplasia, mental retardation, microcephaly, progressive combined immunodeficiency, and aplastic anemia. The syndrome is genetically heterogeneous. Some patients demonstrate *DKC1* gene mutations and are therefore allelic to dyskeratosis congenita.

Ballew BJ, et al: Updates on the biology and management of dyskeratosis congenita and related telomere biology disorders. Expert Rev Hematol 2013; 6: 327.

Fernández García MS, Teruya-Feldstein J: The diagnosis and treatment of dyskeratosis congenita. J Blood Med 2014; 5: 157.

Gramatges MM, Bertuch AA: Short telomeres: from dyskeratosis congenita to sporadic aplastic anemia and malignancy. Transl Res 2013; 162: 353.

Keeling B, et al: Dyskeratosis congenita. Dermatol Online J 2014; 20: 9.

FANCONI SYNDROME

Also known as familial pancytopenia or familial panmyelophthisis, Fanconi syndrome may be associated with diffuse pigmentation of the skin (hypopigmentation, hyperpigmentation, and café au lait macules), absence of the thumbs, aplasia of the radius, severe hypoplastic anemia, thrombocytopenia, retinal hemorrhage, strabismus, generalized hyperreflexia, and testicular hypoplasia. The syndrome is associated with increased risk of myelomonocytic leukemia, SCC, and hepatic tumors. Human papillomavirus DNA is often found in the SCCs. Both cutaneous and pulmonary manifestations of associated Sweet syndrome have been reported. Some patients manifest short stature, failure to thrive, absent thumbs, short palpebral fissures, and typical skin abnormalities, but no hematologic abnormalities.

Fanconi syndrome is inherited in an autosomal recessive manner. Analysis has shown five complementation groups (FA-A, FA-B, FA-C, FA-D, and FA-E) and therefore five associated genes. The genes play an important role in hematopoiesis, and abnormal gene expression has been shown to increase apoptosis.

Auerbach AD: Fanconi anemia and its diagnosis. Mutat Res 2009; 668: 4.
Chatham-Stephens K, et al: Metachronous manifestations of Sweet's syndrome in a neutropenic patient with Fanconi anemia. Pediatr Blood Cancer 2008; 51: 128.
Dokal I, et al: Inherited aplastic anaemias/bone marrow failure syndromes. Blood Rev 2008; 22: 141.

ECTODERMAL DYSPLASIAS

The ectodermal dysplasias are a clinically and genetically heterogenous group of genodermatoses in which the cardinal features are the abnormal, absent, incomplete, or delayed development during embryogenesis of one or more of the epidermal or mucosal appendages (hair, sebaceous glands, nails, teeth, or mucosal glands). Well over 100 ectodermal dysplasias have been described; those with the most prominent dermatologic features are reviewed here. Craniofacial reconstruction and dental implants can improve quality of life for some patients with ectodermal dysplasia.

Hypohidrotic Ectodermal Dysplasia (Anhidrotic Ectodermal Dysplasia, Christ-Siemens-Touraine Syndrome)

The classic triad of this disorder consists of hypotrichosis, anodontia, and hypohidrosis or anhidrosis. Patients with the disorder have cheekbones that are high and wide, whereas the lower half of the face is narrow (similar to congenital syphilis). The supraorbital ridges are prominent, and the nasal bridge is depressed, forming a saddle nose. The tip of the nose is small and upturned, and the nostrils are large and conspicuous. The eyebrows are scanty, and the eyes slant upward with prominent darkening around the eyes similar to denny morgan lines in atopic dermatitis. The lips are thickened, with the upper lip particularly protrusive. At the buccal commissures, there may be radiating furrows (pseudorhagades), and on the cheeks there may be telangiectasias. Sebaceous gland hyperplasia may be noted on the cheeks and forehead. Absence of mammary glands and nipples has been reported.

Generalized hypotrichosis is present with thin, sparse hair on the scalp. The skin is soft, thin, dry, and smooth. There is partial or total anodontia with peg shaped/conical teeth similar to those seen in incontinentia pigmenti. The nails may be thinned, brittle, and ridged. Mental retardation has been reported but may be a consequence of hyperthermic episodes in childhood.

The inheritance pattern is almost always X-linked recessive. Three genes, ectodysplasin (*EDA1*), EDA-receptor (*EDAR*), and EDAR-associated death domain (*EDARADD*), have been described.

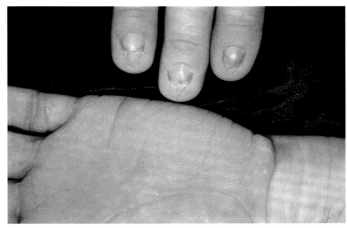

Fig. 27.39 Hidrotic ectodermal dysplasia.

All are involved in nuclear factor (NF)–κB activation. Female carriers may have segmental expression that can be demonstrated with a starch iodide test for sweating. Both autosomal recessive and dominant modes of inheritance have been described.

X-linked anhidrotic ectodermal dysplasia with immunodeficiency is caused by mutations in the gene encoding NF-κB modulator, *NEMO*, or inhibitor of κB kinase (*IKK-γ*). Stop codon mutations are associated with a severe phenotype with associated osteopetrosis and lymphedema. Patients may demonstrate an impaired immunity to mycobacterial infections such as mycobacterium avium complex hyper-IgM syndrome, impaired natural killer cell cytotoxicity, and various associated autoimmune diseases.

Hidrotic Ectodermal Dysplasia

The hidrotic type of congenital ectodermal (Clouston syndrome) manifests with alopecia, nail dystrophy, palmoplantar hyperkeratosis (Fig. 27.39), and eye changes, such as cataracts and strabismus. Some patients have features resembling pachyonychia congenita. Inheritance is autosomal dominant. Eccrine sweat glands function normally, and facial features are normal Widespread poromas and palmoplantar syringofibroadenomas have been described. The defective gene has been identified as *GJB6*, encoding the gap junction protein connexin 30.

AEC Syndrome (Hay-Wells Syndrome)

Ankyloblepharon (fusion or partial fusion of the lids), ectodermal defects, and cleft lip and/or palate constitute the AEC syndrome. It is caused by p63 mutations and inherited autosomal dominantly. Ankyloblepharon is present at birth. Sparse hair, dental defects, cleft palate and lip, dystrophic nails, hypospadias, syndactyly, absent lacrimal puncta, stenotic auditory canals, and short stature may be present. An erosive scalp dermatitis occurs at an early age and can also be seen in KID syndrome (see later in this chapter). The scalp dermatitis is often extensive and difficult to treat, and it persists or recurs (Fig. 27.40). Low-frequency ultrasound has been successful in treating scalp wounds unresponsive to other measures.

EEC Syndrome

Ectodermal dysplasia, ectrodactyly, and cleft lip/palate are defining features of EEC syndrome. The EEC patient lacks scalp dermatitis but has mild hypohidrosis, and ectrodactyly (congenital absence of all or part of a digit, also seen in Goltz syndrome) is a prominent feature (Fig. 27.41). Some patients with EEC also have features of

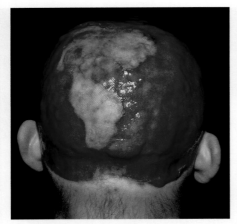

Fig. 27.40 AEC syndrome with scalp dermatitis.

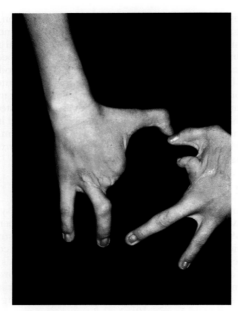

Fig. 27.41 Ectrodactyly in EEC syndrome.

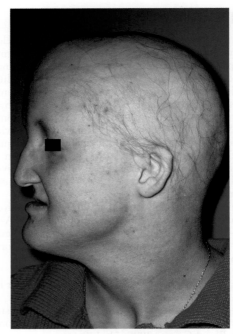

Fig. 27.42 Rapp-Hodgkin syndrome.

mucous membrane pemphigoid with mucosal anti-BMZ BP-180 autoantibodies and severe bilateral cicatrizing conjunctivitis with blindness. Folliculitis with scarring may be noted during puberty, and ocular keratitis can be a prominent feature. As with the AEC syndrome, EEC syndrome is associated with mutations in the *p63* gene.

Rapp-Hodgkin Ectodermal Dysplasia Syndrome

Characteristic features of Rapp-Hodgkin ectodermal dysplasia syndrome include anomalies of hair (pili torti, pili canaliculi, alopecia, erosive folliculitis, thinning of eyebrows/lashes), cleft lip/palate, onychodysplasia, dental caries, hypodontia, craniofacial abnormality (Fig. 27.42), hypohidrosis, otitis media (hearing deficits), and hypospadias. It is usually inherited in an autosomal dominant manner. The syndrome is allelic to AEC and EEC, with *p63* mutations demonstrated in all three syndromes.

Other Ectodermal Dysplasias

Salient features include corkscrew hairs (exaggerated pili torti), scalp keloids, follicular plugging, keratosis pilaris, xerosis, eczema, palmoplantar keratodermia, syndactyly, onychodysplasia, and conjunctival neovascularization. Typical facies, anteverted pinnae, malar hypoplasia, cleft lip/palate, and dental abnormalities may also be found.

Odonto-Tricho-Ungual-Digital-Palmar Syndrome

First described by Mendoza et al., the salient clinical features are natal teeth, trichodystrophy, prominent interdigital folds, simian-like hands with transverse palmar creases, and ungual digital dystrophy, inherited as an autosomal dominant trait. Hypoplasia of the first metacarpal and metatarsal bones and distal phalanges of the toes may also occur.

Lenz-Majewski Syndrome

Lenz-Majewski syndrome is characterized by hyperostosis, craniodiaphyseal dysplasia, dwarfism, cutis laxa, proximal symphalangism, syndactyly, brachydactyly, mental retardation, enamel hypoplasia, and hypertelorism.

Lelis Syndrome

The Lelis syndrome is a form of ectodermal dysplasia with acanthosis nigricans, palmoplantar hyperkeratosis, hypotrichosis, hypohidrosis, nail dystrophy, early loss of adult teeth, and mental retardation.

Nectinopathies

Cleft lip/palate–ectodermal dysplasia and ectodermal dysplasia–syndactyly syndrome are caused by recessive mutations in the *PVRL1* and *PVRL4* genes, respectively. These genes encode nectins 1 and 4, which act in cooperation with cadherins to promote cellular adhesion.

Brancati F, et al: Nectinopathies. G Ital Dermatol Venereol 2013; 148: 59.

Felipe AF, et al: Corneal changes in ectrodactyly–ectodermal dysplasia–cleft lip and palate syndrome. Int Ophthalmol 2012; 32: 475.

Kawai T, et al: Diagnosis and treatment in anhidrotic ectodermal dysplasia with immunodeficiency. Allergol Int 2012; 61: 207.

Knaudt B, et al: Skin symptoms in four ectodermal dysplasia syndromes including two case reports of Rapp-Hodgkin syndrome. Eur J Dermatol 2012; 22: 605.

Mendoza HR, et al: A newly recognized autosomal dominant ectodermal dysplasia syndrome: The odonto-tricho-ungual-digital-palmar syndrome. American journal of medical genetics 1997; 71(2): 144–9.

Ng BG, et al: Mutations in the glycosylphosphatidylinositol gene *PIGL* cause CHIME syndrome. Am J Hum Genet 2012; 90: 685.

PACHYDERMOPERIOSTOSIS (IDIOPATHIC HYPERTROPHIC OSTEOARTHROPATHY, TOURAINE-SOLENTE-GOLE SYNDROME)

Pachydermoperiostosis is characterized by thickening of the skin in folds and accentuation of creases on the face and scalp, clubbing of the fingers, and periostosis of the long bones. The changes are especially prominent on the forehead, where the horizontal lines are deepened and the skin becomes shiny (Fig. 27.43). The eyelids, particularly the upper lids, are thickened. Likewise, there is thickening of the ears and lips, and the tongue is enlarged. The scalp may be thickened and may show cutis verticis gyrata (pachydermie vorticelle). The extremities, especially the elbows, knees, and hands, are enlarged and spade shaped. The fingers become club shaped. The palms are rough, and the thenar and hypothenar eminences are enlarged. Hyperhidrosis is common. Hyperkeratotic linear lesions of the palms and soles may be present. These lines are rippled, resembling sand of the "wind-blown desert." Movements of the muscles may be painful. An association with gynecomastia and osteoporosis has been described.

There are inherited and acquired forms of pachydermoperiostosis. The acquired form may occur with chronic pulmonary, mediastinal, and cardiac diseases that are associated with chronic hypoxia in peripheral tissues. Some cases have been associated with bronchogenic carcinoma. When such an association occurs, enlargement of the forehead, hands, and fingers may antedate recognition of the tumor or may develop after the tumor is identified as present. Bronchogenic carcinoma–associated pachydermoperiostosis occurs almost exclusively in men over age 40, whereas inherited Touraine-Solente-Gole syndrome usually occurs as an autosomal dominant disorder with onset in late adolescence. It is not associated with malignant disease. More prominent signs are seen in males. Autosomal recessive inheritance with cleft palate and congenital heart defects has been described. Frontal rhytidectomy has been used to treat associated leonine facies, and bone manifestations have shown some response to oral bisphosphonate therapy and arthroscopic synovectomy. *HPGD* gene mutations affecting 15-hydroxyprostaglandin dehydrogenase (15-PGDH) and mutations in the prostaglandin transporter gene *SLCO2A1* have been described.

CUTIS VERTICIS GYRATA

Cutis verticis gyrata is characterized by folds and furrows on the scalp, usually in an anteroposterior direction. Most frequently, the vertex is involved, but other areas may have the distinctive furrowing. There may be 2–20 folds. The hair itself is normal.

Cutis verticis gyrata has been reported primarily in males, with a male/female ratio of 6:1. Onset is usually at puberty, with more than 90% of patients developing it before age 30. The condition may be familial when it occurs as a component of pachydermoperiostosis. It has been reported to result from developmental anomalies, inflammation, trauma, tumors, nevi, amyloidosis, syphilis, myxedema, Ehlers-Danlos syndrome, Turner syndrome, Klinefelter syndrome, fragile X syndrome, vemurafenib, and the insulin resistance syndrome. Cutis verticis gyrata may be found in patients with mental retardation, seizures, and schizophrenia. Biopsy findings can be normal or may show thick collagen bundles and hypertrophy of adnexal structures. Rarely, a cerebriform intradermal nevus may be mistaken for this disorder. In severely involved cases, excision with grafting or scalp reduction may be indicated.

George L, et al: Frontal rhytidectomy as surgical treatment for pachydermoperiostosis. J Dermatolog Treat 2008; 19: 61.

Harding JJ, et al: Cutis verticis gyrata in association with vemurafenib and whole-brain radiotherapy. J Clin Oncol 2014; 32: e54.

Sasaki T, et al: Identification of mutations in the prostaglandin transporter gene *SLCO2A1* and its phenotype-genotype correlation in Japanese patients with pachydermoperiostosis. J Dermatol Sci 2012; 68: 36.

Taha HM, Orlando A: Butterfly-shape scalp excision. J Plast Reconstr Aesthet Surg 2014; 67: 1747.

APLASIA CUTIS CONGENITA

Aplasia cutis congenita (ACC) is a congenital absence of at least the skin but the defect may extend all of the way through the skull if on the scalp. ACC may be from a primary failure of skin formation or from in utero destruction of skin that had formed. The most typical location for ACC is the scalp but there are other stereotypical locations associated with certain syndromes or intrauterine events.

Scalp ACC is divided into membranous and nonmembranous forms. Membranous ACC is notable at birth with a thin membrane often overlying a small nodule that can be filled with clear or serosanguineous fluid. These lesions are usually round or oval and may be due to failed fusion of embryonic planes, because they can also occur off midline and even on the face. Lesions of membranous aplasia cutis may have a "hair collar sign," which refers to a ring of long, dark terminal hair encircling the lesion. Membranous ACC can be a marker of cranial dysraphism or a remnant connection to the CNS such as an atretic encephalocele or meningocele. Therefore midline vertex or posterior scalp lesions and any membranous aplasia cutis with a hair collar sign warrants an MRI to rule out a connection to the CNS and evaluate for a remnant neural lesion.

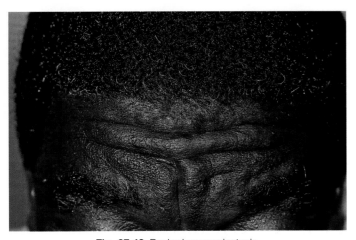

Fig. 27.43 Pachydermoperiostosis.

Nonmembranous aplasia cutis is usually more stellate and then leads to scarring, which may indicate that it was caused by destruction of skin. Imaging is recommended for stellate lesions to rule out bony defects. If large, there can be hemorrhage or infection. Scalp aplasia cutis can be autosomal dominantly inherited.

If there is intrauterine demise of a twin (fetus papyraceus) there can be a resultant cutaneous infarction in the living twin that has a characteristic "H" pattern on the abdomen with aplasia cutis and resultant scarring horizontally across the abdomen with vertical band extending superiorly and inferiorly on the sides forming an "H." Aplasia cutis can occur due to medications such as methimazole. Distal radial epiphyseal dysplasia has been associated with localized ACC.

FOCAL PREAURICULAR DERMAL DYSPLASIA

Focal preauricular dermal dysplasia is a form of ACC not typically associated with any extracutaneous anomalies.

SYNDROMES ASSOCIATED WITH APLASIA CUTIS

Adams-Oliver syndrome includes severe ACC of the scalp, which may involve both skin and skull ossification defects, limb defects (brachydactyly, syndactyly of toes two and three, and hypoplastic toenails), extensive cutis marmorata telangiectatica congenita, cryptorchidism, and cardiac abnormalities, including ventricular septal defects, and tetralogy of Fallot. Adams-Oliver is a rare, autosomal dominant inherited neuroectodermal syndrome caused by *NOTCH-1* mutations although various other mutations have been reported in a minority of patients.

The SCALP syndrome is a syndrome with CNS malformations, ACC, limbal dermoid, and a giant congenital pigmented melanocytic nevus with neurocutaneous melanosis. The 19q13.11 deletion syndrome with microcephaly, scalp defects, and developmental delay was recently found to be from a *UBA2* mutation. Scalp-ear-nipple syndrome is characterized by ACC, ear anomalies, and breast anomalies. Johanson-Blizzard syndrome is characterized by hypoplasia of the nasal ala, scalp defects, and oligodontia.

Atasoy HI, et al: Unique variant of Adams-Oliver syndrome with dilated cardiomyopathy and heart block. Pediatr Int 2013; 55: 508.

Bakry O, et al: Adams-Oliver syndrome. J Dermatol Case Rep 2012; 6: 25.

Humphrey SR, et al: A practical approach to the evaluation and treatment of an infant with aplasia cutis congenita. J Perinatol 2017 Oct 19; Epub ahead of print.

Lam J, et al: SCALP syndrome. J Am Acad Dermatol 2008; 58: 884.

Marble M, et al: Missense variant in UBA2 associated with aplasia cutis congenita, duane anomaly, hip dysplasia and other anomalies. Am J Med Genet A 2017; 173: 758.

Stittrich AB, et al: Mutations in *NOTCH1* cause Adams-Oliver syndrome. Am J Hum Genet 2014; 95: 275.

FOCAL DERMAL HYPOPLASIA (GOLTZ SYNDROME)

Goltz syndrome is an X-linked dominant disorder that presents at birth with a blaschkoid pattern of reddish tan, cribriform, atrophic, plaques (Fig. 27.44). The buttocks, axillae, and thighs are often involved. Adipocytes accumulate in the lesions, resulting in yellowish brown nodules herniate through the atrophic areas. Telangiectases are often present, and segmental presentations have been described. Papillomas may occur around the orifices of the mouth, anus, and vulva. They may be misdiagnosed as condylomata acuminata. An early inflammatory vesicular stage has been described, along with cleft lip and palate although a blaschkoid pattern of vesicles is more

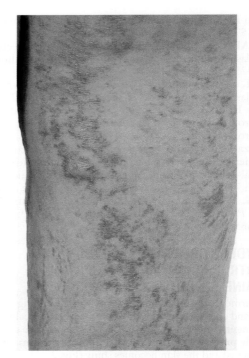

Fig. 27.44 Goltz syndrome.

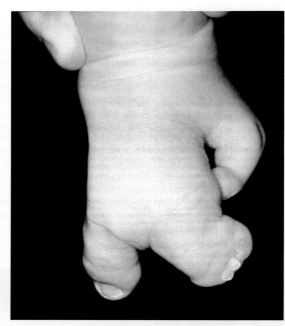

Fig. 27.45 Goltz syndrome.

typical of incontinentia pigmenti. About 80% of patients have skeletal defects such as ectrodactyly (similar to EEC syndrome), syndactyly, oligodactyly, or adactyly (Fig. 27.45). Scoliosis, spina bifida, and hypoplasia of the clavicle have also been reported. From 40%–50% of patients have ocular or dental abnormalities, with coloboma being the most common ocular defect.

Goltz syndrome is X linked dominant, caused by mutations in *PORCN*, a regulator of Wnt signaling. Females are protected by inactivating the affected X chromosome during lionization (similar to other X linked dominant disorders such as incontinentia pigmenti). Therefore a history of spontaneous male abortions and only female offspring is supportive. Males can have postzygotic mutations that lead to blaschkoid or segmental patterns of Goltz. If males have an extra X chromosome (XXY or XXYY), then they could have the full syndrome. Van Allen–Myhre syndrome appears to represent a severe form of Goltz syndrome with split-foot and split-hand anomalies. Treatment of atrophic erythematous patches has been successful using a flashlamp-pumped pulsed dye laser.

MIDAS SYNDROME

MIDAS (microphthalmia, dermal aplasia, and sclerocornea) is also X-linked dominant (mutation in the *HCSS* gene) and presents with linear facial and neck scarring along with microphthalmia. The clinical lesions are somewhat similar to Goltz syndrome, but the distribution of MIDAS is characteristic.

Asano M, et al: A case of almost unilateral focal dermal hypoplasia resulting from a novel mutation in the *PORCN* gene. Acta Derm Venereol 2013; 93: 120.
Lim SK, et al: MIDAS syndrome presenting with linear skin atrophy on the face. Korean J Dermatol 2015; 53: 381.
Stevenson DA, et al: Goltz syndrome and PORCN mosaicism. Int J Dermatol 2014; 12: 1481.

Restrictive Dermopathy

Restrictive dermopathy is a rare, lethal, autosomal recessive inherited laminopathy characterized by abnormal facies, tight skin, sparse or absent eyelashes, and secondary joint changes. Virtually all cases are associated with polyhydramnios, reduced fetal movements, and premature delivery. Infants exhibit a fixed facial expression, with blurring of the groove between nose and cheek, sometimes described as an "Asiatic porcelain doll" appearance. Patients also exhibit micrognathia, mouth in the O position, rigid and tense skin with erosions especially at the flexures, denudations, and multiple joint contractures. Some patients have wide cranial sutures, small pinched nose, low-set ears, microstomia, rocker-bottom feet, scaly skin, and respiratory insufficiency. Pulmonary hypoplasia, microcolon, vessel transposition, natal teeth, ectropion, submucous cleft palate, hypospadias, urethral duplication, dysplasia of clavicles, adrenal hypoplasia, and an enlarged placenta with short umbilical cord may be noted.

Histopathologic features include hyperkeratosis, parakeratosis, abnormal keratohyaline granules, and effacement of the rete ridge pattern. The dermis is attenuated with collagen fibers parallel to the epidermis, resembling a scar or tendon. Elastic fibers are absent. The subcutis demonstrates hypoplastic eccrine and sebaceous glands. The disease is usually caused by mutations in *ZMPSTE24*, causing loss of function of the encoded zinc metalloproteinase STE24 and resulting in accumulation of prelamin A at the nuclear periphery. Dominant and progeroid forms may be related to LMNA mutations.

Starke S, et al: Progeroid laminopathy with restrictive dermopathy–like features caused by an isodisomic LMNA mutation *p.R435C*. Aging (Albany NY) 2013; 5: 445.

WERNER SYNDROME (ADULT PROGERIA)

Werner syndrome is an autosomal recessive, premature aging syndrome characterized by many metabolic and structural abnormalities involving the skin, hair, eyes, muscles, fatty tissues, bones, blood vessels, and carbohydrate metabolism. Cells demonstrate genomic instability. Most of these signs and thus the diagnosis are not fully manifested until age 30. These patients usually die before age 50 from malignant disease or vascular accidents.

The most characteristic findings are premature aging and arrest of growth at puberty, senile cataracts developing in the late twenties and thirties, and premature balding and graying. The skin changes include poikiloderma, scleroderma, atrophy, hyperkeratoses, and leg ulcers. The skin has a diffuse, dark-gray or blackish pigmentation. Painful callosities with ulcerations may occur around the malleoli, Achilles tendons, heels, and toes. The hair thins on the eyebrows, axillae, and pubis. The skin over the cheekbones becomes taut, producing proptosis and beaking of the nose. There is loss of subcutaneous tissue and wasting of muscles, especially the extremities, so that the legs become spindly and the trunk becomes stocky. The vocal cords become thickened, leading to a weak, high-pitched voice. Premature arteriosclerosis and sexual impotence are frequently observed. Hypogonadism in both genders are distinctive in Werner syndrome. Diabetes is common, and areas of calcinosis circumscripta occur. Osteoporosis and aseptic necrosis are frequently found in the small bones of the hands.

A high rate of malignancy is associated with Werner syndrome, including a 50-fold increase in melanoma. Thyroid adenocarcinoma, hepatoma, meningioma, leukemia, carcinoma of the breast, fibrosarcoma, and a variety of sarcomas have been reported. Histologic changes in the skin may include atrophy of the epidermis and fibrosis of the dermis.

Werner syndrome is caused by a mutation in the *WRN* gene that is involved in telomere maintenance and thus loss of function may lead to the age-related changes.

PROGERIA (HUTCHINSON-GILFORD SYNDROME)

Progeria, or Hutchinson-Gilford syndrome, is characterized by accelerated aging, dwarfism, alopecia, generalized atrophy of the skin and muscles, enlarged head with prominent scalp veins, and a high incidence of generalized atherosclerosis, usually fatal by the second decade of life. In affected individuals, their large, bald head and lack of eyebrows and eyelashes are distinctive (Fig. 27.46). The skin is wrinkled, pigmented, and atrophic. Progeroid features can be seen in trichothyodystrophy, neonatal progeroid syndrome, restrictive dermopathy, werner syndrome, bloom syndrome and rothmund thompson. The nails are thin and atrophic. Most patients lack subcutaneous fat, which produces the appearance of premature senility. There are usually sclerodermatous plaques on the extremities. The intelligence remains intact. Arteriosclerosis, anginal attacks,

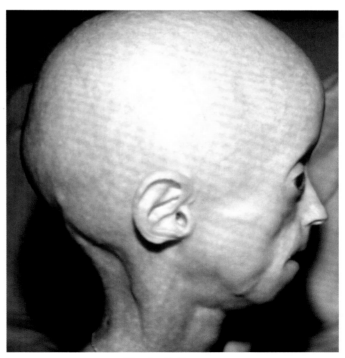

Fig. 27.46 Progeria.

and hemiplegia may occur, followed by death from coronary heart disease at an early age. Mutations in LMNA and mosaicism have been identified. Treatment is symptomatic, mainly control of diabetes mellitus and treatment of leg ulcerations.

Coppedè F: The epidemiology of premature aging and associated comorbidities. Clin Interv Aging 2013; 8: 1023.

Gordon LB, et al: Progeria. Cell 2014; 156: 400.

Goto M, et al: Werner syndrome. Biosci Trends 2013; 7: 13.

Kalinowski A, et al: Interfacial binding and aggregation of lamin A tail domains associated with Hutchinson-Gilford progeria syndrome. Biophys Chem 2014; 195: 43.

Lauper JM, et al: Spectrum and risk of neoplasia in Werner syndrome. PLoS One 2013; 8: e59709.

Oshima J, et al: Werner syndrome. Ageing Res Rev 2017; 33: 105.

DISORGERS WITH PHOTOSENSITIVITY

Xeroderma pigmentosum, Cockayne syndrome, and trichothiodystrophy are caused by mutations in genes involved in nucleotide excision repair (NER). NER repairs DNA lesions throughout the genome, preventing the accumulation of mutations. Therefore these three syndromes share common features of photosensitivity with or without skin cancer or systemic cancer risk. Mutations in a single gene such as ERCC2/XPB or ERCC3/XPD can actually produce the clinical phenotype of any of the three syndromes depending on how they affect the function of the transcription factor TFIIH that is involved in NER.

XERODERMA PIGMENTOSUM

Xeroderma pigmentosum is an autosomal recessive disorder characterized by defective DNA thymidine dimer excision repair, extreme sun sensitivity, freckling, and skin cancer. Mutations in various different genes involved in DNA repair after UV damage and thus lead to similar phenotypes. Sun sensitivity and lentigines are early skin findings (Fig. 27.47), with median onset before age 2 years. Skin cancers often appear before age 10, and an increase in internal cancer has been noted as well. NIH data suggest a

10,000-fold increase in skin cancer before age 20. In a study of 830 patients, 45% had basal cell carcinoma or SCC, and melanoma was noted in 5%. Most of the tumors occur on the head and neck in sun-exposed areas. Skin tumors in xeroderma pigmentosum patients have sunlight-induced mutations in *RAS*, *p53*, and *PTCH* genes. Ocular abnormalities were found in 40% and included photophobia, ectropion, corneal opacity, blepharospasm and neoplasms. Progressive neurologic degeneration is seen in about 20% of patients. Loss of high-frequency hearing can also occur. Xeroderma pigmentosum patients in complementation group C remain free of neurologic problems. Complementation groups are defined by correction of excision repair when fibroblasts from patients in different groups are fused. A variant type with normal excision repair has also been described.

The main intervention that is vital is extremely diligent photoprotection. Vitamin D, nicotinamide, and zinc supplementation may help. Retinoids can prevent the appearance of new cancers, but side effects are significant, and a rebound in the number of cancers occurs when the drug is stopped, suggesting that the tumors are merely suppressed. Individual tumors may be excised or destroyed with cryotherapy. Some may be treated with topical imiquimod or 5-FU. Topical application of recombinant liposomal encapsulated T4 endonuclease V repairs UV-induced cyclobutane-pyrimidine dimers and is a promising form of therapy. Gene therapy is also being pursued. Guidelines for evaluation and management from the XP Society can be found at www.xps.org. A publication from the NIH can be found at www.cc.nih.gov/ccc/patient_education/pepubs/xp7_17.pdf.

The De Sanctis–Cacchione syndrome consists of xeroderma pigmentosum with mental deficiency, dwarfism, and gonadal hypoplasia. It occurs most often in patients in complementation group D.

COCKAYNE SYNDROME (NO SKIN CANCER)

Cockayne syndrome is an autosomal recessive syndrome with sun sensitivity and neurologic degeneration related to mutations in five NER genes: *ERCC8* (Cockayne syndrome A), *ERCC6* (Cockayne syndrome B), *XPB*, *XPD*, and *XPG*. Mutations in *XPB* or *XPD* DNA helicase can result in xeroderma pigmentosum, Cockayne syndrome, or trichothiodystrophy. Cockayne differs from xeroderma pigmentosum in the lack of freckling and in the presence of dwarfism, beaked nose, loss of subcutaneous tissue, deafness, basal ganglia calcification, failure of brain growth, and retinopathy. Dermatologic features include photodermatitis with telangiectasia, atrophy, and scarring. The hands and feet are large and cyanotic. Microcephaly, sunken eyes, severe flexion contractures, dorsal kyphosis, cryptorchidism, cataracts, growth retardation, mental retardation, hypothalamic and cerebellar dysfunction, and retinitis pigmentosa with optic atrophy may be seen. There is progressive neurologic disturbance with a shortened life span.

Patients in complementation groups B, D, and G (XPB, XPD, XPG) have skin features of xeroderma pigmentosum and neurologic features of Cockayne syndrome. Mutations in the associated genes may give rise to clinical manifestations of xeroderma pigmentosum, Cockayne syndrome, or the XP-Cockayne syndrome complex. The XP-Cockayne syndrome patients have an elevated skin cancer risk but the other Cockayne patients do not.

TRICHOTHIODYSTROPHY

Trichothiodystrophy (TTD) is an autosomal recessive disorder originally described as photosensitivity, ichthyosis, brittle hair, intellectual impairment, decreased fertility, and short stature (PIBIDS). There are also nonphotosensitive versions caused by other mutations with the acronym IBIDS. A review of 112 patients noted a wide spectrum of clinical features that varied from patients with only hair involvement to those with profound developmental defects. Common features included intellectual impairment (86%),

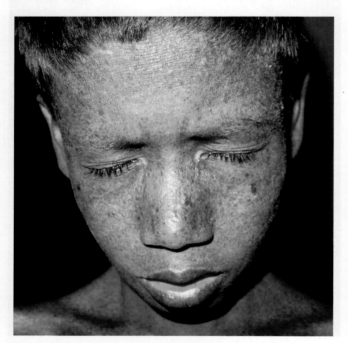

Fig. 27.47 Xeroderma pigmentosum. (Courtesy Dr. Debabrata Bandyopadhyay.)

short stature (73%), ichthyosis (65%), ocular abnormalities (51%), infections (46%), and photosensitivity (42%). More than half the patients had abnormal characteristics at birth, and 19 patients died before age 10.

The hair, with sulfur reduced to 50% of the normal value, has distinctive features under polarizing and light microscopy and scanning EM and can help aid in early diagnosis. With light microscopy, keratin orientation alternates in a **Z** pattern. With polarizing microscopy, the hair shows alternating bright and dark regions that give a striking striped, or tiger tail, appearance, but the pattern may not be evident at birth, and a similar pattern of bright and dark bands has been described in the keratitis ichthyosis deafness syndrome. Hairs demonstrate heterogeneous deficiency in sulfur, with the greatest loss in areas of trichoschisis (clean fractures). Trichorrhexis nodosa–like fractures may also be seen. In addition, the hair is extremely flattened and folds over itself like a thick ribbon. The hair shaft outline is irregular and slightly undulating, and the melanin granules are distributed in a wavy pattern. With scanning EM, the surface shows marked ridging and fluting, and the cuticle scales may be absent or greatly reduced.

The three genes mutated in TTD are *ERCC2*, *ERCC3*, and *GTF2HF*, which are involved in DNA repair, encoding parts of a transcription repair factor TFIIH. The UV sensitivity and defective NER are similar to those of xeroderma pigmentosum patients, but these patients do not experience an increased incidence of skin cancer. Two of the three described complementation groups match xeroderma pigmentosum groups B and D, with the *XPD* gene accounting for most photosensitive trichothiodystrophy. A combined xeroderma pigmentosum/trichothiodystrophy complex has been described. Patients with trichothiodystrophy without xeroderma pigmentosum do not have an increase in skin cancer formation.

Aamann MD, et al: Cockayne syndrome group B protein stimulates NEIL2 DNA glycosylase activity. Mech Ageing Dev 2014; 135: 1.

DiGiovanna JJ, et al: Shining a light on xeroderma pigmentosum. J Invest Dermatol 2012; 132: 785.

Faghri S, et al: Trichothiodystrophy: a systematic review of 112 published cases characterises a wide spectrum of clinical manifestations. Journal of medical genetics 2008; 45(10): 609–21.

Ferrando J, et al: Further insights in trichothiodistrophy. Int J Trichology 2012; 4: 158.

Grossberg AL: Update on pediatric photosensitivity disorders. Curr Opin Pediatr 2013; 25: 474.

Hasan S, Saeed S: Xeroderma pigmentosum—a rare genodermatosis. J Pigment Disord 2015; 2: 230.

Lanzafame M, et al: From laboratory tests to functional characterisation of Cockayne syndrome. Mech Ageing Dev 2013; 134: 171.

Lehmann AR, et al: Xeroderma pigmentosum. Orphanet J Rare Dis 2011; 6: 70.

Natale V, et al. Xeroderma pigmentosum–Cockayne syndrome complex. Orphanet J Rare Dis 2017; 12: 65.

Niedernhofer LJ, et al: Xeroderma pigmentosum and other diseases of human premature aging and DNA repair. Mech Ageing Dev 2011; 132: 340.

Saygi S, et al: A boy with developmental delay probably due to trichothiodystrophy. Eur J Paediatr Neurol 2017; 21: e75.

BLOOM SYNDROME (BLOOM-TORRE-MACHACEK SYNDROME)

Bloom syndrome is characterized by photosensitive telangiectatic erythema in the butterfly area of the face (which can be very similar to RTS) along with dwarfism. The earlier onset and the presence of cataracts help differentiate Bloom from RTS. Telangiectatic erythematous patches resembling lupus erythematosous develop in the first 2 years of life (Fig. 27.48). Bullous, crusted

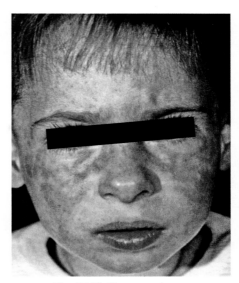

Fig. 27.48 Bloom syndrome.

lesions may be present on the lips. Exacerbation of skin lesions occurs during the summer. Cockayne and EPP display similar photosensitivity. Other changes that may be noted are café au lait spots, ichthyosis, acanthosis nigricans, syndactyly, irregular dentition, lens opacities, prominent ears, hypospadias, and cryptorchidism. Bloom patients have a high-pitched voice. The stunted growth is characterized by normal body proportions, no endocrine abnormalities (except diabetes mellitus), and low birth weight at full term. Dolichocephaly and narrow, delicate facies are present. Immune functions are abnormal, and GI and respiratory infections often occur. Cancer of all cell types and sites is increased in frequency. Leukemia, lymphoma, adenocarcinoma of the sigmoid colon, and oral and esophageal SCC, as well as other malignancies, have been associated with Bloom syndrome. About one quarter of patients under age 20 develop a neoplasm. Regular use of a broad-spectrum sunscreen, as well as photoprotection, is recommended.

Bloom is caused by mutations in *BLM* gene, which codes for a RecQ DNA helicase. *BLM* interacts with WRN, the DNA helicase mutated in Werner syndrome, and is part of a large *BRCA-1*–containing complex containing DNA repair factors. BLM interacts directly with ATM (likely explaining the telangiectasias in each), the protein product of the gene mutated in ataxia-telangiectasia, and together they recognize abnormal DNA structures.

Arora H, et al: Bloom syndrome. Int J Dermatol 2014; 53: 798.

Thomas ER, et al: Surveillance and treatment of malignancy in Bloom syndrome. Clin Oncol (R Coll Radiol) 2008; 20: 375.

ROTHMUND-THOMSON SYNDROME (POIKILODERMA CONGENITALE)

Rothmund-Thomson syndrome (RTS) is a rare autosomal recessive disorder. Poikiloderma begins at 3–6 months of age, with tense, pink, edematous patches on the cheeks, hands, feet, and buttocks, sparing the chest, back, and abdomen (acute phase). Sensitivity to sunlight may be manifested by the development of bullae or intense erythema after brief sun exposure. This is followed by fine, reticulated or punctate atrophy associated with telangiectasia and reticulated pigmentation (chronic phase) (Fig. 27.49). The skin lesions are characteristic. The arms and legs are affected, with sparing of the antecubital and popliteal fossae. Associated cutaneous neoplasms include SCC, Bowen disease, basal cell carcinoma, and melanoma, but the risk for osteosarcoma of bone is particularly high (>30%). Patients with Rothmund-Thomson syndrome may

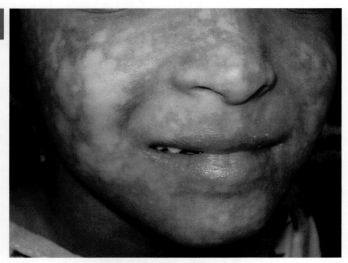

Fig. 27.49 Rothmund-Thomson syndrome.

have a broad range of noncutaneous lesions. Short stature (66%), small hands with radial ray defects, saddle nose, absence or sparseness of eyebrows and eyelashes (73%), alopecia of the scalp (50%), and numerous bone defects (75%) are often observed. Hypogonadism, dystrophic nails, and defective dentition are seen in a significant proportion of patients (25%–60%). Cataracts occur in a small percentage of patients in childhood or young adult life, and glomerulonephritis has been reported. The syndrome is related to biallelic mutations of the *RECQL4* gene. Thus at least a subset of patients with Rothmund-Thomson syndrome has abnormal DNA helicase activity, as do patients with Werner and Bloom syndromes.

POIKILODERMA WITH NEUTROPENIA

Clericuzio-type poikiloderma with neutropenia (PN) is also characterized by a poikilodermatous eruption that usually starts in the first year and importantly is associated with neutropenia and sinopulmonary infections. They can also have PPK, nail deformities, and skeletal abnormalities. PN should be considered in patients who present with poikiloderma and RTS is being considered. PN is caused by mutations in *USB1*.

Canger EM, et al: Oral findings of Rothmund-Thomson syndrome. Case Rep Dent 2013; 2013: 935716.
Manavi S, Mahajan VK: Rothmund-Thomson syndrome. Indian Dermatol Online J 2014; 5: 518.
Suter AA, et al: Rothmund-Thomson syndrome. Mol Genet Genomic Med 2016; 4: 359.

HEREDITARY SCLEROSING POIKILODERMA AND MANDIBULOACRAL DYSPLASIA

Hereditary sclerosing poikiloderma is an extremely rare autosomal dominant disorder. The skin changes consist of generalized poikiloderma appearing in childhood (but not at birth), with hyperkeratotic and sclerotic cutaneous bands extending across the antecubital spaces, axillary vaults, and popliteal fossae. In addition, the palms and soles may show sclerosis resembling shiny scotch-grain leather. Aortic stenosis, clubbing of the fingers, and localized calcinosis of the skin have also been noted. The cases described by Weary were subsequently reported later in life as mandibuloacral dysplasia, a rare autosomal recessive syndrome characterized by mandibular hypoplasia, delayed cranial suture closure, dysplastic clavicles, abbreviated club-shaped terminal phalanges, myopathy, lipodystrophy, acro-osteolysis, atrophy of the skin of the hands and feet, and typical facial changes. Mandibuloacral dysplasia must be distinguished from progeria and Werner syndrome.

A distinct subtype has been described in two generations of a South African family. The characteristics included poikiloderma, tendon contracture, and pulmonary fibrosis, with apparent autosomal dominant inheritance. Sparse, fine hairs are present on the scalp, face, and body.

Khumalo NP, et al: Poikiloderma, tendon contracture and pulmonary fibrosis. Br J Dermatol 2006; 155: 1057.
Lombardi F, et al: Compound heterozygosity for mutations in LMNA in a patient with a myopathic and lipodystrophic mandibuloacral dysplasia type A phenotype. J Clin Endocrinol Metab 2007; 92: 4467.

SCLEROATROPHIC SYNDROME OF HURIEZ

Huriez syndrome, a very rare autosomal dominant disorder, is a palmoplantar keratoderma characterized by scleroatrophy of the hands, with sclerodactyly, along with ridging, clubbing, or hypoplasia of the nails. Patients with Huriez syndrome may also have multiple telangiectasias of the lips and face and flexion contractures of the little finger. Aggressive SCCs occur in the scleroatrophic skin, including that of the palms and soles (13% lifetime risk, 5% mortality rate in affected persons). Affected patients have reduced Langerhans cells in affected skin, but normal dermal dendritic cells.

DISORDERS WITH CRANIOFACIAL ABNORMALITIES

Franceschetti-Klein Syndrome (Mandibulofacial Dysostosis)

This syndrome includes palpebral antimongoloid fissures, hypoplasia of the facial bones, macrostomia, vaulted palate, malformations of both the external and internal ear, buccal-auricular fistula, abnormal development of the neck with stretching of the cheeks, accessory facial fissures, and skeletal deformities. Patients who have the complete syndrome usually die in infancy, but patients with the abortive type may live to an old age. Franceschetti-Klein syndrome is allelic to the Treacher Collins syndrome and caused by the Treacher Collins–Franceschetti *(TCOF1)* gene.

Treacher Collins Syndrome

Treacher Collins syndrome includes midface hypoplasia with micrognathia, microtia, conductive hearing loss, and cleft palate. It is inherited as an autosomal dominant trait and caused by mutations in the *TCOF1* gene, which encodes a protein called treacle.

Oculoauriculofrontonasal Syndrome

This syndrome is sporadic in nature, although autosomal recessive inheritance has been suggested by some authors. Features include hemifacial microsomia, microtia, ocular hypertelorism, upper palpebral colobomata, preauricular tags, lateral face clefting, and nasal clefting.

Popliteal Pterygium Syndrome

Pterygia or skinfolds may extend from the thigh down to the heel and thus prevent extension or rotation of the legs. Crural pterygia, cryptorchidism, bifid scrotum, agenesis of the labia majora, cleft lip and palate, adhesions between the eyelids, syndactyly, and talipes equinovarus may be present. Autosomal dominant inheritance has been described, and popliteal pterygium syndrome is allelic to the van der Woude syndrome.

van der Woude Syndrome

The van der Woude syndrome is an autosomal dominant craniofacial disorder characterized by hypodontia, pits of the lower lip, and cleft palate due to mutations in the *IRF6* gene. Other reported associations include natal teeth, ankyloglossia, syndactyly, equinovarus foot deformity, and congenital heart disease. Lower lip pits may be found in other congenital disorders, such as popliteal pterygium syndrome, and occasionally in orofaciodigital syndrome type I (oral frenula and clefts, hypoplasia of alae nasi, and digital asymmetry). Surgical correction is the treatment of choice.

Apert Syndrome (Acrocephalosyndactyly)

Apert syndrome is autosomal dominant inherited and is characterized by craniosynostosis and fusion of the digits (syndactyly). Patients present with synostosis of the feet, hands, carpi, tarsi, cervical vertebrae, and skull. The facial features are distorted and the second, third, and fourth fingers are fused into a bony mass with a single nail. Occulocutaneous albinism and severe acne vulgaris have been reported with Apert syndrome, although some of the acneiform lesions actually represent follicular hamartomas. Neurologic defects may be caused in part by brain compression by the abnormal skull. Mutations in the fibroblast growth factor receptor *(FGFR2)* gene are responsible for Apert, Crouzon, and Pfeiffer syndromes. Nevus comedonicus has been shown to be due to a post zygotic mutation in *FGFR2*.

Pfeiffer Syndrome

Pfeiffer syndrome is autosomal dominant inherited and consists of osteochondrodysplasia and craniosynostosis.

Crouzon Syndrome

Crouzon syndrome includes craniosynostosis and acanthosis nigricans. It is associated with mutations in the *FGFR2* gene. The crouzonodermoskeletal syndrome with choanal atresia and hydrocephalus is caused by mutations in *FGFR3*, a gene associated with achondroplastic dwarfism. Affected patients can also present with acanthosis nigricans

Carpenter Syndrome

Carpenter syndrome is an acrocephalopolysyndactyly syndrome with craniosynostosis and acral deformities that include syndactyly.

Whistling Face Syndrome

In this rare disorder, also known as distal arthrogryposis type 2, the child appears to be whistling all the time. This configuration is the result of microstomia, deep-set eyes, flattened midface, coloboma, contracted joint muscles of the fingers and hands, and alterations of the nostrils. Ulnar deviation of the fingers, kyphoscoliosis, and talipes equinovarus may be present.

Asch S, et al: New insights into whorls and swirls. Pediatric dermatology 2018; 35(1): 21–9.

Herman TE, et al: Crouzono-dermo-skeletal syndrome, Crouzon syndrome with acanthosis nigricans syndrome. J Perinatol 2014; 34: 164.

Hirai H, et al: Acanthosis nigricans in a Japanese boy with hypochondroplasia due to a K650T mutation in *FGFR3*. Clin Pediatr Endocrinol 2017; 26: 223.

Raposo-Amaral CE, et al: Patient-reported quality of life in highest-functioning Apert and Crouzon syndromes. Plast Reconstr Surg 2014; 133: 182e.

Roscioli T, et al: Genotype and clinical care correlations in craniosynostosis. Am J Med Genet C Semin Med Genet 2013; 163: 259.

OTHER SYNDROMES THAT INCLUDE HAIR ABNORMALITIES

Hallerman-Streiff Syndrome

People with Hallerman-Streiff syndrome have characteristic "bird facies" (micrognathia with a small shin, a pointed nose, and microphthalmia along with a proportionately larger posterior part of their head). They can have congenital cataracts, hypotrichosis, and dental abnormalities, including absent teeth leading to malocclusion. The hair is diffusely sparse and brittle. Baldness may occur frontally or at the scalp margins, but sutural alopecia—hair loss following the lines of the cranial sutures—is characteristic of this syndrome. Nystagmus, strabismus, and other ocular abnormalities occur. Cleft palate and syndactyly may be present, representing overlap with oculodentodigital dysplasia associated with *GJA1* gene mutation.

Polyostotic Fibrous Dysplasia (Albright Disease)

Polyostotic fibrous dysplasia may present as slowly progressive, lifelong unilateral hair loss (scalp, pubic, axillary, and palpebral).

Cronkhite-Canada Syndrome

Cronkhite-Canada syndrome is characterized by alopecia, skin pigmentation, onychodystrophy, malabsorption, and generalized GI polyposis. Patients often present with diarrhea. The hyperpigmentation often involves the palms and soles. Recently the alopecia was proposed to be alopecia areata because it can affect body hair and may respond to systemic steroids.

Marinesco-Sjögren Syndrome

Marinesco-Sjögren syndrome consists of cerebellar ataxia, mental retardation, congenital cataracts, inability to chew food, thin brittle fingernails, and sparse hair. The dystrophic hairs do not have the normal layers (cortex, cuticle, medulla), and 30% of the hair shafts show narrow bands of abnormal, incomplete keratinization.

Multiple Familial Trichoepitheliomas

Generalized trichoepitheliomas, alopecia, and myasthenia gravis may be a variant of the generalized hair follicle hamartoma syndrome. There is a report of a localized variant of this syndrome. Histologically, there is replacement of the hair follicles by trichoepithelioma-like epithelial proliferations associated with hyperplastic sebaceous glands. It is caused by a mutation in the CYLD gene (similar to Brooks Spiegler and familial cylindromatosis).

Crow-Fukase (POEMS) Syndrome

This acquired syndrome is characterized by polyneuropathy, organomegaly, endocrinopathy, M-protein, and skin changes (POEMS) such as diffuse hyperpigmentation, dependent edema, skin thickening, hyperhidrosis, glomerluoid hemangiomas and hypertrichosis (see Chapter 28).

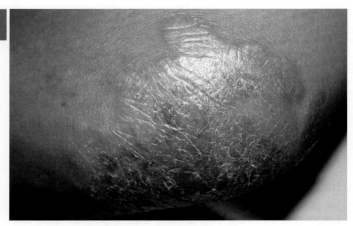

Fig. 27.50 Noninfectious granuloma in cartilage-hair hypoplasia.

Cartilage-Hair Hypoplasia (Mckusick-Type Metaphyseal Chondrodysplasia)

Cartilage-hair hypoplasia encompasses short-limbed dwarfism and abnormally fine and sparse hair in children. These children are especially susceptible to viral infections (varicella-zoster virus and herpes simplex virus) and recurrent respiratory infections. They can get sarcoidal-like granulomas (Fig. 27.50) likely due to inefficient handling of live rubella virus vaccine (similar to ataxia telangiectasia and other immunodeficiencies). A high incidence of non-Hodgkin lymphoma, leukemia, SCC, and basal cell carcinoma has been reported. A functional defect of small lymphocytes, with impaired cell-mediated immunity, may occur. Most patients are anergic to skin-test panels and have increased numbers of natural killer cells. The major mutation involves the *RMRP* gene, which encodes a component of mitochondrial RNA-processing endoribonuclease.

Cartilage-hair hypoplasia has been associated with Omenn syndrome (*RAG1/RAG2I* mutations), a variant of severe combined immunodeficiency disease, which includes erythroderma, eosinophilia, and susceptibility to various pathogens. Mutations in recombination-activating genes 1 and 2 or the protein Artemis have been associated with Omenn syndrome.

Trichorhinophalangeal Syndrome

This genetic disorder consists of fine and sparse scalp hair, thin nails, pear-shaped broad nose, and cone-shaped epiphyses of the middle phalanges of some fingers and toes. Supernumerary teeth have been reported. There is an autosomal dominant and also a recessive inheritance type. Trichorhinophalangeal syndrome can result from mutations in *TRPS1* gene. Type II (Langer-Giedion syndrome) includes mental retardation and multiple exostoses and is a contiguous gene syndrome caused by a one-copy deletion spanning the genes *TRPS1*, *RAD21*, and *EXT1*. Type III resembles a severe form of type I with short stature.

Papillon-Lefèvre Syndrome

Papillon-Lefèvre syndrome is characterized by hyperkeratosis palmaris et plantaris, periodontosis, and sparsity of the hair and is reviewed in Chapter 11.

Klippel-Feil Syndrome

Klippel-Feil syndrome consists of a low posterior scalp hairline extending onto the shoulders, with a short neck, limiting movement of the neck and suggestive of webbing. The cervical vertebrae are fused. This syndrome is caused by faulty segmentation of the mesodermal somites between the third and seventh weeks in utero. Strabismus, nystagmus, cleft palate, bifid uvula, and high palate are other features. Ear abnormalities include microtia, external ear canal stenosis, and chronic ear inflammation. Klippel-Feil syndrome occurs mostly in girls.

McKusick Syndrome

Features of McKusick syndrome include short-limbed dwarfism and fine, sparse, hypoplastic, and dysmorphic hair.

GAPO Syndrome

Growth retardation, alopecia, psuedoanondontia, and optic atrophy (GAPO) is a syndrome in which children have a very aged appearance along with alopecia caused by an ANTXR1 mutation.

Atrichia With Papules

This rare autosomal recessive disorder, often seen in patients of south Asian descent, is characterized by loss of hair beginning shortly after birth and the development of cutaneous cystic papules. The cyst epithelium demonstrates keratins 15 and 17, suggesting derivation from the follicular bulge and the presence of stem cells. Vitamin D receptor gene mutations can also present with congenital total alopecia, but the patients have severe vitamin D deficiency so this must be considered in the differential diagnosis. Both the hairless gene and the vitamin D receptor gene produce zinc-finger proteins and may have overlapping functions.

Biggs CM, et al: Diverse autoantibody reactivity in cartilage-hair hypoplasia. J Clin Immunol 2017; 37: 508.

Candamourty R, et al: Trichorhinophalangeal syndrome type 1. J Nat Sci Biol Med 2012; 3: 209.

Casey G, et al: Hereditary vitamin D–resistant rickets presenting as alopecia. Pediatr Dermatol 2014; 31: 519.

Chattopadhyay E, et al: A novel mutation at *ANTXR1* in an Indian patient with growth retardation–alopecia–pseudoanodontia–optic atrophy syndrome. Oral Surg Oral Med Oral Pathol Oral Radiol 2017; 124: e261.

David D, et al: Co-segregation of trichorhinophalangeal syndrome with a t(8;13)(q23.3;q21.31) familial translocation that appears to increase *TRPS1* gene expression. Hum Genet 2013; 132: 1287.

Ettinger M, et al: Skin signs of primary immunodeficiencies—how to find the genes to check. Br J Dermatol 2017 Aug 9; Epub ahead of print.

Lv H, et al: Three mutations of *CYLD* gene in Chinese families with multiple familial trichoepithelioma. Am J Dermatopathol 2014; 36: 605.

Maas S, Shaw A, Bikker H, et al: Trichorhinophalangeal syndrome. 2017 Apr 20. In: Adam MP, Ardinger HH, Pagon RA, et al. [Eds.] GeneReviews® [Internet]. Seattle (WA): University of Washington, Seattle.

Min BJ, et al: An interstitial, apparently-balanced chromosomal insertion in the etiology of Langer-Giedion syndrome in an Asian family. Eur J Med Genet 2013; 56: 561.

Nickles K, et al: Long-term results after treatment of periodontitis in patients with Papillon-Lefèvre syndrome. J Clin Periodontol 2013; 40: 789.

Ong S, et al: Alopecia areata incognita in Cronkhite-Canada syndrome. Br J Dermatol 2017; 177: 531.

Perelygina L, et al: Rubella persistence in epidermal keratinocytes and granuloma M2 macrophages in patients with primary immunodeficiencies. J Allergy Clin Immunol 2016; 138: 1436.

Wang S, et al: Atrichia with papular lesions in a Chinese family caused by novel compound heterozygous mutations and literature review. Dermatology 2013; 226: 68.

Wen XH, et al: Cronkhite-Canada syndrome. World J Gastroenterol 2014; 20: 7518.

KERATOSIS PILARIS

Keratosis pilaris (KP) is a very common, chronic, autosomal dominantly inherited skin condition characterized by small, acuminate, follicular papules with a horny plug in each follicle. Mild KP may be limited to the posterior upper arms. The thighs are the next most common site, but lesions may occur on the cheeks, eyebrows, forearms, buttocks, trunk, and legs. Facial involvement may be mistaken for acne vulgaris and may leave small, pitted scars, even when the condition does not scar elsewhere. Because facial KP is common in prepubertal children it is important to distinguish from acne to avoid unnecessary concern for precocious puberty that would be warranted for true acne in a child under 8. KP may or may not be erythematous. Sometimes the keratotic plugs are the most prominent feature of the eruption, whereas at other times most of the lesions are punctate erythematous papules. Occasionally, inflammatory acneiform pustules and papules may appear. Variants of KP with more prominent scarring are included under the heading of keratosis pilaris atrophicans.

Forcible removal of one of the plugs leaves a minute, cup-shaped depression at the apex of the papule, which is soon filled by new keratotic material. The lesions tend to be arranged in poorly defined groups, dotting the otherwise normal skin in a fairly regular pattern. Fillagrin mutations lead to KP in association with hyperlinear palms and risk for atopic dermatitis.

Other conditions associated with KP are trisomy 21, ichthyosis follicularis, atrichia with papular lesions, mucoepidermal dysplasia, CFC syndrome (KP, curly hair, sparse hair with pulmonary valve stenosis, hypertrophic cardiomyopathy, or atrial septal defect), ectodermal dysplasia with corkscrew hairs, and KID syndrome. KP rubra has prominent erythema and widespread areas of skin involvement, but no atrophy or hyperpigmentation.

Treatment is difficult, but some patients respond to topical retinoids. Often the therapies that improve the keratotic component exacerbate the redness. Ammonium lactate 12% or urea-based moisturizers can produce some smoothing of the lesions but seldom result in improvement of the erythema. Topical calcipotriene is effective in some patients. Pulsed dye laser has been used for the erythema, especially if severe on the face.

ERYTHROMELANOSIS FOLLICULARIS FACIEI ET COLLI

This is characterized by follicular papules along with hyperpigmentation on the lateral cheeks extending to the neck seen mostly in males. The hyperpigmentation and extension to the neck help differentiate and it is most commonly described in patients with type III, IV, and V skin patients. A case has been described with reticulate pigmentation of the extremities.

FOLLICULAR ATROPHODERMA

Follicular atrophoderma consists of follicular indentations without hairs, notably occurring on extensor surfaces of the hands, legs, and arms. Scrotal (fissured) tongue may also be found. It has been described repeatedly in association with other genetically determined abnormalities, including X-linked dominant chondrodysplasia punctata, Bazex syndrome (follicular atrophoderma type), and keratosis palmoplantaris disseminata. Bazex (Bazex-Dupré-Christol) syndrome is characterized by congenital hypotrichosis, follicular atrophoderma, multiple milia, hypohidrosis, and basal cell carcinomas. Both trichorrhexis nodosa and pili bifurcati have been described in patients with the syndrome.

KERATOSIS PILARIS ATROPHICANS

Keratosis pilaris atrophicans presents with keratotic papules that result in atrophy and alopecia. It is seen in three syndromes: keratosis pilaris atrophicans faciei (ulerythema oophrogenes),

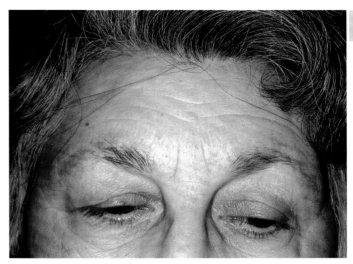

Fig. 27.51 Ulerythema ophryogenes.

atrophoderma vermiculata, and keratosis pilaris follicularis spinulosa decalvans. Keratosis pilaris atrophicans has been reported as being associated with woolly hair and Noonan syndrome. Overlap between the three entities may occur. Keratosis pilaris atrophicans faciei is characterized by persistent erythema and small, horny, follicular papules with onset during childhood on involution there are pitted, atrophic scars that lead to alopecia. The disorder involves the eyebrows, and in some the cheeks, forehead, and even the scalp. The term *ulerythema ophryogenes* is used to describe cases with involvement limited to the lateral third of the eyebrows. Lesions may also begin on the cheeks or temples, rather than the eyebrows. The follicles become reddened (Fig. 27.51), then develop papules, and finally follicular atrophy.

Histologically, follicular hyperkeratosis of the upper third of the hair follicle is seen. A small, depressed scar forms when the lesion heals. It may occur with atopy or woolly hair and may be seen in Noonan syndrome and the CFC syndrome. Transmission is autosomal dominant. Response to therapy is often limited, but some success has been noted with keratolytics and retinoids. Pulsed dye laser therapy has led to improvement in erythema, but not skin roughness.

Ichthyosis Follicularis (Ichthyosis Follicularis, Alopecia, and Photophobia Syndrome)

Ichthyosis follicularis, alopecia, and photophobia (IFAP) is characterized by noncicatricial universal alopecia, severe photophobia, and generalized cutaneous follicular projections that are flesh colored and spiny. There is xerosis of nonspiny skin, and absence of sebaceous glands has been noted histologically. Hepatosplenomegaly, undescended testicles, nail dystrophy, inguinal hernia, short stature, seizures, psychomotor developmental delay, digital anomalies, and ptosis have been reported. Males outnumber females 5:1. The main considerations in the differential diagnosis are KID syndrome and keratosis follicularis spinulosa decalvans (KFSD). Ichthyosis follicularis results from mutations in the *MBTPS2* gene impairing cholesterol homeostasis. Patients can be treated with topical keratolytics and emollients. A partial response to acitretin therapy has been noted in some patients. Intensive lubrication of the ocular surface is essential. Cardiopulmonary complications remain the major cause of death.

Keratosis Follicularis Spinulosa Decalvans (Siemens-1 Syndrome)

In keratosis follicularis spinulosa decalvans (KFSD), keratosis pilaris begins on the face and progresses to involve the scalp, limbs, and trunk. There is hyperkeratosis of the palms and soles. Cicatricial alopecia of the scalp and eyebrows is characteristic. Atopy, photophobia, and corneal abnormalities are frequently associated. Patients are often itchy and recently elevated substance P was found in a patient that may lead to a future therapeutic target. Deafness, physical and mental retardation, recurrent infections, nail abnormalities, acne keloidalis nuchae, tufted hair folliculitis, and aminoaciduria have also been purported associations. The disorder is genetically heterogeneous. The X-linked dominant form is caused by *MBTPS2* mutation that is allelic to IFAP, thus explaining the significant overlap. Autosomal dominant inheritance has also been described.

Al-Saif FM, et al: Erythromelanosis follicularis faciei et colli with reticulated hyperpigmentation of the extremities. Clin Case Rep 2017; 5: 1576.

Alcántara González J, et al: Keratosis pilaris rubra and keratosis pilaris atrophicans faciei treated with pulsed dye laser. J Eur Acad Dermatol Venereol 2011; 25: 710.

Arif T, et al: Erythromelanosis follicularis faciei et colli. Pediatr Dermatol 2017 Nov 21; Epub ahead of print.

Doche I, et al: Substance P in keratosis follicularis spinulosa decalvans. JAAD Case Rep 2015; 1: 327.

Janjua SA, et al: Keratosis follicularis spinulosa decalvans associated with acne keloidalis nuchae and tufted hair folliculitis. Am J Clin Dermatol 2008; 9: 137.

Marqueling AL, et al: Keratosis pilaris rubra. Arch Dermatol 2006; 142: 1611.

Mégarbané H, et al: Ichthyosis follicularis, alopecia, and photophobia (IFAP) syndrome. Orphanet J Rare Dis 2011; 6: 29.

DISORDERS WITH ATROPHODERMA

Atrophodermia Vermiculata

Atrophodermia vermiculata is also known as atrophoderma vermiculata, atrophodermia ulerythematosa, folliculitis ulerythematosa reticulata, and honeycomb atrophy. It is characterized by symmetric involvement of the face by numerous small, closely crowded areas of atrophy separated by narrow ridges, producing a cribriform or honeycomb surface. This worm-eaten (vermiculate) appearance results from atrophy of the follicles and surrounding skin. Each atrophic area is an abrupt, pitlike depression 1–3 mm in diameter. Among the ridges, a few milia may be seen.

The skin covering the ridges is even with the normal skin but contrasts with it by being somewhat waxy, firmer, and apparently stretched. The cause of the disease is undetermined, but familial occurrence has been noted, and it may be associated with other diseases, such as congenital heart block, other cardiac anomalies, neurofibromatosis, oligophrenia, or Down syndrome.

Histologically, the epidermis is slightly atrophic, with diminution in size of the interpapillary projections. In the dermis, the capillaries are dilated, and the vessels have a moderate lymphocytic perivascular infiltration. Follicles may be enlarged, tortuous, dilated, and hyperkeratotic.

Rombo Syndrome

Rombo syndrome is a rare disorder characterized by atrophodermia vermiculata, cyanosis of the hands and feet, milia, telangiectases, hypotrichosis, multiple basal cell carcinomas, and trichoepitheliomas. The associated vermicular atrophoderma produces a coarse, grainy skin texture. Rombo syndrome is inherited in an autosomal dominant manner. It must be distinguished from Bazex syndrome, Rasmussen syndrome (milia, trichoepithelioma, cylindroma), and multiple trichoepitheliomas.

H SYNDROME

The "H syndrome" is an inherited syndrome characterized by hyperpigmentation, hypertrichosis, and indurated patches of skin involving the legs and most specifically inner thighs. Flexion contractures (hallux valgus) occur in over half. Genital masses, lymphadenopathy, and ichthyotic skin changes can also occur. Hearing loss, hypogonadism, hepatosplenomegaly, short height, and heart anomalies are some of the systemic findings. The patients exhibit growth hormone deficiency and hypergonadotropic hypogonadism with azoospermia. Biopsies of involved skin demonstrate acanthosis with dermal and subcutaneous infiltration by histiocytes, plasma cells, and mast cells.

Molho-Pessach V, et al: The H syndrome. J Am Acad Dermatol 2008l; 59: 79.

MELAS SYNDROME

MELAS syndrome (mitochondrial myopathy, encephalopathy, lactic acidosis, strokelike episodes) is a rare neurodegenerative mitochondrial disorder inherited in the maternal line. Diffuse erythema with reticular pigmentation and vitiligo may occur. Caution is required during anesthesia for procedures, because severe acidosis, neurologic deterioration, and cardiorespiratory compromise may occur with a single dose of propofol.

El-Hattab AW, et al: MELAS syndrome. Mol Genet Metab 2015; 116: 4.

Kubota Y, et al: Skin manifestations of a patient with MELAS syndrome. J Am Acad Dermatol 1999; 41: 469.

Potestio CP, et al: Improvement in symptoms of the syndrome of mitochondrial encephalopathy, lactic acidosis, and stroke-like symptoms (MELAS) following treatment with sympathomimetic amines—possible implications for improving fecundity in women of advanced reproductive age. Clin Exp Obstet Gynecol 2014; 41: 343.

28   Dermal and Subcutaneous Tumors

In this chapter proliferations derived from vascular endothelial cells, fibroblasts, myofibroblasts, smooth muscle cells, Schwann cells, and lipocytes are reviewed. Also discussed are several neoplasms of cells invading or aberrantly present in the dermis, such as metastatic cancer, endometriosis, and meningioma.

CUTANEOUS VASCULAR ANOMALIES

Vascular anomalies are overgrowths of various types of blood or lymphatic vessels. They can either occur in isolation or as part of a syndrome caused by a localized or generalized genetic mutation.

The International Society for the Study of Vascular Anomalies (ISSVA) created a classification system that has become the standard way of categorizing vascular lesions (http://www.issva.org/UserFiles/file/Classifications-2014-Final.pdf). Vascular lesions can be divided into vascular tumors that are dynamic and can exhibit rapid growth and malformations that are more static but can still grow. Recently antiproliferative medical therapy such as sirolimus has been found to be effective for some vascular anomalies, indicating that many of the malformations are actually more dynamic than originally thought.

VASCULAR TUMORS

Benign Tumors

Infantile Hemangioma

Infantile hemangiomas (IHs) are the most common benign tumors of childhood, occurring in approximately 4%–5% of children. Importantly, IHs are either not detectable at birth or present with a patch of vasoconstriction called the "premonitory sign," or a slightly bruised or telangiectatic. Many other vascular tumors such as kaposiform hemangioendotheliomas, congenital hemangiomas, fibrosarcomas, and rhabdomyosarcomas can be fully formed tumors at birth, and this can help differentiate them from IH. As the vessels of the IH form, a rim of vasoconstriction can often be seen at the edge even if it was not present from the start.

Risk factors for IH include low birth weight, female gender, multiplets (twin, triplets), prematurity, and maternal age over 30, although low birth weight seems to be the strongest predictor and the other factors may be confounded by the low birth weight associated with them. IH happen in all ethnicities and in all cutaneous locations. The majority of IHs occur sporadically and there is no known genetic predisposition for hemangiomas.

The pathogenesis of IHs is complex and not fully elucidated. CD133+ stem cells within the hemangioma differentiate into mature blood vessels that express GLUT-1, a glucose transporter normally restricted to endothelial cells with blood-tissue barrier function, as in brain and placenta. The vessels proliferate, then involute. Some suggest the stem cells could originate from placental trophoblast. Histologically, IHs are composed of primitive endothelial cells that are similar to placenta. Ultrastructurally, they lack typical Weibel-Palade bodies but do have crystalloid inclusions typical of embryonic endothelium and stain for GLUT-1. They also stain for Fc-γ-RII, Lewis Y antigen (LeY), and merosin. Early hemangiomas show evidence of endothelial progenitor cells that

stain with CD133 and CD34. In late stages, the endothelium flattens, and the lumina are more apparent because of increased blood flow. In time, fibrosis becomes pronounced as involution progresses.

IHs can present anywhere on the body and can be divided based on multiple features. Superficial IHs are easily seen on top of the skin and often have a bright red or maroon look when proliferating (Fig. 28.1). Deep hemangiomas are under the skin and often have a blue hue but are soft. Mixed hemangiomas have features of superficial and deep hemangiomas. Localized hemangiomas are round or oval and have well-defined margins. Segmental or patterned hemangiomas have less distinct borders and appear to grow in embryologic segments. Segmental hemangiomas can be associated with multiple syndromes as outlined later.

IHs go through a characteristic growth pattern with rapid growth occurring most commonly in the first 6 months, although they can grow up to 12 months. The most rapid growth of IH is between 5.5 and 7.5 weeks of life (no matter what the age of gestation) and 90% are finished significantly growing by 4 months, although larger lesions can continue to grow up to a year of life and very rarely longer. Therefore therapy, when needed, is ideally started early in life to prevent the rapid growth that can lead to tissue distortion. IHs then regress and although the majority of the regression happens by age 4 (Fig. 28.2), continued improvement can occur up to and past age 10.

Complications of hemangiomas are related mostly to their location and typically due to physical distortion of the tissue or ulceration. Lesions around the eye can lead to amblyopia or astigmatism and should be co-managed with an ophthalmologist. Nasal tip lesions can lead to permanent distortion of the nasal tissue, collapse of the columella, or obstruction of the nasal passages, impairing breathing and almost always require early therapy to prevent this. Hemangiomas (especially segmental) in the jawline or neck ("beard" distribution) can be associated with airway involvement with IH (Fig. 28.3). These patients present with inspiratory stridor in early infancy, often when there is severe airway occlusion or when there is a superimposed infection leading to airway inflammation. Airway IHs are often misdiagnosed as croup, especially because systemic steroids given for croup will shrink the hemangioma and thus ameliorate the symptoms. A lateral neck x-ray can show airway constriction, but direct visualization by an otorhinolaryngologist is necessary if an airway hemangioma is suspected. Perineal hemangiomas, lip hemangiomas, and those with a large or rapidly growing superficial component are at higher risk for ulceration (Fig. 28.4). Segmental hemangiomas can ulcerate even if there is very little cutaneous component.

The decision to treat a hemangioma is in part based on how completely a hemangioma will regress without therapy. A hemangioma with a very sharp angle at the skin (similar to a mushroom cap) will leave more redundant tissue than a hemangioma with a gentle slope. Central forehead, central cheek, nasal tip, and lip IHs are more likely to leave permanent distortion due to the need for these areas to have more taught skin, and treatment is often necessary to prevent this. The skin may appear normal after involution, but larger and more pedunculated lesions are more likely to leave atrophy, telangiectasia, or anetoderma-type redundancy. If a hemangioma ulcerates, there is invariably a scar.

There is a variant of IH that is present at birth as a flat patch of telangiectasia or vasoconstriction but proliferates very little or not at all. These IHs have been named infantile hemangiomas

587

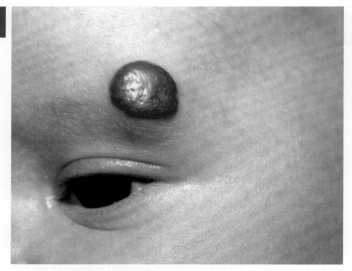

Fig. 28.1 Infantile hemangioma. (Courtesy Steven Binnick, MD.)

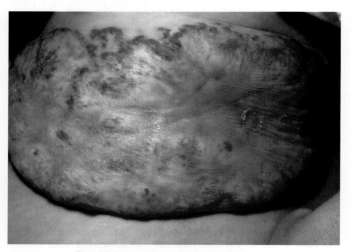

Fig. 28.2 Involuting infantile hemangioma.

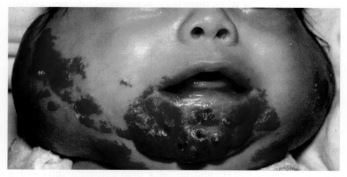

Fig. 28.3 Infantile hemangioma in beard distribution.

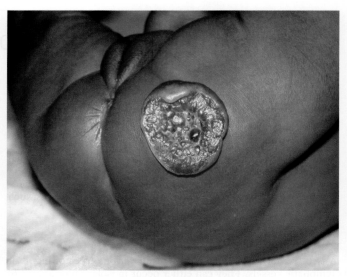

Fig. 28.4 Infantile hemangioma with ulceration.

differentiate from capillary malformations because they also have associated risk of hemangioma syndromes such as PHACE and LUMBAR syndrome (see later in this chapter) depending on location. Therapy for IH-MAG is often not necessary, but the same therapies that work for regular IHs will work for IH-MAG.

Simple observation may be appropriate for many hemangiomas, allowing the lesions to regress spontaneously. Parents should be informed of the appropriate time frame and the pros and cons should be explained. Indications for therapy include ulceration and threatened interference with vital functions (e.g., feeding, vision, respiration, passage of urine or stool). Specifically, there is a risk of occlusion amblyopia, astigmatism, and myopia from periorbital hemangiomas, as well as interference with limb function, tissue destruction, or cardiovascular compromise from high-output cardiac failure. Strong consideration should be given to treatment of hemangiomas that may lead to permanent disfigurement or long-term psychological consequences, such as large hemangiomas of the ear, nose, glabellar area, or lips.

For therapy, β-blockers are used most frequently, but systemic treatment can rarely be complicated by bradycardia or hypoglycemia, and regular feedings are critical before and during treatment. Propranolol is now approved by the U.S. Food and Drug Administration (FDA) for hemangiomas in children over 45 weeks of age (e.g., 40 weeks of normal gestation plus 5 weeks of infancy would equal 45 weeks). Atenolol and other more selective β-blockers have been used in patients who have concerns about propranolol in terms of its risk of bronchoconstriction and sleep disturbances. Propranolol crosses the blood-brain barrier, so some have argued that other β-blockers may have a lower risk of cognitive or behavioral impairment, although long-term studies do not seem to show any learning disabilities in children who have been given propranolol for hemangiomas. Side effects of propranolol include hypotension, bradycardia, and hypoglycemia. Symptoms of hypoglycemia may be masked by the propranolol because it blocks the tachycardia and sweating that often alerts someone to his or her hypoglycemia. It is extremely important that the child has been fed immediately before the propranolol administration to avoid hypoglycemia. If children are vomiting or having diarrhea or not feeding well, the medicine should be held. Protocols for starting propranolol typically involve checking a baseline heart rate and blood pressure and then starting oral propranolol at 1 mg/kg/day divided twice daily at least 10 hours apart (0.5 mg/kg/dose). If the vital signs are normal 1 and 2 hours after starting this dose, it is continued for a week and then the patient is uptitrated

with minimal or arrested growth (IH-MAG) or "abortive" hemangiomas. IH-MAG are manifested by a congenital patch of telangiectatic blood vessels and often the premonitory sign around them. They are GLUT-1 positive and may have small areas of typical hemangioma that show up within the original telangiectatic patch, and they tend to regress in the same time frame as IH but can also ulcerate. IH-MAG are important to recognize and to 2 mg/kg/day divided twice daily. In the same manner and if clinically indicated this can be repeated a week later up to 3 mg/kg/day divided twice daily. Regrowth of treated hemangiomas is frequently seen and seems to be more prominent the sooner the propranolol is stopped. Most authors will treat children until around 12–15 months of age and if there is rebound, the medication can be restarted. There are rarely children who need to stay on propranolol for multiple years and even more rarely children whose hemangiomas regrow somewhat a year or more after stopping the medicine.

Some hemangiomas respond to topical β-blockers. Topical timolol, although off label, is extremely effective for superficial hemangiomas and can help heal ulcerations. The timolol gel-forming solution 0.5% is typically used, but caution is advised in premature infants and ulcerations. Timolol is approximately 10 times more potent per drop than propranolol and some advocate that similar precautions should be taken as for propranolol. Timolol is absorbed especially through the scalp and likely through mucous membranes or ulcerations. One drop is applied to the hemangioma 2 or 3 times per day.

Oral prednisolone at a dose of 2–4 mg/kg/day has also been used for IH but has mostly been replaced by propranolol. In the patients who respond well to treatment, the enlarging hemangioma stops growing in 3–21 days. The prednisolone is continued for 30–90 days. Systemic steroids are still used if propranolol is contraindicated or in conjunction with propranolol in hemangiomas that need to be treated emergently. The use of both medications concomitantly is extremely effective but when tapering the prednisolone, hypoglycemia has been reported. Intralesional corticosteroid treatment has been used but carries some risk of embolization and occlusion of ocular vessels. Injection regularly produces pressures exceeding the systemic arterial pressure, leading to possible embolization. Selective arterial embolization may be necessary for extremely large lesions such as in life-threatening situations.

Treatment with recombinant interferon is not used because of the risk of spastic diplegia. Topical imiquimod, low-frequency ultrasound, and ultrapotent topical steroids have been used historically before the realization of the efficacy of β-blockers. Both neodymium-doped yttrium-aluminum-garnet (Nd:YAG) and potassium titanyl phosphate (KTP) lasers have been used to deliver intralesional therapy.

There are two hemangioma syndromes that are also associated with large segmental hemangiomas of specific locations. Segmental hemangiomas on the head, neck, and proximal upper shoulder/neck areas, especially if over 5 cm in length, can be associated with PHACE syndrome. Larger hemangiomas seem to have higher risk. PHACE denotes the association of posterior fossa brain malformations (primarily the Dandy-Walker malformation), large segmental hemangiomas, arterial anomalies, coarctation of the aorta and other cardiac defects, and eye abnormalities. Most patients do not exhibit all of the features of PHACE. Midline defects of the chest and abdomen such as sternal clefting or complete sternal absence, as well as supraumbilical raphe, can be seen, so an S is sometimes added to the acronym: PHACE(S). The face can be divided into four embryologic segments: S1 is the forehead lateral to the medial canthus including the upper eyelid, S2 is the midcheek, S3 is the jawline, and S4 is a stripe down the central face from forehead to chin. A fifth segment has been recently proposed that involves the ocular orbit because an isolated hemangioma of the orbit can be associated with PHACE. PHACE workup involves evaluating for all of the possible anomalies, therefore the following should be done:

1. An echocardiogram with special attention to the ascending aorta. Cardiac defects described include coarctation, aortic arch abnormalities, aberrant subclavian artery origin, vascular ring (less common), and interrupted or double aortic arch.

2. Magnetic resonance imaging (MRI) of the brain for evaluation of the posterior fossa and including fine cuts of the orbits if there is concern for an orbital hemangioma: posterior fossa abnormalities (Dandy-Walker), hypoplasia of medulla or pons, absent pituitary, or intracranial hemangioma.

3. Evaluation of the cervical and intracerebral blood vessels with MRI/magnetic resonance angiogram (MRA) of the head and neck: abnormal carotid, subclavian, or brachiocephalic arteries.

4. Ophthalmologic evaluation: "morning glory" disc, abnormal or persistent fetal vasculature.

Further imaging of the chest may be needed if the hemangioma extends down, as well as consultation with appropriate subspecialties depending on the findings of the imaging. Evaluate for any associated endocrinologic abnormalities, including hypopituitarism, hypogonadism, hypothyroidism, or growth hormone deficiency. Headaches have been reported at higher levels. Patients should also be followed for normal neurodevelopment.

Propranolol use is debated in PHACE. Some patients with PHACE have had stroke after starting propranolol. Ideally imaging is done before start to rule out significant enough vascular changes that there may be a higher risk of stroke. However, most agree that if the hemangioma is high risk (vision threatening, airway, ulcerating), lower-dose propranolol can be started while starting the process of imaging.

LUMBAR syndrome (also called SACRAL and PELVIS) is the constellation of a large segmental perineal hemangioma with associated spinal dysraphism, renal anomalies, bony anomalies, and gastrointestinal (GI) anomalies. The acronym LUMBAR syndrome has been used to describe the association of lower body hemangioma, urogenital anomalies, myelopathy, bony deformities, anorectal malformations, arterial anomalies, and renal anomalies. In patients with a segmental hemangioma in the perineum, imaging with ultrasound or MRI should be considered to rule out abnormalities of the urogenital or renal systems. Segmental hemangiomas, especially if larger than 5 cm involving the area above the intergluteal cleft (often seen as a part of LUMBAR), are an extremely high-risk marker of spinal cord tethering. Ultrasound may not be sensitive to diagnose some abnormalities, and MRI is recommended in those patients so that any necessary repair can happen before permanent damage.

Children with five or more hemangiomas may have hemangiomas involving internal organs, most commonly the liver. Liver ultrasound is recommended in these patients. The individual lesions are smaller in size ranging from 1–10 mm and there can rarely be hundreds of lesions. Visceral lesions may be present in the central nervous system (CNS), lungs, liver, or other organs, leading to obstructive jaundice, internal bleeding, or respiratory failure. Having a few small lesions in the liver may not have any sequelae and can often be monitored to ensure resolution. More extensive involvement of the liver can lead to shunting of cardiac output leading to high-output failure. Therapy can be rapidly beneficial to improve cardiac function. Hemangiomas secrete type III deiodinase, which is an enzyme that converts active T3 and T4 to reverse T3. If there is a large enough volume of hemangiomas, an infant can become floridly hypothyroid requiring intravenous repletion. Single large hemangiomas in the liver are typically congenital hemangiomas (see later section).

Borok J, et al: Safety and efficacy of topical timolol treatment of infantile haemangioma. Br J Dermatol 2017 Aug 3; Epub ahead of print.

Brosig CL, et al: Neurodevelopmental outcomes in children with PHACE syndrome. Pediatr Dermatol 2016; 33: 415.

Chamlin SL, et al: Multicenter prospective study of ulcerated hemangiomas. J Pediatr 2007; 151: 684.

Garzon MC, et al: PHACE syndrome. J Pediatr 2016; 178: 24.

Hochman M: Infantile hemangiomas. Facial Plast Surg Clin North Am 2014; 22: 509.

Hoff SR, et al: Head and neck vascular lesions. Otolaryngol Clin North Am 2015; 48: 29.

Iacobas I, et al: LUMBAR. J Pediatr 2010; 157: 795.

Kanada KN: A prospective study of cutaneous findings in newborns in the United States. J Pediatr 2012; 161: 240.

McCuaig CC, et al: Therapy of ulcerated hemangiomas. J Cutan Med Surg 2013; 17: 233.

Munden et al: Monitoring propranolol treatment in periocular infantile haemangioma. Eye (Lond) 2014; 28: 1281.

Pope E, et al: Oral versus high-dose pulse corticosteroids for problematic infantile hemangiomas. Pediatrics 2007; 119: e1239.

Püttgen K, et al: Topical timolol maleate treatment of infantile hemangiomas. Pediatrics 2016; 138: e20160355.

Shehata N, et al: Late rebound of infantile hemangioma after cessation of oral propranolol. Pediatr Dermatol 2013; 30: 587.

Yu J, et al: Prevalence and clinical characteristics of headaches in PHACE syndrome. J Child Neurol 2016; 31: 468.

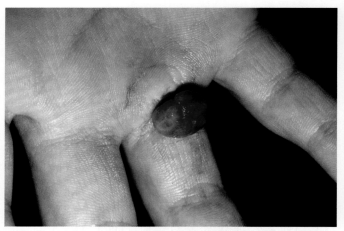

Fig. 28.5 Pyogenic granuloma. (Courtesy Steven Binnick, MD.)

Rapidly Involuting Congenital Hemangioma and Noninvoluting Congenital Hemangioma

Rapidly involuting congenital hemangioma (RICH) and noninvoluting congenital hemangioma (NICH) are rare GLUT-1–negative vascular tumors that present fully grown at birth and either involute rapidly or fail to involute. Activating mutations in *GNA11* and *GNAQ* have been demonstrated in these congenital lesions. Because many lesions only partially involute, some are deemed partially involuting congenital hemangioma (PICH). Children with RICH or NICH and IH have been described, but because IH is so common this is likely coincidence. Clinically most NICH lesions are flatter plaques and most RICH lesions are more raised and nodular. Systemic steroids and propranolol have been tried without success. If therapy is necessary for an ulcerated or bleeding lesion surgery or embolization has been used successfully.

A new type of congenital hemangioma with fetal involution has been proposed. This may be a RICH that involutes partially or entirely before birth. These lesions leave behind atrophy once resolved.

Ayturk UM, et al: Somatic activating mutations in *GNAQ* and *GNA11* are associated with congenital hemangioma. Am J Hum Genet 2016; 98: 789.

Lu H, et al: A rare atypical rapidly involuting congenital hemangioma combined with vascular malformation in the upper limb. World J Surg Oncol 2016; 14: 229.

Maguiness S, et al: Rapidly involuting congenital hemangioma with fetal involution. Pediatr Dermatol 2015; 32: 321.

Sur A, et al: Multiple successful angioembolizations for refractory cardiac failure in a preterm with rapidly involuting congenital hemangioma. AJP Rep 2016; 6: e99.

Pyogenic Granuloma

A pyogenic granuloma is a small, eruptive, usually solitary, sessile or pedunculated, friable papule (Fig. 28.5). The lesion is common in children but may occur at any age, especially during pregnancy or with medication use as described later. Pyogenic granuloma occurs most often on an exposed surface: on the hands, forearms, or face, or at sites of trauma. The lesions can also occur in the mouth, especially on the gingiva, most often in pregnant women (granuloma gravidarum). On the sole of the foot or nail bed, it may be mistaken for a melanoma. Pyogenic granulomas bleed easily on the slightest trauma and, if cut off superficially, promptly recur. Recurring lesions may have one or many satellite lesions.

Pyogenic granulomas may be seen in patients treated with isotretinoin, capecitabine, vemurafenib, or indinavir. Isotretinoin treatment of acne vulgaris can be complicated by numerous exuberant pyogenic granuloma–like lesions of the trunk or periungual lesions. Some data suggest that patients with pyogenic granuloma have a statistically higher prevalence of *Bartonella* seropositivity compared with controls, but a definite etiologic role has not been established.

Histologically, pyogenic granuloma is a lobular capillary hemangioma, with lobules separated by connective tissue septa. With time, the epidermis becomes thinned, then eroded. Heavy secondary staphylococcal colonization is common. Intravascular pyogenic granuloma appears as a lobular capillary proliferation within a vein.

Treatment is by curettage or shave excision, followed by destruction of the base by fulguration or aluminum chloride. Silver nitrate alone may be sufficient to treat smaller lesions but may leave a silver tattoo, and it does not allow histopathologic evaluation to rule out a bleeding amelanotic lesion such as a melanoma. Topical timolol, imiquimod under occlusion, and sclerotherapy with monoethanolamine oleate or sodium tetradecyl sulfate have been used successfully. At times, a recalcitrant lesion may require excision or laser ablation. The drug-induced variety will regress after lowering of the dose or discontinuation of the medication. Systemic corticosteroids have been used to treat recurrent giant pyogenic granulomas.

Samatha Y, et al: Management of oral pyogenic granuloma with sodium tetradecyl sulphate. NY State Dent J 2013; 79: 55.

Sammut SJ, et al: Pyogenic granuloma as a cutaneous adverse effect of vemurafenib. N Engl J Med 2014; 371: 1265.

Locally Aggressive or Borderline Vascular Tumors

These tumors can proliferate more aggressively and show borderline malignant potential.

Hemangioendotheliomas

Hemangioendotheliomas (HEs) are a group of tumors that span the spectrum from benign to low-grade malignancy.

Kaposiform Hemangioendothelioma

Kaposiform hemangioendothelioma (KHE) is an uncommon vascular tumor that affects infants and young children. Rare cases have been reported in adults. It was first designated KHE in 1993. Although it frequently occurs in the retroperitoneum, KHE may

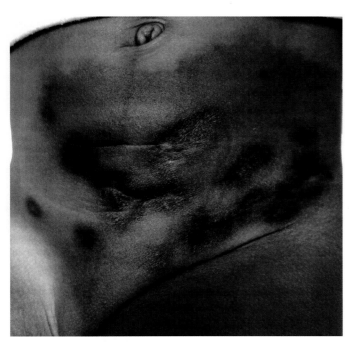

Fig. 28.6 Kaposiform hemangioendothelioma.

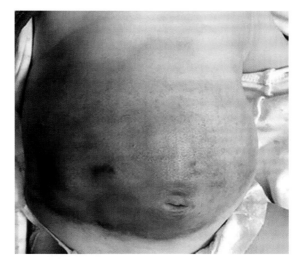

Fig. 28.7 Kasabach-Merritt syndrome.

present as multinodular soft tissue masses, purpuric macules, plaques, and multiple telangiectatic papules (Fig. 28.6). The lesions extend locally and usually involve the skin, soft tissues, and even bone. The cutaneous variant may be associated with lymphangiomatosis. KHE is locally aggressive and may be complicated by platelet trapping and consumptive coagulopathy (Kasabach-Merritt syndrome), but distant metastases have not yet been reported. It has also been reported in association with Milroy-Nonne disease (primary hereditary lymphedema).

Histologically, there are combined features of cellular IH and Kaposi sarcoma. Additionally, in some tumors, lymphangiomatosis is seen sharply separated from the vascular lesion. There is a multilobular appearance that closely resembles that of tufted angioma, but in KHE, lesions are larger and less circumscribed and involve the deep soft tissue and even bone. Transition between these tumors has been described.

The prognosis depends on the depth and location of the lesion. Significant morbidity and mortality may result from compression and invasion of surrounding structures. If localized to the skin, lesions may be successfully excised. However, because of their tendency for deep and infiltrative growth, this is usually not possible. Combination of systemic corticosteroids and vincristine is often used but is being replaced by rapamycin (sirolimus).

Kasabach-Merritt Syndrome

In Kasabach-Merritt syndrome (KMS) there is platelet trapping within the vascular tumor and this leads to activation of the clotting cascade and disseminated intravascular coagulation (DIC). Low-grade KMS can be happening subtly but can worsen rapidly with acute, extreme swelling and purple discoloration to the lesion and this can be life threatening. The fibrinogen and platelet counts are low, the activated partial thromboplastin time and prothrombin time will be prolonged, and the D-dimer is elevated, indicating DIC. Before the onset of the acute event, the infant will often have a reddish or bluish plaque or tumor on the limb or trunk or, in rare instances, no visible lesion at all. The lesions usually have an associated lymphatic component, and most are KHEs. KMS also occurs in tufted angiomas and multifocal lymphangioendotheliomatosis, lesions that both demonstrate lymphatic differentiation.

Venolymphatic and lymphatic malformations can also cause platelet trapping with resultant DIC. KMS is rarely reported with angiosarcoma. Some patients with VMs will have a chronic low-grade consumptive coagulopathy that occurs throughout life, and RICH lesions can trap platelets but not induce KMS; these should not be confused with KMS. The original reports of KMS occurring in IHs are incorrect.

Infants with KMS suddenly develop a painful violaceous mass in association with purpura and thrombocytopenia (Fig. 28.7). The most striking sign is the bleeding tendency, especially in the hemangioma itself or into the chest or abdominal cavities. The spleen may be enlarged. Hemoglobin, platelets, fibrinogen, and factors II, V, and VIII are all reduced. Prothrombin time and partial thromboplastin time are prolonged, and fibrin split products may be elevated. Cases of microangiopathic hemolytic anemia have also been described. Repeated episodes of bleeding may occur, and although these may be spontaneous, bleeding can be precipitated by surgery, directed either at the hemangioma or elsewhere. The mortality rate may be as high as 30%, with most deaths secondary to bleeding complications.

KMS may be a self-limited disorder but often requires therapy. Systemic corticosteroids seem to work quickly, but often maintenance therapy is needed to prevent recurrence. Sirolimus has also become a favored therapy due to its efficacy and rapid benefit. Low-dose aspirin (5–10 mg/kg/day) can be used to decrease the platelet trapping and seems to help prevent KMS in some patients. This is a reasonable maintenance plan, but in children, care must be taken to avoid concomitant vaccination with live vaccines (especially influenza and varicella) and stopping aspirin if either primary infection is suspected to avoid Reye syndrome. Some have argued that the dose of aspirin is lower than the threshold to cause Reye syndrome. Adding ticlopidine may provide more benefit.

Historically, interferon (IFN) alfa-2a, vincristine, vinblastine, cyclophosphamide, actinomycin D, embolization, ε-aminocaproic acid, antiplatelet agents, irradiation, excision, and compression therapy have been used, alone or in combination.

Drolet BA, et al: Consensus-derived practice standards plan for complicated kaposiform hemangioendothelioma. J Pediatr 2013; 163: 285.

Margolin JF, et al: Medical therapy for pediatric vascular anomalies. Semin Plast Surg 2014; 28: 79.

O'Rafferty C, et al: Recent advances in the pathobiology and management of Kasabach-Merritt phenomenon. Br J Hameatol 2015; 171: 38.

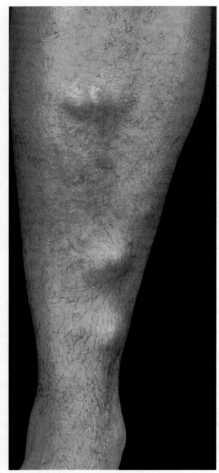

Fig. 28.8 Spindle cell hemangioendotheliomas (spindle cell hemangiomas). (Courtesy Dr. Timothy Gardner.)

Spindle Cell Hemangioma (Spindle Cell Hemangioendothelioma)

Spindle cell hemangioma is a vascular tumor that typically presents in a child or young adult with blue nodules of firm consistency on a distal extremity (Fig. 28.8). Usually, multifocal lesions occur within an anatomic region. Histologically, a well-circumscribed dermal nodule will contain dilated vascular spaces with fascicles of spindle cells between them. Areas of the tumor will have an open alveolar pattern resembling hemorrhagic lung tissue. Phleboliths are common. A thrombosed, large, adjacent vessel with recanalization may be identified. The lesions appear to represent benign vascular proliferations in response to trauma to a larger vessel. They may recur after excision.

Epithelioid Hemangioendothelioma

Epithelioid hemangioendothelioma usually presents as a solitary, slow-growing papule or nodule on a distal area of an extremity and behaves as a low-grade malignancy (Fig. 28.9). There is a male preponderance, and onset is frequently before the individual is 25 years of age. Histologically, there are two components: dilated vascular channels and solid epithelioid and spindle-cell elements with intracytoplasmic lumina. It is caused by a fusion of *WWTR1-CAMTA1*; therefore *CAMTA1* nuclear expression can differentiate it from other tumors. Wide excision is recommended with evaluation of regional lymph nodes, which are the usual site of metastases.

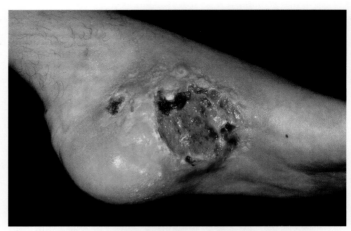

Fig. 28.9 Large, ulcerated epithelioid hemangioendothelioma.

In the minority of cases in which distant metastatic lesions develop, chemotherapy, radiation, or both may be employed.

Retiform Hemangioendothelioma

Retiform hemangioendothelioma is another form of low-grade malignancy that presents as a slow-growing exophytic mass, dermal plaque, or subcutaneous nodule on the upper or lower extremities of young adults. Histologically, there are arborizing blood vessels reminiscent of normal rete testis architecture. Human herpesvirus 8 (HHV-8) deoxyribonucleic acid (DNA) sequences have been reported in this tumor. Wide excision is recommended, although local recurrences are common. To date, no widespread metastases have occurred, although regional lymph nodes may develop tumor infiltrates.

Epithelioid Sarcoma–Like (Pseudomyogenic) Hemangioendothelioma

The epithelioid sarcoma–like variant demonstrates sheets of spindle, epithelioid, and rhabdomyoblastic cells. They can occur on the palms or soles and mimic a recalcitrant wart. This variant also behaves as a low-grade malignancy.

Endovascular Papillary Angioendothelioma (Dabska Tumor)

Endovascular papillary angioendothelioma, a rare low-grade angiosarcoma, presents as a slow-growing tumor on the head, neck, or extremity of infants or young children. It shows multiple vascular channels with papillary plugs of endothelial cells surrounding central, hyalinized cores that project into the lumina, sometimes forming a glomeruloid pattern. The entity is controversial; similar histologic features have been observed in other vascular tumors, such as angiosarcoma, retiform hemangioendothelioma, and glomeruloid hemangioma. The tumor may be a distinct entity or may demonstrate a histologic pattern seen in other vascular tumors. Wide excision and excision of the regional lymph nodes, when involved, are usually curative.

Doyle LA, et al: Nuclear expression of CAMTA1 distinguishes epithelioid hemangioendothelioma from histologic mimics. Am J Surg Pathol 2016; 40: 94.

Flucke U, et al: Epithelioid hemangioendothelioma. Diagn Pathol 2014; 9: 131.

Liau JY, et al: Composite hemangioendothelioma presenting as a scalp nodule with alopecia. J Am Acad Dermatol 2013; 69: e98.

McNab PM, et al: Composite hemangioendothelioma and its classification as a low-grade malignancy. Am J Dermatopathol 2013; 35: 517.
Requena L, et al: Cutaneous epithelioid sarcomalike (pseudomyogenic) hemangioendothelioma. JAMA Dermatol 2013; 149: 459.

Tufted Angioma (Angioblastoma)

The tufted angioma lesion usually develops in infancy or early childhood on the neck and upper trunk. Adult onset has also been described. The lesions present as poorly defined, dull-red plaques with a mottled appearance, varying from 2–5 cm in diameter. Some show clusters of smaller angiomatous papules superimposed on the main macular area (Fig. 28.10), and associated hypertrichosis has been noted. The lesions are usually sporadic, although familial cases have been reported. Histologic examination reveals small, circumscribed angiomatous tufts and lobules scattered in the dermis in a so-called cannonball pattern. Tumors with features of both tufted angioma and KHE have been described, and transformation between the tumors has also been noted. Immunostaining can be helpful in distinguishing these tumors. Tufted angioma is characterized by a proliferation of CD34+ endothelial cells with few actin-positive cells. KHE shows CD34 staining only in the luminal endothelial cells. In IH, GLUT-1 is positive.

Most lesions slowly extend with time, being progressive but benign in nature. Occasional spontaneous regression is documented. Therapy is dependent on the activity of the lesion. For small flat lesions aspirin may be enough but should be used with caution at low doses and stopped around the time of live vaccines such as varicella in young children to avoid Reye syndrome. For larger, growing lesions, especially with Kasabach-Merritt phenomenon, systemic steroids are rapidly effective. Vincristine is classically used, but sirolimus has proven to be very effective. Aspirin may then be used to maintain benefit more long-term. Treatment with pulsed dye laser, intense pulsed light, excision, and radiation has been successful. Lesions associated with KMS have also been treated with embolization, prednisone, and vincristine.

The term *angioblastoma* has also been used for a rare pediatric tumor often associated with destruction of regional structures,

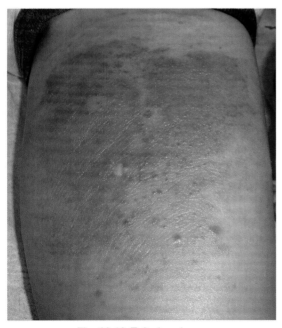

Fig. 28.10 Tufted angioma.

including bone. Basic fibroblast growth factor has been reported to be elevated, and some patients have responded to treatment with IFN alfa-2b.

Adams DM, et al: Efficacy and safety of sirolimus in the treatment of complicated vascular anomalies. Pediatrics 2016; 137: e20153257.
Fahrtash F, et al: Successful treatment of kaposiform hemangioendothelioma and tufted angioma with vincristine. J Pediatr Hematol Oncol 2010; 32: 506.
Javvaji S, et al: Response of tufted angiomas to low-dose aspirin. Pediatr Dermatol 2013; 30: 124.
Sabharwal A, et al: Acquired tufted angioma of upper lip. Head Neck Pathol 2013; 7: 291.
Wang L, et al: Congenital disseminated tufted angioma. J Cutan Pathol 2013; 40: 405.
Yamamoto Y, et al: Successful treatment of tufted angioma with propranolol. J Dermatol 2014; 41: 1120.

Hemangiopericytoma

True hemangiopericytomas are rare. The term is now reserved for lesions that demonstrate differentiation toward pericytes and cannot be otherwise classified. Most lesions formerly classified as hemangiopericytoma are now classified as solitary fibrous tumor or giant cell angiofibroma. Remaining lesions can often be classified as glomangiopericytoma/myopericytoma or infantile myofibromatosis.

Clinically, hemangiopericytomas are nontender, bluish red tumors that occur on the skin or in the subcutaneous tissues on any part of the body. The firm, usually solitary nodule may be up to 10 cm in diameter. Histologically, the tumor is composed of endothelium-lined vessels that are filled with blood and surrounded by cells with oval or spindle-shaped nuclei (pericytes). The pericytes often form a concentric perivascular pattern. Staghorn-like ectatic spaces are often encountered. Wide local excision is the treatment of choice, but radiation therapy may produce excellent palliation.

Lesions Formerly Classified as Hemangiopericytomas

Various soft tissue tumors can present with a hemangiopericytoma-like staghorn vascular pattern, the most common being solitary fibrous tumor. Solitary fibrous tumor is usually CD34+ and has a wide distribution in the skin, mucosa, and viscera. When excision cannot be accomplished, targeted therapy, including imatinib, may be helpful. Myofibromas demonstrate nodular, pale-blue, hypocellular zones with surrounding hypercellular zones that contain staghorn vessels. Some examples lack the hypocellular zones and present only with a hemangiopericytoma-like pattern. Myopericytoma is a rare mesenchymal neoplasm that typically involves the extremities. The tumor demonstrates concentric perivascular spindle cells with myoid differentiation. Glomangiopericytoma is a closely related tumor composed of perivascular spindle cells with myoid differentiation; it combines features of glomus tumors and a hemangiopericytoma-like vascular pattern.

Stacchiotti S, et al: Targeted therapies in rare sarcomas. Hematol Oncol Clin North Am 2013; 27: 1049.
Watanabe K, et al: CD34-negative solitary fibrous tumour resistant to imatinib. BMJ Case Rep 2013 Jul 5; 2013.

Other Vascular Tumors

Cherry Angiomas (Senile Angiomas, de Morgan Spots)

These round, slightly elevated, ruby-red papules 0.5–6 mm in diameter are the most common vascular anomalies. It is a rare

30-year-old person who does not have a few, and the number increases with age. Probably every 70-year-old person has some senile angiomas. Most are on the trunk; they are rarely seen on the hands, feet, or face. Early lesions may mimic petechiae. When lesions are surrounded by a purpuric halo, amyloidosis should be suspected. Eruptive lesions have been described after nitrogen mustard therapy. Light electrodesiccation or laser ablation with intense pulsed light and long-pulse Nd:YAG laser systems can be effective. Shave excision can also be performed, but most patients accept reassurance and do not request removal.

Fodor L, et al: A side-by-side prospective study of intense pulsed light and Nd:YAG laser treatment for vascular lesions. Ann Plast Surg 2006; 56: 164.
Ma HJ, et al: Eruptive cherry angiomas associated with vitiligo. J Dermatol 2006; 33: 877.

Targetoid Hemosiderotic Hemangioma

In 1988 Santa Cruz and Aronberg described a lesion characterized by a central brown or violaceous papule surrounded by an ecchymotic halo (Fig. 28.11). The term *hobnail hemangioma* has been proposed because many lesions are not targetoid. These acquired hemangiomas occur in young to middle-aged individuals and are present on the trunk or extremities. Because of their dark purple/black color they clinically simulate melanoma. The color likely represents trauma to a preexisting vascular lesion, with thrombosis and subsequent recanalization. Histologically, a biphasic growth pattern is seen, with central, superficial, dilated vascular structures lined by prominent hobnail endothelial cells, and collagen-dissecting, narrow vessels in deeper parts of the lesion. The endothelial cells commonly stain for CD31, but not CD34. D2-40 staining suggests lymphangiomatous proliferation.

Gutte RM, Joshi A: Targetoid hemosiderotic hemangioma. Indian Dermatol Online J 2014; 5: 559.

Glomeruloid Hemangioma

Glomeruloid hemangioma is a distinctive benign vascular neoplasm first described in 1990 and reported in patients with POEMS (Crow-Fukase) syndrome and Castleman disease. Some have also been associated with idiopathic thrombocytopenic purpura and Sjögren syndrome. Similar lesions have been reported in patients who are otherwise healthy.

The POEMS syndrome consists of polyneuropathy (severe sensorimotor), organomegaly (heart, spleen, kidneys), endocrinopathy,

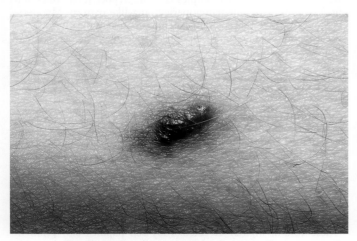

Fig. 28.11 Targetoid hemosiderotic hemangioma.

M component (M protein, monoclonal gammopathy), and skin changes (hyperpigmentation, hypertrichosis, thickening, sweating, clubbed nails, leukonychia, angiomas). Small, firm, red to violaceous papules appear on the trunk and proximal extremities in approximately one third of patients. Histologically, the lesions may be microvenular hemangiomas, cherry angiomas, multinucleated cell angiohistiocytomas, or glomeruloid hemangiomas. The latter consist of ectatic vascular structures containing aggregates of capillary loops within a dilated lumen, simulating the appearance of a renal glomerulus. Sequestered degenerating red blood cells are a characteristic finding. Two types of endothelial cell have been noted within the lesions: a capillary-type endothelium with large vesicular nuclei, open chromatin pattern, and a large amount of cytoplasm; and sinusoidal endothelium with small basal nuclei, dense chromatin, and scant cytoplasm. Lesions associated with POEMS syndrome demonstrate increased expression of vascular endothelial growth factor (VEGF) and its receptor, Flt-1.

Jacobson-Dunlop E, et al: Glomeruloid hemangiomas in the absence of POEMS syndrome. J Cutan Pathol 2012; 39: 402.

Eccrine Angiomatous Hamartoma

Eccrine angiomatous hamartoma usually appears as a solitary nodular lesion on the acral areas of the extremities, particularly the palms and soles, but identical lesions also occur on areas of the body that normally have few eccrine glands. This lesion appears at birth or in early childhood and is often associated with pain and hyperhidrosis. The lesion is a dome-shaped, tender, bluish nodule. Hypertrichosis may be present. When it is stroked or pinched, drops or beaded rings of perspiration may be seen.

Histologically, there is a combination of lobules of mature eccrine glands and ducts with thin-walled blood vessels. Excessive mucin, fat, smooth muscle, nerve infiltration, and terminal hairs may be present. The lesion has been associated with spindle cell hemangioma, arteriovenous malformation (AVM), and verrucous hemangioma. Excision may be necessary because of pain.

Halder C, et al: Eccrine angiomatous hamartoma. Indian J Dermatol 2014; 59: 403.
Shin J, et al: Eccrine angiomatous hamartoma. Ann Dermatol 2013; 25: 208.

Vascular Malformations

Malformations are abnormal structures that result from an aberration in embryonic development or trauma. The abnormality may be caused by an anatomic malformation or a functional alteration (as in nevus anemicus). Anatomic malformations are subdivided according to the type of vessel involved: capillary, venous, arterial, lymphatic, or combined. The term *capillary malformation* is best used as a term encompassing a variety of entities, including salmon patch, certain telangiectasias, port wine stains (PWSs), and cutis marmorata telangiectatica congenita. The characteristics of capillary malformations help differentiate various syndromes.

Happle R: What is a capillary malformation? J Am Acad Dermatol 2008; 59: 1077.
Lee MS, et al: Diffuse capillary malformation with overgrowth. J Am Acad Dermatol 2013; 69: 589.

Capillary Malformations

There are multiple different forms of capillary malformations (CMs), and each type can be seen in isolation or in association with a syndrome. CMs notably develop eczematous changes more easily over the top and will become darker red or purple with Valsalva maneuver or temperature changes. Differentiating the type of CM can help with diagnosis of the specific syndrome. Each of the different types of CM will be described and then the vascular syndromes that can present with CM will be discussed. Histologically, PWSs are made of dilated capillaries in the subpapillary network. Laser therapy has been used with satisfactory results, but a number of treatments are required, and recurrence years later usually requires some retreatment. The flashlamp pulsed dye 585- or 595-nm laser has the best record of safety and efficacy. Pulse durations are adjusted based on the size of the blood vessel and response to therapy. For darker-skinned patients, multiple pulse stacking with multiple cryogen spurts provides better epidermal protection. Long-pulse pulsed alexandrite lasers work best for hypertrophic, purple lesions, whereas pulsed dye lasers work best for flat, pink lesions. A frequency-doubled (532-nm) Nd:YAG laser that allows for shorter pulse widths, large spot sizes, and high fluences resulted in up to 75% improvement in color at 1 month after a single treatment. Topical sirolimus added to standard pulsed dye laser may augment therapy. The CMs associated with capillary malformation–arteriovenous malformation (CM-AVM) may have arterial flow and therefore laser may exacerbate them.

Nevus Simplex

Nevus simplex is a type of CM that is light pink, is easily blanchable, often has a splattered appearance, is located in characteristic locations along the neural axis, and tends to fade over time. There have been many names used historically, including nevus flammeus and PWSs, but the nomenclature has been clarified by Frieden et al. recently. Nevus simplex malformations are common birthmarks in children, occurring in approximately 80% of children. They may persist in at least 5% of the population. Colloquial terms are used for certain types: "stork bite" is a pink-red macule situated on the posterior midline between the occipital protuberance and the tip of the spine of the fifth cervical vertebra (Fig. 28.12); "angel's kiss" is located on the glabella. Other typical locations are upper eyelid (15% of babies), along the nasal philtrum and ala, the temples, vertex scalp, upper back, and along the lumbar spine. Lesions in the lumbar area in isolation are typically not associated with spinal dysraphism but in association with other features can be a marker and necessitate imaging. Frieden proposed the term *nevus simplex complex* when children have very widespread lesions. Nevus simplex malformations tend to fade over time and are only rarely associated with syndromes (reviewed later in

chapter): Beckwith-Wiedemann, Roberts SC, Nova, odontodysplasia, or megalencephaly CM syndrome.

Port Wine Stains

Port wine stains (PWSs) occur in an estimated 3 per 1000 children. The stains are present at birth and vary in color from pink to dark or bluish red. The lesions are usually unilateral, and although the face and neck are common locations (Fig. 28.13), they can be located anywhere on the skin and may be widespread and involve as much as half the body. With facial lesions, the mucous membrane of the mouth may be involved. Although the surface of a PWS is usually smooth, small vascular nodular outgrowths or warty excrescences may develop over decades thus justifying early preventive intervention. These lesions often become more bluish or purple with age.

Rarely, PWS may appear as an acquired condition, usually with onset after trauma. The early inflammatory stage of morphea can also start with a purple patch that is mistaken for a PWS.

Reticulated Port Wine Stains

Reticulated PWSs are faint red-pink patches that have indistinct borders but often accentuate dramatically with Valsalva maneuver or temperature changes. They tend to be widespread and can be mistaken for cutis marmorata telangiectatica congenita (CMTC) (both lesions can occur in the same patient). Therefore some of the previous association between CMTC and systemic findings are likely mislabeled. Reticulated PWSs have been associated with various syndromes, including diffuse CM with overgrowth and some patients with PiK3Ca-related overgrowth syndromes (PROS), especially those with the megalencephaly capillary malformation (MCAP) phenotype.

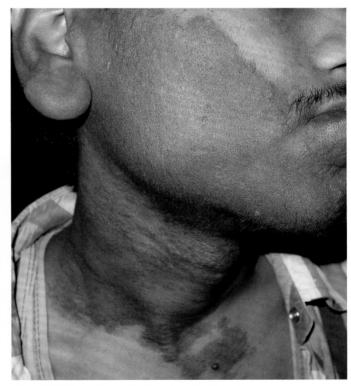

Fig. 28.13 Port wine stain. (Courtesy Dr. Debarbrata Bandyopadhyay.)

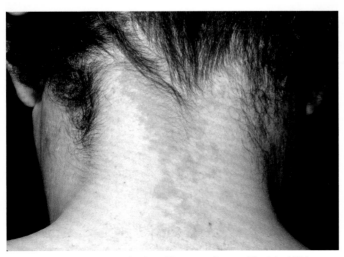

Fig. 28.12 Nevus simplex. (Courtesy Steven Binnick, MD.)

Geometric Port Wine Stain

PWS can sometimes be dark purple and geometric with a sharp distinct cutoff. This CM phenotype is more associated with underlying venous or venolymphatic malformations such as can be seen in the following syndromes: Proteus syndrome; Klipell-Trenaunay syndrome; congenital lipomatous overgrowth with vascular anomalies, epidermal nevi, and skeletal, scoliosis, and spinal abnormalities (CLOVES) syndrome; and CLAPO syndrome. The geometric CM can have vascular and keratotic vascular papules within it.

Cutis Marmorata Telangiectatica Congenita

Cutis marmorata telangiectatica congenita (CMTC) has been recategorized as a type of capillary malformation. CMTC is characterized by the presence of a red-purple, livedo-appearing, reticulated, vascular network with a segmental distribution, usually involving the extremities (Fig. 28.14). The mottling is pronounced and is made more distinct by crying, vigorous activity, and cold. There is often associated atrophy giving a "pseudoathletic" look that outlines the muscles. CMTC can be difficult to differentiate from a reticulated PWS, but typically CMTC has more uniformity and is more netlike. Lesions tend toward improvement with time but may not fully resolve. If located around the eye, some have advocated for ophthalmologic evaluation. The condition occurs sporadically, and there is a female preponderance. CMTC can be associated with phakomatosis pigmentovascularis and the Adams-Oliver syndrome (limb abnormalities, scalp defects, skull ossification defects).

SYNDROMES ASSOCIATED WITH CAPILLARY MALFORMATIONS

Sturge-Weber Syndrome

PWS on the upper face may be a marker for Sturge-Weber syndrome (SWS; encephalotrigeminal angiomatosis) (Fig. 28.15). There is debate as to what pattern these PWSs are following and what locations portend the highest risk. Originally PWSs were described as following nerve distributions (V1, V2, etc.), but more recently it has been proposed that they actually follow similar embryologic segments to hemangiomas (S1, S2, etc.). With either delineation, it seems that the involvement of the forehead and the more of the face involved (as long as the PWS includes some part of the V1/S1 distribution) is the highest risk. Therefore a PWS that covers the forehead, upper cheek, and lower cheek has a higher risk than a PWS that covers only the forehead. The leptomeningeal component of SWS is present in only 10% of patients with all or most of one V1 branch of the trigeminal nerve involved. If bilateral V1 or V1/V2/V3 are involved the rate of SWS is significantly higher. Leptomeningeal angiomatosis may clinically manifest as epilepsy, mental retardation, hemiplegia, hemisensory defects, and homonymous hemianopsia. Characteristic calcifications are present in the outer layers of the cerebral cortex; these consist of double-contoured "tram tracks" that follow the brain convolutions. The most important initial evaluation of an infant with a PWS that involves the eyelid is by an ophthalmologist to rule out congenital glaucoma because this can be vision threatening. Ocular abnormalities, such as glaucoma, buphthalmos (infantile glaucoma, related to abnormal development of angle formed by cornea and iris), retinal detachment, and blindness can occur in SWS. These may be present without leptomeningeal involvement.

SWS results from the persistence of the primitive embryonal vascular plexus that develops during the sixth fetal week around the cephalic neural tube and in the region destined to become facial skin. Normally, the plexus regresses during the ninth week, but in SWS it persists. Mutations in *GNAQ* and *GNA11* have been implicated, although it is unclear if the mutation alone is sufficient to cause SWS.

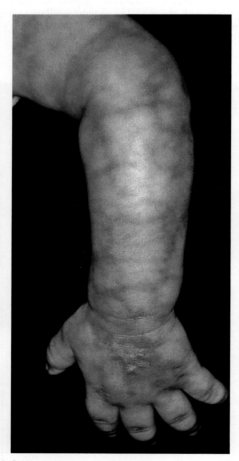

Fig. 28.14 Cutis marmorata telangiectatica congenitale. (Courtesy Brooke Army Medical Center Teaching File.)

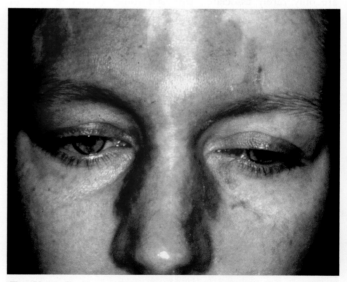

Fig. 28.15 Capillary malformation (port wine stain) with Sturge-Weber syndrome.

Because the risk of SWS is fairly low even with a PWS on the forehead, historically not all infants underwent imaging because the management did not necessarily change. It has now been demonstrated that early institution of aspirin may help prevent seizures, cognitive delays, and hemiparesis. Therefore early imaging to rule out SWS is warranted in patients who have a significant risk to be able to know whom to offer aspirin. Although calcifications are the most notable CNS finding and can be seen on computed tomography (CT) scan, they can develop later, so an MRI is the most sensitive test in infancy.

PiK3CA-Related Overgrowth Syndromes (PROS)

Mutations in *PIK3CA* cause multiple different syndromes with varied findings of CM with overgrowth. Depending on which mutation occurs and how much tissue is involved (due to mosaicism) patients can have various phenotypes: MCAP or CLOVES syndrome. Collectively, because there is some overlap, these (along with fibroadipose hyperplasia and hemimegalencephaly) are collectively known as *PIK3CA*-related overgrowth syndromes (PROS). Klippel-Trenaunay syndrome and KTS–Parkes-Weber syndrome are also caused by postzygotic mutations in *PiK3CA*. *PIK3CA* mutations have also recently been found in patients with CLAPO syndrome characterized by a CM of the lower lip and asymmetric overgrowth and head/neck lymphatic malformation.

Megalencephaly Capillary Malformation

MCAP was originally called M-CMTC and therefore CMTC was historically incorrectly associated with multiple congenital anomalies. The cutaneous lesions in MCAP are actually reticulated PWS (as described earlier) and not CMTC. Other features are an upper lip/nasal philtrum PWS, megalencephaly, a sandal toe deformity with 2-3 syndactyly of the toes, polymicrogyrisa, and skin elasticity. Patients should be followed for signs of hydrocephalus, and brain MRI is recommended. Renal ultrasound every 3 months until age 8 to rule out Wilms tumor has also been recommended.

CLOVES

The lipomatous overgrowth in CLOVES is typically very prominent at birth. Affected patients also often have large venous or venolymphatic malformations, as well as AVMs that can involved the skin but also importantly the CNS. Epidermal nevi can be localized or widespread. There is usually significant overgrowth of hands and/or feet. Patients can have spinal cord tethering in addition to renal agenesis. Patients require multidisciplinary care, including neurosurgery and orthopedic surgery and other specialties depending on their symptoms. Imaging to establish the presence of CNS vascular lesions or other anomalies helps guide therapy. Recently systemic rapamycin has been shown to be helpful in shrinking complicated vascular anomalies, including lymphatic malformations.

Klippel-Trenaunay Syndrome (KTS) and KTS–Parkes-Weber

Klippel-Trenaunay syndrome (KTS) is characterized as a triad of nevus flammeus, venous and lymphatic malformations, and soft tissue hypertrophy of the affected extremity (Fig. 28.16). The lower limb is affected in approximately 95% of patients. When there is an associated arteriovenous (AV) fistula, Parkes-Weber is appended to the diagnosis.

The earliest and most common presenting sign is a geometric CM. The deeper venous malformation (VM) in this sporadic syndrome may be confined to the skin, but it often extends to muscle and bone. The involved limb is usually larger and longer

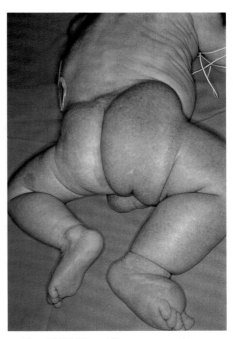

Fig. 28.16 Klippel-Trenaunay syndrome.

than normal. Venous thromboembolism has been reported, with an incidence as high as 22%. In other patients, the deep venous system is hypoplastic. Other, less frequent features include intermittent claudication, venous ulcers, increased skin temperature, diffuse hair loss, hypertrichosis, lymphedema, altered sweating, lacrimation, or salivation. Gait abnormalities are common. Intradural spinal cord AVMs, epidural hemangioma, and epidural angiomyolipoma have been reported to occur at the same segmental level as cutaneous lesions of KTS. Clinical evaluation consists of color duplex ultrasonography to evaluate the patency of the deep venous system, MRI for visualization of hypertrophic muscle and bone, arteriography when an AV fistula is suspected, and conventional radiography of both extremities. Early venography may be performed, if the deep venous system is not hypoplastic, to determine whether there are defects that might be amenable to surgical correction. When AV shunting is found the term *KTS–Parkes-Weber* is used.

Flashlamp-pumped pulsed dye laser treatments may be used for the nevus flammeus component. The varicosities and malformations may respond to microfoam sclerosis, endovenous thermal ablation, or surgical stripping. Edema is managed through elevation, graded compression pumps, fitted garments, and diuretics. Surgery may be performed to correct the inequality in limb length, to relieve deep venous obstruction, or to correct an associated AV fistula. Skin ulcers have responded to sunitinib. The Klippel-Trenaunay Support Group website can be found at www.k-t.org.

Diffuse Capillary Malformation with Overgrowth

Diffuse capillary malformation with overgrowth is a clinical phenotype proposed to describe patients with widespread PWS (often reticulated) with some usually nondebilitating proportionate overgrowth. Patients had normal neurologic function but require orthopedic follow-up for limb discrepancies.

Capillary Malformation–Arteriovenous Malformation

CM-AVM syndrome is an autosomal dominant disorder caused by heterozygous *RASA1* mutations and resulting in multifocal

CMs and high risk for fast-flow lesions. The CMs in CM-AVM may have arterial flow. Affected individuals have widespread "thumbprint" or café au lait–like oval CMs but can also have AVMs in the brain and spine. Therefore imaging of the brain and complete spine to rule out AVMs is recommended. Cobb syndrome (cutaneous meningospinal angiomatosis) is characterized by a port wine hemangioma or other vascular malformation in a dermatome supplied by a segment of the spinal cord containing a VM or AVM and may also be from *RASA1* mutations.

Capillary Malformation–Arteriovenous Malformation 2

CM-AVM2 is a newly described similar phenotype caused by *EPHRIN B4* mutation but an apparently lower risk of CNS AVMs.

Microcephaly Capillary Malformation Syndrome

Microcephaly capillary malformation syndrome is characterized by microcephaly with seizures and severe developmental delay, along with similar small discrete CMs as are seen in CM-AVM.

Proteus Syndrome

Proteus syndrome is characterized by vascular malformations that include nevus flammeus, hemihypertrophy, macrodactyly, verrucous epidermal nevus, soft tissue subcutaneous masses, and cerebriform overgrowth of the plantar surface. It is caused by an *AKT-1* mutation and is reviewed in Chapter 27.

Beckwith-Wiedemann Syndrome

Patients with Beckwith-Wiedemann syndrome have prominent nevus simplex especially on the glabella in addition to a protruding large tongue, posterior ear pits on the helix, omphalocele or other anterior abdominal wall defects, and hypoglycemia. Other rare syndromes associated with nevus simplex include Nova syndrome (patients have hydrocephalus), odontodysplasia (patients have defects in dentin and failed rupture of teeth), and Roberts-SC syndrome (symmetric limb defects and developmental delay).

TAR Syndrome

TAR syndrome is defined by congenital thrombocytopenia and bilateral absence or hypoplasia of the radius, and some patients have been reported to have port wine stain.

Adams DM, et al: Efficacy and safety of sirolimus in the treatment of complicated vascular anomalies. Pediatrics 2016; 137: e20153257.

Amyere M, et al: Germline loss-of-function mutations in *EPHB4* cause a second form of capillary malformation-arteriovenous malformation (CM-AVM2) deregulating RAS-MAPK signaling. Circulation 2017; 136: 1037.

Cerrati EW, et al: Surgical treatment of head and neck port-wine stains by means of a staged zonal approach. Plast Reconstr Surg 2014; 134: 1003.

Griffin TD, et al: Port wine stain treated with a combination of pulsed dye laser and topical rapamycin ointment. Lasers Surg Med 2016; 48: 193.

Hackett CB, et al: Basal cell carcinoma of the ala nasi arising in a port wine stain treated using Mohs micrographic surgery and local flap reconstruction. Dermatolog Surg 2014; 40: 590.

Jagtap S, et al: Sturge-Weber syndrome. J Child Neurol 2013; 28: 725.

Kim C, et al: Histopathologic and ultrasound characteristics of cutaneous capillary malformations in a patient with capillary malformation–arteriovenous malformation syndrome. Pediatr Dermatol 2015; 32: 128.

Lacerda Lda S, et al: Differential diagnoses of overgrowth syndromes. Radiol Res Pract 2014; 2014: 947451.

Laquer VT, et al: Microarray analysis of port wine stains before and after pulsed dye laser treatment. Lasers Surg Med 2013; 45: 67.

Lee MS, et al: Diffuse capillary malformation with overgrowth. J Am Acad Dermatol 2013; 69: 589.

Lian CG, et al: Novel genetic mutations in a sporadic port-wine stain. JAMA Dermatol 2014; 150: 1336.

Martinez-Lopez A, et al: CLOVES syndrome. Clin Genet 2017; 91: 14.

McDonell LM, et al: Mutations in *STAMBP*, encoding a deubiquitinating enzyme, cause microcephaly–capillary malformation syndrome. Nat Genet 2013; 45: 556.

Memarzadeh A, et al: Limb length discrepancy in cutis marmorata telangiectatica congenita. Br J Dermatol 2014; 170: 681.

Mirzaa G, Conway R, Graham JM Jr, et al: PIK3CA-related segmental overgrowth. 2013 Aug 15. In: Adam MP, Ardinger HH, Pagon RA, et al. [Eds.] GeneReviews [Internet]. Seattle: University of Washington, Seattle.

Nguyen S, et al: Skin ulcers in Klippel-Trenaunay syndrome respond to sunitinib. Transl Res 2008; 151: 194.

Ortiz AE, et al: Port-wine stain laser treatments and novel approaches. Facial Plast Surg 2012; 28: 611.

Pleimes M, et al: Characteristic congenital reticular erythema. J Pediatr 2013; 163: 604.

Reddy KK, et al: Treatment of port-wine stains with a short pulse width 532-nm Nd:YAG laser. J Drugs Dermatol 2013; 12: 66.

Redondo P, et al: Microfoam treatment of Klippel-Trenaunay syndrome and vascular malformations. J Am Acad Dermatol 2008; 59: 355.

Rodriguez-Laguna L, et al: CLAPO syndrome. bioRxiv 2017; 154591.

Shirley MD, et al: Sturge-Weber syndrome and port-wine stains caused by somatic mutation in *GNAQ*. N Engl J Med 2013; 368: 1971.

Swarr DT, et al: Expanding the differential diagnosis of fetal hydrops. Prenat Diagn 2013; 33: 1010.

Yiş U, et al: Capillary malformation–arteriovenous malformation syndrome with spinal involvement. Pediatr Dermatol 2014; 31: 744.

VENOUS MALFORMATION

Venous malformations (VMs) present as rounded, blue or purple, spongy nodules. They often occur on the head and neck and may involve both the skin and the mucous membranes. There is usually a deep component with a connection to the venous circulation. Calcified phleboliths and localized hyperhidrosis may occasionally be present, and the lesions can sometimes be painful. In addition to typical VMs that are caused by a *TEK* mutation, there are other malformations categorized as VMs (glomuvenous malformations, cerebrocavernous malformations) Some lesions are amenable to sclerotherapy or surgical resection, but results are mixed. Compression may be helpful. Customized, snug-fitting garments are preferable to elastic bandages.

Several Syndromes Associated with Venous Malformations

Common and familial VMs in addition to blue rubber bleb nevus syndrome (BRBS) are caused by a *TEK* mutation (*TEK* encodes the protein TIE-2). It is proposed that VMCM is due to a germline mutation and BRBS is caused by a somatic mutation (see following subsections). Patients with VMCM seem to have a germline mutation and then a second hit mutation in the *TEK* gene causes the VMs. In BRBS a progenitor cell may acquire a mutation in both *TEK* genes and then spread to other areas leading to multifocal lesions.

Multiple Cutaneous and Mucosal Venous Malformations (VMCM Syndrome)

VMCM patients have multiple small blue soft VMs. D-Dimer is sometimes elevated in VMCM but not in glomangiomas. The lesions of VMCM are small and unlike BRBS are not hyperkeratotic or firm.

Blue Rubber Bleb Nevus Syndrome

BRBS is characterized by cutaneous and GI venous malformations. There is often a dominant lesion that is much larger than the others. The skin lesions have a cyanotic, bluish appearance with a soft, elevated, nipple-like center, but deeper lesions may also occur. They can be emptied by firm pressure, leaving them flaccid. The lesions are located predominantly on the trunk and arms but also the palms and soles. Nocturnal pain may occur. Lesions can be found throughout the GI tract (Fig. 28.17) but are numerous in the small intestine, and rupture of a lesion may produce melena. Occasionally, other organs may express VMs, and symptomatic CNS lesions have been described. Localized coagulopathy (DIC) can occur. Treatment of bleeding or painful lesions is destruction or excision. Minimally invasive surgical techniques are well suited to the treatment of numerous lesions. For patients who continue to have bleeding episodes that require blood transfusions, octreotide, a somatostatin analog known to decrease splanchnic blood flow, may be effective. ε-Aminocaproic acid has also been used.

Bannayan-Riley-Ruvalcaba Syndrome

Bannayan-Riley-Ruvalcaba syndrome is described later in this chapter.

Maffucci Syndrome

Maffucci syndrome is characterized by multiple vascular malformations with dyschondroplasia caused in most patients by mutations

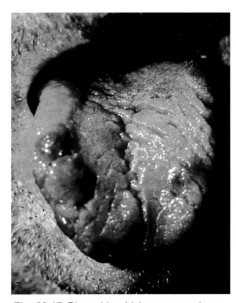

Fig. 28.17 Blue rubber bleb nevus syndrome.

in *IDH1* or *IDH2*. The dyschondroplasia is manifested by uneven bone growth as a result of the defects of ossification, with enchondromatosis that results in multiple and frequent fractures in the period of bone growth. During the prepubertal years, 1–2 cm nodules appear on the small bones of the hand or foot. Later, larger nodules, the enchondromas, appear on the long bones. Much later, similar lesions appear on the trunk. Sarcomatous degeneration occurs in 50% of patients. The distribution of the lesions is mostly unilateral. Multiple VMs of the skin and mucous membranes are present in this nonhereditary mesodermal dysplasia disorder. Lymphangiomas may also occur. Pigmentary changes, such as vitiligo and café au lait macules, have been noted. In Ollier disease, the enchondromatosis is present without the cutaneous abnormalities.

Cerebral Cavernous Malformations

Cerebral cavernomas are vascular malformations in the brain that may be inherited in an autosomal dominant manner. The causative mutations are in *CCM1 (KRIT1)*, *CCM2*, or *PDCD10*. Cutaneous malformations are sometimes present, including hyperkeratotic cutaneous capillary VMs.

Glomuvenous Malformation

VM should be distinguished from glomuvenous malformation (GM, glomangioma). GM is made up of glomus cells and is caused by mutations in glomulin. GM can be pink at initial presentation but evolve to blue-black with a cobblestone appearance and minimal hyperkeratosis. Involvement of an extremity is typical, and the GMs are often painful if compressed because they are made of glomus cells. The lesion often shrinks with external pressure and is typically painful in the morning due to congestion. Increased pain may be noted at puberty, during menstruation, with pregnancy, or with oral contraceptives. Sclerotherapy is more effective in VM than in GM.

Glomus Tumor

The solitary glomus or neuromyoarterial tumor (also known as a solitary glomangioma) is most frequently a skin-colored or slightly dusky blue, firm nodule 1–20 mm in diameter. The characteristic location is subungual, but tumors may occur on the fingers and arms, or elsewhere. Subungual tumors show a bluish tinge through the translucent nail plate. The tumor is usually extremely tender, and paroxysmal pain occurs frequently. Sensitivity is likely to be present constantly, and when touched the tumor responds with severe radiating pain. However, nontender glomus tumors are encountered. Digital lesions are more common in women, and there is a male predominance of nondigital lesions. Hereditary multiple glomus tumors may represent an autosomal dominant mosaic trait and may be congenital. There appears to be an association between glomus tumor and neurofibromatosis. High-resolution MRI, high-resolution ultrasonography (5–9 MHz), and color duplex sonography may be used to define the limits of the tumor before surgery is undertaken. Progressive growth may lead to ulceration.

Histologically, glomus tumors contain numerous vascular lumina lined by a single layer of flattened endothelial cells. Peripheral to the endothelial cells are layers of glomus cells. Generally, these are round and arranged in distinct rows resembling strings of black pearls. Rarely, the cells have a somewhat spindled morphology. Multiple glomus tumors tend to have only one or two layers of glomus cells. Glomangiomyomas have a prominent muscularis media in addition to one or two layers of glomus cells. Both solitary and multiple glomus tumors are related to the arterial segment of the cutaneous glomus, the Sucquet-Hoyer canal. The glomus cells are modified vascular smooth muscle cells and stain with vimentin rather than desmin. Smooth muscle actin is often positive.

Treatment of solitary glomus tumors is best carried out by complete excision, which immediately produces relief from pain. The subungual tumors are most difficult to locate and eradicate because they are usually small, seldom more than a few millimeters in diameter.

Rare reports of glomangiosarcomas describe large, deeply located extremity lesions that consist of sarcomatous areas intermingled with areas of benign glomus tumor.

Amyere M, et al: Common somatic alterations identified in Maffucci syndrome by molecular karyotyping. Mol Syndromol 2014; 5: 259.

de Vos IJ, et al: Review of familial cerebral cavernous malformations and report of seven additional families. Am J Med Genet A 2017; 173: 338.

Fayad LM, et al: Venous malformations. Skeletal Radiol 2008; 37: 895.

Ham KW, et al: Glomus tumors. Arch Plast Surg 2013; 40: 392.

Harrison B, Sammer D: Glomus tumors and neurofibromatosis. Plast Reconstr Surg Glob Open 2014; 2: e214.

Soblet J, et al: Blue rubber bleb nevus (BRBN) syndrome is caused by somatic *TEK (TIE2)* mutations. J Investig Dermatol 2017; 137: 207.

Yanai T, et al: Immunohistochemical demonstration of cyclooxygenase-2 in glomus tumors. J Bone Joint Surg Am 2013; 95: 725.

ARTERIOVENOUS FISTULAS

An *arteriovenous fistula* (AV) is a route from artery to vein, bypassing the capillary bed. AV fistulas may be congenital or acquired. Congenital AV fistulas occur mostly on the extremities and may be recognized, or at least suspected, in the presence of varicose veins, ulcerations, and CMs. They may occur internally as a component of Osler-Weber-Rendu disease (hereditary hemorrhagic telangiectasia). Acquired AV fistulas are usually the result of trauma (Fig. 28.18) but may be created intentionally for hemodialysis access.

The skin over AV fistulas is warmer, hair may grow faster, and the affected limb may be larger than the other; thrills and bruits may be discerned in some cases. Changes may result from stasis, a vascular steal syndrome, edema, a vascular mass, increased sweating, or paresthesias. At times, reddish purple nodules or a plaque may be present with a clinical resemblance to Kaposi sarcoma; this has been called pseudo–Kaposi sarcoma (Stewart-Bluefarb syndrome).

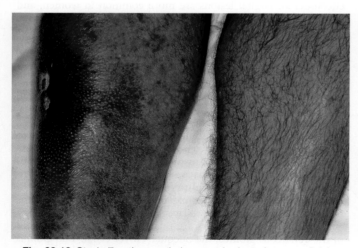

Fig. 28.18 Stasis-like changes below acquired arteriovenous fistula.

It may occur because of congenital malformations, in which case a unilateral purplish discoloration of the skin over or distal to the AV anomaly begins to appear in the second or third decade of life. This type accounts for 80% of cases; the remainder are secondary to fistulas caused by trauma. Iatrogenic AV fistulas, such as those produced to facilitate hemodialysis, may also bring about skin changes, including reactive angioendotheliomatosis. Histologically, there is an increase in thick-walled vessels lined by plump endothelial cells, extravasated erythrocytes, and deposits of hemosiderin. Proliferating endothelial cells may occlude the lumen.

Cirsoid aneurysms (angioma arteriale racemosum) are uncommon congenital AV fistulas of the scalp or face. They may appear on the skin as a pulsating mass that may extend over the neck and scalp and may penetrate into the cranium, or they may simply manifest as a solitary blue or red papule in the midadult period. Abdominal AV fistulas may be associated with lower extremity edema, cyanosis, pulsatile varicose veins, and scrotal edema.

Diagnosis of an AV fistula is established by plethysmography, thermography, determination of oxygen saturation of venous blood, or arteriography.

Treatment of traumatically induced AV fistulas by excision is curative. Because the congenital malformation variety consists of multiple small distal lesions, surgical intervention is not feasible in many patients. Color echo-Doppler ultrasonography–guided sclerotherapy with polidocanol microfoam has been used successfully in this setting. Sodium tetradecyl sulfate and ethanolamine oleate have both been used as sclerosants in various forms of AV malformation. Pressure and elevation as supportive measures may limit ulceration, infection, and other secondary complications.

Rosenberg TL, et al: Arteriovenous malformations of the head and neck. Otolaryngol Clin North Am 2018; 51: 185.

Rutherford RB: Noninvasive evaluation for congenital arteriovenous fistulas and malformations. Semin Vasc Surg 2012; 25: 49.

Scruggs J, et al: Cutaneous manifestations of abdominal arteriovenous fistulas. Cutis 2011; 87: 284.

OTHER LESIONS

Nevus anemicus is a congenital disorder characterized by macules of varying size and shape that are paler than the surrounding skin (Fig. 28.19) and cannot be made red by trauma, cold, or heat. The nevus resembles vitiligo, but there is a normal amount of melanin. Wood's light does not accentuate it, and diascopy causes it to merge into the surrounding blanched skin. The patches are usually well defined with irregular edges. Nevus anemicus can be an important early marker of neurofibromatosis in a young child, before other stigmata have appeared. Nevus anemicus can also be found in tuberous sclerosis or as one component of phakomatosis pigmentovascularis. In nevus anemicus, a flare does not develop after rubbing the skin but does develop after rubbing the adjacent normal skin. The underlying defect is an increased sensitivity of the blood vessels to catecholamines. On biopsy and with confocal microscopy, lesional skin resembles normal skin.

Nevus oligemicus presents as a patch of livid skin that is cooler than the normal skin as a result of decreased blood flow. Vasoconstriction of deep vessels is thought to be the underlying defect.

Sinusoidal hemangioma is a vascular malformation that usually presents in adults as a bluish purple nodule, less than 4 cm in diameter, on the trunk or breasts. Multiple lesions may occur, and a facial location has also been reported. Histologically, it appears as a lobular, circumscribed mass with dilated, interconnected vascular channels filled with blood.

Ferrari F, et al: Juvenile xanthogranuloma and nevus anemicus in the diagnosis of neurofibromatosis type 1. JAMA Dermatol 2014; 150: 42.

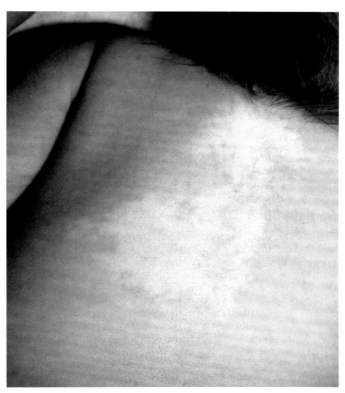

Fig. 28.19 Nevus anemicus.

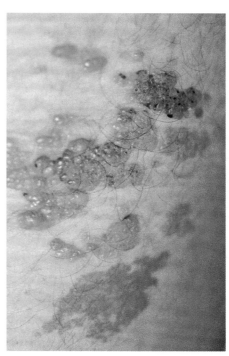

Fig. 28.20 Microcystic lymphatic malformation adjacent to café au lait macule.

Marque M, et al: Nevus anemicus in neurofibromatosis type 1. J Am Acad Dermatol 2013; 69: 768.

Prominent Inferior Labial Artery

The arteries supplying the lips are normally tortuous to accommodate the movements of the mouth. Howell and Freeman reported a potentially troublesome arterial anomaly of the lower lip characterized by the appearance of a pulsating papule in the lower vermilion, 1 or 2 cm from the oral commissure, formed by an especially tortuous segment of the inferior labial artery. A similar anomaly may involve the upper lip. Caliber-persistent labial artery may be misdiagnosed as squamous cell carcinoma, and the biopsy may produce significant bleeding. On the lip, it is best to "palpate for pulsation prior to puncture."

Howell JB, Freeman RG: The potential peril from caliber-persistent arteries of the lips. J Am Acad Dermatol 2002; 46: 256.

LYMPHATIC MALFORMATIONS

Microcystic Lymphatic Malformation (Lymphangioma Circumscriptum)

The old term for microcystic lymphatic malformation (MLM) was lymphangioma circumscriptum; however, this is not a tumor but rather a congenital malformation of the superficial lymphatics. An MLM presents as groups of deep-seated, vesicle-like papules (Fig. 28.20), resembling frog spawn, at birth or shortly thereafter. The lesions are usually yellowish but may be pink, red, or dark when bled into. This creates the illusion that they are rapidly changing. When the papules are punctured, they exude clear, colorless lymph. The papules are arranged irregularly in groups that may be interconnected by sparsely scattered lymph cysts. The entire process, however, as a rule is localized to one region. The sites of predilection are the abdomen, axillae, genitalia, and mouth, particularly the tongue. The scrotum is subject to multifocal lymphatic malformations presenting as clear, thick-walled, vesicle lesions. At times, the surface is verrucous, in which case the color may be brownish, and the lesions may be mistaken for warts. Lesions resembling molluscum contagiosum have also been described.

Frequently, the lesions consist of a combination of blood and lymph elements, so that purple areas are sometimes seen scattered within the vesicle-like papules. The lesions are also frequently associated with a deep component that occupies the subcutaneous tissues and muscles. Over time, these lymphatic malformations show only slight changes.

As with angiokeratomas, lymphangiomas may be seen adjacent to café au lait macules. This may represent a twin spotting phenomenon. Acquired lesions occur in the setting of chronic lymphedema. Lesions occurring after radiation therapy overlap with atypical vascular lesion (AVL). A peculiar penicillamine-induced dermopathy may result from damage to the underlying supporting structures of the dermis and allow dilation of lymph vessels within areas of trauma, such as the dorsal hands and knees. Central facial involvement may be seen in variegate porphyria, and sites of chronic high-potency steroid application may develop lymphangiectasia.

Excision and grafting, fulguration, or coagulation is frequently unsatisfactory because of recurrences resulting from vascular connections between the surface lesions and deep-seated lymphatic cisterns. The deeper component should be evaluated by MRI or other suitable radiologic imaging to delineate the extent of deep involvement before planned procedures. Vaporization with the carbon dioxide (CO_2) laser may be successful if deeper components are not present. Pulsed dye laser, intense pulse light systems, sclerosants, and electrosurgical techniques have also been reported as effective. Keloid formation has been described after laser vaporization of genital lymphangiomas. Sclerotherapy has been reported as successful, and radiotherapy has been used successfully in select refractory cases.

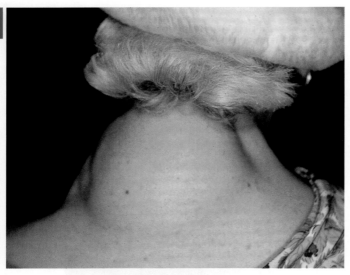

Fig. 28.21 Cystic hygroma.

Emer J, et al: A case of lymphangioma circumscriptum successfully treated with electrodessication following failure of pulsed dye laser. Dermatol Online J 2013; 19: 2.

Kupetsky EA, Pugliano-Mauro M: Lymphangioma circumscriptum. Dermatol Surg 2014; 40: 928.

Yang X, et al: Highly selective electrocoagulation therapy. Dermatol Surg 2014; 40: 899.

Macrocystic Lymphatic Malformation

Macrocystic lymphatic malformations are deep-seated, typically multilocular, poorly defined, soft tissue masses that are painless and covered by normal skin. They are most common in the oral cavity and on the extremities and have been described in Maffucci syndrome. Cystic hygromas are clinically better circumscribed, occurring usually in the neck (Fig. 28.21), axilla, or groin. The posterior neck lesions may be associated with Turner syndrome, other chromosomal aneuploidy conditions, hydrops fetalis, or other congenital abnormalities. Cytogenic analysis of children born with cystic hygromas is indicated, because aneuploidy may recur in subsequent pregnancies. Transabdominal or transvaginal sonography can visualize these lesions in utero. Usually, the lesions will recur after surgical treatment because of their depth, but injection sclerotherapy with agents such as OK-432 (picibanil) may result in regression. Sildenafil has been reported as an effective nonsurgical treatment in the setting of pediatric orbital lymphangioma.

Gandhi NG, et al: Sildenafil for pediatric orbital lymphangioma. JAMA Ophthalmol 2013; 131: 1228.

Guruprasad Y, et al: Cervical cystic hygroma. J Maxillofac Oral Surg 2012; 11: 333.

Lymphangiomatosis

Diffuse or multifocal dilated lymphatic channels involving the skin, soft tissues, bone, and parenchymal organs are a rare congenital condition. If an extremity is affected, the prognosis is good; however, when vital internal organs are involved, the prognosis is poor. Skin lesions are presenting signs in 7% of patients with thoracic lymphangiomatosis. These patients have a high incidence of complications, including chylothorax (49%), pulmonary infiltrates (45%), bone lesions (39%), splenic lesions (19%), cervical involvement (15%), and DIC (9%). Splenic lymphangiomatosis has been associated with Proteus syndrome. Diffuse pulmonary lymphangiomatosis has been successfully treated with bevacizumab.

KAPOSIFORM LYMPHANGIOMATOSIS

Kaposiform lymphangiomatosis is a newly described entity made of spindled lymphatic endothelial cells that grow progressively and is in between a tumor and a malformation. The intrathoracic disease is prominent and it can present in the skin with subcutaneous masses or ecchymosis. Histopathology shows spindled cells that are arranged in parallel, strands and sheets that anastomose, and is less well defined than KHE. Kasabach-Merritt–like coagulopathy has been reported. There is significant mortality but sirolimus therapy shows promise.

Gorham-Stout Syndrome

Gorham-Stout syndrome is characterized by lymphangiomatosis and chylous effusions, with osteolytic changes resulting in "vanishing bones." The cutaneous lymphatic malformation may be the initial sign of the disease, which typically appears in young children, usually in areas adjacent to involved bones. If a patient has a lymphatic malformation that becomes painful, Gorham should be considered. Although multiple areas of the skeletal system may be involved, usually only a single bone is destroyed. The bone is completely or partially replaced with fibrous tissue. Sirolimus therapy has been helpful in some patients. Response to pegylated IFN alfa-2b was noted in a 9-year-old boy with systemic disease. Response to bisphosphonates has also been noted.

Multifocal Lymphangioendotheliomatosis

Patients with multifocal lymphangioendotheliomatosis present at birth with hundreds of red-brown plaques as large as several centimeters. Similar lesions occur in the GI tract and are associated with severe bleeding with a significant risk of mortality. Severe thrombocytopenia occurs in affected children with a coagulopathy (Kasabach-Merritt–like) that can be life threatening. There are reports of children with very few skin lesions and severe thrombocytopenia and reports of children with classic skin lesions but no thrombocytopenia. Treatment with corticosteroids and/or IFN alfa results in little to no improvement, but recently sirolimus has shown significant benefit. One patient was reported who did well with a liver transplant. The histology is distinctive, with delicate, thin-walled vessels lined by hobnailed endothelium with papillary tufting. The endothelial cells demonstrate a high proliferative fraction with Ki-67 staining and are reactive with LYVE-1, suggesting lymphatic differentiation.

Acquired Progressive Lymphangioma (Benign Lymphangioendothelioma)

This is a group of slow-growing lymphangiomas that present as bruiselike lesions or erythematous macules in children or middle-aged adults. Rarely, the lesion is yellow or alopecic. The histologic appearance is that of delicate, endothelium-lined spaces dissecting between collagen bundles. A similarity to the plaque stage of Kaposi sarcoma (KS) may be striking. Simple excision is curative. Topical and systemic steroids in addition to surgery have been effective.

Al-Jamali J, et al: Gorham-Stout syndrome of the facial bones. Oral Surg Oral Med Oral Pathol Oral Radiol 2012; 114: e23.

Aman J, et al: Successful treatment of diffuse pulmonary lymphangiomatosis with bevacizumab. Ann Intern Med 2012; 156: 839.

Croteau SE, et al: Kaposiform lymphangiomatosis. J Pediatr 2014; 164: 383.

Droitcourt C, et al: Multifocal lymphangioendotheliomatosis with thrombocytopenia. Pediatrics 2015; 136: e517.

Hagendoorn J, et al: Novel molecular pathways in Gorham disease. Pediatr Blood Cancer 2014; 61: 401.

Nikolaou VS, et al: Vanishing bone disease (Gorham-Stout syndrome). World J Orthop 2014; 5: 694.

Ricci KW et al: A phase 2 clinical trial assessing efficacy and safety of the mTOR inhibitor sirolimus in the treatment of generalized lymphatic anomaly, kaposiform lymphangiomatosis, and Gorham-Stout disease. Am J Respir Crit Care Med 2015; 191: A5454.

Salman A, et al: Acquired progressive lymphangioma. Pediatr Dermatol 2017; 34: e302.

Yang CH, et al: Orthotopic liver transplant for multifocal lymphangioendotheliomatosis with thrombocytopenia. Pediatr Transplant 2016; 20: 456.

Phakomatosis Pigmentovascularis

Patients with a combination of vascular malformations and melanocytic (Fig. 28.22) or epidermal nevi are grouped into this disorder. The revised classification includes only four types: phakomatosis cesioflammea (blue nevus/dermal melanosis and nevus flammeus), phakomatosis spilorosa (nevus spilus and a pale-pink vascular spot), phakomatosis cesiomarmorata (blue spots and cutis marmorata telangiectatica congenita), and unclassifiable cases not corresponding to the previous patterns. These may all be phenotypes of a common disorder, and a recent report shows *GNAQ* or *GNA11* mutations. Associated systemic findings may include intracranial and visceral vascular anomalies, ocular abnormalities, choroidal melanoma, and hemihypertrophy of the limbs. Phakomatosis cesioflammea is the most common type (85%), and half of patients with this type have serious manifestations. Bilateral deafness and malignant hypertension have also been described. Some authors have suggested that particularly extensive and aberrant mongolian spots may be a marker for more severe systemic involvement. Phakomatosis spilorosa has been associated with multiple granular cell tumors.

Phacomatosis pigmentokeratotica is now classified separately as a syndrome that includes speckled lentiginous nevi and nevus sebaceous and may be on the same spectrum as Schimmelpenning syndrome (nevus sebaceous syndrome). There can be associations of seizures, epibulbar dermoids, and potential malignancies. Phacomatosis pigmentokeratotica has been shown to be caused by an *HRAS* or *KRAS* mutation and can be considered a RASopathy (see Chapter 27).

Arnold AW, et al: Phacomatosis melanorosea without extracutaneous features. Eur J Dermatol 2012; 22: 473.

Groesser L, et al: Phacomatosis pigmentokeratotica is caused by a postzygotic *HRAS* mutation in a multipotent progenitor cell. J Investig Dermatol 2013; 133: 1998.

Om A, et al: Phacomatosis pigmentokeratotica. Pediatr Dermatol 2017; 34: 352.

Thomas AC, et al: Mosaic activating mutations in *GNA11* and *GNAQ* are associated with phakomatosis pigmentovascularis and extensive dermal melanocytosis. J Investig Dermatol 2016; 136: 770.

Dilation of Preexisting Vessels

Spider Angioma (Vascular Spider, Spider Nevus, Nevus Araneus)

The lesion of spider angioma is suggestive of a red spider. The ascending central arteriole represents the "body" of the spider, and the radiating fine vessels suggest the multiple legs. These small telangiectases occur singly or severally, most frequently on the face, neck, and dorsal hands, indicating they may be induced by sun exposure.

Young children and pregnant women show these lesions most frequently. In pregnant women, palmar erythema is usually present with the vascular spiders. The presence of vascular spiders in otherwise healthy children is common.

Vascular spiders also occur in patients with cirrhosis, hepatitis C, malignant disease of the liver, and other hepatic dysfunctions. The common denominator has been shown to be an elevated blood estrogen level. Elevations in VEGF and basic fibroblastic growth factor are also significant predictors for spider angiomas in cirrhotic patients. When vascular spiders occur with palmar erythema and pallid nails with distal hyperemic bands, cirrhosis of the liver should be considered. AV hemangioma has also been reported to be associated with chronic liver disease.

The vascular spiders of childhood may involute without treatment, although several years may elapse before this occurs. In pregnant women, most lesions will involute soon after delivery. If active therapy will be performed pulse dye laser is effective without scarring, but electrodesiccation may produce good results in experienced hands.

Venous Lakes

Venous lakes (phlebectases) are small, dark-blue, slightly elevated blebs (Fig. 28.23). They are easily compressed and are located on the face, ears, lips, neck, forearms, and backs of the hands. These manifestations of chronic sun damage are extremely dilated, blood-filled spaces lined with thin, elongated endothelial cells and usually surrounded by prominent solar elastosis. Venous lakes may be treated by light electrocautery, laser ablation, fulguration, infrared coagulation, intralesional injection of 1% polidocanol, and cryotherapy.

Capillary Aneurysms

These flesh-colored solitary lesions, resembling an intradermal nevus, may suddenly grow larger and darker and become blue-black or black as a result of thrombosis. Capillary aneurysms are surrounded by a zone of erythema. The lesions may be clinically indistinguishable from malignant melanoma. Histologically, these are thrombotic, dilated capillaries lying just below the epidermis. Shave excision in stages will expose the clot and eliminate the uncertainty.

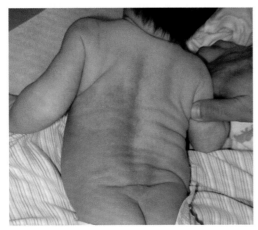

Fig. 28.22 Phacomatosis pigmentovascularis. (Courtesy of Department Dermatology, Keio University School of Medicine, Tokyo, Japan.)

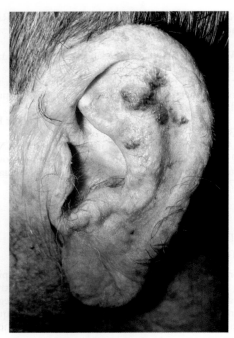

Fig. 28.23 Venous lake.

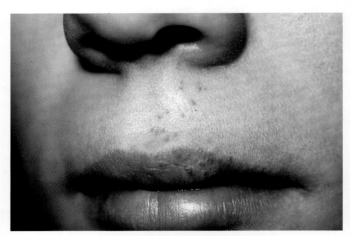

Fig. 28.24 Unilateral nevoid telangiectasia.

Telangiectasia

Telangiectases are fine, linear vessels coursing on the surface of the skin; collectively, they are named telangiectasia. Telangiectasia may occur in normal skin at any age, in both genders, and can occur anywhere on the skin and mucous membranes but if abundant or with other symptoms, they can be important markers of systemic disease. Fine telangiectases may be seen on the alae nasi of most adults. They are prominent in areas of chronic actinic damage seen in fair-skinned persons. Persons long exposed to wind, cold, or heat are also subject to telangiectasia.

Telangiectases can be found in such conditions as radiodermatitis, xeroderma pigmentosum, lupus erythematosus (LE), dermatomyositis, scleroderma and the CREST syndrome, rosacea, cirrhosis of the liver, acquired immunodeficiency syndrome (AIDS), poikiloderma, basal cell carcinoma, necrobiosis lipoidica diabeticorum, sarcoid, lupus vulgaris, adenoma sebaceum, keloid, angioma serpiginosum, angiokeratoma corporis diffusum, ataxia-telangiectasia, pregnancy, and Bloom syndrome. These entities are discussed in other sections with the disease states in which they occur.

Altered capillary patterns on the fingernail folds (cuticular telangiectases) are indicative of collagen vascular disease, such as LE, scleroderma, or dermatomyositis. Tortuous glomeruloid loops are characteristic of LE, whereas dilated loops and avascular areas are typical of scleroderma and dermatomyositis. Reticular telangiectatic erythema may occur overlying implantable cardioverter-defibrillators.

Electrodessication and laser ablation can be effective. Pulsed dye laser and other vascular lasers, such as the 532-nm Nd:YAG laser, are usually well tolerated and associated with a low risk of scarring. Larger vessels require a longer pulse duration. Contact or cryospray cooling can reduce the incidence of complications. Pulse stacking (multiple pulses of low fluences) has been used to reduce the incidence of side effects, such as purpura, hyperpigmentation, hypopigmentation, and scar formation.

Hereditary Hemorrhagic Telangiectasia

Hereditary hemorrhagic telangiectasia (HHT, Osler-Weber-Rendu disease) is a genetic syndrome caused by mutations in either *ENG*, *ACVRL1*, *GDF2*, or *SMAD4*. The telangiectasias are widespread and usually involve the mucosa. They can be very tiny or much larger patches that can bleed easily. Patients often present with severe nose bleeds in childhood or GI bleeding less commonly. Patients with mutations in *SMAD4* and have GI polyps. There are AVMs that can affect the skin, CNS, liver, GI tract, or lungs. Genetic testing can help prove the diagnosis and screening with pulmonary, CNS and liver imaging is recommended in affected patients to rule out AVMs in these locations. In addition to other causes of telangiectasias outlined earlier, CM-AVM and CM-AVM2 are in the differential.

Generalized Essential Telangiectasia

Generalized essential telangiectasia (GET) is characterized by the dilation of veins and capillaries over a large segment of the body without preceding or coexisting skin lesions. The telangiectases may be distributed over the entire body or localized to some large area, such as the legs, arms, and trunk. The lesions may be discrete or confluent. Distribution along the course of the cutaneous nerves may occur. This type of telangiectasia is rarely associated with systemic disease, although patients with a similar appearance may have autoimmune disease. One report documented GI bleeding from a "watermelon" stomach in a woman with GET.

Most frequently, GET develops in women in their forties and fifties. The initial onset is on the lower legs and then spreads to the upper legs, abdomen, and arms. The dilations persist indefinitely. Generally, this is a sporadic condition, although it has been described in families as an autosomal dominant trait, in which case it has been termed *hereditary benign telangiectasia*.

It has been reported that GET may be differentiated from telangiectasia associated with systemic disease by assessing alkaline phosphatase activity. Telangiectatic vessels in GET do not have alkaline phosphatase activity in the endothelium of the terminal arteriole and the arterial portion of the capillary loops.

Individual areas may be treated with laser ablation. High-energy, high-frequency, long-pulse Nd:YAG laser and the 585-nm flashlamp-pumped pulsed dye laser have been reported to produce good results. Tetracycline, ketoconazole, and treatment of a chronic sinus infection have led to involution in individual reports.

Unilateral Nevoid Telangiectasia

In unilateral nevoid telangiectasia, fine, threadlike telangiectases develop in a unilateral, sometimes dermatomal, distribution (Fig. 28.24). The areas most often involved are the trigeminal and C3 and C4 or adjacent areas, with the right side involved slightly more often than the left. In some cases the condition is congenital, but more often it is acquired. Increased estrogen appears to play a role in the onset of acquired cases (e.g., pregnancy, puberty in women, adrenarche in men), and hepatitis/alcohol-related cases have been reported. Bilateral nevoid telangiectasia has been reported to be more common in older people, men and in the setting of some other illness such as liver disease or diabetes. Lesions have responded to pulsed dye laser treatment.

Angiokeratomas

Angiokeratomas are collections of blood vessels with an overlying hyperkeratotic surface. Angiokeratoma corporis diffusum (Fabry disease) is discussed in Chapter 26.

Angiokeratoma Circumscriptum

Angiokeratoma circumscriptum is a malformation of dermal and subcutaneous capillaries and veins that remains unclassified in the ISSVA classification. The lesions are purple or red and well defined, occurring mainly on the lower extremities, but can also occur on the chest or forearm. Lesions are often congenital and over time, a verrucous component appears. Linear segmental lesions have been described. Superficial ablative therapy is typically followed by recurrence, regardless of whether ablation is performed by excision, laser, cryotherapy, or electrocautery. In contrast, full-thickness excision is generally effective and may be used in combination with laser therapy if necessary.

Angiokeratoma of Mibelli

The lesions of angiokeratoma of Mibelli consist of 1–5 mm red vascular papules, the surfaces of which become hyperkeratotic over time. The papules are dull red or purplish black, verrucous, and rounded and are usually situated on the dorsum of the fingers and toes, the elbows, and the knees. Frequently, these are called telangiectatic warts. The patient often has cold, cyanotic hands and feet. Autosomal dominant inheritance has been described, and an association with chilblains is common. The condition is most frequently discovered in prepubertal children.

Histologically, hyperkeratosis, increased thickness of the granular layer, and dilation of the subpapillary vessels to form lacunae are the chief features.

The differential diagnosis of angiokeratomas of the dorsal hands in children includes acral pseudolymphomatous angiokeratoma in children (APACHE). However, APACHE is unilateral and sporadic in nature, without associated cold sensitivity; histologic examination reveals a dense, nodular, lymphohistiocytic infiltrate with occasional plasma cells, eosinophils, and multinucleated giant cells. It is a variant of pseudolymphoma and not primarily a vascular lesion. Similar lesions may occur in adolescents and adults, and the terms acral angiokeratoma-like pseudolymphoma and T-cell–rich angiomatoid polypoid pseudolymphoma of the skin have been used to describe these varied presentations.

Angiokeratoma may be treated with electrocautery, fulguration, CO_2 laser ablation, long-pulse vascular laser therapy, or cryotherapy, with fairly good results.

Angiokeratoma of the Scrotum (Fordyce)

Angiokeratomas have a predilection for the scrotum (Fig. 28.25) and sometimes the vulva in middle-aged and elderly individuals. There is often a diffuse redness of the involved area. Urethral or clitoral lesions may also be seen. Infrequently, the keratotic part may be accidentally scratched leading to considerable bleeding. Histologically, the many communicating lacunae in the subpapillary layer are lined with endothelium and connected underneath by dilated veins. The primary therapy is reassurance, but therapy

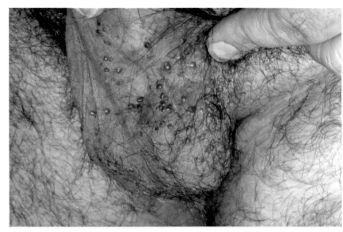

Fig. 28.25 Angiokeratoma of Fordyce.

with shave excision, cautery, laser ablation, or fulguration can be used.

Brown KR, et al: Superficial venous disease. Surg Clin North Am 2013; 93: 963.

Dayrit JF, et al: T-cell-rich angiomatoid polypoid pseudolymphoma of the skin. J Cutan Pathol 2011; 38: 475.

Kim EJ, et al: Demographic and clinical differences between unilateral and bilateral forms of naevoid telangiectasia. Br J Dermatol 2015; 172: 1651.

McDonald J, Pyeritz RE: Hereditary hemorrhagic telangiectasia. 2000 Jun 26 [Updated 2017 Feb 2]. In: Adam MP, Ardinger HH, Pagon RA, et al. [Eds.] GeneReviews [Internet]. Seattle: University of Washington, Seattle.

Turan H, et al: Acquired unilateral nevoid telangiectasia syndrome accompanied by chronic hepatitis B virus infection. Acta Dermatovenerol Croat 2013; 21: 133.

Wang L, et al: Solitary angiokeratoma on palms and soles. J Dermatol 2013; 40: 653.

Zeng Y, et al: Treatment of angiokeratoma of Mibelli alone or in combination with pulsed dye laser and long-pulsed Nd:YAG laser. Dermatol Ther 2014; 27: 348.

HYPERPLASIAS

Angiolymphoid Hyperplasia with Eosinophilia

Angiolymphoid hyperplasia with eosinophilia (ALHE) is a benign vascular growth that usually presents with pink to red-brown, dome-shaped, dermal papules or nodules of the head or neck (Fig. 28.26). There is a predilection for the scalp, especially the retro-auricular area. ALHE may also occur in the mouth and on the trunk, extremities, penis, and vulva. Grouped lesions merge to form plaques or grapelike clusters. There is a female preponderance, and the average age of onset is 32 years. Symptoms can include pain or pruritus, which may occur after trauma. An underlying AV shunt can be present. Histologically, central thick-walled vessels with hobnail endothelium are noted. Surrounding hyperplasia of smaller vessels and nodular lymphoid aggregates with eosinophils are present.

Lesions do not spontaneously regress. Treatment with surgical excision is successful in 65% of cases. The lesions may recur if the underlying AV shunt is not excised. Intralesional corticosteroids, pulsed dye laser therapy with conventional or ultralong pulsed systems, Nd:YAG laser, cryotherapy, pentoxifylline, indomethacin, imiquimod, and electrodesiccation have been successful in some patients. Difficult cases have been controlled with IFN alfa-2b,

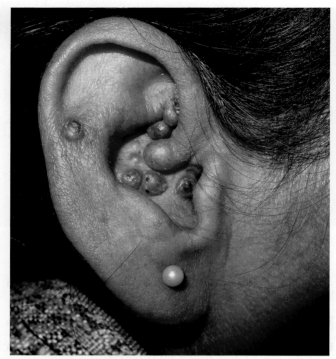

Fig. 28.26 Angiolymphoid hyperplasia with eosinophilia. (Courtesy Dr. Debabrata Bandyopadhyay.)

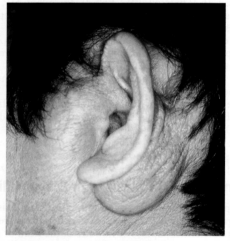

Fig. 28.27 Kimura disease. (Courtesy Department of Dermatology, Keio University School of Medicine.)

isotretinoin, or vinblastine, and partial responses to intralesional bleomycin have been reported.

It is important to distinguish ALHE from Kimura disease (Fig. 28.27). Kimura disease is an inflammatory disorder that presents as massive subcutaneous swelling in the periauricular and submandibular region in young Asian men. Histologically, prominent germinal centers with eosinophils are present in the subcutaneous tissue. Although blood vessels are abundant, changes are less prominent than in ALHE. Additionally, Kimura disease is associated with allergic conditions such as asthma, rhinitis, and eczema, and it is frequently accompanied by lymphadenopathy, peripheral blood eosinophilia, and elevated IgE level. Although clonal T-cell gene

rearrangement has been reported in both ALHE and Kimura disease, heteroduplex polymerase chain reaction (PCR) has disproved clonality in some cases positive on conventional PCR. Treatment of Kimura disease is either with watchful waiting for the expected regression or with surgery, radiation, or systemic steroids. Coexistence of ALHE and peripheral T-cell lymphoma has been reported.

Akdeniz N, et al: Intralesional bleomycin for angiolymphoid hyperplasia. Arch Dermatol 2007; 143: 841.
Carlesimo M, et al: Angiolymphoid hyperplasia with eosinophilia treated with isotretinoin. Eur J Dermatol 2007; 17: 554.
Choi JE, et al: Successful treatment of Kimura's disease with a 595-nm ultra-long pulsed dye laser. Acta Derm Venereol 2008; 88: 315.
Griauzde J, Srinivasan A: Imaging of vascular lesions of the head and neck. Radiol Clin North Am 2015; 53: 197.
Hoff SR, et al: Head and neck vascular lesions. Otolaryngol Clin North Am 2015; 48: 29.

Intravascular Papillary Endothelial Hyperplasia

Masson described this intravascular papillary proliferation that may mimic angiosarcoma. The lesions appear as red or purplish, 5-mm to 5-cm papules or deep nodules on the head, neck, or upper extremities. The condition represents recanalization of a thrombosed vessel. It can occur de novo or as part of a preexisting vascular lesion. Histologic examination reveals intravascular papillary projections lined by endothelial cells. Thrombi may still be present, and the papillary projections may have a fibrinous or hyaline core. High-resolution ultrasound imaging may be useful in establishing the diagnosis, although the diagnosis is usually made by biopsy. Excision is curative.

Beutler BD, Cohen PR: Case presentation intravascular papillary endothelial hyperplasia of the vulva. Dermatol Online J 2016; 22.
Kim TH, et al: Intravascular papillary endothelial hyperplasia (Masson's tumour) in the vulva. Eur J Obstet Gynecol Reprod Biol 2013; 169: 413.

Angioma Serpiginosum

Angioma serpiginosum, first described by Hutchinson in 1889, is characterized by minute, copper-colored to bright-red angiomatous puncta that tend to become papular. These puncta occur in groups that enlarge through the constant formulation of new points at the periphery, whereas those at the center fade. In this manner, linear arrays, small rings, or serpiginous patterns are formed. No purpura is present, but a netlike or diffuse erythema forms the background. In the areas undergoing involution, a delicate tracery of rings and lines, a fine desquamation, and at times a semblance of atrophy are seen. Slight lichenification and scaling may be evident in the papular lesions. Dermoscopy shows small red dots and globules. The eruption predominates on the lower extremities. Although it affects both genders at all ages, 90% of cases occur in girls under 16. It is usually slowly progressive and chronic, and although involution may occur, it is probably never complete. Treatment with a pulsed dye laser will improve or eliminate such lesions. Angioma serpiginosum following Blaschko's lines, with associated esophageal papillomatosis, has been reported as an X-linked dominant condition with mild features of Goltz syndrome (see Chapter 27).

Angioma serpiginosum must be differentiated from the progressive pigmentary disease of Schamberg. In the latter, pinpoint areas of purpura, the so-called cayenne pepper spots, form macules that tend to coalesce and form diffusely pigmented patches. The pigment is hemosiderin. Purpura annularis telangiectodes (Majocchi) is often bilateral and is characterized by acute outbreaks of telangiectatic points that spread peripherally and form small rings. In lichenoid purpuric and pigmentary dermatosis of Gougerot and Blum, the primary lesion is a minute, lichenoid, reddish brown papule that is sometimes hemorrhagic. It has a tendency toward central involution and residual pigmentation.

In angioma serpiginosum, the most important histologic finding is dilated and tortuous capillaries in the dermal papillae and the upper dermis. No inflammatory infiltrate or extravasation of red blood cells is observed. The dilated capillaries show no alkaline phosphatase activity, in contrast to normal capillaries.

Blinkenberg EO, et al: Angioma serpiginosum with oesophageal papillomatosis is an X-linked dominant condition that maps to Xp11.3–Xq12. Eur J Hum Genet 2007; 15: 543.
Freites-Martinez A, et al: Angioma serpiginosum. An Bras Dermatol 2015; 90: 26.
Marks V, et al: Reflectance confocal microscopy features of angioma serpiginosum. Arch Dermatol 2011; 147: 878.

Microvenular Hemangioma

The recently described microvenular hemangioma is an acquired, benign vascular neoplasm that presents as an asymptomatic, slowly growing, 0.5–2.0 cm, reddish lesion on the trunk or extremities of adults (average age 32). Multiple and eruptive variants have been described. Dermoscopic examination reveals multiple, well-demarcated, red globules. Monomorphous, elongated blood vessels with small lumina involve the entire reticular dermis. In many areas, the endothelial cells are surrounded by pericytes. The endothelial cells are podoplanin (D2-40) negative. GLUT-1 may be focally positive. The main differential diagnosis is Kaposi sarcoma. Along with glomeruloid hemangioma, microvenular hemangioma may sometimes be present in POEMS syndrome. Excision, if needed, is usually curative.

Napekoski KM, et al: Microvenular hemangioma. J Cutan Pathol 2014; 41: 816.

Proliferating Angioendotheliomatosis

Diseases designated angioendotheliomatosis have historically been divided into two groups: a reactive, involuting type and a malignant, rapidly fatal type. "Malignant angioendotheliomatosis" has been shown to be intravascular (angiotropic) lymphoma rather than a true vascular lesion.

The reactive type of angioendotheliomatosis is uncommon. It can be idiopathic or occur in patients who have subacute bacterial endocarditis, Chagas disease, pulmonary tuberculosis, cryoproteinemia, severe atherosclerotic disease, periodontal disease, antiphospholipid antibodies, and medications (trabectedin and pegfilgrastim). Patients present with red-purple patches, plaques, nodules, petechiae, and ecchymoses, usually of the lower extremities. Some may present with a livedoid pattern or lesions resembling atrophie blanche. Diffuse dermal angiomatosis is a variant associated with ischemia or atherosclerosis. The lesion occurs most often on the thigh, breast, or pannus in areas of vascular insufficiency (Fig. 28.28) and may clear with revascularization. It has also been described in association with an AV fistula and with anticardiolipin antibodies.

Histologically, the vessels in benign reactive angioendotheliomatosis are dilated and are filled with proliferating endothelial cells, usually without atypia. Some cases demonstrate a proliferation of capillaries in the dermis, with diffuse, lobular, or mixed patterns. Fibrin microthrombi are common, and some cases show amyloid deposits or positive immunohistochemical staining for HHV-8 in lesional endothelial cell nuclei. The course in this type is characterized by involution over 1–2 years. Therapy

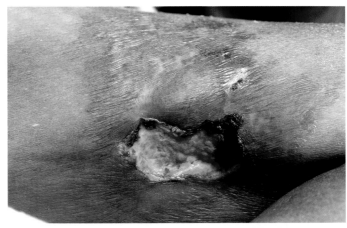

Fig. 28.28 Diffuse dermal angiomatosis.

for the underlying condition has been considered as hastening involution.

The malignant type of "angioendotheliomatosis" is actually a large-cell, intravascular lymphoma and is discussed in Chapter 32.

Kawaoka J, et al: Coexistence of diffuse reactive angioendotheliomatosis and neutrophilic dermatosis heralding primary antiphospholipid syndrome. Acta Derm Venereol 2008; 88: 402.
Li V, et al: A rare case of reactive angioendotheliomatosis secondary to cryoglobulinaemia. Br J Dermatol 2015; 173: 132.
Mayor-Ibarguren A, et al: Diffuse reactive angioendotheliomatosis secondary to the administration of trabectedin and pegfilgrastim. Am J Dermatopathol 2015; 37: 581.
Nikam B, et al: Reactive angioendotheliomatosis as a presenting cutaneous manifestation of Hughes syndrome. Lupus 2015; 24: 1557.

MALIGNANT NEOPLASMS

Kaposi Sarcoma

Moritz Kaposi described this vascular neoplasm in 1872 and called it "multiple benign pigmented idiopathic hemorrhagic sarcoma." Since his description, the disease has been reported in five separate clinical settings, with different presentations, epidemiology, and prognoses, as follows:

1. Classic KS, an indolent disease seen chiefly in middle-aged men of Southern and Eastern European origin
2. African cutaneous KS, a locally aggressive process affecting middle-aged Africans in tropical Africa
3. African lymphadenopathic KS, an aggressive disease of young patients, primarily children under age 10
4. KS in patients immunosuppressed by AIDS
5. Lymphoma or immunosuppressive therapy

Clinical Features
Classic Kaposi Sarcoma. The early lesions appear most often on the toes or soles as reddish, violaceous, or bluish black macules and patches that spread and coalesce to form nodules or plaques. These have a rubbery consistency. There may be brawny edema of the affected leg. Macules or nodules may appear, usually much later, on the arms and hands, and rarely may extend to the face, ears, trunk, genitalia, or buccal cavity, especially the soft palate. The course is slowly progressive and may lead to great enlargement of the lower extremities as a result of lymphedema. However,

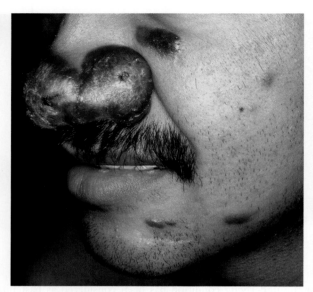

Fig. 28.29 Kaposi sarcoma in an HIV-infected patient.

there may be periods of remission, particularly in the early stages of the disease, when nodules may undergo spontaneous involution. After involution, there may be an atrophic and hyperpigmented scar.

African Cutaneous Kaposi Sarcoma. Nodular, infiltrating, vascular masses occur on the extremities, mostly of men between ages 20 and 50. This form of KS is endemic in tropical Africa and has a locally aggressive but systemically indolent course.

African Lymphadenopathic Kaposi Sarcoma. Lymph node involvement, with or without skin lesions, may occur in children under age 10. The course is aggressive, often terminating fatally within 2 years of onset.

AIDS-Associated Kaposi Sarcoma. Cutaneous lesions begin as one or several red to purple-red macules, rapidly progressing to papules, nodules, and plaques. There is a predilection for the head (Fig. 28.29), neck, trunk, and mucous membranes. A fulminant, progressive course with nodal and systemic involvement is expected. KS may be the presenting manifestation of human immunodeficiency virus (HIV) infection.

Immunosuppression-Associated Kaposi Sarcoma. The lesion's morphology resembles that of classic KS; however, the site of presentation is more variable.

Internal Involvement. The GI tract is the most frequent site of internal involvement in classic KS. The small intestine is probably the viscus most often involved. In addition, the lungs, heart, liver, conjunctiva, adrenal glands, and lymph nodes of the abdomen may be affected. Skeletal changes are characteristic and diagnostic. Bone involvement is always an indication of widespread disease. Changes noted are rarefaction, cysts, and cortical erosion.

African cutaneous KS is frequently accompanied by massive edema of the legs and frequent bone involvement.

African lymphadenopathic KS has been reported among Bantu children, who develop massive involvement of the lymph nodes, especially the cervical nodes, preceding the appearance of skin lesions. The children also develop lesions on the eyelids and conjunctiva, from which masses of hemorrhagic tissue hang down. Eye involvement is often associated with swelling of the lacrimal, parotid, and submandibular glands, with a picture similar to Mikulicz syndrome.

In AIDS-associated KS, 25% of patients have cutaneous involvement alone, whereas 29% have visceral lesions only. The most

frequent sites of visceral involvement are the lungs (37%), GI tract (50%), and lymph nodes (50%). Visceral involvement ultimately occurs in more than 70% of patients with AIDS-associated KS. Other immunosuppressed patients with KS may have visceral involvement in a variable percentage of cases.

Epidemiology. KS is worldwide in distribution. In Europe, there are foci of classic KS in Galicia, near the Polish-Russian border, and extending southward to Austria and Italy. In New York City, KS has occurred mostly in elderly Galician Jewish and southern Italian men. In Africa, KS occurs largely south of the Sahara Desert. Northeast Congo and Rwanda-Burundi areas have the highest prevalence, and to a lesser extent, West and South Africa.

The prevalence of AIDS-related KS has decreased since the 1980s. Most cases are in men who have sex with men (MSM). Very few reports have documented the exceptional occurrence of KS in patients with AIDS who acquired their infection from intravenous drug use, or in Haitians, children, or people with hemophilia. Patients at risk for developing KS associated with other causes of immunosuppression include those with iatrogenic suppression from oral prednisone or other chronic immunosuppressive therapies, as may be given to transplant patients. Endemic disease in southern Europe is strongly associated with oral corticosteroid use and diabetes and is inversely associated with cigarette smoking.

KS is associated with an increased risk of developing second malignancies, such as malignant lymphomas (Hodgkin disease, T-cell lymphoma, non-Hodgkin lymphoma), leukemia, and myeloma. The risk of lymphoreticular malignancy is about 20 times greater in KS patients than in the general population.

Etiopathogenesis. KS is formed by proliferation of abnormal vascular endothelial cells. HHV-8 is found in KS lesional tissue irrespective of clinical type. Primary effusion lymphoma, solid lymphoma, and Castleman disease are other confirmed associations with HHV-8 infection.

Histology. Histopathology of KS varies considerably according to the stage of the disease. Early lesions demonstrate irregularly shaped, ectatic vessels with scattered lymphocytes and plasma cells. The endothelial cells of the capillaries are large and protrude into the lumen, resembling buds. Later lesions show proliferation of vessels around preexisting vessels and adnexal structures. The preexisting structure may jut into the vascular space, forming a promontory sign. Dull-pink globules, extravasated erythrocytes, and hemosiderin are present. Nodular lesions are composed of spindle cells with erythrocytes that appear to line up between spindle cells with no apparent vascular space.

Treatment. All types of KS are radiosensitive. Radiation therapy has been used with considerable success, whether in small fractionated doses, in larger single doses to limited or extended fields, or by electron beam radiation. Local excision, cryotherapy, alitretinoin gel (Panretin), locally injected chemotherapy or IFN, and laser ablation have been used for troublesome, localized lesions.

Vincristine solution, 0.1 mg/mL injected intralesionally, not more than 3 mL at one time and at intervals of 2 weeks, produces involution of tumors, some for as long as 8 months. These studies indicate that adequate control of KS lesions may be achieved, at least for periods of 6–12 months. The development of resistance to medication seems to be inevitable.

Many other agents have been found to be effective; among the best are IFN, vinblastine, and actinomycin D. The response rate initially is high, but recurrent lesions, which are common, are generally less responsive. Systemic therapy is usually needed if more than 10 new KS lesions develop in 1 month, or if there is symptomatic lymphedema, symptomatic pulmonary disease, or symptomatic visceral involvement.

In the setting of HIV, protease inhibitors have been shown to have antiangiogenic effects; however, the results of nonnucleoside reverse transcriptase inhibitor–based regimens are not inferior to protease inhibitor–based therapy in the prevention of KS. This suggests that regression of KS is mediated by an overall improvement in immune function and not by the effects of specific antiretrovirals. Liposomal anthracyclines and paclitaxel have been approved by the FDA as first-line and second-line monotherapy, respectively, for advanced KS.

Rapamycin (sirolimus), an inhibitor of the mammalian target of rapamycin (mTOR), is an effective immunosuppressant for the prevention of transplant rejection, with benefits as a treatment for KS. Dual inhibition of PI3Kα and mTOR by PI-103 appears promising.

Course

Classic KS progresses slowly, with rare lymph node or visceral involvement. Death usually occurs years later from unrelated causes. African cutaneous KS is aggressive, with early nodal involvement, and death from KS is expected within 1–2 years. AIDS-related KS, although widespread, is almost never fatal; almost all patients die of intercurrent infection. The course of the disease is variable in patients who develop immunosuppression-related KS from causes other than AIDS. Removal of the immunosuppression may result in resolution of the KS without therapy. Among transplant patients, a change from a calcineurin inhibitor to sirolimus often results in regression of KS lesions. KS-associated immune reconstitution syndrome can run a severe course with lung involvement and thrombocytopenia associated with worse outcomes.

Beatrous SV, et al: Cutaneous HIV-associated Kaposi sarcoma. Dermatol Online J 2017; 23.

Bender Ignacio R, et al: Evolving Paradigms in HIV Malignancies: Review of Ongoing Clinical Trials. J Natl Compr Canc Netw. 2018; 16(8): 1018-1026. doi: 10.6004/jnccn.2018.7064. Review. PubMed PMID: 30099376; PubMed Central PMCID: PMC6109631.

PDQ Adult Treatment Editorial Board. Kaposi Sarcoma Treatment (PDQ®): Health Professional Version. 2018 Jul 27. PDQ Cancer Information Summaries [Internet]. Bethesda (MD): National Cancer Institute (US); 2002. Available from http://www.ncbi.nlm.nih.gov/books/NBK65897/PubMed PMID: 26389335.

Volkow P, et al: Clinical characteristics, predictors of immune reconstitution inflammatory syndrome and long-term prognosis in patients with Kaposi sarcoma. AIDS Res Ther 2017; 14: 30.

Atypical Vascular Lesion

Atypical vascular lesion (AVL) occurs after mastectomy and radiation. Staghorn-like, thin-walled vessels are present, but endothelial atypia is minimal. Lesions may represent a precursor to malignancy. *MYC* amplification is noted in postirradiation angiosarcomas but not in primary cutaneous angiosarcoma or in other radiation-associated vascular proliferations, such as AVL.

Udager AM, et al: MYC immunohistochemistry in angiosarcoma and atypical vascular lesions. Pathology 2016; 48: 697.

Angiosarcoma

Angiosarcomas of the skin occur in four clinical settings. First and most common are those that occur in the head and neck of elderly people. The male/female ratio is 2:1. The lesion often begins as a poorly defined bluish macule that may be mistaken for a bruise. Distinguishing features are the frequent occurrence of a peripheral erythematous ring, satellite nodules, presence of

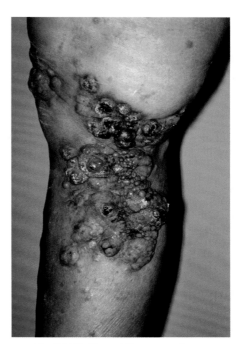

Fig. 28.30 Stewart-Treves syndrome.

intratumoral hemorrhage, and the lesion's tendency to bleed spontaneously or after minimal trauma. The tumor progressively enlarges asymmetrically, often becomes multicentric, and develops indurated bluish nodules and plaques. The sudden development of thrombocytopenia may herald metastatic disease or an enlarging primary tumor.

Solid sheets of atypical epithelioid cells may be present, but more often the pattern is that of subtle infiltration in the dermis, producing the appearance of cracks between collagen bundles. The spaces are lined by hyperchromatic nuclei. Immunoperoxidase staining for endothelial markers such as ERG (an endothelial transcription factor), CD31, CD34, and *Ulex europeus* lectin aids in the diagnosis, and most malignant vascular tumors are positive for podoplanin (D2-40).

The prognosis is worse in men and those older than 70. Surgical excision, and adjuvant radiotherapy radiotherapy are the best options for limited disease. Chemotherapy and radiation therapy for extensive disease are often only palliative, especially when dealing with scalp lesions and high-grade lesions. Doxorubicin-ifosfamide chemotherapy produces a modest response rate. Paclitaxel is now often used as a first-line palliative systemic therapy, achieving an objective response rate of 56%. Pazopanib has been used for taxane-resistant disease. Sirolimus and IFN both show promise for scalp and facial angiosarcomas. Because of the multicentricity of lesions, the frequent occurrence on the face or scalp, and the rapid growth with early metastasis, death occurs in most patients within 2 years.

The second classic clinical situation in which angiosarcoma develops is in chronic lymphedematous areas, as occurs in the upper arm after mastectomy, the so-called Stewart-Treves syndrome (Fig. 28.30). This tumor appears approximately 11–12 years after surgery in an estimated 0.45% of patients. The prognosis is poor for these patients, with a mean survival of 19–31 months and 5-year survival rate of 6%–14%. Metastases to the lungs are the most frequent cause of death. Early amputation offers the best hope.

A third setting includes tumors that develop in previously irradiated sites. If the condition for which radiation therapy was given was a benign one, the average interval between radiation and development of angiosarcoma is 23 years. If the preceding illness was a malignant condition, the interval is shortened to 12 years. Again, the prognosis is poor, with survival generally between

6 months and 2 years after diagnosis. Many patients with the Stewart-Treves syndrome received radiation, and radiation may play a pathogenic role.

Angiosarcomas develop in settings other than those previously described, and this small miscellaneous subset comprises the fourth category. An angiosarcoma producing granulocyte colony-stimulating factor was associated with prominent peripheral leukocytosis.

Harker D, et al: MYC amplification in angiosarcomas arising in the setting of chronic lymphedema of morbid obesity. J Cutan Pathol 2017; 44: 15.

Lee BL, et al: Investigation of prognostic features in primary cutaneous and soft tissue angiosarcoma after surgical resection. Ann Plast Surg 2017; 78: S41.

Ogata D, et al: Pazopanib treatment slows progression and stabilizes disease in patients with taxane-resistant cutaneous angiosarcoma. Med Oncol 2016; 33: 116.

Sholl LM, et al: Radiation-associated neoplasia. Histopathology 2017; 70: 70.

FIBROUS TISSUE ABNORMALITIES

Keloid

A keloid is a firm, irregularly shaped, fibrous, hyperpigmented, pink or red excrescence. The growth usually arises as the result of a cut, laceration, or burn—or less often an acne pustule on the chest or upper back—and spreads beyond the limits of the original injury, often sending out clawlike (cheloid) prolongations. The overlying epidermis is smooth, glossy, and thinned from pressure. The early, growing lesion is red and tender and has the consistency of rubber. It is often surrounded by an erythematous halo, and the keloid may be telangiectatic. Lesions may be tender, painful, and pruritic and may rarely ulcerate or develop draining sinus tracts.

Keloids are often multiple (Fig. 28.31). They may be as tiny as pinheads or as large as an orange. Those that follow burns and scalds are large. Lesions are often linear, frequently having bulbous expansions at each end. The surface may be larger than the base, so that the edges are overhanging. The most common location is the sternal region, but keloids also occur frequently on the neck, ears, extremities, or trunk and rarely on the face, palms, or soles. The earlobes are often involved as a result of ear piercing, but involvement of the central face is rare. Keloids are much more common and grow to larger dimensions in black persons than others.

Why certain individuals develop keloids remains unsolved. Trauma is usually the immediate causative factor, but this induces

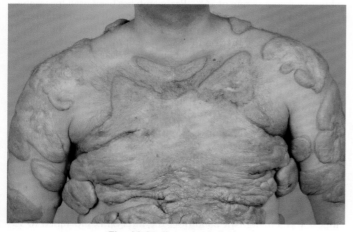

Fig. 28.31 Extensive keloids.

keloids only in those with a predisposition for their development. There is also a regional predisposition.

Histologically, a keloid is a dense and sharply defined nodular growth of myofibroblasts and collagen with a whorl-like arrangement resembling hypertrophic scar. Centrally, thick hyalinized bundles of collagen are present and distinguish keloids from hypertrophic scars. Elastic tissue is scanty, as in a scar. Through pressure, the tumor causes thinning of the normal papillary dermis and atrophy of adjacent appendages, which it pushes aside. Mucopolysaccharides are increased, and often there are numerous mast cells.

Keloids are usually distinctive. They may be distinguished from hypertrophic scars by their clawlike projections, which are absent in the hypertrophic scar; the extension of the keloid beyond the confines of the original injury; and the presence of thick, hyalinized collagen bundles histologically. Frequently, spontaneous improvement of the hypertrophic scar occurs over months, but not in the keloid. Atypical lesions should be biopsied because carcinoma en cuirasse may mimic keloid.

Initial treatment is usually by means of intralesional injection of triamcinolone suspension alone or in combination with 5-fluorouracil (5-FU), methotrexate, verapamil, and/or long-pulsed Nd:YAG laser or light-emitting diode. Using a 30-gauge needle on a 1-mL tuberculin Luer syringe, triamcinolone suspension is injected into various parts of the lesion; 40 mg/mL is generally used for initial treatment, although as the lesion softens, 10–20 mg/mL may be sufficient to produce involution with less risk of surrounding hypopigmentation and atrophy related to lymphatic spread of the corticosteroid. Injections are repeated at intervals of 6–8 weeks, as required. Flattening and cessation of itching are reliably achieved by this approach and in some cases may even be achieved with topical corticosteroids. The lesions are never made narrower, however, and hyperpigmentation generally persists. 5-FU can produce responses in refractory keloids but is associated with a somewhat higher risk of hyperpigmentation, pain, and ulceration after injection. Bleomycin is being investigated alone and in combination with triamcinolone. Transforming growth factor (TGF)–β is known to be involved in keloid formation, and triamcinolone acetonide–induced decreases in cellular proliferation and collagen production are associated with a statistically significant decrease in the level of TGF-β1 in both normal and keloid fibroblast cell lines. Anti–TGF-β1 therapy looks promising, as does nuclear factor (NF)–κB inhibition and green tea polyphenol epigallocatechin-3-gallate.

Other approaches to treatment include flashlamp pulsed dye laser treatment, which is also associated with reduced expression of TGF-β1. Cryosurgery (including contact, intralesional needle cryoprobe, and spray), intralesional etanercept, and calcium channel blockers have some demonstrated efficacy in the treatment of keloids. Fibroblasts derived from the central part of keloids grow faster than peripheral keloid and nonkeloid fibroblasts. Verapamil has been shown to decrease interleukin-6 (IL-6) and VEGF in these cultured cells and to inhibit cell growth.

If surgical removal by excision is feasible, and if narrowing of the keloid is a vitally important goal, the keloid may be excised. After the excision, intralesional injection of triamcinolone or IFN alfa-2b may be combined with postoperative irradiation or topical application of imiquimod. Silicone sheeting, gel, and pressure are other adjunctive methods used to limit recurrences. Results with these modalities have been mixed, and a Cochrane review concluded that the quality of evidence supporting silicone sheeting is generally poor. Keloids demonstrate an increased number of mast cells, and silicone gel–sheet treatment has been shown to reduce lesional mast cell numbers and decrease itching. Banding at the base of the keloid with a suture ligature for 5 weeks has been used successfully to treat pedunculated lesions.

Pierced-ear keloids occur with considerable frequency. When the keloid is young, intralesional injection of triamcinolone is frequently sufficient to control the problem. In old keloids, excision of the lesion using lidocaine with triamcinolone, followed by injections at 2-week intervals, produces good results. CO_2 laser excision has also been successful in old, mature keloids in this site.

Alexandrescu D, et al: Comparative results in treatment of keloids with intralesional 5-FU/kenalog, 5-FU/verapamil, enalapril alone, verapamil alone, and laser. J Drugs Dermatol 2016; 15: 1442.
Ali FR, et al: Laser treatment of keloid scars. Dermatol Surg 2017; 43: 318.
Awad SM, et al: Suppression of transforming growth factor-beta1 expression in keloids after cryosurgery. Cryobiology 2017; 75: 151.
Chen XE, et al: Combined effects of long-pulsed neodymium-yttrium-aluminum-garnet laser, diprospan and 5-fluorouracil in the treatment of keloid scars. Exp Ther Med 2017; 13: 3607.
Hsu KC, et al: Review of silicone gel sheeting and silicone gel for the prevention of hypertrophic scars and keloids. Wounds 2017; 29: 154.
Huang L, et al: A study of the combination of triamcinolone and 5-fluorouracil in modulating keloid fibroblasts in vitro. J Plast Reconstr Aesthet Surg 2013; 66: e251.
Lee HS, et al: Low-level light therapy with 10 nm light emitting diode suppresses collagen synthesis in human keloid fibroblasts. Ann Dermatol 2017; 29: 149.
Mankowski P, et al: Optimizing radiotherapy for keloids. Ann Plast Surg 2017; 78: 403.
O'Brien L, et al: Silicone gel sheeting for preventing and treating hypertrophic and keloid scars. Cochrane Database Syst Rev 2013; 9: CD003826.
Saha AK, et al: A comparative clinical study on role of 5-fluorouracil versus triamcinolone in the treatment of keloids. Indian J Surg 2012; 74: 326.

Dupuytren Contracture

Dupuytren contracture is a fibromatosis of the palmar aponeurosis. The lesion arises most frequently in men between ages 30 and 50 as multiple firm nodules in the palm. Usually, three to five nodules about 1 cm in diameter develop, proximal to the fourth finger. Later, the fibromatosis produces contractures, which may be disabling. The condition occurs at times with alcoholic cirrhosis, diabetes mellitus, muscular dystrophy, and chronic epilepsy. It is also associated with Peyronie disease, plantar fibromatosis, and knuckle pads. In some cases there is a familial predisposition. The fibrous nodules are composed of myofibroblasts that express androgen receptors. 5α-Dihydrotestosterone induces an increase in Dupuytren fibroblast proliferation. In contrast to deep fibromatoses, which behave more aggressively, superficial fibromatoses lack β-catenin and adenomatous polyposis coli (APC) gene mutations.

Early disease may respond well to intralesional triamcinolone, collagenase, or percutaneous needle fasciotomy, but surgical excision of the involved palmar fascia may be the only way to liberate severely contracted fingers. Androgen blockade represents a potential avenue of pharmacologic therapy. As with keloids, TGF-β2 inhibition appears promising.

Plantar Fibromatosis

The plantar analog of Dupuytren contracture, plantar fibromatosis (Ledderhose disease), occurs as slowly enlarging nodules on the soles that ultimately cause difficulty in walking or even weight bearing. The diagnosis is usually made clinically, but both biopsy and MRI can be used to confirm the diagnosis. The usual surgical treatment is wide excision of the plantar fascia. Subtotal excision is associated with a high rate of recurrence. Although adjuvant radiotherapy is effective in decreasing the recurrence rate, it has a significant complication rate, with functional impairment. As with other forms of fibromatosis, intralesional injection of triamcinolone acetonide or collagenase may represent nonsurgical alternatives.

Peyronie Disease

Plastic induration of the penis is a fibrous infiltration of the intercavernous septum of the penis. This fibrosis results in the formation of nodules or plaques. As a result of these plaques, a fibrous chordee is produced, and curvature of the penis occurs on erection, sometimes so severe as to make intromission difficult or impossible. In some patients, pain may be severe. The association of Peyronie disease with Dupuytren contracture has been recognized.

Injection of IFN alfa-2b, verapamil, or collagenase has been used. Intralesional triamcinolone suspension injected or iontophoresed into the plaques and nodules has shown mixed results. Oral therapies include tocopherol (vitamin E), para-aminobenzoate, colchicine, tamoxifen, and acetyl-L-carnitine, but data supporting oral therapy are weak. Surgical correction tailored to the degree of deformity is often successful. Extracorporeal shock wave therapy may reduce penile pain but may worsen curvature.

Bear BJ, et al: Treatment of recurrent Dupuytren contracture in joints previously effectively treated with collagenase *Clostridium histolyticum.* J Hand Surg Am 2017; 42: 391.e1.
Lauritzson A, Atroshi I: Collagenase injections for Dupuytren's disease. BMJ Open 2017; 7: e012943.

Lipofibromatosis

Lipofibromatosis is a rare tumor of infancy that typically presents as a poorly demarcated, slow-growing soft tissue mass on an extremity. It is sometimes associated with other defects, such as syndactyly, cleft lip and palate, trigonocephaly, and atrial septal defect. Histologically, mature fat is separated by collagenous septa containing fibroblasts and myofibroblasts. A subtle honeycomb pattern of fibrosis may be noted at the edge of the fat lobule.

Boos MD, et al: Lipofibromatosis. Pediatr Dermatol 2014; 31: 298.

Knuckle Pads

Knuckle pads (heloderma) are well-defined, round, plaquelike, fibrous thickenings that develop on the extensor aspects of the proximal interphalangeal joints of the toes and fingers (Fig. 28.32), including the thumbs. They develop at any age and grow to about 10–15 mm in diameter over a few weeks or months, then persist permanently. They are flesh colored or somewhat brown, with normal or slightly hyperkeratotic epidermis overlying and adherent to them. They are a part of the skin and are freely movable over underlying structures.

Knuckle pads are sometimes associated with Dupuytren contracture, clubbing, or camptodactylia (irreducible flexion contracture of one or more fingers). Some cases are familial, and some are related to trauma or frequent knuckle cracking. Autosomal dominant associations of knuckle pads, mixed hearing loss, keratoderma, and leukonychia have been reported, including Bart-Pumphrey syndrome (*GB72* mutations). Knuckle pads have also been associated with autosomal dominant epidermolytic palmoplantar keratoderma with a mutation in keratin 9.

Histologically, the lesions are fibromas. They are differentiated clinically from the nodular type of neurodermatitis and from the small, hemispheric pitted papules that may develop over the knuckles after frostbite or in acrocyanosis, and from rheumatic nodules. Treatment with intralesional injection of corticosteroids may be beneficial. As with keloids, intralesional 5-FU may be beneficial.

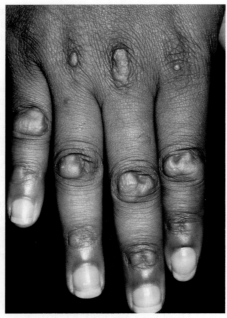

Fig. 28.32 Knuckle pads. (Courtesy Curt Samlaska, MD.)

Luber AJ, et al: Characterization of knuckle (Garrod) pads using optical coherence tomography in vivo. Cutis 2015; 96: E10.

Pachydermodactyly

Pachydermodactyly represents a benign fibromatosis of the fingers. There is a fullness of the medial and lateral digit just proximal to the proximal interphalangeal joint. This asymptomatic process most often is first noted in adolescence and usually involves multiple fingers. It can be misdiagnosed as juvenile idiopathic arthritis. Five types have been described: classic, localized, transgrediens (abnormality extends to metacarpophalangeal areas), familial, and pachydermodactyly associated with tuberous sclerosis. Some cases may result from repetitive ticlike obsessive-compulsive behaviors. Increased collagen or mucin accounts for the swelling. Patients with pachydermodactyly associated with repetitive tics respond to treatment for the obsessive-compulsive disorder.

El-Hallak M, et al: Pachydermodactyly mimicking juvenile idiopathic arthritis. Arthritis Rheum 2013; 65: 2736.

Desmoid Tumor

Desmoid tumors occur as large, deep-seated, well-circumscribed masses arising from the muscular aponeurosis. They most frequently occur on the abdominal wall, especially in women during or soon after pregnancy. Desmoid tumors have been divided into five types: abdominal wall, extraabdominal, intraabdominal, multiple, and those occurring in Gardner syndrome/familial adenomatous polyposis. They recur locally and can kill if they invade, surround, or compress vital structures. The most dangerous desmoid tumors are therefore those at the root of the neck and the intraabdominal type. MRI will aid in the evaluation of soft tissue extension and recurrence after treatment. Mutations in the β-catenin gene correlate with local recurrence. Treatment may be with wide local excision, radiotherapy, or hormonal manipulation. High-dose tamoxifen in combination with sulindac has been effective. Mesenteric desmoid tumors have been treated with antiangiogenic therapy with toremifene and IFN alfa-2b. Imatinib mesylate appears promising.

Skubitz KM: Biology and treatment of aggressive fibromatosis or desmoid tumor. Mayo Clin Proc 2017; 92: 947.

Collagenous Fibroma (Desmoplastic Fibroblastoma)

This slow-growing, deep-set, benign fibrous tumor is usually located in the deep subcutis, fascia, aponeurosis, or skeletal muscle of the extremities, limb girdles, or head and neck regions, including mucosa. It is characterized by hypocellularity and dense bands of hyalinized collagen that may infiltrate into skeletal muscle. Despite this, recurrence is unlikely after excision. Chromosomal translocation (2; 11)(q31; q12) and trisomy 8 have been reported. Tumor cells stain for vimentin and may stain for actin, but have been negative for CD34, S-100 protein, keratin, CD68, desmin, and β-catenin.

Pereira TD, et al: Desmoplastic fibroblastoma (collagenous fibroma) of the oral cavity. J Clin Exp Dent 2016 Feb 1; 8: e89.

Aponeurotic Fibroma

Aponeurotic fibroma has also been called juvenile aponeurotic fibroma (calcifying fibroma). It is a tumor-like proliferation characterized by the appearance of slow-growing, cystlike masses that occur on the limbs, especially the hands and feet. Histologically, the distinctive lesions are sharply demarcated and composed of collagenous stroma showing acid mucopolysaccharides infiltrated by plump mesenchymal cells with oval nuclei. Hyalinized areas are also present, suggesting chondroid or osteoid metaplasia. An aid to the diagnosis is stippled calcification, readily seen on radiographs. Surgical excision is the treatment of choice and can be guided by MRI.

Shim SW, et al: MRI features of calcifying aponeurotic fibroma in the upper arm. Skeletal Radiol 2016; 45: 1139.

Infantile Myofibromatosis

Infantile myofibromatosis is the most common fibrous tumor of infancy. Eighty percent of patients have solitary lesions, with half of these occurring on the head and neck. About 60% are present at or soon after birth.

Congenital generalized fibromatosis is an uncommon condition that presents at birth or soon after. It is characterized by multiple, firm, dermal and subcutaneous nodules. Skeletal lesions, primarily of the metaphyseal regions of the long bones, occur in 50% of patients. If only the skin and bones develop fibromas, the prognosis is excellent, with spontaneous resolution of the lesions and with no complications expected in the first 1–2 years of life. Some refer to this limited disease as "congenital multiple fibromatosis." Females more frequently contract the generalized disease.

The fibromas may involve the viscera, including the GI tract, breast, lungs, liver, pancreas, tongue, serosal surfaces, lymph nodes, or kidney. Autosomal dominant inheritance has been reported, and mutations in *PDGFRB* and *NOTCH3* have been described. Histologically, fascicles of spindle cells occur in a whorled pattern. These nodules are composed of myofibroblasts.

Mortality rate in the more widespread subset is high; 80% die of obstruction or compression of vital organs. Patients who survive past 4 months have spontaneous regression of their disease. Translocation-associated cases may respond to tyrosine kinase inhibitors imatinib and sunitinib with or without low-dose chemotherapy.

Diffuse Infantile Fibromatosis

This process occurs within the first 3 years of life and is usually confined to the muscles of the arms, neck, and shoulder area. There is multicentric infiltration of muscle fibers with fibroblasts resembling those in aponeurotic fibromas. Calcification does not occur. Recurrence after excision occurs in about one third of patients.

Aggressive Infantile Fibromatosis

The clinical presentation of this locally recurring, nonmetastasizing lesion involves single or multiple, fast-growing masses that are present at birth or that occur within the first year of life. Infantile fibromatosis may be seen in any location, although the arms, legs, and trunk are the usual sites. Histologically, it is hypercellular and mimics malignancy.

Mota F, et al: Infantile myofibromatosis—a clinical and pathological diagnostic challenge. Dermatol Online J 2017; 23.
Murray N, et al: The spectrum of infantile myofibromatosis includes both non-penetrance and adult recurrence. Eur J Med Genet 2017; 60: 353.

Hyaline Fibromatosis Syndrome (Juvenile Hyaline Fibromatosis and Infantile Systemic Hyalinosis)

Juvenile hyaline fibromatosis and infantile systemic hyalinosis are allelic autosomal recessive conditions characterized by multiple subcutaneous skin nodules, hyaline deposition, gingival hypertrophy, osteolytic bone lesions, and joint contractures. Nodular tumors of the scalp, face, and extremities usually appear in early childhood. Pink confluent papules may occur on the paranasal folds, periauricular area (Fig. 28.33), and perianal region. The gene has been mapped to chromosome 4q21 and the anthrax toxin receptor 2 gene (*ANTXR2*). Histologically, fibroblasts with fine, intracytoplasmic eosinophilic granules are embedded in a homogeneous eosinophilic dermal ground substance. Ultrastructurally, the fibroblasts demonstrate defective synthesis of collagen, deposited as fibrillogranular material.

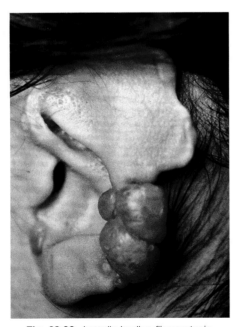

Fig. 28.33 Juvenile hyaline fibromatosis.

Baltacioglu E, et al: Juvenile hyaline fibromatosis. Indian J Dermatol 2017; 62: 210.

Infantile Digital Fibromatosis (Infantile Digital Myofibroblastoma, Inclusion Body Fibroma)

Infantile digital fibromatosis is a rare neoplasm of infancy and childhood that usually occurs on the dorsal or lateral aspects of the distal phalanges of the toes and fingers. The thumb and great toe are usually spared. These asymptomatic, firm, red, smooth nodules occur during the first year of life, 47% in the first month. Rare congenital lesions have been noted. The lesions do not metastasize but may infiltrate deeply. Histologically, the epidermis is normal, but the dermis is infiltrated with proliferating myofibroblasts and collagen bundles. Eosinophilic cytoplasmic inclusions in many of the fibroblasts are characteristic. Treatment by surgical excision has a high risk of recurrence, and conservative, nonsurgical management is often appropriate. Spontaneous regression is generally noted, but the lesion may cause functional impairment and may infiltrate deeply before regression occurs. Mohs micrographic surgery has been performed successfully using both trichrome staining and smooth muscle actin staining to demonstrate the inclusion bodies within tumor cells.

Marks E, et al: Infantile digital fibroma. Arch Pathol Lab Med 2016; 140: 1153.

Fibrous Hamartoma of Infancy

Fibrous hamartoma of infancy is a single dermal or subcutaneous firm nodule of the upper trunk that is present at birth or shortly thereafter. Overlying skin changes are uncommon but may include increased hair, alteration in pigmentation, and eccrine gland hyperplasia with hyperhidrosis. Most cases are solitary, but multiple tumors have been reported; 91% of lesions are noted within the first year of life, and 23% are congenital. The male/female ratio is 2.4:1. Most lesions occur in the axillary region, upper arm, upper trunk, inguinal region, and external genital area. An association with Williams syndrome has been reported. Biopsy shows an organoid pattern with different types of tissue organized in whorls or bands. In early lesions, lobules of mature fat are interspersed between myxoid and fibrous areas. Myxoid zones have primitive mesenchymal cells with stellate nuclei. Fibrosing areas demonstrate delicate collagen bundles and many elongated fibroblast nuclei. Very rarely, fibrosarcomatous features may be present. EGFR exon 20 insertion/duplication mutations have been described. The overlying skin may demonstrate abortive hair follicles, and many eccrine units may be present. Complex chromosomal translocations have been reported. Over time, both the myxoid and the fibrosing areas develop into cell-poor fibrous areas with thick collagen bundles. There is no recurrence after excision.

Al-Ibraheemi A, et al: Fibrous hamartoma of infancy. Mod Pathol 2017; 30: 474.
Park JY, et al: EGFR exon 20 insertion/duplication mutations characterize fibrous hamartoma of infancy. Am J Surg Pathol 2016; 40: 1713.

Fibromatosis Colli

In fibromatosis colli, there is a fibrous tissue proliferation infiltrating the lower third of the sternocleidomastoid muscle at birth. Fine-needle aspiration is useful to confirm the diagnosis. Spontaneous remission occurs within a few months. Occasionally, some patients are left with a wryneck deformity; however, this complication is amenable to surgery.

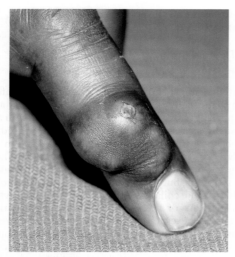

Fig. 28.34 Giant cell tumor of the tendon sheath.

Tenosynovial Giant Cell Tumor (Giant Cell Tumor of the Tendon Sheath and Pigmented Villonodular Tenosynovitis)

This giant cell tumor is most frequently attached to the tendons of the fingers (Fig. 28.34), hands, and wrists and has a predilection for the flexor surfaces. It is firm, 1–3 cm in diameter, and does not spontaneously involute. It recurs after excision in approximately 25% of cases. Fibroma of the tendon sheath represents a variant of the giant cell tumor that lacks giant cells. The fibroma tends to occur more in younger men (average age at onset 30) than the giant cell variety. When a proliferation similar to giant cell tumor of the tendon sheath occurs in deeper tissues, it is referred to as pigmented villonodular tenosynovitis. The pigment is hemosiderin.

Histologically, the giant cell tumor consists of lobules of densely hyalinized collagen. The characteristic osteoclast-like giant cells have deeply eosinophilic cytoplasm that molds to adjacent cells. Oval gray fibroblast nuclei are present throughout the lesion. Lipophages and siderophages may be numerous, and hemosiderin deposition may impart a brown color to the lesions on gross examination. The fibroma of the tendon sheath generally lacks lipophages and siderophages as well as giant cells, with the lobules composed of dense, fibrocollagenous tissue with oval gray fibroblast nuclei.

The rate of recurrence depends on the presence or absence of a pseudocapsule, lobulation of the tumor, extraarticular location, and presence of satellite lesions. Local recurrence has been treated with more extensive surgery, and imaging studies can define the extent of the tumor. Radiation therapy has been reported anecdotally.

Gouin F, et al: Localized and diffuse forms of tenosynovial giant cell tumor (formerly giant cell tumor of the tendon sheath and pigmented villonodular synovitis). Orthop Traumatol Surg Res 2017; 103: S91.

Ainhum

Ainhum is also known as dactylolysis spontanea, bankokerend, and sukhapakla. It is a disease affecting the toes, especially the fifth toe, characterized by a linear constriction around the affected digit that ultimately leads to the spontaneous amputation of the distal part. It occurs chiefly among black men in Africa. Usually, ainhum is unilateral but may be bilateral.

The disease begins with a transverse groove in the skin on the flexor surface of the toe, usually beneath the first interphalangeal articulation. The furrow is produced by a ringlike fibrosis and an induration of the dermis. It deepens and extends laterally around the toe until the two ends meet, so that the digit becomes constricted, as if in a ligature. The constricted part becomes swollen, soft, and after a time, greatly distended. Ulceration may result in a malodorous discharge, with pain and gangrene. The course of the disease is slow, but in 5–10 years, spontaneous amputation occurs, generally at a joint.

The cause is unknown. The condition may result from chronic trauma and exposure to the elements by walking barefoot in the tropics. Fissuring followed by chronic inflammation and fibrosis may then result.

Treatment in early cases by cutting the constricting band is unsuccessful. In advanced cases, amputation of the affected member is advisable. Surgical correction by Z-plasty has produced good results. Intralesional injection of betamethasone (15 injections total) has also been successful.

Pseudoainhum

Pseudoainhum has been a term used in connection with certain hereditary and nonhereditary diseases in which annular constriction of digits occurs. Hereditary disorders include hereditary palmoplantar keratodermas, especially Vohwinkel syndrome and mal de Meleda, pachyonychia congenita, Ehlers-Danlos syndrome, erythropoietic protoporphyria, and keratoderma with universal atrichia. Nonhereditary disorders associated with constriction of digits include ainhum, Hansen disease, cholera, ancylostomiasis, scleroderma, Raynaud syndrome, pityriasis rubra pilaris, psoriasis, Olmsted syndrome, Reynold syndrome (scleroderma and primary biliary cirrhosis with antimitochondrial antibodies), syringomyelia, ergot poisoning, gout, and spinal cord tumors. Factitial pseudoainhum may be produced by self-application of a rubber band, string, or other ligature. Congenital cases have been reported that may affect digits or limbs. Pseudoainhum may occur as a familial condition or may be secondary to amniotic bands. Treatment includes surgery or intralesional injection of corticosteroids, as in ainhum. Retinoids may be used in responsive diseases.

Connective Tissue Nevi

Connective tissue nevi are uncommon lesions that may present as acquired isolated plaques, as multiple lesions (acquired or congenital), or as one finding in a more generalized disease. Biopsy findings include abnormal collagen bundles and altered amounts elastin. These lesions characteristically occur on the trunk, most often in the lumbosacral area (Fig. 28.35). Although solitary lesions occur, they are often multiple and may show a linear or zosteriform arrangement. Individual lesions are slightly elevated plaques 1–15 cm in diameter, varying in color from light yellow to orange, with a surface texture resembling shagreen leather. In Proteus syndrome, the connective tissue nevi are present as plantar, or occasionally palmar, masses with a cerebriform surface. Connective tissue nevi of the acquired type have been classified as eruptive collagenomas, isolated collagenomas, or isolated elastomas, depending on the number of lesions and the predominant dermal fibers present. They cannot be differentiated clinically.

Hereditary types of connective tissue nevi include dermatofibrosis lenticularis disseminata in the Buschke-Ollendorff syndrome, familial cutaneous collagenoma, and the shagreen patches seen in tuberous sclerosis. Buschke-Ollendorff syndrome is an autosomal dominant inherited disorder in which widespread dermal papules and plaques develop asymmetrically over the trunk and limbs. Elastic fiber thickening, highly variable fiber diameter, and desmosine increases threefold to sevenfold above normal have been described in these patients. The associated feature of osteopoikilosis is asymptomatic but is diagnostic of the syndrome in x-ray evaluation. Focal sclerotic densities are seen, primarily in the long

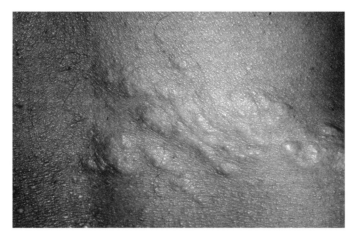

Fig. 28.35 Connective tissue nevus.

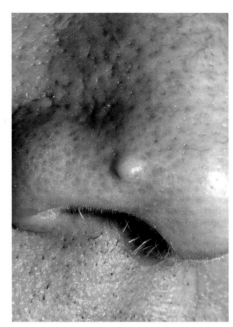

Fig. 28.36 Fibrous papule of the nose. (Courtesy Curt Samlaska, MD.)

bones, pelvis, and hands. Buschke-Ollendorff syndrome is highly variable, and familial inheritance of elastic tissue nevi without evidence of osteopoikilosis has been reported.

Papular elastorrhexis is characterized by multiple white, evenly scattered papules, usually occurring on the trunk. Elastic fibers are decreased and may appear thin and fragmented. Most reported cases are sporadic, but familial occurrence has been described.

Patients with familial cutaneous collagenomas may present with numerous symmetric, asymptomatic dermal nodules on the back. The age of onset is usually in the middle to late teens. In patients with the inherited disease, multiple endocrine neoplasia type I (MEN-I) multiple collagenomas were reported in 23 of 32 patients. These were less than 3 mm in diameter and were on the upper torso, neck, and shoulders. They occurred in association with many other cutaneous findings, including angiofibromas, café au lait macules, and lipomas. Atrioseptal defect has also been reported in association with familial collagenomas.

The collagenomas of tuberous sclerosis are associated with adenoma sebaceum, periungual fibromas, and ash-leaf macules. Because at least half the cases of tuberous sclerosis result from new mutations, all patients with connective tissue nevi should be carefully studied for evidence of tuberous sclerosis, even in the absence of a family history of the disease. Isolated plantar collagenoma may exhibit a cerebriform appearance and resemble plantar fibromas of Proteus syndrome.

Eruptive collagenomas may be widespread or localized. Mucinous nevus is a form of connective tissue nevus characterized by increased ground substance without increases in collagen or elastin. Histologically, collagen bundles are widely separated by mucin and may be attenuated. Overlying follicular induction similar to that seen in dermatofibromas may be present. Both eruptive collagenoma and mucinous nevus have been described as a manifestation of syphilis.

Batra P, et al: Eruptive collagenomas. Dermatol Online J 2010; 16: 3.
McCuaig CC, et al: Connective tissue nevi in children. J Am Acad Dermatol 2012; 67: 890.

Elastofibroma Dorsi

Elastofibroma dorsi is a benign tumor usually located in the deep soft tissues in the subscapular region, but sometimes at other sites. The tumor is firm and unencapsulated and measures up to several centimeters in diameter. It is believed to represent an unusual response to repeated trauma. Histologically, the tumor consists of abundant compact sclerotic collagen mixed with large, swollen, irregular elastic fibers, often appearing as globules of elastic tissue. It usually appears on nuclear medicine scans, suggesting it is not as uncommon as once believed. CT and MRI can define the extent of the lesion, and excision is curative.

Deveci MA, et al: Elastofibroma dorsi. Acta Orthop Traumatol Turc 2017; 51: 7.

Angiofibromas

These skin-colored to reddish papules show fibroplasia and varying degrees of vascular proliferation in the upper dermis. Angiofibromas may occur as a solitary nonhereditary form, the fibrous papule of the nose; as multiple nonhereditary lesions, the pearly penile papules; or as multiple hereditary forms, as in tuberous sclerosis, Birt-Hogg-Dube syndrome (in combination with the specific lesion, the fibrofolliculoma), and MEN-I. Reports of agminated or segmental angiofibromas may represent a segmental form of tuberous sclerosis. The multiple hereditary types may respond to rapamycin and are discussed in other chapters.

Cellular angiofibroma typically occurs in the genital region of older women. It consists of small spindle cells arranged in short fascicles and relatively abundant, small, rounded vessels. Cellular angiofibromas may express estrogen and progesterone receptors as well as CD34.

Fibrous Papule of Nose (Fibrous Papule of Face, Benign Solitary Fibrous Papule)

These lesions occur in adults as dome-shaped, sessile, skin-colored, white or reddish papules, 3–6 mm in diameter, on or near the nose (Fig. 28.36). Fibrous papule is usually solitary, but a few lesions can occur. It may be confused with a nevocytic nevus, neurofibroma, granuloma pyogenicum, or a basal cell carcinoma. As with other angiofibromas, fibrous papules demonstrate concentric fibrosis surrounding vessels and adnexal structures. Stellate dermal dendrocytes are often prominent. Clear cell, granular, and epithelioid variants have been described. They stain for factor XIIIa. Large, pyramidal, junctional melanocytes are often noted overlying the lesion, and a superficial shave biopsy may be mistaken for a melanocytic lesion. Conservative excision is curative; recurrence is rare. Multiple lesions should prompt a search for other stigmata of tuberous sclerosis.

Pearly Penile Papules

This is the term given to pearly-white, dome-shaped angiofibromas occurring circumferentially on the coronal margin and sulcus of the glans penis. The lesions may be firm or soft and filiform. Occasionally, lesions are also present on the penile shaft. Pearly penile papules are not uncommon. Patients usually present at age 20–30, concerned that these are condylomata, or are referred as having treatment-resistant venereal warts. These lesions should be distinguished from papillomas, hypertrophic sebaceous glands, and condyloma acuminatum. No treatment is necessary, only reassurance. If treatment is desired, laser ablation or shave excision is effective.

Acral Fibrokeratoma

Acral fibrokeratoma, often called acquired digital fibrokeratoma, is characterized by a pinkish, hyperkeratotic, hornlike projection occurring on a finger, toe, palm, or sole. The projection usually emerges from a collarette of elevated skin. The average age of the patient is 40. The lesion resembles a rudimentary supernumerary digit, cutaneous horn, or neuroma. Onset during immunosuppressive therapy has been reported, and grouped lesions may occur. Multiple periungual lesions are associated with tuberous sclerosis.

Histologic sections show a central core of thick collagen bundles interwoven closely in a vertical position. This is surrounded by capillaries and a fine network of reticulum fibers. Stellate dermal dendrocytes may be present, as in fibrous papule. Simple surgical excision or laser ablation at the level of the skin surface is effective. The term *acquired reactive digital fibroma* has been proposed for a unique form of posttraumatic dermal nodular fibrous proliferation present on the digits. The lesions are composed of haphazard fascicles of spindle cells that express vimentin and occasionally CD34.

Marchini M, et al: Tuberous sclerosis complex. N Engl J Med 2017; 376: e42.
Wheless JW, et al: A novel topical rapamycin cream for the treatment of facial angiofibromas in tuberous sclerosis complex. J Child Neurol 2013; 28: 933.

Familial Myxovascular Fibromas

Multiple verrucous papules on the palms and fingers have been described that on biopsy show focal neovascularization and mucin-like changes in the papillary dermis. Clinically, these lesions closely resemble warts. They have been reported in several family members, with a probable autosomal dominant inheritance.

Superficial Acral Fibromyxoma (Digital Fibromyxoma)

Superficial acral fibromyxoma typically appears in the superficial soft tissues of the acral extremity of an adult. Most are painless. Histologically, they are characterized by a moderately cellular proliferation of bland, spindled and stellate fibroblasts with a loose storiform or fascicular growth pattern. Mucin and small blood vessels are prominent. Spindle cells typically express CD34, CD99, and epithelial membrane antigen. CD10 and nestin expression have also been reported. Conventional and Mohs excision have been used.

Hankinson A, et al: Superficial acral fibromyxoma (digital fibromyxoma). Dermatol Surg 2016; 42: 897.

Subungual Exostosis

Subungual exostosis is closely related to solitary osteochondroma, and both are found beneath the distal edge of the nail, most frequently of the great toe. Rarely, the terminal phalanges of other toes, particularly the little toe, or even the fingers, may be involved. The exostosis is seen mainly in women between ages 12 and 30. The first appearance is a small pinkish growth projecting slightly beyond the inner free edge of the nail. The overlying nail becomes brittle and either breaks or is removed, after which the tumor, being released, mushrooms upward and distally above the level of the nail. It grows slowly to a maximum diameter of about 8 mm. Pressure of the shoe on the lesion causes great pain.

Subungual exostosis must be differentiated from pyogenic granuloma, verruca vulgaris, pterygium inverum unguis, ingrowing nail, and glomus tumor. If subungual exostosis is suspected, the diagnosis can be confirmed by radiographic examination. Complete excision or curettage is the proper method of treatment. Secondary intention healing is generally good. Vacuum-assisted closure has been used for large wounds.

Russell JD, et al: Subungual exostosis. Cutis 2016; 98: 128.

Chondrodermatitis Nodularis Chronica Helicis

This small, nodular, tender, chronic inflammatory lesion occurs on the helix of the ear. Most patients are men. The lesions are not uncommon, and sometimes as many as 12 nodules may arrange themselves along the edge of the upper helix. The lesions are 2–4 mm in diameter, well defined, slightly reddish, and extremely tender. At times, the surface is covered by an adherent scale or a shallow ulcer. After the masses have reached a certain size, growth ceases, but the lesions persist unchanged for years. There is no tendency to malignant change. Similar lesions may occur on the anthelix, predominantly in women.

Chondrodermatitis nodularis chronica helicis is produced by ischemic necrosis of the dermis and generally occurs on the side the patient favors during sleep. The patient may have a history of frostbite, chronic trauma, or chronic actinic exposure with concomitant actinically induced lesions of the face and dorsal hands.

Histologically, a zone of eosinophilic necrosis of collagen is flanked by granulation tissue. Overlying acanthosis and hyperkeratosis and central ulceration may be present. The histologic changes resemble those of a decubitus ulcer, but on a smaller scale. Occasionally, bizarre reactive fibroblasts are noted, as in atypical decubital fibroplasia.

Topical nitroglycerin is effective in some patients with chondrodermatitis nodularis chronica helicis, and pressure-induced ischemia can be reduced with the use of a self-adhering foam before sleep. Refractory lesions may be removed by shave technique, or the underlying cartilage may be excised or fenestrated to reduce pressure on the overlying skin during sleep. Photodynamic therapy has also been used. The patient may be encouraged to change sleeping positions, but many find this difficult. Pillows with an ear slot are also available.

Kechichian E, et al: Management of chondrodermatitis nodularis helicis. Dermatol Surg. 2016; 42: 1125.
Shah S, Fiala KH: Chondrodermatitis nodularis helicis. Dermatol Ther 2017; 30.

Oral Submucous Fibrosis

A distinctive fibrosis of the oral mucosa has become common in the western Pacific basin and South Asia among persons whose diet is heavily seasoned with chili or who chew betel, a compound of the nut of the areca palm, the leaf of the betel pepper, and lime.

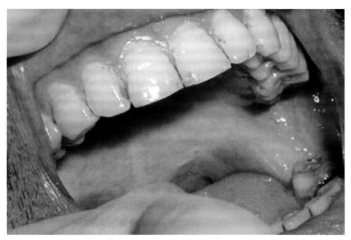

Fig. 28.37 Oral submucous fibrosis. (Courtesy Dr. Shyam Verma.)

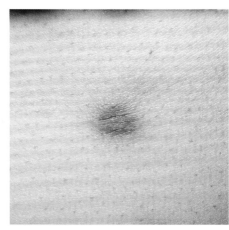

Fig. 28.38 Dermatofibroma. (Courtesy Dr. Lawrence Lieblich.)

The irritation produced first causes a thickening of the palate, tonsillar pillars, and fauces secondary to dermal and muscular fibrosis (Fig. 28.37). As the disease progresses, opening of the mouth and protrusion of the tongue develop, such that eating, swallowing, and speech are impaired. Later, ulceration and leukoplakic areas occur, and finally, in approximately 7% of patients, malignant transformation to squamous cell carcinoma (SCC) develops. Treatment consists of the intralesional injection of triamcinolone or dexamethasone alone or with hyaluronidase or the antioxidant spirulina. In advanced cases, surgical excision and grafting or laser ablation has been used. Discontinuance of the offending substance and physical therapy are also needed.

Arakeri G, et al: Oral submucous fibrosis. J Oral Pathol Med 2017; 46: 413.

Fascial Hernia

Evanescent herniations in the form of nodules appear in the skin where the deep and superficial veins meet as they go through the fascia. These herniated nodules, seen most frequently on the lower extremities, become prominent when the underlying muscles contract, and pain may occur with prolonged exertion. Treatment is not indicated unless the area is chronically painful. Light compression may be effective.

Perineal Skin Tag (Infantile Perianal Pyramidal Protrusion)

Perineal skin tags may be congenital or acquired. They are generally asymptomatic but may require surgical intervention if inflamed or traumatized. A similar appearance may occur as a manifestation of lichen sclerosus.

Cutaneous Pseudosarcomatous Polyp and Umbilical Polyp

Cutaneous pseudosarcomatous polyps and umbilical pseudosarcomatous polyps are benign proliferations with a taglike configuration but also dramatic cytologic atypia and pleomorphism. The cells stain positive for vimentin and variably for CD34 and factor XIIIa. Their clinical behavior is benign.

Acrochordon (Fibroepithelial Papilloma, Skin Tag)

Small, flesh-colored to dark-brown, pinhead-sized and larger, sessile and pedunculated papillomas commonly occur on the neck, often in association with small seborrheic keratoses. These tags are also seen frequently in the axillae and on the eyelids and less often on the trunk and groins, where the soft, pedunculated growths often hang on thin stalks. These flesh-colored, teardrop-shaped tags feel like small bags. Occasionally, as a result of twisting of the pedicle, one will become inflamed, tender, and even gangrenous. Both genders have the same incidence, with almost 60% of individuals acquiring acrochordons by age 69. Skin tags often increase in number when the patient is gaining weight or during pregnancy and may be related to the growth hormone–like activity of insulin. They may be associated with diabetes mellitus. In patients preselected for GI complaints, skin tags appear to be more prevalent in those with colonic polyps. This association has not been proved for the general population.

Histologically, acrochordons are characterized by epidermis enclosing a dermal fibrovascular stalk. Smaller lesions often demonstrate seborrheic keratosis–like acanthosis and horn cysts.

Small lesions can be clipped off at the base with little or no anesthesia. Aluminum chloride may be applied for hemostasis if needed. Light electrodesiccation can also be effective. For larger lesions, anesthesia and snip excision are preferred.

An entity that is frequently reported as perianal acrochordons or skinfolds has now been named infantile perianal pyramidal protrusions. This occurs in young children, usually girls, in the midline anterior to the anus. It reduces with time, and no treatment is necessary. Child abuse, genital warts, hemorrhoids, granulomatous lesions of inflammatory bowel disease, or rectal prolapse must be considered in the differential diagnosis of these lesions.

Skin tag–like basal cell carcinomas in childhood should suggest a diagnosis of nevoid basal cell carcinoma syndrome (NBCCS). Biopsy should be performed on acrochordons in children because the lesions are uncommon in this age group and may be the presenting sign of NBCCS.

Dermatofibroma (Fibrous Histiocytoma)

This common skin lesion's appearance is usually sufficiently characteristic to permit clinical diagnosis. Dermatofibroma is generally a single, round or ovoid papule or nodule, about 0.5–1 cm in diameter, that is reddish brown, sometimes with a yellowish hue (Fig. 28.38). The sharply circumscribed nodule is more evident on palpation than expected from inspection. The larger lesions may present an abrupt elevation at the border to form an exteriorized tumor resting on a sessile base.

Dermatofibroma may be elevated or slightly depressed. The hard lesion is adherent to the overlying epidermis, which may be thinner from pressure or even indented, so that there is a dell-like depression over the nodule. In such cases only the depression is seen, but on palpation the true nature of the lesion is found. Fitzpatrick proposed the term *dimple sign* for the depression created over a dermatofibroma when it is grasped gently between thumb and forefinger.

Dermatofibromas seldom occur in children and are encountered mostly in middle-aged adults. Their size generally varies from 4–20 mm, although giant lesions greater than 5 cm occur. After they reach this size, growth ceases, and the harmless lump remains stationary. The principal locations are on the lower extremities, above the elbows, or on the sides of the trunk. Systemic lupus erythematosus, treatment with prednisone or immunosuppressive drugs, chronic myelogenous leukemia, and HIV infection have been associated with the development of multiple dermatofibromas. It is suspected that many dermatofibromas are initiated by injuries to the skin, such as insect bites or blunt trauma.

Histologic examination reveals a dermal mass composed of close whorls of fibrous tissue in which there are numerous spindle or histiocytic cells. The cells have features of fibroblasts and myofibroblasts but are probably of primitive mesenchymal origin. Immunohistochemical studies show that most cells are positive for factor XIIIa and CD10, and negative for MAC387, S-100, and CD34. The tumor is not well circumscribed and may extend into adjacent structures and surround individual collagen bundles at the periphery (collagen trapping). Overlying acanthosis is typical, and induction of primitive epithelial germs or mature follicular structures may be noted. Basal cell carcinoma–like changes often overlie dermatofibromas, but true basal cell carcinoma is quite rare.

At times, large histiocytic cells within the lesion are strikingly atypical ("monster cells"). Occasionally, granular cytoplasm may predominate. Hemosiderin may be present, and foam cells and lipid deposits may be seen. The presence of Touton giant cells containing hemosiderin is pathognomonic of dermatofibroma. There is a great variation in the vascular components. Rarely, the vascularization is pronounced and suggests a form of hemangioma (sclerosing hemangioma). Deep, penetrating dermatofibromas may grow into the subcutaneous tissue through the fibrous septa or with a pushing front of tumor. They lack the extensive lacy and lamellar infiltrative growth pattern of dermatofibrosarcoma protuberans. Deep, fascial, fibrous histiocytomas may involve the fat or muscle at times. Signet ring and plaque-type variants have been described. A pigmented variant has shown histologic overlap with Bednar tumor (pigmented dermatofibrosarcoma protuberans). The lesion stained positive for CD34, a marker usually absent in dermatofibromas.

The clinical appearance of the lesion and its location, chiefly on the lower extremities, are distinctive. Clinically, granular cell tumor, dermatofibrosis lenticularis disseminata, clear cell acanthoma, and melanoma are some of the lesions to be considered. At times, only a biopsy can differentiate these. Progressive enlargement beyond 2 or 3 cm in diameter suggests a malignant fibrous histiocytoma or dermatofibrosarcoma protuberans, and excisional biopsy is indicated.

These lesions usually are asymptomatic and do not require treatment. Involution may occur after many years if the lesion is left alone. Simple reassurance is suggested.

Epithelioid Cell Histiocytoma

Usually solitary but occasionally multiple, these lesions appear as dome-shaped papules composed of bland epithelioid cells. These histiocytomas typically stain for factor XIIIa, and many consider them to be closely related to dermatofibromas.

Dermal Dendrocyte Hamartoma

Dendrocyte hamartoma presents as a rounded, medallion-like lesion on the upper trunk; it is composed of fusiform CD34-positive,

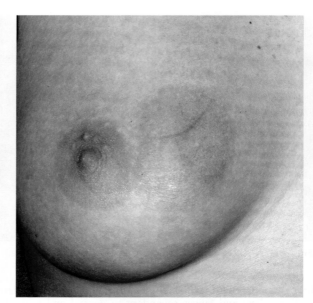

Fig. 28.39 Dermal dendrocyte hamartoma.

factor XIIIa-negative cells in the middle and reticular dermis. The lesions are asymptomatic, brown or erythematous in color, and may have a slightly atrophic, wrinkled surface (Fig. 28.39). The major differential diagnosis is congenital atrophic dermatofibrosarcoma protuberans (DFSP), but to date there has been no evidence of chromosomal abnormalities, such as the t(17; 22)(q22; q13) translocation with the DFSP fusion gene *COL1A1-PDGFB*.

Nodular Fasciitis (Nodular Pseudosarcomatous Fasciitis)

Also known as subcutaneous pseudosarcomatous fibromatosis, this benign mesenchymal neoplasm occurs most often on the arms. Clinically, a firm, solitary, sometimes tender nodule develops in the deep fascia and often extends into the subcutaneous tissue. It usually measures 1–4 cm in diameter. The lesion appears suddenly over a few weeks, without apparent cause, in normal, healthy persons. Gender distribution is equal, and the average age at onset is 40.

Microscopic findings consist of well-defined, loose nodules of stellate and spindled cells that may have a myxoid "tissue culture" appearance. Capillary proliferation is typical, and erythrocyte extravasation between spindle cells is common. Nodular lymphoid infiltrates are often noted within the lesion. On electron microscopic examination, the component cells in the neoplasm have proved to be myofibroblasts. A characteristic t(17; 22)(p13; q13), balanced translocation has been described resulting in *MYH9-USP6* gene fusion.

Dermal, intravascular, and infiltrative variants with ganglionlike cells (proliferative fasciitis) have been described. These are designated when the nodular masses arise in the dermis, in intimate association with blood vessels, or show ganglionlike giant cells and infiltration of collagen. Some lesions respond to intralesional triamcinolone and do not require excision. Recurrence is rare, and the prognosis is excellent. Cranial fasciitis of childhood is an uncommon variant of nodular fasciitis, manifesting as a rapidly enlarging mass in the subcutaneous tissue of the scalp, which may invade the cranium. It occurs in infants and children, resembles nodular fasciitis histologically, and usually does not recur after surgical excision. Some lesions have demonstrated dysregulation of the Wnt/β-catenin pathway.

Proliferative fasciitis and proliferative myositis are closely related entities. Proliferative fasciitis demonstrates irregular extension into the fibrous septa with collagen trapping and ganglionlike nuclei. Proliferative myositis has a similar appearance but extends into adjacent muscle.

Pseudosarcomatous ischemic fasciitis (atypical decubital fibroplasia) is a manifestation of pressure-induced necrosis. The histologic appearance is similar to that of chondrodermatitis nodularis of the ear, only on a much larger scale. A wide zone of fibrinoid necrosis is bordered by granulation tissue and large, atypical fibroblast nuclei that resemble radiation fibroblasts.

Oh BH, et al: Treatment of nodular fasciitis occurring on the face. Ann Dermatol 2015; 27: 694.

Solitary Fibrous Tumor

Solitary fibrous tumors occur in the mediastinum but may also be found in many other parts of the body. They have a diffuse, "patternless" growth pattern and stain strongly positive for CD34. Some express progesterone receptor. Their behavior is unpredictable, and complete excision is recommended. Spindle cell lipomas with few or no lipocytes ("low-fat" and "nonfat" spindle cell lipomas) may be misinterpreted as solitary fibrous tumors because they are also CD34 positive.

Kim JM, et al: Comparison and evaluation of risk factors for meningeal, pleural, and extrapleural solitary fibrous tumors. Pathol Res Pract 2017; 213: 619.

Plexiform Fibrohistiocytic Tumor

The rare plexiform fibrohistiocytic tumor arises primarily on the upper extremities of children and young adults. There is a strong female predisposition. It presents as a slowly growing, painless growth in the subcutaneous tissue. There is usually extension into the dermis or the underlying skeletal muscle. Histologically, it is a distinctly biphasic tumor, with a fibroblastic component mixed with aggregates of mononuclear histiocyte-like cells and multinucleated osteoclast-like cells. The multinucleated cells label for vimentin and CD68, whereas the spindle cells express smooth muscle actin but not factor XIIIa. There is considerable histologic overlap with cellular neurothekeoma. Both tumors are uniformly positive for NKIC3 and CD10. MiTF is strongly and diffusely positive in cellular neurothekeoma but negative in the plexiform fibrohistiocytic tumor, suggesting that the two are distinct. Although most patients are cured with excisional surgery, some tumors will recur locally, and infrequently, regional and systemic metastases can occur.

Lynnhtun K, et al: Plexiform fibrohistiocytic tumour. Histopathology 2012; 60: 1156.

Dermatofibrosarcoma Protuberans

Dermatofibrosarcoma protuberans (DFSP) is characterized by bulky, protuberant, neoplastic masses. Between 50% and 60% occur on the trunk, with less common involvement of the proximal extremities and the head and neck. The disease begins with one or multiple elevated, erythematous, firm nodules or plaques, often associated with a purulent exudate or with ulceration. Patients, usually middle-age, complain of a firm, painless lump in the skin that has been slowly increasing in size for several years. The course is slowly progressive, with pain becoming prominent as the lesion grows, and frequent recurrence after initial conservative surgical intervention (Fig. 28.40). In untreated patients, severe pain and contractures may result. There is minimal tendency to metastasize, although wide dissemination has been reported.

Histologically, DFSP shows a subepidermal fibrotic plaque with uniform spindle cells and variable vascular spaces. In many

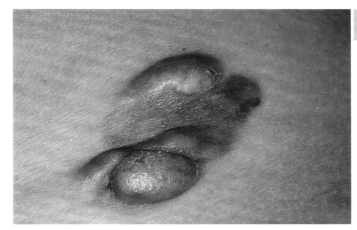

Fig. 28.40 Recurrent dermatofibrosarcoma protuberans.

cases, there is a pronounced matlike woven pattern of spindle cells. Cytogenetic studies typically demonstrate a t(17; 22)(22; q13) fusion involving the *COL1A1* gene on chromosome 17 and the *PDGFB* gene on chromosome 22. Giant cells may be present in small numbers. Pigmented DFSPs, in which the cells contain melanin, predominantly affect persons of color and are called Bednar tumors. CD34 and nestin positivity are characteristic and serve as markers to distinguish DFSP from dermatofibroma. Nestin expression correlates with the degree of invasion. S-100 is negative and may be used to separate spindle cell melanoma from a Bednar tumor. Recurrent DFSP can be myxoid and resembles the diffuse type of neurofibroma histologically. A juvenile variant, called giant cell fibroblastoma, is characterized by a loose arrangement of spindle cells and by multinucleated giant cells adjacent to dilated spaces that resemble dilated lymphatic vessels.

The differential diagnosis, especially in the early stage, is that of keloid, large dermatofibroma, or medallion-like dermal dendrocytoma. CD34+ myxoid dermatofibrohistiocytoma of the skin occurs as an indolent posttraumatic tumor. It resembles myxoid DFSP.

Mohs surgical excision technique is the treatment of choice for DFSP. In a series of 50 patients, recurrence rate was 2%; with wide local excision, recurrence is 11%–50%. A preoperative MRI may assist in planning successful clearance. Radiation has been used as adjunctive therapy and imatinib mesylate has been effective in some unresectable tumors.

Li Y, et al: Clinical features, pathological findings and treatment of recurrent dermatofibrosarcoma protuberans. J Cancer 2017; 8: 1319.
Thway K, et al: Dermatofibrosarcoma protuberans. Ann Diagn Pathol 2016; 25: 64.

Atypical Fibroxanthoma

Atypical fibroxanthoma (AFX) of the skin is a low-grade malignancy that occurs chiefly on the sun-exposed parts of the head or neck in white persons over age 50. Most cases appear to be related to undifferentiated pleomorphic sarcoma (UPS) (malignant fibrous histiocytoma), which AFX resembles histologically. Its smaller size and more superficial location account largely for its more favorable prognosis. Some cases probably represent spindled or anaplastic SCC that has lost the ability to express keratin. Clinically, the tumor begins as a small, firm nodule, often with an eroded or crusted surface without characteristic morphologic features (Fig. 28.41). A distinct clinical variant has a different

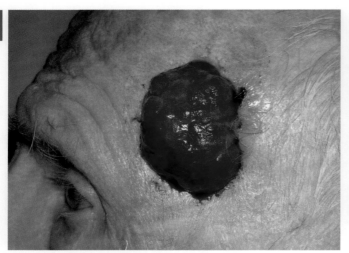

Fig. 28.41 Atypical fibroxanthoma. (Courtesy Chris Miller, MD.)

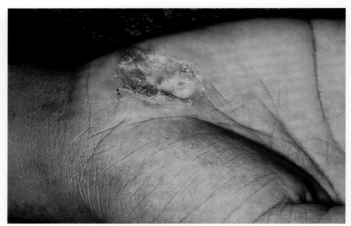

Fig. 28.42 Epithelial sarcoma.

presentation as a slowly enlarging tumor on a covered area, in patients with an average age of 39. This variant accounts for 25% of cases.

The lesion develops in the dermis and is separated from the epidermis by a thin band of collagen. The tumor consists of bizarre spindle cells mingled with atypical histiocytic cells. The cytoplasm may be vacuolated and resembles the xanthoma cell. Mitotic figures, prominent eosinophilic nucleoli, and the presence of a biphasic tumor cell population are characteristic findings, but purely spindle cell variants also occur. S-100 staining decorates colonizing dendritic cells, but not the tumor cells, and prekeratin staining is negative; this helps distinguish AFX from SCC. Variants with clear cells, granular cells, and osteoclast-type cells have been described. Tumor cells stain for CD10, S-100A6, and procollagen I, but none of these markers is specific for AFX.

The treatment of choice is complete surgical excision. Mohs microsurgery results in fewer recurrences and smaller defects than conventional excision. Although the prognosis is excellent, local recurrence after inadequate excision is common, and cases of metastasizing AFX have been reported.

Hanlon A, et al: LN2, CD10, and ezrin do not distinguish between atypical fibroxanthoma and undifferentiated pleomorphic sarcoma or predict clinical outcome. Dermatol Surg 2017; 43: 431.

Undifferentiated Pleomorphic Sarcoma (Malignant Fibrous Histiocytoma)

The undifferentiated pleomorphic type is the most common soft tissue sarcoma of middle and late adulthood. It arises deeply and is more likely to appear in deep fascial planes than in subcutaneous tissue. One third occur on the thigh or buttock. Peak incidence is in the seventh decade. These sarcomas sometimes arise in an area of radiodermatitis or in a chronic ulceration.

Several histologic variants have been described, including myxoid, inflammatory, and giant cell types. Gene expression profiling is now being used to define subtypes of pleomorphic sarcoma. Cell staining is positive for vimentin and factor XIIIa. Pleomorphic cellular elements and bizarre mitotic figures are characteristic. AFXs are smaller and more superficial tumors of the dermis, compared with the deeper location of UPS. Epithelioid sarcoma lacks the large, bizarre, multinucleated cells often seen in UPS.

The prognosis in UPS is related to the site; deeper and more proximally located tumors have a poorer prognosis. The myxoid variant is less likely to metastasize. An especially poor prognosis attends tumors arising in sites of radiodermatitis. Local recurrence after excision occurs in 25%, 35% metastasize, and overall survival is 50%. Mohs surgical removal may result in fewer recurrences.

The angiomatoid type may have a different presentation on the extremities of children, as a slowly growing dermal or subcutaneous mass. It has been separated because it has a relatively good prognosis.

Cutaneous Myxofibrosarcoma

Myxofibrosarcoma is the term used for myxoid variants of UPS. The diagnosis of cutaneous myxofibrosarcoma is often delayed because the tumor may appear indolent clinically and may mimic an interstitial granuloma histologically. Areas of atypical spindle cells within a prominent myxoid stroma and pleomorphic multinucleated cells suggest the diagnosis. The main differential diagnosis is myxoid liposarcoma. The margins are often poorly defined, and preoperative MRI can be helpful in surgical planning.

Pasquali S, et al: Neoadjuvant chemotherapy in soft tissue sarcomas. Ther Adv Med Oncol 2017; 9: 415.

Epithelioid Sarcoma

Epithelioid sarcoma occurs chiefly in young adults, with onset usually from ages 20–40. Two thirds of cases are in men. Almost all lesions are on the extremities, with half on the hands or wrists (Fig. 28.42). They have been reported from a wide variety of locations, however, including the genital region ("proximal type").

The tumor grows slowly among fascial structures and tendons, often with central necrosis of the tumor nodules and ulceration of the overlying skin. Initial clinical diagnoses may include granuloma annulare, rheumatoid nodule, or ganglion cyst. Histologically, irregular nodular masses of large, deeply acidophilic, polygonal cells merge with spindle cells in a biphasic pattern. Central necrosis within masses of epithelioid cells may give the impression of a palisaded granuloma. Absence of staining for CD68 (KP-1) and coexpression of keratins and vimentin confirm the diagnosis. Loss of INI1 expression is also helpful diagnostically, but has no prognostic implications.

Wide local excision of small, early lesions may achieve a cure. Recurrence after attempted excision is seen in three of four patients, and late metastasis in 45%. There is a propensity for lymph node and lung metastases, and in one series of eight patients, 5-year and 10-year survival rates of 25% were reported. Women have a

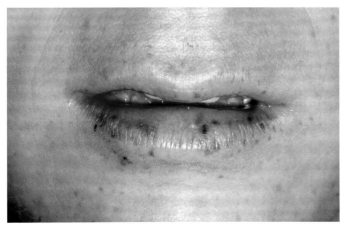

Fig. 28.43 Carney syndrome.

more favorable prognosis; the proximal lesions have a worse prognosis.

Chbani L, et al: Epithelioid sarcoma. Am J Clin Pathol 2009; 131: 222.

Myxomas

Cutaneous myxomas may be solitary and may appear as flesh-colored nodules on the face, trunk, or extremities. They may also occur as part of Carney complex. This has also been reported under the acronyms NAME (nevi, atrial myxoma, myxoid neurofibromas, ephelides) and LAMB (lentigines, atrial myxoma, mucocutaneous myxomas, blue nevi) and simply as cutaneous lentiginosis with atrial myxoma.

The Carney complex consists of patients who have two or more of the following:

1. Cardiac myxomas (79%)
2. Cutaneous myxomas (not myxoid neurofibromas) (45%)
3. Mammary myxoid fibromas (30%)
4. Spotty mucocutaneous pigmentation, including lentiginoses (not ephelides) and blue nevi, often of a distinctive epithelioid variety (65%)
5. Adrenocortical adenoma/primary pigmented nodular adrenocortical disease (45%), which results in Cushing syndrome
6. Testicular tumors (56% of male patients)
7. Pituitary growth hormone–secreting tumors (10%).

A peculiar type of schwannoma featuring melanin and psammoma bodies may also be present.

The cutaneous myxomas occur as small (<1 cm), multiple, skin-colored papules with a predilection for development by a mean age of 18 years, and a tendency to occur on the ears, eyelids, and nipples. The lentigines are prominent on the face, lips, conjunctival mucosa, rectal mucosa, and genital mucosa (Fig. 28.43). Cardiac myxomas may occur in any of the four chambers of the heart and are recurrent in 20%. They may embolize to the skin, producing acral necrotic lesions.

Recognition of this syndrome, with diagnosis and removal of the atrial myxomas, can be lifesaving. The first-degree family members should be examined because this is an autosomal dominant inherited condition. The disease has been mapped to two loci, and a third is likely. Mutations in the gene coding for the protein kinase A type Ia regulatory subunit (*PPKAR1A*) on chromosome 17 have been documented in about half the families.

A malignant counterpart, the myxosarcoma, is a tumor that arises in the subcutaneous fat and underlying soft tissues. There is a tendency for local recurrence after wide and deep excision. Metastases are rare.

Aggressive Angiomyxoma

Aggressive angiomyxoma is an uncommon soft tissue neoplasm that usually involves the vulvoperineal and pelvic regions of young women. Any angiomyxoid tumor in this area is suspect for aggressive behavior. The tumor is mucinous and deeply infiltrative but does not demonstrate nuclear atypia or mitosis. The rate of local recurrence is high despite wide surgical resection, and MRI can be helpful in preoperative planning.

Mastocytosis

Mastocytosis is a general term applied to local and systemic accumulations of mast cells. Mast cells are bone marrow–derived CD34+ cells. These cells carry preformed mediators, such as histamine, heparin, and various cytokines, which, when released, may cause symptoms such as flushing, urticaria, diarrhea, abdominal pain, headache, dyspnea, syncope, and palpitations.

Mastocytosis is divided into childhood-onset and adult-onset disease. The condition varies in these two age-groups in terms of clinical presentation, prognosis, and pathogenic factors. Studies have revealed mutations in the *c-KIT* proto-oncogene in many adult-onset cases. Its protein product is the transmembrane tyrosine kinase KIT receptor (CD117), whose ligand is stem cell factor (also known as mast cell growth factor). Both clonality studies and mutational analysis indicate that many adult cases of mastocytosis result from a neoplastic proliferation of mast cells, with a mutation at codon 816 in the *c-KIT* gene. This mutation is activating, resulting in the proliferation of mast cells. A second mutation, a chromosomal deletion on 4q12, results in the juxtaposition of platelet-derived growth factor receptor-α and FIP1L1. This fusion gene activates hematopoietic cells and is pathogenic in a subset of patients with systemic mastocytosis (SM) and eosinophilia. This subset of patients has also been considered as having a type of "hypereosinophilic syndrome." Thus the vast majority of adults with mastocytosis have systemic disease that may be viewed as a fundamentally myelodysplastic disorder.

Children often do not express any *c-KIT* mutation; nor do the uncommon familial cases. The disease in the latter is usually transmitted by autosomal dominant inheritance with reduced expressivity, although other patterns may occur. The mutations leading to familial disease have not been defined. It appears that spontaneous childhood disease may occur from cytokine-derived hyperplasias, from mutations other than the activating 816 type, or from mutations yet to be described. Some pediatric cases, however, are known to have inactivating mutations of *c-KIT*, and a few have the adult-type activating mutations. Childhood disease is defined as occurring before age 15. The majority of children develop their disease before age 2, and in most of them, the condition spontaneously involutes.

Clinical Classification

Mast cell disease is divided into two broad categories—cutaneous and systemic. Cutaneous mastocytosis describes cases with involvement of only the skin and includes most cases of childhood mastocytosis and infrequent adult cases. Childhood cases usually fall into one of three categories of cutaneous mastocytosis. The most common (60%–80% of patients) is urticaria pigmentosa or so-called "maculopapular" cutaneous mastocytosis; fewer (10%–35%) patients present with solitary mastocytosis; the remainder have the rare forms of diffuse cutaneous mastocytosis or the telangiectatic type. A classification has been proposed by Akin and Metcalfe, which incorporates the World Health Organization (WHO) criteria (Box 28.1).

BOX 28.1 Classification of Mastocytosis

CUTANEOUS AND SYSTEMIC MASTOCYTOSIS
1. Indolent systemic mastocytosis (ISM)
   - Isolated bone marrow mastocytosis
   - Smoldering systemic mastocytosis (SSM)
2. Systemic mastocytosis with associated hematopoietic disease (SM-AHD, AHNMD [*associated* hematologic non–mast cell disorder]): systemic mastocytosis with leukemia, myelodysplastic syndrome/disease, or non-Hodgkin lymphoma
3. Aggressive systemic mastocytosis (ASM)
4. Mast cell leukemia
5. Mast cell sarcoma
6. Extracutaneous mastocytoma

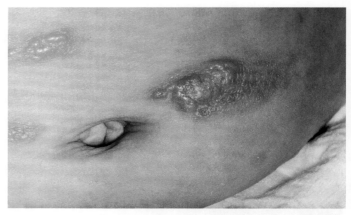

Fig. 28.44 Bullous mastocytosis.

The vast majority of adult patients with mastocytosis are classified as having systemic mastocytosis, because they typically have clonal proliferation of the bone marrow–derived mast cells. Of adult patients with SM not associated with hematopoietic disease, 60% have indolent mastocytosis and 40% have aggressive mastocytosis. Patients with aggressive SM usually lack skin lesions. Mast cell leukemia and sarcoma are very rare. Many patients who present to the dermatologist with only skin lesions will have the indolent variety. Symptoms and signs of systemic disease are classified as those related to organ infiltration by mast cells and those caused by mediator release from mast cells. Direct organ involvement is most frequently bone pain from lytic bone lesions, hepatosplenomegaly, lymphadenopathy, or cytopenia from bone marrow involvement. For the dermatologist, the most important symptoms are those related to mediator release, usually acting on the GI tract, respiratory tree, or blood vessels. These include pruritus, flushing, urticaria, angioedema, headache, nausea, vomiting, abdominal cramps, diarrhea, gastric/duodenal ulcer, malabsorption, asthma-like symptoms, presyncope, syncope, and anaphylaxis. These may occur spontaneously or may result from massive histamine release after ingestion of known mast cell degranulators, such as alcohol, morphine, codeine, or extended rubbing of the skin. *Hymenoptera* stings may induce anaphylaxis. Mast cells also produce heparin, which may result in hematemesis, epistaxis, melena, and ecchymoses. Osteoporosis may also occur from chronic heparin release, resulting in fractures.

Cutaneous Mastocytosis

Cutaneous mastocytosis is relatively common, representing about 1 in 500 initial consultations to pediatric dermatologists.

Solitary Mastocytoma

About 10%–40% of childhood mastocytosis presents as the solitary lesion, which may be present at birth or may develop during the first weeks of life. It originates as a brown macule that urticates on stroking. It may develop into a papule, a raised round or oval plaque, or a tumor. The size is usually less than 1 cm, but occasionally it may reach two or three times this diameter. The surface is usually smooth but may have a peau d'orange appearance. Although the mastocytoma may occur anywhere on the body, it favors the dorsum of the hand near the wrist. Edema, urtication, vesiculation, and even bulla formation may be observed in the lesion. Even a solitary lesion may produce systemic symptoms, usually flushing.

Although the generalized form may begin with a single lesion, dissemination usually occurs within 3 months of its appearance. Most solitary mastocytomas involute spontaneously by age 10 or earlier. They also respond favorably to excision or to the application of a hydrocolloid dressing to prevent the rubbing that triggers

mediator release and symptomatology. Progression to malignant disease does not occur.

Generalized Eruption, Childhood Type (Urticaria Pigmentosa)

The generalized form of cutaneous mastocytosis represents 60%–90% of childhood cases. In this type the eruption usually begins during the first weeks of life, presenting with rose-colored, pruritic, urticarial, slightly pigmented macules, papules, or nodules. The lesions are oval or round and vary in diameter between 5 and 15 mm and may coalesce. The color varies from yellowish brown to yellowish red. Occasionally, the lesions are a pale-yellow color, and this has been called xanthelasmoidea. Vesicle and bulla formation is a frequent prominent feature early in the disease (Fig. 28.44). Indeed, vesicles and bullae may be the initial presenting signs, but they usually persist no longer than 3 years. In the older age-groups, vesiculation rarely occurs.

At their onset, lesions are similar to urticaria, except that they are not evanescent. The lesions persist and gradually become chamois or slate colored (Fig. 28.45). When they are firmly stroked or vigorously rubbed, urticaria with a surrounding erythematous flare (Darier sign) usually develops. Dermatographism of clinically uninvolved skin is present in one third to one half of patients. For many years, the brown, waxy skin lesions may persist before they begin to involute. Pigmentation and all evidence of the disease usually disappear within a few years, generally before puberty. The eruption, however, may infrequently persist into adult life. Although systemic involvement is possible, malignant systemic disease is extremely rare.

Diffuse Cutaneous Mastocytosis

In this rare form with diffuse involvement, the entire integument may be thickened and infiltrated with mast cells to produce a peculiar orange color, giving rise to the term *homme orange*. There is an infiltrated doughy or boggy consistency to the skin, and lichenification may be present. In the neonatal period, diffuse cutaneous blistering may occur, leading to the diagnosis of epidermolysis bullosa or some other primary bullous disorder. This is termed *bullous mastocytosis*.

Systemic Mastocytosis

SM is diagnosed by fulfilling the one major criterion and one minor criterion, or three minor criteria. The major criterion is the finding of dense infiltrates of mast cells (aggregates of 15 or more) in bone marrow or other extracutaneous tissues. The four minor criteria are as follows:

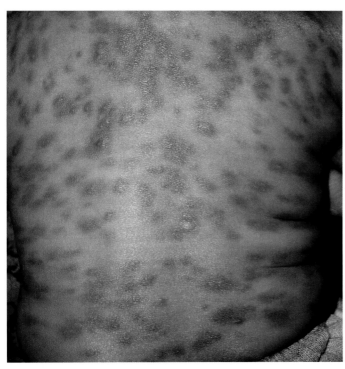

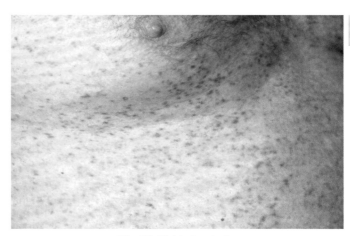

Fig. 28.46 Mastocytosis.

Fig. 28.45 Urticaria pigmentosa.

1. Atypical mast cell morphology
2. Aberrant mast cell surface phenotype (CD25 or CD2)
3. Serum/plasma tryptase greater than 20 ng/mL
4. A codon 816 *c-KIT* mutation in peripheral blood, bone marrow, or lesional tissue

Patients with a history of *Hymenoptera*-induced anaphylaxis and an elevated tryptase level should be evaluated for systemic mastocytosis.

The most common type of SM in adults is indolent systemic mastocytosis. These patients lack evidence of an associated non–mast cell hematologic disorder; lack end-organ dysfunction such as ascites, malabsorption, cytopenias, and pathologic fractures; and lack mast cell leukemia. The disorder is then diagnosed through physical and histopathologic examination of skin lesions. Several different patterns of cutaneous involvement have been described.

Generalized Eruption, Adult Type

The generalized eruption is the most common pattern of mastocytosis presenting to the dermatologist. The most common lesions are macules, papules, or nodules disseminated over most of the body, but especially on the upper arms, legs, and trunk. The upper arms and upper inner thighs may be the only areas involved on presentation. These may be reddish purple (Fig. 28.46), rust colored, or brown. The brown lesions may closely resemble common nevi. They may urticate on rubbing, as seen in children with urticaria pigmentosa.

Erythrodermic Mastocytosis

There is generalized erythroderma, and the skin has a leather-grain appearance. Urtication can be produced over the entire surface.

Telangiectasia Macularis Eruptiva Perstans

This is a persistent, pigmented, asymptomatic eruption of macules usually less than 0.5 cm in diameter, with a slightly reddish brown tinge. Despite the name, little or no telangiectasia may evident. Darier sign may not be demonstrable, because the number of mast cells in the skin may not be greatly increased.

Classification and Prognosis in Adult Systemic Mastocytosis

The 2008 WHO classification includes indolent SM, aggressive SM, SM associated with a clonal non–mast cell lineage disease, and mast cell leukemia. Patients with SM with an associated hematologic non–mast cell lineage disorder (SM-AHNMD) are typically older adults with signs and symptoms of systemic disease. A variety of associated non–mast cell hematologic conditions, including polycythemia vera, hypereosinophilic syndrome, chronic myelogenous or monocytic leukemia, lymphocytic leukemia, primary myelofibrosis, and Hodgkin disease, may be seen. Typically, this type does not have skin lesions. The prognosis in these patients is that of their underlying hematologic condition. Smoldering SM is characterized by a slow progression and lack of end-organ dysfunction from mast cell infiltration. It describes patients with 30% or more infiltration of the bone marrow cavity by mast cells, a serum tryptase level greater than 200 ng/mL, and hepatosplenomegaly. Aggressive SM has a more fulminant course and describes the condition of patients with end-organ dysfunction caused by mast cell infiltration: bone marrow failure, liver dysfunction, splenomegaly with hypersplenism, pathologic fractures, and GI involvement with malabsorption and weight loss. This group of patients has a poor prognosis. Mast cell leukemia occurs when the atypical mast cells (multilobular or multiple nuclei) represent 10% of circulating cells or 20% of bone marrow cells. The prognosis is poor.

Mast Cell Sarcoma and Extracutaneous Mastocytoma

These are rare findings of isolated tumors of either atypical mast cells in mast cell sarcoma or benign-appearing mast cells in extracutaneous mastocytoma. They occur in sites other than the skin or bone marrow. Mast cell sarcomas are aggressive, locally destructive lesions, in contrast to the benign mastocytomas, which carry a good prognosis.

Biochemical Studies

Mast cells produce tryptase. Serum tryptase has become the preferred laboratory test to demonstrate evidence of increased mast cell burden, replacing urinary histamine and urinary histamine metabolites. The test is of prognostic significance in some patients. Tryptase is measured as a total serum tryptase level. This should be obtained when the patient is in a normal state of health, because anaphylaxis will increase tryptase transiently. Mastocytosis patients may have a persistently and significantly elevated tryptase level. Results above 20 ng/mL are a minor criterion for the diagnosis of systemic mastocytosis.

Histopathology

The typical skin lesion shows a dense dermal aggregate of mononuclear cells with abundant amphophilic cytoplasm. When these large mononuclear cells are stained with Giemsa or toluidine blue, the metachromatic granules are observed. A Leder stain will stain the cells diffusely red. When blisters are present, the roof of the vesicle or bulla is subepidermal. The mast cells collect in a band below the vesicle. Infiltration of local anesthetic adjacent to the lesion rather than directly into it and the use of anesthetic without epinephrine may help to avoid mast cell degranulation. Monoclonal antibodies against tryptase and CD117 (KIT) are available and are very sensitive.

Diagnosis

The typical case of cutaneous mastocytosis is easily diagnosed by the presence of solitary or multiple pigmented macules, papules, or nodules that urticate when irritated by stroking or scratching. The diagnosis is confirmed by biopsy of the lesion with demonstration of increased numbers of mast cells. The bullous and vesicular lesions may be more difficult to diagnose clinically; however, scrapings from the base of the bulla when stained with Giemsa or Wright stain will show mast cells in profusion.

Once the diagnosis of skin lesions of mastocytosis is made, the decision to assess for bone marrow involvement is key. Although therapy to reduce the disease burden of proliferating clonal mast cells is not effective, bone marrow examination will provide information about the extent of the disease and the presence or absence of a non–mast cell hematologic disorder, and it will assist in the counseling on prognosis. All adult patients and children with the unexplained presence of an abnormal complete blood cell count (CBC), hepatomegaly, splenomegaly, lymphadenopathy, or serum baseline tryptase of greater than 20 ng/mL should be offered a bone marrow examination. Both serum tryptase levels and markers of bone turnover, including C-telopeptide and osteoprotegerin, are associated with extent of disease.

In asymptomatic adults whose only sign or symptom of mastocytosis is skin lesions, and who choose not to have a bone marrow examination, serum tryptase and CBC should be repeated at least yearly during a complete history and physical examination. Elevation of the tryptase level, a drop in the platelet count or hemoglobin, a rise in the monocytes, or the onset of organomegaly should trigger a bone marrow examination. In children with early-onset disease, the prognosis is good; usually, tryptase evaluation or mutational analysis is reserved for those with the findings just listed, or with persistent localized bone pain, severe GI symptoms, or biochemical evidence of hepatic insufficiency.

Differential Diagnosis. Clinically, a small solitary mastocytoma most frequently resembles a pigmented nevus or juvenile xanthogranuloma. Urtication establishes the diagnosis. The disseminated lesions are also distinctive enough to cause little or no difficulty in the diagnosis. The nodular form may resemble xanthomas; however, the presence of urtication is distinctive. The vesicular and bullous lesions are to be distinguished from various hereditary and nonhereditary bullous diseases. The main histologic similarity is to Langerhans cell histiocytosis.

Prognosis

Most cases of early-onset, skin-limited disease in children clear completely. The solitary mastocytoma involutes spontaneously, usually within 3 years of onset. In children and adults with indolent systemic mastocytosis, the prognosis is also good. This is the most common category of patients presenting for diagnosis in the dermatology clinic. Patients with AHNMD have the prognosis of the associated disease. In the newly described patients with smoldering systemic mastocytosis, the prognosis is intermediate and not yet well defined. Patients with aggressive systemic mastocytosis, mast cell leukemia, or mast cell sarcoma have a poor prognosis.

Treatment

Symptomatic relief of histamine-mediated symptoms may be achieved in many cases by the use of antihistamines. Both H1 and H2 blockers and antiserotonin drugs, such as cyproheptadine, may alleviate urtication, pruritus, and flushing. Nifedipine, 10 mg three times daily, may also be effective in isolated cases. Psoralen with ultraviolet A (PUVA) or medium-dose UVA1 therapy alone produces excellent clearing of the skin in most cases. Most patients will have sustained benefit for at least 6 months after treatment. Approximately 25% will have a remission lasting longer than 5 years, and in others the frequency of phototherapy may be tapered to once or twice a month, and patients still remain clear. Intralesional triamcinolone or potent topical corticosteroids under occlusion may also clear cutaneous lesions; however, the lesions do recur after discontinuance. Also, concern about local atrophy, striae, and systemic absorption limits the utility of this treatment.

The importance of avoiding physical stimuli such as extremes of temperature, pressure/friction, and chemical degranulators of mast cells cannot be overemphasized. The application of a hydrocolloid dressing over an isolated mastocytoma in an infant may reduce the flushing it produces. The chemicals that patients with mastocytosis must avoid include opiates, aspirin, alcohol, quinine, scopolamine, gallamine, decamethonium, reserpine, amphotericin B, polymyxin B, and D-tubocurarine. *Hymenoptera* stings may induce anaphylaxis; the patient (and parents of an affected child) should be taught to recognize the signs of anaphylactic shock, given a premeasured dose of epinephrine (EpiPen) for emergency use, and educated on its use. After such an event, it is prudent to treat for several days with 20–40 mg of prednisone to avoid recurrent attacks.

Control of diarrhea in SM may be achieved by orally administered disodium cromoglycate. GI ulcers may be treated with proton pump inhibitors and H2 antagonists. The treatment of systemic mast cell disease is of limited efficacy. For patients with indolent SM and severe osteoporosis, IFN alfa may be considered. In patients with smoldering systemic mastocytosis, watchful waiting is recommended, although IFN alfa, with or without glucocorticoids, may be considered for progressive "B" findings. In aggressive systemic mastocytosis, IFN alfa may also be used, with or without glucocorticoids. 2-Chlorodeoxyadenosine (as used in Langerhans cell histiocytosis) can also be effective in aggressive systemic mastocytosis. A gain-of-function D816V point mutation in the transmembrane receptor KIT kinase domain is found in the majority of patients with systemic mastocytosis. Patients with the mutation do not generally respond to imatinib mesylate. Patients with SM who have the *FIP1L1–PDGFRA* translocation, who lack the *c-KIT* mutation, or who have novel mutations may respond to imatinib, and it may even prove helpful in patients with associated leukemia. CD1a-positive familial cutaneous mastocytosis without germline or somatic mutations in *c-KIT* has been described. Cladribine (an adenosine deaminase inhibitor) has been used successfully for cytoreductive therapy in the setting of systemic mastocytosis. Bone marrow transplantation for the most severely affected patients with SM is being investigated.

Husain Z, et al: Management of poorly controlled indolent systemic mastocytosis using narrowband UVB phototherapy. Cutis 2017; 99: E30.

Lortholary O, et al: Masitinib for treatment of severely symptomatic indolent systemic mastocytosis: a randomised, placebo-controlled, phase 3 study. Lancet 2017; 389: 612.

Valent P, et al: Advances in the classification and treatment of mastocytosis. Cancer Res 2017; 77: 1261.

ABNORMALITIES OF NEURAL TISSUE

Solitary Neurofibroma

The typical solitary cutaneous neurofibroma is usually 3–6 mm in diameter. It is soft, flaccid, translucent, and pinkish white. Frequently, the soft small tumor can be invaginated, as if through a ring in the skin, by pressure with the finger (this is called "buttonholing").

When only one or two lesions are present, they are typically spontaneous tumors without internal manifestations. When three or more are present, a diagnosis of neurofibromatosis should be considered. Infrequently, large pendulous masses occur, in which numerous, tortuous, thickened nerves can be felt; this has been likened to a "bag of worms." These plexiform neurofibromas, which often have overlying pigmentation, usually occur in neurofibromatosis (see Chapter 27).

Histologically, the lesion demonstrates wavy spindled nuclei and fine collagen fibers. The stroma is often myxoid and contains many mast cells. Cholinesterase activity is markedly positive in the neurofibromas; the Schwann cells are S-100 positive; neurofilament protein staining demonstrates scattered axons; and CD34 demonstrates a characteristic fingerprint pattern. Shave removal is usually adequate therapy for symptomatic lesions.

Granular Cell Tumor

About one third of reported granular cell tumors occur on the tongue (Fig. 28.47), one third involve the skin, and one third occur in the internal organs. The tumor is usually a well-circumscribed, solitary, firm nodule ranging from 5–30 mm, with a brownish red or flesh tint, depending on nearness to the surface. Its surface is often rough or verrucous, corresponding to pseudo-epitheliomatous hyperplasia overlying the tumor. Rarely, the lesions may ulcerate. They are multiple in 10%–15% of cases.

The solitary lesion may be located anywhere on the body, but almost half of all tumors appear on the head or neck. Usually, patients are in their third to fifth decade. About two thirds of patients are black, and two thirds are women. In most cases, the tumor grows very slowly, and when completely removed, does not usually recur. However, local or multicentric recurrence may at times cause confusion in determining whether a granular cell tumor is malignant.

The histologic picture is distinctive. The cells are large, pale, and irregularly polygonal, with a poorly defined cellular membrane, and contain coarsely granular cytoplasm with scattered giant lysosomal granules. Some of the cells are multinucleated or contain vacuoles or small pyknotic or eosinophilic inclusions. At times, the arrangement is in cords or sheets, in irregular alveolar masses, or even organoid. Pseudoepitheliomatous hyperplasia is a regular feature. The cells stain positively with vimentin, neuron-specific enolase, S-100, myelin protein, p75 nerve growth factor, calretinin, NKI/C3, and PGP9.5. Hybrid forms that overlap with perineurioma have been described.

Malignant granular cell tumor is uncommon. Most are much larger than the benign granular cell tumors, with an average diameter of 9 cm; benign lesions average less than 2 cm. Most malignant granular cell tumors demonstrate cytologic atypia, but some are quite bland cytologically. Other factors that correlate with malignant behavior are an infiltrative growth pattern, history of local recurrence, older patient age, presence of necrosis, increased mitotic activity, spindling of tumor cells, and nuclear staining with the proliferation marker Ki67 (MIB 1) in more than 10% of tumor nuclei. Mutant p53 protein has been identified in more than half of malignant granular cell tumors studied. About one third are aneuploid, one third hyperdiploid, and one third diploid. In contrast, almost all benign tumors are diploid.

Because of the difficulties in distinguishing benign from some malignant granular cell tumors, complete excision is advisable whenever possible. Malignant granular cell tumors often have an infiltrative growth pattern and perineural extension. Mohs micrographic surgery may be helpful in ensuring complete excision.

Arcot R, et al: Peripheral and cranial nerve sheath tumors—a clinical spectrum. Indian J Surg 2012; 74: 371.

Cardis MA, et al: Granular cell differentiation. J Dermatol 2017; 44: 251.

Paul SP, et al: An unusual granular cell tumour of the buttock and a review of granular cell tumours. Case Rep Dermatol Med 2013; 2013: 109308.

Perineurioma

The normal perineurium is composed of flattened cells that surround the nerve. Perineuriomas are derived from these cells. Cutaneous lesions appear as nondescript papules clinically. Sclerosing perineuriomas demonstrate concentric lamellar fibrosis and are epithelial membrane antigen (EMA) positive. Reticular, granular, and lipomatous variants have been described.

Macarenco RS, et al: Extra-acral cutaneous sclerosing perineurioma with CD34 fingerprint pattern. J Cutan Pathol 2017; 44: 388.

Michal M, et al: Whorling cellular perineurioma. Ann Diagn Pathol 2017; 27: 74.

Neuroma Cutis

Cutaneous neuromas include traumatic neuromas, multiple mucosal neuromas, and solitary palisaded encapsulated neuromas. Segmental neuromas have also been described.

Traumatic neuromas result from the overgrowth of nerve fibers in the severed ends of peripheral nerves. The lesion may be tender

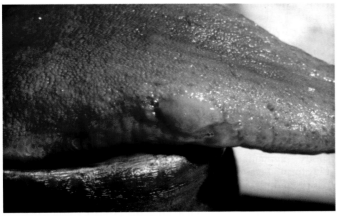

Fig. 28.47 Granular cell tumor.

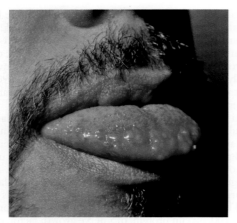

Fig. 28.48 Multiple mucosal neuromas.

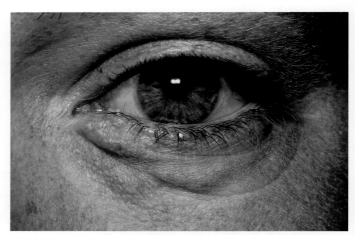

Fig. 28.49 Schwannoma. (Courtesy Dr. Curt Samlaska.)

or painful, and when scarring has occurred or the distal stump has been removed, a phantom limb syndrome may result. These often occur on the fingers, at sites of amputation of supernumerary digits, or on the sole, usually at the third metatarsal space.

Multiple mucosal neuromas occur as part of the autosomal dominant inherited, multiple mucosal neuroma syndrome (MEN-2b). These patients have a marfanoid habitus, thickened protruding lips, and multiple neuromas of the oral mucosa (lips, tongue, gingiva), conjunctiva, and sometimes sclera (Fig. 28.48). A few have multiple cutaneous neuromas, usually limited to the face. There is a strong association with medullary carcinoma of the thyroid, bilateral pheochromocytomas, and diffuse GI tract ganglioneuromatosis. Disease is caused by a mutation in the *RET* proto-oncogene. Infants at risk should be screened for this mutation and total thyroidectomy performed if positive.

The palisaded, encapsulated neuroma of the skin is a solitary, large, encapsulated tumor, usually of the face. It is a slow-growing, flesh-colored, dome-shaped, firm lesion, usually appearing around the mouth or nose. It closely resembles a basal cell carcinoma or an intradermal nevus.

Brau-Javier CN, et al: Acquired segmental neuromas. PR Health Sci J 2013; 32: 101.

Rodríguez-Peralto JL, et al: Benign cutaneous neural tumors. Semin Diagn Pathol 2013; 30: 45.

Neurothekeoma (Nerve Sheath Myxoma)

Neurothekeoma refers to a tumor of the nerve sheath and is composed of cords and nests of large cells packed among collagen bundles close to small nerves. Mitotic figures and nuclear atypia are sometimes seen, but the tumor is benign. These benign intradermal or subcutaneous tumors are divided histologically into two distinct subtypes: the classic or myxoid variant and the cellular type. An intermediate or mixed variety is also recognized. The myxoid variant (nerve sheath myxoma) is characterized by islands of stellate and spindled cells in a mucinous matrix. The cells stain strongly for S-100 protein. Myxoid neurothekeoma occurs in middle-age adults, primarily on the head, neck, and upper extremities. It is twice as common in women. The cellular type occurs in childhood, with a high female preponderance, and has a predilection for the head, neck, or shoulders. The cellular type does not stain for S-100 protein but does stain for S-100A6, PGP9.5, MiTF, and NK1C3. It is unclear if these tumors really demonstrate nerve sheath differentiation, but for now they are grouped with the myxoid neurothekeomas. Examples of cellular neurothekeoma with high mitotic rate and atypia mimic

malignant spindle cell tumors. They have a significant rate of recurrence but at this point are not known to have a clear metastatic potential.

Cardoso J, et al: Cellular neurothekeoma with perineural extension. J Cutan Pathol 2012; 39: 662.

El Kehdy J, et al: Solitary nodule on the base of the nose in an adolescent girl. Pediatr Dermatol 2012; 29: 659.

Fetsch JF, et al: Neurothekeoma. Am J Surg Pathol 2007; 31: 1103.

Hornick JL, et al: Cellular neurothekeoma. Am J Surg Pathol 2007; 31: 329.

Schwannoma (Neurilemmoma)

Peripheral schwannomas are usually solitary nerve sheath tumors, most often seen in women. They occur almost exclusively in deep tissues, along the main nerve trunks of the extremities, especially the flexor surface of the arms, wrists, and knees. They are also seen on the scalp, sides of the neck, and tongue. The solitary tumor is a nodule of 3–30 mm in diameter (Fig. 28.49). It is soft or firm and pale pink or yellowish; it may or may not be painful. Schwannomas involve many other organs, and brain tumors such as meningiomas, gliomas, and astrocytomas may occur.

In some cases, the tumors are multiple, and these may be seen with neurofibromatosis type 1 (NF-1) or more often NF-2, or as an entity independent of neurofibromatosis. The independent type may be congenital or may have a delayed onset. It may be sporadic or familial. Three clinical patterns are described: elevated, dome-shaped nodules; pale-brown, indurated macules; and multiple papules coalescing into plaques 2–100 mm in diameter, with a predilection for the trunk. Cases have occurred that appeared to be unassociated with NF-2, but on further investigation of the individual or family, revealed other signs of NF-2 and the gene abnormality on chromosome 22.

Plexiform schwannomas may occur as single or multiple lesions, localized to a single anatomic site or more generalized, and arise in the dermis or subcutaneous tissue. They may occur as a solitary lesion or may be associated with NF-1, NF-2, or multiple schwannomas. Another subtype of schwannoma is the melanotic psammomatous type seen in association with Carney syndrome, featuring spotty pigmentation, myxomas, and endocrine overactivity. Plexiform melanocytic schwannoma may demonstrate mitotic figures and pleomorphic nuclei and must be differentiated from malignant melanoma. Important clues include the presence of focal Verocay bodies, as well as an EMA-positive capsule derived from perineurium.

Histologically, the classic forms are well encapsulated with characteristic subcapsular edema and two types of tissue, referred to as Antoni types A and B. Hard schwannomas are firm on gross examination and are composed of Antoni A tissue—palisades of basophilic Schwann cell nuclei separated by brightly eosinophilic zones (Verocay bodies). Soft schwannomas are diffusely edematous. They are composed mostly of Antoni B tissue, a degenerative change characterized by loose, edematous connective tissue and ectatic blood vessels. S-100, vimentin, and myelin basic protein stains are positive in hard schwannomas. Staining is variable in soft schwannomas. A Bodian or neurofilament protein stain reveals very few or no nerve fibers within the bulk of the tumor, although a compressed nerve may be present at one edge of the mass in a subcapsular location. "Ancient schwannomas" may demonstrate remarkable nuclear atypia, which represents a benign degenerative change. Mitoses are absent. Ancient schwannomas should not be confused with malignant peripheral nerve sheath tumor ("malignant schwannoma"), a tumor that arises in long-standing neurofibromas in the setting of NF-1. Excision is almost invariably curative, except in the malignant variety, for which combined wide resection and radiotherapy is needed.

Yeh I, et al: Plexiform melanocytic schwannoma. J Cutan Pathol 2012; 39: 521.

Infantile Neuroblastoma

Neuroblastoma is the most common malignant tumor of early childhood. Cutaneous nodules are most often seen in younger patients, being present in 32% of infants with the disease. These occur as multiple, 2–20 mm, firm, blue nodules that, when rubbed, blanch and form a halo of erythema. The blanching persists for 1–2 hours and is followed by a refractory period of several hours. Biopsy shows clusters of basophilic cells with a high nuclear/cytoplasmic ratio, surrounded by eosinophilic, fine fibrillar material. Elongated nuclei are often noted focally. Two other findings that may be present are periorbital ecchymoses (the so-called raccoon eyes) and heterochromia of the irises.

For infants with skin involvement, the prognosis is generally good, with either spontaneous remission or spontaneous transformation into benign ganglioneuromas expected. Prognostic factors other than age, based on molecular genetic characteristics such as the status of the oncogene *MYCN* and chromosome 1p deletion, are helping to stratify prognosis and therapeutic recommendations.

Monclair T, et al: The International Neuroblastoma Risk Group (INRG) staging system. J Clin Oncol 2009; 27: 298.

Ganglioneuroma

Ganglioneuroma has only rarely been described in the skin as an isolated entity. These tumors are composed of mature ganglion cells commingled with fascicles of spindle cells. They arise most often in von Recklinghausen neurofibromatosis or with neuroblastomas and usually occur in childhood. The tissue stains positively for both argyrophilic and argentaffin granules.

Furmanczyk PS, et al: Cutaneous ganglioneuroma associated with overlying hyperkeratotic epidermal changes. Am J Dermatopathol 2008; 30: 600.
Murphy M, et al: Cutaneous ganglioneuroma. Int J Dermatol 2007; 46: 861.

Nasal Glioma (Cephalic Brainlike Heterotopias)

Nasal gliomas are rare, benign, congenital tumors. When they occur extranasally, they are easily confused with hemangiomas. The tumor is usually a firm, incompressible (unlike hemangioma

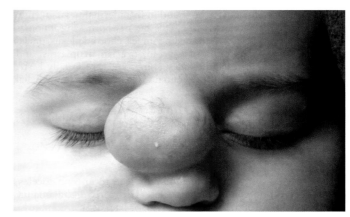

Fig. 28.50 Nasal glioma. (Courtesy Scott Bartlett, MD.)

and encephalocele), reddish blue to purple lesion occurring on the nasal bridge or midline near the root (Fig. 28.50). It does not transilluminate or enlarge with crying, unlike some encephaloceles. It may also occur intranasally.

Nasal gliomas differ from encephaloceles in that the latter are connected to the subarachnoid space by a sinus tract, whereas the former usually lose this connection before birth. Clinically, these cannot be absolutely differentiated, so a biopsy should not be performed. Skull radiographs, MRI, ultrasound, and Doppler flow studies may be performed, to help define the lesion and detect possible skull involvement. Neurosurgical consultation is advisable.

Histologically, the nodule consists of glial tissue associated with glial giant cells, fibrous tissue, and numerous blood vessels. It is unencapsulated. The lesion does not involute spontaneously.

Bellet JS: Developmental anomalies of the skin. Semin Perinatol 2013; 37: 20.
Gnagi SH, Schraff SA: Nasal obstruction in newborns. Pediatr Clin North Am 2013; 60: 903.

Cutaneous Meningioma

Primary cutaneous meningioma represents a continuum with rudimentary meningocele. It results from the presence of meningocytes outside the calvarium. If actual brain remnants are present, the lesion is called a rudimentary cephalocele. Small, hard, fibrous, calcified nodules occur along the spine, in the scalp, on the forehead, or rarely in the external ear canal. Most occur over the scalp, and some have an underlying connection to the CNS or an underlying bony abnormality. They usually come to medical attention in the first year of life. On the scalp, they may present with a dark tuft of hair or an alopecic area surrounded by a dark collar of hair (hair collar sign).

Type I lesions present at birth and develop from ectopic arachnoid cells. Type II lesions usually present in adults and demonstrate arachnoid cells surrounding nerve bundles. Type III lesions are caused by direct extension or metastasis from dural neoplasms. Cutaneous meningiomas may develop in the scalp secondary to an intracranial meningioma, either through erosion of the skull or by extension through an operative defect of the skull. Last, they may also arise from cranial or spinal nerves. Clinically, these lesions have no distinctive appearance. They are firm subcutaneous nodules adherent to the skin.

Diagnosis is made by histologic examination. The tumors consist of vascular-like anastomosing spaces with spindle cells forming whorls around collagen bundles. Lamellar, calcified psammoma bodies are often present. Psammoma bodies are not specific for meningiomas and may also be found in intradermal nevi, juvenile xanthogranuloma, pituitary of the fetus and newborn, schwannomas associated with Carney syndrome, meninges, choroid plexus, pineal gland, papillary carcinoma of thyroid, ovarian neoplasms, and mammary intraductal papilloma. Meningiomas are usually EMA and p63 positive, creating the potential for confusion with epithelial lesions.

Fox MD, et al: Cutaneous meningioma. J Cutan Pathol 2013; 40: 891.

Encephalocele and Meningocele

Primary defects in the neural tube may lead to encephaloceles, meningoceles, or meningomyeloceles. They present in infancy along the midline of the face, scalp, neck, or back as soft, compressible masses that may transilluminate or enlarge with crying. Tufts of long, dark hair or alopecia with a surrounding collar of dark hair may overlie them.

Many cutaneous lesions of the midline of the back, most frequently at the base of the spine, suggest that malformations of the spinal cord and associated structures are present. Cutaneous manifestations of spinal dysraphism include depressed or polypoid lesions; dyschromic or hairy lesions; dermal or subcutaneous lesions; vascular malformations; or neoplasms of many types. Midline masses require intensive radiologic and neurosurgical evaluation before biopsy because of the possible connection to the CNS. MRI is the imaging modality of choice. Approximately 10% of patients will have evidence of occult spinal dysraphism if one abnormality is present, whereas the majority will have dysraphism if two or more abnormalities are present.

Chordomas, Parachordomas, and Myoepitheliomas

Parachordomas are closely related to myoepitheliomas and mixed tumor of skin and salivary gland. They generally occur as an isolated neoplasm. Both benign and malignant parachordomas occur in skin and can be differentiated by the degree of cellularity, atypia, and number of mitoses. Chordomas are soft tissue neoplasms that present as firm, smooth nodules in the sacrococcygeal region or at the base of the skull in middle-aged patients. They arise from notochord remnants. The pathologic appearance for each of these tumors is that of an incompletely encapsulated tumor with nests and cords of large epithelioid cells with multivacuolated physaliferous cells. Chordomas may metastasize late in their course to various sites, including the skin. Wide excision with postoperative radiation therapy is the treatment of choice.

Ali S, et al: Parachordoma/myoepithelioma. Skeletal Radiol 2013; 42: 431.
Rekhi B, et al: Histopathological, immunohistochemical and molecular spectrum of myoepithelial tumours of soft tissues. Virchows Arch 2012; 461: 687.

ABNORMALITIES OF FAT TISSUE

Lipomas

Lipomas, subcutaneous tumors composed of fat tissue, may occur as a solitary sporadic lesion or as multiple lesions with or without a familial component. There are multiple histologic subtypes, and these frequently have an associated clinical correlation. Most have specific chromosomal alterations that help in their identification in difficult cases. Protease inhibitors given for HIV disease may induce lipomas, angiolipomas, or benign symmetric lipomatosis, as well as lipodystrophy.

Lipomas are most often found on the trunk. They also occur frequently on the neck, forearms, and axillae. They are soft, single or multiple, small or large, lobulated, compressible growths, over which the skin on traction often becomes dimpled, although otherwise unchanged. Lipomas usually stop growing after attaining a certain size, then remain stationary indefinitely. Frontalis-associated lipomas of the forehead are relatively large lesions arising either within or deep to the frontalis muscle.

A lipoma located in the midline of the sacral region may be a marker for spinal dysraphism or other embryologic malformation. Other midline lesions, such as tufts of hair ("fawn's tail"), hemangiomas (Cobb syndrome), skin tags, sinuses, or pigmented lesions, should also raise suspicion for occult embryologic malformations. MRI is the most sensitive imaging modality. If spinal dysraphism is diagnosed, early treatment may be possible before irreversible damage has occurred. Do not attempt to biopsy a sacrococcygeal lipoma; call a neurosurgeon into consultation. It may be a lipomeningocele with communicating sinuses to the dura.

Histologically, the lipoma is an encapsulated, lobulated tumor containing normal fat cells held together by strands of connective tissue. Occasionally, eccrine sweat glands may be associated, and then they are called adenolipomas. Alterations in chromosomes 12q13–15 and chromosomes 13q12–22 may be detected in benign lipomas.

Lipomas may be left untreated, unless they are large enough to be objectionable. They may be excised, removed with liposuction, extruded through a 3-mm incision after being freed with a cutting curette, or segmentally extracted through a stab incision. More advanced surgical technique is necessary to remove the deep lesions on the forehead, which may lie below the fascial plane. Injection with phosphatidylcholine has also been reported as successful.

Multiple lipomas may occur in groups of two to hundreds of confluent painless tumors of various sizes over any part of the body (Fig. 28.51). These lesions are sometimes painful when growing rapidly. When present in certain patterns, special designations are applied. Madelung disease (benign symmetric lipomatosis or multiple symmetric lipomatosis) occurs most often in middle-aged men, who may develop multiple, large, painless, coalescent lipomas around the neck, shoulders, and upper arms. Familial multiple lipomatosis is a dominantly inherited syndrome in which multiple asymptomatic lipomas of the forearms and thighs appear in the third decade of life. The shoulders and neck are spared, and the lipomas are encapsulated and movable. Diffuse lipomatosis is characterized by an early age of onset, usually before 2 years; diffuse infiltration of muscle by an unencapsulated mass of histologically mature lipocytes; and progressive enlargement and extension

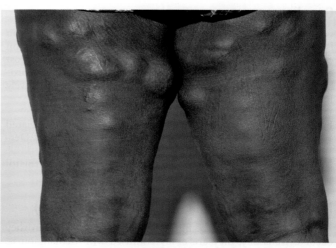

Fig. 28.51 Multiple lipomas.

of the tumor mass. It usually involves a large portion of the trunk or an extremity. Some cases are associated with distant lipomas or hemangiomas or with hypertrophy of underlying bone.

Dercum disease (adiposis dolorosa) is seen most often in obese or corpulent menopausal women who develop symmetric, tender, circumscribed fatty lesions. These are often accompanied by weakness and psychiatric disturbances. Relief of pain lasting for weeks after intravenous infusions of lidocaine, 1.3 g/day for 4 days, has been reported.

Several other conditions are characterized by multiple abnormalities, including lipomas. Encephalocraniocutaneous lipomatosis is a rare neurocutaneous syndrome characterized by unilateral porencephalic cysts with cortical atrophy, ipsilateral facial and scalp lesions, ocular abnormalities, cranial asymmetry, and neurologic complications. The skin changes consist of unilateral lipomatous scalp tumors with overlying alopecia and connective tissue nevi. Ipsilateral lipodermoids, choristomas, and calcifications are the eye findings. CNS abnormalities include unilateral cerebral atrophy, dilated ventricles, porencephaly, cerebral calcifications, and lipomas of the leptomeninges. Seizures and mental retardation may occur. Some patients may have overlapping features of Proteus syndrome: multiple lipomas, epidermal nevi, cerebriform lesions of the plantar surfaces, vascular malformations, macrodactyly, hemihypertrophy, exostoses, and scoliosis.

Bannayan-Riley-Ruvalcaba syndrome is characterized by multiple subcutaneous lipomas and vascular malformations, lentigines of the penis and vulva, verrucae, and acanthosis nigricans. There is overlap in some of these cases with Cowden syndrome. Both syndromes have been associated with allelic mutations of the *PTEN* gene.

Multiple endocrine neoplasia type I has been associated with skin lesions consisting of multiple facial angiofibromas, collagenomas, café au lait spots, lipomas, confetti-like hypopigmented macules, and multiple gingival papules, in addition to the tumors of the parathyroid glands, endocrine pancreas, and anterior pituitary.

Fröhlich syndrome consists of multiple lipomas, obesity, and sexual infantilism.

Gardner syndrome consists of multiple osteomas, fibromas, desmoid tumors, lipomas, fibrosarcomas, epidermal inclusion cysts, and leiomyomas, associated with intestinal polyposis exclusively in the colon and rectum. The coexistence of cutaneous cysts, leiomyomas, and osteomas (mostly on the skull) with intestinal polyposis is frequently not recognized until malignant degeneration of one of the polyps occurs and surgical removal brings the syndrome to notice. Half of such patients develop carcinoma of the colon before age 30, and almost all these patients die before age 50, unless they have surgical treatment. In general, total colectomy is advised. Bony exostoses occur in 50% of patients and usually involve the membranous bones of the face and head. Cysts occur in 63% of patients and again, most frequently involve the face and scalp. These are epidermal inclusion cysts; two thirds have within them foci of pilomatrical differentiation. Pigmented lesions of the ocular fundus occurred in 90% of 41 patients with Gardner syndrome and 46% of 43 first-degree relatives. They are usually multiple and bilateral and, having been seen in a 3-month-old infant, are probably congenital. Gardner syndrome is transmitted as an autosomal dominant disease. The defect is a mutation in the *APC* gene located at chromosome 5q21. In some families, polyposis and carcinoma may occur without the skin and bone tumors. Lipomas have also been noted in the Carney complex, along with myxomas and pigmented lesions.

Subtypes

Angiolipomas present as painful subcutaneous nodules, having all the other features of a typical lipoma. Multiple subcutaneous angiolipomas are common and have no invasive or metastatic potential. They may be associated with CMs and may be induced by protease inhibitor therapy of HIV disease.

The angiolipoleiomyoma (angiomyolipoma of the skin) affects the acral skin of middle-aged men. No signs of tuberous sclerosis or renal angiomyolipoma are present. Mature adipocytes, thick-walled blood vessels, and smooth muscle cells in fascicles around blood vessels are present.

Neural fibrolipoma is an overgrowth of fibrofatty tissue along a nerve trunk that often leads to nerve compression. Patients are usually age 30 or younger and note a slowly enlarging subcutaneous mass with associated tenderness, decreased sensation, or paresthesia. The median nerve is most often involved. At times, macrodactyly appears, with elongation and splaying of the phalanges. MRI will provide the diagnosis, but unfortunately, there is no effective treatment.

Chondroid lipomas are deep-seated, firm, yellow tumors that characteristically occur on the legs of women. Histologically, there is a thin capsule around mature lipocytes that have a single large vacuole and multivacuolated, S-100/vimentin-positive cells within a chondromyxoid matrix.

The spindle cell lipoma is an asymptomatic, slow-growing subcutaneous tumor that has a predilection for the posterior back, neck, and shoulders of older patients. It is usually solitary, although multiple lesions may occur. Some patients have a familial background of similar lesions. The neoplasm consists of lobulated masses of mature adipose tissue with areas of spindle cell proliferation. The spindle cells stain positive for CD34. Abnormalities of chromosomes 16 and 13 have been reported. The spindled component of young spindle cell lipomas may be myxoid or cellular. The nuclei may be wavy and accompanied by mast cells, as in a neurofibroma. Examples with minimal fat may be misdiagnosed as solitary fibrous tumors. In old spindle cell lipomas (fibrolipomas), the spindle cell component has matured into dense collagen bundles.

Pleomorphic lipomas, as with spindle cell lipomas, occur mostly on the back or neck of older individuals. There are floret giant cells with overlapping nuclei. Occasional lipoblast-like cells and atypical nuclei may be present and require differentiation from a liposarcoma. There is loss of chromosome 16q material. Despite this alarming appearance, the lesions behave in a perfectly benign manner. Pleomorphic lipomas lack the size, depth, infiltrative growth, and arborizing vascular pattern of liposarcoma. The term *atypical lipomatous tumor* is used to describe well-differentiated, low-grade liposarcoma. Extensive or deeply infiltrating tumors should be reviewed by a clinician experienced in soft tissue pathology.

The intradermal spindle cell/pleomorphic lipoma is distinct in that it most often affects women and has a wide distribution, occurring with relatively equal frequency on the head and neck, trunk, and the upper and lower extremities. Histologically, these lesions are unencapsulated and have infiltrative margins. Again, the spindle cells stain positive for CD34.

Hibernoma (lipoma of brown fat) is a form of lipoma composed of finely vacuolated fat cells of embryonic type. Hibernomas have a distinctive brownish color and a firm consistency and usually occur singly. These tumors are benign. They occur chiefly in the mediastinum and the interscapular region of the back, but they also occur on the scalp, sternal region, and legs. They are usually about 3–12 cm in breadth, and the onset is most often in adult life. Abnormalities of chromosomes 10 and 11 have been reported in the lesions. Epidural lipomatosis, collections of fat in the epidural space, may cause acute chord compression in the course of systemic corticosteroid treatment. A case of this distinctive, uncommon side effect proved to be the result of deposits of brown fat.

Dalal KM, et al: Diagnosis and management of lipomatous tumors. J Surg Oncol 2008; 97: 298.

Pinto CI, et al: Madelung's disease. AEsthetic Plast Surg 2017; 41: 359.

Nevus Lipomatosus Superficialis

Soft, yellowish papules or cerebriform plaques, usually of the buttock or thigh, less often of the ear or scalp, with a wrinkled rather than warty surface, characterize nevus lipomatosus superficialis. The distribution may be either zonal (as in the multiple lesions reported by Hoffmann and Zurhelle) or solitary. Solitary lesions appear as plaque, or linear array, but some resemble broad, fatty acrochordons. Onset before age 20 is the rule. Most do not require treatment, but diagnostic biopsy is sometimes performed, and intralesional phosphatidylcholine has been reported as successful.

Sendhil Kumaran M, et al: Nevus lipomatosus superficialis unseen or unrecognized. J Cutan Med Surg 2013; 17: 335.

Folded Skin With Scarring ("Michelin Tire Baby" Syndrome)

In this rare syndrome, the infant has numerous deep, conspicuous, symmetric, ringed creases around the extremities, resembling stacked tires (Fig. 28.52). The underlying skin may manifest a smooth muscle hamartoma, a nevus lipomatosis, or elastic tissue abnormalities. It may occur as an autosomal dominant or recessive trait, as a sporadic condition, as an isolated finding or in association with congenital facial and limb abnormalities, or with severe neurologic defects.

Ulucan H, et al: Circumferential skin folds and multiple anomalies. Clin Dysmorphol 2013; 22: 87.

Benign Lipoblastoma

Frequently confused with a liposarcoma, benign lipoblastoma affects infants and young children exclusively, with approximately 90% of cases occurring before 3 years of age. It most often involves the soft tissues of the upper and lower extremities. A circumscribed and a diffuse form can be distinguished. The circumscribed form is superficially located and clinically comparable to a lipoma. The diffuse form is more deeply situated and is analogous to diffuse lipomatosis. Microscopically, both forms consist of lobulated immature adipose tissue composed of lipoblasts, a plexiform capillary pattern, and a richly myxoid stroma. Cytogenetic studies for rearrangements of chromosome 8q11–q13 or fluorescence in situ hybridization (FISH) analysis for the *PLAG1–HAS2* fusion gene help to distinguish this tumor from liposarcoma, a distinction that can be difficult histologically. Complete local excision is the treatment of choice; however, recurrences may occur in as many as one quarter of patients.

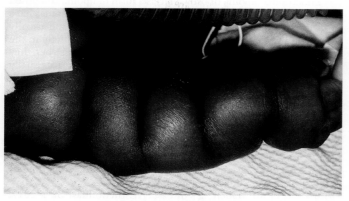

Fig. 28.52 "Michelin tire baby."

Choi HJ, et al: Pediatric lipoblastoma of the neck. J Craniofac Surg 2013; 24: e507.

Deen M, et al: A novel *PLAG1-RAD51L1* gene fusion resulting from a t(8;14)(q12;q24) in a case of lipoblastoma. Cancer Genet 2013; 206: 233.

Liposarcoma

Liposarcomas are the most common soft tissue sarcoma. They usually arise from the intermuscular fascia, and only rarely from the subcutaneous fat. They do not arise from preexisting lipomas. The usual course is an inconspicuous swelling of the soft tissue that undergoes an imperceptibly gradual enlargement. When a fatty tumor becomes larger than 10 cm in diameter, liposarcoma should be seriously considered. The upper thigh is the most common site. Other frequent sites are the buttocks, groin, and upper extremities. Adult males are mainly affected.

Liposarcomas may be well differentiated; subtypes include the adipocytic, sclerosing, inflammatory, spindle cell, and dedifferentiate variants. In this category, there are aberrations of chromosome 12. Myxoid and round cell–variant liposarcoma often shows poorly differentiated histology. In most cases, there is a reciprocal translocation t(12; 16)(q13; q11). The third major class is pleomorphic liposarcoma. Dermal lesions may resemble pleomorphic lipoma but are S100 positive and contain lipoblasts.

Treatment is adequate radical excision of the lesion. In patients with well-differentiated superficial lesions, the prognosis is good; for deeper, high-grade lesions, the extension between fascial planes and presence of small satellite nodules require carefully planned surgery, which may be assisted by MRI guidance. For metastatic liposarcomas, radiation therapy may be effective.

Al-Zaid T, et al: Dermal pleomorphic liposarcoma resembling pleomorphic fibroma. J Cutan Pathol 2013; 40: 734.

ABNORMALITIES OF SMOOTH MUSCLE

Leiomyoma

Cutaneous leiomyomas are smooth muscle tumors characterized by painful nodules that occur singly or multiply. They may be separated conveniently into solitary and multiple cutaneous leiomyomas arising from arrectores pilorum muscles (piloleiomyomas); solitary genital leiomyomas arising from the dartoic, vulvar, or mammillary muscle; and solitary angioleiomyomas arising from the muscles of veins.

Solitary Cutaneous Leiomyoma

The typical lesion is a deeply circumscribed, rounded nodule 2–15 mm in diameter. It is freely movable. The overlying skin may have a reddish or violaceous tint. Although the lesion is insensitive at first, painful paroxysms may occur. Once pain commences, it tends to intensify.

Multiple Cutaneous Leiomyomas

These brownish, grouped, papular lesions vary from 2–23 mm in diameter and are the most common variety of leiomyoma (Fig. 28.53). Two or more sites of the skin surface may be involved. The firm, smooth, superficial, sometimes translucent, and freely movable nodules are located most frequently on the trunk and extremities. They often form linear or dermatomal patterns, either alone or with scattered isolated nonsegmental lesions elsewhere. These leiomyomas may occur on the tongue or, less often, elsewhere in the mouth as well. The usual age at onset is the teens to the fourth decade. Eruptive lesions have been described in chronic lymphocytic leukemia.

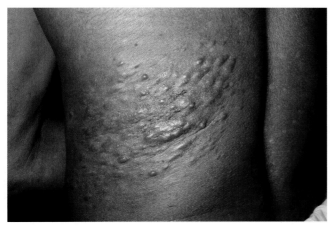

Fig. 28.53 Multiple leiomyomas. (Courtesy Dr. Debabrata Bandyopadhyay.)

Multiple leiomyomas are inherited in an autosomal dominant manner as part of Reed syndrome. Women with this inherited type often have uterine leiomyomas as well. This is part of an inherited syndrome in which some patients also have a predisposition to type II papillary renal carcinomas or renal collecting duct cancer. Mutations in the fumarate hydratase gene are present in 75% of patients with Reed syndrome; these mutations may also be inherited in an autosomal recessive manner. Fully affected children have severe neurologic impairment. The adult carriers may develop leiomyomas. Sporadic leiomyoma, leiomyosarcomas, renal cancers, and uterine leiomyomas have a very low frequency of fumarate hydratase gene mutations.

Genital Leiomyomas

These lesions are located on the scrotum, on the labia majora, or rarely on the nipples. They may be intracutaneous or subcutaneous in location. Most genital leiomyomas are painless and solitary. Alport syndrome is an X-linked dominant syndrome consisting of hematuric nephropathy, deafness, and maculopathy caused by mutations in type IV collagen. Some of these patients will have diffuse leiomyomatosis, which may affect the esophagus, tracheobronchial tree, perirectal area, and genital tract and vulva. Bilateral nipple leiomyomas have been associated with *BRAF* inhibition therapy.

Angioleiomyoma (Vascular Leiomyoma)

Angioleiomyoma arises from the muscle of veins. Pain, either spontaneous or provoked by pressure or cold, occurs in about half the cases. Vascular leiomyoma is found mostly on the lower leg in middle-aged women. Solid tumors occur three times more frequently in women, and cavernous tumors occur four times more often in men. Solid lesions on the extremities are usually painful; tumors of the head are rarely painful. In AIDS patients, multiple skin and visceral angioleiomyomas may occur. These tumors' cells possess the Epstein-Barr virus genome.

Histologically, the leiomyoma is made up of bundles and masses of smooth muscle fibers. Varying amounts of collagen are intermingled. The smooth muscle cells are finely fibrillated and contain a glycogen vacuole adjacent to the nucleus. The nuclei are typically long, thin, and cigar shaped.

Angiolipoleiomyoma

Fitzpatrick et al. reported eight patients with acquired, solitary, asymptomatic acral nodules. Seven were men, and all were adults.

Histologically, they had well-circumscribed subcutaneous tumors composed of smooth muscle cells, blood vessels, connective tissue, and fat.

Treatment

Leiomyomas are benign. Solitary painful lesions may be excised. When they are multiple and familial, monitoring for renal cell or collecting duct carcinoma is important. When multiple lesions are present and painful, as may occur especially in the winter, relief of pain may be achieved by giving doxazosin, an oral α_1-adrenoceptor antagonist. This is better tolerated than phenoxybenzamine, an α-adrenergic blocker, which also has been reported to provide pain relief. Nifedipine (10 mg three times daily or long acting forms 30–90 mg daily), amlodipine, gabapentin, oral nitroglycerin, and α-blockers have also had variable success. An ice cube applied over the lesions often induces pain, and the effectiveness of therapy may be assessed by the length of time it takes for the ice cube to cause pain. Botulinum toxin type A (Botox) injection has also been reported as effective.

Aggarwal S, et al: Disseminated cutaneous leiomyomatosis treated with oral amlodipine. Indian J Dermatol Venereol Leprol 2013; 79: 136.

Kontochristopoulos G, et al: A case of Reed's syndrome. Case Rep Dermatol 2014; 6: 189.

Stewart L, et al: Association of germline mutations in the fumarate hydratase gene and uterine fibroids in women with hereditary leiomyomatosis and renal cell cancer. Arch Dermatol 2008; 144: 1584.

Congenital Smooth Muscle Hamartoma

Congenital smooth muscle hamartoma is typically a skin-colored or lightly pigmented patch or plaque with hypertrichosis. It is often present at birth, usually on the trunk, with the lumbosacral area involved in two thirds of patients. Older patients may have perifollicular papules. They vary in size from 2 × 3 to 10 × 10 cm. The "Michelin tire baby" syndrome may result from a diffuse smooth muscle hamartoma. One patient presented with a linear reddish purple plaque. The incidence is approximately 1 in 2600 newborns. Transient elevation on rubbing may be seen (pseudo-Darier sign) in 80% of patients. An association with multiple adult myofibromas has been reported, as has association with congenital melanocytic nevus.

Histologically, numerous thick, long, well-defined bundles of smooth muscle are seen in the dermis at various angles of orientation. There may be an increase in hair follicles, and some cases have been associated with congenital or blue nevi.

In some patients, there is clinical and histologic overlap with Becker nevus. Classically, Becker nevus is a unilateral (rarely bilateral) acquired hyperpigmentation, usually beginning as a tan macule on the shoulder or pectoral area of a teenage male. Over time, hypertrichosis develops within it. Biopsy of such lesions shows acanthosis, papillomatosis, and increased basal cell pigmentation. Occasional congenital lesions manifesting hyperpigmentation and hypertrichosis have shown biopsy findings consistent with those of a Becker nevus (no smooth muscle proliferation), and lesions with a typical late-onset history compatible with Becker nevus have occasionally shown smooth muscle hamartoma–like changes in the dermis. Other cases of late-onset smooth muscle hamartomas are occasionally reported that are not hyperpigmented or hypertrichotic. No treatment is necessary.

Tzu J, et al: Combined blue nevus–smooth muscle hamartoma. J Cutan Pathol 2013; 40: 879.

Leiomyosarcoma

Superficial leiomyosarcomas, originating in the dermis or subcutaneous tissue, account for approximately 2% of all soft tissue sarcomas. An association with Reed syndrome has been reported. Occasionally, a lesion may present in the skin that is a metastasis from an internal source. The cutaneous leiomyosarcoma appears in the dermis as a solitary nodule. It may originate from the arrector pili or genital dartoic muscle. This has a good prognosis. Recurrence rates with Mohs surgery are approximately 15%, with metastases a rare event. Subcutaneous leiomyosarcomas, on the contrary, have a guarded prognosis, because hematogenous metastases occur in approximately 35% of patients. These prove fatal in about one third of patients. Lung metastases are common, so chest imaging is an important part of monitoring these patients.

The clinical appearance of leiomyosarcomas is not distinctive, and thus the diagnosis is established by the histopathologic findings. These differ from the leiomyoma by dense cellularity, nuclear pleomorphism, numerous mitotic figures, and disarray of the smooth muscle bundles. Collagen is found only in the septa. Desmin, smooth muscle actin, and h-caldesmon are helpful in differentiating leiomyosarcoma from other spindle cell or pleomorphic tumors.

The preferred method of treatment is wide local excision with a 1-cm margin. The Mohs surgical approach is useful in limiting recurrences and sparing tissue. Radiation therapy and chemotherapy are generally not effective.

Deneve JL, et al: Cutaneous leiomyosarcoma. Cancer Control 2013; 20: 307.
Wang C, et al: Reed syndrome presenting with leiomyosarcoma. JAAD Case Rep 2015; 1: 150.
Weiler L, et al: Isolated cutaneous leiomyosarcoma revealing a novel germline mutation of the fumarate hydratase gene. Br J Dermatol 2016; 175: 1104.

MISCELLANEOUS TUMORS AND TUMOR-ASSOCIATED CONDITIONS

Cutaneous Endometriosis

Endometriosis of the skin is characterized by the appearance of brownish papules at the umbilicus or in lower abdominal scars after gynecologic surgery in middle-aged women. The usually solitary tumor ranges from a few to 60 mm (average 5 mm) in diameter. The tender or painful lesion is bluish black from the bleeding that occurs cyclically in many patients. Histopathologic findings are glandular structures with a columnar epithelium and a surrounding fibromyxoid stroma typically containing extravasated red blood cells and hemosiderin. Decidualized endometriosis demonstrates glassy-pink epithelioid cells surrounding contracted lumina. Treatment of choice is surgical excision. Preoperative treatment with danazol or leuprolide may reduce its size.

Cameron M, et al: Postmenopausal cutaneous endometriosis. Breast J 2017; 23: 356.
DeClerck BK, et al: Cutaneous decidualized endometriosis in a nonpregnant female. Am J Dermatopathol 2012; 34: 541.

Teratoma

Teratomas may develop in the skin but are most common in the ovaries or testes. Occurrence with a myelomeningocele has been reported. They have no characteristic clinical features, but on microscopic examination many types of tissue, representative of all three germ layers, are present. Hair, teeth, and functioning thyroid tissue are examples of fully differentiated tissues that may develop. Occasionally, malignancy may occur.

Bellet JS: Developmental anomalies of the skin. Semin Perinatol 2013; 37: 20.

Metastatic Carcinoma

Malignant tumors are able to grow at sites distant from the primary site of origin; thus dissemination to the skin may occur with any malignant neoplasm. These infiltrates may result from direct invasion of the skin from underlying tumors, may extend by lymphatic or hematogenous spread, or may be introduced by therapeutic procedures.

From 5%–10% of patients with cancer develop skin metastases. The reported incidence figures vary widely according to the type of study undertaken and the site of primary tumor studied. The frequency of involvement of the skin is low when other sites are considered, such as the lung, liver, lymph nodes, and brain.

Usually, metastases occur as numerous firm, hard, or rubbery masses, with a predilection for the chest, abdomen, or scalp, in an adult over age 40 who has had a previously diagnosed carcinoma. However, many variations exist in morphology, number of lesions, site of growth, age at onset, and timing of metastases. They are most often intradermal papules, nodules, or tumors that are firm, skin colored to reddish, purplish, black, or brown; may be fixed to underlying tissues; and rarely ulcerate.

Several unusual morphologic patterns occur. Carcinoma en cuirasse is a diffuse infiltration of the skin that imparts an indurated and hidebound leathery quality to skin. This sclerodermoid change, also referred to as scirrhous carcinoma, is produced by fibrosis and single rows of tumor cells. This type primarily occurs with breast carcinoma. Carcinoma telangiectaticum is another unusual type of cutaneous metastasis from breast carcinoma that presents as small, pink to purplish papules, pseudovesicles, and telangiectases.

Inflammatory carcinoma (carcinoma erysipelatoides) is characterized by erythema, edema, warmth, and a well-defined leading edge, similar to erysipelas in appearance (Fig. 28.54). This is usually caused by breast carcinoma but has been reported with many other primary tumors. Histologically, there is minimal to no inflammation, but rather neoplastic cells within dilated superficial dermal vessels.

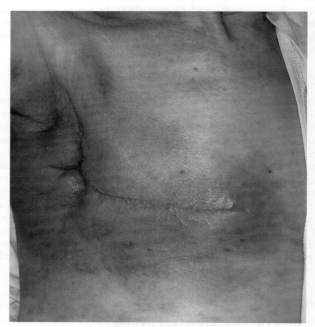

Fig. 28.54 Carcinoma erysipeloides.

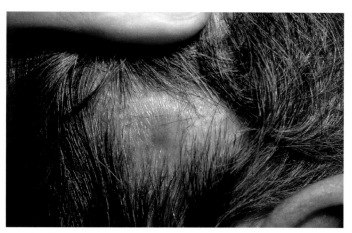

Fig. 28.55 Alopecia neoplastica secondary to breast carcinoma.

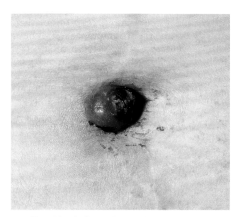

Fig. 28.56 Sister Mary Joseph nodule.

Alopecia neoplastica may present as a cicatricial localized area of hair loss (Fig. 28.55). On biopsy it is usually seen to be caused by breast metastases in women and by lung or kidney carcinoma in men. Metastatic breast cancer may be darkly pigmented, as may Paget disease of the breast.

The so-called Sister Mary Joseph nodule is formed by localization of metastatic tumors to the umbilicus (Fig. 28.56). The most common primary sites are the stomach, large bowel, ovary, and pancreas. Zosteriform, linear, or chancroidal ulcerations of the genitalia and verrucous nodules of the legs are other, rarely reported clinical presentations.

The primary tumor is usually diagnosed before the appearance of metastases, and dissemination to the skin is often a late finding. Metastases to other, more frequently involved organs, such as the lung and liver, have usually occurred. A poor prognosis is thus the rule. Skin infiltrates may, however, be the first harbinger of a malignant visceral neoplasm and are often the first clinically apparent metastatic site.

The principal anatomic sites to which metastases localize are the chest, abdomen, and scalp, with the back and extremities being relatively uncommon areas. Involvement of the skin is likely to be near the area of the primary tumor. Thus chest lesions are usually caused by breast carcinoma in women and lung carcinoma in men, abdominal or perineal lesions by colonic carcinoma, and the face by SCC of the oral cavity. Extremity lesions, when they occur, are most often caused by melanoma.

Because of its overall high prevalence, breast cancer is the type most frequently metastatic to the skin in women, and melanoma,

followed by lung cancer, is the type seen most often in men. Colon carcinoma is also common because of its high incidence in both genders. Renal cell carcinoma, although less common, has a predilection for scalp metastases. Metastatic lesions are uncommon in children, but when they do occur, neuroblastoma and leukemia are the most frequent causes.

Lymphangiosarcoma (Stewart-Treves syndrome) develops in a site of chronic lymphedema, such as in breast cancer patients who have had lymph node resection. Antikeratin antibodies are useful in identifying metastatic breast carcinoma, whereas CD34, CD31, and *Ulex europeus* lectin are positive in Stewart-Treves angiosarcoma. Differential staining with keratins 7 and 20 can help suggest the site of origin in cases of cutaneous metastatic adenocarcinoma.

Sittart JA, et al: Cutaneous metastasis from internal carcinomas. An Bras Dermatol 2013; 88: 541

Paraneoplastic Syndromes

Some cancers produce findings in the skin indicating that an underlying internal malignancy may be present. These may range from a specific eruption characteristic of a particular type of cancer, such as necrolytic migratory erythema, to a nonspecific cutaneous reaction pattern, such as that caused by an internal malignancy. Although many of these syndromes are discussed in other chapters, a few are mentioned here as illustrative examples of this phenomenon.

Bazex syndrome, or acrokeratosis paraneoplastica, is characterized by violaceous erythema and scaling of the fingers, toes, nose, and aural helices. Nail dystrophy and palmoplantar keratoderma may be seen. These cases are secondary to primary malignant neoplasms of the upper aerodigestive tract or metastatic cancer to lymph nodes, often in the cervical region.

The glucagonoma syndrome is characterized by weight loss, glucose intolerance, anemia, glossitis, and necrolytic migratory erythema. Erythematous patches with bullae and light-brown papules with scales involving the face, groin, and abdomen characterize the skin eruption. This is seen with glucagon-secreting tumors of the pancreas.

Erythema gyratum repens is a gyrate serpiginous erythema with characteristic wood grain–pattern scales; it is almost always associated with an underlying malignancy. Hypertrichosis lanuginosa acquisita, or malignant down, is the sudden growth of profuse, soft, nonmedullated, nonpigmented, downy hair in an adult. The most common sites of associated carcinoma reported were the lung and colon.

The sign of Leser-Trélat is the sudden appearance of multiple pruritic seborrheic keratoses, associated with an internal malignancy. Trousseau sign, or migratory thrombophlebitis, is usually associated with pancreatic carcinoma (Fig. 28.57). A form of pemphigus, paraneoplastic pemphigus, is most frequently associated with lymphoma, chronic lymphocytic leukemia, and Castleman disease.

Several cutaneous diseases that are not associated with internal malignancy with the frequency of the previous conditions, but that may be a sign of internal malignancy in some cases, are exfoliative erythroderma (lymphoproliferative disease), acanthosis nigricans (adenocarcinoma), multicentric reticulohistiocytosis, Sweet syndrome (acute myelogenous leukemia), nodular fat necrosis (pancreatic carcinoma), Paget disease (underlying adnexal or breast carcinoma, or adenocarcinoma of genitourinary tract or colon), dermatomyositis in patients over age 40, palmar fasciitis and polyarthritis syndrome, and acquired ichthyosis (lymphoproliferative).

A variant of acquired ichthyosis, pityriasis rotunda, manifests circular, brown, scaly patches from 1–28 cm in diameter and varying in number from 1 to 20. They may occur on the trunk or extremities. These symptomless patches may be a clue to the diagnosis of hepatocellular carcinoma in South African black patients. Tripe

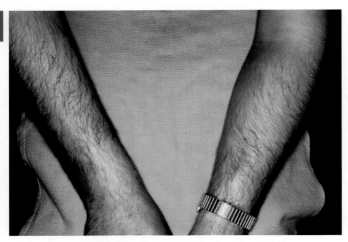

Fig. 28.57 Superficial migratory thrombophlebitis

palms, considered by some to be acanthosis nigricans of the palms, are associated with carcinoma in more than 90% of cases. Filiform hyperkeratosis of the palms may present in patients who develop cancer.

Da Silva JA, et al: Paraneoplastic cutaneous manifestations. An Bras Dermatol 2013; 88: 9.
Durieux V, et al: Autoimmune paraneoplastic syndromes associated to lung cancer. Lung Cancer 2017; 106: 102.
Holbrechts S, et al: Autoimmune paraneoplastic syndromes associated to lung cancer. Lung Cancer 2017; 106: 93.
Moore RL, et al: Epidermal manifestations of internal malignancy. Dermatol Clin 2008; 26: 17.
Pipkin CA, et al: Cutaneous manifestations of internal malignancies. Dermatol Clin 2008; 26: 1.
Shah A, et al: Neoplastic/paraneoplastic dermatitis, fasciitis, and panniculitis. Rheum Dis Clin North Am 2011; 37: 573.
Steele HA, et al: Mucocutaneous paraneoplastic syndromes associated with hematologic malignancies. Oncology (Williston Park) 2011; 25: 1076.

Carcinoid

Carcinoid involves the lungs, heart, and GI tract, as well as the skin. The outstanding feature of the skin is flushing, usually lasting 5–10 minutes. It most prominently involves the head and neck, but also produces a diffuse, scarlet color, with mottled red patches on the thorax and abdomen. Striking color changes may occur, with salmon red, bluish white, and other colors appearing simultaneously on various portions of the skin. Cyanosis may also be present. As the episodic flushing continues over months to years, telangiectases and plethora appear, as though the patient has polycythemia vera. Gyrate and serpiginous patches of erythema and cyanosis flare up and subside, not only on the face, but also on all parts of the body and extremities.

Pellagroid changes may appear as a result of shunting of dietary tryptophan away from the kynurenine-niacin pathway and into the 5-hydroxyindole pathway. Periorbital swelling, edema of the face, neck, and feet, and sclerodermatous changes may occur. Disseminated deep dermal and subcutaneous metastatic nodules from a primary bronchial carcinoid tumor have been documented. The clinical features of the carcinoid syndrome become evident only after hepatic metastases have occurred, or when the primary tumor is a bronchial carcinoid, or if the carcinoid arises in an ovarian teratoma, where the venous drainage bypasses the hepatic circulation.

The release of excessive amounts of serotonin and bradykinin into the circulation produces attacks of flushing of the skin, weakness, abdominal pain, nausea, vomiting, sweating, bronchoconstriction, palpitation, diarrhea, and collapse. These attacks may last a few hours. Right-sided cardiac valvular fibrosis occurs in 60% of chronically affected patients. Symptoms may be induced in these patients by the injection of epinephrine, at which time kinin peptide is released. Alcohol, hot beverages, exercise, and certain foods, among other factors, may induce flushing. The patient will provide the relevant triggers by history.

Etiologic Factors

Carcinoid, also called argentaffinoma, is a tumor that arises from the argentaffin Kulchitsky chromaffin cells in the appendix or terminal ileum, as well as in other parts of the GI tract, from the lungs as bronchial adenomas, and rarely from ovarian or testicular teratomas. Some of these produce large amounts of serotonin (5-hydroxytryptamine), a derivative of tryptophan, and others do not. The primary lesion is more active in the production of serotonin than are the metastases. The tumor frequently metastasizes to the draining lymph glands or to neighboring organs, especially the liver, and rarely to more distal sites.

Laboratory Findings

The diagnosis may be established by finding a high level of 5-hydroxyindolacetic acid (5-HIAA) in the urine. The normal urinary excretion of 5-HIAA is 3–8 mg/day, but in the presence of carcinoid it may reach 300 mg. Urinary values greater than 25 mg/day are diagnostic of carcinoid. Any value above the normal output is considered suspicious. The ingestion of bananas may cause significant elevations of 5-HIAA in the urine within a few hours, because banana pulp contains serotonin (4 mg/banana) and catecholamines. Tomatoes, red plums, pineapples, avocados, and eggplants also contain serotonin, but in much smaller amounts.

A screening test for 5-HIAA is the addition of nitrosonaphthol to the urine. A purple color is produced when 40 mg/day of 5-HIAA is excreted. Other serotonin metabolites besides 5-HIAA are found in the urine. The blood also contains serotonin in amounts of 0.2–0.4 mg%. In the presence of carcinoid, the amount may be 10 times normal.

Metastatic carcinoid may appear in the skin. A high index of suspicion is needed, because metastatic carcinoid has been reported to mimic apocrine poroma on shave biopsy.

Treatment

In the rare cases where there is only a primary tumor without metastases, this should be removed. Excision of metastatic lesions in the liver may also be considered. If this is impossible, long-acting somatostatin analogs provide good long-term symptomatic control of the flushing and diarrhea. Injections are given monthly. Vitamin supplementation with niacin and avoidance of known trigger factors to flushing are recommended. Restriction of tryptophan-containing foods for short periods may limit serotonin production.

Jabbour SA: Skin manifestations of hormone-secreting tumors. Dermatol Ther 2010; 23: 643.

Shah KR, et al: Cutaneous manifestations of gastrointestinal disease. J Am Acad Dermatol 2013; 68: 189.e1.

29 Epidermal Nevi, Neoplasms, and Cysts

EPIDERMAL NEVI

Epidermal nevi are hamartomatous growths of the epidermis that are present at birth in about half of patients or develop early in childhood. The term *epidermal nevus* includes several entities, including keratinocytic epidermal nevi, nevus sebaceus, and nevus comedonicus, depending on which epidermal cell or structure comprises the lesion. Epidermal nevi of all types are considered an expression of cutaneous mosaicism with genetic mutation in the affected skin. Lesions follow the lines of Blaschko, suggesting that they represent postzygotic mutations. Some syndromes have also been included in this classification, such as Proteus, CHILD, and phakomatosis pigmentokeratotica (a RASopathy with reported HRAS and KRAS mutations), and both localized lesions and systematized presentations may be caused by the same genetic mutations. In general, larger lesions, more widespread lesions, and lesions of the head and neck are more likely to have associated internal complications. The combination of an epidermal nevus and an associated internal problem is termed *epidermal nevus syndrome*. For each histologic type, the frequency and nature of associated systemic problems may be characteristic. Overall, about 1 in 1000 children have an epidermal nevus of some type.

Keratinocytic Epidermal Nevi

Keratinizing epidermal nevi are the most common type of epidermal nevus and are described by a great variety of terms, such as *linear epidermal nevus, hard nevus of Unna, soft epidermal nevus,* and *nevus verrucosus (verrucous nevus).* If the lesion is widespread on half the body, the term *nevus unius lateris* has been used. The term *ichthyosis hystrix* is used if the lesions are bilateral and widespread.

The most common pattern of keratinocytic epidermal nevus is linear epidermal nevus. The individual lesions are verrucous, skin-colored, dirty-gray, or brown papules, which coalesce to form a serpiginous plaque (Fig. 29.1). Interspersed in the localized patch may be horny excrescences and rarely comedones. The age of onset of epidermal nevi is generally at birth, but they may also develop within the first 10 years of life. They follow the lines of Blaschko.

The histologic changes in the epidermis are hyperplastic and affect chiefly the stratum corneum and stratum malpighii. There is variable hyperkeratosis, acanthosis, and papillomatosis. Up to 62% of biopsies of epidermal nevi have this pattern, so-called nonepidermolytic epidermal nevi. About 16% show epidermolytic hyperkeratosis. At times, other histologic patterns may be found, including a psoriatic type, an acrokeratosis verruciformis–like type, and a Darier disease–like type. It is assumed that each of these types would be associated with a specific mutation in the affected skin that, if widespread, would give rise to the cutaneous disorder with the same histology. For example, epidermal nevi that show epidermolytic hyperkeratosis would have the same gene mutation as the disorder of cornification, bullous congenital ichthyosiform erythroderma (i.e., keratins K1 and K10). In fact, patients with this type of epidermal nevus may have gonadal mosaicism that can result in offspring with the full-blown disorder. In a significant portion of the classic and common keratinocytic epidermal nevi that simply shows hyperkeratosis, papillomatosis, and acanthosis

histologically, there is an activating gene mutation in fibroblast growth factor receptor 3 *(FGFR3), HRAS,* or *PIK3CA,* a downstream effector of FGFR signaling. FOXN1 is highly expressed in these lesions. These same gene mutations are found in sporadic seborrheic keratoses, which, not surprisingly, have the same histology.

Keratinocytic epidermal nevi may be associated with skeletal abnormalities and central nervous system (CNS) manifestations. CNS manifestations appear to be more common when the lesions are large and located on the head and neck. Large keratinocytic epidermal nevi of the trunk and extremities are more frequently associated with skeletal abnormalities. Because both nevus sebaceus and keratinocytic epidermal nevi were included in the original and large reports of epidermal nevus syndrome, the precise characterization of the "keratinocytic epidermal nevus syndrome" remains to be defined.

Both Proteus syndrome and CLOVE syndrome (congenital lipomatous overgrowth, vascular malformations, and epidermal nevi) can have skin lesions of epidermal nevus. CLOVE is distinguished from Proteus syndrome by congenital overgrowth of a ballooning nature, which grows proportionately with the patient and typically affects the feet.

The CHILD syndrome and verruciform xanthoma are both characterized by the presence histologically of elongated and widened dermal papillae filled with xanthoma-like cells. Epidermal hyperplasia, with acanthosis, papillomatosis, parakeratosis, and hyperkeratosis, is also present (the features of a keratinocytic epidermal nevus). In rare cases, instead of half the body being affected, large quadrants of the body, favoring folds, are the sites of the epidermal growths (ptychotropism). CHILD and verruciform xanthoma (in some cases) contain mutations in the *NSDHL* gene, located on the X chromosome and required for cholesterol biosynthesis.

Epidermal nevus syndrome associated with *FGFR3* mutation is characterized by widespread epidermal nevus and developmental brain defects. Epidermal nevus syndrome may also be associated with vitamin D–resistant hypophosphatemic rickets, perhaps from circulating fibroblast growth factor 23 (FGF-23) acting as a phosphaturic.

Rarely, malignancies occur in keratinocytic epidermal nevi or in other organs. Any newly appearing lesion within a stable epidermal nevus should be biopsied to exclude this possibility. Management of keratinocytic epidermal nevi is difficult because, unless the treatment extends into the dermis (and thus may cause scarring), the lesion recurs. The use of a combination of 5% 5-fluorouracil (5-FU) plus 0.1% tretinoin creams once daily may be beneficial, and the response may be enhanced by occlusion. Cryotherapy can be quite effective, with good cosmetic results. Corticosteroids or a combination of a topical corticosteroid and calcipotriene may be beneficial. Carbon dioxide (CO_2) and erbium:yttrium-aluminum-garnet (Er:YAG) laser treatment may also be effective. If the lesion is small, simple excision can be considered.

Akingboye A, et al: Papillary transitional cell bladder carcinoma and systematized epidermal nevus syndrome. Cutis 2017; 99: 61.

Gantner S, et al: CHILD syndrome with mild skin lesions. J Cutan Pathol 2014; 41: 787.

Koh MJ, et al: Systematized epidermal nevus with epidermolytic hyperkeratosis improving with topical calcipotriol/betametasone

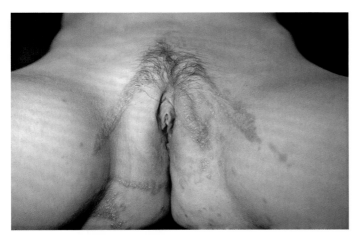

Fig. 29.1 Linear epidermal nevus.

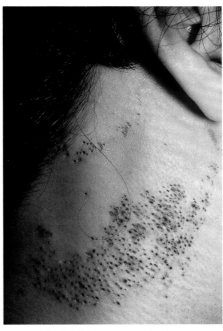

Fig. 29.2 Nevus comedonicus.

dipropionate combination ointment. Pediatr Dermatol 2013; 30: 370.

Om A, et al: Phacomatosis pigmentokeratotica. Pediatr Dermatol 2017; 34: 352.

Yarak S, et al: Squamous cell carcinoma arising in a multiple verrucous epidermal nevus. An Bras Dermatol 2016; 91: 166.

Nevus Comedonicus

Nevus comedonicus is characterized by closely arranged, grouped, often linear papules that have at their center dilated follicular openings with keratinous plugs resembling comedones. Cysts, abscesses, fistulas, and scars develop in about half the cases, which have been described as "inflammatory" nevus comedonicus. As with other epidermal nevi, lesions may be localized to a small area or may have an extensive distribution. They are most frequently unilateral, although bilateral cases are also seen. Lesions occur mostly on the trunk and follow the lines of Blaschko. The lesions may develop any time from birth to age 15 but are usually present by age 10. Follicular tumors, including trichofolliculoma and pilar sheath acanthoma, can appear within the lesion. An "epidermal nevus syndrome" or "nevus comedonicus syndrome" has been reported with electroencephalogram (EEG) abnormalities, ipsilateral cataract, corneal changes, and skeletal anomalies (hemivertebrae, scoliosis, and absence of fifth ray of hand).

The pilosebaceous follicles are dilated and filled with keratinous plugs (Fig. 29.2). On the palms, pseudocomedones are present. Histologic examination reveals large dilated follicles filled with orthokeratotic horny material and lined by atrophic squamous epithelium. The interfollicular epidermis is papillomatous, as seen in typical epidermal nevi. Hair follicle differentiation, well-formed follicular structures, and normal sebaceous glands are not common in well-formed lesions.

Somatic mutations in *NEK9* are frequently associated. Apert syndrome is characterized by skeletal anomalies and acne. It is caused by a mutation in *FGFR2*. A mutation has also been found in *FGFR2* in at least one case of nevus comedonicus, suggesting that nevus comedonicus may be a mosaic form of Apert syndrome.

Treatment of lesions not complicated by inflammatory cysts and nodules is primarily cosmetic. Pore-removing cosmetic strips and comedone expression may improve the cosmetic appearance. Topical tretinoin may be beneficial, as may Er:YAG or CO_2 laser. Patients with inflammatory lesions are much more difficult to manage. If the area affected is limited, surgical excision may be considered. Oral isotretinoin, chronically at the minimum effective dose (0.5 mg/kg/day, or less if possible), may partially suppress the formation of cysts and inflammatory nodules; however, many

cases of nevus comedonicus fail to respond. The comedonal lesions do not improve with oral isotretinoin.

Chiriac A, et al: Extensive unilateral nevus comedonicus without genetic abnormality. Dermatol Online J 2016 Sep 15; 22.

Ferrari B, et al: Nevus comedonicus. Pediatr Dermatol. 2015; 32: 216.

Levinsohn JL, et al: Somatic mutations in NEK9 cause nevus comedonicus. Am J Hum Genet 2016; 98: 1030.

Polat M, et al: Bilateral nevus comedonicus of the eyelids associated with bladder cancer and successful treatment with topical tretinoin. Dermatol Ther 2016; 29: 479.

Tchernev G, et al: Nevus comedonicus. Dermatol Ther (Heidelb) 2013; 3: 33.

Zhu C, et al: Ultrapulse carbon dioxide laser treatment for bilateral facial nevus comedonicus. Dermatol Ther 2017; 30.

Epidermal Nevus Syndrome

Epidermal nevus syndrome does not represent a single entity, but rather multiple syndromes characterized by keratinocytic or organoid nevi, at times associated with internal organ involvement. Each variant has characteristic cutaneous findings and at times relatively specific internal findings. There are at least five variants of organoid epidermal nevus syndrome:

1. Schimmelpenning syndrome (Fig. 29.3). Nevus sebaceus coexists with cerebral, ocular, and skeletal defects. Lesions of the head and neck may lack prominent sebaceous hyperplasia. Coloboma and lipodermoid of the conjunctiva can occur. Vitamin D–resistant hypophosphatemic rickets may be present.

2. Phacomatosis pigmentokeratotica. Nevus sebaceus and papular nevus spilus coexist. The nevus sebaceus may have a flat, erythematous central area with an elevated margin showing features of a nonorganoid epidermal nevus. Multiple angiomas may be found in the nevus spilus component. True basal cell carcinomas develop in the nevus sebaceus of this syndrome. CNS complications can occur, along with hyperhidrosis, weakness, and sensory or motor neuropathy. Vitamin D–resistant rickets may also be present.

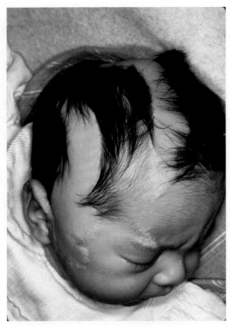

Fig. 29.3 Schimmelpenning syndrome.

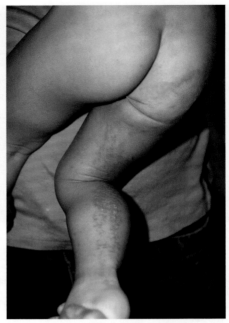

Fig. 29.4 Inflammatory linear verrucous epidermal nevus.

3. Nevus comedonicus syndrome. Nevus comedonicus with ipsilateral ocular, skeletal, or neurologic defects defines this syndrome.
4. Angora hair nevus syndrome. A linear epidermal nevus is covered with long, white hair growing from dilated follicular pores. CNS, eye, and skeletal abnormalities may be found.
5. Becker nevus syndrome. Becker nevus is associated with ipsilateral hypoplasia of the breast.

Keratinocytic nevi are seen in at least four epidermal nevus syndromes:

1. Proteus syndrome.
2. Type 2 segmental Cowden disease. A linear soft, thick, papillomatous keratinocytic nevus in the absence of cerebriform hyperplasia of the palms and soles, but with segmental glomerulosclerosis. It is caused by loss of heterozygosity in an embryo carrying a *PTEN* germline mutation. Associated anomalies include lipomas, connective tissue nevi, vascular nevi, hemihypertrophy, seizures, hydrocephalus, and gastrointestinal (GI) polyps.
3. CHILD syndrome. X-linked dominant, male lethal trait. It is caused by a mutation in *NSDHL*. Chondrodysplasia punctata is characteristic. There is a marked affinity of the nevus for the body folds (ptychotropism). There is a tendency to spontaneous involution.
4. Fibroblast growth factor receptor 3 epidermal nevus syndrome (Garcia-Hafner-Happle syndrome). A velvety-type nonepidermolytic epidermal nevus and cerebral defects identify this syndrome.

Less well-defined syndromes include the following:

1. Nevus trichilemmocysticus. Multiple trichilemmal cysts along Blaschko's lines are associated with osteomalacia and fractures.
2. Didymosis aplasticosebacea. Sebaceous nevus coexists with aplasia cutis, usually in close proximity to each other.
3. SCALP syndrome: sebaceous nevus, CNS malformations, aplasia cutis congenita, limbal dermoid, and pigmented nevus. It is a

combination of didymosis aplasticosebacea and a large melanocytic nevus.
4. Gobellos syndrome: systematized, linear, velvety, orthokeratotic nevus with hypertrichosis and follicular hyperkeratosis. Multiple bony defects are present.
5. Bafverstedt syndrome: horny excrescences in a linear pattern with mental retardation and seizures. Diffuse ichthyosis-like hyperkeratosis covers the entire body, including the palms and soles.
6. NEVADA syndrome: keratinocytic, verrucous nevus with angiodysplasia.
7. CLOVE syndrome: congenital lipomatous overgrowth, vascular malformation, and epidermal nevus. Extensive truncal vascular malformations and overgrown feet are characteristic.

Asch S, Sugarman JL: Epidermal nevus syndromes. Handb Clin Neurol 2015; 132: 291.

Happle R: The group of epidermal nevus syndromes. J Am Acad Dermatol 2010; 63: 25.

Inflammatory Linear Verrucous Epidermal Nevus

The term inflammatory linear verrucous epidermal nevus (ILVEN) may encompass as many as four separate conditions, with some representing mosaicism for erythrokeratodermia variabilis et progressiva. The most common form is the classic ILVEN, or "dermatitic" epidermal nevus. At least three quarters of these cases appear before age 5 years, most before age 6 months. Later onset in adulthood has been reported. ILVEN is characteristically pruritic and pursues a chronic course. Lesions follow the lines of Blaschko. The individual lesions comprising the affected region are erythematous papules and plaques with fine scale (Fig. 29.4). The lesions are morphologically nondescript and, if the distribution is not recognized, could be easily overlooked as an area of dermatitis or psoriasis. Multiple, widely separated areas may be affected, usually on only one side of the body; this may also be bilateral, analogous to other epidermal nevi. Familial cases have been reported. Rarely, systemic involvement, with musculoskeletal and neurologic sequelae (developmental delay, epilepsy), has been reported.

Histologically, classic ILVEN demonstrates abruptly alternating areas of hypergranulosis with orthokeratosis, and parakeratosis with agranulosis. An inflammatory infiltrate of lymphocytes is present in the upper dermis. At times, the histology may simply be that of a subacute dermatitis. Although the histologic diagnosis of psoriasis can be considered, the correct diagnosis can be established if the dermatopathologist is made aware of ILVEN as a consideration. If there is a question, the presence of involucrin expression in the parakeratotic areas can distinguish ILVEN from psoriasis.

Three other types of inflammatory nevus have been included in this group. Some cases of "linear" lichen planus have been considered as "epidermal nevi," because they typically follow lines of Blaschko. CHILD syndrome, also considered a type of "inflammatory" epidermal nevus, is usually clinically distinct, demonstrating its characteristic hemidysplasia. The most confusing entity has been the "nevoid" or "linear" psoriasis. These cases are of two types. The first type is a child with a family history of psoriasis who has a nevoid lesion at or near birth. The child later develops psoriasis that "koebnerizes" into the ILVEN lesion, suggesting it is a "locus minoris resistensiae" for psoriasis. Treatment of the psoriasis clears the psoriasis overlying the ILVEN, but not the ILVEN. Arthritis developed in one such patient. In the second type, psoriasis initially presents in one band or area. Histologically, it resembles psoriasis. Most of these patients develop typical psoriasis later in life, suggesting a mosaicism that allowed expression of the psoriasis earlier in the initially affected area.

Inflammatory LVEN is differentiated from other epidermal nevi by the presence of erythema and pruritus clinically and by histologic features. Lichen striatus can be distinguished by its histology and natural history. Topical corticosteroids and topical retinoids appear to have limited benefit in ILVEN. However, topical vitamin D (calcipotriol and calcitriol) and topical anthralin have been beneficial. Surgical modalities include excision, cryotherapy, and laser. In cases of "nevoid," "linear," or "blaschkolinear" psoriasis, acitretin, narrow-band (NB) ultraviolet (UV) B therapy, and calcipotriene have been beneficial, but etanercept has failed.

Conti R, et al: Inflammatory linear verrucous epidermal nevus. J Cosmet Laser Ther 2013; 15: 242.

Hammami Ghorbel H, et al: Treatment of inflammatory linear verrucous epidermal nevus with 2940 nm erbium fractional laser. J Eur Acad Dermatol Venereol 2014; 28: 824.

Umegaki-Arao N, et al: Inflammatory linear verrucous epidermal nevus with a postzygotic GJA1 mutation is a mosaic erythrokeratodermia variabilis et progressiva. J Invest Dermatol 2017; 137: 967.

Wollina U, et al: ILVEN—Complete remission after administration of topical corticosteroid. Georgian Med News 2017; 263: 10.

HYPERKERATOSIS OF THE NIPPLE AND AREOLA

Hyperkeratosis of the nipple and areola (HNA) is an uncommon, benign, asymptomatic, acquired condition of unknown pathogenesis. Women represent 80% of cases, and HNA presents in their second or third decade. In men, the time of presentation is variable. Most cases are bilateral, although unilateral cases can occur. In about half the cases, both the areola and the nipple are involved. Breastfeeding is usually not affected. Clinically, there is verrucous thickening and brownish discoloration of the nipple and/or areola. Histologically, orthokeratotic hyperkeratosis occurs, with occasional keratinous cysts in the filiform acanthotic epidermis. The course is chronic. Treatment with cryotherapy, electrosurgical superficial

removal of hyperkeratosis, excision and reconstruction, low-dose acitretin, topical steroids, radiofrequency ablation and calcipotriol have benefitted some patients. A similar clinical manifestation has been seen in graft-versus-host disease (GVHD), malignant acanthosis nigricans, and candidiasis of the nipple associated with mucocutaneous candidiasis. Painful areolar hyperkeratosis may be seen as a complication of sorafenib therapy. HNA must be distinguished from acanthosis nigricans, pregnancy-associated hyperkeratosis of the nipple, nipple eczema with lichenification, and Darier disease. Isolated papules or small plaques in this location probably represent seborrheic keratoses affecting the nipple or areola. The relationship of HNA and areolar melanosis is unclear; these conditions have significant clinical similarity, except for the absence of hyperkeratosis in those lesions described as areolar melanosis.

Alonso-Corral MJ, et al: Nevoid hyperkeratosis of the nipple and the areola. Dermatol Online J 2016 Feb 17; 22.

Boussofara L, et al: Bilateral idiopathic hyperkeratosis of the nipple and areola. Acta Dermatovenerol Alp Panonica Adriat 2011; 20: 41.

Foustanos A, et al: Surgical approach for nevoid hyperkeratosis of the areola. J Cutan Aesthet Surg 2012; 5: 40.

Higgins HW, et al: Pregnancy-associated hyperkeratosis of the nipple. JAMA Dermatol 2013; 149: 722.

CLEAR CELL ACANTHOMA (PALE CELL ACANTHOMA)

Clear cell acanthoma is also known as Degos acanthoma. The typical lesion is a circumscribed, red, moist, shiny nodule with some crusting and peripheral scale (Fig. 29.5); it is usually about 1–2 cm in diameter. A collarette of scale is usually observed, and there may be pigmented variants. Exophytic nodules have been reported. The favorite site is on the shin, calf, or occasionally the thigh, although other sites (e.g., abdomen, scrotum) have been reported. The lesion is asymptomatic and slow growing and can occur in either gender, usually after age 40. Solitary lesions are most common, but multiple nodules have been described, including the setting of Cowden syndrome. Rarely, an eruptive form of the disease occurs, producing up to 400 lesions. Squamous cell carcinoma (SCC) arising from clear cell acanthoma has also been reported. Lesions occurring in plaques of psoriasis on the buttocks have been described, and clear cell acanthoma on the nipple has been associated with chronic eczema, suggesting a possible inflammatory etiology.

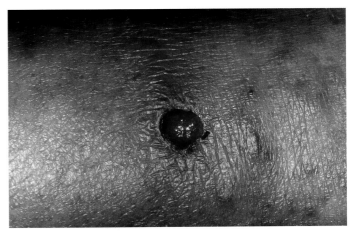

Fig. 29.5 Clear cell acanthoma.

The acanthotic epidermis consists of pale, edematous cells and is sharply demarcated. The basal cell layer is normal. Neutrophils are scattered within the acanthoma and in groups below and within the stratum corneum, a finding similar to the micropustules of psoriasis. The dermal blood vessels are dilated and tortuous, as seen in psoriasis. The clear keratinocytes abound in glycogen, staining positive with periodic acid–Schiff (PAS). Several centers have reported identification of human papillomavirus (HPV) in clear cell acanthomas, making distinction of these lesions from warts difficult. Clear cell acanthoma must be differentiated from eccrine poroma, which appears most frequently on the hair-free part of the foot, and from clear cell hidradenoma, which occurs most often on the head, especially the face and eyelids. Treatment is surgical, with cryotherapy, CO_2 laser, or excision.

Hidalgo-García Y, et al: Clear cell acanthoma of the areola and nipple. Actas Dermosifiliogr 2016; 107: 793.

Potenziani S, et al: Multiple clear cell acanthomas and a sebaceous lymphadenoma presenting in a patient with Cowden syndrome. J Cutan Pathol 2017; 44: 79.

Shahriari N, et al: In vivo reflectance confocal microscopy features of a large cell acanthoma. Dermatol Pract Concept 2016; 6: 67.

Shirai A, et al: Multiple clear cell acanthoma associated with multiple Bowen's disease. Int J Dermatol 2014; 53: e386.

Tempark T, Shwayder T: Clear cell acanthoma. Clin Exp Dermatol 2012; 37: 831.

WAXY KERATOSES OF CHILDHOOD (KERINOKERATOSIS PAPULOSA)

Waxy keratoses of childhood is a genodermatosis that is either sporadic or familial. It may be generalized or segmental. Clinically, the lesions are keratotic, flesh-colored papules that affect the trunk and extremities. They appear before age 3 years. Histologically, there is papillomatosis with focal "church-spire" tenting of the epidermis and marked hyperkeratosis. The natural history of this rare disorder is unknown. Clinically and histologically, the lesions must be distinguished from warts.

Gönül M, et al: A case of waxy keratoses of childhood. Dermatology 2008; 217: 143.

Happle R, et al: Kerinokeratosis papulosa with a type 2 segmental manifestation. J Am Acad Dermatol 2004; 50: S84.

Mehrabi D, et al: Waxy keratoses of childhood in a segmental distribution. Pediatr Dermatol 2001; 18: 415.

MULTIPLE MINUTE DIGITATE HYPERKERATOSIS

Multiple minute digitate hyperkeratosis (MMDH) is a rare disorder. About half of cases are familial, inherited in an autosomal dominant manner, and the other half are sporadic. This condition has also been called digitate keratoses, disseminated spiked hyperkeratosis, minute aggregate keratosis, and familial disseminated piliform hyperkeratosis. Clinically, hundreds of tiny, asymptomatic digitate keratotic papules appear on the trunk and proximal extremities. They are not associated with follicular structures. Histologically, each lesion represents a spiked, digitate, or tented area of acanthotic epidermis with overlying orthohyperkeratosis. Similar lesions can be seen after inflammation and radiation therapy. The relationship of the familial/sporadic cases and the postinflammatory condition is unclear. In some adult patients, an underlying malignancy is found.

Caccetta TP, et al: Multiple minute digitate hyperkeratosis. J Am Acad Dermatol 2012; 67: e49.

Pimentel CL, et al: Multiple minute digitate hyperkeratosis. J Eur Acad Dermatol Venereol 2002; 16: 422.

ACANTHOLYTIC ACANTHOMA, EPIDERMOLYTIC ACANTHOMA, ACANTHOLYTIC DYSKERATOTIC ACANTHOMA

These three acanthomas represent benign, usually solitary, but at times multiple papules that are nondescript and may be mistaken for basal cell carcinoma (BCC), SCC, or HPV infection. Histologic examination shows epidermal hyperplasia with acantholysis resembling pemphigus vulgaris, pemphigus foliaceus, or Hailey-Hailey disease. The condition multiple epidermolytic acanthoma usually occurs in the genital area and histologically resembles Hailey-Hailey disease. This probably represents a localized variant of that condition.

Jang BS, et al: Multiple scrotal epidermolytic acanthomas successfully treated with topical imiquimod. J Dermatol 2007; 34: 267.

Kazlouskaya V, et al: Solitary epidermolytic acanthoma. J Cutan Pathol 2013; 40: 701.

Minakawa S, et al: Acantholysis caused repeated hemorrhagic bullae in a case of acantholytic acanthoma. J Dermatol 2012; 39: 1107.

WARTY DYSKERATOMA

Warty dyskeratomas are usually solitary and are found on the head and neck (70%), trunk (20%), or extremities. Rare oral lesions occur. The lesion is a brown-red papule or nodule with a soft, yellow, central keratotic plug. Histologically, a cuplike depression filled with a keratotic plug is most common. The epithelium lining the invagination shows the features of Darier disease, with intraepidermal clefts, acantholytic cells, and pseudovilli. Keratin pearls, corps ronds, and grains may be seen. Cystic lesions with prominent keratinous cysts can occur, especially in the vulva. Cutaneous lesions appear to originate from a hair follicle. Warty dyskeratoma must be distinguished histologically from keratoacanthoma and acantholytic SCC. Acantholytic acanthoma has a similar histology, but dyskeratosis is absent, distinguishing it from warty dyskeratoma. Treatment is surgical.

Lencastre A, et al: Warty dyskeratoma. J Am Acad Dermatol 2016; 75: e97.

Torres KM, et al: Cystic acantholytic dyskeratosis of the vulva. Indian Dermatol Online J 2016; 7: 272.

SEBORRHEIC KERATOSIS

Seborrheic keratoses are incredibly common and usually multiple. They present as oval, slightly raised, tan or light-brown to black, sharply demarcated papules or plaques, rarely more than 3 cm in diameter (Fig. 29.6). They appear "stuck on" the skin, as if they could be removed with the flick of a fingernail. They are located mostly on the chest and back but also frequently involve the scalp, face, neck, and extremities. An inframammary accumulation is common. Occasionally, genital lesions are seen. The palms and soles are spared; "seborrheic keratoses" in these areas are usually eccrine poromas. The surface of the warty lesions often becomes crumbly, resembling a loosely attached crust. When this is removed, a raw, moist base is revealed. Seborrheic keratoses may be associated with itching. Some patients have hundreds of these lesions on the trunk. Although it had been thought that the age of onset is generally in the fourth to fifth decade, in Australia the prevalence of seborrheic keratoses was 20% in males and 25% in females age 15–25. Typical lesions of the trunk are much more common in white persons; however, the "dermatosis papulosa nigra" variant of the central face is common in African Americans and Asians.

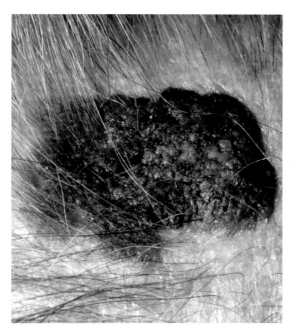

Fig. 29.6 Seborrheic keratosis. (Courtesy Steven Binnick, MD.)

The pathogenesis of seborrheic keratoses is unknown. Clinically, they usually originate de novo or appear initially as a lentigo. A sudden eruption of many seborrheic keratoses may follow an exfoliative erythroderma, erythrodermic psoriasis, or an erythrodermic drug eruption. These lesions may be transient. Seborrheic keratoses are more common in areas of sun exposure, including favoring the driver's side in truck drivers. In about one third or more of cases, solar lentigines and seborrheic keratoses both have gain-of-function mutations in *FGFR3* and *PIK3CA*, the genes mutated in keratinocytic epidermal nevi. This supports the concept that some seborrheic keratoses begin as flat lesions that cannot be distinguished from solar lentigines.

Histologically, most seborrheic keratoses demonstrate acanthosis, varying degrees of papillomatosis, hyperkeratosis, and at times, keratin accumulations within the acanthotic epidermis (pseudo–horn cysts). The epidermal cells lack cytologic atypia, except at times in the irritated variant, where typical mitoses may occur. Six histologic types are distinguished: hyperkeratotic, acanthotic, adenoid or reticulated, clonal, irritated, and melanoacanthoma. Poor correlation exists between the clinical appearance and the observed histology, unlike for inverted follicular keratosis, dermatosis papulosa nigra, and stucco keratosis, where the histologic features are characteristic and match the clinical lesion. Melanoacanthoma differs from regular seborrheic keratosis by the presence of numerous dendritic melanocytes within the acanthotic epidermis. Oral melanoacanthoma, which has also been called melanoacanthosis, is clinically a reactive pigmented lesion seen primarily in young black patients (see Chapter 34). Many cases of inverted follicular keratosis represent irritated seborrheic keratoses. Some view granular parakeratotic acanthomas a variant of irritated seborrheic keratosis, and others see it as a separate entity.

The differential diagnosis usually poses no problems in most cases, but clinically atypical lesions can be a challenge. The most difficult, especially for the nondermatologist, is to differentiate the solitary black seborrheic keratosis from melanoma. The regularly shaped verrucous lesion is often different from the smooth-surfaced and slightly infiltrating pattern of melanoma. Dermoscopy can sometimes be of great value; at other times, however, seborrheic keratoses may demonstrate dermatoscopic features typical of melanocytic lesions, and the presence of horn cysts does not exclude a melanocytic lesion. Actinic keratoses are usually erythematous, more sharply rough, and slightly scaly. The edges are not sharply demarcated, and they occur most often on the face, bald scalp, and backs of the hands. Nevi may be closely simulated. Clonal seborrheic keratoses demonstrate intraepidermal nests suggestive of intraepidermal epithelioma of Jadassohn. Rarely, Bowen disease, SCC, BCC, trichilemmal carcinoma, or melanoma arises within typical-appearing seborrheic keratosis. Some of these may represent collision lesions, not cancers arising from seborrheic keratoses. It is prudent to biopsy any lesion that appears atypical, because even the most seasoned dermatologist has been humbled by the occasional diagnosis of melanoma in low-suspect lesions.

Seborrheic keratoses are easily removed with liquid nitrogen, curettage, or both, to avoid the need for local anesthesia to perform the curettage. The spray freezes the lesion to make it brittle enough for easy removal with the curette. Scarring is not produced by this method. Light freezing with liquid nitrogen alone is also effective, and most patients prefer it to simple curettage with local anesthesia mainly because of decreased wound care. Light fulguration and shave removal are other acceptable methods. A novel topical agent is in clinical trials.

SIGN OF LESER-TRÉLAT

The sudden appearance of numerous seborrheic keratoses in an adult may be a cutaneous sign of internal malignancy. Sixty percent of the neoplasms have been adenocarcinomas, primarily of the GI tract. Other common malignancies are lymphoma, breast cancer, and SCC of the lung, but many other types have been reported. To be considered a case of Leser-Trélat, the keratoses should begin at approximately the same time as the development of the cancer, have a rapid onset, and run a parallel course in regard to growth and remission. The lesions are often pruritic, and acanthosis nigricans and tripe palms may accompany the appearance of the seborrheic keratoses of Leser-Trélat.

Al Ghazal P, et al: Leser-Trélat sign and breast cancer. Lancet 2013; 381: 1653.
Da Rosa AC, et al: Three simultaneous paraneoplastic manifestations (ichthyosis acquisita, Bazex syndrome, and Leser-Trélat sign) with prostate adenocarcinoma. J Am Acad Dermatol 2009; 61: 538.
Heidenreich B, et al: Genetic alterations in seborrheic keratoses. Oncotarget 2017; 8: 36639.

DERMATOSIS PAPULOSA NIGRA

Dermatosis papulosa nigra occurs in about 35% of black persons and is also relatively common in Asians. It usually begins in adolescence, appearing first as minute, round, skin-colored or hyperpigmented macules or papules that develop singly or in sparse numbers on the malar regions or on the cheeks below the eyes. It has been described in patients as young as age 3. The lesions increase in number and size over time, so that over the course of years, the patient may have hundreds of lesions (Fig. 29.7). These are distributed over the periorbital regions initially but may occur on the rest of the face as well as the neck and upper chest. Lesions do not spontaneously resolve. They closely simulate seborrheic keratoses. The lesions are asymptomatic and do not develop scaling, crusting, or ulceration.

Microscopically, the chief alterations are in the epidermis. Irregular acanthosis, papillomatosis, and deposits of uncommonly large amounts of pigment throughout the rete, particularly in the basal layer, are characteristic. Many believe this to be a form of seborrheic keratosis. This concept is supported by the finding of *FGFR3* mutations in the lesions of dermatosis papulosis nigra, similar to those found in seborrheic keratoses.

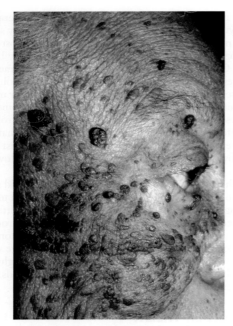

Fig. 29.7 Dermatosis papulosa nigra.

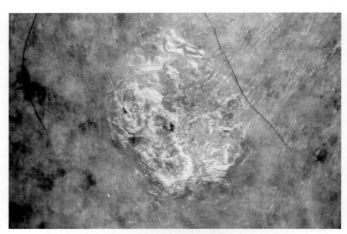

Fig. 29.8 Benign lichenoid keratoses.

Treatment is made difficult by the tendency for the development of dyspigmentation. Light curettage with or without anesthesia; light, superficial liquid nitrogen application; and light electrodesiccation are effective but may result in hyperpigmentation or hypopigmentation. KTP, CO_2, and Nd:YAG lasers have been reported effective but not superior to simple electrodesiccation. Aggressive treatment should be avoided to minimize dyspigmentation and scarring.

STUCCO KERATOSIS

Stucco keratoses have been described as "stuck on" lesions occurring on the lower legs, especially in the vicinity of the Achilles tendon. They are also seen on the dorsa of the feet, forearms, and dorsal hands. The palms, soles, trunk, and head are never affected. Varying in diameter from 1–5 mm, the lesions are loosely attached and thus can easily be scratched off. They vary in number from a few to more than 50. Stucco keratoses are common in the United States and Australia. They occur mostly in men over 40 years old. Histologically, the picture is that of a hyperkeratotic type of seborrheic keratosis, with no hypergranulosis and no wart particles seen on electron microscopy. The presence of *PIK3CA* mutations in stucco keratoses suggests they are a variant of seborrheic keratosis. The treatment, if required, consists of emollients, which soften the skin and cause the scaly lesions to fall off. Ammonium lactate 12% lotion may be effective in improving the appearance of the lesions. Stucco keratoses must be distinguished from Flegel disease.

Ali FR, et al: Carbon dioxide laser ablation of dermatosis papulosa nigra. Lasers Med Sci 2016; 31: 593.
Bruscino N, et al: Dermatosis papulosa nigra and 10,600-nm CO_2 laser, a good choice. J Cosmet Laser Ther 2014; 16: 114.
Garcia MS, et al: Treatment of dermatosis papulosa nigra in 10 patients. Dermatol Surg 2010; 36: 1968.
Hafner C, et al: *FGFR3* and *PIK3CA* mutations in stucco keratosis and dermatosis papulosa nigra. Br J Dermatol 2010; 162: 508.
Veraitch O, et al: Early-onset dermatosis papulosa nigra. Br J Dermatol 2016; 174: 1148.

HYPERKERATOSIS LENTICULARIS PERSTANS (FLEGEL DISEASE)

Rough, yellow-brown, keratotic, flat-topped papules 2–5 mm in diameter and found primarily on the dorsal feet and lower legs are characteristic. The palms, soles, and oral mucosa may rarely be involved. Familial cases have been reported.

The histologic findings are distinctive, with hyperkeratosis and parakeratosis overlying a thinned epidermis and irregular acanthosis at the periphery. A bandlike inflammatory infiltrate occurs in the papillary dermis. Topical emollients, topical keratolytics, topical corticosteroids, zinc bandages, topical 5-FU, and psoralen plus ultraviolet A (PUVA) therapy have been reported useful. Oral retinoids may result in improvement but are difficult to justify in this chronic, asymptomatic condition except in rare severe cases. Both benefit and failure with topical vitamin D analogs have been reported. The lesions do not recur after shallow shave excision.

Krishnan A, Kar S: Hyperkeratosis lenticularis perstans (Flegel's disease) with unusual clinical presentation. J Dermatol Case Rep 2012; 6: 93.
Valdebran M, et al: Dermoscopic findings in hyperkeratosis lenticularis perstans. J Am Acad Dermatol 2016; 75: e211.

BENIGN LICHENOID KERATOSES (LICHEN PLANUS–LIKE KERATOSIS)

Benign lichenoid keratoses are usually solitary, dusky-red to violaceous, papular lesions up to 1 cm in diameter and at times larger (Fig. 29.8). They occur most often on the distal forearms, hands, or chest of middle-aged white women. The lesions are typically biopsied because the clinical features are identical to those of a superficial BCC. A slight violaceous hue or the presence of an adjacent solar lentigo can raise the suspicion of lichen planus–like keratosis. Multiple lesions may simulate a photodermatitis, such as lupus erythematosus (LE). Evolution from preexisting solar lentigines is often noted histologically or by history, and the presence of the same underlying genetic mutations (*FGFR3, PIK3CA,* and *RAS*) supports this concept.

Histologically, the lesion may be indistinguishable from idiopathic lichen planus. Whereas idiopathic lichen planus rarely demonstrates parakeratosis, plasma cells, or eosinophils, these may be present in lichen planus–like keratosis. The remnants of a solar lentigo may be seen at the periphery. These features, plus the clinical information that this represents a solitary lesion, suggest the correct diagnosis. Clinical correlation is essential because similar histologic findings may be seen in lichenoid drug eruptions, acral LE, and lichenoid regression of melanoma. Direct immunofluorescence is

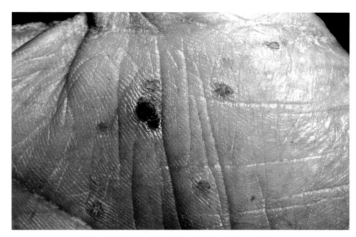

Fig. 29.9 Arsenical keratosis of the palm.

positive, with clumped deposits of immunoglobulin M in a lichen planus–like pattern at the dermoepidermal junction (DEJ). This differs from the continuous granular immunoglobulin deposition of acral LE. Cryotherapy with liquid nitrogen is effective.

Chan AH, et al: Differentiating regressed melanoma from regressed lichenoid keratosis. J Cutan Pathol 2017; 44: 338.

Kim HS, et al: Clinical and histopathologic study of benign lichenoid keratosis on the face. Am J Dermatopathol 2013; 35: 738.

ARSENICAL KERATOSES

Arsenical keratoses are keratotic, pointed, 2–4 mm, wartlike lesions on the palms, soles, and sometimes ears of persons who have a history of drinking contaminated well water or taking medications containing arsenic trioxide, usually for asthma (e.g., Fowler's solution, Bell's Asthma Mixture), atopic dermatitis, or psoriasis, often years previously (Fig. 29.9). These lesions resemble palmar pits but may have a central hyperkeratosis. When the keratosis is picked off with the fingernails, a small, dell-like depression is seen.

Bowen disease (BD) and invasive arsenical SCC may be present, with the latent period being 10 and 20 years, respectively. The profound increase in BD and SCC appears to be characteristic of patients with arsenic exposure from well water. In patients exposed to arsenic through elixirs, BCCs are more characteristically seen. The latency period for development of BCC is also 20 years. Lesions are most common on the scalp and trunk. Arsenical keratoses may be a marker for increased lung and urothelial carcinoma.

Hsu LI, et al: Use of arsenic-induced palmoplantar hyperkeratosis and skin cancers to predict risk of subsequent internal malignancy. Am J Epidemiol 2013; 177: 202.

Ruiz de Luzuriaga AM, et al: Arsenical keratoses in Bangladesh. Dermatol Clin 2011; 29: 45.

Son SB, et al: Successful treatment of palmoplantar arsenical keratosis with a combination of keratolytics and low-dose acitretin. Clin Exp Dermatol 2008; 33: 202

NONMELANOMA SKIN CANCERS AND THEIR PRECURSORS

More nonmelanoma skin cancers (NMSCs) are diagnosed annually in the United States than all other cancers combined. In 2006 more than 3.5 million new NMSC cases were estimated to occur, and the incidence is rising. One in two men and one in three women

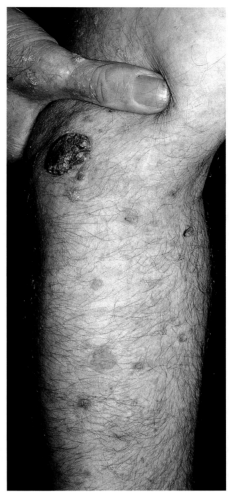

Fig. 29.10 Actinic keratosis/Bowen disease in transplant recipient.

in the United States will develop NMSC in their lifetime, usually after age 55. Although these result in only about 2000–2500 deaths annually, because of their sheer numbers, NMSCs represent about 5% of all Medicare cancer expenditures. Those at risk for skin cancer are fair-skinned individuals who tan poorly and who have had significant chronic or intermittent sun exposure. Red hair phenotype with loss-of-function mutations in the melanocortin-1 receptor may be a risk factor as well. Additional risk factors include a history of skin cancer, prior radiation therapy, PUVA treatment, arsenic exposure, and systemic immunosuppression (Fig. 29.10). Once an individual has developed an NMSC, the risk for a second is increased 10-fold. Over the 3-year period after the initial NMSC diagnosis, more than 40% of BCC and SCC patients develop a BCC, and 18% of SCC patients develop another SCC. By 5 years, as many as 50% of women and 70% of men will develop a second NMSC. The rate of developing NMSCs is no different 3 years or 10 years after the initial NMSC diagnosis. Patients with a history of NMSC should be examined regularly for NMSCs.

Ultraviolet radiation (UVR) is the major cause of nongenital NMSCs and actinic keratoses. The effect of UVR appears to be mediated through mutation of the *p53* gene, which is found mutated in a substantial percentage of NMSCs and actinic keratoses. Most skin cancers are highly immunogenic, but the immune response is suppressed by continued actinic exposure. Both chronic sun exposure and intermittent intense exposure are risk factors for the development of NMSCs. It is believed that avoiding sun exposure reduces the risk for NMSC. The use of sunscreens in the prevention of NMSCs has been controversial; they may inadvertently lead to prolonged intentional sun exposure, negating their possible beneficial effect. Nonetheless, dermatologists and their societies recommend a program of sunscreen use together with sun avoidance to patients at risk for skin cancer. This includes avoiding midday sun, seeking shade, wearing protective clothing, and regularly applying a sunblock of sun protection factor (SPF) 15–30 with both UVB and UVA coverage. This program was pioneered in Australia and has led to improvements in some skin cancer rates there.

Marcil I, Stern RS: Risk of developing a subsequent nonmelanoma skin cancer in patients with a history of nonmelanoma skin cancer. Arch Dermatol 2000; 136: 1524.

Olsen, CM, et al: Turning the tide? Changes in treatment rates for keratinocytic cancers in Australia 2000 through 2011. J Am Acad Dermatol 2014; 71: 21.

Rogers, HW, et al: Incidence estimate of nonmelanoma skin cancer in the United States, 2006. Arch Dermatol 2010; 146: 283.

Wysong, A, et al: Nonmelanoma skin cancer visits and procedure patterns in a nationally representative sample. Dermatol Surg 2013; 39: 596.

ACTINIC KERATOSIS (SOLAR KERATOSIS)

Actinic keratoses represent in situ dysplasias resulting from sun exposure. They are found chiefly on the chronically sun-exposed surfaces of the face (Fig. 29.11), ears, balding scalp, dorsal hands, and forearms. They are usually multiple, discrete, flat or elevated, verrucous or keratotic, red, pigmented, or skin colored. Usually, the surface is covered by an adherent scale, but sometimes it is smooth and shiny. On palpation, the surface is rough, like sandpaper, and at times lesions are more easily felt than seen. The patient may complain of tenderness when the lesion is rubbed or shaved over with a razor. The lesions are usually relatively small, measuring 3 mm to 1 cm in diameter, most being less than 6 mm. Rarely, lesions may reach 2 cm in size, but a lesion larger than 6 mm should be considered an actinic keratosis only if confirmed by biopsy or if it completely resolves with therapy. The hypertrophic type, which may lead to cutaneous horn formation, is most frequently present on the dorsal forearms and hands.

Actinic keratoses are the most common epithelial precancerous lesions. Although lesions typically appear in persons over age 50, actinic keratoses may occur in the twenties or thirties in patients who live in areas of high solar irradiation and have fair skin. Patients with actinic keratoses have a propensity for the development of nonmelanoma cutaneous malignancies. Actinic keratoses can be prevented by the regular application of sunscreen and by a low-fat diet. Beta carotene is of no benefit in preventing actinic keratoses.

Six types of actinic keratosis can be recognized histologically: hypertrophic, atrophic, bowenoid, acantholytic, pigmented, and lichenoid. The epidermis may be acanthotic or atrophic. Keratinocyte maturation may be disordered, with overlying parakeratosis sometimes present. The basal cells are most frequently dysplastic, although in more advanced lesions, dysplasia may be seen throughout the epidermis, simulating BD (bowenoid actinic keratosis).

The clinical diagnosis of actinic keratosis is usually straightforward. Early lesions of chronic cutaneous LE, erosive and pustular dermatosis of the scalp, and pemphigus foliaceus are sometimes confused with actinic keratoses. Seborrheic keratoses, even when lacking pigmentation, are usually more "stuck on" in appearance and more sharply marginated than actinic keratoses. Dermoscopy may aid in this distinction. It is difficult to distinguish hypertrophic actinic keratoses from early SCC, and a low threshold for biopsy is recommended. Similarly, actinic keratoses, which present as red patches, cannot easily be distinguished from BD or superficial BCC. If there is a palpable dermal component, or if on stretching the lesion there is a pearly quality, a biopsy should be considered. Any lesion larger than 6 mm, and any lesion that has failed to resolve with appropriate therapy for actinic keratosis, should also be carefully evaluated for biopsy.

Because some percentage of actinic keratoses will progress to NMSC, their treatment is indicated. There are many effective therapeutic modalities. Cryotherapy with liquid nitrogen is most effective and practical when there are a limited number of lesions. A bulky cotton applicator dipped into liquid nitrogen or a handheld nitrogen spray device can be used. If the cotton-tipped applicator method is used, the liquid nitrogen into which the applicator is dipped should be used for only one patient, because there is a theoretic risk of cross-contamination from one patient to another. Infectious agents are not killed by freezing, so many dermatologists now use the spray devices. We recommend using a small-opening tip with continuous bursts of nitrogen spray in a circular motion, depending on the size of the lesion, attempting an even frosting. Only the lesion should be frosted, and the duration of cryotherapy must be carefully controlled. A long freeze that results in significant epidermal-dermal injury produces white scars, which are easily seen on the fair skin of those at risk for actinic keratoses. When correctly performed, healing usually occurs within 1 week on the face, but may require up to 4 weeks on the arms and legs. Caution should be exercised when treating below the knee, because wound healing in these regions is particularly poor, and a chronic ulcer can result. Also, caution is required in persons at risk for having a cryoprotein, such as hepatitis C virus–infected patients and those with connective tissue disease or lymphoid neoplasia, who may have an excessive reaction to cryotherapy. It is better on the first visit to "undertreat" until the tolerance of a patient's skin to cryotherapy is known. Application of 0.5% 5-FU for 1 week before cryotherapy improves the response.

For extensive, broad, or numerous lesions, topical chemotherapy is recommended. Any lesion that could represent an NMSC should be biopsied before beginning topical chemotherapy or photodynamic therapy (PDT) for actinic keratoses. The two agents most frequently used are 5-FU cream, 0.5%–5%, or imiquimod 5% cream. Topical tretinoin and adapalene do not have the efficacy of these two agents but can be used for prolonged periods and represent an option for patients with a few early lesions. They are also useful for pretreatment of hyperkeratotic lesions before a course of 5-FU. Also, 3% diclofenac in 2.5% hyaluronan gel can be effective when used for 60 days for actinic keratoses. Topical

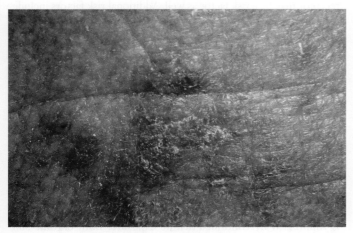

Fig. 29.11 Actinic keratosis.

resiquimod and ingenol mebutate are newer topical therapeutic options and trichloracetic acid peels may still be useful in some patients. The inflammatory reaction with these agents parallels efficacy, but some data suggest a trend toward less irritation without diminished efficacy if dimethicone lotion is applied before ingenol mebutate.

The frequency and duration of treatment are determined by the individual's reaction and the anatomic site of application. 5-FU is applied once daily in most cases. For the face, 0.5% 5-FU tends to give a predictable response, which is slightly less severe than that produced by the 1%–5% concentrations. Some patients prefer the stronger concentration for a briefer period, while others favor a slower onset of the reaction and a more prolonged course. For the 5% cream, treatment duration rarely needs to exceed 2–3 weeks. For the 0.5% cream, the treatment course is typically 3–6 weeks. Usually, the central face will respond more briskly than the temples and forehead, which may require a longer duration of treatment. If the reaction is brisk, a midstrength corticosteroid ointment can be helpful or the treatment can be stopped and restarted at a lower concentration. Depending on the individual's sensitivity, an erythematous burning reaction will occur within several days. Treatment is stopped when a peak response occurs, characterized by a change in color from bright to dusky red, reepithelialization, and crust formation. Healing usually occurs within another 2 weeks of stopping treatment, depending on the treatment site. Certain areas of the face are prone to intense irritant dermatitis when exposed to 5-FU, and tolerance can be improved if the patient avoids application to the glabella, melolabial folds, and chin. For the scalp, the 0.5% concentration may be adequate, but prolonged or multiple treatment courses often are required if this low concentration is used. The 5% cream produces a more predictable, although brisk, reaction. A thick cutaneous horn can prevent penetration of 5-FU, and hypertrophic actinic keratoses on the scalp, dorsal hand, and forearm may respond poorly unless the area is pretreated with an agent to remove excessive keratin overlying the lesions. Pretreatment with tretinoin for 2–3 weeks can improve efficacy and shorten the duration of subsequent 5-FU treatment. It has been observed that 5-FU "seeks out" lesions that may not be clinically apparent. The use of topical 5-FU to the face can also reverse photoaging. Clinically inapparent BCCs may be detected during or on completion of the treatment. Rarely, patients who have had multiple courses of 5-FU topical chemotherapy will develop a true allergic contact dermatitis to the 5-FU. This is manifested by the redness, edema, or vesiculation extending beyond the area of application and by the patient developing pruritus rather than tenderness of the treated areas. Patch testing can be confirmatory.

Imiquimod is an interferon (IFN) inducer and eradicates actinic keratoses by producing a local immunologic reaction against the lesions. The ideal protocol for application of imiquimod may not yet be determined. About 80% of patients respond to imiquimod, and 20% may not respond at all, perhaps because that they lack some genetic component required to induce an inflammatory cascade when imiquimod is applied. If it is applied three times a week, patients develop an inflammatory reaction similar to that seen with daily application of 5-FU. The severity of the reaction is somewhat unpredictable, with a small subset of patients, especially fair-skinned women, developing a severe burning and crusting reaction after only one or a few applications. In others, no reaction at all occurs. With twice-weekly application, the treatment course is prolonged, up to 16 weeks. Severe erythema occurs in 17.7% and scabbing/crusting in 8.4% of patients so treated. The median percentage reduction in actinic keratoses is 83.3% with this treatment protocol. However, only 7% of patients treating actinic keratoses on the arms and hands with imiquimod three times per week achieved complete clearance. Applying it more frequently leads to increased toxicity. Overall, although the reaction is less predictable with imiquimod, it is also typically less severe than

with high-concentration 5-FU. The adverse event rates are similar to those with low-concentration (0.5%) 5-FU. Another regimen is to apply imiquimod for long periods at a reduced frequency, once or twice weekly. Applications can be in alternating 1-month cycles or continuous for many months. This may allow management of some patients who require treatment but cannot tolerate any significant changes in appearance. Ultimately, the choice between topical 5-FU and imiquimod will be based on patient preference, prior physician and patient experience with the modalities, and the cost. Imiquimod is significantly more expensive per gram than any form of 5-FU. A meta-analysis comparing efficacy studies of the two agents dosed in various concentrations and regimens suggested imiquimod may have higher efficacy for actinic keratosis on the face and scalp. A recent Cochrane review concluded that 5-FU, imiquimod, ingenol mebutate, and diclofenac are similarly efficacious but have different adverse events and cosmetic outcomes. Direct comparative trials between these agents would be of great value in determining the optimal and most cost-effective strategy for the treatment of extensive actinic keratosis, and the cost of treatment can vary widely depending on the modality chosen.

Surgical management of actinic keratoses with chemical peels, laser resurfacing, and PDT are discussed in Chapters 37 and 38.

Bower C: Field treatment of actinic keratosis on the scalp. Br J Dermatol 2017; 176: 1425.

Gupta AK, et al: Interventions for actinic keratoses. Cochrane Database Syst Rev 2012; 12: CD004415.

Hanke CW, et al: Safety and efficacy of escalating doses of ingenol mebutate for field treatment of actinic keratosis on the full face, full balding scalp, or chest. J Drugs Dermatol 2017; 16: 438.

Holzer G, et al: Randomized controlled trial comparing 35% trichloroacetic acid peel and 5-aminolaevulinic acid photodynamic therapy for treating multiple actinic keratosis. Br J Dermatol 2017; 176: 1155.

Jim On S, et al: Regression analysis of local skin reactions to predict clearance of actinic keratosis on the face in patients treated with ingenol mebutate gel. J Drugs Dermatol 2017; 16: 112.

Khanna R, et al: Patient satisfaction and reported outcomes on the management of actinic keratosis. Clin Cosmet Investig Dermatol 2017; 10: 179.

Kirby JS, et al: Variation in the cost of managing actinic keratosis. JAMA Dermatol 2017; 153: 264.

Micali G, et al: Topical pharmacotherapy for skin cancer. Part II. Clinical applications. J Am Acad Dermatol 2014; 70: 979. e1.

Tolley K, et al: Pharmacoeconomic evaluations in the treatment of actinic keratoses. Int J Immunopathol Pharmacol 2017; 30: 178.

Walker JL, et al: 5-Fluorouracil for actinic keratosis treatment and chemoprevention. J Invest Dermatol 2017; 137: 1367.

CUTANEOUS HORN (CORNU CUTANEUM)

Cutaneous horns are encountered most frequently on the dorsal hands and scalp. Lesions may also occur on the hands, penis, ears (Fig. 29.12), and eyelids. They are skin-colored, horny excrescences 2–60 mm long, sometimes divided into several antler-like projections.

These lesions are most often benign, with the hyperkeratosis being superimposed on an underlying seborrheic keratosis, verruca vulgaris, angiokeratoma, molluscum contagiosum, or trichilemmoma in about 60% of cases. However, 20%–30% may overlie premalignant keratosis, and 20% may overlie SCCs or BCCs. The risk for a cutaneous horn overlying a malignancy is much higher in fair-complexioned elderly persons. Hyperkeratotic actinic plaques less than 1 cm in diameter on the dorsum of the hand, wrist, or

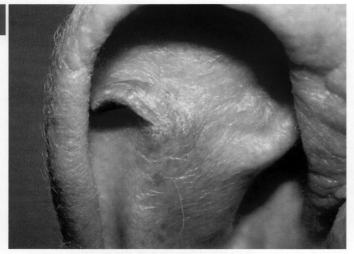

Fig. 29.12 Cutaneous horn of the ear.

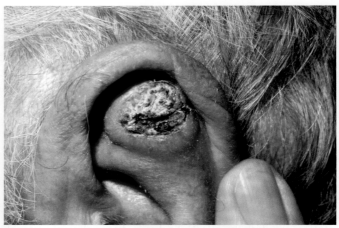

Fig. 29.13 Keratoacanthoma. (Courtesy Steven Binnick, MD.)

forearms in white patients have been shown to have a malignancy rate of 50%. One third of penile horns are associated with underlying malignancies. Excisional biopsy with histologic examination of the base is necessary to determine the best therapy, which would be dictated by the diagnosis of the underlying lesion and by the apparent adequacy of removal.

Mantese SA, et al: Cutaneous horn. An Bras Dermatol 2010; 85: 157.

KERATOACANTHOMA

Clinical Features

There are four types of keratoacanthoma: solitary, multiple, eruptive, and keratoacanthoma centrifugum marginatum. The exact biologic behavior of keratoacanthoma remains controversial. In the past, it had been considered a reactive condition or pseudomalignancy that could be treated expectantly. Now, the favored view is that keratoacanthomas are low-grade SCCs, which in many cases will regress. The regression may be partially mediated by immunity but takes the form of terminal differentiation. The course of these tumors is unpredictable. Even those that ultimately involute can cause considerable destruction before they regress. Any lesions that have the histologic features of keratoacanthoma and appear in an immunosuppressed host should be managed as an SCC, with complete eradication.

Sunlight appears to play an important role in the etiology, especially in the solitary types, with light-skinned persons being predominantly affected. Cases of keratoacanthoma after trauma, hypertrophic lichen planus, discoid LE, tattoos, fractional thermolysis, and imiquimod erosions, and along the distal ends of surgical excisions, suggest that an isomorphic phenomenon is common. The keratoacanthomas appear about 1 month after the traumatic injury. All these associated conditions result in damage to the dermis, especially along the DEJ, and necessitate wound healing. The biologic behavior of these lesions is unknown, but they have added to the controversy of keratoacanthoma as a reactive versus a malignant process. Eruptive keratoacanthomas and SCCs have appeared during treatment for metastatic melanoma with the *BRAF* inhibitor vemurafenib as well as with anti-PD1 agents such as pembrolizumab. In Muir-Torre syndrome, sebaceous tumors and keratoacanthomas occur in association with multiple internal malignancies. A second, less common cancer scenario is the keratoacanthoma–visceral carcinoma syndrome (KAVCS); only a

handful of cases have been reported. Patients have multiple or large keratoacanthomas that appear at the same time as an internal malignancy, always of the genitourinary tract. The relationship of Muir-Torre syndrome (MTS) to KAVCS awaits identification of the genetic basis of both syndromes.

Solitary Keratoacanthoma

The solitary keratoacanthoma is a rapidly growing papule that enlarges from a 1-mm macule or papule to as large as 25 mm in 3–8 weeks. When fully developed, it is a hemispheric, dome-shaped, skin-colored nodule that has a smooth crater filled with a central keratin plug (Fig. 29.13). The smooth shiny lesion is sharply demarcated from its surroundings. Telangiectases may run through the lesion. Subungual keratoacanthomas are tender subungual tumors that usually cause significant nail dystrophy. Subungual lesions often do not regress spontaneously and induce early underlying bony destruction, characterized on radiograph as a crescent-shaped lytic defect without accompanying sclerosis or periosteal reaction.

The solitary keratoacanthoma occurs mostly on sun-exposed skin, with the central portion of the face, backs of the hands, and arms most often involved. Less frequently, other sites are involved, such as the buttocks, thighs, penis, ears, and scalp. Elderly fair-skinned individuals most frequently develop keratoacanthomas. Lesions of the dorsal hands are more common in men, and keratoacanthomas of the lower legs are more common in women. The most interesting feature of this disease is the rapid growth for 2–6 weeks, followed by a stationary period for another 2–6 weeks, and finally a spontaneous involution over another 2–6 weeks, leaving a slightly depressed scar. The stationary period and involuting phase are variable; some lesions may take 6 months to 1 year to resolve completely. An estimated 5% of treated lesions recur. Invasion along nerve trunks has been documented and may result in recurrence after a seemingly adequate excision.

Histopathology

The histologic findings of keratoacanthoma and a low-grade SCC are so similar that it is frequently difficult to make a definite diagnosis on the histologic findings alone. When a properly sectioned specimen is examined under low magnification, the center of the lesion shows a crater filled with eosinophilic keratin. Over the sides of the crater, which seems to have been formed by invagination of the epidermis, a "lip" or "marginal buttress" of epithelium extends over the keratin-filled crater. At the base and sides of the crater, the epithelium is acanthotic and composed of keratinocytes, which are highly keratinized and have an eosinophilic, glassy cytoplasm. Surrounding the keratinocyte proliferation, a dense inflammatory infiltrate is frequently seen. Neutrophilic microabscesses are common within the tumor, and trapping of elastic fibers is often identified at the periphery of the tumor. These features favor a diagnosis of keratoacanthoma. The most definitive histologic feature is evidence of terminal differentiation, where the scalloped outer border of the tumor has lost its infiltrative character and is reduced to a thin rim of keratinizing cells lining a large, keratin-filled crater. The presence of acantholysis within the tumor is incompatible with a diagnosis of keratoacanthoma. It is also important to distinguish keratoacanthoma from marked pseudoepitheliomatous hyperplasia, as seen in prurigo nodularis. Unfortunately, histology does not completely correlate with biologic behavior. The diagnosis of benign-behaving keratoacanthoma versus a potentially aggressive SCC may not always be possible. Even if the classic histologic features of keratoacanthoma are seen, the diagnosis of SCC should be considered if the lesion does not behave as expected.

Treatment

Although keratoacanthomas spontaneously involute, it is impossible to predict how long this will take. The patient may be faced with destructive growth of a tumor for as long as 1 year. More importantly, SCC cannot always be excluded clinically. Therefore excisional biopsy of the typical keratoacanthoma of less than 2 cm in diameter should be considered in most cases. If the history is characteristic, or multiple lesions have appeared simultaneously, less aggressive interventions may be considered. Nonsurgical therapy may also be considered in certain sites to preserve function or improve cosmetic outcome.

Intralesional injections of 5-FU solution, 50 mg/mL (undiluted from ampule) at weekly intervals; bleomycin, 0.5 mg/mL; or methotrexate, 25 mg/mL, can be effective. For a typical lesion, four injections along the base at each pole are recommended. Low-dose systemic methotrexate can be considered if multiple lesions are present and there is no contraindication. For clinically typical lesions, these modalities may be tried before resorting to surgical removal, especially if the latter presents any problem. Excision is recommended if there is not at least 50% involution of the lesion after 3 weeks. Radiation therapy may also be used on giant keratoacanthomas when surgical excision or electrosurgical methods are not feasible.

Eruptive Keratoacanthomas of the Lower Leg

In older patients, especially older women, keratoacanthomas on the lower legs are often multiple and erupt in great numbers when one is treated surgically. The old quip is that "you kill one and five come to the funeral." An effective approach is to treat the lesions with 5-FU cream under Unna boot occlusion. Topical imiquimod, intralesional 5-FU, intralesional methotrexate, psoriatic doses of oral methotrexate, and oral acitretin can also be useful.

Multiple Keratoacanthomas (Ferguson Smith Type)

This type of keratoacanthoma is frequently referred to as the Ferguson Smith type of multiple self-healing keratoacanthoma. These lesions are identical clinically and histologically to the solitary type. There is frequently a family history of similar lesions. The condition has been traced to two large Scottish kindreds. Affected families from other countries have also been reported. Beginning on average at about age 25, but possibly as early as the second decade, patients develop crops of keratoacanthomas that begin as small red macules and rapidly become papules that evolve to typical keratoacanthomas. Lesions may number from a few to

hundreds, but generally only 3–10 lesions are noted at any one time. Sun-exposed sites are favored, especially the ears and nose, and in most cases scalp lesions occur. In addition, these patients typically develop keratoacanthomas at sites of trauma, often at the ends of surgical excisions. Lesions grow over 2–4 weeks, reaching a size of 2–3 cm, then remain stable for 1–2 months before slowly involuting. They leave a prominent crateriform scar. If the early lesions are aggressively treated with cryotherapy, shave removal, or curettage, the scar may be less marked than that induced by spontaneous involution. Treatment with an oral retinoid can be effective in stopping the appearance of new lesions and causing involution of existing ones.

Generalized Eruptive Keratoacanthomas (Grzybowski Variant)

The generalized eruptive keratoacanthoma is very rare and sporadic, with most patients having no affected family members. The usual age of onset is between 40 and 60. The patients are usually in good health and are not immunosuppressed. The cause of this condition is unknown. HPV has not been detected in most patients in whom it was sought. The clinical features are characteristic and unique. The Grzybowski type of multiple keratoacanthoma is characterized by a generalized eruption of numerous dome-shaped, skin-colored papules 2–7 mm in diameter. Multiple larger typical keratoacanthomas may also appear. Thousands of lesions may develop. The eruption is usually generalized, but spares the palms and soles. The oral mucous membranes and larynx can be involved. Severe pruritus may be a feature. Clinically, pityriasis rubra pilaris or widespread lichen planopilaris are often considered. Bilateral ectropion, narrowing of the oral aperture, and severe facial disfigurement can result. Linear arrangement of some lesions, especially over the shoulders and arms, has also been noted. Despite the multiplicity of lesions, no case of "metastasis" from a skin lesion or increased risk of internal malignancy has been reported in the Grzybowski variant of keratoacanthoma. Dr. Grzybowski's original patient died of a myocardial infarction 16 years after diagnosis. Oral treatment with retinoids, methotrexate, and cyclophosphamide can prove effective.

Keratoacanthoma Centrifugum Marginatum

This uncommon variant of keratoacanthoma is usually solitary, although multiple lesions can occur. Keratoacanthoma centrifugum marginatum is characterized by progressive peripheral expansion and concomitant central healing, leaving atrophy. Spontaneous involution, as may be seen in other variants of keratoacanthoma, does not occur. Lesions range from 5–30 cm in diameter (Fig. 29.14). The dorsum of the hands and pretibial regions are favored sites. Oral treatment with etretinate and methotrexate with prednisone has been effective in isolated cases.

Annest NM, et al: Intralesional methotrexate treatment for keratoacanthoma tumors. J Am Acad Dermatol 2007; 56: 989.

Anzalone CL, Cohen PR: Generalized eruptive keratoacanthomas of Grzybowski. Int J Dermatol 2014; 53: 131.

Baykal C, et al: Management of keratoacanthoma in patients with xeroderma pigmentosum. J Eur Acad Dermatol Venereol 2016; 30: e91.

Bieber AK, et al: Systemic methotrexate for prurigo nodularis and keratoacanthomas in actinically damaged skin. JAAD Case Rep 2016; 2: 269.

Hawilo A, et al: Keratoacanthoma centrifugum marginatum. Skinmed 2017; 15: 69.

John AM, et al: Muir-Torre syndrome (MTS). J Am Acad Dermatol 2016; 74: 558.

Kwiek B, et al: Keratoacanthoma (KA). J Am Acad Dermatol 2016; 74: 1220.

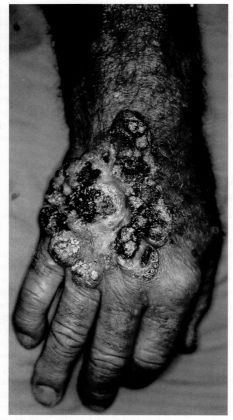

Fig. 29.14 Keratoacanthoma centrifugum marginatum.

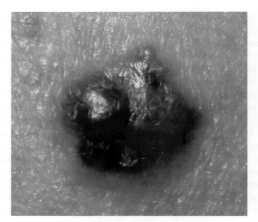

Fig. 29.15 Basal cell carcinoma.

Ogita A, et al: Histopathological diagnosis of epithelial crateriform tumors. J Dermatol 2016; 43: 1321.

Rhee do Y, et al: Successful treatment of multiple vemurafenib-induced keratoacanthomas by topical application of imiquimod cream. J Dermatolog Treat 2016; 27: 448.

Takai T: Advances in histopathological diagnosis of keratoacanthoma. J Dermatol 2017; 44: 304.

Veerula VL, et al: Multiple keratoacanthomas occurring in surgical margins and de novo treated with intralesional methotrexate. Cutis 2016; 98: E12.

BASAL CELL CARCINOMA

Basal cell carcinoma (BCC) is the most common cancer in the United States, Australia, New Zealand, and many other countries with a largely white, fair-skinned population with moderate sun exposure. In Hawaii, the incidence of BCC is 14-fold higher in persons of European ancestry (especially Celtic) than in Japanese, and 34-fold higher than in Filipinos. Still, persons of color can develop BCCs, especially fair-skinned Asians and Hispanics who have accumulated significant lifetime sun exposure from occupational sources, usually farm work. White Hispanics have less skin cancer awareness, use sun protection less frequently, and are more likely to use tanning beds than darker-skinned Hispanics. They represent a prevalent at-risk population for skin cancer over the next decades.

Intermittent intense sun exposure, as identified by prior sunburns; radiation therapy; a positive family history of BCC; immunosuppression; a fair complexion, especially red hair; easy sunburning (skin types I or II); and blistering sunburns in childhood are risk factors for the development of BCC. Indoor tanning is a strong risk factor for early-onset BCC, particularly among women.

Of interest, actinic elastosis and wrinkling are not risk factors for the development of BCC. In fact, BCCs are relatively rare on the dorsal hand, where sun exposure is high, whereas actinic keratoses and SCCs abound. SCC is three times more common than BCC on the dorsum of the hand. These findings suggest that the mechanism by which UVR induces BCC is not related solely to the total amount of UVR received. In contrast to actinic keratoses and SCCs, prevention with regular use of sunscreens is more difficult to demonstrate. The ratio of BCC to SCC decreases as one moves from northern (≈10) to southern (≈2) United States. Once a person has had a BCC, his or her risk for a subsequent BCC is high: 44% in the next 3 years.

Many clinical morphologies of BCC exist. Clinical diagnosis depends on the clinician being aware of the many forms BCC may take. Because these clinical types may also have different biologic behavior, histologic classification of the type of BCC may also influence the therapy chosen.

Nodular Basal Cell Carcinoma (Classic Basal Cell Carcinoma)

The classic or nodular BCC constitutes 50%–80% of all BCCs. Nodular BCC is composed of one or a few small, waxy, semi-translucent nodules forming around a central depression that may or may not be ulcerated, crusted, and bleeding. The edge of larger lesions has a characteristic rolled border. Telangiectases course through the lesion. Bleeding on slight injury is a common sign. As growth progresses, crusting appears over a central erosion or ulcer, and when the crust is knocked or picked off, bleeding occurs, and the ulcer becomes apparent. This ulcer is characterized by chronicity and gradual enlargement over time. The lesions are asymptomatic, and bleeding is the only difficulty encountered. The lesions are most frequently found on the face (Fig. 29.15) (85%–90% on head and neck) and especially on the nose (25%–30%). The forehead, ears, periocular areas, and cheeks are also favored sites. However, any part of the body may be involved.

Cystic Basal Cell Carcinoma

These dome-shaped, blue-gray cystic nodules are clinically similar to eccrine and apocrine hidrocystomas.

Morpheaform, or Cicatricial Basal Cell Carcinoma

This type of BCC presents as a white sclerotic plaque, and 95% of these occur on the head and neck. Ulceration, a pearly rolled border, and crusting are usually absent. Telangiectasia is variably present. Therefore the lesion is often missed or misdiagnosed for some time. The differential diagnosis includes desmoplastic trichoepithelioma, a scar, microcystic adnexal carcinoma, and desmoplastic melanoma. The unique histologic feature is the strands of basal cells interspersed amid densely packed, hypocellular connective tissue. Morpheic BCCs constitute 2%–6% of all BCCs. Data suggest use of fluorouracil may be a risk factor for morpheaform versus nonmorpheaform BCC.

Infiltrative Basal Cell Carcinoma

Infiltrative BCC is an aggressive subtype characterized by deep infiltration of spiky islands of basaloid epithelium in a fibroblast-rich stroma. Clinically, it lacks the scarlike appearance of morpheiform BCC. Histologically, the stroma is hypercellular, the islands are jagged in outline, and squamous differentiation is common.

Micronodular Basal Cell Carcinoma

These tumors are not clinically distinctive, but the micronodular growth pattern makes them less amenable to curettage.

Superficial Basal Cell Carcinoma

Superficial BCC is also termed superficial multicentric BCC. This is a common form of BCC, comprising at least 15% of the total. It favors the trunk (45%) or distal extremities (14%). Only 40% occur on the head and neck. The multicentricity is merely a histologic illusion created by the passing of the plane of section through the branches of a single, multiply branching lesion.

This type of BCC most frequently presents as a dry, psoriasiform, scaly lesion. It is usually a superficial flat growth, which in many cases exhibits little tendency to invade or ulcerate. The lesions enlarge very slowly and may be misdiagnosed as patches of eczema or psoriasis. They may grow to be 10–15 cm in diameter. Close examination of the edges of the lesion will show a threadlike raised border (Fig. 29.16). These erythematous plaques with telangiectasia may occasionally show atrophy or scarring. Some lesions may develop an infiltrative component in their deeper aspect and grow into the deeper dermis. When this occurs, they may induce dermal fibrosis and multifocal ulceration, forming a "field of fire" type of large BCC. Sometimes the lesion will heal at one place with a white atrophic scar and then spread actively to the neighboring skin. A patient can have several of these lesions simultaneously or over time. This form of BCC is the most common pattern seen in patients with human immunodeficiency virus (HIV) infection and BCC.

Pigmented Basal Cell Carcinoma

This variety has all the features of nodular BCC, but in addition, brown or black pigmentation is present (Fig. 29.17). When dark-complexioned persons, such as Latin Americans, Hispanics, or Asians, develop BCC, this is the type they tend to develop. Pigmented BCCs make up 6% of all BCCs. In the management of these lesions, it should be known that, if ionizing radiation therapy is chosen, the pigmentation remains at the site of the lesion.

Rodent Ulcer

Also known as Jacobi ulcer, rodent ulcer is a neglected BCC that has formed an ulceration. The pearly border of the lesion may not be recognized. If it occurs on the lower extremity, it may be misdiagnosed as a vascular ulceration.

Fibroepithelioma of Pinkus

First described by Pinkus as premalignant fibroepithelial tumor, this is usually an elevated, skin-colored, sessile lesion on the lower trunk, lumbosacral area, groin, or thigh and may be as large as 7 cm. The lesion is superficial and resembles a fibroma or papilloma. Histologically, interlacing basocellular sheets extend downward from the surface to form an epithelial meshwork enclosing a hyperplastic mesodermal stroma. As with infundibulocystic BCC, fibroepithelioma is composed of pink epithelial strands with blue basaloid buds. Fibroepithelioma has a more prominent fibromucinous stroma and lacks the horn cysts characteristic of infundibulocystic BCC. Fibroepithelioma often demonstrates sweat ducts within the pink epithelial strands. A slight inflammatory infiltrate may also be present. Simple removal by excision or electrosurgery is the treatment of choice.

Polypoid Basal Cell Carcinoma

The polypoid BCCs present as exophytic nodules of the head and neck.

Porelike Basal Cell Carcinoma

Patients with thick sebaceous skin of the central face may develop a BCC that resembles an enlarged pore or stellate pit. The lesions virtually always occur on the nose, melolabial fold, or lower forehead. Affected patients are generally men, and the majority are smokers. Many years pass from the appearance of the lesion until a diagnostic biopsy is taken, because the lesion is considered inconsequential.

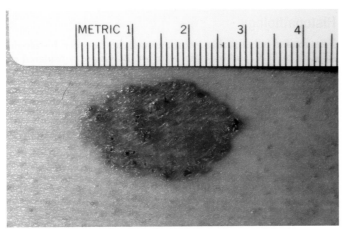

Fig. 29.16 Superficial basal cell carcinoma.

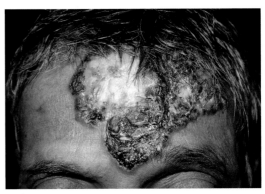

Fig. 29.17 Pigmented basal cell carcinoma. (Courtesy Debabrata Bandyopadhyay, MD.)

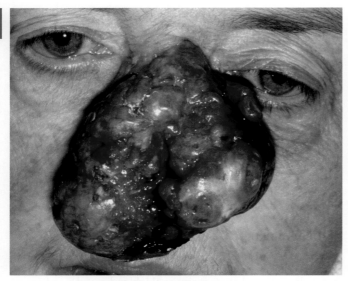

Fig. 29.18 Large basal cell carcinoma.

Aberrant Basal Cell Carcinoma

Even in the absence of any apparent carcinogenic factor, such as arsenic, radiation, or chronic ulceration, BCC may occur in odd sites, such as the scrotum, vulva, perineum, nipple, and axilla.

Solitary Basal Cell Carcinoma in Young Persons

These curious lesions are typically located in the region of embryonal clefts in the face and are often deeply invasive. Complete surgical excision is much safer than curettage for their removal. Cases in children and teenagers, unassociated with the basal cell nevus syndrome or nevus sebaceus, are well documented.

Natural History

Basal cell carcinomas run a chronic course as the lesion slowly enlarges and tends to become more ulcerative (Fig. 29.18). As a rule, the lesions tend to bleed without pain or other symptoms. Some tend to heal spontaneously and form scar tissue as they extend. Peripheral spreading may produce configurate, somewhat serpiginous patches. The ulceration may burrow deep into the subcutaneous tissues or even into cartilage and bone, causing extensive destruction and mutilation. At least half the deaths that occur from BCC result from direct extension into a vital structure rather than metastases.

Metastasis

Metastasis is extremely rare, occurring in 0.0028%–0.55% of BCCs. This low rate is believed to occur because the tumor cells require supporting stroma to survive. The following criteria are now widely accepted for the diagnosis of metastatic BCC:

1. The primary tumor must arise in the skin.
2. Metastases must be demonstrated at a site distant from the primary tumor and must not be related to simple extension.
3. Histologic similarity must exist between the primary tumor and the metastases.
4. The metastases must not be mixed with SCC.

Metastatic BCC is twice as common in men as in women. Immunosuppression does not appear to increase the risk of metastasis of BCC. Most BCCs that metastasize arise on the head and neck and tend to be large tumors that have recurred despite multiple surgical procedures or radiation therapy. The histologic finding of perineural or intravascular BCC increases the risk for metastasis. The regional lymph nodes are the most common site of metastasis, followed by the lung, bone, skin, liver, and pleura. Spread is equally distributed between hematogenous and lymphatic. An average of 9 years elapses between the diagnosis of the primary tumor and metastatic disease, but the interval for metastasis ranges from less than 1 year to 45 years. Although the primary tumor may be present for many years before it metastasizes, once metastases occur, the course is rapidly downhill. After metastasis, fewer than 20% of patients survive 1 year, and fewer than 10% will live for more than 5 years.

Association with Internal Malignancies

Frisch et al. reported a series of 37,674 patients with BCCs followed over 14 years. Comparison of cancer rates for the general population was remarkable, with 3663 new cancers versus 3245 in the control population. Malignant melanoma and lip cancers were most frequently found; however, internal malignancies were also noted to be excessive, involving the salivary glands, larynx, lung, breast, kidney, and lymphatics (non-Hodgkin lymphoma). The rate of non-Hodgkin lymphoma was particularly high. Patients receiving the diagnosis of BCC before age 60 had a higher rate of breast cancer, testicular cancer, and non-Hodgkin lymphoma.

Immunosuppression

Immunosuppression for organ transplantation increases the risk for the development of BCC by about 10-fold. Some increased risk for BCC is also thought to occur in HIV-infected patients and in those receiving immunosuppressive medications for other reasons. Patients with chronic lymphocytic leukemia are also at increased risk for BCC. In the immunosuppressed population, a history of blistering sunburns in childhood is a strong risk factor for the development of BCC after immunosuppression.

Etiology and Pathogenesis

It appears that BCCs arise from immature pluripotential cells associated with the hair follicle. Mutations that activate the hedgehog signaling pathway, which controls cell growth, are found in most BCCs. The affected genes are those for sonic hedgehog, patched 1, and smoothened *(SMO)*. Inactivation of patched 1 is most common, and *SMO* mutations are associated with 10%–20% of sporadic BCCs.

Histopathology

The general belief is that a correlation exists between histologic subtype of BCC and biologic behavior. BCCs are considered as being of low risk or high risk, depending on their probability of causing problems in the future: subclinical extension, incomplete removal, aggressive local invasive behavior, and local recurrence. Therefore the dermatopathology report of a BCC should include a subtype descriptor when possible. Unfortunately, many shave biopsy specimens do not allow for accurate typing, and the presence of an indolent growth pattern superficially does not exclude the possibility of a deeper, more aggressive growth pattern. The common histologic patterns are nodular, superficial, infiltrative, morpheic, micronodular, and mixed. The nodular type is a low-risk type. High-risk types include the infiltrative, morpheic, and micronodular patterns, because of aggressive local invasive behavior and a tendency to recur. Superficial BCC is prone to increased recurrence due to inadequate removal. When evaluating the histologic margin of superficial BCC, tumor stroma involving the margin should be considered a positive margin.

The early lesion shows small, dark-staining, polyhedral cells resembling those of the basal cell layer of the epidermis, with large nuclei and small nucleoli. These occur within the epidermis as thickenings or immediately beneath the epidermis as downgrowths connected with it. After the growth has progressed, regular compact columns of these cells fill the tissue spaces of the dermis, and a connection with the epidermis may be difficult to demonstrate. At the periphery of the masses of cells, the columnar cells may be characteristically arranged like fence posts (palisading). This may be absent when the tumor cells are in cord arrangement or in small nests. Cysts may form. The interlacing strands of tumor cells may present a lattice-like pattern. The dermal stroma is an integral and important part of the BCC. The stroma is loose and fibromyxoid, with a sparse lymphoid infiltrate often present. The stroma can be highlighted by metachromatic toluidine blue staining, which can be useful during Mohs surgery.

Differential Diagnosis

Distinguishing between small BCCs and small SCCs is largely an intellectual exercise. Both are caused chiefly by sunlight, neither is likely to metastasize, and both will require removal, usually by simple surgical excision or curettage. A biopsy is always indicated but may be performed at the definitive procedure, when the likelihood of the diagnosis of NMSC is high and the patient is fully informed and gives consent.

A waxy, nodular, rolled edge is fairly characteristic of BCC (Fig. 29.19). The SCC is a dome-shaped, elevated, hard, and infiltrated lesion. The early BCC may easily be confused with sebaceous hyperplasia, which has a depressed center with yellowish small nodules surrounding the lesion. However, these lesions never bleed and do not become crusted.

Bowen disease, Paget disease, amelanotic melanoma, and actinic and seborrheic keratoses may also simulate BCC. Ulcerated BCC on the shins is frequently misdiagnosed as a stasis ulcer, and a biopsy may be the only way to differentiate the two. Pigmented BBC is frequently misdiagnosed as melanoma or as a pigmented nevus. The superficial BCC is easily mistaken for psoriasis or eczema. The careful search for the rolled edge of the peripheral nodules is important in differentiating BCC from all other lesions.

Treatment

Each lesion of BCC must be thoroughly evaluated individually. Age and gender of the patient as well as the size, site, and type of lesion are important factors to be considered when choosing the proper method of treatment. No single treatment method is ideal for all lesions or all patients. The choice of treatment will also be influenced by the experience and ability of the treating physician in the various treatment modalities. A biopsy should be performed in all patients with suspected BCC to determine the histologic subtype and confirm the diagnosis.

The aim of treatment is for a permanent cure with the best cosmetic results. This is important because the most common location of BCC is the face. Recurrences result from inadequate treatment and are usually seen during the first 4–12 months after treatment. A minimum 5-year follow-up is indicated, however, to continue a search for new lesions, because the development of a second BCC is common.

Treatment of BCC is usually surgical (see Chapter 37), but some forms of BCC are amenable to medical treatment, PDT or radiation therapy. Vismodegiband related inhibitors of smoothened that targets the hedgehog pathway, has antitumor activity and clinically meaningful response in locally advanced or metastatic BCC. Electrochemotherapy, combining bleomycin with short electric pulses, has been used as palliative skin-directed therapy for patients with multiple or large BCC for whom conventional treatments are not viable options.

Topical Therapy

Topical therapy appears to be most effective in the treatment of superficial BCC. For nodular BCCs, the cure rates are only 65%, which is unacceptable given the other options available. On the other hand, superficial BCCs may be cured 80% of the time with topical treatment. Topical 5-FU applied twice daily for at least 6 weeks can yield acceptable results in properly selected (i.e., thin) tumors but is not otherwise very effective, with high recurrence rates. Imiquimod applied three times a week with occlusion, or five times a week without occlusion, is the favored form of topical, patient-applied treatment for superficial BCC. Duration of treatment is 6 weeks but may be extended if the lesion does not appear to have been eradicated. Cosmetic results are excellent, especially for lesions of the anterior chest and upper back, where significant scarring usually results from surgical procedures. PDT has also emerged as a treatment option for BCC. A randomized controlled trial (RCT) found imiquimod to be superior, and 5-FU not to be inferior, to PDT for superficial BCC. Cure rates are higher with surgical excision than with topical therapy.

Apalla Z, et al: Spotlight on vismodegib in the treatment of basal cell carcinoma. Clin Cosmet Investig Dermatol 2017; 10: 171.

Arits AH, et al: Photodynamic therapy versus topical imiquimod versus topical fluorouracil for treatment of superficial basal-cell carcinoma. Lancet Oncol 2013; 14: 647.

Bartos V, et al: Basal cell carcinoma multiplicity. Klin Onkol 2017; 30: 197.

Campana LG, et al: Basal cell carcinoma. J Transl Med 2017; 15: 122.

Godoy CAP, et al: Evaluation of surgical margins according to the histological type of basal cell carcinoma. An Bras Dermatol 2017; 92: 226.

Komatsubara KM, et al: Advances in the treatment of advanced extracutaneous melanomas and nonmelanoma skin cancers. Am Soc Clin Oncol Educ Book 2017; 37: 641.

Mott SE, et al: Approach to management of giant basal cell carcinoma. Cutis 2017; 99: 356.

Odom D, et al: A matching-adjusted indirect comparison of sonidegib and vismodegib in advanced basal cell carcinoma. J Skin Cancer 2017; 2017: 6121760.

O'Donnell BP, et al: A prospective evaluation of the candle wax sign. J Am Acad Dermatol 2017; 77: 163.

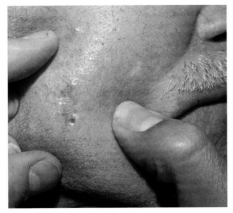

Fig. 29.19 Basal cell carcinoma, accentuation of pearly border when skin is stretched.

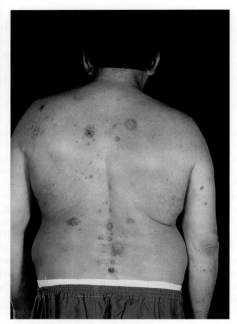

Fig. 29.20 Multiple basal cell carcinomas in nevoid basal cell carcinoma syndrome.

NEVOID BASAL CELL CARCINOMA SYNDROME (GORLIN SYNDROME)

Clinical Features

The nevoid BCC syndrome (NBCCS) or basal cell nevus syndrome is an autosomal dominant inherited disorder. The major diagnostic criteria for NBCCS include the following:

1. Development of multiple BCCs (>5) or a BCC before age 30 (Fig. 29.20)
2. Odontogenic keratocysts of the jaws
3. Pitted depressions on the hands and feet (palmar plantar pits) (two or more)
4. Lamellar calcification of the falx under age 20
5. First-degree relative with NBCCS

Minor criteria are as follows:

1. Childhood medulloblastoma
2. Lympho-mesenteric or pleural cysts
3. Macrocephaly (97th percentile)
4. Cleft lip/palate
5. Vertebral/rib abnormalities
6. Preaxial or postaxial polydactyly
7. Ovarian/cardiac fibromas
8. Ocular abnormalities

The diagnosis of NBBCS is made if the affected individual has two major criteria and one minor criterion, or one major criterion and three minor criteria. Genetic testing has revealed that some persons carrying the genetic mutation do not meet the diagnostic criteria.

Essentially, all cases of NBCCS are caused by mutations in the *PTCH* (or *PTCH1*) gene. One family with a mutation in the *SUFU* gene has been reported. *SUFU* mutations have been reported with medulloblastoma susceptibility. Mutations occur throughout the *PTCH* gene, and no correlation appears to exist between the site of the mutation and the clinical phenotype. Most mutations result in premature termination and production of shortened gene

product. Loss of the *PTCH* gene can also occur by deletions of part of the long arm of chromosome 9, where the *PTCH* gene is located (region q22). This represents about 6% of NBCCS patients.

The clinical findings seen with NBCCS depend on two characteristics: the race of the patient and the form of mutation (nucleotide point mutation or chromosome deletion). Of 105 patients reported in one series, 80% were white. The first tumor developed by the mean age of 23 years for white patients. Palmar pits were seen in 87%. Jaw cysts were found in 74%, with 80% manifested by age 20. The total number of cysts ranged from 1 to 28. Medulloblastomas developed in four patients, and three had cleft lip or palate. Physical findings in this series included "coarse face" (54%), macrocephaly (50%), hypertelorism (42%), frontal bossing (27%), pectus deformity (13%), and Sprengel deformity (11%). In Japanese and African American patients with NBCCS, palmar and plantar pits, odontogenic keratocysts, and skeletal abnormalities are most common, with BCCs not appearing until much later in life. Those patients with NBCCS caused by deletions of chromosome 9q22 have all the stigmata of typical NBCCS patients, and in addition often have severe mental retardation, hyperactivity, overfriendliness with strangers, short stature, and less often, neonatal hypotonia, epicanthic folds, short neck, pectus, scoliosis, and epilepsy.

Skin Tumors

The BCCs occur at an early age or any time thereafter as multiple lesions, usually numerous. The usual age of appearance is 17–35 years. Although any area of the body may be affected, there is a marked tendency toward involvement of the central facial area, especially the eyelids, periorbital area, nose, upper lip, and cheeks. Persons with fair skin (type 1) and prior excessive UV exposure are particularly prone to develop many BCCs. Lesions typically appear as 1–10 mm, hyperpigmented or skin-colored, dome-shaped papules. They have a striking resemblance to typical compound or intradermal nevi. Polypoid BCC or acrochordon-like BCC is a more unusual variant that tends to occur in NBCCS patients in childhood. Among the many BCCs that an NBCCS patient may have, some sit indolently and others may grow more aggressively.

Jaw Cysts

Jaw cysts occur in approximately 90% of patients. They occur as early as age 5 years and rarely after age 30. Both the mandible and the maxilla may show cystic defects on x-ray, with mandibular involvement occurring twice as often. Jaw cysts most commonly present as painless swelling. They usually have a keratinized lining (keratocysts) but uncommonly a cyst may be an ameloblastoma.

Pits of Palms and Soles

An unusual pitting of palms and soles is a distinguishing feature of the disease. This usually becomes apparent in the second decade of life. Up to 87% of patients with NBCCS will have pits. Histologically, they show basaloid proliferation, but the lesions do not progress or behave as a BCC.

Skeletal Defects/Birth Defects

Most NBCCS patients have skeletal anomalies that are easily detected on radiographs. Macrocephaly is the first feature observed and explains the high rate of cesarean delivery of NBCCS-affected neonates. Other skeletal defects include bifid, fused, missing, or splayed ribs; scoliosis; and kyphosis. Radiographic evidence of multiple lesions is highly suggestive of this syndrome; and because most are present congenitally, radiology may be useful in diagnosing this syndrome in patients too young to manifest other abnormalities. Cleft lip/palate is seen in 5% of patients; lamellar calcification of the falx will be evident in 90% of patients by age 20; and polydactyly also occurs. Numerous ocular findings have been reported, and if NBCCS is suspected or confirmed, an ophthalmologic evaluation should be performed. Spina bifida is, fortunately, uncommon.

Histopathology

The histology of BCCs arising in syndromic patients is identical to that arising in nonsyndromic patients, with the solid and superficial types being most common.

Differential Diagnosis

Several other unique types of BCC presentation should not be confused with NBCCS. One type is the linear unilateral BCC syndrome, in which a linear arrangement of close-set papules, sometimes interspersed with comedones, is present at birth. Biopsy reveals BBCs, but they do not increase in size with the age of the patient. A second type, referred to as Bazex syndrome, is an X-linked dominant inherited disease comprising follicular atrophoderma of the extremities, localized or generalized hypohidrosis, hypotrichosis, and multiple BCCs of the face, which often arise at an early age. A third type consists of multiple hereditary infundibulocystic BCCs and is an autosomal dominant syndrome. It is distinguished from NBCCS by the absence of palmar pits and jaw cysts in most cases. Clinically, patients appear to have multiple trichoepitheliomas. Numerous skin-colored pearly papules affect the central face, accentuated in the nasolabial folds. The generalized basaloid follicular hamartoma (BFH) syndrome differs from NBCCS by having basaloid follicular hamartomas instead of BCCs. It is reported from a large kindred in the southeastern United States (see later). Tiny palmar pits are present. Histologically, infundibulocystic BCC and BFH may be indistinguishable, so the two familial syndromes may be difficult to separate. Rombo syndrome, reported in one large Swedish family, has multiple BCCs, vermiculate atrophoderma, and hypotrichosis. A patient with multiple BCCs and myotonic dystrophy has been reported, suggesting yet another genodermatosis associated with multiple BCCs.

Treatment

Genetic counseling is essential. Strict sun avoidance and maximum sun protection, as recommended for xeroderma pigmentosum patients, is advised. Avoidance of ionizing radiation is also paramount, because NBCCS patients are particularly sensitive to radiation; multiple BCCs may appear in the distribution of radiation therapy used to treat medulloblastoma or BCC or other cancers. Treatment involves very regular monitoring and biopsy of suspicious lesions. Topical therapy with tazarotene and imiquimod may be of some use in preventing and treating the superficial tumors. Oral retinoid therapy may reduce the frequency of new BCCs appearing and may slow the growth of existing small BCCs. However, once the oral retinoids are stopped, the lesions again begin to grow. Vismodegib, the hedgehog pathway inhibitor, reduces BCC tumor burden and prevents growth of new BCCs in those with NBCCS; however, poor tolerability of the medication leads to a high rate of discontinuation (≈50%). A topical formulation of a smoothened inhibitor appears to be effective and better tolerated, leading to BCC regression. Surgical treatments are used for most lesions, either curettage and desiccation or excision. At times, megasessions, with removal of multiple tumors under general anesthesia in the operating room, are needed to keep up with the large number of BCCs these patients develop. PDT appears to be particularly beneficial when used to treat areas that have had multiple BCCs in the past.

Ally MS, et al: The use of vismodegib to shrink keratocystic odontogenic tumors in patients with basal cell nevus syndrome. JAMA Dermatol 2014; 150: 542.

da Paz Oliveira G, et al: Clinical and neuroimaging features in Gorlin-Goltz syndrome. Neurology 2017; 88: e53.

Foulkes WD, et al: Cancer surveillance in Gorlin syndrome and rhabdoid tumor predisposition syndrome. Clin Cancer Res 2017; 23: e62.

Gilchrest BA, et al: Photodynamic therapy for patients with basal cell nevus syndrome. Dermatol Surg 2009; 35: 1576.

Mello RN, et al: A multidisciplinary approach to the successful management of Gorlin syndrome. J Surg Case Rep 2017; 2017: rjw224.

Shiohama T, et al: Brain morphology in children with nevoid basal cell carcinoma syndrome. Am J Med Genet A 2017; 173: 946.

SQUAMOUS CELL CARCINOMA

Squamous cell carcinoma (SCC) is the second most common form of skin cancer. Most cases of SCC of the skin are induced by UVR. Chronic, long-term sun exposure is the major risk factor, and areas that have had such exposure (face, scalp, neck, dorsal hands) are favored locations. SCC becomes relatively more common as the annual amount of UVR increases, so SCC is more common in Texas than in Minnesota, for example. Immunosuppression greatly enhances the risk for the development of SCC, approximately 65-fold to 250-fold among organ transplant recipients, with azathioprine exposure especially associated with greater risk for development of cutaneous SCC. Sorafenib and possibly the tumor necrosis factor (TNF) inhibitors may be associated with increased risk of cutaneous SCC. High-risk genital HPVs, primarily 16, 18, 31, and 35, play a role in SCCs that develop on the genitalia and periungually. Chronic ulcers, hidradenitis suppurativa, recessive dystrophic epidermolysis bullosa, lesions of discoid LE, erosive lichen planus, prior radiation exposure, and PUVA therapy also appear to enhance the risk for SCC development. Metastasis, with mortality of 18%, is very uncommon for SCCs arising at sites of chronic sun damage, whereas it is relatively high (20%–30%) in SCCs occurring in the various scarring processes. In recessive dystrophic epidermolysis bullosa, metastatic SCC is the most common cause of death in adulthood. Patients with epidermodysplasia verruciformis (EDV) also develop SCCs on sun-exposed sites, associated with unique HPV types. These unique EDV HPV types (e.g., HPV-5, HPV-8) may also play a role in SCCs that develop in immunosuppressed persons. SCC of the oral mucosa is discussed in Chapter 34. Because the vast majority of cutaneous SCCs are induced by UVR, sun protection, with avoidance of the midday sun, protective clothing, and the regular application of a sunblock of SPF 30 or higher, is recommended. Some researchers have suggested that smoking is also a risk factor for cutaneous SCC, but this is controversial.

Clinical Features

Frequently, SCC begins at the site of actinic keratosis on sun-exposed areas such as the face and backs of the hands. BCCs far outnumber SCCs on facial skin, but SCCs on the hand occur three times more frequently than BCCs (Fig. 29.21). The lesion may be superficial, discrete, and hard and arises from an indurated, rounded, elevated base. It is dull red and contains telangiectases. In the course of a few months, the lesion becomes larger, deeply nodular, and ulcerated. The ulcer is at first superficial and hidden by a crust. When the crust is removed, a well-defined papillary base is seen, and on palpation, a discrete hard disk is felt. In the early phases, this tumor is localized, elevated, and freely mobile over underlying structures; later it gradually becomes diffuse, more or less depressed, and fixed. The growth eventually invades the

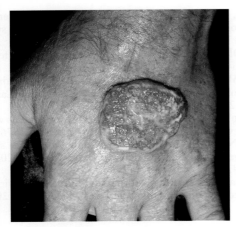

Fig. 29.21 Squamous cell carcinoma.

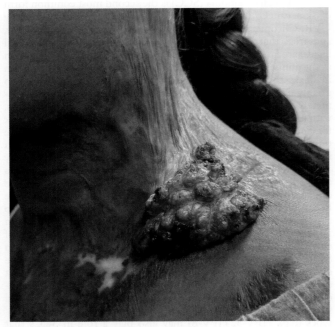

Fig. 29.22 Squamous cell carcinoma via burn scar. (Courtesy Dr. Debabrata Bandyopadhyay.)

underlying tissues. The tumor above the level of the skin may be dome shaped, with a corelike center that later ulcerates. The surface in advanced lesions may be cauliflower-like, composed of densely packed, filamentous projections, between which are clefts filled with a viscous, purulent, malodorous exudate.

In black patients, SCCs are 20% more common than BCCs. The most favored sites are the face and lower extremities, with involvement of non–sun-exposed areas more common. Elderly women (mean age 77) are primarily affected in cases involving the lower legs. Prior direct heat exposure from open fireplaces may be the predisposing factor. In contrast, the most frequently found predisposing conditions in white patients are scarring processes, such as burns (Fig. 29.22), leg ulcers, and hidradenitis suppurativa.

On the lower lip, SCC often develops on actinic cheilitis. From repeated sunburn, the vermilion surface becomes dry, scaly, and fissured. At the beginning, only a local thickening is noticeable. This then becomes a firm nodule. It may grow outward as a sizable tumor or inward with destructive ulceration. A history of smoking

is also a frequent and significant predisposing factor. Lower lip lesions far outnumber upper lip lesions; men greatly outnumber women (12:1); and the median age is the late sixties. SCCs occurring on the lower lip metastasize in 10%–15% of cases. SCC of the lip may also occur in areas of discoid LE in black patients. Neoplastic transformation into SCC may develop in 0.3%–3% of patients with discoid LE of the lip.

Periungual SCC frequently presents with signs of erythema and scaling, which can superficially resemble a wart. The patient may even have periungual warts on other digits. Early on, pain and ulceration are uncommon. Radiographs show that 50% have changes in the terminal phalanx. There is a low rate of metastases (3%), but local excision with Mohs microsurgery is recommended, as it reduces the risk of recurrence. Periungual SCC is strongly associated with genital HPV types, primarily 16, 18, 31, and 35.

Given the numerous presentations of SCC on the skin, there should be a low threshold for biopsy of any suspicious keratotic, ulcerated, or nodular lesion, especially on the background of chronic sun exposure.

Histopathology

SCC is characterized by irregular nests, cords, or sheets of neoplastic keratinocytes invading the dermis to various depths. Thickness is an important risk factor for metastasis, with thickness >2 mm associated with a metastatic rate of 4% and >6 mm with a rate of 16%. Less than 5% of patients with metastatic SCC had a primary cutaneous SCC <2 mm in thickness. Immunosuppression, location on the ear, and increased horizontal size all increase the risk of metastasis by twofold to fourfold. Desmoplasia and tumor thickness also increase local recurrence risk, by 16 and 6 times, respectively. Although histologic differentiation should be reported, it seems less important than these other tumor features in predicting prognosis. In tumors that are poorly differentiated or of primary clear cell morphology, other types of neoplasm must be excluded, such as melanoma. Immunoperoxidase staining for keratins is very useful in this setting. Desmoplastic SCCs by light microscopy have prominent trabecular growth patterns, narrow columns of atypical epithelial cells, and marked desmoplastic stromal reaction. These tumors tend to recur. Acantholytic SCC is a recognized histologic subtype but is of no prognostic importance. The finding of perineural or vascular invasion and recurrence are poor prognostic features.

Differential Diagnosis

The differentiation of SCC from keratoacanthoma is of academic interest in most cases, because simple surgical excision is performed on most of these lesions. However, if nonsurgical modalities are contemplated, a biopsy confirming the diagnosis of keratoacanthoma is recommended. In the setting of immunosuppression, keratoacanthoma-like lesions should be managed as SCCs. The rapid growth and presence of a rolled border with a keratotic central plug suggest the diagnosis of keratoacanthoma, as does explosive growth. An early SCC may be confused with a hypertrophic actinic keratosis, and indeed, the two may be indistinguishable clinically. Biopsy to include the base of the lesion is necessary to make the diagnosis.

Pseudoepitheliomatous hyperplasia (PEH) must be distinguished histologically from true SCC. Marked PEH may be seen in granular cell tumor, bromoderma, blastomycosis, granuloma inguinale, and chronic pyodermas. It is frequently mistaken for SCC in chronic stasis ulcers, ulcerations occurring in thermal burns, lupus vulgaris, leishmaniasis, and even sporotrichosis. PEH arises from adnexal structures, as well as the surface epidermis. Hyperkeratosis and hypergranulosis of adjacent hair follicles are often present. Strands of epidermal cells may extend into the reticular dermis and usually trap elastic fibers, a finding also seen in keratoacanthoma but rarely in conventional SCCs. A potential diagnostic pitfall is the presence of benign PEH adjacent to and overlying invasive SCC. This is particularly common in lesions that have been picked or scratched.

Metastases

The rate of SCC metastasis from all skin sites ranges from 0.5%–5.2%. Lesions at elevated risk of metastasis (and recurrence) are those on the lip, ear, or anogenital skin; those occurring at the site of chronic scar or irradiation; those 2 cm or more in diameter; those more than 4 mm thick; those that are recurrent, have poor histologic differentiation, or perineural invasion; and those occurring in patients with organ transplantation or hematologic malignancy. Such patients may be considered for more aggressive surgical management and adjuvant radiotherapy. Careful attention should be paid to regional lymph nodes draining the site of the SCC. These should be examined at the initial evaluation when the suspicious lesion is identified and at the regular visits that follow the treatment of the SCC.

Patients with SCC are at increased risk of developing other malignancies, such as cancers of the respiratory organs, buccal cavity, pharynx, and small intestine (in men), as well as non-Hodgkin lymphoma and leukemia.

Prevention/Treatment

The primary treatment of SCC of the skin is surgical (see Chapter 37). Oral retinoids may be useful as a preventive strategy in patients with immunosuppression who develop frequent cancers. PDT might be beneficial to reduce the number of SCCs occurring in areas of prior UV damage where SCCs have already occurred, and pembrolizumab may have a role in treating advanced disease. As with BCC, electrochemotherapy has been used as palliative skin-directed therapy for patients a for whom conventional treatments are not viable options. Organ transplant recipients should be educated about sun protection and skin cancer risk, ideally *before* their transplantation, and should have regular skin examinations by a trained dermatologist. The use of sirolimus instead of other immunosuppressives appears to reduce the prevalence of SCCs in organ transplant recipients. Immunosuppressed patients receiving voriconazole for treatment or prophylaxis of invasive fungal infections should be made aware of its role in photocarcinogenesis and its link to increased SCC incidence and should be similarly educated about sun protection measures.

Amaral T, et al: Non-melanoma skin cancer. Expert Opin Pharmacother 2017; 18: 689.

Brantsch KD, et al: Analysis of risk factors determining prognosis of cutaneous squamous-cell carcinoma. Lancet Oncol 2008; 9: 713.

Brougham ND, et al: The incidence of metastasis from cutaneous squamous cell carcinoma and the impact of its risk factors. J Surg Oncol 2012; 106: 811.

Degache E, et al: Major response to pembrolizumab in two patients with locally advanced cutaneous squamous cell carcinoma. J Eur Acad Dermatol Venereol 2017; ePub ahead of print.

Di Monta G, et al: Electrochemotherapy efficacy evaluation for treatment of locally advanced stage III cutaneous squamous cell carcinoma. J Transl Med 2017; 15: 82.

Emadi SE, et al: Common malignant cutaneous conditions among albinos in Kenya. Med J Islam Repub Iran 2017; 31: 3.

Huang SH, et al: Overview of the 8th edition TNM classification for head and neck cancer. Curr Treat Options Oncol 2017; 18: 40.

Kim SK, et al: Outcomes of radiation therapy for advanced T3/T4 non-melanoma cutaneous squamous cell and basal cell carcinoma. Br J Dermatol 2017; ePub ahead of print.

Motaparthi K, et al: Cutaneous squamous cell carcinoma. Adv Anat Pathol 2017; 24: 171.

Muzic JG, et al: Incidence and trends of basal cell carcinoma and cutaneous squamous cell carcinoma. Mayo Clin Proc 2017; 92: 890.

Nahhas AF, et al: A review of the global guidelines on surgical margins for nonmelanoma skin cancers. J Clin Aesthet Dermatol 2017; 10: 37.

Rose AM, et al: Patients with low-risk cutaneous squamous cell carcinoma do not require extended out-patient follow-up. J Plast Reconstr Aesthet Surg 2017; 70: 852.

Stuart SE, et al: Tumor recurrence of keratinocyte carcinomas judged appropriate for Mohs micrographic surgery using appropriate use criteria. J Am Acad Dermatol 2017; 76: 1131.

VERRUCOUS CARCINOMA (CARCINOMA CUNICULATUM)

Verrucous carcinoma is a distinct, well-differentiated, low-grade SCC. It affects mostly elderly men. The primary characteristic of these lesions is their close resemblance, clinically and histologically, to a wart. The lesions present as a bulbous mass with a soft consistency and often multiple sinuses opening to the surface, resembling "rabbit burrows." Lesions of this type are most common on the sole (Fig. 29.23) but also occur in the genital area and on the oral mucosa. In some cases, as in the Buschke-Lowenstein tumor, verrucous carcinomas are induced by HPV. These HPVs may be of the "low-risk" types, such as HPV-6 or HPV-11, or the high-risk types, such as HPV-16 or HPV-18. In other cases, no HPV can be found, and pressure or other factors (but not UV light) are thought to play a role. The natural history is of a

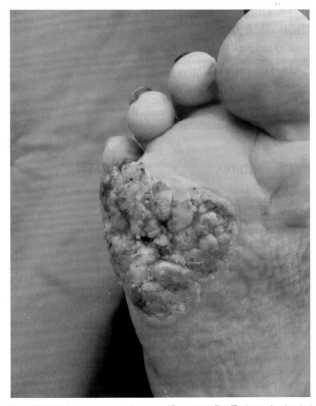

Fig. 29.23 Verrucous carcinoma. (Courtesy Dr. Tatiana Andrade.)

slow-growing mass that over years may invade the bones beneath the tumor.

Histologically, the lesion shows a characteristic picture of bulbous rete ridges topped by an undulating keratinized mass. The squamous epithelium is well differentiated, and cytologic atypia is minimal. The cytoplasm is often apple-pink and may have a glassy appearance. The tumor border is smooth and pushing, rather than spiky and infiltrative.

Excision is the best treatment, and Mohs microsurgery may be a helpful technique. Radiotherapy has been reported to induce anaplastic transformation, and although the risk appears to be low, it is best avoided if other treatment options exist. Lymph node metastasis is rare, and the prognosis is favorable when complete excision is accomplished. Other treatments used for cutaneous verrucous carcinomas with variable success include topical or systemic chemotherapy (bleomycin, 5-FU, cisplatin, methotrexate), CO_2 laser, intralesional IFN alfa, imiquimod, and PDT.

Abbas MA: Wide local excision for Buschke-Löwenstein tumor or circumferential carcinoma in situ. Tech Coloproctol 2011; 15: 313.

Cassarino DS, et al: Cutaneous squamous cell carcinoma. J Cutan Pathol 2006; 33: 191.

Ghosh S, et al: Squamous cell carcinoma developing in a cutaneous lichen planus lesion. Case Rep Dermatol Med 2014; 2014: 205638.

Gordon DK, et al: Verrucous carcinoma of the foot, not your typical plantar wart. Foot (Edinb) 2014; 24: 94.

Koch H, et al: Verrucous carcinoma of the skin. Dermatol Surg 2004; 30: 1124.

Narayana GP, Sandhya I: Verrucous carcinoma of the finger. Indian Dermatol Online J 2014; 5: 218.

Walvekar RR, et al: Verrucous carcinoma of the oral cavity. Oral Oncol 2009; 45: 47.

BOWEN DISEASE (SQUAMOUS CELL CARCINOMA IN SITU)

Bowen disease (BD) is intraepidermal SCC. Multiple possible agents can induce BD, including HPV of certain types, arsenic exposure, and sun exposure. An association with the Merkel cell polyomavirus has been reported in immunosuppressed patients. The origin of the cells developing into BD is unknown but might be a pluripotential epidermal cell. BD may ultimately become invasive. When it does, it may have an aggressive biologic behavior.

Clinical Features

BD may be found on any part of the body as an erythematous, slightly scaly and crusted, noninfiltrated patch from a few millimeters to many centimeters in diameter (Fig. 29.24). The lesion is sharply defined. The scale may be pronounced enough for the lesion to be mistaken for psoriasis, or the plaque may have a stuck-on appearance and be mistaken for a broad, sessile seborrheic keratosis. Papillated keratotic lesions can occur. When BD occurs on the vulvar skin, vaginal mucosa, or perianal areas, it may be deeply pigmented (Fig. 29.25). Infrequently, BD may be pigmented elsewhere. Invasion is often indicated by the development of an exophytic, endophytic, or ulcerative component. A rare but particularly difficult clinical scenario is the elderly female patient with multicentric BD of the shins.

As the lesion slowly enlarges, spontaneous cicatrization may develop in portions of the lesion. When the intraepithelial growth becomes invasive, the lesion may appear ulcerated and fungating. The squamous carcinoma that evolves from BD tends to be more aggressive than SCC arising in actinic keratosis. When SCC in

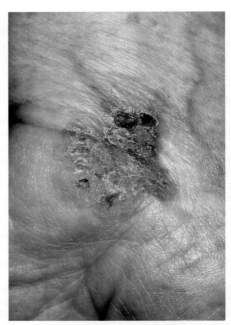

Fig. 29.24 Bowen disease. (Courtesy Steven Binnick, MD.)

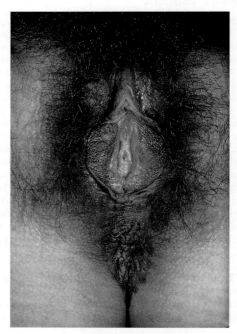

Fig. 29.25 Bowen disease.

situ occurs as a velvety plaque on the glans penis, it is referred to as erythroplasia of Queyrat (see later discussion).

Around or beneath the nail, BD can be difficult to diagnose. It can present as a red (erythronychia) or black/brown (melanonychia) longitudinal band of several millimeters in width. HPV may be associated with these lesions, which should be biopsied.

Histopathology

The atypical keratinocytes may invade the adjacent epidermis in a buckshot or clonal nested pattern. With time, they may replace the entire epidermis, often with deep, full-thickness involvement of adnexal structures, especially the hair follicles. The epidermis shows hyperkeratosis, parakeratosis, and broad acanthosis or anastomosis of adjacent rete ridges. Epidermal maturation is absent, so the epidermis appears disorganized, and individually keratinizing cells and atypical cells are seen at all levels of the epidermis. There is, however, a sharp delineation between dermis and epidermis, and the basement membrane is intact. The upper dermis usually shows a chronic inflammatory infiltrate. Although the cells tend to be anaplastic with a high nuclear/cytoplasmic ratio, variants with smaller nuclei and abundant cytoplasm exist, and transitional areas between the patterns may be seen. Invasive lesions of BD tend to have a squamoid to basaloid appearance, with central necrosis. Adnexal differentiation may be present.

Differential Diagnosis

Frequently, BD is misdiagnosed as psoriasis, superficial multicentric BCC, tinea corporis, nummular eczema, seborrheic keratosis, or actinic keratosis. Paget disease, especially the extramammary type, may mimic BD not only clinically but also histologically. There is no dyskeratosis in Paget disease, and the intervening nonvacuolated epidermal cells are not atypical. Stains for mucin and carcinoembryonic antigen (CEA) are positive in Paget disease and negative in pagetoid BD. BD may be heavily pigmented, especially when occurring in the anogenital region. Lesions of bowenoid papulosis show a histologic spectrum from genital warts with buckshot atypia to full-thickness atypia indistinguishable from BD. If the lesions are multicentric and behave as genital warts, the term bowenoid papulosis may be applied. Treatment is guided completely by the clinical pattern. Genital SCC is induced by high-risk HPV, so bowenoid papulosis represents the initial clinical lesion in the progression from HPV infection to carcinoma. There is no clear boundary where bowenoid papulosis stops and SCC in situ begins.

Treatment

Topical treatment of SCC in situ with cryotherapy and topical 5-FU has been disappointing because of a high recurrence rate. Imiquimod 5% cream, applied once daily for up to 16 weeks, seems to be effective enough to be recommended as a therapeutic option. Response rates have been as high as 90%. It may allow treatment of large lesions that might be difficult to approach surgically. Combination treatment with imiquimod 5% cream, three times a week, and 5% 5-FU, twice daily (except at the times of the imiquimod application), has also been reported effective. Tazarotene could be added to this treatment for hyperkeratotic lesions or to enhance penetration. PDT can be considered. Ingenol mebutate has also been used.

Simple excision of small lesions is a reasonable treatment option. Large, poorly defined lesions, or lesions in which preservation of normal tissue is critical, are indications for Mohs microsurgery. Other surgical techniques to treat SCC in situ are described in Chapter 37. Curettage and desiccation may also be performed, but recurrence may occur if extension down the follicles is not eradicated. Lesions of the lower legs are particularly problematic, because they are often multiple and in elderly persons are often found in conjunction with significant venous insufficiency. Any form of therapy may result in chronic leg ulceration in this setting. Using a compression bandage should be considered after surgery, similar to that applied to a chronic leg ulcer, to help prevent ulceration.

Christensen E, et al: Guidelines for practical use of MAL-PDT in non-melanoma skin cancer. J Eur Acad Dermatol Venereol 2010; 24: 505.

Cohen DK, et al: Photodynamic therapy for non-melanoma skin cancers. Cancers (Basel) 2016; 8.

Grimes C, et al: Use of topical imiquimod in the treatment of VIN. Int J Womens Dermatol 2016; 2: 35.

Mainetti C, et al: Successful treatment of relapsing Bowen's disease with ingenol mebutate. Dermatology 2016; 232: 9.

Makino T, et al: Detection of human papillomavirus type 35 in recurrent Bowen's disease lesions of the fingers. Eur J Dermatol 2017; 27: 198.

Modi G, et al: Combination therapy with imiquimod, 5 fluorouracil, and tazarotene in the treatment of extensive radiation-induced Bowen's disease of the hands. Dermatol Surg 2010; 36: 694.

Morton CA, et al: British Association of Dermatologists' guidelines for the management of squamous cell carcinoma in situ (Bowen's disease) 2014. Br J Dermatol 2014; 170: 245.

Neagu TP, et al: Clinical, histological and therapeutic features of Bowen's disease. Rom J Morphol Embryol 2017; 58: 33.

Perruchoud DL, et al: Bowen disease of the nail unit. J Eur Acad Dermatol Venereol 2016; 30: 1503.

Salleras Redonnet M, et al: Ingenol mebutate gel for the treatment of Bowen's disease. Dermatol Ther 2016; 29: 236.

Truchuelo M, et al: Effectiveness of photodynamic therapy in Bowen's disease. J Eur Acad Dermatol Venereol 2012; 26: 868.

Xue R, et al: Pathologic features of anogenital precancerous high-grade squamous intraepithelial lesion (squamous cell carcinoma in situ). J Cutan Pathol 2016; 43: 735.

Zaar O, et al: Effectiveness of photodynamic therapy in Bowen's disease. J Eur Acad Dermatol Venereol 2017; 31: 1289.

ERYTHROPLASIA OF QUEYRAT

Erythroplasia of Queyrat is SCC in situ of the glans penis or prepuce. SCC in situ on the penile shaft also occurs. Both conditions are caused by high-risk HPV types (16, 18, 31, 35). Clinically, erythroplasia of Queyrat is characterized by single or multiple, fixed, well-circumscribed, erythematous, moist, velvety or smooth, red-surfaced plaques on the glans penis (Fig. 29.26). Uncircumcised men, usually over age 40, are most often affected, and when SCC in situ affects the penile shaft, it is usually distally under the

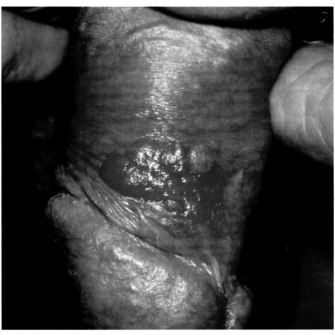

Fig. 29.26 Erythroplasia of Queyrat.

foreskin. The differential diagnosis includes Zoon balanitis, candidiasis, penile psoriasis, irritant balanitis, and extramammary Paget disease. A biopsy is usually indicated to confirm the diagnosis. The intensity of the inflammatory infiltrate under lesions of erythroplasia of Queyrat can be great, and plasma cells can be numerous. This may lead to the histologic misdiagnosis of both erythroplasia and Zoon balanitis occurring simultaneously or sequentially.

Because red lesions on the glans of elderly uncircumcised men are common, the following factors suggest that a biopsy is indicated:

1. The lesion is fixed (does not move or resolve).
2. The patient lacks other stigmata of psoriasis or another skin disease that could affect the glans penis.
3. The patient's sexual partner has cervical dysplasia.
4. The lesion does not resolve with effective topical therapy for irritant balanitis, candidiasis, or psoriasis.

Once the diagnosis of SCC in situ of the penis is made, the patient's sex partner(s) should be referred for evaluation. Sexual partners of men with SCC of the penis are more likely to develop preinvasive and invasive cancer of the cervix or anus.

Progression to invasive SCC is more common in erythroplasia of Queyrat than in BD of the nongenital skin, and the resulting SCCs are more aggressive and tend to metastasize earlier than those that develop in BD of the nongenital skin. There is no evidence of an increase in internal malignancy in patients with erythroplasia.

Topical therapy can be effective in the treatment of erythroplasia of Queyrat and has the advantage that it can identify and treat areas not visible clinically. Topical 5% 5-FU cream applied once daily under occlusion (with the foreskin or a condom) can be effective. It will induce a brisk reaction and superficial erosion, which can be uncomfortable. Treatment is continued for 3–12 weeks, depending on the response. Imiquimod cream 5%, applied between once daily and three times weekly, will similarly induce a significant reaction and may clear the lesion after 3–12 weeks. Careful follow-up is required, especially for the first few years. Surgical modalities such as excision, laser therapy, and PDT are reserved for patients failing topical treatments. Radiation therapy can also be effective.

Fai D, et al: Methyl-aminolevulinate photodynamic therapy for the treatment of erythroplasia of Queyrat in 23 patients. J Dermatolog Treat 2012; 23(5): 330–332.

Schmitz L, et al: Optical coherence tomography imaging of erythroplasia of Queyrat and treatment with imiquimod 5% cream: a case report. Dermatology 2014; 228(1): 24–26.

BALANITIS PLASMACELLULARIS (ZOON BALANITIS)

Balanitis plasmacellularis is also known as balanoposthitis chronica circumscripta plasmacellularis or Zoon balanitis. Zoon balanitis represents about 7% of persistent genital lesions biopsied for diagnosis. It is a benign inflammatory lesion of the glans penis, which histologically demonstrates a plasma cell–rich infiltrate. The plasma cell infiltrate, although characteristic, may not be present in all lesions of this type, and in fact, some researchers believe there is a spectrum of histology in idiopathic, benign, nonscarring balanitis, from lesions containing few plasma cells to lesions containing many plasma cells. Clinically, Zoon balanitis is characterized by a red patch, which is usually sharply demarcated and usually on the inner surface of the prepuce or the glans penis (Fig. 29.27). The lesion is erythematous, moist, and shiny. It occurs as a single lesion but may consist of several confluent macules. It is asymptomatic and does not produce inguinal adenopathy. Uncircumcised men from ages 24–85 are most often affected. As

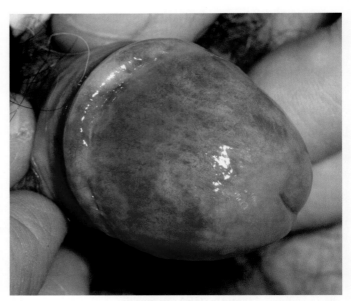

Fig. 29.27 Zoon balanitis.

with erythroplasia of Queyrat, presence of the foreskin constitutes a significant risk factor, and the disease is rarely seen in circumcised men.

Vulvitis chronica plasmacellularis is the counterpart of balanitis in women. The vulva shows a striking, lacquer-like luster. Erosions, punctate hemorrhage, synechiae, and a slate to ochre pigmentation may supervene.

Plasmacytosis circumorificialis is the same disease on the oral mucosa, lips, cheeks, and tongue. The differential diagnosis of Zoon balanitis is penile psoriasis, lichen planus, lichen sclerosus, and SCC in situ. Histologically, the epidermis is atrophic, with flattened diamond-shaped keratinocytes and mild spongiosis. In the papillary dermis, a band of infiltrate consisting almost exclusively of plasma cells is present. Dilated vessels are also seen. This picture is strikingly different from that of the main clinical differential diagnosis, erythroplasia of Queyrat, in which the epidermis is principally involved, with atypia of keratinocytes throughout the entire epithelium. HPV has not been detected.

Topical corticosteroids, alone or in combination with anticandidal treatment, are helpful in patients with Zoon balanitis. Potent topical steroids, pimecrolimus cream 1%, tacrolimus ointment 0.1%, mupirocin and imiquimod cream 5% have all been reported effective in select cases. Circumcision may be curative. Laser ablation and PDT can also be effective.

Bari O, et al: Successful management of Zoon's balanitis with topical mupirocin ointment. Dermatol Ther (Heidelb) 2017; 7: 203.

Borgia F, et al: Zoon's balanitis successfully treated with photodynamic therapy. Photodiagnosis Photodyn Ther 2016; 13: 347.

Daga SO, et al: Zoon's balanitis treated with topical tacrolimus. Urol Ann 2017; 9: 211.

Edwards SK, et al: 2013 European guideline for the management of balanoposthitis. Int J STD AIDS 2014; 25: 615.

Hugh JM, et al: Zoon's balanitis. J Drugs Dermatol 2014; 13: 1290.

Wollina U: Ablative erbium:YAG laser treatment of idiopathic chronic inflammatory non-cicatricial balanoposthitis (Zoon's disease). J Cosmet Laser Ther 2010; 12: 120.

You HS, et al: Dermatoses of the glans penis in Korea. Ann Dermatol 2016; 28: 40.

PSEUDOEPITHELIOMATOUS KERATOTIC AND MICACEOUS BALANITIS

Pseudoepitheliomatous keratotic and micaceous balanitis was described by Lortat-Jacob and Civatte in 1966. The lesions occurring on the glans penis are verrucous excrescences with scaling. Ulcerations, cracking, and fissuring on the surface of the glans are frequently present. The keratotic scale is usually micaceous and resembles psoriasis. Most patients are over age 50 and frequently have been circumcised for phimosis in adult life. Histologically, there is marked hyperkeratosis and parakeratosis, as well as pseudoepitheliomatous hyperplasia. Acanthotic masses give rise to a crater-like configuration. HPV has not been detected. This lesion is probably best considered as a form of verrucous carcinoma. The treatment is usually surgical or cryosurgical and Mohs micrographic surgery may play a role. PDT has also been used. Topical 5-FU has been effective, but the hyperkeratotic scale may make penetration suboptimal. If topical chemotherapy is used, posttreatment biopsies are recommended.

Hanumaiah B, et al: Pseudoepitheliomatous keratotic and micaceous balanitis. Indian J Dermatol 2013; 58: 492.
Murthy PS, et al: Pseudoepitheliomatous, keratotic, and micaceous balanitis. Indian J Dermatol 2010; 55: 190.
Perry D, et al: Pseudoepitheliomatous, keratotic, and micaceous balanitis. Dermatol Nurs 2008; 20: 117.
Sardesai VR, et al: Pseudoepitheliomatous keratotic and micaceous balanitis with malignant transformation. Indian J Sex Transm Dis 2013; 34: 38.
Zhu H, et al: Treatment of pseudoepitheliomatous, keratotic, and micaceous balanitis with topical photodynamic therapy. Int J Dermatol 2015; 54: 245.

PAGET DISEASE OF THE BREAST

Clinical Features

Paget disease (PD) of the nipple affects women primarily (there are very rare male cases). Between 1% and 4% of breast carcinomas present with PD. It is characterized by a unilateral, sharply marginated, erythematous, and at times crusted patch or plaque affecting the nipple and occasionally the areola (Fig. 29.28). At times, it may be hyperpigmented and may mimic melanoma. As the lesion grows, it may spread to the areola, and even beyond, making the areolae appear asymmetric. Over months or years, it may become eroded. The nipple may or may not be retracted. In advanced

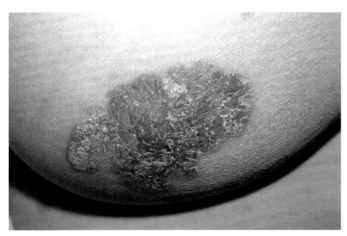

Fig. 29.28 Paget disease of the breast. (Courtesy Steven Binnick, MD.)

cases, a subjacent mass and ipsilateral axillary adenopathy may be palpable. About 5% of patients have PD without confirmed evidence of underlying carcinoma, and the remaining 95% have either an invasive or an intraductal carcinoma in proportions of 35%–65%, depending on the reporting center. In rare cases, even when no underlying carcinoma is found on surgical removal, the sentinel node may be positive.

Histopathology

PD is characterized by the presence of Paget cells: large, round, pale-staining cells with large nuclei. Intercellular bridges are absent. The cells appear singly or in small nests between the squamous cells. Usually, acanthosis is present, the granular layer is preserved, and there is no parakeratosis, but atypical cells may be "spat out" into the stratum corneum. Frequently, a layer of basal cells separates the Paget cells from the basement membrane and is seen crushed beneath the nests of Paget cells. This histologic feature helps distinguish PD from pagetoid melanoma and Bowen disease. In the dermis, an inflammatory reaction is often present. Unusual variants include PD with marked intraepidermal melanin and an acantholytic anaplastic form.

The Paget cell is PAS positive, diastase resistant, almost always HER-2/neu positive, and EMA positive; it stains with CAM 5.2 and CK 7. This staining profile and negativity for S-100 and cytokeratins 5/6 allow clear distinction from pagetoid melanoma and pagetoid Bowen disease. CEA positivity is variable in PD of the breast, being positive in 0%–50% of PD cases compared with virtually 100% of extramammary PD cases. The Toker cell, a normal clear cell of the breast, stains similarly but is HER-2/neu negative. It has been proposed as the precursor cell of PD and may be so for some cases of PD with no underlying breast cancer.

Diagnosis

The presence of unilateral eczema of the nipple recalcitrant to simple treatment should lead to suspicion of PD, and the lesion should be biopsied. The presence of bilateral lesions suggests a benign process, usually atopic dermatitis. Papillary adenoma of the nipple clinically resembles PD, but on biopsy it shows a papillary and adenomatous growth in the dermis with connection to the surface. There is a lining of apocrine-type secretory epithelium. HNA may occasionally be unilateral but histologically reveals only hyperkeratosis, acanthosis, and papillomatosis.

Treatment

Patients with PD of the breast should be referred to a center with expertise in the management of breast cancer. Prognosis depends on the presence of an underlying invasive ductal carcinoma or nodal metastases. Patients presenting with a palpable breast mass typically have more advanced disease and lower 5-year survival. Some data suggest PD itself may be an independent marker of worse prognosis of invasive breast carcinoma (IBC) compared with IBC of similar stage and characteristics without PD.

EXTRAMAMMARY PAGET DISEASE

Extramammary Paget disease (EMPD) is much less common than PD. It affects adults, usually between 65 and 70 years of age. The vulva is the most common location, except perhaps in China, where penoscrotal EMPD is reported in large numbers. Penoscrotal EMPD is uncommon in black persons. EMPD presents most often as a unifocal process, but multifocal lesions may occur, including cases involving as many as four anatomic locations simultaneously. Lesions typically affect apocrine sites, including the vulva, scrotum, perianal area, penis, inguinal folds and axilla, but rare cases can affect other anatomic locations. Axillary lesions

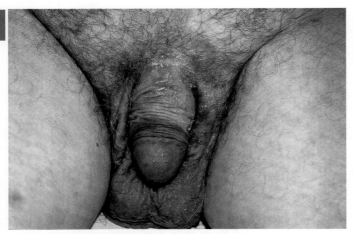

Fig. 29.29 Extramammary Paget disease.

typically appear with or after genital lesions and are more frequent in men. The growths are typically erythematous, well-demarcated plaques measuring several centimeters in diameter (Fig. 29.29). The condition often goes undiagnosed for months to years, as the misdiagnoses of pruritus ani, a fungal infection, contact dermatitis, lichen sclerosus, or intertrigo are made. A nonhealing banal eczematous patch persisting in the anogenital or axillary region should raise concern about EMPD and trigger a biopsy. Intense pruritus is common. Bleeding, nodularity, and induration are late signs. Underpants erythema, or redness in the whole genital area, may be indicative of widespread lymphatic involvement in the pelvic basin and is a poor prognostic sign. Lesions may be hyperpigmented or hypopigmented.

Extramammary PD can be divided into the following four forms:

1. Primary EMPD (arising intraepidermally), with or without invasion
2. EMPD associated with an underlying apocrine carcinoma
3. EMPD associated with an underlying adjacent malignancy
4. EMPD associated with an underlying distant carcinoma

The majority of patients with EMPD do not have underlying carcinoma, and the process apparently begins as an intraepidermal neoplasm, which can then invade (invasive EMPD). The clinical appearance of all types of EMPD is identical. The location of the EMPD determines the percentage of patients who have other associated malignancies. In vulvar EMPD, 4%–17% have an associated adnexal neoplasm, and 11%–20% have a distant carcinoma of the breast, cervix, vagina, bladder, colon, rectum, ovary, liver, gallbladder, or skin. In perianal EMPD, an underlying adnexal carcinoma occurs in 7%–10% of cases, and a distant carcinoma of the rectum, stomach, breast, or ureter is present in 15%–45%. Penoscrotal EMPD has an associated carcinoma of the prostate, bladder, testicles, ureter, or kidney in 11% of cases. In a large series from The Netherlands, underlying malignancy was found in 35% of patients with EMPD. In all patients with EMPD, an extensive and targeted cancer workup should be undertaken, depending on the histologic staining pattern (see next) and the location. Prolonged follow-up and malignancy screening should be considered, because EMPD patients have an increased risk of secondary malignancy at these sites even years after the initial EMPD diagnosis.

Histologically, the findings are similar to those found in mammary PD: acanthosis, hyperkeratosis, parakeratosis, and pale, vacuolated Paget cells in suprabasilar levels of the epithelium. Signet ring Paget cells are present in a small minority of cases.

Paget cells can form nests that compress basal keratinocytes. Conventional histopathologic findings are similar in both primary cutaneous EMPD and most cases in which EMPD is caused by an underlying malignancy. Mucin, stainable by alcian blue or colloidal iron, is present in the majority of cases. The finding of cytoplasmic mucin makes a urothelial origin unlikely.

Significant effort has been put into developing a series of stains that would clearly distinguish PD from EMPD and identify patients who have underlying carcinomas, either local apocrine cancers or distant neoplasms. This involves examining the expression of various cytokeratins, mucins, and other products specific to certain organ systems. RCAS1 may be very sensitive for EMPD cells, and measurement of serum levels of this marker can be used to monitor patients with invasive disease, analogous to following prostate-specific antigen (PSA) in patients with treated prostate cancer. In vulvar and perianal EMPD, two distinct staining patterns have been defined. CK7+/CK20+/GCDFP15 negative is called the type I or endodermal pattern and is associated with EMPD and distant cancers. Ectodermal or cutaneous pattern (type II) stains the atypical cells CD7+/CK20−/GCDFP15 positive. This is associated with a cutaneous origin for the EMPD. In addition, tissue-specific markers may at times identify the distant tumor responsible for the EMPD. Immunohistochemical studies can provide some guidance in distinguishing between these possibilities, largely through identifying antigens that are not found on the cells of primary cutaneous EMPD. The specificity of these studies is limited, but a positive finding of an immunoprofile that differs from that of typical primary EMPD should lead to a thorough investigation. Primary cutaneous EMPD has an immunophenotype similar to that of apocrine epithelium: cytokeratin 7 positive, cytokeratin 20 negative, and CEA positive. Cases caused by spread from an underlying bladder carcinoma are typically uroplakin and p63 positive. Those caused by rectal carcinoma are usually CK7 negative, CDX2 positive, and CK20 positive. Prostatic adenocarcinoma can also result in EMPD and can be identified by staining for PSA or the marker P504S. Unfortunately, PSA positivity can be seen in female patients with EMPD, and not all males with PSA positivity of the EMPD cells have underlying prostate cancer. The p63 staining in vulvar EMPD suggests an underlying urothelial carcinoma. Staining with AKT, CDK2, mTOR, and other proteins in the mTOR pathway suggests that this pathway may be important in the pathogenesis of EMPD.

Extramammary PD can remain within the epithelium or "invade" the dermis. "Invasive" EMPD has a high rate of metastasis and a very poor prognosis. Sentinel node examination of patients with "invasive" EMPD should be considered because it predicts the risk for metastasis.

Surgical removal is the treatment of choice, with Mohs microsurgery having a better outcome than fixed surgical margins. Despite what appears to be adequate clinical margins, recurrence rates are high because of the discontinuous and microscopic wide extension of EMPD. The recurrence rate after micrographic surgery is about 12% and more than 30% for standard 2-cm margins. Positive KI67 and PAS staining of surgical margins may suggest the need for wider excision. Imiquimod has been used with success in multiple reports, but follow-up is limited. Topical 5-FU, radiation therapy, PDT, and laser therapy have also been used. Intralesional IFN alfa-2b was beneficial in one case. Some cases of genital EMPD are HER-2/neu positive and have responded to trastuzumab, a monoclonal antibody directed against HER-2.

Bae JM, et al: Mohs micrographic surgery for extramammary Paget disease. J Am Acad Dermatol 2013; 68: 632.

Dai B, et al: Primary invasive carcinoma associated with penoscrotal extramammary Paget's disease. BJU Int 2015; 115: 153.

Edey KA, et al: Interventions for the treatment of Paget's disease of the vulva. Cochrane Database Syst Rev 2013; 10: CD009245.

Elbendary A, et al: Diagnostic criteria in intraepithelial pagetoid neoplasms. Am J Dermatopathol 2017; 39: 419.

Hendi A, et al: Unifocality of extramammary Paget disease. J Am Acad Dermatol 2008; 59: 811.

Karam A, Dorigo O: Increased risk and pattern of secondary malignancies in patients with invasive extramammary Paget disease. Br J Dermatol 2014; 170: 661.

Perez DR, et al: Management and outcome of perianal Paget's disease. Dis Colon Rectum 2014; 57: 747.

Sanderson P, et al: Imiquimod therapy for extramammary Paget's disease of the vulva. J Obstet Gynaecol 2013; 33: 479.

Wang HW, et al: A prospective pilot study to evaluate combined topical photodynamic therapy and surgery for extramammary Paget's disease. Lasers Surg Med 2013; 45: 296.

CLEAR CELL PAPULOSIS

Clear cell papulosis is an uncommon disorder that presents with multiple, minimally elevated, hypopigmented papules. Most cases have been reported in Asian or Hispanic children. Onset is usually before age 6 and may be as soon as 4 months of age. The eruption favors the pubic region, lower abdomen, and along the milk lines. Histology demonstrates mild acanthosis, decreased epidermal pigmentation, and the presence of single or small clusters of large clear cells in the basal and occasionally suprabasal layers of the epidermis. The cells are positive for EMA, CEA, and CD7, identical to Toker cells.

Tseng FW, et al: Long-term follow-up study of clear cell papulosis. J Am Acad Dermatol 2010; 63: 266.

Wang D, et al: A case report of clear cell papulosis and a review of the literature. Ann Acad Med Singapore 2017; 46: 160.

MERKEL CELL CARCINOMA (TRABECULAR CARCINOMA)

Merkel cell carcinoma (MCC) was first described by Toker in 1972. The cell of origin is the Merkel cell, a slow-acting mechanoreceptor in the basal layer of the epidermis. Although still a rare tumor occurring at an incidence of about 0.44 per 100,000 population, MCC recently increased threefold over 15 years, an increased incidence of 8% per year. Melanoma, by comparison, increased at a rate of only 3% per year over the same period. More than 1500 MCCs occur yearly in the United States. This is a tumor of the elderly population, with 90% of cases found in persons older than 50, 76% in those over 65, and 72% in those over 70. The mean age is 76 in women and 74 in men. About 60% of MCC patients are men, and 95% occur in white people. There is strong evidence that MCC is induced by sun exposure. About 90% of cases occur on sun-exposed sites, with 27% of cases on the face, 9% on the scalp and neck (or 36% on the head and neck), 22% on the upper extremity, 15% on the lower extremity (37% on the extremities), and only 11% on the trunk. About 3% occur on the ear, eyelid, or lip. PUVA therapy is associated with an increased risk for MCC. Immunosuppression by organ transplantation, chronic lymphocytic leukemia, and HIV infection all substantially increase the risk for developing MCC, so that in some series, 8%–15% of patients with MCC have some form of immune impairment.

Clinically, this tumor presents as a rapidly growing, nontender, red to violaceous nodule with a shiny surface (Fig. 29.30) and overlying telangiectasia. Most cases are *not* considered malignant by the dermatologist at biopsy. The acronym AEIOU has been suggested: asymptomatic/lack of tenderness, expanding rapidly, immune suppression, older than 50 years, and ultraviolet-exposed site on a person with fair skin. MCC is an aggressive tumor with a propensity for local recurrence and nodal and distant metastases. At presentation, about one third of cases have regional node

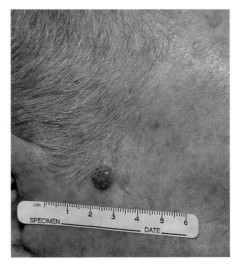

Fig. 29.30 Merkel cell carcinoma.

involvement, and hematogenous spread will eventuate in at least one third of patients. Spontaneous remissions have been reported, primarily in women with head and neck tumors; this is most often associated with reduction of iatrogenic immunosuppression. The regression is rapid, but the MCC can recur after "spontaneous resolution." MCC can present as a metastatic disease without an evident primary tumor; such patients have a significantly better prognosis than those of the same stage with a known primary.

Approximately 80% of MCCs in North America and 25% of MCCs in Australia are associated with a virus, the Merkel cell polyomavirus (MCPyV). The virus is found integrated into the genome of the MCC when present, and all progenitor cells have the same viral genome, suggesting that the viral infection began at the time the neoplasia was developing, or before. MCC patients are more likely to be seropositive for MCPyV. Infection with this virus is widespread, with seroprevalence increasing from 30% in children younger than 5 to almost 80% in persons older than 50. Lymphoid tissue, especially the tonsils, seems to be the reservoir. The virus may behave similar to HPV, with increasing seroprevalence with exposure over time and spontaneous clearance in most adults. MCPyV can be recovered from about 4% of immunocompetent persons and 36% of immunosuppressed patients. This may explain the high risk for MCC with immunosuppression, analogous to the high risk of HPV-related neoplasia in immunosuppressed patients. MCPyV has also been reported in NMSCs in both immunocompetent and immunosuppressed patients. Bowen disease, BCC, and SCC have been associated with viral infection in up to 40% of cases in some laboratories, but these results have not been reproduced and may represent laboratory overidentification. At the University of California, San Francisco, the rate is less than 1%. Normal skin infection has also been reported, and the viral copies in these NMSCs are much fewer than in MCC. The pathogenic role of MCPyV in NMSCs other than MCC is speculative. Visceral tumors and other small cell neuroendocrine tumors of other organ systems do *not* contain MCPyV, substantiating its role in the development of MCC.

Staging predicts prognosis and guides therapy. Sentinel lymph node biopsy (SLNB) should be performed at definitive excision of the primary tumor. One third of patients with no palpable adenopathy have a positive SLNB. The SLNB sample must be stained with CK20 (if the primary tumor is positive) to detect micrometastases. Computed tomography (CT) will detect metastatic disease in only 20% of MCC patients. Whether tumors less than 1 cm in diameter require SLNB is controversial, but even in small tumors, lymph node metastases can be found; in one study, 14% of those with 0.5-cm tumors had regional nodal involvement. Imaging with CT, magnetic resonance imaging (MRI), or positron emission tomography (PET) may be used to search for metastatic disease. Palpable lymph nodes must be sampled to exclude the presence of metastatic disease. MCC patients who harbor MCPyV have a better prognosis (45% vs. 15% 5-year survival), and the MCC is more likely to present on an extremity. Natural killer cell response also correlates with prognosis. MCC should be treated expeditiously; patients have developed metastatic disease in the weeks awaiting definitive surgery.

The treatment of MCC should be directed by persons with expertise in managing this rare tumor. Therapy may need to be individualized, depending on various risk factors present. Many of these patients are elderly and may not be able to tolerate some of the recommended treatments. The goal of therapy for patients with only local disease or regional nodal metastases is cure and local control. This involves the combined use of surgery and radiation therapy in most cases. Radiation therapy alone can be efficacious and is recommended for patients unable to tolerate surgery. Radiation therapy is directed at both the primary site and the draining and/or regional lymph node basins in most cases and should be considered even if the sentinel lymph nodes are negative. Recurrence is seen in 46%–76% of untreated lymph nodes. Even after Mohs surgery, radiation therapy reduces the local recurrence rate from 16% to near 0%. Prophylactic lymph node dissection enhances local control but does not improve survival. It is gradually being replaced with radiation therapy of the affected nodal basin. Locoregional recurrence remains a substantial problem in patients with MCC and is a poor prognostic sign. Therefore the emerging consensus is that addressing the regional lymph nodes is crucial in therapy. Traditional adjuvant chemotherapy has been disappointing because it does not prevent later development of metastatic, regional, or local disease, but avelumab appears very promising. MCC may be initially responsive to chemotherapy, but disease progression occurs. In the setting of metastatic MCC, chemotherapy would be considered palliative. Partial response was seen with use of a multikinase inhibitor, pazopanib.

Histologically, MCC is a dermal tumor that may extend into the subcutaneous tissue. The cells are about 15 μm in diameter and have very scant cytoplasm and hyperchromatic nuclei with a distinctive smudged chromatin pattern. Mitoses and apoptotic cells are numerous. The cells are arranged in sheets and cords. Depth of invasion, lymphovascular involvement, and mitotic index may be poor prognostic histologic features. MCC must be distinguished from small cell lung cancer, lymphoma, neuroblastoma, small cell endocrine carcinoma, Ewing sarcoma, melanoma, and even BCC. Immunoperoxidase confirmation of the diagnosis and exclusion of other small cell tumors is required to establish the diagnosis. The tumor should be CK20 positive and thyroid transcription factor 1 (TTF-1) negative. CK20 staining is of the "perinuclear dot pattern." CK7 tends to stain small cell lung cancer and not MCC. MCC is negative for S-100 and leukocyte common antigen (LCA).

Avelumab impresses in Merkel cell carcinoma. Cancer Discov 2017; 7: OF5.

Albores-Saavedra J, et al: Merkel cell carcinoma demographics, morphology, and survival based on 3870 cases. J Cutan Pathol 2010; 37: 20.

Andres C, et al: Prevalence of MCPyV in Merkel cell carcinoma and non-MCC tumors. J Cutan Pathol 2010; 37: 28.

Faust H, et al: Prospective study of Merkel cell polyomavirus and risk of Merkel cell carcinoma. Int J Cancer 2014; 134: 844.

Gunaratne DA, et al: Definitive radiotherapy for Merkel cell carcinoma confers clinically meaningful in-field locoregional control. J Am Acad Dermatol. 2017; 77: 142.

Huang SH, et al: Overview of the 8th edition TNM classification for head and neck cancer. Curr Treat Options Oncol 2017; 18: 40.

Iyer JG, et al: Relationships among primary tumor size, number of involved nodes, and survival for 8044 cases of Merkel cell carcinoma. J Am Acad Dermatol 2014; 70: 637.

Jouary T, et al: Adjuvant prophylactic regional radiotherapy versus observation in stage I Merkel cell carcinoma. Ann Oncol 2012; 23: 1074.

Kim JA, Choi AH: Effect of radiation therapy on survival in patients with resected Merkel cell carcinoma. JAMA Dermatol 2013; 149: 831.

Kouzmina M, et al: Frequency and locations of systemic metastases in Merkel cell carcinoma by imaging. Acta Radiol Open 2017; 6: 2058460117700449.

Laniosz V, et al: Natural killer cell response is a predictor of good outcome in MCPyV(+) Merkel cell carcinoma. J Am Acad Dermatol 2017; 77: 31.

Nghiem P, et al: Systematic literature review of efficacy, safety and tolerability outcomes of chemotherapy regimens in patients with metastatic Merkel cell carcinoma. Future Oncol 2017; 13: 1263.

Pape E, et al: Radiotherapy alone for Merkel cell carcinoma. J Am Acad Dermatol 2011; 65: 983.

PDQ Adult Treatment Editorial Board: Merkel Cell Carcinoma Treatment (PDQ): Patient Version. PDQ Cancer Information Summaries [Internet]. Bethesda (MD): National Cancer Institute (US); 2002-2017 Jun 16.

Pulitzer M: Merkel cell carcinoma. Surg Pathol Clin 2017; 10: 399.

Vargo JA, et al: RE: Adjuvant radiation therapy and chemotherapy in Merkel cell carcinoma. J Natl Cancer Inst 2017; 109.

SEBACEOUS NEVI AND TUMORS

Nevus Sebaceus (Organoid Nevus)

Nevus sebaceus of Jadassohn presents as a sharply circumscribed, yellow-orange hamartoma, varying from a few millimeters to several centimeters in size. These lesions are usually solitary, congenital, and linear in configuration. The scalp is the most common location (50%), but other areas of the head and neck (45%) are also common. The trunk is involved in 5% or less of cases. The lesions persist throughout life and are usually alopecic. In childhood, they are only slightly papillated or velvety, but in adulthood, with hyperplasia of the sebaceous elements, the lesions become more elevated and cerebriform (Fig. 29.31). Large, pedunculated lesions presenting as exophytic tumors at birth are an unusual phenotype. Recent work has shown that somatic HRAS and KRAS mutations give rise to nevus sebaceus.

Numerous neoplasms, most of them adnexal, have been described arising in nevus sebaceus. The most common tumors are trichoblastoma and syringocystadenoma papilliferum, each occurring in about 5% of nevus sebaceus. HRAS mutation has been implicated in the pathogenesis of trichoblastomas in this setting. Both these tumors present as new, often pigmented papules or nodules arising in the nevus sebaceus. BCC is uncommon, occurring in less than 1% of lesions. Many cases previously diagnosed as BCC are actually trichoblastomas. Many of the tumors are difficult to classify precisely. Development of benign tumors occurs in less than 5% of nevus sebaceus before age 16, and malignant tumors are rare in childhood or adolescence. The risk for tumor development increases with age. Rarely, aggressive malignant adnexal neoplasms may arise, usually in older adults. Familial cases have been described.

Nevus sebaceus may be associated with multiple internal abnormalities, making it one of the cutaneous abnormalities to be included within the epidermal nevus syndrome (see earlier).

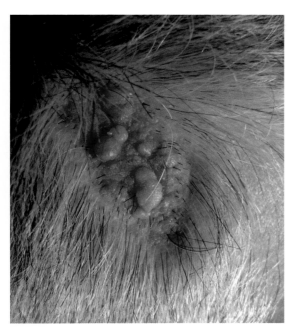

Fig. 29.31 Nevus sebaceus.

Schimmelpenning syndrome is a synonym for sebaceous nevus syndrome (SNS). In cases of SNS, the nevus sebaceus is usually on the scalp and is linear and large (≥10 cm). The sebaceous nevi usually occupy more than one dermatome. Ocular colobomas and choristomas are characteristic. Neurologic findings are present in 7% of all patients with nevus sebaceus and up to two thirds of patients with SNS. Epilepsy is seen in about two thirds of cases, usually beginning in the first year of life. Mental retardation can occur. Although numerous anatomic abnormalities of the brain have been described in SNS, CT and MRI are frequently normal in children with seizures and mental retardation. Urologic and cardiovascular defects have also been reported. A rare variant of SNS is the SCALP syndrome: sebaceous nevus syndrome, CNS malformations, aplasia cutis congenita, limbal dermoid, and pigmented nevus (giant congenital melanocytic nevus). The aplasia cutis and sebaceous nevus are adjacent and on the scalp. SCALP syndrome is also called didymosis aplasticosebacea.

A rare but frequently reported association is that of nevus sebaceus and hypophosphatemic rickets. Most patients have large sebaceous nevi and evidence of "SNS." If the rickets goes unrecognized, permanent bone loss and orthopedic injury result. Serum phosphate is low, and there is excess phosphate in the urine. Serum calcium is normal. It is now clear that the nevus sebaceus itself secretes a factor responsible for phosphorus wasting. FGF-23 and matrix extracellular phosphoglycoprotein (MEPE) are both elevated in the blood of patients with this syndrome, and the levels of these substances parallel the hypophosphatemia. Surgical removal of the nevus sebaceus is the treatment of choice. When the nevus sebaceus is removed, the metabolic abnormalities normalize, and FGF-23 and MEPE levels return to normal. Partial removal can ameliorate the condition. Octreotide can also be used if surgical removal is not possible.

Histologically, in prepubertal lesions, the epithelium is acanthotic and papillomatous. Pilosebaceous structures are immature and resemble the fetal pilar germ. After puberty, the epidermis is more hyperplastic and at times papillomatous. It may resemble a seborrheic keratosis or acanthosis nigricans or may have features of an epidermal nevus. Sebaceous glands are usually abundant, placed high in the dermis, and connect directly to the epidermal surface. Follicular structures, if present, are usually vellous or partially formed. Apocrine glands are present in about half the lesions. The dermis is thickened, with increased vascularity and fibrous connective tissue. Mature lesions have been described as broad, bald, bumpy (papillomatous), and bubbly (sebaceous). The finding of EDV–associated and genital-mucosal HPV DNA in nevus sebaceus is of unclear significance.

Although the risk of development of malignancy exists, it is small, and virtually always occurs after adolescence. For this reason, surgical removal can be delayed until adulthood, when the patient can make an informed decision regarding removal. If the lesion leads to disfigurement, stigmatization, or symptomatology, it may be removed at any age.

Cribier B, et al: Tumors arising in nevus sebaceus. J Am Acad Dermatol 2000; 42: 263.
Depeyre A, et al: A case of basaloid degeneration of nevus sebaceous during childhood. Facial Plast Surg 2016; 32: 576.
Idriss MH, Elston DM: Secondary neoplasms associated with nevus sebaceus of Jadassohn. J Am Acad Dermatol 2014; 70: 332.
Liu Y, et al: Nevus sebaceus of Jadassohn with eight secondary tumors of follicular, sebaceous, and sweat gland differentiation. Am J Dermatopathol 2016; 38: 861.
Saraggi D, et al: Pigmented trichoblastoma developed in a sebaceous nevus. Pathol Res Pract 2017; 213: 860.

Sebaceous Hyperplasia

Onset of sebaceous hyperplasia is usually after age 40, and the prevalence increases with age. The areas of predilection are the forehead, infraorbital regions, and temples. The lesions are small, cream-colored or yellowish, umbilicated papules 2–6 mm in diameter. Dermoscopy can be helpful in confirming the diagnosis and identifies the central crater, the yellow lobules, and the associated telangiectasia. Unusual sites may be affected, such as the areolae, nipples, penis, neck, and chest, where disease occurs as solitary lesions, clustered papules, or beaded lines. Prominent sebaceous hyperplasia occurs in 15% of patients taking cyclosporine and may involve ectopic sites such as the oral mucosa. It often appears many years after the cyclosporine is begun. Histologically, sebaceous hyperplasia demonstrates hyperplasia of one sebaceous gland, with normal-sized surrounding glands. The glands are multilobulated, each dividing into smaller lobules to produce a cluster resembling a bunch of grapes. Clinically, they may mimic an early BCC.

Premature sebaceous hyperplasia, also known as familial presenile sebaceous hyperplasia, presents with extensive sebaceous hyperplasia with onset at puberty and worsening with age. Familial patterns have been reported, inherited in an autosomal dominant manner. It involves the face, neck, and upper thorax but spares the periorificial regions.

Treatment is solely for cosmetic purposes and employs electrosurgery, laser therapy, PDT, or even shallow shave biopsy. Isotretinoin will reduce lesions, but they immediately recur when the drug is stopped, so isotretinoin is probably not indicated for this condition. Long-term successful therapy with isotretinoin requires low-dose maintenance therapy.

Errichetti E, et al: Areolar sebaceous hyperplasia associated with oral and genital Fordyce spots. J Dermatol 2013; 40: 670.
Flux K: Sebaceous neoplasms. Surg Pathol Clin 2017; 10: 367.
Kim HS, et al: Sebaceous hyperplasia of the scrotum and penile shaft. Ann Dermatol 2011; 23: S341.
McDonald SK, et al: Successful treatment of cyclosporine-induced sebaceous hyperplasia with oral isotretinoin in two renal transplant recipients. Australas J Dermatol 2011; 52: 227.
Noh S, et al: A case of sebaceous hyperplasia maintained on low-dose isotretinoin after carbon dioxide laser treatment. Int J Dermatol 2014; 53: e151.

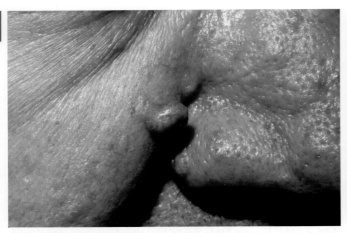

Fig. 29.32 Sebaceous adenomas of Muir Torre syndrome. (Courtesy Steven Binnick, MD.)

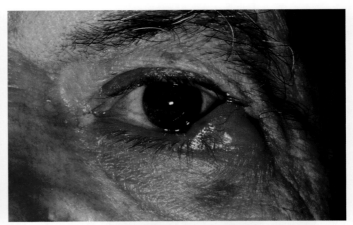

Fig. 29.33 Sebaceous carcinoma in patient with Muir-Torre syndrome.

Sebaceous Adenoma

This slow-growing tumor usually presents as a pink, flesh-colored, or yellow papule or nodule (Fig. 29.32). Sebaceous adenoma occurs primarily on the head and neck (70%) in elderly persons (mean age 60). Histologically, the tumor is composed of multiple, sharply marginated, sebaceous lobules. Each lobule has a basal layer of darker germinative cells, but the maturation is not as well developed as in a normal sebaceous gland. The basaloid cells occupy more than the typical one to two cell layers seen in the normal sebaceous gland or in sebaceous hyperplasia. Multiple openings directly to the overlying epidermis may be found. Sebaceous adenoma may be a cutaneous marker of the Muir-Torre syndrome.

Sebaceoma (Sebaceous Epithelioma)

Clinically, they appear as yellow or orange papules, nodules, or plaques, usually on the scalp, face, and neck. Sebaceous epitheliomas also may be associated with Muir-Torre syndrome. Histologically, the tumor consists of oval nests of irregularly shaped basaloid cells with differentiation toward sebaceous cells. The basaloid cells should outnumber the differentiated sebocytes in a sebaceoma. Also, there may be cystic spaces containing vacuolated, amorphous material.

Reticulated Acanthoma With Sebaceous Differentiation

This rare tumor presents as an enlarging, erythematous to brown plaque, often on the back. Histologically, the tumor has a reticulated seborrheic keratosis–like pattern, being broad and well circumscribed. There are clusters of sebocytes at the bases of the rete ridges. Sebaceous ducts may also be seen. These ductal elements are EMA positive and CEA negative. This tumor can also be associated with Muir-Torre syndrome.

Sebaceous Carcinoma

Sebaceous carcinoma is a rare neoplasm, and 75% of cases occur on the eyelid or around the eye. It most frequently arises on the eyelids from the meibomian or Zeis glands. It usually appears in the tarsal region of the upper eyelids (75%) and represents 1% or more of eyelid malignancies. It is frequently misdiagnosed as a chalazion, delaying appropriate treatment. The scalp, other areas of the face, and the trunk are the next most common areas involved.

Lesions present as a painless subcutaneous nodule or less often a pedunculated growth. Rarely, sebaceous carcinoma has been reported to involve the feet, external genitalia, and oral mucosa. Fatal metastatic disease occurs in 9%–50% of cases (30% of eyelid cases), and 5-year survival for this tumor is 80%. Sebaceous carcinomas arising in nonocular locations can also metastasize, usually to regional lymph nodes. Sebaceous carcinoma may be seen in MTS (Fig. 29.33).

Histologically, the tumor is composed of lobules or sheets of cells that extend deeply into the dermis, subcutaneous fat, or muscle. The tumor cells are pleomorphic and show various degrees of sebaceous differentiation, manifested by a vacuolated rather than clear cytoplasm. Undifferentiated cells with mitotic figures can be found. The cells vary greatly in size and shape. A characteristic feature in ocular tumors is pagetoid or bowenoid spread of the tumor onto the overlying conjunctiva or skin. Sebaceous differentiation may be minimal in this in situ component, leading to the misdiagnosis of SCC in situ.

Treatment is surgical, with Mohs micrographic surgery having the best results; there is an 11% recurrence rate after Mohs and 30% after standard excision. Given the extent of sebaceous carcinomas, oculoplastic reconstruction is usually required. In extraocular cases, complete excision, as for an adnexal carcinoma, and careful follow-up are recommended.

Muir-Torre Syndrome

Sebaceous tumors of the skin were first reported by Muir in 1967 and Torre in 1968 as being associated with the development of internal malignancy, a combination that has been called the Muir-Torre syndrome (MTS). The cutaneous lesions may be sebaceous adenomas, sebaceomas, or sebaceous carcinomas. In MTS, these tumors occur more often on the trunk than they do in the general population, in whom sebaceous tumors favor the head and neck. Keratoacanthomas (KAs) are also common and multiple. The KAs may show sebaceous differentiation. The combination of a sebaceous tumor and a KA should be highly suggestive of MTS. The recognition of the association of sebaceous neoplasms and MTS is highlighted by one report, in which 42% of persons with a sebaceous neoplasm had MTS. Between 22% and 32% of patients with MTS present with the sebaceous neoplasm before development of the internal malignancy. About 60% have already had an internal malignancy by the time the sebaceous neoplasm occurs. Because the mean age of presentation of the sebaceous neoplasm is 63 years, the confirmation of MTS becomes important for genetic counseling of the patient's children. MTS is inherited in an autosomal dominant manner in about 60% of cases; penetrance is high, but expression is variable.

MTS is now recognized to be a subset of the Lynch syndrome, or hereditary nonpolyposis colorectal cancer syndrome (HNCCS). HNCCS and MTS are caused by mutations in mismatch repair (MMR) genes (*MLH1*, *MSH2*, and *MSH6* for MTS and Lynch syndrome, and *PMS2* only in Lynch syndrome). *MSH2* mutations are responsible for 90% of MTS families. The most common malignancy is colonic adenocarcinoma (47%), usually proximal to the splenic flexor. Multiple polyps are not present. Genitourinary tumors (21%), breast cancer (12%), and hematologic disorders (9%) are also common.

The absence of an MMR enzyme results in microsatellite instability (MSI). Although staining for markers such as *MSH-2* and *MSH-6* can prove the presence of MSI within the tumor, this is a common finding in sebaceous neoplasms and most patients will not have germline mutation or clinical evidence of MTS. Clinical history and physical examination are key to the diagnosis. If the Mayo MTS risk score is 2 or greater, genetic testing and counseling may be appropriate:

Mayo Muir-Torre Syndrome (MTS) Risk Score Algorithm	
Variable	**Score**
Age at sebaceous neoplasm diagnosis (years)	
≥60	0
<60	1
Total number of sebaceous neoplasms	
1	0
≥2	2
Personal history of Lynch syndrome–related cancer	
No	0
Yes	1
Family history of Lynch-related cancer	
No	0
Yes	1
Sum of scores creates a total score, referred to as the "Mayo MTS Risk Score." A Mayo MTR Risk Score of ≥2 has a sensitivity of 100% and specificity or 81% for predicting a germline mutation in a Lynch Syndrome mismatch repair gene.	
Information for patients regarding the syndrome and genetic testing can be found at the following sources: https://rarediseases.info.nih.gov/diseases/6821/muir-torre-syndrome/cases/30944; http://www.cancer.net/cancer-types/muir-torre-syndrome; and https://www.myriad.com/patients-families/disease-info/colon-cancer/.	

Once the diagnosis is confirmed, the patient and genetically related family members should be appropriately screened for underlying malignancies of the GI and genitourinary systems. This screening should begin at a much younger age than is standard: 20–25 years for colonoscopy and 30–35 years for transvaginal ultrasound. Other organs are screened if the affected family has such cancers; screening might include upper endoscopy, urine cytology, or abdominal ultrasound. The value of screening for noncolonic carcinomas has not been demonstrated. Genetic counseling should be provided.

Abbas O, Mahalingam M: Cutaneous sebaceous neoplasms as markers of Muir-Torre syndrome. J Cutan Pathol 2009; 36: 613.

Ishiguro Y, et al: Usefulness of PET/CT for early detection of internal malignancies in patients with Muir-Torre syndrome. Surg Case Rep 2017; 3: 71.

Robert ME, et al: A clinical scoring system to identify patients with sebaceous neoplasms at risk for the Muir-Torre variant of Lynch syndrome. Genet Med 2014; 16: 711.

SWEAT GLAND TUMORS

Syringoma

Syringomas are common neoplasms demonstrating sweat duct differentiation. They present as small papules 1–3 mm in diameter and may be yellow, brown, or pink. They are virtually always multiple and most frequently occur on the eyelids and upper cheeks (Fig. 29.34). Syringomas are disproportionately common in these sites in Japanese women. Other sites of involvement include the axillae, abdomen, forehead, penis, and vulva. Genital syringomas may cause genital pruritus and may be mistaken for genital warts. Rarely, they may be unilateral or linear. Symmetric distal extremity involvement has also been reported. Eruptive syringomas are histologically identical to syringomas of the eyelid but appear suddenly as numerous lesions on the neck, chest, axillae, upper arms, in the pubic area (Fig. 29.35), and periumbilically, usually in young persons. Some have suggested that eruptive syringomas represent a proliferative process of inflamed normal eccrine glands, analogous to traumatic neuroma being a proliferation of normal peripheral nerve. The fact that numerous lesions appear after "waxing" in the pubic areas supports this hypothesis. Many individual case reports document unusual clinical variants of

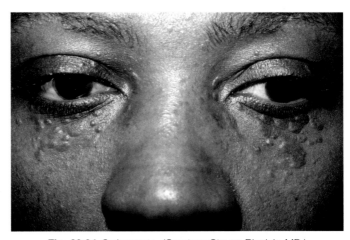

Fig. 29.34 Syringomas. (Courtesy Steven Binnick, MD.)

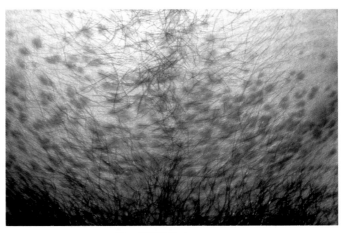

Fig. 29.35 Syringomas.

syringomas. These include types limited to the scalp, associated with alopecia; a unilateral linear or nevoid distribution; those limited to the vulva or penis; those limited to the distal extremities; and the lichen planus–like and milia-like types. Syringomas may calcify and may be mistaken for subepidermal calcified nodules. The rare "plaque-type" syringoma may be mistaken for a microcystic adnexal carcinoma.

Familial cases of syringomas occur. In general, except in eruptive cases, syringomas develop slowly and persist indefinitely without symptoms. Acral lesions are often present. Syringomas occur in 18% of adults with Down syndrome, particularly females. This is approximately 30 times the frequency seen in patients with other syndromes.

Histologically, syringomas are characterized by dilated cystic spaces lined by two layers of cuboidal cells and epithelial strands of similar cells. Some of the cysts have small, comma-like tails, which produce a distinctive picture, resembling tadpoles or the pattern of a paisley tie. There is a dense fibrous stroma. At times, the cells of the syringoma have abundant clear cytoplasm, which represents accumulated glycogen. This has been called "clear cell syringoma." Syringomas stain positive for keratins 5, 6, 14, 6, 16, 19, and 77 on the inner cell layer, and K5 and K14 on the outer cell layer, in a pattern identical to the intraglandular eccrine duct. The microscopic differential diagnosis of "paisley tie" epithelial islands embedded in a sclerotic stroma includes microcystic adnexal carcinoma (sclerosing sweat duct carcinoma), desmoplastic trichoepithelioma, and morpheaform BCC.

Treatment is difficult, but many lesions respond to very light electrodessication or shave removal. For larger lesions, surgical removal may be considered. CO_2 laser treatment by the pinhole method or by fractional thermolysis has been reported as effective.

Akita H, et al: Syringoma of the face treated with fractional photothermolysis. J Cosmet Laser Ther 2009; 11: 216.

Ceulen RP, et al: Multiple unilateral skin tumors suggest type 1 segmental manifestation of familial syringoma. Eur J Dermatol 2008; 18: 285.

Cho SB, et al: Treatment of syringoma using an ablative 10,600-nm carbon dioxide fractional laser. Dermatol Surg 2011; 37: 433.

Cohen PR et al: Penile syringoma. J Clin Aesthet Dermatol 2013; 6: 38.

Ghanadan A, Khosravi M: Cutaneous syringoma. Indian J Dermatol 2013; 58: 326.

Kim JY, et al: Periorbital syringomas treated with an externally used 1,444 nm neodymium-doped yttrium aluminum garnet laser. Dermatol Surg. 2017; 43: 381.

Turan E, et al: A rare association in Down syndrome: milialike idiopathic calcinosis cutis and palpebral syringoma. Cutis 2016; 98: E22.

Hidrocystomas

Hidrocystomas, which may be of eccrine or apocrine differentiation, are 1–3 mm translucent cystic papules that occasionally have a bluish tint. They usually are solitary, occur on the face (Fig. 29.36) or scalp, and are more common in women. In some patients, multiple lesions may be present, and they may be pigmented. They may become more prominent during hot weather. They most often occur periocularly. Multiple hidrocystomas with apocrine secretion on the eyelids are the hallmark of Schopf-Schulz-Passarge syndrome (SSPS), an adult-onset autosomal recessive form of ectodermal dysplasia associated with *WNT10A* mutations. Other features include hypodontia, hypotrichosis, nail dystrophy, and palmoplantar keratoderma. Multiple palmoplantar syringofibroadenomas are present in most cases of SSPS and can present as a palmoplantar keratoderma. Up to 44% of patients have other adnexal tumors. Skin and visceral malignancies are not increased in SSPS.

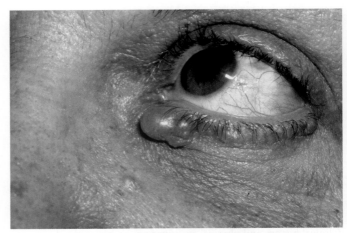

Fig. 29.36 Hidrocystoma. (Courtesy Steven Binnick, MD.)

Microscopically, a single cystic cavity is lined by two layers of small, cuboidal epithelial cells. Apocrine differentiation in the form of decapitation secretion is common. Lesions with papillary proliferations of the lining are classified as cystadenomas. Treatment, if desired, is by excision for solitary lesions. Laser treatment may be effective, both with CO_2 and pulsed dye laser. Topical atropine ointment 1% or scopolamine cream 0.01% (1.2 mL of 0.25% scopolamine eyedrops in 30 g of Eucerin), once daily, has been used with variable success in patients with multiple lesions. Pupil size may increase with these agents. Oral glycopyrrolate, 1 mg twice daily, may be useful in suppressing exercise-induced and hot weather–induced enlargement. Botulinum toxin may also be effective, either injected or applied topically.

Couto Júnior Ade S, et al: Hidrocystoma. An Bras Dermatol 2010; 85: 368.

Gandhi V, et al: Eccrine hidrocystoma successfully treated with topical synthetic botulinum peptide. J Cutan Aesthet Surg 2011; 4: 154.

Jabbar AS, et al: Eccrine hidrocystomas presenting as multiple papules on the cheeks. Dermatol Online J 2013; 19: 19269.

Jakobiec FA, Zakka FR: A reappraisal of eyelid eccrine and apocrine hidrocystomas: microanatomic and immunohistochemical studies of 40 lesions. Am J Ophthalmol 2011; 151: 358.

Madan V, et al: Multiple eccrine hidrocystomas. Dermatol Surg 2009; 35: 1015.

Park HC, et al: Treatment of multiple eccrine hidrocystomas with isotretinoin followed by carbon dioxide laser. J Dermatol 2013; 40: 414.

Singh M, et al: Giant eccrine hidrocystoma of the eyelid. Indian J Dermatol Venereol Leprol 2017; 83: 267.

Tziotzios C, et al: Clinical features and *WNT10A* mutations in 7 unrelated cases of Schopf-Schulz-Passarge syndrome. Br J Dermatol 2014; 171: 1211.

Woolery-Lloyd H, et al: Treatment for multiple periorbital eccrine hidrocystomas: botulinum toxin A. J Drugs Dermatol 2009; 8: 71.

Acrospiromas (Poroma, Hidroacanthoma Simplex, Dermal Duct Tumor, Nodular Hidradenoma, Clear Cell Hidradenoma)

Acrospiromas are benign tumors with acrosyringial differentiation. A poroma presents as a slow-growing, 2–12 mm, slightly protruding, sessile, soft, reddish tumor that occurs most often on the sole (Fig. 29.37) or side of the foot. Palmar lesions may also occur, and, more

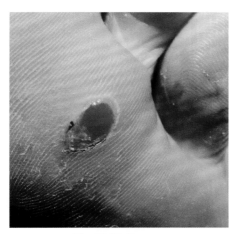

Fig. 29.37 Poroma.

rarely, lesions appear wherever sweat glands are found. The lesion will bleed on slight trauma. A distinctive finding is the cup-shaped shallow depression from which the tumor grows and protrudes. Poromas tend to occur singly, but multiple lesions may also occur. A rare variant is called eccrine poromatosis, in which more than 100 lesions may involve the palms and soles and may be associated with hidrotic ectodermal dysplasia, immunosuppression, or chemotherapy. These may represent acrosyringeal nevi. Dermal duct tumors present deep nodules that may involve any part of the body. Nodular and clear cell hidradenomas are larger nodules that often involve the head or neck but may occur anywhere. Hybrid combinations of different patterns of acrospiroma are very common.

Histologically, poromas demonstrate solid masses of uniform, cuboidal epithelial cells with ample cytoplasm and focal duct differentiation. The cells are smaller than those in the contiguous epidermis and tend to arrange themselves in cords and broad columns extending downward from the normal epidermis. Areas of clear cell and cystic degeneration may be present, and an underlying dermal duct tumor or hidradenoma may be present. Melanocytes may be dispersed throughout the tumor and may be clinically hyperpigmented. The surrounding stroma is highly vascular, with telangiectatic vessels. Hidroacanthoma simplex represents an intraepidermal eccrine poroma. These lesions resemble clonal seborrheic keratoses, except for the presence of focal duct differentiation. Dermal duct tumors are composed of the same small acrosyringeal cells as other acrospiromas. The cells form small dermal islands with ductal differentiation. When the cells form a large nodule, the tumor is referred to as a nodular hidradenoma. When clear cells and cystic degeneration are prominent, the tumor is referred to as a clear cell hidradenoma. A distinctive feature of the latter two tumors is the presence of areas of eosinophilic hyalized stroma. All the cells in a poroma, except entrapped ducts, stain with K5/14. Focally, they are K1/10 positive and uniformly K77 negative. This is the staining pattern of the sweat duct ridge and acrosyringium (intraepidermal portions of sweat duct). The clinical differential diagnosis includes porocarcinoma, pyogenic granuloma, melanoma (amelanotic and melanotic), Kaposi sarcoma, BCC, and seborrheic keratosis. The lesions are benign but often recur after inadequate excision. Malignant degeneration may occur, and atypia is sometimes minimal within tumors that have metastasized. For these reasons, simple complete excision is recommended when feasible.

Malignant Acrospiroma (Malignant Poroma, Porocarcinoma)

This represents the most common form of sweat duct carcinoma. Most malignant acrospiromas appear clinically similar to poromas

but may also manifest as a blue or black nodule, plaque, or ulcerated tumor. Porocarcinoma affects men and women equally at an average age of 70 years. The most frequent sites of involvement are the legs (30%), feet (20%), face (12%), thighs (8%), and arms (7%). Of interest is the rare involvement of the palms and soles, despite these having the greatest concentration of sweat glands. The average age from onset to treatment is 4–8 years. These tumors are of intermediate aggressiveness, with metastases usually occurring to regional lymph nodes and, less often, hematogenously.

Histologically, the tumor may be seen adjoining benign acrospiroma. Atypia may be marked or minimal, with pleomorphic or monomorphous nuclei and abundant or scant eosinophilic cytoplasm. Most frequently, the cells are smaller and more basophilic than those in benign acrospiromas with a high mitotic rate. Focal squamous or sarcomatous differentiation may be present. Pagetoid spread within the adjacent epidermis may be seen. As in benign acrospiromas, clear cell and cystic degeneration may be present. The degree of ductal differentiation is variable. The tumors can be deeply infiltrative. Perineural and lymphovascular involvement by the tumor can be present and should be noted on the dermatopathology report. The epidermis may be invaded by metastatic porocarcinoma. Mohs surgery can be a valuable technique, particularly on the face. As with other cutaneous neoplasms, margins should be free of tumor islands and tumor stroma to be considered negative. Local recurrence approaches 20%, and lymph node metastases occur in about 20% of patients. SNLB could be considered. Distant metastases occur in 10% of cases, often at a distant skin site.

Aaribi I, et al: Successful management of metastatic eccrine porocarcinoma. Case Rep Oncol Med 2013; 2013: 282536.
Battistella M, et al: From hidroacanthoma simplex to poroid hidradenoma. Am J Dermatopathol 2010; 32: 459.
Chang O, et al: Eccrine porocarcinoma of the lower extremity. World J Surg Oncol 2011; 9: 94.
Deckelbaum S, et al: Eccrine poromatosis. Int J Dermatol 2014; 53: 543.
Ishida M, Okabe H: Expression profiles of mTOR pathway proteins in porocarcinoma. Biomed Rep 2013; 1: 28.
Kurashige Y, et al: Eccrine porocarcinoma. Case Rep Dermatol 2013; 5: 259.
Lallas A, et al: Eccrine poroma. J Eur Acad Dermatol Venereol 2016; 30: e61.
Minagawa A, Koga H: Dermoscopy of pigmented poromas. Dermatology 2010; 221: 78.
Nguyen A, Nguyen AV: Eccrine porocarcinoma. Cutis 2014; 93: 43.
Sawaya JL, Khachemoune A: Poroma. Int J Dermatol 2014; 53: 1053.
Schirra A, et al: Eccrine poroma. J Eur Acad Dermatol Venereol. 2016; 30: e167.
Shin HT, et al: Clear cell hidradenoma on the palm. Ann Dermatol 2014; 26: 403.
Skowron F, et al: Primary eccrine porocarcinoma. Ann Dermatol Venereol 2014; 141: 258.

Spiradenoma

Spiradenoma presents clinically as a solitary, 1-cm, deep-seated nodule, occurring most frequently on the ventral surface of the body, especially over the upper half. Normal-appearing skin covers the nodule, which may be skin colored, blue, or pink (Fig. 29.38). Occasionally, multiple lesions may be present and may occur in a linear or segmental pattern. Giant lesions that are very vascular are rarely seen. Lesions may be painful, but not universally. Spiradenoma has a generally benign clinical course and occurs most frequently between ages 15 and 35, although it has also been reported in infancy and childhood. Familial cases have been

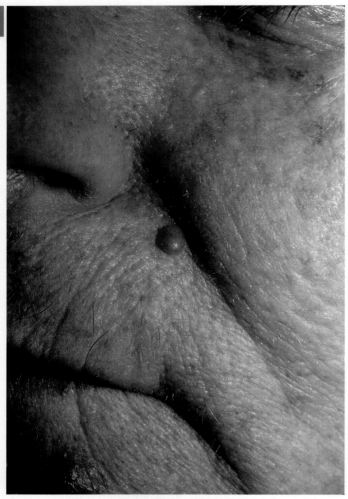

Fig. 29.38 Spiradenoma.

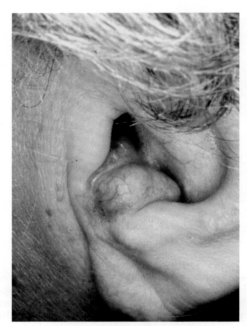

Fig. 29.39 Cylindroma.

Dai B, et al: Spiradenocarcinoma, cylindrocarcinoma and spirad-enocylindrocarcinoma. Histopathology 2014; 65: 658.
Englander L, et al: A rare case of multiple segmental eccrine spiradenomas. J Clin Aesthet Dermatol 2011; 4: 38.
Gordon S, et al: Pediatric segmental eccrine spiradenomas. Pediatr Dermatol 2013; 30: e285.
Sanchez Petitto G, et al: FDG PET/CT in malignant eccrine spiradenoma. Clin Nucl Med 2017; 42: 125.

Cylindroma

Cutaneous cylindroma occurs predominantly on the scalp and face as a solitary lesion (Fig. 29.39). The tumor is firm but rubber-like and pink-blue; it ranges in size from a few millimeters to several centimeters. The solitary cylindroma is considered to be nonhereditary and at times may be found in areas other than the head and neck. Women are affected more than men.

The dominantly inherited form, Brooke-Spiegler syndrome (BSS), appears soon after puberty as numerous rounded masses of various sizes on the scalp. The lesions resemble bunches of grapes or small tomatoes. Lesions appear in the second or third decade of life. Sometimes they cover the entire scalp like a turban. BSS is characterized by the presence of multiple adnexal neoplasms, including cylindroma, trichoepitheliomas, spiradenomas, trichoblastomas, follicular cysts, and milia. Familial cylindroma is now considered a variant of BSS because it harbors the same mutation. There is no genotypic/phenotypic correlation in these two syndromes. BSS is caused by a mutation in the *CYLD* tumor suppressor gene.

Histologically, these are cylindrical masses of epithelial cells surrounded and segmented by thick bands of a hyaline material. Cylindroma may be mistaken for pilar cyst, but the distinctive appearance and consistency make diagnosis easy, especially in the multiple type. Treatment is surgical; success using ablative laser therapy has also been reported.

Chen M, et al: Brooke-Spiegler syndrome associated with cyl-indroma, trichoepithelioma and eccrine spiradenoma. Int J Dermatol 2013; 52: 1602.
Grossmann P, et al: Novel and recurrent germline and somatic mutations in a cohort of 67 patients from 48 families with

described. Rarely, malignant transformation occurs, and the subsequent tumor may also have features of a cylindroma (spiradenocylindrocarcinoma).

Microscopically, spiradenoma demonstrates either a single nodule or multiple basophilic nodules within the dermis. Tumor cells have minimal to no visible cytoplasm. They are often arranged in characteristic small rosettes. Three cell types are present: cells with large, pale-gray nuclei; those with smaller, darker-gray nuclei; and jet-black lymphocytes peppered throughout the nodule. Ductlike structures are often present, as are large, pink hyaline globules that resemble the bright-red hyaline basement membrane material that outlines the islands of cylindromas. In fact, spirad-enomas and cylindromas often occur together in the same patient, and hybrid collision tumors are quite common. These have histori-cally been thought to be of eccrine lineage, but both tumors may instead originate from the hair follicle bulge.

When painful, eccrine spiradenoma may be mistaken for leiomyoma, glomus tumor, neuroma, and angiolipoma. Treatment is simple excision. Spiradenocylindrocarcinoma presents as a solitary nodule that may have experienced an abrupt change in size. Histologically, these lesions have focal areas of atypia, mitoses, and invasion. They may metastasize to regional lymph nodes or hematogenously, and PET/CT scans may be helpful for staging.

Ben Brahim E, et al: Malignant eccrine spiradenoma. J Cutan Pathol 2010; 37: 478.

Brooke-Spiegler syndrome including the phenotypic variant of multiple familial trichoepitheliomas and correlation with the histopathologic findings in 379 biopsy specimens. Am J Dermatopathol 2013; 35: 34.

Rajan N, et al: Transition from cylindroma to spiradenoma in CYLD-defective tumours is associated with reduced DKK2 expression. J Pathol 2011; 3: 309.
Richard A, et al: CO₂ laser treatment of skin cylindromas in Brooke-Spiegler syndrome. Ann Dermatol Venereol 2014; 141: 346.

Mixed Tumor (Chondroid Syringoma)

Cutaneous mixed tumor is an uncommon skin tumor, representing about 1 in 1000 skin lesions removed electively. It favors men between ages 25 and 65. Mixed tumor presents clinically as a firm, intradermal or subcutaneous nodule, virtually always located on the head or neck. These tumors are usually asymptomatic and measure 5–30 mm in diameter, but may be much larger.

Histologically, nests of cuboidal or polygonal epithelial cells in the dermis give rise to tubuloalveolar and ductal structures and occasionally, keratinous cysts. These structures are embedded in a matrix varying from a faint-blue chondroid substance to an acidophilic hyaline material. Myoepithelial and lipomatous elements may also be found in the tumor in addition to the chondroid stroma. Ossification may occur. The treatment is surgical. Mixed tumors may also occur in other organs, especially salivary glands, where they are also known as pleomorphic adenomas. In salivary and rarely in cutaneous chondroid syringoma, tyrosine crystals may be seen in the tumor. Tumors with only focal glandular elements, or with no epithelial elements, have been called "cutaneous myoepitheliomas." They are tumors of the myoepithelial cells; these cells surround the sweat glands and, by their contraction, help deliver the product of the glands to the surface. Both cutaneous mixed tumors and cutaneous myoepitheliomas stain positively with SOX-10, supporting the notion that these tumors exist on a spectrum.

Malignant Mixed Tumor (Malignant Chondroid Syringoma)

The rare malignant mixed tumor favors the trunk and extremities, whereas the benign mixed tumor of the skin favors the head and neck. At presentation, the masses range from 1–10 cm, with a median size of 4 cm. They often grow rapidly. The chance of metastasis is greater than 50%, with a predilection for visceral spread. Metastases usually take the form of an adenocarcinoma, and the chondroid stroma found in primary lesions is often not found. Histologic features that distinguish malignant mixed tumor from chondroid syringoma include cytologic atypia, pleomorphism, increased mitotic activity, and focal necrosis. Treatment is surgical.

Hafezi-Bakhtiari S, et al: Benign mixed tumor of the skin, hypercellular variant. J Cutan Pathol 2010; 37: e46.
Hudson LE, et al: Giant chondroid syringoma of the lower eyelid. Ophthal Plast Reconstr Surg 2017; 33: e43.
Nangia A, et al: Chondroid syringoma with extensive osseous differentiation. Indian J Pathol Microbiol 2014; 57: 344.
Naujokas A, et al: SOX-10 expression in cutaneous myoepitheliomas and mixed tumors. J Cutan Pathol 2014; 41: 353.
Sivamani R, et al: Chondroid syringoma. Dermatol Online J 2006; 12: 8.

Ceruminoma

Ceruminous glands, modified apocrine glands of the external ear, may give rise to both benign and malignant tumors. Distinguishing these may be difficult; thus both the malignant and the benign

tumors have been termed *ceruminomas*. The tumors present as a firm papule or nodule in the external auditory canal. Ulceration and crusting may occur, and continued growth may obstruct the meatus, resulting in hearing loss. Histologically, glands and cysts are present, lined by a tuboglandular proliferation with two layers: an inner layer of ceruminous cells (containing cerumen and with decapitation secretion) and a basal spindled or cuboidal myoepithelial layer. Treatment is excision, which is curative if margins are clear.

Crain N, et al: Ceruminous gland carcinomas. Head Neck Pathol 2009; 3: 1.
Giuseppe M, et al: Adenoma of the ceruminous gland (ceruminoma). Otol Neurotol 2011; 32: e14.
Jan JC, et al: Ceruminous adenocarcinoma with extensive parotid, cervical, and distant metastases. Arch Otolaryngol Head Neck Surg 2008; 134: 66.
Thompson LD, et al: Ceruminous adenomas. Am J Surg Pathol 2004; 28: 308.

Hidradenoma Papilliferum

Hidradenoma papilliferum is a benign adenoma that arises from anogenital mammary-like glands and is located almost exclusively in the vulvar and perianal areas. The tumor is covered by normal skin. On palpation, it is a firm papule less than 1 cm in diameter. Malignant transformation is rare and can resemble a focus of ductal carcinoma in situ. Microscopically, hidradenoma papilliferum is encapsulated and lies in the dermis, having no connection with the epidermis. There is a cystlike cavity lined with villi. The walls of the cavity and the villi are lined, occasionally with a single layer but usually with a double layer of cells: luminal secretory cells and myoepithelial cells. PIK3CA and AKT1 mutations have been identified. This is a benign lesion, and the diagnosis and treatment are accomplished by excisional biopsy.

Duhan N, et al: Hidradenoma papilliferum of the vulva. Arch Gynecol Obstet 2011; 284: 1015.
Elbendary A, et al: Hidradenoma papilliferum with oncocytic metaplasia. Am J Dermatopathol 2016; 38: 444.
Goto K, et al: PIK3CA and AKT1 mutations in hidradenoma papilliferum. J Clin Pathol 2017; 70: 424.
Kurashige Y, et al: Hidradenoma papilliferum of the vulva in association with an anogenital mammary-like gland. J Dermatol 2014; 41: 411.
Moon JW, et al: Giant ectopic hidradenoma papilliferum on the scalp. J Dermatol 2009; 36: 545.
Veeranna S, et al: Solitary nodule over the labia majora. Indian J Dermatol Venereol Leprol 2009; 75: 327.

Syringadenoma Papilliferum (Syringocystadenoma Papilliferum)

This lesion develops in a nevus sebaceus of Jadassohn on the scalp or face in about one third of patients. Around half are present at birth, whereas approximately 25% arise on the trunk and genital and inguinal regions during adolescence. The lesions are rose-red papules of firm consistency (Fig. 29.40); they vary from 1–3 mm and may occur in groups. Vesicle-like inclusions are seen, pinpoint to pinhead in size, filled with clear fluid. Some of the papules may be umbilicated and simulate molluscum contagiosum. Extensive verrucous or papillary plaques may also be present.

Histologically, the tumor shows ductlike structures that extend from the surface epithelium. Numerous papillary projections may extend into the lumina, which may be cystic. The papillary projections are lined by glandular epithelium, often consisting of two rows of cells. The tumor cells stain positive for CEA. The dermal

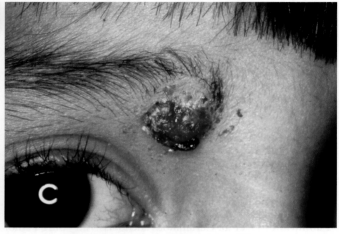

Fig. 29.40 Syringocystadenoma papilliferum.

stroma contains numerous plasma cells. Rarely, malignant transformation may occur. Excision is recommended.

Bruschini L, et al: Syringocystadenoma papilliferum of the external auditory canal. Am J Case Rep 2017; 18: 520.

Cassarino DS, et al: SOX10 immunohistochemistry in sweat ductal/glandular neoplasms. J Cutan Pathol 2017; 44: 544.

Chi CC, et al: Syringocystadenocarcinoma papilliferum. Dermatol Surg 2004; 30: 468.

Dufrechou L, et al: Syringocystadenoma papilliferum arising on the scrotum. Pediatr Dermatol 2013; 30: e12.

Ghazeeri G, Abbas O: Syringocystadenoma papilliferum developing over hyperkeratosis of the nipple in a pregnant woman. J Am Acad Dermatol 2014; 70: e84.

Idriss MH, Elston DM: Secondary neoplasms associated with nevus sebaceus of Jadassohn. J Am Acad Dermatol 2014; 70: 332.

Khurana VK, et al: A case of syringocystadenocarcinoma papilliferum on lower leg. Indian J Dermatol 2013; 58: 405.

Monticciolo NL, et al: Verrucous carcinoma arising within syringocystadenoma papilliferum. Ann Clin Lab Sci 2002; 32: 434.

Mundi JP, et al: Syringocystadenoma. Dermatol Online J 2013; 19: 20722.

Ogunrinade K, et al: Agminated syringocystadenoma papilliferum. Dermatol Online J 2013; 19: 19270.

Sangma MM, et al: Syringocystadenoma papilliferum of the scalp in an adult male. J Clin Diagn Res 2013; 7: 742.

Satter E, et al: Syringocystadenocarcinoma papilliferum with locoregional metastases. Dermatol Online J 2014; 20: 22335.

Schaffer JV, et al: Syringocystadenoma papilliferum in a patient with focal dermal hypoplasia due to a novel *PORCN* mutation. Arch Dermatol 2009; 145: 218.

Steshenko O, et al: Syringocystadenoma papilliferum of the vulva. BMJ Case Rep 2014 May 28; 2014.

Papillary Eccrine Adenoma/Tubular Apocrine Adenoma

Papillary eccrine adenoma/tubular apocrine adenoma (PEA/TAA—sounds like "pita") is an uncommon benign sweat gland neoplasm that presents clinically as dermal nodules located primarily on the extremities of black patients, especially on the dorsal hand or foot. Histologic findings consist of a well-circumscribed, dermal, unencapsulated growth composed of dilated ductlike structures lined by two or more layers of cells. Intraluminal papillations may project into the cystic spaces. Because this lesion tends to recur

locally, complete surgical excision with clear margins is recommended. Hybrid or overlapping lesions with a superficial component resembling syringocystadenoma papilliferum and a deep component resembling tubular adenoma can occur.

Ansai SI, et al: Tubulopapillary cystic adenoma with apocrine differentiation. Am J Dermatopathol 2017; 39: 829.

Kim MS, et al: a case of tubular apocrine adenoma with syringocystadenoma papilliferum that developed in a nevus sebaceus. Ann Dermatol 2010; 22: 319.

Lee HJ, et al: Syringocystadenoma papilliferum of the back combined with a tubular apocrine adenoma. Ann Dermatol 2011; 23: S151.

Martinelli PT, et al: Mohs micrographic surgery for tubular apocrine adenoma. Int J Dermatol 2006; 45: 1377.

Syringofibroadenoma (Acrosyringeal Nevus of Weedon and Lewis)

First described by Mascaro in 1963, five variants of eccrine syringofibroadenoma are now recognized:

1. Solitary
2. Multiple, in Schopf syndrome
3. Multiple, without other skin manifestations
4. Nonfamilial unilateral linear
5. Reactive

The solitary type presents frequently as a hyperkeratotic nodule or plaque involving the extremities. The linear type may be linear, blaschkoid, or zosteriform in appearance, and some cases may represent an acrosyringeal nevus. Multiple lesions have been termed *eccrine syringofibroadenomatosis* (ESFA) and occur in both variants of hidrotic ectodermal dysplasia, Schopf syndrome, and Clouston syndrome. The multiple ESFAs may appear in a mosaic pattern. In Clouston syndrome (due to mutation in the *GJB6* gene), HPV-10 has been detected in the tumors. Multiple lesions have also been reported without other associated cutaneous findings. Many cases represent a reactive epithelial proliferation, whereas others represent a true neoplasm of acrosyringeal cells. Histologically, the strands resemble those of the fibroepithelial tumor of Pinkus, but with broader anastomosing cords without the basaloid buds. "Reactive eccrine syringofibroadenoma" most often occurs on the lower leg and may show adjacent changes of an associated dermatosis. Carcinomatous transformation of ESFA has been reported.

De Andrade AC, et al: Clouston syndrome associated with eccrine syringofibroadenoma. An Bras Dermatol 2014; 89: 504.

Desai CA, et al: Reactive eccrine syringofibroadenoma in hyperkeratotic eczema. Indian Dermatol Online J 2016; 7: 325.

Husein-ElAhmed H, et al: Solitary eccrine syringofibroadenoma arising on the toe. J Dtsch Dermatol Ges 2014; 12: 148.

Xu XL, et al: A case of multiple eccrine syringofibroadenoma mimicking verruca vulgaris. J Dermatol 2013; 40: 665.

Microcystic Adnexal Carcinoma (Sclerosing Sweat Duct Carcinoma)

This tumor generally presents as a very slow-growing plaque or nodule. It occurs most frequently on the head and neck (87%), face (73%), and scalp (10%). Lesions favor the midface and periorbital area, with a predilection for the left side. The upper lip (Fig. 29.41) is involved nine times more often than the lower lip. Given their propensity for sun-exposed sites, long-term sun exposure may play a role in the pathogenesis of microcystic adnexal carcinomas; they have also occurred at sites of prior therapeutic radiation. The lesions are locally aggressive, with local recurrences in 50% of cases. Metastasis rarely occurs. Microcystic adnexal

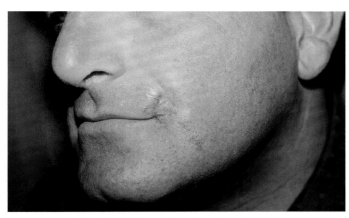

Fig. 29.41 Microcystic adnexal carcinoma.

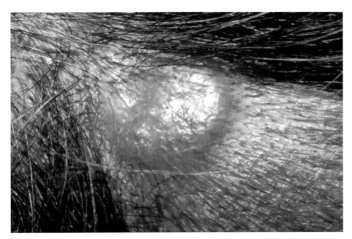

Fig. 29.42 Eccrine carcinoma.

carcinoma occurs most often in Caucasians (90%) but also is reported in Japanese Americans and in African Americans, in whom it may be found in atypical locations. Histologically, the superficial part of the tumor is composed of ducts, keratinous cysts, and small cords of cells, superficially resembling a syringoma. The deeper component consists of nests and strands in a dense stroma. Perineural invasion is common and may be extensive. This explains the frequent recurrence after initial excision. Specific immunohistochemical markers have been proposed to distinguish microcystic adnexal carcinoma from infiltrative BCC, desmoplastic trichoepithelioma, and SCC. Mohs microsurgery is the treatment of choice. Radiation treatment of the tumor is controversial; it may be useful as adjuvant therapy but appears to be inadequate as monotherapy, with potential for recurrence and more aggressive behavior of the tumor.

Aslam A: Microcystic adnexal carcinoma and a summary of other rare malignant adnexal tumours. Curr Treat Options Oncol 2017; 18: 49.

Baxi S, et al: Microcystic adnexal carcinoma of the skin. J Med Imaging Radiat Oncol 2010; 54: 477.

Chen MB, et al: Metastatic microcystic adnexal carcinoma with DNA sequencing results and response to systemic antineoplastic chemotherapy. Anticancer Res 2017; 37: 5109.

Gabillot-Carre M, et al: Microcystic adnexal carcinoma. Dermatology 2006; 212: 221.

Hansen T, et al: Extrafacial microcystic adnexal carcinoma. Dermatol Surg 2009; 35: 1835.

Pugh TJ, et al: Microcystic adnexal carcinoma of the face treated with radiation therapy. Head Neck 2012; 34: 1045.

Vidal CI, et al: p63 Immunohistochemistry is a useful adjunct in distinguishing sclerosing cutaneous tumors. Am J Dermatopathol 2010; 32: 257.

Yu JB, et al: Surveillance, epidemiology, and end results (SEER) database analysis of microcystic adnexal carcinoma (sclerosing sweat duct carcinoma) of the skin. Am J Clin Oncol 2010; 33: 125.

Eccrine Carcinoma (Syringoid Carcinoma)

Eccrine carcinoma is rare and presents as a plaque or nodule on the scalp (Fig. 29.42), trunk, or extremities. Local recurrence is common, but metastases are rare. It is composed of ducts and tubules with atypical basaloid cells. A more cellular tumor with numerous tubules and ducts has been termed *polymorphous sweat gland carcinoma*. Overlap features with microcystic adnexal carcinoma occur, but in general, eccrine carcinoma has a less desmoplastic stroma.

Mucinous Carcinoma

Mucinous carcinoma is typically a round, elevated, reddish, and sometimes ulcerated mass, usually located on the head and neck (75%). Forty percent occur on the eyelid. It grows slowly and is usually asymptomatic. Local recurrence is seen in 36%, but the rate of metastasis and widespread dissemination is low (15%). Rare tumors on the eyelid (derived from glands of Moll) may express estrogen and progesterone receptors, analogous to mucinous carcinoma of the breast. Mucinous gut carcinomas may also metastasize to skin and must be excluded before diagnosing a primary cutaneous mucinous carcinoma.

Histologically, tumors are characterized by the presence of large areas of mucin, in which small islands of basophilic epithelial cells are embedded (blue islands floating in a sea of mucus). Basaloid cells in a cribriform pattern, with ductlike structures, are typical. The recommended treatment is surgical excision; Mohs surgery leads to lower rates of recurrence compared with those treated with traditional surgical excision (13% vs. 34%).

Areán-Cuns C, et al: Primary mucinous carcinoma of the skin. Actas Dermosifiliogr 2017; 108: 884.

Kamalpour L, et al: Primary cutaneous mucinous carcinoma. JAMA Dermatol 2014; 150: 380.

Marra DE, et al: Mohs micrographic surgery of primary cutaneous mucinous carcinoma using immunohistochemistry for margin control. Dermatol Surg 2004; 30: 799.

Aggressive Digital Papillary Adenocarcinoma (Digital Papillary Adenocarcinoma)

This aggressive malignancy involves the digit between the nail bed and the distal interphalangeal joint spaces in most cases, or occurs just proximal to this region. It presents as a solitary cystic nodule. Ulceration and bleeding can occur, and rarely the malignancy may be fixed to underlying tissues. Most patients are men in their fifties. The tumor is locally aggressive, with a 50% local recurrence rate. Metastases, particularly pulmonary, occur in about 15% of cases. The tumor is poorly circumscribed and is composed of tubuloalveolar and ductal structures with areas of papillary projections. The tumor is positive for S-100, and the cystic contents are positive for CEA and EMA. Complete excision is the treatment of choice. Cases previously called aggressive digital papillary "adenoma" are best regarded as adenocarcinoma.

Chen S, Asgari M: Papillary adenocarcinoma in situ of the skin. Dermatol Pract Concept 2014; 4: 23.

Hsu HC, et al: Aggressive digital papillary adenocarcinoma. Clin Exp Dermatol 2010; 35: 113.

Suchak R, et al: Cutaneous digital papillary adenocarcinoma. Am J Surg Pathol 2012; 36: 1883.

Primary Cutaneous Adenoid Cystic Carcinoma

This rare cutaneous tumor usually presents on the chest, scalp, or vulva of middle-aged to older persons. It is similar histologically to adenoid cystic carcinoma of the salivary gland, with a proliferation of small, ductlike islands and larger islands with a "Swiss cheese" or cribriform pattern. Detection of HPV and overexpression of p16 (a tumor suppressor protein also called CDKN2A) has been demonstrated in many of these lesions. Adenoid cystic carcinoma may recur locally or rarely metastasizes. Surgical excision, perhaps with Mohs micrographic surgery, is the treatment of choice.

Boland JM, et al: Detection of human papilloma virus and p16 expression in high-grade adenoid cystic carcinoma of the head and neck. Mod Pathol 2012; 25: 529.

Dores GM, et al: Primary cutaneous adenoid cystic carcinoma in the United States. J Am Acad Dermatol 2010; 63: 71.

Maybury CM, et al: A nodule in the groin: primary cutaneous adenoid cystic carcinoma (pcACC). JAMA Dermatol 2013; 149: 1343.

Ramakrishnan R, et al: Primary cutaneous adenoid cystic carcinoma. Am J Surg Pathol 2013; 37: 1603.

Xu YG, et al: Cutaneous adenoid cystic carcinoma with perineural invasion treated by Mohs micrographic surgery. J Oncol 2010; 2010: 469049.

Apocrine Gland Carcinoma

Apocrine gland carcinoma unrelated to PD is rare. The axilla or anogenital region is the most common site, but occasionally other areas with apocrine glands may be involved. Lesions present as a mass. Widespread metastases occur in at least 40% of cases.

Figueira EC, et al: Apocrine adenocarcinoma of the eyelid. Ophthal Plast Reconstr Surg 2013; 29: 417.

Goldstein R, et al: Advanced vulvar apocrine carcinoma expressing estrogen receptors that responds to tamoxifen therapy. Future Oncol 2012; 8: 1199.

Hollowell KL, et al: Cutaneous apocrine adenocarcinoma. J Surg Oncol 2012; 105: 415.

Kajal B, et al: Apocrine adenocarcinoma of the vulva. Rare Tumors 2013; 5: e40.

Singh H, et al: Apocrine sweat gland carcinoma. Clin Nucl Med 2013; 38: e223.

Terada T, et al: Apocrine carcinoma of the scrotum with extramammary Paget's disease. Int J Dermatol 2013; 52: 504.

HAIR FOLLICLE NEVI AND TUMORS

Pilomatricoma (Calcifying Epithelioma of Malherbe)

Also known as Malherbe calcifying epithelioma and pilomatrixoma, this benign tumor is derived from hair matrix cells. It usually occurs as a single lesion, which is most often found on the face, neck, or proximal upper extremity. Lesions may also be located on the scalp, trunk, and lower extremities. Pilomatricoma is an asymptomatic, deeply seated, 0.5–7 cm, firm nodule covered by normal or pink skin (Fig. 29.43). On stretching, it may show the

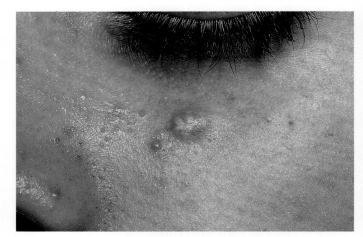

Fig. 29.43 Pilomatricoma, larger lesion with yellow tint.

"tent sign," with multiple facets and angles; on gentle pinching, it may show the "skin crease sign," with a central longitudinal crease. Overlying epidermal atrophy is common, leading to an appearance that may resemble anetoderma or striae. "Giant" and "bullous" presentations have been described. In a review of 239 patients, the youngest was 1 year and the oldest 83 years. There is a bimodal age distribution, in the first and sixth decades. Females are more often affected than males.

Multiple pilomatricomas are uncommon. They are usually seen in association with myotonic dystrophy–Steinert syndrome. They may also occur in Rubinstein-Taybi syndrome, trisomy 9, and Turner syndrome. Patients with Gardner syndrome have epidermoid cysts with focal areas of pilomatricoma-like changes. Rarely, multiple pilomatricomas will be inherited in an autosomal dominant pattern with no other association.

The histopathology shows an encapsulated mass. Basophilic cells with minimal cytoplasm resemble those of the hair matrix. They evolve into eosinophilic "shadow" cells. Calcification occurs frequently. Ossification, melanin deposits, and foreign body reaction with giant cells may all be present. Activating mutations in β-catenin are present in the majority of pilomatricomas. It is expressed in the basophilic but not the shadow cells. "Melanocytic matricoma" is a rare lesion presenting as a small papule, which histologically is composed of metrical cells, some shadow cells, and numerous dendritic melanocytes containing melanin. It appears to be a fairly common variant in the Japanese population.

Clinical differential diagnosis is usually impossible in the adult, but in children, because epidermoid cysts are rare, this diagnosis should be considered for any firm cystic mass of the face and upper body. When palpated, pilomatricomas are firmer and more faceted than epidermoid and pilar cysts. Fine-needle aspiration has led to misdiagnosis, with the basophilic cells being interpreted as carcinoma. Treatment is surgical excision.

Malignant Pilomatricoma (Pilomatrix Carcinoma, Pilomatrical Carcinoma)

Malignant pilomatricomas are rare tumors. Described as being locally aggressive, but with limited metastatic potential, many cases labeled "malignant" may actually have been "proliferating" pilomatricomas. Metastases to regional lymph nodes are most common. Mohs micrographic surgery may be considered to obtain clear margins.

Belliappa P, et al: Bullous pilomatricoma. Int J Trichology 2013; 5: 32.

Brown RE, et al: Diagnostic imaging of benign and malignant neck masses in children. Quant Imaging Med Surg 2016; 6: 591.

Chattopadhyay M, et al: Anetodermic pilomatricoma in a patient with hypermobility syndrome. Clin Exp Dermatol 2014; 39: 218.

Cornejo KM, Deng A: Pilomatrix carcinoma. Am J Dermatopathol 2013; 35: 389.

Gupta M, et al: Aggressive pilomatrixoma. Diagn Cytopathol 2014; 42: 906.

Handler MZ, et al: Prevalence of pilomatricoma in Turner syndrome. JAMA Dermatol 2013; 149: 559.

Hernández-Núñez A, et al: Retrospective study of pilomatricoma. Actas Dermosifiliogr 2014; 105: 699.

Herrmann JL, et al: Pilomatrix carcinoma. J Am Acad Dermatol 2014; 71: 38.

Ieni A, et al: Limits of fine-needle aspiration cytology in diagnosing pilomatrixoma. Indian J Dermatol 2012; 57: 152.

Ishida M, Okabe H: Pigmented pilomatricoma. Int J Clin Exp Pathol 2013; 6: 1890.

Julian CG, et al: A clinical review of 209 pilomatricomas. J Am Acad Dermatol 1998; 39: 191.

Kim IH, Lee SG: The skin crease sign. J Am Acad Dermatol 2012; 67: e197.

Kwon D, et al: Characteristics of pilomatrixoma in children. Int J Pediatr Otorhinolaryngol 2014; 78: 1337.

Lamprou K, et al: Cutaneous hybrid tumor composed of epidermal cyst and cystic pilomatricoma. Int J Trichology 2016; 8: 195.

Niiyama S, et al: Proliferating pilomatricoma. Eur J Dermatol 2009; 19: 188.

Souto MP, et al: An unusual presentation of giant pilomatrixoma in an adult patient. J Dermatol Case Rep 2013; 7: 56.

Trichofolliculoma

Trichofolliculoma is a benign, highly structured tumor of the pilosebaceous unit, characterized by a small, dome-shaped nodule about 5 mm in diameter on the face or scalp. From the center of the flesh-colored nodule, a small wisp of fine, vellus hairs protrudes through a central pore (Fig. 29.44). It may occur at any age but mostly affects adults. Mouse studies suggest that dysregulation of bone morphogenic protein signaling in hair follicle progenitors may contribute to trichofolliculoma formation.

Histologically, the tumor consists of one or more large follicles with smaller, radiating, secondary follicular structures, sometimes referred to as "the mother follicle with her babies." The secondary follicles range from an immature rudimentary matrix to well-formed follicles with papillae, matrix, trichohyaline, and fine hairs ("fingers of fully formed follicles forming fiber"). The tumor may have little stroma or may be embedded in a fibrous orb. Sebaceous glands may be prominent, a variant termed *sebaceous trichofolliculoma*. The follicular structures in trichofolliculomas transition through phases of the hair cycle. In telogen, they may resemble fibrofolliculomas. The presence of hair shafts helps distinguish the two. Folliculosebaceous cystic hamartoma may closely resemble a sebaceous trichofolliculoma. Treatment is surgical removal.

Al-Ghadeer H, et al: Congenital sebaceous trichofolliculoma of the upper eyelid. Ophthal Plast Reconstr Surg 2017; 33: S60.

Romero-Pérez D, et al: Clinicopathologic study of 90 cases of trichofolliculoma. J Eur Acad Dermatol Venereol 2017; 31: e141.

Tanimura S, et al: Two cases of folliculosebaceous cystic hamartoma. Clin Exp Dermatol 2006; 31: 68.

Wu YH: Folliculosebaceous cystic hamartoma or trichofolliculoma? A spectrum of hamartomatous changes inducted by perifollicular stroma in the follicular epithelium. J Cutan Pathol 2008; 35: 843.

Brooke-Spiegler Syndrome (Multiple Familial Trichoepithelioma, Epithelioma Adenoides Cysticum)

This autosomal dominant condition usually presents in childhood or around puberty. Familial cylindroma, multiple familial trichoepithelioma, and Brooke-Spiegler syndrome are all variants of the same condition. The favored term is *Brooke-Spiegler syndrome* (BSS). There is a variable phenotypic expression among and within families and patients. The multiple trichoepitheliomas present as multiple cystic and solid papules on the face, favoring the upper lip, nasolabial folds, and eyelids (Fig. 29.45). The individual lesions are small, round, smooth, shiny, slightly translucent, firm, circumscribed papules or nodules. The individual lesions average 2–4 mm in diameter. The center may be slightly depressed. Most frequently, the lesions are grouped but discrete. On the face, they are often symmetric. Other sites may be the scalp, neck, and trunk. Multiple linear and dermatomal trichoepitheliomas may rarely be seen. Multiple cylindromas and spiradenomas, epidermoid cysts, and milia may occur in association with multiple trichoepitheliomas. BSS is caused by mutations in *CYLD*, which functions as a tumor suppressor gene. It has a critical role in deubiquinating proteins,

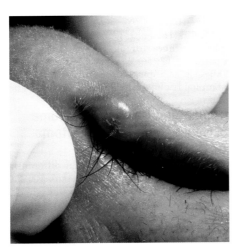

Fig. 29.44 Trichofolliculoma.

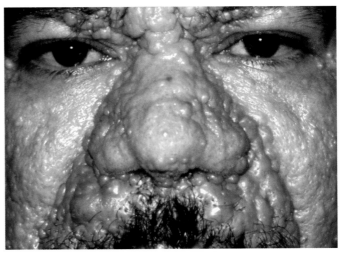

Fig. 29.45 Brooke-Spiegler syndrome.

which is important in controlling their biologic function. Some individuals in these families have primarily trichoepitheliomas, others have primarily cylindromas, and others have a panoply of adnexal tumors, including cylindromas, trichoepitheliomas, and spiradenomas. BSS patients seem to be at particular risk for degeneration of their cylindromas and spiradenomas to carcinomas. Topical sirolimus has been reported as helpful for patients with multiple tumors.

Solitary Trichoepithelioma

The singly occurring trichoepithelioma is nonhereditary and mostly favors the face. However, it may also be found on the scalp, neck, trunk, and proximal extremities. It presents as a firm dermal papule or nodule and must be distinguished from BCC.

Giant Solitary Trichoepithelioma

The lesions may be several centimeters in diameter, occurring most frequently on the thigh or perianal regions. They are found in older adults.

Desmoplastic Trichoepithelioma

This lesion, which is difficult to differentiate from morpheiform BCC histologically, occurs as solitary or multiple lesions on the face. Desmoplastic trichoepitheliomas are firm and slightly indented (central dell sign), with a raised, annular border (Fig. 29.46). Young women are most often affected, and familial solitary and multiple desmoplastic trichoepitheliomas have been described.

Trichoepitheliomas are dermal tumors with multiple nests of basaloid cells, some of which show abortive follicular differentiation. Keratinous cysts, calcification, and amyloid may all be seen. The stroma in most trichoepitheliomas resembles the fibrous sheath of a normal hair follicle. It contains many fine collagen fibers and fibroblasts that surround the tumor islands in a concentric array. Clusters of plump nuclei resembling the cells of the follicular papilla (papillary mesenchymal bodies) are common. In the desmoplastic variety, the tumor is composed of small cords of epithelium embedded in a dense eosinophilic stroma with fewer fibroblasts. The islands often present a "paisley tie" appearance, and the microscopic differential diagnosis includes morpheaform BCC, syringoma, and microcystic adnexal carcinoma. The clinical features may distinguish these entities. Focal calcification, horn cysts, and a central dell favor trichoepithelioma. In desmoplastic trichoepithelioma, clefts form between collagen fibers in the stroma,

whereas in BCC, clefts form between the tumor islands and stroma. Trichoepitheliomas are best classified as benign tumors of the hair germ. As such, they may be considered variants of trichoblastoma. Histologically, trichoepithelioma must be differentiated from keratotic BCC, with which it is frequently confused.

Solitary lesions can be treated by surgical excision. Multiple lesions can be smoothed down by resurfacing the skin with laser surgery, dermabrasion, or electrosurgery. This procedure must be repeated at regular intervals, as the lesions gradually recur.

Trichoblastoma

These benign neoplasms of follicular germinative cells usually present as asymptomatic nodules 0.5–1 cm in size in the deep dermis or subcutaneous tissue. The scalp is the most common location, especially if associated with nevus sebaceus of Jadassohn. Trichoblastomas usually occur in adult men and women, but children can also develop them. The lesions may be pigmented. Trichoblastomas arise in organoid nevi and represent the majority of basaloid neoplasms described as "basal cell carcinomas" in nevus sebaceus. The rare Curry-Jones syndrome, with cutaneous streaky hypopigmentation, hyperpigmented linear atrophic lines on the soles, and many other musculoskeletal, ocular, and GI defects, can feature multiple trichoblastomas. Histologically, trichoblastoma is a dermal or subcutaneous tumor composed of basaloid cells with areas of follicular differentiation. The islands may connect with the overlying epidermis, especially in the setting of an organoid nevus. The stroma is identical to that seen in trichoepithelioma and typically contains papillary mesenchymal bodies. Merkel cells may be prominent within the tumor, and amyloid can be found. Cutaneous lymphadenoma is a variant of trichoblastoma with extensive infiltration of the tumor islands by lymphocytes and histiocytes. The stroma resembles that of other trichoblastomas. A single or double row of basaloid tumor cells is seen at the periphery of each island, whereas the center is composed of histiocytes and lymphocytes. Surgical excision is curative.

Aguilera CA, et al: Heterozygous cylindromatosis gene mutation c.1628_1629delCT in a family with Brook-Spiegler syndrome. Indian J Dermatol 2016; 61: 580.

Grossmann P, et al: Novel and recurrent germline and somatic mutations in a cohort of 67 patients from 48 families with Brooke-Spiegler syndrome including the phenotypic variant of multiple familial trichoepitheliomas and correlation with the histopathologic findings in 379 biopsy specimens. Am J Dermatopathol 2013; 35: 34.

LoPiccolo MC, et al: Comparing ablative fractionated resurfacing, photodynamic therapy, and topical imiquimod in the treatment of trichoblastomas of Brooke-Spiegler syndrome. Dermatol Surg 2011; 37: 1047.

Mollet PU, Muñoz JF: False-negative tumor-free margins following Mohs surgery for aggressive trichoblastoma. Am J Dermatopathol 2012; 34: 255.

Tu JH, et al: Use of topical sirolimus in the management of multiple familial trichoepitheliomas. Dermatol Ther 2017; 30.

Trichilemmoma and Cowden Syndrome (Cowden Disease, Multiple Hamartoma Syndrome)

Trichilemmoma is a benign neoplasm that differentiates toward cells of the outer root sheath. It usually occurs as a small, solitary papule on the face, particularly the nose and cheeks. Sporadic tumors are often caused by activating HRAS mutations. Most lesions are clinically misdiagnosed as BCC or benign keratosis.

Trichilemmomas may also occur as multiple facial lesions. When they do, this is a specific cutaneous marker for Cowden syndrome (CS), an autosomal dominant inherited condition. The prevalence

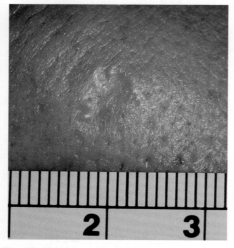

Fig. 29.46 Trichoepithelioma, desmoplastic type.

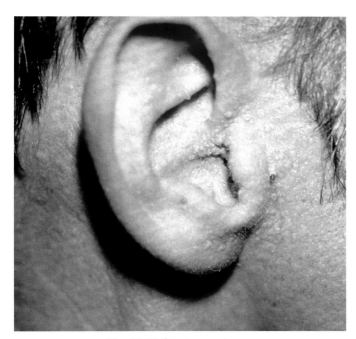

Fig. 29.47 Cowden syndrome.

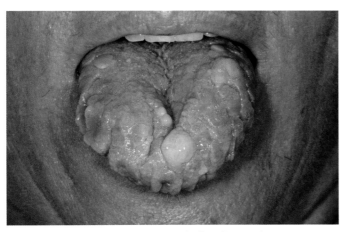

Fig. 29.48 Oral papillomas in Cowden syndrome.

and usually in multiple anatomic locations, favoring the buccal and gingival mucosa. They can coalesce and form the characteristic cobblestone pattern seen in 40% of CS patients. Involvement of the respiratory mucosa can occur, with an acanthosis nigricans–like appearance. The mucosal lesions develop after the cutaneous lesions and have a persistent but benign course. Other cutaneous lesions include lipomas, hemangiomas, xanthomas, acanthosis nigricans, and various hyperpigmented macules. Macrocephaly with head circumference of greater than 97% is a major criterion for the diagnosis.

Malignancies develop in up to 40% of patients with CS. They are major criteria for the diagnosis and include breast, endometrial, and thyroid carcinoma. Breast cancer occurs in 25%–50% of female patients and has been reported in male patients with CS. For breast cancer, the average age at diagnosis is 36 years. About 75% of affected females have fibrocystic disease of the breast. Endometrial cancer occurs in 6% of women with CS and has appeared as early as adolescence. Although not criteria for the diagnosis, multiple GI polyps (in 70%–85%) and GI malignancies also occur. Minor criteria include thyroid lesions (including adenomas or goiter, and thyroiditis, in two thirds of patients), mental retardation, lipomas, fibromas (multiple sclerotic fibromas or storiform collagenomas), and genitourinary tumors. Multiple lipomatosis of the testicles is a common manifestation. The adult form of Lhermitte-Duclos disease, or dysplastic gangliocytoma of the cerebellum, represents the neurologic manifestation of CS. Lhermitte-Duclos disease is another pathognomonic criterion for the diagnosis of CS. A number of mucocutaneous malignancies have been found in patients with CS, including melanoma, BCC, SCC, MCC, and trichilemmal carcinoma.

Mutations in the tumor suppressor gene *PTEN* are responsible for the majority of CS. Patients who do not have a mutation in *PTEN* have mutations in the promoter region for *PTEN* or have methylation and downregulation of *KILLIN*, another tumor suppressor, with resultant rates of breast and renal cancer higher than those seen with *PTEN* mutation. In 10% of cases, the mutation is not in *PTEN* or the promoter and may be in the succinate dehydrogenase genes. Another disorder caused in 65% of cases by mutations in *PTEN* is Bannayan-Riley-Ruvalcaba syndrome (BRRS): autosomal dominant inherited macrocephaly, genital lentigines, motor and speech delay, mental retardation, hamarto-matous polyps, myopathies, lipomas, and hemangiomas. BRRS is now considered a variant of CS that presents earlier in life, and patients having overlap syndromes with features of both CS and BRRS have been described. Some patients with a Proteus-like syndrome also have mutations in *PTEN*. These diseases have been called the "*PTEN* hamartoma tumor syndrome."

Microscopically, trichilemmomas show variable hyperkeratosis and parakeratosis. Tumor lobules extend downward from the epidermis and demonstrate glycogen-rich clear cells, peripheral palisading, and a thick, hyalinized basement membrane.

Facial papillomas can be removed with surgical procedures, but new lesions continue to appear throughout life. Some patients achieve satisfactory cosmetic results from dermabrasion or CO_2 laser. Regular cancer screening and genetic counseling are paramount in CS. Rapamycin prevents the development of mucocutaneous lesions and premature death in the animal model for CS, suggesting that the mTOR pathway is involved in the development of the cutaneous lesions and the later complications of CS.

of CS is 1 in /200,000–250,000. The penetrance is almost complete, with 90% of affected patients having stigmata by age 20. Diagnostic criteria for CS have been established, and certain mucocutaneous manifestations are considered pathognomonic, including trichilem-momas of the face, acral keratoses, papillomatous papules (Fig. 29.47), and mucosal lesions (Fig. 29.48). The trichilemmomas, or "facial papules," are present in 86% of CS patients and appear on average at age 22 but can appear at any age from childhood to advanced age (75 years). Trichilemmomas are generally limited to the head and neck, especially the central face, around the orifices; however, other sites may be involved (e.g., ears). Because not all facial papules have characteristic histology, the presence of "papil-lomatous" lesions is a diagnostic criterion. The other pathogno-monic mucocutaneous benign features are acral keratoses, which present as either verrucous hyperkeratosis on the extensor extremities, or palmoplantar translucent keratoses, in 28% and 20% of CS patients, respectively. Acral neuromatosis may present as translucent papules on the backs and sides of the fingers. The mucous membranes are involved in more than 80% of patients

Al-Daraji WI, et al: Storiform collagenoma as a clue for Cowden disease or *PTEN* hamartoma tumour syndrome. J Clin Pathol 2007; 60: 840.

Bennett KL, et al: Germline epigenetic regulation of *KILLIN* in Cowden and Cowden-like syndrome. JAMA 2010; 304: 2724.

Blumenthal GM, Dennis PA: *PTEN* hamartoma tumor syndromes. Eur J Hum Genet 2008; 16: 1289.

Caux F, et al: Segmental overgrowth, lipomatosis, arteriovenous malformation and epidermal nevus (SOLAMEN) syndrome is related to mosaic *PTEN* nullizygosity. Eur J Hum Genet 2007; 15: 767.

Farooq A, et al: Cowden syndrome. Cancer Treat Rev 2010; 36: 577.

Ferran M, et al: Acral papular neuromatosis. Br J Dermatol 2008; 158: 174.

Ferran M, et al: Bilateral and symmetrical palmoplantar punctate keratoses in childhood. Clin Exp Dermatol 2009; 34: e28.

Flores IL, et al: Oral presentation of 10 patients with Cowden syndrome. Oral Surg Oral Med Oral Pathol Oral Radiol 2014; 117: e301.

Ngeow J, et al: Clinical implications for germline PTEN spectrum disorders. Endocrinol Metab Clin North Am 2017; 46: 503.

Ngeow J, et al: Second malignant neoplasms in patients with Cowden syndrome with underlying germline *PTEN* mutations. J Clin Oncol 2014; 32: 1818.

Ni Y, et al: Germline mutations and variants in the succinate dehydrogenase genes in Cowden and Cowden-like syndromes. Am J Hum Genet 2008; 83: 261.

Orloff MS, Eng C: Genetic and phenotypic heterogeneity in the *PTEN* hamartoma tumour syndrome. Oncogene 2008; 27: 5387.

Orloff MS, et al: Germline *PIK3CA* and *AKT1* mutations in Cowden and Cowden-like syndromes. Am J Hum Genet 2013; 92: 76.

Pilarski R, et al: Cowden syndrome and the PTEN hamartoma tumor syndrome. J Natl Cancer Inst 2013; 105: 1607.

Robinson S, Cohen AR: Cowden disease and Lhermitte-Duclos disease. Neurosurg Focus 2006; 20: E6.

Squarize CH, et al: Chemoprevention and treatment of experimental Cowden's disease by mTOR inhibition with rapamycin. Cancer Res 2008; 68: 7066.

Stathopoulos P, et al: Cowden syndrome. Oral Maxillofac Surg 2014; 18: 229.

Tan MH, et al: A clinical scoring system for selection of patients for *PTEN* mutation testing is proposed on the basis of a prospective study of 3042 probands. Am J Hum Genet 2011; 88: 42.

Tan MH, et al: Lifetime cancer risks in individuals with germline *PTEN* mutations. Clin Cancer Res 2012; 18: 400.

Tsai JH, et al: Frequent activating HRAS mutations in trichilemmoma. Br J Dermatol 2014; 171: 1073.

Umemura K, et al: Gastrointestinal polyposis with esophageal polyposis is useful for early diagnosis of Cowden's disease. World J Gastroenterol 2008; 14: 5755.

Woodhouse J, Ferguson MM: Multiple hyperechoic testicular lesions are a common finding on ultrasound in Cowden disease and represent lipomatosis of the testis. Br J Radiol 2006; 79: 801.

Trichilemmal Carcinoma

Trichilemmal carcinomas are reported to arise on sun-exposed areas, most often the face and ears. They present as a slow-growing papule, indurated plaque, or nodule with a tendency to ulcerate. They may arise in the association of immunosuppression. It may be difficult to distinguish trichilemmal carcinoma from invasive BD (which often shows adnexal differentiation) or a clear cell SCC. Surgical removal is recommended; Mohs micrographic surgery has been used successfully. Local recurrence and metastasis have occurred.

Chai MK, et al: Eyelid trichilemmal carcinoma. Saudi J Ophthalmol 2017; 31: 183.

Hamman MS, Brian Jiang SI: Management of trichilemmal carcinoma. Dermatol Surg 2014; 40: 711.

Kulahci Y, et al: Multiple recurrence of trichilemmal carcinoma of the scalp in a young adult. Dermatol Surg 2010; 36: 551.

Tolkachjov SN, et al: Mohs micrographic surgery in the treatment of trichilemmal carcinoma. J Am Acad Dermatol 2015; 72: 195.

Zhuang SM, et al: Survival study and clinicopathological evaluation of trichilemmal carcinoma. Mol Clin Oncol 2013; 1: 499.

Trichodiscoma, Fibrofolliculoma, Perifollicular Fibromas, Mantleomas, and Birt-Hogg-Dubé Syndrome

These benign tumors form a spectrum of neoplasms combining a follicular element and the specialized periadventitial dermis of the upper portion of the hair follicle. They may represent variations of the same tumor cut in different planes of section. All these lesions clinically appear as 2–4 mm, asymptomatic, skin-colored, dermal papules affecting the face and upper trunk. They may be single but are frequently multiple. When multiple, they are often numerous and are a marker for Birt-Hogg-Dubé syndrome (BHD) (Fig. 29.49). The histomorphology of these hair follicle tumors is identical in patients with BHD and in cases unassociated with BHD. Fibrofolliculoma demonstrates cords and strands of two-cell to four-cell epithelium emanating from a follicular structure. The epithelial elements may anastomose, and sebaceous elements may be present. This follicular structure is surrounded by a collagenous or fibromucinous orb. Trichodiscomas represent a sectioning artifact that demonstrates only the tumor stroma.

The BHD syndrome is inherited in an autosomal dominant manner. It is caused by a mutation in the gene folliculin (*FLCN*), which is located on chromosome 17p. Many of the mutations occur in a hypermutable region of the gene. This gene is conserved in many species and expressed in many tissues, but its exact function is unknown. Recently it has been linked to numerous cell pathways important in cancer biology, including cell growth, metabolism, adhesion, motility, kinesis, and survival. Homozygous loss of function of the folliculin gene is embryonically lethal, suggesting that *FLCN* may indeed play a broad and important role in the cell. Cutaneous lesions are common in patients with BHD, affecting more than 80% of persons 30 years or older. The fibrofolliculomas appear in adulthood and usually precede other stigmata but can be quite subtle. In the vast majority of cases, they are multiple and often very numerous. They can be widespread but always affect the nose, paranasal area, back of the pinna, and behind the ear. Comedo-like papules with keratinous plugs may be seen. Lesions can coalesce into plaques and be grouped. Multiple epidermoid cysts can occur. Hyperseborrhea may be seen, with numerous facial fibrofolliculomas. Skin tags are present in 100%

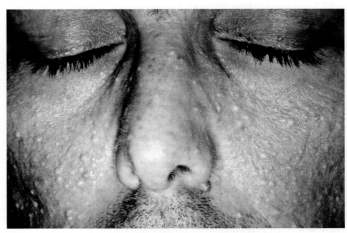

Fig. 29.49 Birt-Hogg-Dubé syndrome.

of patients, most often in the axillae. Small, discrete, soft, mucosa-colored or white papules of the lips, gingiva, tongue, and buccal mucosa are present in about 40% of patients and families with BHD. Biopsies of the oral lesions reveal an acanthotic epithelium overlying a fibrotic process.

In addition to the cutaneous lesions previously noted, patients are at risk for the development of renal tumors and spontaneous pneumothorax. The renal tumor risk is seven times that of the general population and especially affects men (at twice the risk) and those over 40. At least 30% of patients with BHD develop renal tumors, and these can appear after age 20. Renal tumors may be multiple and bilateral, a clinical scenario that should suggest the diagnosis of BHD. Patients with BHD develop renal onco-cytomas and chromophobe renal carcinomas, or a mixed type that is characteristic of BHD. These are otherwise rare histologic variants of renal cell carcinoma. Multiple renal cysts may also occur.

Patients with BHD have greater than 30 times the risk of developing a spontaneous pneumothorax than unaffected persons—a lifetime risk of 24%. Pneumothorax can occur at a young age in BHD; 17% of BHD patients under 40 will have a spontaneous pneumothorax. Median age of pneumothorax occurrence is 38 years. Spontaneous pneumothorax results from multiple pulmonary cysts, which affect 83% of BHD patients. The cysts are at the lung base and subpleural. Recurrent pneumothorax is common and should suggest BHD. Patients do not seem to have progressive pulmonary failure, and severe chronic obstructive pulmonary disease is not associated with *FLCN* mutations. Colonic polyps and neoplasms, which were initially reported to be associated with BHD syndrome, do *not* appear to be increased in BHD syndrome. Thyroid nodules are seen in 90% of affected families and 65% of BHD patients. BHD must be differentiated from familial multiple discoid fibroma, which presents similarly with facial papules but is histologically distinct, lacks systemic complications, and does not involve the *FLCN* gene.

The treatment of the fibrofolliculomas is surgical debulking. In most patients, the lesions are small and can be cosmetically removed by shave removal, curettage, or resurfacing if the lesions are numerous. Smoking is proscribed because it may worsen lung complications. Renal imaging should be periodically performed, but the best method is unclear. CT is more accurate than ultrasound, especially for smaller lesions, but repeat scans lead to unacceptable radiation exposure. MRI is expensive but diagnostically most accurate. Although there is no genotype/phenotype correlation known at this time for *FLCN* mutations, certain families seem to be predisposed to certain complications of BHD. In those families, more aggressive screening for the particularly prevalent complica-tion seems warranted. Because the *FLCN* gene seems to interact with the mTOR pathway, it has been suggested that the use of rapamycin has potential benefit in BHD; however, an RCT showed no benefit.

Furuya M, Nakatani Y: Birt-Hogg-Dubé syndrome. J Clin Pathol 2013; 66: 178.

Gaur K, et al: The Birt-Hogg-Dubé tumor suppressor folliculin negatively regulates ribosomal RNA synthesis. Hum Mol Genet 2013; 22: 284.

Gijezen LM, et al: Topical rapamycin as a treatment for fibrofol-liculomas in Birt-Hogg-Dubé syndrome. PLoS One 2014; 9: e99071.

Houweling AC, et al: Renal cancer and pneumothorax risk in Birt-Hogg-Dubé syndrome; an analysis of 115 *FLCN* mutation carriers from 35 BHD families. Br J Cancer 2011; 105: 1912.

Imada K, et al: Birt-Hogg-Dubé syndrome with clear-cell and oncocytic renal tumour and trichoblastoma associated with a novel *FLCN* mutation. Br J Dermatol 2009; 160: 1350.

Lee JE, et al: Birt-Hogg-Dubé syndrome. Diagn Interv Radiol 2017; 23: 354.

Mallipeddi R, et al: Birt-Hogg-Dubé syndrome with a renal angiomyolipoma. Byrne Australas J Dermatol 2012; 53: 151.

Medvetz DA, et al: Folliculin, the product of the Birt-Hogg-Dubé tumor suppressor gene, interacts with the adherens junction protein p0071 to regulate cell-cell adhesion. PLoS One 2012; 7.

Menko FH, et al: Birt-Hogg-Dubé syndrome. Lancet Oncol 2009; 10: 1199.

Nishii T, et al: Unique mutation, accelerated mTOR signaling and angiogenesis in the pulmonary cysts of Birt-Hogg-Dubé syndrome. Pathol Int 2013; 63: 45.

Pritchard SE, et al: Successful treatment of facial papules with electrodessication in a patient with Birt-Hogg-Dubé syndrome. Dermatol Online J 2014; 20.

Rato M, et al: Birt-Hogg-Dubé syndrome—report of two cases with two new mutations. J Dermatol Case Rep 2017; 11: 12.

Reiman A, et al: Gene expression and protein array studies of folliculin-regulated pathways. Anticancer Res 2012; 32: 4663.

Spring P, et al: Syndrome of Birt-Hogg-Dubé, a histopathological pitfall with similarities to tuberous sclerosis. Am J Dermatopathol 2013; 35: 241.

Starink TM, et al: Familial multiple discoid fibromas. J Am Acad Dermatol 2012; 66: 259.e1.

Tee AR, Pause A: Birt-Hogg-Dubé. Fam Cancer 2013; 12: 367.

Tong Y, et al: Birt-Hogg-Dubé syndrome. Am J Clin Dermatol 2017 Jul 10; ePub ahead of print.

Toro JR, et al: *BHD* mutations, clinical and molecular genetic investigations of Birt-Hogg-Dubé syndrome. J Med Genet 2008; 45: 321.

Vincent A, et al: Birt-Hogg-Dubé syndrome. J Am Acad Dermatol 2003; 49: 698.

Other Hair Follicle Tumors

Dilated Pore (of Winer)

This lesion typically presents as a solitary, prominent, open comedo on the face or upper trunk of an elderly individual. Histologically, it is composed of a greatly dilated follicular pore lined by outer root sheath epithelium. Multiple short, bulbous, acanthotic projec-tions extend from the central infundibulum-like pore.

Pilar Sheath Acanthoma

Pilar sheath acanthoma is most often found on the face, particularly above the upper lip in adults. Patients present with a solitary, 5–10 mm, skin-colored nodule with a central keratinous plug. Histologically, pilar sheath acanthoma differs from a dilated pore by having larger tumor lobules radiating from the central infundibulum-like pore.

Trichoadenoma

Presenting as a solitary growth ranging from 3–15 mm in diameter, this lesion may be clinically mistaken for a seborrheic keratosis, having a vegetative or verrucous appearance. Although most frequently found on the face, it may occur at other sites, especially the buttock, which is the second most common location. Tricho-adenomas also differentiate toward the follicular infundibulum. Histologically, they are quite distinctive, being composed of a collection of ringlike eosinophilic structures that often occur in pairs (resembling eyeglasses). No hair shafts are present.

Basaloid Follicular Hamartoma

Basaloid follicular hamartoma (BFH) is a distinctive benign adnexal tumor that has four described variants: solitary papule, localized plaque of alopecia, linear or blaschkoid unilateral plaque, and

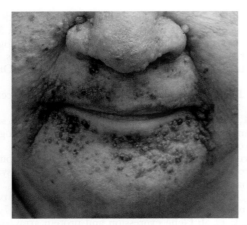

Fig. 29.50 Basaloid follicular hamartoma. (Courtesy Dr. J. English.)

generalized papules. Generalized BFH form has also been termed *generalized hair follicle hamartoma*. Most often affecting the skin of the face and scalp, BFHs are solitary or multiple, skin-colored, 2–3 mm papules (Fig. 29.50) or infiltrating plaques associated with progressive hair loss in the affected areas. Congenital and adult appearances have been described. In some generalized cases, there is an association with alopecia, myasthenia gravis, or circulating autoantibodies (antinuclear and antiacetylcholine receptor antibodies). Cystic fibrosis and generalized follicular hamartomas have been reported in three siblings, suggesting a possible genetic linkage. A familial, autosomal dominant form has been described, with numerous milia; comedo-like lesions; hyperpigmented papules of the face, scalp, ears, neck, and trunk; hypotrichosis; hypohidrosis; and pinpoint palmar pits. It presents in early childhood. Happle-Tinschert syndrome is segmentally arranged BFH, linear atrophoderma with hypopigmentation or hyperpigmentation, enamel defects, ipsilateral hypertrichosis, and skeletal and cerebral anomalies.

Histologically, BFH may be indistinguishable from infundibulocystic BCC. Lesions are characterized by thin, branching eosinophilic strands and thick cords with associated basaloid buds and keratin cysts. Unlike most other pilar tumors, the stroma is loose, fibrillar, or mucinous. In nevoid and generalized forms, apparently normal skin may also demonstrate small islands of basaloid cells. Trichoblastomas may occur within nevoid lesions. *PTCH* gene signaling is upregulated in the cells contacting the dermis in BFH. Generalized BFH syndrome must be distinguished from Bazex-Dupré-Christol syndrome, Brown-Crounse syndrome, Rombo syndrome, basal cell nevus syndrome, and Brooke-Spiegler syndrome. Its differentiation from multiple hereditary infundibulocystic BCC syndrome may be difficult. Treatment essentially consists of recognition of the correct diagnosis, avoidance of unnecessary surgery, and periodic monitoring (malignant growths may arise within BFH, if not transform from it). Oral and topical retinoids and PDT have been reported effective for widespread BFH.

Folliculosebaceous Cystic Hamartoma

Folliculosebaceous cystic hamartoma is a benign hamartoma of epithelial and mesenchymal elements. It presents as a solitary, 0.5–1.5 cm papule or nodule virtually always on the head, with two thirds occurring on or adjacent to the nose. Rare giant lesions up to 15 cm in diameter have been reported. Age of onset ranges from infancy to the sixth decade. Histologically, the lesion is composed of three elements: an intradermal cystic structure lined by squamous epithelium identical to that of the infundibulum; numerous sebaceous lobules radiating from the cystic structure;

and a surrounding stroma with fibrous, adipose, vascular, and neural tissues. Stromal spindle cells are positive for CD34. The tumor may represent a sebaceous trichofolliculoma biopsied during telogen phase.

Tumors of the Follicular Infundibulum

These flat, keratotic papules, and sometimes hypopigmented macules, of the head and neck are usually solitary but may be multiple. They appear in adulthood. The terms *eruptive infundibulomas* and *infundibulomatosis* have been used to describe cases with multiple lesions. In the rare generalized cases, there is a strong clinical resemblance to Darier disease, with accentuation on the neck, central chest, groin, and axillae. Histologically, the solitary and multiple cases are identical. There is a platelike proliferation of epidermal cells growing parallel to the epidermis and connecting to it at multiple sites. Clear, glycogenated cells similar to those of a trichilemmoma, sebaceous differentiation, cystic and ductal structures, and papillary mesenchymal bodies may be seen. Caution is required in interpreting biopsy specimens, as the edge of an infundibulocystic BCC can appear similar.

Alomari A, et al: Solitary and multiple tumors of follicular infundibulum. J Cutan Pathol 2013; 40: 532.
Ansai S, et al: A clinicopathologic study of folliculosebaceous cystic hamartoma. Am J Dermatopathol 2010; 32: 815.
Bavikar RR, et al: Postauricular pilar sheath acanthoma. Int J Trichology 2011; 3: 39.
Bruscino N, et al: Pilar sheath acanthoma simulating basal cell carcinoma. G Ital Dermatol Venereol 2014; 149: 155.
Kubba A, et al: Tumor of follicular infundibulum. Indian J Dermatol Venereol Leprol 2014; 80: 141.
Lo CS, et al: Unilateral segmentally arranged basaloid follicular hamartomas with osteoma cutis and hypodontia. Clin Exp Dermatol 2013; 38: 862.
Mills O, Thomas LB: Basaloid follicular hamartoma. Arch Pathol Lab Med 2010; 134: 1215.
Misago N, et al: A revaluation of folliculosebaceous cystic hamartoma. Am J Dermatopathol 2010; 32: 154.
Shimanovich I, et al: Trichoadenoma of Nikolowski is a distinct neoplasm within the spectrum of follicular tumors. J Am Acad Dermatol 2010; 62: 277.
Waxweiler WT, et al: A novel phenotype with features of basal cell nevus syndrome and basaloid follicular hamartoma syndrome. J Am Acad Dermatol 2011; 65: e17.

EPITHELIAL CYSTS AND SINUSES

Epidermal Cyst (Epidermal Inclusion Cyst, Infundibular Cyst)

Epidermal inclusion cyst is one of the most common benign skin tumors. It presents as a compressible, but not fluctuant, cystic mass from 0.5 cm to several centimeters in diameter (Fig. 29.51). The surface of the overlying skin is usually smooth and shiny from the upward pressure. These nodules are freely movable over underlying tissue and are attached to the normal skin above them by a comedo-like central infundibular structure or punctum. The pasty contents of the cysts are formed mostly of macerated keratin, which has a cheesy consistency and pungent odor. Epidermal inclusion cysts occur most often on the face, neck, and trunk but may be found in almost any location. They frequently result from plugging of the follicular orifice, often in association with acne vulgaris. They may also occur by epidermal implantation. Deep penetrating injuries, such as with a sewing machine needle or stapler, or even with nail biting, may result in epidermoid cysts growing within bone. In persons with dark pigment, the lining of the epidermoid cyst and its contents may be pigmented. Epidermoid cysts rarely appear

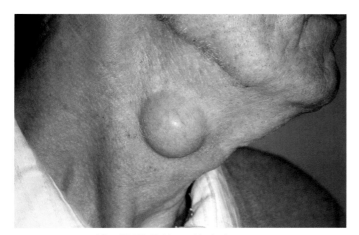

Fig. 29.51 Epidermal inclusion cyst.

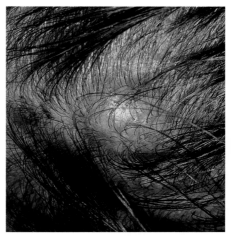

Fig. 29.52 Pilar cyst.

before puberty, and earlier onset should suggest an alternative diagnosis (e.g., pilomatricoma, dermoid cyst, Gardner syndrome). Lesions of the scalp are usually trichilemmal cysts. Rare cysts of the soles are caused by infection by HPV-60.

Epidermoid cysts may rupture and induce a vigorous foreign body inflammatory response, after which they are firmly adherent to surrounding structures and are more difficult to remove. Rupture is associated with the sudden onset of redness, pain, swelling, and local heat, simulating an abscess. Incision and drainage will confirm the diagnosis of inflamed cyst, when the smelly, cheesy material is evacuated. This will also lead to rapid resolution of symptoms. These episodes are often misdiagnosed as "infection" of the cyst, but cultures are usually negative, and antibiotic treatment is not required. Intralesional triamcinolone may hasten resolution of the symptoms. Rarely, malignancies such as SCC, BCC, and melanoma have arisen within epidermoid cysts. Rapidly enlarging cysts should be considered for excision, and histology should be reviewed carefully.

The epidermoid cyst is a keratinizing cyst, the wall of which is stratified squamous epithelium containing keratohyalin granules. It is differentiated from the pilar cyst by the different pattern of keratinization, although hybrid cysts with infundibular, trichilemmal, and even pilomatrical differentiation can be seen. Idiopathic scrotal calcinosis is the end stage of calcification of epidermoid cysts of the scrotum. Pilomatrical differentiation within an epidermoid cyst should suggest Gardner syndrome.

Surgical excision is curative, but the complete cyst and any associated "daughter" cysts must be removed. Enucleation of the cyst through a small incision or a hole made with a 4-mm biopsy punch or a laser may be attempted. A suture looped several times through the cyst and overlying skin can be used to exert traction on the cyst facilitating removal. A curette may be used to scrape out and snag all the fragments of the cyst wall. Alternatively, the lining of the cyst can be eradicated by cauterizing it with 20% trichloroacetic acid. Inflamed cysts may also be treated in this way, but the inflammation makes complete removal of the cyst more difficult. If any fragment of the cyst wall is left behind, the cyst may recur.

Proliferating Epidermoid Cyst

These tumors, derived from epidermoid cysts, occur more often in men (64%), and the most frequent sites are the pelvic/anogenital areas (36%), scalp (21%), upper extremities (18%), and trunk (15%). In rare cases, carcinomatous changes can be seen on histology, with anaplasia, high mitotic rate, and deep invasion. Proliferating epidermoid cysts are locally aggressive, but distant metastasis is rare.

Malignant oncholemmal cyst may describe a rare slow-growing tumor arising from a subungual keratinous cyst.

Baek SO, et al: Giant epidermal inclusion facial cyst. J Craniofac Surg 2011; 22: 1149.
Bajoghli A, et al: Melanoma arising from an epidermal inclusion cyst. J Am Acad Dermatol 2013; 68: e6.
Chang RS, et al: Spectrum of hybrid cysts and their clinical significance. Am J Dermatopathol 2017 Sep 12; ePub ahead of print.
Ghigliotti G et al: Usefulness of dermoscopy for the diagnosis of epidermal cyst. Clin Exp Dermatol 2014; 39: 649.
Jayalakshmy PS, et al: Pigmented epidermal cyst with dense collection of melanin. Indian Dermatol Online J 2012; 3: 131.
Sau P, et al: Proliferating epithelial cysts. J Cutan Pathol 1995; 22: 394.
Song SW, et al: Minimally invasive excision of epidermal cysts through a small hole made by a CO_2 laser. Arch Plast Surg 2014; 41: 85.

Pilar Cyst (Trichilemmal Cyst, Isthmus-Catagen Cyst)

The trichilemmal cyst, also known as a wen, is similar clinically to the epidermoid cyst, except that about 90% of pilar cysts occur on the scalp (Fig. 29.52). Women over age 60 are predominantly affected. The cyst may be found rarely on the face, trunk, and extremities. An overlying punctum is not present, and lesions tend to be more mobile and firmer than epidermoid cysts. Hereditary trichilemmal cysts (autosomal dominant) link to the short arm of chromosome 3 but not to β-catenin or MLH1.

The trichilemmal cyst is lined by stratified squamous epithelium, which is derived from the outer root sheath. The lining cells demonstrate trichilemmal keratinization, increasing in size as they approach the cyst cavity and abruptly keratinizing without forming a granular cell layer. The cyst contents are homogeneous; they usually calcify and rarely ossify. Hybrid cysts with features of both an epidermoid cyst and a pilar cyst can be seen.

Treatment is the same as for the epidermoid cyst. Pilar cysts are much more easily enucleated, so more limited incision is required to remove the lesion.

Proliferating Trichilemmal Cyst/Malignant Trichilemmal Cyst

A spectrum of lesions ranges from typical pilar cysts with focal areas of epithelial proliferation to solid proliferating growths with

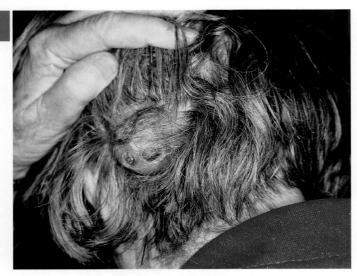

Fig. 29.53 Pilar cyst, proliferating type.

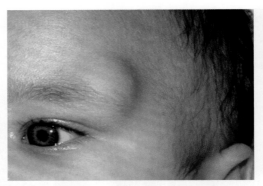

Fig. 29.54 Dermoid cyst. (Courtesy Scott Bartlett, MD.)

atypia that are best considered SCCs. The typical proliferating pilar cyst or proliferating pilar tumor is a large (up to 25 cm) exophytic neoplasm confined almost exclusively to the scalp and back of the neck. These lesions are approximately five times more common in women, and the mean age of patients is 65 years. They gradually enlarge and may ulcerate (Fig. 29.53). The vast majority of lesions are cured by local excision. Some lesions may recur and, less often, they may be locally aggressive. Focal areas of atypia and mitoses may be seen in benign-behaving, proliferating pilar tumors. In uncommon cases, there are focal areas that show frank SCC. These lesions should be called "malignant proliferating pilar tumor." Areas of SCC are characterized by increased cellularity, atypia, frequent mitoses, and, most important, invasion of the surrounding stroma. These tumors may behave aggressively. The clinical features that should suggest potential aggressive behavior are nonscalp location, recent rapid growth, size greater than 5 cm, and an infiltrative growth pattern clinically and histologically. In KID (keratosis, ichthyosis, deafness) syndrome, the development of malignant proliferating pilar tumor may occur in young adulthood and may be fatal.

Proliferating trichilemmal cysts are composed of proliferations of squamous cells with trichilemmal differentiation, forming scroll-like structures or small cysts. Lesions are usually well circumscribed. Focal cellular atypia, mitoses, and necrosis may be present and do not necessarily predict aggressive behavior. Cases with aggressive growth and metastases usually have cytologic atypia, as well as an invasive growth pattern. The presence of a clearly benign component and a second anaplastic component growing outward suggests the development of a carcinoma. Proliferating pilar cysts and their malignant counterparts express hair cytokeratins (cytokeratin 7), and malignant trichilemmal tumors express CD34, suggesting fetal hair root phenotype and trichilemmal differentiation.

Aneiros-Fernandez J, et al: Giant proliferating trichilemmal malignant tumor. Indian J Dermatol Venereol Leprol 2011; 77: 730.

Chaichamnan K, et al: Malignant proliferating trichilemmal tumors with CD34 expression. J Med Assoc Thai 2010; 93: S28.

Dewanda NK, Midya M: Baker's dozen on the scalp. J Cutan Aesthet Surg 2014; 7: 67.

Eiberg H, et al: Mapping of hereditary trichilemmal cyst (*TRICY1*) to chromosome 3p24–p21.2 and exclusion of β-catenin and MLH1. Am J Med Genet 2005; 133A: 44.

Eskander A, et al: Squamous cell carcinoma arising in a proliferating pilar (trichilemmal) cyst with nodal and distant metastases. J Otolaryngol Head Neck Surg 2010; 39: E63.

Goyal S, et al: Malignant proliferating trichilemmal tumor. Indian J Dermatol 2012; 57: 50.

Khaled A, et al: Malignant proliferating trichilemmal cyst of the scalp. Pathologica 2011; 103: 73.

Pusiol T, et al: Ossifying trichilemmal cyst. Am J Dermpathol 2011; 33: 867.

Rangel-Gamboa L, et al: Proliferating trichilemmal cyst. Int J Trichology 2013; 5: 115.

Seidenari S, et al: Hereditary trichilemmal cysts. Clin Genet 2013; 84: 65.

Sutherland D, et al: Malignant proliferating trichilemmal tumor treated with radical radiotherapy. Cureus 2017; 9: e999.

Dermoid Cyst

Cutaneous dermoid cysts, also called congenital inclusion dermoid cysts, result from local anomalies in embryonic development and occur along embryonic closure zones. On the face, they occur above the lateral end of the eyebrow (external angular dermoid) (Fig. 29.54), at the nasal root, along the midline of the forehead, over the mastoid process, on the floor of the mouth, and anywhere along the midline of the scalp from the frontal to the occipital region. Dermoid cysts may also be found on the chest, back, abdomen, and perianal area. Nasal and external angular dermoids may be seen in multiple members of a family, suggesting a genetic component. Lesions usually present within the first year of life, although only 70% of lesions have been identified by age 5 years. The typical lesion is a few millimeters to several centimeters in diameter and located in the subcutaneous fat. A tethering to the underlying tissues and an underlying bony defect may be noted. They are nonpulsatile, firm, and cystic, and they do not transilluminate. A punctum or opening to the skin surface may be present, but dermoid cysts are not usually attached to the overlying skin. A tuft of hair may project from a pit, signifying the presence of an underlying sinus or cyst. Inflammation of the cyst caused by rupture (with extrusion of hair and a foreign body reaction) or infection may first bring the patient to the physician. Because the dermoid may connect to underlying structures, including the pleura and CNS, infection may spread to the CNS or lungs, with potentially serious consequences. Patients with spina bifida frequently develop dermoid cysts of the repaired portion of their spinal column. Dermoids overlying the lower spine may be associated with tethered cord and late development of ambulatory difficulties. At times, dermoids may be on the lateral buttocks. Dermal sinuses/dermoids may be associated with other findings of occult spinal dysraphism, including hyperpigmented patches, "skin tags," hemangiomas, and hairy nevi.

Histologically, the cyst wall is lined with keratinizing stratified squamous epithelium containing skin appendages, including lanugo hair. Portions of the cyst lining may demonstrate a wavy eosinophilic (shark tooth) pattern resembling that of a steatocystoma.

In a child, attempts at surgical removal or biopsy of a cyst over cleavage planes (including along the midline of the back) should not be attempted without proper assessment to rule out an intraspinal or intracranial communication, but this may not be necessary before removal of lateral eyebrow dermoids. CT or MRI is required. Any underlying bony changes detected by CT scan should be followed up with an MRI scan; cranial penetration by the cyst at times may be difficult to identify by CT. If an intracranial connection is detected, the patient should be referred to a neurosurgeon.

Guruprasad Y, Chauhan DS: Midline nasal dermoid cyst with Tessier's 0 cleft. J Nat Sci Biol Med 2014; 5: 479.

Madke B, et al: Nasal dermoid sinus cyst in a young female. Indian Dermatol Online J 2013; 4: 380.

Maurice SM, Burstein FD: Disappearing dermoid. J Craniofac Surg 2012; 23: e31.

Vega RA, et al: Intradiploic dermoid cyst of the lateral fronto-temporal skull. Pediatr Neurosurg 2013; 49: 232.

Pilonidal Sinus

Pilonidal cyst or sinus occurs in the midline sacral region at the upper end of the cleft of the buttocks. A pit may be all that is visible before puberty. Pilonidal cysts/sinuses usually become symptomatic during adolescence. The lesion becomes inflamed from rupture or less frequently infection. Pilonidal sinus/cyst often occurs with nodulocystic acne, dissecting cellulitis, and hidradenitis suppurativa (the acne tetrad). Histologically, the cyst/sinus is lined by stratified squamous epithelium of the type seen in normal epidermis or follicular infundibulum. Some pilonidal cysts/sinuses are composed of epithelium, which keratinizes without formation of a granular cell layer, analogous to the outer root sheath. Referral to a general surgeon is recommended, because recurrences may follow simple cystectomy and marsupialization. SCCs have been reported to arise from chronic inflammatory pilonidal disease.

Eryılmaz R, et al: Recurrent squamous cell carcinoma arising in a neglected pilonidal sinus. Int J Clin Exp Med 2014; 7: 446.

Muzi MG, et al: Long-term results of pilonidal sinus disease with modified primary closure. Am Surg 2014; 80: 484.

Steatocystoma Simplex

Solitary steatocystoma (simple sebaceous duct cyst, steatocystoma simplex) occurs with equal frequency in adult women and men and occurs on the face, trunk, or extremities. The oral mucosa may also be involved. It is not familial, and solitary lesions are much less common than multiple ones. The cysts are usually 0.5–1.5 cm in size, although rarely, solitary steatocystomas more than 8 cm have been reported. The cyst contains an oily, yellow fluid and may contain vellus hairs. Histologically, the cyst is lined by stratified squamous epithelium. Small, mature, sebaceous lobules are present along the cyst wall and empty into the cyst. The luminal surface of the cyst is eosinophilic, wavy (shark tooth pattern), and ribbon-like, analogous to the sebaceous duct. "Hybrid" cysts may have portions of their lining of the steatocystoma type, with the other portions resembling pilar cyst, epidermoid cyst, or even pilomatricoma. Simple excision is curative.

Sunohara M, et al: Two cases of steatocystoma simplex in infants. Dermatol Online J 2012; 18: 2.

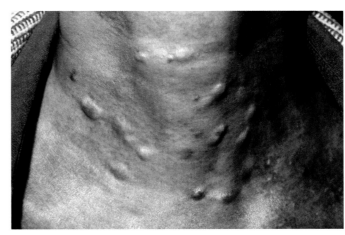

Fig. 29.55 Steatocystoma multiplex. (Courtesy Steven Binnick, MD.)

Steatocystoma Multiplex

Steatocystoma multiplex (SM) consists of multiple, uniform, yellowish, cystic papules usually 2–6 mm in diameter (Fig. 29.55), located principally on the upper anterior portion of the trunk, upper arms, axillae, and thighs. The lesions lack a punctum. The majority of patients present with dermal lesions, but multiple subcutaneous masses resembling multiple lipomas can occur. Lesions usually appear in adolescence or early adulthood, when sebaceous activity is at its peak. Development of SM can first occur in late adulthood. In severe cases, the lesions may be generalized, with sparing only of the palms and soles. At times the lesions may be limited to the face or scalp, a distinct form termed the *facial papular variant.* Lesions limited to the genital area have also been reported. Congenital and adolescent-onset linear lesions are rare. Steatocystoma may be larger (up to 2 cm) and prone to rupture and suppuration (steatocystoma multiplex suppurativum). If these lesions are widespread, the condition can be very disfiguring. Steatocystomas contain a syrup-like, yellowish, odorless, oily material. In the suppurative type, colonization with bacteria can occur, leading to foul odor and social isolation.

Histologically, the lining of the cyst is stratified squamous epithelium, with the cyst lining containing mature sebaceous glands. The epithelial lining is identical to the sebaceous duct. The luminal surface is wavy and eosinophilic and may stain with calretinin (perhaps only in the late-onset facial type). The granular layer is absent, but large basophilic granules may be seen focally in the epithelial cells in the upper layers of the cyst lining. In some cases, hair follicles occur in the cyst wall, and vellus hairs may be present in the cavity. A relationship with eruptive vellus hair cysts (EVHCs) has been suggested because of a similar clinical appearance, time of onset, and overlapping histologic features. It has been proposed that these clinical entities are a spectrum of the same disease process and should be classified as "multiple pilosebaceous cysts."

Often familial, SM demonstrates an autosomal dominant mode of inheritance. Sporadic cases, however, can occur. Keratin 17 missense mutations occur in familial (but not sporadic) SM, usually in a hypermutable site of exon 1 of the gene (the helix initiation motif). K17 is expressed in the nail bed, hair follicles, and sebaceous glands. This same genetic mutation also causes pachyonychia congenita type 2 (PC-2). Patients with PC-2 have milder keratoderma, but also natal teeth, pili torti, angular cheilosis, and hoarseness. These patients have multiple cysts, some of which are steatocystomas and some EVHCs. Milia, flexural abscesses identical to hidradenitis, and scrotal and vulvar cysts can also be seen in these kindreds. Hybrid cysts may occur. It is unclear why patients with hereditary SM and K17 mutations identical to those seen in PC-2 have no other stigmata of PC-2. Oligodontia and partial persistent primary dentition can be seen in some kindreds with SM and K17 mutations.

The definitive treatment of individual lesions is removal. This may be accomplished with small incisions and gentle extraction. However, the sheer number of the cysts usually precludes this type of treatment, and the location on the chest makes healing with cosmetically acceptable scars an issue. Laser incision of the cysts may also be effective. They may remain clinically improved for many months; however, eventual recurrence is the rule. Oral isotretinoin, 0.75–1 mg/kg/day, has been reported to benefit the suppurative variant of steatocystoma. Long-term follow-up has not been reported.

Bakkour W, Madan V: Carbon dioxide laser perforation and extirpation of steatocystoma multiplex. Dermatol Surg 2014; 40: 658.

Bridges AG, et al: Co-occurrence of steatocystoma multiplex, eruptive vellus hair cysts, and trichofolliculomas. Cutis 2017; 100: E23.

Choudhary S, et al: A modified surgical technique for steatocystoma multiplex. J Cutan Aesthet Surg 2010; 3: 25.

Hollmig T, Menter A: Familial coincidence of hidradenitis suppurativa and steatocystoma multiplex. Clin Exp Dermatol 2010; 34: e151.

Jain M, et al: Acral steatocystoma multiplex. Indian Dermatol Online J 2013; 4: 156.

Lee D, et al: Steatocystoma multiplex confined to the scalp with concurrent alopecia. Ann Dermatol 2011; 23: S258.

Moody MN, et al: 1450-nm Diode laser in combination with the 1550-nm fractionated erbium-doped fiber laser for the treatment of steatocystoma multiplex. Dermatol Surg 2012; 38: 1104.

Ofaiche J, et al: Familial pachyonychia congenita with steatocystoma multiplex and multiple abscesses of the scalp due to the *p.Asn92Ser* mutation in keratin 17. Br J Dermatol 2014; 171: 1565.

Papakonstantinou E, et al: Facial steatocystoma multiplex combined with eruptive vellus hair cysts. J Eur Acad Dermatol Venereol 2015; 29: 2051.

Park J, et al: Late onset localized steatocystoma multiplex of the vulva. Indian J Dermatol Venereol Leprol 2014; 80: 89.

Torchia D et al: Eruptive vellus hair cysts. Am J Clin Dermatol 2012; 13: 19.

Waldemer-Streyer RJ, et al: A tale of two cysts: steatocystoma multiplex and eruptive vellus hair cysts. Case Rep Dermatol Med 2017; 2017: 3861972.

Eruptive Vellus Hair Cysts

Eruptive vellus hair cysts (EVHCs) appear as multiple (up to hundreds), 1–4 mm, skin-colored or hyperpigmented, dome-shaped papules of the midchest and proximal upper extremities. They may be congenital but usually have their onset between ages 4 and 18 (in the first and second decades). Disseminated lesions have been reported. A unilateral distribution can occur. Facial lesions can be distinctly hyperpigmented and simulate a primary melanocytic disorder, such as nevus of Ota. The pinna of the ear may rarely be affected. Hidrotic and anhidrotic ectodermal dysplasia and Lowe syndrome have been associated with EVHC and familial cysts have been described with associated preauricular pits, lipomas, joint hypermobility, and cardiac defects. Onset in later adulthood with chronic renal failure has been reported in multiple cases. Clinically, EVHCs tend to be smaller than steatocystomas and may have an area of central hyperkeratosis or umbilication, a feature lacking in steatocystoma. Acne is distinguished by the lack of inflammatory lesions.

Histologically, the cystic epithelium is of the stratified squamous type; the cyst contents are composed of laminated keratin and multiple vellus hairs, and follicle-like invaginations may be present in the cyst wall. Steatocystoma may at times have vellus hairs, and EVHCs may have sebaceous glands in their lining. About 25% of EVHC lesions spontaneously resolve by transepidermal elimination. Topical tazarotene has been effective, but with no long-term follow-up. Similarly, lactic acid 12% and topical tretinoin can lead to improvement. Most treatments are surgical, including extraction, and CO_2 laser. Er:YAG laser is inferior to tazarotene and is associated with recurrence.

Helbig D, et al: Comparative treatment of multiple vellus hair cysts with the 2940 nm Er:YAG and 1540 nm Er:Glass laser. J Cosmet Laser Ther 2011; 13: 223.

Ponzo MG, et al: Case series: a kindred with eruptive vellus hair cysts and systemic features. J Cutan Med Surg 2017; 21: 564.

Torchia D, et al: Eruptive vellus hair cysts. Am J Clin Dermatol 2012; 13: 19.

Milia

Milia are keratinous cysts 1–4 mm in diameter (Fig. 29.56). They are white and easily seen as cystic through the overlying attenuated skin. Milia are common, and multiple clinical patterns of milia have been described. Milia can be considered primary, appearing spontaneously, or secondary, caused by trauma, skin disease, or medication.

Primary milia occur congenitally (or shortly after birth in preterm neonates) in up to 50% of newborns. They favor the face, especially the nose, scalp, upper trunk, and proximal extremities of all races and both genders. They resolve over weeks. Rare kindreds with an autosomal dominant inheritance have profuse, essentially confluent, congenital milia on the face. These also spontaneously resolve. Adults and children frequently develop milia, especially on the cheeks, eyelids, forehead, and genitalia. In infants, milia localized to the areola may be seen. These milia tend to persist. *Multiple eruptive milia* is a term applied to lesions that occur spontaneously in too large a number to be considered benign primary milia of children and adults. Cases favor the head and erupt over weeks to months. This can be idiopathic or familial. Nasal crease milia appear in a horizontal row in the nasal crease in nonatopic persons. Some cases are congenital. Pseudoacne of the nasal crease may be related. Milia en plaque describes a rare disorder characterized by an erythematous plaque containing numerous milia. These lesions are usually on the head and neck, especially the periauricular or periorbital regions. They are most

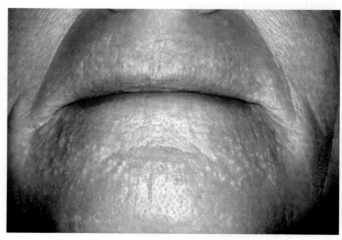

Fig. 29.56 Milia. (Courtesy Steven Binnick, MD.)

common in middle-aged women. One 3-year-old child had widespread depigmented macules and patches with numerous milia in the depigmented areas, termed *generalized milia with nevus depigmentosus.*

Secondary milia can develop as a result of blistering skin diseases, such as epidermolysis bullosa, pemphigus, bullous pemphigoid, porphyria cutanea tarda, herpes zoster, polymorphous light eruption, lupus erythematosus, Stevens-Johnson syndrome, contact dermatitis, and many other conditions. They also tend to occur after trauma, such as dermabrasion, chemical peel, ablative laser therapy, skin grafts, and radiotherapy. Long-term topical corticosteroid therapy and use of occlusive moisturizers may result in the appearance of milia. Cyclosporine and 5-FU have been associated with the development of milia.

Multiple milia have been reported in a number of genodermatoses, such as congenital ectodermal defect; reticular pigmented genodermatosis with milia (Naegeli-Franceschetti-Jadassohn syndrome); congenital absence of dermal ridges, syndactyly, and facial milia; generalized BFH syndrome; basal cell nevus syndrome; atrichia with papular lesions; pachyonychia congenita type 2; Rombo syndrome; Brooke-Spiegler syndrome; Loey-Pietz syndrome; and Bazex syndrome.

Primary milia are small epidermoid cysts, derived from the infundibulum of the vellus hair. As with epidermoid cysts, primary milia are fixed and persistent. Secondary milia may be derived from eccrine ducts or hair follicles as they attempt to reepithelialize eroded epidermis. They are often transient and spontaneously disappear. Milia must be distinguished from milia-like idiopathic calcinosis cutis, miliary osteomas, syringomas with milia-like structures, trichoepitheliomas, comedonal acne, flat warts, and xanthelasma. Lesions of cutaneous T-cell lymphoma with prominent follicular mucinosis may have many milia. Treatment is incision and expression of the contents with a beveled cutting tipped hypodermic needle, 11 blade, or comedo extractor. No anesthesia is needed for most patients. Topical tretinoin (Retin-A) has been reported effective in treating milia en plaque and more generalized forms of milia involving the face. Minocycline has also been used to treat milia en plaque.

Farmer W, et al: Eruptive milia during isotretinoin therapy. Pediatr Dermatol 2017; 34: 728.

Nambudiri VE, et al: Milia en plaque of the nose. Pediatrics 2014; 133: e1373.

Rutter KJ, Judge MR: Profuse congenital milia in a family. Pediatr Dermatol 2009; 26: 62.

Sambrano BL, et al: Eruptive milia secondary to vemurafenib. J Am Acad Dermatol 2013; 69: e258.

Voth H, Reinhard G: Periocular milia en plaque successfully treated by erbium:YAG laser ablation. J Cosmet Laser Ther 2011; 13: 35.

Verrucous Cysts (Cystic Papillomas)

Verrucous cysts resemble epidermoid cysts, except that the lining demonstrates papillomatosis and coarse hypergranulosis. Koilocytes may be present. On the sole, red granules resembling those in myrmecia are often seen. They have been shown to contain HPV and probably form as a result of HPV infection of a follicular unit or sweat duct (see Chapter 19).

Pseudocyst of the Auricle (Auricular Endochondral Pseudocyst)

Pseudocyst of the auricle presents as a fluctuant, tense, noninflammatory swelling on the upper half of the ear (Fig. 29.57). Most affected persons are between ages 20 and 45, and up to 90% are male. Pruritic disorders such as atopic dermatitis and systemic lymphoma, hard pillows in China, carrying heavy objects on the

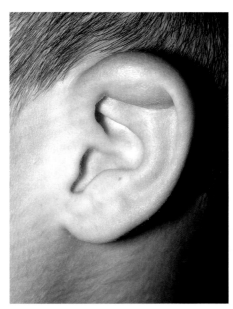

Fig. 29.57 Pseudocyst of the auricle.

shoulder, helmet and earphone wearing, and a slap to the side of the head have all been associated with auricular pseudocysts. This strongly suggests that trauma plays a role, although patients will frequently deny trauma. The fluid collection is between the two layers of the bilaminate cartilage of the pinna. There is no cyst lining, with the affected cartilage showing focal degeneration and granulation tissue. Needle aspiration yields serous or bloody fluid. Simple aspiration is ineffective. Aspiration or drainage, followed by the application of a bolster or pressure dressing for several weeks, is usually effective. Because application of pressure for several weeks is required, a sutured-on bolster with buttons or gauze is easier for the patient than an externally applied dressing. Intracystic injections of corticosteroids, fibrin glue, or minocycline have been used in recurrent cases. Surgical intervention involves removal of the inner anterior portion of the cyst.

Kallini JR, Cohen PR: Rugby injury–associated pseudocyst of the auricle. Dermatol Online J 2013; 19: 11.

Lee JY, et al: Successful treatment of a pseudocyst of the auricle using intralesional sodium tetradecyl sulfate injection. Dermatol Surg 2013; 39: 1938.

Patigaroo SA, et al: Clinical characteristics and comparative study of different modalities of treatment of pseudocyst pinna. Eur Arch Otorhinolaryngol 2012; 269: 1747.

Pusiol T, et al: Invasive squamous cell carcinoma arising from a human papillomavirus genotype 16–associated verrucous cyst. Int J Infect Dis 2010; 14: e378.

Wu MY, et al: Sandwich compression with rubbery tourniquet sheets and cotton balls for auricular pseudocyst. Laryngoscope 2017 Sep 20; ePub ahead of print.

Cutaneous Columnar Cysts

Five types of cyst that occur in the skin are lined by columnar epithelium, as described next.

Bronchogenic Cysts

These small, solitary cysts or sinuses are most often located in the region of the suprasternal notch or over the manubrium sterni. Bronchogenic cysts can also occur on the chin, neck, and abdominal wall. A scapular location is rarely described. Boys are affected four times more often than girls. Lesions are typically subcutaneous and rarely connect to deeper structures. Histologically, the cyst is composed of a wall lined by respiratory epithelium and may contain seromucinous glands and underlying fibromuscular connective tissue or cartilage. Gastric mucosa may also be seen.

Branchial Cleft Cysts

These present as cysts, sinuses, or skin tags along the anterior border of the sternocleidomastoid muscle or near the angle of the mandible. Branchial cysts are lined primarily with stratified squamous epithelium. Lymphoid follicles are often present, and smooth muscle is absent, distinguishing brachial cleft from bronchogenic cysts, although some evidence suggests that these cysts are related.

Thyroglossal Duct Cysts

Thyroglossal duct cysts virtually always occur on the anterior portion of the neck, near the hyoid bone. They present as a sinus, cyst, or recurrent abscess of the neck. Thyroglossal duct cysts are the most common cause of congenital neck anomalies in childhood. Presentation in adult life can occur. Malignancies (papillary adenocarcinoma, follicular adenocarcinoma, mixed papillary/follicular adenocarcinoma, adenocarcinoma, SCCs) arising from cysts have been reported in 1% of cases. Clinically, thyroglossal duct cysts are deep to subcutaneous tissue and usually are not managed by dermatologists.

Cutaneous Ciliated Cysts

Cutaneous ciliated cysts are usually solitary and located on the legs of females. Men account for only 10% of cases. These cysts have also been described in the perineum and vulva (vulvar ciliated cysts). The epithelium lining the cysts is cuboidal to columnar, with pseudostratified areas. Cilia are seen, and the lining cells stain strongly for dynein. This histology is similar to the normal fallopian tube, suggesting that the cysts are of müllerian origin. Ciliated metaplasia of the eccrine duct has been proposed for lesions occurring on the upper half of the body and in men. As with the median raphe cyst, the cavity is often filled with debris.

Median Raphe Cysts

Median raphe cysts of the penis are developmental defects lying in the ventral midline of the perineum from the anus to the urethra, most often on the distal shaft near the glans. They most frequently present as dermal lesions of less than 1 cm in young men and may appear suddenly after sexual intercourse–associated trauma. These cysts may appear as a cord or a series of beads (termed *canal-like*) (Fig. 29.58). They are lined by pseudostratified columnar epithelium with focal areas of mucin-secreting epithelium present. Ciliated cells may be present and, as with ciliated cysts in females, the cavity is typically filled with debris. Melanocytes may

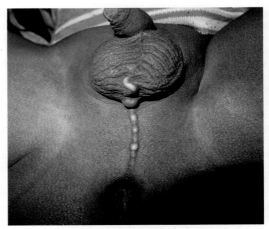

Fig. 29.58 Median raphe cyst. (Courtesy Steven Binnick, MD.)

occasionally be present in the cyst wall, giving the cysts a pigmented appearance. Median raphe cysts do not stain with human milk fat globulin 1, distinguishing them from apocrine cystadenomas. Median raphe cysts do not connect with the urethra and can be treated with surgical excision.

CONGENITAL PREAURICULAR FISTULA

This anomaly occurs as a pit in the preauricular region, often in several members and generations of a family. On each side, just anterior to the external ear, there is a small dimple, pore, or fistulous opening that may extend as far as the middle ear. Most congenital preauricular fistulas are benign and do not require surgery. Complications of surgery are common, and complete excision of both the pit and the sinus tract should be the goal if surgery is attempted.

Geller KA, et al: Thyroglossal duct cyst and sinuses. Int J Pediatr Otorhinolaryngol 2014; 78: 264.

Joehlin-Price AS, et al: PAX-8 expression in cutaneous ciliated cysts. Am J Dermatopathol 2014; 36: 167.

Kawaguchi Y, et al: Infected bronchogenic cyst treated with drainage followed by resection. Ann Thorac Surg 2014; 98: 332.

Krauel L, et al: Median raphe cysts of the perineum in children. Urology 2008; 71: 830.

LaCarrubba F, et al: Canal versus cysts of the penile median raphe. Pediatr Dermatol 2010; 27: 667.

Lee DK, et al: Efficacy of ethanol ablation for thyroglossal duct cyst. Ann Otol Rhinol Laryngol 2015; 124: 62.

Mattingly JK, et al: Cervical bronchogenic cysts. Am J Otolaryngol 2014; 35: 655.

Nishida H, et al: Pigmented median raphe cyst of the penis. J Cutan Pathol 2012; 39: 808.

Pastore V, Bartoli F: "Extended" Sistrunk procedure in the treatment of recurrent thyroglossal duct cysts. Int J Pediatr Otorhinolaryngol 2014; 78: 1534.

Proia G, et al: Papillary carcinoma on a thyroglossal duct cyst. Acta Otorhinolaryngol Ital 2014; 34: 215.

Reserva JL, et al: Cutaneous ciliated cyst of the scalp. Am J Dermatopathol 2014; 36: 679.

Thompson LD, et al: A clinicopathologic series of 685 thyroglossal duct remnant cysts. Head Neck Pathol 2016; 10: 465.

30 Melanocytic Nevi and Neoplasms

Melanocytes originate in the embryonal neural crest and migrate to the epidermis, dermis, leptomeninges, retina, mucous membrane epithelium, inner ear, cochlea, and vestibular system. Nevus cells are a form of melanocyte with a tendency to aggregate into clusters of cells. Nevus cells lack dendritic processes but are otherwise similar to other melanocytes.

EPIDERMAL MELANOCYTIC LESIONS

The melanocytes occurring at the dermoepidermal junction (DEJ) are dendritic cells that supply melanin to the skin. These cells contain pigment granules (melanosomes). Melanocytes stain with the dopa reaction and silver stains because they contain melanin. Immunohistochemical stains, such as S-100, HMB-45, MelanA/Mart-1, MITF, and SOX-10, do not depend on the presence of melanin. These stains have largely replaced silver stains for the identification of melanocytes in biopsy specimens. Melanocytes of the epidermis transfer melanosomes through their thin, dendritic processes, where they are actively taken up by keratinocytes. Melanocyte numbers vary by anatomic site and are increased in sun-damaged skin, but they vary little among racial groups. The type, number, size, dispersion, and degree of melanization of the melanosomes determine the pigmentation of the skin and hair.

Treatment of epidermal pigmented lesions can be directed at pigmented keratinocytes, melanocytes, or melanosomes. Q-switched (QS) lasers target the melanosome. Lasers with a longer pulse duration lasting milliseconds (ms) result in melanocyte destruction. Laser treatment produces consistent lightening of ephelides, but the response is variable for café au lait macules, Becker nevus, and nevus spilus.

Ephelis

The common freckle occurs in light-skinned individuals in response to sun exposure. Histologically, freckles demonstrate pigmented basilar keratinocytes, and a mild increase in the number of melanocytes.

Nevus Spilus

Nevus spilus (speckled lentiginous nevus) presents as a light-brown or tan macule, speckled with smaller, darker macules or papules (Fig. 30.1). It frequently occurs on the trunk and lower extremities, tends to follow Blaschko lines, and is noted in approximately 2% of the population. The nevus spilus may be small, measuring less than 1 cm in diameter, or may be quite large and follow a segmental distribution, referred to as a "zosteriform" lentigo. Multiple sites may be involved in the same individual and may be widely separated by normal skin. Happle has suggested dividing the entity into two forms, a macular type and a papular type. The dark speckles in the macular type are more evenly distributed and represent junctional lentiginous nevi; malignant melanoma has been reported more frequently in this type. Nevus spilus maculosus is consistently found in phakomatosis spilorosea, whereas nevus spilus papulosus demonstrates compound or intradermal nevi and is seen in phakomatosis pigmentokeratotica.

Nevus spilus in combination with a nevus flammeus is called phakomatosis pigmentovascularis (see Chapter 28). Phakomatosis pigmentokeratotica includes a speckled lentiginous nevus, organoid nevus, hemiatrophy, and neurologic findings such as muscular weakness. Generalized nevus spilus has been associated with nevus anemicus and primary lymphedema. Nevus spilus has also been reported in association with nevus depigmentosus and with bilateral nevus of Ito.

Histologically, the flat, tan background may show only basilar hyperpigmentation, such as is present in a café au lait spot, or lentiginous proliferation of the epidermis with bulbous rete ridges. The darker speckles usually contain nevus cells and may occasionally demonstrate blue nevi or Spitz nevi.

Melanoma may rarely occur in nevus spilus and some have given rise to multiple melanomas, suggesting a first-hit postzygotic mutation predisposing to melanoma in some cases. A changing lesion should be biopsied. Removal by QS ruby laser or QS alexandrite laser has been reported as effective but may require many sessions for acceptable results.

Boot-Bloemen MCT, et al: Melanoma in segmental naevus spilus. Acta Derm Venereol 2017; 97: 749.

Brito MH, et al: Synchronous melanomas arising within nevus spilus. An Bras Dermatol 2017; 92: 107.

Kar H, et al: Treatment of nevus spilus with Q switched Nd:YAG laser. Indian J Dermatol Venereol Leprol 2013; 79: 243.

Tavoloni Braga JC, et al: Early detection of melanoma arising within nevus spilus. J Am Acad Dermatol 2014; 70: e31.

Lentigo

Lentigo Simplex

These lesions occur as sharply defined, round to oval, brown or black macules. Lentigines usually arise in childhood but may appear at any age. There is no predilection for areas of sun exposure. Multiple lentigines may appear after clearing of plaques of psoriasis, including during biologic therapy. Histologically, lentigo simplex shows hyperpigmentation of basilar keratinocytes and an increase in the number of melanocytes in the basal layer. Melanophages are usually present in the upper dermis.

Solar Lentigo (Lentigo Senilis)

Solar lentigines are commonly known as "liver spots." They are persistent, benign, discrete, hyperpigmented, round to oval macules occurring on sun-damaged skin. The backs of the hands, cheeks, and forehead are favorite sites in the typical older patient. Red-haired, light-skinned individuals, especially those with high solar exposure, may develop many of these on the shoulders and central upper chest, even at an early age. Solar lentigines may be accompanied by depigmented macules, actinic purpura, and other chronic actinic degenerative changes in the skin. They may evolve into benign lichenoid keratoses and reticulated seborrheic keratoses.

Histologically, the rete ridges appear club shaped or show narrow, budlike extensions. There is a marked increase in pigmentation in the basal cell layer, especially at the tips of the bulbous rete. The number of melanocytes is slightly increased, and the upper dermis often contains melanophages.

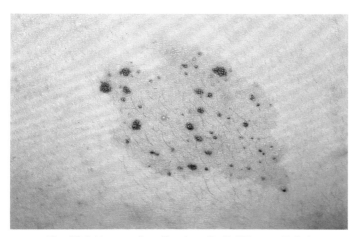

Fig. 30.1 Nevus spilus. (Courtesy Dr. Rui Tavares-Bello.)

Application of liquid nitrogen with a cotton-tipped applicator or cryospray unit is often an effective destructive modality. Argon, QS neodymium-yttrium-aluminum-garnet (Nd:YAG), frequency-doubled Nd:YAG, QS and long-pulse alexandrite, QS ruby, and Er:YAG lasers have been reported as effective. Intense pulsed light has also been used. Postinflammatory pigment alteration is the major complication seen with destructive modalities. Sun protection will reduce the number of new lesions. Bleaching creams containing 4% or 5% hydroquinone, used over several months, will induce temporary lightening. Hydroquinone-cyclodextrin (2%), 4-hydroxyanisole (4-HA), chemical peels, local dermabrasion, topical tretinoin, and adapalene are other treatment options. The combination of 2% 4-HA and 0.01% tretinoin is superior to either active component alone, and a commercial preparation containing these two ingredients plus 2% mequinol has been shown to lighten lesions.

Early lesions of lentigo maligna (melanoma in situ) may be light to medium brown and may mimic solar lentigines. Dermoscopy and confocal microscopy can improve diagnostic accuracy, but when in doubt, a biopsy is appropriate. Lentigo maligna, benign solar lentigo, and pigmented actinic keratosis all occur on sundamaged skin, and collision lesions are common. If a lesion is not homogeneous clinically, representative biopsies should be taken from each color or shade of brown within the lesion.

PUVA Lentigines

Individuals receiving oral methoxsalen photochemotherapy (psoralen plus ultraviolet A, PUVA), may develop persistent pigmented macules with possible melanocytic atypia. These lesions may occur on sites that are normally protected from sunlight. High-dose single exposures to radiation may result in similar radiation lentigines in exposed skin.

Ink Spot Lentigo (Sunburn Lentigo)

Sunburn lentigines typically occur on the shoulders as small, extremely irregular, reticulated, dark-gray to black macules resembling spots of ink on the skin. Histologically, there is a mild increase in the number of melanocytes and increased melanin in both the basilar keratinocytes and the stratum corneum.

Labial, Penile, and Vulvar Melanosis (Melanotic Macules, Mucosal Lentigines)

Melanotic macules are usually light brown on the oral labial mucosa but may be strikingly irregular and darkly pigmented in the genitalia (Fig. 30.2). In females, the labia minora are most often affected,

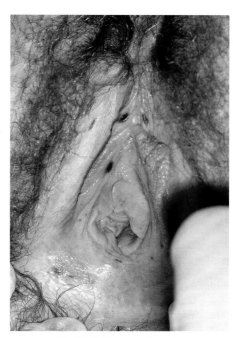

Fig. 30.2 Vulvar melanosis.

and in males, the glans and prepuce. Histologically, these lesions demonstrate broad, "boxcar" rete ridges with prominent basilar hyperpigmentation and a normal to slightly increased number of melanocytes. The melanocytes are usually morphologically normal.

Multiple Lentigines Syndrome

The lesions appear shortly after birth and develop a distinctive speckled appearance that has given rise to the designation LEOPARD syndrome. LEOPARD is Gorlin's mnemonic acronym for lentigines, electrocardiographic abnormalities, ocular hypertelorism, pulmonary stenosis, abnormalities of genitalia, retardation of growth, and deafness. Inheritance is autosomal dominant. Multiple lentigines occur mainly on the trunk, but other areas may also be involved, such as the palms and soles, buccal mucosa, genitalia, and scalp. *PTPN11* gene mutations are seen in both LEOPARD syndrome and Noonan syndrome. Café noir spots noted in these patients are larger and darker than café au lait spots. Histologically, some are melanocytic nevi, whereas others demonstrate histologic features of lentigo simplex.

Moynahan Syndrome

Moynahan syndrome consists of multiple lentigines, congenital mitral stenosis, dwarfism, genital hypoplasia, and mental deficiency.

Generalized Lentiginosis

An occasional patient will have generalized lentiginosis without associated abnormalities.

Centrofacial Lentiginosis

Centrofacial lentiginosis is characterized by lentigines on the nose and adjacent cheeks, variously associated with status dysraphicus, multiple skeletal anomalies, and central nervous system (CNS) disorders. Mucous membranes are spared. Onset is in the first years of life. Lentigines of the central face are also typical of Carney complex.

30

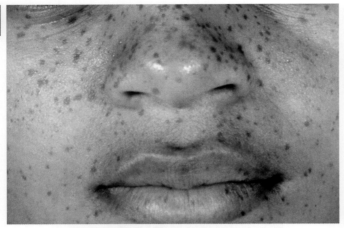

Fig. 30.3 Inherited patterned lentiginosis.

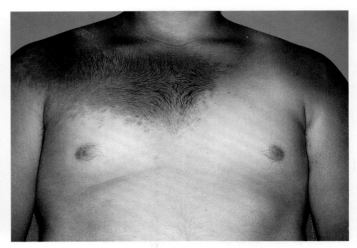

Fig. 30.4 Becker nevus.

Carney Complex

Carney complex is also known as NAME syndrome and LAMB syndrome. This designation comprises cardiocutaneous myxomas, lentigines, blue nevi, and endocrine abnormalities. It is discussed in more detail with myxomas in Chapter 28.

Inherited Patterned Lentiginosis

O'Neill and James reported 10 light-complexioned black patients with autosomal dominant lentigines beginning in infancy or early childhood, but no internal abnormalities (Fig. 30.3). The lentigines are distributed over the central face and lips, with variable involvement of the dorsal hands and feet, elbows, and buttocks. The mucous membranes are spared.

Partial Unilateral Lentiginosis

Partial unilateral lentiginosis is a rare disorder of cutaneous pigmentation characterized by the presence of multiple simple lentigines, wholly or partially involving half the body. Conjunctival involvement has been reported. Agminated lentiginosis appears to be a similar if not identical entity.

Peutz-Jeghers Syndrome

Peutz-Jeghers syndrome is an autosomal dominant syndrome consisting of pigmented macules on the lips, oral mucosa, and perioral and acral areas. Gastrointestinal polyps, especially prominent in the jejunum, are frequently associated. It is discussed further in Chapter 36.

Imhof L, et al: A prospective trial comparing Q-switched ruby laser and a triple combination skin-lightening cream in the treatment of solar lentigines. Dermatol Surg 2016; 42: 853.
Lv XP: Gastrointestinal tract cancers. Oncol Lett 2017; 13: 1499.
Raziee M, et al: Efficacy and safety of cryotherapy vs. trichloroacetic acid in the treatment of solar lentigo. J Eur Acad Dermatol Venereol 2008; 22: 316.
Vachiramon V, et al: Comparison of Q-switched Nd:YAG laser and fractional carbon dioxide laser for the treatment of solar lentigines in Asians. Lasers Surg Med 2016; 48: 354.

Becker Nevus

Becker nevus presents as a hyperpigmented, hypertrichotic patch on the upper trunk (Fig. 30.4) or proximal upper extremity. The lesion usually begins before puberty, and almost all patients are males. The lesion is typically associated with a smooth muscle hamartoma histologically. Usually, the lesion is asymptomatic and of little consequence, but some lesions have also been associated with connective tissue nevus, inflammatory linear verrucous epidermal nevus, basal cell carcinoma (BCC), phakomatosis pigmentovascularis, ipsilateral breast hypoplasia or abnormalities of underlying bone or of vascular, neural, or other soft tissue structures (Becker nevus syndrome). The pathogenesis may be related to postzygotic mutations in beta-actin and increased expression of androgen receptors within lesional skin. Treatment may not be necessary, but some patients desire removal of pigment or terminal hair associated with the lesion. Ablative 10,600-nm fractional laser and hair removal laser therapy have been used with partial success. Topical flutamide has also been used.

Cai ED, et al: Postzygotic mutations in beta-actin are associated with Becker's nevus and Becker's nevus syndrome. J Invest Dermatol 2017; 137: 1795.
Hernandez-Quiceno S, et al: Becker's nevus syndrome in a pediatric female patient. Case Rep Pediatr 2016; 2016: 3856518.
Momen S, et al: The use of lasers in Becker's naevus. J Cosmet Laser Ther 2016; 18: 188.
Patrizi A, et al: Clinical characteristics of Becker's nevus in children. Pediatr Dermatol 2012; 29: 571.
Taheri A, et al: Treatment of Becker nevus with topical flutamide. J Am Acad Dermatol 2013; 69: e147.

MELANOACANTHOMA

Cutaneous melanoacanthoma is an uncommon lesion first described by Bloch. Clinically, it resembles a pigmented seborrheic keratosis or pigmented BCC and tends to occur in older white men. Histologically, it is a benign epidermal neoplasm composed of keratinocytes and dendritic melanocytes. It is best considered a form of seborrheic keratosis. The starburst dermatoscopic appearance can be confused with that of Spitz nevus. Grouped and ulcerated lesions rarely occur.

Oral melanoacanthoma is also a proliferation of two cell types, melanocytes and epithelial cells, but appears to be a reactive lesion. It occurs as a macular or slightly raised pigmented area on the buccal mucosa, predominantly in young adult black women (Fig. 30.5). Rapid onset and spontaneous resolution are typical.

Cantudo-Sanagustín E, et al: Pathogenesis and clinicohistopathological characteristics of melanoacanthoma. J Clin Exp Dent 2016; 8: e327.

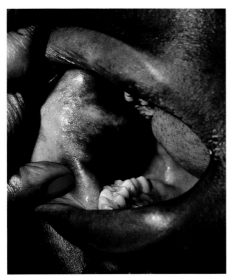

Fig. 30.5 Melanoacanthoma.

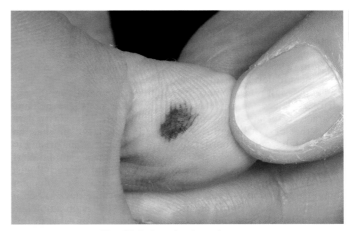

Fig. 30.6 Junctional acral nevus.

Chung E, et al: Clinical and dermoscopic features of cutaneous melanoacanthoma. JAMA Dermatol 2015; 151: 1129.

BENIGN MELANOCYTIC NEVI

Common moles, also known as nevocytic nevi or banal nevi, tend to increase in number during the first three decades of life. They are less common in doubly covered areas, such as the buttocks. They typically begin as sharply defined macular lesions, become papular, then gradually become soft and lose their pigment.

Sun exposure increases the number of moles in the exposed skin. Australians have more moles than Europeans. White persons have more than black persons, and individuals with a light complexion have more nevi than those with a dark complexion. Women have more total nevi and more nevi on the legs. Men have more on the trunk. Black persons have more nevi on the palms, soles, conjunctivae, and nail beds. A study of young British women showed an association of holidays overseas with an increased nevus count. The association was greatest in anatomic sites intermittently exposed to sunlight.

Eruptive nevi may occur in association with bullous diseases, severe sunburn, immunosuppression, or sulfur mustard gas exposure. The cheetah phenotype refers to patients with more than 100 uniform, dark-brown to black pigmented macules 4 mm or smaller. The evaluation of these patients can be challenging, because similar-appearing lesions range from junctional nevi to melanoma histologically.

Melanocytic lesions with a junctional component are more often removed during the summer months, whereas excision of intradermal nevi is relatively constant during the year. This suggests that some change in these lesions draws more attention during the summer months. Nevi may darken during pregnancy, but other changes should prompt consideration of a biopsy.

Clinical and Histologic Features

Features of benign nevi include a diameter of 6 mm or less, perfectly uniform pigmentation, flaccid epidermis, smooth, uniform border, and an unchanging size and color. Benign nevi tend to be round to oval and undergo a predictable course of maturation.

Junctional nevi are sharply circumscribed brown macules, varying in diameter from 1–6 mm. They usually appear between 3 and 18 years of age. During adolescence and adulthood, some become compound or intradermal. Small, well-nested junctional melanocytic proliferations are almost invariably benign. Benign junctional nevi associated with bulbous hyperplasia of the rete ridges are referred to as junctional lentiginous nevi. Lentigo maligna can appear well nested with an appearance similar to that of junctional lentiginous nevi. Any broad junctional melanocytic lesion on sun-damaged skin should be viewed with suspicion.

Compound nevi demonstrate both junctional and intradermal melanocytes. Benign compound nevi are well nested at the junction, with dispersion of individual melanocytes at the base of the lesion. They demonstrate bilateral symmetry but are not symmetric from top to bottom. Instead, with descent into the dermis, the melanocytes become smaller and spindled in appearance. Nests at the junction tend to be round to oval and are about equidistant from one another. Dermal nests are generally smaller than the junctional nests and become progressively smaller deeper in the dermis. Individual cells rather than nests are present at the base. Pigment is most prominent at the junction and becomes progressively less prominent deeper in the dermis. Intradermal nevi look similar to compound nevi, without the junctional nests.

In most benign nevi, there are no melanocytes above the DEJ. Individual melanocytes in a "buckshot" scatter throughout the epidermis are typical of superficial spreading melanoma. Sunburned benign nevi may also demonstrate buckshot intraepidermal scatter of melanocytes, and buckshot scatter may be seen in the central portion of acral nevi and Spitz nevi. Genital nevi often demonstrate large, poorly cohesive nests. They may also resemble dysplastic nevi histologically. A histologic resemblance to dysplastic nevi is also common in nevi from the scalp, ears, dorsal foot, and breast, even in patients with no other evidence of the dysplastic nevus syndrome.

On the palms and soles, the rete pattern follows the dermatoglyphs (Fig. 30.6). Nests in these locations tend to run along the rete ridges. If a benign palmar nevus is bisected across the dermatoglyphs, the nests will appear round to oval. If the same lesion is sectioned parallel to the dermatoglyphs, the nests will appear elongated and may mimic those of melanoma as an artifact of sectioning. Careful communication with the pathologist is essential when submitting an acral melanocytic lesion to the laboratory.

Malignant Degeneration

Almost half of melanomas occur in preexisting nevi, and an increased number of nevi represents a risk factor for melanoma. The signs of malignant transformation in pigmented nevi are recent enlargement, an irregular or scalloped border, asymmetry, changes or variegation in color (especially red, white, or blue), surface changes (scaling, erosion, oozing, crusting, ulceration, or bleeding), development of a palpable thickening, signs of inflammation, or the appearance of satellite pigmentation. Symptoms may include development of pain, itch, or tenderness. The "ugly duckling" sign refers to nevi in an individual generally tending to share a similar appearance. Any mole that does not share the same characteristics should be considered for biopsy. Moles with dark areas that do not lie entirely within the lesion, but produce an extension beyond the border, may represent melanoma arising in association with a preexisting nevus. The clinician should alert the pathologist to the presence of these areas and the pathologist should section through the appropriate area. Perifollicular hypopigmentation is a common finding in benign nevi. When it occurs at the edge of the nevus, it may give the lesion a notched appearance. Dermatoscopic examination may be of value in this setting. Lesions with changing clinical or dermatoscopic features should be biopsied.

Nevi frequently darken with pregnancy or with oral contraceptive use. Nevi from normal persons have no estrogen or progesterone receptors, but there may be positive estrogen receptor binding in nevi from pregnant women, as is also found in malignant melanoma. The development of what appears to be a new pigmented nevus in a patient over age 35 should alert the physician to possible melanoma, because patients without the dysplastic nevus syndrome usually do not develop new nevi at this age.

Treatment

Acquired nevi should be removed if they show signs of malignant transformation. Nevi of the neckline, beltline, or other areas that are irritated may be removed to relieve the patient of the irritation. Nevi may also be removed if they are in a location where it is impractical to observe them. If a solitary, darkly pigmented lesion is present on the oral or genital mucous membrane, a biopsy should be performed, because nevi are uncommon in these locations. Nail matrix nevi and lentigines produce a pigmented nail band. The proximal matrix gives rise to the dorsal nail plate, and the distal matrix gives rise to the ventral nail plate. When the nail is observed end-on, the level of the pigment may be evident and indicates the location of the pigmented lesion in the matrix. A widening band indicates a matrix lesion increasing in diameter. Biopsy of a solitary, expanding, acquired longitudinal pigmented band in an adult is typically necessary to ascertain the cause. Hutchinson's sign (pigmentation of the nailfold) is an indicator of melanoma. Nail matrix melanoma in children is exceptional.

Conjunctival nevi occur, and most can be followed serially if the lesion has been present since childhood or has shown no evidence of growth. Changing pigmented lesions and those acquired after childhood are best evaluated in conjunction with an ophthalmologist. Most conjunctival nevi occur on the bulbar conjunctiva and often about the nasal or temporal corneoscleral limbus. Suspicion of melanoma should arise if a pigmented lesion occurs in the palpebral or forniceal conjunctiva, if lesions are not hinged at the limbus and are immovable, if they extend into the cornea, if there is canalicular obstruction that leads to tearing, or if adjacent dilated vessels are noted.

Combined melanocytic nevi are common. They consist of a banal nevus together with a blue nevus, Spitz nevus, or deep penetrating nevus. Two or more distinct populations of melanocytes are evident.

Melanocytic nevi may occur in lymph nodes and are present in about 10% of sentinel node biopsies. Nodal nevi typically occur in the capsule, in contrast to melanoma metastases, which are typically subcapsular. Nodal nevi are frequently associated with cutaneous nevi in the draining basin, especially nevi with congenital features.

Pseudomelanoma (Recurrent Nevus)

Melanotic lesions clinically resembling a superficial spreading melanoma may occur at the site of a recent shave removal of a melanocytic nevus. Melanocytic nevi occurring in areas of lichen sclerosus or bullous disease often have similar features. On dermatoscopic examination, a regular network and the presence of streaks suggest reactive pigmentation. Any truly suspicious lesion should be removed. Histologically, the junctional component often demonstrates a predominance of nonnested melanocytes, confluence of nests, and nests that vary in size and shape. The presence of a superficial dermal scar with remnants of the original nevus beneath this zone of fibrosis is an important clue to the correct diagnosis. Although atypical in appearance, the junctional proliferation remains entirely confined to the area overlying the scar.

Recurrent Spitz nevus is a particular problem because many of the histologic features of benign Spitz nevi overlap with those of melanoma. In benign recurrent Spitz nevi, the dermal component typically retains cytologic maturation, dispersion at the base of the lesion, and an immunostaining pattern typical for benign nevi. Recurrent blue nevi also present special difficulties. High cellularity, cellular pleomorphism, mitotic figures, and a lymphoid host response may be present. In the absence of marked cytologic atypia, frequent mitotic figures or necrosis en masse, the lesions are likely to be benign. Because of the special problems posed by recurrent Spitz and blue nevi, the initial biopsy of these lesions should be a complete excisional biopsy whenever possible. Congenital nevi have a higher rate of recurrence when surgery is done at a younger age.

Balloon Cell Nevus

Clinically, balloon cell nevi are indistinguishable from ordinary nevi. Histologically, they are composed of large, pale, polyhedral balloon cells. Generally, foci of ordinary nevus cells are also evident. Rarely, the lesions are composed entirely of balloon cells. Balloon cell change has been reported in cellular blue nevus as well. Balloon cell melanoma does exist, but the nuclei are large and pleomorphic, and the architecture of the lesion is that of melanoma. Balloon cell nodal nevi may be seen in sentinel node specimens.

Halo Nevus

Halo nevus is also known as Sutton nevus, perinevoid vitiligo, and leukoderma acquisitum centrifugum. The lesions are characterized by a pigmented nevus with a surrounding depigmented zone (Fig. 30.7). Halo nevi tend to be multiple and occur most frequently

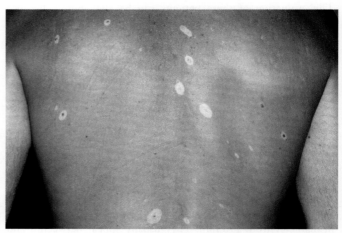

Fig. 30.7 Halo nevi. (Courtesy Steven Binnick, MD.)

on the trunk, mostly in teenagers. The central nevus gradually loses its pigmentation, turns pink, and then disappears, leaving a round to oval area of depigmentation. Over time, the area repigments. Darkening of the central nevus rather than lightening has also been reported in association with the halo phenomenon. Halo nevi have been reported during infliximab therapy. Target-like pigmented nevi present with the appearance of an inverse halo nevus phenomenon.

The infiltrate contains many cytotoxic T cells and may represent immunologically induced rejection. The peripheral blood has been shown to contain activated adhesive lymphocytes that disappear when the lesion is excised. Patients also demonstrate antibodies to melanocytes and cell-mediated immunity to melanoma cells. There may be associated vitiligo.

Regressing melanoma may also have associated leukoderma, but the pattern is usually haphazard and confined to the pigmented lesion. Other lesions that may also have a surrounding zone of leukoderma include blue nevi and neurofibromas.

Histologically, halo nevi demonstrate a band of lymphocytes that extends throughout the lesion, intimately mingling with the melanocytes. In contrast, the lymphoid infiltrate associated with melanoma tends to aggregate at the periphery of the lesion. In early halo nevi, amelanotic melanocytes may be found in the leukodermic halo. Later, melanocytes are absent until repigmentation occurs. A granulomatous infiltrate may rarely be present. The term Myerson's nevus has been applied to eczematous change associated with a nevus. Hypopigmentation may be present.

A full mucocutaneous examination at diagnosis is indicated to exclude a concurrent melanoma, but this is rarely found. The decision to remove the nevus at the center of the halo is based on its morphologic features, as with any other nevus.

Congenital Melanocytic Nevus

Giant Pigmented Nevus (Giant Hairy Nevus, Bathing Trunk Nevus)

Giant pigmented nevi appear as large, darkly pigmented hairy patches in which smaller, darker patches may be interspersed or present as small satellite lesions. The skin may be thickened and verrucous. The trunk is a favored site, especially the upper or lower parts of the back (Fig. 30.8). Giant hairy nevi are present at birth and grow proportionally with the body. Widespread congenital dermal nevus with large nodules may affect the entire body, including the palms, soles, and oral mucous membrane. Some congenital melanocytic nevi have associated placental infiltration by benign melanocytes.

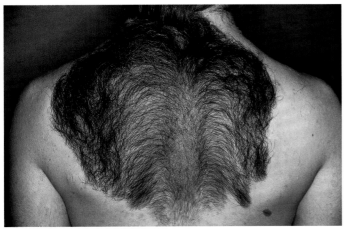

Fig. 30.8 Giant hairy nevus.

The incidence of melanomas developing in giant congenital pigmented nevi is between 2% and 15%. Approximately 60% of these melanomas appear within the first decade of life, and the majority arise in the dermis or subjacent tissue, rather than at the DEJ. About 40% of the malignant melanomas seen in children occur in large congenital nevi. The risk is greatest for axial lesions and those larger than 40 cm. In one study, 94% of large congenital nevi that gave rise to melanoma had satellite nevi.

Large axial lesions may be associated with neurocutaneous melanocytosis. The risk is greatest for large axial lesions with many satellite lesions, and almost half of patients with symptomatic neurocutaneous melanosis develop leptomeningeal melanoma. Neurocutaneous melanosis can be detected by magnetic resonance imaging (MRI).

Histologically, giant congenital nevi extend into the deep dermis and may involve the subcutis, fascia, muscle, and other underlying structures. Nevus cells are found in a patchy perivascular distribution and often extend in a patchy, single-file fashion between collagen bundles. Nests are often seen in association with adnexal structures or nerves. Extensive desmoplasia has been described. Estrogen and progesterone binding has been noted in congenital nevi. These receptors are generally absent from common acquired nevi.

Benign "proliferative" nodules within giant congenital nevi may be confused histologically with malignant change. Features useful in distinguishing the two include lack of high-grade atypia, lack of necrosis, rarity of mitoses, a lack of Ki-67 expression, evidence of transition between the cells of the nodule and those of the adjacent nevus, and lack of compressive expansile growth. Comparative genomic hybridization has demonstrated chromosomal aberrations in atypical nodular proliferations in congenital nevi, but many of these are numerical aberrations of whole chromosomes, suggesting a mitotic spindle defect. These differ from the chromosomal aberrations seen in melanoma.

Treatment decisions must be individualized. Half of all melanomas in giant congenital nevi occur in deep structures. Extensive surgery to remove the upper portions of the lesion reduces, but does not eliminate, the risk of melanoma. In patients with leptomeningeal melanosis, the risk of melanoma remains high. Satellite lesions and extremity lesions have a lower incidence of neoplastic conversion than large axial lesions, and the risk-benefit ratio of extensive surgery on these lesions differs accordingly. Some lesions are not amenable to excision because they involve functionally critical areas.

Serial staged excision is the method of choice whenever possible. Tissue expansion, cultured autologous cultured skin substitutes, and flap closure are especially useful in the head and neck region. Alternative approaches to treatment, such as dermabrasion, curettage, carbon dioxide (CO_2) laser ablation or treatment with QS Nd:YAG, ruby, and alexandrite lasers can lead to improvement in appearance. Therapy may also eliminate some nevus cells, with theoretic lowering of the melanoma risk. It is important to emphasize that most melanomas in giant congenital nevi occur in the dermal component rather than at the DEJ. Any treatment that alters the surface may alter detection of deep melanoma. Malignant transformation has been reported 20 years after dermabrasion. Regardless of the method of choice, lifelong periodic cutaneous examination and general medical evaluation are indicated.

Small and Medium-Sized Congenital Nevocytic Nevus

Small, congenital nevocytic nevi are generally defined as less than 2 cm in greatest diameter, and medium-sized lesions measure more than 2 cm but less than 20 cm. They are found in about 1% of newborns. About half eventually become hairy. Histologically, they share many features with giant congenital nevi but usually do not extend into the subcutaneous tissue. Many of the histologic features associated with congenital nevi also occur in acquired nevi. The risk of melanoma in small to medium-sized congenital nevi is extremely low; it may be no greater or only slightly greater than the risk of melanoma arising in ordinary acquired nevi. One important difference is that malignant degeneration may occur in the deep dermal component of small congenital nevi, rather than at the DEJ. Most of the melanomas that do occur do so after puberty. Excision is recommended for changing lesions and may be considered for those of cosmetic concern and in areas difficult to observe.

Green MC, et al: Management considerations for giant congenital melanocytic nevi in adults. Mil Med 2014; 179: e463.

Ma T, et al: Tissue expansion in the treatment of giant congenital melanocytic nevi of the upper extremity. Medicine (Baltimore) 2017; 96: e6358.

Mutti LA, et al: Giant congenital melanocytic nevi. An Bras Dermatol 2017; 92: 256. Vourc'h-Jourdain M, et al: Large congenital melanocytic nevi. J Am Acad Dermatol 2013; 68: 493.

Viana ACL, et al: A prospective study of patients with large congenital melanocytic nevi and the risk of melanoma. An Bras Dermatol 2017; 92: 200.

Spindle and Epithelioid Cell Nevus (Spitz Nevus)

Spitz nevi typically appear as pink, smooth-surfaced, raised, round, firm papules (Fig. 30.9). Most frequently, Spitz nevi occur during the first two decades of life, although they occur in adulthood in about one third of cases. Infrequently, multiple lesions present as agminate (clustered) (Fig. 30.10) or disseminated lesions in children and adults. Although they usually contain no visible pigment, some lesions are pigmented. Occasionally, Spitz nevi can be blue-black in color. A starburst pattern is characteristic on dermatoscopic examination. Although dermoscopy and confocal microscopy are being used in this setting, both false-positive and false-negative studies occur, and histologic examination remains the "gold standard" for evaluation of suspicious lesions.

As with other nevi, Spitz nevi may be junctional, compound, or intradermal. Compound nevi are most common and are characterized by compact hyperkeratosis, hypergranulosis, and pseudoepitheliomatous hyperplasia. The cells are large, with round to spindled nuclei. Epithelioid cells have large vesicular nuclei with prominent nucleoli and ample pink cytoplasm. Adjacent to the nucleus, the cytoplasm typically has a more amphophilic hue, giving it a characteristic two-tone appearance, similar to the cytoplasm of the cells in reticulohistiocytic granuloma. The nests tend to be oval and oriented in a vertical direction, as are the nuclei within the nests, so that they appear to be "raining down" the adjacent rete ridges. Clefts are typically present adjacent to some of the nests, and superficial vascular ectasia is characteristic. Dull-pink globules (Kamino bodies) are seen within the epidermis. These represent trapped basement membrane zone material and stain similar to collagen with a trichrome stain as well as with immunostains for type IV collagen. Buckshot scatter of melanocytes may be noted within the epidermis overlying the center of the lesion, but the lesion is sharply circumscribed, and cells disperse as individual units between collagen bundles at the base of the lesion. Rosette-like structures may occur. In a review of 349 Spitz nevi, the presence of epithelioid and spindled cells was the only feature present in 100% of cases. Other findings, in descending order, included maturation (72%), inflammatory infiltrate (70%), epidermal hyperplasia (66%), melanin (50%), telangiectasias (40%), Kamino bodies (34%), desmoplastic stroma (26%), mitosis (23%), pagetoid extension (13%), and hyalinization of the stroma (8%).

Melanomas may have many of the previous features, but generally lack Kamino bodies, and often demonstrate broad lateral extension, deep mitoses, and large nests at the base of the lesion. Cytologic features that favor a diagnosis of melanoma over Spitz nevus include pleomorphism, mitotic figures, notching of the nuclear envelope, and a peppered moth chromatin pattern. In questionable cases, adjunctive studies may be of value. S-100A6 shows strong and diffuse expression in Spitz nevi. Other melanocytic nevi often express S-100A6 weakly or not at all. Melanomas may express S-100A6, but the expression tends to be weak and patchy in the dermal component and is often negative in the junctional component. HMB-45 typically stains Spitz nevi in a top-heavy fashion, whereas melanomas stain uniformly top to bottom. MIB-1 (Ki-67), a proliferation marker, may also be helpful as an adjunct to the histopathologic diagnosis of Spitz nevi. MIB-1–positive nuclei are rare in the deep portion of a Spitz nevus, whereas they are often numerous in melanoma. Comparative genomic

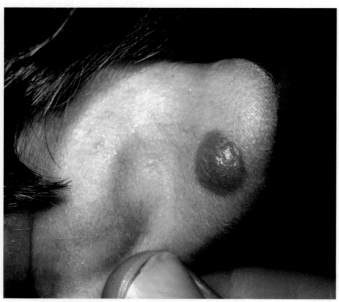

Fig. 30.9 Spitz nevus. (Courtesy Steven Binnick, MD.)

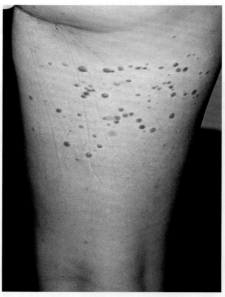

Fig. 30.10 Agminated Spitz nevi. (Courtesy Brooke Army Medical Center Teaching File.)

hybridization demonstrates chromosomal aberrations in the majority of melanomas, but most Spitz nevi show no aberrations. A minority of Spitz nevi show an isolated gain of chromosome 11p, the site of *HRAS*, but this aberration is not observed in melanoma. Specific gains or losses can be demonstrated with fluorescent in situ hybridization (FISH) probes. Studies of the mitogen-activated protein kinase (MAPK) pathway and genomic gains and losses may also prove helpful in this setting.

Junctional Spitz nevi usually show some degree of buckshot scatter of melanocytes and share many histologic features with melanoma. Lesions that lack sharp lateral circumscription are more likely to represent melanoma. Intradermal Spitz nevi lack overlying hyperkeratosis, hypergranulosis, or pseudoepitheliomatous hyperplasia, but the cells disperse as individual units at the deep margin. Dermal spitzoid lesions that remain nested at the deep margin are likely to represent melanoma. Desmoplastic Spitz nevi may be compound or intradermal, and are characterized by a dense, hypocellular collagenous stroma.

Pigmented spindle cell nevus is regarded by many as a variant of Spitz nevus. The lesions tend to be pigmented macules on the legs of young women. The cells are smaller and uniformly spindled, but other histologic features are similar to those of Spitz nevi. In contrast to Spitz nevi, they stain poorly with S-100A6. Desmoplastic Spitz nevi are moderately to strongly positive for p16, whereas most desmoplastic melanomas are negative, but studies have produced conflicting results regarding the usefulness of this antibody. Neuropilin-2 looks promising as an adjunctive study. Both Spitz nevi and spitzoid melanoma have a lower incidence of *BRAF* and *NRAS* mutations than common acquired nevi and conventional melanomas. *HRAS* mutations are typical of Spitz nevi but are rare to absent in spitzoid melanoma. *HRAS*-duplicated Spitz nevi are large, with large nuclei. *BAP1*-mutated nevi (Wiesner nevi) are composed of dermal nests of large epithelioid melanocytes with pleomorphism and lack of maturation, simulating melanoma. Immunoperoxidase staining for *BAP1* is negative, whereas staining for VE1 (V600E) *BRAF* mutation is positive. *BAP1* mutation is associated with the familial uveal melanoma syndrome, which includes large numbers of Wiesner nevi, mesothelioma, and renal cell carcinoma. *BAP1* mutation can also be seen in melanoma (especial blue nevus–like melanoma), so lack of *BAP1* staining alone is not sufficient to prove that the lesion is benign.

Although new molecular techniques may allow better differentiation, because of the histologic overlap with melanoma, the biopsy technique for suspected Spitz nevi should be complete excision whenever possible. Critical differentiating histologic features include sharp lateral circumscription and dispersion at the base of the lesion. An incomplete excision will fail to demonstrate either the lateral or the deep aspect of the tumor, and these diagnostic features will not be evident. When a lesion is incompletely excised, most authorities recommend reexcision of the site to ensure complete removal. At times, however, the dogma that all Spitz nevi should be completely excised must be tempered in the patient's best interest. An otherwise typical Spitz nevus that extends to the deep margin on a young child's nose may be difficult to excise without disfigurement. The risks of anesthesia must also be weighed against the likelihood that the lesion is anything but a benign Spitz nevus. Data suggest that children and teenagers with atypical spitzoid neoplasms and positive sentinel nodes have a less aggressive clinical course than those with unambiguous melanoma, but this may merely reflect mixed outcomes of benign and malignant lesions that were classified together.

Abboud J, et al: The diagnosis and management of the Spitz nevus in the pediatric population. Syst Rev 2017; 6: 81.

Busam KJ, et al: Multiple epithelioid Spitz nevi or tumors with loss of *BAP1* expression. JAMA Dermatol 2013; 149: 335.

Dika E, et al: Spitz nevi and other spitzoid neoplasms in children. Pediatr Dermatol 2017; 34: 25.

Gerami P, et al: Risk assessment for atypical spitzoid melanocytic neoplasms using FISH to identify chromosomal copy number aberrations. Am J Surg Pathol 2013; 37: 676.

Lott JP, et al: Clinical characteristics associated with Spitz nevi and spitzoid malignant melanomas. J Am Acad Dermatol 2014; 71: 1077.

Luo S, et al: Spitz nevi and other spitzoid lesions. Part I. J Am Acad Dermatol 2011; 65: 1073.

Luo S, et al: Spitz nevi and other spitzoid lesions. Part II. J Am Acad Dermatol 2011; 65: 1087.

Massi D, et al: Atypical Spitz tumors in patients younger than 18 years. J Am Acad Dermatol 2015; 72: 37.

Menezes FD, et al: Spitz tumors of the skin. Surg Pathol Clin 2017; 10: 281.

Urso C: On the nature of atypical Spitz tumors. Arch Pathol Lab Med 2016; 140: 1316.

Valdebran M, et al: Nuclear and cytoplasmic features in the diagnosis of banal nevi, Spitz nevi, and melanoma. J Am Acad Dermatol 2016; 75: 1032.

Atypical Nevus (Dysplastic Nevus, Clark Nevus)

In 1978 Clark et al. described families with unusual nevi and multiple inherited melanomas, a condition they referred to as the "B-K mole syndrome" (after Family B and Family K). About the same time, Lynch et al. recognized similar findings in other families and designated this the "familial atypical multiple mole–melanoma" (FAMM) syndrome. The most widely accepted term for the marker lesions is *dysplastic nevus*, with the patient's condition called the *dysplastic nevus syndrome* (DNS). The lesions may also be referred to as atypical nevi, Clark nevi, or nevi with architectural disorder. Patients with dysplastic nevi who have at least two blood relatives with dysplastic nevi and melanoma have the worst prognosis for development of melanoma. These individuals may have a 100% lifetime risk of melanoma. An associated increased risk of developing pancreatic carcinoma is present in some families. Some studies have indicated that ocular melanomas may occur in these patients.

The genetic basis for familial melanoma is being elucidated. One quarter to one third of patients have germline mutations on chromosome 9p in the *CDKN2A* tumor-suppressor gene (also known as *p16*, *MTS1*, and *p16INK4A*). It encodes for an inhibitor of a cyclin-dependent kinase 4 (CDK4), which functions to suppress proliferation. Patients with mutations that impair the function of the p16 suppressor protein, referred to as the p16M alleles, have a concomitant predisposition to pancreatic cancer. In other families in whom this is not present and who have 16W alleles, the predisposition to melanoma does not correlate with an elevated risk of pancreatic cancer. Mutations in the *CDK4* gene have also been found to be responsible for a lesser number of cases of familial melanomas. The products of this gene interact with the same cell growth cycle process as p16.

Moles with a histology similar to dysplastic nevi also occur frequently in patients without a personal or family history of melanoma, with 5%–20% of patients having at least one clinically dysplastic nevus, depending on the criteria used. During the growth phase, many nevi demonstrate junctional extension beyond the dermal component. This "shouldering" phenomenon is also one of the criteria for dysplastic nevi, and many growing nevi will have some histologic features of dysplastic nevi. The same is true for many congenital nevi, genital nevi, and those on the breast, dorsal foot, and scalp, none of which appears to be a marker for DNS.

Dysplastic nevi differ from common acquired nevi in several respects. Clinically, dysplastic nevi are characterized by a variegated tan, brown, and pink coloration, with the pink hues seen mainly in the macular portion of the nevus. A macular component is always present and may comprise the entire lesion but frequently surrounds a papular center. The nevi are larger than common

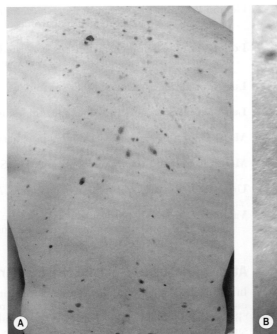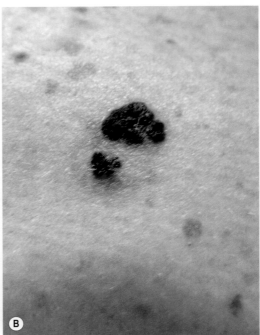

Fig. 30.11 (A) Dysplastic nevi, "ugly duckling" sign, left shoulder. (B) Close-up of left shoulder lesion, superficial spreading melanoma.

nevi, usually 5–12 mm in diameter (common nevi usually measure 6 mm or less). The shape of dysplastic nevi is often irregular, with indistinct borders. Atypical nevi are most often seen on the back (Fig. 30.11), and exposure to sun promotes the development of these lesions in individuals with DNS.

The lesions appear to be precursors for melanoma, as well as serving as a marker for an increased risk of de novo melanoma. Most of the melanomas that occur in these patients will arise in normal-appearing skin. Nuclear minichromosome maintenance protein expression is low in banal nevi (≈1%), higher in dysplastic nevi (≈6%), and highest in cutaneous melanomas (≈50% of cells). Survivin is present in 85.2% of dysplastic nevi. Criteria for histologic diagnosis of dysplastic nevi vary. The U.S. National Institutes for Health (NIH) consensus conference published the following as characteristic histologic features: basilar melanocytic hyperplasia with bulbous elongation of the rete ridges; spindle-shaped or epithelioid melanocytes arranged horizontally and aggregating in nests that fuse with adjacent rete ridges; lamellar and concentric superficial dermal fibrosis; and cytologic atypia (usually present but not essential for diagnosis). In compound dysplastic nevi, the junctional component generally extends at least three rete ridges beyond the dermal component. Grading of atypia is variable from one observer to another. Much of the atypia is focal and localized to the periphery (shoulder region) of the lesion. Atypia that extends throughout the lesion is more significant, and lesions with high-grade atypia may be difficult to distinguish from melanoma. Lesions with the architecture of a dysplastic (Clark) nevus but cytologic features of a Spitz nevus have been referred to as "spark" nevus (Spitz/Clark), "spastic" nevus (Spitz/dysplastic), or "ditz" (dysplastic/Spitz).

When a patient with clinically dysplastic nevi is seen, initial examination should include a total body inspection, including the scalp. A family history should be obtained with special attention paid to items such as moles, skin cancer, and melanoma. In general, excision of individual atypical nevi should be limited to those suspicious for melanoma. There should be prudent sun avoidance and sunscreen use. Patients should be educated in self-examination and encouraged to examine themselves monthly. Physician examination every year is also prudent. Baseline dermatologic photography may aid surveillance examinations. This is particularly helpful for detecting new lesions. Digital epiluminescence microscopic surveillance of atypical nevi may also be of value. Indications for removal of a lesion include an increase in diameter, focal enlargement, radial streaming, peripheral black dots, and clumping within the pigment network. Individual patients often demonstrate a consistent nevus phenotype clinically and on dermatoscopic examination. Lesions that differ from this "signature pattern" should generally be removed for histologic examination.

In patients with dysplastic nevi and a positive family or personal history of melanoma, physician examination every 3–6 months is recommended, with excision of nevi that change in clinical appearance and new lesions suspicious for melanoma.

Narrow excisional biopsies of dysplastic nevi often fail to remove the subclinical junctional component of the lesion. The pathologist is left to comment on a specimen with melanocytic atypia at a positive margin. When the lesions recur, they often appear atypical both clinically and histologically. Recurrent lesions may easily be misinterpreted as melanoma by someone unfamiliar with the preceding lesion. In general, the most appropriate biopsy technique for a dysplastic nevus is a broad saucerization that extends 0.5–2 mm beyond the clinically evident border of the lesion. After wound contraction, the added margin results in little difference in the appearance of the final scar, and the risk of a recurrent lesion is much lower. Especially on the upper shoulders and limb girdle area, saucerized biopsies often result in scars with a better appearance than those produced by suture closure. When faced with a positive lateral margin, it is best to reexcise lesions with high grade atypia. The reexcision may take the form of a wider saucerization. Lesions with low grade atypia may be observed.

Duffy K, et al: The dysplastic nevus. Part I. J Am Acad Dermatol 2012; 67: 1.e1.

Duffy K, et al: The dysplastic nevus. Part II. J Am Acad Dermatol 2012; 67: 19.e1.

Hiscox B, et al: Recurrence of moderately dysplastic nevi with positive histologic margins. J Am Acad Dermatol 2017; 76: 527.

Maghari A: Dysplastic (or atypical) nevi showing moderate or severe atypia with clear margins on the shave removal specimens are most likely completely excised. J Cutan Med Surg 2017; 21: 42.

Strazzula L, et al: The utility of re-excising mildly and moderately dysplastic nevi. J Am Acad Dermatol 2014; 71: 1071.

Epidermolysis Bullosa–Associated Nevus

Patients with epidermolysis bullosa (EB) may develop eruptive nevi and large, acquired melanocytic nevi with a clinical and dermoscopic appearance that resembles melanoma. Long-term follow-up suggests benign behavior. Biopsy findings with EB-associated nevus can be similar to those of a persistent/recurrent nevus.

Cash SH, et al: Epidermolysis bullosa nevus. Arch Dermatol 2007; 143: 1164.

Lattouf C, et al: Epidermolysis bullosa simplex, Dowling-Meara type with eruptive nevi. Int J Dermatol 2012; 51: 1094.

MELANOMA (MALIGNANT MELANOMA)

Except in the setting of giant congenital nevi, melanomas typically originate from melanocytes at the DEJ. Almost half will develop in preexisting nevi, but the rest will develop on previously normal-appearing skin. Usually, there is a prolonged, noninvasive, radially oriented growth phase in which the lesion enlarges asymmetrically. Eventually, a tumor nodule develops, reflecting a vertical growth phase. Although the presence of a vertical growth phase may represent an independent risk factor for metastasis, the single greatest risk factor is the depth of invasion.

The "ABCD" criteria for melanoma are imperfect but are simple for lay individuals to understand and have proved helpful for the detection of melanoma. The letters stand for asymmetry, border irregularity, color variegation, and a large diameter (>6 mm). Epiluminescence microscopy is a noninvasive technique for examining pigmented lesions that makes subsurface structures visible. In the hands of experienced users, it can be a helpful technique.

The incidence of melanoma has increased in light-skinned people. Melanoma is not usually encountered in the darker races, and acral lesions account for a greater share of melanomas in dark-skinned individuals. The lowest incidence is found among Asians. The incidence of melanoma is low until after puberty. Children rarely manifest congenital or acquired melanoma. Congenital melanoma may occur because of transplacental transmission from an affected mother, as a primary intrauterine lesion, as a melanoma that occurs on a congenital nevus in utero, or as prenatal metastatic lesions from neurocutaneous melanosis. All these have a poor prognosis. In children, melanomas occur at least half the time from preexisting normal skin, where the clues to diagnosis are the same as in adults, but recognition is often delayed because of the overall low incidence in the pediatric population. Melanomas may also develop in preexisting nevi, most importantly deep within giant congenital nevi.

During pregnancy, pigmented nevi often become uniformly darker and may enlarge symmetrically. Estrogen and progesterone receptors develop on the melanocytes, and these changes are likely to be hormonally induced. If, however, changes occur that would normally incite worry about melanoma, such as irregular pigmentation or asymmetric growth, a biopsy should be performed. Women who develop melanoma during pregnancy have a shorter disease-free interval after excision; however, there is no adverse survival effect.

Etiologic Factors

A light complexion, light eyes, blond or red hair, the occurrence of blistering sunburns in childhood, heavy freckling, and a tendency to tan poorly and sunburn easily indicate increased risk for melanoma. Large numbers of common nevi, the presence of large nevi, and the presence of clinically dysplastic lesions all increase the risk of melanoma. Axial giant congenital nevi or mutations in the p16 *CDK4* gene are potent risk factors. The risk of developing multiple primary melanomas is elevated if the patient has a family history of melanoma, has clinically or histologically atypical nevi, has more than 50 benign nevi, and does not use sunscreen. Sunscreens should be applied daily to sun-exposed areas, but must be used in conjunction with sun avoidance. Mutations of the *BRAF* gene are frequent in melanomas on nonchronically sun-exposed skin in Caucasians. Acral and mucosal lentiginous melanomas are associated with mutations of the *KIT* gene and amplifications of the gene for cyclin D1 or the *CDK4* gene. Amplifications of the gene for cyclin D1 are also detected in normal-looking melanocytes adjacent to these melanomas, suggesting field cancerization, as has been postulated for head and neck carcinomas in which early mutations impart a selective growth advantage, leading to expansion of the population of cells and creating a field of cells ripe for secondary mutations.

Other implicated factors include PUVA, tanning lamps, xeroderma pigmentosum, burn scars, and immunodeficiency. An association between administration of levodopa therapy for Parkinson disease and the onset of melanoma remains unproved.

Melanoma Types

Clinicopathologic types of melanoma include lentigo maligna, superficial spreading melanoma, acral-lentiginous melanoma, nodular melanoma, desmoplastic melanoma, mucosal melanoma, ocular melanoma, primary CNS melanoma, and primary soft tissue malignant melanoma. Clinically, melanomas may be pedunculated, polypoid, amelanotic, or hyperkeratotic. Some authors recognize animal-type melanoma as a distinct subtype. It resembles dendritic melanoma seen in horses and demonstrates low nuclear expression of glutathione *S*-transferase.

Lentigo Maligna (Lentiginous Melanoma on Sun-Damaged Skin)

Lentigo maligna begins as a tan macule that extends peripherally, with gradual, uneven darkening over years. It is more common in older patients with heavily sun-damaged skin and in sunny climates. It appears to be increasing in frequency, and some data suggest it is now the most common form of melanoma. The spread and darkening are usually so slow that the patient pays little attention to this insidious lesion. After a radial growth period of 5–20 years, a vertical growth phase of invasive melanoma can develop (Fig. 30.12). The lesion is then referred to as lentigo maligna melanoma. A palpable nodule within the original macular lesion is the best evidence that this has occurred, although there may be darkening or bleeding as well. Lentiginous types of melanoma also give rise to desmoplastic melanoma, which may appear as a papule, firm plaque, or inconspicuous area of induration.

The lentiginous melanomas (lentigo maligna and acral-lentiginous melanoma) proliferate principally at the DEJ, with little buckshot scatter into the overlying epidermis. Because the junctional involvement is often only one cell thick, lentiginous melanomas often extend laterally far beyond the clinically apparent margin. The lateral subclinical extension frequently exceeds the "standard" 5-mm margin for in situ melanoma, and asymmetric growth is common.

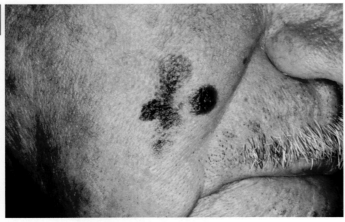

Fig. 30.12 Lentigo maligna melanoma.

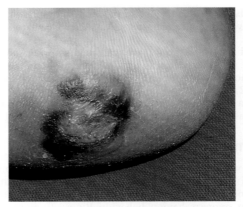

Fig. 30.14 Acral melanoma. (Courtesy Shyam Verma, MBBS, DVD.)

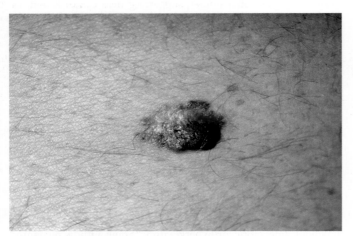

Fig. 30.13 Superficial spreading malignant melanoma.

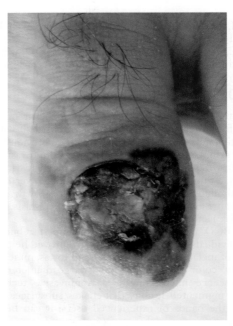

Fig. 30.15 Acral melanoma.

Superficial Spreading Melanoma

Superficially spreading melanoma once was the most common form of melanoma and affects adults of all ages, with the median age in the fifth decade. Unlike lentigo maligna, it occurs most often on intermittently exposed skin. The upper back in both genders and the legs in women are the most common sites. There is a tendency to multicoloration, not just with different shades of tan, but variegated black, red, brown, blue, and white (Fig. 30.13). Lesions may arise de novo or in association with a preexisting nevus. Areas of color change within a nevus, especially dark areas that extend beyond the border of the remainder of the lesion, are suspicious for melanoma arising in a nevus. As a vertical growth phase develops, a papule or nodule usually appears. Skin markings disappear as the lesion expands. Regression may appear as variation in pigmentation or a scalloped margin. The radial growth phase is characterized by buckshot scatter of melanocytes throughout the epidermis. Because of this, the borders tend to be more sharply defined than those of lentiginous types of melanoma.

Acral-Lentiginous Melanoma

Acral-lentiginous melanoma is the most common type of melanoma in dark-skinned and Asian populations. This is because the frequency of the other types is low in these patients, not because the incidence of acral-lentiginous melanoma is any higher than in white persons. The median age of patients is 50 years, with equal gender distribution. The most common site of melanoma in black persons is the foot, with 60% of patients having subungual or plantar lesions (Fig. 30.14). All lentiginous melanomas demonstrate a junctional growth pattern and tend to have indistinct margins. Over time, a vertical growth phase develops. Periungual hyperpigmentation and Hutchinson sign may be seen; a black discoloration of the proximal nailfold at the end of a pigmented streak (melanonychia striata) is an ominous sign suggesting melanoma in the matrix of the nail.

The early changes of acral-lentiginous melanoma may be light brown and uniformly pigmented. The thumb and hallux are more frequently involved than the other digits. In time, the lesion becomes darker and nodular and may ulcerate. Metastases to the epitrochlear and axillary nodes are common, because diagnosis is often delayed. Subungual melanoma (Fig. 30.15) may be misdiagnosed as onychomycosis, verruca vulgaris, chronic paronychia, subungual hyperkeratosis, pyogenic granuloma, Kaposi sarcoma, glomus tumor, or subungual hematoma. Nests in acral nevi tend to follow dermatoglyphs. If ink is applied to an acral melanocytic lesion and then wiped off (leaving ink in the furrows), the presence of pigment between the inked furrows suggests the possibility of melanoma. A biopsy demonstrating large dendritic melanocytes with dendrites that vary in diameter in an acral location suggests acral-lentiginous melanoma, even in the absence of irregular junctional nests or confluent melanocytic growth.

Mucosal Melanoma

Primary melanoma of the mucous membranes is rare and typically demonstrates a lentiginous (junctional) growth pattern. In the mouth, especially the palate, the lesion is usually pigmented and may be ulcerated. It may occur in the nasal mucosa as a polypoid tumor. On the lip, it is apt to be an indolent ulcer. Melanoma of the vulva is manifested by a tumor and is often ulcerated, with bleeding and pruritus. It is most often detected after metastasis to the groin has occurred.

Nodular Melanoma

These lesions arise without a clinically apparent radial growth phase, but usually, large atypical melanocytes can be found in the epidermis beyond the region of vertical growth. Primary dermal melanomas in congenital nevi are also nodular and lack a radial growth phase. Nodular melanoma constitutes about 15% of all melanomas. It occurs twice as often in men as in women, primarily on sun-exposed areas of the head, neck, and trunk. The tumors may be smooth and dome shaped, fungating, friable, or ulcerated. Bleeding is usually a late sign.

Polypoid Melanoma

This is a variant of nodular melanoma, presenting as a pedunculated tumor. At its base, the polypoid melanoma does not appear to descend for any appreciable distance into the dermis. Nevertheless, the 5-year survival rate is only 42%, compared with 57% for other nodular melanomas. The prognosis relates to the thickness (a measure of the volume of the tumor) and the presence of a vertical growth phase.

Desmoplastic Melanoma

This deeply infiltrating type of melanoma usually has a spindle cell pattern histologically in which collagen fibers extend between the tumor cells. Desmoplastic melanoma most often occurs on the head or neck of older men (Fig. 30.16), often within a subtle lentigo maligna. The lesions may also occur on the digits, in association with a subtle acral-lentiginous melanoma. One third of cases present with only a palpable dermal irregularity and are amelanotic. The biopsy demonstrates a spindle cell proliferation with a dense fibrous stroma. Atypia is variable. The lesions are typically neurotropic and demonstrate extensive growth along the perineurium beyond the bulk of the tumor. Nodular lymphoid

aggregates are frequently present and are an important clue to the diagnosis. S-100 protein and SOX-10 are the most reliable immunostains. HMB-45 and Mart-1 are usually negative. Pure desmoplastic melanomas have a low risk of metastasis, but hybrid tumors carry a much greater risk.

Amelanotic Melanoma

Nonpigmented melanoma differs from other melanomas only in its lack of pigment. The lesion is pink (Fig. 30.17), erythematous, or flesh colored, and often mimics BCC or granuloma pyogenicum. Amelanotic melanoma is the typical variant seen in albino persons. Dermatoscopic features may still be of diagnostic value, even in amelanotic melanomas.

Soft Tissue Melanoma and Clear Cell Sarcoma

Primary soft tissue melanoma is rare and distinguished from clear cell sarcoma by the presence of *BRAF* mutations and the absence of the characteristic t(12; 22)(q12; q12) translocation that is seen in clear cell sarcoma. As with melanoma, clear cell sarcoma contains melanosomes and stains positively for S-100 and HMB-45. It occurs most frequently on the lower extremities of young people. The average age at onset is 27. The history is of an enlarging, often painful mass on an extremity, with the foot or ankle involved 43% of the time. The tumors arise in and are bound to the aponeuroses, tendons, or fascia and only infrequently invade the overlying skin. Histologically, there are compact nests and fascicles of polygonal or fusiform cells, with a clear cytoplasm present between dense fibrous tissue septa that connect with tendinous or aponeurotic tissue. Multinucleated cells are common. Frequently, there are translocations of chromosomes 12 and 22. Metastases are often present at first diagnosis, and the prognosis is poor. Local recurrence or distant metastases after the initial excision are frequent and result in death in more than 50% of reported cases. Treatment is with wide excision and lymph node dissection. Radiotherapy and chemotherapy are used as an adjunct in some cases. The lesion appears to arise from neural crest cells.

Differential Diagnosis

Melanoma may clinically simulate a wide variety of lesions, including pigmented BCC, darkly pigmented seborrheic keratosis, pyogenic granuloma, and Kaposi sarcoma. Melanomas may appear pearly, may contain horn cysts, and may exhibit a collarette, and none of these is sufficient to forego a biopsy. Other melanoma-simulating

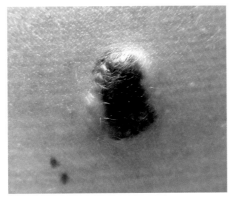

Fig. 30.16 Desmoplastic melanoma.

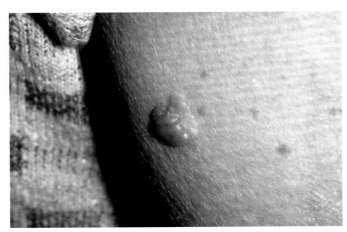

Fig. 30.17 Amelanotic melanoma.

lesions include subungual traumatic hematoma, cherry angioma, pigmented Bowen disease, and pigmented Paget disease.

Biopsy

Complete removal with a 1–3 mm margin of skin is the preferred method of biopsy for a lesion suspected to be melanoma. Saucerization technique is frequently used for macular lesions. Although the National Comprehensive Cancer Network (NCCN) recommends avoiding wider margins to permit accurate lymphatic mapping for sentinel node biopsy, some evidence suggests that accurate mapping is usually still possible even after wide excision.

In lesions too large for simple excision, an incisional or punch biopsy, deep enough to permit measurement of thickness, has no effect on prognosis. When melanoma is suspected in a giant pigmented nevus, an incisional biopsy should be performed. Biopsy of lentigo maligna is problematic because the lesions tend to be quite large and arise in cosmetically sensitive areas. Skip areas are common in these lesions and may lead to misdiagnosis. Areas of the tumor may undergo lichenoid regression and resemble benign lichenoid keratosis. Collision with other pigmented lesions, such as benign solar lentigo, pigmented large cell acanthoma, and pigmented actinic keratosis, is common. Because of the potential for sampling error, small biopsies frequently result in misdiagnosis. If the lesion is heterogeneous, multiple areas may need to be sampled.

Histopathology

Biopsies should be read by a dermatopathologist or other pathologist experienced in pigmented lesions. The report should include thickness and an assessment of the deep and peripheral margins. The presence of ulceration should be noted. Several studies demonstrate that concordance for assessment of Clark's level is poor, and reporting of Clark's level has largely been replaced by reporting of the mitotic rate. The presence of satellite metastasis is a powerful adverse prognostic indicator and should be noted in the report. Other factors that may be important to note include regression, tumor-infiltrating lymphocytes, vertical growth phase, angiolymphatic invasion, neurotropism, and histologic subtype.

Whereas benign nevi are well nested at the DEJ, melanomas usually demonstrate junctional areas where nonnested melanocytes predominate. Benign nevi demonstrate dispersion of individual melanocytes at the base of the lesion, whereas melanomas remain nested at the base. Melanomas are typically asymmetric, whereas metastatic and nodular melanomas may present as perfectly symmetric spheres. Benign nevi demonstrate bilateral symmetry and show maturation (smaller, more neuroid cells) with descent into the dermis. Most melanomas lack bilateral symmetry and show minimal maturation with descent into the dermis. In nevi, nests at the DEJ tend to be round to oval, situated at the tips and sides of rete ridges, and are about equidistant from one another. In melanoma, junctional nests are often elongated or have irregular shapes. They are randomly distributed and often involve the arches over the dermal papillae, as well as the tips and sites of the rete ridges. Confluent runs of melanocytes are frequently seen at the DEJ and often continue down the adnexal structures. In nevi, dermal nests are generally smaller than the junctional nests and become progressively smaller deeper in the dermis. In melanoma, dermal nests generally fail to become smaller in the deeper dermis. In nevi, pigment is most prominent at the junction and becomes progressively less prominent deeper in the dermis. Melanomas often retain pigment deep in the lesion. In superficial spreading melanoma, individual melanocytes are present in buckshot scatter throughout the epidermis. Lentiginous types of melanoma tend to proliferate at the DEJ with little associated buckshot scatter. Invasive melanoma is often associated with a lymphoid infiltrate that forms a band at the periphery of the lesion. Plasma cells may

be numerous. A vertical growth phase is identified by the presence of dermal mitoses, a dermal nest larger than the largest junctional nest, or invasion of the reticular dermis or solar elastotic band. Melanoma depth is measured from the granular layer or base of the ulcer. If invasion has occurred from follicular extension of the tumor, the lesion is measured from the inner root sheath. Rare variants of melanoma include balloon cell melanoma and dendritic "equine-type" or blue nevus–like melanoma.

Some types of benign nevus mimic individual features of melanoma. Sunburned nevi, acral nevi, and Spitz nevi may demonstrate buckshot intraepidermal scatter of melanocytes. Blue nevi typically are pigmented to the base of the lesion and extend into the dermis as a bulbous projection with minimal maturation and no dispersion of cells at the base. The silhouette, sclerotic stroma, and bland cytology are key to the diagnosis.

Comparative genomic hybridization has shown that chromosomal aberrations are common in melanoma. They occur earlier in the progression of acral melanoma than in melanomas on the trunk. In general, melanomas tend to have abnormalities involving chromosomes 9, 10, 7, and 6. Acral melanomas are more likely to have aberrations involving chromosomes 5p, 11q, 12q, and 15, and many amplifications are found at the cyclin D1 locus. Lentigo maligna melanomas are more likely to show losses of chromosomes 17p and 13q. Chromosomal aberrations are rare in benign banal nevi. A minority of Spitz nevi may show an isolated gain involving the entire short arm of chromosome 11. As individual gene mutations are defined, next generation sequencing will be used more widely to characterize histologically ambiguous lesions.

Metastasis

Early metastases typically occur by way of the lymphatic channels, and regional lymphadenopathy may be the first sign. Satellite metastases appear as pigmented nodules around the site of the excision (Fig. 30.18). Later, metastases occur through the bloodstream and may become widespread. The chief site for metastatic melanoma is the skin, but all other organs are at risk. CNS metastasis is the most common cause of death. Although most metastatic spread occurs in the first 5 years after diagnosis, late-onset metastases occur, especially in premenopausal women. Melanemia, melanuria, and cachexia are likely to occur in terminal disease. In extreme cases, the entire integument may become deeply pigmented (generalized melanosis), with melanin in melanophages, endothelial cells, and tissue histiocytes. Occasionally, patients present with metastatic melanoma from an unknown source. Full-body skin examination may reveal a depigmented or irregularly pigmented atrophic patch consistent with a regressed primary lesion. Such

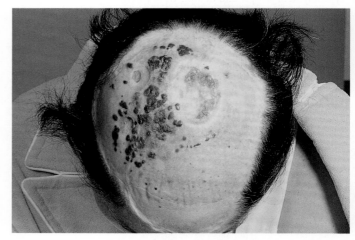

Fig. 30.18 Metastatic malignant melanoma.

BOX 30.1 Summary of American Joint Committee on Cancer Melanoma Staging

T0: No evidence of primary tumor ("melanoma of unknown primary" or completely regressed melanoma)

Tis: Melanoma in situ

pTx: Tumor thickness cannot be determined (tangential sectioning or the epidermis is not visualized.)

IMPORTANT NOTES ABOUT MEASURING TUMOR DEPTH

Tumor thickness is now recorded to the nearest 0.1 mm (instead of the nearest 0.01 mm).

Important pathologic staging implications:
0.75 mm–0.84 mm now recorded as 0.8 mm (pT1b)
0.95 mm–1.04 mm now recorded as 1.0 mm (pT1b)

Breslow thickness for pathologic staging includes the thickness measured in the biopsy or excision, whichever is deepest. (Per American Joint Committee on Cancer [AJCC], the two are not added, but the authors of this book recognize that the two depths added together may be a reasonable guide to therapy. Similarly, per AJCC, the depth of regression is not measured, but we believe this depth may be useful to clinicians. Per AJCC, the entire depth of a purely desmoplastic melanoma is measured, but we would caution that purely desmoplastic melanoma behaves differently from conventional melanoma with a lower risk of metastasis.)

If the biopsy is transected, Breslow thickness is recorded as "AT LEAST." The depth of an associated nevus is not measured.

T1: Up to 1.0 mm in thickness
 T1a: <0.8 mm without ulceration
 T1b: <0.8 mm with ulceration or
 • 0.8–1.0 mm

T2: 1.01–2.0 mm in thickness
 • T2a: No ulceration
 • T2b: Ulceration

T3: 2.01–4.0 mm in thickness
 • T3a: No ulceration
 • T3b: Ulceration

T4: >4.0 mm in thickness
 • T4a: No ulceration
 • T4b: Ulceration
 • pNXa At least one node detected *microscopically*

• pNXb At least one node detected *clinically* and others detected microscopically
• pNXc: Microsatellite, satellite, or in-transit metastases
 • Microsatellite: focus of metastatic melanoma detected microscopically, adjacent to or deep to the primary melanoma
 • Satellite: focus of metastatic melanoma in the skin or subcutis detected *clinically* within 2 cm but discontinuous from the primary tumor
 • In-transit metastasis: clinically evident metastasis in the skin or subcutis located >2 cm from the primary tumor

N0: No regional lymph node metastasis

N1: Metastasis in one lymph node
• N1a: Clinically occult
• N1b: Clinically apparent
• N1c: No regional node, but microsatellite, satellite, or in-transit metastases noted

N2: Two to three regional nodes or a node with microsatellite, satellite, or in-transit metastases
• N2a: All clinically occult
• N2b: At least one of the nodes clinically apparent

N2c: One node positive plus microsatellite, satellite, or in-transit metastases

N3: Four or more nodes, or microsatellite, satellite, or in-transit metastases with at least two positive nodes or matted nodes
• N3a: All clinically occult
• N3b: At least one of the nodes clinically apparent or any matted nodes
• N3c: Two or more positive nodes or any matted nodes plus microsatellite, satellite, or in-transit metastases

M0: No distant metastases

M1: Distant metastases
• M1a: Skin or nodes
• M1b: Lung
• M1c: All other non–central nervous system (CNS) sites
• M1c: CNS
• For each M designation, 0 indicates lactic acid dehydrogenase (LDH) is normal, 1 indicates elevated LDH

patients are estimated to have a 40% chance of 5-year survival. Estrogen receptors may play a role in melanoma progression and metastasis, with lower levels of expression of receptors in thicker lesions.

Staging

The American Joint Committee on Cancer (AJCC) developed a staging system for cutaneous melanoma. The system's categories depend on definitions for primary tumors, lymph node involvement, and distant metastases (Box 30.1; www.cancerstaging.net). The American Academy of Dermatology (AAD) guideline regarding management and follow-up of melanoma can be found at www.aad.org.

Prognosis

The prognosis for a patient with stage I melanoma is primarily related to tumor thickness. Cure rates by stage are as follows:

• Stage I (T1 or T2a, N0, M0): >80%
• Stage II (T2b–T4, N0, M0): 60%–80%
• Stage III (N1–N3, M0): 10%–60%
• Stage IV (M1): <10%

Many variables have been reported to influence survival, but some may not be independent variables, and those routinely reported in staging have changed over time:

• Presence of tumor-infiltrating lymphocytes; a brisk response is best.
• Mitotic rate; 0 is best, and >6/mm^2 is worst.
• Ulceration has an adverse effect.
• Location; hair-bearing limbs yield a better prognosis than when lesions are present on the trunk, head, neck, palm, or sole.
• Gender; women have a better prognosis than men.
• Age; younger patients have a better prognosis.
• Presence of leukoderma at distal sites improves the prognosis.
• Regression is associated with a poorer prognosis.

Multivariant analysis shows that some factors are not independently predictive and others are of variable significance in different series. Pregnancy does not have an adverse effect on survival in patients with clinically localized melanoma. Tumor thickness, ulceration, and lymph node involvement have the greatest predictive value and are used to determine therapy.

The presence or absence of melanoma in regional lymph nodes is the single most important prognostic factor for melanoma. Sentinel lymph node dissection using lymphoscintigraphy with

^{99m}Tc-labeled colloids is widely used for the staging of clinically node-negative melanomas. The success rate in localizing the sentinel lymph node approaches 98% at centers experienced in the technique. When combined with the vital blue dye technique, the success rate can approach 99%. About 20% of patients with melanoma between 1.5 and 4 mm in depth will have metastasis in their sentinel node(s). For desmoplastic and neurotropic melanoma (mean Breslow depth, 4.0 mm; median, 2.8 mm), published data suggest that up to 12% have at least one positive sentinel lymph node, although recent data suggest those with metastases are likely to be hybrid tumors rather than pure desmoplastic melanomas. Tumor thickness and ulceration are the major independent predictors of sentinel lymph node metastases. Age and axial tumor location are also significant. Patients with larger metastases to the sentinel node (metastatic deposits >2 mm in diameter) have significantly decreased survival.

Local recurrence related to a positive margin should not be equated with local recurrence representing dermal in-transit lymphatic metastasis. The latter is associated with a poor prognosis, whereas the former may be cured in many cases by reexcision.

Workup and Follow-Up

There is no definite proof that any routine laboratory work or imaging study affects longevity, and no routine laboratory or imaging studies should be done for stage 0 or 1a melanoma. Some advocate only ordering studies as prompted by signs or symptoms regardless of stage. Other guidelines recommend limited studies varying by stage. The AAD guideline states that baseline laboratory tests and imaging studies are generally not recommended in asymptomatic patients with a new diagnosis of primary melanoma regardless of thickness. It also notes that surveillance laboratory tests and imaging studies in asymptomatic patients have a low yield but are associated with relatively high false-positive rates.

A pelvic computed tomography (CT) scan should be performed in those with palpable inguinofemoral lymphadenopathy. The highest yield for CT scans is in the area adjacent to nodal disease. As glucose metabolism is increased in malignant tumors, positron emission tomography (PET) using the glucose analog fluorine-18-fluorodeoxyglucose (F18-FDG) can be used to detect metastases in patients with signs or symptoms. Although evidence supporting any routine imaging studies in the absence of signs or symptoms is scant, some authorities consider them for the first few years in patients with very-high-risk disease.

Periodic skin examinations are important to detect second primary tumors as well as metastatic disease. The AAD guideline notes that no clear data regarding follow-up interval exist but recommends at least annual history and physical examination, and that patient self-examination remains the most important means of detecting recurrent disease or a new primary melanoma. Because tumor recurrence occurs sooner in patients with thick melanomas than those with thin melanomas, some authors have suggested follow-up schedules based on AJCC staging, to include annual examinations for patients with stage I disease, examinations every 6 months for 2 years and then annually for those with stage IIa disease, and examinations every 4 months for 2 years, every 6 months in the third year, and annually thereafter for those with stage IIb to stage IIc disease. A palpable node is an indication for fine-needle aspiration (FNA).

Treatment

Early excision remains the most important determinant of outcome. Most published guidelines are based on data that relate largely to superficial spreading melanoma and may not be applicable to all melanomas. For any melanoma, simple complete excision should be performed. Wider margins reduce the risk of local recurrence, but scant evidence suggests that they affect mortality rate, which is more closely related to distant metastasis than to local/regional recurrence. A margin of 0.5 cm is currently recommended for excision of a melanoma in situ, although narrower margins may be performed in the interest of sparing vital tissue. A 1.0-cm margin is recommended for superficial spreading melanomas 1.0 mm or less in thickness, a 1–2 cm margin for those 2 mm or less, and a 2-cm margin for those thicker than 2.0 mm. In the case of lentigo maligna, mucosal, and acral-lentiginous melanoma, subclinical extension of the in situ tumor usually exceeds 0.5 cm, and asymmetric growth is common. In such cases, a symmetric "standard" margin may do a disservice to the patient. It may result in a positive lateral margin and difficult closure because excessive uninvolved skin was sacrificed. Mohs micrographic surgery may be useful in this setting. Although hematoxylin-eosin (H&E)–stained frozen sections have been used, immunostains such as MelanA, MITF, or SOX-10 are easier to interpret. Staged excision with permanent sections is another option. In patients who are poor surgical candidates or those with large lesions involving the face or genitalia, nonsurgical treatments such as topical imiquimod and radiotherapy may be useful alternatives. Nail apparatus melanoma may necessitate amputation of a digit or skin grafting. This is another setting where Mohs micrographic surgery may be considered as a tissue-sparing technique. It may also be helpful in the management of desmoplastic melanoma, especially when neurotropism is present.

Sentinel node biopsy (SNB) should be discussed with patients whose melanomas are 0.8–1 mm or greater in thickness. SNB should be considered for thinner lesions in patients who have ulceration, dermal mitosis, or other features of a vertical growth phase, Clark level IV or V invasion, regression, or a positive deep margin on initial biopsy. Dual-basin drainage from the trunk is not independently associated with an increased risk of nodal metastases, but each basin must be identified and sampled. Those with a positive SNB or nodal metastasis confirmed by FNA should receive counseling regarding dissection of the remainder of the nodal basin, but recent studies suggest that completion dissection may not be associated with a survival benefit. An analysis of SNB results in 422 Swedish patients with a mean thickness of 3.2 mm suggests that SN-negative patients have better disease-free survival (P <0.0001), but the false-negative rate may be as high as 14%.

Oncogenic mutations in *KIT* occur in mucosal and acral melanomas, as well as those on chronically sun-damaged skin. Imatinib may have a role in treating tumors in these sites. For other melanomas, targeted therapies include *BRAF* inhibitors that delay the progression of melanoma and immune checkpoint inhibitors that allow the immune system to destroy the tumor.

Ipilimumab blocks the CTLA-4 protein, reducing tumor tolerance. It has shown impressive results in a minority of patients with melanoma. Inhibitors of the programmed death-1 (PD-1) pathway, including nivolumab and pembrolizumab, are immune checkpoint inhibitors that are now widely used. The RAS-RAF-MEK-ERK pathway is a critical signal transduction pathway in melanoma, and alterations in this pathway, including *BRAF* and *NRAS* mutations, are important drivers of melanomagenesis. *BRAF* inhibition with vemurafenib can produce time-limited responses. The mechanism of action of vemurafenib involves selective inhibition of mutated-*BRAF* V600E kinase, leading to reduced signaling through the aberrant MAPK pathway. MEK inhibitors have potential in the treatment of advanced melanoma harboring other genetic mutations, such as *NRAS* and *GNAQ/GNA11*. *GNAQ/GNA11* with secondary BAP mutation is commonly noted in uveal and blue nevus–like melanoma.

Combinations of inhibitors have the potential to overcome tumor resistance. Side effects of therapy can be significant. Typical vemurafenib side effects include arthralgia, fatigue, alopecia, photosensitivity, pruritus, hand-foot syndrome, eruptive benign and malignant squamous proliferations, and panniculitis. PD-1 inhibitors have been associated with immunobullous disease, especially pemphigoid, and eruptive keratoacanthomas as well as cytopenias, diarrhea and nausea. For in-transit metastases, surgical excision, interferon (IFN), hyperthermic isolated limb perfusion with melphalan, CO_2 laser ablation, and intralesional bacille Calmette-Guérin (BCG) are used. Dinitrochlorobenzene in the setting of in-transit melanoma metastases has been reported to induce local remission but did not prevent metastatic lymph node and liver involvement. For stage IV disease, treatment options include resection, radiation, dacarbazine, temozolomide, interleukin-2, paclitaxel, and combination chemotherapy.

Adjuvant therapy should be discussed with patients who have positive nodes or node-negative melanoma that is 4 mm thick, ulcerated, or Clark's level IV or V. IFN alfa-2b is U.S. Food and Drug Administration (FDA) approved as adjuvant therapy. Although meta-analysis suggests that IFN therapy may increase relapse-free survival, an advantage for overall survival is uncertain. Systemic symptoms may require discontinuation of therapy in some patients, and lipodystrophy has been reported with IFN therapy. The results of trials have been mixed. Reports of long-term survival after resection of distant melanoma metastases suggest that cytoreductive surgery may play a role in select patients.

Clinical vaccine trials are ongoing, and some have shown promising results. However, despite numerous trials, only a few patients have been shown to exhibit strong antigen-specific cellular responses. CD137 is a promising target for immunotherapy. Antiangiogenic agents also show promise when used in combination with cytotoxic agents.

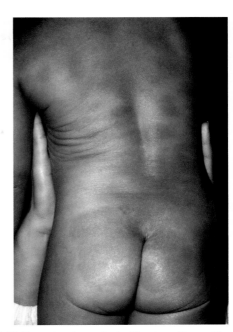

Fig. 30.19 Dermal melanocytosis. (Courtesy Steven Binnick, MD.)

Ali FR, et al: Integration of reflectance confocal microscopy into clinical practice for the management of lentigo maligna. Clin Exp Dermatol 2017; 42: 593.

Broussard L, et al: Melanoma Cell Death Mechanisms. Chonnam Med J. 2018 Sep;54(3):135-142. doi: 10.4068/cmj.2018.54.3.135. Epub 2018 Sep 27. Review. PubMed PMID: 30288368; PubMed Central PMCID: PMC6165917.

Carlson JA: On the cusp of a revolution: melanoma molecular diagnostics. J Am Acad Dermatol 2013; 69: 646.

Carlson JA, et al: Next-generation sequencing reveals pathway activations and new routes to targeted therapies in cutaneous metastatic melanoma. Am J Dermatopathol 2017; 39: 1.

Chiaravalloti AJ, et al: A deep look into thin melanomas: What's new for the clinician and the impact on the patient. Int J Womens Dermatol. 2018 Jun 11;4(3):119-121. doi: 10.1016/j.ijwd.2018.01.003. eCollection 2018 Sep. Review. PubMed PMID: 30175212; PubMed Central PMCID: PMC6116825.

da Silveira Nogueira Lima JP, et al: A systematic review and network meta-analysis of immunotherapy and targeted therapy for advanced melanoma. Cancer Med 2017; 6: 1143.

Dimitriou F, et al: The World of Melanoma: Epidemiologic, Genetic, and Anatomic Differences of Melanoma Across the Globe. Curr Oncol Rep. 2018 Sep 24;20(11):87. doi: 10.1007/s11912-018-0732-8. Review. PubMed PMID: 30250984.

DiSano JA, et al: Pregnancy after a melanoma diagnosis in women in the United States. J Surg Res. 2018 Nov;231:133-139. doi: 10.1016/j.jss.2018.05.026. Epub 2018 Jun 17. PubMed PMID: 30278920.

Ditto A, et al: Treatment of genital melanoma. Int J Gynecol Cancer 2017; 27: 1063.

Faries MB, et al: Completion dissection or observation for sentinel-node metastasis in melanoma. N Engl J Med 2017; 376: 2211.

Ito T, et al: Acral lentiginous melanoma. J Am Acad Dermatol 2015; 72: 71.

Lim SY, et al: Mechanisms and strategies to overcome resistance to molecularly targeted therapy for melanoma. Cancer 2017; 123: 2118.

PDQ Adult Treatment Editorial Board: Melanoma Treatment (PDQ®): Health Professional Version. 2018 Sep 28. PDQ Cancer Information Summaries [Internet]. Bethesda (MD): National Cancer Institute (US); 2002-. Available from http://www.ncbi.nlm.nih.gov/books/NBK66034/PubMed PMID: 26389469.

Rastrelli M, et al: Melanoma. In Vivo 2014; 28: 1005.

Reddy BY, et al: Somatic driver mutations in melanoma. Cancer 2017; 123: 2104.

Schadendorf D, et al: Melanoma. Lancet. 2018 Sep 15;392 (10151):971-984. doi: 10.1016/S0140-6736(18)31559-9. Review. PubMed PMID: 30238891.

Suzuki NM, et al: Histologic review of melanomas by pathologists trained in melanocytic lesions may change therapeutic approach in up to 41.9% of cases. An Bras Dermatol. 2018 Sep-Oct;93(5):752-754. doi: 10.1590/abd1806-4841.20187209. PubMed PMID: 30156634; PubMed Central PMCID: PMC6106672.

Trinidad CM, et al: Update on eighth edition American Joint Committee on Cancer classification for cutaneous melanoma and overview of potential pitfalls in histological examination of staging parameters. J Clin Pathol. 2018 Oct 1. pii: jclinpath-2018-205417. doi: 10.1136/jclinpath-2018-205417. [Epub ahead of print] PubMed PMID: 30275100.

DERMAL MELANOCYTIC LESIONS

Dermal Melanocytosis

This occurs as a bluish gray macule that varies in diameter from 2–8 cm. It occurs typically in the sacral region of the newborn, in 80%–90% of Asian, southern European, American black, and Native American persons. The Mayan Indians uniquely take great pride in it as an indicator of pure Mayan inheritance. It may be situated in other locations. Multiple spots may occur in a widespread distribution (Fig. 30.19), and overlapping spots have been described. These have been called generalized dermal melanocytosis or dermal melanocytic hamartomas. They may occur in phakomatosis pigmentovascularis types II, IV, and V and have been described in the setting of Sjögren-Larsson syndrome. Extensive mongolian spots have been associated with Hunter syndrome and trisomy 20 mosaicism.

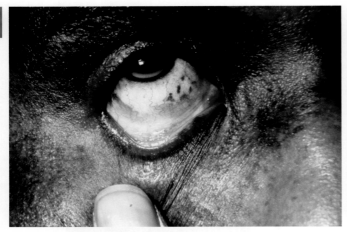

Fig. 30.20 Nevus of Ota.

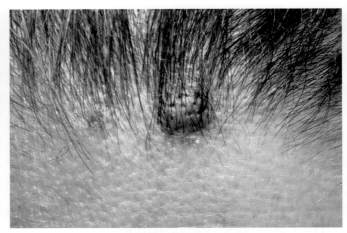

Fig. 30.21 Blue nevus.

Histologically, the mongolian spot shows elongated dendritic dermal melanocytes, widely scattered among normal collagen bundles in the deep dermis. It usually disappears during childhood, although rarely, it may persist into adulthood. Picosecond lasers as well as QS ruby and Nd:YAG lasers have been used to treat mongolian spots. Application of bleaching creams should be considered before treatment to reduce overlying pigmentation. The outcome of laser treatment tends to be better for lesions treated before age 20.

Nevus of Ota (Oculodermal Melanocytosis)

The nevus of Ota is also known as nevus fuscoceruleus ophthalmomaxillaris. It is usually present at birth in the two thirds of patients who have ocular involvement. Other lesions may not appear until the teen years. The conjunctiva and skin around the eye supplied by the first and second branch of the trigeminal nerve may be involved, as well as the sclera (Fig. 30.20), ocular muscles, retrobulbar fat, periosteum, and buccal mucosa. On the skin, brown, slate-gray, or blue-black macules slowly grow larger and deeper in color. Nevus of Ota persists throughout life; 80% occur in females, and 5% are bilateral. Glaucoma or ipsilateral sensorineural hypoacusia may also occasionally complicate nevus of Ota. Malignant melanoma rarely occurs, and malignant degeneration occurs more frequently in white patients. The most common site of malignancy is the choroid.

Histologically, elongated dendritic dermal melanocytes are seen scattered in the upper portion of the dermis. Acquired unilateral nevus of Ota–like macules are known as "sun nevus." Some express hormone receptors. Picosecond and QS lasers have been used successfully to treat nevus of Ota. Nd:YAG laser at 1064 nm is suitable for use in a wide range of skin types. Acquired dermal melanocytosis (acquired bilateral nevus of Ota–like macules or Hori nevus) is recalcitrant to laser therapy compared with nevus of Ota. Good results have been reported after treatment with QS ruby laser. Initial topical bleaching with 0.1% tretinoin and 5% hydroquinone ointment containing 7% lactic acid can be used to reduce epidermal melanin before laser treatment. Epidermal cooling has been advocated in the past, but some data suggest an increased incidence of hyperpigmentation with epidermal cooling. QS ruby laser has also been used after epidermal ablation using a scanned CO_2 laser. Lesions of phakomatosis pigmentovascularis have been treated successfully with QS ruby and alexandrite lasers, with flashlamp-pumped pulsed dye laser for the vascular component. Intense pulse light systems have been combined with the QS ruby laser for complex dyspigmentation among Asian patients. Fractional photothermolysis using a fractionated 1440-nm Nd:YAG laser has also been reported as successful.

Nevus of Ito

Also known as nevus fuscoceruleus acromiodeltoideus, the nevus of Ito has the same features as nevus of Ota, except that nevus of Ito occurs in the distribution of the posterior supraclavicular and lateral cutaneous brachial nerves, to involve the shoulder, side of the neck, and supraclavicular areas.

Kagami S, et al: Laser treatment of 26 Japanese patients with mongolian spots. Dermatol Surg 2008; 34: 1689.

Kouba DJ, et al: Nevus of Ota successfully treated by fractional photothermolysis using a fractionated 1440-nm Nd:YAG laser. Arch Dermatol 2008; 144: 156.

Ohshiro T, et al: Picosecond pulse duration laser treatment for dermal melanocytosis in Asians. Laser Ther 2016; 25: 99.

Blue Nevus

Blue nevi appear as well-defined blue papules or nodules (Fig. 30.21). Histologically, they share the silhouette of a bulbous finger-like or wedge-shaped protrusion into the dermis. All variants show minimal maturation and no dispersion of melanocytes in the deep portion of the lesion. All except epithelioid blue nevi and some cellular blue nevi are associated with a dense sclerotic stroma. They usually occur as combined nevi: combinations of various types of blue nevus, blue nevus combined with banal nevus, or blue nevus combined with Spitz nevus.

Blue Nevus of Jadassohn-Tiche (Common Blue Nevus, Nevus Ceruleus)

The typical lesion is a steel-blue papule or nodule that begins in early life. Some may be large and congenital. The slowly growing lesion is rarely more than 2–10 mm in diameter and occurs mostfrequently on the dorsal hands, feet, and face. Histologically, the lesion is composed of dendritic dermal melanocytes and melanophages. The sclerotic stroma is particularly prominent in this variant.

Cellular Blue Nevus

Usually, a cellular blue nevus is a large, firm, blue or blue-black nodule. It is most frequently seen on the buttock and sacrococcygeal region and occasionally is present at birth. Women have cellular blue nevus 2.5 times more often than men, and the average age of the patient seen with this lesion is 40 years. Infrequently, these lesions may invade underlying structures, such as the skull in scalp lesions. Occasionally, cellular blue nevi may occur on the eyelids.

Histologically, in addition to deeply pigmented melanophages, islands of cells are observed with large, fusiform vesicular nuclei, prominent nucleoli, and abundant pale cytoplasm. The cellular islands contain little or no pigment or stroma. Important diagnostic criteria for benign blue nevi include a low mitotic rate, absence of necrosis, low Ki-67–positive proliferative fraction, and uniform HMB-45 labeling. Cytologic atypia may be present in benign blue nevi, but mitotic figures should not be seen. Such "ancient" blue nevi frequently demonstrate edematous stromal areas and hyaline changes in vessels, suggesting a degenerative phenomenon.

Epithelioid Blue Nevus

Epithelioid blue nevi are mostly seen in patients with the Carney complex (myxomas, spotty skin pigmentation, endocrine overactivity, and schwannomas). They occur on the extremities and trunk and less frequently on the head and neck. They may also be noted in the absence of Carney complex and may occur on the genital mucosa. The lesions are composed of large polygonal and epithelioid melanocytes often laden with melanin. These cells are admixed with heavily pigmented dendritic melanocytes, spindled melanocytes, and melanophages. Some melanocytes are situated among the dermal collagen bundles singly, in short rows, and small groups. The nuclei are vesicular with very pale chromatin and a single, prominent nucleolus. They may demonstrate moderate pleomorphism and rare mitotic figures. In contrast to other blue nevi, they lack the usual sclerotic stroma. Some authors have grouped epithelioid blue nevi with dendritic (equine-type) and epithelioid melanomas under the designation "pigmented epithelioid melanocytoma," which they regard as a borderline malignancy or low-grade melanoma. One problem with this designation is the lack of data suggesting that the lesions in patients with the Carney complex behave in a malignant manner. More than 50% of patients with Carney complex harbor mutations in the protein kinase A regulatory subunit 1α *(PRKAR1A)* gene, and the protein kinase is absent in the associated epithelioid blue nevi. Some evidence suggests that molecular studies could be useful to classify these lesions more accurately in regard to biologic behavior. Loss of BAP-1 is common as a late event in the pathogenesis of blue nevus–like melanoma, and can be determined via routine immunohistochemistry.

Deep Penetrating Nevus

This unique type of nevus is frequently seen in combination with other forms of blue nevus. The fascicles of cells have small,

hyperchromatic nuclei with a smudged chromatin pattern and inconspicuous nucleoli. Adjacent melanophages are noted with deep penetrating nevus.

Amelanotic Blue Nevus (Hypomelanotic Blue Nevus, "Gray Nevus")

In the amelanotic or hypomelanotic variant of cellular blue nevus, mild cytologic atypia and pleomorphism may be present. Mitotic activity (up to 3 mitoses/mm) may also be observed. It is important to recognize the amelanotic blue nevus so as not to confuse it with a malignant lesion.

Malignant Blue Nevus

The term *malignant blue nevus* has been used to refer to melanomas arising in a blue nevus, usually a cellular blue nevus. It has also been used for de novo melanoma resembling a cellular blue nevus. The term *blue nevus–like melanoma* may be a better descriptor. When melanoma occurs in a blue nevus, an abrupt transition can be seen between the nevus and the melanoma. The melanoma demonstrates a sheetlike growth pattern, mitoses, necrosis, and nuclear atypia.

Treatment

Excision is the mainstay of treatment for blue nevi. Successful results have been reported with the QS ruby laser. Treatment of the malignant variety is the same as for a malignant melanoma. Intratumoral therapy with IFN beta has also been used.

Bax MJ, et al: Pigmented epithelioid melanocytoma (animal type melanoma). J Am Acad Dermatol 2017; 77: 328.

Borgenvik TL, et al: Blue nevus-like and blue nevus-associated melanoma. ANZ J Surg 2017; 87: 345.

Gavriilidis P, et al: Pigmented epithelioid melanocytoma. BMJ Case Rep 2013 Mar 22; 2013.

Murali R, et al: Blue nevi and related lesions. Adv Anat Pathol 2009; 16: 365.

31 Macrophage/Monocyte Disorders

Granulomatous reactions generally represent patterns of chronic inflammation that may take a long time to develop and a long time to respond to treatment. Granulomatous inflammation can occur in the setting of inflammatory disorders (autoimmune, autoinflammatory), medication reactions, malignancies, and infections.

PALISADED GRANULOMATOUS DERMATOSES

Granuloma Annulare

Granuloma annulare (GA) is a relatively common idiopathic disorder of the dermis and subcutaneous tissue. It occurs in all races and at all ages but affects women twice as often as men. Most cases spontaneously resolve, leaving entirely normal skin, but loss of elastic tissue may occur, leaving atrophic lesions resembling middermal elastolysis or anetoderma. Long-term follow-up of at least 20 years in patients with GA reveals that lesions usually heal, and that the patients remain healthy and do not develop unusual diseases. GA may recur in a significant subset of patients, particularly with generalized lesions. GA may exhibit the isomorphic response of Koebner, may affect healed areas of herpes zoster, and may be restricted to sun-exposed areas. GA lesions will sometimes spontaneously resolve when biopsied. Case reports and retrospective reviews of associations demonstrate that GA can be a reactive condition associated with a variety of underlying disorders and medications. In most patients, however, GA is a benign, self-limited condition affecting only the skin. Variants in the GA spectrum have been subdivided with distinct names based on clinical morphologic patterns or specific histologic features, and some suggest these variants warrant consideration as separate entities.

Many morphologies of GA exist, though the vast majority of patients have localized disease, a subset have generalized disease, and children may have subcutaneous lesions. Other clinical morphologies are rare. Usually, patients exhibit primarily one clinical type during the course of their illness, except in the subcutaneous form, in which typical papular or localized GA may also occur.

Localized Granuloma Annulare

The localized form of GA tends to affect children and young to middle-aged adults. Usually, only one or a few lesions are present at any one time. Localized GA usually appears on the lateral or dorsal surfaces of the fingers or hands or dorsal feet, and occasionally on the elbows or ankles (Figs. 31.1 to 31.3). Rarely, other sites, such as the eyelid or even a Becker nevus, may be affected. Lesions are erythematous to violaceous, thinly bordered plaques or papules that slowly spread peripherally while undergoing central involution, so that roughly annular lesions are formed. The overlying skin usually remains completely normal. Lesions may coalesce and sometimes form scalloped patterns or firm plaques. The lesions never ulcerate and on resolving, virtually always leave no residua. They develop slowly and often involute spontaneously. Although more than 50% of patients clear within 2 years, lesions will recur in 40%. Data regarding disease associations are limited to small series, but autoimmune thyroiditis has been described women

with localized GA, though it is unclear if there is a disease-specific relationship or if both entities are simply more common in women of a particular demographic.

Generalized Granuloma Annulare

Although both disseminated and generalized GA have been described, many use the terms interchangeably. Originally, disseminated GA described patients with more than 10 lesions, and generalized GA described patients with multiple lesions involving the trunk and upper/lower extremities. Some now use *disseminated* if patients have predominantly papular lesions and *generalized* if patients have multiple annular plaques. These distinctions are based on very small case series and the prognostic, treatment, or histopathologic significance is unclear. Generalized GA affects mostly women in the fifth and sixth decades but is also a common pattern in adolescents and children. The association of generalized GA with diabetes mellitus has been questioned, although in some childhood cases diabetes and GA appeared at the same time. Similarly, dyslipidemia (elevated cholesterol, triglycerides, or low density lipoprotein (LDL) cholesterol) has been reported with generalized GA. The eruption of generalized GA presents as a diffuse but symmetric, papular or annular eruption. Lesions may number in the hundreds. Lesions favor the nape of the neck, upper trunk, and proximal extremities and rarely exceed 5 cm in diameter (Fig. 31.4). The palms, soles, and eyelids may be affected. The face and genital area are usually spared. In occasional cases, sun exposure seems to be a trigger (see actinic granuloma later, under Annular Elastolytic Giant Cell Granuloma). Some patients are completely asymptomatic, whereas others complain of pruritus. Spontaneous clearing usually occurs but at variable times, and relapses may occur after clearance. The average duration is 3 to 4 years but may be as short as 4 months or longer than 10 years.

Patch-Type or Macular Granuloma Annulare

Macular GA is significantly more common in women, usually at age 30–70. Flat or only slightly palpable erythematous or red-brown lesions occur, especially on the upper medial thighs and in bathing-trunk distribution. Individual lesions average at least several centimeters in diameter but may be much larger. On careful palpation, small papules can be felt in some patients, and on stretching the skin the papules or small annular lesions can be seen.

Subcutaneous Granuloma Annulare (Deep Granuloma Annulare, Pseudorheumatoid Nodule)

Subcutaneous GA is most common in children, with boys affected twice as frequently as girls. Childhood cases appear at any age from 1 year to adolescence, with one congenital case reported. Lesions tend to occur on the lower legs, especially the dorsal foot, but may also occur on the distal upper extremity or scalp. Multiple lesions are usually present. There is often a history of trauma to the affected area preceding the appearance of a lesion. Typically, lesions are skin-colored, deep dermal or subcutaneous nodules up to several centimeters in diameter (Fig. 31.5). Superficial papular lesions are present in about one quarter of patients with subcutaneous GA. Lesions in general are asymptomatic and resolve over a few years. The major clinical problem occurs when the initial

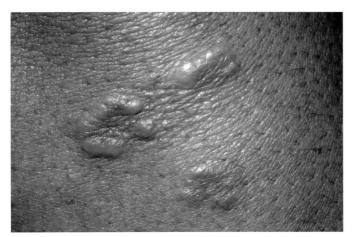

Fig. 31.1 Granuloma annulare.

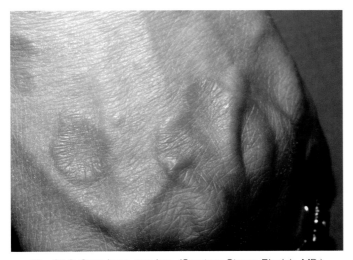

Fig. 31.2 Granuloma annulare. (Courtesy Steven Binnick, MD.)

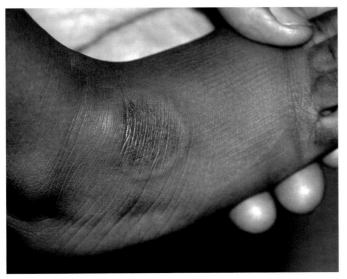

Fig. 31.3 Granuloma annulare. (Courtesy Paul Honig, MD.)

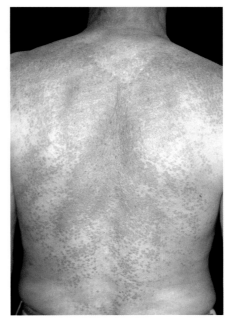

Fig. 31.4 Disseminated granuloma annulare.

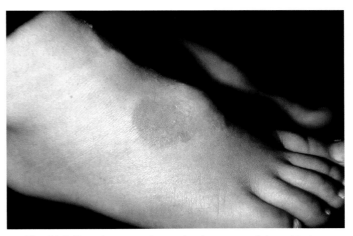

Fig. 31.5 Granuloma annulare, subcutaneous and dermal lesion.

pathologic interpretation is "rheumatoid nodule" and an unnecessary extensive rheumatologic workup is performed. An unusual variant remains localized to the penis or scrotum, an atypical location for GA in general. Adult women without rheumatoid arthritis may develop similar lesions around the joints.

Perforating Granuloma Annulare

Perforating GA usually appears on the dorsal hands and presents as papules with a central keratotic core (Fig. 31.6). This core represents transepidermal elimination of the degenerated material in the center of GA lesions and clinically can resemble a pustule. It has been suggested that in patients with atypical forms of GA it may be prudent to evaluate for underlying hematologic dyscrasia.

Palmar Granuloma Annulare/Acute-Onset Painful Acral Granuloma Annulare

This clinical variant of GA does not resemble other forms of the disease, and the diagnosis is often missed clinically. Palmar or

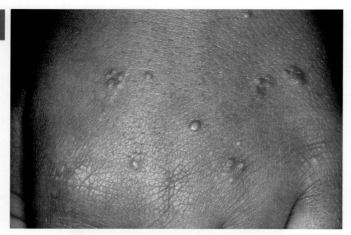

Fig. 31.6 Perforating granuloma annulare. (Courtesy Curt Samlaska.)

acral GA can be chronic but is often acute. Males and females present with the sudden onset of painful lesions on the hands and feet and a scattering of lesions at other sites. The lateral, dorsal, and marginal hands and, to less extent, the feet are affected. Lesions are tender to palpation and, when present on the palms, are dusky and may vaguely resemble erythema multiforme. Patients may have associated arthralgias and diarrhea, and they feel feverish, features of a "cytokine storm." The erythrocyte sedimentation rate (ESR) may be elevated, even above 50 mm/hr. Lesions resolve over months, at times after systemic corticosteroid or hydroxychloroquine therapy. The authors have seen one such case associated with Hodgkin disease.

Granuloma Annulare in HIV Disease

GA may occur in persons with human immunodeficiency virus (HIV) infection at all stages of disease, possibly due to cutaneous immune dysregulation. Lesions are typically papular, and generalized GA is more common (60%) than localized GA (40%). Photodistributed and perforating lesions may also occur.

Granuloma Annulare and Malignant Neoplasms

The occurrence of GA and a cancer in the same patient is rare, but it has been reported many times. Most of these patients are older. Half the cases occur in lymphoma/leukemia patients and half in those with solid tumors. The diagnosis of the neoplasm usually predates the diagnosis of GA but can precede it. In some cases, lesions are described as "atypical" in that they may be painful (see earlier), or present with less common clinical morphologic variants, such as palmar lesions.

Other Conditions Associated With Granuloma Annulare

GA has been reported after a bee sting, after waxing induced pseudofolliculitis in a patient, and after injections at a medical spa for mesotherapy or bacille Calmette-Guérin (BCG) immunization. Two groups of infectious diseases have been described as having GA-like lesions either histologically or clinically: borreliosis and tuberculosis (TB). Both Lyme disease in the United States and *Borrelia* infections in Europe have been described rarely as demonstrating interstitial granulomatous inflammation; clinically, however, at least in Europe, the lesions resemble morphea rather than GA. Despite laboratory evidence of infection, treatment of the patient with appropriate antibiotics may not lead to resolution of the skin lesions. A tuberculid can closely resemble disseminated GA, although histologically, caseous necrosis may be seen in the center of the granulomas. Treatment for TB leads to resolution of the skin lesions. In the appropriate patient, evaluation for TB and antituberculous treatment may be indicated. Medications can trigger interstitial granulomatous cutaneous reactions, including GA and mimickers resembling GA (see Interstitial Granulomatous Drug Reaction, later in this chapter). Tumor necrosis factor (TNF) inhibitor–induced GA has been reported, and newer anticancer agents (*BRAF* inhibitors and especially checkpoint inhibitors) have been reported to cause granulomatous lesions, including GA.

Granuloma Annulare and Eye Disease

Anterior and chronic intermediate uveitis has been described in patients with localized GA. The uveitis can be unilateral or bilateral, may be mild and may respond to topical therapy, or may be aggressive, resulting in visual impairment. The frequency of uveitis in patients with GA seems to be too low to recommend that all patients with GA be screened by an ophthalmologist. However, GA patients should be questioned about visual symptoms, including reduced visual acuity. If these are present, ophthalmologic evaluation would be appropriate. Patients with granulomatous skin lesions and uveitis may also have sarcoidosis, and careful review of the histology and consideration for further screening may be warranted.

Histology

Because there are many clinical patterns of GA, skin biopsies are often performed to confirm the diagnosis. In general, two histopathologic patterns often coexist in the same patient. The classic pattern of GA is a palisading granuloma characterized by histiocytes and epithelioid cells surrounding a central zone of altered collagen. There is often mucin deposition within the foci of altered collagen. Fibrin and nuclear dust may also be present in the degenerated foci. Lesions are most often located in the upper and middle reticular dermis but may involve the deep dermis or subcutaneous tissue. At the periphery of lesions, a leukocytoclastic vasculitis may rarely be found. Immunoglobulin M (IgM) and C3 in the blood vessels of the skin lesions are found in about half of patients.

The second pattern of GA is characterized by an interstitial pattern of inflammation, which may be seen in isolation or adjacent to well-formed palisaded lesions. This histologic variant is more common than the classic palisading granuloma. A patchy dermal infiltrate of histiocytes and other mononuclear cells with occasional neutrophils is interspersed between collagen bundles. The patchy distribution within the dermis is best appreciated at scanning magnification. Interstitial mucin is often present in the affected areas. Although these features are sufficient to confirm the diagnosis of GA, further sectioning may reveal typical palisaded granulomas.

Treatment

Patients regularly report that a biopsy of the lesion will cause its involution. Because the lesions are often asymptomatic and spontaneous involution occurs, no treatment is required in many mild cases. Numerous modalities have been reported to improve GA, suggesting that no one treatment is uniformly efficacious and the "treatment of choice." It is best to develop a therapeutic ladder for both localized and generalized cases of GA. For localized cases, the intralesional injection of triamcinolone suspension is effective and is a reasonable initial treatment. Many patients relapse within 3–7 months. Superpotent topical corticosteroids or topical calcineurin inhibitors, or imiquimod, may occasionally be effective in some patients, especially those with more macular lesions. Excimer laser, fractional photothermolysis, or photodynamic therapy can be efficacious for localized disease.

Generalized GA patients represent a major therapeutic challenge. For any treatment, 3–6 months of therapy appears necessary for efficacy or failure to be demonstrated. The two therapeutic modalities more widely reported in the literature are phototherapy and antimalarial agents. Phototherapy with psoralen ultraviolet A (PUVA) was used in initial reports, with more recent reports suggesting that narrow-band ultraviolet B (NB-UVB) may be used with benefit as well. Phototherapy should be used with caution in patients with photodistributed GA or features suggestive of possible annular elastolytic giant cell granuloma. Antimalarials have been used for decades, with initial reports describing improvement with chloroquine, and more recent data demonstrating good response rates to hydroxychloroquine, though chloroquine has successfully been used in patients who failed hydroxychloroquine.

Although systemic corticosteroids may be very effective, the high doses required and the usual immediate relapse as the steroids are tapered make this approach untenable in most situations. In addition, because dyslipidemia or metabolic syndrome may be present, systemic corticosteroids may be relatively contraindicated. Many systemic agents have been reported as effective, but few have been tested in large numbers of patients or in blinded or controlled trials. With all treatments, the GA may clear, only to recur when therapy is stopped. Antibiotics such as doxycycline; the combination of rifampin, ofloxacin, and minocycline, once monthly; pentoxiphylline, 400 mg three times daily; or high-dose nicotinamide, potassium iodide, oral calcitriol, or dapsone, 100 mg/day, can be effective. Fumaric acid esters over 1–18 months have also shown efficacy. The combination of fumaric acid esters with PUVA appears to give the highest level of response with phototherapy. Oral retinoids, especially isotretinoin, can be considered at a dose of 0.5 mg/kg or slightly more. Oral vitamin E has been used in one study of 21 patients with some improvement. For patients with severe disease, TNF inhibitors can be considered. Etanercept, infliximab, and adalimumab have all been reported to be effective. It is of interest that these medications can also cause GA. Systemic agents, such as cyclosporine, interferon (IFN) gamma, and hydroxyurea, have been reported to be effective in small series of patients. The potential toxicity of these medications limits their use to patients with significant GA.

Adams DC, Hogan DJ: Improvement of chronic generalized granuloma annulare with isotretinoin. Arch Dermatol 2002; 138: 1518.

Badavanis G, et al: Successful treatment of granuloma annulare with imiquimod cream 5%. Acta Derm Venereol 2005; 85: 547.

Balin SJ, et al: Myelodysplastic syndrome presenting as generalized granulomatous dermatitis. Arch Dermatol 2011; 147: 331.

Barzilai A, et al: Pseudorheumatoid nodules in adults: a juxta-articular form of nodular granuloma annulare. Am J Dermatopathol 2005; 27: 1.

Baskan EB, et al: A case of granuloma annulare in a child following tetanus and diphtheria toxoid vaccination. J Eur Acad Dermatol Venereol 2005; 19: 639.

Brey NV, et al: Acute-onset, painful acral granuloma annulare. Arch Dermatol 2006; 142: 49.

Brey NV, et al: Association of inflammatory eye disease with granuloma annulare? Arch Dermatol 2008; 144: 803.

Cunningham L, et al: The efficacy of PUVA and narrowband UVB phototherapy in the management of generalised granuloma annulare. J Dermatolog Treat 2016; 27: 136.

Czarnecki DB, et al: The response of generalized granuloma annulare to dapsone. Acta Dermatol Venereol (Stockh) 1986; 66: 82.

Dahl MV: Testing lipid levels in granuloma annulare. Arch Dermatol 2012; 148: 1136.

Garg S, Baveja S: Generalized granuloma annulare treated with monthly rifampicin, ofloxacin and minocycline combination therapy. Indian J Dermatol 2013; 58: 197.

Garg S, Baveja S: Monthly rifampicin, ofloxacin, and minocycline therapy for generalized and localized granuloma annulare. Indian J Dermatol Venereol Leprol 2015; 81: 35.

Giunta A, et al: Granuloma annulare. G Ital Dermatol Venereol 2017; 152: 193.

Grewal SK, et al: Antimalarial therapy for granuloma annulare. J Am Acad Dermatol 2017; 76: 765.

Gualco F, et al: Interstitial granuloma annulare and borreliosis. J Eur Acad Dermatol Venereol 2007; 21: 1117.

Karsai S, et al: Fractional photothermolysis for the treatment of granuloma annulare. Lasers Surg Med 2008; 40: 319.

Keimig EL: Granuloma annulare. Dermatol Clin 2015; 33: 315.

Klein A, et al: Off-label use of fumarate therapy for granulomatous and inflammatory skin diseases other than psoriasis vulgaris. J Eur Acad Dermatol Venereol 2012; 26: 1400.

Lee SB, et al: Vemurafenib-induced granuloma annulare. J Dtsch Dermatol Ges 2016; 14: 305.

Levin NA, et al: Resolution of patch-type granuloma annulare lesions after biopsy. J Am Acad Dermatol 2002; 46: 426.

Levy J, et al: Granuloma annulare as an isotopic response to zoster. J Cutan Med Surg 2014; 18: 413.

Lukacs J, et al: Treatment of generalized granuloma annulare. J Eur Acad Dermatol Venereol 2015; 29: 1467.

Marcus DV, et al: Granuloma annulare treated with rifampin, ofloxacin, and minocycline combination therapy. Arch Dermatol 2009; 145: 787.

Min MS, et al: Treatment of recalcitrant granuloma annulare with adalimumab. J Am Acad Dermatol 2016; 74: 127.

Nebesio CL, et al: Lack of an association between granuloma annulare and type 2 diabetes mellitus. Br J Dermatol 2002; 146: 122.

Patrizi A, et al: Childhood granuloma annulare. G Ital Dermatol Venereol 2014; 149: 663.

Pavlovsky M, et al: NB-UVB phototherapy for generalized granuloma annulare. Dermatol Ther 2016; 29: 152.

Piette EW, Rosenbach M: Granuloma annulare: clinical and histologic variants, epidemiology, and genetics. J Am Acad Dermatol 2016; 75: 457.

Piette EW, Rosenbach M: Granuloma annulare: pathogenesis, disease associations and triggers, and therapeutic options. J Am Acad Dermatol 2016; 75: 467.

Poppe H, et al: Treatment of disseminated GA with oral vitamin E. Dermatology 2013; 227: 83.

Simpson B, et al: Triple antibiotic combination therapy may improve but not resolve granuloma annulare. Dermatol Ther 2014; 27: 343.

Thornsberry LA, English JC 3rd: Etiology, diagnosis and therapeutic management of granuloma annulare. Am J Clin Dermatol 2013; 14: 279.

Toro JR, et al: Granuloma annulare and human immunodeficiency virus infection. Arch Dermatol 1999; 135: 1341.

Verne SH, et al: Laser treatment of granuloma annulare. Int J Dermatol 2016; 55: 376.

Weinberg JM, et al: Granuloma annulare restricted to Becker's nevus. Br J Dermatol 2004; 151: 245.

Wollina U, Langner D: Treatment of disseminated granuloma annulare recalcitrant to topical therapy. J Eur Acad Dermatol Venereol 2012; 26: 1319.

Wu W, et al: Dyslipidemia in granuloma annulare. Arch Dermatol 2012; 148: 1131.

Zhong W, et al: Perforating granuloma annulare. J Eur Acad Dermatol Venereol 2016; 30: 1246.

Annular Elastolytic Giant Cell Granuloma (Meischer), Annular Elastolytic Granuloma, and Actinic Granuloma (O'brien)

Annular elastolytic giant cell granuloma (AEGCG) and actinic granuloma are unified by their histopathologic appearance. Annular elastolytic granuloma (AEG) has been proposed as an alternative term to describe this spectrum of cases. Perhaps some cases called facial annular sarcoidosis and non–diabetes-associated necrobiosis lipoidica (NL) of the face can been included in this category. It is currently unclear whether these simply represent variants of GA, occurring most frequently on sun-damaged skin, or are distinct diseases.

Two patterns of AEGCG have been reported. The first is a single, asymptomatic, atrophic-appearing, yellow, thin plaque on the forehead (Meischer granuloma). Fine wrinkling and loss of elasticity characterize the skin within the ring. Clinically, this pattern resembles facial NL more than GA. The second variant consists of multiple extensor upper extremity and sometimes trunk lesions, occurs more frequently in women, and favors sun-exposed areas. In these cases, the lesions have an active erythematous-to-yellow/orange border with central clearing or whiter centers (Fig. 31.7). A papular variant has been described. Although the vast majority of cases occur in adults, children and even an infant have been affected. Most patients are otherwise well, though reports exist of rare associations with temporal arteritis. However, AEGCG has been described in association with acute myelogenous leukemia (which resolved with remission and recurred with relapse of the leukemia) and pleomorphic cutaneous T-cell lymphoma. At times, as in GA, the lesions of AEGCG may heal with loss of elastic tissue and clinical features of skin laxity and anetoderma. The condition is chronic.

Actinic granuloma, as described by O'Brien, may represent the same disorder as AEGCG. It presents as papules and plaques on sun-exposed skin. Lesions are frequently numerous and may coalesce to cover much of the exposed skin. A history of onset after significant sun exposure and the distribution on physical examination should lead to suspicion of the diagnosis. A few lesions may occur on sun-protected sites or may spill over from affected areas to more photoprotected sites. Rarely, open comedones, scarring, and milia formation may be present clinically. Actinic granuloma may be associated with transepidermal elimination of damaged connective tissue or loss of elastic tissue surrounding the follicular ostia, leading to a Favre-Racouchot–like appearance. Repigmentation of gray hairs and improvement in solar damage within the center of lesions, have been described. This condition affects older adults (usually over age 50) and can be intensely pruritic. Actinic granuloma is not associated with diabetes mellitus, but in numerous reports, it occurred in patients with temporal arteritis. It is speculated that the vasculitis is also caused by actinic injury to the connective tissue surrounding the temporal artery. Notably both GA lesions and temporal arteritis have been reported following varicella-zoster virus infection as well. Conjunctival involvement has been reported.

Histologically, all these conditions show a characteristic histology. The dermal infiltrate of macrophages is largely interstitial, and well-formed palisaded granulomas are uncommon. Multinucleated giant cells, often quite large, are numerous. Mucin is scant or lacking. The macrophages characteristically contain fragments of actinically damaged elastic tissue (elastophagocytosis). When this typical histology is seen in concert with the classic clinical features previously noted, it may be reasonable to make these specific diagnoses. These conditions cannot, however, be diagnosed on clinical or histologic grounds alone. Some cases with the clinical features of AEGCG or actinic granuloma will show histology more characteristic of typical GA or even sarcoidosis, suggesting a spectrum of both clinical and histologic features in these patients. Other granulomatous disorders can also demonstrate elastophagocytosis on histology as well.

Treatment of AEGCG (annular elastolytic granuloma) and actinic granuloma has been difficult. Aggressive sun protection should be encouraged for patients with lesions primarily on sun-exposed skin. Topical and intralesional corticosteroids and topical calcineurin inhibitors can be used for individual lesions. Many patients respond to systemic corticosteroids, but relapse immediately when the steroids are tapered or discontinued. Oral antimalarials are at times effective, as is dapsone. Insulin improved diabetic control and the actinic granuloma in one patient. Other anecdotal treatments include oral retinoids, tetracycline-class antibiotics, fumaric acid, PUVA, pentoxiphylline, tranilast, cyclosporine, and methotrexate. TNF inhibitors have been beneficial for recalcitrant cases.

Neutrophilic sebaceous adenitis presents with asymptomatic annular plaques on the face of men more than women. Fewer than 10 cases have been reported. It may be photosensitive. The condition resolves spontaneously after weeks to months without scarring. Histologically, in early lesions there is a neutrophilic, multifocal infiltrate around sebaceous glands with necrosis of some sebocytes. In later lesions the inflammation is primarily lymphohistiocytic. In addition to granuloma annulare/annular elastolytic giant cell granuloma, tinea facei, pemphigus foliaceus, a gyrate erythema, and lupus erythematosus are in the clinical differential diagnosis.

Berliner JG, et al: The sarcoidal variant of annular elastolytic granuloma. J Cutan Pathol 2013; 40:917.

Can B, et al: Successful treatment of annular elastolytic giant cell granuloma with hydroxychloroquine. Int J Dermatol 2013; 52: 509.

De Oliveira FL, et al: Hybrid clinical and histopathological pattern in annular lesions. Case Rep Dermatol Med 2012; 2012: 102915.

Errichetti E, et al: Annular elastolytic giant cell granuloma treated with topical pimecrolimus. Indian J Dermatol Venereol Leprol 2014; 80: 475.

Fernandez-Florez A, et al: Repigmentation of gray hairs in lesions of annular elastolytic giant cell granuloma. Cutis 2015; 96: E19.

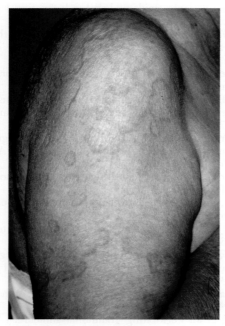

Fig. 31.7 Annular elastolytic granuloma.

Goldminz AM, Gottlieb AB: Noninfectious granulomatous dermatitides. Part 2 of 3. Semin Cutan Med Surg 2013; 32:e1.

Haimovic A, et al: Annular elastolytic giant cell granuloma successfully treated with adalimumab subsequently complicated by drug-induced lupus. J Drugs Dermatol 2017; 16: 169.

Monserrat Garcia MT, et al: Annular elastolytic giant cell granuloma in sun-protected sites responds to dapsone. Actas Dermosifiliogr 2016; 107: 531.

Nanbu A, et al: Annular elastolytic giant cell granuloma successfully treated with minocycline. Acta Derm Venereol 2015; 95: 756.

Panzarelli A, et al: Annular elastolytic giant cell granuloma and temporal arteritis following herpes zoster. Skinmed 2015; 13: 321.

Ruocco E, et al: Annular elastolytic giant cell granuloma and temporal arteritis following herpes zoster. Skinmed 2015; 13: 267.

Interstitial Granulomatous Drug Reaction

Interstitial granulomatous drug reaction (IGDR) is an uncommon but increasingly recognized pattern of adverse reactions to medication. Cases reported as GA induced by a medication often have an "interstitial" pattern and lack mucin, and some of the same medications cause both IGDR and "GA," so medication-induced GA and IGDR are considered together here. Some authors have suggested the unifying term *reactive granulomatous dermatitis*, to include the spectrum of disorders ranging from palisaded neutrophilic and granulomatous dermatitis, to interstitial dermatitis, to interstitial granulomatous drug reaction, as each of those entities requires similar workup and has a similar list of potential drug-inducing culprits. Most patients with IGDR have been taking the medication for months to years, though the reaction may occur more quickly. A wide variety of medications have been implicated, including calcium channel blockers (most common cause reported), lipid-lowering agents, angiotensin-converting enzyme (ACE) inhibitors, diuretics, nonsteroidal antiinflammatory drugs (NSAIDs), antihistamines, anticonvulsants including gabapentin, antidepressants, allopurinol and febuxostat, darifenacin, sorafenib, ganciclovir, trastuzumab, strontium ranelate, sennoside (common over-the-counter laxative), Chinese herbs, and even soy. Immunomodulatory medications, including thalidomide, leflunomide, lenalidomide, anakinra, IFNs alpha and beta, and TNF inhibitors have been implicated in causing IGDR in many cases. Rarely, drug-induced hypersensitivity syndrome (DIHS/DRESS) will display the histology of IGDR.

Clinically, the lesions are erythematous-to-mauve or violaceous annular thing plaques or patches with an indurated border and sometimes a tendency to central lightening. Lesions favor the creases (groin, axillae, popliteal fossae) but may also affect the trunk, proximal extremities, and rarely the palms and soles. Lesions may uncommonly be photodistributed, affecting the face and dorsal extensor forearm and hands. Pruritus is minimal or absent. Mucous membranes are spared. Histologically, there is a diffuse dermal infiltrate that is perivascular but has a prominent interstitial component. The inflammatory infiltrate is centered in the lower dermis; it contains neutrophils, eosinophils, histiocytes, and small multinucleated giant cells (sometimes just two or three nuclei). Degenerated collagen bundles may be surrounded by histiocytes, neutrophils, and eosinophils, resembling "Churg-Strauss" granulomas, and mucin is usually scant or absent. Unique features that should suggest IGDR over GA include an interface component and "atypical" lymphocytes in the infiltrate. The histologic differential diagnosis includes interstitial granulomatous dermatitis, palisaded neutrophilic and granulomatous dermatitis, and interstitial GA. Lesions resolve over months once the offending agent is stopped.

Cassone G, Tumiati B: Granuloma annulare as a possible new adverse effect of topiramate. Int J Dermatol 2014; 53: 259.

Chen YC, et al: Interstitial granulomatous drug reaction presenting as erythroderma: remission after discontinuation of enalapril maleate. Br J Dermatol 2008; 158: 1143.

Cornillier H, et al: Interstitial granulomatous dermatitis occurring in a patient with SAPHO one month after starting leflunomide, and disappearing with ustekinumab. Eur J Dermatol 2016;26:614-5.

Coutinho I, et al: Interstitial granulomatous dermatitis. Am J Dermatopathol 2015; 37: 614.

Deng A, et al: Interstitial granulomatous dermatitis associated with the use of tumor necrosis factor alpha inhibitors. Arch Dermatol 2006; 142: 198.

Fernando SL, et al: Drug-induced hypersensitivity syndrome with superficial granulomatous dermatitis-a novel finding. Am J Dermatopathol 2009; 31: 611.

Georgesen C, et al: Interstitial granulomatous dermatitis associated with gabapentin. Dermatitis 2014; 25: 374.

Goldminz AM, Gottlieb AB: Noninfectious granulomatous dermatitides. Part 3 of 3. Semin Cutan Med Surg 2013; 32: e7.

Hernandez N, et al: Generalized erythematous-violaceous plaques in a patient with a history of dyslipidemia. Int J Dermatol 2013; 52: 393.

Kim MS, et al: Allopurinol-induced DRESS syndrome with a histologic pattern consistent with interstitial granulomatous drug reaction. Am J Dermatopathol 2014; 36: 193.

Laura A, et al: Interstitial granulomatous drug reaction due to febuxostat. Indian J Dermatol Venereol Leprol 2014; 80: 182.

Magro CM, et al: The interstitial granulomatous drug reaction. J Cutan Pathol 1998; 25: 72.

Ratnarathorn M, et al: Disseminated granuloma annulare: a cutaneous adverse effect of anti-TNF agents. Indian J Dermatol 2011; 56: 752.

Rosenbach M, English JC 3rd: Reactive granulomatous dermatitis. Dermatol Clin 2015; 33: 373.

Tan ES, et al: Interstitial granulomatous drug reaction induced by quetiapine. Clin Exp Dermatol 2016; 41: 210.

Granuloma Multiforme (Leiker)

Granuloma multiforme (GM) is seen most frequently in central Africa, where it is a common disorder, and rarely elsewhere. It affects adults over age 40 and is more common in women. Lesions are most frequently found on the upper trunk and arms and in sun-exposed areas. GM begins as small papules that evolve within 1 year into round or oval plaques up to 15 cm in diameter. The active edge of lesions may be elevated to as much as 4 mm in height and the center slightly depressed and hypopigmented. Pruritus can occur, and coalescing lesions may form unusual polycyclic shapes. The course is chronic. GM is, most importantly, separated from tuberculoid leprosy. Histologically, GM resembles GA, but multinucleated giant cells are prominent. Giant cells typically contain phagocytosed connective tissue, and elastic tissue is decreased in the areas affected by the granulomas. GM shares many features with AEGCG and actinic granuloma, or GA of sun-exposed skin, and in fact may be considered identical to these disorders.

Kumari R, et al: Granuloma multiforme. Indian J Dermatol Venereol Leprol 2009; 75: 296.

NECROBIOTIC XANTHOGRANULOMA

Necrobiotic xanthogranuloma (NXG) is a rare multisystem disease with prominent skin findings. The cause is unknown, though there is a strong association with paraproteinemia. Some consider it to exist along a spectrum of "adult orbital xanthogranulomatous disease" (AOXGD), which also includes adult-onset xanthogranuloma

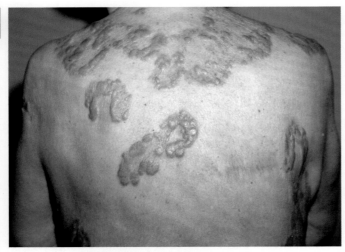

Fig. 31.8 Necrobiotic xanthogranuloma.

(AOX), and adult-onset asthma with periocular xanthogranuloma (AAPOX). NXG is gradually progressive, affecting men and women equally, and beginning on average at about age 50 (range 25–80 or older). The most common site affected is the periorbital area (>80% of patients). Multicentric involvement is typical. Lesions may be localized or initially present in scars. The characteristic skin lesions are violaceous plaques and nodules with a prominent yellow (xanthomatous) component. Periorbitally, early lesions may be mistaken for xanthelasma, but NXG lesions are more deep, firm, and indurated and may extend into the orbit and ulcerate. The trunk and proximal extremities may have violaceous to orange-red plaques with an active red border and an atrophic center with superficial telangiectasias (Fig. 31.8). These plaques may grow to 25 cm in diameter. The skin lesions ulcerate in 50% of cases, leading to atrophic scarring. Acral nodules may also occur, some localized solely to the subcutaneous tissue. Extensive lesions limited to the vulvar region have been described. Extracutaneous involvement most often affects the eyes. Patients may complain of burning, itching, or pain around or in the eyes. Diplopia and inflammation in various compartments of the eye can occur, including conjunctivitis, keratitis, scleritis, uveitis, iritis, ectropion, or proptosis. Ulceration and scarring of the plaques and distortion of the eye may lead to visual occlusion. Blindness may result. Lymphadenopathy, hepatosplenomegaly, and mucosal, myocardial, and pulmonary lesions may occur. As with other granulomatous processes, the granulomas may be metabolically active and produce 1α-hydroxylase, leading to increased 1,25-dihydroxyvitamin D and hypercalcemia. Most importantly, there is a monoclonal IgG (usually κ) paraproteinemia in 80% of cases, though other paraproteins have been reported including rarely an IgA paraproteinemia. Thrombocytopenia, neutrophilia, neutropenia, and eosinophilia may be present. The bone marrow may show leukopenia, plasmacytosis (25%–50% of patients), or frank myeloma (10%–20%). In some patients, a myelodysplastic syndrome may be present or may develop (chronic lymphocytic lymphoma, Hodgkin or non-Hodgkin lymphoma). Many patients are diagnosed with "monoclonal gammopathy of unknown significance" (MGUS), as 5%–10% of patients over 70 may display a paraprotein. It is important to confer with patients' hematologists about the significance of the NXG and relationship between the disease and myeloma. The NXG predates the development of the myeloma or myelodysplastic syndrome by an average of 2.5–5 years, but has been reported as long as 20 years preceding an eventual diagnosis of myeloma.

Histologically, there are extensive zones of degenerated collagen surrounded by palisaded macrophages. These macrophages are

of various forms: foamy, Touton cells, epithelioid, and giant cells, sometimes with more than 50 nuclei. Peripheral foamy cytoplasm is common. Atypical multinucleated giant cells with multiple nuclei clustered at one end of the cell (polarized nuclei) are seen in 80% or more of cases. The process extends into the fat, obliterating fat lobules. Cholesterol clefts and extracellular lipid deposits may be prominent, but not universally present and are not required for the diagnosis. Within this process is a perivascular and interstitial infiltrate of lymphocytes and plasma cells. Lymphoid follicles are present. In the skin, the lymphoid aggregates are polytypic. The histologic differential diagnosis includes NL and other histiocytoses. NXG has more atypical and Touton giant cells, lymphoid nodules, and cholesterol clefts. As in plane xanthomas seen with paraproteinemia, the associated monoclonal gammopathy of undetermined significance (MGUS) appears to enhance the intracellular accumulation of cholesterol within the macrophages/histiocytes.

The treatment is usually directed at the paraprotein or underlying malignancy. Treatment of the malignancy may lead to resolution of the NXG lesions. Other treatments have included intralesional or topical corticosteroids, laser therapy, systemic corticosteroids, topical mechlorethamine, hydroxychloroquine, dapsone, IFN alpha, systemic chemotherapeutic agents (e.g., chlorambucil, cyclophosphamide, melphalan, fludarabine), plasmapheresis, or local radiation therapy (for eye lesions). Numerous reports have documented response to high-dose intravenous immunoglobin (which may in fact be treating the underlying paraproteinemia). In addition, rituximab, extracorporeal photophoresis, and thalidomide have induced remissions. Infliximab, azathioprine, and methotrexate have also been used. Simple excision is an option, but lesions may recur.

Abdul-Hay M: Immunomodulatory drugs for the treatment of periorbital necrobiotic xanthogranuloma. Clin Adv Hematol Oncol 2013; 11: 680.

Ali FR, Young HS: Ophthalmological considerations in necrobiotic xanthogranuloma. Clin Exp Dermatol 2016; 41: 563.

Bhari N, et al: Necrobiotic xanthogranuloma with multiple myeloma. Clin Exp Dermatol 2015; 40: 811.

DeLuca IJ, Grossman ME: Vulvar necrobiotic xanthogranuloma. J Am Acad Dermatol 2014; 71: e247.

Hallerman C, et al: Successful treatment of necrobiotic xanthogranuloma with intravenous immunoglobin. Arch Dermatol 2010; 146: 957.

Higgins LS, et al: Clinical features and treatment outcomes of patients with necrobiotic xanthogranuloma associated with monoclonal gammopathies. Clin Lymphoma Myeloma Leuk 2016; 16: 447.

Koch PS, et al: Erythematous papules, plaques and nodular lesions on the trunk and within preexisting scars. JAMA Dermatol 2013; 149: 1103.

Lam K, et al: Bilateral necrobiotic xanthogranuloma of the eyelids followed by a diagnosis of multiple myeloma 20 years later. Ophthal Plast Reconstr Surg 2013; 29: e118.

Liszewski W, et al: Treatment of refractory necrobiotic xanthogranulomas with extracorporeal photopheresis and intravenous immunoglobulin. Dermatol Ther 2014; 27: 268.

Miguel D, et al: Treatment of necrobiotic xanthogranuloma—a systematic review. J Eur Acad Dermatol Venereol 2017; 31: 221.

Minami-Hori M, et al: Adult orbital xanthogranulomatous disease. Clin Exp Dermatol 2011; 36: 628.

Nambudiri VE, et al: Successful multimodality treatment of recalcitrant necrobiotic xanthogranuloma using electron beam radiation and intravenous immunoglobulin. Clin Exp Dermatol 2016; 41: 179.

Rodriguez O, et al: Necrobiotic xanthogranuloma treated with topical nitrogen mustard. JAMA Dermatol 2016; 152: 589.

Rubinstein A, et al: Successful treatment of necrobiotic xantho-granuloma with intravenous immunoglobulin. J Cutan Med Surg 2013; 17: 347.

Sfeir JG, et al: Hypercalcemia in necrobiotic xanthogranuloma. J Bone Miner Res 2017; 32: 784.

Wei YH, et al: Necrobiotic xanthogranuloma. Dermatol Ther 2015; 28: 7.

Wood AJ, et al: Necrobiotic xanthogranuloma. Arch Dermatol 2009; 145: 279.

SARCOIDOSIS

Sarcoidosis is a chronic multisystem inflammatory disease characterized by granuloma formation in most affected tissues. Sarcoidosis occurs worldwide, in patients of every age, ethnicity, and socioeconomic class, though prevalence and disease patterns vary. In Europe, it is most prevalent in Scandinavia, especially in Sweden, with a prevalence of 64 per 100,000 population. In the United Kingdom, the rate is 20 per 100,000, and in France and Germany, about 10 in 100,000, with lower rates in Spain and Japan of 1.4 in 100,000. In the United States the southeastern states and certain urban centers (New York City; Detroit; Washington, DC) show the highest prevalence, and there is a marked racial variation, with a rate of 10.9 per 100,000 for white persons and 35.5 per 100,000 for African Americans. Women are affected slightly more often than men, with the highest incidence in African American women between ages 30 and 39. The lifetime risk for the development of sarcoidosis is 0.85% for white and 2.4% for black U.S. residents. The disease begins most frequently between ages 20 and 40, with a second peak at ages 65–69. Patients with late-onset sarcoidosis are five times more frequently women than men, have uveitis, and have specific skin lesions in one third of cases.

Interleukin-2 (IL-2)– and IFN-γ–secreting CD4+ helper T (Th) cells are important in causing lesions, as are other Th1 and Th17 cytokines. Several genetic associations have been made with sarcoidosis, but the underlying cause still remains a mystery. HLA-DRB1 variants are associated with an increased risk. HLA-DQB1*0201 and HLA-DRB1*0301 are strongly associated with acute disease and a good prognosis. HLA-B8/DR3 may be associated with Lofgren syndrome. Mutations in the promoter region of TNF are associated with erythema nodosum (EN) in sarcoidosis in Caucasians, and a variant in intron 1 of the lymphotoxin alpha (LTA) gene is associated with EN in female Caucasian sarcoidosis patients. Polymorphisms in the IL-23 receptor are associated with sarcoidal uveitis. ANXA11, BTNL2, and CCR5 gene polymorphisms have also been identified in specific populations as conferring risk for sarcoidosis.

Cutaneous involvement is present in 25%–30% of patients with sarcoidosis and may be classified as specific, which reveals granulomas on biopsy, or nonspecific, which represents reactive inflammation such as EN which when biopsied does not show classic sarcoidal granulomas. In about 20% of patients, the skin lesions appear before the systemic disease; in 50%, the skin and systemic lesions appear simultaneously; and in 30%, the skin lesions appear after the systemic disease, sometimes by as much as 10 years. This is often coincidental with the tapering of systemic corticosteroids for pulmonary sarcoidosis. The cutaneous manifestations of sarcoidosis are varied, and numerous morphologic lesion types have been described, including common morphologies (papules, nodules, plaques, subcutaneous nodules, tattoo- or scar-associated lesions, hypopigmented lesions) and less common morphologies (ichthyosiform, erythrodermic, ulcerative). Involvement of the face, particularly around the nose, eyes, and mouth, is common. Lesions can develop around prior scars, tattoos, or remote foreign body deposits (such as on the knees). Lupus pernio describes plaque or nodular sarcoidosis of the nose and central face which can develop scale, deeply infiltrate, damage underlying structures, and be disfiguring. Lesions of special sites such as genital, mucosal, alopecic, and nail disease may also uncommonly occur. Sarcoidal lesions are usually multiple, firm, and elastic when palpated. They extend to involve the entire thickness of the dermis. The overlying epidermis may be slightly thinned, discolored, telangiectatic, or scaly. The color may be pink, red, or violaceous in some patients, but is frequently faint, showing dull tints of red, purple, brown, or yellow, according to the stage of development, and perhaps varying by the underlying skin tone. Usually, the lesions are asymptomatic, but approximately 10%–15% of patients itch. There is a racial difference in the frequency of cutaneous lesions in sarcoidosis. Among white patients, EN is as common as the specific cutaneous manifestations, and both types of cutaneous involvement occur in about 10% of white patients with sarcoidosis. In black patients, EN is much less common; however, specific cutaneous manifestations occur in 50% or more of patients. The skin lesions in general do not correlate with the extent or nature of systemic involvement or with prognosis. The exceptions are EN, which is associated with a good prognosis, and subcutaneous sarcoidosis and lupus pernio. The morphologic types of sarcoidosis are discussed next, and when possible, the relationship to systemic sarcoidosis.

Erythema Nodosum in Sarcoidosis

Erythema nodosum is the most common nonspecific cutaneous finding in sarcoidosis. EN rarely occurs in sarcoidosis beginning after age 65. Sarcoidosis may first appear with fever, polyarthralgias, uveitis, bilateral hilar adenopathy, fatigue, and EN. This combination, known as Lofgren syndrome, occurs frequently in Scandinavian whites and is rare in American blacks. The typical red, warm, and tender subcutaneous nodules of the anterior shins are distinctive and are most frequently seen in young women. The face, upper back, and extensor surfaces of the upper extremities may less frequently be involved. There is a strikingly elevated ESR, frequently above 50 mm/hr. EN is associated with a good prognosis, with the sarcoidosis involuting within 2 years of onset in 80% of patients. Conversely, the absence of EN is a risk factor for persistent disease activity. Sweet syndrome may also rarely be seen in association with sarcoidosis as a nonspecific finding.

Papular Sarcoid

Papules are the most common morphology of cutaneous sarcoidosis and are usually less than 1 cm in diameter. Lesions may be localized or generalized, in which case small papules predominate (Fig. 31.9). This is also known as miliary sarcoid. The papules are especially numerous over the face, eyelids, neck, and shoulders. Plaques may occur by the expansion or coalescence of papules. In time, the lesions involute to faint macules. Hyperkeratosis may rarely be prominent, giving the lesions a verrucous appearance. "Papular sarcoidosis of the knee" is distinctive, in that disease may be limited to this site. In this region, the sarcoidal granulomas often contain foreign bodies, potentially representing remote childhood injury. In Caucasians, it often occurs in the context of Lofgren syndrome (see earlier) and has a good prognosis. Papular lesions along the alar rim in African Americans, in contrast, may be the first evidence of lupus pernio (see later) and portend a poor prognosis.

Annular Sarcoidosis

Papular lesions may coalesce or be arranged in annular patterns, usually with a red-brown hue (Fig. 31.10). On palpation, the lesions are indurated. Central clearing with hypopigmentation, atrophy, and scarring may occur. Lesions favor the head and neck and are usually associated with chronic sarcoidosis. Alopecia may result in the center of the lesion. Annular plaques of sarcoidosis can

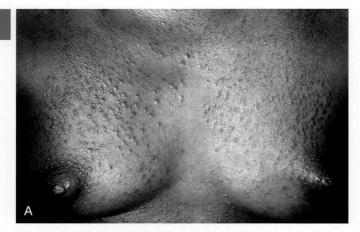

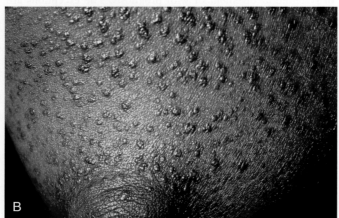

Fig. 31.9 (A and B) Sarcoidosis.

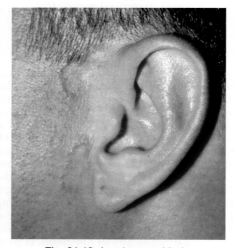

Fig. 31.10 Annular sarcoidosis.

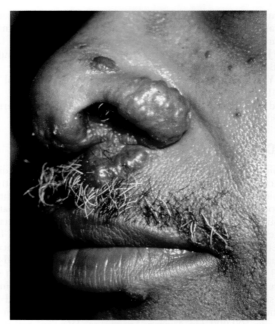

Fig. 31.11 Lupus pernio.

extremities. Although they appear macular, a dermal or subcutaneous component is often palpable.

Lupus Pernio

Lesions typically are brown to violaceous, smooth, shiny plaques on the head and neck, especially the nose (Fig. 31.11), cheeks, lips, forehead, and ears. They can be very disfiguring. Involvement of the nasal mucosa and underlying bone may occur and lead to nasal perforation and collapse of the nasal bridge resembling granulomatosis with polyangiitis. Upper aerodigestive tract involvement is also common. Ear, nose, and throat (ENT) evaluation is recommended. In three quarters of lupus pernio patients, chronic fibrotic respiratory tract involvement is found. In 43%, lupus pernio is associated with granulomas in the bones (punched-out cysts), most often of the fingers. Chronic ocular lesions occur in 37% of patients. Sarcoid involving the sinus is associated with lupus pernio in 50% of cases. Lupus pernio is typically seen in women in their fourth or fifth decade. The skin lesions rarely involute spontaneously. At times, lupus pernio may resemble rhinophyma. It is important to make the correct diagnosis, because ulceration of sarcoidal lesions may occur with laser treatment, even with pulsed dye laser. Patients with lupus pernio tend to have a chronic, recalcitrant course, and may require specific treatment based on this morphology (see later).

Ulcerative Sarcoidosis

Ulcerative sarcoidosis is very rare, affecting about 0.5% of patients with sarcoidosis. It affects primarily blacks, but it is also well recognized in Japanese. It is two to three times more common in women than men. In one third of cases, it is the presenting finding of sarcoidosis, except in Japan, where it is usually a late finding in patients with known sarcoidosis. The ulcerations may occur de novo or in sarcoidal plaques. Lesions favor the lower extremities, but most patients have lesions in more than one anatomic region. Trauma may be the inciting event. The clinical appearance may not be specific, but skin biopsies are diagnostic. Lupus pernio may also be present. Many patients have multisystem sarcoidosis, although infrequently, no other evidence of sarcoidosis is found.

preferentially develop in sun-exposed areas. This should be distinguished from annular elastolytic granulomas (see earlier).

Hypopigmented Sarcoidosis

Hypopigmentation may be the earliest sign of sarcoidosis and is usually diagnosed in darkly pigmented races. Lesions vary from a few millimeters to more than 1 cm in diameter and favor the

Biopsies may show necrosis in the center of sarcoidal granulomas. NL and ulcerative sarcoidosis share overlapping clinical features and the histology may overlap in some cases. Occasionally differentiating the two requires evaluation for extracutaneous disease, which is present in sarcoidosis and absent in NL. Methotrexate, which can be therapeutic in sarcoidosis, may also lead to ulceration in sarcoidosis patients.

Subcutaneous Sarcoidosis

Subcutaneous sarcoidosis is also known as Darier-Roussy sarcoid and consists of a few to numerous 0.5–3 cm, deep-seated nodules on the trunk and extremities; only rarely do they appear on the face. The overlying epidermis may be normal (30%), erythematous (50%), or slightly violaceous (10%). The lesions are usually asymptomatic. About 90% of patients will have multiple lesions, and the upper extremity is most frequently affected (virtually 100% of patients). Lesions on the upper extremity have a tendency to form indurated linear bands from the elbow to the hand on the cubital side of the forearm. The amount of subcutaneous involvement in the upper extremity may be so extensive as to simulate chronic cellulitis. A biopsy is usually required to confirm the diagnosis. Although it has been described that 90% of patients with subcutaneous sarcoid also will have systemic involvement, usually bilateral hilar adenopathy, it should be noted that sarcoidosis is by definition a multiorgan disease, and hilar adenopathy is the most common lung finding—it remains unclear whether specific cutaneous morphologies such as subcutaneous lesions confer prognosis, beyond that noted for lupus pernio.

Plaques

These distinctive lesions are flat-surfaced, slightly elevated plaques (Fig. 31.12) that appear with greatest frequency on the cheeks, limbs, and trunk symmetrically. Superficial nodules may be superimposed, and coalescence of plaques may lead to serpiginous lesions. Involvement of the scalp may lead to permanent alopecia. The finding of alopecia in an annular plaque with a raised border should raise the diagnostic consideration of sarcoidosis.

Erythrodermic Sarcoidosis

Erythrodermic sarcoidosis is an extremely rare form of sarcoidosis. A diffuse infiltrative erythroderma of the skin usually begins as erythematous, scaling patches that merge to involve large portions of the body. A biopsy is confirmatory, but the diagnosis can be clinically suspected if small, "apple jelly" papules are seen on

diascopy throughout the erythroderma. Diffuse granulomatous dermatitis in the setting of myelodysplastic disorders should be excluded.

Ichthyosiform Sarcoidosis

Ichthyosiform sarcoidosis resembles ichthyosis vulgaris or acquired ichthyosis, with fine scaling usually on the distal extremities (Fig. 31.13). It is virtually always seen in nonwhite persons, especially African Americans. Almost all patients have or will develop systemic disease. In 75% of patients, the skin lesions follow or occur at the same time as the diagnosis of systemic sarcoidosis. Although the lesions have no palpable component, a biopsy will reveal dermal noncaseating granulomas.

Alopecia

Alopecia on the scalp caused by sarcoidosis can have multiple morphologies. Plaques may extend into and involve the scalp, leading to scarring hair loss. More rarely, macular lesions from one to several centimeters in diameter appear on the scalp and closely resemble alopecia areata. This form may be permanent or reversible. Diffuse alopecia, scaly plaques resembling seborrheic dermatitis, and cicatricial lesions resembling discoid lupus erythematosus or pseudopelade may also occur. A biopsy of all forms of alopecic sarcoid will reveal dermal granulomas and sometimes loss of follicular structures. Scalp sarcoidosis is virtually always

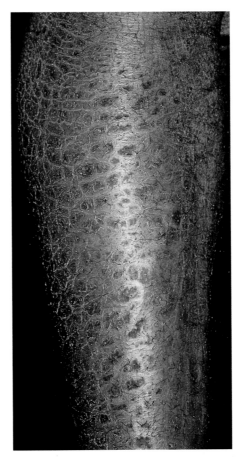

Fig. 31.13 Sarcoidosis, ichthyosiform type; biopsy showed noncaseating granuloma, although there was no palpable dermal component to the lesions.

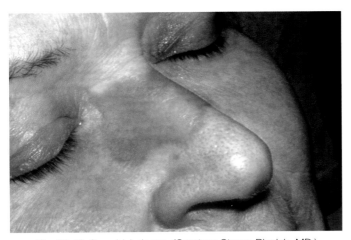

Fig. 31.12 Sarcoidal plaque. (Courtesy Steven Binnick, MD.)

seen in African or African American women. In cases where sarcoidosis affects the scalp, causing alopecia, the patient almost always has other cutaneous lesions, and the vast majority of cases will demonstrate systemic involvement. Syringotropic involvement may lead to hypohidrosis.

Morpheaform Sarcoidosis

Extremely rarely, specific cutaneous lesions of sarcoidosis may be accompanied by substantial fibrosis and simulate morphea. Less than 10 cases have been described to date. Most often, the lesions are localized and resemble linear morphea. Skin biopsy will demonstrate noncaseating granulomas. African American women are most frequently affected. This form of sarcoidosis responds favorably to antimalarial therapy.

Sarcoidosis in Scars (Scar Sarcoid) and Tattoos

Infiltration and elevation of tattoos and old, flat scars are two variants of scar sarcoid. Previously flat scars become raised and may become erythematous or violaceous (Fig. 31.14). These lesions may be confused with hypertrophic scars. Infiltration of tattoos may be the first manifestation of sarcoidosis and can be confused with a granulomatous hypersensitivity reaction to the tattoo pigment. Papulonodular reactions within black tattoos in particular appear to be common, but sarcoidosis can develop in any color of any tattoo. Granulomas within tattoos may be a granulomatous hypersensitivity reaction, a mycobacterial infection, or a sign of sarcoidosis. Cosmetic tattooing, as may be performed in a dermatology office, may result in sarcoidal granulomas in patients with pulmonary sarcoidosis. Hyaluronic acid injections can also be complicated by the development of sarcoidal lesions in patients with sarcoidosis. As noted later, patients with hepatitis C virus (HCV) infection receiving IFN therapy are at high risk for developing sarcoidosis and can develop disfiguring sarcoidal reactions after cosmetic filler injections. Similar granulomatous reactions may occur in the earlobe after ear piercing and represent granulomatous allergic dermatitis to metals introduced by the procedure or the earring. Titanium, nickel, cobalt, zinc, gold, and palladium can all be the allergen.

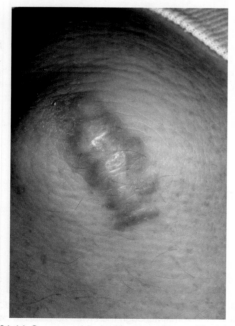

Fig. 31.14 Scar sarcoidosis. (Courtesy Steven Binnick, MD.)

From 22% to 77% of biopsies from patients with cutaneous sarcoidosis will contain polarizable foreign material, suggesting that scar sarcoidosis is very common. The foreign material seems to be a nidus that favors the development of sarcoidal granulomas. Scar sarcoid sometimes occurs in patients with acute disease and EN, especially if the lesions are small papules on the knees. It may also occur in patients with chronic sarcoidosis. The presence of polarizable material in a granulomatous process does not confirm the diagnosis of "foreign body granuloma," but rather should result in evaluation of the patient for evidence of systemic sarcoidosis. When foreign material is found, infection must be carefully excluded if no other features of sarcoidosis are found.

Nail Sarcoidosis

Sarcoidosis of the nail can affect any compartment of the nail, causing onycholysis, subungual hyperkeratosis (nail bed involvement), brittle nails, pitting, ridging, or rough nails (trachyonychia), distal matrix involvement, and even pterygium (nail matrix destruction). Nails may be hyperpigmented. Sarcoidal dactylitis and phalangeal bone disease as well as intrathoracic sarcoidosis often accompany nail sarcoidosis. "Drumstick" dactylitis is associated with lupus pernio.

Mucosal Sarcoidosis

The lesions in the mouth are characterized by pinhead-sized papules that may be grouped and fused together to form a flat plaque. The hard palate, tongue, buccal mucosa, or posterior pharynx may be involved. They may simulate Fordyce spots. In lupus pernio, the nasal mucosa is frequently involved. Rarely, in ulcerative sarcoidosis, the oral mucosa may be involved. Sarcoidosis may also infiltrate the gingiva, causing "strawberry gums" that simulate granulomatosis with polyangiitis (Wegener).

Systemic Sarcoidosis

Sarcoidosis may involve virtually every internal organ, and its presentations are protean. Many cases of sarcoidosis are asymptomatic, and only when routine radiographs of the chest reveal some abnormality is sarcoidosis suspected. Fever may be the only symptom of the disease or may be accompanied by weight loss, fatigue, and malaise.

Intrathoracic lesions, including parenchymal lung lesions and hilar adenopathy, are the most common manifestation of the disease, occurring in 90% of cases of sarcoidosis. All patients with cutaneous sarcoidosis, even without any respiratory symptoms, should be evaluated with chest radiograph and pulmonary function tests annually. Pulmonary radiograph changes are staged as follows:

Stage 0: normal
Stage I: bilateral hilar and/or paratracheal adenopathy
Stage II: adenopathy with pulmonary infiltrates
Stage III: pulmonary infiltrates only
Stage IV: pulmonary fibrosis

The panda sign correlates with gallium uptake in the nasopharynx and lacrimal and parotid glands; the lambda sign correlates with uptake in the paratracheal lymph nodes. These characteristic findings can be used as presumptive evidence for sarcoidosis. Lymphadenopathy, especially of the mediastinal and hilar nodes, and generalized adenopathy, or adenopathy confined to the cervical or axillary areas, may be an initial sign of sarcoidosis or may occur during the course of the disease. Notably there appears to be a slight association between sarcoidosis and lymphoma, and patients with diagnosed sarcoidosis and new lymph node changes warrant thorough evaluation. Polyarthralgias may be seen with acute sarcoidosis or as a component of chronic disease. Chronic arthritis may occur. Osseous involvement is often present in chronic disease

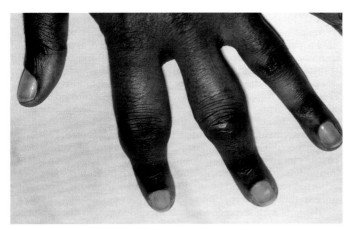

Fig. 31.15 Osseous sarcoidosis. (Courtesy Steven Binnick, MD.)

(Fig. 31.15). The most characteristic changes are found radiographically in the bones of the hands and feet, particularly in the phalanges. These consist of round, punched-out, lytic, cystic lesions. These are seen frequently in patients with lupus pernio. The bone lesions represent epithelioid granulomas.

Ocular involvement is present in 25%–30% of patients, so all patients with sarcoidosis, even if asymptomatic, should have routine ophthalmologic examinations. Any eye findings should be treated because even asymptomatic ocular sarcoidosis can lead to blindness. Anterior uveitis is the most common ocular manifestation. The lacrimal gland may be involved unilaterally or bilaterally by painless nodular swellings. Lesions of the iris are nodular and painless. There may also be lesions of the retina, choroid, sclera, and optic nerve. Optic neuritis with vision or color vision loss is an emergency. Ophthalmic disease is highly correlated with systemic involvement. Conjunctival biopsy is positive in about 50% of patients with sarcoidosis, making it an easy site to sample and confirm the diagnosis.

Parotid gland and lacrimal gland enlargement with uveitis and fever may occur in sarcoidosis; this is known as uveoparotid fever or Heerfordt syndrome and usually lasts 2–6 months if not treated. Facial nerve palsy and central nervous system (CNS) disease are frequently seen in Heerfordt syndrome. Mikulicz syndrome is bilateral sarcoidosis of the parotid, submandibular, sublingual, and lacrimal glands.

Clinically apparent hepatic involvement occurs in about 20% of patients; however, a blind liver biopsy will reveal granulomas in 60% of cases, and autopsy studies suggest 50%–70% of patients have hepatic granulomas. Hepatomegaly with elevation of serum alkaline phosphatase, biliary cirrhosis with hypercholesterolemia, and portal hypertension with esophageal varices are some of the manifestations. Liver biopsy showing hepatic granulomas is an excellent means of confirming the diagnosis of sarcoidosis.

Renal disease may be caused by direct involvement with granulomas or secondary to hypercalcemia. Hypercalcemia results from the macrophages in the granulomas having large amounts of 25-hydroxyvitamin D–1α-hydroxylase, which converts 25-hydroxyvitamin D to the more active 1,25-dihydroxyvitamin D. Patients may appear "vitamin D deficient" if both forms of vitamin D are not checked. Nephrolithiasis may result.

Cardiac involvement occurs in 5%–10% of cases, but in a higher percentage of autopsy cases. The most common symptom is "sudden death." Baseline cardiac evaluation with a detailed cardiac history and electrocardiogram (ECG) is recommended in all patients. ECG abnormalities, or a history of palpations, should prompt referral to a cardiologist for consideration of a Holter monitor or dedicated cardiac imaging, such as cardiac magnetic resonance imaging (MRI) or positron emission tomography (PET) scan. Fatal arrhythmias and heart failure can develop.

Neurosarcoidosis occurs in 5%–10% of patients. It can present in numerous ways, from focal cranial nerve involvement (most often facial nerve palsy) to aseptic meningitis, seizures, psychiatric changes, stroke, and space-occupying lesions. Neurosarcoidosis tends to be chronic and relapsing, with a higher mortality rate. Vision loss in sarcoidosis after heat exposure is called the Uhthoff phenomenon. MRI with or without gadolinium is useful for detecting CNS lesions of sarcoidosis and following therapy.

Patients with sarcoidosis may have other concurrent or comorbid diagnoses, including an elevated risk of lymphoma. Thyroid disorders are common in sarcoidosis (5% or more), and the nonspecific symptoms of thyroid disease can be mistaken for sarcoidosis-related complaints. There appears to be an association between sarcoidosis and psoriasis. Patients with sarcoidosis may have an increased risk of skin cancer, both nonmelanoma (squamous cell carcinoma and basal cell carcinoma) and melanoma, though this likely varies by skin type and has not been replicated in large, population-based studies. Eruptive, large, atypical dermatofibromas have been reported in a patient with sarcoidosis.

Measuring ACE levels in sarcoidosis patients has little utility. ACE levels may be elevated in all granulomatous diseases, including infectious granulomatous disorders. An elevated ACE level is suggestive of, but not diagnostic for, granulomatous inflammation. A normal ACE level cannot be used to rule out sarcoidosis, and an elevated level does not necessarily indicate the presence of multisystem involvement. An ACE level more than three times the upper limit of normal may be suggestive of sarcoidosis. The use of fluorine-18-fluorodeoxyglucose (F18-FDG) PET is more accurate in identifying extent of involvement and is being studied as a tool for monitoring response to treatment. Ultrasound has been used to quantify granuloma burden and may represent a future tool to monitor disease response.

Pediatric Sarcoidosis

Childhood sarcoidosis is rare. The clinical features are very age dependent. Older children, age 10–15, typically have lung, lymph node, and eye involvement. Calcium abnormalities are present in 30% of children with sarcoidosis. Older children develop specific sarcoidal skin lesions at the same rate as adults, about 30% of the time. One presentation resembles granulomatous periorificial dermatitis.

Blau syndrome is caused by mutations in the *NOD2* gene and is associated with early-onset sarcoidosis (age <5 years). It is more common in white patients. The triad of skin, joint, and eye involvement is characteristic and often confused with juvenile rheumatoid arthritis. Skin lesions are typically small papules and are the first clinical feature in more than half of patients, starting at a median age of 1 year. The skin lesions are often generalized and may be flat topped, giving them a lichenoid appearance. They are red-brown to tan and can occur in clusters or linear arrays. The face may have confluent lesions. Lung involvement is rare and can be helpful to distinguish this from sarcoidosis.

Histopathology

The histology of sarcoidosis in all affected tissues is identical. The characteristic finding is that of the "naked tubercle," composed of collections of large, pale-staining, epithelioid histiocytes. There may be small foci of necrosis in the center of the granulomas, and multinucleate giant cells, sometimes with inclusions (asteroid bodies, Schaumann bodies), may be present. Although classically there are few lymphocytes around the granulomas, they may be numerous. The granulomas may be nodular, diffuse, or tubular along neurovascular structures. Perifollicular and other periadnexal involvement can be seen in sarcoidosis.

The histologic differential diagnosis is broad, and the diagnosis of sarcoidosis cannot be definitively made histologically. Allergic granulomas caused by metals are histologically identical to sarcoidosis. Other foreign body granulomas (especially as a result of silica), granulomatous rosacea, granulomatous secondary syphilis, tuberculoid leprosy, atypical mycobacterial infections, and leishmaniasis may closely simulate sarcoidosis.

The diagnosis of sarcoidosis is established by the demonstration of involvement consistent with sarcoidosis in two different organ systems. This is usually done histologically, or by characteristic findings with radiologic techniques, including gallium scans, PET, and MRI. If cutaneous sarcoidal granulomas are identified in a patient with no prior history of sarcoidosis, the first diagnostic test should be a chest radiograph. If this is abnormal, further pulmonary evaluation is indicated. Ophthalmologic evaluation should also be performed. Because many patients with sarcoidosis may develop ocular involvement that may be asymptomatic, every patient should see an ophthalmologist. Blind biopsy of the minor salivary glands may demonstrate sarcoidal granulomas in about 50% of patients with systemic sarcoidosis. Otherwise, there are organ-specific guidelines to evaluate patients for the potential presence of sarcoidosis. Histologic evaluation of any involved tissue may be considered. The site for biopsy may be guided by PET scans, which, if characteristic, can be used to support the diagnosis. As the skin is the most accessible organ, and cutaneous sarcoidosis can present with varied clinical characteristics, dermatologists should have a low threshold to biopsy potential lesions to spare patients more invasive procedures.

Sarcoidosis in the Setting of Immunologic Abnormalities

Numerous reports document sarcoidosis occurring in patients with various forms of spontaneous or iatrogenic immunologic aberrations. Patients with ataxia-telangiectasia, severe combined immunodeficiency, and common variable immunodeficiency—three primary immunodeficiencies with both B-cell and T-cell defects—are predisposed to sarcoidal granulomas in the skin. Histologically, these have a low CD4/CD8 ratio, in contrast to classic sarcoidosis, which is rich in CD4+ T cells. Sarcoidosis may be associated with lymphoma, especially Hodgkin disease (sarcoidosis-lymphoma syndrome). B-cell lymphoma, chronic myeloid and lymphoid leukemia, and mucosa-associated lymphoid tissue (MALT) lymphoma have all been described in patients with sarcoidosis. Sarcoidosis patients are about 40%–60% more likely to develop malignancy, including solid tumors such as skin cancers (threefold risk), renal cancer, and nonthyroid endocrine tumors. In addition, adenopathy in patients with lymphoma or solid tumors may demonstrate sarcoidal granulomas without tumor. This is important to know when a patient with a cancer develops an enlarged node, and sampling of the node becomes important to avoid unnecessary therapy. Sézary syndrome with extensive cutaneous granulomas has been described.

Alteration of the immune system with medications can lead to the development of systemic sarcoidosis. These typically cause a constellation of pulmonary and cutaneous disease. Etanercept, adalimumab, and infliximab (the TNF inhibitors) have all been reported to trigger sarcoidosis. This is ironic, because they are also often therapeutic in sarcoidosis (analogous to the situation with TNF inhibitors and psoriasis). Numerous reports document the appearance of sarcoidosis in association with IFN alfa therapy, usually for the treatment of HCV infection. HCV alone may also trigger sarcoidosis. Cutaneous lesions (60% of patients), pulmonary findings (75%), or both, as well as other features of sarcoidosis, occur in 5% of patients treated with IFN alfa for HCV. The addition of ribavirin may increase the risk. In more than 80% of patients, the sarcoidosis resolves after the treatment is discontinued. Treatment of HIV infection with highly active antiretroviral therapy

(HAART) has led to the appearance of sarcoidosis or tattoo granulomas, apparently by enhancing the number and function of Th cells. Sarcoidosis is now well recognized as a feature of immune reconstitution syndrome (IRIS). Hematopoietic stem cell transplantation (HSCT), both allogenic or autologous, has been associated with the appearance of pulmonary sarcoidosis. If HSCT is performed for malignant disease, the presence of hilar adenopathy may be interpreted as recurrent or metastatic disease, and inappropriate treatment may be given. Other medications causing sarcoidosis include alemtuzumab (anti-CD52 monoclonal antibody for cutaneous T-cell lymphoma [CTCL]), omalizumab, vemurafenib (*BRAF* inhibitor), and ipilimumab (anti-CTLA4 monoclonal antibody for malignant melanoma). PD-1 inhibitors have been reported to cause a range of granulomatous reactions, from skin-only to multiorgan disease resembling sarcoidosis.

Patients with sarcoidosis are at increased risk to develop other immune-mediated and chronic inflammatory diseases, including systemic lupus erythematosus, autoimmune chronic hepatitis, multiple sclerosis, celiac disease, thyroid disease, and ulcerative colitis (but not Crohn disease, though there are reports of the two coexisting).

Differential Diagnosis

Granulomatous secondary syphilis may closely simulate sarcoidosis both clinically and histologically. Blau syndrome, an autosomal dominant granulomatous disease, is similar to childhood sarcoidosis (see earlier). It can be distinguished from sarcoidosis by the lack of pulmonary involvement. Granulomatous CTCL can usually be distinguished histologically and by the presence of pulmonary involvement in sarcoidosis.

Treatment

Numerous therapies have been reported as beneficial in cutaneous sarcoidosis, usually after anecdotal observation. Virtually no information exists regarding what types of therapy are best for which of the various cutaneous manifestations. The cutaneous disease may spontaneously remit without treatment. Because most skin lesions are asymptomatic, the major indication for treatment is cosmetic. Treatment begins by evaluating the patient for systemic disease. If found, the treatment of the systemic disease may clear the skin lesions. Otherwise, a stepwise approach to management based on extent, severity, and rapidity of progression can be considered.

Systemic corticosteroids are almost always beneficial in cutaneous sarcoidosis. Unfortunately, the doses required to control cutaneous disease may be too high (usually in excess of 15 mg/day) to be ideal for long-term use. For limited skin disease, intralesional injection of 2.5–10 mg/mL (or higher) of triamcinolone acetonide suspension is very effective. For thinner lesions, superpotent topical corticosteroids or topical tacrolimus may be effective. Local procedures can be beneficial for some forms of sarcoidosis. Pulsed dye laser, used repeatedly, PDT, phototherapy, and even CO_2 laser remodeling may be effective in the appropriate cases. Although lasers have been reported as beneficial, they should be used with caution as skin trauma can induce new lesions, and existing lesions may worsen or ulcerate after laser. Phototherapy and photodynamic therapy have been described as helpful, but the benefit is often transient and relapses are common once therapy is stopped. In severe lupus pernio, nasal skin excision followed by flap reconstruction can lead to dramatic improvement.

Antibiotic treatment tetracycline antibiotics (minocycline is more effective and has better data, but doxycycline may be better tolerated and does not risk pigmentary changes; both are dosed at 100 mg twice daily) may be considered in patients with skin lesions in whom systemic disease does not require treatment. About two thirds to three quarters of patients will respond to minocycline, and one quarter of patients have complete resolution of their skin lesions. A more aggressive antibiotic regimen called CLEAR—combined levofloxacin, 500 mg/day; ethambutol, 25 mg/kg/day, up to 1200 mg; azithromycin, 250 mg/day; and rifampin, 10 mg/kg/day, or up to 300 mg/day—has been reported in a single small study. Maximum response occurs after several months of therapy.

Antimalarials, both chloroquine and hydroxychloroquine, have been used to treat extensive cutaneous sarcoidosis, in doses of 250 mg/day or 200–400 mg/day, respectively. About three quarters of patients appear to respond partially or completely. In some cases, the associated CNS disease or hypercalcemia also improves. These agents may also be used to reduce the dose of systemic steroids required. Antimalarial therapy can be combined with antibiotic treatment. Pentoxifylline has been shown to be of mild benefit in pulmonary sarcoidosis and anecdotally may help some patients with mild skin disease. Apremilast has been shown to be beneficial in a small study of 17 patients with skin disease.

Methotrexate, in doses of 15–25 mg per week, is also efficacious and seems to help patients with severe lupus pernio or ulcerative sarcoidosis who are otherwise difficult to treat. Methotrexate-induced hepatitis occurs in 15% of patients with sarcoidosis treated. Leflunomide may be given similar to methotrexate and may be used in patients with gastrointestinal intolerance for methotrexate. Response rates are about 75%. The retinoids, principally isotretinoin, have been reported as beneficial in some patients, usually at doses of 0.5–1.0 mg/kg. Response is only seen after 6 weeks or more. Thalidomide, 50–200 mg/day, has led to improvement of the skin lesions after several months, though a recent randomized trial of 40 patients failed to show benefit, and with the advent of the biologic agents, thalidomide is used less often. Venous thrombosis may complicate thalidomide therapy, especially if doses above 100 mg/day are used, and it is a teratogen. Thalidomide is an option when methotrexate is contraindicated. Lenalidomide has also been reported as beneficial. Azathioprine and mycophenolate mofetil are often used for extracutaneous disease, but appear less effective than methotrexate for skin disease, though they do have some benefit. Cyclophosphamide has been used for refractory disease, and rituximab has been used for recalcitrant pulmonary disease. The combination of thalidomide, an immunosuppressive agent, with an antimalarial may be effective when these agents fail individually.

TNF is an important cytokine in the formation of granulomas. Not surprisingly, TNF inhibitors, particularly infliximab and adalimumab, can be effective in refractory cutaneous and systemic sarcoidosis. Etanercept was studied in pulmonary sarcoid and the trial was stopped early, and is the biologic with most reports of TNF-induced sarcoidosis; most experts avoid its use in sarcoidosis, in favor of other agents. Adalimumab and infliximab are both highly effective in treating skin sarcoidosis. Golimumab showed a nonstatistically significant trend toward improvement in one large double blind placebo controlled trial. Infliximab appears to be particularly beneficial in controlling severe lupus pernio; only 10%–30% of patients respond to other agents, and 80% or more will respond to infliximab. Combination therapy with thalidomide, an immunosuppressive agent, a TNF inhibitor, and an antimalarial may be used in severe, refractory cutaneous disease. Fumaric acid esters has improved cutaneous sarcoidosis and may be considered when other agents fail.

Systemic corticosteroid therapy is indicated for acute systemic involvement with fever and weight loss, in active eye disease, for sarcoidal involvement of the myocardium, in active pulmonary disease with functional disability, in hypersplenism, in hypercalcemia, and for symptomatic CNS involvement. Acthar gel may be beneficial in recalcitrant cases of advanced systemic sarcoidosis or refractory lupus pernio, including in some patients who fail to respond to TNF inhibitors.

Adam A, et al: Sarcoidosis associated with vemurafenib. Br J Dermatol 2013; 169: 181.

Ahmed I, Harshad SR: Subcutaneous sarcoidosis. J Am Acad Dermatol 2006; 54: 55.

Amber KT, et al: TNF-α: a treatment target or cause of sarcoidosis? J Eur Acad Dermatol Venereol 2015; 29: 2104.

Arostequi JI, et al: *NOD2* gene-associated pediatric granulomatous arthritis. Arthritis Rheum 2007; 56: 3805.

Baughman RP, et al: Efficacy and safety of apremilast in chronic cutaneous sarcoidosis. Arch Dermatol 2012; 148: 262.

Baughman RP, Lower EE: Goldilocks, vitamin D, and sarcoidosis. Arthritis Res Ther 2014; 16: 111.

Baughman RP, et al: Infliximab for chronic cutaneous sarcoidosis. Sarcoidosis Vasc Diffuse Lung Dis 2016; 32: 289.

Berg SA, et al: Sarcoidosis and squamous cell carcinoma. Cutis 2016; 98: 377.

Bhagat R, et al: Pulmonary sarcoidosis following stem cell transplantation. Chest 2004; 126: 642.

Bohelay G, et al: Striking leflunomide efficacy against refractory cutaneous sarcoidosis. J Am Acad Dermatol 2013; 70: e111.

Bonifazi M, et al: Sarcoidosis and cancer risk. Chest 2015; 147: 778.

Buss G, et al: Two cases of interferon-alpha-induced sarcoidosis koebnerized along venous drainage lines. Dermatol 2013; 226: 289.

Chakravarty SD, et al: Sarcoidosis triggered by interferon-beta treatment of multiple sclerosis. Semin Arthritis Rheum 2012; 42: 206.

Choi HJ, et al: Papular sarcoidosis limited to the knees. Int J Dermatol 2006; 45: 169.

Chung J, Rosenbach M: Extensive cutaneous sarcoidosis and coexistant Crohn disease with dual response to infliximab. Dermatol Online J 2014; 21.

Cohen PR, Carlos CA: Granuloma annulare mimicking sarcoidosis. Am J Dermatopathol 2015; 37: 547.

Cotliar J, et al: Pembrolizumab-associated sarcoidosis. JAAD Case Rep 2016; 2: 290.

Drake WP, et al: Oral antimycobacterial therapy in chronic cutaneous sarcoidosis. JAMA Dermatol 2013; 149: 1040.

Droitcourt C, et al: A randomized, investigator-masked, double-blind, placebo-controlled trial on thalidomide in severe cutaneous sarcoidosis. Chest 2014; 146: 1046.

Esteves TC, et al: Prognostic value of skin lesions in sarcoidosis. Eur J Dermatol 2015; 25: 556.

Ginarte M, et al: Morpheaform sarcoidosis. Acta Derm Venereol 2006; 86: 264.

Goldbach H, et al: Multiple eruptive dermatofibromas in a patient with sarcoidosis. Cutis 2016; 98: E15.

Green JJ, Lawrence N: Generalized ulcerative sarcoidosis induced by therapy with the flashlamp-pumped pulsed dye laser. Arch Dermatol 2000; 137: 507.

Haimovic A, et al: Sarcoidosis. Part I. Cutaneous disease. J Am Acad Dermatol 2012; 66: 699.e1.

Haimovic A, et al: Sarcoidosis. Part II. Extracutaneous disease. J Am Acad Dermatol 2012; 66: 719.e1.

Hayakawa J, et al: A syringotropic variant of cutaneous sarcoidosis. J Am Acad Dermatol 2013; 68: 1016.

Heidelberger V, et al: Efficacy and tolerance of anti-TNF-α agents in cutaneous sarcoidosis. JAMA Dermatol 2017; 153: 681.

Ji J, et al: Cancer risk in hospitalized sarcoidosis patients. Ann Oncol 2009; 20: 1121.

Judson MA, et al: The WASOG sarcoidosis organ assessment instrument. Sarcoidosis Vasc Diffuse Lung Dis 2014; 31: 19.

Kapoor S: Cutaneous and systemic malignancies in patients with sarcoidosis. Ann Acad Med Singapore 2009; 38: 179.

Khalid U, et al: Sarcoidosis in patients with psoriasis. PLoS One 2014; 9: e109632.

Kluger N: Sarcoidosis on tattoos. Sarcoidosis Vasc Diffuse Lung Dis 2013; 30: 86.

Lamrock E, Brown P: Development of cutaneous sarcoidosis during treatment with tumour necrosis alpha factor antagonists. Australas J Dermatol 2012; 53: e87.

Lheure C, et al: Sarcoidosis in patients treated with vemurafenib for metastatic melanoma. Dermatology 2015; 231: 378.

Maña J, et al: Granulomatous cutaneous sarcoidosis. Sarcoidosis Vasc Diffuse Lung Dis 2013; 30: 268.

Marcoval J, et al: Subcutaneous sarcoidosis: clinicopathological study of 10 cases. Br J Dermatol 2005; 153: 790.

Martinez Leborans L, et al: Cutaneous sarcoidosis in a melanoma patient under ipilimuamb therapy. Dermatol Ther 2016; 29: 306.

Martusewics-Boros MM, et al: What comorbidities accompany sarcoidosis? Sarcoidosis Vasc Diffuse Lung Dis 2015; 32: 115.

Mermin D, et al: A case of hyaluronic acid injections triggering cutaneous sarcoidosis at previously treated sites. J Eur Acad Dermatol Venereol 2017; 31: e55.

Motswaledi MH, et al: Oral sarcoidosis. Aust Dent J 2014; 59: 389.

Noe MH, Rosenbach M: Cutaneous sarcoidosis. Curr Opin Pulm Med 2017; 23: 482.

Pariser RJ: A double-blind, randomized, placebo-controlled trial of adalimumab in the treatment of cutaneous sarcoidosis. J Am Acad Dermatol 2013; 68: 765.

Pascual JC, et al: Sarcoidosis after highly active antiretroviral therapy in a patient with AIDS. Clin Exp Dermatol 2004; 29: 156.

Rosenbach M: The dermatologist's role in sarcoidosis. JAMA Dermatol 2013; 149: 760.

Sage RJ, et al: Preventing vitamin D toxicity in patients with sarcoidosis. J Am Acad Dermatol 2011; 64: 795.

Sanchez M, et al: Sarcoidosis. Dermatol Clin 2015; 33: 389.

Sepehri M, et al: Papulo-nodular reactions in black tattoos as markers of sarcoidosis. Dermatology 2016; 232: 679.

Shinya C, et al: Cutaneous sarcoidosis presenting with pinhead-sized papules. Eur J Dermatol 2008; 18: 191.

Sodhi A, Aldrich T: Vitamin D supplementation: not so simple in sarcoidosis. Am J Med Sci 352: 252.

Stagaki E, et al: The treatment of lupus pernio. Chest 2009; 135: 468.

Steen T, English JC: Oral minocycline in treatment of cutaneous sarcoidosis. JAMA Dermatol 2013; 149: 758.

Torres LK, Faiz SA: Tattoos and sarcoidosis. N Engl J Med 2014; 370: e34.

Ungprasert P, et al: Epidemiology of cutaneous sarcoidosis, 1976-2013. J Eur Acad Dermatol Venereol 2016; 30: 1799.

Wanat KA, Rosenbach M: A practical approach to cutaneous sarcoidosis. Am J Clin Dermatol 2014; 15: 283.

Wanat KA, Rosenbach M: Cutaneous sarcoidosis. Clin Chest Med 2015; 36: 685.

Wanat KA, et al: Sarcoidosis and psoriasis. JAMA Dermatol 2013; 149: 848.

Wu CH, et al: Comorbid autoimmune diseases in patients with sarcoidosis. J Dermatol 2017; 44: 423.

Yung S, et al: Cutaneous sarcoidosis in a patient with severe asthma treated with omalizumab. Can Respir J 2015; 22: 315.

Zouboulis CC, et al: Multi-organ sarcoidosis treatment with fumaric acid esters. Dermatol 2014; 228: 202.

HISTIOCYTOSES

These disorders are characterized by infiltrates that contain either Langerhans cells (the X-type histiocytoses) or non–Langerhans cell histiocytes (the non-X histiocytoses). There are three large families of histiocytoses based on the classification schema proposed by Zelger and Burgdorf and refined by Weitzman and Jaffe. These families are:

1. Langerhans cell (X-type) histiocytosis (LCH)
2. Non-LCH histiocytoses of the juvenile xanthogranuloma (JXG) family (which have the phenotype of dermal dendritic cells, being positive for factor XIIIa, fascin, MS-1, and CD68);
3. Multicentric reticulohistiocytosis (MRH) and sinus histiocytosis with massive lymphadenopathy (SHML; Rosai- Dorfman disease), which are thought not to be in the JXG family of non-X histiocytoses.

In the end, the final diagnosis is established by typical clinical features, a compatible histology, and an evolution typical for that disorder. Recently, mutations in *BRAF* have been described, commonly in *LCH* and *ECD*, along with emerging reports of *PTEN* gene mutation and increased expression of *PD-L1* across the spectrum of these entities, shedding more light on the etiopathogenesis of these disorders, and providing rationale for the use of novel targeted therapeutics.

Because more than 100 different disorders related to histiocytes and macrophage/dendritic cell disorders have been described, each representing a rare disorder, a revised classification system of this spectrum of rare disorders has been proposed. This classification system includes five categories: (1) Langerhans related, (2) cutaneous and mucocutaneous, (3) malignant histiocytoses, (4) Rosai-Dorfman disease, and (5) hemophagocytic lymphohistiocytosis and macrophage activation syndrome. The histiocytic infiltrative disorders are included later in this chapter; Rosai-Dorfman (SHML) is discussed in Chapter 32. Hemophagocytic lymphohistiocytosis (HLH) is an overwhelming "cytokine storm" that can occur as a complication of multiple disorders, including infections, malignancy, and rheumatologic disorders. The term *macrophage activation system (MAS)* has been used when HLH develops in the setting of certain rheumatologic disorders, particularly juvenile idiopathic arthritis. Patients have an underlying disease, high fever, organomegaly, cytopenias, a markedly elevated ferritin, elevated triglycerides and LDH, and hemophagocytosis on bone marrow aspirate. Because of the intense cytokine inflammation, interleukin inhibitors are being explored as potential therapeutic options for this intense reactive inflammatory condition.

Non-Langerhans Cell (X-type) Histiocytosis

Zelger and Burgdorf proposed classifying this group of disorders as the "xanthogranuloma family." Their classification scheme relies on the morphology of the monocyte/macrophage composing the lesion. Weitzman and Jaffe refined this concept and outlined the immunohistochemical features of the cells involved. These classification schemas are useful for this uncommon group of disorders. However, because the histiocytes within any disorder can change their appearance, no one specific morphologic cell type absolutely characterizes these disorders.

The non-X histiocytoses are divided clinically into three groups: those involving primarily or only the skin (JXG); those that affect the skin but have a major systemic component (Erdheim-Chester disease); and those that are primarily a systemic disease with occasional skin lesions as a part of the disease (Rosai-Dorfman; SHML). At any level of differentiation or appearance of the histiocyte, there may be a disease in any category. Conceptually, this allows one to think of the JXG group of non-X histiocytoses as lying along a spectrum: benign cephalic histiocytosis, JXG, Erdheim-Chester disease, generalized eruptive histiocytosis, xanthoma disseminatum, and progressive nodular histiocytosis. Most diseases at the beginning of the spectrum are localized, benign disorders; as one progresses through the diseases, they tend to become more generalized but are still benign; at the end of the spectrum lie diseases that may have visceral involvement and are less likely to involute. This parallels the histologic appearance of the infiltrating histiocyte, which progresses from scalloped to vacuolated to xanthomatized and finally spindled. In any disease, however, many morphologies of the histiocyte may be seen.

Emile JF, et al: Revised classification of histiocytoses and neoplasms of the macrophage-dendritic cell lineages. Blood 2016; 127: 2672.

Gatalica Z, et al: Disseminated histiocytoses biomarkers beyond BRAFV600E. Oncotarget 2015; 6: 19819.

Grom AA, et al: Macrophage activation syndrome in the era of biologic therapy. Nat Rev Rheumatol 2016; 12: 259.

Haroche J, et al: Histiocytoses. Lancet Oncol 2017;18: e113.

Weitzman S, Jaffe R: Review: uncommon histiocytic disorders. Pediatr Blood Cancer 2005; 45: 256.

Zelger B, Burgdorf WHC: The cutaneous "histiocytoses." In Advances in Dermatology. St Louis: Mosby, 2001.

Juvenile Xanthogranuloma

Juvenile xanthogranuloma is the most common non-LCH. The vast majority of lesions (70%) are diagnosed within the first year of life. Approximately one third of lesions are congenital. The mean age of onset is 22 months, and the median, 5 months, demonstrating the proclivity for early onset. About 80% of cases are solitary (Fig. 31.16). Boys are more often affected than girls. In adults, lesions tend to occur in the late twenties to early thirties, and the gender distribution is equal. JXG is 10 times more common in white than in black persons, but it occurs in all races. Multiple cutaneous lesions affect male children much more frequently (12:1).

JXGs begin as well-demarcated, firm, rubbery, round to oval dermal papules or nodules often less than a centimeter. Early lesions are pink to red with a yellow tinge and become tan-brown over time. On dermoscopy, the lesions have an orange-yellow background, a subtle erythematous border with branched and linear vessels running from the edge to the center of the lesion, and "clouds" of paler yellow areas representing areas of xanthomatized histiocytes; a "setting sun" pattern of yellow center with linear branching vessels at the periphery has been described. Most lesions are asymptomatic. The head and neck are the most common locations, followed by the upper trunk and upper extremities. Lesions have been divided into three types: small papular (2–5 mm; Fig. 31.17); large nodular (5–20 mm; Fig. 31.18); and giant xanthogranuloma (>20 mm). The small-type lesions are more numerous than the large type. Nodules may coalesce into giant plaques. Often, however, one patient will have both types of lesion, and the proposed increased risk for ocular involvement in the micronodular type and other internal involvement in the macronodular type has been refuted. Skin lesions regress spontaneously within 3–6 years in children. In adults, lesions are usually persistent. Hyperpigmentation, atrophy, or anetoderma may remain after lesions resolve.

Multiple atypical presentations have been described. These include hyperkeratotic nodules; macronodular tumors 2–10 cm in diameter; clustered (agminated) forms; linear lesions; flat, plaquelike lesions; and pedunculated or cylindrical exophytic lesions. Atypical sites of involvement include the genitalia, change to, lips, oral cavity, palms, soles, earlobes, and fingers. The most common location for JXGs after the dermis is the subcutaneous tissue, again most often on the head and neck. About 15% of JXGs present in this manner, usually as a solitary mobile mass up to 3 cm in diameter. Subcutaneous JXG typically appears before age 1 and often before age 3 months. Oral JXG may develop in infancy or childhood and is most frequently a solitary lesion of the tongue, lip, or palate.

Extracutaneous JXG is uncommon and occurs as visceral involvement, in association with either multiple cutaneous lesions or a solitary extracutaneous lesion. Visceral disease of both types accounts for only 4% of childhood JXGs and for 5%–10% of all

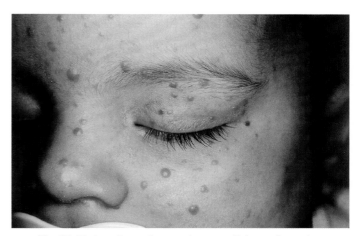

Fig. 31.17 Juvenile xanthogranuloma, multiple small papules.

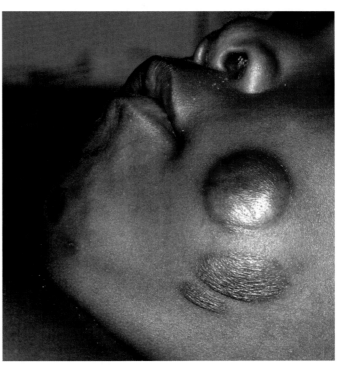

Fig. 31.18 Large juvenile xanthogranuloma.

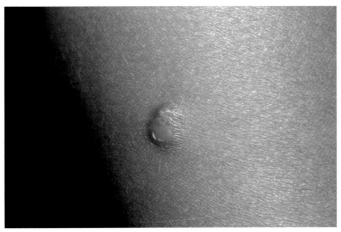

Fig. 31.16 Juvenile xanthogranuloma. (Courtesy Curt Samlaska, MD.)

JXG cases. Ocular involvement occurs in about 0.3%–0.4% of children with multiple JXGs, and only 41% of children with ocular JXGs have skin lesions. Skin lesions appear after eye lesions in 45% of cases. In 92%, eye lesions occur during the first 2 years of life. The most common location is the iris, where JXG can present as a tumor, unilateral glaucoma, unilateral uveitis with spontaneous hyphema, or as heterochromia iridis. The eyelid or posterior eye may also be involved. Ocular screening is recommended for children with multiple cutaneous lesions before age 2 years.

Mass lesions of the nasal, orbital, and paranasal sinus region can occur and cause erosion of the orbit and extend to the skull. Other extracutaneous sites and their presentations, in order of frequency, include the lung (respiratory distress and nodular opacities on chest radiograph), liver (hepatomegaly and, rarely, fatal giant cell hepatitis), testis (mass), and rarely, the CNS, kidney, spleen, and retroperitoneum. Other evaluations for extracutaneous JXGs are not indicated unless there are symptoms or findings suggesting their presence. Extracutaneous lesions also spontaneously regress. If surgical intervention is required, extracutaneous lesions tend not to recur, even if they are incompletely excised. Rarely, the burden of visceral JXGs may be so great that the patient's life is threatened. These cases have been called disseminated JXG, systemic JXG, or systemic xanthogranuloma. In 25% of these patients, no skin lesions are found, or the skin lesions may appear after the systemic disease is identified. Progressive CNS, liver, or bone marrow involvement usually mandates aggressive therapy and is usually managed with the protocols used to treat LCH. Bone marrow involvement can also produce HLH syndrome with profound cytopenias. Locally aggressive tumors may be radiated.

The JXGs have been reported in association with neurofibromatosis (NF-1) and juvenile myelomonocytic leukemia (JMML). Patients with NF-1 and JXG were reported to be 20–32 times more likely to develop JMML, but this association has recently been questioned. One large review of 739 patients with NF-1 over a 20-year period revealed that 14 had a malignancy, and JXGs were found in 4 of 14 and 6 of 29 controls, suggesting that JXGs do not confer an increased risk for malignancy in patients with NF-1. Because JMML occurs in infancy or early childhood, café au lait macules often are the only findings of NF-1 at the time. Sometimes, all three conditions affect the same patient, with males having a 3 : 1 predominance and usually a maternal history of NF-1. Children with JXG should be examined for stigmata of NF-1. If these stigmata are found, especially in a boy with a maternal history of NF-1, the pediatrician should be alert to the possible, although uncommon, occurrence of JMML. Nevus anemicus may be seen in children with JXG and NF-1. The presence of nevus anemicus in a young infant with JXG should put the health care team on alert that this patient may have NF-1. Rarely, JXG in childhood may be associated with mastocytosis or childhood acute lymphoblastic leukemia. The leukemia and the JXG can have the same clonality, and the JXG lesions may occur after the treatment of the leukemia or, less often, concurrently. Similarly, Wiskott-Aldrich syndrome has been reported with multiple JXGs. Multiple xanthogranulomas are rare in adults, and it is quite unusual for them to occur in an eruptive manner. At least six cases have been associated with hematologic malignancy (chronic lymphocytic leukemia, essential thrombocytosis, large B-cell lymphoma, adult T-cell lymphoma/leukemia, and monoclonal gammopathy). Systemic involvement with JXG in adults is also rare and usually requires histologic confirmation.

Lesions appear histologically as nonencapsulated but circumscribed proliferations in the upper and middle reticular dermis and may extend more deeply into the subcutaneous tissue or abut directly on the epidermis with no grenz zone. Epidermotropism does not occur. As classically proposed, the histopathology varies in accordance with the age of the lesion. Very early lesions are composed of mononuclear cells with abundant amphophilic cytoplasm that is poorly lipidized or vacuolated. Later, the cells become more vacuolated and multinucleated forms appear. In mature lesions, foam cells, multinucleated foam cells (Touton giant cells) and foreign body giant cells are present. Touton giant cells are characteristic of JXG but not specific for it. The inflammatory infiltrate consists of lymphocytes, eosinophils, and neutrophils and lacks plasma cells. Fibrosis occurs in the older lesions. The histology just described is characteristic of cutaneous JXGs. Soft tissue and visceral JXGs present with more monomorphous cytology, may have very few of the characteristic Touton giant cells, and can have a prominent spindle cell appearance. Immunohistochemistry is especially valuable in confirming the diagnosis of extracutaneous JXG. The cells of JXG of all anatomic locations stain with factor XIIIa, vimentin, fascin, MS-1, and CD68, but not with CD1a, S-100, or other specific markers for Langerhans cells.

The treatment for most cases of JXG is observation. By age 6 years, most lesions have resolved, often leaving normal or only slightly hyperpigmented skin. In adults, spontaneous involution is slower, and local removal with surgery could be considered. Injection of bevacizumab intravitreally may be used to treat JXG of the iris.

It is noteworthy that the patterns of involvement by JXG and LCH are similar, with childhood onset and primary cutaneous involvement; when visceral disease occurs, the liver, bone, and lungs are usually involved. Without histologic confirmation, isolated JXG of the bone would be most likely diagnosed as isolated LCH, a much more common condition. These clinical similarities between JXG and LCH may occur because both diseases are caused by antigen-presenting dendritic cells. JXG is a proliferation of dermal dendrocytes, and LCH is a proliferation of Langerhans cells. The clinical features favoring JXG include lack of crusting or scale and the distribution and uniformity of size of lesions. Histologic evaluation is definitive in difficult cases, because JXGs are negative for the Langerhans cell marker CD1a. Unlike LCH, JXGs are usually negative for S-100, although a few S-100–positive cells may be seen in a JXG. JXG may appear in a patient who also has LCH. One patient has been reported with JXG associatyed with a a PI3KCD mutation but JXG lacks BRAF mutations seen in LCH. Benign cephalic histiocytosis may be difficult to distinguish both clinically and histologically, although its lesions tend to be flatter and are mainly on the head and neck. Papular xanthoma can be distinguished histologically. Clinically, mastocytosis will urticate when scratched (Darier sign) and can be distinguished histologically. Solitary JXG appearing in a child must be distinguished from a Spitz nevus, which usually requires a biopsy.

Ashkenazy N, et al: Successful treatment of juvenile xanthogranuloma using bevacizumab. J AAPOS 2014; 18: 295.

Berti S, et al: Giant congenital juvenile xanthogranuloma. Arch Dis Child 2013; 98: 317.

Bowling JC, et al: Solitary anogenital xanthogranuloma. Clin Exp Dermatol 2005; 30: 716.

Chantorn R, et al: Severe congenital systemic juvenile xanthogranuloma in monozygotic twins. Pediatr Dermatol 2008; 25: 470.

Chiba K, et al: Diagnostic and management difficulties in a case of multiple intracranial juvenile xanthogranuloma. Childs Nerv Syst 2013; 29: 1039.

De Oliveria Rocha B, et al: Erythematous yellowish plaque on the face of a child. Int J Dermatol 2013; 52: 295.

Dehner LP: Juvenile xanthogranulomas in the first two decades of life. Am J Surg Pathol 2003; 27: 579.

Ferrari F, et al: Juvenile xanthogranuloma and nevus anemicus in the diagnosis of neurofibromatosis type 1. JAMA Dermatol 2014; 150: 42.

Folster-Holst R: Severe systemic juvenile xanthogranuloma is an indication for systemic therapy. Br J Dermatol 2017; 176: 302.

Haroche J, Abla O: Uncommon histiocytic disorders. Hematology Am Soc Hematol Educ Program 2015; 571.

Hau JT, Langevin K: Coalescing nodules on the trunk of an infant. Dermatol Online J 2016; 22.**Haughton AM, et al:** Disseminated juvenile xanthogranulomatosis in a newborn resulting in liver transplantation. J Am Acad Dermatol 2008; 58: S12.

Hirata M, et al: A case of adult limbal xanthogranuloma. Jpn J Ophthalmol 2007; 51: 302.

Jesenak M, et al: Wiskott-Aldrich syndrome caused by a new mutation associated with multifocal dermal juvenile xantho-granulomas. Pediatr Dermatol 2013; 30: 91.

Lehrke HD, et al: Intracardiac juvenile xanthogranuloma with presentation in adulthood. Cardiovasc Pathol 2014; 23: 54.

Liy-Wong C, et al: The relationship between neurofibromatosis type 1, juvenile xanthogranuloma, and malignancy. J Am Acad Dermatol 2017; 76: 1084.

Mallory M, et al: Café-au-lait macules and enlarging papules on the face. J Am Acad Dermatol 2013; 68: 348.

Murphy JT, et al: Juvenile xanthogranuloma. J Pediatr Hematol Oncol 2014; 36: 641.

Ng SY: Segmental juvenile xanthogranuloma. Pediatr Dermatol 2014; 31: 615.

Ngendahayo P, de Saint Aubain N: Mitotically active xantho-granuloma. Am J Dermatopathol 2012; 34: e27.

Pretel M, et al: Dermoscopic "setting sun" pattern of juvenile xanthogranuloma. J Am Acad Dermatol 2015; 72: S73.

Savasan S, et al: Successful bone marrow transplantation for life-threatening xanthogranuloma disseminatum in neuro-fibromatosis type-1. Pediatr Transplant 2005; 9: 534.

Shoo BA, et al: Xanthogranulomas associated with hematologic malignancy in adulthood. J Am Acad Dermatol 2008; 59: 488.

Strehl JD, et al: Juvenile xanthogranulomas developing after treatment of Langerhans cell histiocytosis. Int J Clin Exp Pathol 2012; 5: 720.

Benign Cephalic Histiocytosis

Benign cephalic histiocytosis (BCH) is a rare condition affecting boys and girls of all races equally. The usual onset is between 2 months and 3 years of age (rarely up to 5 years), with 50% of cases beginning between 5 and 12 months. The disease begins initially on the head in virtually all cases, often the cheeks, eyelids, forehead, and ears. Lesions may later appear on the neck and upper trunk and, less often, more caudad. There are always multiple lesions, but often few in number (5–20), although they can number more than 100. Individual lesions are slightly raised, reddish-yellow papules 2–4 mm in diameter (Fig. 31.19). Lesions may coalesce to give a reticulate appearance. The lesions cause no symptoms. The mucosa and viscera are not involved. Lesions spontaneously involute over 2–8 years, leaving behind hyperpigmented macules. Some cases of BCH have evolved to become JXGs, and one patient later developed generalized eruptive histiocytoma many years after the involution of BCH. This supports the concept outlined earlier that these conditions lie along a spectrum, and all derive from the same cell type, a dermal dendritic cell. Histologically, there is a diffuse dermal infiltration of monomorphous macrophages, which stain positive for CD68 and factor XIIIa and negative with S-100 and CD1a.

Koca R, et al: Benign cephalic histiocytosis: a case report. Ann Dermatol 2011; 23: 508.

Patsatsi A, et al: Benign cephalic histiocytosis. Pediatr Dermatol 2014: 31: 547.

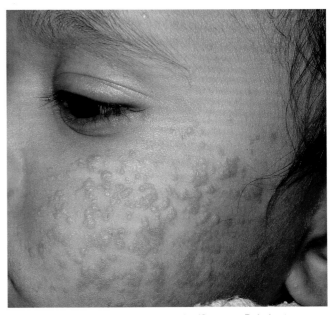

Fig. 31.19 Benign cephalic histiocytosis. (Courtesy Debabrata Bandyopadhyay, MD.)

Generalized Eruptive Histiocytoma (Generalized Eruptive Histiocytosis)

Generalized eruptive histiocytosis (GEH) is a very rare disease, usually presenting in young adulthood. The diagnostic criteria follow:

1. Widespread, erythematous, essentially symmetric papules, especially involving the trunk and proximal extremities, sparing the flexors, and rarely involving the mucous membranes (there is no visceral involvement)
2. Progressive development of new lesions, often in crops, over several years with eventual spontaneous involution to hyper-pigmented macules
3. Benign histologic picture of monomorphous, vacuolated macrophages

Lesions appear in crops and may be grouped or clustered. They are skin colored, brown, or violaceous. GEH is rare in childhood. It may be difficult to distinguish from widespread BCH in childhood, if indeed it is a separate condition. In adults and children, GEH may suddenly appear several weeks after a bacterial or viral illness; in adults it may be associated with underlying malignancy, usually leukemia or lymphoma. GEH is distinguished from xanthoma disseminatum by the lack of visceral disease, the benign course, and by the scalloped appear-ance of the macrophages in xanthoma disseminatum. Histologi-cally, there is a dermal infiltrate of monomorphous vacuolated macrophages and mononuclear histiocytes. The GEH cells stain positive for vimentin, CD68, and usually factor XIIIa, and negative for S-100 and CD1a. The natural history of GEH is unpredictable, with complete resolution in some cases and persistence in others. Some cases have progressed to widespread xanthogranulomas, xanthoma disseminatum, or progressive nodular histiocytosis, again supporting the concept that these diseases all fall along a spectrum and derive from the same cell type. In childhood no treatment may be required. In adulthood treatment with PUVA or isotretinoin could be considered. GEH has been described as both a reactive condi-tion, or clonally related to an underlying hematoproliferative disorder. GEH has been reported in association with chronic myelomonocytic leukemia, FIP1L1-PDGFRA–positive chronic eosinophilic leukemia, and an *NTRK1* gene rearrangement.

Attia A, et al: Generalized eruptive histiocytoma. J Dermatol Case Rep 2011; 3:53.

Klemke C, et al: Atypical generalized eruptive histiocytosis associated with acute monocytic leukemia. J Am Acad Dermatol 2003; 49: 233.

Pinney SS, et al: Generalized eruptive histiocytosis associated with a novel fusion in LMNA-NTRK1. Dermatol Online J 2016; 22.

Seward JL, et al: Generalized eruptive histiocytosis. J Am Acad Dermatol 2004; 50: 116.

Shon W, et al: Atypical generalized eruptive histiocytosis clonally related to chronic myelomonocytic leukemia with loss of Y chromosome. J Cutan Pathol 2013; 40: 725.

Ziegler B, et al: Generalized eruptive histiocytosis associated with FIP1L1-PDGFRA-positive chronic eosinophilic leukemia. JAMA Dermatol 2015; 151: 766.

Xanthoma Disseminatum (Montgomery Syndrome)

Xanthoma disseminatum (XD) is a very rare, potentially progressive non-LCH that preferentially affects males in childhood or young adulthood (2:1 male/female ratio). XD is characterized by the insidious onset of small, yellowish red to brown papules and nodules that are discrete and disseminated. They characteristically involve the eyelids (Fig. 31.20) and flexural areas of the axillary and inguinal folds and the antecubital and popliteal fossae. Over years, the lesions increase in number, forming coalescent xanthomatous plaques and nodules. About 30%–50% of cases have mucous membrane involvement, most often of the oropharynx (causing dysphagia), larynx (causing dysphonia and airway obstruction), and conjunctiva and cornea (causing blindness). Diabetes insipidus, usually transient, occurs in 40% (30% at presentation). CNS involvement, with epilepsy, hydrocephalus, and ataxia, can occur. Synovitis, inflammatory arthritis, and osteolytic bone lesions have been described. The natural history of the disease is variable. About one third of XD patients undergo spontaneous complete remission, one third have partial remission, and one third have persistent or progressive disease. Patients who have a spontaneous complete remission do not have evidence of systemic disease other than diabetes insipidus. Spontaneous remission often leaves areas of atrophy or anetoderma, caused by local loss of elastic tissue.

The serum lipids are abnormal in 20% of XD cases, which may lead to confusion with hyperlipidemic xanthomatosis. Histologic examination of early lesions shows surprisingly nonfoamy, scalloped macrophages. Later, lesions show xanthoma cells, Touton giant cells, and frequently a mild inflammatory cell infiltrate of lymphocytes, plasma cells, and neutrophils. The macrophages stain with CD68 and factor XIIIa.

Disseminated xanthosiderohistiocytosis is a variant of XD in which the lesions have a keloidal consistency; they have annular borders, a cephalad distribution, and extensive iron and lipid deposition in the macrophages and connective tissue.

Progressive XD can produce considerable morbidity and can even be fatal. Therefore aggressive therapy may be indicated. Lipid-lowering therapy has improved lesions in a few patients. 2-Chlorodeoxyadenosine, has shown benefit in some patients. Statins, fenofibrate, doxycycline, cyclosporine, and cyclophosphamide have been used with varying efficacy in limited reports. Cladribine has been reported as beneficial in one case. An IL-1 receptor antagonist was used for one patient with multisystem involvement and recalcitrant disease, based on reports of beneficial responses in patients with ECD. F18-FDG PET or computed tomography (CT) can be useful in defining extent of disease and response to treatment of visceral lesions. Surgical removal, or laser therapy has been described for individual lesions, including a nonablative 1450-nm diode laser.

Attia AM, et al: Xanthoma disseminatum. J Postgrad Med 2014; 60: 69.

Campero M, et al: Cerebral and cutaneous involvements of xanthoma disseminatum successfully treated with an IL-1 receptor antagonist. Dermatology 2016; 232: 171.

Gupta P, et al: Xanthoma disseminatum associated with inflammatory arthritis and synovitis. Pediatr Dermatol 2015; 32: e1.

Gupta V, et al: Xanthoma disseminatum. J Eur Acad Dermatol Venereol 2016; 30: e43.

Hsu MC, et al: Nonablative 1,450-nm diodelaser treatment for xanthoma disseminatum. Dermatol Surg 2014; 40: 1423.

Jin S, et al: A case of xanthoma disseminatum. Br J Dermatol 2014; 170: 1177.

Khezri F, et al: Xanthoma disseminatum. Arch Dermatol 2011; 147: 459.

Kim WJ, et al: Successful treatment of xanthoma disseminatum with combined lipid lowering agents. Ann Dermatol 2012; 24: 380.

Lee HC, et al: Unusual flexural papules in a male patient with diabetes. Clin Exp Dermatol 2012; 37: 931.

Park HY, et al: A case of xanthoma disseminatum with spontaneous resolution over 10 years. Dermatology 2011; 222: 236.

Park M, et al: Xanthoma disseminatum. Acta Dermatovenerol Croat 2014; 22: 150.

Progressive Nodular Histiocytosis

Progressive nodular histiocytosis (PNH) is a very rare disorder that affects men and women equally and usually begins between ages 40 and 60 years. The characteristic clinical feature is the development of two types of lesion: superficial papules and deeper, larger, subcutaneous nodules. The superficial lesions are small xanthomatous papules up to 5 mm in diameter. They are diffusely distributed on the body, but spare the flexors (unlike xanthoma disseminatum, which favors the flexors). The larger deep lesions can be up to 5 cm in diameter and are associated with pain, ulceration, and disfigurement. Smaller lesions may evolve to the larger lesions over time. On the face, lesions may coalesce, giving the patient a leonine facies and creating ectropion. New lesions progressively appear, and spontaneous resolution

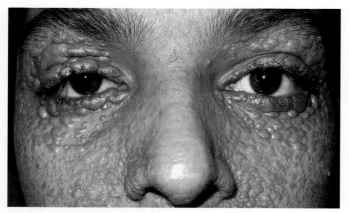

Fig. 31.20 Xanthoma disseminatum. (Courtesy Debabrata Bandyopadhyay, MD.)

of individual lesions can be seen, but general involution of all the lesions does not occur. Mucosal lesions are unusual but can involve the conjunctiva and larynx. Iron deficiency anemia can occur because the histocytes in the nodules may accumulate iron, reducing available body iron stores. Histologically, the superficial lesions show foamy macrophages, and the deeper lesions show a densely cellular proliferation of spindle-shaped histiocytes with multinucleated giant cells. It is the development of these deep lesions composed of primarily spindled histiocytes that is the diagnostic feature of PNH. Local excision may be used for symptomatic lesions.

Amin SM, et al: Progressive nodular histiocytosis with normal karyotypic analysis. Dermatol Online J 2013; 19: 18577.
Glavin FL, et al: Progressive nodular histiocytosis: a case report with literature review, and discussion of differential diagnosis and classification. J Cutan Pathol 2009; 36: 1286.
Hilker O, et al: Progressive nodular histiocytosis. J Dtsch Dermatol Ges 2013; 11: 301.
Nakayashiki N, et al: Effective surgical treatment of progressive nodular histiocytosis. J Plast Surg Hand Surg 2014; 48: 80.
Nofal A, et al: Progressive nodular histiocytosis. Int J Dermatol 2011; 50: 1546.

Papular Xanthoma

Papular xanthoma (PX) is a rare form of non-LCH that is poorly defined. The disease can occur at any age, but usually appears in early childhood or after adolescence. PX usually presents as a solitary lesion favoring men 4:1 over women. The primary lesion is a small, yellow papule 1–10 mm in diameter. If multiple, lesions are generalized, not grouped, and do not favor the flexors. No abnormalities are found on lipid profile examination. Erosive arthritis (resembling MRH) has been reported in one child and one adult. Histologically, there are aggregates of xanthomatized foamy macrophages in the dermis, with Touton giant cells. Inflammatory cells are scant or absent. Cells stain positive for markers of monocytes/macrophages such as CD68, but are negative for factor XIIIa. The differential diagnosis includes normolipemic plane xanthomas and normolipemic papuloeruptive xanthomatosis. In infants the natural history is for spontaneous involution. In one adult patient, treatment with doxycycline was effective. Recently there have been two reports of plaquelike papular xanthoma as solitary, red-yellow plaques with a superficial infiltrate of foamy macrophages and Touton cells with a clear grenz zone.

Andrew R, et al: Papular xanthomas with destructive arthritis. J Am Acad Dermatol 2013; 69: e309.
Breier F, et al: Papular xanthoma. J Cutan Pathol 2002; 29: 200.
Coutinho I, et al: Plaque-like papular xanthoma. J Eur Acad Dermatol Venereol 2016; 30: 332.
Emberger M, et al: Plaque-like papular xanthoma, an unusual, localized variant of non-Langerhans cell disease. Eur J Dermatol 2013; 23: 278.

Erdheim-Chester Disease

A rare non-LCH, Erdheim-Chester disease (ECD) is primarily a visceral disorder with cutaneous lesions in 20%–30% of patients (half at presentation). ECD can begin at any age from childhood to the ninth decade. The characteristic feature is bilateral and symmetric sclerosis of the metaphyseal and diaphyseal regions of the long bones. These radiologic findings are considered pathognomonic. Diabetes insipidus may occur, from involvement of the pituitary and retroperitoneal fibrosis affecting the kidneys. Despite a normal gross appearance, many internal organs are affected. The course is progressive with infiltration of many visceral organs,

followed by fibrosis. This is often fatal, usually from pulmonary fibrosis and cardiac failure; 1-year and 5-year survival rates are 96% and 68%, respectively. Skin lesions typically present as red-brown or xanthomatous, 2–15 mm papules or nodules. Lesions favor the eyelids (as with xanthomas), axilla, groin, neck, trunk (inframammary areas), and face (similar to lesions seen in XD). As in LCH, a significant percentage of patients (≈50%) have the *BRAF* V600E mutation, with recent reports demonstrating increased PD-L1 expression as well. Some patients have simultaneously both LCH and ECD (called mixed histiocytosis), apparently driven by these mutations. Less often, patients have had *NRAS* mutations. Initial treatment is with IFN alfa; in unresponsive patients, anakinra or infliximab (cytokine blockade) may be beneficial. In patients who progress despite these treatments, a *BRAF* inhibitor (vemurafenib) or *NRAS* inhibitor (if a mutation is detected) could be considered, though *BRAF*-inhibitor use is rapidly growing and may be used earlier in treatment, including as first-line therapy in patients with *BRAF* V600E mutations and moderate to severe disease. *MEK* inhibitors are also being actively evaluated for their efficacy as both monotherapy and in conjunction with *BRAF* inhibitors. Cladribine and imatinib are options if no mutation is detected.

Aitken SJ, et al: An *NRAS* mutation in a case of Erdheim-Chester disease. Histopathology 2015; 66: 316.
Cangi MG, et al: *BRAF* V600E mutation is invariably present and associated to oncogene-induced senescence in Erdheim-Chester disease. Ann Rheum Dis 2015; 74: 1596.
Cavalli G, et al: The multifaceted clinical presentations and manifestations of Erdheim-Chester disease. Ann Rheum Dis 2013; 72: 1691.
Ferrero E, et al: TNF-α Erdheim-Chester disease pericardial effusion promotes endothelial leakage in vitro and is neutralized by infliximab. Rheumatology 2014; 53: 198.
Haroche J, et al: High prevalence of *BRAF* V600E mutations in Erdheim-Chester disease but not in other non–Langerhans cell histiocytosis. Blood 2012; 120: 2700.
Haroun F, et al: Erdheim-Chester Disease. Anticancer Res 2017; 37: 2777.
Hervier B, et al: Association of both Langerhans cell histiocytosis and Erdheim-Chester disease linked to the *BRAF*-V600E mutation. Blood 2014; 124: 1119.
Hervier B, et al: Treatment of Erdheim-Chester disease with long-term high-dose interferon alfa. Semin Arthritis Rheum 2012; 41: 907.
Killu AM, et al: Erdheim-Chester disease with cardiac involvement successfully treated with anakinra. Int J Cardiol 2013; 167: e115.
Kornik RI, et al: Diabetes insipidus, bone lesions, and new-onset red-brown papules in a 42-year-old man. J Am Acad Dermatol 2013; 68: 1034.
Vagilio A, Diamond EL: Erdheim-Chester disease. Blood 2017; 130: 1282.

Progressive Mucinous Histiocytosis in Women

Progressive mucinous histiocytosis is a rare autosomal dominant or X-linked hereditary disorder described primarily in women though it can rarely affect males. The skin lesions consist of a few to numerous skin-colored to red-brown papules, ranging from pinhead to pea sized, which tend to appear on the face, arms, forearms, hands, and legs. Affected family members may display differing clinical morphologic patterns. Onset is in the second decade of life, with slow progression and no tendency to spontaneous involution. One report described a boy with dermal nodules which resolved but then develop persistent plaques of PMH. Visceral and mucosal lesions have not been reported. Histologically, in the middermis there is a proliferation of spindle-shaped and epithelioid monocytes. Superficial telangiectatic vessels and increased mast cells are found. Abundant mucin is demonstrated by alcian blue staining, indicating the presence of acid mucopolysaccharides. This condition can be distinguished from the other non–Langerhans cell histiocytoses by its familial pattern, lack of lipidized and multinucleated cells, and presence of mucin. Immunoperoxidase studies most consistently show positivity for CD68 and negativity for CD1a, S-100, and CD34. One report required electron microscopy to confirm the diagnosis.

Hemmati I, et al: Progressive mucinous histiocytosis. J Cutan Med Surg 2010; 14: 245.
Nguyen NV, et al: Hereditary progressive mucinous histiocytosis. Pediatr Dermatol 2015; 32: e273.
Requena C, et al: Hereditary progressive mucinous histiocytosis. J Cutan Pathol 2017; 44: 781.
Schlegel C, et al: Hereditary progressive mucinous histiocytosis. Acta Derm Venereol 2010; 90: 65.

Reticulohistiocytosis

Two distinct forms of reticulohistiocytosis occur: reticulohistiocytoma and MRH. The two forms have identical histology but distinct clinical manifestations.

Reticulohistiocytoma. Reticulohistiocytoma usually occurs as a solitary, firm dermal lesion less than 1 cm in diameter. Lesions favor the trunk and extremities. Solitary lesions and multiple lesions without systemic involvement, in contrast to MRH, have been described, mainly in adult men and rarely in children.

Multicentric Reticulohistiocytosis. A multisystem disease, MRH usually begins about age 50 (range 6–86 years). It is twice as common in women as men and affects all races. The primary manifestations are skin lesions and a potentially destructive arthritis. In 40% of cases the joint disease occurs first, in 30% the skin lesions precede the joint symptoms, and in 40% the joint and skin disease appear simultaneously.

Clinically, there may be a few to a few hundred firm, skin-colored to red-brown papules and nodules, mostly 2–10 mm in diameter, but some reaching several centimeters in size. These occur most frequently on the fingers and hands, with a tendency to cause paronychial lesions (Fig. 31.21). In about half of MRH patients, lesions will be arranged around nailfolds, giving a "coral bead" appearance, which may be associated with nail dystrophy. The upper half of the body, including the arms, scalp, face, ears, and neck, are also common sites. About 90% of patients have lesions on the face and hands. Nodular and papular involvement of the pinnae (Fig. 31.22) and a symmetric distribution of the lesions, especially over joints, are characteristic. The nodules on the arms, elbows, and knees may resemble rheumatoid nodules. Diffuse erythematous lesions can occur, at times simulating erythroderma. Patients may present initially with macular or minimally infiltrated erythema on sun-exposed sites, simulating a photodermatitis or dermatomyositis. Small papules are often present, which are useful in confirming the diagnosis of MRH. Lesions may ulcerate. Xanthelasma occurs in 30% of patients. Atypical patchy areas of hypopigmentation over the face and upper limbs have been noted. About 10% of MRH patients may complain of pruritus. The itching is not localized to the skin lesions and may precede their appearance.

Mucous membrane involvement is seen in one third of MRH patients and is most common on the lips and tongue; other sites are the gingiva, palate, buccal mucosa, nasopharynx, larynx, and sclera. Lesions of the esophagus can lead to dysphagia. One third have hypercholesterolemia and xanthelasma. Rheumatoid factor is usually negative.

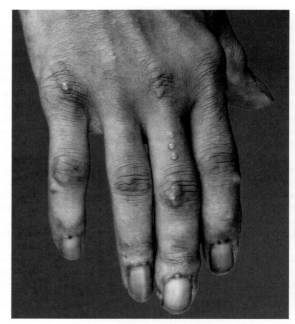

Fig. 31.21 Multicentric reticulohistiocytosis.

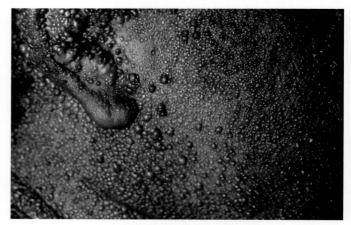

Fig. 31.22 Multicentric reticulohistiocytosis.

Osteoarticular changes are the most important aspect of MRH. No association exists between the extent, size, or severity of the skin eruption and the course of the joint disease. The associated arthropathy is an inflammatory, symmetric, polyarticular arthritis that can affect many joints, including the hands, knees, shoulders, wrists, hips, ankles, elbows, feet, and spine. The arthritis can be rapidly destructive and mutilating, with absorption and telescopic shortening of the phalanges and digits—doigts en lorgnette (opera-glass fingers). In earlier reports, at least 50% of cases developed arthritis mutilans, but this has been reduced to about 11%. The infiltrating cells in the skin and joints are identical on microscopic examination and immunophenotypic evaluation. The clinical course varies. In many cases, there is complete involution after about 8 years. The joint destruction is permanent, however, and is a cause of severe disability. The joint involvement may resemble rheumatoid arthritis and psoriatic arthritis. Weight loss and fever occur in one third of patients.

About 15% of patients with MRH have associated autoimmune disorders. Thyroiditis, Sjögren syndrome, ulcerative colitis, and vitiligo have all been reported. About 25% of reported cases have had an associated malignancy. Given this high rate of malignancy, every patient with MRH should have a careful history and physical examination and a complete age-appropriate cancer screening, repeated at regular intervals (similar to the protocol followed for patients with dermatomyositis). No specific tumor type has been associated; cancers reported with MRH include breast, gastrointestinal tract, genitourinary tract, and melanoma, as well as leukemia and lymphoma. The skin lesions usually appear before diagnosis of the malignancy, but synchronous behavior of the skin lesions and underlying malignancy is only occasionally reported. In one case TB was identified, and treatment of the TB led to resolution of the MRH.

Other organs and tissues may be involved, such as bone, muscle, lymph nodes, liver, myocardium, pericardium, lungs, pleura, and stomach. Myocardial involvement may be fatal. Usual interstitial pneumonia or typical MRH cells may be seen in pulmonary lesions.

Histologically, the skin lesions are usually centered in the middermis and tend to occupy much or all of the dermis. The infiltrating cells are mononuclear and multinucleate monocytes/macrophages. The giant cells are most characteristic, with an abundant smooth or slightly granular, eosinophilic or amphophilic, "ground-glass" cytoplasm. Their cytoplasm is darker in the center than at the periphery. These cells stain positive for periodic acid–Schiff (PAS) after diastase digestion. The overlying epidermis may be thinned but is usually separated from the dermal process by a narrow zone of collagen (grenz zone). Characteristically, there is a polymorphous infiltrate of lymphocytes, neutrophils, eosinophils, and plasma cells within the lesions. On immunohistochemistry, monocyte/macrophage cells stain positive for CD68, vimentin, and CD163. In MRH, the cells in the skin and joints stain positive for acid phosphatase that is tartrate resistant (TRAP) and cathepsin K, markers for osteoclasts. This may explain the response of MRH to bisphosphonates, which cause apoptosis of osteoclasts and are taken up by cells in the reticuloendothelial system.

Given the aggressive nature of the arthritis, early and adequate treatment should be considered. However, associated malignancy is common and can be worsened by immunosuppressive therapy. The same would be true if the patient had underlying asymptomatic TB. Initially, the patient should be screened for these two conditions, and these should be adequately treated if found. In patients free of neoplasia and TB, the treatment is individualized. Spontaneous remissions are common, making efficacy of treatment difficult to determine. The major goal of treatment is to prevent the destruction of the joints that are the cause of disability. TNF inhibitors and bisphosphonates are frequently employed as part of the therapeutic management, often in combination with other agents. If systemic therapy is considered, two approaches can be taken, one building off of TNF inhibitors, the other building off of bisphosphonates. The two agents may be used together as well. One approach is the use of the combination of systemic corticosteroids, methotrexate (or leflunomide), and a TNF inhibitor. Of the TNF inhibitors, infliximab has proved more effective than etanercept and should probably be the initial agent used. The other approach is to use a combination of immunosuppressives and a bisphosphonate. The infiltrating cells in MRH seem phenotypically to be osteoclastic in behavior, so this therapy is logical and appears to be joint sparing. In refractory cases, use of a bisphosphonate and TNF inhibitor with methotrexate and systemic corticosteroids could be considered. Tocilizumab has been used, as the granulomatous lesions involve TNF-α, IL-1, and IL-6 inflammation. For patients with skin lesions only, therapy is not required. PUVA, antimalarials, topical nitrogen mustard, and low-dose methotrexate, a bisphosphonate, or a TNF inhibitor could be considered if symptoms are severe.

UV light has been reported to induce lesions of the disease, and patients with photodistributed lesions or a dermatomyositis-like presentation should avoid light treatment.

Arai S, et al: Multicentric reticulohistiocytosis presenting with the cutaneous features of photosensitivity dermatitis. J Dermatol 2012; 39: 180.

Bennassar A, et al: Multicentric reticulohistiocytosis with elevated cytokine serum levels. J Dermatol 2011; 38: 905.

Goto H, et al: Successful treatment of multicentric reticulohistiocytosis with alendronate. Arthritis Rheum 2003; 48: 3538.

Hsiung SH, et al: Multicentric reticulohistiocytosis presenting with clinical features of dermatomyositis. J Am Acad Dermatol 2003; 48: S11.

Kalajian AH, Callen JP: Multicentric reticulohistiocytosis successfully treated with infliximab. Arch Dermatol 2008; 144: 1350.

Lonsdale-Eccles AA, et al: Successful treatment of multicentric reticulohistiocytosis with leflunomide. Br J Dermatol 2009; 161: 470.

Lovelace K, et al: Etanercept and the treatment of multicentric reticulohistiocytosis. Arch Dermatol 2005; 141: 1167.

Macía-Villa CC, Zea-Mendoza A: Multicentric reticulohistiocytosis. Clin Rheumatol 2016; 35: 527.

Mavragani CP, et al: Alleviation of polyarticular syndrome in multicentric reticulohistiocytosis with intravenous zoledronate. Ann Rheum Dis 2005; 64: 1521.

Miettinen M, Fetsch JF: Reticulohistiocytoma (solitary epithelioid histiocytoma). Am J Surg Pathol 2006; 30: 521.

Millar A, et al: Multicentric reticulohistiocytosis. Rheumatology (Oxford) 2008; 47: 1102.

Motegi S, et al: Successful treatment of multicentric reticulohistiocytosis with adalimumab, prednisolone, and methotrexate. Acta Derm Venereol 2016; 96: 124.

Pachecho-Tena C, et al: Treatment of multicentric reticulohistiocytosis with tocilizumab. J Clin Rheumatol 2013; 19: 272.

Satoh M, et al: Treatment trial of multicentric reticulohistiocytosis with a combination of prednisolone, methotrexate and alendronate. J Dermatol 2008; 35: 168.

Selmi C, et al: Multicentric reticulohistiocytosis. Curr Rheumatol Rep 2015; 17: 511.

Taniguichi T, et al: Ultraviolet light–induced Köbner phenomenon contributes to the development of skin eruptions in multicentric reticulohistiocytosis. Acta Derm Venereol 2011; 91: 160.

Webb-Detiege T, et al: Infiltration of histiocytes and multinucleated giant cells in the myocardium of a patient with multicentric reticulohistiocytosis. J Clin Rheumatol 2009; 15: 25.

West KL, et al: Multicentric reticulohistiocytosis. Arch Dermatol 2012; 148: 228.

Zhao H, et al: TNF antagonists in the treatment of multicentric reticulohistiocytosis. Mol Med Rep 2016; 14: 209.

Indeterminate Cell Histiocytosis

Indeterminate cell histiocytosis (ICH) is a rare histiocytosis composed of cells that stain variably with markers for Langerhans cells (S-100 and CD1a) but are negative for langerin (CD207) and do not demonstrate Langerhans cell granules on electron microscopy. The cells may be CD68 positive, suggesting a monocyte/macrophage lineage. The exact origin of these cells is unclear. One recent series of three cases demonstrated *ETV3-NCOA2* translocations, suggesting that ICH is a distinct entity. *ETV3* encodes a transcriptional repressor involved in macrophage growth arrest, and *NCOA2* encodes a transcription factor for balance between white and brown adipose tissue. ICH affects both children and adults. Solitary and multiple lesions may occur, and the color of lesions varies from yellow to red-brown. Lesions may be papules, plaques, or nodules 3 mm to 10 cm in size. These clinical features are not specific and resemble the papular lesions seen in many forms of non-LCH. Conjunctival involvement has been reported. Solitary malignant tumors with similar immunohistochemistry have been described, clinically resembling atypical fibroxanthoma. ICH seems to have a benign course in the vast majority of patients, and no therapy is required. UVB, PUVA, and total-skin electron beam therapy have resulted in clearing of skin lesions. Pravastatin, thalidomide (alone or with isotretinoin), and methotrexate have been effective. Many patients have been treated with numerous chemotherapeutic agents similar to those used for LCH, but therapeutic response has been equivocal. Acute myelogenous leukemia has followed some of these courses of chemotherapy. Solitary lesions with malignant histology should be managed with surgical excision, ensuring adequate margins. The utility of adjunctive therapy and sentinel lymph node sampling is not known. Postscabietic nodules and rarely post–pityriasis rosea lesions may contain a proliferation of cells that are immunohistologically identical to indeterminate cells.

Bakry OA, et al: Indeterminate cell histiocytosis with naïve cells. Rare Tumors 2013; 5: e13.

Brown RA, et al: *ETV3-NCOA2* in indeterminate cell histiocytosis. Blood 2015; 126: 2344.

Burns MV, et al: Treatment of indeterminate cell histiocytosis with pravastatin. J Am Acad Dermatol 2010; 64: e85.

Caputo R, et al: Chemotherapeutic experience in indeterminate cell histiocytosis. Br J Dermatol 2005; 153: 206.

Ferran M, et al: Acquired mucosal indeterminate cell histiocytoma. Pediatr Dermatol 2007; 24: 253.

Fournier J, et al: Successful treatment of indeterminate cell histiocytosis with low-dose methotrexate. J Dermatol 2011; 38: 937.

Logemann N, et al: Indeterminate cell histiocytosis successfully treated with narrowband UVB. Dermatol Online J 2013; 19: 20031.

Malhomme de la Roche H, et al: Indeterminate cell histiocytosis responding to total skin electron beam therapy. Br J Dermatol 2008; 158: 838.

Tóth B, et al: Indeterminate cell histiocytosis in a pediatric patient. Pathol Oncol Res 2012; 18: 535.

Vener C, et al: Indeterminate cell histiocytosis in association with later occurrence of acute myeloblastic leukaemia. Br J Dermatol 2007; 156: 1357.

Wollenberg A, et al: Long-lasting "Christmas tree rash" in an adolescent. Acta Derm Venereol 2002; 82: 288.

Sea-Blue Histiocytosis

Sea-blue histiocytosis may occur as a familial inherited syndrome or as an acquired secondary or systemic infiltrative process. The characteristic and diagnostic cell is a histiocytic cell containing cytoplasmic granules that stain blue-green with Giemsa and blue with May-Gruenwald stain. The disorder is characterized by infiltration of these cells into the marrow, spleen, liver, lymph nodes, and lungs, as well as the skin in some patients. Skin lesions include papules or nodules, facial waxy plaques, eyelid swelling, and patchy-gray pigmentation of the face and upper trunk. Similar histologic findings have occurred in patients with myelogenous leukemia, light-chain deposition disease, adult Niemann-Pick disease (type B), sphingomyelinase deficiency, or mutations in the apolipoprotein E gene, and following the prolonged use of intravenous fat supplementation or liposomal amphotericin B. The unifying feature in all these conditions is an abnormal lipid metabolism by the infiltrating histiocytes. This condition has been seen in the infiltrate of a patient with CTCL.

Bermejo N, et al: Sea-blue histiocytosis in bone marrow of a patient with chronic thrombocytopenia. Acta Haematol 2015; 133: 277.

Bigorgne C, et al: Sea-blue histiocyte syndrome in the bone marrow secondary to total parenteral nutrition. Leukemia Lymphoma 1998; 28: 523.

Caputo R, et al: Unusual variants of non–Langerhans cell histiocytosis. J Am Acad Dermatol 2007; 57: 1031.

Michot JM, et al: Very prolonged liposomal amphotericin B use leading to a lysosomal storage disease. Int J Antimicrob Agents 2014; 43: 566.

Naghashpour M, Cualing H: Splenomegaly with sea-blue histiocytosis, dyslipidemia, and nephropathy in a patient with lecithin-cholesterol acyltransferase deficiency. Metabolism 2009; 58: 1459.

Newman B, et al: Aggressive histiocytic disorders that can involve the skin. J Am Acad Dermatol 2007; 56: 302.

Langerhans Cell Histiocytosis (X-Type Histiocytoses)

The X-type group of histiocytoses is caused by Langerhans cells. A rare disease, LCH is characterized by proliferation of Langerhans cells. Many organs can be affected. The prognosis is based on the locations of involvement. Patients who have involvement of the reticuloendothelial system (bone marrow, liver, and spleen) have higher-risk disease and accordingly the worst prognosis, whereas those with only skin, bone, or pituitary involvement have the best. Age of onset is an important determinant of the natural history of the disease, and therefore childhood and adult forms of LCH are considered separately. Adults are more likely to have mucocutaneous lesions, twice as likely to reactivate (63% vs. 37%), and more likely to die of their disease (24% vs. 11%). Patients may begin with any pattern of disease and evolve or relapse to another pattern. This is especially true of younger children. Up to 50% of children under age 1 year diagnosed with skin-limited LCH progress to have multisystem disease. Repeated evaluation and close follow-up are required.

The spectrum of disease is broad, with solitary, usually benign and autoinvoluting lesions at one end and multicentric, multiorgan visceral and skin disease at the other. The Langerhans cells seem to be myeloid dendritic cells and not necessarily epidermal Langerhans cells. Most cases of LCH demonstrate clonality and telomere shortening. In addition, *BRAF* 600E and *ARAF* mutations have been detected in a majority of cases. All these features would suggest LCH as a "neoplastic" condition. Adult patients with LCH may have myeloid and solid cancers supporting a "neoplastic" phenotype. In the case of associated leukemias, the leukemic cells may share the same surface markers and may be clonally related. However, preliminary evidence shows that IL-17A is elevated, and IL-17A receptor status determines extent of disease. This suggests that LCH represents a "hybrid" condition with features of both neoplasia and immunologic dysregulation. This helps explain the variable outcome from spontaneous involution to progressive and fatal disease.

Histologically, in all cases of LCH in the skin there is a dense dermal infiltrate of Langerhans cells. This can be superficial and immediately below the epidermis (usually corresponding to small papules or scaly patches clinically), folliculocentric, or deep and diffuse (in papular and nodular lesions). The Langerhans cells are recognized by their abundant, amphophilic cytoplasm and eccentric round or kidney bean–shaped nucleus, in addition to appropriate staining as outlined later. There is frequently exocytosis of the abnormal cells into the overlying epidermis. If this is extensive, macroscopic vesicles can be seen, and erosion can occur secondarily. The dermal infiltrate is accompanied by many other inflammatory cells, including neutrophils, eosinophils, lymphocytes, and plasma cells. Dermal edema and hemorrhage are characteristically present.

In larger and older lesions, the infiltrating histiocytic cells become foamy, and fibrosis may be present. These older lesions may lack immunoreactivity for specific Langerhans cell markers and can resemble JXG. The histologic features of the Langerhans cells, such as nuclear atypia and mitotic indices, do not predict prognosis and are not reproducible. Immunohistochemistry is useful in confirming the diagnosis. The infiltrating cells in LCH are positive for S-100, CD1A, and Langerin (CD207), which is a protein expressed in the Birbeck granule. Electron microscopy is rarely required to diagnose LCH because of this panel of Langerhans cell, "characteristic" markers.

International standardization of terminology and treatment protocols has resulted in improved management of patients and has allowed for investigational protocols rapidly to determine efficacy of treatments identified by recent scientific advancements, such as use of vemurafenib with the identification of *BRAF* V600E mutations.

Congenital Self-Healing Reticulohistiocytosis (Hashimoto-Pritzker Disease)

Congenital self-healing reticulohistiocytosis (CSHR) is an auto-involuting, self-limited form of LCH. It can be considered as one end of the spectrum of LCH. CSHR is usually present at birth or appears very soon thereafter, although a case in an 8-year-old child has been reported. CSHR has been described in two forms: a solitary and a multinodular variant. Solitary or generalized lesions can affect any part of the cutaneous surface. Lesions range from 0.2–2.5 cm in diameter. Lesions may grow postnatally. Exceptionally large tumors up to 8 cm in diameter can occur. At presentation, the lesions can be papules or nodules, with or without erosion or ulceration. Individual lesions are red, brown, pink, or dusky (Fig. 31.23). Lesions may rarely appear as hemorrhagic bullae. Infections such as herpes simplex and bacterial infections can also cause hemorrhagic papules and blisters and must be ruled out by culture. Lesions greater than 1 cm characteristically ulcerate as they resolve. Lesions are asymptomatic and spontaneously involute over the first 6 months, leaving normal skin or atrophic scarring from the ulcerated nodules. Internal involvement has been reported on the mucosa and even in the lungs (which also have spontaneously involuted), making distinction of CSHR and autoinvoluting LCH difficult. Histologically, the skin lesions are composed of Langerhans cells, and no histologic features identify this variant of LCH. Because LCH with systemic involvement may present in identical fashion, systemic evaluation is recommended, including a physical examination, complete blood count, liver function tests, and radiologic evaluation of the bones. The affected child must be followed regularly because, as in other forms of LCH, recurrences (especially within the first year) occur in about 10% of cases.

Childhood Langerhans Cell Histiocytosis. In childhood LCH, boys are slightly more often affected than girls. The incidence in children is about 2.6 cases per 1 million, with a greater rate in children under 1 year of age (7 per 1 million), 2 cases per 1 million in ages 1–4, and about 1 case per 1 million in ages 5–14. Children conceived through in vitro fertilization before 2002 appear to have increased risk for development of LCH. Neonatal disease occurs in 6% of cases but at times is unrecognized, especially if asymptomatically involving an internal organ (not affecting its function). Overall, in childhood LCH, bone lesions are present in about two thirds of cases and skin disease in about one third. Only 10% of cases have neither skin nor bone involvement. In children under 1 year of age the skin is involved in three quarters of cases, with ear and bone being involved in about one third. The prognosis for children under 1 year is worse because two thirds of children under 1 year have multisystem disease, with half having involvement of liver, lungs, or bone marrow. In children age 1–4, bone disease is most common, but two thirds or more have multisystem disease. In children age 5–14, bone disease is almost always seen, and multisystem disease is seen in less than 20%.

Adult Langerhans Cell Histiocytosis. In adults the peak age of presentation is between 20 and 35 years, with multisystem disease in one third to two thirds of adults with LCH. Bones are the most common organ involved, and 12% of adult LCH patients have disease limited to one or several bones. Skin and mucosal involvement is the second most common manifestation in adults. Diabetes insipidus occurs in 20% of patients, and other endocrine abnormalities can result from hypothalamic-pituitary involvement. These remain a problem after the LCH is treated and require constant monitoring.

Clinical Presentation

Skin Lesions. About 10% of children have single-organ disease involving only the skin, and 50% of children with multisystem LCH have skin involvement. Almost 90% of children less than 1 year old with multisystem LCH have skin lesions. The pattern of skin disease does not predict the presence or extent of systemic disease. The most common form of skin disease in children is tiny red, red-brown or yellow papules that have a characteristic hemorrhagic top and associated petechial component that are widespread but favor the intertriginous areas, behind the ears, and the scalp (Figs. 31.24 and 31.25). There is a superficial resemblance to seborrheic dermatitis, especially in infants, but the focal hemorrhage differentiates it. The papules are often folliculocentric. Lesions may erode or weep. In children, this pattern is frequently associated with multisystem disease. In a rare variant of this LCH pattern (more commonly seen in infants), vesicles appear (Fig. 31.26). The vesicles rupture easily, resulting in widespread erosions. This presentation may be confused with other bullous diseases, especially congenital candidiasis, herpesvirus infections, bullous impetigo, bullous mastocytosis, primary immunobullous diseases, and epidermolysis bullosa, and cultures should be done to differentiate (especially in neonates, in whom infectious diseases can be lethal). The vesicles result from large intraepidermal collections of Langerhans cells, and a Tzanck smear may demonstrate this. A less common presentation is with slightly larger papules, up to 1 cm in diameter. These lesions tend to be yellow-red and resemble xanthomas or xanthogranulomas. They can be numerous and widespread. A rare variant resembling lichen planopilaris has been reported. Congenital lesions with hemorrhage have been reported as resembling "blueberry muffin" babies, but the biopsies show typical LCH.

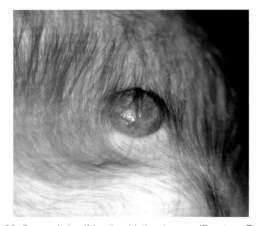

Fig. 31.23 Congenital self-healing histiocytomas. (Courtesy Paul Honig, MD.)

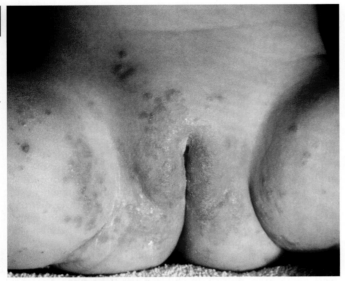

Fig. 31.24 Langerhans cell histiocytosis.

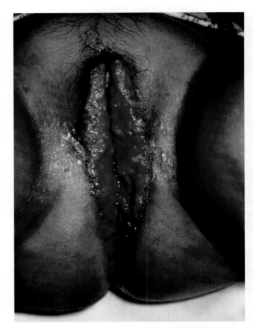

Fig. 31.27 Adult Langerhans cell histiocytosis.

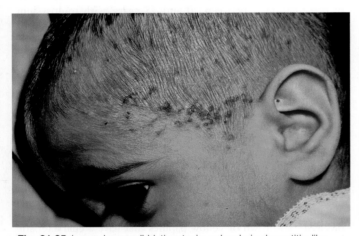

Fig. 31.25 Langerhans cell histiocytosis, seborrheic dermatitis–like eruption with hemorrhage.

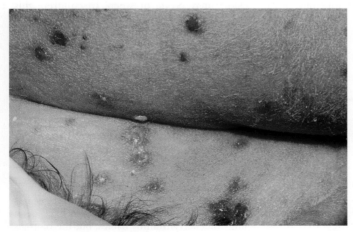

Fig. 31.26 Langerhans cell histiocytosis, bullous lesions.

Although uncommon, nail changes can occur, including nail dystrophy, nail bed purpura, loss of the nail plate, and paronychia. Both fingernails and toenails may be affected. Most patients with nail involvement have multisystem disease. LCH restricted to the genitalia is rare, but vulvar, inguinal, and perianal disease may be the initial manifestation of LCH. It tends to be painful and ulcerative and may simulate hidradenitis suppurativa or cutaneous Crohn disease, because axillary and scalp involvement may also be present.

In adults the skin lesions can be papular or diffuse, sometimes with both forms of lesion present at different sites. Acneiform lesions of the chest and back, identical clinically to acne vulgaris, can occur. Xanthomatous lesions may be seen. A pattern repeatedly reported in the skin of adults with LCH is a red, erosive, intertriginous eruption (Fig. 31.27), with a close resemblance to deficiency dermatitis or cutaneous Crohn disease. Similar to pediatric lesions there is usually a hemorrhagic or petechial component. It favors the groin and inframammary areas, especially in elderly women. Nodular lesions of scabies can closely simulate LCH. This includes the finding of Langerhans or indeterminate cells in the dermal infiltrate on electron microscopy and S-100 and CD1a staining. The larger papules resemble JXG and xanthomas.

Oral Mucosa Lesions. The oral mucosa may be involved in children with LCH. Mucosal ulcerations are painful and often affect the buccal mucosa. They primarily affect the buccal mucosa. Alveolar bone lesions are the most common oral lesions, and these osteolytic lesions can lead to significant periodontitis. Gingival ulceration can result (Fig. 31.28). Teeth detach from the underlying bone and on x-ray appear to be "floating." Palpable masses and gingival lesions should be sought and a dental evaluation completed in all patients. Cervical adenopathy is common. Bilateral parotid swelling may occur.

Bony Lesions. The most commonly involved organ in pediatric LCH is the bone (Fig. 31.29). The lesions may be asymptomatic or may cause pain. The skull is most often involved, followed by the long bones, then the flat bones. Bony lesions tend to occur in older children and young adults. Lesions are treated with curettage, intralesional corticosteroids, or radiation. Endocrine dysfunction occurs, usually in the form of diabetes insipidus,

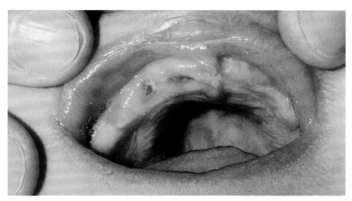

Fig. 31.28 Langerhans cell histiocytosis, gingival lesions.

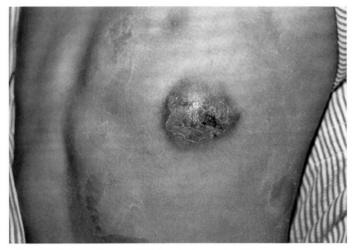

Fig. 31.29 Langerhans cell histiocytosis, eosinophilic granuloma of rib that eroded through to the skin.

which is more common in patients with bone disease of the skull and in those with extensive disease. Diabetes insipidus is one of the common long-term sequelae of children recovering from LCH.

Visceral Involvement. The bone marrow may be affected, resulting in cytopenias. This may present as purpura in the skin. The liver may be involved directly by infiltration with Langerhans cells or may be affected indirectly by enlarged nodes in the porta hepatis, leading to obstructive disease. Either pattern can lead to biliary cirrhosis. Pulmonary disease with diffuse micronodular infiltrates and cysts occurs less frequently in children than in adults with LCH.

Pulmonary LCH occurs on average in the 3rd decade. A diffuse micronodular pattern on chest radiograph may progress to cyst formation (honeycomb lung), large bullae, and pneumothorax. More than 90% of adults with pulmonary LCH are tobacco or marijuana smokers. Pneumothorax occurs in 25% of cases. High-resolution CT is useful for diagnosis. Lung transplantation may be required. It is unclear if isolated pulmonary LCH is a reactive process or a variant of LCH.

Treatment and Prognosis. In LCH, outcome and therefore therapeutic choice is determined by the extent of involvement and, more important, the function of affected organs. Children younger than 1 year with multisystem disease have the worst prognosis, with mortality rate approaching 50%; children age 1–4 years have a 30% or lower mortality rate; and mortality rate is only 6% in children 5 years or older. Involvement of the ear and lung is a poor prognostic finding in patients with multisystem disease. Early initial response to multidrug chemotherapy in childhood multisystem LCH is an important predictor of survival, with survival of 92% of responders and 11% of nonresponders after 6 weeks of treatment. Baseline and repeated evaluation is important. Lesions in one organ system may resolve while disease progresses in another organ. Skin lesions may spontaneously resolve, only for the disease to recur, even years later, so patients must be followed regularly.

For treatment and prognosis, patients are classified as having single-system LCH or multisystem LCH. Those with multisystem LCH are further stratified into those with involvement of high-risk "organs" (bone marrow, liver, spleen, and CNS) and those without involvement of these organ systems. Patients with multisystem disease should be referred to an oncologist for evaluation and treatment. Due to the *BRAF* 600E mutation, the *BRAF* inhibitor vemurafenib has shown excellent efficacy. Most often, vinblastine and a corticosteroid are used as initial treatment, but reactivation remains a problem. Patients with localized skin disease can be managed by the dermatologist. Topical steroids, topical nitrogen mustard, PUVA, NB-UVB (or excimer laser), thalidomide methotrexate and azathioprine can be considered, depending on the extent of skin disease. Also, 5% imiquimod may be effective for limited skin lesions. Oral retinoids (acetretin and isotretinoin) can be used adjunctively with other treatments if there are no contraindications.

Associated lymphomas, solid tumors, and myelodysplasias have occurred in patients with LCH, with acute lymphoblastic leukemia and myelodysplastic syndrome preceding the appearance of LCH, and acute myelogenous leukemia and acute lymphoblastic leukemia following it. In some cases of cutaneous and systemic lymphomas, aggregates of Langerhans cells are seen in the tissue affected by the lymphoma. Whether this represents the coexistence of LCH and lymphoma, or a reactive proliferation of Langerhans cells within the tissue affected by the lymphoma, is unknown.

Aggarwal V, et al: Congenital Langerhans cell histiocytosis with skin and lung involvement. Indian J Pediatr 2010; 77: 811.

Åkefeldt SO, et al: Langerhans cell histiocytosis in children born 1982–2005 after in vitro fertilization. Acta Paediatrica 2012; 101: 1151.

Bechan GI, et al: Telomere length shortening in Langerhans cell histiocytosis. Br J Haematol 2008; 140: 420.

Black A, et al: Seventy-nine-year-old man with Langerhans cell histiocytosis treated with cladribine. J Am Acad Dermatol 2010; 65: 681.

Brown NA, et al: High prevalence of somatic MAP2K1 mutations in *BRAF* V600E negative Langerhans cell histiocytosis. Blood 2014; 124: 1655.

Campanati A, et al: Purely cutaneous Langerhans' cell histiocytosis in an adult woman. Acta Derm Venereol 2009; 89: 299.

Chen AJ, et al: Congenital self-healing reticulohistiocytosis. Australas J Dermatol 2016; 57: 76.

Christie LJ, et al: Lesions resembling Langerhans cell histiocytosis in association with other lymphoproliferative disorders. Hum Pathol 2006; 37: 32.

Delprat C, Aricò M: Blood spotlight on Langerhans cell histiocytosis. Blood 2014; 124: 867.

Edelbroek JR, et al: Langerhans cell histiocytosis first presenting in the skin of adults. Br J Dermatol 2012; 167: 1287.

Fahrner B, et al: Long-term outcome of hypothalamic pituitary tumors in Langerhans cell histiocytosis. Pediatr Blood Cancer 2012; 58: 606.

Fernandes LB, et al: Langerhans cells histiocytosis with vulvar involvement and responding to thalidomide therapy. An Bras Dermatol 2011; 86: S78.

Fleta-Asin B, et al: Progressive cutaneous lesions in an elderly woman with systemic failure. Int J Dermatol 2012; 51: 1175.

Girschikofsky M, et al: Management of adult patients with Langerhans cell histiocytosis. Orphanet J Rare Dis 2013; 8: 72.

Golpanian S, et al: Pediatric histiocytosis in the United States. J Surg Res 2014; 190: 221.

Hancox JG, et al: Adult onset folliculocentric Langerhans cell histiocytosis confined to the scalp. Am J Dermatopathol 2004; 26: 123.

Harmon CM, et al: Langerhans cell histiocytosis. Arch Pathol Lab Med 2015; 139: 1211.

Haroche J, et al: Dramatic efficacy of vemurafenib in both multisystemic and refractory Erdheim-Chester disease and Langerhans cell histiocytosis harboring the *BRAF* V600E mutation. Blood 2013; 121: 1495.

Haupt R, et al: Langerhans cell histiocytosis (LCH). Pediatr Blood Cancer 2013; 60: 175.

Hoang MT, et al: Recurrent perianal red plaque with superficial erosions and pustular exudate in a 16-month-old boy. Clin Exp Dermatol 2012; 38: 203.

Huang JT, et al: Langerhans cell histiocytosis mimicking molluscum contagiosum. J Am Acad Dermatol 2011; 67: e117.

Kansal R, et al: Identification of the V600D mutation in exon 15 of the *BRAF* oncogene in congenital, benign Langerhans cell histiocytosis. Genes Chromosomes Cancer 2013; 52: 99.

Kapur P, et al: Congenital self-healing reticulohistiocytosis (Hashimoto-Pritzker disease). J Am Acad Dermatol 2007; 56: 290.

Kim BE, et al: Clinical features and treatment outcomes of Langerhans cell histiocytosis. J Pediatr Hematol Oncol 2014; 36: 125.

Kim JE, et al: Solitary congenital erosion in a newborn. Ann Dermatol 2014; 26: 250.

Kurt S, et al: Diagnosis of primary Langerhans cell histiocytosis of the vulva in a postmenopausal woman. Case Rep Obstet Gynecol 2013; 2013: 962670.

Larsen L, et al: Congenital self-healing reticulohistiocytosis. Dermatology Online J 2012; 18: 2.

Lindahl LM, et al: Topical nitrogen mustard therapy in patients with Langerhans cell histiocytosis. Br J Dermatol 2012; 166: 642.

Lourda M, et al: Detection of IL-17A-producing peripheral blood monocytes in Langerhans cell histiocytosis patients. Clin Immunol 2014; 153: 112.

Maia RC, et al: Langerhans cell histiocytosis. Hematology 2015; 20: 83.

Mataix J, et al: Nail changes in Langerhans cell histiocytosis. Pediatr Dermatol 2008; 25: 247.

Mir A, et al: Perifollicular Langerhans cell histiocytosis. Dermatol Online J 2012; 18: 6.

Morimoto A, et al: Recent advances in Langerhans cell histiocytosis. Pediatr Int 2014; 56: 451.

Murakami I, et al: IL-17A receptor expression differs between subclasses of Langerhans cell histiocytosis, which might settle the IL-17A controversy. Virchows Arch 2013; 462: 219.

Nakashima T, et al: Congenital self-healing LCH. Pediatr Int 2010; 52: e224.

O'Kane D, et al: Langerhans cell histiocytosis associated with breast carcinoma successfully treated with topical imiquimod. Clin Exp Dermatol 2009; 34: e829.

Oliveira A, et al: Langerhans cell histiocytosis. Dermatol Online J. 2012; 18: 8.

Pedrosa AF, et al: Primary Langerhans cell histiocytosis of the vulva. Int J Dermatol 2014; 53: e240.

Podjasek JO, et al: Adult-onset systemic Langerhans cell histiocytosis mimicking inflammatory bowel disease. Int J Dermatol 2014; 53: 305.

Ruiz-Villaverde R, et al: Erythroderma as an initial presentation of Langerhans cell histiocytosis involving the sinus. Actas Dermosifiliogr 2014; 105: 630.

Sahm F, et al: BRAFV600E mutant protein is expressed in cells of variable maturation in Langerhans cell histiocytosis. Blood 2012; 120: e28.

Satter EK, et al: Diffuse xanthogranulomatous dermatitis and systemic Langerhans cell histiocytosis. J Am Acad Dermatol 2009; 60: 841.

Shaffer MP, et al: Langerhans cell histiocytosis presenting as blueberry muffin baby. J Am Acad Dermatol 2005; 53: S143.

Shannon K, Hermiston M: A(nother) RAF mutation in LCH. Blood 2014; 123: 3063.

Slott Jensen ML, et al: Congenital self-healing reticulohistiocytosis: an important diagnostic challenge. Acta Paediatr 2011; 100: 784.

Szturz P, et al: Lenalidomide proved effective in multisystem Langerhans cell histiocytosis. Acta Oncol 2012; 51: 412.

Von Stebut E, et al: Successful treatment of adult multisystemic Langerhans cell histiocytosis with psoralen-UV-A, prednisone, mercaptopurine, and vinblastine. Arch Dermatol 2008; 144: 649.

Wang P, et al: Extensive cutaneous Langerhans cell histiocytosis in an elderly woman. J Dermatol 2011; 38: 794.

Wheller L, et al: Unilesional self-limited Langerhans cell histiocytosis. J Cutan Pathol 2013; 40: 595.

Yazc N, et al: Langerhans cell histiocytosis with involvement of nails and lungs in an adolescent. J Pediatr Hematol Oncol 2008; 30: 77.

Yoje SL, et al: Langerhans cell histiocytosis in acute leukemias of ambiguous or myeloid lineage in adult patients. Mod Pathol 2014; 27: 651.

Yurkovich M, et al: Solitary congenital self-healing Langerhans cell histiocytosis. Dermatol Online J 2013; 19: 3.

32 Cutaneous Lymphoid Hyperplasia, Cutaneous T-Cell Lymphoma, Other Malignant Lymphomas, and Allied Diseases

CUTANEOUS LYMPHOID HYPERPLASIA (LYMPHOCYTOMA CUTIS, LYMPHADENOSIS BENIGNA CUTIS, PSEUDOLYMPHOMA)

Benign cutaneous lymphoid hyperplasia can be caused by medications, injected foreign substances, infections, and arthropod bites, or it may be idiopathic. If there is a histologic resemblance to lymphoma, the term *pseudolymphoma* is often used. By standard techniques, most cases of cutaneous lymphoid hyperplasia will be found to lack clonality. Cases of monoclonal B-cell and T-cell cutaneous lymphoid hyperplasia do occur. Thus a finding of monoclonality does not equate to the diagnosis of malignancy or lymphoma, and it does not predict biologic behavior.

Two clinical patterns of cutaneous lymphoid hyperplasia exist. The nodular form consists of nodular and diffuse dermal aggregates of lymphocytes, macrophages, and dendritic cells (DCs). The clinicohistologic differential diagnosis is cutaneous B-cell lymphoma. The diffuse type is usually associated with drug exposure or photosensitivity (actinic reticuloid). Histologically, it must be distinguished from cutaneous T-cell lymphoma.

Cutaneous Lymphoid Hyperplasias—Nodular B-Cell Pattern

The nodular pattern of cutaneous lymphoid hyperplasia is the most common pattern. It usually presents in adults and is two to three times more common in women. It favors the face (cheek, nose, or earlobe), and the majority of cases present as a solitary (Fig. 32.1) or localized cluster of asymptomatic, erythematous to violaceous papules or nodules. Less frequently, lesions may affect the trunk (36%) or extremities (25%). At times, the lesions may coalesce into a plaque or may be widespread in one region, where they present as miliary papules. Systemic symptoms are absent and, except for rare cases with regional lymphadenopathy, there are no other physical or laboratory abnormalities. It is usually idiopathic but can be caused by tattoos, *Borrelia* infections, herpes zoster scars, antigen injections, acupuncture, drug reactions, and persistent insect bite reactions.

Borrelia-induced cutaneous lymphoid hyperplasia occurs more commonly in young women. It tends to involve the earlobe and nipple. In contrast, borrelial immunocytoma (classified as a subtype of marginal zone lymphoma) appears as tense pink nodules on the legs of older men. The lack of borrelial pseudolymphoma in the United States compared with Europe may relate to the presence of different borrelial species in Europe, specifically *Borrelia afzelii*, that cause borreliosis. Lesions occur at the site of the tick bite or close to the edge of a lesion of erythema migrans. They may appear up to 10 months after infection. Lesions may be multiple and favor the earlobes, nipple/areola, nose, and, in men, the scrotal area and vary from 1–5 cm in diameter. Usually there are no symptoms, but associated regional lymphadenopathy may be present. Late manifestations of *Borrelia* infection are uncommon. The diagnosis is suspected from a history of a tick bite or erythema migrans, the location (earlobe or nipple), and the histologic picture. The diagnosis is confirmed by an elevated anti-*Borrelia* antibody (present in 50% of cases) and the finding of borrelial DNA in the affected tissue. The treatment is penicillin. Rare cases progress to true lymphoma.

Histologic examination of nodular cutaneous lymphoid hyperplasia reveals a dense, nodular infiltrate that occupies primarily the dermis and lessens in the deeper dermis and subcutaneous fat (i.e., it is "top-heavy"). The process is usually separated from the epidermis by a clear grenz zone. The infiltrate is composed chiefly of mature small and large lymphocytes, histiocytes, plasma cells, DCs, and eosinophils. In the deeper portions, well-defined germinal centers are usually seen, with central large lymphoid cells with abundant cytoplasm and tingible body macrophages, and a peripheral cuff of small lymphocytes. A plasma cell–predominant variant has been described. Reactive hyperplasia of adnexal epithelium is common and characteristic, but it may also occasionally be seen in true lymphomas. Germinal centers are symmetric and surrounded by a mix of B and T cells. BCL-6 and CD10 expression is limited to the germinal centers, which also have an intact CD21+ network of DCs. Typically, more than 90% of the cells in the germinal center express the proliferative marker Ki-67 (MIB-1). There is no evidence of light-chain restriction by in situ hybridization. CD30+ cells may occasionally be prominent, raising concern about the development of a CD30+ lymphoproliferative disorder.

Because most lesions are asymptomatic, treatment is often not required. If the process has been induced by a medication, use of the medication should be discontinued. Infection should be treated and localized foci of infection removed. Intralesional steroidal agents are sometimes beneficial, but lesions may recur in a few months. Potent topical corticosteroids may also be tried for superficial lesions. Intralesional corticosteroids, cryosurgery, thalidomide (100 mg/day for a few months), interferon (IFN) alfa, IFN alfa-2b, laser ablation, and surgical excision can all produce good results. Low-dose radiation therapy is usually very effective and may be used on refractory facial lesions that cannot be satisfactorily removed surgically.

Cutaneous Lymphoid Hyperplasias—Bandlike T-Cell Pattern

Cutaneous lymphoid hyperplasias may histologically show a bandlike and perivascular dermal infiltrate, at times with epidermotropism. The lesions may be idiopathic or may be caused by photosensitivity (formerly called actinic reticuloid; now called chronic actinic dermatitis), medications (usually anticonvulsants, but also many others), or contact dermatitis (so-called lymphomatoid contact dermatitis). Clinically these patients have lesions that resemble mycosis fungoides: widespread erythema with scaling. Thicker plaques may occur as well, and these cases are frequently caused by medications. The treatment is to stop any implicated medication. If stopping the medication is ineffective, topical and intralesional corticosteroids, psoralen plus ultraviolet A (PUVA) therapy, and, for persistent localized lesions, radiotherapy may be considered. Histologically, a T-cell–rich band of lymphocytes is present. Epidermotropism, atypia, and even clonality may suggest

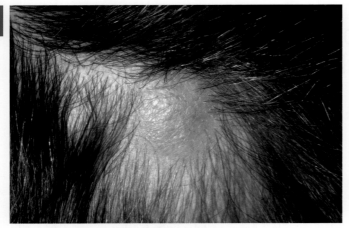

Fig. 32.1 Cutaneous lymphoid hyperplasia, nodular B-cell pattern.

mycosis fungoides, but the lesions resolve when the drug or other inciting agent is withdrawn.

Jessner Lymphocytic Infiltrate of the Skin

The existence of this entity has recently been challenged, and the condition may best be classified as a variant of lupus erythematosus (LE). Clinically Jessner infiltrate is a persistent papular and plaquelike eruption that is photosensitive and occurs primarily on the face. Histologically there is a superficial and deep perivascular and periadnexal lymphocytic infiltrate. Interface dermatitis is absent. The infiltrating lymphocytes are suppressor T cells (CD8+). Features that suggest this may be distinct from other forms of cutaneous LE include the absence of an interface dermatitis, lack of mucin, and negative direct immunofluorescence (DIF). Tumid LE also lacks interface dermatitis but has ample mucin. Polymorphous light eruption (PMLE) is distinguished from Jessner infiltrate by having edematous papules and plaques that are more transient and by the presence of dermal edema. In PMLE the infiltrating cells are also CD8+. True cases of lymphocytic infiltration of the skin may still exist. To distinguish them clearly from LE and PMLE, the lesions must contain predominantly CD8+ suppressor T cells, must lack dermal mucin and dermal edema, and must be fixed (not transient as with PMLE); patients must have negative DIF and serologic testing for LE. Both Jessner lymphocytic infiltrate and chronic cutaneous LE respond to antimalarials.

Mitteldorf C, et al: Cutaneous pseudolymphoma. Surg Pathol Clin. 2017; 10: 455.
Romero-Pérez D, et al: Cutaneous pseudolymphomas. Actas Dermosifiliogr 2016; 107: 640.
Shetty SK, et al: Pseudolymphoma versus lymphoma. J Oral Maxillofac Pathol 2016; 20: 328.
Staser K, et al: Injection-site cutaneous pseudolymphoma induced by a GM-CSF-producing tumor cell vaccine. JAMA Dermatol 2017; 153: 332.

CUTANEOUS LYMPHOMAS

Because cutaneous Hodgkin disease is very rare, the term *non-Hodgkin lymphoma* has little meaning when speaking of a lymphoma in the skin, because virtually all cutaneous lymphomas are "non-Hodgkin lymphomas." Cutaneous lymphoma can be considered to be either primary or secondary. Primary cutaneous lymphomas are those that occur in the skin, and where no evidence of extracutaneous involvement is found for some period after the appearance of the cutaneous disease. Secondary cutaneous lymphoma includes cases that have simultaneous or preceding evidence of extracutaneous involvement. These cases are best classified and managed as lymph node–based lymphomas with skin involvement. This conceptual separation is not ideal, but it has been important in developing classification schemes and determining prognosis in cutaneous lymphomas.

For many years, classification of lymphomas has been based on their histologic appearance, and lesions from all organ systems were classified histomorphologically in an identical manner to lymphomas arising in lymph nodes. It had been recognized that these classification schemes have major shortcomings when applied to extranodal lymphomas. Specifically, they did not uniformly predict clinical behavior. The new World Health Organization (WHO) classification scheme recognizes distinct forms of primary cutaneous lymphoma.

Cutaneous lymphomas are classified based on their cell type. There are B-cell lymphomas and T-cell lymphomas, but B-cell lymphomas can be T-cell rich. In the latter cases, atypia is restricted to the B-cell population, and immunoglobulin gene rearrangements are detected. Histologic features used in the classification system include cell size (large vs. small), nuclear morphology (cleaved or noncleaved), and immunophenotype. Because appropriate classification may be prognostically important, experienced dermatopathology consultation should be sought in cases of cutaneous lymphoma.

Primary Cutaneous T-Cell Lymphomas

A major insight into cutaneous lymphoma was the finding that the majority of lymphomas in the skin were of T-cell origin. This is logical, because T cells normally traffic through the skin and are important in "skin-associated lymphoid tissue." Unfortunately, dermatologists frequently use the term *cutaneous T-cell lymphoma* (CTCL) synonymously with *mycosis fungoides* (MF). Although MF represents the large majority of primary CTCLs, up to 30% of primary CTCLs are not MF. The following discussion is divided into MF and related conditions, Sézary syndrome, lymphomatoid papulosis, and non-MF primary CTCLs.

Mycosis Fungoides

Mycosis fungoides (MF) is a malignant neoplasm of T-lymphocyte origin, almost always a memory T-helper (Th) cell. The incidence has been cited as 1 in 300,000 per year, but has been increasing. MF affects all races. In the United States black persons are relatively more often affected than white persons. MF is twice as common in men as in women.

Natural History. In most cases, MF is a chronic, slowly progressive disorder. It usually begins as flat patches (patch stage) favoring the bathing suit area and lower trunk. Biopsy may not be diagnostic at this stage, but the inability to diagnose early cases has more to do with the limits of diagnostic capabilities than a transformation from some nonneoplastic (premycotic) condition to MF, and these cases are best considered MF from the onset. Pruritus, sometimes severe, is usually present at this stage. Over time, sometimes years, the lesions become more infiltrated, and the diagnosis is usually confirmed with repeated histologic evaluation. Infiltrated plaques occur eventually (plaque stage). In some cases, tumors may eventually appear (tumor stage). Some MF patients may present with or progress to erythroderma. Most rarely, patients may present with tumors de novo, the so-called d'emblée form. With immunophenotyping, many MF cases are now recognized as non-MF T-cell lymphomas. Eventually, in some patients noncutaneous involvement is detected. This is usually first identified in lymph nodes. Peripheral blood involvement and visceral organ involvement may also occur.

In general, MF affects elderly patients and has a long evolution. However, once tumors develop or lymph node involvement occurs, the prognosis is guarded, and MF can be fatal. In most fatal cases, the patient dies of septicemia. Early, aggressive chemotherapy in an attempt to "cure" MF is associated with excessive morbidity and mortality rates and is not indicated.

Evaluation and Staging. Staging information can be found at http://www.cancer.gov/types/lymphoma/hp/mycosis-fungoides-treatment-pdq. Because MF is a systemic disease from the onset (because lymphocytes naturally traffic throughout the body), concepts used for solid tumors, such as tumor burden and metastasis, cannot be readily applied. The TNMB system scores involvement in the skin (T), lymph node (N), viscera (M), and peripheral blood (B) and is in evolution. Skin involvement is divided into less than 10% (T1), more than 10% (T2), tumors (T3), and erythroderma (T4). Node involvement is normal clinically and pathologically (N0), palpable but pathologically not MF (N1), not palpable but pathologically MF (N2), or clinically and pathologically involved (N3). Viscera and blood are either not involved (M0 and B0) or involved (M1 and B1).

- Stage IA is T1, N0, M0.
- Stage IB is T2, N0, M0.
- Stage IIA is T1–T2, N1, M0.
- Stage IIB is T3, N0–N1, M0.
- Stage IIIA is T4, N0, M0.
- Stage IIIB is T4, N1, M0.
- Stage IVA is T1–T4, N2–N3, M0.
- Stage IVB is T1–T4, N0–N3, M1.

The "B" or blood status does not alter staging of the disease. The International Society for Lymphomas/European Organization of Research and Treatment of Cancer staging has differed by putting all clinically normal nodes into N0 and indicating the presence or absence of a clone in node or blood.

Example:

N1a: Clone negative
N1b: Clone positive

A staging workup would include a complete history and physical examination, with careful palpation of lymph nodes and mapping of skin lesions; a complete blood cell count (CBC) with assays for circulating atypical cells (Sézary cells); serum chemistries, including renal and liver function tests with lactate dehydrogenase; a chest radiograph evaluation; and a skin biopsy. If palpable, lymph nodes should be examined histologically. Fine-needle aspiration is not an ideal mode of evaluation, because early lymph node involvement may be localized to certain areas of the affected nodes and often requires architectural evaluation for detection. If any abnormalities are detected through these evaluations, they should be pursued. Computed tomography (CT) can be performed to assess chest, abdominal, and pelvic lymph nodes and visceral organs. These tests are useful in patients with stage II to IV disease, but are not indicated in patients with stage IA disease. Whether patients with stage IB disease should undergo these tests is unknown.

Stage IA patients have a life expectancy identical to that of a control population; only 8%–9% progress to more advanced disease, and only 2% die of their disease. By contrast, patients with T2 disease have shorter survival than controls (median survival of 11.7–15.6 years); 24% of T2 patients progress to more advanced disease. T3 patients have a median survival of 3.2–8.4 years, and T4 patients, 1.8–3.7 years. Palpable adenopathy is associated with a median survival of only 7.7 years, whereas patients without adenopathy have survival of 21.8 years. Lymphadenopathy, tumors, and cutaneous ulceration are cardinal prognostic factors; no patient dies without having developed one of these, and patients with all three (in any order) survive a median of 1 year.

Fig. 32.2 Mycosis fungoides, patch stage.

Clinical Features. In the early patch/plaque stage, the lesions are macular or slightly infiltrated patches or plaques varying in size, with many measuring 5 cm or more. Folliculotropic disease can resemble lichen nitidus or lichen spinulosis. Except for the folliculotropic and childhood variants, lesions greater than 5 cm are virtually always present. In contrast, most histologic simulators present with smaller skin lesions. The eruption may be generalized or may begin localized to one area and then spread. The lower abdomen, buttocks, upper thighs, and breasts of women are preferentially affected. The lesions may have an atrophic surface or may present as true poikiloderma with atrophy, mottled dyspigmentation, and telangiectasia. Poikiloderma vasculare atrophicans most often represents a clinical form of patch-stage MF. Likewise, large-plaque parapsoriasis and cases of small-plaque parapsoriasis with poikilodermatous change are early patch-stage lesions of MF. In contrast, typical digitate dermatosis rarely if ever evolves into MF. "Invisible" MF is generalized skin involvement that is not visible to the naked eye but can be documented histologically. With current diagnostic methods, this can usually be confirmed. In general, the patch-stage lesions (Fig. 32.2) resemble eczema. Ovoid, annular, polycyclic, or arciform configurations can occur. Less common forms are the verrucous or hyperkeratotic form, the hypopigmented form (which predominates in dark-skinned children) (Fig. 32.3), lesions resembling a pigmented purpura, and the vesicular, bullous, or pustular form. Subtle lesions of MF may manifest clinically during anti–tumor necrosis factor (TNF) therapy.

In the plaque stage lesions are more infiltrated and may resemble psoriasis (Fig. 32.4), a subacute dermatitis, or a granulomatous dermal process such as granuloma annulare. The palms and soles may be involved, with hyperkeratotic, psoriasiform, and fissuring plaques. The infiltration of the plaques, at first recognized by light palpation, may be present in only a few of the lesions. It is a manifestation of diagnostic importance. Different degrees of infiltration may exist, even in the same patch, and sometimes it is more pronounced peripherally, the central part of the plaque being depressed to the level of the surrounding skin. The infiltration becomes more marked and leads to discoid patches or extensive plaques, which may be as wide as 30 cm.

Eventually, through coalescence of the various plaques, the involvement becomes widespread, but there are usually patches of apparently normal skin interspersed. When the involvement is advanced, painful superficial ulcerations may occur. During this phase, enlarged lymph nodes usually develop. They are nontender, firm, and freely movable.

The tumor stage is characterized by large, variously sized and shaped nodules on infiltrated plaques (Fig. 32.5) and on apparently

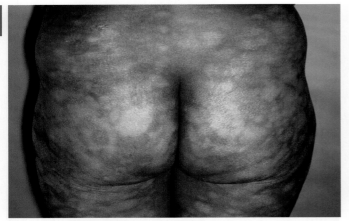

Fig. 32.3 Mycosis fungoides, patch stage.

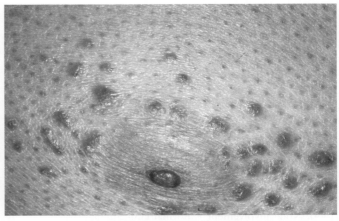

Fig. 32.6 Follicular mycosis fungoides.

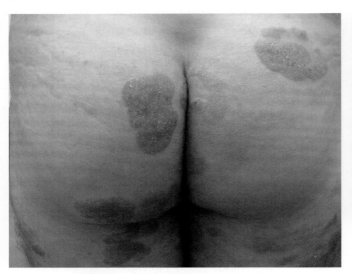

Fig. 32.4 Mycosis fungoides, plaque stage.

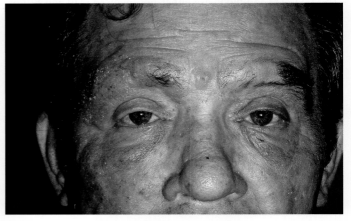

Fig. 32.7 Alopecia mucinosa.

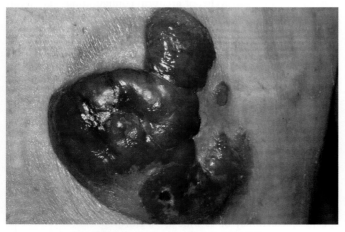

Fig. 32.5 Mycosis fungoides, tumor stage.

normal skin. These nodules tend to break down early and to form deep oval ulcers, whose bases are covered with a necrotic grayish substance and which have rolled edges. The lesions generally have a predilection for the trunk, although they may be seen anywhere on the skin or may involve the mouth and upper respiratory tract. Infrequently, tumors may be the first sign of MF.

The erythrodermic variety of MF is a generalized exfoliative process that often exhibits islands of spared skin. The hair is scanty, nails are dystrophic, palms and soles are hyperkeratotic, and at times, generalized hyperpigmentation may occur. Erythroderma may be the presenting feature.

Alopecia Mucinosa. The infiltrating cells of MF can demonstrate a predilection for involving the hair follicle (Fig. 32.6). This may be observed simply by folliculotropism of the cells (pilotropic or follicular MF) or by the appearance of follicular mucinosis (Fig. 32.7). In all cases of follicular mucinosis, the histologic specimen should be carefully examined and the diagnosis of MF considered. Among patients older than 40 who have follicular mucinosis, a large percentage will have MF or go on to develop it. However, the finding of a T-cell clone in lesions of follicular mucinosis without MF is not predictive of the development of CTCL.

Selective tropism of the CTCL cells to the sweat glands and ducts is termed *syringotropic* CTCL (Fig. 32.8). This is often seen in conjunction with follicular involvement. Syringolymphoid hyperplasia may be seen in these cases histologically and may mimic eccrine carcinoma. Cases previously called "syringolymphoid hyperplasia with alopecia" are now considered to be cutaneous T-cell lymphoma. Clinically, the lesions present as discrete follicular and nonfollicular erythema, along with alopecia, milia, and follicular cysts. The initial clinical diagnosis in such cases is often discoid lupus erythematosus. The prognosis in MF with adnexal involvement is as predicted by the staging system for other MF forms.

CHAPTER 32 Cutaneous Lymphoid Hyperplasia, Cutaneous T-Cell Lymphoma, Other Malignant Lymphomas, and Allied Diseases **735**

32

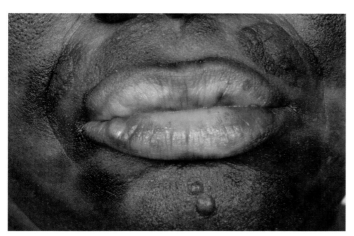

Fig. 32.8 Syringotropic mycosis fungoides.

Patients with granulomatous MF have a poorer prognosis and a poorer response to skin-directed therapy.

Systemic Manifestations. MF as a form of malignant lymphoma may progress to include visceral involvement. Lymph node involvement is most common; it predicts progression of MF in at least one quarter of patients and reduces survival to about 7 years. Any other evidence of visceral involvement is a poor prognostic sign. An abnormal result on liver-spleen scan, chest radiograph or CT evaluation, abdominal or pelvic CT scans, or bone marrow biopsy is associated with a survival of about 1 year. The prognosis is worse in non-Caucasian patients with early-onset MF, especially African American women.

Pathogenesis. MF is a neoplasm of memory Th cells in most cases. Rare cases of suppressor cell (CD8+) MF have been reported. These CD8+ cases may behave indolently, like MF, or aggressively. The aggressive subset tends to present with plaques rather than patches. The events leading to the development of the malignant T cells are unknown. Some speculate that it is caused by chronic exposure to an antigen, but this has yet to be confirmed. Patients with atopic dermatitis appear to be at increased risk for development of MF, suggesting that persistent stimulation of T cells may lead to development of a malignant clone.

The inflammatory nature of the skin lesions has led to investigation of the interactions of the malignant T cells and both keratinocytes and antigen-presenting cells (APCs, including Langerhans cells) in MF. MF skin lesions have many features of skin that is immunologically "activated." MF cells express cutaneous lymphocyte antigen (CLA), the ligand for E selectin, which is expressed on the endothelial cells of inflamed skin. This allows the malignant cells to traffic into the skin from the peripheral blood. CCR4, another homing molecule, is expressed on MF cells, and the ligand for this receptor is on basal keratinocytes. APCs are increased in MF lesions and have increased functional capacity to activate T cells. There is increased expression of major histocompatibility complex (MHC) class II antigens on the surface of the APCs. Through cytokines, infiltration of neoplastic and reactive T cells is increased. The pattern in early MF is more Th1-like, and the nonneoplastic infiltrating cells (tumor-infiltrating lymphocytes, TILs) may play a role in downregulating and controlling the neoplastic cells. There are more CD8+ cells in these early lesions, and these TILs may control the malignant clone. In fact, MF patients with more than 20% CD8+ cells in their skin survive longer than those with less than 15%. In more advanced MF and in Sézary syndrome, perhaps through interleukin (IL)–4 and IL-10, a Th2 environment exists. This downregulates suppressor

cell function and allows the malignant clone to proliferate. In addition, the Th2-dominant environment reduces effective Th-cell function, explaining the increased risk of infection and secondary cancer in patients with advanced CTCL. Correcting the aberrant immune response in advanced CTCL is the basis of some treatment approaches.

Common chromosomal alterations in MF include gain of 7q36 and 7q21–7q22 and loss of 5q13 and 9p21. This characteristic pattern differs from that seen in Sézary syndrome, suggesting that the two disorders are distinct. As MF advances, the number of circulating malignant T cells increases, and they can be detected by flow cytometry as CD4+,CD7– or CD4+,CD26– circulating cells.

Histopathology. Perhaps more than in any other situation in dermatopathology, the ability to diagnose MF histologically correlates closely with the skill, training, and experience of the reviewing pathologist. When the clinician is considering a diagnosis of MF, consultation with a skilled dermatopathologist should be strongly considered if original histologic reports are nonconfirmatory or nonspecific.

In patch-stage lesions, subtle epidermotropism of lymphocytes resembles a vacuolar interface dermatitis with a lymphocyte in every vacuole. As lesions progress, there is a distinct bandlike distribution of lymphocytes with epidermotropism. At this stage, a large, dark lymphocyte is present in every vacuole. The lymphocytes within the epidermis may be numerous or few but are typically larger, darker, and more angulated than those in the dermis. Papillary dermal fibrosis is typically present. The superficial perivascular lymphoid infiltrate that surrounds the postcapillary venule is typically more prominent above the vessel than below the vessel ("bare underbelly" sign).

Plaques of MF show a more prominent, superficial bandlike lymphoid infiltrate and a deeper perivascular dermal component than patch-stage lesions. Papillary dermal fibrosis is more prominent, and the subpapillary plexus is shifted downward. Epidermotropism is much more marked and is typically associated with minimal spongiosis. This helps distinguish patch-stage MF from spongiotic dermatitis. Vesicular variants are an exception to this rule. In vesicular variants, spongiosis is prominent and results in intraepidermal and subcorneal vesiculation. Eosinophils are common in folliculotropic MF (with or without follicular mucinosis) but are uncommon in other MF forms.

In thick plaques and tumors, epidermotropism may be substantially diminished. The diagnosis of MF is confirmed by the presence of dense sheets of infiltrating lymphocytes in the dermis and subcutaneous fat. These cells may have cerebriform nuclei. Cardinal features that should suggest a diagnosis of MF include the following:

- Solitary or small groups of lymphocytes in the basal cell layer
- Epidermotropism of lymphocytes, with disproportionately scant spongiosis
- More lymphocytes within the epidermis than would normally be seen in an inflammatory dermatosis, with little accompanying acanthosis or spongiosis
- Lymphocytes in the epidermis larger than those in the dermis
- Papillary dermal fibrosis with bundles of collagen arranged haphazardly
- Prominent folliculotropism or syringotropism of the lymphocytes, especially with intrafollicular mucin deposition (follicular mucinosis)

Features that should suggest a diagnosis of inflammatory dermatosis over MF include the following:

- Prominent upper dermal and papillary edema
- Marked epidermal spongiosis
- Accumulation of the intraepidermal inflammatory cells in flask-shaped collections, with the top open to the stratum corneum

Immunohistochemistry is of some value in assessing MF. MF cells characteristically are CD4+, but lose the CD7 and CD26 antigens. Loss of CD7 expression within the large, dark lymphocytes in the epidermis, with normal expression in the benign recruited lymphocytes in the infiltrate below, suggests a diagnosis of MF. DNA hybridization or a Southern blot test is frequently performed in equivocal cases to detect clonal rearrangement of the T-cell receptor (TCR). An identical rearrangement at multiple sites suggests MF. In early lesions of MF, the number of infiltrating cells may be insufficient for a clone to be detected, so a negative test does not exclude the diagnosis of MF. Testing with fresh tissue is somewhat more sensitive than with fixed tissue using current methods. Similar techniques can be used to evaluate lymph nodes in MF patients. Lymph node involvement can be detected by these molecular methods, whereas routine histologic evaluation yields normal results. Patients with more advanced disease are more likely to have clones in their lymph nodes, and the presence of clonality is predictive of shorter survival.

Differential Diagnosis. In the early patch stage, MF may be difficult to diagnose. The skin lesions usually resemble a nondescript form of eczema with some scale. Interestingly, despite the itching, scratch marks and lichenification are usually absent. MF presenting as papuloerythroderma of Ofuji is an obvious exception. The multiple morphologies of MF make the differential diagnosis vast. Plaquelike lesions may resemble subacute dermatitis or psoriasis. Tumors must be differentiated from other forms of lymphoreticular malignancy and metastases.

Treatment. Many forms of therapy induce remissions of variable length. The therapeutic choice depends on extent of disease, the patient's overall health and physical status, the physician's experience and preference, and the availability of various options. The new topical biologic response modifier resiquimod has shown dramatic effects in many patients and may become first-line therapy. Other agents are still commonly used, as the disease presents with a wide spectrum. Topical corticosteroids, topical nitrogen mustard or 1,3-bis-(2-chloroethyl)-l-nitrosourea (carmustine, BCNU), bexarotene gel 1%, and PUVA or narrow-band UVB are generally good choices for stages IA, IB, and IIA disease. Patch-stage MF has responded to alefacept. Total-skin electron beam (TSEB) therapy can be used for refractory stage IIA and IIB cases. Single-agent chemotherapy or photophoresis can be used as initial management for stage III patients. Low-dose methotrexate may control the skin lesions of MF but has been associated with development of a secondary aggressive lymphoma in a few patients. Pegylated liposomal doxorubicin and combinations of IFN alfa, retinoids (bexarotene or isotretinoin), photophoresis, IFN gamma, skin-directed PUVA, sargramostim (granulocyte-macrophage colony-stimulating factor), alemtuzumab, and perhaps IL-2, IL-12, and IFN alfa may be effective in stage IV disease, as well as for patients who have failed the therapies previously cited for stages IIB and III MF. Multiagent systemic chemotherapy is used much less often with the advent of immunomodulatory treatments for MF. Chemotherapy should be considered only when all other treatment options have failed. Treatment of early-stage disease is in general restricted to skin-directed treatments. More advanced disease is treated with different modalities at different institutions. Combinations of agents are often used, and the combinations and their order of use vary among institutions. In general, therapies that also enhance the patient's immune system are favored in persons with more advanced disease. Complete remission of MF has been noted after a severe reaction to combined therapy with bexarotene, vorinostat, and high-dose fenofibrate. The reaction included fever, extensive skin necrosis, and granuloma formation.

Biologic Response Modifiers (Multimodality Immunomodulatory Therapy). Resiquimod and imiquimod may completely change the treatment of CTCL, as therapy directed at a few lesions can produce widespread regression of the disease. IFN alfa and IFN gamma have been shown to have efficacy against MF. IFN alfa is associated with a positive response in about 60% of patients and a complete response in 19%. Toxicity is significant and includes fever, chills, myalgias, neutropenia, and depression. Low-dose IFN-alfa and IFN-gamma treatments and granulocyte-macrophage colony-stimulating factor (GM-CSF) are now used in adjunctive fashion in combination with retinoid therapy, phototherapy, and other modalities. This is termed *multimodality immunomodulatory therapy.*

Topical Corticosteroids. The availability of superpotent class I topical corticosteroids has led to a reassessment of their possible role in the management of early MF (patch stage, T1 and T2). Zackheim et al. reported a 63% complete remission rate for patients with T1 disease and a total response rate of 94%. In T2 patients, complete response was seen in only 25% but total response in 82%. The predominant side effect was a temporary and reversible suppression of the hypothalamic-pituitary axis in about 13% of patients.

Topical Nitrogen Mustard. Anhydrous gel or ointment-based mustard products are being used more often, but aqueous mustard is still used as well, with a 10-mg vial of mechlorethamine hydrochloride dissolved in 60 mL of tap water and applied to the entire skin surface, except the face, axillae, and genitalia, with a 2-inch paint brush or gauze pad. The last milliliter may be diluted to half-strength or greater dilution for application to the face, axillae, and genitalia. Such treatment leads to complete responses in 80% of patients with stage IA disease, 68% in stage IB, 61% in stage IIA, 49% in stage IIB, and 60% in stage III patients. About 10% of patients obtain a durable and long-lasting remission of more than 8 years. The major side effects of topical nitrogen mustard (NH2) therapy are cutaneous intolerance, which occurs in almost 50% of patients, and allergic contact dermatitis, which occurs in 15%. Short (1 hour) contact does not reduce this rate of sensitization. This can be reduced by the use of an ointment formulation, but response rates have been reported to be inferior with the ointment form. At least half of patients will relapse when therapy is stopped, but they frequently will respond again to NH2.

The duration of maintenance therapy after achieving remission varies in different centers. Some treat for an additional 6 months, and others taper treatment over 1 year or more, or continue treatment indefinitely.

Topical BCNU (Carmustine). Topical BCNU, 2 mg/mL in 150-mL aliquots, dissolved in ethanol, is dispensed to the patient. From this stock solution, the patient takes 5 mL and adds it to 60 mL of water at room temperature. This is applied once a day to the whole body, sparing the folds, genitals, hands, and feet (if they do not have lesions). If the extent of disease is limited, only the affected areas are treated. The average treatment course is 8–12 weeks. If, after 3–6 months, the patient's condition is not responding, the concentration may be doubled and the treatment repeated for 12 weeks. For small or persistent lesions, the straight stock solution may be applied daily. Patients tolerate BCNU better than nitrogen mustard, contact sensitization is uncommon, and responses are more rapid. CBC should be monitored monthly during treatment, but marrow suppression occurs in less than 10% of patients treated with the low concentrations. Telangiectasia, which may be persistent and severe, can occur after prolonged BCNU therapy or after an adverse cutaneous reaction to the medication.

Ultraviolet Therapy. Both UVB (narrow- or broad-band) and PUVA (systemic or bath) have been effective in the management of MF. About 75% of patients with patch-stage disease will have a complete clinical remission with UVB therapy. Home therapy is successful. PUVA has been used more extensively and, because of its deeper penetration, is perhaps better suited to the treatment of a disorder with a dermal component. Complete clearing is seen in 88% of patients with limited patch/plaque disease and in 52%

CHAPTER 32 Cutaneous Lymphoid Hyperplasia, Cutaneous T-Cell Lymphoma, Other Malignant Lymphomas, and Allied Diseases **737**

32

of patients with extensive disease. Tumor-stage MF patients do not typically clear, and erythrodermic patients have poor tolerance for PUVA. Up to 50% of patients with a complete response to PUVA may have a remission of up to 10 years. Retinoids and IFN alfa may be added to PUVA. Retinoids may reduce the total number of PUVA treatments required. Low-dose IFN alfa plus PUVA may be used in patch-stage patients in whom topical therapy and PUVA alone are ineffective. The excimer laser may be used once or twice a week to deliver the phototherapy if the patient has a limited number of lesions. On average, 5–6 weeks of treatment is required, and remissions of up to 2 years or more can be achieved.

Extracorporeal photochemotherapy (photophoresis, ECP) is a therapeutic modality in which the circulating cells are extracted and treated with UVA outside the body; the patient ingests psoralen before the treatment. Complete responses are seen in about 20% of MF patients, and a partial response occurs in a similar percentage. In the original reports, the overall response rate for erythrodermic patients was 80%, but many of these patients failed to have at least the 50% clearing required to be considered a partial response. In one comparative trial, standard PUVA was significantly more effective than photophoresis alone, and photophoresis was judged ineffective in plaque-stage (T2) MF. ECP is now used in combination with other agents, especially IFN alfa, and appears to have better efficacy. Insulin-dependent diabetic patients respond poorly.

Photodynamic Therapy. Photodynamic therapy (PDT) with methyl-aminolevulinic acid has been used successfully for paucilesional MF. Responses were seen in 75% of patients, and patient satisfaction was high. Other photosensitizing agents are being evaluated.

Radiation. TSEB therapy in doses in excess of 3000 Gy is very effective in the management of MF. Stage T1 patients have a 98% complete response; stage T2, 71%; stage T3, 36%; and stage T4, 64%. Long-term remissions occur in about 50% of T1 patients and 20% of T2 patients. Erythrodermic patients tolerate TSEB therapy poorly; other modalities should be attempted initially. Adjuvant therapy with a topical agent or PUVA can be considered if the patient relapses, as frequently occurs. The most common side effects of TSEB therapy are erythema, edema, worsening of lesions, alopecia, and nail loss. Persistent hyperpigmentation and chronically dry skin are also problems after TSEB therapy. Orthovoltage radiation may be used to control tumors or resistant thick plaques in patients whose conditions have been otherwise controlled with another modality.

Retinoids. Both isotretinoin and etretinate have efficacy in the treatment of MF. A clinical response is noted in about 44% of patients. Dosage of isotretinoin is about 1 mg/kg/day to start and may be increased up to 3 mg/kg/day as tolerated. Retinoids may be effective in stage IB (T2) and stage III patients, and as a palliative treatment in those with stage IVA disease. Bexarotene (Targretin), a synthetic retinoid that is bound preferentially by the retinoid X receptor (RXR), is thought to work by inducing apoptosis in the malignant T cells. It is available as a topical gel and as an oral tablet. Topical therapy is used in patients with stage IA to IIA CTCL. Patients improve about 50% with this treatment. Oral bexarotene at a dose of 300 mg/m² also has a response rate of about 50% in early-stage CTCL. This dose is complicated by hypercholesterolemia, marked hypertriglyceridemia (at times complicated by pancreatitis), central hypothyroidism, and leukopenia. It may be combined with PUVA and other forms of treatment at a lower dose.

Systemic Chemotherapy. Multidrug chemotherapy often exacerbates the ongoing immune imbalance and may prevent the patient's immune system from attacking the malignant T cells. For this reason, and because of the enhanced efficacy of combination immunomodulatory treatment regimens, systemic chemotherapy is now very uncommonly used for MF. Methotrexate alone, in doses from 5–125 mg/wk, is effective for the management of T3 patients. In these patients Zackheim et al. reported that 41% had

a complete response, and an additional 17% a partial response, giving a total response of 58%. The median overall survival was 8.4 years, and 69% of patients were alive at 5 years. For advanced MF, higher doses of methotrexate with citrovorum-factor rescue were successful in obtaining a response, which was then maintained with lower doses of methotrexate, not requiring rescue. Similarly, vorinostat (and other histone deacetylase inhibitors), pentostatin, etoposide, fludarabine, and 2-chlorodeoxyadenosine have been used. Curcumin is being studied, as are forodesine, a novel inhibitor of purine nucleoside phosphorylase, and pralatrexate, a novel targeted antifolate agent.

Fusion Toxin. The toxin DAB389IL-2 is the fusion of a portion of the diphtheria toxin to recombinant IL-2. This selectively binds to cells expressing the IL-2 receptor and leads to their death. A series of MF patients who expressed the IL-2 receptor demonstrated a response rate of 37%, including a complete response in 14%. These patients had failed conventional therapies. Patients in stages I to III achieved response, but no patient with stage IV disease did so. Fever, chills, hypotension, nausea, and vomiting were common, and at high doses a vascular leak syndrome occurred. This agent is reserved for advanced-stage patients who have failed other modalities.

Ahn CS, et al: Mycosis fungoides. Am J Dermatopathol 2014; 36: 933.

Berg S, et al: Multidisciplinary management of mycosis fungoides/Sézary syndrome. Curr Hematol Malig Rep 2017; 12: 234.

Boulos S, et al: Clinical presentation, immunopathology, and treatment of juvenile-onset mycosis fungoides. J Am Acad Dermatol 2014; 71: 1117.

Hoppe RT: Remarkable advances in the management of mycosis fungoides and the Sezary syndrome. Oncol Res Treat 2017; 40: 242.

Kelati A, et al: Defining the mimics and clinico-histological diagnosis criteria for mycosis fungoides to minimize misdiagnosis. Int J Womens Dermatol 2017; 3: 100.

Lewis DJ, et al: Complete resolution of mycosis fungoides tumors with imiquimod 5% cream. J Dermatolog Treat 2017; 28: 567.

Vaidya T, et al: Mycosis Fungoides. 2018 Oct 1. StatPearls [Internet]. Treasure Island (FL): StatPearls Publishing; 2018 Jan-. Available from http://www.ncbi.nlm.nih.gov/books/NBK519572/PubMed PMID: 30137856.

Vonderheid EC, et al: CD4(+)CD26(–) lymphocytes are useful to assess blood involvement and define B ratings in cutaneous T cell lymphoma. Leuk Lymphoma 2018; 59: 330.

Pagetoid Reticulosis

Localized epidermotropic reticulosis, pagetoid reticulosis, or Woringer-Kolopp disease is an uncommon lymphoproliferative disorder considered be a form of mycosis fungoides. Other terms suggested for these cases have included acral mycosis fungoides or mycosis fungoides palmaris et plantaris. In large, MF clinics, such cases represent about 0.6% of all MF cases. Pagetoid reticulosis is divided into classic Woringer-Kolopp, which usually describes solitary lesions, and cases with multiple lesions (Ketron-Goodman variant). The unique features of Woringer-Kolopp disease are clinical. The disease presents as a solitary lesion that is often located on an extremity and frequently has a keratotic rim. If there is more than a single lesion, the lesions often tend to involve both the palms and the soles. Frequently, over months to years, the lesion gradually enlarges, reaching more than 10 cm in size. In some cases, the lesions spontaneously come and go over many years. About 20% of cases occur in patients who are younger than 15 years. The long duration without progression has been a clinical hallmark of Woringer-Kolopp disease. Histologically, there is prominent epidermotropism of lymphocytes, with many lining up in the basal cell layer. This histologic pattern correlates with

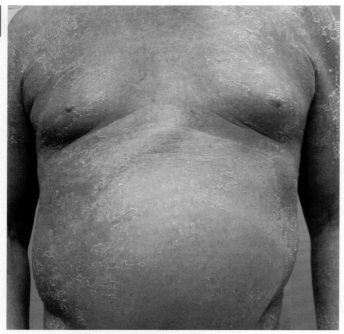

Fig. 32.9 Sézary syndrome. (Courtesy Alain Rook, MD.)

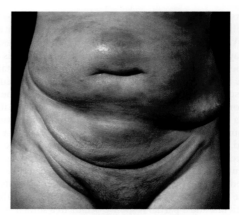

Fig. 32.10 Granulomatous slack skin.

strong αEβ7- and α4β7-integrin expression by the infiltrating cells. This integrin expression is also seen in the epidermotropic cells of classic MF and contact dermatitis. In MF, most cases are CD4+, but in the acral MF cases, they may be CD4+, CD8+, or negative for both. TCR gene rearrangements can be detected in many cases of Woringer-Kolopp disease. Therapeutically, local excision and radiation therapy have been "curative" in many patients. Topical and systemic PUVA and PDT have also proved effective. Local recurrence is possible.

Sézary Syndrome

Sézary syndrome is the leukemic phase of mycosis fungoides. The characteristic features are generalized erythroderma (Fig. 32.9), superficial lymphadenopathy, and atypical cells in the circulating blood. Although patients with classic MF may progress to Sézary syndrome, patients with Sézary syndrome usually are erythrodermic from the onset. The skin shows a generalized or limited erythroderma of a typical fiery red color. Associated features can include leonine facies, eyelid edema, ectropion, diffuse alopecia, hyperkeratosis of the palms and soles, and dystrophic nails. Some patients develop lesions identical to vitiligo, especially on the lower legs. Symptoms include severe pruritus and burning, with episodes of chills. Prognosis is poor, with an average survival of about 5 years.

Superficial lymphadenopathy is usually found in the cervical, axillary, and inguinal areas. Leukocytosis up to 30,000 cells/mm³ is usually present. In the peripheral blood, skin infiltrate, and lymph nodes, Th cells with deeply convoluted nuclei are found, the so-called Sézary cells. Chromosomal aberrations are common but differ from the typical pattern seen in MF. Resistance to Fas-ligand and TNF-related apoptosis has been demonstrated.

In a fair number of Sézary patients, the cutaneous histology may be nonspecific, showing a spongiotic dermatitis. Additional hematologic evaluation may be necessary to confirm the diagnosis in the erythrodermic patient. T-cell gene rearrangement studies are frequently used to confirm the diagnosis of Sézary syndrome. In addition, an increased CD4/CD8 ratio in the blood, with an increase in the number of CD3+/CD4+/CD7−/CD26− circulating cells, is suggestive of leukemic MF.

The erythroderma of Sézary syndrome must be distinguished from chronic lymphocytic leukemia (CLL), psoriasis, atopic dermatitis, photodermatitis, seborrheic dermatitis, contact dermatitis, drug reaction, and pityriasis rubra pilaris. This is done primarily by histopathologic and immunopathologic examination. In Sézary syndrome, the infiltrating T cells in the skin have a Th2 phenotype, and Th2 cytokines are produced by these cells. This explains the reduced delayed-type hypersensitivity, elevated immunoglobulin E (IgE), and eosinophilia seen in these patients.

Sézary syndrome is difficult to treat. Low-dose methotrexate has a reasonable response rate of about 50% and an overall survival of 101 months, suggesting a survival benefit with its use. Photophoresis, used in combination with other agents, is effective in some patients, but the median survival time is only 39–60 months (see earlier). TSEB radiation has produced some complete cutaneous responses, as well as improvement in the blood burden of malignant cells. Zanolimumab has also been used in this setting.

Granulomatous Slack Skin

Granulomatous slack skin is a rare variant lymphoma that typically presents in middle-aged adults and gradually progresses over years. It occurs more often in men. Lesions are erythematous, atrophic, bulky, infiltrated, pendulous, and redundant plaques in the axillae and groin (Fig. 32.10). Unusual presentations may resemble Hansen disease or acquired ichthyosis. Histologically, there is a lymphohistiocytic infiltrate extending through the dermis into the subcutaneous fat. Focal collections of huge, multinucleated cells with 20–30 nuclei arranged in a wreathlike pattern are characteristic. Elastophagocytosis is prominent and elastic tissue is absent in areas of inflammation. Lymphocytes are also found within the multinucleate giant cells and are arranged around them. Epidermotropic lymphocytes are also seen. Immunohistologically, the cells are CD4+. T-cell gene rearrangements can be detected. In most patients, the condition evolves into mycosis fungoides, but about one third of patients with granulomatous slack skin develop Hodgkin disease after years to decades.

Lymphomatoid Papulosis

Lymphomatoid papulosis (LyP) is an uncommon, but not rare, disorder. It occurs at any age, including childhood, but is most common in adults with a mean age of 44. In typical cases, the lesions and course are very similar to Mucha-Habermann disease (pityriasis lichenoides et varioliformis acuta), except that the lesions tend to be slightly larger and fewer in number and have a greater propensity to necrosis. Symptoms are usually minimal. The primary lesion is a red papule up to about 1 cm in diameter (Fig. 32.11). The lesions evolve to papulovesicular, papulopustular, or

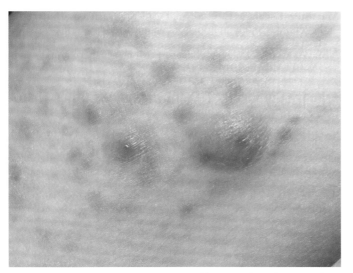

Fig. 32.11 Lymphomatoid papulosis. (Courtesy Alain Rook, MD.)

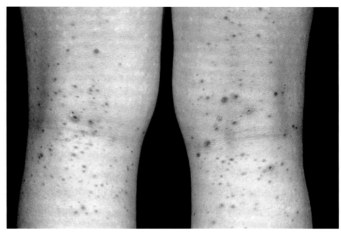

Fig. 32.12 Pityriasis lichenoides et varioliformis acuta.

hemorrhagic, then necrotic papules over days to weeks. They typically heal spontaneously within 8 weeks, somewhat longer in larger lesions. Lesions are usually generalized, although cases limited to one anatomic region have been reported.

There may be crops of lesions or a constant appearance of a few lesions. In most patients, however, the condition tends to be chronic, and lesions are present most of the time if no treatment is given. The average number of lesions present at any one time is usually 10–20, but cases with more than 100 lesions occur. Lesions heal with varioliform, hyperpigmented, or hypopigmented scars. Cases previously reported as solitary, large nodules of LyP would now be classified as CD30+ large cell lymphomas or as overlaps between LyP and lymphoma, termed borderline cases. Localized agminated LyP may be seen in areas typical for mycosis fungoides.

The diagnosis of LyP is confirmed histologically.

Type A lesions contain atypical large cells with abundant cytoplasm and prominent nuclei, with prominent eosinophilic nucleoli. If these cells contain two nuclei, they closely resemble Reed-Sternberg cells. In type B lesions, the atypical cells are smaller, with a smaller cerebriform, hyperchromatic nucleus. These resemble the atypical cells of MF. In both types of lesion, atypical mitotic figures may be observed. Immunophenotypically, the large atypical cells mark as T cells, usually Th type. The atypical cells, especially those of the type A lesions, stain for the activation marker Ki-1 or CD30. Bcl-2 expression occurs in about 50% of cases. When clonal rearrangement studies are performed, clonal rearrangements may be found in up to 40% of LyP lesions, but this finding is not predictive of the behavior of that lesion or the case in general. Type C lesions overlap with primary cutaneous large cell lymphoma, with no clear distinction between the two. Type D, CD8+ LyP is a rare variant in which CD8+ T cells proliferate, mimicking cytotoxic lymphoma. Type E has been proposed as an angioinvasive type resembling angiodestructive lymphoma histologically, but with a self-healing course. The follicular type resembles folliculotropic MF with a relapsing course. LyP with chromosomal arrangement of DUSP22-IRF4 on 6p25.3 has a biphasic pattern with small cerebriform lymphocytes infiltrating the epidermis and larger atypical CD30+ lymphocytes forming dense nodules in dermis.

LyP types A and B are associated with lymphoma in up to 20% of patients. The lymphoma may occur before, concurrently with, or after the appearance of the LyP. In most cases LyP precedes development of lymphoma, sometimes by a long period—up to

20 years. The associated lymphoma is most often MF (40%), a CD30+ T-cell lymphoma (30%), or Hodgkin disease (25%). Patients with pure type B lesions are much less likely to develop lymphoma than patients with type A lesions. Lesions of LyP may occur on a background of MF and must be distinguished from CD30+ large cell transformation of MF. Papular lesions of LyP tend to occur in crops. Even though the LyP lesions may demonstrate the same clonal rearrangements as the MF, they often continue to appear in crops, even when the MF lesions respond to therapy.

Therapy may not be necessary; no evidence shows that treatment of LyP prevents development of secondary lymphoma. Superpotent topical corticosteroids have been beneficial in some childhood cases. Topical bexarotene may abort early lesions, and oral bexarotene may suppress lesion formation. PUVA systemically or topically may be effective, although maintenance treatment is usually required. Both narrow- and broad-band UVB may be successful. Of all the systemic agents, methotrexate gives the most dependable response, with up to 90% of LyP patients improving significantly. It is given in weekly doses similar to those used for rheumatoid arthritis, usually 7.5–15 mg/wk. Higher doses may be required in some patients. Response is rapid. Some patients treated with methotrexate may have remissions of the LyP. In most, however, maintenance therapy is required.

Kempf W: A new era for cutaneous CD30-positive T-cell lymphoproliferative disorders. Semin Diagn Pathol 2017; 34: 22.

Kempf W, et al: Lymphomatoid papulosis—making sense of the alphabet soup. J Dtsch Dermatol Ges 2017; 15: 390.

Sauder MB, et al: CD30(+) lymphoproliferative disorders of the skin. Hematol Oncol Clin North Am 2017; 31: 317.

Pityriasis Lichenoides Et Varioliformis Acuta (Mucha-Habermann Disease)

Pityriasis lichenoides et varioliformis acuta (PLEVA) is a disorder characterized by papulonecrotic lesions, often in children or young adults. Individual lesions are erythematous macules, papules, or papulovesicles. Lesions tend to be brownish red and evolve through stages of crusting, necrosis, and varioliform scarring. Lesions tend to appear in crops and may number from a few to more than 100 (Fig. 32.12). In general, PLEVA patients have more and smaller lesions than patients with LyP. The trunk is favored, but even the palms and soles may infrequently be involved. The patient feels otherwise well. The natural history is benign, with spontaneous involution occurring over 1–3 years. In children, diffuse cases resolved more quickly than cases that were purely central; cases with primarily peripheral lesions took almost twice as long to resolve.

Histologically, PLEVA is characterized by a neutrophilic scale-crust, interface dermatitis with a lymphocyte in every vacuole, variable epidermal necrosis, erythrocyte extravasation, intravascular margination of neutrophils, and a dense perivascular lymphoid infiltrate in the superficial and deep dermis in a wedge-shaped pattern. T-cell gene rearrangements may be detected, but the significance of this finding is unclear at this time. Treatment of PLEVA may include oral erythromycin or tetracyclines and phototherapy (broad- or narrow-band UVB, PUVA, or PDT). Topical tacrolimus may be effective. Low-dose methotrexate, 5.0–15 mg/wk, may be required in severe cases, including the febrile variant. A rapid response to azithromycin has been reported. Etanercept has been reported as effective, but infliximab has been reported to cause pityriasis lichenoides.

An unusually severe form of PLEVA, febrile ulceronecrotic Mucha-Habermann disease, is characterized by the acute onset of diffuse, coalescent, large, ulceronecrotic skin lesions associated with high fever and constitutional symptoms. The condition may begin as typical PLEVA, but the ulceronecrotic lesions usually begin to appear within a few weeks. Skin necrosis may be extensive, especially in the intertriginous regions. Associated symptoms include gastrointestinal (GI) and central nervous system (CNS) symptoms, pneumonitis, myocarditis, and even death (in adult cases). The condition favors boys age 18 or younger. This severe form of PLEVA usually lasts several months with successive outbreaks, then resolves or converts to more classic PLEVA. Reported triggers include viral infections and radiocontrast injection. Systemic corticosteroids are often used in the acute phase, followed by methotrexate. Dapsone has been used for maintenance and as a steroid-sparing agent. Infliximab and intravenous immune globulins have been used, but TNF agents have also triggered the disease.

Pityriasis Lichenoides Chronica

Pityriasis lichenoides chronica (PLC) is a chronic form of pityriasis lichenoides related to PLEVA by its common histology. Lesions are crops of evanescent erythematous, scaly papules and small macules that commonly heal with hypopigmentation. Lesions of PLC favor the lateral trunk and proximal extremities. Patients may have from 10 to hundreds of lesions, but usually fewer than 50. The condition is most common in children, but may occur at any age.

Histologically, the changes in PLC are similar to PLEVA but much more subtle and include interface dermatitis with a lymphocyte in every vacuole. In all forms of pityriasis lichenoides, T-cell gene rearrangement studies may demonstrate monoclonality. Treatment with phototherapy (natural sunlight, UVB, UVA1, or PUVA) is most effective. Topical corticosteroids and tacrolimus are sometimes effective. Generally, PLC is a benign disease, but rare patients have progressed to develop CTCL. The authors recommend that patients with PLC be followed regularly; changes in lesion morphology, including induration, erosion, atrophy, persistent erythema, or poikiloderma, should trigger repeat pathologic evaluation.

Fernández-Guarino M, et al: Treatment of adult diffuse pityriasis lichenoides chronica with narrowband ultraviolet B: experience and literature review. Clin Exp Dermatol 2017; 42: 303.

Kreuter A, et al: Complete resolution of febrile ulceronecrotic Mucha-Habermann disease following infliximab therapy. J Dtsch Dermatol Ges 2016; 14: 184.

Maranda EL, et al: Phototherapy for pityriasis lichenoides in the pediatric population. Am J Clin Dermatol 2016; 17: 583.

Martinez-Escala ME, et al: γδ T-cell-rich variants of pityriasis lichenoides and lymphomatoid papulosis. Br J Dermatol 2015; 172: 372.

Nofal A, et al: Febrile ulceronecrotic Mucha-Habermann disease. Int J Dermatol 2016; 55: 729.

Primary Cutaneous T-Cell Lymphomas Other Than Mycosis Fungoides

CD30 is a marker found on some activated, but not resting T and B cells. It also marks the Reed-Sternberg cells of Hodgkin disease and is expressed in large cell transformation of mycosis fungoides. Monoclonal antibodies Ki-1/Ber H2 are used to identify CD30 positivity. A cutaneous lymphoma is considered to be CD30+ if there are large clusters of CD30+ cells or more than 75% of the anaplastic T cells are CD30+. The prognosis of CD30+ primary cutaneous anaplastic large cell lymphoma is excellent, with a spontaneously regressing and relapsing course being typical. Disease localized to the legs has a worse prognosis. Large cell transformation of MF and systemic CD30+ lymphoma with cutaneous involvement have a poor prognosis. Those cases of systemic disease that express anaplastic lymphoma kinase (ALK-1) associated with a 2:5 translocation have a somewhat better prognosis. Primary cutaneous large T-cell lymphomas that are CD30+ are typically ALK-1 negative and have a very good prognosis, but systemic disease that is ALK-1 negative has a very poor prognosis.

Individual lesions of primary cutaneous disease may require no treatment, as a spontaneous regressing/relapsing course is expected. Persistent lesions often respond to irradiation, and the typical relapsing course may remit with low-dose methotrexate. The group of T-cell lymphomas that are not large cell and CD30+ are classified in the WHO system as peripheral T-cell lymphomas.

CD56 is another important immunophenotypic marker for cutaneous lymphomas, including a subset of subcutaneous panniculitis-like T-cell lymphoma, natural killer (NK)/T-cell lymphoma, and CD8+ aggressive epidermotropic cytotoxic T-cell lymphoma.

CD30+ Cutaneous T-Cell Lymphoma (Primary Cutaneous Anaplastic Large Cell Lymphoma)

Clinically, the CD30+ CTCLs present as solitary or localized skin lesions that have a tendency to ulcerate. They are rare in children and occur with slightly greater frequency in males. Lesions are usually firm, red to violaceous tumors up to 10 cm in diameter (Fig. 32.13). Tumors may grow in a matter of weeks. There is no favored anatomic site. Onset has been reported during glatiramer acetate treatment of multiple sclerosis.

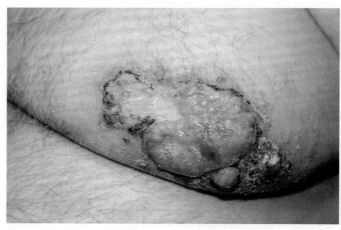

Fig. 32.13 CD30+ anaplastic T-cell lymphoma. (Courtesy Alain Rook, MD.)

Spontaneous regression and relapses in the skin are common, but the development of extracutaneous, bone marrow, or lymph node involvement is uncommon. The "pyogenic lymphoma" of the skin is a neutrophil-rich CD30+ lymphoma with skin lesions that clinically resemble Sweet syndrome, pyoderma gangrenosum, halogenoderma, leishmaniasis, or deep fungal infection. IL-8 overexpression by the anaplastic CD30+ cells causes the neutrophilic infiltration. Histologically, there is a dense dermal nonepidermotropic infiltrate with atypical tumor cells whose large nuclei have one or several prominent nucleoli and abundant cytoplasm. Other than low-dose methotrexate, chemotherapy generally has little role in the treatment of this disease. Local hyperthermia has been used successfully, as has inhibition of the mammalian target of rapamycin.

Non–Mycosis Fungoides CD30– Cutaneous Large T-Cell Lymphoma

Non-MF CD30– large CTCLs usually present as solitary or generalized plaques, nodules, or tumors of short duration. There is no preceding patch stage, which distinguishes it from MF. The prognosis is poor, with 5-year survival of 15%. The malignant cells are pleomorphic, large or medium cell types or are immunoblastic. Some cases previously called d'emblée MF are better classified in this group. Multiagent chemotherapy is commonly required.

Pleomorphic T-Cell Lymphoproliferative Disorder (Small/Medium-Sized Cutaneous T-Cell Lymphoma)

This group comprises about 3% of all primary cutaneous lymphomas. Pleomorphic small/medium-sized CTCL is distinguished from the large cell type by having less than 30% large pleomorphic cells. It is distinguished from MF by clinical features (lack of patch or plaque lesions). These primary cutaneous lymphomas usually present with one or several red-purple papules, nodules, or tumors 5 mm to 15 cm in size. Immunophenotypically, they are usually of Th-cell origin, and clonal rearrangements of the TCR gene are usually present. A CD4 phenotype, as opposed to a CD8 phenotype, is associated with a more favorable prognosis, but a CD4/CD56 phenotype has a poorer prognosis. Most cases are indolent, but radiation, chemotherapy, retinoids, IFNs, and monoclonal antibodies have been used in widespread or progressive disease.

Follicular T-Cell Lymphoma (Provisional Entity)

This entity is regarded by some as a monomorphic variant of the preceding. It presents as a nodular infiltrate of BCL-6+ follicular helper T-cells. There is no epidermotropism. Patients may present with multiple papules, nodules, and plaques, sometimes localizing to intertriginous sites. Most cases run an indolent course but are relatively resistant to therapy.

Primary Cutaneous Acral CD8+ T-Cell Lymphoma (Indolent CD8+ Lymphoid Proliferation of the Ear—Provisional Entity)

This is another indolent lymphoproliferative disorder, typically localized to the ear, or rarely other parts of the face. As with the previously discussed disorders, there is no epidermotropism. The nodule is composed of small to medium-sized monomorphic CD8+ T cells.

ANGIOIMMUNOBLASTIC T-CELL LYMPHOMA AND ANGIOIMMUNOBLASTIC LYMPHADENOPATHY WITH DYSPROTEINEMIA

Angioimmunoblastic lymphoma is an uncommon lymphoproliferative disorder. Patients are middle-aged or elderly and present with fever (72%), weight loss (58%), hepatomegaly (60%), polyclonal hyperglobulinemia (65%), and generalized adenopathy (87%). Pruritus occurs in 44% and a rash in 46%. The skin eruption is usually morbilliform in character, resembling an exanthem or a drug reaction. Petechial, purpuric, nodular, ulcerative, and erythrodermic eruptions have also been reported and may mimic infection. In about 30% of cases the eruption is associated with the ingestion of a medication. The eruptions usually resolve with oral corticosteroids, misleading the clinician into believing that the eruption was benign. Reversible myelofibrosis has been described. Recent evidence suggests that the neoplastic cells are derived from germinal center Th cells because they express genes unique to this population, including BCL-6, programmed death–1 (*PD-1*) and *CXCL13*.

Histopathologically, there is a patchy and perivascular dermal infiltrate of various types of lymphoid cells, plasma cells, histiocytes (enough rarely to give a "granulomatous" appearance), and eosinophils. The lymphoid cells are usually Th cells (CD4+). Some portion of the lymphoid cells is atypical in most cases, suggesting the diagnosis. Blood vessels are increased and the endothelial cells are prominent, often cuboidal. Unfortunately, these changes may not be adequate to confirm the diagnosis. However, clonal T-cell gene rearrangement is found in three quarters of these skin lesions and is the same as the clone in the lymph node. Immunophenotyping of the skin lesions does not give a consistent pattern. At times, the skin lesions will show leukocytoclastic vasculitis on biopsy. Lymph node biopsy is usually required to confirm the diagnosis and exclude progression to lymphoma.

Angioimmunoblastic lymphadenopathy with dysproteinemia (AILD) appears to develop in a stepwise manner. Initially, there is an immune response to an unknown antigen. This immune reaction persists, leading to oligoclonal T-cell proliferation. Monoclonal evolution may occur, eventuating in lymphoma (angioimmunoblastic lymphoma, AILD-L). These are usually T-cell lymphomas, but B-cell lymphomas can also occur. In the case of AILD-L, skin lesions may contain the neoplastic cells (secondary lymphoma cutis). In up to 50% of cases, multiple unrelated neoplastic cell clones have been identified. Clones identified in the skin may be different from clones found in lymph node. Trisomy 3 or 5 or an extra X chromosome may be found. AILD is an aggressive disease, with mortality rates of 48%–72% in various series (average survival 11–60 months). The cause of death is usually infection. Epstein-Barr virus and human herpesvirus (HHV)-6 and HHV-8 have been implicated in AILD.

Treatment of AILD has included systemic corticosteroids, methotrexate plus prednisone, combination chemotherapy, fludarabine, 2-chlorodeoxyadenosine, IFN alfa, and cyclosporine. Early treatment with systemic steroids during an oligoclonal or prelymphomatous stage may induce a long-lasting remission. Asymptomatic patients may not be treated initially but must be watched very closely. More aggressive chemotherapy achieves better remission. Nonetheless, recurrence rates are high, and average survival is 1–3 years.

Lennert Lymphoma (Lymphoepithelioid Lymphoma)

Lennert lymphoma is a rare CD4+ systemic T-cell lymphoma. Cutaneous lesions occur in less than 10% of patients and present as papules, plaques, or nodules. The skin lesions may not represent lymphoma cutis because palisaded granulomatous and nonspecific dermal infiltrates may occur. The clinicohistologic appearance may closely resemble granuloma annulare. The course is low-grade until the lymphoma transforms to a high-grade, large-cell lymphoma.

Subcutaneous (Panniculitis-Like) T-Cell Lymphoma

Clinically, patients are usually young adults who present with subcutaneous nodules (Fig. 32.14), usually on the lower extremities.

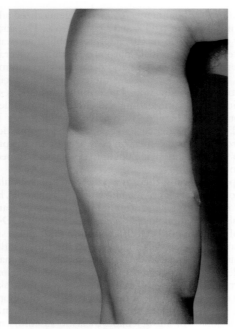

Fig. 32.14 Subcutaneous T-cell lymphoma.

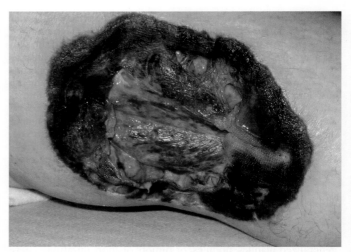

Fig. 32.15 Natural killer T-cell lymphoma. (Courtesy Alain Rook, MD.)

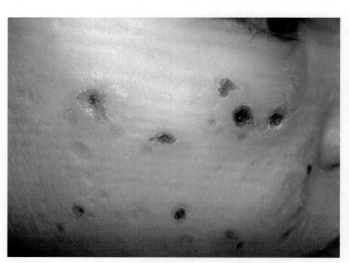

Fig. 32.16 Hydroa vacciniforme–like natural killer T-cell lymphoma.

The alpha/beta phenotype is generally associated with indolent disease, and gamma/delta lymphoma, which is associated with a more aggressive course, is now considered a separate provisional entity in the WHO classification. Weight loss, fever, and fatigue are common and may herald the onset of a rapidly progressive hemophagocytic syndrome.

Histologically, there is a lacelike infiltration of the lobules of adipocytes, mimicking panniculitis, especially lupus profundus. A characteristic feature is rimming of neoplastic cells around individual adipocytes with nuclear molding and atypia. Immunophenotypically, the neoplastic cells mark as T cells (CD2+, CD3+). Most cases are derived from α/β T cells and are CD56–. Subcutaneous γ/δ T-cell lymphomas are classified separately. They are typically CD56+. Karyorrhectic debris, dermal involvement, and epidermotropism are clues to the diagnosis of γ/δ T-cell lymphoma. Multiagent chemotherapy is commonly required, at times with stem cell support. Denileukin diftitox (Ontak) has been reported to produce a favorable response.

Nasal/Nasal-Type NK/T-Cell Lymphoma (Angiocentric Lymphoma)

Natural killer/T-cell lymphoma most frequently presents in extranodal tissue and is characterized by a high incidence of nasal involvement. It is more common in Asia, where it affects primarily women with a mean age of 40. In Korea it is reported to be the most common form of cutaneous lymphoma after mycosis fungoides. It is uncommon in the United States. Nasal NK/T-cell lymphoma presents clinically as dermal or subcutaneous papules or nodules that may ulcerate (Fig. 32.15). Lesions are usually widespread and involve the lower extremities. A hydroa vacciniforme-type affects children in Central and South America and Asia. The lesions present as ulcerative papulovesicles with scarring involving the face and extremities (Fig. 32.16). Skin lesions are exacerbated by sun exposure and are reproduced with UVA irradiation. Hypersensitivity to mosquito bites is frequent, and the prognosis for those who develop Epstein-Barr–associated NK-cell/T-cell lymphoma is poor despite therapy. (See Chapter 3.)

Histologically, the dermis and subcutaneous fat are infiltrated with intermediate-sized, atypical granular lymphocytes, within and around the walls of small and medium-sized vessels. Epidermotropism may be noted. The lymphoma cells express a spectrum of T- and NK-cell immunophenotypic markers, variably expressing CD2, CD3, CD4, CD8, and the NK-cell marker CD56. CD56 is not cell lineage specific, and a subset of CD56 cutaneous lymphoma cases is classified under the SPTCL category. Epstein-Barr virus is present in the NK variants and variably present in the T-cell variants. T-cell clonality is detected if the T-cell immunophenotype is present. The prognosis is poor.

Brown RA, et al: Primary cutaneous anaplastic large cell lymphoma. J Cutan Pathol 2017; 44: 570.

Junkins-Hopkins Md JM: Aggressive cutaneous T-cell lymphomas. Semin Diagn Pathol 2017; 34: 44.

Kempf W: A new era for cutaneous CD30-positive T-cell lymphoproliferative disorders. Semin Diagn Pathol 2017; 34: 22.

Sauder MB, et al: CD30(+) lymphoproliferative disorders of the skin. Hematol Oncol Clin North Am 2017; 31: 317.

Adult T-Cell Leukemia/Lymphoma

Infection with human lymphotropic virus type 1 (HTLV-1) may lead to acute T-cell leukemia/lymphoma (ATL) in 0.01%–0.02%

of infected persons. This virus is endemic in Japan, Southeast Asia, the Caribbean region, Latin America, and equatorial Africa. ATL usually has an acute onset, with leukocytosis, lymphadenopathy, and HOTS (hypercalcemia, osteolytic bone lesions, T-cell leukemia, and skin lesions). Lesions resemble mycosis fungoides, except that patches are uncommon, and plaques and nodules predominate. Histologically, the skin lesions contain lichenoid infiltrates of medium-sized lymphocytes with convoluted nuclei. Epidermotropism and involvement around and within adnexa occur. Granuloma formation may occur in the dermis. ATL cells are usually CD4+/CD7− and show T-cell gene rearrangements.

CUTANEOUS B-CELL LYMPHOMA

Primary cutaneous B-cell lymphomas (Fig. 32.17) occur less often than cutaneous T-cell lymphomas; 25% of cases of primary cutaneous non-Hodgkin lymphomas are B cell in origin.

The great majority of primary cutaneous B-cell lymphomas are composed of cells with the morphologic characteristics of the B cells normally found in the marginal zone or germinal centers of lymph nodes. Secondary cutaneous involvement can occur with all forms of B-cell lymphoma based primarily in lymph node or other sites. The clinical features are similar to those of primary cutaneous lymphoma, with violaceous papules or nodules (Fig. 32.18). In secondary cutaneous B-cell lymphomas, the prognosis is generally poor. It is therefore critical to evaluate any patient suspected of having primary cutaneous B-cell lymphoma to exclude involvement at another site. Radiation is commonly used for indolent forms of primary cutaneous B-cell lymphoma, but excision, intralesional rituximab, intralesional corticosteroids, and systemic chemotherapy have also been used. Higher-grade lymphomas, such as leg-type lymphoma, primary cutaneous follicle center lymphoma occurring on the leg, and precursor B-cell lymphoblastic lymphoma, are typically treated with systemic chemotherapy regimens, including combinations of anthracycline-containing chemotherapies and rituximab.

Primary Cutaneous Marginal-Zone Lymphoma (PCMZL, Malt-Type Lymphoma, Including Primary Cutaneous Immunocytoma)

These lymphomas present as solitary or multiple dermal or subcutaneous nodules or tumors, primarily on the upper part of the body, trunk, or extremities. Widespread lesions suggest secondary skin involvement by systemic lymphoma. Women are affected by PCMZL more than men. Immunocytomas are associated with European *Borrelia* and occur as tense, shiny, pink to red nodules on the legs of older patients, typically men.

Histologically, the infiltrate may be nodular or diffuse. The neoplastic cells are medium-sized gray cells with predominantly cleaved nuclei that proliferate within the space surrounding and between benign germinal centers. Plasma cells are typically present and may be numerous. Light-chain restriction is easiest to identify in the plasma cell population by means of in situ hybridization. Immunophenotypically, the cells are CD20+, CD79+, and BCL-2+. The prognosis is excellent, with 5-year survival close to 100%. Local radiation therapy, or excision if lesions are few, is recommended. In some *Borrelia*-endemic areas in Europe, immunocytomas are common. They present on the legs of older men and are characterized by sheets of plasmacytoid B cells with Dutcher bodies. Treatment is similar to other forms of PCMZL.

Primary Cutaneous Follicle Center Cell Lymphoma (PCFCCL, Diffuse and Follicular Types)

Clinically, most patients with PCFCCL present with single or multiple papules, plaques, or nodules, with surrounding erythema, in one anatomic region. About two thirds of cases present on the trunk, about 20% on the head and neck (vast majority on scalp), and about 15% on the leg. PCFCCLs are more common in men than women. Males outnumber females 4:1 in trunk lesions, whereas women disproportionately have head and leg lesions. Untreated, the lesions gradually increase in size and number, but extracutaneous involvement is uncommon. The prognosis is excellent; 5-year survival with treatment approaches 100%. Secondary cutaneous involvement of systemic follicular lymphoma has a poor prognosis.

Histologically, the neoplasm is composed of centroblasts (uncleaved nuclei with peripheral nucleolus) and centrocytes (cleaved nuclei with peripheral nucleolus). The diffuse form is more common than the follicular form. In the diffuse form, the neoplastic cells retain the normal BCL-6+ phenotype of a follicle center cell, but typically lose expression of CD10. The follicular growth pattern is composed of irregularly shaped, asymmetric follicles that crowd together like pieces of a jigsaw puzzle. The

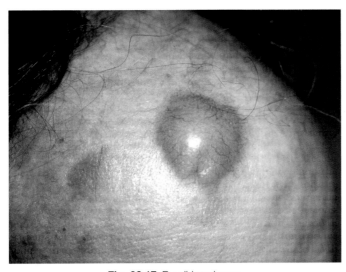

Fig. 32.17 B-cell lymphoma.

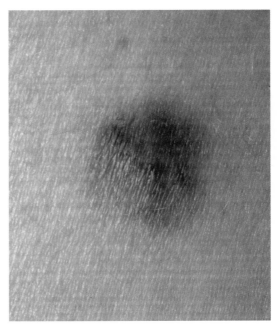

Fig. 32.18 Secondary cutaneous lymphoma.

cells typically stain for both BCL-6 and CD10, and these stains demonstrate neoplastic cells that have "wandered" beyond the confines of the follicle center. Elongated "carrot-shaped" nuclei are often present within the follicular centers, and CD21 staining shows defects in the net of DCs in the follicle center.

In early lesions, the neoplastic cells are smaller, and a substantial portion of normal T cells surround and mix with the neoplastic B cells. Over time, the neoplastic B cells become a more predominant portion of the infiltrate, the neoplastic cells are larger, and tumor-infiltrating T cells diminish. Immunophenotypically, the neoplastic cells stain with B-cell markers (CD20), and clonal rearrangement of the immunoglobulin gene can be demonstrated by polymerase chain reaction (PCR), but is difficult to demonstrate via in-situ hybridization. Lack of adenopathy, and lack of involvement of the bone marrow help to exclude nodal follicle center lymphoma. Nodal follicular lymphoma usually expresses BCL-2, and there is a t(14:18) translocation in more than 80% of cases. The translocation and BCL-2 expression are lacking in 80% of primary cutaneous follicular lymphoma.

Radiation therapy totaling 30–40 Gy and including all erythematous skin and a 2-cm margin of normal skin is very effective for lesions of the head and trunk. A combination of intralesional IFN alfa, 5-MU every 4 weeks, and topical bexarotene gel 1% twice has also been used. Anthracycline-based chemotherapy or rituximab may be used for relapses, as well as for more aggressive lesions of the leg. In Europe, a few cases of PCFCCL are associated with *Borrelia* infection and may arise in lesions of acrodermatitis chronica atrophicans.

Diffuse Large B-Cell Lymphoma (Primary Cutaneous Large B-Cell Lymphoma)

Clinically, lesions present as solitary or localized red or purple papules, nodules, or plaques. In general, solitary or localized lesions are typical of primary disease, and widespread lesions suggest secondary cutaneous involvement of primary nodal lymphoma. Lesions on the head and neck have an excellent prognosis. Lesions on the leg have a poorer prognosis, with a 5-year survival of about 50%, and are considered in some classifications as a separate entity (Fig. 32.19).

The diffuse large B-cell lymphoma is composed of large lymphocytes. Tumors consisting of sheets of centroblasts and immunoblasts (noncleaved nuclei with peripheral or central nucleoli, respectively) should be stained for MUM1, a marker for leg-type lymphoma. If the tumor cells express MUM1, the prognosis is

worse. Immunophenotypically, cells usually express CD20 and monotypic immunoglobulin, and leg-type lymphoma expresses BCL-2. Secondary cutaneous involvement with nodal large B-cell lymphoma is also associated with a poor prognosis.

Richter transformation of CLL into a high-grade lymphoma occurs in 3%–10% of CLL patients. Its onset is often heralded by fever, night sweats, and weight loss. The lymphoma usually arises in the lymph nodes or bone marrow, but can also present in the skin or internal organs.

Intravascular Large B-Cell Lymphoma (Malignant "Angioendotheliomatosis," Angiotropic Large Cell Lymphoma)

Clinically, these patients present with variable cutaneous morphologies, often subtle and nonspecific. Some intravascular large B-cell lymphomas resemble classic lymphoma with violaceous papules or nodules. Others more closely resemble intravascular thrombotic disorders, with livedo reticularis–like lesions or telangiectatic patches. Sclerotic plaques may also occur. Even normal skin can show the characteristic changes on biopsy. Patients often present with fever of unknown origin. CNS symptoms are prominent, with progressive dementia or multiple cerebrovascular ischemic events that may precede skin findings by many months.

Histologically, the features are characteristic and diagnostic. Dermal and subcutaneous vessels are dilated and filled with large neoplastic cells. Focal extravascular accumulations may be seen. The neoplastic cells are CD20+ and CD79a+ and monotypic for immunoglobulin. Clonal Ig gene rearrangements may be detected. Despite the large number of intravascular cells in the skin and other affected organs, the peripheral blood smears and bone marrow may be normal histologically. The prognosis is very poor, and multiagent chemotherapy is typically required. Rare cases of intravascular lymphoma may be of T-cell origin, but the behavior is similar to that of the B-cell variant.

EBV+ Mucocutaneous Ulcer (2016 WHO Provisional Entity)

EBV+ mucocutaneous ulcer is an indolent, often self-limited EBV+ B-cell proliferation affecting the oropharyngeal mucosa or skin. It is associated with immunosuppression and is seen in patients age 70 and older. In contrast to EBV+ diffuse large B-cell lymphoma, it does not progress to systemic disease. Patients present with a sharply circumscribed ulcer with a polymorphous infiltrate containing variable numbers of medium to large-sized immunoblast-like cells and pleomorphic Reed-Sternberg–like EBV+, CD30+ cells with a B-cell immunophenotype (most cases express CD79a).

Plasmacytoma (Multiple Myeloma)

Most cutaneous plasma cell infiltrates with light chain restriction represent marginal zone lymphoma overrun with plasma cells. True cutaneous plasmacytomas are seen most often in the setting of myeloma, occurring in 2% of myeloma patients. Plasmacytomas may also occur by direct extension from an underlying bone lesion (Fig. 32.20). They may appear at sites of trauma, such as biopsies or intravenous catheters (inflammatory oncotaxis). Most often, secondary cutaneous plasmacytomas occur in the patient with advanced myeloma, and the prognosis is poor.

Anetoderma may show plasmacytoma on biopsy. A rare manifestation of a solitary plasmacytoma of bone is an overlying erythematous skin patch that may be 10 cm or more in diameter. The chest is the most common location. Lymphadenopathy is present, and some of the patients have or develop POEMS syndrome (polyneuropathy, organomegaly, endocrinopathy, monoclonal protein, skin changes). This syndrome has been called

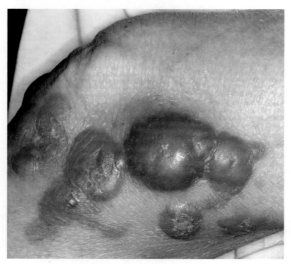

Fig. 32.19 B-cell lymphoma of the leg.

CHAPTER 32 Cutaneous Lymphoid Hyperplasia, Cutaneous T-Cell Lymphoma, Other Malignant Lymphomas, and Allied Diseases **745**

32

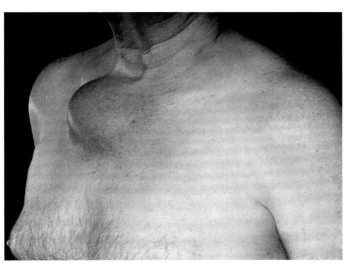

Fig. 32.20 Plasmacytoma extending from the sternum.

adenopathy and extensive skin patch overlying a plasmacytoma (AESOP).

Histologically, plasmacytomas are nodular and diffuse collections of plasma cells with varying degrees of pleomorphism and atypia. The degree of atypia may predict prognosis. The cells are monotypic for Ig production and produce the same light chain as the myeloma. The immunoglobulin produced is most often IgG or IgA, and rarely IgD or IgE. CD79 is positive, but CD19 and CD20 are negative.

In addition to plasmacytomas, patients with myeloma may develop a vast array of cutaneous complications, including normolipemic plane xanthomas, necrobiotic xanthogranuloma, amyloidosis, vasculitis, and calcinosis cutis. An unusual but characteristic skin finding in myeloma is multiple follicular spicules of the nose, forehead, cheeks, and chin. They are yellowish and firm to palpation and can be removed without bleeding. Numerous small ulcerations may occur on the trunk. Both the spicules and the ulcers contain an eosinophilic material composed of the abnormal monoclonal protein produced by the malignant cells. The spicules are not made of keratin. Clinically similar cutaneous spicules composed of keratin can be seen in vitamin A deficiency, chronic renal failure, acquired immunodeficiency syndrome (AIDS), Crohn disease, and other malignant diseases.

The appropriate treatment of plasmacytomas is determined by the presence or absence of associated systemic disease. Solitary or paucilesional primary cutaneous plasmacytomas have been treated successfully with local surgery and radiation therapy. Systemic chemotherapy may be required if these modalities fail.

Cutaneous and Systemic Plasmacytosis

Cutaneous plasmacytosis and systemic plasmacytosis occur primarily in Asians, slightly favoring men. They typically occur between ages 20 and 55. These conditions are characterized by polyclonal proliferations of plasma cells and hyperglobulinemia and were originally considered variants of Castleman disease. Cutaneous plasmacytosis affects only the skin, but patients may have lymphadenopathy and systemic symptoms of fever and malaise. Systemic plasmacytosis usually involves two or more organ systems, in addition to the skin, lung, bone marrow, and liver. Dyspnea may result from interstitial pneumonia. Infrequently, cases of systemic plasmacytosis may progress to lymphoma. The course is chronic and relatively benign unless pulmonary involvement ensues, and response to various cytostatic and immunosuppressive treatments

has been poor. PUVA and topical tacrolimus have been reported to be effective for skin lesions. The skin lesions in cutaneous and systemic plasmacytosis are identical, consisting of multiple brown-red plaques, mostly of the central upper trunk but also the face. The lesions, 1–3 cm in diameter, are often considered simply as postinflammatory hyperpigmentation until they are palpated. Histologically, they show a dense perivascular infiltrate of mature plasma cells, which stain for both κ and λ light chains (polyclonality). The disease may be a manifestation of IgG4-related disease, a clinical entity characterized by elevated levels of serum IgG4 and tissue infiltration of IgG4+ plasma cells in various organ systems. Elevated IL-6 has been reported in some patients.

IgG4-Related Skin Disease

IgG4-related skin disease presents with mass-forming lymphoplasmacytic cutaneous infiltrates, often with eosinophils, including some forms of granuloma faciale and many cases of marginal zone lymphoma. IgG4 is elevated in serum, and many IgG4+ cells can be identified in the affected tissue. These findings are not specific for the disease, however, and clinicopathologic correlation is essential. Erythematous and itchy plaques and nodules typically involve the head and neck, particularly the periauricular region, cheeks, and jawline. Systemic infiltrates may involve the lymph nodes, lacrimal and salivary glands, or parenchymal organs such as the kidney and pancreas. Retroperitoneal fibrosis may occur. Accumulated data suggest no association with systemic malignancy. Randomized controlled trials are lacking, but the associated autoimmune pancreatitis typically responds to oral corticosteroids, and both rituximab and dapsone have been reported as effective in individual patients.

HODGKIN DISEASE

The vast majority of reports of cutaneous Hodgkin disease actually represent type A lymphomatoid papulosis. These two diseases have a considerable number of overlapping features. The type A cells of LyP have similar morphology and share immunophenotypic markers with Reed-Sternberg cells. LyP can be seen in patients with Hodgkin disease. Primary cutaneous Hodgkin disease without nodal involvement is thus difficult to prove and is extremely rare, if it exists.

Most cases of Hodgkin disease of the skin usually originate in the lymph nodes, from which extension to the skin is either retrograde through the lymphatics or direct. Lesions present as papules or nodules, with or without ulceration. Lesions resembling scrofuloderma may occur. Miliary dissemination to the skin can occur in advanced disease.

Nonspecific cutaneous findings are common in patients with Hodgkin disease. Generalized, severe pruritus may precede other findings of Hodgkin disease by many months or may occur in patients with a known diagnosis. Secondary prurigo nodules and pigmentation may occur as a result of scratching. An evaluation for underlying lymphoma should be considered in any patient with severe itching, no primary skin lesions, and no other cause identified for the pruritus. Acquired ichthyosis, exfoliative dermatitis, and generalized and severe herpes zoster are other cutaneous findings in patients with Hodgkin disease.

MALIGNANT HISTIOCYTOSIS (HISTIOCYTIC MEDULLARY RETICULOSIS)

Most cases considered to be malignant histiocytosis in the past are now considered to be other forms of lymphoma or lymphomas with large components of reactive histiocytes. Very rare cases of true malignancies of histiocytes may still occur and can have cutaneous lesions, most characteristically erythematous nodules. Often the bone marrow examination in these patients is initially normal, but cases are rapidly progressive and fatal, and the bone marrow becomes involved.

Brunet V, et al: Retrospective study of intravascular large B-cell lymphoma cases diagnosed in Quebec. Medicine (Baltimore) 2017; 96: e5985.

Cerroni L: Past, present and future of cutaneous lymphomas. Semin Diagn Pathol 2017; 34: 3.

Dabaja B: Renaissance of low-dose radiotherapy concepts for cutaneous lymphomas. Oncol Res Treat 2017; 40: 255.

di Fonzo H, et al: Intravascular large B cell lymphoma presenting as fever of unknown origin and diagnosed by random skin biopsies. Am J Case Rep 2017; 18: 482.

Eberle FC, et al: Intralesional anti-CD20 antibody for low-grade primary cutaneous B-cell lymphoma. J Dtsch Dermatol Ges 2017; 15: 319.

Hope CB, et al: Primary cutaneous B-cell lymphomas with large cell predominance-primary cutaneous follicle center lymphoma, diffuse large B-cell lymphoma, leg type and intravascular large B-cell lymphoma. Semin Diagn Pathol 2017; 34: 85.

Nicolay JP, et al: Cutaneous B-cell lymphomas—pathogenesis, diagnostic workup, and therapy. J Dtsch Dermatol Ges 2016; 14: 1207.

Servitje O, et al: Primary cutaneous marginal zone B-cell lymphoma. J Am Acad Dermatol 2013; 69: 357.

Suárez AL, et al: Primary cutaneous B-cell lymphomas. Part I. J Am Acad Dermatol 2013; 69: 329.e1.

Suárez AL, et al: Primary cutaneous B-cell lymphomas. Part II. J Am Acad Dermatol 2013; 69: 343.e1.

Sundram U: Cutaneous Lymphoproliferative Disorders: What's New in the Revised 4th Edition of the World Health Organization (WHO) Classification of Lymphoid Neoplasms. Adv Anat Pathol. 2018 Sep 7. doi: 10.1097/PAP.0000000000000208. [Epub ahead of print] PubMed PMID: 30199396.

LEUKEMIA CUTIS

Clinical Features

Cutaneous eruptions seen in patients with leukemia may be divided into specific lesions (leukemia cutis) and nonspecific lesions (reactive and infectious processes). Overall, about 30% of biopsies from patients with leukemia will show leukemia cutis. All forms of leukemia can be associated with cutaneous findings, but skin disease is more common in certain forms of leukemia. Myeloid leukemia with monocytic differentiation involves the skin more often than other types of myeloid leukemia. CD68 and lysozyme immunostains can be helpful in distinguishing this form of leukemia. Dermatologic manifestations are frequently seen in patients with acute myelogenous leukemia (AML) and myelodysplastic syndrome (MDS). AML includes types M1 to M5. In AML and MDS patients, only about 25% of skin biopsies will show leukemia cutis, the remainder showing complications of the leukemia. These include infections, graft-versus-host disease, drug reactions, or the reactive conditions associated with leukemia sometimes referred to as leukemids. By contrast, in patients with acute lymphocytic leukemia (ALL), chronic myelogenous leukemia (CML), and CLL, about 50% of biopsies will show leukemia cutis. Lesion presentation may be subtle and may include macular erythema, hyperpigmentation, or morbilliform rash.

Specific Eruptions

The most common morphology of leukemic infiltrations of the skin in all forms of leukemia is multiple papules or nodules (60% of cases) or infiltrated plaques (26%). These lesions are usually flesh colored, erythematous, or violaceous (plum colored) (Figs. 32.21 and 32.22). They are rubbery on palpation, and ulceration

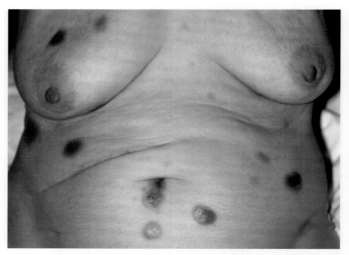

Fig. 32.21 Acute myelomonocytic leukemia cutis.

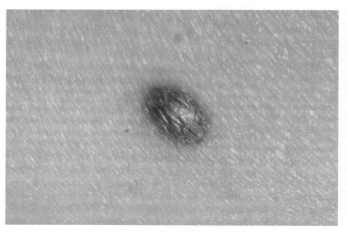

Fig. 32.22 Leukemia cutis.

is uncommon. Extensive involvement of the face may lead to a leonine facies.

Less common manifestations of leukemia cutis are subcutaneous nodules resembling erythema nodosum or panniculitis, arciform lesions (in juvenile CML), ecchymoses, palpable purpura, erythroderma, ulcerations (which may resemble pyoderma gangrenosum or venous stasis ulceration), and urticaria-like, urticaria pigmentosa–like (in ALL), and guttate psoriasis–like lesions. Rare manifestations are a lesion resembling Sister Mary Joseph nodule and cutaneous sarcoidal lesions. Myelogenous leukemia may be complicated by lesions resembling stasis dermatitis or chilblains. Gingival infiltration causing hypertrophy is common in, and relatively unique to, patients with acute myelomonocytic leukemia (Fig. 32.23).

Leukemia cutis most often occurs concomitant with or after the diagnosis of leukemia. The skin may also be a site of relapse of leukemia after chemotherapy, especially in patients who present with leukemia cutis. Infrequently, leukemia cutis may be identified while the bone marrow and peripheral blood are normal. These patients are classified as "aleukemic leukemia cutis" because they have normal bone marrow evaluations and no circulating blasts. A Leder stain, myeloperoxidase, or lysozyme may be used to identify the atypical cells as myeloid. Systemic involvement occurs within 3 weeks to 20 months (average 6 months). Leukemia cutis is a poor prognostic finding in leukemia patients, with 90% having extramedullary involvement and 40% with meningeal infiltration.

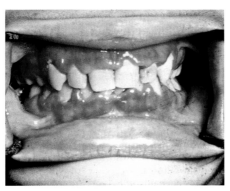

Fig. 32.23 Gingival involvement in leukemia.

The term *congenital leukemia* applies to cases appearing within the first 4–6 weeks of life. Leukemia cutis occurs in 25%–30% of such cases, the vast majority being congenital myelogenous leukemia. The typical morphology is multiple, red or plum-colored nodules. In about 10% of patients with congenital leukemia cutis (or 3% of all cases of congenital leukemia), the skin involvement occurs while the bone marrow and peripheral blood are normal. Systemic involvement is virtually always identified in 5–16 weeks. Unlike in other forms of leukemia, cutaneous infiltration does not worsen prognosis in congenital leukemia. Congenital leukemia cutis has been complicated by disseminated linear calcinosis cutis. Early-onset aleukemic leukemia cutis can occasionally undergo spontaneous regression. One report involved a child with mastocytosis who also developed a leukemia clone with a t(5; 17)(q35; q12), nucleophosmin (NPM)–retinoic acid receptor-α (RARA) fusion gene.

Granulocytic Sarcoma (Chloroma)

Granulocytic sarcomas are rare tumors of immature granulocytes. They occur in about 3% of patients with myelogenous leukemia. Granulocytic sarcoma is seen in four settings: in patients with known AML; in patients with CML or MDS as a sign of an impending blast crisis; in undiagnosed patients as the first sign of AML; or after bone marrow transplantation (BMT) as the initial sign of relapse. Most lesions occur in the soft tissues, periosteum, or bone. Skin lesions represent 20%–50% of reported cases. They may be solitary or multiple and appear as red, mahogany, or violaceous firm nodules with a predilection for the face, scalp, or trunk.

The name "chloroma" comes from the green color of fresh lesions, which can be enhanced by rubbing with alcohol; this is caused by the presence of myeloperoxidase. This appearance is variable, so the preferred term is now *granulocytic sarcoma*.

Blastic Plasmacytoid Dendritic Cell Neoplasm (Formerly Blastic NK-Cell Lymphoma, CD4, CD56+ Hematodermic Neoplasm)

The majority of patients are men, with a mean age of about 60 years. All patients present with multiple, rapidly expanding plaques and/or nodules on noncontiguous sites. Lesions are characteristically purple. The course is aggressive in most patients, with rapid cutaneous relapse after chemotherapy and systemic involvement. Histologically, the cells infiltrate the dermis or subcutaneous fat, and the neoplastic cells tend to form in single file within dermal collagen. There is usually a grenz zone below the epidermis. The lymphoma cells are small/medium to large, blastic lymphocytes. Angiocentricity may be noted but is not prominent. Immunophenotyping is usually CD3–, CD4+/CD56+. MIB-1 shows a proliferation activity greater than 50%, and T-cell gene rearrangements

are negative. In general, results with radiation therapy and chemotherapy have been poor. BMT may play an important role in therapy.

Hairy Cell Leukemia

Skin involvement is rare in hairy cell leukemia. Violaceous papules and nodules, which are the characteristic morphology of other forms of leukemia cutis, are extremely rare in hairy cell leukemia. Rather, a diffuse erythematous, nonpruritic eruption occurs, often in the setting of a systemic mycobacterial infection or a drug reaction. This may progress to erythroderma or a severe blistering eruption. Stopping the medication usually leads to resolution of the eruption. This is especially common in patients treated with 2-chlorodeoxyadenosine and allopurinol; the former treatment alone does not lead to these severe skin reactions, suggesting that the allopurinol is the cause. Patients with hairy cell leukemia also develop lesions of pustular vasculitis of the dorsal hands, a neutrophilic dermatitis closely related to bullous Sweet syndrome. This is sometimes referred to as a "vasculitis" in the oncology literature.

Nonspecific Conditions Associated With Leukemia (Leukemids)

Leukemia and its treatment are associated with a series of conditions that may also be seen in patients without leukemia, but that are seen frequently enough in leukemic patients to be recognized as a complication of leukemia or its treatment.

When a dermatologist or dermatopathologist is consulted to evaluate a patient with leukemia and skin lesions, the differential diagnosis usually includes four groups of conditions: drug reactions, leukemia cutis, an infectious complication, and a reactive condition. Drug reactions include all forms of reactions but are usually erythema multiforme, morbilliform reactions, or acral erythema. Infections may present in many ways but are usually purpuric papules, pustules, or plaques, if they are caused by bacteria or fungi. Ulceration is typical. Herpes simplex and herpes zoster should be considered in all erosive, ulcerative, or vesicular lesions. The reactive conditions include a group of neutrophilic dermatoses with considerable clinical overlap (e.g., Sweet syndrome, pyoderma gangrenosum, neutrophilic hidradenitis, leukocytoclastic vasculitis). Transient acantholytic dermatosis and eosinophilic reactions resembling insect bites may occur, most often in patients with CLL, in whom a pruritic and unremitting exfoliative erythroderma is a unique feature. A granulomatous rosacea-like leukemid and cutaneous reactive angiomatosis have also been described in patients with leukemia.

Evaluation of these patients must be complete, and extensive diagnostic tests and empiric treatment are often pursued until the diagnosis is established. In the acute setting, a clinical diagnosis is made based on morphology. Possible infectious complications are covered by appropriate antibiotics, especially if the patient is febrile or the diagnosis of a herpesvirus infection is made. A skin biopsy is often diagnostic. For herpes infections, a PCR or direct fluorescent antibody test should be done because the results are virus specific and rapid, so appropriate treatment can be given quickly. Once the diagnostic tests return, the therapy is tailored to the appropriate condition. Except for herpes infections, a skin biopsy is often required. If infection is considered, a portion of the biopsy should be sent for culture.

CUTANEOUS MYELOFIBROSIS

Myelofibrosis is a chronic myeloproliferative disorder characterized by a clonal proliferation of defective multipotential stem cells in the bone marrow. Overproduction and premature death of atypical megakaryocytes in the bone marrow produce excess amounts of platelet-derived growth factor (PDGF), a potent stimulus for fibroblast proliferation and collagen production. Extramedullary hematopoiesis (EMH) is a hallmark of myelofibrosis. Myelofibrosis may coexist with signs of mastocytosis. Blast cells and committed stem cells escape the marrow in large numbers, enter the circulation, and form tumors of the same atypical clone in other organs, especially the spleen, liver, and lymph nodes. EMH in the skin of neonates is usually caused by intrauterine viral infections. In adults, cutaneous EMH has rarely been reported, characteristically associated with myelofibrosis. Skin lesions are dermal and subcutaneous nodules. Histologically, the cutaneous lesions are composed of dermal and subcutaneous infiltrates of mature and immature myeloid cells, erythroid precursors (in only half of cases), and megakaryocytic cells (which may predominate). There is marked production of collagen fibers in the cutaneous lesions by the mechanism previously described. Myelofibrosis must be distinguished from CML, because both have elevated white blood cell counts with immature myeloid forms, defective platelet production, and marrow fibrosis. Both may terminate in blast crisis, and myelofibrosis may rarely convert to CML. CML is associated with the Philadelphia chromosome, whereas chromosomal abnormalities occur in 40% of myelofibrosis cases on various chromosomes.

HYPEREOSINOPHILIC SYNDROME

Idiopathic hypereosinophilic syndrome (HES) is defined as eosinophilia with more than 1500 eosinophils/mm^3 for more than 6 months, with some evidence of parenchymal organ involvement; there must also be no apparent underlying disease to explain the hypereosinophilia and usually no evidence of vasculitis. About 90% of patients reported have been men, mostly between ages 20 and 50. Childhood cases are rare. Presenting symptoms include fever (12%), cough (24%), fatigue, malaise, muscle pains, and skin eruptions. Two pathogenic variants of HES have been defined: m-HES (myeloproliferative HES) and l-HES (lymphocytic HES). Patients with m-HES are overwhelmingly males, and anemia, thrombocytopenia, elevated serum B$_{12}$ levels, mucosal ulcerations, splenomegaly, and endomyocardial fibrosis are the clinical features. Isolated Loeffler's endocarditis has been reported as a presenting sign. Eosinophil clonality and interstitial deletion on 4q12 result in fusions of *FIP1qL1* and *PDGFRa* genes, forming an F/P fusion protein displaying constitutive activity, are pathogenically related to m-HES cases. Increased mast cells and elevated tryptase levels with myeloid precursors in peripheral blood and myelofibrosis may be found, suggesting that mast cells may be pathogenically related to this form of HES. Leukemia may develop in patients with m-HES patients. The l-HES variant has been associated with circulating T-cell clones of CD4+ phenotype, which secrete Th2 cytokines, especially IL-5. Women and men are equally affected by l-HES, and cutaneous manifestations are observed in virtually all patients. Skin manifestations include urticaria, angioedema, pruritus, eczema, and erythroderma. Splinter hemorrhages and necrotic skin lesions are seen in some HES patients as well. Endomyocardial fibrosis is uncommon, but pulmonary and digestive symptoms are common. Some cases of l-HES are clinically identical to Gleich syndrome or episodic angioedema and hypereosinophilia. Over time, some patients with l-HES will develop lymphoma.

Treatment is determined by classifying cases appropriately as m-HES or l-HES. Patients with m-HES may be treated with corticosteroids, hydroxyurea, IFN alfa, and chemotherapeutic agents. Imatinib mesylate (Gleevac, 100 mg/day or less) can be highly effective for m-HES patients with the F/P mutation because it inhibits the phosphorylation of the F/P protein and leads to apoptosis of cells producing this protein. Imatinib has rapidly become first-choice treatment for this subset of patients. Response may be dramatic, with eosinophil levels improving, and skin and GI manifestations clearing in days. For l-HES patients, systemic glucocorticoids, and perhaps IFN alfa with glucocorticoids, can

be used and are usually effective. Monoclonal anti–IL-5 antibody, cyclosporine, anti–IL-2Rα, infliximab, and CTLA-4-Ig may be treatment options. If lymphoma supervenes, intense chemotherapy and allogenic stem cell transplantation can be considered.

Brunetti L, et al: Blastic plasmacytoid dendritic cell neoplasm and chronic myelomonocytic leukemia. Leukemia 2017; 31: 1238.

Hu Z, et al: Blastic plasmacytoid dendritic cell neoplasm associated with chronic myelomonocytic leukemia. Blood 2016; 128: 1664.

Lefèvre G, et al: The lymphoid variant of hypereosinophilic syndrome. Medicine (Baltimore) 2014; 93: 255.

Plötz SG, et al: Clinical overview of cutaneous features in hypereosinophilic syndrome. Curr Allergy Asthma Rep 2012; 12: 85.

Sullivan JM, et al: Treatment of blastic plasmacytoid dendritic cell neoplasm. Hematology Am Soc Hematol Educ Program 2016; 2016: 16.

Tomé A, et al: Pediatric blastic plasmacytoid dendritic cell neoplasm. J Pediatr Hematol Oncol 2017; 39: 323.

Ulrickson ML, et al: Gemcitabine and docetaxel as a novel treatment regimen for blastic plasmacytoid dendritic cell neoplasm. Am J Hematol 2017; 92: E75.

SINUS HISTIOCYTOSIS WITH MASSIVE LYMPHADENOPATHY (ROSAI-DORFMAN DISEASE)

Sinus histiocytosis with massive lymphadenopathy (SHML), or Rosai-Dorfman disease, usually appears in patients in the first or second decade of life as a febrile illness accompanied by massive cervical (and often other) lymphadenopathy, polyclonal hyperglobulinemia, leukocytosis, anemia, and elevated erythrocyte sedimentation rate. Males and black persons are especially susceptible. Extranodal involvement occurs in 40% of cases, with skin being the most common site. About 10% of patients with SHML have skin lesions, and 3% have disease detectable only in the skin. The terms *cutaneous sinus histiocytosis* and *cutaneous Rosai-Dorfman disease* have been applied to these patients. Skin lesions consist of isolated or disseminated, yellow-brown papules, pustules, or nodules (Fig. 32.24) or macular erythema. Large annular lesions,

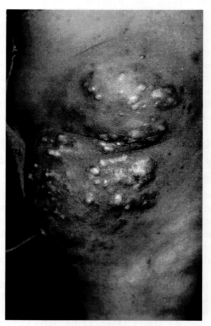

Fig. 32.24 Rosai-Dorfman disease.

resembling granuloma annulare, may occur. Most patients with cutaneous Rosai-Dorfman disease are older (age 40–60).

Histologically, there is a superficial and deep perivascular infiltrate of lymphocytes and plasma cells. Nodular and diffuse infiltration of the dermis by large, foamy histiocytes is present. An important diagnostic feature is the finding of intact lymphocytes (and less often plasma cells) in the cytoplasm of the histiocytic cells; this is called emperipolesis. Foamy histiocytes may be seen in dermal lymphatic channels. The cutaneous histology in some cases may be very nonspecific, except for the finding of emperipolesis, and only on evaluation of lymph node or other organ involvement does the diagnosis become clear. Immunohistochemistry and electron microscopy may be very useful, because the infiltrating cells are positive for CD4, factor XIIIa, and S-100 but do not contain Birbeck granules.

The cause of SHML is unknown, but numerous reports have identified HHV-6 in involved lymph nodes. The condition usually clears spontaneously, so no treatment is required. Numerous agents have been used therapeutically, with variable success, but are indicated only if the condition puts the patient at risk for death or a significant complication (usually by compressing a vital organ). Treatments have included radiation, systemic corticosteroids, and thalidomide. Single-agent and multiagent chemotherapy is met with mixed to poor response. To treat skin lesions, cryotherapy, topical corticosteroids, acitretin, and intralesional corticosteroids may be tried.

Bunick CG, et al: Cutaneous Rosai-Dorfman disease of the right ear responsive to radiotherapy. J Am Acad Dermatol 2012; 67: e225.

Fumerton R, et al: Refractory cutaneous Rosai-Dorfman disease responsive to cryotherapy. Cutis 2011; 87: 296.

Kutlubay Z, et al: Rosai-Dorfman disease. Am J Dermatopathol 2014; 36: 353.

Sun NZ, et al: Cutaneous Rosai-Dorfman disease successfully treated with low-dose methotrexate. JAMA Dermatol 2014; l150: 787.

POLYCYTHEMIA VERA (ERYTHREMIA)

Polycythemia vera (PCV) is characterized by an absolute increase of circulating red blood cells, with a hematocrit level of 55%–80%.

Leukocyte and platelet counts are also increased. The skin changes are characteristic. The skin tends to be red, especially on the face, neck, and acral areas. The mucous membranes are engorged and bluish. The phrase "red as a rose in summer and indigo blue in winter" has been ascribed to Osler in describing PCV. Telangiectases, bleeding gums, and epistaxis are frequently encountered. Cyanosis, purpura, petechiae, hemosiderosis, rosacea, and koilonychia may also be present.

In 50% of patients with PCV, aquagenic pruritus occurs. In about two thirds, this is of limited severity and does not require treatment. The pruritus is typically triggered after a bath or shower, and the feeling induced may be itching, burning, or stinging. It usually lasts 30–60 minutes and is independent of the water temperature. Pruritus unassociated with water exposure may also occur. There is a concurrent elevation of blood and skin histamine. Pruritus is present in about 20% of patients at presentation and develops in the remaining 30% over the course of their disease. Patients with pruritus have lower mean corpuscular volumes and higher leukocyte counts. Some have suggested that iron deficiency plays a role in PCV-associated pruritus, so a ferritin level and a trial of iron therapy may be indicated. Platelet counts are no different between PCV patients who itch and those who do not.

The treatment of PCV-associated pruritus may be difficult. Initial therapy would include first- or second-generation H1 antihistamines. Hydroxyzine was reported as the most effective antihistamine by a group of PCV patients. H2 blockers can be added. Narrow-band UVB therapy has been reported to be effective in 80% of patients. Topical therapy is of limited benefit, but paroxetine (Paxil), 20–60 mg/day, may be dramatically effective. Phlebotomy may be useful in patients with elevated hematocrit, and imatinib mesylate appears effective in many patients.

Pecci A, et al: Cutaneous involvement by post-polycythemia vera myelofibrosis. Am J Hematol 2014; 89: 448.

33 Diseases of the Skin Appendages

DISEASES OF THE HAIR

Normal human hairs can be classified according to cyclic phases of growth. Anagen hairs are growing hairs; catagen hairs are those undergoing transition from the growing to the resting stage; and telogen hairs are resting hairs, which remain in the follicles for variable periods before they fall out (teloptosis). The lag period between loss of the telogen hair and growth of a new anagen hair has been called kenogen.

Anagen hairs grow for about 3 years (1000 days), with a range between 2 and 6 years. The follicular matrix cells grow, divide, and become keratinized to form growing hairs. Catagen hairs are in a transitional phase, lasting 1 or 2 weeks, in which all growth activity ceases, with the eventual formation of the telogen "club" hair. Many apoptotic cells are present in the outer root sheath of the catagen hair as it involutes. Telogen club hairs are resting hairs, which continue in this state for 3–5 months (≈100 days) before they are released.

Of human hairs plucked from a normal scalp, 85%–90% are anagen hairs, and 10%–15% are telogen hairs. Catagen hairs normally constitute less than 1% of scalp hairs. The scalp normally contains an estimated 100,000 hairs, and the average number of hairs shed daily is 100–150. The hair growth rate of terminal hairs is about 0.37 mm/day. Contrary to popular belief, neither shaving nor menstruation has any effect on hair growth rate. The average uncut scalp hair length is estimated to be 25–100 cm, although exceptional hairs may be as long as 170 cm (70 inches).

Lanugo hair is the fine hair present on the body of the fetus. This is replaced by the vellus and terminal hairs. Vellus hairs are fine and usually light colored and have a narrow hair shaft thinner than the width of the inner root sheath. Terminal hairs are coarse, thick, and dark, except in blond-haired persons. Hair occurs on all skin surfaces except the palms, soles, labia minora, lips, nails, glans, and prepuce. Terminal hairs are typically present on a man's face, chest, and abdomen, but vellus hairs usually predominate on these sites in women.

Causes of alopecia are generally divided into the broad categories of cicatricial and noncicatricial alopecia. The evaluation should take into account the patient's age and ethnicity. Examination of hair shafts can establish a diagnosis of trichodystrophy. Hair counts, hair pull, and hair pluck (trichogram) can establish the degree of hair shedding, the type of hair that is shed, and the anagen/telogen ratio. Biopsies can also determine the anagen/telogen ratio and provide information regarding the potential for regrowth, as well as providing a diagnosis. Biopsies are particularly valuable in the evaluation of cicatricial alopecia. Often, a correct diagnosis hinges on a synthesis of clinical, histologic, serologic, and immunofluorescent data.

Noncicatricial Alopecia

Alopecia Areata

Clinical Features. Alopecia areata (in French, pelade) is characterized by rapid and complete loss of hair in one or more round or oval patches, typically 1–5 cm in diameter, usually on the scalp (Fig. 33.1), bearded area, eyebrows, eyelashes, and, less frequently, other hairy areas of the body. A few resting hairs may be found within the patches. Early in the course, there may be sparing of gray hair, and white hairs are rarely affected. Sudden whitening of hair may represent widespread alopecia areata in a patient with salt-and-pepper hair. In about 10% of alopecia areata patients, especially in long-standing cases with extensive involvement, the nails develop uniform pits that may form transverse or longitudinal lines. Trachyonychia, onychomadesis, and red or spotted lunulae occur, but less often. Dermoscopic examination typically demonstrates diffuse, round, or polycyclic perifollicular yellow dots.

Complete loss of scalp hair is referred to as alopecia totalis, and complete loss of all hair as alopecia universalis. Loss may occur confluently along the temporal and occipital scalp (ophiasis) or on the entire scalp except for this area (sisaipho). Rarely, alopecia areata may present in a diffuse pattern that may mimic pattern alopecia. Clues to the correct diagnosis include a history of periodic regrowth, nail pitting (Fig. 33.2), and the presence of tapered fractures or "exclamation point" hairs. Alopecia areata generally presents as an anagen effluvium, with an inflammatory insult to the hair matrix resulting in tapering of the hair shaft and fracture of anagen hairs. As the hair miniaturizes or converts from anagen to telogen, the remaining lower portion of the hair rises above the level of the scalp, producing the exclamation point hair.

Alopecia areata is associated with a higher incidence than usual of atopic dermatitis, Down syndrome, lichen planus, and autoimmune diseases, such as systemic lupus erythematosus (SLE), thyroiditis, diabetes mellitus, myasthenia gravis, and vitiligo. However, most cases of alopecia areata occur without associated disease, and routine screening for these disorders is of little value unless prompted by signs or symptoms.

Migratory poliosis of the scalp may represent a forme fruste of alopecia areata. Patients with this disorder present with migrating circular patches of white hair, but never lose hair. The histology resembles alopecia areata.

Etiologic Factors. Oligoclonal and autoreactive T lymphocytes are present in the peribulbar inflammatory infiltrate, and many patients respond to immunomodulating drugs. Affected alopecia areata scalp skin grafted on to nude mice with severe combined immunodeficiency demonstrates loss of infiltrating lymphocytes and hair growth. In this model, injecting T lymphocytes with scalp homogenate can reproduce the alopecia. Follicular melanocytes substitute for scalp homogenates to produce alopecia areata in this model, providing evidence that follicular melanocytes are the targets for activated T cells in this disease. This hypothesis is also supported by the observations that white hair is rarely affected and regrowing hair is often depigmented.

The early phase of hair loss appears to be mediated by type 1 cytokines, including interleukin (IL)–2, interferon (IFN)–γ, and tumor necrosis factor (TNF)–α. The hair bulb normally represents an area of relative immune privilege during anagen, as evidenced by a very low level of expression of major histocompatibility complex (MHC) class Ia antigens. This immune privilege may prevent antigen recognition by autoreactive CD8+ T cells. Alopecia areata may be related to collapse of this immune privilege.

Overall, almost 25% of patients have a positive family history; there are reports of twins with alopecia areata. Patients with "early onset, severe, familial clustering alopecia areata" have a unique and highly significant association with the human leukocyte antigens (HLAs) DR4, DR11, and DQ7. The "later onset, milder severity,

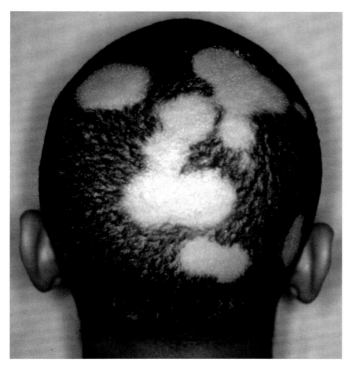

Fig. 33.1 Alopecia areata.

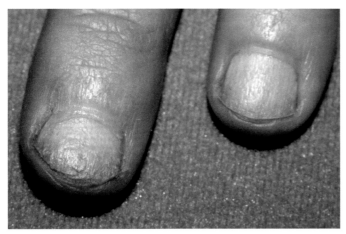

Fig. 33.2 Nails of a patient with alopecia areata. (Courtesy Steven Binnick, MD.)

better prognostic" subsets of patients have a lower frequency of familial disease and do not share these HLAs. Familial alopecia areata associated with hereditary thrombocytopenia related to mutations in genes on chromosome 17 has been described. R620W (c.1858C>T, a variant of the protein tyrosine phosphatase nonreceptor 22 gene, *PTPN22*) is associated with a variety of autoimmune disorders, including alopecia areata. It is associated with early onset of disease, widespread hair loss, and a positive family history.

Histology. In early alopecia areata, there is a lymphoid infiltrate in the peribulbar area of anagen or early catagen follicles. Eosinophils may be present in the infiltrate, and lymphocyte-mediated damage to the bulb produces melanin pigment incontinence in the surrounding stroma. The presence of many catagen hairs and pigment casts within the follicular canal can cause histologic

confusion with trichotillomania. The follicles eventually miniaturize, appearing as small, dystrophic anagen hairs high in the dermis, often with a persistent lymphocytic peribulbar infiltrate. Fibrous tract remnants beneath the miniaturized bulbs of alopecia areata may contain lymphoid cells, eosinophils, and melanin pigment. With time, the lymphocytes disappear, but focal eosinophils and pigment remain. Finally, only focal melanin pigment remains in the fibrous tract remnants. Every histologic feature of alopecia areata may be seen in syphilis. The presence of plasma cells is suggestive of syphilis, but plasma cells are also lacking in about one third of syphilis biopsies. Plasma cells may be present in biopsies from any form of inflammatory alopecia if the biopsy is taken from the occipital scalp, because this site readily recruits plasma cells.

Differential Diagnosis. The sharply circumscribed patch of alopecia with exclamation point hairs at the periphery and the absence of scarring are indicative of alopecia areata. Tinea capitis, androgenetic alopecia, early lupus erythematosus (LE), syphilis, congenital triangular alopecia, alopecia neoplastica, and trichotillomania should be kept in mind when alopecia areata is considered. In endemic areas of Southwest Asia, *Pheidole* ants shear hair shafts during the night, resulting in overnight loss of clumps of hair. The resulting round patches of hair loss closely mimic alopecia areata.

Treatment. The natural course of the hair loss is highly variable. Some patches will regrow in a few weeks without any treatment. In a series of 63 consecutive responders to a follow-up questionnaire, hair had spontaneously regrown in all but four after 1 year and in all but one after 2 years. The great majority had recovered in 3 months after their only office visit. Therefore anecdotal reports of success must be interpreted carefully in the light of the high rate of spontaneous recovery.

Intralesional injections of corticosteroid suspensions are the treatment of choice for localized, cosmetically conspicuous patches, such as those occurring in the frontal hairline or involving an eyebrow. Injections of triamcinolone, 2–10 mg/mL, are typically given intradermally or in the superficial subcutaneous tissue. Large volumes and higher concentrations of triamcinolone present a greater risk of atrophy. Injection under significant pressure or with a small-bore syringe increases the likelihood of retinal artery embolization. High-strength topical corticosteroids may be used as a safer first-line therapy but are less reliable than injections. Several investigators have reported the use of pulsed oral corticosteroids in rapidly progressing or widespread disease. However, long-term treatment is frequently needed to maintain growth, and the attendant risks should be carefully weighed against the benefits. In a study of 66 patients age 9–60 years, monthly methylprednisolone was administered at a dose of 500 mg/day for 3 days, or 5 mg/kg twice daily over 3 days in children. More than 60% of patients with widespread patchy alopecia responded. Half the patients with alopecia totalis had a good response, whereas a quarter of those with universal alopecia responded. Patients with ophiasic alopecia areata did not respond. Predictors of response include disease duration of 6 months or less, younger than 10 years at disease onset, and multifocal disease.

Oral and topical Janus kinase (JAK) inhibitors, including tofacitinib and ruxolitinib, have demonstrated excellent responses in many patients. The roles of phosphodiesterase 4 inhibitors and platelet-rich plasma are unclear. Induction of contact sensitivity to squaric acid dibutyl ester, dinitrochlorobenzene (DNCB), and diphencyprone can be useful in refractory cases. Topical or oral methoxsalen (psoralen) and ultraviolet A (PUVA) therapy is an option for refractory or widespread lesions. Short-contact topical anthralin 1% cream (applied for 15–20 minutes and then shampooed off) can be of benefit. Topical minoxidil may be combined with other treatments or used as a single agent. Psoriatic doses of methotrexate and sulfasalazine in doses up to 1.5 g three times daily may be beneficial. Cyclosporine has been used alone or combined with other modalities, including PUVA. Biologics have produced mixed, and largely disappointing, results, and alopecia areata has developed during biologic therapy for other conditions. The 308-nm xenon chloride excimer laser (300–2300 mJ/cm²/session) has been reported to produce regrowth after 11 and 12 sessions over 9–11 weeks. Periocular pigmentation and iris darkening are associated with use of travoprost, bimatoprost, and latanoprost for eyelash disease. Therapeutic results are mixed. Botanicals, including peony glucosides and glycyrrhizin, demonstrate some promise. In a mouse model, a fusion protein of parathyroid hormone and a bacterial collagen-binding domain produced hair regrowth.

Alopecia areata can cause tremendous psychological stress. Education about the disease process, cosmetically acceptable alternatives (especially information about wigs), and research into innovative therapies should all be made available to the patient. In addition to the information conveyed by the dermatologist, an excellent resource is the National Alopecia Areata Foundation (www.naaf.org, info@naaf.org).

Prognosis. The tendency is for spontaneous recovery in alopecia areata patients who are postpubertal at onset. At first the regrowing hairs are downy and light in color; later they are replaced by stronger and darker hair with full growth. Predictors of a poor prognosis are the presence of atopic dermatitis, childhood onset, widespread involvement, ophiasis, duration of longer than 5 years, and onychodystrophy. Acute diffuse and total alopecia is a newly defined subtype of alopecia areata that occurs in young adults and has a good prognosis.

Açıkgöz G, et al: Pulse methylprednisolone therapy for the treatment of extensive alopecia areata. J Dermatolog Treat 2014; 25: 164.

Apfelbacher CJ: Research questions for the treatment of alopecia areata have been prioritized. Br J Dermatol 2017; 176: 1128.

Ayatollahi A, et al: Platelet rich plasma for treatment of non-scarring hair loss. J Dermatolog Treat 2017; 28: 574.

Barrón-Hernández YL, et al: Bimatoprost for the treatment of eyelash, eyebrow and scalp alopecia. Expert Opin Investig Drugs 2017; 26: 515.

Bayart CB, et al: Topical Janus kinase inhibitors for the treatment of pediatric alopecia areata. J Am Acad Dermatol 2017; 77: 167.

Craiglow BG, et al: Tofacitinib for the treatment of alopecia areata and variants in adolescents. J Am Acad Dermatol 2017; 76: 29.

Gupta AK, et al: What is new in the management of alopecia areata. Skinmed 2016; 14: 375.

Ibrahim O, et al: Treatment of alopecia areata with tofacitinib. JAMA Dermatol 2017; 153: 600.

Jang YH, et al: Systematic review and quality analysis of studies on the efficacy of topical diphenylcyclopropenone treatment for alopecia areata. J Am Acad Dermatol 2017; 77: 170.

Lai VWY, et al: Systemic treatments for alopecia areata: A systematic review. Australas J Dermatol 2018. doi: 10.1111/ajd.12913. [Epub ahead of print] Review. PubMed PMID: 30191561.

Landis ET, Pichardo-Geisinger RO: Methotrexate for the treatment of pediatric alopecia areata. J Dermatolog Treat 2017 Jun 30; ePub ahead of print.

Lim SK, et al: Low-dose systemic methotrexate therapy for recalcitrant alopecia areata. Ann Dermatol 2017; 29: 263.

Liu LY, et al: Tofacitinib for the treatment of severe alopecia areata and variants. J Am Acad Dermatol 2017; 76: 22.

Ngwanya MR, et al: Higher concentrations of dithranol appear to induce hair growth even in severe alopecia areata. Dermatol Ther 2017; 30. E12500.

Triyangkulsri K, et al: Role of janus kinase inhibitors in the treatment of alopecia areata. Drug Des Devel Ther 2018; 12: 2323-2335. doi: 10.2147/DDDT.S172638. eCollection 2018. Review. PubMed PMID: 30100707; PubMed Central PMCID: PMC6067625.

Telogen Effluvium

Telogen effluvium presents with excessive shedding of normal telogen club hairs. This excessive shedding of telogen hairs most often occurs 3–5 months after the premature conversion of many anagen hairs to telogen hairs induced by surgery, parturition, fever, drugs, dieting, or traction. Local patches of early telogen conversion may be induced by papulosquamous diseases affecting the scalp. Alternatively, follicles may remain in prolonged anagen rather than normally cycling into telogen. This occurs during pregnancy. On delivery, many follicles are then released simultaneously into telogen, and shedding occurs 3–5 months later. Prolongation of telogen also occurs during pregnancy and results in an initial wave of hair loss soon after delivery or heralding early termination of a pregnancy. Shortening of the anagen phase occurs in pattern (androgenetic) alopecia and in chronic telogen effluvium. A greater proportion of hairs in telogen at any one time results in a chronic increase in telogen shed. Administration of topical minoxidil may produce a telogen effluvium by premature termination of telogen necessary to initiate anagen in responding follicles. This causes early telogen release and a brief telogen effluvium.

Whatever the cause of the telogen loss, the hair is lost "at the root." Each hair will have a visible depigmented club-shaped bulb and will lack a sheath (Fig. 33.3).

Telogen shed may be estimated by the pull test: grasping 40 hairs firmly between thumb and forefinger, followed by a slow pull that causes minimal discomfort to the patient. A count of more than 4–6 club hairs is abnormal, but the result is influenced by recent shampooing (2–3 hairs being abnormal in a freshly shampooed scalp), combing, and the phase of telogen effluvium (whether resolving or entering a chronic phase). The clip test may also be useful; 25–30 hairs are cut just above the scalp surface and

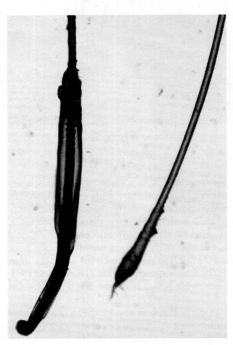

Fig. 33.3 Anagen and telogen hair. Anagen hair has a pigmented bulb and is surrounded by a gelatinous root sheath; telogen hair has a nonpigmented bulb and lacks a root sheath.

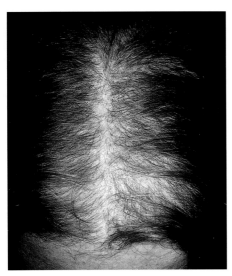

Fig. 33.4 Telogen effluvium secondary to "crash" dieting.

mounted. Indeterminate and telogen hairs are short and of small diameter. Many hairs of this type may be present in telogen effluvium or pattern alopecia. Trichogram evaluation (50 hairs plucked with Kelly clamp with rubber drains over teeth) can also provide information on the anagen/telogen ratio.

Age, gender, race, and genetic factors influence the normal average daily hair loss in an individual. Again, a full head of hair numbers about 100,000; of these, approximately 100–150 are lost daily. In telogen effluvium, estimates of loss vary from 150 to more than 400. Patients may be instructed to collect and count the hair daily; however, they should make sure they collect all small hairs and those that come out in washing and in the bed, as well as those present on the comb or brush. When the pull test is positive, hair shed counts are not needed. An alternative is to collect all hairs lost during a 1-minute combing session. For this technique, developed by Dr. Jeffrey Miller, the patient combs for 1 minute before shampooing on 3 consecutive days. The patient is instructed to comb from the vertex to the anterior hairline. The normal range of lost hairs with this technique is 10–15. Loss of more than 50 is common in telogen effluvium. Serial 1-minute hair counts can be performed to monitor progress.

Telogen effluvium may be related to protein or other nutrient deprivation (Fig. 33.4). Assessment of dietary habits and determination of iron saturation and ferritin are the simplest ways to determine nutritional status. Iron replacement is advisable if saturation or ferritin is low, but in one study, iron replacement alone did not result in resolution of telogen effluvium. Iron may merely serve as a marker for overall nutritional status. Patients with evidence of deficiency should be given supplements to correct the identified deficiency and encouraged to eat a varied diet. Sources of blood loss, such as menstrual bleeding and gastrointestinal (GI) blood loss, should be investigated. Hypothyroidism, allergic contact dermatitis to hair dyes, and renal dialysis with secondary hypervitaminosis A may also be associated with telogen effluvium. Drug-induced telogen effluvium has been noted with the use of aminosalicylic acid, amphetamines, bromocriptine, captopril, carbamazepine, cimetidine, coumarin, danazol, enalapril, etretinate, levodopa, lithium carbonate, metoprolol, metyrapone, pramipexole, propranolol, pyridostigmine, and trimethadione. Postnatal telogen effluvium of infants may occur between birth and the first 4 months of age. Usually, regrowth occurs by 6 months of age. Telogen counts by Kligman in six infants varied from 64%–87%. He also found a tendency for the alopecia to occur in the male-pattern distribution. Idiopathic chronic telogen effluvium has been described by Whiting in a group of 355 patients (346 women and 9 men) with diffuse generalized thinning of scalp hair. Most were 30–60 years old, and their hair loss started abruptly, with increased shedding and thinning. There was a fluctuating course and diffuse thinning of the hair all over the scalp, accompanied by bitemporal recession. This chronic form is related to shortening of the anagen phase and may respond to 5% minoxidil solution.

Trichodynia is a common symptom in patients with telogen effluvium, as it is in pattern hair loss. Trichodynia may also coexist with signs of depression, obsessive personality disorder, or anxiety.

If a 4-mm punch biopsy is performed, 25–50 hairs are normally present for inspection in transverse (horizontal) sections. If more than 12%–15% of terminal follicles are in telogen, this indicates a significant shift from anagen to telogen. Pattern (androgenetic) alopecia demonstrates miniaturization, variable hair shaft diameter, and an increased proportion of telogen hairs. Traction alopecia and trichotillosis (trichotillomania) result in an increased number of catagen and telogen hairs. Pigment casts, empty anagen follicles, trichomalacia, and catagen hairs help distinguish these entities from simple telogen effluvium.

No specific therapy is required for most patients with telogen effluvium. In the majority of cases, the hair loss will stop spontaneously within a few months, and the hair will regrow. Drug-induced telogen effluvium responds to discontinuation of the offending agent. The prognosis is good if a specific event can be pinpointed as a probable cause. Papulosquamous scalp disorders may precipitate telogen hair loss and should be addressed. Iron and thyroid status should be determined if the course is prolonged or if history or physical examination suggests an abnormality. Patients should be encouraged to eat a balanced diet. In a mouse model, sonic stress can produce catagen. This model may be useful in the study of agents for the treatment of telogen effluvium.

Martínez-Velasco MA, et al: The hair shedding visual scale. Dermatol Ther (Heidelb) 2017; 7: 155.

Mubki T, et al: Evaluation and diagnosis of the hair loss patient. Part I. J Am Acad Dermatol 2014; 71: 415.e1.

Rebora A: Intermittent chronic telogen effluvium. Skin Appendage Disord 2017; 3: 36.

Shin S, et al: Suprabulbar thinning of hair in telogen effluvium. Yonsei Med J 2017; 58: 682.

Anagen Effluvium

Anagen effluvium usually results from hair shaft fracture. It is frequently seen following the administration of cancer chemotherapeutic agents, such as the antimetabolites, alkylating agents, and mitotic inhibitors. These agents result in temporary shutdown of the hair matrix with resultant tapering of the shaft (Pohl-Pinkus constrictions). Trichograms reveal tapered fractures. Only anagen hairs are affected. The 10% of scalp hairs in telogen have no matrix and are unaffected. The loss tends to be diffuse but not complete. Severe loss is frequently seen with doxorubicin, the nitrosureas, and cyclophosphamide. When high doses are given, loss of anagen hairs becomes most apparent clinically in 1–2 months. Hair loss after chemotherapy is usually, but not always, reversible. Permanent alopecia after chemotherapy resembles pattern alopecia histologically. A pressure cuff applied around the scalp during chemotherapy and scalp hypothermia have been reported to prevent such anagen arrest; because the scalp may be a site of metastasis, however, it may be better not to spare the scalp from the effects of chemotherapy. Topical minoxidil has been shown to shorten the period of baldness by an average of 50 days.

In addition to the cytotoxic chemotherapeutic agents, various agents, such as isoniazid (INH), thallium, and boron, may induce anagen effluvium. Anagen effluvium with tapered fractures also occurs in alopecia areata and syphilis. In these diseases, an inflammatory insult to the hair bulb results in tapered fractures.

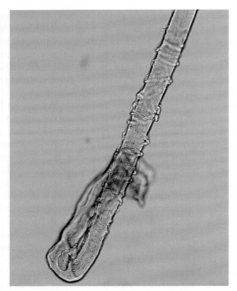

Fig. 33.5 Loose anagen hair with "rumpled sock" cuticle.

Anagen loss may also occur at the root. Loose anagen syndrome, described by Price in 1989, is a disorder in which anagen hairs may be pulled from the scalp with little effort. It occurs mostly in blond girls and usually improves with age. The syndrome appears to be related to a defect in the hair cuticle. Instead of anchoring the hair firmly, the cuticle simply folds back like a rumpled sock (Fig. 33.5), allowing the hair shaft to be extracted. Woolly hair can be associated with loose anagen hair syndrome. A keratin mutation, E337K in K6HF, was identified in three of nine families studied. Colobomas have also been associated with loose anagen hair.

Anagen hairs may be easily extracted from active areas of LE and lichen planopilaris. They usually lack the root sheath that normally surrounds a plucked anagen hair. Anagen effluvium has also been described in lesions of pemphigus.

Pattern Alopecia (Androgenetic Alopecia)

Male-Pattern Baldness. Male-pattern alopecia (common baldness) shows itself during the teens, twenties, or early thirties with gradual loss of hair, chiefly from the vertex and frontotemporal regions. The process may begin at any time after puberty, and the presence of "whisker" or kinky hair may be the first sign of impending male-pattern alopecia. The anterior hairline recedes on each side, in the Geheimratswinkeln ("professor angles"), so that the forehead becomes high. Eventually, the entire top of the scalp may become devoid of hair. Several patterns of this type of hair loss occur, but most common is the biparietal recession with loss of hair on the vertex. The rate of hair loss varies among individuals. Sudden hair loss may occur in the twenties and then proceed relentlessly, though very slowly, for a number of years. The follicles produce finer and lighter hairs with each hair cycle until terminal hairs are eventually replaced by vellus hairs. During evolution of the process, hair shafts vary significantly in diameter. The parietal and occipital areas are usually spared permanently from this process of progressive miniaturization.

Early-onset male-pattern alopecia is related to the androgen receptor gene. There is no doubt that inherited factors and the effect of androgens such as dihydrotestosterone on the hair follicle are important. Arguments for polygenic inheritance include the high prevalence, gaussian curve of distribution in the population, increased risk with number of affected relatives, increased risk in relatives of severely affected women compared with mildly affected

women, and greater import of an affected mother than an affected father. The possibility that the early onset (before age 30) and later onset (after 50) forms may be inherited separately by single genes is also hypothesized.

Male-pattern alopecia is dependent on adequate androgen stimulation and appears to be related to the androgen receptor gene. Eunuchs do not develop baldness if they are castrated before or during adolescence. If they are given androgen therapy, baldness may develop. The 5α-reduction of testosterone is increased in the scalp of balding individuals, yielding increased dihydrotestosterone. Androgen-inducible transforming growth factor (TGF)–β1 derived from dermal papilla cells appears to mediate hair growth suppression. In congenital 5α-reductase deficiency, the type 2 isoenzyme is lacking, and baldness does not occur. Pattern alopecia does occur in males with X-linked ichthyosis, indicating that steroid sulfatase is not critical for the production of alopecia.

Progressive shortening of the anagen phase of hair growth is noted as the hair shaft diameter decreases, so hairs not only are narrowing, but also are becoming shorter. A higher proportion of telogen hairs in the affected area results in greater telogen shed. There may also be an increase in the duration of the lag phase between telogen and anagen (the kenogen lag phase).

Histologically, a decrease in anagen and increase in telogen follicles is present. Follicular miniaturization and variability in shaft diameter are noted. These features are particularly evident in transverse sections. Below the level of the miniaturized or telogen follicle, a vascular or fibromucinous fibrous tract remnant is present. These tracts appear numerous in cross section. Many mast cells may be noted in the fibrous tract remnant, but inflammatory cells are absent. Sebaceous glands may be enlarged, and hair thinning may be associated with solar elastosis. Sparse lymphoid inflammation with spongiosis may be noted at the level of the follicular infundibulum. This may represent associated seborrheic folliculitis. A sparse lymphoid infiltrate may also be noted at the level of the hair bulge.

Miniaturized human hair follicles grafted on to immunodeficient mice can quickly regenerate and grow as well as or better than terminal follicles from the same individual. This suggests that even advanced pattern alopecia may be reversible. Partial reversal of pattern alopecia has been noted after chemotherapy or treatment of psoriasis with methotrexate. Unfortunately, available pharmacologic interventions produce little effect in advanced pattern alopecia.

Men with spinal and bulbar muscular atrophy (Kennedy disease), an X-linked neurodegenerative disease caused by an expansion of a polymorphic tandem CAG repeat within the androgen receptor gene, have a decreased incidence of pattern alopecia.

Minoxidil, an oral hypotensive drug that causes hypertrichosis when given systemically, is available as topical solutions (Rogaine). Minoxidil promotes the survival of dermal papilla cells, prolongs anagen phase, and results in enlargement of shaft diameter. Clinically, apparent success is best in early cases (<10 years) of limited extent (bald area <10 cm in diameter on vertex) in whom pretreatment hair density is greater than 20 hairs/cm². Minoxidil is available without a prescription as a solution or foam. Those who respond must continue to use minoxidil indefinitely to maintain a response.

Finasteride, a type 2 5α-reductase inhibitor, given as a 1-mg tablet daily, is effective in preventing further hair loss and in increasing the hair counts to the point of cosmetically appreciable results in men age 18–41 with mild to moderate hair loss at the vertex, in the anterior midscalp, and in the frontal region. Finasteride has been shown to stop hair loss in up to 90% of men for at least 5 years. Approximately 65% of men demonstrate hair regrowth. As with minoxidil, continued use of finasteride is required to sustain benefits. Hair patterning on the temples is not improved. Hair growth will be evident only after 6 months or more of therapy.

If no effect is seen after 12 months, further treatment is unlikely to be of benefit. In one study, regimens that included finasteride were more effective than minoxidil alone, and therapeutic efficacy was enhanced by combining the two drugs. Short-term side effects related to finasteride are infrequent; however, the need to take this medication indefinitely suggests that study of long-term side-effect profiles is critical. A prostate cancer prevention trial with a different dosage form of the same drug showed a decrease in the incidence of cancer. However, those cancers that did occur in the treatment group had a higher average Gleason score, possibly because only lower-grade cancers were prevented.

Dutasteride blocks both type 1 and type 2 5α-reductase and is effective in the treatment of male-pattern hair loss. Other treatments that show some promise in preliminary studies include fluridil (topical antiandrogen that suppresses human androgen receptor), topical adenosine, and hormone-enriched topical cell culture medium. Hair transplantation using micrografts of hair follicles from the occipital area to the anterior scalp may satisfactorily recreate hairlines and give excellent cosmetic results. The role of platelet-rich plasma and microneedling is being defined.

Female-Pattern Alopecia (Androgenetic Alopecia in Women)

Women generally have diffuse hair loss throughout the apical scalp with the part wider anteriorly. There is typically sparing of the frontal hairline, although a subset of women exhibits a "male" pattern of temporal recession. Although maintenance of the frontal hairline is the rule in women, a progressive decrease in hair density from the vertex to the front of the scalp does occur. The same basic changes—reduced hair density and diameter and diminished anagen and increased telogen hair—occur in women as in men. Sebaceous gland hyperplasia may be present but is less common than in men. Transverse histologic sections demonstrate variability in the size of hair follicles (anisotrichosis).

The cause is now believed to be a genetic predisposition with an excessive response to androgens. Both women and men with pattern alopecia have higher levels of 5α-reductase and androgen receptor in frontal hair follicles than in occipital follicles. Evidence also suggests a hierarchy of androgen sensitivity within follicular units. Follicular miniaturization relates to unrepaired DNA damage and a reduced proliferation rate of matrix keratinocytes. Smoking may be an independent risk factor. Most women with pattern alopecia have normal menses and fertility. If other evidence of androgen excess is present, such as hirsutism, menstrual irregularities, or acne, or if the onset is sudden, evaluation as outlined for hirsutism (see later) should be performed. Topical minoxidil, and oral antiandrogens, such as spironolactone and cyproterone acetate, have been used to treat androgenetic alopecia in women. In one study, cyproterone acetate (CPA) was more effective than minoxidil when there were other signs of hyperandrogenism, hyperseborrhea, and menstrual abnormalities, and when the body mass index was high. When these other factors were absent, minoxidil was the more effective treatment.

Treatment with finasteride is of limited benefit for most women, although the subset with temporal recession may show some benefit. Finasteride treatment is contraindicated in women who may become pregnant. Hair transplantation, wigs, or interwoven hair may give satisfactory cosmetic results. In a pilot study, topical melatonin appeared to prolong anagen phase and may prove to be of some benefit. In some women, telogen effluvium may produce worsening of preexisting pattern alopecia. Reversible causes of telogen effluvium, such as seborrheic dermatitis, nutrient deficiency, and thyroid disease, should be addressed. As in men, the role of platelet-rich plasma and microneedling is being defined.

Adil A, et al: The effectiveness of treatments for androgenetic alopecia. J Am Acad Dermatol 2017; 77: 136.

Alves R, et al: Platelet-rich plasma in combination with 5% minoxidil topical solution and 1 mg oral finasteride for the treatment of androgenetic alopecia. Dermatol Surg 2018; 44: 126.

Czyzyk A, et al: Severe hyperandrogenemia in postmenopausal woman as a presentation of ovarian hyperthecosis. Gynecol Endocrinol 2017; 33: 836.

Dey-Rao R, et al: Genome-wide gene expression dataset used to identify potential therapeutic targets in androgenetic alopecia. Data Brief 2017; 13: 85.

Garg S, et al: Platelet-rich plasma—an "elixir" for treatment of alopecia. Stem Cell Investig 2017; 4: 64.

Girijala RL, et al: Platelet-rich plasma for androgenic alopecia treatment: A comprehensive review. Dermatol Online J 2018; 24(7). pii: 13030/qt8s43026c. PubMed PMID: 30261560.

Ho C, Hughes J: Alopecia, androgenetic. [Updated 2017 Mar 6]. In: StatPearls [Internet]. Treasure Island (FL): StatPearls Publishing.

Rodrigues BL, et al: "Treatment of male pattern alopecia with platelet-rich plasma: a double blind controlled study with analysis of platelet number and growth factor levels". J Am Acad Dermatol 2018. pii: S0190-9622(18)32643-4. doi: 10.1016/j.jaad.2018.09.033. [Epub ahead of print] PubMed PMID: 30287324.

Rudnicka L, et al: Dyslipidemia in patients with androgenetic alopecia. J Eur Acad Dermatol Venereol 2017; 31: 921.

Shah KB, et al: A comparative study of microneedling with platelet-rich plasma plus topical minoxidil (5%) and topical minoxidil (5%) alone in androgenetic alopecia. Int J Trichology 2017; 9: 14.

Trichotillosis

Trichotillosis (trichotillomania) is the compulsive practice of plucking hair from the scalp, brows, or eyelashes. Typical areas are irregular patches of alopecia that contain hairs of varying length (Fig. 33.6). The scalp has a rough texture, resulting from the short remnants of broken-off hairs. It is seen mostly in girls younger than 10, although boys and all adults may engage in the

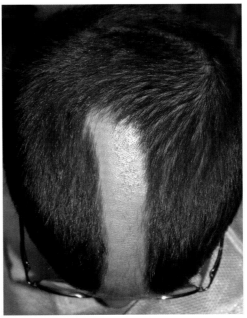

Fig. 33.6 Trichotillosis.

practice as well. Some patients relate exquisite pain localized to a follicle that can only be relieved by plucking the hair.

When speaking with a patient with characteristic areas of alopecia, rather than asking "if," one should ask "how" removal of the hair is done. If this fails to uncover a history of hair pulling, shaving a 3-cm² area in the involved part of the scalp will result in hairs too short for plucking, and normal regrowth in the "skin window" within 3 weeks. Finally, a biopsy, especially if cut horizontally, may demonstrate empty anagen follicles, catagen hairs, pigment casts within the infundibulum, trichomalacia, and hemorrhage. Alopecia areata shares many of these histologic features, and care must be taken to search for the presence of peribulbar lymphocytes or inflammatory cells within the fibrous tract remnants.

Trichotillosis is usually a manifestation of an obsessive-compulsive disorder but may also be associated with depression or anxiety. It may be associated with compulsive swallowing of the plucked hairs (trichophagia) and may result in formation of a gastric bezoar (Rapunzel syndrome). Behavior modification, psychotherapy, and appropriate psychopharmacologic medication (e.g., clomipramine, olanzapine) may be helpful. *N*-acetylcysteine was effective in a study in adults, but a separate study showed disappointing results in children. Valproic acid, quetiapine, and naltrexone have been reported as effective in some patients. Bimatoprost has been used when eyelashes are involved.

Barroso LAL, et al: Trichotillomania. An Bras Dermatol 2017; 92: 537.

Bloch MH, et al: *N*-acetylcysteine in the treatment of pediatric trichotillomania. J Am Acad Child Adolesc Psychiatry 2013; 52: 231.

Falkenstein MJ, et al: Predictors of relapse following treatment of trichotillomania. J Obsessive Compuls Relat Disord 2014; 3: 345.

Grant JE, et al: Placebo response in trichotillomania. Int Clin Psychopharmacol 2017; 32: 350.

Grant JE, et al: The opiate antagonist, naltrexone, in the treatment of trichotillomania. J Clin Psychopharmacol 2014; 34: 134.

Harrison JP, et al: Pediatric trichotillomania. Curr Psychiatry Rep 2012; 14: 188.

Peabody T, et al: Clinical management of trichotillomania with bimatoprost. Optom Vis Sci 2013; 90: e167.

Rothbart R, et al: Pharmacotherapy for trichotillomania. Cochrane Database Syst Rev 2013; 11: CD007662.

Rothbart R, Stein DJ: Pharmacotherapy of trichotillomania (hair pulling disorder). Expert Opin Pharmacother 2014; 15: 2709.

Weidt S, et al: Trichotillomania. Neuropsychiatr Dis Treat 2017; 13: 1153.

Other Forms of Noncicatricial Alopecia

Alopecia syphilitica may have a typical moth-eaten appearance on the occipital scalp (Fig. 33.7), may show a generalized thinning of the hair, or may resemble alopecia areata. Other areas, such as the eyebrows, eyelashes, and body hair, may be involved. The alopecia may be the first sign of syphilis.

Follicular mucinosis (alopecia mucinosa) most often occurs on the scalp or beard area and manifests as a boggy, red plaque or hypopigmented patch with hair loss. Comedo-like lesions may exude mucin when expressed. Biopsy demonstrates deposition of mucin in the outer root sheath and sebaceous glands. The mucin stains as hyaluronic acid, rather than epithelial sialomucin. Primary cases (unassociated with underlying disease) usually occur as localized lesions of the head or neck. Young people are primarily affected and may demonstrate clonality even in lesions that do not progress clinically. The secondary type is associated with mycosis fungoides–type cutaneous T-cell lymphoma or a chronic inflammatory skin disease. Lesions associated with mycosis fungoides are generally widespread and chronic and occur in older

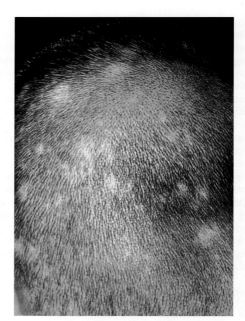

Fig. 33.7 Syphilitic alopecia. (Courtesy Brooke Army Medical Center Teaching File.)

patients. Intralesional steroids and phototherapy have been reported as useful.

Vascular or neurologic alopecia, most often of the lower extremities, may be seen in diabetes mellitus or atherosclerosis. In meralgia paresthetica, there may be alopecia of the anesthetic area of the outer thigh.

Endocrinologic alopecia may occur in various endocrinologic disorders. In hypothyroidism, the hair becomes coarse, dry, brittle, and sparse. The proportion of telogen hairs has been shown to be three to seven times higher than the normal 10%. In hyperthyroidism, the hair becomes extremely fine and sparse. Oral contraceptives (OCs) have been implicated in some cases of androgenetic alopecia. It develops in predisposed women who are usually taking androgenic progestogens. It is advisable to discontinue the androgen-dominant pill and substitute an estrogen-dominant OC. Some women develop telogen effluvium 2–4 months after discontinuing anovulatory agents, which is analogous to postpartum alopecia.

Congenital alopecia occurs as total or partial loss of hair, or a lack of initial growth, accompanied usually by other ectodermal defects of the nails, teeth, and bone. The hair is light and sparse and grows slowly. Congenital triangular alopecia (Fig. 33.8) and aplasia cutis congenita are examples of congenital localized absence of hair. Hidrotic ectodermal dysplasia is a diffuse abnormality of hair associated with dental and nail changes.

Lipedematous alopecia consists of thickening of the scalp that gives the impression of thick cotton batting. The hair may be normal or shortened and sparse. Biopsy shows an increase in thickness of the subcutaneous fat and variable lymphoid inflammation. This disease appears to affect black persons primarily.

Borgia F, et al: Follicular mucinosis with diffuse scalp alopecia treated with narrow-band UVB phototherapy. G Ital Dermatol Venereol 2016; 151: 212.

Gibson LE, et al: Follicular mucinosis in childhood. J Am Acad Dermatol 2013; 69: 1054.

Yasar S, et al: Clinical and pathological features of 31 cases of lipedematous scalp and lipedematous alopecia. Eur J Dermatol 2011; 21: 520.

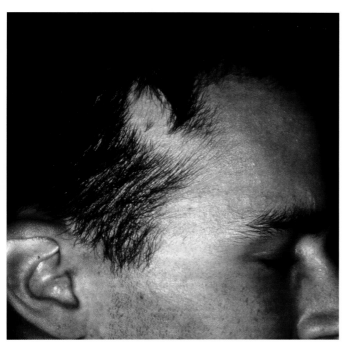

33

Fig. 33.8 Congenital triangular alopecia.

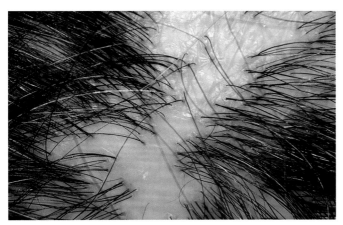

Fig. 33.9 Loss of follicular ostia in scarring alopecia.

CICATRICIAL ALOPECIA

Cicatricial alopecia appears as areas of hair loss with absence of follicular ostia (Fig. 33.9). Acute lesions may appear as erythematous plaques, perifollicular papules, keratotic follicular spines, or pustules. Deep inflammatory lesions may be boggy or may resemble noncicatricial areata clinically. The inflammatory nature of the lesion may only be evident on biopsy.

Discoid lupus erythematosus (DLE), lichen planopilaris, sarcoidosis, and folliculitis decalvans are the most common inflammatory causes of cicatricial alopecia. Chronic bacterial and fungal infections may produce inflammatory alopecia that mimics primary scarring alopecia. For example, fungal folliculitis may mimic LE.

Biopsy can confirm the diagnosis and provide prognostic information regarding the potential for new growth. A 4-mm punch biopsy will provide the pathologist with an adequate specimen. Smaller specimens are of limited value. The punch should be placed parallel to the direction of hair growth to avoid transecting follicles, and the punch should be advanced to the deep

subcutaneous fat. The biopsy site will typically bleed profusely, but a 4-mm-wide strip of gel foam advanced into the defect will generally provide rapid hemostasis. Sutures are rarely necessary, and because the scar from a sutured biopsy site generally stretches back to the original dimensions of the biopsy, suturing provides little benefit to the patient.

The biopsy should be taken from a well-established lesion that is still active, rather than from the advancing edge. Dermoscopy may be helpful in selecting the biopsy site. The pathologist may prefer vertical or transverse (horizontal) sectioning of the specimen. Each has advantages. Every follicular unit in the specimen will be demonstrated in transverse sections. Vertical sections are superior for demonstrating changes in the surface epidermis, dermoepidermal junction (DEJ), superficial dermis, and subcutaneous fat. In general, the features of androgenetic (pattern) alopecia, telogen effluvium, and trichotillomania are better demonstrated in transverse (horizontal) sections through the specimen. Alopecia areata and syphilitic alopecia are well demonstrated in transverse sections if serial step sections are obtained to demonstrate deeper planes of section, or if the block is cut horizontally in a bread-loaf fashion before embedding. They are equally well demonstrated with serial vertical sections through the block. LE and lichen planopilaris are more easily demonstrated in serial vertical sections.

The diagnostic yield can be enhanced by pairing vertical and transverse sections. If two biopsies are done, one specimen can be bisected vertically for direct immunofluorescence (DIF) and hematoxylin and eosin (H&E) processing. It is most easily split by laying it on its side and bisecting it with a No. 15 blade pushed cleanly through the specimen in a single downward motion. Sawing at the specimen will not produce a satisfactory result. One-half the bisected specimen is placed in formalin and the other half in immunofluorescent media. The second specimen can be bisected for transverse sections in the clinic or left for the laboratory to bisect after processing. If to be bisected in the clinic, it should be placed on its side. The 15 blade should be pushed downward through the specimen in a single motion at the level of the mid-dermis. All pieces for vertical and transverse sections may be placed in a single bottle to be embedded in a single cassette. If a single biopsy specimen is submitted for H&E sections, it can be bisected vertically, then one-half bisected transversely 1 mm above the fat (Tyler technique). This provides the advantages of both vertical and transverse sections with a single specimen.

In LE, the biopsy must be from a lesion of several months' duration to demonstrate hyperkeratosis, follicular plugging, basement membrane zone thickening, and dermal mucin. Only biopsies from established lesions of lupus will demonstrate reliable immunofluorescence.

When biopsies of the most active area of alopecia have failed to yield a definite diagnosis, a biopsy from a scarred area may provide additional information. Scars show loss of elastic tissue with the Verhoeff–van Gieson stain. The pattern of elastic tissue loss is the "footprint" of the preceding inflammatory process (Figs. 33.10 and 33.11), and remains the gold standard for evaluation of scarring alopecia, although polarized microscopy and immunofluorescence of H&E-stained sections can also be useful. Lichen planopilaris and folliculitis decalvans both affect the infundibulum. Both result in wedge-shaped superficial dermal scars. DLE results in scarring of both the follicular units and the intervening dermis. Morphea does not produce a scar, but rather hyalinization of collagen bundles with preservation of the elastic fibers. In idiopathic pseudopelade, the fibrous tract remnants are widened, but the elastic tissue sheath at the periphery of the fibrous tract is preserved.

Most patients with cicatricial alopecia experience gradual progression of the alopecia, and the prolonged course of the disease may lead to inappropriate therapeutic complacency. The progressive destruction of hairs will result in ever-expanding areas of permanent alopecia. Therefore cicatricial alopecia must be treated aggressively and early to avoid permanent disfigurement. Surgical revision of

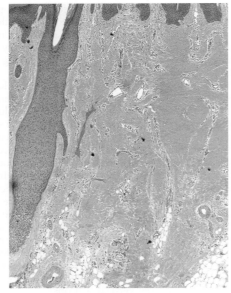

Fig. 33.10 Scarring alopecia (hematoxylin-eosin [H&E] stain).

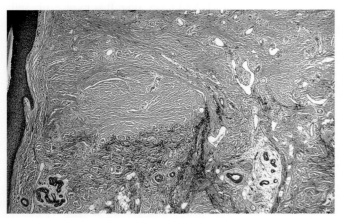

Fig. 33.11 Scarring alopecia (elastic stain). Normal elastic fibers (black) indicate the nonscarred portions of the dermis.

the hairless plaque is an option for stable end-stage alopecia, but unless the underlying disease is controlled, surgery may only lead to a flare of the underlying disease with progression of hair loss. Therapy may be forestalled by the inability to establish a definite diagnosis. To help guide therapy for patients who defy diagnosis, work groups of the North American Hair Research Society have proposed a classification scheme based on the type and pattern of inflammation. Some forms of destructive alopecia are lymphocyte mediated; others are suppurative processes. The type of infiltrate and the portion of the pilosebaceous unit affected can be used to guide therapy. This classification system may also allow patients to enroll in clinical trials, even in the absence of a definite diagnosis.

Elston DM: Elastic fibers in scars and alopecia. Am J Dermato-pathol 2017; 39: 556.

Fung MA, et al: Elastin staining patterns in primary cicatricial alopecia. J Am Acad Dermatol 2013; 69: 776.

Horenstein MG, et al: Follicular density and ratios in scarring and nonscarring alopecia. Am J Dermatopathol 2013; 35: 818.

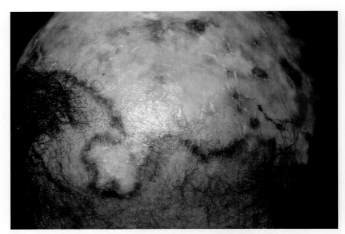

Fig. 33.12 Discoid lupus erythematosus. (Courtesy Steven Binnick, MD.)

LYMPHOID-MEDIATED DISORDERS

Lupus Erythematosus

Chronic cutaneous (discoid) lupus of the scalp (DLE) is a common cause of cicatricial alopecia. In active disease, anagen hairs may be easily extracted from the involved area. Usually, erythema, atrophy, follicular plugging, and mottled hyperpigmentation and hypopigmentation are present (Fig. 33.12). Patients with chronic cutaneous lupus of the scalp may have accompanying SLE or skin lesions of DLE on other parts of the body. The external ear canal and concha should always be examined because they are common sites for discoid lesions. Occasionally, alopecia occurs in a plaque of tumid lupus. Lupus panniculitis may occasionally result in alopecia in the absence of surface skin changes. SLE is often associated with discoid lesions of the scalp. Patients with SLE may also have short miniaturized "lupus hairs" on the anterior scalp.

Biopsy of early lesions of DLE is often nondiagnostic. Patchy lymphoid inflammation and perifollicular mucinous fibrosis may be the only histologic findings. Focal vacuolar interface dermatitis may or may not be noted. Active established lesions, present for several months, have a higher diagnostic yield. Active established lesions usually demonstrate hyperkeratosis, follicular plugging, vacuolar interface dermatitis, basement membrane zone thickening, pigment incontinence, and dermal mucin. Perivascular and periadnexal lymphoid infiltrates are patchy and involve the eccrine coil and fibrous tract remnants. Fibrous tract involvement creates dense vertical columns of lymphocytes. The underlying subcutaneous tissue may demonstrate nodular lymphoplasmacytic infiltrates and fibrin or hyaline rings around necrotic fat. Hypertrophic lesions of chronic cutaneous LE often demonstrate lichenoid dermatitis. DIF typically demonstrates continuous granular deposition of immunoglobumin (Ig)G, IgA, IgM, and C3 at the DEJ ("full house" pattern). This pattern is particularly helpful in distinguishing lichenoid hypertrophic LE from lichen planopilaris. Burnt-out lesions of DLE demonstrate loss of elastic fibers throughout the dermis, which differs from the focal peri-infundibular wedge-shaped scars of lichen planopilaris. In SLE, follicular atrophy may be associated with pronounced dermal mucinosis.

Chronic cutaneous lupus may respond to intralesional or potent topical corticosteroids, but systemic therapy is frequently required. Antimalarials, retinoids, dapsone, thalidomide, sulfasalazine, mycophenolate mofetil, and methotrexate have been used successfully. Topical tazarotene and topical calcineurin inhibitors are generally disappointing.

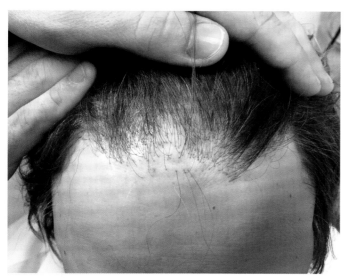

Fig. 33.13 Frontal fibrosing alopecia. (Courtesy Len Sperling, MD.)

Lichen Planopilaris and Frontal Fibrosing Alopecia

Lichen planopilaris presents with perifollicular erythema and progressive scarring. Small follicular papules may be noted, or the lesion may resemble the ivory-white irregular patches of pseudopelade. In some patients, typical polygonal flat-topped papules are present on the wrists and ankles, and lacy white lesions are noted on the oral and genital mucosa. Widespread follicular papules may be present on the trunk or extremities. In most patients, however, only the scalp is involved. Frontal fibrosing alopecia is a variant of lichen planopilaris. Most patients are older women with bandlike frontotemporal alopecia, hypopigmentation and atrophy (Fig. 33.13), often with "genitalized" kinky hairs. The kinky hairs resemble those in progressive acquired kinking of the hair (a manifestation of early male pattern alopecia) suggesting a hormonal influence. The current epidemic was first described by Dr. Kossard in Australia, but a similar condition was described by the Swedish physician Axel Munthe in 1929, and recounted in his memoirs "The Story of San Michele."

Graham-Little–Piccardi-Lasseur syndrome includes cicatricial alopecia on the scalp, keratosis pilaris in the skin of the trunk and extremities, and noncicatricial hair loss in the pubis and axillae. It has been described in association with complete androgen insensitivity syndrome, a condition that also presents with non-cicatricial alopecia in the axillary and pubic hair.

Diagnostic biopsies demonstrate lichenoid interface dermatitis of the follicular unit and sometimes the intervening epidermis. The entire fibrous tract may be filled with cytoid bodies (Fig. 33.14). The changes usually occur focally and may be best visualized with serial vertical sections. Perifollicular mucinous fibrosis is common, and focal perifollicular lymphoid infiltrates tend to involve the infundibulum (infiltrates of LE tend to involve isthmus). DIF may be negative or may reveal cytoid bodies and shaggy linear fibrin at the DEJ.

Lichen planopilaris responds to oral and intralesional corticosteroids. Topical corticosteroids or topical calcineurin inhibitors may be adequate in a few patients, but resulting scalp atrophy with prominence of capillary plexus may be misinterpreted as erythema signifying active disease. As in lupus, topical tazarotene and topical macrolactams are generally disappointing. Oral retinoids, antimalarials and excimer laser can be effective, but some reports have noted progression of alopecia with antimalarials despite a reduction in erythema. It is therefore important to follow the size of the alopecic patches, presence of easily extractable anagen hairs,

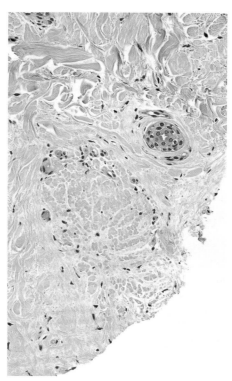

Fig. 33.14 Lichen planopilaris. Note cytoid bodies completely filling the fibrous tract remnant.

and presence of follicular spines as well as erythema and pruritus. The peroxisome proliferator activated receptor-γ agonist piogli-tazone is effective at halting progression in many patients. A 3-month trial of 15 mg followed by 3 months at 30 and 45 mg (if there is no response) should be attempted before the treatment is deemed a failure. Patients should be followed for peripheral edema and other signs of heart failure, but in the authors' experience, the drug is well tolerated by the majority of patients for the length of time it is employed. Mycophenolate mofetil is generally reliable for patients with refractory disease, and excimer laser can be helpful in refractory disease. Tofacitinib therapy is promising. Biologics have been suggested as therapy, but onset of lichen planopilaris has been noted during etanercept therapy. Dutasteride is often effective as first line therapy in the setting of frontal fibrosing alopecia, and is generally paired with piaglitazone. Oral retinoid therapy has been reported as effective for controlling the facial papules often associated with the disease.

Central Centrifugal Cicatricial Alopecia

Central centrifugal cicatricial alopecia (CCCA) is seen most often in African American women, is slowly progressive, usually begins in the crown, and advances to the surrounding areas (Fig. 33.15). The term is often used as a broad category that includes "hot comb alopecia," idiopathic pseudopelade, and central elliptical alopecia. Some patients will demonstrate crops of crusts at the periphery of the patches, a feature of folliculitis decalvans. Treat-ment of CCCA is difficult and often unsatisfactory. Discontinuation of chemical and heat processing and reduction of traction are recommended. Patients with overlapping features of folliculitis decalvans may respond to long-term antibiotic therapy and topical corticosteroids. In such overlapping cases, the histology shows a lymphocytic infiltrate during the chronic stage, but periodic crops of pustules demonstrate a neutrophilic folliculitis.

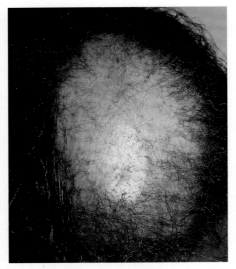

Fig. 33.15 Central centrifugal cicatricial alopecia.

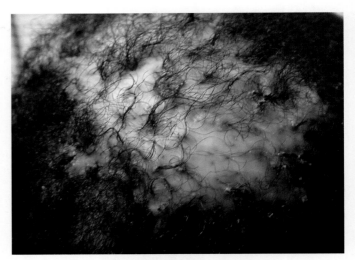

Fig. 33.16 Folliculitis decalvans.

NEUTROPHIL-MEDIATED DISORDERS

Folliculitis Decalvans

Folliculitis decalvans presents with crops of pustules that result in cicatricial alopecia. Successive crops of pustules, crusts, or erosions lead to expansion of the alopecic patches (Fig. 33.16). Staphylococci are sometimes cultured from the lesions, and some authors have suggested that folliculitis decalvans merely represents a chronic staphylococcal infection. It is more likely that follicular destruction is the result of an abnormal suppurative immune response. Staphylococci and other organisms probably play a role in inciting the response. Erlotinib-induced folliculitis decalvans has been reported. The lesions often respond to long-term treatment with a tetracycline. The improvement may reflect the antineutrophil effects of the drug or its antimicrobial effects. Many patients also respond to other forms of antistaphylococcal therapy, but the lesions generally recur after the antibiotic is discontinued. In contrast, long-term tetracycline treatment generally results in a continued response. Some sustained responses have been noted after combination therapy with rifampin and clindamycin. Rifampin alone may promote the emergence of bacterial resistance. Selenium sulfide shampoo and topical corticosteroids may be useful as adjunctive therapy. Oral retinoids, oral and topical fusidic acid, oral zinc sulfate, photodynamic therapy (PDT) and topical tacrolimus have been reported as successful, and anti-TNF biologics have been used for refractory disease.

A variant of folliculitis decalvans occurs in African American patients who present with pseudofolliculitis of the beard, acne keloidalis nuchae, and scarring alopecia in the vertex and parietal scalp. The scalp demonstrates ingrown hairs, crops of pustules or crusts, and permanent scarring alopecia. Although pseudofolliculitis barbae is generally accepted to be the result of ingrown hairs, the pathogenesis of acne keloidalis nuchae remains in question. Histologically, ingrown hairs are common in advanced lesions. Early lesions may not demonstrate the hair. Some patients merely develop small papules on the nape of the neck, whereas others develop pustules, crusts, and progressive alopecia. This latter group overlaps with folliculitis decalvans, and patients generally respond to treatment with a topical corticosteroid and an oral tetracycline.

Acne Necrotica

Acne necrotica presents with discrete excoriated follicular papules in the scalp. Biopsy demonstrates an inflammatory crust and

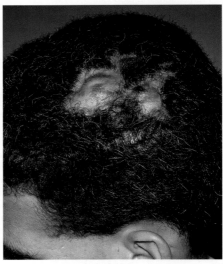

Fig. 33.17 Dissecting cellulitis.

suppurative folliculitis. Usually, there is no associated scarring alopecia, but occasional cases overlap with folliculitis decalvans.

Erosive Pustular Dermatitis of the Scalp

Pustular dermatitis often presents as expanding eroded patches on the scalp with moist granulation tissue. The lesions often follow trauma or a surgical procedure and tend to be chronic and progressive. They respond best to class I topical corticosteroids. PDT has also been used effectively.

Dissecting Cellulitis (Perifolliculitis Capitis Abscessens et Suffodiens of Hoffman)

Dissecting cellulitis often coexists with acne conglobata and hidradenitis suppurativa. It may also occur with folliculitis decalvans. The lesions are deep, boggy, and suppurative (Fig. 33.17). They may respond to tetracyclines, retinoids, and intralesional corticosteroids.

Tufted Folliculitis

Tufted folliculitis presents with doll's hair–like bundling of follicular units (Fig. 33.18). It is seen in a wide range of scarring conditions,

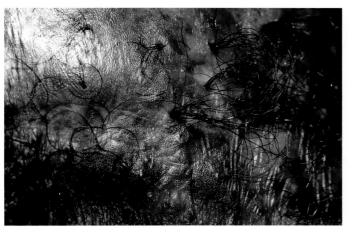

Fig. 33.18 Tufted doll's hairs, cicatricial alopecia.

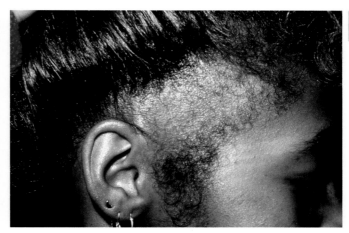

Fig. 33.19 Traction alopecia.

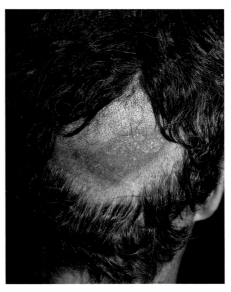

Fig. 33.20 Pressure alopecia with scalp demonstrating pressure-induced geometric pressure necrosis.

including chronic staphylococcal infection, chronic LE, lichen planopilaris, Graham-Little syndrome, folliculitis decalvans, acne keloidalis nuchae, immunobullous disorders, and dissecting cellulitis. Compound hairs (two or more hairs sharing a common infundibulum) occur physiologically on the occipital scalp and legs and should not be confused with tufted folliculitis.

OTHER FORMS OF PERMANENT ALOPECIA

Pseudopelade of Brocq

Also known as alopecia cicatrisata, this pseudopelade is a rare form of cicatricial alopecia in which destruction of the hair follicles produces multiple round, oval, or irregularly shaped, hairless, cicatricial patches of varying sizes. They are usually coin sized and are white or slightly pink in color, with a smooth, shiny, marble-like or ivory, atrophic, "onion skin" surface. Interspersed in the patches may be a few spared follicles with hairs growing from them. A clinical inflammatory stage is completely absent. No pustules, crusts, or broken-off hairs are present. The onset, as a rule, is insidious, with one or two lesions appearing on the vertex. The condition affects females three times more often than males and has a prolonged course. In advanced cases, large irregular patches are formed by coalescence of some of the many small macules, a pattern referred to as "footprints in the snow." The alopecia is permanent and the disease slowly progressive. Most cases of pseudopelade demonstrate scarring in a wedge-shaped pattern in the superficial dermis and represent an end stage of lichen planopilaris. A distinct subset called idiopathic pseudopelade accounts for most patients with CCCA. In these patients, the dermis is contracted into a thin band of dense collagenous tissue. Elastic fibers are intact and quite thick as a result of elastic recoil related to dermal contraction. Fibrous tract remnants are wide and hyalinized with an intact elastic sheath. Lymphoid and neutrophilic inflammation is absent, but loss of the inner and outer root sheaths with subsequent hair fiber granuloma formation is noted. Sebaceous glands are decreased or absent, as they are in most forms of permanent alopecia. DIF is negative.

Traction Alopecia

Traction alopecia occurs from prolonged tension on the hair, either from wearing the hair tightly braided or in a ponytail, pulling the hair to straighten it, rolling curlers too tightly, or from the habit of twisting the hairs with the fingers. Traction alopecia most often involves the periphery of the scalp, especially the temples and above the ears, but a fringe of hair is characteristically present at the frontal and temporal hairline (Fig. 33.19).

Sarcoidosis

Sarcoidosis of the scalp presents with diffuse or patchy hair loss. The involved scalp is often indurated, and a raised peripheral border may be present. The lesions are often red-brown in color and may have an "apple jelly" appearance on diascopy. Biopsy reveals noncaseating granulomas. Treatment is the same as for other forms of sarcoidosis.

Pressure Alopecia

Pressure alopecia occurs in adults after prolonged pressure on the scalp during general anesthesia, with the head fixed in one position. It may also occur in chronically ill persons after prolonged bed rest in one position (Fig. 33.20), which causes persistent pressure on one part of the scalp. It probably arises because of pressure-induced ischemia.

Tumor Alopecia

Tumor alopecia refers to hair loss in the immediate vicinity of either benign or malignant tumors of the scalp. Syringomas, nerve

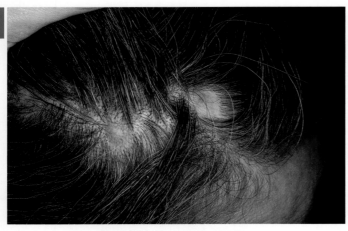

Fig. 33.21 Alopecia neoplastica.

sheath myxomas, and steatocystoma multiplex are benign tumors that may be limited to the scalp and may cause alopecia. Alopecia neoplastica is the designation given to hair loss from metastatic tumors, most often from breast or renal carcinoma (Fig. 33.21).

Keratosis Pilaris Atrophicans

Keratosis pilaris atrophicans includes many forms of keratosis pilaris with cicatricial alopecia. Variants include keratosis pilaris atrophicans faciei, atrophoderma vermiculatum, keratosis follicularis spinulosa decalvans, and ichthyosis follicularis.

Keratosis pilaris atrophicans faciei (ulerythema ophryogenes, keratosis pilaris rubra atrophicans faciei, folliculitis rubra, lichen pilare, xerodermie pilaire symmétrique de la face) begins in infancy as follicular papules with perifollicular erythema. Initially, the lesions are restricted to the lateral eyebrows. With time, they spread to involve the cheeks and forehead. There may be associated keratosis pilaris on the extremities and buttocks. The condition may also be associated with an atopic diathesis, ectodermal dysplasia, or Noonan syndrome.

Atrophoderma vermiculatum (acne vermoulanti, honeycomb atrophy, folliculitis ulerythematosa reticulata, ulerythema acneiforme, folliculitis ulerythematous reticulata, atrophodermia reticulata symmetrica faciei, atrophoderma reticulatum) presents with erythematous follicular papules on the cheeks in childhood. With time, the lesions develop into pitlike depressions (reticulate atrophy). Autosomal dominant inheritance has been described. This condition generally spares the scalp and eyebrows.

Keratosis follicularis spinulosa decalvans is a rare X-linked disorder described by Siemens in 1926. The gene has been mapped to Xp21.2–p22.2. It begins in infancy with keratosis pilaris localized on the face, then evolves to more diffuse involvement. Progressive cicatricial alopecia occurs on the scalp, eyebrows, and sometimes eyelashes. The alopecia starts during childhood, and active disease may remit during the early teenage years. Corneal and conjunctival inflammation, corneal dystrophy, and blepharitis occur, and photophobia is usually a prominent finding.

Ichthyosis follicularis also demonstrates extensive spiny follicular hyperkeratosis, permanent alopecia, and photophobia. Palmar plantar keratosis, nail deformities, atopy, and recurrent cheilitis have been described.

ATRICHIA WITH PAPULAR LESIONS

Atrichia with papular lesions is a rare autosomal recessive disorder with early onset of atrichia, followed by a papular eruption appearing within the first years of life. The condition has been linked to chromosome 8p21, and mutations have been detected in what

is now referred to as the hairless gene. It is discussed in more detail in Chapter 27.

Bastida J, et al: Treatment of folliculitis decalvans with tacrolimus ointment. Int J Dermatol 2012; 51: 216.

Callender VD, et al: Hair breakage as a presenting sign of early or occult central centrifugal cicatricial alopecia. Arch Dermatol 2012; 148: 1047.

Dlova NC, et al: Central centrifugal cicatricial alopecia. J Investig Dermatol Symp Proc 2017; 18: S54.

Donovan JC, et al: Transversely sectioned biopsies in the diagnosis of end-stage traction alopecia. Dermatol Online J 2013; 19: 11.

Elston CA, et al: Elastic staining versus fluorescent and polarized microscopy in the diagnosis of alopecia. J Am Acad Dermatol 2013; 69: 288.

Elston D: The "Tyler technique" for alopecia biopsies. J Cutan Pathol 2012; 39: 306.

Fertig R, et al: Frontal fibrosing alopecia treatment options. Intractable Rare Dis Res 2016; 5: 314.

Keith DJ, et al: Erlotinib-induced folliculitis decalvans. Clin Exp Dermatol 2013; 38: 924.**Lin J, et al:** Hypopigmentation in frontal fibrosing alopecia. J Am Acad Dermatol 2017; 76: 1184.

Loganathan E, et al: Complications of hair restoration surgery. Int J Trichology 2014; 6: 168.

Loh SH, et al: Pressure alopecia. J Am Acad Dermatol 2015; 72: 188.

MacDonald A, et al: Frontal fibrosing alopecia. J Am Acad Dermatol 2012; 67: 955.

Mihaljević N, et al: Successful use of infliximab in a patient with recalcitrant folliculitis decalvans. J Dtsch Dermatol Ges 2012; 10: 589.

Miteva M, et al: Dermoscopy guided scalp biopsy in cicatricial alopecia. J Eur Acad Dermatol Venereol 2013; 27: 1299.

Navarini AA, et al: Low-dose excimer 308-nm laser for treatment of lichen planopilaris. Arch Dermatol 2011; 147: 1325.

Nic Dhonncha E, et al: The role of hydroxychloroquine in the treatment of lichen planopilaris. Dermatol Ther 2017; 30.

Pirmez R, et al: Successful treatment of facial papules in frontal fibrosing alopecia with oral isotretinoin. Skin Appendage Disord 2017; 3: 111.

Rácz E, et al: Treatment of frontal fibrosing alopecia and lichen planopilaris. J Eur Acad Dermatol Venereol 2013; 27: 1461.

Rodney IJ, et al: Hair and scalp disorders in ethnic populations. J Drugs Dermatol 2013; 12: 420.

Rossi A, et al: Unusual patterns of presentation of frontal fibrosing alopecia. J Am Acad Dermatol 2017; 77: 172.

Shao H, et al: Follicular unit transplantation for the treatment of secondary cicatricial alopecia. Can J Plast Surg 2014; 22: 249.

Spring P, et al: Lichen planopilaris treated by the peroxisome proliferator activated receptor-γ agonist pioglitazone. J Am Acad Dermatol 2013; 69: 830.

Taylor SC, et al: Hair and scalp disorders in adult and pediatric patients with skin of color. Cutis 2017; 100: 31.

Trüeb RM: A comment on frontal fibrosing alopecia (Axel Munthe's syndrome). Int J Trichology 2016; 8: 203.

Yang CC, et al: Tofacitinib for the treatment of lichen planopilaris: A case series. Dermatol Ther 2018; e12656. doi: 10.1111/dth.12656. [Epub ahead of print] PubMed PMID: 30264512.

Ye Y, et al: Non-scarring patchy alopecia in patients with systemic lupus erythematosus differs from that of alopecia areata. Lupus 2013; 22: 1439.

HAIR COLOR

Melanin in the hair follicles is produced in the cytoplasm of the melanocytes. Organelles involved include the endoplasmic reticulum, ribosomes, and Golgi apparatus. Melanocytes producing hair pigment are associated with the hair matrix, and melanogenesis occurs only during anagen. This cyclic melanin synthesis distinguishes follicular melanogenesis from the continuous melanogenesis of the epidermis. With age, cyclic melanocytic activity in the follicular unit declines. By age 40, most individuals show evidence of graying. Graying results primarily from a reduction in tyrosinase activity within hair bulb melanocytes. Defective migration of melanocytes from a diminishing reservoir in the outer root sheath may play a role. Physiologic graying may also be related to reactive oxygen species–mediated damage to nuclear and mitochondrial DNA in bulbar melanocytes. The melanocortin 1 receptor gene *(MCR1)* is closely related to red hair, freckling, and sun sensitivity.

The pigment in black and dark-brown hair is composed of eumelanin, whereas in blond and red hair, it is pheomelanin. In black hair, the melanocytes contain the densest melanosomes. Brown hair differs only by its smaller melanosomes. Light-brown hair consists of a mixture of the melanosomes of dark hair and the incomplete melanosomes of blond hair. Many of the melanosomes in blond hair develop only on the matrix fibers and not in the spaces between the fibers.

Red hair shows incomplete melanin deposits on the matrix fibers, to produce a blotchy-appearing melanosome. Pheomelanin is distinguished by its relatively high content of sulfur, which results from the addition of cysteine to dopaquinone along the biosynthetic pathway of melanin synthesis.

In gray hair (canities), melanogenic activity is decreased as a result of fewer melanocytes and melanosomes, as well as a gradual loss of tyrosinase activity. Graying of the scalp hair is genetically determined and may start at any age. Usually, it begins at the temples and progresses with time. The beard usually follows, with the body hair graying last. Premature whitening of scalp hair is usually caused by vitiligo, sometimes without recognized, or actually without, lesions of glabrous skin.

Early graying (before age 20 in white or before age 30 in black persons) is usually familial; however, it may occur in progeria and in Rothmund-Thomson, Böök (PHC), and Werner syndromes, as well as after radiation exposure.

In poliosis, gray or white hair occurs in circumscribed patches. This may occur in Waardenburg syndrome and piebaldism, Tietz syndrome, Alezzandrini syndrome, neurofibromatosis, and tuberous sclerosis. Poliosis is also found in association with regressing melanoma, vitiligo, and Vogt-Koyanagi syndrome and may be seen in alopecia areata when the new hairs grow. Migratory poliosis without hair loss may represent a forme fruste of alopecia areata.

Green hair has been traced to copper in the water of a swimming pool. This occurs only in blond or light hair and may be treated with topical ethylenediamine tetraacetic acid (EDTA), penicillamine-containing shampoos, or 1.5% aqueous 1-hydroxyethyl diphosphonic acid. Tars and chrysarobin stain light-colored hair brown.

Changes in hair color occur in various disorders. The hair is blond in phenylketonuria and homocystinuria. Light hair is also seen in oasthouse urine disease (familial methionine malabsorption syndrome), Menkes steely (kinky) hair syndrome, and albinism. In Griscelli and Chédiak-Higashi syndromes, the hair has a silvery sheen. In kwashiorkor, hair assumes a red-blond color and may demonstrate periodic banding (flag sign, segmental heterochromia). Alternating light and dark bands may also occur in iron deficiency anemia and with courses of sunitinib. In vitamin B_{12} deficiency and with IFN therapy, whitening may occur. The disorder has been called canities segmentata sideropenica and responds completely to iron supplementation. Triparanol is associated with hypopigmented hair. By changing vellus to terminal hairs, minoxidil causes darkening of hair. Another hypotensive agent, diazoxide, gives the hair a reddish tint. Chloroquine therapy may cause hair whitening, usually in redheads and blonds, but not in brunettes. Pigmentation of the eyelashes and irides has been described with latanoprost. Xanthotrichia (yellow hair) has been noted with selenium sulfide and dihydroxyacetone.

Many black patients with acquired immunodeficiency syndrome (AIDS) have experienced softening, straightening, lightening, and thinning of their hair. Patients with human immunodeficiency virus 1 (HIV-1) infection may also experience elongated eyelashes and telogen effluvium.

Liu F, et al: Colorful DNA polymorphisms in humans. Semin Cell Dev Biol 2013; 24: 562.
Praetorius C, et al: A polymorphism in *IRF4* affects human pigmentation through a tyrosinase-dependent MITF/TFAP2A pathway. Cell 2013; 155: 1022.

HAIR STRUCTURE DEFECTS

Examination of hairs for structural defects is greatly facilitated by a method devised by Shelley: putting a piece of double-stick tape on a microscope slide and aligning 5-cm segments of hair in parallel on it. Dermoscopy can be useful in assessing hair morphology. Microscopic mounts of hairs are best examined under a dissecting microscope or polarized light. Gold coating and scanning electron microscopy (SEM) can also be done on hairs so mounted. Hairs from multiple body sites may need to be sampled. This has been documented in Netherton syndrome, where scalp hair can be normal while eyebrow hair demonstrates the characteristic hair shaft defect.

Hair Casts (Pseudonits)

Hair casts represent remnants of the inner root sheath. They often occur in great numbers and may mimic nits in the scalp. Whereas nits are firmly cemented to the hair shaft, however, hair casts slide freely along the shaft. Taeb et al. reviewed 36 published cases and distinguished two groups: girls age 2–8 years with diffuse involvement and no scalp disease, and children and adults with psoriasis, lichen planus, seborrheic dermatitis, traction, or trichotillomania. Keipert made a similar distinction, separating a large group of cases with some keratinizing disorder of the scalp and dark, oddly shaped masses of keratin adherent to or surrounding the hairs, which he called "parakeratotic" hair casts; and lighter-colored tubular casts 2–4 mm long, which he called "peripilar" hair casts. Taeb et al. found 0.025% tretinoin lotion to be effective. False hair casts may occur as a result of hair spray or deodorant concretions. Immunoglobulin casts and cutaneous spicules have been noted in multiple myeloma.

Pili Torti

Also known as "twisted hairs," pili torti is a malformation of hair characterized by twisting of the hair shaft on its own axis (Fig. 33.22). The hair shaft is segmentally thickened, and light and dark segments are seen. Scalp hair, eyebrows, and eyelashes may be affected. The hairs are brittle and easily broken.

In the classic type, unassociated with other disorders, onset is usually in early childhood; by puberty, it has usually improved. Clinically, pili torti may be associated with patchy alopecia and short, broken hairs. It usually follows a dominant inheritance pattern, although recessive and sporadic cases have been reported. Acquired cases have been described in young women with anorexia nervosa. Pili torti may be seen with associated abnormalities. The Björnstad syndrome consists of congenital deafness of the cochlear type, with pili torti. Both autosomal dominant and autosomal recessive inheritance patterns have been described. *BCS1L* mutations cause the Björnstad syndrome. The gene encodes an adenosine triphosphatase (ATPase) necessary for the assembly of complex III in mitochondria. *BCS1L* mutations also cause lethal conditions, including the complex III deficiency and the

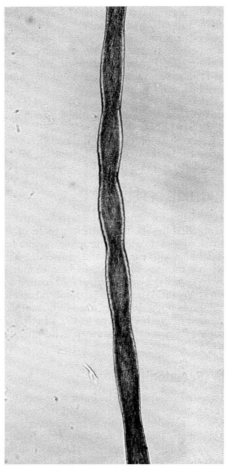

Fig. 33.22 Pili torti.

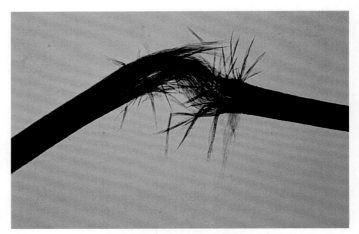

Fig. 33.23 Trichorrhexis nodosa.

GRACILE syndrome, with severe multisystem and neurologic manifestations.

Pili torti also may occur in citrullinemia (argininosuccinate synthetase deficiency), Menkes steely (kinky) hair syndrome, Bazex follicular atrophoderma syndrome, ectodermal dysplasias, Crandall syndrome (pili torti, nerve deafness, hypogonadism), Netherton syndrome (along with bamboo hair), with isotretinoin and etretinate therapy, in anorexia nervosa, and in trichothiodystrophy.

Laron syndrome is an autosomal recessive disease with primary insulin-like growth factor 1 deficiency and primary growth hormone insensitivity. Affected children have sparse hair and frontal recession. Pili torti et canaliculi, tapered hair, and trichorrhexis nodosa have been noted.

Pili torti and loose anagen hairs have been described during treatment with erlotinib.

Menkes Steely (Kinky) Hair Syndrome

Pili torti and often monilethrix and trichorrhexis nodosa are all common in the hairs in this sex-linked recessively inherited disorder. It has also been called steely hair disease because the hair resembles steel wool. The characteristic ivory color of the hair appears between 1 and 5 months of age. Drowsiness, lethargy, convulsive seizures, severe neurologic deterioration, and periodic hypothermia ensue, with death at an early age. Hairs become wiry, sparse, fragile, and twisted about their long axis. Osteoporosis and dental and ocular abnormalities are common. The skin is pale and the face pudgy, and the upper lip has an exaggerated "Cupid's bow" configuration. The occipital horn syndrome, primarily a connective tissue disorder,

is a milder variant of Menkes syndrome. Patients have a deficiency of serum copper and copper-dependent enzymes, resulting from mutations in the *ATP7A* gene. The gene encodes a trans–Golgi membrane–bound copper transporting P-type ATPase. Loss of this protein activity blocks the export of dietary copper from the GI tract and causes the copper deficiency. Low serum copper and ceruloplasmin levels are characteristic, but are not seen in all patients; levels are particularly variable in the first weeks of life. Other tests helpful for screening include the ratio of catechols, such as dihydroxyphenylalanine, to dihydroxyphenylglycol. High levels of the catechols dopa, dihydrophenylacetic acid, and dopamine and low levels of dihydroxyphenylglycol are characteristic. Studies of copper egress in cultured fibroblasts have also been used.

Early detection allows for genetic counseling and institution of copper histidine treatment, which has shown promising results in some infants. Pamidronate treatment is associated with an increase in bone mineral density in children with Menkes disease. In zebra fish, antisense morpholino oligonucleotides directed against the splice-site junctions of two mutant calamity alleles were able to correct the molecular defect. Also, L-threo-dihydroxyphenylserine can correct neurochemical abnormalities in a mouse model. This is a promising area for research.

Trichorrhexis Nodosa

The affected hair shafts fracture easily and may have small white nodes arranged at irregular intervals. These nodes are the sites of fraying of the hair cortex. The splitting into strands produces a microscopic appearance suggestive of a pair of brooms stuck together end to end by their bristles. The hairs soon break at these nodes (Fig. 33.23). The number of these nodes along one hair shaft varies from one to several, depending on its length. These fractured hairs are found mostly on the scalp, often in just a small area or areas, but other sites, such as the pubic area, axillae, and chest, may be involved.

Several categories or types of trichorrhexis nodosa have been described. Proximal trichorrhexis nodosa involves the proximal shafts of the hairs of black patients who traumatize their hair with styling or chemicals. The involved hairs break a few centimeters from the skin surface, resulting in patches of short hair. It appears to occur in genetically predisposed patients. Distal trichorrhexis nodosa affects primarily Asians and white patients; it occurs several inches from the scalp and is associated with trichoptilosis, or longitudinal splitting, known as "split ends." Acquired localized trichorrhexis nodosa is a common type in which the defect occurs in a localized area a few centimeters across. Diseases that accompany localized trichorrhexis nodosa in which pruritus is a prominent symptom (perhaps caused by scratching and rubbing) include

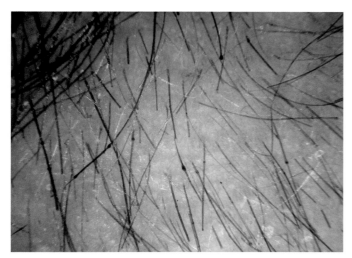

Fig. 33.24 Trichorrhexis invaginata in Netherton syndrome.

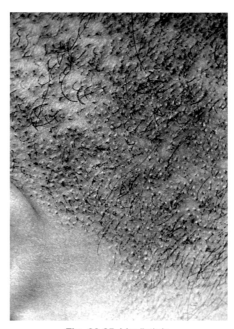

Fig. 33.25 Monilethrix.

circumscribed neurodermatitis, contact dermatitis, and atopic dermatitis.

The occurrence of trichorrhexis nodosa in some patients with argininosuccinicaciduria has suggested an etiologic connection. Trichorrhexis nodosa has been described in Menkes steely hair syndrome, Netherton syndrome, hypothyroidism, ectodermal dysplasia, the syndrome of intractable infant diarrhea, biotinidase deficiency, and trichothiodystrophy. Trichoschisis, a clean transverse fracture across the hair shaft, is more often present in trichothiodystrophy. The curly hair that may result from isotretinoin therapy has been attributed to extensive trichorrhexis nodosa. Because trauma may induce this hair shaft abnormality, the specificity of this finding in the previous conditions may simply be fortuitous. Treatment is directed toward the avoidance of trauma to the hair.

Trichorrhexis Invaginata

Also known as "bamboo hair," trichorrhexis invaginata is caused by intussusception of the hair shaft at the zone where keratinization begins. The invagination is caused by softness of the cortex in the keratogenous zone. The softness may be caused by inadequate conversion of –SH to S–S proteins in the cortex. The patient with bamboo hair will have nodose ball-and-socket deformities, with the socket forming the proximal and the ball part forming the distal portion of the node along the hair shaft. This type of hair is associated with Netherton syndrome (Fig. 33.24). Occasionally, only the proximal half of the abnormality is seen; this has been called "golf tee hairs."

Trichorrhexis invaginata associated with congenital ichthyosiform erythroderma or ichthyosis linearis circumflexa constitutes Netherton syndrome. Atopic manifestations and high IgE levels are typically present. The bamboo hairs may be present not only on the scalp but also on the eyebrows, eyelashes, and rarely in other hairy areas. Hair sparsity is noted all over the body. The bamboo hairs may become normal within a few years. Other reported findings include pili torti, trichorrhexis nodosa, moniliform hairs, urticaria, angioedema, growth retardation, recurrent infections, multiple epithelial neoplasms, and mental retardation. An autosomal recessive mode of inheritance has been suggested, although reported cases involving women far outnumber men. Pathogenic mutations have been identified in serine protease inhibitor Kazal-type 5 *(SPINK5)* on chromosome 5q32, a gene encoding lymphoepithelial Kazal-type-related inhibitor (LEKTI), a serine protease inhibitor involved in skin barrier formation and immunity. PUVA therapy has been reported to help the circumflex linear ichthyosis, and etretinate has both exacerbated and improved skin findings.

Menne et al. reported the bamboo hair defect in very thin, probably vellus, hairs in a 7-year-old boy with short, thin, brittle scalp hairs and no eyebrows. They termed this a "canestick deformity."

Pili Annulati (Ringed Hair, Spangled Hair)

Pili annulati is an unusual disease in which the hair seems banded by alternating segments of light and dark color when seen in reflected light. The light bands are caused by clusters of abnormal air-filled cavities, which scatter light, and reduplicated lamina densa in the region of the root bulb. Hair growth is normal in patients with pili annulati, although it is rarely associated with trichorrhexis nodosa–like breaks of the hair shaft. There are no other associated abnormalities of skin or other organ systems. It is inherited by autosomal dominant mode, begins in infancy, and requires no treatment, because the spangled appearance of the hair is not unattractive. The condition has been reported to disappear following recovery from alopecia totalis.

Pili Pseudoannulati

This anomaly of human hair mimics pili annulati. The two differ in that the light bands in pili annulati are caused by internal effects, whereas the bright segments in pili pseudoannulati are caused by reflection and refraction of light by flattened, twisted surfaces of hair. The pseudo type is a variant of normal hair.

Monilethrix

Monilethrix, also known as "beaded hairs," is a rare hereditary disease. It is characterized by dryness, fragility, and sparseness of the scalp hair (Fig. 33.25), with fusiform or spindle-shaped swellings of the hair shaft separated by narrow atrophic segments. The hair tends to break at the delicate internodes. There is an occasional rupture at the node and longitudinal fissuring of the shaft, which also involves the nodes.

The disease is often associated with keratosis pilaris of the extensor surfaces, temples, and back of the neck. Hair on regions other than the scalp may be affected. Leukonychia may occur. Inheritance of monilethrix is an autosomal dominant trait. It has been described in association with Menkes syndrome. Mutations in the gene for desmoglein 4 are seen in monilethrix and in localized autosomal recessive hypotrichosis, a disorder that shares clinical features with monilethrix but lacks the characteristic hair shaft changes. Several cases of monilethrix have been linked to the type II keratin gene cluster on chromosome 12q13. Causative heterozygous mutations of a highly conserved glutamic acid residue of the type II hair keratins hHb6 and hHb1 occur. Both hHb1 and hHb6 are largely coexpressed in cortical trichocytes of the hair shaft, confirming that monilethrix is a disease of the hair cortex. The hair may improve during pregnancy, but after delivery, the hair returns to its original state. Improvement may also occur with age, and there may be seasonal improvement during the summer. Improvement with acitretin has been reported.

Intermittent Hair Follicle Dystrophy

Birnbaum et al. reported a disorder of the hair follicle leading to increased fragility of the shaft, with no identifiable biochemical disturbance. The prevalence of this disorder is unknown.

Bubble Hair Deformity

Bubble hairs appear as areas of hair with altered texture. Fragility has been reported. The hairs may be curved or straight and stiff. Small, bubble-like defects are found within the hair shafts on light microscopy and electron microscopy. The condition is produced by overheating of wet hair with a malfunctioning hair dryer, analogous to the popping of popcorn. All damp hair will develop bubbles of gas when exposed to high heat.

Basit S, et al: Genetics of human isolated hereditary hair loss disorders. Clin Genet 2015; 88: 203.

Bindurani S, et al: Monilethrix with variable expressivity. Int J Trichology 2013; 5: 53.

Calvieri S, Rossi A: Alopecia in genetic diseases. G Ital Dermatol Venereol 2014; 149: 1.

Donsante A, et al: L-threo-dihydroxyphenylserine corrects neurochemical abnormalities in a Menkes disease mouse model. Ann Neurol 2013; 73: 259.

Falco M, et al: Novel compound heterozygous mutations in *BCS1L* gene causing Bjornstad syndrome in two siblings. Am J Med Genet A 2017; 173: 1348.

Leitner C, et al: Pitfalls and pearls in the diagnosis of monilethrix. Pediatr Dermatol 2013; 30: 633.

Lünnemann L, et al: Hair-shaft abnormality in a 7-year-old girl. JAMA Dermatol 2013; 149: 357.

Ozuguz P, et al: Generalized hair casts due to traction. Pediatr Dermatol 2013; 30: 614.

Pirmez R, et al: Loose anchoring of anagen hairs and pili torti due to erlotinib. Int J Trichology 2016; 8: 186.

Shao L, Newell B: Light microscopic hair abnormalities in children. Pediatr Dev Pathol 2014; 17: 36.

Singh G, et al: Prognosis and management of congenital hair shaft disorders with fragility—part I. Pediatr Dermatol 2016; 33: 473.

Singh G, et al: Prognosis and management of congenital hair shaft disorders with fragility—part II. Pediatr Dermatol 2016; 33: 481.

Tümer Z: An overview and update of *ATP7A* mutations leading to Menkes disease and occipital horn syndrome. Hum Mutat 2013; 34: 417.

Werner K, et al: Pili annulati associated with hair fragility. Cutis 2013; 91: 36.

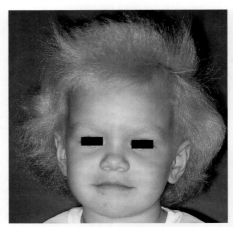

Fig. 33.26 Uncombable hair syndrome.

Uncombable Hair Syndrome

First reported in 1973 by Dupré et al. as cheveux incoiffables ("undressable hairs") and by Stroud and Mehergan as "spun-glass hair," the microscopic abnormality of a triangular cross-sectional appearance with a longitudinal groove gives the disease its other name, pili triangulati et canaliculi.

Clinically, the defect is noted in the first few years of life as dry, blond, shiny hair that stands straight out from the scalp and cannot be combed (Fig. 33.26). On light microscopy, it may appear quite normal when viewed lengthwise, but on horizontal sectioning and on SEM, it shows the longitudinal grooves that make it abnormally rigid. These depressions are sometimes seen in unaffected persons, and thus 50% of hairs need to be affected for the condition to be clinically detectable.

Autosomal dominant, autosomal recessive, and sporadic forms have been described. Uncombable hair has been associated with angel-shaped phalangoepiphyseal dysplasia. It has also been seen in combination with retinal dystrophy, juvenile cataract, and brachydactyly. It has also been reported in a patient who acquired the abnormality at age 39 after an episode of diffuse alopecia treated with spironolactone. Although there are usually no associated ectodermal defects, isolated cases have been reported in which uncombable hair is one component of several clustered findings. Until more experience is available in the literature, grouping these cases into new syndromes is premature.

Some patients have responded clinically to biotin, 0.3 mg orally three times daily. Some cases improve spontaneously in late childhood.

Calderon P, et al: Uncombable hair syndrome. J Am Acad Dermatol 2009; 61: 512.

Kinking Hair

Acquired progressive kinking of the hair, first described and named by Wise and Sulzberger in 1932, involves a structural abnormality of kinking and twisting of the hair shaft at irregular intervals. The main recognized variant of this disorder begins in men in their late teens or early twenties on the frontotemporal or vertex regions, then progresses to both the parietal and the frontal area. Usually straight, light-brown hair becomes curly, frizzy, and lusterless.

When this occurs in the androgen-dependent areas of young men, it is a precursor of male-pattern hair loss; usually these men have a strong family history of androgenetic alopecia. Treatment with topical minoxidil has not prevented development of hair thinning. "Whisker" hairs, the short dark hairs that grow anterior to the ears in young people who eventually develop androgenic

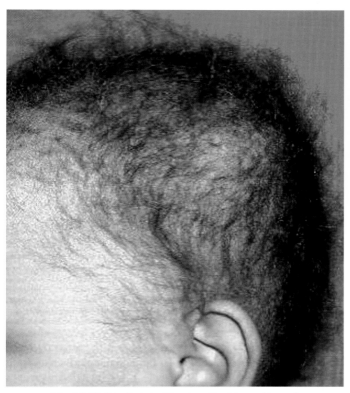

Fig. 33.27 Woolly hair. (Courtesy Dr. Shyam Verma.)

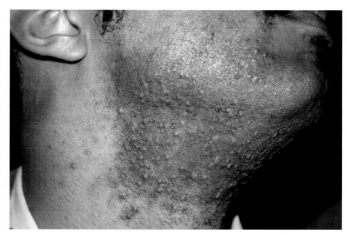

Fig. 33.28 Pseudofolliculitis barbae. (Courtesy Steven Binnick, MD.)

alopecia, is believed to be a variant of acquired kinking of the hair.

Acquired hair kinking has been described in other clinical situations. Some reports detail prepubertal patients or women, as well as men, in whom kinking develops in non–androgen-dependent areas such as the eyebrows or lashes. In these reports, alopecia has not developed, and the curly, frizzy hair may remain present or may revert to its previous condition.

Widespread kinking of the hair may be induced by drugs, notably retinoids, and it may also occur in patients with AIDS.

Woolly Hair

Woolly hair is present at birth and is usually most severe during childhood (Fig. 33.27), when it is often impossible to brush the hair. In adult life, there is a variable amelioration in the condition. A clear distinction exists between the appearance of the affected and nonaffected members of a family. Both autosomal dominant and autosomal recessive inheritance have been described. Woolly hair nevus has partial scalp involvement by woolly hair, which has a greatly reduced diameter. Naxos disease is an autosomal recessive syndrome with arrhythmogenic right ventricular cardiomyopathy, diffuse nonepidermolytic palmoplantar keratoderma, and woolly hair. Hair abnormalities are a reliable marker for subsequent heart disease. The disease is caused by a mutation in the gene encoding plakoglobin. Carvajal syndrome is a familial cardiocutaneous syndrome consisting of woolly hair, palmoplantar keratoderma, and heart disease. It is caused by a recessive deletion mutation in desmoplakin.

Woolly hairs tend to unite into tight locks, whereas the hairs of black persons remain individual. The hair may not grow beyond a length of 12 cm, but may attain a normal appearance in adult life. In the familial group, the eyebrows and hairs on the arms, legs, and pubic and axillary regions may be short and pale. There are no associated cutaneous or systemic diseases. A Dutch kindred

has been described with premature loss of curly brittle hair, premature loss of carious teeth, nail dystrophy, and acral keratoderma. It has been designated the curly hair–acral keratoderma–caries syndrome.

The microscopic findings of woolly hair include a decreased diameter, an ovoid shape on cross section, a pili torti–like twisting about a longitudinal axis, trichorrhexis nodosa, and pili annulati.

Plica Neuropathica (Felted Hair)

Plica neuropathica is a curling, looping, intertwisting, and felting or matting of the hair in localized areas of the scalp. Predisposing factors include kinky hairs, changes in hair care, and a neurotic mental state. Plica polonica is a former name for this condition.

MacDonald A, et al: Acquired progressive kinking of hair affecting the scalp and eyelashes in an adult woman. Clin Exp Dermatol 2011; 36: 882.
Song KH, et al: Acquired progressive kinking of the hair in a Korean female adolescent. J Dermatol 2013; 40: 80.
Urbina F: Eyelash involvement in acquired progressive kinking of the hair. Clin Exp Dermatol 2012; 37: 562.

Pseudofolliculitis Barbae

Pseudofolliculitis barbae ("razor bumps") consists of hairs that, after appearing at the surface, curve back and pierce the skin as ingrowing hairs. This results in inflammatory papules and pustules, which may scar (Fig. 33.28). In severe cases, large deforming keloids may result in the beard area. Pseudofolliculitis of the beard is seen in more than 50% of black men, who must sometimes give up shaving to alleviate the disorder. A single nucleotide polymorphism, giving rise to a disruptive Ala12Thr substitution in the 1A α-helical segment of the companion layer–specific keratin K6hf, appears to be partially responsible for the phenotype. White persons are infrequently affected; however, it is more common in renal transplant recipients. Tenderness responds to midstrength topical corticosteroids. The use of clippers or chemical depilatories, glycolic acid lotion, and adjunctive antibiotic therapy may be helpful. Benzoyl peroxide 5%/clindamycin 1% gel has been shown to be effective in double-blind evaluation. Laser hair removal with the long-pulse neodymium:yttrium-aluminum-garnet (Nd:YAG) laser is suitable for a wide range of skin types, and topical eflornithine can prolong responses. The diode laser and PDT have also been used.

Alexis A, et al: Folliculitis keloidalis nuchae and pseudofolliculitis barbae. Dermatol Clin 2014; 32: 183.

Diernaes JE, et al: Successful treatment of recalcitrant folliculitis barbae and pseudofolliculitis barbae with photodynamic therapy. Photodiagnosis Photodyn Ther 2013; 10: 651.

Emer JJ: Best practices and evidenced-based use of the 800 nm diode laser for the treatment of pseudofolliculitis barbae in skin of color. J Drugs Dermatol 2011; 10: s20.

Xia Y, et al: Topical eflornithine hydrochloride improves the effectiveness of standard laser hair removal for treating pseudofolliculitis barbae. J Am Acad Dermatol 2012; 67: 694.

Pili Multigemini

This rare malformation is characterized by the presence of bifurcated or multiple divided hair matrices and papillae, giving rise to the formation of multiple hair shafts within the individual follicles (Fig. 33.29). Pili multigemini sometimes follows lines of Blaschko. Mehregan et al. reported a patient with cleidocranial dysostosis and extensive pili multigemini over the heavily bearded chin and cheek areas. There is no treatment.

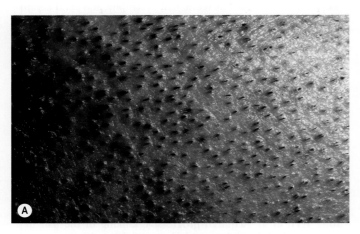

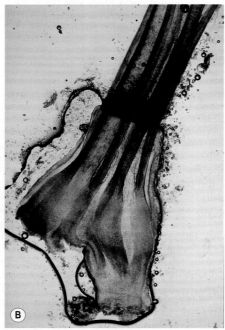

Fig. 33.29 (A) Pili multigemini of beard. (B) Multiple hair shafts in single follicle.

Pili Bifurcati

In this disorder, bifurcation is found in short segments along the shafts of several hairs. Each branch of the bifurcation is covered with its own cuticle. It has been seen in association with the trisomy 8 mosaic syndrome. Pili bifurcati differs from pili multigemini, in which a single follicular matrix produces two different-sized hair shafts with separate cuticles that do not fuse again. Trichoptilosis is characterized by split distal ends that are never surrounded by a complete cuticle.

Lester L, et al: The prevalence of pili multigemini. Br J Dermatol 2007; 156: 1362.

Trichostasis Spinulosa

Trichostasis spinulosa is a common disorder of the hair follicles that clinically gives the impression of blackheads (Fig. 33.30), but the follicles are filled with funnel-shaped, horny plugs within which are bundles of vellus hairs. The hairs are round at their proximal ends and shredded distally. The disease occurs primarily on the nose and forehead, but may also occur on the trunk and may be accompanied by pruritus. Dermoscopy or microscopy can be used to establish the diagnosis. The condition may be more common in patients in renal failure.

Trichostasis spinulosa results from retention of telogen hairs, which are derived from a single hair matrix. It is primarily caused by a hyperkeratosis of the follicular infundibulum, which leads to a partial obstruction of the follicular orifice and thus does not permit shedding of small telogen hairs.

The plugs may be removed with hydroactive adhesive (Biore) pads. Keratolytics are also effective after using a wax depilatory. The pulsed diode and alexandrite lasers have been used successfully, and application of 0.05% tretinoin solution, applied daily for 2 or 3 months, may also produce satisfactory results.

Badawi A, et al: Treatment of trichostasis spinulosa with 0.5-millisecond pulsed 755-nm alexandrite laser. Lasers Med Sci 2011; 26: 825.

Deshmukh SD, et al: Trichostasis spinulosa presenting as itchy papules in a young lady. Int J Trichology 2011; 3: 44.

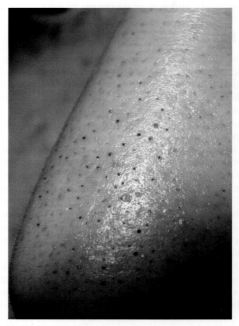

Fig. 33.30 Trichostasis spinulosa. (Courtesy Steven Binnick, MD.)

Gündüz O, et al: Trichostasis spinulosa confirmed by standard skin surface biopsy. Int J Trichology 2012; 4: 273.

Trichodysplasia Spinulosa (Viral-Associated Trichodysplasia)

Trichodysplasia spinulosa is seen in immunosuppressed patients and is associated with a polyomavirus. The condition is characterized by follicular distention with keratotic spines, especially on the face. Electron microscopy, immunohistochemistry, and viral load measurements indicate an etiologic role for the virus. Leflunomide and cidofovir have each been used therapeutically. Physical extraction has also proved successful.

Barton M, et al: Trichodysplasia spinulosa in a 7-year-old boy managed using physical extraction of keratin spicules. Pediatr Dermatol 2017; 34: e74.
Kassar R, et al: Leflunomide for the treatment of trichodysplasia spinulosa in a liver transplant recipient. Transpl Infect Dis 2017; 19.
Leitenberger JJ, et al: Two cases of trichodysplasia spinulosa responsive to compounded topical cidofovir 3% cream. JAAD Case Rep 2015; 1: S33.

HYPERTRICHOSIS

Hypertrichosis is an overgrowth of hair not localized to the androgen-dependent areas of the skin. Several forms exist. Many cases are induced by medications, including minoxidil, cyclosporine, and efalizumab. The excessive hair growth can be managed with bleaching, trimming, shaving, plucking, waxing, chemical depilatories, and electrosurgical epilation. Treatment with long-pulse Nd:YAG, diode, ruby, and long- and short-pulse alexandrite lasers as well as with intense pulsed light sources can be effective. Skin type must be considered when choosing a laser system. The greatest experience in dark skin types has been with the long-pulse Nd:YAG laser.

Localized Acquired Hypertrichosis

Eyelash trichomegaly can occur with erlotinib, latanoprost, and intentionally with bimatoprost. Dermal tumors, such as melanocytic nevi, smooth muscle hamartomas, meningiomas, and Becker nevi, may have excessive terminal hair growth. Repeated irritation, trauma, occlusion under a cast, eczematous states, topical steroid use, linear melorheostotic scleroderma, lymphedema associated with filariasis, the Crow-Fukase (POEMS) syndrome, and pretibial myxedema may be other situations with a localized increase in hair growth. Porphyrias generally show a localized hypertrichosis over the malar area, such as in porphyria cutanea tarda or variegate porphyria. In the Gunther variety of erythropoietic porphyria, however, the hypertrichosis may be generalized or more diffuse.

Localized Congenital Hypertrichosis

Hypertrichosis cubiti (hairy elbows) consists of long vellus hair on the extensor surfaces of the distal third of the upper arm and the proximal third of the forearm bilaterally. It is a progressive, excessive growth of lanugo hairs that often begins in infancy; the hairs may reach a length of 10 cm. Later, they become coarser, but regression has been observed during adolescence. There appear to be familial cases and a sporadic form. Short stature and some developmental abnormalities are present in some patients; however, endocrine studies or other evaluations are not necessary. The condition appears to be of cosmetic significance only.

Other causes of localized congenital hypertrichosis include congenital nevocytic nevi, anterior cervical hypertrichosis, and simple nevoid hypertrichosis. Localized hypertrichosis may be a

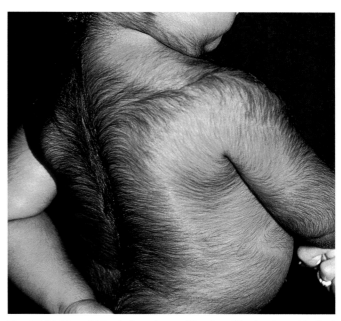

Fig. 33.31 Hypertrichosis lanuginosa. (Courtesy Brooke Army Medical Center Teaching File.)

sign of underlying spinal dysraphism when it occurs over the sacral midline, or a sign of an underlying neoplasm.

Generalized Congenital Hypertrichosis (Congenital Hypertrichosis Lanuginosa)

This rare type of excessive and generalized hairiness is a fully penetrant, X-linked dominant trait. The entire body is covered with fine vellus hairs 2–10 cm long (Fig. 33.31). The scalp hair appears to be normal. Except for the palms and soles, all other areas are covered. Congenital hypertrichosis lanuginosa may be associated with dental anomalies and gingival fibromatosis. This type of hairiness has attracted considerable attention over the centuries. Hair removal by laser may be quite useful.

Other cases of congenital generalized hypertrichosis may be secondary to drug ingestion by the mother. The fetal hydantoin syndrome is characterized by hypertrichosis, depressed nasal bridge, large lips, a wide mouth, and a short, webbed neck. The fetal alcohol syndrome includes hypertrichosis, a small face, capillary hemangiomas, and physical and mental retardation. A case of generalized hypertrichosis and multiple congenital defects was reported in a baby born to a mother who used minoxidil throughout pregnancy. Fetal valproate syndrome is characterized by generalized hypertrichosis sparing the palms and soles, coarse facies, gum hypertrophy, hypotonia, club feet and hands, and abnormal dermatoglyphics.

Generalized or Patterned Acquired Hypertrichosis

These cases include those caused by acquired hypertrichosis lanuginosa, those associated with various syndromes, and those secondary to drug intake. Acquired hypertrichosis lanuginosa is an ominous sign of internal malignancy (Fig. 33.32). Syndromes associated with increased hair growth include lipoatrophic diabetes, stiff skin syndrome, Down syndrome, Rubenstein-Taybi syndrome, Laband syndrome, Cornelia de Lange syndrome, Hurler syndrome, leprechaunism, Winchester syndrome, Schynzel-Giedier syndrome, presymptomatic Leigh syndrome (neurometabolic mitochondrial disorder), and hypertrichosis with acromegalic

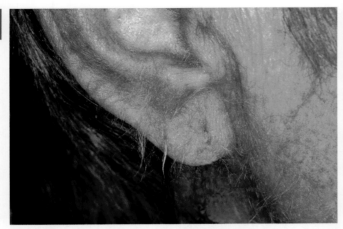

Fig. 33.32 Hypertrichosis lanuginosa associated with an internal malignancy (malignant down).

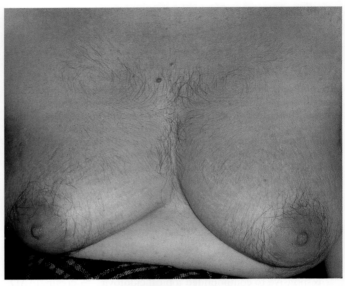

Fig. 33.33 Hirsutism.

features. Drugs associated with hypertrichosis include minoxidil, cyclosporine, diphenylhydantoin, diazoxide, streptomycin, penicillamine, corticosteroids, danazol, psoralens, hexachlorobenzene, PUVA, topical bimatoprost, topical corticosteroids, and topical androgens.

Baertling F, et al: Hypertrichosis in presymptomatic mitochondrial disease. J Inherit Metab Dis 2013; 36: 1081.

Berry RS, et al: Congenital dermatofibrosarcoma with associated hypertrichosis. J Cutan Pathol 2013; 40: 990.

Goel N, et al: Familial congenital generalized hypertrichosis. Indian J Dermatol Venereol Leprol 2013; 79: 849.

Ma HJ, et al: Acquired localized hypertrichosis induced by internal fixation and plaster cast application. Ann Dermatol 2013; 25: 365.

HIRSUTISM

Clinical Features

Hirsutism is an excess of terminal hair growth in women in a pattern more typical of men. Androgen-dependent growth areas affected include the upper lip, cheeks, chin, central chest, breasts, lower abdomen, and groin (Fig. 33.33). This altered growth pattern of the hair may be associated with other signs of virilization, which include temporal balding, masculine habitus, deepening of the voice, clitoral hypertrophy, and amenorrhea. Acne is an additional sign of hyperandrogenism.

Pathogenesis

When virilization accompanies hirsutism, especially when progression is rapid, a neoplastic cause is likely. In the absence of virilization, a neoplastic cause is extremely unlikely. Most medically significant hirsutism is related to the polycystic ovarian syndrome (PCOS, hyperinsulinemic hyperandrogenism with anovulation). In a study of 873 patients with medically significant hirsutism, PCOS was present in 82%. Idiopathic hirsutism was present in 4.7%, and 6.75% of the patients had elevated androgen levels and hirsutism with normal ovulation.

Ethnic variation should be considered when evaluating hirsutism. Women of Southwest Asian, Eastern European, and southern European heritage usually have facial, abdominal, and thigh hair; whereas Asian and Indian women generally have little terminal hair growth in these areas.

In women, androgen biosynthesis occurs in the adrenal gland and ovary. Testosterone and the androgen precursor androstenedione are secreted by the ovary. The adrenal contributions are preandrogens: dehydroepiandrosterone (DHEA), DHEA sulfate, and androstenedione. These require peripheral conversion in the skin and liver to testosterone. Testosterone is converted to dihydrotestosterone, the androgen that promotes androgen-dependent hair growth, in the hair follicle by 5α-reductase. Receptor molecules in the end organ are necessary for binding and hormone action at that level. Because testosterone is normally bound to carrier molecules in the plasma at a 99% level, and it is the unbound testosterone that is active, the levels of free testosterone correlate with clinical evidence of androgen excess.

Hirsutism may result from excessive secretion of androgens from either the ovary or the adrenal gland. The excessive secretion may be from functional excesses or rarely from neoplastic processes. Ovarian causes include PCOS (Stein-Leventhal syndrome) and a variety of ovarian tumors, both benign and malignant. PCOS is defined by anovulation (fewer than nine periods a year or periods longer than 40 days apart) with clinical evidence of hyperandrogenism. Ovarian cysts are not required for the diagnosis, and laboratory and imaging studies are not required to establish the diagnosis, according to the U.S. National Institutes of Health (NIH) consensus criteria. Rotterdam criteria for diagnosing PCOS require the presence of two of the following criteria: androgen excess, ovulatory dysfunction, or polycystic ovaries. The pathogenesis of PCOS may relate to insulin resistance, with resultant elevated insulin levels leading to ovarian overproduction of androgens. Prevalence rates of PCOS for black and white women in the United States are 8.0% and 4.8%, respectively.

Ovarian tumors include unilateral benign microadenomas, arrhenoblastomas. Leydig cell tumors, hilar cell tumors, granular/theca cell tumors, and luteomas are rare causes of hirsutism. In tumor-associated hirsutism, the onset is usually rapid, occurs with other signs of virilization, and begins between ages 20 and 40.

Adrenal causes include congenital adrenal hyperplasia (CAH) and adrenal tumors, such as adrenal adenomas and carcinomas. The adrenogenital syndrome or CAH is an autosomal dominant disorder that may result from deficiency of the enzyme 21-hydroxylase (most common form), 11β-hydroxylase, or 3β-hydroxy steroid dehydrogenase. Onset is generally in childhood, with ambiguous genitalia, precocious growth, and virilism. Nonclassic (adult-onset) CAH may present with hirsutism.

Pituitary causes include Cushing disease, acromegaly, and prolactin-secreting adenomas. Patients with prolactin-secreting microadenomas have a 20% incidence of hirsutism and acne. Prolactin elevations may be seen in patients with PCOS. Other settings where prolactin levels may be elevated and that may lead to hirsutism include hypothyroidism, phenothiazine intake, and hepatorenal failure.

Other causes of hirsutism include the exogenous intake of androgens. End-organ hypersensitivity may be a mechanism in patients with a normal evaluation. Drugs such as minoxidil, diazoxide, corticosteroids, and phenytoin, which have been reported to cause hirsutism, generally cause hypertrichosis—a generalized increase in hair that is not limited to the androgen-sensitive areas.

Evaluation

Most hirsutism is related to ethnic heritage or PCOS. 21-Hydroxylase–deficient nonclassic adrenal hyperplasia, the hyperandrogenic insulin-resistant acanthosis nigricans syndromes, and androgen-secreting tumors are relatively uncommon causes. A careful history and physical examination are essential. The history should focus on onset and progression, virilization, menstrual and pregnancy history, and family/racial background. Physical examination may reveal signs of Cushing disease, hypothyroidism, or acromegaly. Other signs to be evaluated are the distribution of muscle mass and body fat, clitoral dimensions, voice depth, and galactorrhea.

Laboratory evaluation is controversial. In the authors' opinion, testing is of value only when it affects management. If this is accepted, there is no mandatory hormonal testing for stable hirsutism in patients who have no signs of virilization. A diagnosis of PCOS can be made clinically and does not require laboratory confirmation. Determination of serum lipids and testing for glucose intolerance may be the most important laboratory evaluations in patients with PCOS because these have the greatest impact on management and long-term prognosis. When the history and physical examination suggest the possibility of a neoplasm, laboratory evaluation should include a total testosterone level. A DHEA sulfate level is usually performed if an adrenal cause is suspected. A 24-hour urine cortisol test is the gold standard for the diagnosis of Cushing disease. Measurement of thyroid-stimulating hormone (TSH), growth hormone, and somatomedin C levels are indicated if the history and physical examination suggest hypothyroidism or acromegaly.

Dexamethasone suppression tests are recommended by some authorities, but the results often do not affect management. A baseline 17-hydroxyprogesterone (17-HP) and adrenocorticotropic hormone (ACTH) stimulation test can screen for late-onset CAH, but steroid replacement has not been proved to result in better outcomes than empiric treatment with antiandrogens. Baseline 17-HP may be normal in some women with nonclassic 21-hydroxylase deficiency, and ACTH stimulation may result in overdiagnosis of the syndrome. An exaggerated 17-HP response to ACTH stimulation is common in PCOS at a pharmacologic dose (250 μg) but not at a physiologic dose (1 μg) of ACTH. An ovarian origin of hirsutism can be identified by a buserelin test in 30% of patients with hirsutism and by dexamethasone in 22% of patients, but data proving that buserelin challenge results in better outcomes are lacking. A prolactin level will screen for prolactin-secreting tumors but will also lead to further expensive testing in many patients ultimately diagnosed with PCOS. A prolactin level should be obtained in any patient with galactorrhea but is of limited value as a routine screening test for patients with hirsutism alone.

If signs of acromegaly, Cushing disease, or virilization are present clinically, referral to an endocrinologist is recommended. The presence of major menstrual irregularities is also an indication for referral to an endocrinologist or gynecologist. Although 90% of women with hirsutism have an elevated testosterone level, increases greater than 200 ng/dL and rapid onset or progressive virilization suggest serious underlying disease. A major elevation in the DHEA sulfate level (>7000 ng/mL) suggests an adrenal neoplasm, and imaging of the adrenal gland is recommended. Many patients with late-onset CAH will have normal screening DHEA sulfate. Patients with prolactin levels above 20 ng/mL should likewise be referred for further evaluation with magnetic resonance imaging (MRI) or computed tomography (CT). Polymorphisms in the gene coding for sex hormone–binding globulin have been identified in some families with hirsutism, but such testing does not affect management.

Treatment

Various forms of mechanical, chemical, and laser epilation can be performed for hirsutism, as for hypertrichosis. Spironolactone with various OCs, CPA plus ethinyl estradiol, gonadotropin-releasing hormone agonists (e.g., leuprolide, nafarelin), flutamide, finasteride, and topical eflornithine have been used successfully alone and in various combinations to treat hirsutism. The optimal combination and dosage remain to be determined, but in one study, 20 μg of ethinyl estradiol was as effective as 30 μg when used in association with drospirenone. The Endocrine Society clinical practice guideline recommends hormonal OCs as the first-line management for menstrual abnormalities and hirsutism in patients with PCOS. The guideline notes that hormonal OCs and metformin are the best treatment options in adolescents with PCOS, that thiazolidinediones have an unfavorable risk-benefit ratio compared with other treatments, and that statins require further study.

Finasteride at doses of 2.5–5 mg/day has been shown to decrease hair number and diameter in women with hirsutism. The combination of spironolactone, 100 mg/day, plus finasteride, 5 mg/day, has been shown to be superior to spironolactone, 100 mg/day, alone. An analysis of the current literature suggested that spironolactone alone, 100 mg/day, is superior to finasteride alone, 5 mg/day, and to low-dose CPA alone, 12.5 mg/day for the first 10 days of a cycle, in the treatment of hirsutism. Spironolactone is typically used at a dose of 100 mg twice daily, so further studies are needed comparing this higher dose with other modes of therapy. In a prospective, randomized study of Diane 35 (CPA, 2 mg, and ethinyl estradiol, 35 μg), Diane 35 plus spironolactone, and spironolactone alone, all treatments were well tolerated. Combination therapy resulted in superior measured endocrine responses, but the authors concluded that spironolactone alone was the most cost-effective treatment. The choice of an OC is also controversial. Third-generation OCs result in a significant increase in sex hormone–binding globulin and a decrease in free testosterone, but both second-generation and third-generation OCs are clinically effective in treating hirsutism. When flutamide is used, initial treatment with 250 mg/day is followed by a long maintenance treatment period using 125 mg/day.

Metformin therapy has been shown to control menstrual cycles and improve fertility in women with PCOS. It causes a decline in testosterone and insulin levels. Oligomenorrheic women with an increased luteinizing hormone to follicle-stimulating hormone (LH/FSH) ratio and lower testosterone levels respond best. Spironolactone, 50 mg/day, was superior to metformin, 1000 mg/day, in the treatment of hirsutism and menstrual cycle frequency in a study of 82 adolescent and young women with PCOS. Doses of 200 mg/day are typically used to treat hirsutism. At this dose, menstrual irregularities induced by the drug are common, and it may be best used in combination with an OC. Good correlation has been noted between an increase in ovulation frequency with clomiphene citrate and the chance of pregnancy in women with PCOS. Other options include acarbose, gonadotrophins, and laparoscopic ovarian drilling. Infertility is best managed by a specialist in this field. Empiric treatment with an antiandrogen may be as effective as steroid replacement for the management of hirsutism in patients with nonclassic CAH.

Bates GW Jr, et al: Polycystic ovarian syndrome management options. Obstet Gynecol Clin North Am 2012; 39: 495.

Bitzer J, et al: The use of cyproterone acetate/ethinyl estradiol in hyperandrogenic skin symptoms—a review. Eur J Contracept Reprod Health Care 2017; 22: 172.

Buzney E, et al: Polycystic ovary syndrome. J Am Acad Dermatol 2014; 71: 859.e1.

Codner E, et al: Metformin for the treatment of hyperandrogenism in adolescents with type 1 diabetes mellitus. Horm Res Paediatr 2013; 80: 343.

Heidelbaugh JJ: Endocrinology update: hirsutism. FP Essent 2016; 451: 17.

Jayasena CN, Franks S: The management of patients with polycystic ovary syndrome. Nat Rev Endocrinol 2014; 10: 624.

Legro RS, et al: Diagnosis and treatment of polycystic ovary syndrome. J Clin Endocrinol Metab 2013; 98: 4565.

Loriaux DL: An approach to the patient with hirsutism. J Clin Endocrinol Metab 2012; 97: 2957.

Mihailidis J, et al: Endocrine evaluation of hirsutism. Int J Womens Dermatol 2017; 3: S6.

Pasquali R, et al: Therapy in endocrine disease: treatment of hirsutism in the polycystic ovary syndrome. Eur J Endocrinol 2013; 170: R75.

Pignatelli D: Non-classic adrenal hyperplasia due to the deficiency of 21-hydroxylase and its relation to polycystic ovarian syndrome. Front Horm Res 2013; 40: 158.

Roe AH, et al: Using the Androgen Excess-PCOS Society criteria to diagnose polycystic ovary syndrome and the risk of metabolic syndrome in adolescents. J Pediatr 2013; 162: 937.

Romualdi D, et al: Clinical efficacy and metabolic impact of two different dosages of ethinyl-estradiol in association with drospirenone in normal-weight women with polycystic ovary syndrome. J Endocrinol Invest 2013; 36: 636.

Ruan X, et al: Use of cyproterone acetate/ethinylestradiol in polycystic ovary syndrome. Eur J Contracept Reprod Health Care 2017; 22: 183.

Sangeeta S: Metformin and pioglitazone in polycystic ovarian syndrome. J Obstet Gynaecol India 2012; 62: 551.

Setji TL, Brown AJ: Polycystic ovary syndrome. Am J Med 2014; 127: 912.

Shrimal A, et al: Long-pulsed Nd:YAG laser and intense pulse light-755 nm for idiopathic facial hirsutism. J Cutan Aesthet Surg 2017; 10: 40.

Somani N, Turvy D: Hirsutism. Am J Clin Dermatol 2014; 15: 247.

Unluhizarci K, et al: Hirsutism. Front Horm Res 2013; 40: 103.

TRICHOMYCOSIS AXILLARIS

Discrete nodules 1–2 mm in size and attached firmly to the hair shafts of the axillary or pubic areas characterize trichomycosis. The color of the nodules may be yellow, red, or black (Fig. 33.34). Hyperhidrosis of the affected regions is usually present. A yellowish discoloration of the axillae is sometimes noted. Large numbers of *Corynebacterium* are present in the concretions. Trichomycosis axillaris may coexist with erythrasma and pitted keratolysis. Treatment with a topical antibiotic preparation (e.g., clindamycin or erythromycin) or naftifine, which has antibacterial properties, combined with any modality that will decrease the hyperhidrosis, is effective, but shaving is faster.

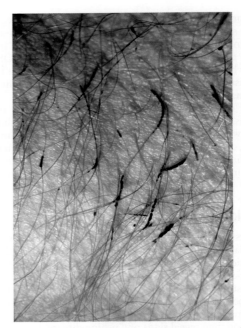

Fig. 33.34 Trichomycosis axillaris.

Rho NK, et al: A corynebacterial triad: prevalence of erythrasma and trichomycosis axillaris in soldiers with pitted keratolysis. J Am Acad Dermatol 2008; 58: S57.

Rojas Mora E, et al: Trichomycosis axillaris. Actas Dermosifiliogr 2017; 108: 264.

ASSOCIATED HAIR FOLLICLE DISEASES

Tinea Amiantacea (Pityriasis Amiantacea)

Thick, asbestos-like (amiantaceous), shiny scales on the scalp characterize pityriasis amiantacea. The silvery-white or dull-gray crusting may be localized or, less often, generalized over the entire scalp. The proximal parts of the hairs are matted together by the laminated crusts. There are no structural changes in the hair, but in some patches where the crusting is thick, there may be some purulent exudate under the crust and temporary alopecia such as occurs after some cases of furunculosis of the scalp.

The cause is most often severe or untreated seborrheic dermatitis or psoriasis, although it may occur paradoxically during tumor necrosis factor-alpha inhibitor therapy. In a prospective study of 85 patients, psoriasis was documented in 35% and processes suggesting seborrheic dermatitis or atopic dermatitis occurred in another 35%. Tinea capitis was the eventual diagnosis in 13%. *Staphylococcus* was found in 96.5% of patients, compared with 15% of controls. The patient should shampoo daily or every other day with selenium sulfide suspension or a tar- or steroid-containing shampoo for 2 weeks. Prior application of peanut oil or a keratolytic a few hours before shampooing facilitates removal of the scales and crusts. With such debridement, followed by topical steroid solution in Caucasians or steroid ointment in African Americans, the secondary bacterial infection usually resolves without the need for oral antistaphylococcal therapy.

Abdel-Hamid IA, et al: Pityriasis amiantacea. Int J Dermatol 2003; 42: 260.

Amorim GM, Fernandes NC: Pityriasis amiantacea. An Bras Dermatol 2017; 91: 694.

Ettler J, et al: Pityriasis amiantacea. Clin Exp Dermatol 2012; 37: 639.

Folliculitis Nares Perforans

Perforating folliculitis of the nose is characterized by small pustules near the tip of the inside of the nose. The lesion becomes crusted, and when the crust is removed, the bulbous end of the affected vibrissa is found to be embedded in the inspissated material. The affected hairs are typical of those occurring inside the nostril. *Staphylococcus aureus* may at times be cultured from the pustules. The hair should be removed and antibiotic ointment such as mupirocin applied.

White SW, et al: Pseudofolliculitis vibrissae. Arch Dermatol 1981; 117: 368.

Acquired Perforating Dermatosis

Perforating folliculitis, Kyrle disease, and acquired perforating collagenosis are designations that have been supplanted by the more inclusive term *acquired perforating dermatosis*. The condition is not uncommon and is most often associated with renal failure or diabetes, or both. Between 4% and 10% of dialysis patients develop umbilicated dome-shaped papules on the legs, or less often on the trunk, neck, arms, or scalp, with variable itchiness (Figs. 33.35 and 33.36). Early lesions may be pustular; late lesions resemble prurigo nodularis both clinically and histologically. A central hyperkeratotic cone projects into the dermis, so that when it is removed, a pitlike depression remains. Usually the papules

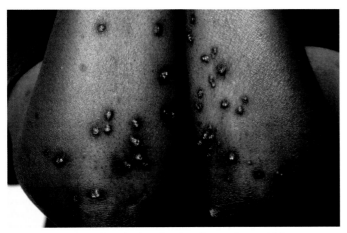

Fig. 33.35 Acquired perforating disease in renal failure.

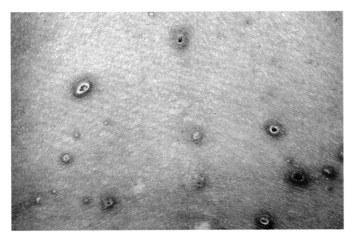

Fig. 33.36 Reactive perforating disease in renal failure. (Courtesy Steven Binnick, MD.)

are discrete, but they may coalesce to form circinate plaques. Coalescing verrucous plaques are frequently seen, especially on the lower extremities. Koebner phenomenon may also be observed, in which case plaques or elevated verrucous streaks are formed, primarily in the antecubital and popliteal spaces. Atrophic scars are seen on involution of these lesions.

Histologically, the epidermis becomes edematous, the granular layer disappears, and parakeratosis develops. Eventually, the epidermis becomes atrophic, with disruption of the sites over the papillae. Through these sites, necrobiotic connective tissue, degenerating inflammatory cells, and collagen bundles are extruded into a cup-shaped epidermal depression.

Acquired perforating dermatosis is thought to be a response to trauma, usually scratching or rubbing in response to the pruritus of the associated renal failure or dry skin. Other predisposing conditions reported include HIV infection, sclerosing cholangitis or other liver diseases, hypothyroidism, hyperparathyroidism, Hodgkin disease, healed areas of herpes zoster, and reactions to laser hair removal, telaprevir, or indinavir and several biologic and targeted therapeutic agents (e.g., gefitinib, infliximab, etanercept, bevacizumab, sorafenib, and natalizumab).

Ultraviolet treatment, either PUVA or Ultraviolet B (UVB), helps the pruritus of renal disease and improves the perforating disorder. Hydration of the skin with a soaking tub bath in plain water, followed immediately (without drying) by triamcinolone ointment just before bedtime, is also useful. Topical retinoic acid (0.1% cream), tacalcitol, doxycycline, amitriptyline, photodynamic therapy, isotretinoin, and etretinate have been effective in flattening lesions. HIV-infected patients may respond well to thalidomide. The disease may remit promptly after renal transplantation.

Akoglu G, et al: Clinicopathological features of 25 patients with acquired perforating dermatosis. Eur J Dermatol 2013; 23: 864.

Kim SW, et al: A clinicopathologic study of thirty cases of acquired perforating dermatosis in Korea. Ann Dermatol 2014; 26: 162.

Pernet C, et al: Telaprevir-induced acquired perforating dermatosis. JAMA Dermatol 2014; 150: 1371.

Reactive Perforating Collagenosis

Reactive perforating collagenosis is an inherited condition characterized by pinhead-sized, skin-colored papules that grow to a diameter of 4–6 mm and develop a central area of umbilication in which keratinous material is lodged. The discrete papules may be numerous and may involve sites of frequent trauma, such as the backs of the hands, forearms, elbows, and knees. The lesion reaches a maximum size of about 6 mm in 4 weeks and then regresses spontaneously in 6–8 weeks. This is believed to be caused by a peculiar reaction of the skin to superficial trauma. Koebnerization is often observed. Young children are most frequently affected. Most reports support an autosomal recessive mode of inheritance; however, it may also be inherited by autosomal dominance. No specific treatment is indicated because the lesions involute spontaneously. Tretinoin 0.1% cream may be effective.

Kandhari R, et al: Familial reactive perforating collagenosis in three siblings. Indian J Dermatol Venereol Leprol 2014; 80: 86.

Kline A, Relic J: Disseminate and recurrent infundibulofolliculitis in childhood. Pediatr Dermatol 2015; 32: e5.

Pai VV, et al: Familial reactive perforating collagenosis. Indian J Dermatol. 2014; 59: 287.

Traumatic Anserine Folliculosis

Traumatic anserine folliculosis is a curious gooseflesh-like follicular hyperkeratosis that may result from persistent pressure and lateral friction of one skin surface on another. Such friction is often caused by habitual pressure on the elbows, chin, jaw, or neck, often while watching television. Two thirds of patients who develop this are atopic.

Padilha-Gonalves A: Traumatic anserine folliculosis. J Dermatol 1979; 6: 365.

Erythromelanosis Follicularis Faciei Et Colli

Erythromelanosis follicularis faciei et colli is an erythematous pigmentary disease involving the follicles. A reddish brown, sharply demarcated, symmetric discoloration involves the preauricular and maxillary regions. At times, the pigmentation may be blotchy. In addition, follicular papules and erythema are present. Under diascopic pressure, the reddish brown area, containing telangiectases, becomes pale, and the light-brown pigmentation becomes more apparent. Pityriasiform scaling and slight itching may occur. Keratosis pilaris on the arms and shoulders is frequently found. It preferentially affects Asian and Indian patients.

Histologically, a slight hyperkeratosis occurs, with epidermal hyperpigmentation and dilation of the upper dermal vessels. The hair follicles may be enlarged in the infundibular area, and the sebaceous glands may be hypertrophic. A lymphocytic infiltration surrounds the adnexa. Successful treatment with topical tacalcitol or a dual-wavelength laser system has been reported.

Kim WJ, et al: Topical tacalcitol ointment can be a good therapeutic choice in erythromelanosis follicularis faciei et colli. J Am Acad Dermatol 2012; 67: 320.
Li YH, et al: Treatment of erythromelanosis follicularis faciei et colli using a dual-wavelength laser system. Dermatol Surg 2010; 36: 1344.

Disseminate and Recurrent Infundibulofolliculitis

Hitch and Lund described a disseminate follicular eruption on the torso of an African American man that involved all the pilosebaceous structures. The lesions were irregularly shaped papules pierced by a hair. They likened the eruption to cutis anserina viewed through a magnifying glass. The eruption is mildly pruritic at times and is chronic, with recurrent exacerbations. The papules are uniform and 1 or 2 mm in diameter. They involve all the follicles in the affected areas, which are usually the upper trunk and neck, although the entire trunk and proximal extremities may be involved. Rarely, pustules may occur.

Histologically, the infundibular portion of the follicles is chiefly affected, and the lesions are inflammatory rather than hyperkeratotic. Edema, lymphocytic and neutrophilic infiltration, and slight fibroblastic infiltration surround the affected follicles. Treatment with topical steroids, isotretinoin, or PUVA may be effective.

Hinds GA, et al: A case of disseminate and recurrent infundibulofolliculitis responsive to treatment with topical steroids. Dermatol Online J 2008; 14: 11.

Lichen Spinulosus

Lichen spinulosus (keratosis spinulosa) is primarily a disease of children and is characterized by minute, filiform horny spines, which protrude from follicular openings independent of any papules. The spines are discrete and grouped. The lesions appear in crops and are symmetrically distributed. There is a predilection for the neck, buttocks, abdominal wall, popliteal spaces, and extensor surfaces of the arms. Minimal or no itching is present. Occasional cases of a generalized form in adults with HIV infection or alcoholism have been reported.

Histologic evaluation shows simple inflammatory changes and follicular hyperkeratosis. The lesions may respond to keratolytics and emollients, such as salicylic acid, lactic acid, or urea gels or ointments. Tretinoin or tacalcitol creams are other alternatives. The lesions tend to involute at puberty.

Uehara A, et al: Successful treatment of lichen spinulosus with topical adapalene. Eur J Dermatol 2015; 25: 490.
Venkatesh A, et al: Generalized lichen spinulosus in a 4-year-old boy without systemic disease. Arch Dermatol 2012; 148: 865.

DISORDERS OF THE SWEAT GLANDS

Hyperhidrosis

Hyperhidrosis, or excessive sweating, may be localized to one or several areas or may be more generalized. True generalized hyperhidrosis is rare; even hyperhidrosis caused by systemic diseases is usually accentuated in certain regions.

Palmoplantar Hyperhidrosis (Essential Hyperhidrosis)

Palmoplantar hyperhidrosis is usually localized to the palms, soles, and/or axillae and may worsen during warm temperatures. Patients with palm and sole hyperhidrosis often have axillary hyperhidrosis, but only 25% of patients with axillary hyperhidrosis have palmoplantar hyperhidrosis. The hands may be cold and may show a dusky hue. The soggy keratin of the hyperhidrotic soles is frequently affected by pitted keratolysis and has a foul odor. Sweating may be constant or intermittent; in the latter case, anxiety, stress, or fear may trigger it. This type of sweating can be autosomal dominantly inherited. Its onset is in childhood for the palmar and plantar type and adolescence for axillary disease. It tends to improve with age. Sweating typically ceases during sleep.

Gustatory Hyperhidrosis

Certain individuals regularly experience excessive sweating of the forehead, scalp, upper lip, perioral region, or sternum a few moments after eating spicy foods, tomato sauce, chocolate, coffee, tea, or hot soups. Gustatory sweating may be idiopathic or caused by hyperactivity of the sympathetic nerves (Pancoast tumor or postoperatively), sensory neuropathy (diabetes mellitus or subsequent to zoster), parotitis or parotid abscess, and surgery or injury of the parotid gland (auriculotemporal syndrome of von Frey). Frey syndrome occurs in one third or more of patients after parotid surgery. Fortunately, only 10% of affected patients require treatment.

Other Localized Forms of Hyperhidrosis

Localized sweating can occur over lesions of blue rubber bleb nevus syndrome, glomus tumors, and hemangiomas (sudoriferous hemangioma), and in POEMS syndrome, Gopalan (burning feet) syndrome, complex regional pain syndrome resulting from spinal cord tumors (especially when unilateral palmar hyperhidrosis is the complaint), and pachydermoperiostosis.

Generalized Hyperhidrosis

Febrile diseases, vigorous exercise, or a hot, humid environment (e.g., tropical milieu) may induce generalized hyperhidrosis. Hyperthyroidism, acromegaly, diabetes mellitus, pheochromocytoma, hypoglycemia, salicylism, substance abuse, lymphoma, carcinoid syndrome, pregnancy, and menopause may also produce generalized hyperhidrosis. Additional causes of hyperhidrosis include concussion, Parkinson disease, other disturbances of the sympathetic nervous system, and metastatic tumors producing a complete transection of the spinal cord. Drugs such as anticholinesterases, antidepressants of the selective serotonin reuptake inhibitor or tricyclic types, antiglaucoma agents, bladder stimulants, opioids, and sialogogs may cause hyperhidrosis.

Treatment. Therapy of generalized hyperhidrosis focuses on treating the underlying systemic disease. Virtually all cases of hyperhidrosis seen by dermatologists are of the palmoplantar or axillary types, and the treatments discussed here relate primarily to these conditions.

Topical Medication. Topical aluminum chloride or aluminum chlorhydroxide are the agents most often used for hyperhidrosis. For the axillae, application of a 10%–35% solution nightly to a very dry axilla (blown dry with hair dryer) is usually very effective. To limit irritation, lower concentrations should be tried first. Also, it should be washed off in 6–8 hours. Occlusion is usually not required. In palmar hyperhidrosis, the application of aluminum chloride nightly in up to a 50% concentration, alone or occluded with plastic gloves, has produced good results for some patients. After topical treatment is effective when performed nightly, the frequency may be reduced to once or twice a week with continued benefit.

Botulinum Toxin. Injection of botulinum A toxin the palms, soles, or axillae dramatically reduces sweating at the treated areas to at least 25% and often to less than 10% of baseline rates. Dosages vary according to the type of botulinum toxin used and the site of treatment. (See Chapter 39 for a discussion of this treatment.) Complications are rare but include some grip weakness when higher doses are used in the palms. This problem, the expense, and the painful injections limit its use especially in the palms and soles. The hypohidrosis continues for an average of 7 months, with some patients continuing to have substantial benefit at 16 months after one injection. Repeated injections generally do not lose efficacy and result in a similar, although at times longer, response and complication rates. This form of treatment should be offered to all patients who fail topical treatments before surgical modalities are considered. Frey syndrome remits for 1–1.5 years in almost every patient treated. This treatment may be considered for other rare forms of localized hyperhidrosis. Botulinum toxin B is also effective, but with more limited duration of response.

Localized Devices. Iontophoresis with plain tap water is an alternative local therapy. It is frequently effective, using either a Drionic device or a Fischer unit. Treatments generally require 20- to 30-minute sessions each day or twice a day. Once response has occurred, treatments may be used intermittently (even to once every 2 weeks) for maintenance. Use of glycopyrrolate 0.01%, botulinum toxin, and aluminum chloride 2% in the iontophoresis medium may hasten the response.

Microwave technology that causes selective heating of the lower layers of the skin destroys the eccrine and apocrine glands thermally. Reported patient satisfaction is high. Transient edema, erythema, and pain, as well as longer-term adverse effects such as fibrous bands and muscle weakness, may occur.

Radiofrequency delivered via microneedles and laser treatment of hyperhidrosis appear to be effective, but require more study to judge response rates and adverse effects.

Internal Medication. The use of anticholinergic agents such as propantheline bromide, oxybutynin (available in extended-release formulation, which may result in lower efficacy), and glycopyrrolate may be helpful. The dosage of each is regulated by the patient's tolerance and response. Often sweating is suppressed just as anticholinergic side effects reach intolerable levels, and this approach has to be abandoned. Side effects of acetylcholine-blocking agents may also cause or aggravate such conditions as glaucoma and convulsions. The effects on sweating generally last 4–6 hours, and many patients prefer to use the medication to ensure dryness for special occasions only, rather than as continuous treatment.

Other agents reported to reduce localized hyperhidrosis include diltiazem and clonidine.

Surgical Treatment. Axillary hyperhidrosis may be effectively controlled by excision of the most actively sweating portion of the axillary skin, followed by undercutting and subcutaneous resection of the sweat glands for 1–2 cm on each side of the elliptical excision. This procedure is virtually always effective. Alternatively, liposuction or surgical ultrasonic aspiration removal may be used. The most important preoperative consideration is the accurate mapping of the most active sweating areas of the axillae. The responsible eccrine glands are not necessarily located in the same areas as the axillary hair and are often in a reasonably limited area. Mapping may be performed with cobalt chloride or starch iodide. In a comparative trial the effectiveness of botulinum toxin injections were superior to suction-curettage surgery.

Upper thoracic sympathectomy has been found to be effective in excessive palmar sweating when all other measures have failed. Sympathetic denervation of the upper extremities is performed through endoscopy by reversibly clipping or electrocautery of portions of the third through fifth rib levels. The levels interrupted depend on the type of hyperhidrosis being treated and a risk benefit discussion with the patient. Acute surgical complications occur in less than 2% of patients but include chronic pain, infection, pneumothorax, hemothorax, bleeding, pneumonia, and even death. Sweating of the hands can be stopped or improved; however, long-term adverse effects such as compensatory and gustatory hyperhidrosis occur in many patients, compromising satisfaction. These may be severe and as debilitating as the original problem. Topical glycopyrrolate may help alleviate compensatory hyperhidrosis, but it does not decrease with time. Horner syndrome may rarely result.

Baker DM: Topical glycopyrrolate reduces axillary hyperhidrosis. J Eur Acad Dermatol Venereol 2016; 30: 2131.

Cerfolio RJ, et al: The Society of Thoracic Surgeons expert consensus for the surgical treatment of hyperhidrosis. Ann Thorac Surg 2011; 91: 1642.

Chai HY, et al: Efficacy of iontophoresis with glycopyrronium bromide for treatment of primary palmar hyperhidrosis. J Eur Acad Dermatol Venereol 2012; 26: 1167.

Cheshire WP, et al: Drug-induced hyperhidrosis and hypohidrosis. Drug Saf 2008; 31: 109.

Dagash H, et al: Tap water iontophoresis in the treatment of pediatric hyperhidrosis. J Pediatr Surg 2017; 52: 309.

Doolittle J, et al: Hyperhidrosis. Arch Dermatol Res 2016; 308: 743.

Dyring-Andersen B, et al: Unilateral hyperhidrosis and hypothermia. Br J Dermatol 2016; 174: 1147.

Fatemi Naeini F, et al: A novel option for treatment of primary axillary hyperhidrosis. J Postgrad Med 2015; 61: 141.

Feldmeyer L, et al: Short- and long-term efficacy and mechanism of action of tumescent suction curettage for axillary hyperhidrosis. J Eur Acad Dermatol Venereol 2015; 29: 1933.

Gorenstein LA, Krasna MJ: Less common side effects of sympathetic surgery. Thorac Surg Clin 2016; 26: 453.

Hsu TH, et al: A systematic review of microwave-based therapy for axillary hyperhidrosis. J Cosmet Laser Ther 2017; 19: 275.

Hussain AB, et al: Shelley procedure in axillary hyperhidrosis. Clin Exp Dermatol 2016; 41: 229.

Ibrahim O, et al: The comparative effectiveness of suction-curettage and onabotulinumtoxin-A injections for the treatment of primary focal axillary hyperhidrosis. J Am Acad Dermatol 2013; 69: 88.

Laje P, et al: Thoracoscopic bilateral T3 sympathectomy for primary focal hyperhidrosis in children. J Pediatr Surg 2017; 52: 313.

Leclère FM, et al: Efficacy and safety of laser therapy on axillary hyperhidrosis after one year follow-up. Lasers Surg Med 2015; 47: 173.

Lecloufet M, et al: Duration of efficacy increases with the repetition of botulinum toxin A injections in primary palmar hyperhidrosis. J Am Acad Dermatol 2014; 70: 1083.

Montaser-Kouhsari L, et al: Comparison of intradermal injection with iontophoresis of abobotulinum toxin A for the treatment of primary axillary hyperhidrosis. J Dermatolog Treat 2014; 25: 337.

Nasr MW, et al: Comparison of microwave ablation, botulinum toxin injection, and liposuction-curettage in the treatment of axillary hyperhidrosis. J Cosmet Laser Ther 2017; 19: 36.

Ohshima Y, Tamada Y: Classification of systemic and localized sweating disorders. Curr Probl Dermatol 2016; 51: 7.

Romero FR, et al: Palmar hyperhidrosis. An Bras Dermatol 2016; 91: 716.

Schick CH: Pathophysiology of hyperhidrosis. Thorac Surg Clin 2016; 26: 389.

Schick CH, et al: Radiofrequency thermotherapy for treating axillary hyperhidrosis. Dermatol Surg 2016; 42: 624.

Seo SH, et al: Tumescent superficial liposuction with curettage for treatment of axillary hyperhidrosis. J Eur Acad Dermatol Venereol 2008; 22: 30.

Shayesteh A, et al: Primary hyperhidrosis. J Dermatol 2016; 43: 928.

Sugrue G, Mookadam F: Uncommon cause of Horner's syndrome. BMJ Case Rep 2016 Aug 26; 2016.

Wolosker N, et al: Management of compensatory sweating after sympathetic surgery. Thorac Surg Clin 2016; 26: 445.

Anhidrosis and Hypohidrosis

Anhidrosis is the absence of sweating. Hypohidrosis, or reduced sweating, is part of the spectrum of these disorders. Dysfunction in any step in the normal physiologic process of sweating can lead to decreased or absent sweating. It may be localized or generalized. Generalized anhidrosis occurs in anhidrotic ectodermal dysplasia, miliaria profunda (tropical asthenia), Sjögren syndrome, Fabry syndrome, hereditary sensory neuropathy (type IV) with anhidrosis, and in some patients with diabetic neuropathy, thyroid dysfunction, and multiple myeloma. Crisponi/CISS1 syndrome has a manifestation of anhidrosis in early childhood that converts to paradoxic cold-induced sweating around puberty. It is caused by mutations in *CRLF1* or *CLCF1*. The many drugs that may cause hypohidrosis include anticholinergics, tricyclic antidepressants, antiepileptics, antihistamines, antihypertensives, antipsychotics, antiemetics, antivertigo drugs, bladder antispasmodics, gastric antisecretory drugs, muscle relaxants, neuromuscular paralytics, and opioids. Anhidrosis may follow infections, may be part of a neurodegenerative disorder, may occur as a symptom related to toxin exposure, may be a paraneoplastic phenomenon, or may be secondary to autoimmune inflammation. Atopic dermatitis is frequently associated with reduced sweating and pruritus when sweating is triggered. Patients with psoriasis may have similar symptoms, but less frequently. There remains an idiopathic category; this variant may respond to oral steroid treatment. Remission is possible but not universal. Immunosuppressants have been ineffective.

Anhidrosis with pruritus is a rare syndrome of young adults. Severe itching occurs whenever the person is stimulated to sweat. No sweat is delivered to the skin surface, but when the body temperature is raised by about 0.5°C, fine papules appear at each eccrine orifice. The associated pruritus is so severe that the patient feels completely incapacitated and distracted. Cooling immediately resolves the symptoms. This may represent one form of tropical asthenia or a mild form of the autonomic neuropathies described

later. The natural history is unknown, but spontaneous resolution may occur after several years. These patients are frequently misdiagnosed as having cholinergic urticaria.

Segmental anhidrosis may be associated with tonic pupils (Holmes-Adie syndrome); this is called Ross syndrome. Patients have heat intolerance and segmental areas of anhidrosis on the trunk, arms, or legs. Loss of deep tendon reflexes in the arms, trunk, and legs is consistently seen. Compensatory segmental hyperhidrosis of functionally intact areas may occur. A selective degeneration of the cholinergic sudomotor neurons is the hypothesized abnormality.

Autonomic neuropathies associated with antibodies to nicotinic acetylcholine receptors may cause a variety of symptoms related to dysfunction of systems controlled by autonomic nerves. There is a spectrum of abnormalities ranging from severe autonomic failure characterized by orthostatic hypotension, GI dysmotility, anhidrosis, bladder dysfunction, and sicca syndrome to isolated anhidrosis and heat intolerance. In this condition, a biopsy may reveal an inflammatory infiltrate surrounding the eccrine glands, and some patients respond to pulse steroids or immunosuppressants. It may also spontaneously resolve.

Anhidrosis localized to skin lesions occurs regularly over plaques of tuberculoid leprosy. This is also true of segmental vitiligo (but not the generalized type), in the hypopigmented streaks of incontinentia pigmenti, in lesions of syringolymphoid hyperplasia with alopecia and anhidrosis, and on the face and neck of patients with the rare Bazex syndrome, consisting of follicular atrophoderma, basal cell carcinomas, and hypotrichosis, an X-linked dominant disorder.

Alhashem AM, et al: Crisponi/CISS1 syndrome. Am J Med Genet A 2016; 170A: 1236.

Cheshire WP, et al: Drug-induced hyperhidrosis and hypohidrosis. Drug Saf 2008; 31: 109.

Nolano M, et al: Ross syndrome. Brain 2006; 129: 2119.

Sandroni P, et al: Other autonomic neuropathies associated with ganglionic antibodies. Auton Neurosci 2009; 146: 13.

Satoh T: Clinical analysis and management of acquired idiopathic generalized anhidrosis. Curr Probl Dermatol 2016; 51: 75.

Tay LK, Chong WS: Acquired idiopathic anhidrosis. J Am Acad Dermatol 2014; 71: 499.

Vernino S, et al: Autonomic ganglia, acetylcholine receptor antibodies, and autoimmune ganglionopathy. Auton Neurosci 2009; 146: 3.

Vijayashree R, et al: Syringolymphoid hyperplasia with alopecia and anhidrosis in a 12-year-old boy. Int J Dermatol 2011; 50: 1552.

Yilmazer S, et al: Generalized anhidrosis. Neurosciences 2013; 18: 178.

Bromhidrosis

Also known as fetid sweat, osmidrosis, and malodorous sweating, bromhidrosis is chiefly encountered in the axillae. Bacterial decomposition of apocrine sweat, producing fatty acids with distinctive offensive odors, is considered to be the cause. Often, patients who complain of offensive axillary sweat actually have no offensive odor; the complaint represents a delusion, paranoia, phobia, or a lesion of the central nervous system. Intranasal foreign body and chronic mycotic infection in the sinuses are additional causes. True bromhidrosis is usually not recognized by the patient.

Fish odor syndrome (trimethylaminuria) should be considered in patients presenting with complaints of offensive odor. It is caused by excretion of trimethylamine, which has a rotten-fish odor, in the eccrine sweat, urine, saliva, and other secretions. This chemical is produced from carnitine and choline in the diet and is normally metabolized in the liver. An autosomal dominant defect in the ability to metabolize trimethylamine because of a defect in flavin-containing monooxygenase 3 is the cause of this syndrome. Dietary reduction of foods high in carnitine and choline is beneficial.

Antibacterial soaps and many commercial deodorants are quite effective in controlling axillary malodor. Frequent bathing, changing of underclothes, shaving of the axillae, and topical application of aluminum chloride (Drysol) are all helpful measures. Botulinum toxin A injections in the axilla have controlled body odor in this site as well as in the pubic area. Other remedies as described under essential hyperhidrosis are rarely indicated.

Plantar bromhidrosis is produced by bacterial action on eccrine sweat–macerated stratum corneum. Hyperhidrosis is the main associated factor, and pitted keratolysis is often present. Careful washing with an antibacterial soap and use of dusting powders on the feet are helpful in eliminating bromhidrosis. Use of topical antibiotics, such as clindamycin, may be beneficial. Previously described measures to control plantar hyperhidrosis may be instituted. Botulinum toxin A should be effective.

Li ZR, et al: Excision of apocrine glands with preservation of axillary superficial fascia for the treatment of axillary bromhidrosis. Dermatol Surg 2015; 41: 640.
Semkova K, et al: Hyperhidrosis, bromhidrosis, and chromhidrosis. Clin Dermatol 2015; 33: 483.
Ulman CA, et al: Fish odor syndrome. Dermatol Online J 2014; 20: 1260.
Zhao H, et al: Treatment of axillary bromhidrosis through a mini-incision with subdermal vascular preservation. Int J Dermatol 2016; 55: 919.

Chromhidrosis

Chromhidrosis, or colored sweat, is an exceedingly rare functional disorder of the apocrine sweat glands, frequently localized to the face or axilla. It has been less often noted on the abdomen, chest, breasts, thighs, groin, genitalia, and lower eyelids. The colored sweat may be yellow (most common), blue, green, or black. The colored secretion appears in response to adrenergic stimuli, which cause myoepithelial contractions. Colored apocrine sweat fluoresces and is caused by lipofuscin. Treatment with botulinum toxin A or topical capsaicin has been reported to be effective.

Eccrine chromhidrosis is caused by the coloring of the clear eccrine sweat by dyes, pigments, or metals on the skin surface. Examples are the blue-green sweat seen in copper workers and the "red sweat" seen in flight attendants from the red dye in the labels on life vests. Brownish staining of the axillae and undershirt may occur in ochronosis. Yellow sweat has been reported to be secondary to long-term intake of bisacodyl. Bile secretion in eccrine sweat occurs in patients with liver failure and marked hyperbilirubinemia. Small, round, brown or deep-green macules occur on the palms and soles.

Blalock TW, et al: A case of generalized red sweating. Dermatol Online J 2014 Dec 14; 21.
Gaffney DC, Cooper HL: Coloured sweat in two brothers. Australas J Dermatol 2016; 57: e23.
Ghosh SK, et al: A curious case of blue-green discoloration in a middle-aged Indian man. Dermatol Online J 2015; 21.
Triwongwaranat D, et al: Green pigmentation on the palms and soles. JAMA Dermatol 2013; 149: 1339.
Wang A, et al: Chromhidrosis. Am J Dermatopathol 2014; 36: 853.
Yöntem A, et al: Blue-colored sweating. Turk J Pediatr 2015; 57: 290.

Fox-Fordyce Disease

Fox-Fordyce disease is rare, occurring mostly in women during adolescence or soon afterward. It may occasionally be familial in

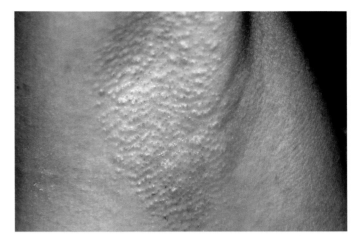

Fig. 33.37 Fox-Fordyce disease. (Courtesy Steven Binnick, MD.)

nature. It is characterized by conical, flesh-colored or grayish, intensely pruritic, discrete follicular papules in areas where apocrine glands occur (Fig. 33.37). The axillae and areolae are the primary sites of involvement, but the umbilicus, pubes, labia majora, and perineum may be affected. Apocrine sweating does not occur in affected areas, and hair density may be decreased. In some cases, there is no itching. About 90% of cases occur in women between ages 13 and 35, but the disease also may present postmenopausally, after laser hair removal, or in males. Pregnancy invariably leads to improvement.

Histologically, Fox-Fordyce disease is characterized by obstruction of the follicular ostia by orthokeratotic cells. An inflammatory infiltrate of lymphocytes surrounds the upper third of the hair follicles and upper dermal vessels. An associated spongiosis of the infundibulum occurs at the entrance of the apocrine duct into the hair follicle. In one case, detached apoeccrine cells obstructed the duct. Foam cells have been noted as a histologic marker, because many of these findings are either nonspecific or difficult to demonstrate. Localized axillary xanthomatosis has been postulated to be either a variant of Fox-Fordyce disease or a type of verruciform xanthoma.

No form of therapy is universally effective for patients with Fox-Fordyce disease. OCs, topical tretinoin or adapalene, topical pimecrolimus or weak corticosteroid creams, intralesional steroids or botumlinim toxin, topical clindamycin solution, benzoyl peroxide, isotretinoin, fractional lasers, and UV phototherapy have all been effective in small numbers of patients. Excision or liposuction-assisted curettage may be successful in axillary sites.

Al-Qarqaz F, et al: Fox-Fordyce disease treatment with fractional CO_2 laser. Int J Dermatol 2013; 52: 1572.
Bormate AB Jr, et al: Perifollicular xanthomatosis as a hallmark of axillary Fox-Fordyce disease. Arch Dermatol 2008; 144: 1020.
González-Ramos J, et al: Successful treatment of refractory pruritic Fox-Fordyce disease with botulinum toxin type A. Br J Dermatol 2016; 174: 458.
Han HH, et al: Successful treatment of areolar Fox-Fordyce disease with surgical excision and 1550-nm fractionated erbium glass laser. Int Wound J 2016; 13: 1016.
Milcic D, et al: Clinical effects of topical pimecrolimus in a patient with Fox-Fordyce disease. Australas J Dermatol 2012; 53: e34.
Sammour R, et al: Fox-Fordyce disease. J Eur Acad Dermatol Venereol 2016; 30: 1578.

Granulosis Rubra Nasi

Granulosis rubra nasi is a rare familial disease of children, occurring on the nose, cheeks, and chin. It is characterized by diffuse redness, persistent hyperhidrosis, and small, dark-red papules that disappear on diascopic pressure. The tip of the nose is red or violet. A few small pustules may occur. Hyperhidrosis precedes the erythema. The tip of the nose is cold and is not infiltrated. The disease usually disappears spontaneously at puberty, leaving no trace. The cause is unknown. Histologically, blood vessels are dilated, and an inflammatory infiltrate is seen around the sweat ducts. Treatment is with local preparations for relief of the inflammation, with involution expected at puberty. Botulinum toxin A has been effective in one case.

Grazziotin TC, et al: Treatment of granulosis rubra nasi with botulinum toxin type A. Dermatol Surg 2009; 35: 1298.
Sargunam C, et al: Granulosis rubra nasi. Indian Dermatol Online J 2013; 4: 208.

Hidradenitis

Hidradenitis is a term used to describe diseases in which the histologic abnormality is primarily an inflammatory infiltrate around the eccrine glands. This group includes neutrophilic eccrine hidradenitis and idiopathic plantar hidradenitis (recurrent palmoplantar hidradenitis). Hidradenitis suppurativa is discussed in Chapter 13.

Neutrophilic Eccrine Hidradenitis

Ninety percent of patients with neutrophilic eccrine hidradenitis (NEH) have a malignancy. NEH has been described primarily in patients with acute myelogenous leukemia (AML); however, other leukemias, lymphomas, and infrequently solid tumors may be present. It usually begins about 10 days after the start of treatment. Although the majority of patients have been treated with cytarabine, NEH has not been uniformly linked to any chemotherapeutic or targeted therapy agent and may occur in untreated patients. Patients with AML in remission have been reported to develop NEH, with associated sclerodermoid changes that herald a relapse of the leukemia. Granulocyte colony-stimulating factor, imatinib mesylate, BRAF inhibitors, combination highly active retroviral therapy combination zidovudine, decitabine, acetaminophen, and various antibiotics have also been implicated as triggers for this neutrophilic dermatosis.

The lesions are typically erythematous and edematous papules and plaques of the extremities, trunk, face (periorbital), and palms (in decreasing frequency). Pigmentation, purpura, or pustules may be present within the papules and plaques. Fever and neutropenia are often present. Histologically, there is a dense neutrophilic infiltrate around and infiltrating eccrine glands. Necrosis of sweat glands may be present, with or without the inflammatory infiltrate. Syringosquamous metaplasia may occur. This finding can also occur in fibrosing alopecia, in burn scars, adjacent to various nonmelanoma skin cancers and ischemic and surgical ulcers, in alopecia mucinosa, and in ports of radiation therapy.

The lesions may recur with repeated courses of chemotherapy, but many do not. Resolution over 1–4 weeks (average 10 days) usually occurs. Nonsteroidal antiinflammatory drugs or oral corticosteroids may hasten the healing. Prophylactic administration of dapsone prevented recurrence in one patient.

Infections may also precipitate neutrophilic hidradenitis as a recurrent, pruritic, papular eruption. *Serratia, Enterobacter cloacae, Nocardia,* and *S. aureus* have been implicated, and appropriate antibiotics for bacterial agents are curative. The diagnosis is confirmed by histologic evaluation and culture of affected tissue (surface cultures may not be adequate). Additionally, many HIV-infected patients have developed neutrophilic eccrine hidradenitis. An idiopathic generalized variant has occurred in four healthy Asian children ages 6–16 months. Spontaneous resolution is reported.

Recurrent Palmoplantar Hidradenitis

Recurrent palmoplantar hidradenitis is primarily a disorder of healthy children and young adults. Lesions are primarily painful, subcutaneous nodules on the plantar surface, resembling erythema nodosum. Rarely, palmar lesions also occur. In some children, *Pseudomonas* infection may be the cause (pseudomonal hot foot syndrome; see Chapter 14, *P. aeruginosa* folliculitis). Children may present refusing to walk because of plantar pain. The condition is typically recurrent and may be triggered by exposure to wet shoes or cold, damp weather. The use of oral and topical steroidal preparations may be beneficial.

Abbas O, et al: Question: Can you identify this condition? Palmoplantar eccrine hidradenitis. Can Fam Physician 2010; 56: 666.
Andreu-Barasoain M, et al: Generalized idiopathic neutrophilic eccrine hidradenitis in a 7-month-old child. J Am Acad Dermatol 2012; 67: e133.
Herms F, et al: Neutrophilic eccrine hidradenitis in two patients treated with BRAF inhibitors. Br J Dermatol 2017; 176: 1645.
Oscoz-Jaime S, et al: Neutrophilic eccrine hidradenitis in a patient treated with highly activity antiretroviral therapy. Med Clin (Barc) 2017; 148: 93.

DISEASES OF THE NAILS

Several general references are available that review a wide spectrum of nail changes.

André J, et al: Nail pathology. Clin Dermatol 2013; 31: 526.
Baran R, et al: Diseases of the nails and their management. Hoboken: Wiley, 2012.
Baran R, et al: Nail therapies. Boca Raton: CRC Press, 2012.
Baswan S, et al: Understanding the formidable nail barrier. Mycoses 2017; 60: 284.
Chernoff KA, Scher RK: Nail disorders. Clin Dermatol 2016; 34: 736.
Choi JN: Dermatologic adverse events to chemotherapeutic agents, part 2. Semin Cutan Med Surg 2014; 33: 40.
Chu DH, et al: Diagnosis and management of nail disorders in children. Pediatr Clin North Am 2014; 61: 293.
Flint WW, et al: Nail and skin disorders of the foot. Med Clin North Am 2014; 98: 213.
Haneke E: Nail surgery. Clin Dermatol 2013; 31: 516.
iKhan S, et al: Genetics of human isolated hereditary nail disorders. Br J Dermatol 2015; 173: 922.
Kyllo RL, Anadkat MJ: Dermatologic adverse events to chemotherapeutic agents, part 1. Semin Cutan Med Surg 2014; 33: 28.
Park JH, et al: Nail neoplasm. J Dermatol 2017; 44: 279.
Robert C, et al: Nail toxicities induced by systemic anticancer treatments. Lancet Oncol 2015; 16: e181.
Stephen S, et al: Diagnostic applications of nail clippings. Dermatol Clin 2015; 33: 289.
Tosti A, et al: Color atlas of nails. New York: Springer, 2010.
Uraloglu M, et al: Congenital nail abnormalities. Ann Plast Surg 2014; 73: 346.
Zaiac MN, et al: Nail abnormalities associated with systemic pathologies. Clin Dermatol 2013; 31: 627.

Nail-Associated Dermatoses

Numerous dermatoses are associated with characteristic, sometimes specific, nail changes. Many are considered in other chapters.

Lichen Planus of Nails

The reported incidence of nail involvement in lichen planus varies from 5%–10%. Lichen planus of the nails occurs without skin changes, but most with nail disease will have lichen planus at other locations. Although it may occur at any age, most frequently it begins during the fifth or sixth decade of life. The nail plate may be greatly thinned, and at times, distinct papules of lichen planus may involve the nail bed. Twenty-nail dystrophy (trachyonychia) may be the sole manifestation of lichen planus. Other nail changes are irregular longitudinal grooving and ridging of the nail plate, thinning of the nail plate, pterygium formation, shedding of the nail plate with atrophy of the nail bed, subungual keratosis, or even onychopapilloma, erythronychia (red streaks), subungual hyperpigmentation, and nail degloving (Figs. 33.38 and 33.39).

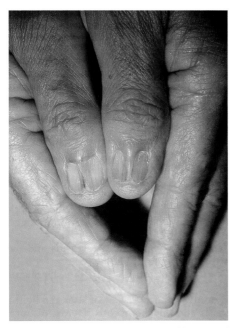

Fig. 33.38 Pterygium caused by lichen planus. (Courtesy Dr. Lawrence Lieblich.)

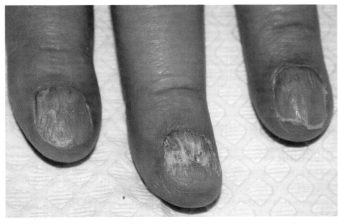

Fig. 33.39 Nail lichen planus.

This last sign involves partial or total shedding of the nail or the entire nail apparatus. The surrounding skin may also slough. This may be caused by trauma, ischemia and gangrene, or severe dermatologic disease such as toxic epidermal necrolysis or lichen planus.

The histologic changes of lichen planus may be evident in any individual nail constituent or a combination of them. The constituent most frequently involved is the matrix.

Treatment with intralesional injection of corticosteroids may be effective. Digital nerve blocks should be considered before infiltration of the matrix or nail bed. Topical corticosteroids under polyethylene occlusive dressings are usually inadequate; however, when applied with tazarotene it may be successful. Oral prednisone (0.5–1 mg/kg for 3 weeks) or oral retinoids in combination with topical corticosteroids applied to the involved sites has been successful in some patients. Tosti et al. reported that children with typical lichen planus of the nails responded to 0.5–1 mg/kg per month of intramuscular triamcinolone acetonide given for 3–6 months, until the proximal half of the nail was normalized. Disease recurred in only two patients during the follow-up period. Although twenty-nail dystrophy was not treated, patients spontaneously improved; those with idiopathic atrophy of the nails were unchanged. (See Chapter 12 for additional therapeutic considerations.)

Baran R, et al: Nail degloving, a polyetiologic condition with 3 main patterns. J Am Acad Dermatol 2008; 58:232.

Brauns B, et al: Intralesional steroid injection alleviates nail lichen planus. Int J Dermatol 2011; 50: 626.

Goettmann S, et al: Nail lichen planus. J Eur Acad Dermatol Venereol 2012; 26: 1304.

Jellinek NJ: Longitudinal erythronychia. J Am Acad Dermatol 2011; 64: 167e1.

Nakamura R, et al: Dermatoscopy of nail lichen planus. Int J Dermatol 2013; 52: 684.

Piraccini BM, et al: Nail lichen planus. Eur J Dermatol 2010; 20: 489.

Richert B, et al: Nail bed lichen planus associated with onychopapilloma. Br J Dermatol 2007; 156: 107.

Tosti A, et al: Nail lichen planus in children. Arch Dermatol 2001; 137: 1027.

Psoriatic Nails

Nail involvement in psoriasis is common, with the reported incidence varying from 10%–78%. Older patients, those with active exacerbations of disease, and those with psoriatic arthritis are more likely to express nail abnormalities. The nail plate may have pits (Fig. 33.40), or much less often, furrows or transverse depressions (Beau lines), crumbling nail plate, or leukonychia, with a rough or smooth surface. Splinter hemorrhages are found in the nail bed, with reddish discoloration of a part or all of the nail bed, and horny masses. In the hyponychium, subungual hyperkeratosis, oil spots (Fig. 33.41), and a yellowish green discoloration may occur in the area of onycholysis. Onychomycosis may be closely simulated. The severity of nail disease may correlate with the severity of skin and joint disease. Pustular psoriasis may produce onycholysis, with lakes of pus in the nail bed or in the perionychial areas. Rarely, anonychia may result. Other papulosquamous diseases may affect the nails similar to psoriasis, with the exception of nail pitting. Reiter disease, pityriasis rubra pilaris, Sézary syndrome, and acrokeratosis paraneoplastica produce hypertrophic nails with subungual hyperkeratosis.

Psoriatic nail disease may be a solitary finding or may be part of a widespread skin and nail involvement. The treatment options selected depend on the degree of cutaneous and nail involvement (see Chapter 10 for additional information and therapeutic options). Successful systemic treatment of psoriasis will usually also improve or clear the nail changes. Methotrexate, PUVA, cyclosporine,

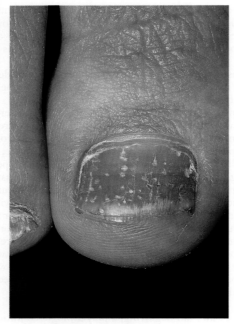

Fig. 33.40 Pitting caused by psoriasis.

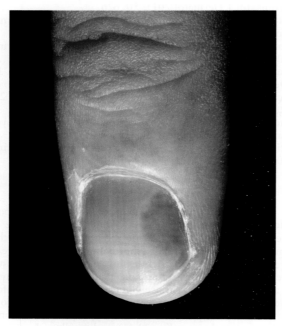

Fig. 33.41 Oil spot in a psoriatic nail.

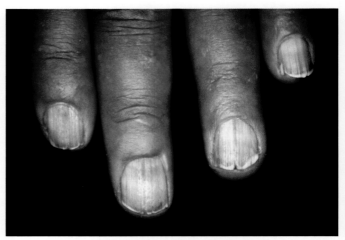

Fig. 33.42 Darier disease of the nail.

Armstrong AW, et al: Treatments for nail psoriasis. J Rheumatol 2014; 41: 2306.

Crowley JJ, et al: Treatment of nail psoriasis. JAMA Dermatol 2015; 151: 87.

Demirsoy EO, et al: Effectiveness of systemic treatment agents on psoriatic nails. J Drugs Dermatol 2013; 12: 1039.

de Vries AC, et al: Interventions for nail psoriasis. Cochrane Database Syst Rev 2013; 1: CD007633.

Diluvio L, et al: Childhood nail psoriasis. Pediatr Dermatol 2007; 24: 332.

Manhart R, Rich P: Nail psoriasis. Clin Exp Rheumatol 2015; 33: S7.

Maranda EL, et al: Laser and light therapies for the treatment of nail psoriasis. J Eur Acad Dermatol Venereol 2016; 30: 1278.

Pasch MC: Nail psoriasis. Drugs 2016; 76: 675.

Pourchot D, et al: Nail psoriasis. Pediatr Dermatol 2017; 34: 58.

Raposo I, Torres T: Nail psoriasis as a predictor of the development of psoriatic arthritis. Actas Dermosifiliogr 2015; 106: 452.

Sandre MK, Rohekar S: Psoriatic arthritis and nail changes. Semin Arthritis Rheum 2014; 44: 162.

Schons KR, et al: Nail psoriasis. An Bras Dermatol 2014; 89: 312.

Wiznia LE, et al: A clinical review of laser and light therapy for nail psoriasis and onychomycosis. Dermatol Surg 2017; 43: 161.

Darier Disease

Longitudinal, subungual, red or white streaks, associated with distal wedge-shaped subungual keratoses, are the nail signs diagnostic for Darier-White disease (Fig. 33.42). Keratotic papules on the dorsal portion of the nailfold may clinically resemble acrokeratosis verruciformis, but histologically, they have features of Darier disease. Other nail findings include splinter hemorrhages and leukonychia. All these findings are less pronounced on the toenails.

Halteh P, et al: Darier disease. Postgrad Med J 2016; 92: 425.

Clubbing

Clubbing is divided into two types: idiopathic and acquired, or secondary. The changes occur not only in the nails but also in the terminal phalanges. The nails bulge and are curved in a convex arc in both transverse and longitudinal directions (Fig. 33.43). The eponychium is thickened. The angle formed by the dorsal

biologics, or acitretin may be effective. All local therapies have limitations. Intralesional injection of triamcinolone acetonide suspension, 3–5 mg/mL, with a 30-gauge needle is frequently helpful. Digital nerve block facilitates adequate injection. A variety of lasers, phototherapy, and PDT are other procedural treatments with reported efficacy. Topical 5-fluorouracil (5-FU) applied to the proximal nailfold has been reported to be effective. It is best to avoid the free edge of the nail when applying 5-FU because it may cause distal onycholysis. Topical cyclosporine, tacrolimus and topical tazarotene 0.1% gel may also be helpful. Topical calcipotriol improves about 50% of patients with localized pustular psoriasis of the nails and may be used as a maintenance treatment after successful intervention with systemic retinoids.

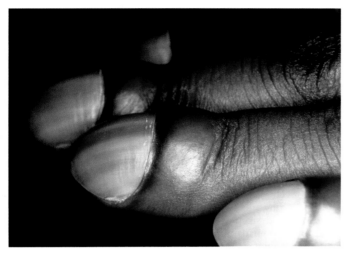

Fig. 33.43 Clubbing.

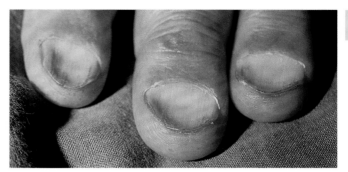

Fig. 33.44 Koilonychia.

Shell Nail Syndrome

Cornelius described a shell nail in association with bronchiectasis. The nail resembles a clubbed nail, but the nail bed is atrophic instead of being a bulbous proliferation of the soft tissue.

Cornelius CE: Shell nail syndrome. Arch Dermatol 1969; 100: 118.

Koilonychia (Spoon Nails)

Spoon nails are thin and concave, with the edges everted so that if a drop of water were placed on the nail, it would not run off (Fig. 33.44). Koilonychia may result from faulty iron metabolism and is one of the signs of Plummer-Vinson syndrome, as well as of hemochromatosis. Spoon nails have been observed in coronary disease, syphilis, polycythemia, and acanthosis nigricans. Familial forms are also known to occur. Other associations include psoriasis, lichen planus, Raynaud syndrome, scleroderma, acromegaly, hypothyroidism and hyperthyroidism, monilethrix, palmar hyperkeratoses, and steatocystoma multiplex. A significant number of cases are idiopathic. Manual trauma in combination with cold exposure may result in seasonal disease. Sherpas people living in the Nepalese Himalayas, who often serve as porters on mountain-climbing expeditions. Chronic cold exposure, in combination with hypoxemia, may contribute to the high frequency with which koilonychia is observed among them and people living in the Leh Ladahk region of India.

Walker J, et al: Koilonychia. J Eur Acad Dermatol Venereol 2016; 30: 1985.
Yanamandra U, et al: Ladakhi koilonychia. BMJ Case Rep 2014 Jan 16; 2014.

Congenital Onychodysplasia of Index Fingers

Congenital onychodysplasia of the index fingers is defined by the presence of the condition at birth, index finger involvement (unilateral or bilateral), variable distortion of the nail or lunula, and polyonychia, micronychia, anonychia, hemionychogryphosis, or malalignment. It may also involve adjacent fingers, such as the middle fingers and thumbs. An underlying bone dysplasia may be present beneath the involved nail. Cases have occurred in an autosomal dominant pattern; other proposed causes include in utero ischemia or exposure to teratogens.

Hussein TP, et al: Malformations of the index nails. Clin Exp Dermatol 2009; 34: 890.
Park SW, et al: Treatment of congenital onychodysplasia of the index finger with specialized nail device. Clin Exp Dermatol 2013; 38: 791.

surface of the distal phalanx and the nail plate (Lovibond angle) is approximately 160 degrees; with clubbing, however, this angle is obliterated and becomes 180 degrees or greater. There is no diamond-shaped window when the dorsal surfaces of the corresponding finger of each hand are opposed (Schamroth sign). The soft tissues of the terminal phalanx are bulbous and are mobile when pressure is applied over the matrix. Thickening of the nail bed is present and can be assessed reliably by a plain radiograph of the index finger.

Idiopathic clubbing is either the isolated dominantly inherited type or the pachydermoperiostosis type with its associated findings. In the hereditary isolated type, mutations of the human *HPGD* gene encoding NAD(+)-dependent 15-hydroxyprostaglandin dehydrogenase and the prostaglandin transporter SLCO2A1 have been identified. Secondary (acquired) clubbing is usually a consequence of pulmonary, cardiac, thyroid, hepatic, or GI disease. About 36% of HIV-infected patients have clubbed nails. Typically, there is periostitis, with periosteal new bone formation in the phalanges, metacarpals, and distal ulna and radius. This is called hypertrophic osteoarthropathy and is responsible for the painful clubbing. It typically occurs in men with bronchogenic carcinoma. Unilateral or asymmetric clubbing may also occur in Takayasu arteritis and sarcoidosis.

Anoop TM, et al: Differential clubbing and cyanosis. N Engl J Med 2011; 364: 666.
Callemeyn J, et al: Clubbing and hypertrophic osteoarthropathy. Acta Clin Belg 2016; 71: 123.
Carlson S, Rauchenstein J: Hypertrophic osteoarthropathy. J Am Osteopath Assoc 2015; 115: 745.
Ciment AJ, Ciment L: Regression of clubbing after treatment of lung cancer. N Engl J Med 2016; 375: 1171.
Dever LL, et al: Digital clubbing in HIV-infected patients. AIDS Patient Care STDS 2009; 23: 19.
Pallarés-Sanmartin A, et al: Validity and reliability of the Schamroth sign for the diagnosis of digital clubbing. JAMA 2010; 304: 159.
Spicknall KE, et al: Clubbing. J Am Acad Dermatol 2005; 52: 1020.
Tüysüz B, et al: Primary hypertrophic osteoarthropathy caused by homozygous deletion in *HPGD* gene in a family. Rheumatol Int 2014; 34: 1539.
Zhang Z, et al: Two novel mutations in the SLCO2A1 gene in a Chinese patient with primary hypertrophic osteoarthropathy. Gene 2014; 534: 421.

Trachyonychia

The nails may become opalescent, thin, dull, fragile, and finely ridged longitudinally (and as a result, distally notched). When this involves all 20 nails, it is referred to as *twenty-nail dystrophy*. This latter presentation may be seen at any age from 1½ years to adulthood, although it is most frequently diagnosed in children. It can be idiopathic or may be caused by alopecia areata, psoriasis, lichen planus, atopy, ichthyosis vulgaris, or other inflammatory dermatoses. Familial forms exist. In some cases, spongiosis may be found on nail biopsy. Trachyonychia has also been reported associated with autoimmune processes such as selective IgA deficiency, vitiligo, sarcoidosis, and graft-versus-host disease. Unilateral involvement may occur in complex regional pain syndrome. Thus it is caused by a heterogeneous group of inflammatory conditions. Tazarotene alone or in association with topical corticosteroids may improve the condition. Childhood cases may resolve spontaneously; in one study, 82% cleared within 6 years.

Gordon KA, et al: Trachyonychia. Indian J Dermatol Venereol Leprol 2011; 77: 640.
Kumar MG, et al: Long-term follow-up of pediatric trachyonychia. Pediatr Dermatol 2015; 32: 198.
Sakata S, et al: Follow up of 12 patients with trachyonychia. Australas J Dermatol 2006; 47: 166.

Onychauxis

In onychauxis, the nails are thickened but without deformity (simple hypertrophy). Simple thickening of the nails may be the result of trauma, acromegaly, Darier disease, psoriasis, or pityriasis rubra pilaris. Some cases are hereditary. Treatment involves periodic partial or total debridement of the thickened nail plate by mechanical or chemical (40% urea paste) means. Matricectomy and nail ablation are options, as they are in onychogryphosis, congenital nail dystrophies, and chronic painful nails, such as recalcitrant ingrown toenails or splits within the medial or lateral third of the nail.

Baran R, et al: Matricectomy and nail ablation. Hand Clin 2002; 18: 696.
Singh G, et al: Nail changes and disorders among the elderly. Indian J Dermatol Venereol Leprol 2005; 71: 386.

Onychogryphosis

Hypertrophy may produce nails resembling claws or a ram's horn. Onychogryphosis may be caused by trauma or peripheral vascular disorders but is most often caused by neglect (failure to cut the nails for very long periods). It is most often seen in elderly persons. Liquid nitrogen applied to the thick nail just before trimming makes it easier. Some recommend avulsion of the nail plate with surgical destruction of the matrix with phenol or the CO_2 laser, if the blood supply is good.

Yang TH, Tsai HH: Performing cryotherapy on onychogryphotic nails before nail trimming. J Am Acad Dermatol 2016; 75: e69.

Onychophosis

A common finding in the elderly population, onychophosis is a localized or diffuse hyperkeratotic tissue that develops on the lateral or proximal nailfolds, within the space between the nailfolds and the nail plate. It may involve the subungual area, as a direct result of repeated minor trauma, and most frequently affects the first and fifth toes. The use of comfortable shoes should be encouraged. The areas involved should be debrided and treated with keratolytics. Emollients are also helpful.

Singh G, et al: Nail changes and disorders among the elderly. Indian J Dermatol Venereol Leprol 2005; 71: 386.

Anonychia

Absence of nails, a rare anomaly, may be the result of a congenital ectodermal defect, ichthyosis, severe infection, prenatal phenytoin exposure, severe allergic contact dermatitis, self-inflicted trauma, Raynaud phenomenon, lichen planus, epidermolysis bullosa, or severe exfoliative diseases. Permanent anonychia has been reported as a sequel of Stevens-Johnson syndrome. It may also be found in association with congenital developmental abnormalities, such as microcephaly, and wide-spaced teeth (autosomal recessive inheritance), autosomal dominant Cooks syndrome (brachydactyly anonychia), which has been associated with duplications of the noncoding elements of Sox9, DOOR syndrome (deafness, onycho-osteodystrophy, mental retardation), and the glossopalatine syndrome (abnormal mouth, tongue being attached to temporomandibular joint).

Anonychia may also present as an autosomal recessive disorder with anonchyia as the solitary finding. It has been found to be caused by a mutation in the gene for R-spondin 4. R-spondins are secreted proteins that activate the Wnt/β-catenin signaling pathway. R-spondin 4 is exclusively expressed in the mesenchyme underlying the digit tip epithelium in embryonic mice.

Ishii Y, et al: Mutations in R-spondin 4 underlie inherited anonychia. J Invest Dermatol 2008; 128: 867.
Kurth I, et al: Duplications of noncoding elements 5′ of *SOX9* are associated with brachydactyly-anonychia. Nat Genet 2009; 41: 862.
Qureshi A, et al: Congenital anonychia. J Hand Surg Eur Vol 2016; 41: 348.
Singal A, Daulatabad D: Nail tic disorders. Indian J Dermatol Venereol Leprol 2017; 83: 19.
Wasif N, et al: A novel nonsense mutation in *RSP04* gene underlies autosomal recessive congenital anonychia in a Pakistani family. Pediatr Dermatol 2013; 30: 139.

Onychoatrophy

Faulty underdevelopment of the nail may be congenital or acquired. The nail is thinned and small. Vascular disturbances, epidermolysis bullosa, onychotillomania, lichen planus, Darier disease, multicentric reticulohistiocytosis, and Hansen disease may cause onychoatrophy. Onychoatrophy is also seen in congenital syndromes such as Apert, Goltz, Turner, Ellis–van Creveld, nail-patella, dyskeratosis congenita, cartilage-hair hypoplasia, progeria, hypohidrotic ectodermal dysplasia, incontinentia pigmenti, popliteal web, trisomy 13, trisomy 18, and as a side effect of etretinate therapy.

Onychomadesis

Onychomadesis is a periodic idiopathic shedding of the nail beginning at its proximal end (Fig. 33.45). The temporary arrest of the function of the nail matrix may cause onychomadesis. Neurologic disorders, peritoneal dialysis, cutaneous T-cell lymphoma, Kawasaki disease, pemphigus vulgaris, drug allergy, hand, foot, and mouth disease, varicella infection, Cronkite-Canada syndrome, and keratosis punctata palmaris et plantaris have been reported causes. It may appear as a periodic finding in runners. Immobilization from casting for fractures may cause onychomadesis. Medications such as antineoplastic agents, valproic acid, azithromycin, and retinoids may cause onychomadesis as well. It may be an idiopathic finding in adults and neonates.

Apalla Z, et al: Onychomadesis after hand-foot-and-mouth disease outbreak in northern Greece. Int J Dermatol 2015; 54: 1039.

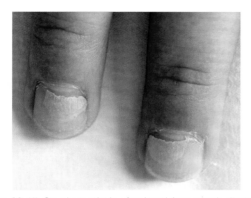

Fig. 33.45 Onychomadesis after hand-foot-mouth disease.

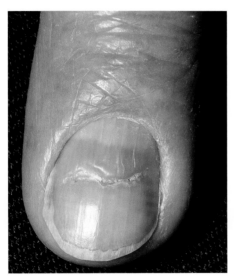

Fig. 33.46 Beau lines.

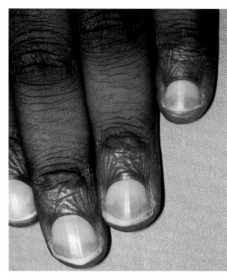

Fig. 33.47 Half and half nails.

Hardin J, Haber RM: Onychomadesis. Br J Dermatol 2015; 172: 592.
Salgado F, et al: Shedding light on onychomadesis. Cutis 2017; 99: 33.

Beau Lines

Beau lines are transverse furrows that begin in the matrix and progress distally as the nail grows (Fig. 33.46). They are ascribed to the temporary arrest of function of the nail matrix. Although usually found to be bilateral, unilateral Beau lines may occur. Various systemic and local traumatic factors may cause the lines. They may result from almost any systemic illness or major injury, such as a broken hip. Some specific associations are childbirth, measles, paronychia, acute febrile illnesses, high-altitude exposure, and drug reaction. When the process is intermittent, the nail plate may resemble corduroy. Shelley "shoreline" nails appear to be a severe expression of essentially the same transient growth arrest. Beau lines have been reported in all 20 nails of a newborn.

Park J, et al: Images in clinical medicine. Multiple Beau's lines. N Engl J Med 2010; 362: e63.
Ryu H, et al: Beau's lines of the fingernails. Am J Med Sci 2015; 349: 363.

Half and Half Nails

Half and half nails show the proximal portion of the nail white and the distal half red, pink, or brown, with a sharp line of demarcation between the two halves (Fig. 33.47). About 76% of hemodialysis patients and 56% of renal transplant patients have at least one type of nail abnormality. Half and half nails are the most common, affecting 20% of hemodialysis patients. Absence of lunula, splinter hemorrhage, and half and half nails were significantly more common in hemodialysis patients, whereas leukonychia was significantly more common in transplant patients.

Galperin TA, et al: Cutaneous manifestations of ESRD. Clin J Am Soc Nephrol 2014; 9: 201.
Manaktala PS, et al: Half and half nails (Lindsay's nails) in chronic renal disease. J Assoc Physicians India 2014; 62: 44.

Muehrcke Lines

Muehrcke described narrow, white transverse bands occurring in pairs as a sign of chronic hypoalbuminemia. The lines may resolve when serum albumin is raised to or near normal (Fig. 33.48). Unlike Mees lines, the disturbance appears to be in the nail bed, not in the nail plate. Similar lines have been reported in patients with normal albumin levels who are receiving chemotherapy. In a case of unilateral Muehrcke lines associated with trauma, it was suggested that edema effects this change by inducing microscopic separation of the normally tightly adherent nail from its bed.

Short N, et al: Muehrcke's lines. Am J Med 2010; 123: 991.
Stanifer J, et al: Muehrcke's lines as a diagnostic clue to increased catabolism and a severe system disease state. Am J Med Sci 2011; 342: 331.

Mees Lines

Mees described single or multiple white transverse bands in 1919 as a sign of inorganic arsenic poisoning (Fig. 33.49). They have also been reported in thallium poisoning, septicemia, dissecting aortic aneurysm, parasitic infections, chemotherapy, as an idiopathic finding, and in both acute and chronic renal failure.

Chauhan S, et al: Mees' lines. Lancet 2008; 372: 1410.
Hadi A, Stern D: Acquired idiopathic true transverse leukonychia. Skinmed 2017, 15: 315.

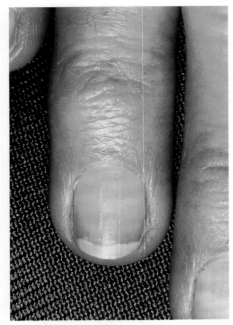

Fig. 33.48 Muehrcke lines.

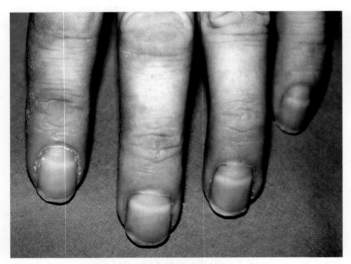

Fig. 33.49 Mees lines.

Lu CI, et al: Short-term thallium intoxication. Arch Dermatol 2007; 143: 93.

Terry Nails

In Terry nails, the distal 1–2 mm of the nail shows a normal pink color (Fig. 33.50), whereas the entire nail plate or proximal end has a white appearance as a result of telangiectases in the nail bed. These changes have been noted in 25% of hospitalized patients, most often those with cirrhosis, chronic congestive heart failure, and adult-onset diabetes, and in very elderly patients.

Baran B, et al: Terry's nail. Hepatobiliary Pancreat Dis Int 2013; 12: 109.
Nia AM, et al: Terry's nails. Am J Med 2011; 124: 602.

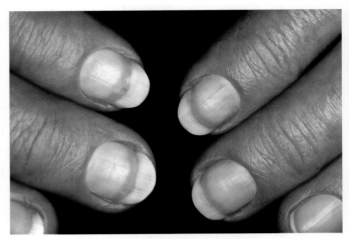

Fig. 33.50 Terry nail.

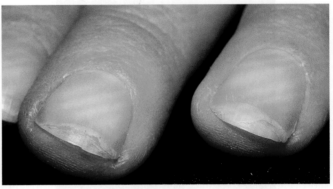

Fig. 33.51 Onychoschizia.

Onychorrhexis (Brittle Nails)

Brittleness with breakage of the nails may result from frequent soap and water exposure, nail polish remover, hypothyroidism, anorexia or bulimia, or with epidermal growth factor receptor inhibitor, ibrutinib, or oral retinoid therapy. It affects up to 20% of the population, women twice as often as men. In a series of 35 patients treated with biotin, 63% showed clinical improvement. The nail plate thickness in patients treated with biotin increases by 25%. Daily application of white petrolatum after soaking in water is also helpful.

Nanda S, et al: Utility of gel nails in improving the appearance of cosmetically disfigured nails. J Cutan Aesthet Surg 2014; 7: 26.
Stulhofer Buzina D, et al: Adverse reaction to cetuximab, an epidermal growth factor receptor inhibitor. Acta Dermatovenerol Croat 2016; 24: 70.
Van de Kerkhof PC: Brittle nail syndrome. J Am Acad Dermatol 2005; 53: 644.

Onychoschizia

Splitting of the distal nail plate into layers at the free edge is a very common problem among women and in 30% of newborns. It represents a dyshesion of the layers of keratin, likely as a result of dehydration (Fig. 33.51). Longitudinal splits may also occur. Patients with biotinidase deficiency may manifest onychoschizia, along with total or partial alopecia and an eczematous or desquamating periorificial eruption. Hypotonia, seizures, and developmental delay in children and depression in adults are the most common systemic abnormalities. Lack of treatment may result in loss of hearing and vision.

Nail polish should be discontinued; nail buffing can be substituted. Use of gel nails is well accepted and effective. Frequent application of emollients may be helpful. Biotin has also been shown to be effective in doses up to 2.5 mg/day, or two to four times that much in deficient patients.

Chinazzo M, et al: Nail features in healthy term newborns. J Eur Acad Dermatol Venereol 2017; 31: 371.

Stippled Nails

Small, pinpoint depressions in an otherwise normal nail characterize this type of nail change. This may be an early change seen in psoriasis. Stippled nails are also seen with some cases of alopecia areata, in early lichen planus, psoriatic or rheumatoid arthritis, chronic eczematous dermatitis, perforating granuloma annulare, and in some individuals with no apparent disease. The deeper, broader pits are more specific for psoriasis. The pitting in alopecia areata tends to be shallower and more regular, suggesting a "Scotch plaid" (tartan) pattern. Patients with such changes usually have more severe alopecia areata than those without this finding.

Tosti A, et al: Prevalence of nail abnormalities in children with alopecia areata. Pediatr Dermatol 1994; 11: 12.
You HR, Kim SJ: Factors associated with severity of alopecia areata. Ann Dermatol 2017; 29: 565.

Racquet Nails (Nail en Raquette)

In racquet nails, the end of the thumb is widened and flattened, the nail plate is flattened as well, and the distal phalanx is abnormally short (Fig. 33.52). Racquet nails occur on one or both thumbs and are usually inherited as an autosomal dominant trait. Acquired cases have been documented in hyperparathyroidism and Erasmus syndrome (systemic sclerosis following silica exposure).

Baran R, et al: Acquired racquet nails. J Eur Acad Dermatol Venereol 2014; 28: 257.
Vetrichevvel TP, et al: Acquired racquet nails in Erasmus syndrome. Int J Dermatol 2010; 49: 932.

Chevron Nail (Herringbone Nail)

This entity is a rare, transient fingernail ridge pattern of children. The ridges arise from the proximal nailfold and converge in a V-shaped pattern toward a midpoint distally.

Delano S, et al: Chevron nails. Pediatr Dermatol 2014; 31: e24.

Hapalonychia

Softened nails result from a defect in the matrix that makes the nails thin and soft so that they can be easily bent. This type of nail change is attributed to malnutrition and debility. It may be associated with myxedema, rheumatoid arthritis, anorexia, bulimia, Hansen disease, Raynaud phenomenon, oral retinoid therapy, or radiodermatitis.

Baran R, et al: Baran and Dawber's diseases of the nails and their management. Oxford: Blackwell Scientific, 2012.

Platonychia

The nail is abnormally flat and broad. It may be seen as part of an autosomal dominant condition in which multiple nail abnormalities are present in many members of a large family.

Hamm H, et al: Isolated congenital nail dysplasia. Arch Dermatol 2000; 136: 1239.

Nail-Patella Syndrome (Hereditary Osteo-Onychodysplasia, Fong Syndrome)

Nail-patella syndrome comprises numerous anomalies and is characterized by the absence or hypoplasia of the patella and congenital nail dystrophy. Triangular lunulae are characteristic (Fig. 33.53). Other bone features are thickened scapulae, hyperextensible joints, radial head abnormalities, and posterior iliac horns. The skin changes may also include webbing of the elbows. Eye changes such as cataracts, glaucoma, and heterochromia of the iris may also be present. Hyperpigmentation of the pupillary margin of the iris ("Lester iris") is a characteristic finding in about half the cases. Patients with nail-patella syndrome may exhibit glomerulonephritis with urinary findings of albuminuria, hematuria, and casts of all kinds, especially hyaline casts. They may be predisposed to developing hemolytic-uremic syndrome, edema, and hypertension. About 60% of patients have renal abnormalities, and 20% develop renal failure. It is an autosomal dominant trait; mutations of the human *LMX1B* gene result in this syndrome.

Fernandes GC, et al: Nail-patella syndrome. J Clin Rheumatol 2011; 17: 402.
Figueroa-Silva O, et al: Nail-patella syndrome. J Eur Acad Dermatol Venereol 2016; 30: 1614.
Ghoumid J, et al: Nail-patella syndrome. Eur J Hum Genet 2016; 24: 44.

Onychophagia

Nail biting is a common compulsive behavior that may greatly shorten the nail bed, sometimes damages the matrix, and at times

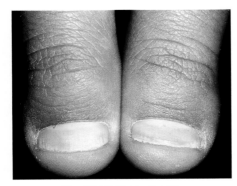

Fig. 33.52 Racquet nails.

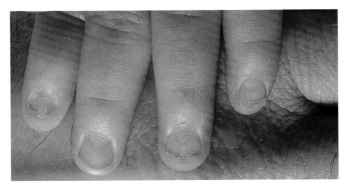

Fig. 33.53 Nail-patella syndrome. (Courtesy Dr. Marshall Guill.)

leads to longitudinal melanonychia or pterygium formation. It is a difficult habit to cure. If there is strong motivation, habit reversal training with awareness training, competing response training, and social support may help. Psychopharmacologic intervention with medications, such as serotonin reuptake inhibitors, *N*-acetylcysteine, and hypnosis are other options.

Halteh P, et al: Onychophagia. J Dermatolog Treat 2017 28: 166.
Singal A, Daulatabad D: Nail tic disorders. Indian J Dermatol Venereol Leprol 2017; 83: 19.
Smith L, et al: What future role might *N*-acetyl-cysteine have in the treatment of obsessive compulsive and grooming disorders? J Clin Psychopharmacol 2016; 36: 57.
Woods DW, Houghton DC: Evidence-based psychosocial treatments for pediatric body-focused repetitive behavior disorders. J Clin Child Adolesc Psychol 2016; 45: 227.

Onychotillomania

Onychotillomania is a compulsive neurosis in which the patient picks constantly at the nails or tries to tear them off. This obsessive-compulsive disorder may be treated by habit reversal training, hypnosis, or psychopharmacologic agents.

Pacan P, et al: Onychophagia and onychotillomania. Acta Derm Venereol 2014; 94: 67.
Rieder EA, Tosti A: Onychotillomania. J Am Acad Dermatol 2016; 75: 1245.

Onycholysis

Onycholysis is a spontaneous separation of the nail plate, usually beginning at the free margin and progressing proximally. Rarely, the lateral borders may be involved, with spread confined to this area. Less often, separation may begin proximal to the free edge, in an oval area 2–6 mm broad, with a yellowish brown hue ("oil spot"). This is a lesion of psoriasis; distal onycholysis is also often caused by psoriasis. The nail itself is smooth and firm with no inflammatory reaction. Underneath the nail, a discoloration may occur from the accumulation of bacteria, most frequently *Pseudomonas*, or yeast, usually *Candida*. Color changes, such as green (a result of pyocyanin from *Pseudomonas*), black, or blue may be seen. One or more nails may be affected.

Onycholysis is noted most often in women, probably secondary to traumatically induced separation. It is common in patients with hand dermatitis. Keratinization of the distal nail bed, chronic exposure to irritants, untreated dermatitis, and secondary infection with *Candida albicans* are potential reasons for the failure of the nail to reattach itself.

The many systemic causes include hyper/hypothyroidism, pregnancy, porphyria, pellagra, and syphilis. Onycholysis has also been associated with atopic dermatitis, eczema, lichen planus, congenital abnormalities of the nails, trauma induced by clawing, pinching, stabbing (manicuring), and foreign body implantation. It may be caused by mycotic, pyogenic, or viral (herpes) infections. Women should be checked for vaginal candidiasis, because that anatomic location may be the source of the infection opportunistically invading and aggravating onycholysis. Chemical causes may include the use of solvents, nail polish base coat, nail hardeners containing formalin derivatives, artificial fingernails, and allergic or irritant contact dermatitis from their use. Rarely, photo-onycholysis may occur during or soon after therapy with tetracycline derivatives, psoralens, fluoroquinolones, or chloramphenicol and subsequent exposure to sunlight. Chemotherapeutic agents, targeted cancer therapies, and systemic retinoids may induce onycholysis. On rare occasions, it may be a sign of subungual exostoses, squamous cell carcinoma, or metastasis. Autosomal dominant hereditary forms are also known. Toenail onycholysis is almost entirely mechanical in etiology, from pressure with closed toe shoes.

Trauma and chemical irritants should be completely avoided and the nail bed kept completely dry. The affected portion of the nail should be kept clipped away. Drying by exposing the nail bed with a hairdryer will rid the area of *Pseudomonas* and assist greatly in eliminating *Candida*. The combination of drying and topical corticosteroids to minimize inflammation will often allow for reattachment of the nail and improvement or cure. Usually, this process takes 3–6 months or more.

Iorizzo M: Tips to treat the 5 most common nail disorders. Dermatol Clin 2015; 33: 175.
Robert C, et al: Nail toxicities induced by systemic anticancer treatments. Lancet Oncol 2015; 16: e181.
Zaias N, et al: Finger and toenail onycholysis. J Eur Acad Dermatol Venereol 2015; 29: 848.

Median Nail Dystrophy (Dystrophia Unguis Mediana Canaliformis, Solenonychia)

Median nail dystrophy consists of longitudinal splitting or canal formation in the midline of the nail. The split, which often resembles a fir tree, occurs at the cuticle and proceeds outward as the nail grows (Fig. 33.54). Trauma has been suspected of being the chief cause. Repeated typing with the nail tip on a personal digital assistant (PDA) has been reported to cause a median nail dystrophy. Some cases will resolve with avoidance of trauma or occlusive therapy with tacrolimus ointment; however, many will persist for years despite scrupulous care. The deformity may result from a papilloma or glomus tumor in the nail matrix, producing a structure resembling a tube (solenos) distal to it. Familial cases and an onset with isotretinoin or retonavir therapy are other associations.

Alli N, Dogan S: Short-term isotretinoin-induced elkonyxis and median nail dystrophy. Cutan Ocul Toxicol 2016; 35: 85.
Borges-Costa J, et al: Median nail dystrophy associated with ritonavir. Int J Dermatol 2013; 52: 1581.
Kim BY, et al: Treatment of median canaliform nail dystrophy with topical 0.1% tacrolimus ointment. J Dermatol 2010; 37: 573.

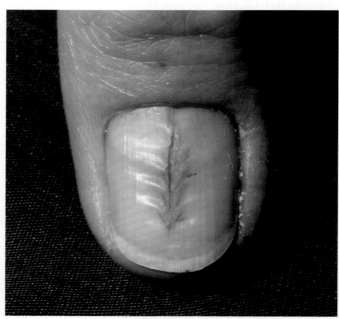

Fig. 33.54 Median nail dystrophy. (Courtesy Steven Binnick, MD.)

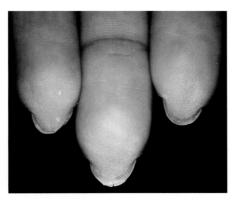

Fig. 33.55 Pterygium inversum unguis.

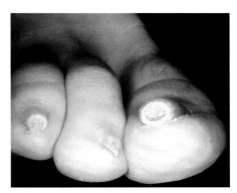

Fig. 33.56 Pincer nails.

Pterygium Unguis

Pterygium unguis forms as a result of scarring between the proximal nailfold and matrix. The classic causative example is lichen planus. It has been reported to result from sarcoidosis, porokeratosis of Mibelli, peripheral circulatory disturbances, and Hansen disease. Onychomatricoma may infrequently simulate pterygium, but histologic examination will confirm the nature of this benign tumor. Successful treatment with the fractionated carbon dioxide laser has been reported.

Ho D, et al: Successful treatment of traumatic onychodystrophy and associated pterygium unguis with fractionated carbon dioxide laser. J Drug Dermatol 2016; 15: 1461.
Perrin C, et al: Onychomatricoma with dorsal pterygium. J Am Acad Dermatol 2008; 59: 990.

Pterygium Inversum Unguis

Pterygium inversum unguis is characterized by adherence of the distal portion of the nail bed to the ventral surface of the nail plate (Fig. 33.55). The condition may be present at birth or acquired and may cause pain with manipulation of small objects, typing, and close manicuring of the nail. It results from the extension of the zone of the nail bed that normally contributes to the formation of the nail plate. This eventually leads to a more ventral and distal extension of the hyponychium. The most common forms of pterygium inversum unguis are the acquired secondary types caused by systemic connective tissue diseases, particularly progressive systemic sclerosis and SLE.

Baek JH, et al: A case of acquired idiopathic pterygium inversum unguis. Ann Dermatol 2014; 26:374.
Marie I, et al: Nail involvement in systemic sclerosis. J Am Acad Dermatol 2017; 76: 1115.

Hangnail

Hangnail is an overextension of the eponychium (cuticle), which becomes split and peels away from the proximal or lateral nailfold. These lesions are painful and annoying; persistent cuticle biting frequently develops. Trimming these away with scissors is the best solution. The use of emollient creams to keep the cuticle soft is also recommended.

Lee HJ, et al: Minor cutaneous features of atopic dermatitis in South Korea. Int J Dermatol 2000; 39: 337.

Pincer Nails

Pincer nails, trumpet nails, or omega (from the shape of the Greek letter) nails are alternative terms for a common toenail disorder in which the lateral edges of the nail slowly approach one another, compressing the nail bed and underlying dermis (Fig. 33.56). It may less often occur in the fingernails and, surprisingly, is usually asymptomatic. Infrequently, pain, recurrent or chronic infections, or even underlying osteomyelitis may complicate this condition. It may be an autosomal dominant inherited condition, may be acquired after trauma, or associated with Kawasaki disease, renal disease, Clouston syndrome, LE, or use of β-adrenergic blockers or pamidronate.

Some treatment success has been obtained using commercial plastic braces after flattening of the nail. Urea ointment under occlusion, various surgical approaches, and chemical matricectomy with phenol and surgical nail bed repair have also been reported to be effective.

Cho YJ, et al: Correction of pincer nail deformities using a modified double Z-plasty. Dermatol Surg 2015; 41: 736.
Failla V, et al: Pincer nails associated with pamidronate. Clin Exp Dermatol 2010; 36: 305.
Markeeva E, et al: Combined surgical treatment of a pincer nail with chemical matricectomy, median nail incision, and splinting. J Dtsch Dermatol Ges 2015; 13: 256.
Okada K, et al: Novel treatment using thioglycolic acid for pincer nails. J Dermatol 2012; 39: 996.

Onychocryptosis (Unguis Incarnatus, Ingrown Nail)

Ingrown toenail is one of the most frequent nail complaints. It occurs chiefly on the great toes, where there is an excessive lateral nail growth into the nailfold, leading to this painful, inflammatory condition. The lateral margin of the nail acts as a foreign body and may cause exuberant granulation tissue. Unguis incarnatus may be caused by wearing improperly fitting shoes and by improper trimming of the nail at the lateral edges so that the anterior portion cuts into the flesh as it grows distally. Drugs such as targeted cancer therapies, isotretinoin, lamivudine, and indinavir may induce periungual granulation tissue, mimicking onychocryptosis.

In mild cases, soaking the foot in warm soapy water and insertion of a cotton pad, dental floss, or a flexible plastic tube beneath the distal corner of the offending nail may make surgery unnecessary. When surgical intervention is necessary, simple removal of the lateral portion of the nail plate can produce significant relief. Another simple procedure involves removal of the overhanging lateral nailfold so that the nail does not cut into it. When healed, the nail edge resembles that of the thumb, and an excellent functional result occurs. The nail is not altered, because it is not touched.

Partial or complete nail avulsion with ablation of the nail matrix will prevent recurrence. Ablation can be accomplished surgically, with phenol, 10% sodium hydroxide, or with a CO_2 laser. When phenol is used, the proximal nailfold should be incised and reflected to avoid burning it. As an alternative, the nailfold can be left in place and injected with a corticosteroid to reduce the subsequent inflammation. Liquid nitrogen spray to the area of tissue and nail involved for a freeze time of 20–30 seconds has been successful in some patients. This may be painful, however, and is reserved for patients who are not candidates for other surgical approaches.

Haricharan RN, et al: Nail-fold excision for the treatment of ingrown toenail in children. J Pediatr 2013; 162: 398.
Park DH, et al: The management of ingrowing toenails. BMJ 2012; 344: e2089.
Romero-Pérez D, et al: Onychocryptosis. Int J Dermatol 2017; 56: 221.
Rounding C, Bloomfield S: Surgical treatments for ingrowing toenails. Cochrane Database Syst Rev 2005; CD001541.
Taheri A, et al: A conservative method to gutter splint ingrown toenails. JAMA Dermatol 2014; 150: 1359.

Retronychia

Retronychia is an unusual event associated with ingrowing of the nail plate into the proximal nailfold. This then induces a chronic paronychia. The great toe of women are most commonly involved. The cause is usually trauma, usually of the great toe. An incomplete shedding of the nail plate results in the new, growing nail pushing the old, partially detached nail plate up and backward into the proximal nailfold. Avulsion is curative.

Braswell MA, et al: Beau lines, onychomadesis, and retronychia. J Am Acad Dermatol 2015; 73: 849.
Gerard E, et al: Risk factors, clinical variants and therapeutic outcome of retronychia. Eur J Dermatol 2016; 26: 377.
Piraccini BM, et al: Retronychia in children, adolescents, and young adults. J Am Acad Dermatol 2014; 70: 388.
Ventura F, et al: Retronychia—clinical and pathophysiological aspects. J Eur Acad Dermatol Venereol 2016; 30: 16.

NAIL DISCOLORATIONS

Mendiratta V, et al: Nail dyschromias. Indian J Dermatol Venereol Leprol 2011; 77: 652.
Ruben BS: Pigmented lesions of the nail unit. Semin Cutan Med Surg 2010; 29: 148.

Leukonychia or White Nails

Five forms of white nail are recognized: leukonychia punctata, leukonychia striata, longitudinal leukonychia, leukonychia partialis, and leukonychia totalis. The punctate variety is common in normal persons with otherwise normal nails (Fig. 33.57). Leukonychia striata, or transverse white parallel line, may be hereditary, of traumatic origin, or associated with systemic diseases such as HIV or Kawasaki, or with acetretin and anticancer drugs. Longitudinal white lines are seen in Hailey-Hailey disease and with oncychopapillomas. Partial leukonychia may occur with tuberculosis, nephritis, selenium deficiency, complex regional pain syndrome, Hodgkin disease, chilblains, metastatic carcinoma, or Hansen disease, or it may be idiopathic.

Leukonychia totalis may be hereditary, of a simple autosomal dominant type. Mutations in the *PLCD1* gene are responsible. Both mutations in GJA1 and loss of function mutations in CAST may be associated with leukonychia and other associated abnormalities of the skin. It may also be associated with electron beam therapy, typhoid fever, Hansen disease, cirrhosis, ulcerative colitis, HIV, nail biting, use of emetine or vorinostat, complex regional pain syndrome, anticancer therapies, and trichinosis. Leukonychia may result from abnormal keratinization, with persistence of

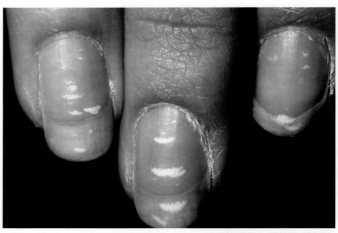

Fig. 33.57 Transverse leukonychia. (Courtesy Curt Samlaska, MD.)

keratohyalin granules in the nail plate. A syndrome comprising leukonychia totalis, multiple sebaceous cysts, and renal calculi in several generations has been reported. Other reports have linked total leukonychia with deafness or with koilonychia; however, it is most often inherited as an isolated finding.

Hasunuma N, et al: True leukonychia in Crohn disease. JAMA Dermatol 2014; 150: 779.
Lin Z, et al: Loss-of-function mutations in CAST cause peeling skin, leukonychia, acral punctate keratoses, cheilitis, and knuckle pads. Am J Hum Genet 2015; 96: 440.
Mutoh M, et al: A syndrome of leukonychia, koilonychia and multiple pilar cysts. Acta Derm Venereol 2015; 95: 249.
Nomikos M, et al: Mutations in PLCδ1 associated with hereditary leukonychia display divergent PIP2 hydrolytic function. FEBS J 2016; 283: 4502.
Robert C, et al: Nail toxicities induced by systemic anticancer treatments. Lancet Oncol 2015; 16: e181.
Wang H, et al: Exome sequencing reveals mutation in GJA1 as a cause of keratoderma-hypotrichosis-leukonychia totalis syndrome. Hum Mol Genet 2015; 24: 243.

Longitudinal Erythronychia

Longitudinal red bands in the nail plate that commence in the matrix and extend to the point of separation of the nail plate and nail bed may occur on multiple nails with inflammatory conditions, such as lichen planus, graft-versus-host disease, amyloidosis, acrokeratosis verruciformis of Hopf, or Darier disease, or as an isolated finding. When only a localized single or bifid streak is present on a single digit, this may signal a benign or malignant tumor of the matrix. The fingernails of middle-aged persons are most often affected, with the thumbnail usually involved. There may be a benign lesion such as a glomangioma, a distal keratosis, as with Darier disease, human papillomavirus (HPV) infection, or an onychopapilloma; however, malignancies such as squamous cell carcinoma or amelanotic melanoma may be present. Excision of this distal keratosis, however, usually does not result in cure or diagnostic findings; biopsy of the affected matrix is necessary. When the presentation is polydactylous, biopsy is rarely done. In solitary monodactylous, single or bifid bands in men over 50 a biopsy should be seriously considered. If observation is the decision, as in longitudinal melanonychia, if the band broadens over time, excisional biopsy is indicated, because this may be secondary to an amelanotic melanoma or squamous cell carcinoma. In patients with painful lesions excision will result in cure and diagnosis.

Beggs S, et al: Onychopapilloma presenting as longitudinal erythronychia in an adolescent. Pediatr Dermatol 2015; 32: e173.
Jellinek NJ, Lipner SR: Longitudinal erythronychia. Dermatol Surg 2016; 42: 310.
Lipner SR, Scher RK: Evaluation of nail lines. Cleve Clin J Med 2016; 83: 385.

Melanonychia

Black or brown pigmentation of the normal nail plate is termed melanonychia. The entire nail may be involved or multiple longitudinal or transverse bands on several nails may occur. It is when there is a solitary acquired longitudinal band that concern for malignancy is paramount. The nail pigment may be present as a normal finding on many digits in black patients. Longitudinal black or brown banding of the nails has been reported to occur in 77%–96% of black persons and 11% of Asians. Other causes include trauma, systemic disease, or medication; or as a postinflammatory event from such localized events as lichen planus or fixed drug reaction. Pigmentation of the nails may occur with acanthosis nigricans, Addison disease, Peutz-Jeghers syndrome, or vitamin B_{12} deficiency; after adrenalectomy for Cushing syndrome; as a part of Laugier-Hunziker syndrome (pigmentation of nails associated with buccal and lip hyperpigmentation); with PUVA or ionizing radiation treatment; and as drug-induced melanocyte activation with such medications as chemotherapy, antimalarials, minocycline, antivirals (zidovudine [Fig. 33.58] or lamivudine), or metals (gold, arsenic, thallium, mercury). Drugs may induce both transverse and longitudinal bands, with anticancer therapies causing most transverse bands. Friction may cause longitudinal pigmented bands in the toenails, and subungual hemorrhage or black nail caused by *Proteus mirabilis* or a variety of fungi may enter into the differential diagnosis of a dark nail.

When only one nail is affected by melanonychia striata—a single, longitudinal, brown or black band (Fig. 33.59)—a tumor of the nail matrix is the most important consideration. The location in the matrix can be inferred from the location of the pigment in the nail plate when viewed end-on. Dorsal nail plate pigmentation results from a proximal matrix lesion. Ventral nail-plate pigmentation is the result of a lesion in the distal matrix. A nevus, lentigo, onychopapilloma, onychomaticoma or squamous cell carcinoma may cause melanonychia striata in addition to melanoma.

Tosti et al. studied 100 white adult patients with a single band of longitudinal melanonychia of unknown cause. Biopsies revealed melanocytic hyperplasia in 65, nevi in 22, melanocytic activation in 8, and melanoma in 5. Decker et al.'s series has nearly the same frequency of melanoma. Although features below are helpful clinically, a biopsy in any adult with the appearance of a longitudinal band of pigment in only one nail without a clear relation to a definite cause should be seriously considered. Reasons to biopsy include a band that has a triangular shape (wider at proximal than distal part), a blurred lateral border of the band, a lack of homogeneity of the pigmentations (bands or lines of different color), a band over 6 mm in width, or pigmentation of the periungual skin (Hutchinson sign). The latter is not pathognomonic, however, because Bowen disease may produce this appearance, and pigmentation of the nail matrix and proximal nail bed may reflect through the nailfold (pseudo-Hutchinson sign). Finally, dermoscopic features that suggest melanoma are a brown coloration of the background and the presence of irregular coloration, spacing, or thickness of longitudinal lines or disruption of their parallelism. Retracting the proximal nailfold to expose the origin of the streak at the matrix allows selection of the best biopsy site. The recommended biopsy includes the whole lesion; this may be accomplished by the tangential matrix excision, which may leave minimal scarring in some patients, or more certainly, this is accomplished by longitudinal excision.

Recommendations for prepubertal children, however, are different. Longitudinal melanonychia that appears in children is usually benign in nature, and it is recommended that, because an ungual melanocytic band can appear at an age when other nevi appear, the majority can be followed. If the lesion is alarming in its appearance, however, especially if widening or darkening, sampling the whole lesion by tangential matrix or longitudinal excision is necessary.

Cooper C, et al: A clinical, histopathologic, and outcome study of melanonychia striata in childhood. J Am Acad Dermatol 2015; 72: 773.
Decker A, et al: Frequency of subungual melanoma in longitudinal melanonychia. Dermatol Surg 2017; 43: 798.
Jin H, et al: Diagnostic criteria for and clinical review of melanonychia in Korean patients. J Am Acad Dermatol 2016; 74: 1121.

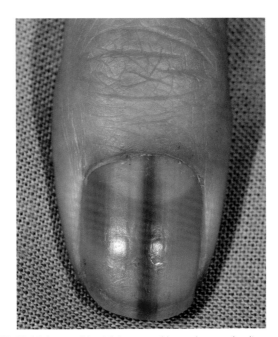

Fig. 33.59 Melanonychia striata caused by melanoma in situ. (Courtesy Adam Rubin, MD.)

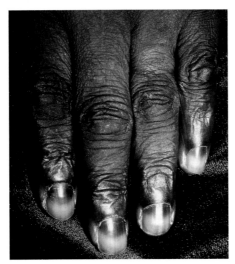

Fig. 33.58 Zidovudine-induced hyperpigmentation of the nail.

Lalosevic J, et al: Laugier-Hunziker syndrome. An Bras Dermatol 2015; 90: 223

Mannava KA, et al: Longitudinal melanonychia. Hand Surg 2013; 18: 133.

Ohn J, et al: Dermoscopic feature of nail matrix nevus (NMN) in adults and children. J Am Acad Dermatol 2016; 75: 535.

Piraccini BM, et al: Tips for diagnosis and treatment of nail pigmentation with practical algorithm. Dermatol Clin 2015; 33: 185.

Richert B, et al: Tangential excision of pigmented nail matrix lesions responsible for longitudinal melanonychia. J Am Acad Dermatol 2013; 69: 96.

Sawada M, et al: Proposed classification of longitudinal melanonychia based on clinical and dermoscopic criteria. Int J Dermatol 2014; 53: 581.

Shimizu A, et al: Detection of human papillomavirus type 67 in subungual Bowen's disease presenting as longitudinal melanonychia. Acta Derm Venereol 2015; 95: 745.

Tosti A, et al: Dealing with melanonychia. Semin Cutan Med Surg 2009; 28: 49.

Green Nails

When onycholysis is present, a green discoloration may occur in the onycholytic area as a result of an infection with *Pseudomonas aeruginosa* (see Chapter 14). The color change may also occur as transverse green stripes. The stripes are ascribed to intermittent episodes of infection. Green nails may also result from copper in tap water.

Gish D, Romero BJ: Green fingernail. J Fam Pract 2017; 66: E7.

Staining of Nail Plate

Nicotine, dyes (including hair dyes and nail polish), potassium permanganate, mercury compounds, hydroquinone, elemental iron, mepacrine, photographic developer, anthralin, chrysarobin, glutaraldehyde, or resorcin may cause nail plate staining. This is only a partial list; Mendiratta and Jain provide a complete listing. A helpful diagnostic maneuver to distinguish nail plate staining from exogenous sources and nail plate pigmentation from melanin or endogenous chemicals is to scrape the surface of the nail plate several times firmly with a glass slide or scalpel blade. Exogenous stains frequently scrape off completely if the agent has not penetrated the entire nail plate. If the stain follows the curvature of the lunulae, it is probably endogenous; if it follows the curvature of the proximal and lateral nailfolds, it is exogenous.

Hardin ME, et al: Nicotine staining of the hair and nails. J Am Acad Dermatol 2015; 73: e105.

Mendiratta V, et al: Nail dyschromias. Indian J Dermatol Venereol Leprol 2011; 77: 652.

Red Lunulae

Dusky erythema confined to the lunulae has been reported in association with alopecia areata. About 20% of patients with SLE have been reported to have this abnormality. Red lunulae may also be seen in patients taking oral prednisone for severe rheumatoid arthritis or dermatomyositis, as well as in cardiac failure, cirrhosis, lymphogranuloma venereum, psoriasis, vitiligo, chronic urticaria, lichen sclerosus et atrophicus, CO_2 poisoning, chronic obstructive pulmonary disease, twenty-nail dystrophy, and reticulosarcoma. The cause may be vascular congestion.

Cohen PR: Red lunulae. J Am Acad Dermatol 1992; 26: 292.

Elmansour I, et al: Nail changes in connective tissue diseases. Pan Afr Med J 2014; 18: 150.

Spotted Lunulae

This distinctive change occurs with alopecia areata.

Cohen PR: The lunula. J Am Acad Dermatol 1996; 34: 943.

Purpura of Nail Beds

Purpura beneath the nails usually results from trauma. Causes of toe involvement include physical pressure on the toes, such as that seen in surfboarding caused by a windsurfer trying to maintain balance, or exogenous pressure exerted from poorly fitting shoes. Nail bed purpura may simulate a melanoma if the patient does not communicate the acuteness at onset.

Pierson JC, et al: Pen push purpura. Cutis 1993; 51: 422.

Blue Nails

A blue discoloration of the lunulae is seen in argyria and cases of hepatolenticular degeneration (Wilson disease). The blue color in the latter is probably related to the changes in copper metabolism by the patient. It has also been reported in hemoglobin M disease and hereditary acrolabial telangiectases. Lunular blue color, as well as blue discoloration of the whole nail bed, occurs with some therapeutic agents, especially 5-FU, minocycline, imipramine, mepacrine and other antimalarials, hydroxyurea, phenolphthalein, and azidothymidine. Blue discoloration may also result from subungual hematoma, blue nevi, and melanotic whitlow. Blue nails are a normal variant finding in black people.

Casamiguela KM, Cohen PR: Chemotherapy-associated tongue hyperpigmentation and blue lunula. J Drugs Dermatol 2013; 12: 223.

Kalouche H, et al: Blue lunulae. Australas J Dermatol 2007; 48: 182.

Kim Y, et al: A case of generalized argyria after ingestion of colloidal silver solution. Am J Ind Med 2009; 52: 246.

Yellow Nail Syndrome

The yellow nail syndrome is characterized by marked thickening and yellow to yellowish green discoloration of the nails. It is often associated with systemic disease, most often lymphedema and compromised respiration. The nails are typically overcurved both transversely and longitudinally, grow very slowly (<0.2 mm/wk), are often subject to onycholysis, and lose both lunulae and cuticles (Fig. 33.60). Lymphedema, pleural effusions, chronic pulmonary infections, and chronic sinusitis most frequently precede the nail changes. Other less frequently associated conditions include autoimmune disorders, immunodeficiency states, use of gold or D-penicillamine, and malignancies. In the latter cases, treatment of the underlying lymphoma or solid tissue tumor has resulted in improvement of the nail findings. Individual clinical responses have been seen with oral zinc or 800 IU/day of D-α-tocopherol alone or in combination with itraconazole. Although 30%–50% of patients experience spontaneous improvement in the condition of their nails, fluconazole taken in combination with vitamin E cured or improved all 13 patients treated by Baran et al.

Al Hawsawi K, et al: Yellow nail syndrome. Pediatr Dermatol 2010; 27: 675.

Baran R, et al: Combination of fluconazole and alpha-tocopherol in the treatment of yellow nail syndrome. J Drugs Dermatol 2009; 8: 276.

Piraccini BM, et al: Yellow nail syndrome. J Dtsch Dermatol Ges 2014; 12: 131.

Shetty S, Bhaskaranand N: Yellow nail syndrome. Indian Pediatr 2016; 53: 1133.

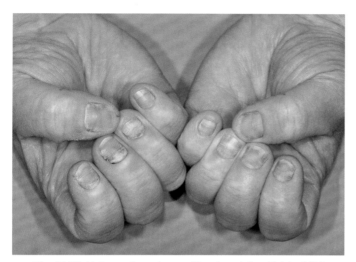

Fig. 33.60 Yellow nail syndrome. (Courtesy Adam Rubin, MD.)

Zaiac MN, et al: Nail abnormalities associated with systemic pathologies. Clin Dermatol. 2013; 31: 627.

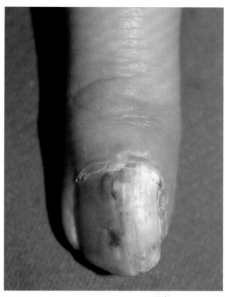

Fig. 33.61 Onychomatricoma. (Courtesy Adam Rubin, MD.)

Neoplasms of the Nail Unit

Various benign and malignant neoplasms may occur in or overlying the nail matrix and in the nail bed. Signs heralding such neoplasms are paronychia, ingrown nail, onycholysis, pyogenic granuloma, nail plate dystrophy, longitudinal leukonychia or erythronychia, bleeding, and discolorations. Symptoms of pain, itching, and throbbing may also occur with various neoplasms.

Benign tumors of the nail unit include verruca, pyogenic granuloma, fibromas such as superficial acral fibromyxomas and angiofibromas (Koenen tumors), nevus cell nevi, onychopapillomas, onychomatircomas, onychocytic matricomas, glomangiomas, and epidermoid and onycholemmal cysts. Pyogenic granuloma–like lesions may occur during treatment with isotretinoin, lamivudine, indinavir, the epidermal growth factor receptor inhibitor family of drugs, or other targeted cancer therapies. Glomangioma is readily recognized by exquisite tenderness in the nail bed. Onychopapillomas are benign tumors of the nail bed that usually present as longitudinal erythronychia. Onychomatricoma is a benign tumor of the nail matrix. It presents as a yellow, thickened plate growing out from under the proximal nailfold and then extending distally in a longitudinal band (Fig. 33.61). There is an increased transverse curvature of the nail, and splinter hemorrhages often are seen in the proximal nail. On dermatoscopic examination will reveal multiple cavities in a honeycomb pattern. Infrequently, it can appear as a cutaneous horn emanating from the proximal nailfold, with dorsal pterygium formation. Biopsy at the matrix origin will permit diagnosis and differentiate it from onychocytic carcinoma.

Bowen disease (Fig. 33.62) and squamous cell carcinoma (Fig. 33.63) of the nail bed are uncommon. Radiographs may reveal lytic changes in the distal phalanx. Metastases are rare. Mohs surgery is the treatment of choice. When these lesions occur on more than one digit, they are proved to be secondary to HPV infection. Bowen disease may be pigmental. When keratoacanthoma occurs, there is often lysis of underlying bone, which fills in after excision of the tumor. Basal cell carcinoma may occur but is uncommon in this location.

Subungual melanoma is frequently diagnosed late in the course of growth (Fig. 33.64), because it simulates onychomycosis or subungual hematoma, with which it is confused. Amelanotic melanoma may occur and may be mistaken for granuloma pyogenicum. Although melanoma is rare among Japanese, periungual

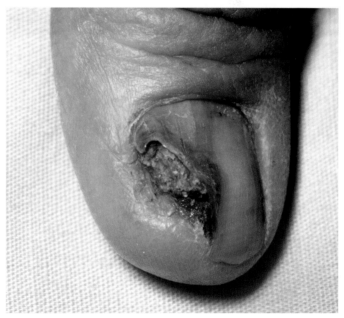

Fig. 33.62 Bowen disease of the nail bed.

and subungual melanoma is more frequently found in Japanese than in other ethnic populations. Melanoma in this location is discussed in Chapter 30 and in the melanonychia section of this chapter.

Onycholemmal carcinoma is a slowly growing, malignant tumor of the nail bed epithelium. It is composed of small cysts filled with eosinophilic amorphous keratin. The cyst wall is lined with atypical keratinocytes. No granular layer is seen. Also, solid nests and strands of atypical keratinocytes fill the dermis and may invade the bone. Mohs excision or even disarticulation of the digit may be necessary.

Evaluation of these masses may be carried out by plain x-ray films, looking for bone lysis or other changes. MRI by both T1-weighted spin-echo images and turbo spin-echo T2-weighted images may offer excellent diagnostic information about these

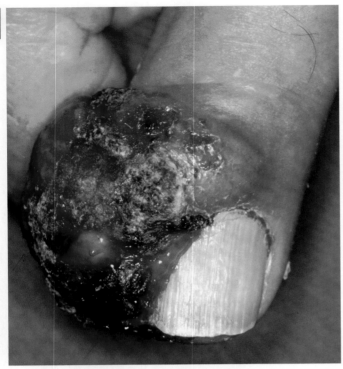

Fig. 33.63 Squamous cell carcinoma.

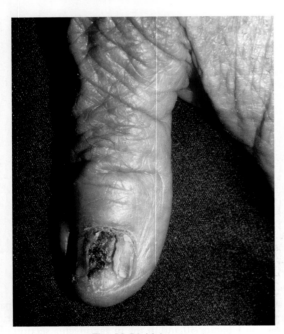

Fig. 33.64 Melanoma.

tumors as well. Histologic examination remains the diagnostic gold standard.

Bony lesions may simulate some of these conditions. Enchondroma of the distal phalanx often presents as a paronychia. Subungual exostoses may also present as an inflammatory process, but more often resemble a verruca at the start. Most of these are on the great toe. Tender swelling of the distal finger with nail distortion and radiographic evidence of solitary lytic changes can be caused by intraosseous epidermoid cysts, and radiographic

evaluation will aid in the diagnosis of these entities. Tender swelling of the distal finger with nail distortion and radiographic evidence of solitary lytic changes can be caused by intraosseous epidermoid cysts.

Beggs S, et al: Onychopapilloma presenting as longitudinal erythronychia in an adolescent. Pediatr Dermatol 2015; 32: e173.

Busquets J, et al: Subungual onycholemmal cyst of the toenail mimicking subungual melanoma. Cutis 2016; 98: 107.

Chanprapaph K, et al: Epidermal growth factor receptor inhibitors. Dermatol Res Pract 2014; 2014: 734249.

Chaser BE, et al: Onycholemmal carcinoma. J Am Acad Dermatol 2013; 68: 290.

Cohen PR: Longitudinal erythronychia. Am J Clin Dermatol 2011; 12: 231.

DaCambra MP, et al: Subungual exostosis of the toes: Clin Orthop Relat Res 2014; 472: 1251.

De Vasconcelos P, et al: Subungual keratoacanthoma in a pianist. G Ital Dermatol Venereol 2016; 151: 455.

Di Chiacchio N, et al: Onychomatricoma. Br J Dermatol 2015; 173: 1305.

Figueiras Dde A, et al: Paronychia and granulation tissue formation during treatment with isotretinoin. An Bras Dermatol 2016; 91: 223.

Ishida M, et al: Subungual pigmented squamous cell carcinoma presenting as longitudinal melanonychia. Int J Clin Exp Pathol 2014; 7: 844.

Ito T, et al: Onychopapilloma manifesting longitudinal melanonychia. J Dermatol 2015; 42: 1199.

Koç O, et al: Subungual glomus tumour. Australas Radiol 2007; 51 Spec No: B107.

Lam C, et al: Longitudinal melanonychia of the toenail. JAMA Dermatol 2014; 150: 449.

Lecerf P, et al: A retrospective study of squamous cell carcinoma of the nail unit diagnosed in a Belgian general hospital over a 15-year period. J Am Acad Dermatol 2013; 69: 253.

Lee WJ, et al: Nail apparatus melanoma. J Am Acad Dermatol 2015; 73: 213.

Lesort C, et al: Dermoscopic features of onychomatricoma. Dermatology 2015; 231: 177.

Okon LG, et al: A case of onychomatricoma. J Am Acad Dermatol 2017; 76: S19.

Ormerod E, de Berker D: Nail unit squamous cell carcinoma in people with immunosuppression. Br J Dermatol 2015; 173: 701.

Park JH, et al: Nail neoplasms. J Dermatol 2017; 44: 279.

Perrin C: Tumors of the nail unit. Part I. Am J Dermatopathol 2013; 35: 621.

Perrin C: Tumors of the nail unit. Part II. Am J Dermatopathol 2013; 35: 693.

Perrin C, et al: Acquired localized longitudinal pachyonychia and onychomatrical tumors. Am J Dermatopathol 2016; 38: 664.

Perruchoud DL, et al: Bowen disease of the nail unit. J Eur Acad Dermatol Venereol 2016; 30: 1503.

Romano RC, et al: Malignant melanoma of the nail apparatus. Int J Surg Pathol 2016; 24: 512.

Russell JD, et al: Subungual exostosis. Cutis 2016; 98: 128.

Samlaska CP, et al: Intraosseous epidermoid cysts. J Am Acad Dermatol 1992; 27: 454.

Schwager ZA, et al: Superficial acral fibromyxoma and other slow-growing tumors in acral areas. Cutis 2015; 95: E15.

Stephen S, et al: Diagnostic applications of nail clippings. Dermatol Clin 2015; 33: 289.

Tang N, et al: A retrospective study of nail squamous cell carcinoma at 2 institutions. Dermatol Surg 2016; 42: S8.

Topin-Ruiz S, et al: Surgical treatment of subungual squamous cell carcinoma by wide excision of the nail unit and skin graft reconstruction. JAMA Dermatol 2017; 153: 442.

Tosti A, et al: Clinical, dermoscopic, and pathologic features of onychopapilloma. J Am Acad Dermatol 2016; 74: 521.

Wang L, et al: Invasive onychocytic carcinoma. J Cutan Pathol 2015; 42: 361.

Wollina U: Bowen's disease of the nail apparatus. Wien Med Wochenschr 2015; 165: 401.

Wynes J, et al: Pigmented onychomatricoma. J Foot Ankle Surg 2015; 54: 723.

Lesions on the mucous membranes may be more difficult to diagnose than lesions on the skin, and not merely because they are less easily and less often seen. There is less contrast of color and greater likelihood of alterations in the original appearance because of secondary factors, such as maceration from moisture, abrasion from food and teeth, and infection. Vesicles and bullae rapidly rupture to form grayish erosions, and the epithelium covering papules becomes a soggy, lactescent membrane, easily rubbed off to form an erosion. Grouping and distribution are less distinctive in the mouth than on the skin, and in some cases it is necessary to establish the diagnosis by observing the character of any associated cutaneous lesions or by noting subsequent developments.

CHEILITIS

Cheilitis Exfoliativa

The term *cheilitis exfoliativa* has been used to designate a primarily desquamative, mildly inflammatory condition of the lips, of unknown cause, and also a clinically similar reaction secondary to other disease states. The former is a persistently recurring lesion that produces scaling and sometimes crusting; it most often affects the upper lip. The recurrent exfoliation leaves a temporarily erythematous and tender surface.

In the latter form, the lips are chronically inflamed and covered with crusts that from time to time tend to desquamate, leaving a glazed surface on which new crusts form. Fissures may be present, and there may be burning, tenderness, and some pain. The lower lip is more often involved, with the inflammation limited to the vermilion part. The cheilitis may be secondary to seborrheic dermatitis, atopic dermatitis (AD), psoriasis, retinoid therapy, pyorrhea, long-term actinic exposure, or the habit of lip licking. Infrequently, the initial or only manifestation of AD may be a chronic cheilitis. Irritating or allergenic substances in lipsticks, dentifrices, and mouthwashes may be causative factors. Dyes in lipsticks may photosensitize. Candidiasis may be present. Cheilitis may be part of Plummer-Vinson or Sjögren syndrome. Cheilitis is seen in patients with acquired immunodeficiency syndrome (AIDS), and it is a known common complication of protease inhibitor therapy. These and other, uncommon causes of cheilitis are discussed in more detail within the specific entities.

The only uniformly effective treatment of cheilitis exfoliativa is the elimination of causes when they can be found. Topical tacrolimus ointment, pimecrolimus cream, or low-strength corticosteroid ointments and creams are usually helpful. Excimer laser therapy or the handheld ultraviolet B (UVB) unit may be useful. If the underlying etiology is determined, specific therapy may be instituted. When there are fissures, petrolatum or zinc oxide ointment applied liberally and often may heal them.

Almazrooa SA, et al: Characterization and management of exfoliative cheilitis. Oral Surg Oral Med Oral Pathol Oral Radiol Endod 2013; 116: e485.

Bhatia BK, et al: Excimer laser therapy and narrowband ultraviolet B therapy for exfoliative cheilitis. Int J Womens Dermatol 2015; 1: 95.

Allergic Contact Cheilitis

The vermilion border of the lips is much more likely to develop allergic contact sensitivity reactions than is the oral mucosa. Allergic cheilitis is characterized by dryness, fissuring, edema, crusting, and angular cheilitis. Over 90% of patients are women and over half of the reactions are caused by lipsticks. Although patch testing with standard allergens will reveal a relevant positive in approximately 25%–30% of patients, about one in five will only react to their own product. It may result from use of topical medications (Fig. 34.1), dentifrices and other dental preparations, antichap agents, lipsticks, and sunscreen-containing lip balms; from contact with cosmetics, nail polish, rubber, and metals; or from eating foods such as mangoes. Fragrance and nickel are the most commonly identified individual sensitizers.

Treatment includes discontinuation of exposure to the offending agent and administration of topical tacrolimus, pimecrolimus, or corticosteroid preparations.

Aerts O, et al: Contact dermatitis caused by pharmaceutical ointments containing "ozonated" olive oil. Contact Dermatitis 2016; 75: 123.

Alrowaishdi F, et al: Allergic contact cheilitis caused by carnauba wax in a lip balm. Contact Dermatitis 2013; 69: 311.

Barrientos N, et al: Contact cheilitis caused by candelilla wax contained in lipstick. Contact Dermatitis 2013; 69: 126.

Bourgeois P, Goossens A: Allergic contact cheilitis caused by menthol in toothpaste and throat medication. Contact Dermatitis 2016; 75: 113.

Budimir V, et al: Allergic contact cheilitis and perioral dermatitis caused by propolis. Acta Dermatovenerol Croat 2012; 20: 187.

de Groot A: Contact allergy to (ingredients of) toothpastes. Dermatitis 2017; 28: 95.

O'Gorman S, Torgerson RR: Contact allergy in cheilitis. Int J Dermatol 2016; 55: e386.

Panasoff J: Cheilitis caused by to mint-containing toothpastes. Contact Dermatitis 2016; 75: 260.

Sarre ME, et al: Allergic contact cheilitis caused by polysilicone-15 (Parsol SLX) in a lip care balm. Contact Dermatitis 2014; 70: 119.

Tan S, et al: Allergic contact dermatitis to *Myroxylon pereirae* (balsam of Peru) in papaw ointment causing cheilitis. Australas J Dermatol 2011; 52: 222.

Actinic Cheilitis

Actinic cheilitis is an inflammatory reaction of the lips to chronic excessive sunlight exposure over many years. The lower lip, which is usually the only one involved, becomes scaly, fissured, atrophic (Fig. 34.2), and at times eroded and swollen; leukoplakia and squamous cell carcinoma (SCC) may develop. Painful erosions may occur; actual ulceration is very rare unless carcinoma has developed. Hereditary polymorphous light eruption can resemble chronic actinic cheilitis, but it has no malignant potential.

Avoiding sun exposure and the use of sunscreen containing lip pomades suffice to minimize further damage. A biopsy should be performed on any suspicious, thickened areas that persist; preferably, a shave technique should be used to avoid scarring.

Cryosurgical treatment may be effective, particularly for localized lesions. In cases with diffuse involvement, application of topical

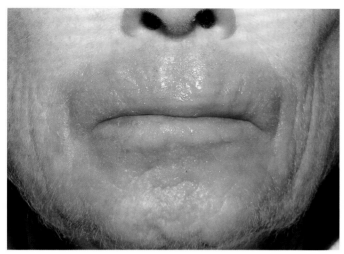

Fig. 34.1 Allergic contact cheilitis to topical steroids. (Courtesy Glen Crawford, MD.)

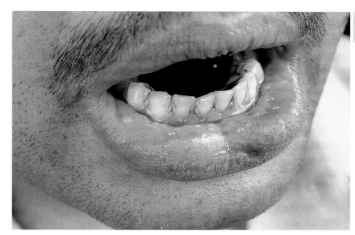

Fig. 34.3 Cheilitis glandularis. (Courtesy Dr. Shyam Verma.)

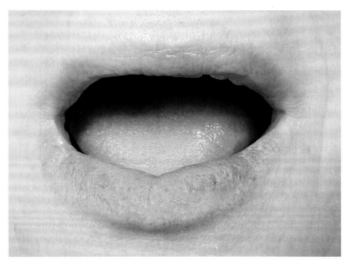

Fig. 34.2 Actinic cheilitis. (Courtesy Joseph Sobanko, MD.)

5-fluorouracil (5-FU), imiquimod, ingenol, or photodynamic therapy (PDT) may be curative. Treatment with a thulium fraction-ated or ablative erbium laser, dermabrasion, or electrodesiccation may be required for severe disease and provides excellent results. Long-term follow-up is necessary. Should treatment fail, vermil-ionectomy of the lower lip may be necessary. Excision of the exposed vermilion mucous membrane with advancement of the labial mucosa to the skin edge of the outer lip is effective, but this is performed less frequently since the advent of laser therapy. Refer to Chapter 29 for more information on actinic cheilitis.

Cohen JL: Erbium laser resurfacing for actinic cheilitis. J Drugs Dermatol 2013; 12: 1290.

Dufresne RG Jr, et al: Dermabrasion for actinic cheilitis. Dermatol Surg 2008; 34: 848.

Flórez Á, et al: Management of actinic cheilitis using ingenol mebutate gel. J Dermatolog Treat 2017; 28: 149.

Ghasri P, et al: Treatment of actinic cheilitis using a 1,927-nm thulium fractional laser. Dermatol Surg 2012; 38: 504.

Muthukrishnan A, Bijai Kumar L: Actinic cheilosis. BMJ Case Rep 2017 Mar 20; 2017.

Vieira RA, et al: Actinic cheilitis and squamous cell carcinoma of the lip. An Bras Dermatol 2012; 87: 105.

Yazdani Abyaneh MA, et al: Photodynamic therapy for actinic cheilitis. Dermatol Surg 2015; 41: 189.

Cheilitis Glandularis

Cheilitis glandularis is characterized by swelling and eversion of the lower lip, patulous openings of the ducts of the mucous glands, cysts, and at times, abscess formation. There is general enlargement of the lips (Fig. 34.3). Mucus exudes freely to form a gluey film that dries over the lips and causes them to stick together during the night. When the lip is palpated between the thumb and index finger, the enlarged mucous glands feel like pebbles beneath the surface. The lower lip is the site of predilection. Middle-aged men are most often affected. Cheilitis glandularis is a chronic inflammatory reaction that is caused by an exuberant response to chronic irritation, or to atopic, factitious, or actinic damage.

On biopsy, there is a moderate histiocytic, lymphocytic, and plasmacytic infiltration in and around the glands. Cheilitis glan-dularis has been reported to eventuate in SCC, but these cases may be attributed to chronic sun exposure, which frequently precedes cheilitis glandularis.

Treatment depends on the nature of the antecedent irritation; in most cases, treatment as described for actinic cheilitis is appropri-ate. Surgical debulking may be necessary. Intralesional triamcinolone may be beneficial in some patients, as may the combination of minocycline and tacrolimus ointment.

Kumar P, Mandal RK: Cheilitis glandularis. Indian J Dermatol Venereol Leprol 2015; 81: 430.

Nico MM, et al: Cheilitis glandularis. J Am Acad Dermatol 2010; 62: 233.

Angular Cheilitis

Angular cheilitis is synonymous with perlèche. Fissures radiate downward and outward from the labial commissures. It is an intertriginous dermatitis caused by excessive wetness or dryness. It is often complicated by secondary infection with *Candida albicans* or *Staphylococcus aureus*.

The disease usually occurs in elderly people who wear dentures, but it may develop simply from an overhanging of the upper lip and cheek, and recession and atrophy of the alveolar ridges in old age. Measuring the facial dimensions with a ruler and tongue blade will help with objective assessment of the importance of decreased vertical facial dimension in the development of perlèche. If the distance from the base of the nose to the lower edge of the mandible is greater than or equal to 6 mm less than the distance from the center of the pupil to the parting line of the lips, the vertical dimension is decreased. In these circumstances, drooling is usually a factor. In children, angular cheilitis occurs frequently in thumb suckers, gum chewers, and lollipop eaters. Other inciting factors include riboflavin deficiency, anorexia nervosa, Down syndrome, intraoral candidiasis, especially in patients with diabetes, AIDS, chronic mucocutaneous candidiasis, Sjögren syndrome, orthodontic treatment, drug-induced xerostomia, and AD.

Opening the "bite" by improving denture fit, capping teeth, replacing lost teeth, or increasing denture height, combined with topical use of nystatin and iodochlorhydroxyquin in hydrocortisone ointment, is usually effective when the condition is associated with anatomically predisposing factors. Stubborn cases typically respond to a slightly stronger corticosteroid, such as desonide, in combination with a topical anticandidal agent. Injection of collagen or insertion of Softform implants to obliterate the angular creases may be beneficial. Therapy for underlying diseases should be maximized. If *S. aureus* is present, mupirocin ointment may be needed. Excision of the region, followed by a rotating flap graft, is another therapeutic option, but surgery should be reserved for resistant cases.

Adedigba MA, et al: Patterns of oral manifestations of HIV/AIDS among 225 Nigerian patients. Oral Dis 2008; 14: 341.
Lu DP: Prosthodontic management of angular cheilitis and persistent drooling. Compend Contin Educ Dent 2007; 28: 572.
Park KK, et al: Angular cheilitis. Part 1. Cutis 2011; 87: 289.
Park KK, et al: Angular cheilitis. Part 2. Cutis 2011; 88: 27.
Sharifzadeh A, et al: Oral microflora and their relation to risk factors in HIV+ patients with oropharyngeal candidiasis. J Mycol Med 2013; 23: 105.
Sharon V, et al: Oral candidiasis and angular cheilitis. Dermatol Ther 2010; 23: 230.

Plasma Cell Cheilitis

This is also referred to as plasma cell orificial mucositis or, when the gingival is the site of involvement, plasma cell gingivitis. It is characterized by a sharply outlined, infiltrated, dark red plaque with a lacquer-like glazing of the surface of the involved area. This lesion has the same microscopic features as Zoon balanitis plasmacellularis. There is plasma cell infiltration in a bandlike pattern. Plasma cell cheilitis is not a response that is specific for any stimulus but rather represents a reaction pattern to any one of a variety of stimuli. Successful therapies include application of topical tacrolimus ointment or clobetasol propionate ointment twice daily, or use of the 308 nm excimer light.

Plasmoacanthoma

Plasma cell cheilitis and plasmoacanthoma have been reported in the same patient and are believed to represent a spectrum of the same disease. Plasmoacanthoma is a verrucous tumor with a plasma cell infiltrate involving the oral mucosa, particularly along the angles. Other locations may occur, such as the perianal, periumbilical, or inguinal areas and toe webs. *C. albicans* has been found within the tissue, suggesting that it may be implicated as a cause of this disease. Excision, destruction, anticandidal preparations, and intralesional steroids are all options for treatment.

Abhishek K, Rashmi J: Plasma cell gingivitis associated with inflammatory cheilitis. Ethiop J Health Sci 2013; 23: 183.
da Cunha Filho RR, et al: "Angular" plasma cell cheilitis. Dermatol Online J 2014; 20.

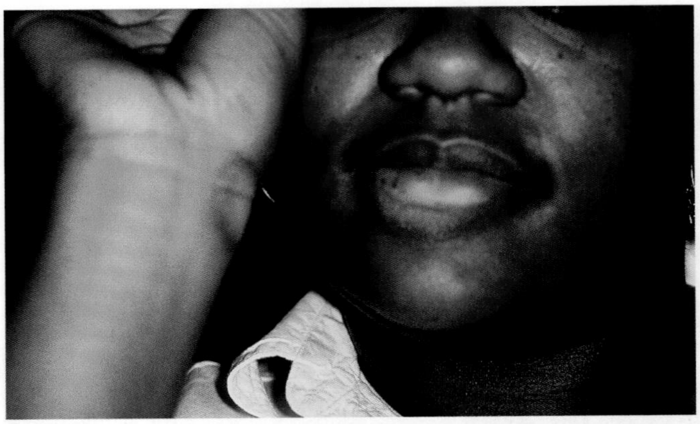

Fig. 34.4 Fixed drug eruption.

Senol M, et al: Intertriginous plasmacytosis with plasmoacanthoma. Int J Dermatol 2008; 47: 265.
Yoshimura K, et al: Successful treatment with 308-nm monochromatic excimer light and subsequent tacrolimus 0.03% ointment in refractory plasma cell cheilitis. J Dermatol 2013; 40: 471.

Drug-Induced Ulcer of the Lip

Painful or tender, well-defined ulcerations without induration on the lower lip may heal after withdrawal of oral medications. The causative drugs may be phenylbutazone, chlorpromazine, phenobarbital, methyldopa, or thiazide diuretics. Solar exposure appears to be a predisposing causative influence; in some cases, this reaction may represent a fixed drug photoeruption. On rare occasions, fixed drug eruptions may also involve the lip, usually caused by naproxen, one of the oxicams, or trimethoprim-sulfamethoxazole (Fig. 34.4).

Abdollahi M, et al: A review of drug-induced oral reactions. J Contemp Dent Pract 2003; 4: 10.
Pemberton MN, et al: Fixed drug eruption to oxybutynin. Oral Surg Oral Med Oral Pathol Oral Radiol Endod 2008; 106: e19.

Other Forms of Cheilitis

Several diseases discussed elsewhere may affect the lips, including lichen planus, lupus erythematosus, erythema multiforme, AD, and psoriasis. A high percentage of patients with Down syndrome have cheilitis of one or both lips. Lip biting may be a factor.

ORAL AND CUTANEOUS CROHN DISEASE

Crohn disease is a chronic granulomatous disease of any part or parts of the bowel. Patients with Crohn disease may develop inflammatory hyperplasia of the oral mucosa, with metallic dysgeusia and gingival bleeding. Reported typical changes include diffuse oral swelling, focal mucosal hypertrophy and fissuring (cobblestoning), persistent ulceration, polypoid lesions, indurated fissuring of the lower lip, angular cheilitis, granulomatous cheilitis, or pyostomatitis vegetans. Oral involvement occurs in 10%–20% of patients with Crohn disease, and 90% have granulomas on biopsy. Males with early-onset disease are most often affected. Concomitant involvement of the anal and esophageal mucosa is common. Direct extension to perianal skin may occur.

Many cases of Crohn disease with other cutaneous manifestations have been reported, notably pyoderma gangrenosum (more closely associated with ulcerative colitis) and erythema nodosum, Sweet syndrome, polyarteritis nodosa, pellagra, pernicious anemia, an acrodermatitis-like eruption, urticaria, and necrotizing vasculitis.

Metastatic Crohn disease denotes noncaseating granulomatous skin lesions in patients with Crohn disease. In the absence of bowel involvement, the diagnosis cannot be made. The morphologic appearances seen include genital swelling or condyloma-like lesions, leg ulceration, pyogenic granuloma–like lesions of the retroauricular skin, and erythematous nodules, plaques, or ulcers in other locations. At times step sectioning or multiple biopsies may be necessary to reveal the granulomas.

Treatment of the gastrointestinal (GI) manifestations with sulfasalazine, metronidazole, systemic corticosteroids, infliximab or other anti–tumor necrosis factor (TNF) agents, or immunosuppressive medications such as cyclosporine, azathioprine, mycophenolate mofetil, and methotrexate can improve the cutaneous findings. Several delivery systems use only the active ingredient of sulfasalazine, mesalamine, including Asacol, Pentasa, Rowasa, and olsalazine, and may be useful in treating the skin involvement of Crohn disease. A mouthwash containing triamcinolone acetonide, tetracycline, and lidocaine may provide symptomatic and objective improvement. Cutaneous ulcerated granulomas and erythematous plaques caused by Crohn disease may respond to high-potency topical corticosteroids or tacrolimus ointment. Curettage and zinc by mouth have resulted in healing in several reported patients. Dietary manipulation is another measure that can be helpful in select individuals. The course is often prolonged over several years.

Alemanno G, et al: Rare cutaneous manifestations associated with Crohn's disease. Int J Colorectal Dis 2014; 29: 765.

Kurtzman DJ, et al: Metastatic Crohn's disease. J Am Acad Dermatol 2014; 71: 804.

Laftah Z, et al: Vulval Crohn's disease. J Crohns Colitis 2015; 9: 318.

Marzano AV, et al: Cutaneous manifestations in patients with inflammatory bowel diseases. Inflamm Bowel Dis 2014; 20: 213.

Shah NP, et al: Treatment of a Crohn's disease-related facial lesion with topical tacrolimus. Oral Surg Oral Med Oral Pathol Oral Radiol 2014; 118: e71.

Thrash B, et al: Cutaneous manifestations of gastrointestinal disease. J Am Acad Dermatol 2013; 68: 211.

Yuksel I, et al: Mucocutaneous manifestations of inflammatory bowel disease. Inflamm Bowel Dis 2009; 15: 546.

PYOSTOMATITIS VEGETANS

Pyostomatitis vegetans, an inflammatory stomatitis, is most often seen in association with ulcerative colitis but may also occur in other inflammatory bowel diseases, such as Crohn disease. Edema and erythema with deep folding of the buccal mucosa characterize pyostomatitis vegetans, together with pustules, small vegetating projections, erosions, ulcers, and fibrinopurulent exudates (Fig. 34.5). Eroded pustules fuse into shallow ulcers, resulting in characteristic "snail-track" ulcers. It has also been associated with sclerosing cholangitis. Several cases have been reported with no underlying systemic disorder. At times, crusted erythematous papulopustules that coalesce into asymmetric annular plaques may occur with or after the oral lesions. These associated skin lesions favor the axillae, groin, and scalp and are termed *pyodermatitis vegetans*. Topical corticosteroids or tacrolimus ointment may be effective; systemic corticosteroids or infliximab, however, are usually necessary.

Histologically, there are dense aggregates of neutrophils and eosinophils.

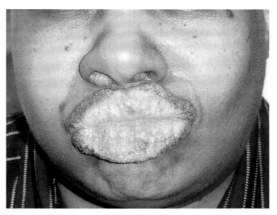

Fig. 34.5 Pyostomatitis vegetans. (Courtesy Scott Norton, MD.)

Clark LG, et al: Pyostomatitis vegetans (PSV)–pyodermatitis vegetans (PDV). J Am Acad Dermatol 2016; 75: 578.

Crippa R, et al: Oral manifestations of gastrointestinal diseases in children. Part 2. Eur J Paediatr Dent 2016; 17: 164.

Dupuis EC, et al: Pyoblepharitis vegetans in association with pyodermatitis-pyostomatitis vegetans. J Cutan Med Surg 2016; 20: 163.

Fantus SA, et al: Vegetating plaques on the lips. Am J Dermatopathol 2015; 37: 699.

Muhvic-Urek M, et al: Oral pathology in inflammatory bowel disease. World J Gastroenterol 2016; 22: 5655.

Wu YH, et al: Pyostomatitis vegetans. J Formos Med Assoc 2015; 114: 672.

CHEILITIS GRANULOMATOSA

Cheilitis granulomatosa is characterized by a sudden onset and progressive course, terminating in chronic enlargement of the lips. Usually, the upper lip becomes swollen first; several months may elapse before the lower lip becomes swollen. Usually, only enlargement is present, without ulceration, fissuring, or scaling. The swelling remains permanently. It may be a part of the Melkersson-Rosenthal syndrome when associated with facial paralysis and plicated tongue.

The cause is unknown. Histologically, cheilitis granulomatosa is characterized by an inflammatory reaction of lymphocytes, histiocytes, and plasma cells and by tuberculoid granulomas consisting of epithelioid and Langerhans giant cells. At times, intralymphatic granulomas are found and may account for the clinical swelling. In the differential diagnosis, solid edema, angioedema, cheilitis glandularis, sarcoidosis, oral Crohn disease, lymphangioma, hemangioma, and neurofibroma, infectious granulomas, contact allergy, reaction to silicone fillers, and Ascher syndrome must be considered. Ascher syndrome consists of swelling of the lips with edema of the eyelids (blepharochalasis) and is inherited.

Cheilitis granulomatosa may be the presenting sign in a patient who will develop Crohn disease or sarcoidosis at a later time.

Treatment with intralesional injections of corticosteroids is usually successful but temporary. Combining this modality with oral antiinflammatory agents for long-term control, such as doxycycline, dapsone, colchicine, sulfasalazine, hydroxychloroquine, anti-TNF agents, or topical tacrolimus ointment, is an excellent strategy. In the firmly established case, surgical repair of the involved lip through a mucosal approach and, in some cases, concomitant intralesional corticosteroid treatment provide the best results.

Alvarez-Garrido H, et al: Crohn's disease and cheilitis granulomatosa. J Am Acad Dermatol 2011; 65: 239.

Gonzalez-Garcia C, et al: Intralymphatic granulomas as a pathogenic factor in cheilitis granulomatosa/Melkersson-Rosenthal syndrome. Am J Dermatopathol 2011; 33: 594.

Lynde CB, et al: Cheilitis granulomatosa treated with intralesional corticosteroids and anti-inflammatory agents. J Am Acad Dermatol 2011; 65: e101.

MELKERSSON-ROSENTHAL SYNDROME

Melkersson in 1928 and Rosenthal in 1930 described a triad consisting of recurring facial paralysis or paresis, soft nonpitting edema of the lips, and scrotal tongue. Attacks usually start during adolescence, with permanent or transitory paralysis of one or both facial nerves, repeated migraines, and recurring edema of the upper lip, cheeks, and occasionally the lower lip and circumoral tissues. Swelling of the skin and mucous membranes of the face and mouth is the dominant finding and most important diagnostic feature (Fig. 34.6). In order of frequency, the swelling occurs first on the upper lip, then the lower lip, and then other regions. Chronic eyelid swelling may occur.

Extrafacial swellings appear on the dorsal aspect of the hands and feet and in the lumbar region. The pharynx and respiratory tract may be involved, with thickening of the mucous membrane. The relapsing condition produces an overgrowth of connective tissue, edema, and atrophy of the muscle fibers, with permanent deformities of the lips, cheeks, and tongue.

The cause of Melkersson-Rosenthal syndrome is unknown. The association at times with megacolon, otosclerosis, and craniopharyngioma supports the theory of a neurotrophic origin. It may be familial. Histopathologic evaluation shows a tuberculoid type of granuloma with lymphedema and a banal perivascular infiltrate. Intralymphatic granulomas may account for the swelling.

Melkersson-Rosenthal syndrome is frequently seen in an incomplete form, and other granulomatous diseases may present as swellings of the lips or orofacial tissues. It is worthwhile calling these, as a group, "orofacial granulomatosis" so that various underlying disease states or etiologic factors will not be missed when evaluating such patients. The differential diagnosis is the same as cheilitis granulomatosa (discussed earlier).

Intralesional injections of corticosteroids may be beneficial therapy. Again, combining this with oral antiinflammatory agents for long-term control, such as doxycycline, dapsone, colchicine, sulfasalazine, hydroxychloroquine, anti-TNF agents, or topical tacrolimus ointment, is an excellent strategy. Clofazimine and thalidomide are reported to be useful, but availability and side effects limit their use. Surgery alone may be used, or surgery combined with intralesional corticosteroid injections and oral medications may be more successful than any of the three alone. Compression therapy is another adjuvant intervention that may add improvement without side effects. Decompression of the facial nerve may be indicated in patients with recurrent attacks of facial palsy. Odontogenic infection has been reported to initiate this condition, and antibiotic therapy for this may lead to remission.

Al-Hamad A, et al: Orofacial granulomatosis. Dermatol Clin 2015; 33: 433.

Belliveau MJ, et al: Melkersson-Rosenthal syndrome presenting with isolated bilateral eyelid swelling. Can J Ophthalmol 2011; 46: 286.

Bohra S, et al: Clinicopathological significance of Melkersson-Rosenthal syndrome. BMJ Case Rep 2015 Jul 31; 2015.

Feng S, et al: Melkersson-Rosenthal syndrome. Acta Otolaryngol 2014; 134: 977.

Li Z et al: Compression therapy. Eur J Dermatol 2011; 21: 1003.

Miest R, et al: Orofacial granulomatosis. Clin Dermatol 2016; 34: 505.

FORDYCE DISEASE (FORDYCE SPOTS)

Fordyce spots are ectopically located sebaceous glands, clinically characterized by minute, orange or yellowish, pinhead-sized macules or papules in the mucosa of the lips, cheeks, and less often the gums. Similar lesions may occur on the areolae, glans penis, and labia minora. Prominent lip involvement may result in a lipstick-like mark left on the rim of a glass mug after consuming a hot beverage (Meffert sign). Involvement of the labial mucosa with pseudoxanthoma elasticum may simulate Fordyce spots. Because the anomaly is asymptomatic and inconsequential, treatment should be undertaken only if there is a significant cosmetic problem. The carbon dioxide (CO_2) laser, electrodesiccation and curettage, bichloracetic acid, PDT, and isotretinoin are therapeutic options.

Chen PL, et al: Fordyce spots of the lip responding to electrodesiccation and curettage. Dermatol Surg 2008; 34: 960.

Errichetti E, et al: Areolar sebaceous hyperplasia associated with oral and genital Fordyce spots. J Dermatol 2013; 40: 670.

STOMATITIS NICOTINA

Also known as smoker's keratosis and smoker's patches, stomatitis nicotina is characterized by distinct, umbilicated papules on the palate. The ostia of the mucous ducts appear as red pinpoints surrounded by milky-white, slightly umbilicated, asymptomatic papules. The intervening mucosa becomes white and thick and tends to desquamate in places, leaving raw, beefy-red areas. Ulceration and the formation of aphthous ulcers may occur. Stomatitis nicotina is attributed to heavy smoking in middle-aged men, although it has also been reported in nonsmokers who habitually drink hot beverages. Heat may be the causative event. Indeed, the most severe cases are associated with the type of tobacco use that produces intense heat—pipe and reverse smoking. Treatment consists of abstaining from the use of tobacco or the ingestion of hot liquids.

Samatha Y, et al: Clinicopathologic evaluation of lesions associated with tobacco usage. J Contemp Dent Pract 2014; 15: 466.

Vellappally S, et al: Smoking related system and oral diseases. Acta Medica 2007; 50: 161.

TORUS PALATINUS

Torus palatinus is a bony protuberance in the midline of the hard palate, marking the point of junction of the two halves of the

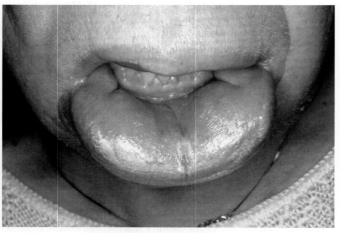

Fig. 34.6 Melkersson-Rosenthal syndrome.

palate. It is asymptomatic. Exostoses also frequently occur in the floor of the mouth, involving the inner surface of the mandible.

Bennett WM: Torus palatinus. N Engl J Med 2013; 368: 1434.
Ladizinski B, Lee KC: A nodular protuberance on the hard palate. JAMA 2014; 311: 1558.

FISSURED TONGUE

Also known as furrowed tongue, scrotal tongue, or lingua plicata, fissured tongue is a congenital and sometimes familial condition in which the tongue is generally larger than normal, and plicate superficial or deep grooves are usually arranged so that there is a longitudinal furrow along the median raphe, reminiscent of scrotal rugae (Fig. 34.7).

Fissured tongue is seen in Melkersson-Rosenthal syndrome and in many patients with Down syndrome. Individual case reports have been seen in association with pachyonychia congenita, pemphigus vegetans, and Cowden syndrome. Geographic tongue occurs together with fissured tongue in 50% of patients, and both are more often present in psoriasis patients than nonpsoriatic patients.

The condition gives rise to no difficulty, and treatment is not necessary, except that the deep furrows should be kept clean by use of mouthwashes. Herpetic geometric glossitis may mimic fissured tongue, but it is painful, affects predominantly immuno-compromised individuals, and is centered on the back of the dorsal tongue.

Dafar A, et al: Factors associated with geographic tongue and fissured tongue. Acta Odontol Scand 2016; 74: 210.
Madani FM, et al: Normal variations of oral anatomy and common oral soft tissue lesions. Med Clin North Am 2014; 98: 1281.
Pedersen AML, et al: Oral mucosal lesions in older people. Oral Dis 2015: 21: 721.
Pereira CM, et al: Herpetic geometric glossitis. Indian J Pathol Microbiol 2010; 53: 133.
Picciani BL, et al: Geographic tongue and fissured tongue in 348 patients with psoriasis. ScientificWorldJournal 2015; 2015: 564326.

GEOGRAPHIC TONGUE

Geographic tongue, also known as benign migratory glossitis, it is a manifestation of atopy, and in others, of psoriasis. It has been reported as being acquired in patients with AIDS or as a result of lithium therapy. In most, however, it is an isolated finding.

The dorsal surface of the tongue is the site usually affected. Geographic tongue begins with a small depression on the lateral border or the tip of the tongue, smoother and redder than the rest of the surface. This spreads peripherally, with the formation of sharply circumscribed, ringed or gyrate, red patches, each with a narrow, yellowish white border, making the tongue resemble a map. The appearance changes from day to day; patches may disappear in one place and manifest in another. The disease is characterized by periods of exacerbation and quiescence. The appearance may also remain unchanged in the same site for long periods. The condition is frequently unrecognized because it produces no symptoms except for the occasional complaint of glossodynia.

There are two clinical variants of geographic tongue. In one type, discrete, annular "bald" patches of glistening, erythematous mucosa with absent or atrophic filiform papillae are noted. Another type shows prominent circinate or annular, white raised lines that vary in width up to 2 mm. The clinical appearance and histo-pathologic findings of the tongue lesions in pustular psoriasis, reactive arthritis (Reiter syndrome), and geographic tongue are

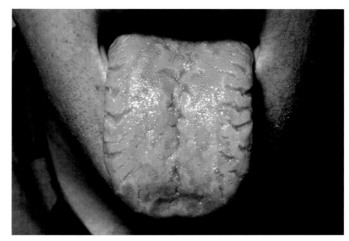

Fig. 34.7 Fissured tongue.

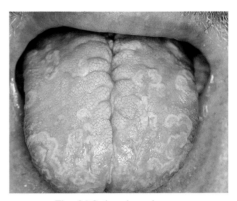

Fig. 34.8 Annulus migrans.

identical; when the tongue lesions occur with psoriasis or reactive arthritis, the name annulus migrans has been suggested for this entity (Fig. 34.8).

Histologically, the main features are marked transepidermal neutrophil migration with the formation of spongiform pustules in the epidermis and an upper dermal mononuclear infiltrate. Although treatment is not usually necessary, a 0.1% solution of tretinoin applied topically has produced clearing within 4–6 days, and tacrolimus ointment may improve it.

Mangold AR, et al: Diseases of the tongue. Clin Dermatol 2016; 34: 458.
Picciani BL, et al: Geographic tongue and psoriasis. An Bras Dermatol 2016; 91: 410.
Purani JM, Purani HJ: Treatment of geographic tongue with topical tacrolimus. BMJ Case Rep 2014 Aug 1; 2014.
Varoni E, Decani S: Geographic tongue. N Engl J Med 2016; 374: 670.

BLACK HAIRY TONGUE

Black or brown hairy tongue occurs on the dorsum of the tongue anterior to the circumvallate papillae, where black, yellowish, or brown patches form, consisting of hairlike intertwining filaments several millimeters long (Fig. 34.9). The "hairs" result from a benign hyperplasia of the filiform papillae of the anterior two thirds of the tongue, resulting in retention of long, conical filaments of orthokeratotic and parakeratotic cells. It occurs much more frequently in men than in women.

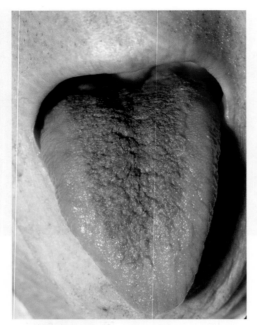

Fig. 34.9 Black hairy tongue. (Courtesy Steven Binnick, MD.)

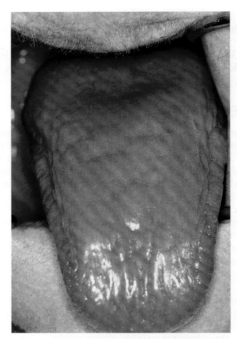

Fig. 34.10 Smooth tongue in Plummer-Vinson syndrome.

Black hairy tongue may be associated with several conditions that may be predisposing factors in its causation: smoking, use of oral antibiotics, interferon treatment, xerostomia, psychotropic drugs, and presence of *Candida* on the surface of the tongue.

This lesion may be differentiated both clinically and histologically from oral hairy leukoplakia, which is seen in human immunodeficiency virus (HIV)–infected patients. Hairy leukoplakia is usually seen on the lateral surface of the tongue, at first in corrugated patches, then with time, as solid white plaques that are adherent. Microscopic examination reveals acanthosis, parakeratosis, irregular projections of keratin, and vacuolated keratinocytes with Epstein-Barr virus (EBV) present within them.

A toothbrush may be used to scrub off the projections, either alone, with 1%–2% hydrogen peroxide, or after application of tretinoin gel, 40% aqueous solution of urea, or papain (meat tenderizer). Such predisposing local factors as smoking, antibiotics, and oxidizing agents should be eliminated, if possible, and scrupulous oral hygiene maintained.

Arab JP, et al: Black hairy tongue during interferon therapy for hepatitis C. Ann Hepatol 2015; 14: 414.

Balaji G, et al: Linezolid induced black hairy tongue. Indian J Pharmacol 2014; 46: 653.

Gurvits GE, Tan A: Black hairy tongue syndrome. World J Gastroenterol 2014; 20: 10845.

Thompson DF, et al: Drug-induced black hairy tongue. Pharmacotherapy 2010; 30: 585.

SMOOTH TONGUE

Also known as atrophic glossitis, the smooth glossy tongue is often painful and results from atrophy of the filiform and eventually the fungiform papillae (Fig. 34.10). It begins with the tip and lateral surfaces of the tongue becoming intensely red, well-defined irregular patches in which the filiform papillae are absent or thinned and the fungiform papillae are swollen. The disease is chronic, and the patches are painful and sensitive, so eating may be difficult and taste impaired. With time, the entire tongue becomes smooth,

and a leukoplakia may result. Treatment of pernicious anemia with vitamin B_{12} therapy will result in improvements in the appearance and sensitivity of the tongue.

Atrophic glossitis is also a distinctive sign of pellagra; it results from a deficiency of niacin or its precursor, tryptophan. The sides and tip of the tongue are erythematous and edematous, with imprints of the teeth. Eventually, the entire tongue assumes a beefy-red appearance. Small ulcers appear, and all the mucous membranes of the mouth may be involved. Later, the papillae become atrophied to produce a smooth, glazed tongue, as seen in pernicious anemia. Burning or pain in the ulcers may be present. Increased salivary flow early in the disease may lead to drooling and angular cheilitis. In malabsorption syndrome, riboflavin deficiency, anorexia nervosa, alcoholism, and sprue, similar changes may be noted. Vitamin B complex is curative.

Patients with iron deficiency anemia, alone or with esophageal webs (Plummer-Vinson syndrome), and those with folic acid deficiency, syphilis, amyloidosis, celiac disease, Sjögren syndrome, or Riley-Day syndrome, may all manifest smooth tongue. Candidiasis may result in tongue pain and a partial or total atrophic appearance, along with a red or magenta color, on the dorsum of the tongue. In such patients, anticandidal therapy results in rapid improvement.

Cunha SF, et al: Papillary atrophy of the tongue and nutritional status of hospitalized alcoholics. An Bras Dermatol 2012; 87: 84.

Demir N, et al: Dermatological findings of vitamin B_{12} deficiency and resolving time of these symptoms. Cutan Ocul Toxicol 2014; 33: 70.

Lee HJ, et al: A smooth, shiny tongue. N Engl J Med 2009; 360: e8.

Mangold AR, et al: Diseases of the tongue. Clin Dermatol 2016; 34: 458.

ERUPTIVE LINGUAL PAPILLITIS

Lacour and Perrin first described this acute, self-limiting inflammatory stomatitis in 1997. It affects children of both genders

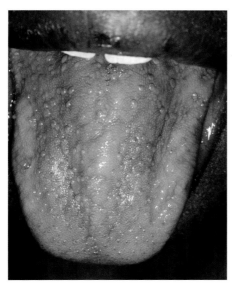

Fig. 34.11 Eruptive lingual papillitis.

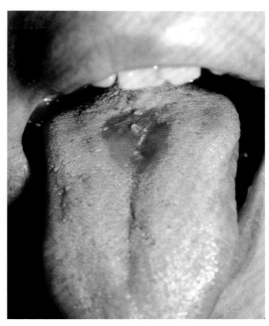

Fig. 34.12 Median rhomboid glossitis. (Courtesy Steven Binnick, MD.)

equally, with a mean age at onset of 3½ years. It has a seasonal distribution, with the majority of cases occurring in the spring. Fever (40%), difficulties in feeding (100%), and intense salivation (60%) are common symptoms. The tongue examination reveals inflammatory hypertrophy of the fungiform papillae on the tip and dorsolateral sites (Fig. 34.11). Additional signs include submandibular or cervical adenopathy (40%) and angular cheilitis (10%). Associated skin eruptions have not been described. Spontaneous involution occurs in a mean of 7 days (range 2–15 days). Recurrence is noted in 13%. Eruptive lingual papillitis is thought to result from a viral infection, and the 50% transmission among family members further supports this theory.

Mondal A, et al: Eruptive lingual papillitis. Indian Pediatr 2014; 51: 243.
Roux O, et al: Eruptive lingual papillitis with household transmission. Br J Dermatol 2004; 150: 299.

MEDIAN RHOMBOID GLOSSITIS

Median rhomboid glossitis is characterized by a shiny, oval or diamond-shaped elevation, invariably situated on the dorsum in the midline immediately in front of the circumvallate papillae (Fig. 34.12). The surface is abnormally red and smooth. In some cases, a few pale-yellow papules surmount the elevation. On palpation, the lesion feels slightly firm, but it usually causes no symptoms. It persists indefinitely, with minimal or no increase in size. There is no relationship to cancer.

Median rhomboid glossitis may result from abnormal fusion of the posterior portion of the tongue, but it is almost always chronically infected with *Candida*. If there is palatal inflammation above the inflamed part of the tongue, AIDS should be suspected and an HIV test obtained. Histologically, the changes are those of a simple, chronic inflammation with fibrosis, and usually with fungal hyphae in the parakeratin layer. Treatment with clotrimazole troches or oral antifungals, such as itraconazole, may lead to improvement.

Basak P, et al: A smooth patch on the tongue. N Engl J Med 2010; 363: 1949.
Panta P, Erugula SR: Median rhomboid glossitis—developmental or candidal? Pan Afr Med J 2015; 21: 221.

EOSINOPHILIC ULCER OF THE ORAL MUCOSA

Eosinophilic ulcer occurs most frequently on the tongue but may occur anywhere in the oral mucosa. It is characterized by an ulcer with indurated and elevated borders that is usually covered by a pseudomembrane. It develops rapidly, most often on the posterior aspect of the tongue, and spontaneously resolves in a few weeks. A traumatic cause has been postulated for this benign, self-limited disorder. The histopathologic findings show a predominantly eosinophilic infiltrate with some histiocytes and neutrophils.

In some multifocal, recurrent cases, CD30+ cells have been reported. These patients may have the oral counterpart of primary cutaneous CD30+ lymphoproliferative disease, or may simply be a simulator of this disorder. In one positive case, EBV staining was positive; the lesion resolved in 4 weeks. HIV-infected patients may develop ulcerations of the oral mucosa, resulting from a variety of infectious agents, such as herpes simplex virus (HSV), candidiasis, and histoplasmosis. However, 5 of the 16 patients reported had no evidence of infection and simply showed eosinophilic infiltrates below the ulcer.

Abdel-Naser MB, et al: Oral eosinophilic ulcer, an Epstein-Barr virus–associated CD30+ lymphoproliferation? Dermatology 2011; 222: 113.
Damevska K, et al: Eosinophilic ulcer of the oral mucosa. Am J Dermatopathol 2014; 36: 594.
Didona D, et al: Eosinophilic ulcer of the tongue. An Bras Dermatol 2015; 90: 88.
Lee EY, et al: Clinical characteristics of odontogenic cutaneous fistulas. Ann Dermatol 2016; 28: 417.

CAVIAR TONGUE

This is a purplish venous ectasias commonly found on the undersurface of the tongue after age 50. They are attributed to elastic tissue deterioration with aging and may be associated with Fordyce angiokeratomas of the scrotum. Phleboliths or thrombophlebitis may occasionally complicate this condition.

Viswanath V, et al: Caviar tongue. Indian J Dermatol Venereol Leprol 2011; 77: 78.

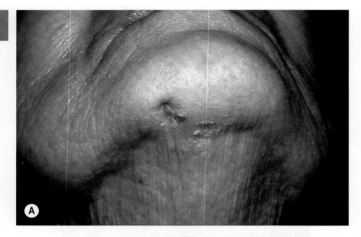

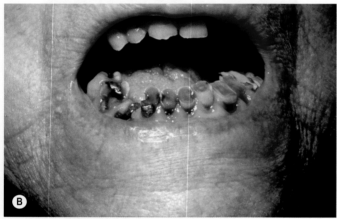

Fig. 34.13 (A) Cutaneous dental sinus. (B) Poor oral hygiene in the patient shown in (A).

CUTANEOUS SINUS OF DENTAL ORIGIN (DENTAL SINUS)

In dental (or odontogenous) sinus, chronic periapical infection around a tooth produces a burrowing, practically asymptomatic, occasionally palpable, cordlike sinus tract that eventually appears beneath the surface of the gum, palate, or periorificial skin. It forms a fistulous opening with an inflamed red nodule at the orifice. It may appear anywhere from the inner ocular canthus to the neck, but is most often seen on the chin or along the jawline (Fig. 34.13). Bilateral involvement has been reported. Dental radiography is diagnostic. Pyogenic granuloma, actinomycosis, SCC, osteomyelitis of the mandible, congenital fistulas, the deep mycoses, bisphosphonate-related osteonecrosis of the jaw, and foreign body reactions must be considered in the differential diagnosis. Treatment requires the removal of the offending tooth or root canal therapy of the periapical abscess.

Bodner L, et al: Cutaneous sinus tract of dental origin in children. Pediatr Dermatol 2012; 29: 421.

Gupta, et al: A clinical predicament—diagnosis and differential diagnosis of cutaneous facial sinus tracts of dental origin. Oral Surg Oral Med Oral Pathol Oral Radiol Endod 2011; 112: e132.

Truong SV, et al: Bisphosphonate-related osteonecrosis of the jaw presenting as a cutaneous dental sinus track. J Am Acad Dermatol 2010; 62: 672.

NEOPLASMS

Many tumors may involve the oral cavity. Most are discussed elsewhere in this book, and several are uncommon entities that affect specialized oral structures, such as the many subtypes of benign and malignant proliferations that occur in the major and minor salivary glands. These are not covered further here, and only a few select neoplasms are presented.

Leukoplakia

Clinical Features

Leukoplakia presents as a whitish thickening of the epithelium of the mucous membranes, occurring as lactescent superficial patches of various shapes and sizes that may coalesce to form diffuse sheets. The surface is generally glistening and opalescent, often reticulated, and may even be somewhat pigmented. The white pellicle is adherent to the underlying mucosa, and attempts to remove it forcibly cause bleeding. At times, it is a thick, rough, elevated plaque. The lips, gums, cheeks, and edges of the tongue are the most common sites, but the lesion may arise on the anus and genitalia. Leukoplakia is found chiefly in men over age 40.

Biopsy of these white lesions may reveal orthokeratosis or parakeratosis with minimal inflammation, or there may be evidence of varying degrees of dysplasia. A benign form is usually a response to chronic irritation and has very little chance of conversion into the precancerous dysplastic form. Premalignant leukoplakia, with atypical cells histologically, is present in only about 10%–20% of leukoplakia. Unfortunately, it is not possible to predict clinically which lesions will be worrisome histologically, except that if ulceration, red areas, or erosions are scattered throughout, the lesion is most likely precancerous. Therefore biopsy is indicated.

When the lesion occurs on the lip, leukoplakia is closely related to chronic actinic cheilitis, which consists of a circumscribed or diffuse keratosis, almost invariably on the lower lip. It is preceded by an abnormal dryness of the lip and may be caused by smoking (especially pipe smoking) or chronic sun exposure. This type of leukoplakia is distinguished from SCC of the lip by the absence of infiltration, from lichen planus and psoriasis of the lips and mouth by the absence of lesions elsewhere, and from lupus erythematosus by the absence of telangiectases. Biopsy is necessary, however, to differentiate these conditions fully.

Intraoral leukoplakia appears to progress to SCC in no more than 1% of lesions per year. In time, an extensive, thick, white pellicle may cover the tongue or oral mucosa. In old lesions, the epithelium may be desquamated, and there may be fissures or ulcerations. Such changes are associated with more or less hyperemia and tenderness, and with a tendency to bleed after slight trauma. If transformation to carcinoma occurs, it generally follows a lag time of 1–20 years, although immunosuppressed transplant patients may have a rapid course of transformation.

Oral hairy leukoplakia is a term used to describe white, corrugated plaques that occur primarily on the sides of the tongue. It was initially described as a manifestation of AIDS. Its appearance in these patients has decreased. It may be seen in patients with local or systemic immunosuppression such as those on steroid inhalers, on immunosuppressant or chemotherapy, therapy, or with leukemia. (Fig. 34.14). This is a virally induced lesion, discussed in Chapter 19, which has a characteristic histology.

Leukoplakia of the vulva usually occurs in obese women after menopause as grayish white, thickened, pruritic patches that may become fissured and edematous from constant rubbing and scratching. Secondary infection with edema, tenderness, and pain may occur. It is differentiated from lichen planus by the absence of discrete, rectangular, or annular flat papules of violaceous hue in the mucosa outside the thickened patches, about the anus, on the buccal mucosa, or on the skin. Leukoplakia of the vulva is

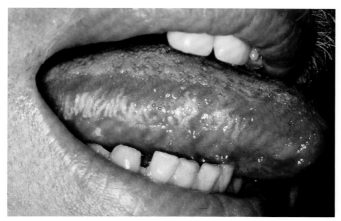

Fig. 34.14 Oral hairy leukoplakia of HIV.

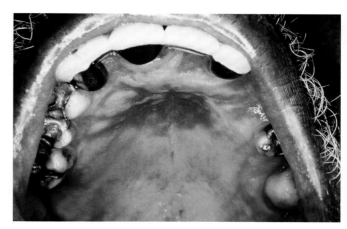

Fig. 34.15 Erythroplakia.

most frequently confused with lichen sclerosus et atrophicus and other vulval atrophies. On the penis, although leukoplakia may occur, a similar precancerous process called erythroplasia (of Queyrat) is usually seen instead.

Etiology

Numerous factors are involved in the cause of leukoplakia. It may develop as a result of tobacco smoking; use of smokeless tobacco; areca, qat, or betel nut chewing; reverse smoking; alcohol; poorly fitting dentures; sharp and chipped teeth; treatment with BRAF inhibitors; or improper oral hygiene. Extensive involvement of the lips and oral cavity with leukoplakia may exist for years with no indication of carcinoma. On the other hand, small, inflamed patches may be the site of a rapidly growing tumor, which, with relatively insignificant local infiltration, may involve the cervical lymphatics. Carcinoma in leukoplakia usually begins as a localized induration, often around a fissure, or as a warty excrescence or a small ulcer. There is a 6%–10% transformation rate of intraoral leukoplakia into SCC. Predictors of a higher risk of SCC development include older age; female gender; nonsmokers; large size; presence on the lateral or ventral tongue, floor of the mouth, or retromolar/soft palate complex; erythroleukoplakia; and a nonhomogeneous morphology.

The degree of epithelial atypia may be considered in staging the risk of developing malignancy. Aneuploid leukoplakia has a high rate of transformation into aggressive SCC, and the cancers derived from it are more likely to be lethal.

Treatment

It must be remembered that cancer develops frequently on histologically dysplastic leukoplakia, and thus its complete removal should be the goal in each case—first by conservative measures, then by surgery or destruction, if necessary. The use of tobacco should be stopped and proper dental care obtained. Fulguration, simple excision, cryotherapy, PDT, and CO_2 laser ablation are effective methods of treatment. Medical therapies that have been the subject of randomized clinical trials may lead to temporary resolution of the lesions, but relapses and adverse effects are common, and there is no evidence that they prevent the transformation to malignancy.

Leukoplakia With Tylosis and Esophageal Carcinoma

Leukoplakia associated with tylosis and esophageal carcinoma is extremely rare but may occur.

Epidermization of the Lip

Relatively smooth leukokeratosis of the lower vermilion, blending evenly into the skin surface distally and having a steep, sharp, irregular proximal margin, may easily be mistaken clinically for precancerous leukoplakia. Histologically, it shows only hyperkeratosis, without parakeratosis or cellular atypia. A shallow shave excision suffices to cure it and to rule out precancerous leukoplakia; no fulguration is required.

Erythroplakia

The term erythroplakia is applied to leukoplakia that has lost (or has not developed) the thick keratin layer that makes leukoplakia white; it is the usual pattern in mucocutaneous junctions. A focal red patch with no apparent cause should be suspected of being precancerous when found on the floor of the mouth, soft palate, or buccal mucosa or under the tongue (Fig. 34.15). Histologically, there is cellular atypia, pleomorphism, hyperchromatism, and increased mitotic figures. Carcinoma in situ or invasive carcinoma is found in 90% of lesions.

Oral Florid Papillomatosis

Oral florid papillomatosis is a confluent papillomatosis covering the mucous membranes of the oral cavity. The distinctive picture is that of a white mass resembling a cauliflower, covering the tongue and extending on to the other portions of the mucous membranes, including the oropharynx, larynx, and trachea. Usually, there is no lymphadenopathy.

The course of the disease is progressive. Many lesions eventuate in SCC, whereas others continue for many years, with the patient dying of some intercurrent disease. Oral florid papillomatosis should be regarded as a verrucous carcinoma, which has been defined as a distinctive, slowly growing, fungating tumor representing a well-differentiated SCC in which metastases occur very late or not at all. The histologic features are those of papillomatosis, acanthosis, and varying degrees of dysplasia of the epithelium, without disruption of the basement membrane. It is reasonable to expect the eventual development of epidermoid carcinoma in most patients. Esophageal involvement and keratotic papules of the extremities may occur. In the differential diagnosis, leukoplakia, proliferative verrucous leukoplakia, candidiasis, acanthosis nigricans, and condyloma acuminatum should be considered. The recommended treatment is surgical excision; however, it is often followed by recurrence and spread.

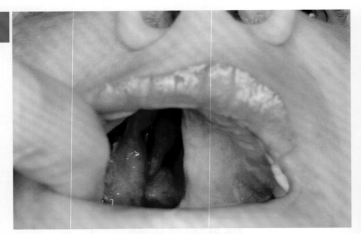

Fig. 34.16 Proliferative verrucous leukoplakia; three sites of squamous cell carcinoma: lip and twice in palate.

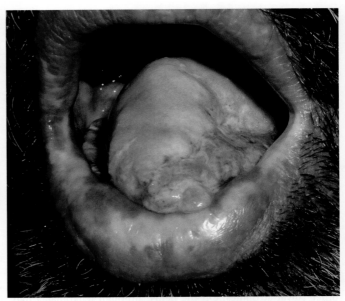

Fig. 34.17 Squamous cell carcinoma secondary to chewing betel nut. (Courtesy Shyam Verma, MBBS, DVD.)

Proliferative Verrucous Leukoplakia

Proliferative verrucous leukoplakia is a slowly progressive condition that begins as multifocal sites of hyperplasia of the oral mucous membranes and proceeds to thicken and enlarge until SCC results (Fig. 34.16). Women outnumber men 4:1. Initially flat, usually white patches are present, but the lesions relentlessly become warty, exophytic masses. About 70% of patients develop SCC, most frequently of the palate and gingiva, with 40% of the total patients dying of it. There has been an irregular association with human papillomavirus (HPV)–16 infection, and risk factors for SCC of the oral cavity are usually not present. Treatment is difficult because of the multifocal nature of the lesions. Aggressive early surgical therapy is best. Many patients develop recurrence after only a short interval.

Squamous Cell Carcinoma

SCC is the most common oral malignancy and constitutes 2%–3% of all new cancers. With almost 30,000 yearly cases in the United States, SCC is the tenth most common malignancy. It occurs primarily in older men. The most frequent sites are the lower lip, tongue, soft palate, and floor of the mouth. SCC of the lip develops from actinic damage, with 95% of the cases involving the lower lip. Intraoral lesions frequently develop from leukoplakia or erythroplakia, at sites of frequent irritation, or from long-standing mucosal inflammatory disease such as ulcerative lichen planus. About 20% of oral squamous cell cancers have an associated focus of leukoplakia; these tend to be diagnosed at a less advanced stage than those where no associated leukoplakia exists. Tobacco smoking, use of smokeless tobacco; areca, qat, or betel nut chewing (Fig. 34.17); and reverse smoking are risk factors for the development of intraoral SCC. Alcohol has not been shown to be an independent risk factor. Many are positive for HPV-16 or HPV-18. The risk factors may also include xeroderma pigmentosa (tip of tongue), dyskeratosis congenita, dystrophic epidermolysis bullosa, erosive lichen planus, and oral submucous fibrosis. Unfortunately, the survival rate has remained at 50% for many years because disease is often discovered late, after it has metastasized to the cervical lymph nodes. Exfoliative cytology is a practical and accurate aid to oral cancer screening. Surgical excision is the treatment of choice; the roles of sentinel lymph node dissection and adjuvant chemotherapy and/or radiation are all controversial issues undergoing active study. Head and neck surgeons, radiation oncologists, dentists, and rehabilitation specialists should provide a team approach to oral SCC treatment.

Abadie WM, et al: Optimal management of proliferative verrucous leukoplakia. Otolaryngol Head Neck Surg 2015; 153: 504.

Akrish S, et al: Oral squamous cell carcinoma associated with proliferative verrucous leukoplakia compared with conventional squamous cell carcinoma. Oral Surg Oral Med Oral Pathol Oral Radiol 2015; 119: 318.

Bagan JV, et al: Malignant transformation of proliferative verrucous leukoplakia to oral squamous cell carcinoma. Oral Oncol 2011; 47: 732.

Carrard VC, et al: Proliferative verrucous leukoplakia. Med Oral Patol Oral Cir Bucal 2013; 18: e411.

Chambers AE, et al: Twenty-first-century oral hairy leukoplakia. Oral Surg Oral Med Oral Pathol Oral Radiol 2015; 119: 326.

Gillenwater AM, et al: Proliferative verrucous leukoplakia. Head Neck 2014; 36: 1662.

Hall LD, et al: Epstein-Barr virus. J Am Acad Dermatol 2015; 72: 1.

Liu W, et al: Oral cancer development in patients with leukoplakia. PLoS One 2012; 7: e34773.

Lodi G, et al: Interventions for treating oral leukoplakia to prevent oral cancer. Cochrane Database Syst Rev 2016; 7: CD001829.

Maia HC, et al: Potentially malignant oral lesions. Einstein (Sao Paulo) 2016; 14: 35.

Rhodus NL, et al: Oral cancer. Dent Clin North Am 2014; 58: 315.

Vale DA, et al: Retrospective analysis of the clinical behavior of oral hairy leukoplakia in 215 HIV-seropositive patients. Braz Oral Res 2016; 30: e118.

Vigarios E, et al: Oral squamous cell carcinoma and hyperkeratotic lesions with BRAF inhibitors. Br J Dermatol 2015; 172: 1680.

Villa A, Woo SB: Leukoplakia—a diagnostic and management algorithm. J Oral Maxillofac Surg 2017; 75: 723.

Yang SW, et al: Outcome of excision of oral erythroplakia. Br J Oral Maxillofac Surg 2015; 53: 142.

Yanik EL, et al: Leukoplakia, oral cavity cancer risk, and cancer survival in the U.S. elderly. Cancer Prev Res (Phila) 2015; 8: 857.

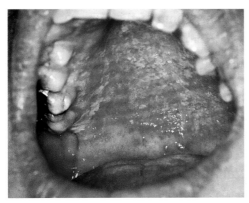

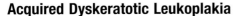

Fig. 34.18 Acquired dyskeratotic leukoplakia.

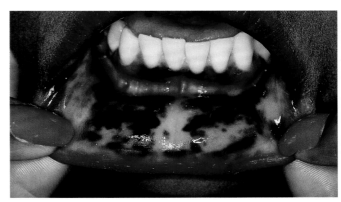

Fig. 34.19 Oral melanosis.

Acquired Dyskeratotic Leukoplakia

James and Lupton reported a patient with acquired dyskeratotic leukoplakia that manifested as distinctive white plaques on the palate, gingivae, and lips (Fig. 34.18). There were similar lesions of the genitalia. Histologically, there was a unique finding of clusters of dyskeratotic cells in the prickle cell layer in all affected sites. Aggressive laser treatment was followed by recurrence. Use of etretinate afforded some improvement, but the condition continued unabated more than 20 years.

James WD, et al: Acquired dyskeratotic leukoplakia. Acta Dermatol 1988; 124: 117.
Kim JH, et al: Acquired dyskeratotic leukoplakia of the lip and conjunctiva. Int J Dermatol 2015; 54: 332.

White Sponge Nevus

The mouth, vagina, or rectum may be the site of this spongy, white overgrowth of the mucous membrane, with acanthosis, vacuolated prickle cells, and acidophilic condensations in the cytoplasm of keratinocytes, which electron microscopy has shown to be aggregated tonofilaments. The buccal mucosa is the most common site of involvement. There are no extramucosal lesions. Progression of the disorder generally stops at puberty. The disease is inherited as an autosomal dominant disorder. A mutation in the mucosal keratin pair K4 and K13 has been identified as the inherited defect. HPV-16 DNA has been present in some patients, the significance of which remains to be determined. Antibiotics, particularly tetracycline, may give significant improvement. A 0.25% aqueous preparation of tetracycline as a mouth rinse, 5 mL swished in the mouth for 1 min twice daily, has been successful.

Bumbăcea RS, et al: Familial case of white sponge nevus. Acta Dermatovenerol Croat 2015; 23: 228.
Cai W, et al: Current approaches to the diagnosis and treatment of white sponge nevus. Expert Rev Mol Med 2015; 17: e9.
Kimura M, et al: Mutation of keratin 4 gene causing white sponge nevus in a Japanese family. Int J Oral Maxillofac Surg 2013; 42: 615.

Melanocytic Oral Lesions

A wide variety of melanocytic lesions appear on the mucous membranes. Nevi of the oral mucosa in general are extremely uncommon. Among the melanocytic nevi of the cellular type, the intramucosal type occurs most frequently, with the compound nevus next and the junction nevus occurring only rarely. Ephelis,

lentigo, blue nevus, Spitz nevus, and labial melanotic macules are other types of focal hyperpigmentation. Ephelides darken on sun exposure and are usually limited to the lower lip. The blue nevus has dendritic cells in the submucosa. Lentigines show acanthosis of rete ridges on biopsy. Oral melanotic macules are solitary, sharply demarcated, flat, pigmented lesions that occur chiefly in young women, do not change on sun exposure, and show only acanthosis and basal-layer melanin on biopsy.

Oral melanoacanthoma is a simultaneous proliferation of keratinocytes and melanocytes. It is most frequently observed in young black patients (average age 23) on the buccal mucosa. It seems to be a reactive process, usually after trauma and resolving spontaneously in 40% of patients. It has been reported to be multifocal, as was likely the case with a patient reported by James et al. A 30-year-old woman developed numerous distinct pigmented oral macules. The condition progressed rapidly to a diffuse oral hyperpigmentation (Fig. 34.19). This appeared to be caused by an undefined inflammation, and slow partial resolution occurred after several years of observation.

Melanoma occurs infrequently, mostly in older patients. It is recognized by being larger than the usual benign pigmented lesion and more irregular in shape, with a tendency to ulcerate and bleed. A peripheral areola of erythema and satellite pigmented spots may be present. There is a striking predilection for palatal (or less often gingival) involvement. The overall prognosis is poor (<5% survival at 5 years) because the lesions are usually deeply invasive by the time they are discovered. Whereas oral nevi are uncommon, biopsy of solitary pigmented oral lesions is indicated when the clinical diagnosis is uncertain. Biopsy of a pigmented tumor will occasionally reveal an SCC.

Cardoso LB, et al: Oral compound nevus. Dermatol Online J 2014; 20.
Feller L, et al: A review of the aetiopathogenesis and clinical and histopathological features of oral mucosal melanoma. Scientific World Journal 2017; 2017: 9189812.
Fernandes D, et al: Pigmented lesions on the mucosa. Oral Surg Oral Med Oral Pathol Oral Radiol 2015; 119: 374.
Gondak RO, et al: Oral pigmented lesions. Med Oral Patol Oral Cir Bucal 2012; 17: e919.
Gupta AA, et al: Oral melanoacanthoma. J Oral Maxillofac Pathol 2012; 16: 441.
James WD, et al: Inflammatory acquired oral hyperpigmentation. J Am Acad Dermatol 1987; 16: 220.
Kauzman A, et al: The blue nevus. Gen Dent 2014; 62: e22.
Lambertini M, et al: Oral melanoma and other pigmentations. J Eur Acad Dermatol Venereol 2017 Sep 1; ePub ahead of print.
Matsumoto N, et al: Pigmented oral carcinoma in situ. Oral Surg Oral Med Oral Pathol Oral Radiol 2014; 118: e79.

Ojha J, et al: Intraoral cellular blue nevus. Cutis 2007; 80: 189.
Shen ZY, et al: Oral melanotic macule and primary oral malignant melanoma. Oral Surg Oral Med Oral Pathol Oral Radiol Endod 2011; 112: e21.
Vaccaro M, et al: Spitz nevus. Pediatr Dermatol 2016; 33: e154.

Melanosis

Pigmentation of the oral cavity tends to occur most frequently in black persons. In other races, the darker the skin, the more mucosal pigmentation may be expected. Oral melanosis may occur with Albright syndrome, Peutz-Jeghers syndrome, Carney complex, Laugier-Hunziker disease, and Addison disease or, rarely, as an idiopathic process with no associated disease.

The differential diagnosis of oral hyperpigmentation should include the amalgam tattoo, a focal, brownish blue macule arising from fragments of dental silver or amalgam implanting into the buccal mucosa or gingiva (Fig. 34.20). Heavy-metal poisoning may also induce such lesions. Bismuth, lead, and cisplatin may produce a pigmented line along the gums near their margin. A multitude of drugs will cause pigmentation; the most common include amodiaquine, chloroquine, imatinib, oral contraceptives, phenothiazines, phenolphthalein, quinacrine, quinidine, thallium, nicotine (tobacco), and zidovudine.

Alawi F: Pigmented lesions of the oral cavity. Dent Clin North Am 2013; 57: 699.
Meleti M, et al: Oral pigmented lesions of the oral mucosa and perioral tissues. Oral Surg Oral Med Oral Pathol Oral Radiol Endod 2008; 105: 606.
Moraes RM, et al: Graphite oral tattoo. Dermatol Online J 2015; 21.

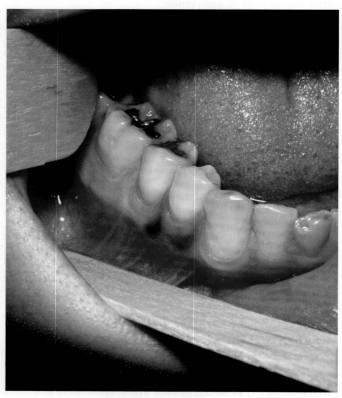

Fig. 34.20 Amalgam tattoo.

Osseous Choristoma of the Tongue

Osseous choristoma of the tongue presents as a nodule on the dorsum of the tongue containing mature lamellar bone without osteoblastic or osteoclastic activity. This does not recur after simple excision.

Adhikari BR, et al: Osseous choristoma of the tongue. J Med Case Rep 2016; 10: 59.
Ginat DT, Portugal L: Lingual osseous choristoma. Ear Nose Throat J 2016; 95: 260.

Peripheral Ameloblastoma

This is a neoplasm of the gingivae, which appears most often on the lower jaw. The mean age at onset is the early fifties and men outnumber women. Peripheral ameloblastoma presents as a growing, pink to red, sessile or pedunculated mass. Excision is followed by recurrence in 19% of the cases, but the lesion is benign. It can simulate basal cell carcinoma histologically.

Chhina S, Rathore AS: Peripheral ameloblastoma of gingiva with cytokeratin 19 analysis. BMJ Case Rep 2015 Jun 4; 2015.

TRUMPETER'S WART

Trumpeter's wart is a firm, fibrous, hyperkeratotic, pseudoepitheliomatous nodule on the upper lip of a trumpet player. A similar callus may grow on the lower lip of trombone players.

Gambichler T, et al: Skin conditions in instrumental musicians. Contact Dermatitis 2008; 58: 217.

EPULIS

The term *epulis* means any benign lesion situated on the gingiva. The majority of these are reactive processes that display varying degrees of fibrosis, inflammation, and vascular proliferation on biopsy. Giant cell epulis (peripheral giant cell granuloma) is a solitary, bluish red, 10–20 mm tumor occurring on the gingiva between or around deciduous bicuspids and incisors. Lesions may be induced by dental implants. Similar lesions may occur in the autosomal dominant inherited syndrome, cherubism. Histologically, epulides resemble giant cell tumor of the tendon sheath.

Banthia R, et al: Peripheral giant cell granuloma. Gen Dent 2013; 61: e12.
Roginsky VV, et al: Familial cherubism. Int J Oral Maxillofac Surg 2009; 38: 218.
Yee J: Congenital epulis in a newborn. Minn Med 2014; 97: 39.

Pyogenic Granuloma

Pyogenic granuloma is an exuberant overgrowth of granulation tissue, frequently occurring in the oral cavity, most often involving the gingiva. It may also occur on the buccal mucosa, lips, tongue, or palate. It is a red to reddish purple, soft, nodular mass that bleeds easily and grows rapidly, but is usually not painful. It often develops during pregnancy. Surgical excision, pulsed dye, erbium:yttrium-aluminum-garnet (Er:YAG) or neodymium:YAG laser, and cryosurgery offer effective methods of treatment.

Cardoso JA, et al: Oral granuloma gravidarum. J Appl Oral Sci 2013; 21: 215.
Cheney-Peters D, Lund TC: Oral pyogenic granuloma after bone marrow transplant in the pediatric/adolescent population. J Pediatr Hematol Oncol 2016; 38: 570.

Daif ET: Correlation of age, sex, and location with recurrence of oral giant pyogenic granuloma after surgical excision. J Craniofac Surg 2016; 27: e433.

Kaya A, et al: Oral pyogenic granuloma associated with a dental implant treated with an Er:YAG laser. J Oral Implantol 2015; 41: 720.

Kocaman G, et al: The use of surgical Nd:YAG laser in an oral pyogenic granuloma. J Cosmet Laser Ther 2014; 16: 197.

Thompson LD: Lobular capillary hemangioma (pyogenic granuloma) of the oral cavity. Ear Nose Throat J 2017; 96: 240.

GRANULOMA FISSURATUM

Granuloma fissuratum is a circumscribed, firm, whitish, fissured, fibrous granuloma occurring in the labioalveolar fold. The lesion is discoid, smooth, and slightly raised, about 1 cm in diameter. The growth is folded like a bent coin, so that the fissure in the bend is continuous on both sides with the labioalveolar sulcus. Symptoms are slight. It is an inflammatory fibrous hyperplasia that usually results from chronic irritation caused by poorly fitting dentures. In the dental literature, it is called epulis fissuratum, particularly when there is a deep cleft traversing the lesion. Treatment is by surgical extirpation, CO_2 laser ablation, or electrodesiccation after biopsy.

Mohan RP, et al: Epulis fissuratum. BMJ Case Rep 2013 Jul 17; 2013.

ANGINA BULLOSA HEMORRHAGICA

The sudden appearance of one or more blood blisters of the oral mucosa characterizes angina bullosa hemorrhagica. There is no associated skin or systemic disease. The blisters may be recurrent, occur most often in the soft palate, and usually present in middle-aged or elderly patients. No treatment is necessary.

Shoor H, et al: Angina bullosa haemorrhagica. BMJ Case Rep 2013 Dec 11; 2013.

Singh D, et al: Angina bullosa haemorrhagica. BMJ Case Rep 2013 Feb 8; 2013.

MUCOCELE

The term *mucocele* refers to a lesion resulting from trauma or obstruction of the minor salivary ducts. The most common type is the mucous extravasation phenomenon, which is usually seen inside the lower lip because it is caused by trauma from biting (Fig. 34.21). The inside of the upper lip and buccal mucosa are infrequently involved. It presents as a soft, rounded, translucent projection and usually has a bluish tint. The lesion varies from 2–10 mm in diameter. It is painless, fluctuant, and tense. Incision, or sometimes merely compression, releases sticky, straw-colored fluid (or bluish fluid if hemorrhage has occurred into it). Usually, the lesions are solitary; however, multiple superficial mucoceles have been reported to occur with graft-versus-host disease and lichenoid inflammation. In these patients, topical corticosteroids may help prevent recurrences.

The cause of mucocele is rupture of the mucous duct, with extravasation of sialomucin into the submucosa to produce cystic spaces with inflammation. Granulation tissue formation is followed by fibrosis. Excisional biopsy will document the diagnosis and eliminate the problem. Cryotherapy and laser ablation have also been reported to be successful.

There are mucous retention cysts in which true obstruction of the duct leads to an epithelial-lined cavity. These are seen more in the posterior portions of the oral mucosa. A ranula (from *Rana*, the frog genus) is a mucocele of the floor of the mouth.

Two other cysts may be present in the mouth. The parotid duct cyst occurs in musicians who use wind instruments; it develops opposite the upper second molar on the buccal mucosa. The dermoid cyst may occur on the floor of the mouth, especially in the sublingual area.

Carlson ER: Diagnosis and management of salivary lesions of the neck. Atlas Oral Maxillofac Surg Clin North Am 2015; 23: 49.

Carlson ER, Ord RA: Benign pediatric salivary gland lesions. Oral Maxillofac Surg Clin North Am 2016; 28: 67.

Vieira EM, et al: Unusual dermoid cyst in oral cavity. Case Rep Pathol 2014; 2014: 389752.

ACUTE NECROTIZING ULCERATIVE GINGIVOSTOMATITIS (TRENCH MOUTH, VINCENT DISEASE)

Acute necrotizing ulcerative gingivitis (ANUG) is characterized by a rapid onset of characteristic punched-out ulcerations appearing on the interdental papillae and marginal gingivae. A dirty-white pseudomembrane may cover the ulcerations (Fig. 34.22). The lesions may spread rapidly and involve the buccal mucosa, lips, and tongue, as well as the tonsils, pharynx, and entire respiratory tract. The slightest pressure causes pain and bleeding. There is a characteristic foul, fetid odor that is always present. ANUG may

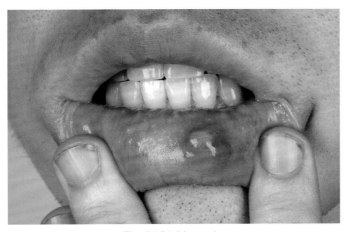

Fig. 34.21 Mucocele.

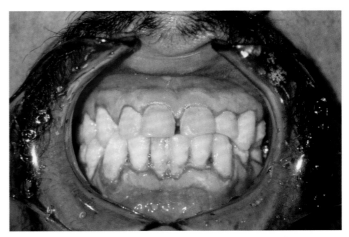

Fig. 34.22 Acute necrotizing ulcerative gingivostomatitis. (Courtesy Department of Oral Medicine, University of Pennsylvania School of Dentistry.)

lead to loss of attachment of the gingiva and alveolar bone (necrotizing ulcerative periodontitis).

Trench mouth begins in a nidus of necrotic tissue, which provides an anaerobic environment for the infection by fusospirochetal organisms (*Bacteroides fusiformis*) in association with *Borrelia vincentii* and other organisms. Poor dental hygiene, smoking, poor nutrition, ingestion of methylenedioxymethamphetamine (ecstasy), and immunosuppression are predisposing factors. It may be seen as a component of the oral infections and inflammatory lesions that occur in immunocompromised HIV-infected patients.

Acute herpetic gingivostomatitis, or primary HSV infection, may be confused with ANUG. Young children are susceptible to this severe febrile stomatitis with lymphadenitis. It is not primarily gingival in location and does not cause necrosis of the interdental papillae. Noma is a form of fusospirillary gangrenous stomatitis occurring in children with low resistance and poor nutrition. The onset is often triggered by measles. At the onset, there is ulceration of the buccal mucosa; this rapidly assumes a gangrenous character and extends to involve the skin and bones, with resultant necrosis. It may end in the patient's death.

Treatment of ANUG consists of thorough dental hygienic measures under the supervision of a dentist. Penicillin with debridement is the treatment of choice. Use of a 3% hydrogen peroxide mouthwash is also helpful.

Atout RN, Todescan S: Managing patients with necrotizing ulcerative gingivitis. J Can Dent Assoc 2013; 79: d46.

Feller L, et al: Necrotizing periodontal diseases in HIV-seropositive subjects. J Int Acad Periodontol 2008; 10: 10.

Hu J, et al: Acute necrotising ulcerative gingivitis in an immunocompromised young adult. BMJ Case Rep 2015 Sep 16; 2015.

Tonna JE, et al: A case and review of noma. PLoS Negl Trop Dis 2010; 4: e869.

ACATALASEMIA

Acatalasemia (Takahara disease) is a rare disease in which the enzyme catalase is deficient in the liver, muscles, bone marrow, erythrocytes, and skin. There are several forms. The absence of catalase leads to progressive gangrene of the mouth, with recurrent ulcerations resulting from increased susceptibility to infection by anaerobic organisms.

Almost 60% of patients with acatalasemia develop alveolar ulcerations, beginning in childhood. The mild type of the disease is characterized by rapidly recurring ulcers. In the moderate type, alveolar gangrene develops, with atrophy and recession of the alveolar bone, so that the teeth fall out spontaneously. In the severe type, widespread destruction of the jaw occurs. After puberty, all lesions heal, even in individuals who have the severe type.

There is no gross difference in appearance between the blood of an acatalasic patient and that of a normal individual, but when hydrogen peroxide is added to a sample of blood, acatalasic blood immediately turns blackish brown, and the peroxide does not foam. Normal blood remains bright and causes the peroxide to foam exuberantly because of the presence of erythrocyte catalase.

Acatalasia is a rare peroxisomal disorder and is inherited as an autosomal recessive trait. Treatment consists of extraction of the diseased teeth and the use of antibiotics to control the harmful effects of the causative bacteria.

Goth L, et al: Inherited catalase deficiency. Mutat Res 2013; 753: 147.

Wang Q, et al: Long-term follow-up evaluation of an acatalasemia boy with severe periodontitis. Clin Chim Acta 2014; 433: 93.

CYCLIC NEUTROPENIA

Cyclic, or periodic, neutropenia is characterized by a decrease of circulating neutrophils and dermatologic manifestations. At regular intervals (21 days), neutropenia and mouth ulcerations develop, usually accompanied by fever, malaise, and arthralgia. Ulcerations of the lips, tongue, palate, gums, and buccal mucosa may be extensive. The ulcers are irregularly outlined and are covered by a grayish white necrotic slough. The anterior teeth may show a grayish brown discoloration. Premature alveolar bone loss and periodontitis occur. In addition, opportunistic cutaneous infections, such as abscesses, furuncles, noma, pyomyositis, and cellulitis, may develop during the neutropenic stage. Urticaria and erythema multiforme have been reported.

There is a cyclic depression of neutrophils occurring at intervals of 12–30 days (average 21 days) and lasting 5–8 days. The neutrophils in the peripheral blood regularly fall to low levels or completely disappear. Some cases have been associated with agammaglobulinemia. The cause of cyclic neutropenia is a germline mutation of the gene encoding neutrophil elastase (*ELANE*). This is thought to produce apoptosis of bone marrow progenitor cells. Both autosomal dominant disease and sporadic cases have this abnormality. Severe congenital neutropenia is caused by a mutation in the same gene but at a different site. The latter condition predisposes to the development of myelodysplasia and acute myelogenous leukemia, whereas cyclic neutropenia does not.

The differential diagnosis includes other periodic fever syndromes, such as the periodic fever, aphthous stomatitis, pharyngitis, and adenopathy (PFAPA) syndrome; Mediterranean fever; Hibernian fever and hyperimmunoglobulin D syndrome; TNF receptor–associated periodic syndrome (TRAPS); and pyogenic sterile arthritis, pyoderma gangrenosum, and acne (PAPA) syndrome. All share a predisposition to the development of aphthous-like oral ulcerations. The autoinflammatory syndromes are discussed in detail in Chapter 7.

Use of recombinant human granulocyte colony-stimulating factor (G-CSF) has been successful in the treatment of cyclic neutropenia patients. If side effects limit use of this therapy, cyclosporine has been reported to be effective as well. Administering antibiotics during infections seems to expedite recovery. Careful attention to oral hygiene, including plaque control, helps improve mouth lesions and reduces the risk of infections. Death may occur from pneumonia, sepsis, gangrenous pyoderma, or granulocytopenia.

Ashok N, et al: A review on noma. Glob J Health Sci 2015; 8: 53.

Boo YJ, et al: Cyclic neutropenia with a novel gene mutation presenting with a necrotizing soft tissue infection and severe sepsis. BMC Pediatr 2015; 15: 34.

Chen Y, et al: Cyclic neutropenia presenting as recurrent oral ulcers and periodontitis. J Clin Pediatr Dent 2013; 37: 307.

Cush JJ: Autoinflammatory syndromes. Dermatol Clin 2013; 31: 471.

Horwitz MS, et al: *ELANE* mutations in cyclic and severe congenital neutropenia. Hematol Oncol Clin North Am 2013; 27: 19.

Nguyen TV, et al: Autoinflammation. J Am Acad Dermatol 2013; 68: 834.

Tripathi SV, et al: Autoinflammatory diseases in dermatology. Dermatol Clin 2013; 31: 387.

RECURRENT INTRAORAL HERPES SIMPLEX INFECTION

Recurrent intraoral infection with HSV is characterized by numerous small, discrete vesicles occurring in one or a few

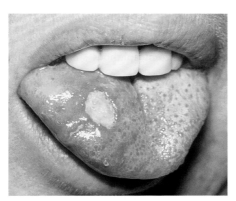

Fig. 34.23 Chronic herpes in patient receiving cancer chemotherapy.

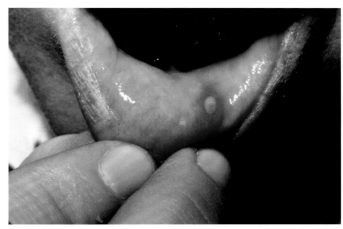

Fig. 34.24 Aphthous stomatitis. (Courtesy Steven Binnick, MD.)

clusters. The site of involvement is a key feature in suspecting the diagnosis. The keratinized or masticatory mucosa—the palate, gingiva, and tongue—is affected. The grouped vesicles rupture rapidly to form punctate erosions with a red base. Smears from the base prepared with Wright stain will show giant multinucleated epithelial cells. Immunofluorescent tests and viral cultures are also confirmatory.

The differential diagnosis of this uncommon manifestation of HSV includes oral herpes zoster, herpangina, and oral aphthosis. The latter two involve nonattached mucosa, whereas recurrent HSV involves mucosa fixed to bone. Differentiation from zoster is made on clinical grounds or by culture and immunofluorescent testing.

Chronic progressive ulcerative and nodular intraoral herpes are seen occasionally in HIV-infected patients or those with leukemia or neutropenia (Fig. 34.23). The presentation may mimic mucosal toxicity to chemotherapy. Solitary painful erosions of the tongue or attached mucosa should be tested for HSV in such patients. Additionally, herpetic geometric glossitis may occur, with linear longitudinal, cross-hatched, or branching fissures of the dorsal tongue, usually along the central area. This condition may be quite painful and may limit oral intake. Although the glossitis usually affects only immunocompromised patients, at least one immunocompetent patient has been affected.

Mirowski GW, et al: Herpetic geometric glossitis in an immunocompetent patient with pneumonia. J Am Acad Dermatol 2009; 61: 139.
Stoopler ET, et al: Recurrent intraoral herpes. J Emerg Med 2016; 51: 324.

RECURRENT APHTHOUS STOMATITIS (CANKER SORES, APHTHOSIS)

Clinical Features

Aphthous stomatitis is a painful, recurrent disease of the oral mucous membrane. It begins as small, red, discrete, or grouped papules, which in a few hours become necrotizing ulcerations. They are small, round, shallow, white ulcers (aphthae), generally surrounded by a ring of hyperemia (Fig. 34.24). As a rule, they are tender; they may become so painful that they interfere with speech and mastication. They are mostly about 5 mm in diameter but may vary in size from 3–10 mm. When larger, they are called major aphthae. A third subcategory, herpetiform aphthae, consists of small, 1- to 3-mm lesions grouped into a coalescing larger plaque, which may take 1–4 weeks to resolve. Usually, one to five lesions occur per attack; however, they may occur in any number. They are located in decreasing frequency on the buccal and labial mucosa, edges of the tongue, buccal and lingual sulci, and soft palate. There is a marked predilection for the nonkeratinized mucosa (any not bound to underlying periosteum). This fact, and because they are rarely confluent, even when they occur as small crops of 1- or 2-mm lesions (herpetiform aphthae), help to distinguish them from the uncommon, recurrent intraoral HSV infection. Aphthae may also occur on the vagina, vulva, penis, anus, and even the conjunctiva. When they involve the oral and genital mucosa and number three or more, the term *complex aphthosis* is applied.

The lesions tend to involute in 1–2 weeks, but recurrences are common. These recurrences may be induced by trauma (e.g., self-biting, toothbrush injury, dental procedures), spicy foods, citrus, fresh pineapple, walnuts, allergy, emotional stress, or hormonal changes in women, as in menstruation, pregnancy, menarche, and menopause. A familial predisposition has also been described as familial epidemic aphthosis.

Recurrent aphthous stomatitis is the most common lesion of the oral mucosa, affecting 10%–20% of the population. It typically starts in the second or third decade, and patients may experience recurrent bouts of lesions several times yearly for many decades. When present in neonates or young children, autoinflammatory syndromes should be considered. In PFAPA syndrome, the high fevers and associated findings occur with striking periodicity every 4 weeks, last 4–6 days, and resolve only to recur the following month. The children are otherwise well. One or two doses of prednisone (2 mg/kg) abort the attack, and tonsillectomy may cure it. Aphthous oral ulcerations may also be seen in the autoinflammatory syndromes, such as familial Mediterranean fever, TRAPS, hyperimmunoglobulinemia D and periodic fever, PAPA syndrome, and deficiency of the interleukin-1 receptor antagonist (DIRA) syndrome.

Ulcerations such as these may also be the presenting sign in Behçet syndrome, HIV infection, malabsorption syndromes, gluten-sensitive enteropathy, pernicious anemia, cyclic neutropenia, neutropenia, ulcerative colitis, and Crohn disease. History, physical examination, complete blood count, and long-term follow-up documenting the recurrent course, in the absence of other symptoms, will secure the diagnosis. Some patients have aphthosis associated with low folate, vitamin B_{12}, or iron levels, so testing should include this evaluation.

Etiologic Factors

Although individual patients often suspect that one of the factors just mentioned is responsible for precipitating recurrence of the lesions, investigators favor infectious or immunologic causation. The true cause is unknown.

Histologically, the lesion consists of a lymphocytic inflammatory infiltration with occasional plasma cells and eosinophils, which suggests delayed hypersensitivity.

Diagnosis

Aphthous stomatitis must be differentiated from mucous patches of early syphilis, candidiasis, Vincent angina, the avitaminoses (particularly pellagra and scurvy), erythema multiforme, pemphigus, cicatricial pemphigoid, lichen planus, primary HSV infection of the mouth, recurrent labial herpes, and recurrent intraoral HSV infection.

Treatment

No permanent cure is available for aphthosis. Several topical agents will lessen the pain. A mixture of equal parts of elixir of Benadryl and Maalox, held in the mouth for 5 minutes before meals, is soothing. Kaolin may also be added to the mixture. Lidocaine (Xylocaine Viscous) 2% solution, keeping 1 teaspoonful in the mouth for several minutes, is also helpful in allaying pain. Another useful topical anesthetic is dyclonine hydrochloride (Dyclone) 0.5% applied to the lesions. A large number of reasonably effective over-the-counter remedies are also available. Triggers, such as spicy foods, citrus, walnuts, pineapple, and other irritating substances, should be avoided.

Other measures may be used to shorten the course and induce healing of lesions. Chlorhexidine mouthwashes are used twice daily with any of the other treatments described. A mixture of equal parts of fluocinonide ointment and Orabase, applied to the ulcers three or four times daily, is effective in aiding the healing of existing ulcers; however, it does not prevent new ulcers. Some patients object to the thick, sticky texture of Orabase and prefer fluocinonide gel. Clobetasol ointment can also be very effective. Intralesional corticosteroids and short, 3- or 4-day courses of oral corticosteroids may help, particularly for indolent or large lesions. Nonsteroidal alternatives include 5 mL of an oral suspension containing 250 mg of tetracycline; this is held in the mouth for 2 minutes and then swallowed. This is done four times daily for 1 week. Amlexanox 5% oral paste (Aphthasol) is a useful topical therapy both to induce healing and to relieve pain. Sucralfate suspension, alone or compounded with a topical corticosteroid, may be useful, as described in peptic ulcer disease and the ulcerations of Behçet disease.

To try to prevent new lesions, known triggers for the individual patient should be avoided as much as possible. Colchicine at 0.6 mg/day for 1 week, then increasing to 1.2 or even 1.8 mg/day, is recommended. If this is ineffective or GI or other side effects limit dosage, dapsone may be added to colchicine or substituted for it. It is given in steadily increasing doses of 25 mg for 3 days, then 50 mg for 3 days, then 75 mg for 3 days, then 100 mg for 7 days. If the blood count is normal, no side effects are present, and the disease is not controlled, further increases to 125 mg or even 150 mg may be given. Thalidomide and lenalidomide are other effective alternatives, but caution regarding teratogenicity and neurotoxicity is necessary if this is considered. One method is thalidomide, 300 mg/day to start, 200 mg/day after 10 days, and 100 mg/day after 2 months. Relapses are treated with 100 mg/day for 12 days.

Several investigators have reported finding low folate, iron, or B_{12} levels in about 20% of aphthosis patients investigated, but others do not see this with such high frequency. Still, it is worth investigating, because correction of the abnormality clears or improves the condition in most patients who have an abnormality. Two studies document improvement with cyanocobalamin, even in those without abnormality.

Akintoye SO, Greenberg MS: Recurrent aphthous stomatitis. Dent Clin North Am 2014; 58: 281.

Brocklehurst P, et al: Systemic interventions for recurrent aphthous stomatitis (mouth ulcers). Cochrane Database Syst Rev 2012; 9: CD005411.

Cui RZ, et al: Recurrent aphthous stomatitis. Clin Dermatol 2016; 34: 475.

Femiano F, et al: Guidelines for diagnosis and management of aphthous stomatitis. Pediatr Infect Dis J 2007; 26: 728.

Glucan E, et al: Cyanocobalamin may be beneficial in the treatment of recurrent aphthous stomatitis even when vitamin B_{12} levels are normal. Am J Med Sci 2008; 336: 379.

Kalampokis I, Rabinovich CE: Successful management of refractory pediatric-onset complex aphthosis with lenalidomide. J Clin Rheumatol 2014; 20: 221.

Manthiram K, et al: Family history in periodic fever, aphthous stomatitis, pharyngitis, adenitis (PFAPA) syndrome. Pediatrics 2016; 138,

Mays JW, et al: Oral manifestations of systemic autoimmune and inflammatory diseases. J Evid Based Dent Pract 2012; 12: 265.

Montgomery-Cranny JA, et al: Management of recurrent aphthous stomatitis in children. Dent Update 2015; 42: 564.

Stoopler ET, Sollecito TP: Recurrent oral ulcers. JAMA 2015; 313: 2373.

MAJOR APHTHOUS ULCER

In Sutton disease, a major aphthous ulcer begins as a small, shotlike nodule on the inner lip, buccal mucosa, or tongue that breaks down into a painful, sharply circumscribed ulcer with a deeply punched-out and depressed crater. It may at times begin in the faucial pillars or oropharynx (Fig. 34.25). It may persist for 2–12 weeks before healing with a soft, pliable scar. There are seldom more than one to three lesions present at one time. However, remissions tend to be short, and new lesions may appear before old ones have healed.

The cause is unknown, but evidence favors an immunologic or infectious etiology. These painful lesions are frequently present in immunocompromised HIV-infected patients who may experience similar lesions in the esophagus, rectum, anus, and genitals. Treatment is difficult, and the general measures discussed under recurrent aphthae should be employed. Intralesional or systemic corticosteroids in short courses may be effective and are often given. If recurrences are such that systemic steroids are prescribed for more than two or three short courses per year, alternative oral medications, such as colchicine, dapsone, or thalidomide, may be tried.

Boldo A: Major recurrent aphthous ulceration. Conn Med 2008; 72: 271.

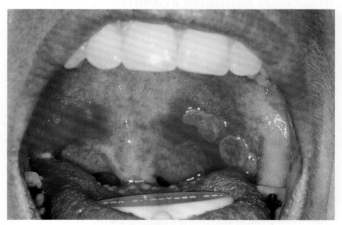

Fig. 34.25 Major aphthae.

Picciani BL, et al: Regression of major recurrent aphthous ulcerations using a combination of intralesional corticosteroids and levamisole. Clinics 2010; 65: 650.

BEHÇET SYNDROME (OCULO-ORAL-GENITAL SYNDROME)

Clinical Features

Behçet syndrome consists of recurrent oral aphthous ulcerations that recur at least three times in one 12-month period in the presence of any two of the following: recurrent genital ulceration, retinal vasculitis or anterior or posterior uveitis, cutaneous lesions (erythema nodosum; pseudofolliculitis or papulopustular lesions; or acneiform nodules in postadolescent patients who are not receiving corticosteroid treatment), or a positive pathergy test.

Oral lesions occur on the lips, tongue (Fig. 34.26), buccal mucosa, soft and hard palate, tonsils, and even in the pharynx and nasal cavity. The lesions are single or multiple, 2–10 mm or larger in diameter, and sharply circumscribed, with a dirty-grayish base and a surrounding bright-red halo. Other patients show deep ulcerations that leave scars resembling those caused by Sutton major aphthous ulcers. The lesions are so painful that eating may be difficult. A foul mouth odor is in most cases very noticeable.

Genital lesions occur in men on the scrotum and penis or in the urethra and in women on the vulva, cervix, or vagina; lesions may be found in both genders on the genitocrural fold, anus, or perineum or in the rectum. These ulcerations are similar to those seen in the mouth. In addition, macules, papules, and folliculitis may develop on the scrotum. Lesions in women may lead to deep destruction of the vulva. Swellings of the regional nodes and fever may accompany oral and genital attacks.

The ocular lesions start with intense periorbital pain and photophobia. Retinal vasculitis is the most classic eye sign and the major cause of blindness. Conjunctivitis may be an early accompaniment of uveitis, and hypopyon may be a late one. Iridocyclitis is frequently seen. Both eyes are eventually involved. Untreated disease leads to blindness from optic atrophy, glaucoma, or cataracts.

Neurologic manifestations are mostly in the central nervous system and resemble most closely those of multiple sclerosis. Remissions and exacerbations are the rule. Thrombophlebitis occurs with some frequency. Thrombosis of the superior vena cava may also occur. Arthralgia is most often present in the form of polyarthritis.

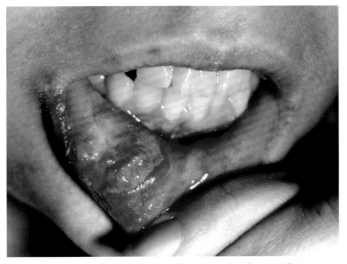

Fig. 34.26 Behçet disease. (Courtesy Ken Greer, MD.)

Unfortunately, the international criteria include nonspecific common cutaneous lesions (pseudofolliculitis, papulopustular or acneiform lesions). Demonstration of either leukocytoclastic vasculitis or a neutrophilic vascular reaction on histologic examination of a lesion would make the cutaneous criteria more specific.

There is a relatively high prevalence of Behçet disease in the Far East and Mediterranean countries, whereas in the United States and Western Europe it is much less common. In large series of patients from areas of high prevalence, men with an age of onset in the thirties predominate. They tend to have a worse prognosis than women. In the United States most reported patients are young women with a high frequency of mucocutaneous lesions and a low prevalence of ocular involvement. This may reflect referral bias or could indicate that the disease is less severe and female predominant in the United States.

On histologic examination, the early lesions show a leukocytoclastic vasculitis. There is perivascular infiltration, which is chiefly lymphocytic in older lesions, with endothelial proliferation that obliterates the lumen. The cause of Behçet disease has been postulated to have an infectious, immunologic, and/or genetic basis, but the evidence is still inconclusive for any of these.

Diagnosis

Usually, the disease starts with a single oral ulceration, which is followed by others. It may take years before additional lesions develop. Again, the diagnosis requires two classic signs in addition to oral ulcerations. In women, anal and genital lesions predominate, often with subsequent involvement of the eyes.

Behçet disease must be differentiated from herpetic or aphthous stomatitis, pemphigus, oral cancer, and Stevens-Johnson syndrome (erythema multiforme). A skin puncture or pathergy test may be used to investigate patients further; however, it is not reliable in that it may be negative in otherwise well-documented cases. It is done by injecting 0.1 mL of normal saline solution into the skin or by simply pricking the skin with a sterile needle. A pustule appears at the site within 24 hours. If results are negative, the test should be repeated at two to five points before results are accepted. Pathergy has been observed in patients with Behçet disease, pyoderma gangrenosum, Sweet syndrome, and bowel-associated dermatosis–arthritis syndrome.

Treatment

Usually, the ulcerations heal spontaneously. Chlorhexidine mouthwashes twice daily and toothpastes and restricted use of the toothbrush should be prescribed when there are oral lesions. For treating the symptoms and healing of the aphthae, local treatments as described for aphthae may be used. Sucralfate suspension has been studied in Behçet oral and genital ulcers and was found to decrease pain and healing time. On the whole, the therapeutic problem of aphthosis is not the healing of the individual lesions but the prevention of new attacks. For that purpose, several options exist, none of which is optimal. Colchicine, 0.6 mg twice daily, may be started for 2 weeks. In the absence of response and GI side effects, the dose may be increased to three times daily. Although this may not totally alleviate the mucocutaneous lesions, it may decrease their recurrence rate by 50% or more. Dapsone may be substituted or added to this for improvement of response. The usual therapeutic final dose is 100 mg/day. Thalidomide has been found to be effective in many patients. One dosing method is thalidomide, 200 mg twice daily for 5 days, and 100 mg twice daily for 15–60 days. It has no effect on iridocyclitis. Again, long-term treatment will usually be complicated by neurotoxicity, and the teratogenicity of thalidomide is well known.

Methotrexate, in a weekly oral dose of 7.5–20 mg, should be reserved for severe refractory cases, as should more aggressive systemic treatments such as systemic corticosteroids, azathioprine, chlorambucil, cyclosporine, interferon alfa, TNF antagonists, apremilast, anakinra, tocilizumab, rituximab, and cyclophosphamide. In general these more aggressive therapeutics have been tested in small trials or case series for treatment of ocular, neurologic, pulmonary, digestive, or vascular manifestations.

The long-term outlook is for intermittent recurrent flares that may be lifelong. Blindness, neurologic impairment, and vascular thromboses are potential serious complications of Behçet syndrome.

Alpsoy E: Behçet's disease. J Dermatol 2016; 43: 620.

Davari P, et al: Clinical features of Behçet's disease. J Dermatolog Treat 2016; 27: 70.

Hatemi G, et al: One year in review 2017: Behçet's syndrome. Clin Exp Rheumatol 2017; 35 Suppl 108: 3.

Koné-Paut I: Behçet's disease in children, an overview. Pediatr Rheumatol Online J 2016; 14: 10.

Ozguler Y, Hatemi G: Management of Behçet's syndrome. Curr Opin Rheumatol 2016; 28: 45.

Pramod JR: Textbook of oral medicine, 3rd ed. New Delhi: Jaypee Brothers Medical Publishers, 2014.

Rotondo C, et al: Mucocutaneous involvement in Behçet's disease. Mediators Inflamm 2015; 2015: 451675.

Scully C: Oral and maxillofacial medicine, 3rd ed. New York: Churchill Livingstone, 2013.

Sollecito TP, Stoopler ET (Eds.): Clinical approaches to oral mucosal disorders. Dent Clin North Am 2013; 57: 561.

Vitale A, et al: New therapeutic solutions for Behçet's syndrome. Expert Opin Investig Drugs 2016; 25: 827.

35 Cutaneous Vascular Diseases

RAYNAUD PHENOMENON AND RAYNAUD DISEASE

Raynaud phenomenon is characterized by episodic, recurrent vasospasm of the fingers and toes resulting in white, blue, and red discoloration provoked by cold or stress. When it occurs in the presence of an associated disease, usually collagen vascular disease and often systemic sclerosis/scleroderma, it is called secondary Raynaud phenomenon. Raynaud disease (or primary Raynaud disease) occurs in the absence of associated illness. Although no significant structural changes occur in primary Raynaud disease, in secondary Raynaud phenomenon, especially when associated with connective tissue disease, sustained and recurrent vasospasm may lead to vessel wall damage.

In a series of 165 patients with Raynaud phenomenon, 51 had primary Raynaud disease. A defined connective tissue disease was present in about one third of the remaining patients, but 54 had undefined connective tissue disease (35 with positive antinuclear antibody [ANA] titer). In another study of 142 patients with idiopathic Raynaud phenomenon followed for more than 10 years, 14% progressed to a definite connective tissue disease. The initial presence of ANAs, thickening of fingers, older age at onset, and female gender were predictors of connective tissue disease. In a larger study of 3035 patients with primary Raynaud phenomenon, age of onset after 40 and progressively worsening Raynaud attacks were predictive of eventual diagnosis of a connective tissue disease (and reclassification as secondary Raynaud phenomenon), a development that occurred in 37.2% of patients after a mean of 4.8 years of follow-up. Sequential nailfold capillary microscopy and autoantibody determinations can predict development of systemic sclerosis in those with Raynaud phenomenon. The absence of nailfold capillaroscopic findings, conversely, predicts the presence of primary Raynaud disease (no associated systemic illness). Laser Doppler perfusion imaging or Doppler ultrasonography may enhance the evaluation of vascular damage from Raynaud disease. Technetium digital blood flow scintigraphy and skin temperature measurement of the fingers and toes by digital thermography may aid in the early diagnosis of Raynaud phenomenon of either the primary or secondary type.

Many of the studies on pathogenesis and therapy in Raynaud phenomenon are conducted on patients with systemic sclerosis/scleroderma, so it may not be possible to translate these findings to patients with primary Raynaud disease. However, cold exposure is a major trigger of vasospasm in all Raynaud patients. The exaggerated sympathetic response to cold may be caused by both excessive vasoconstrictor tone and a weak systemic vasodilation process, centrally mediated at least in part. The abnormal sympathetic response may also explain why some patients say that "stress" triggers Raynaud attacks. High homocysteine levels have been detected in patients with both primary and secondary Raynaud phenomenon. Patients with systemic sclerosis and Raynaud disease have elevated levels of endothelin 1 (ET-1), which correlates with both nailfold capillaroscopic findings and more advanced disease.

Secondary Raynaud Phenomenon

Raynaud phenomenon is produced by an intermittent constriction of the small digital arteries and arterioles. The digits have sequential pallor, cyanosis, and rubor. The involved parts are affected by ischemic paroxysms, which cause them to become pale, cold to the touch, and numb. The phenomenon is more frequently observed in cold weather. When exposed to cold, the digits become white (ischemic), then blue (cyanotic), and finally red (hyperemic). Over time, the parts may fail to regain their normal circulation between attacks and become persistently cyanotic and painful. If this phenomenon persists over a long period, punctate superficial necrosis of the fingertips develops; later, even gangrene may occur.

Secondary Raynaud phenomenon occurs most frequently in young to middle-aged women. It occurs with scleroderma, dermatomyositis, lupus erythematosus (LE, particularly those with anti-Sm and anti-RNP antibodies), mixed connective tissue disease, Sjögren syndrome, rheumatoid arthritis, and paroxysmal hemoglobinuria. Scleroderma was the underlying diagnosis in more than half of patients in one series. Occlusive arterial diseases, such as embolism, thromboangiitis obliterans, arteriosclerosis obliterans, and large-vessel vasculitis (Takayasu arteritis), may be present. In addition, various diseases of the nervous system, including cervical rib, scalenus anticus syndrome, and complex regional pain syndrome (reflex sympathetic dystrophy), may produce the disorder. Physical trauma, such as hand-transmitted vibration, as occurs with pneumatic hammer operation, can induce a syndrome identical to Raynaud and has been termed *vibration white finger* or *hand-arm vibration syndrome*. Pianists and typists may also develop this phenomenon. Raynaud phenomenon is a well-recognized complication after cold injury, especially frostbite. Pharmacologic agents, such as bleomycin, cisplatin-based chemotherapy, ergot, β-adrenergic blockers (including eye drops), cyclosporine, interferon (IFN)–α and IFN-β, vinyl polychloride exposure, and cocaine, may also be the cause. A French national pharmacovigilance database revealed 175 reports of Raynaud phenomenon among 307,128 adverse drug reports. Women were 61% of cases, and 8% of affected patients had a prior history of Raynaud. New agents reported included ribavirin, gemcitabine, hepatitis vaccine, isotretinoin, leflunomide, hydroxycarbamide, rofecoxib, telmisartan, and zolmitriptan. The clumping of red blood cells (RBCs) is believed to be responsible for the induction of Raynaud phenomenon, with high titers of circulating cold agglutinins. It may occur in cryoglobulinemia and polycythemia vera. Patients with cancer may develop Raynaud as a paraneoplastic phenomenon. Endocrine disorders, such as acromegaly, pheochromocytoma, carcinoid, and hypothyroidism, may present with or be associated with Raynaud phenomenon. Raynaud of the nipple is a variant of Raynaud disease that is difficult to diagnose. It presents with severe pain during lactation and must be distinguished from nipple candidiasis and eczema. Patients report the onset of symptoms during pregnancy and, when asked, will say that the symptoms are triggered by cold and accompanied by biphasic or triphasic color changes of the nipple. Nifedipine can be highly effective in this condition and is safe for use during lactation; minimal drug is found in the breast milk.

Simple tests and physical examination will generally distinguish Raynaud disease from secondary Raynaud phenomenon. Sclerodactyly, digital pitted scars, puffy fingers with telangiectasias, positive ANA, subcutaneous calcifications, basilar lung fibrosis, and changes on nailfold capillary microscopy (avascular "skip" areas with irregularly dilated capillary loops) are signs of connective tissue disease.

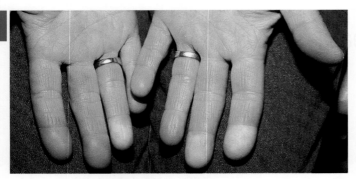

Fig. 35.1 Raynaud disease.

Raynaud Disease (Primary Raynaud Disease)

Raynaud disease is a primary disorder of cold sensitivity primarily seen in young women. The intermittent attacks of pallor, cyanosis, hyperemia, and numbness of the fingers are identical to those in secondary Raynaud phenomenon (Fig. 35.1). The disease is usually bilateral, and gangrene occurs in less than 1% of cases.

The diagnosis requires the absence of the diseases enumerated under secondary Raynaud phenomenon. An international panel proposed the following consensus criteria for differentiation of Raynaud disease from secondary Raynaud phenomenon: normal capillaroscopy; absence of physical findings suggestive of secondary causes, such as sclerodactyly, calcinosis, and ulcerations; no history of existing connective tissue disease; and negative or low-titer ANA (e.g., 1:40). Although some suggest that Raynaud disease should be present for 2 years before being classified as a primary process, it may take as long as 11 years for some systemic disorders to manifest. Overall, fewer than half of patients presenting with Raynaud symptoms will prove to have a connective tissue disease. The prognosis is good for patients with primary Raynaud disease.

Treatment

Treatments have often been studied but only in patients with secondary Raynaud phenomenon and digital ulceration associated with connective tissue disease, so not all treatments can be assumed to be effective in primary Raynaud disease or Raynaud secondary to other causes. If an underlying cause is found, treatment of the associated condition will often lead to improvement of Raynaud phenomenon. In both primary and secondary Raynaud, exposure to cold should be avoided. This includes avoidance of exposure to cold not only of the extremities but also of other parts of the body, because vasospasm may be induced by reduction of core body temperature, and Raynaud attack of atypical sites, such as the tongue, may occur. Warm gloves should be worn whenever possible. Trauma to the fingertips should be avoided. Smoking is absolutely contraindicated. A Raynaud attack may be broken at times by swinging the affected arm in a wide circle from the shoulder—the "windmill" maneuver. The use of standard nitroglycerin paste has had minimal efficacy and can produce systemic side effects. A new form of topical nitroglycerin, MQX-503, significantly improved skin blood flow without serious adverse events in a recent randomized controlled trial (RCT). Alternative treatments, including ginkgo and other herbal medications, have limited efficacy compared with the standard treatments and cannot be recommended for patients with significantly symptomatic disease.

Calcium channel blockers are the first-line therapy used in Raynaud disease because of their efficacy and low side-effect profile. Prolonged-release amlodipine or nifedipine is usually recommended. Some studies indicate that up to two thirds of treated patients will respond favorably. However, a Cochrane review of RCTs of calcium channel blockers for primary Raynaud disease concluded that their benefit was minimal, translating to 1.72 fewer attacks per week compared with placebo. Sildenafil and other phosphodiesterase-5 inhibitors are moderately effective in reducing Raynaud severity score, as well as the frequency and duration of Raynaud episodes, and may improve digital ulcer healing. These have become the second-line agents of choice. The angiotensin receptor antagonist losartan reduced the frequency and severity of attacks to a greater extent than nifedipine in an RCT. Conversely, angiotensin-converting enzyme (ACE) inhibitors failed to show benefit in an RCT and are therefore not recommended. Data on selective serotonin reuptake inhibitors (SSRIs; fluoxetine or ketanserin) are mixed, but SSRIs may be useful in refractory cases or when other agents are not tolerated. Intravenous (IV) biweekly *N*-acetylcysteine was effective in reducing the number of attacks in an observational study, relatively free of side effects. The use of statins, specifically atorvastatin, in patients with Raynaud caused by systemic sclerosis/scleroderma was associated with a reduction in Raynaud-associated symptoms, possibly through the vasoprotective actions of statins. Statin administration was associated with reduced circulating markers of vascular injury, which are usually elevated in scleroderma patients. Bosentan, an endothelin receptor (ETA and ETB) antagonist, significantly reduces the frequency of Raynaud attacks and reduces new digital ulcers. Iloprost, a prostaglandin analog, has substantial efficacy in scleroderma-associated Raynaud disease and digital ulceration, but it is only slightly better than nifedipine and significantly more expensive. Oral prostaglandins appear to lack similar efficacy, except perhaps at high doses.

In cases refractory to these medical treatments, surgical modalities can be considered. Botulinum toxin injections in the palm around each involved neurovascular bundle may lead to dramatic and at times immediate pain reduction. Ulcerations of the affected digits heal after the injections. The duration of response is often months to years, and injections can be repeated with similar efficacy. A review of 10 papers reporting 128 patients in the literature revealed 75%–100% improved, with ulcer healing in 75%–100% of reported patients, with 14.1% experiencing temporary hand weakness. Fat grafting or fat transfer to the hand has also been reported effective in a pilot study. Local digital sympathectomy can be effective and avoids amputation of chronically ulcerated digits. Cervical sympathectomy and endoscopic thoracic sympathectomy may give initial relief, but Raynaud symptoms often recur after 12–18 months. However, despite the return of symptoms, digital ulceration is greatly reduced. Compensatory hyperhidrosis is a common complication of thoracic sympathectomy.

Bank J, et al: Fat grafting to the hand in patients with Raynaud phenomenon. Plast Reconstr Surg 2014; 133: 1109.

Barrett ME, et al: Raynaud phenomenon of the nipple in breastfeeding mothers. JAMA Dermatol 2013; 149: 300.

Blagojevic J, Matucci-Cerinic M: Are statins useful for treating vascular involvement in systemic sclerosis? Nat Clin Pract Rheumatol 2009; 5: 70.

Boulon C, et al: Letter by Boulon and Constans regarding article "Relation of nailfold capillaries and autoantibodies to mortality in patients with Raynaud phenomenon." Circulation 2016; 133: e668.

Bouquet E, et al: Unexpected drug-induced Raynaud phenomenon. Therapie 2017; 72: 547.

Bovenzi M: A longitudinal study of vibration white finger, cold response of digital arteries, and measure of daily vibration exposure. Int Arch Occup Environ Health 2009; 83: 259.

Caglayan E, et al: Vardenafil for the treatment of Raynaud phenomenon. Arch Intern Med 2012; 172: 1182.

Cappelli L, et al: Management of Raynaud phenomenon and digital ulcers in scleroderma. Rheum Dis Clin North Am 2015; 41: 419.

Cohen JC, et al: Raynaud's phenomenon of the tongue. J Rheumatol 2013; 40: 336.

Coveliers HM, et al: Thoracic sympathectomy for digital ischemia. J Vasc Surg 2011; 54: 273.

Cutolo M, et al: Long-term treatment with endothelin receptor antagonist bosentan and iloprost improves fingertip blood perfusion in systemic sclerosis. J Rheumatol 2014; 41: 881.

De Angelis R, et al: Raynaud's phenomenon. Clin Rheumatol 2003; 22: 279.

Ennis H, et al: Calcium channel blockers for primary Raynaud's phenomenon. Cochrane Database Syst Rev 2014; 1: CD002069.

Funauchi M, et al: Effects of bosentan on the skin lesions. Rheumatol Int 2009; 29: 769.

Gargh K, et al: A retrospective clinical analysis of pharmacological modalities used for symptomatic relief of Raynaud's phenomenon in children treated in a UK paediatric rheumatology centre. Rheumatology (Oxford) 2010; 49: 193.

Gliddon AE, et al: Prevention of vascular damage in scleroderma and autoimmune Raynaud's phenomenon. Arthritis Rheum 2007; 56: 3837.

Goundry B, et al: Diagnosis and management of Raynaud's phenomenon. BMJ 2012; 344: e289.

Herrick AL: Modified-release sildenafil reduces Raynaud's phenomenon attack frequency in limited cutaneous systemic sclerosis. Arthritis Rheum 2011; 63: 775.

Hummers LK, et al: A multi-centre, blinded, randomised, placebo-controlled, laboratory-based study of MQX-503, a novel topical gel formulation of nitroglycerine, in patients with Raynaud phenomenon. Ann Rheum Dis 2013; 72: 1962.

Jenkins SN, et al: A pilot study evaluating the efficacy of botulinum toxin A in the treatment of Raynaud phenomenon. J Am Acad Dermatol 2013; 69: 834.

Koenig M, et al: Autoantibodies and microvascular damage are independent predictive factors for the progression of Raynaud's phenomenon to systemic sclerosis. Arthritis Rheum 2008; 58: 3902.

Kowal-Bielecka O, et al: EULAR recommendations for the treatment of systemic sclerosis. Ann Rheum Dis 2009; 68: 620.

Lambova SN, Muller-Ladner U: The role of capillaroscopy in differentiation of primary and secondary Raynaud's phenomenon in rheumatic diseases. Rheumatol Int 2009; 29: 1263.

Lim MJ, et al: Digital thermography of the fingers and toes in Raynaud's phenomenon. J Korean Med Sci 2014; 29: 502.

Maverakis E, et al: International consensus criteria for the diagnosis of Raynaud's phenomenon. J Autoimmun 2014; 48-49: 60.

Merritt WH: Role and rationale for extended periarterial sympathectomy in the management of severe Raynaud syndrome. Hand Clin 2015; 31: 101.

Mohokum M, et al: The association of Raynaud's syndrome with cisplatin-based chemotherapy. Eur J Intern Med 2012; 23: 594.

Mondelli M, et al: Sympathetic skin response in primary Raynaud's phenomenon. Clin Auton Res 2009; 19: 355.

Mueller M, et al: Relation of nailfold capillaries and autoantibodies to mortality in patients with Raynaud phenomenon. Circulation 2016; 133: 509.

Nagy Z, et al: Nailfold digital capillaroscopy in 447 patients with connective tissue disease and Raynaud's disease. J Eur Acad Dermatol Venereol 2004; 18: 62.

Neumeister MW, et al: Botox therapy for ischemic digits. Plast Reconstr Surg 2009; 124: 191.

Pavlidis L, et al: Fat grafting to the hand in patients with Raynaud phenomenon. Plast Reconstr Surg 2015; 135: 229e.

Pavlov-Dolijanovic S, et al: Late appearance and exacerbation of primary Raynaud's phenomenon attacks can predict future development of connective tissue disease. Rheumatol Int 2013; 33: 921.

Pope J, et al: Iloprost and cisaprost for Raynaud's phenomenon in progressive systemic sclerosis. Cochrane Database Syst Rev 2000; 2: CD000953.

Prete M, et al: Raynaud's phenomenon. Autoimmun Rev 2014; 13: 655.

Rosato E, et al: Laser Doppler perfusion imaging is useful in the study of Raynaud's phenomenon and improves the capillaroscopic diagnosis. J Rheumatol 2009; 36: 2257.

Schiopu E, et al: Randomized placebo-controlled crossover trial of tadalafil in Raynaud's phenomenon secondary to systemic sclerosis. J Rheumatol 2009; 36: 2264.

Segreto F, et al: The role of botulinum toxin A in the treatment of Raynaud phenomenon. Ann Plast Surg 2016; 77: 318.

Stewart M, Morling JR: Oral vasodilators for primary Raynaud's phenomenon. Cochrane Database Syst Rev 2012; 7: CD006687.

Sunderkotter C, et al: Comparison of patients with and without digital ulcers in systemic sclerosis. Br J Dermatol 2009; 160: 835.

ERYTHROMELALGIA

Also called erythermalgia and acromelalgia, erythromelalgia has a population-based incidence of 1.3 per 100,000 per year with a female predominance: 2.0 per 100,000 in women and 0.6 per 100,000 in men. Erythromelalgia is characterized by paroxysmal vasodilation of the feet, with burning, localized pain, redness, and high skin temperature. Infrequently, the hands (Fig. 35.2), face, and ears may be involved. The burning paroxysms may last from a few minutes to several days and are usually triggered by an increase in environmental temperature or by exercise. The average patient has 1–2 attacks per week, but in some patients the attacks are much more frequent. Cooling and limb elevation can reduce the symptoms, but often relief can only be obtained by immersing the burning feet in ice water. More than 20% of patients will have evidence of cold injury, and more than 1% will have gangrene or undergo amputation. Quality of life is severely affected by the condition.

Erythromelalgia can be considered primary, secondary, or familial. For treatment purposes, secondary cases of erythromelalgia should be carefully divided into those associated with myeloproliferative

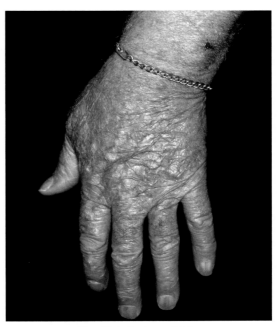

Fig. 35.2 Erythromelalgia.

diseases, often with elevated platelet counts, and other disorders. Myeloproliferative diseases associated with erythromelalgia include polycythemia vera, thrombotic thrombocytopenic purpura (TTP), and various forms of thrombocythemia. Administration of romiplostim, a thrombopoiesis-stimulating protein, has resulted in erythromelalgia. Low-dose aspirin is effective therapy for erythromelalgia associated with platelet abnormalities. If this fails, other methods to reduce the platelet count, such as administration of hydroxyurea, should be considered.

Acquired erythromelalgia has been reported secondary to topical exposure to isopropyl alcohol and after mushroom poisoning with *Clitocybe acromelalga* and *Clitocybe amoenolens*. Medications that have induced erythromelalgia include calcium channel blockers (both nifedipine and verapamil), ergot derivatives such as bromocriptine and pergolide, and cyclosporine. There may be a long period of treatment (years) with these agents before the appearance of the erythromelalgia. Chronic vibration and tobacco use have also been suggested as possible risk factors. Stopping the medication usually leads to improvement of symptoms within weeks.

In the vast majority of cases seen by dermatologists, erythromelalgia is probably a neurologic disorder. It can be seen in various neurologic conditions or diseases associated with neurologic sequelae, such as peripheral neuropathy, myelitis, multiple sclerosis, autoimmune small-fiber axonopathy, or diabetes mellitus. Erythromelalgia is sometimes associated with Raynaud phenomenon; both are disorders of abnormal neurovascular function. One series of 46 patients described concurrent Raynaud in 80% of patients. In many patients, no associated neurologic disease may be detected by routine neurologic examination, but careful neurologic testing will reveal evidence of a small-fiber neuropathy in the majority of such cases.

Inherited, familial, or hereditary erythromelalgia usually has its onset in childhood or adolescence (early or late onset). Familial cases have an autosomal dominant inheritance pattern. Familial erythromelalgia is now known to be an "inherited neuronal ion channelopathy." The mutation is in the gene *SCN9A*, which encodes a peripheral sodium channel $Na_V1.7$. This is a mainly peripheral sodium channel with robust expression in dorsal root ganglion neurons and sympathetic ganglion neurons, especially those with nociceptive function. This sodium channel acts as a "threshold" channel and sets the gain in nociceptors. Many mutations in the affected gene have been mapped. Gene mutations causing erythromelalgia occur in areas that affect the structure of the actual channel by substituting amino acids in this critical location. The mutations causing erythromelalgia are gain-of-function mutations that lead to a hyperpolarizing shift of activation, allowing $Na_V1.7$ to open at lower potentials, enhancing excitability. Furthermore, high temperatures have been shown in vitro to cause a significant depolarizing shift in the mutant channels. Mutational analysis of one patient with careful nerve signaling evaluation demonstrated increased activity-dependent slowing of C-fibers. Mutational-guided therapy was used in two other patients with gain-of-function mutations in $Na_V1.7$, with carbamazepine attenuating the pain in both cases. Novel drugs such as PF-05089771 and TV-45070 have $Na_V1.7$ selectivity and may be promising future agents for patients with primary erythromelalgia.

The amount of gain of function correlates with age of onset of the disease; more significant mutations have earlier onset. The nature of the mutation also affects the binding of medications to the channel, so various mutations may have different responses to the same medication, depending on whether that mutation allows the drug to bind to the channel. Other gain-of-function mutations in *SCN9A* cause "paroxysmal extreme pain disorder" (formerly called familial rectal pain syndrome). This disorder has prominent autonomic manifestations that include skin flushing, sometimes with only half the face turning red (harlequin color change), syncope with bradycardia, and severe burning pain, most often rectal, ocular, or mandibular. One mutation in $Na_V1.7$ produced a clinical syndrome with features of both erythromelalgia and paroxysmal extreme pain disorder. Autosomal recessive nonsense mutations that cause loss of function of the $Na_V1.7$ channel result in the inability to sense pain. These patients are otherwise neurologically normal.

Interestingly, the association of secondary erythromelalgia with autoimmune conditions has led to the supposition that autoantibodies to the $Na_V1.7$ sodium channel may be present. Immunomodulatory therapy such as intravenous immune globulin (IVIG) has been used successfully in some patients with autoimmune disease and erythromelalgia. When severe, erythromelalgia is a life-altering disease, and aggressive management is warranted. Patients may benefit from referral to special clinics for pain management or pain rehabilitation. At times, simple measures such as immersion in cool water may stop pain crises. Biofeedback can be of benefit. In general, no more than 50% of patients with erythromelalgia of the neuropathic type will respond to any one medication, so the treatment must be tailored to each patient, and often combinations of agents are used. Topical amitriptyline 1% and ketamine 0.5% in a gel are safe topical options and are especially reasonable for affected thin-skinned areas, such as the face or ears, where penetration would be optimal. Topical midodrine 0.2% has been used successfully. Oral amitriptyline, sertraline, nortriptyline, pregabalin, and venlafaxine have shown benefit in some patients. Mexiletine, which has a normalizing effect on pathologic gating properties of the $Na_V1.7$ sodium channel mutation, has been reported effective in some patients, as have carbamazepine and the combination of carbamazepine and gabapentin. Corticosteroids have been used in select patients with erythromelalgia, and in one series appeared to be beneficial if used early, following a clear trigger (infectious, traumatic, or surgical) at the onset of erythromelalgia. Neurosurgical intervention has been used in the most severely affected, carefully selected patients who have failed medical management.

Red Ear Syndrome

Red ear syndrome describes a rarely reported disorder characterized by relapsing attacks of redness and burning affecting both ears, usually only one ear at a time. The attacks are more common in the winter and are precipitated by touching, movements, and exposure to warmth. Associated conditions include neural disorders of the trigeminal and glossopharyngeal nerves, migraines, and LE. It is unclear if red ear syndrome is a disease sui generis or is actually erythromelalgia of the ears. Treatment with oral and topical tricyclic antidepressants has been beneficial. Red ear syndrome must be distinguished from the springtime variant of polymorphous light eruption seen in young males with cold exposure, relapsing polychondritis (the lobe is also involved in red ear syndrome), cellulitis, and borrelial lymphocytoma.

Alhadad A, et al: Erythromelalgia. Vasa 2012; 41: 43.

Catterall WA, et al: Inherited neuronal ion channelopathies. J Neurosci 2008; 28: 11768.

Cerci FB, et al: Intractable erythromelalgia of the lower extremities successfully treated with lumbar sympathetic block. J Am Acad Dermatol 2013; 69: e270.

Chen MC, et al: Erythema associated with pain and warmth on face and ears. J Headache Pain 2014; 15: 18.

Cheng X, et al: Mutation I136V alters electrophysiological properties of the Na(v)1.7 channel in a family with onset of erythromelalgia in the second decade. Mol Pain 2008; 4: 1.

Cook-Norris RH, et al: Pediatric erythromelalgia. J Am Acad Dermatol 2012; 66: 416.

Cregg R, et al: Mexiletine as a treatment for primary erythromelalgia. Br J Pharmacol 2014; 171: 4455.

Crunkhorn S: Pain: blocking pain in inherited erythromelalgia. Nat Rev Drug Discov 2016; 15: 384.

David MD, et al: Topically applied midodrine 0.2%, an α1-agonist, for the treatment of erythromelalgia. JAMA Dermatol 2015; 151: 1025.

Drenth JP, et al: Primary erythermalgia as a sodium channelopathy. Arch Dermatol 2008; 144: 320.

Eberhardt M, et al: Inherited pain: sodium channel Na$_V$1.7 *A1632T* mutation causes erythromelalgia due to a shift of fast inactivation. J Biol Chem 2014; 289: 1971.

Eismann R, et al: Red ear syndrome. Dermatology 2011; 223: 196.

Estacion M, et al: Na$_V$1.7 gain-of-function mutations as a continuum. J Neurosci 2008; 28: 11079.

Fisher TZ, et al: A novel Na$_V$1.7 mutation producing carbamazepine-responsive erythromelalgia. Ann Neurol 2009; 65: 733.

Geha P, et al: Pharmacotherapy for pain in a family with inherited erythromelalgia guided by genomic analysis and functional profiling. JAMA Neurol 2016; 73: 659.

Genebriera J, et al: Results of computer-assisted sensory evaluation in 41 patients with erythromelalgia. Clin Exp Dermatol 2012; 37: 350.

Han JH, et al: Paraneoplastic erythromelalgia associated with breast carcinoma. Int J Dermatol 2012; 51: 878.

Iqbal J, et al: Experience with oral mexiletine in primary erythromelalgia in children. Ann Saudi Med 2009; 29: 316.

Kalava K, et al: Response of primary erythromelalgia to pregabalin therapy. J Clin Rheumatol 2013; 19: 284.

Kalgaard OM, et al: Prostacyclin reduces symptoms and sympathetic dysfunction in erythromelalgia in a double-blind randomized pilot study. Acta Derm Venereol 2003; 83: 442.

Kist AM, et al: *SCN10A* mutation in a patient with erythromelalgia enhances C-fiber activity dependent slowing. PLoS One 2016; 11: e0161789.

Kluger N, et al: Romiplostim-induced erythromelalgia in a patient with idiopathic thrombocytopenic purpura. Br J Dermatol 2009; 161: 482.

Lambru G, et al: The red ear syndrome. J Headache Pain 2013; 14: 83.

Lin KH, et al: Effectiveness of botulinum toxin A in treatment of refractory erythromelalgia. J Chin Med Assoc 2013; 76: 296.

Moody S, et al: Secondary erythromelalgia successfully treated with intravenous immunoglobulin. J Child Neurol 2012; 27: 922.

Nanayakkara PWB, et al: Verapamil-induced erythermalgia. Neth J Med 2007; 65: 349.

Natkunarajah J, et al: Treatment with carbamazepine and gabapentin of a patient with primary erythermalgia (erythromelalgia) identified to have a mutation in the *SCN9A* gene, encoding a voltage-gated sodium channel. Clin Exp Dermatol 2009; 34: e640.

Pagani-Estevez GL, et al: Erythromelalgia. J Am Acad Dermatol 2017; 76: 506.

Parker LK, et al: Clinical features and management of erythromelalgia. Clin Exp Rheumatol 2017; 35: 80.

Patel M, et al: Facial erythromelalgia. J Am Acad Dermatol 2014; 71: e250.

Pipili C, Cholongitas E: Erythromelalgia in a diabetic patient managed with gabapentin. Diabetes Res Clin Pract 2008; 79: e15.

Poterucha TJ, et al: Topical amitriptyline combined with ketamine for the treatment of erythromelalgia. J Drugs Dermatol 2013; 12: 308.

Raieli V, et al: Prevalence of red ear syndrome in juvenile primary headaches. Cephalalgia 2011; 31: 597.

Reed KB, Davis MDP: Incidence of erythromelalgia. J Eur Acad Dermatol Venereol 2009; 23: 13.

Ryan S, et al: Red ear syndrome. Cephalalgia 2013; 33: 190.

Tang Z, et al: Primary erythromelalgia. Orphanet J Rare Dis 2015; 10: 127.

Young FB: When adaptive processes go awry: gain-of-function in *SCN9A*. Clin Genet 2008; 73: 34.

LIVEDO RETICULARIS, LIVEDO RACEMOSA

Livedo reticularis is the term used to describe a netlike, mottled or reticulated, pink or reddish blue discoloration of the skin, mostly on the extremities, especially the legs. It is more prominent with exposure to cold and may vanish with warming. It is usually seen on the lower extremities in young children and women. The pathogenic basis is reduced blood flow and lowered oxygen tension in the venous plexus of the skin. Cutis marmorata is another name for livedoid physiologic mottling of skin exposed to cold. For clinical purposes, it is best to separate livedo reticularis (a benign condition in most cases) from fixed livedo reticularis, better known as livedo racemosa. Livedo racemosa forms irregular networks and broken circular segments that are fixed and do not vary appreciably with temperature changes (Fig. 35.3). The lesions are usually asymptomatic. If necrosis or purpura occurs over the livedoid areas, the terms *necrotizing livedo* and *retiform purpura*, respectively, may be used. Livedo racemosa and livedo with purpura or necrosis are almost always associated with significant systemic disease that requires treatment. Unfortunately, the literature does not always accurately separate these entities, and patients may present with variable livedo (resembling livedo reticularis) and later develop more fixed lesions. In addition, some patients who have more variable livedo may have serious underlying disease that may require evaluation and treatment. These patients may not be easily identifiable initially on physical examination features alone. In this section, the term *livedo* will be used to describe this cutaneous finding and its association with other conditions. When livedo reticularis is seen, the clinician should consider the following categories of diseases as possibly causal: physiologic, hypercoagulable states (including myelodysplasias, cancer, and antiphospholipid, cryoglobulinemia, and Sneddon syndromes), vasculitis (especially medium and large vessel), emboli, medications, and neurologic disorders.

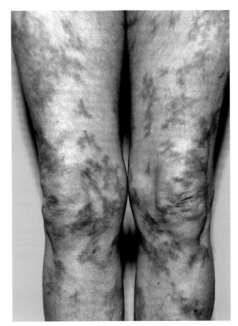

Fig. 35.3 Livedo racemosa.

Drugs may cause livedo. Amantadine (Symmetrel) can cause livedo reticularis. Quinidine and quinine may be associated with a photosensitivity that is livedoid in appearance, but on biopsy an interface dermatitis will be present. Minocycline can cause livedo, and this is a marker for the development of an antineutrophil cytoplasmic antibody (ANCA)–positive vasculitis in these patients. The medication must be stopped immediately. Other medications associated with livedo include gemcitabine, heparin (perhaps associated with heparin-induced antiplatelet antibodies), IFN-β, and bismuth. Cholesterol emboli after intravascular procedures or surgery may present with livedo, often in the setting of renal injury and eosinophilia (see later). The sheaths used for intravascular procedures may be coated with a hydrophilic polymer that may embolize and cause livedo (histopathology can reveal the polymer in the vessels).

Neurologic disorders can create livedo reticularis by altering innervation and, consequently, blood flow in the skin. Brain injury, multiple sclerosis, diabetes mellitus, poliomyelitis, and Parkinson disease are some examples.

Many of the syndromes with fixed livedo (livedo racemosa) have important systemic implications. These conditions can be either primary thrombotic processes or vascular inflammatory processes. It is important to consider in each case that if the vessels of the skin are affected, the vessels in other organs, specifically the central nervous system (CNS) and kidneys, may also be affected. Sneddon syndrome is a rare condition that occurs in young to middle-aged women. These patients present with livedo, report a history of migraines, and then develop cerebrovascular infarcts. The prognosis is poor. Frequently, patients have antiphospholipid antibodies (up to 85%) and may have enough features to be diagnosed with systemic lupus erythematosus (SLE). They would be accurately diagnosed as having antiphospholipid antibody syndrome. Other connective tissue diseases, such as dermatomyositis, rheumatoid arthritis, and systemic sclerosis, may have antiphospholipid antibodies and thus feature livedo. For this reason, patients with SLE and livedo are likely to have more severe disease manifestations, such as renal disease, vasculitis, and antiphospholipid antibodies, even in the absence of full-blown Sneddon syndrome. Headache may be the presenting symptom in these patients, and the misdiagnosis of migraine may initially be considered. Not all patients with Sneddon syndrome can be diagnosed as having antiphospholipid antibody syndrome, however, and their optimal evaluation and management is unclear. Other significant disorders with livedo as a skin manifestation include thrombotic processes (hypercoagulable states, type I cryoglobulinemia), microangiopathic hemolytic anemias (TTP, hemolytic uremic syndrome, disseminated intravascular coagulation), medium- and large-vessel vasculitides, and septicemia. Moyamoya disease is a rare, chronic cerebrovascular occlusive condition characterized by progressive stenosis of the arteries in the circle of Willis. Patients present with ischemic strokes or cerebral hemorrhages. Both idiopathic moyamoya disease and disease connected with factor V Leiden mutation have been associated with livedo reticularis. Divry–van Bogaert syndrome, with livedo racemosa, seizures, and significant CNS disease, may be related to moyamoya or Sneddon syndrome.

Oxalosis may lead to livedo reticularis from deposition of oxalate crystals in and around blood vessel walls. The characteristic crystals are seen on biopsy. Calciphylaxis, with calcium deposits in vessels and tissue, may cause livedo. Other possible causes of livedo include cryofibrinogenemia, Graves disease (associated with anticardiolipin antibodies), atrial myxoma, tuberculosis (perhaps as a complication of vascular inflammation: vascular-based tuberculid), and syphilis.

Danowski KM, et al: Hydrophilic polymer embolization. J Cutan Pathol 2014; 41: 813.

Dean SM: Livedo reticularis and related disorders. Curr Treat Options Cardiovasc Med 2011; 13: 179.

Gibbs MB, et al: Livedo reticularis. J Am Acad Dermatol 2005; 52: 1009.

Lenert P, et al: ANA(+) ANCA(+) systemic vasculitis associated with the use of minocycline. Clin Rheumatol 2013; 32: 1099.

Quaresma MV, et al: Amantadine-induced livedo reticularis. An Bras Dermatol 2015; 90: 745.

Sangle SR, et al: The prevalence of abnormal pulse wave velocity, pulse contour analysis and ankle-brachial index in patients with livedo reticularis. Rheumatology (Oxford) 2013; 52: 1992.

Tektonidou MG, et al: Antiphospholipid syndrome nephropathy in patients with systemic lupus erythematosus and antiphospholipid antibodies. Arthritis Rheum 2004; 50: 2569.

Tietjen GE, et al: Livedo reticularis and migraine. Headache 2002; 42: 352.

Cholesterol Emboli

Cholesterol emboli resulting from severe atherosclerotic disease, usually of the abdominal aorta, may cause unilateral or bilateral livedo of the lower extremities. The livedo may not be present with the patient supine and may only be present when the legs are dependent. Patients frequently have concomitant cyanosis (blue toes), purpura, nodules, ulceration, or gangrene (Fig. 35.4). Pain often accompanies the skin lesions. Acute renal failure occurs in up to 75%, and about one third of patients will have characteristic skin lesions. An eosinophilia on complete blood count (CBC) is present in 80% of cases. Older men with severe atherosclerotic disease are at greatest risk. They are often receiving anticoagulant therapy, and many have recently undergone vascular surgery or instrumentation. Slightly more than 1% of left-sided heart catheterizations are complicated by cholesterol emboli. The differential diagnosis includes vasculitis, septic staphylococcal emboli resulting from endocarditis or an infected aneurysm, and polyarteritis nodosa. Cholesterol emboli can involve all organs except the lungs; therefore disease burden can range from mild to overwhelming. Mortality rate can be significant, as high as 90% among those with multisystem involvement, in whom renal failure, bowel infarction, and other devastating complications can occur. Livedo reticularis of recent onset in an elderly person warrants

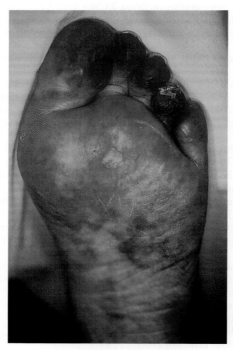

Fig. 35.4 Cholesterol emboli.

consideration of this diagnosis. Deep biopsy with serial sections may demonstrate the characteristic cholesterol clefts within thrombi. Frozen-section evaluation with polarized microscopy is particularly sensitive. Retinal emboli occur in up to 25% of patients, so funduscopic examination can also aid in diagnosis. Low-dose corticosteroids may be useful for treatment of cholesterol emboli–associated renal insufficiency.

Fukumoto Y, et al: The incidence and risk factors of cholesterol embolization syndrome, a complication of cardiac catheterization. J Am Coll Cardiol 2003; 42: 211.

Jucgla A, et al: Cholesterol embolism. J Am Acad Derm 2006; 55: 786.

Masuda J, et al: Use of corticosteroids in the treatment of cholesterol crystal embolism after cardiac catheterization. Intern Med 2013; 52: 993.

Evaluation of the Patient With Possible Cutaneous Vascular Disorders

In the evaluation of patients who present with livedo, purpura, or ulceration, a broad differential diagnosis must be considered. The diseases considered should include primary pathology of the cutaneous vasculature. In general, these vascular disorders of the skin are divided into two main groups: vasculitis and vasculopathy. Vasculitis includes disorders in which the primary damage in the blood vessels results from inflammatory cells infiltrating and damaging vessel walls. As a consequence of inflammation within vessels, the clotting cascade is triggered, and subsequent thrombosis may be seen in and adjacent to involved vessels. In vasculopathy, the primary process is thrombosis. This is usually caused by a hypercoagulable state. Once thrombosis occurs, inflammatory cells enter the vessel and vessel wall in an attempt to reestablish local circulation. Thus late in a primary thrombotic process, vascular inflammation is seen and can be misinterpreted as "vasculitis." Emboli can result in a similar histologic picture, because late embolic lesions may also be inflammatory and histologically misleading. All these processes—vasculitis, vasculopathy, and emboli—alter cutaneous blood flow and can be accompanied by livedo. If vessels lose competence, they leak, creating purpura. If vasculitis, vasculopathy, or embolus is severe enough or affects a large enough vessel, the viability of the overlying skin is compromised, and necrosis and ulceration may occur.

Because these entities resemble one another both clinically and histologically, accurate diagnosis is difficult for even the most skilled dermatologist. Careful sampling of early lesions, with large and deep biopsies, if necessary, may be required to find the "primary" vascular pathology. Because vasculitis can be a focal process, step sections may be required to find the diagnostic features. In addition, the diagnosis proposed must be interpreted in the context of other elements of the patient's medical condition, such as medications, infections, underlying diseases, and involvement of other organ systems besides the skin.

Hirschmann JV, Raugi GJ: Blue (or purple) toe syndrome. J Am Acad Dermatol 2009; 60: 1.

LIVEDOID VASCULOPATHY

Synonyms for livedoid vasculopathy include livedoid vasculitis, atrophie blanche, segmental hyalinizing vasculitis, livedo reticularis with summer/winter ulceration, and painful purpuric ulcers with reticular pattern of the lower extremities ("PURPLE"). It is a hyalinizing, thrombo-occlusive vascular disease characterized by clotting of medium-sized arterioles. The disorder is chronic, recurrent, and painful. Clinically, purpuric macules and papules cluster around the lower legs, ankles, and dorsal feet. These lesions may develop a hemorrhagic crust, then break down to form

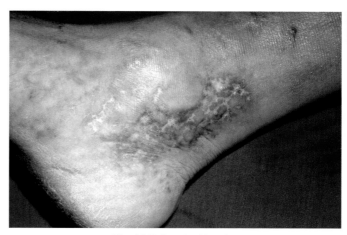

Fig. 35.5 Atrophy blanche.

irregular, superficial ulcers bordered by violaceous erythema. Over many months, the ulcers heal with porcelain-white, atrophic scars with peripheral telangiectasias, termed *atrophie blanche* (Fig. 35.5). Other cutaneous findings, such as livedo reticularis, may also be present. About two thirds to three quarters of patients are female; mean age of onset is 45 years. The condition is bilateral in 80% of patients, and ulceration occurs in 70%.

This clinical presentation must be distinguished from other disorders that can cause purpura and ulcers. The differential diagnosis is broad because many conditions can cause livedo reticularis with ulceration of the lower extremities. Atrophie blanche–like lesions are a fairly common end result of ulceration and are therefore not specific for livedoid vasculopathy.

Conditions that mimic livedoid vasculopathy and must be excluded include, most important, the vasculitides—cutaneous small-vessel vasculitis, cryoglobulinemic vasculitis, ANCA-associated vasculitis, and polyarteritis nodosa. Vasculitis involving medium-sized cutaneous vessels can present with ulceration and atrophic, stellate scarring. The presence of other systemic manifestations typical for these conditions should help differentiate them from livedoid vasculopathy. Venous insufficiency, arterial insufficiency, and traumatic ulceration may heal with atrophie blanche and therefore mimic livedoid vasculopathy. Features such as lower extremity edema, hemosiderosis, and venous varicosities may suggest the presence of venous insufficiency, whereas absent pulses, cool extremities, diminished hair growth, and severe pain are typical of arterial insufficiency. A history of trauma should be obtained. A history of characteristic ulcers should be used to distinguish livedoid vasculopathy from other disorders that can lead to atrophic scarring. Dermatoscopic features include central crusted ulcers or ivory white areas with peripheral reticulated pigmentation, and increased vascular structures. Ultimately, in the absence of any contraindication, biopsy should be used to confirm the diagnosis and exclude other causes of ulceration, especially vasculitis.

Biopsy of an affected area must be sufficiently deep to sample medium-sized vessels in the deep dermis or subcutis. Typical findings include hyalinized, thickened dermal blood vessels with fibrin deposition and focal thrombosis. Perivascular hemorrhage and mild perivascular lymphocytic infiltrate can be seen. Notably, no leukocytoclasis or true vasculitis is seen. Results of direct immunofluorescence (DIF) studies are nonspecific. Biopsies of older lesions of atrophie blanche may be most notable for epidermal atrophy and flattening of the rete ridges, as well as recanalization of occluded vessels. In about 15% of patients, an initial biopsy does not reveal diagnostic histology, and a second is required. After two biopsies, diagnostic pathology is found in 98% of patients.

Livedoid vasculopathy is a vasoocclusive condition, a hypercoaguable state with spontaneous thrombosis leading to local hypoxia and skin ulceration. A variety of risk factors for thromboembolism have been identified in association with livedoid vasculopathy. These include genetic and acquired disorders predisposing to thrombosis such as factor V Leiden mutation; protein C or S deficiency; hyperhomocysteinemia, which results in increased clotting; increased plasminogen activator inhibitor (PAI)–1, an important inhibitor of the fibrinolytic system; methylenetetrahydrofolate reductase gene mutation; increased platelet aggregation; low tissue-type plasminogen activator (tPA) levels; enhanced fibrin formation; high levels of lipoprotein A; antithrombin III deficiency; antiphospholipid antibodies; physiologic decrease in levels of protein C and S, as in pregnancy; and other underlying hypercoaguable states (e.g., connective tissue diseases, malignancies).

A review of 45 patients with livedoid vasculopathy included 29 with hypercoaguable workup, 12 of whom (41%) had abnormalities, some multiple. In addition, a number of patients were noted to have connective tissue disease, solid-organ carcinoma, or hematologic malignancy. Livedoid vasculopathy was associated with a comorbid disease or procoagulant state in 58% (26/45). This likely represents an underestimate because exhaustive coagulation screening was not performed in most patients. In a prospective study of 34 patients, 52% (18 patients) screened had laboratory evidence of a coagulopathy, of whom 32% (11) responded to anticoagulant therapy. Some patients diagnosed with "idiopathic" livedoid vasculopathy, in whom no associated abnormality is found, actually have underlying hypercoaguable states discernible only after subsequent, more thorough, workup. As testing for coagulation abnormalities evolves, a greater percentage of livedoid vasculopathy cases will likely be associated with underlying disorders.

Livedoid vasculopathy has been associated with deep venous thrombosis, pulmonary embolism, and cerebrovascular accident (stroke), among other systemic thromboembolic events. Limited data exist to guide management, but in general, treatment of livedoid vasculopathy should be directed at treating the underlying hypercoaguable state, if any. In patients with coagulopathy or personal or family history of thromboembolism, more aggressive therapy may be warranted. A therapeutic ladder for treatment of livedoid vasculopathy begins with local wound care and compression for edema, along with basic measures to decrease risk of thromboembolism (e.g., smoking cessation), followed by the addition of relatively low-risk pharmacologic interventions (e.g., pentoxifylline or aspirin, or vasodilatory agents), before moving on to anticoagulants (e.g., warfarin, low-molecular-weight heparin, rivaroxaban), and other agents with a less favorable risk profile, if needed. Rivaroxaban was studied in a single-arm, open-label study of 28 patients and reduced pain, with minor bleeding in 24% of treated patients and one case of severe menorrhagia. Exceptions to this order might include the introduction of hydroxychloroquine for connective tissue disease, folic acid and vitamin B complex for methylenetetrahydrofolate reductase mutation, danazol or stanozolol for cryofibrinogenemia, and warfarin for antiphospholipid antibody syndrome or a history of systemic thromboembolism. Colchicine has also been used in limited reports. Elevated lipoprotein (a), a risk factor for cardiovascular disease, has been reported in some patients with livedoid vasculopathy, and one study demonstrated danazol improving lipoprotein (a) and healing livedoid vasculopathy–related ulcers. Controlled trials are needed to define better the role of these agents in the treatment of livedoid vasculopathy, as well as the possible role of therapy in preventing systemic thromboembolic complications. Systemic immunosuppression is usually not beneficial for livedoid vasculopathy, because its pathogenesis is thrombo-occlusive, not inflammatory. A dramatic response to high-dose corticosteroids, for example, suggests an alternate diagnosis. IVIGs have been reported as beneficial but are highly viscous and can induce thrombotic events as well.

Alavi A, et al: Livedoid vasculopathy. J Am Acad Dermatol 2013; 69: 1033.

Alavi A, et al: Atrophie blanche. Adv Skin Wound Care 2014; 27: 518.

Callen JP: Livedoid vasculopathy. Arch Dermatol 2006; 142: 1481.

Criado PR, et al: Livedoid vasculopathy and high levels of lipoprotein (a). Dermatol Thera 2015; 28: 248.

Davis MD, Wysokinski WE: Ulcerations caused by livedoid vasculopathy associated with a prothrombotic state. J Am Acad Dermatol 2008; 58: 512.

Deng A, et al: Livedoid vasculopathy associated with plasminogen activator inhibitor-1 promoter homozygosity (4G/4G) treated successfully with tissue plasminogen activator. Arch Dermatol 2006; 142: 1466.

Di Giacomo TB, et al: Frequency of thrombophilia determinant factors in patients with livedoid vasculopathy and treatment with anticoagulant drugs. J Eur Acad Dermatol Venereol 2010; 24: 1340.

Errichetti E, Stinco G: Recalcitrant livedoid vasculopathy associated with hyperhomocysteinaemia responding to folic acid and vitamin B_6/B_{12} supplementation. Acta Derm Venereol 2016; 96: 987.

Gotlib J, et al: Heterozygous prothrombin *G20210A* gene mutation in a patient with livedoid vasculitis. Arch Dermatol 2003; 139: 1081.

Hairston BR, et al: Treatment of livedoid vasculopathy with low-molecular-weight heparin: report of 2 cases. Arch Dermatol 2003; 139: 987.

Hairston BR, et al: Livedoid vasculopathy. Arch Dermatol 2006; 142: 1413.

Hu SC, et al: Dermoscopic features of livedoid vasculopathy. Medicine (Baltimore) 2017; 96: e6284.

Irani-Hakime NA, et al: Livedoid vasculopathy associated with combined prothrombin G20210A and factor V (Leiden) heterozygosity and MTHFR C677T homozygosity. J Thromb Thrombolysis 2008; 26: 31.

Kim EJ, et al: Pulsed intravenous immunoglobulin therapy in refractory ulcerated livedoid vasculopathy. Dermatol Ther 2015; 28: 287.

Kirsner RS: New hope for patients with livedoid vasculopathy. Lancet Haematol 2016;3(2):e56-7.

Meiss F, et al: Livedoid vasculopathy. Eur J Dermatol 2006; 16: 159.

Monshi B, et al: Efficacy of intravenous immunoglobulins in livedoid vasculopathy. J Am Acad Dermatol 2014; 71: 738.

Rampf J, et al: Methylenetetrahydrofolate-reductase polymorphism associated homocysteinemia in a patient with livedo vasculopathy. Br J Dermatol 2006; 155: 850.

Vasudevan B, et al: Livedoid vasculopathy. Indian J Dermatol Venereol Leprol 2016; 82: 478.

Weishaupt C, et al: Anticoagulation with rivaroxaban for livedoid vasculopathy (RILIVA). Lancet Haematol 2016; 3: e72.

Yong AA, et al: Livedoid vasculopathy and its association with factor V Leiden mutation. Singapore Med J 2012; 53: e258.

CALCIPHYLAXIS

Calciphylaxis (calcific uremic arteriolopathy) is an increasingly reported and frequently fatal syndrome that occurs most often in the setting of chronic renal failure but may also occur with normal renal function (nonuremic calciphylaxis). In calciphylaxis, progressive calcification of the media of arterioles leads to vessel injury, intimal fibrosis, and thrombosis, followed by ischemic necrosis of the skin and soft tissue. About 1%–4% of patients on hemodialysis and 4% of patients on peritoneal dialysis develop calciphylaxis. About half of patients are diabetic, and more than half have a body mass index (BMI) greater than 30; every gain in BMI of 1 point over 30 increases the risk for calciphylaxis by 10%. Women outnumber men 3 : 1 to 4 : 1. Other identified risk factors include liver disease, hypoalbuminemia, protein C deficiency, and exposure to warfarin or systemic glucocorticoids. Warfarin in particular is a recognized risk factor, both for uremic and nonuremic calciphylaxis. A strong association between calciphylaxis and thrombophilia has been recently reported in multiple studies, and patients with calciphylaxis should be evaluated for underlying hypercoaguable disorders.

The pathogenesis of calciphylaxis remains poorly understood. Precipitation of calcium phosphate in vessel walls is generally thought to be mediated by elevated serum calcium, phosphate, and parathyroid hormone (PTH) levels, as are seen in chronic renal failure. Indeed, PTH levels are often elevated in affected patients, and the disease can be seen in the setting of primary hyperparathyroidism, as well as the secondary hyperparathyroidism of chronic renal failure. Calcium-phosphate product is greater than 70 in about 20% of calciphylaxis patients. However, a case control study showed no statistical difference in serum calcium, phosphate, PTH, or calcium-phosphate product in patients with calciphylaxis compared with other dialysis patients. Calcium and phosphate are measured at a moment in time, and often calciphylaxis is diagnosed in hospitalized patients who are actively being dialyzed, but who may have missed treatments before admission—thus the measured $Ca \times P$ product at time of diagnosis may not be representative of the typical levels. Additionally, experts have suggested that a normal $Ca \times P$ product may result from a patient's inability to maintain those ions in solution, and a higher risk of intravascular calcification. Calcium ingestion, as in the form of calcium-containing phosphate binders, did increase risk. Increasingly, a potential role of vitamin K in the pathogenesis has been suggested, as matrix Gla protein is a vitamin K–dependent inhibitor of extraosseous calcification, and warfarin, which downregulates vitamin K–dependent proteins, is a known risk factor, particularly for nonuremic calciphylaxis.

Calciphylaxis may be best thought of as a disease resulting from exposure of a susceptible host with dysfunctional calcium homeostasis to a particular "challenging" agent or precipitating factor, such as metal salts, fluctuation in renal function, or vascular inflammation. For calcification to occur, vascular smooth muscle cells must transform into osteoblast-like cells. Skin lesions in calciphylaxis exhibit significant upregulation of bone morphogenic protein 2 (BMP-2) and increased expression of inactive uncarboxylated matrix Gla protein (Glu-MGP), osteopontin, fibronectin, laminin, and collagen I, indicating extensive remodeling of the subcutaneous extracellular matrix. Calciphylaxis has repeatedly been seen in patients with Polyneuropathy, organomegaly, endocrinopathy, monoclonal plasmaproliferative disorder, skin changes (POEMS) syndrome, suggesting a possible link to vascular endothelial growth factor (VEGF).

Calciphylaxis begins as fixed livedo reticularis (livedo racemosa), which is frequently firm or hard to the touch and very tender. Areas within the livedo become increasingly violaceous, often with areas of lighter, almost white, blanched skin (due to ischemia), and eventually the area becomes purpuric, bullous, and necrotic. Affected tissue has reduced oxygenation. Lesions affect the legs below the knees in the majority of patients. More proximal lesions and those of the fatty areas of the thighs, buttocks, and abdomen occur in about two thirds (Fig. 35.6). Severe pain is a cardinal feature of calciphylaxis, often requiring narcotic analgesia for control. Ischemic myopathy may occur in severe cases, and muscle pain may precede the appearance of the skin lesions. Penile calciphylaxis is a particularly painful variant. The glans penis develops a deep necrotic ischemic ulceration. Penectomy is often required for pain management. Calciphylaxis of the temporal artery may resemble temporal arteritis.

Necrotic skin lesions are resistant to healing, and infection of open wounds with septicemia is the most common cause of death. The mortality rate of calciphylaxis patients is about 50%–60% at 6–12 months and 80% at 2 years; more proximal lesions portend a worse prognosis, and for patients with both proximal and distal

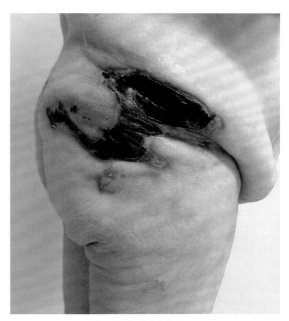

Fig. 35.6 Calciphylaxis.

disease, the 1-year mortality rate is 90%. Mortality rate doubles in those with ulcerative lesions. Patients with warfarin-associated nonuremic calciphylaxis appear to have a better prognosis.

Skin biopsy is still the gold standard for diagnosis of calciphylaxis, though opinions differ on whether it should be considered mandatory, as there are concerns that biopsy can induce ulceration and increase the risk for infection. If performed, biopsy should be adjacent to the necrotic area where there is erythema or early purpura, and it should be deep and large enough to identify diagnostic features. This may require an incisional rather than a simple punch biopsy. Vascular calcification is common in all patients with chronic renal failure, so this alone cannot confirm the diagnosis. In addition, there should be evidence of tissue damage (necrosis), extravascular calcification, and thrombosis in the arterioles of the dermis and subcutaneous tissue. Dermal angioplasia is frequently seen, likely due to reactivity to local tissue ischemia. Because the sensitivity of biopsy may be poor, and the clinical presentation often strongly suggests the diagnosis, the true importance of skin biopsy in calciphylaxis is uncertain. Plain x-ray films of affected areas may reveal a characteristic netlike pattern of calcification, though this may not distinguish from atherosclerotic changes. Computed tomography, ultrasound, and even mammography have been used to identify superficial vascular calcifications and may be used to suggest calciphylaxis in an appropriate clinical setting. Nuclear imaging with bone scintigraphy may also demonstrate features suggestive of calciphylaxis, though the sensitivity may vary at different centers.

Much of the treatment for calciphylaxis is directed at altering abnormal calcium metabolism. Because of its high mortality rate, patients are frequently treated with multiple agents at once, making the efficacy of any single agent particularly difficult to determine. Potential exacerbating or triggering agents, such as calcium and iron, should be stopped. In particular, vitamin K antagonists such as warfarin should be stopped, and patients who require anticoagulation should be transitioned to alternate agents. Combination therapy is increasingly favored, and retrospective data appear to support its use. Low-calcium dialysate, non–calcium carbonate phosphate binders, cinacalcet, bisphosphonates, and IV sodium thiosulfate have all been used with some success, with IV sodium thiosulfate now the mainstay of most treatment regimens. Nephrologists should consider transitioning patients on peritoneal dialysis to hemodialysis. Medically treating hyperparathyroidism, if present, is suggested. Parathyroidectomy is best reserved for patients refractory to the previous regimens who have continued marked PTH elevation. One study suggested improved outcomes in patients with stage 5 chronic kidney disease and hyperparathyroidism who underwent parathyroidectomy. Pain control is essential, and patients should be monitored closely for signs of infection. Intralesional sodium thiosulfate, if tolerated (injections are quite painful), has been reported as beneficial in small reports for localized calciphylaxis, and may be an option for patients where IV treatment is not possible, such as nonuremic patients who do not receive dialysis. Beneficial treatment with oral sodium thiosulfate has been reported in a limited number of cases as well. Pentoxifylline has been used anecdotally to improve blood flow and aid in ulcer healing. Other vasodilators, such as alprostadil, have also been reported as beneficial in case reports. Patients with calciphylaxis treated with sodium thiosulfate may have a higher fracture risk, suggesting a potential dual benefit for bisphosphonates, warranting further study. Notably, renal transplantation has resolved calciphylaxis.

Once ulcer or eschar develops, supportive care to ensure no biofilm or superficial bacterial colonization occurs, and topical antibiotics, enzymatic debridement, and careful wound care are all essential to healing any ulcerated areas and preventing secondary infection and sepsis. Hyperbaric oxygen therapy may be a useful adjunctive therapy for ulcer healing. Once ulcerations are present, gentle debridement is associated with healing and increased survival. Becaplermin has been reported to help heal one patient with calciphylaxis ulcers. Surgical debridement has been suggested to improve mortality rate in retrospective studies, with the caveat that patients who were treated surgically tended to have more mild disease and/or fewer comorbidities. There is an actively enrolling clinical trial evaluating vitamin K as a treatment for calciphylaxis, and some suggest repleting low levels if present.

Bhat S, et al: Complete resolution of calciphylaxis after kidney transplantation. Am J Kidney Dis 2013; 62: 132.

Bonchak JG, et al: Calciphylaxis. Int J Dermatol 2016; 55: e275.

Brandenburg VM, et al: Calcific uraemic arteriolopathy (calciphylaxis). Nephrol Dial Transplant 2017; 32: 126.

Brandenburg VM, et al: Lack of evidence does not justify neglect: how can we address unmet medical needs in calciphylaxis? Nephrol Dial Transplant 2016; 31: 1211.

Carter A, et al: Calciphylaxis with evidence of hypercoagulability successfully treated with unfractionated heparin. Clin Exp Dermatol 2016; 41: 275.

Chen TY, et al: Histopathology of calciphylaxis. Am J Dermatopathol 2017; 39: 795.

Dobry AS, et al: Fractures in calciphylaxis patients following intravenous sodium thiosulfate therapy. J Eur Acad Dermatol Venereol 2017; 31: e445.

Jeong HS, Dominguez AR: Calciphylaxis. Am J Med Sci 2016; 351: 217.

Halasz CL, et al: Calciphylaxis. J Am Acad Dermatol 2017; 77: 241.

Hanafusa T, et al: Intractable wounds caused by calcific uremic arteriolopathy treated with bisphosphonates. J Am Acad Dermatol 2007; 57: 1021.

Hayashi M: Calciphylaxis. Clin Exp Nephrol 2013; 17: 498.

Heck D, et al: POEMS syndrome, calciphylaxis, and focal segmental glomerulosclerosis—VEGF as a possible link. BMC Neurol 2014;14: 210.

Kramann R, et al: Novel insights into osteogenesis and matrix remodelling associated with calcific uraemic arteriolopathy. Nephrol Dial Transplant 2013; 28: 856.

McCarthy JT, et al: Survival, risk factors, and effect of treatment in 101 patients with calciphylaxis. Mayo Clin Proc 2016; 91: 1384.

Nigwekar SU, et al: Sodium thiosulfate therapy for calcific uremic arteriolopathy. Clin J Am Soc Nephrol 2013; 8: 1162.

Nigwekar SU, et al: Calciphylaxis. Am J Kidney Dis 2015; 66: 133.

Ning MS, et al: Sodium thiosulfate in the treatment of non-uremic calciphylaxis. J Dermatol 2013; 40: 649.

Ossorio-Garcia L, et al: Multimodal treatment of calciphylaxis with sodium thiosulfate, alrpostadil, and hyperbaric oxygen. Actas Dermosifiliogr 2016; 107: 695.

Paul S, et al: The role of bone scintigraphy in the diagnosis of calciphylaxis. JAMA Dermatol 2017; 153: 101.

Salmhofer H, et al: Multi-modal treatment of calciphylaxis with sodium-thiosulfate, cinacalcet and sevelamer including long-term data. Kidney Blood Press Res 2013; 37: 346.

Schliep S, et al: Successful treatment of calciphylaxis with pamidronate. Eur J Dermatol 2008; 18: 554.

Shetty A, Klein J: Treatment of calciphylaxis. Adv Perit Dial 2016; 32: 51.

Shmidt E, et al: Net-like pattern of calcification on plain soft-tissue radiographs in patients with calciphylaxis. J Am Acad Dermatol 2012; 67: 1296.

Strazzula L, et al: Intralesional sodium thiosulfate for the treatment of calciphylaxis. JAMA Dermatol 2013; 149: 946.

Tian F, et al: The cutaneous expression of vitamin K-dependent and other osteogenic proteins in calciphylaxis. J Am Acad Dermatol 2016; 75: 840.

Twu O, et al: Use of becaplermin for nondiabetic ulcers. Dermatol Ther 2016; 29: 104.

Vedvyas C, et al: Calciphylaxis. J Am Acad Dermatol 2012; 67: e253.

Weenig RH, et al: Calciphylaxis. J Am Acad Dermatol 2007; 56: 569.

Yu WY, et al: Warfarin-associated nonuremic calciphylaxis. JAMA Dermatol 2017; 153: 309.

MARSHALL-WHITE SYNDROME AND BIER SPOTS

Bier spots are pale, irregularly shaped macules about 10 mm in size, usually found on the upper and lower extremities of young adults. The spots are a type of vascular mottling that can be elicited by placing the limbs in a dependent position; they resolve when the limbs are raised and disappear when the surrounding skin is blanched. They likely represent areas of localized vasoconstriction surrounded by relative vasodilation. Although primarily idiopathic, asymptomatic, and transient, there are case reports of Bier spots in association with such disorders as cryoglobulinemia and scleroderma renal crisis and with pregnancy. Awareness of the condition can prevent misdiagnosis of a pigmentary disorder.

Fan YM, et al: Bier spots. J Am Acad Dermatol 2009; 61: e11.

Mahajan VK, et al: Bier spots. Indian Dermatol Online J 2015; 6: 128.

PURPURA

Purpura is the term used to describe extravasation of blood into the skin or mucous membranes. It presents as distinctive, brownish red or purplish macules a few millimeters to many centimeters in diameter. Several terms are used to describe various clinical manifestations of purpura.

Petechiae are superficial, pinhead-sized (<3 mm), round, hemorrhagic macules, bright red at first, then brownish or rust colored. They are most often seen in dependent areas, occur in crops, regress over days, and usually imply a disorder of platelets rather than of coagulation factors, which typically give rise to ecchymoses or hematomas rather than petechiae.

Ecchymoses are commonly known as bruises. These extravasations signify a deeper, more extensive interstitial hemorrhage that forms a flat, irregularly shaped, blue-purple patch. Such patches gradually turn yellow and finally fade away.

Vibices (singular, vibex) are linear purpuric lesions.

Hematoma designates a pool-like collection of extravasated blood in a dead space in tissue that, if of sufficient size, produces swelling that fluctuates on palpation. Hematomas are usually walled off by tissue planes.

Pathogenesis

Purpura may result from hypercoagulable and hypocoagulable states, vascular dysfunction, idiopathic thrombocytopenic purpura, TTP, disseminated intravascular coagulation (DIC), drug-induced thrombocytopenia, bone marrow failure, congenital or inherited platelet function defects, acquired platelet function defects (aspirin, renal or hepatic disease, gammopathy), and thrombocytosis secondary to myeloproliferable diseases. Most of these disorders produce findings of nonpalpable purpura. Ecchymosis predominates in procoagulant defects, such as hemophilia, pharmacologic anticoagulation, vitamin K deficiency, and advanced hepatic disease resulting in impaired synthesis of clotting factors. There is often a component of trauma. Increased ecchymosis can be the result of poor dermal support of blood vessels, most often localized to the area of trauma, and may result from actinic (senile) purpura, topical or systemic corticosteroid therapy, scurvy, systemic amyloidosis, Ehlers-Danlos syndrome, or pseudoxanthoma elasticum.

Prothrombotic disorders form characteristic "retiform" purpura or purpura associated with livedo reticularis. These include disorders in which fibrin, cryoglobulin, or other material occludes vessels. Representative causes include monoclonal cryoglobulinemia, cryofibrinogenemia, DIC, purpura fulminans, protein C or S deficiency, warfarin-induced necrosis, heparin necrosis, cholesterol emboli, oxalate crystal occlusion, and antiphospholipid syndrome.

Evaluation

A history and physical examination are often sufficient to evaluate for purpura. A family history of bleeding or thrombotic disorders, duration of symptoms, use of drugs and medications that might affect platelet function and coagulation, and review of medical conditions that may result in altered coagulation should be documented. Physical examination should stress the size, type, and distribution of purpura; a search for telangiectasias; a joint examination; and an evaluation of skin elasticity, unusual scars, and unusual body habitus. Correlation of purpura morphology with pathogenesis allows for a more focused approach.

A CBC and differential can be used to assess for microangiopathic anemia, screen for myeloproliferative disorders, and assess the number and morphology of platelets. A bleeding time is the preferred method of assessing platelet function. The partial thromboplastin time (PTT) and prothrombin time (PT) are tests to evaluate abnormal coagulation states.

THROMBOCYTOPENIC PURPURA

Thrombocytopenic purpura may be classified into two large categories: states resulting from accelerated platelet destruction and states resulting from deficient platelet production. Accelerated platelet destruction may be immunologic or nonimmunologic. The former may be caused by antibodies (autoimmune or drug-induced thrombocytopenia), isoantibodies (congenital or post-transfusion), immune complex disease, or other immunologic processes, such as erythroblastosis fetalis, neonatal lupus, scleroderma, other connective tissue diseases, or acquired immunodeficiency syndrome (AIDS). The group of thrombocytopenias with accelerated platelet destruction also includes TTP and DIC.

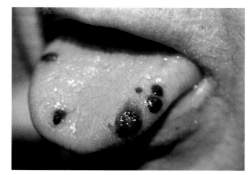

Fig. 35.7 Immune thrombocytopenic purpura.

Deficient platelet production may be related to diseases such as aplastic anemia and leukemia.

Immune Thrombocytopenic Purpura (Immune Thrombocytopenia)

Immune thrombocytopenic purpura (ITP) was also known as "idiopathic" thrombocytopenic purpura or Werlhof disease. It is an autoimmune disease characterized by an isolated thrombocytopenia (platelet count <100,000). The causative antibodies are directed at molecules on the platelet surface, leading to their premature sequestration and destruction, primarily in the spleen. ITP is called primary in the absence of another cause, or secondary if there is a causal association, such as "secondary ITP (SLE-associated)." Bleeding symptoms are minimal or absent in a large proportion of cases. Cutaneous manifestations can include an acute or gradual onset of petechiae or ecchymoses on the skin and mucous membranes, especially in the mouth. Epistaxis, conjunctival hemorrhages, hemorrhagic bullae in the mouth (Fig. 35.7), and gingival bleeding may occur. Melena and hematemesis are also present, as well as menorrhagia, which may be the first sign of the disease in young women. Chronic leg ulcers occasionally develop.

Bleeding can occur when the platelet count is less than 50,000/mm³. Posttraumatic hemorrhage, spontaneous hemorrhage, and petechiae may appear. The risk of serious hemorrhage is greatly increased at levels below 10,000/mm³. The most serious complication is intracranial hemorrhage. ITP may be fatal, but most mortality in adults results from treatment complications. Bleeding time is usually prolonged and coagulation time normal, whereas clot retraction time is abnormal and capillary fragility increased. Increased numbers of megakaryocytes are found in the bone marrow.

The age of onset determines the clinical manifestations and course. In children, onset is often acute and follows a viral illness in 50%–60% of patients. Parvovirus B19 is frequently complicated by thrombocytopenia, which may be ITP or simply a consequence of reduced bone marrow production of platelets. The average lag between purpura and the preceding infection is usually 2 weeks (range 1–4 weeks). Most of these cases resolve spontaneously. Because children are at much less risk of developing serious hemorrhagic complications, a more conservative management approach may be taken. A few patients will develop chronic thrombocytopenia, and deaths, usually from cerebral hemorrhage, have been reported. In a series of 332 children with ITP, 58 (17%) had episodes of major hemorrhage. One death resulted from sepsis. In another series of 427 cases, 323 (72%) had mild to benign disease. About 85% of children who undergo splenectomy experience remission. More than half of the remaining patients spontaneously remit within 15 years.

The chronic form of ITP occurs most often in adults, is persistent, and has a female/male ratio of 2:1 to 4:1. Secondary ITP is more common in adults. Human immunodeficiency virus (HIV) infection, hepatitis C, and autoimmune disease are the most common associated disorders. Treatment of associated disease may lead to improvement of the thrombocytopenia. Breast cancer has been associated with ITP, with a parallel course in one third of cases. Other malignancies have also been associated with ITP. *Helicobacter pylori* infection as a cause of ITP is controversial, but testing for *H. pylori* antibodies and treatment for infection carry limited toxicity and thus could be considered.

In elderly patients, ITP is more difficult to manage. Patients more frequently have major bleeding complications, more complications from immunosuppressive agents, especially corticosteroids, and more complications from splenectomy. Corticosteroids have a particularly low response rate in elderly ITP patients. Danazol has demonstrated reasonable safety and efficacy in the elderly population.

The differential diagnosis of ITP includes drug-induced thrombocytopenia, myelodysplasia, TTP, and congenital/hereditary thrombocytopenia. The goal of treatment for ITP is to raise the platelet count above 20,000–30,000 and to stop all bleeding symptoms. Platelet transfusions are indicated if there is significant bleeding or if the platelet count is dangerously low. If the platelet count is greater than 20,000–30,000, the patient may be closely monitored. The treatment of ITP has changed with the availability of new approaches. Initial treatment is a short course of high-dose corticosteroids, either for 1–2 weeks or as monthly pulses. IVIG or anti-(Rh)D, also known as IV Rh immune globulin (IG), may be given with this treatment. Platelet survival is increased if transfused immediately after immunoglobulin infusion. If the patient relapses or has persistent symptoms, systemic corticosteroids are given with rituximab, anti-(Rh)D, IVIG, or a thrombopoietin agonist such as eltrombopag or romiplostim. Splenectomy can be considered a second-line treatment, although age over 60 makes this treatment less desirable. Danazol can be added as a second-line agent, especially in the elderly patient. When second-line treatments have failed in patients with chronic and persistent or worsening disease, immunosuppression with mycophenolate mofetil (MMF), azathioprine, cyclosporine, vincristine, lymphoma-type chemotherapeutic regimens, and even autologous transplantation could be considered.

Aktepe OC, et al: Human parvovirus B19 associated with idiopathic thrombocytopenic purpura. Pediatr Hematol Oncol 2004; 21: 421.

Aledort LM, et al: Prospective screening of 205 patients with ITP, including diagnosis, serological markers, and the relationship between platelet counts, endogenous thrombopoietin, and circulating antithrombopoietin antibodies. Am J Hematol 2004; 76: 205.

Cines DB, Blanchette VS: Immune thrombocytopenic purpura. N Engl J Med 2002; 346: 995.

Daou S, et al: Idiopathic thrombocytopenic purpura in elderly patients. Eur J Intern Med 2008; 19: 447.

George JN: Definition, diagnosis and treatment of immune thrombocytopenic purpura. Haematologica 2009; 94: 759.

Godeau B: Immune thrombocytopenic purpura. Presse Med 2014; 43: e47.

Kuter DJ, et al: Efficacy of romiplostim in patients with chronic immune thrombocytopenic purpura. Lancet 2008; 371: 395.

Noonavath RN, et al: *Helicobacter pylori* eradication in patients with chronic immune thrombocytopenic purpura. World J Gastroenterol 2014; 20: 6918.

Ozkan MC, et al: Immune thrombocytopenic purpura. Curr Med Chem 2015; 22: 1956.

Rodeghiero F, et al: Standardization of terminology, definitions and outcome criteria in immune thrombocytopenic purpura of adults and children. Blood 2009; 113: 2386.

Drug-Induced Thrombocytopenia

Thrombocytopenic purpura resulting from drug-induced antiplatelet antibodies may be caused by agents such as heparin, sulfonamides (antibiotics and hydrochlorothiazide), digoxin, quinine, quinidine, chlorothiazide, penicillin, cephalosporins, minocycline, acetaminophen, nonsteroidal antiinflammatory drugs (NSAIDs), statins, fluconazole, protease inhibitors, H2 blockers, antiplatelet agents, rifampin, and lidocaine. More broadly, drug-induced immune thrombocytopenia overall can be caused by over 100 drugs, particularly carbamazepine, ibuprofen, quinidine, quinine, oxaliplatin, rifampin, sulfamethoxazole, trimethoprim, and vancomycin. Chemotherapeutic agents, including checkpoint inhibitors, can frequently cause thrombocytopenia.

Heparin-induced thrombocytopenia (HIT) is associated with life-threatening arterial and venous thrombosis and, to a lesser extent, hemorrhagic complications. The platelet count usually begins to fall 4–14 days after starting heparin, more frequently in a patient with prior exposure to the medication. Platelet counts drop to about 50% of their pre-HIT level, usually with a nadir of about 50,000, and rarely 10,000. HIT is mediated by an antibody to the platelet factor 4 (PF4)–heparin complex. The antibody cross-links FcγRII receptors on the platelet surface, resulting in platelet activation, aggregation, and simultaneous activation of blood-coagulation pathways. Tests for HIT antibodies include immunoassays such as enzyme-linked immunosorbent assay (ELISA) and functional tests.

Treatment for drug-induced thrombocytopenia consists of removal of the offending agent. All forms of heparin, including heparin flushes, should be discontinued. Because the HIT antibody continues to activate platelets after heparin cessation, patients with HIT have a persistently high risk of thrombosis and an ongoing need for anticoagulation. A nonheparin anticoagulant (e.g., argatroban, bivalirudin, fondaparinux) should be begun immediately unless there is a strong contraindication to anticoagulation, such as active bleeding or high bleeding risk. Warfarin can cause microthrombosis in these patients, so it should be avoided until after the patient is stably anticoagulated with another agent and the platelet count has recovered to 150,000 or higher. The total duration of anticoagulation should be at least 2–3 months in the absence of a thrombotic event and 3–6 months if thrombosis has occurred.

Chong BH, Isaacs A: Heparin-induced thrombocytopenia. Thromb Haemost 2009; 101: 279.

Curtis BR: Drug-induced immune thrombocytopenia. Immunohematology 2014; 30: 55.

Goldfarb MJ, Blostein MD: Fondaparinux in acute heparin-induced thrombocytopenia. J Thromb Haemost 2011; 9: 2501.

Linkins LA, et al: Treatment and prevention of heparin-induced thrombocytopenia. Chest 2012; 141: e495S.

Reese JA, et al: Identifying drugs that cause acute thrombocytopenia. Blood 2010; 116: 2127.

Shantsila E, et al: Heparin-induced thrombocytopenia. Chest 2009; 135: 1652.

THROMBOTIC MICROANGIOPATHY

The diagnosis of a thrombotic microangiopathy is made in the presence of a microangiopathic hemolytic anemia and thrombocytopenia, in the absence of another plausible explanation. TTP and hemolytic uremic syndrome are the two major diseases in this group. Certain drugs, such as cyclosporine, quinine, ticlopidine, clopidogrel, mitomycin C, docetaxel, trastuzumab, and bleomycin, have been associated with a thrombotic microangiopathy.

Thrombotic Thrombocytopenic Purpura

Classically, TTP consists of the pentad of microangiopathic hemolytic anemia, thrombocytopenic purpura, neurologic abnormalities, fever, and renal disease. However, only the minority of patients (20%–30%) present classically; many patients do not have renal disease, and CNS findings are not required for the diagnosis. The diagnosis of TTP requires only a Coombs-negative microangiopathic hemolytic anemia and thrombocytopenia with platelet aggregation in the microvasculature. Most patients will develop neurologic findings. Fever is present in 75%. Multiple ecchymoses and retiform purpura may be found on the skin. The presence of schistocytes on a blood smear is the morphologic hallmark of the disease, and a schistocyte count greater than 1% in the absence of other known causes of thrombotic microangiopathy strongly suggests a diagnosis of TTP. Tests may show a decreased hematocrit and decreased platelets, an elevated lactate dehydrogenase level, and elevated indirect bilirubin. A delay in diagnosis may lead to a mortality rate as high as 90%. For this reason, the presence of microangiopathic hemolytic anemia and thrombocytopenia in the absence of an obvious cause (e.g., DIC) is justification enough to begin empiric therapy. Biopsies demonstrate hemorrhage and fibrin occlusion of vessels. Inflammation is absent. Studies of plasma samples from patients with active TTP show the presence of unusually large von Willebrand factor (vWF) multimers. The underlying cause of TTP is a congenital or acquired deficiency of the vWF-cleaving protease, ADAMTS13. vWF is secreted by the endothelial cell in long multimers, which should be cleaved into monomers by ADAMTS13 and released into the circulation. Instead, multimers circulate and extend from the surface of the endothelial cells in the microvasculature. Platelets adhere to these multimers and the surface of the endothelial cell, leading to microvascular thrombosis.

The two forms of TTP are idiopathic and congenital (Upshaw-Schulman syndrome). Congenital TTP is less common (<10% of cases) and usually presents in infancy or childhood with jaundice and thrombocytopenia. Some patients with a congenital deficiency of ADAMTS13 do not present until adulthood or may even remain asymptomatic. The course is frequently relapsing TTP at regular intervals. Idiopathic TTP is a rare disease, about 10 cases per 1 million population per year. Women represent 70% of cases, and those of African descent have a ninefold greater risk of developing idiopathic TTP. Idiopathic TTP is caused by an autoantibody directed against ADAMTS13 that can be detected in up to 85% of cases. Neurologic symptoms are the most frequent presentation, ranging from confusion to seizures to coma.

Plasma exchange with fresh frozen plasma is the treatment of choice for TTP. Before it was instituted, 80% of these patients died; now, 80% survive. Plasma exchange clears the vWF multimers, reduces the autoantibody, and replenishes the inhibited ADAMTS13. If plasma exchange is not immediately available, simple plasma infusion can be performed until it can be instituted. Plasma exchange is usually continued daily until clinical symptoms improve and the platelet count is above 150,000, generally about 5–10 total exchanges. In conjunction with plasma exchange, glucocorticoids may be given, although their success is variable. Platelet transfusions should be avoided except in the setting of life-threatening (i.e., CNS) bleeding. Cyclosporine, cyclophosphamide, and rituximab have been used in refractory cases, with promising results. Splenectomy can also be considered. Congenital TTP is usually much easier to treat, with only small amounts of normal plasma infusion required to provide the missing ADAMTS13 and stop the clotting.

Hemolytic Uremic Syndrome

Hemolytic uremic syndrome (HUS) has many similarities to TTP but is now considered a distinct entity, both clinically and pathogenically. HUS is usually a disease of childhood. Patients have a microangiopathic hemolytic anemia, often after a diarrheal illness caused by Shiga toxin (Stx)–producing *Escherichia coli*. The annual incidence is 6.1 cases per 100,000 population. It is the most common cause of acute renal injury requiring transplantation in children age 1–5. *Streptococcus pneumoniae* infection can also precipitate HUS. Cases of HUS not following such infections are called "atypical HUS."

Fever is usually absent in HUS patients. Renal insufficiency occurs in all patients and is the hallmark of HUS. Neurologic disease can occur but affects less than half of patients. Skin involvement is unusual but may take the form of retiform purpura and petechiae.

The pathogenic mechanism of typical HUS is endothelial damage caused by the bacterial toxin and subsequent complement activation on the endothelial surface. The affected vessels are thickened, endothelial cells are detached, and the vascular lumen is narrowed and occluded by platelet thrombi. The renal vessels are at particular risk, because the subendothelial membrane is exposed and vulnerable to complement-mediated damage. In atypical and familial HUS, similar complement activation via the alternative pathway (through C3b) occurs on endothelial surfaces, leading to endothelial damage and intravascular thrombosis.

In atypical and familial HUS, mutations in the alternative complement cascade have been identified. Complement factor H (CFH) mutations are most common, and many patients are heterozygotes. The abnormal CFH complexes with the normal CFH, inactivating it. CFH is the major downregulator of the alternative complement cascade as it degrades C3b. Loss of CFH activity allows for unopposed C3b activity and complement activation. Other mutations are in complement factor I (CFI), which cleaves c3B and C4b. Mutations in membrane cofactor protein (MCP), a cofactor for CFI, in C3 itself, in complement factor B (component of C3b), and in thrombomodulin can also cause atypical HUS. The type of mutation determines the clinical course of atypical HUS, with CFH, CFI, CFB, and thrombomodulin mutations having rates of death or end-stage renal disease of more than 50%. HUS recurs in more than three quarters of patients with CFH and CFI mutations. Some patients are compound heterozygotes with mutations in two of the genes previously noted. About 6% of patients have an autoantibody to CFH and have "autoimmune HUS."

Although atypical or familial HUS is a disorder caused by a genetic deficiency in most cases, onset may not occur until middle age. About 67% of atypical HUS occurs during childhood, with almost all patients with anti-CFH antibodies diagnosed before age 16. Oral contraceptive (OC) use may trigger HUS in 8% of patients with CFH and 20% of patients with CFI mutations.

The treatment of HUS is primarily supportive, including management of renal failure. Plasma exchange may be used but unfortunately does not have the same degree of benefit in HUS as in TTP. Eculizumab, a humanized monoclonal antibody to C5, is effective for the treatment of complement-mediated HUS caused by CFH and CFI mutations and is the first treatment approved by the U.S. Food and Drug Administration (FDA) for atypical HUS. Some data suggest eculizumab may also be beneficial for Stx-associated HUS, but this remains controversial. The cost of the medication, about $400,000 (U.S.) per year, may be prohibitive.

Corticosteroids, azathioprine, vincristine, MMF, and rituximab may be used in atypical HUS. The role of kidney transplantation in atypical HUS is unclear because of the high rate of recurrence and loss of the graft. The likelihood for a successful outcome after transplantation depends on mutation type.

Ardissino G, et al: Skin involvement in atypical hemolytic uremic syndrome. Am J Kidney Dis 2014; 63: 652.

Azoulay E, et al: Expert statements on the standard of care in critically ill adult patients with atypical hemolytic uremic syndrome. Chest 2017; 152: 424.

Beloncle F, et al: Splenectomy and/or cyclophosphamide as salvage therapies in thrombotic thrombocytopenic purpura. Transfusion 2012; 52: 2436.

Benhamou Y, et al: Development and validation of a predictive model for death in acquired severe ADAMTS13 deficiency–associated idiopathic thrombotic thrombocytopenic purpura. Haematologica 2012; 97: 1181.

Bouw MC, et al: Thrombotic thrombocytopenic purpura in childhood. Pediatr Blood Cancer 2009; 53: 537.

Burns ER, et al: Morphologic diagnosis of thrombotic thrombocytopenic purpura. Am J Hematol 2004; 75: 18.

Cataland SR, Wu HM: How I treat: the clinical differentiation and initial treatment of adult patients with atypical hemolytic uremic syndrome. Blood 2014; 123: 2478.

Delmas Y, et al: Outbreak of *Escherichia coli* O104:H4 haemolytic uraemic syndrome in France. Nephrol Dial Transplant 2014; 29: 565.

Feys HB, et al: ADAMTS13 in health and disease. Acta Haematol 2009; 121: 183.

Freedman SB, et al: Shiga toxin-producing *Escherichia coli* infection, antibiotics, and risk of developing hemolytic uremic syndrome. Clin Infect Dis 2016; 62: 1251.

Froissart A, et al: Efficacy and safety of first-line rituximab in severe, acquired thrombotic thrombocytopenic purpura with a suboptimal response to plasma exchange. Crit Care Med 2012; 40: 104.

George JN: How I treat patients with thrombotic thrombocytopenic purpura. Blood 2010; 116: 4060.

Kielstein JT, et al: Best supportive care and therapeutic plasma exchange with or without eculizumab in Shiga-toxin-producing *E. coli* O104:H4 induced haemolytic-uraemic syndrome. Nephrol Dial Transplant 2012; 27: 3807.

Legendre CM, et al: Terminal complement inhibitor eculizumab in atypical hemolytic-uremic syndrome. N Engl J Med 2013; 368: 2169.

Lotta LA, et al: *ADAMTS13* mutations and polymorphisms in congenital thrombotic thrombocytopenic purpura. Hum Mutat 2010; 31: 11.

Marques MB: Thrombotic thrombocytopenic purpura and heparin-induced thrombocytopenia. Clin Lab Med 2009; 29: 321.

Menne J, et al: Validation of treatment strategies for enterohaemorrhagic *Escherichia coli* O104:H4 induced haemolytic uraemic syndrome: case-control study. BMJ 2012; 345: e4565.

Nayer A, Asif A: Atypical hemolytic-uremic syndrome. Am J Ther 2016; 23: e151.

Scully M, et al: Guidelines on the diagnosis and management of thrombotic thrombocytopenic purpura and other thrombotic microangiopathies. Br J Haematol 2012; 158: 323.

Siau K, Varughese M: Thrombotic microangiopathy following docetaxel and trastuzumab chemotherapy. Med Oncol 2010; 27: 1057.

Tsai HM: Thrombotic thrombocytopenic purpura and the atypical hemolytic-uremic syndrome: an update. Hematol Oncol Clin North Am 2013; 27: 565.

Yilmaz M, et al: Cyclosporin A therapy on idiopathic thrombotic thrombocytopenic purpura in the relapse setting. Transfusion 2013; 53: 1586.

NONTHROMBOCYTOPENIC PURPURA (DYSPROTEINEMIC PURPURA)

Cryoglobulinemia and Cryofibrinogenemia

The term *cryoglobulinemia* refers to the presence in the serum of proteins that precipitate at temperatures below 37°C and redissolve on rewarming. These tend to be chronic conditions, unless the underlying disease process is treated. Abnormal serum proteins behaving as cryoglobulins and cryofibrinogens may be IgG, IgM, or both. Type I cryoglobulinemia results from monoclonal immunoglobulins, usually IgM and less frequently IgG, IgA, or light chains caused by an underlying lymphoproliferative disorder, usually multiple myeloma or macroglobulinemia. Type II cryoglobulinemia results from monoclonal IgM (rarely IgG and IgA) immunoglobulins, which have rheumatoid factor (RF)–like activity and form complexes to the constant, fragment crystallizable (Fc) region of polyclonal IgG. This can occur in many connective tissue diseases and may also be caused by the B-cell proliferation seen in hepatitis C virus (HCV) infection. Type III cryoglobulinemia (mixed cryoglobulinemia), in which the cryoglobulins are polyclonal and of various classes, is associated with HCV infection in more than 90% of cases, but may be seen with connective tissue disorders or other infections, such as osteomyelitis or endocarditis. Together, types II and III cryoglobulinemia constitute 80% of cases.

Purpura is most likely to occur on exposed surfaces after cold exposure. This may occur in the summer as well as the winter, possibly due to indoor air conditioning, and has been reported in the intensive care unit in acutely febrile patients treated with cooling packs and ice. It may be of sudden onset and may clear rapidly once the patient is kept warm. Marked brown hyperpigmentation of the dorsal feet, at times in a livedoid pattern, may suggest this diagnosis. Cryoglobulinemia can be the cause of chronic leg ulcers. An unusual clinical presentation of type I cryoglobulinemia in association with multiple myeloma is follicular hyperkeratosis of the central face, especially the nose.

Systemic complications in type I cryoglobulinemia relate primarily to hyperviscosity and thrombosis. Manifestations of type II and III disease are multisystem and similar to those of other types of small- to medium-vessel vasculitis, including arthralgias and myalgias, glomerulonephritis, interstitial pulmonary infiltrates, and neuropathy.

In monoclonal disease, the biopsy reveals amorphous, jelly-like, eosinophilic material in the vessel lumen. In types II and III cryoglobulinemia, a skin biopsy reveals classic leukocytoclastic vasculitis (Fig. 35.8) and, less often, features of polyarteritis nodosa.

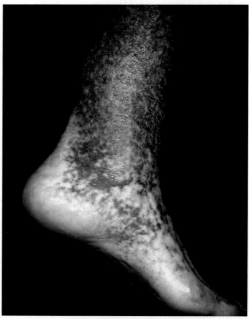

Fig. 35.8 Cryoglobulemic vasculitis.

Asymptomatic disease need not be treated. Most patients should be advised to maintain body warmth, both with layers over the core and with appropriate gear to protect the extremities. With symptomatic disease, the aim of therapy is to treat, eliminate, or control the underlying condition and to suppress the associated immune response. For type I cryoglobulinemia, this means addressing the associated myeloproliferative disorder, and for cryoglobulinemia associated with HCV, that means antiviral therapy. Reduction of the HCV viral load is the long-term solution in HCV-associated cases and can result in disappearance of the cryoglobulins. Improved treatment options for HCV are increasingly available, and direct antiviral therapy has led to improvement in HCV-associated cryoglobulinemia. The overall treatment approach varies significantly based on the underlying disease. Systemic corticosteroids, colchicine, thalidomide, immunosuppressants such as cyclophosphamide or azathioprine, and IVIG have all been used. Rituximab is increasingly reported as beneficial, even in cases of infection-associated cryoglobulinemia, and may be necessary to control cryoglobulinemia-related manifestations before or concurrent with antiviral therapy. Plasmapheresis is indicated for severe or refractory disease. Simple plasma exchange can be helpful, but cryofiltration apheresis is the best method to remove cryoproteins in the treatment of cryoprecipitate-induced diseases. Often plasmapheresis or exchange is combined with another therapy to prevent rapid reappearance of the cryoglobulin.

Compared with cryoglobulinemia, cryofibrinogenemia is less often symptomatic and generally more readily treatable. Patients most often present with purpura, skin necrosis, and arthralgias; ulceration and gangrene can result. The precipitating cryofibrinogen is a cold-insoluble complex of fibrin, fibrinogen, and fibrin split products with albumin, cold-insoluble globulin, factor VIII, and plasma proteins. Associated collagen vascular disorders, infections, and malignancies are significantly more common in patients with both cryofibrinogens and cryoglobulins than in those with isolated cryofibrinogenemia. Cryofibrinogen has been associated with calciphylaxis in the setting of renal disease and livedoid vasculopathy when accompanied by other prothrombotic risks. Familial primary cryofibrinogenemia manifests as painful purpura, with slow-healing ulcerations and edema of both feet during the winter months. Therapy beyond cold avoidance is with aspirin, corticosteroids, or stanazol for moderate disease. Immunosuppressive and antithrombotic therapies are given for severe disease. Response rates are high, but relapses are common.

Cacoub P, et al: Cryoglobulinemia vasculitis. Am J Med 2015; 128: 950.

Colantuono S, et al: Efficacy and safety of long-term treatment with low-dose rituximab for relapsing mixed cryoglobulinemia vasculitis. Clin Rheumatol 2017; 36: 617.

Da Silva Fucuta Pereira P, et al: Long-term efficacy of rituximab in hepatitis C virus–associated cryoglobulinemia. Rheumatol Int 2010; 30: 1515.

De Rosa FG, et al: Observations on cryoglobulin testing. I. J Rheumatol 2009; 36: 1953.

De Rosa FG, et al: Observations on cryoglobulin testing. II. J Rheumatol 2009; 36: 1956.

Emery JS, et al: Efficacy and safety of direct acting antivirals for the treatment of mixed cryoglobulinemia. Am J Gastroenterol 2017; 112: 1298.

Ferri C, et al: Mixed cryoglobulinemia. Semin Arthritis Rheum 2004; 33: 355.

Ghetie D, et al: Cold hard facts of cryoglobulinemia. Rheum Dis Clin North Am 2015; 41: 93.

Harati A, et al: Skin disorders in association with monoclonal gammopathies. Eur J Med Res 2005; 10: 93.

Mazzaro C, et al: Efficacy and safety of peginterferon alfa-2b plus ribavirin for HCV-positive mixed cryoglobulinemia. Clin Exp Rheumatol 2011; 29: 933.

Michaud M, Pourrat J: Cryofibrinogenemia. J Clin Rheumatol 2013; 19: 142.

Molinero C, et al: Cryoglobulinemia precipitated by targeted temperature management. Intensive Care Med 2015; 41: 1355.

Muchtar E, et al: How I treat cryoglobulinemia. Blood 2017; 129: 289.

Ramos-Casals M, et al: The cryoglobulinaemias. Lancet 2012; 379: 348.

Roccatello D, et al: Improved (4 plus 2) rituximab protocol for severe cases of mixed cryoglobulinemia. Am J Nephrol 2016; 43: 251.

Saadoun D, et al: Efficacy and safety of sofosbuvir plus daclatasvir for treatment of HCV-associated cryoglobulinemia vasculitis. Gastroenterology 2017; 153: 49.

Sidana S, et al: Clinical presentation and outcomes of patients with type 1 monoclonal cryoglobulinemia. Am J Hematol 2017; 92: 668.

Sinha D, et al: Cryofiltration in the treatment of cryoglobulinemia and HLA antibody-incompatible transplantation. Ther Apher Dial 2012; 16: 91.

Terrier B, et al: The spectrum of type I cryoglobulinemia vasculitis. Medicine (Baltimore) 2013; 92: 61.

Visentini M, et al: Efficacy of low-dose rituximab for the treatment of mixed cryoglobulinemia vasculitis. Autoimmune Rev 2015; 14: 889.

Yang CH, et al: Long-term plasmapheresis in conjunction with thalidomide and dexamethasone for the treatment of cutaneous ulcers and neovascular glaucoma in recalcitrant type I cryoglobulinemia. JAMA Dermatol 2014; 150: 426.

Waldenström Hyperglobulinemic Purpura (Purpura Hyperglobulinemica)

Waldenström hyperglobulinemic purpura presents with episodic showers of petechiae that may burn or sting, occurring mainly on the lower extremities. The dorsa of the feet are intensely involved, and the petechiae diminish on the ascending parts of the feet (Fig. 35.9). A diffuse "peppery" distribution is typically noted, resembling Schamberg disease. The petechiae may be induced or aggravated by prolonged standing or walking or by wearing constrictive garters or stockings.

Serum protein electrophoresis demonstrates a broad-based peak (polyclonal hypergammaglobulinemia). The bulk of the protein

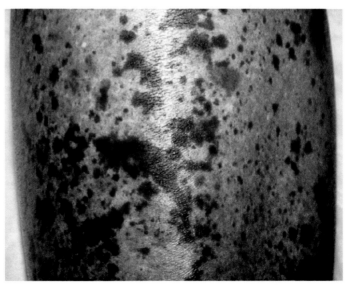

Fig. 35.9 Waldenström hyperglobulinemic purpura.

increase is IgG, although occasionally, increased amounts of IgA are also found. IgM is usually normal or decreased. RF in varying amounts is present in almost all patients. Antithyroglobulins, increased erythrocyte sedimentation rate (ESR), leukopenia, antinuclear factors, and proteinuria may be found. Almost 80% of patients with hypergammaglobulinemic purpura of Waldenström have antibodies to Ro/SSA.

Hyperglobulinemic purpura occurs most frequently in women between ages 18 and 40 and is often seen with Sjögren syndrome and rheumatoid arthritis. Adverse fetal outcomes in these women may be associated with the presence of SSA or SSB autoantibodies. Hyperglobulinemic purpura may also be a primary, chronic, benign illness. When it is associated with hepatitis C, it has a predilection for men and has manifestations that usually last longer than those associated with Sjögren syndrome.

In about one third of patients, leukocytoclastic vasculitis is present. These patients have a higher prevalence of articular involvement, peripheral neuropathy, Raynaud phenomenon, renal involvement, ANA, RF, and anti-Ro/SSA antibodies. The course of the disease is essentially benign but chronic. Rare deaths are related to associated cryoglobulin disease. Hyperglobulinemic purpura may be a manifestation or harbinger of connective tissue or hematopoietic diseases, and rarely, progression to myeloma has been reported.

Patients often improve with support stockings. Corticosteroids should be reserved for severe disease. Indomethacin and hydroxychloroquine may be of value in the treatment of milder disease, especially in patients who have connective tissue disease or are SSA/B (Ro/La) positive. Aspirin and colchicine have been used with some success.

Waldenström Macroglobulinemia

Waldenström macroglobulinemia (WM) is a lymphoplasmacytic lymphoma of B lymphocytes characterized by elevated levels of circulating IgM. Mutations in MYD88 and CXCR4 genes have been described. Disease manifestations relate to hyperviscosity and vascular complications resulting from the circulating paraprotein, as well as from neoplastic lymphoplasmacytic infiltration of important structures such as the bone marrow, lymph nodes, spleen, and other organs. Lymphadenopathy, hepatosplenomegaly, and anemia are characteristic.

Immunoglobulin M is responsible for some of the skin manifestations of the disorder. Elderly men are predominantly affected, and there is a strong familial predisposition. The cutaneous manifestations of WM can be divided into two categories: nonspecific and specific. Nonspecific manifestations are related to the hyperviscosity syndrome created by the circulating IgM and include purpura of the skin and mucous membranes. The purpura may be surmounted by tense giant bullae. Bleeding of the gums and epistaxis can occur. The IgM may behave as a cryoglobulin, resulting in purpura, livedo, cutaneous ulcerations, and vasculitis. Urticaria (some patients satisfy the diagnostic criteria for Schnitzler syndrome or progress from that disorder), disseminated xanthoma, and amyloid deposition can be seen. Specific skin lesions are of two types: specific skin deposits of aggregates of IgM (cutaneous macroglobulinosis) and cutaneous infiltrates with neoplastic lymphoid cells. The specific skin lesions usually occur once the diagnosis of WM is already known, but infrequently the skin lesions are the first clue to the diagnosis. The specific IgM deposits present clinically as subepidermal blisters (clinically and histologically resembling bullous amyloidosis) or translucent 1–3 mm papules. They are found most often on the lower extremity, even on the sole. Slight hyperkeratosis may be seen over the papules.

Histologically, the papules are composed of dermal nodular, homogeneous, and fissured pink deposits that tend to involve newly formed vessels. They are periodic acid–Schiff (PAS) positive but negative for Congo red. DIF identifies the dermal globules as being composed of IgM and is a useful diagnostic approach. When WM results in cutaneous lymphoid aggregates, the presentation is very nonspecific. Small, red-brown to violaceous macules, papules, nodules, or plaques may be present, usually on the face. Rosacea is often initially entertained as a diagnosis. Widespread skin involvement with a "deck-chair sign" (sparing the abdominal skinfolds) has been reported.

The natural history of WM is that of an indolent myelodysplasia. Treatment is directed at reducing the volume of neoplastic cells and should be managed by an oncologist. Most asymptomatic patients are followed or treated only when clinical disease occurs. Chlorambucil, cyclophosphamide, fludarabine, systemic corticosteroids, and rituximab or bortezomib, used alone or in combination, are initial therapeutic options. Rituximab, in combination with cyclophosphamide and dexamethasone, has been used as well. Rituximab is not used as a monotherapy in WM patients with hyperviscosity because they may experience a flare of their disease. Plasmapheresis can be effective in controlling acute symptoms of hyperviscosity syndrome. Ibrutinib has been shown to be safe and highly effective. With the emergence of monoclonal antibodies, proteasome inhibitors, and tyrosine kinase inhibitors, multiple targeted therapeutic options exist. Studies are ongoing for targeted agents to affect the MYD88 pathway.

Autier J, et al: Cutaneous Waldenström's macroglobulinemia with "deck-chair" sign treated with cyclophosphamide. J Am Acad Dermatol 2005; 52: 45.

Camp BJ, Magro CM: Cutaneous macroglobulinosis. J Cutan Pathol 2012; 39: 962.

Castillo JJ, et al: Novel approaches to targeting MYD88 in Waldenstrom macroglobulinemia. Expert Rev Hematol 2017; 10: 739.

Chan I, et al: Cutaneous Waldenström's macroglobulinaemia. Clin Exp Dermatol 2003; 28: 491.

Harnalikar M, et al: Keratotic vascular papules over the feet: a case of Waldenström's macroglobulinaemia–associated cutaneous macroglobulinosis. Clin Exp Dermatol 2010; 35: 278.

Libow LF, et al: Cutaneous Waldenström's macroglobulinemia. J Am Acad Dermatol 2001; 45: S202.

Oberschmid B, et al: M protein deposition in the skin: a rare manifestation of Waldenström macroglobulinemia. Int J Hematol 2011; 93: 403.

Paludo J, et al: Dexamethasone, rituximab, and cyclophosphamide for relapsed and/or refractory and treatment naïve patients with Waldenstrom macroglobulinemia. Br J Haematol 2017; 179: 98.

Tedeschi A, et al: Fludarabine plus cyclophosphamide and rituximab in Waldenström macroglobulinemia. Cancer 2012; 118: 434.

Yun S, et al: Waldenstrom macroglobulinemia. Clin Lymphoma Myeloma Leuk 2017; 17: 252.

PURPURA SECONDARY TO CLOTTING DISORDERS

Hereditary disorders of blood coagulation usually result from a deficiency or qualitative abnormality of a single coagulation factor, as in hemophilia or von Willebrand disease. Acquired disorders usually result from multiple coagulation factor deficiencies, as in liver disease, biliary tract obstruction, malabsorption, or drug ingestion. Acquired clotting disorders may also involve platelet abnormalities, as in DIC. Hemorrhagic manifestations are common and may be severe, especially in hereditary forms. Ecchymoses and subcutaneous hematomas are common, especially on the legs. Severe hemorrhage may follow trauma, and hemarthrosis is frequent. Other hemorrhagic manifestations include respiratory obstruction resulting from hemorrhage into the tongue, throat, or neck; epistaxis; gastrointestinal (GI) and genitourinary tract bleeding; and, rarely, CNS hemorrhage.

Carpenter SL, et al: Evaluating for suspected child abuse. Pediatrics 2013; 131: e1357.

Kruse-Jarres R, et al: Identification and basic management of bleeding disorders in adults. J Am Board Fam Med 2014; 27: 549.

DRUG-INDUCED, FOOD-INDUCED, AND RECREATIONAL ACTIVITY–ASSOCIATED PURPURA

Drug-induced purpura may be related to platelet destruction, vessel fragility, interference with platelet function, or vasculitis. Drug-induced thrombocytopenic purpura is discussed earlier in this chapter. Purpurogenic drugs include aspirin and other NSAIDs, allopurinol, thiazides, gold, sulfonamides, cephalosporins, hydralazine, phenytoin, quinidine, ticlopidine, and penicillin. Combinations of diphenhydramine and pyrithyldione can induce purpuric mottling and areas of necrosis. Cocaine-induced thrombosis with infarctive skin lesions is associated with skin popping. "Paintball" purpura has been described after recreational paintball contests. Hyperemesis or mechanical ventilation can cause a periorbital purpura, and anecdotal reports exist of patients performing "inversion" yoga developing periorbital purpura.

Topical EMLA cream can induce purpura within 30 minutes of application, a result of a toxic effect on the capillary endothelium. Purpura has been associated with the use of acetaminophen in patients with infectious mononucleosis. Small-vessel vasculitis, including urticarial vasculitis, has been caused by the ingestion of tartrazine dye. Pseudoephedrine can induce a pigmented purpura–like reaction. Patch testing reproduces the eruption. Purpuric contact dermatitis is rare and usually caused by rubber chemical or textile dyes.

PURPURIC AGAVE DERMATITIS

Agave americana is a large, thick, long-leaved, subtropical plant with a striking blue-gray color. It is often used in ornamental beddings in the southwestern United States. The plant grows up to 2 m (6½ feet) in diameter and may overgrow the surrounding landscape. These plants are deep rooted and difficult to remove, and some individuals attempt removal using a chainsaw. A striking purpuric dermatosis occurs in a pattern corresponding to the splatter of the plant's sap. Histologically, there is vascular damage at the level of the capillary and postcapillary venule, with a sparse infiltrate of neutrophils and karyorrhectic debris, suggesting low-grade leukocytoclastic vasculitis. Papulovesicular lesions have also been described. The plant's sap contains calcium oxalate crystals, as well as various acrid oils and saponins. The causative component is unknown.

GOLFER'S AND EXERCISE-RELATED "VASCULITIS"

This syndrome occurs mostly in hot weather and affects primarily older men (>50). Golfing or exercise with prolonged walking is the trigger. The syndrome is characterized by asymptomatic or pruritic, burning, or stinging, purpuric, macular or slightly raised papules and plaques, predominantly just above the sock line near the ankles. Mild ankle swelling may be present. The lesions resolve in under 3 days in most patients. Histologically, true LCV (see discussion later in this chapter) is not seen, but erythrocytes and neutrophils are present in the affected tissue. About half the patients are taking antithrombotic agents. This syndrome probably represents a form of purpura caused by anticoagulation and prolonged erect posture rather than a true vasculitis.

Aboutalebi S, Stetson CL: Paintball purpura. J Am Acad Dermatol 2005; 53: 901.

Barabash-Neila R, et al: *Agave americana* causing irritant contact dermatitis with a purpuric component. Actas Dermosifiliogr 2011; 102: 74.

D'Addario SF, et al: Minocycline-induced immune thrombocytopenia presenting as Schamberg's disease. J Drugs Dermatol 2003; 2: 320.

Diaz-Jara M, et al: Pigmented purpuric dermatosis due to pseudoephedrine. Contact Dermatitis 2002; 46: 300.

Genillier-Foin N, Avenel-Audran M: Purpuric contact dermatitis from *Agave Americana*. Ann Dermatol Venereol 2007; 134: 477.

Kelly RI, et al: Golfer's vasculitis. Australas J Dermatol 2005; 46: 11.

Roldán-Marín R, de-la-Barreda Becerril F: Petechial and purpuric eruption induced by lidocaine/prilocaine cream. J Drugs Dermatol 2009; 8: 287.

Sagdeo A, et al: Purpuric eruption on the feet of a healthy young woman. JAMA Dermatol 2013; 149: 751.

Sanyal S, et al: Golfer's purpura. J Eur Acad Dermatol Venereol 2016; 30: 1403.

Verma GK, et al: Purpuric contact dermatitis from footwear. Contact Dermatitis 2007; 56: 362.

PURPURA FULMINANS

Purpura fulminans is a rapidly progressive and fatal syndrome of intravascular thrombosis, circulatory collapse, and cutaneous infarction. Also known as purpura gangrenosa, there are three forms of the disease:

1. Infectious (associated with bacterial or viral infection and DIC)
2. Neonatal/hereditary (deficiency of protein C or S, or antithrombin III)
3. Idiopathic (generally following a febrile illness, leading to acquired protein S deficiency)

The most common form is that associated with an infectious illness, usually bacterial septicemia (most often meningococcemia) but sometimes a viral infection (varicella). Asplenic patients, who are at risk for pneumococcal or meningococcal sepsis, are predisposed to purpura fulminans. Neonates with homozygous protein C or protein S deficiencies may have purpura fulminans (Fig. 35.10). Some patients develop transient deficiencies of proteins C and S in response to infection. A number of reported cases of purpura fulminans have been associated with infections and factor V Leiden mutation, with normal protein C and protein S levels. Meningococcemia, streptococcal sepsis, *Capnocytophaga* sepsis (from a dog bite), staphylococcal septicemia, and urosepsis are the most common causes. Rickettsial disease and malaria may present as purpura fulminans. Active human herpesvirus 6 (HHV-6) replication

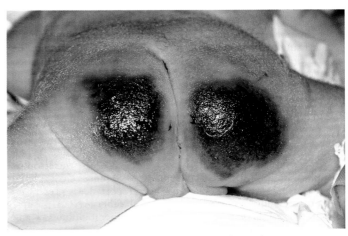

Fig. 35.10 Neonatal purpura fulminans secondary to homozygous protein C deficiency.

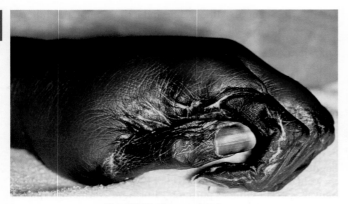

Fig. 35.11 Purpura fulminans.

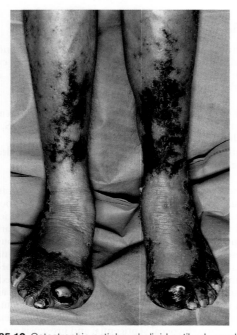

Fig. 35.12 Catastrophic antiphospholipid antibody syndrome.

Management is usually supportive, with treatment of the underlying disease process (e.g., antibiotics for septicemia) and replacement therapy using fresh frozen plasma. Protein C and antithrombin replacement is useful in treating patients shown to have deficiencies. Plasmapheresis has been used in nonbacterial cases. Heparin anticoagulation can be used. Despite these measures, amputation (often multiple extremities) and death continue to occur in patients with severe disease. The use of pressors to maintain blood pressure during the septic episode may contribute to reduced peripheral circulation and peripheral tissue damage, and choice of specific vasoactive agent should be discussed with the intensive care team, potentially preferentially avoiding alpha agonists. Fasciotomy during the initial management of these patients may reduce the depth of soft tissue involvement and the extent of amputation.

Boccara O, et al: Nonbacterial purpura fulminans and severe autoimmune acquired protein S deficiency associated with human herpesvirus-6 active replication. Br J Dermatol 2009; 161: 181.

Choudhary S, et al: Antiphospholipid antibody syndrome presenting with purpura fulminans. Int J Dermatol 2013; 52: 1026.

Cooper JS, et al: Hyperbaric oxygen. Undersea Hyperb Med 2014; 41: 51.

Culpeper KS, et al: Purpura fulminans. Lancet 2003; 361: 384.

Davis MD, et al: Presentation and outcome of purpura fulminans associated with peripheral gangrene in 12 patients at Mayo Clinic. J Am Acad Dermatol 2007; 57: 944.

Ghosh SK, et al: Purpura fulminans. West J Emerg Med 2009; 10: 41.

Ghosh SK, et al: Symmetrical peripheral gangrene. J Eur Acad Dermatol Venereol 2010; 24: 214.

Lerolle N, et al: Assessment of the interplay between blood and skin vascular abnormalities in adult purpura fulminans. Am J Respir Crit Care Med 2013; 188: 684.

Miladi A, et al: Angioimmunoblastic T-cell lymphoma presenting as purpura fulminans. Cutis 2015; 95: 113.

Price VE, et al: Diagnosis and management of neonatal purpura fulminans. Semin Fetal Neonatal Med 2011; 16: 318.

Rompoti N, et al: Purpura fulminans related to paroxysmal nocturnal haemoglobinuria. Eur J Dermatol 2016; 26: 397.

Staquet P, et al: Detection of *Neisseria meningitidis* DNA from skin lesion biopsy using real-time PCR. Intensive Care Med 2007; 33: 1168.

Talwar A, et al: Spectrum of purpura fulminans. Indian J Dermatol Venereol Leprol 2012; 78: 228.

Thornsberry LA, et al: The skin and hypercoagulable states. J Am Acad Dermatol 2013; 69: 450.

Zenz W, et al: Use of recombinant tissue plasminogen activator in children with meningococcal purpura fulminans. Crit Care Med 2004; 32: 1777.

DISSEMINATED INTRAVASCULAR COAGULATION

Up to two thirds of patients with DIC have skin lesions, which may be the initial manifestation of the syndrome. Minute, widespread petechiae; ecchymoses; ischemic necrosis of the skin; and hemorrhagic bullae are the usual findings. Purpura fulminans may supervene and progress to symmetric peripheral gangrene. DIC may be initiated by a variety of disorders, including septicemic hypotension, hypoxemia, acidosis, malignancies, chemotherapy, obstetric crises, antiphospholipid antibody syndrome, SLE, arthropod envenomation, and leukemia. Long-term treatment with granulocyte colony-stimulating factor (G-CSF) has also been reported to precipitate DIC. Children with kaposiform hemangioendotheliomas are at risk for consumptive coagulopathy (Kasabach-Merritt syndrome).

The disease results from widespread intravascular coagulation in which certain coagulation factors are consumed faster than

with acquired protein S deficiency and purpura fulminans has been described.

Purpura fulminans presents as the sudden appearance of large ecchymotic areas, especially prominent over the extremities, progressing to acral hemorrhagic skin necrosis (Fig. 35.11). The term *symmetric peripheral gangrene* is used to describe cases when acral gangrene is present. Fever, shock, and DIC usually accompany the skin lesions, which on biopsy show noninflammatory necrosis with platelet-fibrin thrombi occluding the blood vessels.

Other diseases, such as the fibrinolysis syndrome, may have purpura fulminans as part of the symptom complex. An acquired form has been reported secondary to alcohol and acetaminophen ingestion, as well as from diclofenac or propylthiouracil. When purpura fulminans occurs in the setting of SLE, the catastrophic antiphospholipid antibody syndrome (CAPS) must be considered (Fig. 35.12). Purpura fulminans has been reported as a presenting feature of Churg-Strauss syndrome and other ANCA-positive vasculitides, and of paroxysmal nocturnal hemoglobinuria and angioimmunoblastic T-cell lymphoma. Retiform purpura associated with abuse of levamisole-tainted cocaine can mimic purpura fulminans.

they can be replaced. Laboratory findings include decreased platelets, decreased fibrinogen (only in severe cases; normal in 57% of cases), elevated PT/PTT (50%–60% of cases), increased fibrin degradation products, and elevated D-dimers. Control of the underlying disease is the paramount consideration, and often, antibiotics or surgical drainage of loculated infection may lead to spontaneous resolution of DIC. Bleeding is treated with platelet transfusion in the presence of thrombocytopenia and fresh frozen plasma to correct coagulation factor abnormalities. Heparin is considered when thrombosis in the form of venous, arterial, or widespread microvascular thrombosis (purpura fulminans) is present. Thromboprophylaxis with low-molecular-weight heparin should be considered until there is bleeding or platelets less than 30×10^9. Protein C concentrate may benefit patients with severe sepsis and DIC. Use of recombinant human soluble thrombomodulin, tranexamic acid, and dermatan sulfate have been considered, but data remain limited.

Boral BM, et al: Disseminated intravascular coagulation. Am J Clin Pathol 2016; 146: 670.
Levi M, Meijers JC: Disseminated intravascular coagulation. Blood Rev 2011; 25: 33.
Levi M, et al: Guidelines for the diagnosis and management of disseminated intravascular coagulation. Br J Haematol 2009; 145: 24.
Marti-Carvajal AJ, et al: Treatment for disseminated intravascular coagulation in patients with leukemia. Cochrane Database Syst Rev 2015; 6: CD008562.
Squizzato A, et al: Supportive management strategies for disseminated intravascular coagulation. Thromb Haemost 2016; 115: 896.
Trachil J: Disseminated intravascular coagulation. Expert Rev Hematol 2016; 9: 803.

CONGENITAL FIBRINOGEN DISORDERS

Deficiencies of fibrinogen are classified as reductions in quantity (afibrinogenemia or hypofibrinogenemia) or in quality (dysfibrinogenemia). Afibrinogenemia occurs at a rate of about 1 case per 1 million population. It may present at birth with umbilical cord bleeding. Epistaxis, menorrhagia, hemarthrosis (much less than in hemophilia and with far fewer musculoskeletal sequelae), trauma, and surgery-related bleeding can occur. The severity of the bleeding tendency is highly variable from patient to patient, and some have no bleeding problems. Pregnancy complications include recurrent miscarriage and peripartum hemorrhage. Ironically, because of the loss of the antithrombotic effect of fibrinogen, thrombotic events are increased in afibrinogenemia. Arterial and venous thrombosis can occur. Patients with hypofibrinogenemia are seen more often; in general, they are less symptomatic and only occasionally require treatment. Hypofibrinogenemia may be associated with pregnancy losses and rarely with liver disease due to accumulation of abnormal fibrinogen in the endoplasmic reticulum of hepatocytes. Dysfibrinogenemia is asymptomatic in 55% of patients, 25% exhibit bleeding tendencies, and 20% tend to develop thrombosis. This group represents only 0.8% of patients with deep venous thrombosis, so screening for this condition is not cost-effective unless there is a family history. Mutations in the fibrinogen gene cluster cause all three of these fibrinogen disorders.

Acharya SS, Dimichele DM: Rare inherited disorders of fibrinogen. Haemophilia 2008; 14: 1151.
Bornikova L, et al: Fibrinogen replacement therapy for congenital fibrinogen deficiency. J Thromb Haemost 2011; 9: 1687.
De Moerloose P, et al: Congenital fibrinogen disorders. Semin Thromb Hemost 2013; 39: 585.
Vu D, Neerman-Arbez M: Molecular mechanisms accounting for fibrinogen deficiency. J Thromb Haemost 2007; 5: 125.

BLUEBERRY MUFFIN BABY

Originally coined to describe the characteristic appearance of the purpuric lesions observed in newborns with congenital rubella, the term *blueberry muffin baby* is associated with many disorders that produce extramedullary erythropoiesis. The eruption consists of generalized, dark-blue to magenta, nonblanchable, indurated, round to oval, hemispheric papules ranging from 1–7 mm. Lesions favor the head, neck, and trunk. Etiologic factors include congenital infections (toxoplasmosis, rubella, cytomegalovirus, herpes simplex, parvovirus B19), hemolytic disease of the newborn (Rh incompatibility, blood group incompatibility), hereditary spherocytosis, twin transfusion syndrome, recombinant erythropoietin administration, neuroblastoma, rhabdomyosarcoma, extraosseal Ewing sarcoma, Langerhans cell histiocytosis, and congenital leukemia. Patients with multiple vascular disorders, such as hemangiopericytoma, hemangioma, blue rubber bleb nevus, and glomangioma, may be mistaken for a blueberry muffin baby. Evaluation should include a peripheral blood cell count, hemoglobin level, serologies for congenital TORCH infections, viral cultures, and a Coombs test. A skin biopsy may also be helpful in determining the cause.

Brisman S, et al: Blueberry muffin rash as the presenting sign of Aicardi-Goutieres syndrome. Pediatr Dermatol 2009; 26: 432.
Gaffin JM, Gallagher PG: Blueberry muffin baby (extramedullary hematopoiesis) due to congenital cytomegalovirus infection. Arch Pediatr Adolesc Med 2007; 161: 1102.
Holland KE, et al: Neonatal violaceous skin lesions. Adv Dermatol 2005; 21: 153.
Krenova Z, et al: Extraosseal Ewing sarcoma as a rare cause of the blueberry muffin baby syndrome. Am J Dermatopathol 2011; 33: 733.
Lasek-Duriez A, et al: Blueberry muffin baby and Langerhans' congenital cell histiocytosis. Ann Dermatol Venereol 2014; 141: 130.
Pandey V, et al: Late-onset blueberry muffin lesions following recombinant erythropoietin administration in a premature infant. J Pediatr Hematol Oncol 2012; 34: 534.

MISCELLANEOUS PURPURIC MANIFESTATIONS

Deep Venous Thrombosis

Deep venous thrombosis (DVT) is a common medical condition that can result in immediate (pulmonary embolism) or long-term (venous insufficiency, postphlebitic syndrome) consequences. Risk factors include female gender, obesity, immobilization, low atmospheric pressure, winter season, and the presence of cancer. In 35% of cancer-associated cases, the thrombosis is the first sign of the cancer. The use of erythropoiesis-stimulating agents doubles the risk of venous thromboembolism (VTE) for cancer patients. Hereditary mutations that result in a hypercoagulable state also increase the risk for VTE. The left leg is more often affected than the right. The mean age is 52 years. Significant superficial vein thrombosis is considered a risk factor for DVT, with at least 18% of patients with a superficial vein involved also having a DVT. The risk of pulmonary embolism from DVT is the major concern. From 5%–10% of DVTs occur in the upper extremities and may develop around IV catheters.

On examination, a palpable cord, calf tenderness, unilateral edema, warmth, redness, and venous dilation may suggest the diagnosis. Pretest probability of DVT can be calculated with a simple tool such as the Wells score, and selective use of D-dimer can help exclude DVT. Ultrasound is used to confirm the diagnosis. Preventive strategies include exercise, weight control, and pharmacologic prophylaxis for high-risk patients (e.g., postoperative, after stroke). Symptomatic proximal DVT is treated with at least 3 months of therapeutic anticoagulation to reduce the risk of pulmonary embolism. Thrombolysis may be considered as well.

Bates SM, et al: Treatment of deep-vein thrombosis. N Engl J Med 2004; 351: 268.

Canonico M, Scarabin PY: Hormone therapy and risk of venous thromboembolism among postmenopausal women. Climacteric 2009; 12: 76.

Dennis M, et al: Effectiveness of intermittent pneumatic compression in reduction of risk of deep vein thrombosis in patients who have had a stroke (CLOTS 3). Lancet 2013; 382: 516.

Di Minno MN, et al: Prevalence of deep vein thrombosis and pulmonary embolism in patients with superficial vein thrombosis. J Thromb Haemost 2016; 14: 964.

Doggen CJ: High coagulant factors and venous thrombosis. Blood 2009; 114: 2854.

Hansrani V, et al: The diagnosis and management of early deep vein thrombosis. Adv Exp Med Biol 2017; 906: 23.

Kearon C, et al: Antithrombotic therapy for VTE disease. Chest 2012; 141: e419S.

Linkins LA, et al: Selective D-dimer testing for diagnosis of a first suspected episode of deep venous thrombosis. Ann Intern Med 2013; 158: 93.

Rajasekhar A, Streiff MB: How I treat central venous access device-related upper extremity deep vein thrombosis. Blood 2017; 129: 2727.

Raskob GE, et al: Apixaban versus enoxaparin for thromboprophylaxis after hip or knee replacement. J Bone Joint Surg B 2012; 94: 257.

Schulman S, et al: Treatment of acute venous thromboembolism with dabigatran or warfarin and pooled analysis. Circulation 2014; 129: 764.

Van der Velde EF, et al: Comparing the diagnostic performance of 2 clinical decision rules to rule out deep vein thrombosis in primary care patients. Ann Fam Med 2011; 9: 31.

Watson L, et al: Thrombolysis for acute deep vein thrombosis. Cochrane Database Syst Rev 2016; 11: CD002783.

Superficial Thrombophlebitis

Superficial venous thrombosis is an inflammatory thrombotic condition that classically presents with painful induration and erythema, often in a cordlike, linear or branching configuration. Patients may also exhibit indurated subcutaneous nodules and overlying purpura or brown discoloration indicative of postinflammatory hyperpigmentation.

Primary hypercoagulable states that may be associated with superficial thrombophlebitis include deficiencies of antithrombin III, heparin cofactor II, protein C, protein S, and factor XII; disorders of tPA; abnormal plasminogen; dysfibrinogenemia; and lupus anticoagulant. Secondary hypercoagulable states include varicosities; malignancy (Trousseau syndrome), which classically is of a migratory nature (Fig. 35.13); pregnancy; OC use; infusion of prothrombin complex concentrates; Behçet disease; thromboangiitis obliterans; acute thrombophlebitis of superficial veins of the breast (Mondor disease); septic thrombophlebitis; psittacosis; secondary syphilis; and IV catheters, IV drugs (sugar solutions, protein hydrolysates, calcium, potassium, hypertonic concentrates, diazepam, nitrogen mustard, acridinylaniside, dacarbazine, and carmustine), and street drugs (cocaine, bulking agents such as paregoric, quinine, dextrose, sucrose, and lactose).

In the evaluation of superficial thrombophlebitis, the physician should consider the possibility of underlying deep venous disease. Superficial femoral vein involvement should alert the physician to underlying deep venous disease requiring anticoagulation. Lesser

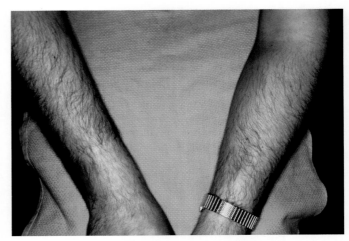

Fig. 35.13 Migrating superficial thrombophlebitis.

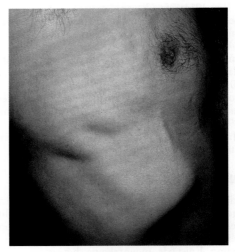

Fig. 35.14 Mondor disease.

saphenous vein thrombophlebitis is also frequently associated with underlying DVT. Elliptical biopsies across the palpable cord may be required to exclude other considerations, such as sarcoidal granulomas, cutaneous polyarteritis nodosa, Kaposi sarcoma, and vasculotropic metastasis.

Treatment is directed at the underlying cause. Leg elevation and local heat will help to promote the dissolution of clots, which may take up to 8–12 weeks to resolve. Heparin therapy may reduce the incidence of thromboembolic complications in high-risk individuals.

Mondor Disease

Mondor disease occurs three times more frequently in women than in men. Most patients are between 30 and 60 years of age. The sudden appearance of a cordlike thrombosed vein along the anterolateral chest wall is characteristic (Fig. 35.14). It is at first red and tender and subsequently changes into a painless, tough, fibrous band. There are no systemic symptoms. Both sides of the chest have the same rate of involvement. Mondor disease may be associated with strenuous exercise, pregnancy, IV drug abuse, jellyfish stings, breast cancer, and breast surgery. The condition represents a localized thrombophlebitis of the veins of the thoracoepigastric area. The veins involved are the lateral thoracic, thoracoepigastric, and superior epigastric. In the end stage, a thick-walled vein remains that has a hard, ropelike appearance and occasionally may result in a furrowing of the breast. Infrequently, a vein coursing up the inside of the upper arm and across or into the axilla may be thrombosed, leading to the "axillary web syndrome." Similar stringlike phlebitis findings have been described in the penis, antecubital fossa, groin, and abdomen. Treatment is symptomatic, with hot, moist dressings and analgesics or NSAIDs. The disease process runs its course in 3 weeks to 6 months.

Alvarez-Garrido H, et al: Mondor's disease. Clin Exp Dermatol 2009; 34: 753.

Di Nisio M, et al: Treatment for superficial thrombophlebitis of the leg. Cochrane Database Syst Rev 2013; 4: CD004982.

Manimala NJ, Parker J: Evaluation and treatment of penile thrombophlebitis (Mondor's disease). Curr Urol Rep 2015;16: 39.

Quéré I, et al: Superficial venous thrombosis and compression ultrasound imaging. J Vasc Surg 2012; 56: 1032.

Samlaska CS, James WD: Superficial thrombophlebitis. I. J Am Acad Dermatol 1990; 22: 975.

Samlaska CS, James WD: Superficial thrombophlebitis. II. J Am Acad Dermatol 1990; 23: 1.

Vijayalakshmi AA, Anand S: Mondor's disease. N Engl J Med 2017; 376: e47.

Postcardiotomy Syndrome

Between 2 and 3 weeks after pericardiotomy, fever, pleuritis, pericarditis, or arthritis may appear together with petechiae on the skin and palate. Postcardiotomy syndrome may be confused with infectious mononucleosis and bacterial endocarditis.

Orthostatic Purpura (Stasis Purpura)

Prolonged standing or even sitting with the legs lowered (as in a bus, airplane, or train) may produce edema and a purpuric eruption on the lower extremities. Elevation of the legs and the use of elastic stockings are helpful preventive strategies.

Obstructive or Traumatic Purpura

Purpura may be evoked by mechanical obstruction to the circulation, with resulting stress on the small vessels. This may be encountered in cardiac decompensation or after convulsions, vomiting episodes, Valsalva maneuver, pertussis, or sexual climax. Nonpalpable purpura has been reported in association with the use of a mucus-clearing device, which requires the patient to exhale forcefully through a flutter valve (flutter valve purpura). Local obstruction of the blood flow with purpura may result from compression of the veins by tumors or a gravid uterus or by occlusions from thrombosis.

Purpuric lesions in children lead to suspicion of the battered child (Fig. 35.15). Bruises and ecchymoses on the genital area, buttocks, left ear or cheek, or hands suggest an abused child. Linear lesions on accessible areas raise suspicion of factitial disease. Ecchymoses of bizarre shapes may also correspond to trauma inflicted during religious rituals or cultural practices, such as coin rubbing and cupping performed as remedies for common diseases. "Cupping" can lead to patterned circles of purpura after the use of suction to attach a cup to the skin. "Passion purpura" on the palate may result from fellatio. On the neck or upper arms, it results from biting and sucking and is better known as a "hickey." Facial, cheek, and periorbital purpura can be postictal and may be mistaken for spousal abuse. Bathtub suction-induced purpura occurs on the lower back location in a U-shaped distribution. It may be mistaken for abuse.

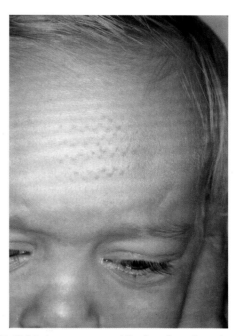

Fig. 35.15 Child abuse; purpura of the face from the sole of a shoe.

Baselga E, et al: Purpura in infants and children. J Am Acad Dermatol 1997; 37: 673.

Jaffe FA: Petechial hemorrhages. Am J Forensic Med Pathol 1994; 15: 203.

Jenkinson H, DiCicco B: Sporty spots. JAMA Dermatol 2018; 154: 66.

Knoell KA, et al: Flutter valve purpura. J Am Acad Dermatol 1998; 9: 292.

Landers MC, et al: Bathtub suction-induced purpura. Pediatr Dermatol 2004; 21: 146.

Reis JJ, et al: Postictal hemifacial purpura. Seizure 1998; 7: 337.

Paroxysmal Nocturnal Hemoglobinuria

Paroxysmal nocturnal hemoglobinuria (PNH) is an acquired intravascular hemolytic anemia that usually occurs in young adults, median age 40 years. It is an acquired clonal disorder resulting from a somatic mutation in a multipotent hematopoietic stem cell that produces all the bone marrow–derived cell lines (neutrophils, lymphocytes, platelets, and erythrocytes). The clinical manifestations of PNH are intravascular hemolysis, smooth muscle dystonia caused by depletion of tissue nitric oxide (abdominal pain, esophageal spasm, fatigue, erectile dysfunction), and life-threatening venous thrombosis. Some cases occur after recovery from aplastic anemia. Widespread cutaneous thrombosis can occur, with initial retiform, angulated, erythematous-to-purpuric cutaneous plaques progressing to hemorrhagic bullae. Stellate purpura of the ear has been observed, resembling cryoglobulinemia or levamisole-associated purpura. Vascular thrombi are found on biopsy. The cause of PNH is a mutation in an X-linked gene, phosphatidylinositol glycan class A *(PIGA)*. The gene product is the first step in the biosynthesis of all glycosyl-phosphatidylinositol (GPI) anchors on the surface of hematopoietic cells. Erythrocytes in PNH lack two GPI-anchored proteins, CD55 and CD59, which function is to prevent complement activation on the erythrocyte surface. CD55 accelerates the rate of breakdown of membrane-bound C3 convertase, and CD59 reduces the number of membrane attack complexes that are formed. Without these proteins, amplification of the complement system is uncontrolled, leading to intravascular destruction of RBCs. The diagnosis of PNH can be made by detecting the loss of CD55 and CD59 through monoclonal antibody tests. The FLAER (fluorescent aerolysin) flow cytometry test is now often used to diagnose PNH. Hematopoietic stem cell transplantation may be curative. Eculizumab, a humanized monoclonal antibody against C5, inhibits terminal complement activation. It stabilizes hemoglobin levels and reduces transfusion requirements in PNH patients and improves overall survival.

Kamranzadeh Fumani H, et al: Allogeneic hematopoietic stem cell transplantation for paroxysmal nocturnal hemoglobinuria. Hematol Oncol 2017; 35: 935.

Kelly RJ, et al: Long-term treatment with eculizumab in paroxysmal nocturnal hemoglobinuria. Blood 2011; 117: 6786.

Loschi M, et al: Impact of eculizumab treatment on paroxysmal nocturnal hemoglobinuria. Am J Hematol 2016; 91: 366.

Ninomiya H, et al: Interim analysis of post-marketing surveillance of eculizumab for paroxysmal nocturnal hemoglobinuria in Japan. Int J Hematol 2016; 104: 548.

Parker C: Eculizumab for paroxysmal nocturnal haemoglobinuria. Lancet 2009; 373: 759.

Parker C: Update on the diagnosis and management of paroxysmal nocturnal hemoglobinuria. Hematology Am Soc Hematol Educ Program 2016; 208.

Risitano AM: Paroxysmal nocturnal hemoglobinuria in the era of complement inhibition. Am J Hematol 2016; 91: 359.

White JM, et al: Haemorrhagic bullae in a case of paroxysmal nocturnal haemoglobinuria. Clin Exp Dermatol 2003; 28: 504.

Paroxysmal Hand Hematoma (Achenbach Syndrome)

Spontaneous focal hemorrhage into the palm or the volar surface of a finger may result in transitory localized pain, followed by rapid swelling and localized bluish discoloration. The lesion resolves spontaneously within a few days. Spontaneous hemorrhage from an arteriole appears to be responsible. The acute nature, purpuric findings, and rapid resolution are distinguishing features of Achenbach syndrome.

Thies K, et al: Achenbach's syndrome revisited. Vasa 2012; 41: 366.

Easy Bruising Syndromes

Young women who bruise easily despite normal coagulation profiles and normal platelet counts may have antiplatelet antibodies. Otherwise, specific platelet function defects should be suspected. Bernard-Soulier syndrome is a rare inherited disorder characterized by giant platelets, thrombocytopenia, and a prolonged bleeding time. It is caused by genetic defects of the glycoprotein Ib–IX complex that constitutes the vWF receptor. Sebastian syndrome consists of giant platelets, leukocyte inclusions, and thrombocytopenia. Fechtner syndrome is a rare type of familial thrombocytopenia associated with large platelets, leukocyte inclusions, and features of Alport syndrome. The May-Hegglin anomaly consists of easy bruising with giant platelets and Döhle-like cytoplasmic inclusions in granulocytes. The inclusions appear as electron-dense long rods and needles oriented along the long axis of the spindle. All four of these syndromes are caused by abnormalities in the *MYH9* gene. Glanzmann thrombasthenia, with dysfunctioning αIIβ3 receptor, is a platelet storage pool defect causing similar clinical findings.

Andrews RK, Berndt MC: Bernard-Soulier syndrome. Semin Thromb Hemost 2013; 39: 656.

Balderramo DC, et al: Sebastian syndrome. Haematologica 2003; 88: ECR17.

Balduini CL, Savoia A: Genetics of familial forms of thrombocytopenia. Hum Genet 2012; 131: 1821.

Hussein BA, et al: May-Hegglin anomaly and pregnancy. Blood Coagul Fibrinolysis 2013; 24: 554.

Landi D, et al: Report of a young girl with *MYH9* mutation and review of the literature. J Pediatr Hematol Oncol 2012; 34: 538.

Matzdorff AC, et al: Perioperative management of a patient with Fechtner syndrome. Ann Hematol 2001; 80: 436.

Nurden AT, et al: Genetic testing in the diagnostic evaluation of inherited platelet disorders. Semin Thromb Hemost 2009; 35: 204.

Nurden P, Nurden AT: Congenital disorders associated with platelet dysfunctions. Thromb Haemost 2008; 99: 253.

Savoia A, et al: Clinical and genetic aspects of Bernard-Soulier syndrome. Haematologica 2011; 96: 417.

Painful Bruising Syndrome (Autoerythrocyte Sensitization, Gardner-Diamond Syndrome, Psychogenic Purpura)

Painful bruising syndrome is a distinctive localized purpuric reaction occurring primarily in young to middle-aged women who usually manifest personality disorders. They may have depression, anxiety, or hysterical or masochistic character traits or may be unable to deal with hostile feelings. A recurrent type of eruption, psychogenic purpura is characterized by extremely painful and tender, poorly defined ecchymoses on the extremities (Fig. 35.16) and sometimes on the face or trunk. The lesions evolve in a few hours and resolve within 5–8 days. New lesions may appear in crops. Emotional upsets are generally associated with the appearance of these painful purpuric lesions. Some patients will report a premonition as to when they will develop new lesions a few hours before by the tingling and burning sensation at the site of a future lesion. Extracutaneous somatic symptoms are common, such as headache, paresthesias, transient paresis, syncope, diplopia, abdominal distress, diarrhea, nausea and vomiting, and arthralgia.

Gardner and Diamond reported that intracutaneous injections of erythrocyte stroma evoked typical lesions. Since then, many have reported similar reactions to autologous whole blood, packed or washed RBCs, or fractions of erythrocyte stroma. These are difficult to assess because similar reactions have been reported to substances as diverse as hemoglobin, phosphatidyl serine, histamine, histidine, trypsin, purified protein derivative (PPD), autologous serum, and platelets. Blinded controlled testing, trying to avoid factitial trauma, has given mixed responses. Abnormalities in

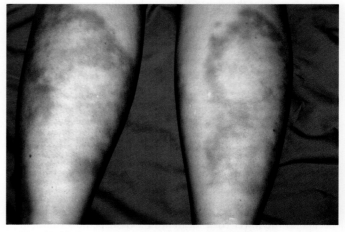

Fig. 35.16 Psychogenic purpura. (Courtesy Steven Binnick, MD.)

tPA-dependent fibrinolysis, thrombocytosis, and anticardiolipin antibodies have also been implicated. Most now believe this syndrome is psychosomatic and artifactual. Pain may lead to rubbing at the site which may lead to ecchymosis formation. The most effective treatment is to address the underlying psychological dysfunction. Improvement of the underlying psychopathology usually leads to disappearance of the cutaneous manifestations.

Hagemeier L, et al: Gardner-Diamond syndrome. Br J Dermatol 2011; 164: 672.

Jafferany M: Auto-erythrocyte sensitization syndrome (Gardner-Diamond syndrome) in a 15-year-old adolescent girl. Int J Dermatol 2013; 52: 1284.

Park JH, et al: Gardner-Diamond syndrome. Dermatol Online J 2016; 22.

PIGMENTARY PURPURIC ERUPTIONS (PROGRESSIVE PIGMENTARY DERMATOSIS, PROGRESSIVE PIGMENTING PURPURA, PURPURA PIGMENTOSA CHRONICA)

The pigmented purpuric eruptions (PPEs) are a group of common dermatoses (capillaritis) of unknown pathogenesis. The most common variant of progressive pigmentary dermatosis is Schamberg disease. The typical lesions are thumbprint-sized and composed of aggregates of pinhead-sized petechiae resembling grains of cayenne pepper on a background of golden-brown hemosiderin staining. Dermoscopy can reveal a spectrum of changes, including coppery-red pigmentation, linear vessels or linear brown lines, variable red dots, and/or red or brown globules. The lesions usually begin on the lower legs, with slow proximal extension (Fig. 35.17). These lesions seldom itch. The favored sites are on the lower shins and ankles, but lesions may be more widespread and occasionally affect the upper extremities or trunk.

Majocchi disease is also known as purpura annularis telangiectodes. The early lesions are 1–3 cm annular patches composed of dark-red telangiectases with petechiae and hemosiderin staining. Central involution and peripheral extension produce ringed, semicircular, target-like, or concentric rings. The eruption begins symmetrically on the lower extremities, spreads up the legs, and

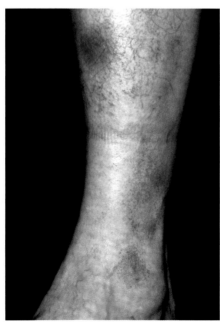

Fig. 35.17 Schamberg disease.

may extend on to the trunk and arms. Involution of individual patches is slow and, because new lesions continue to form, may continue indefinitely. The lesions are asymptomatic.

Gougerot-Blum syndrome (pigmented purpuric lichenoid dermatitis) is characterized by minute, rust-colored to violaceous, lichenoid papules that tend to fuse into plaques of various hues between red, violaceous, and brown (purpura with lichenoid dermatitis). Favorite locations are the legs, thighs, and lower trunk. The chief difference between this and Schamberg disease is the deeper color and the presence of induration, both of which relate to the presence of a lichenoid band of lymphoid inflammation. Similar lesions have also occurred during IFN therapy for hepatitis C.

Ducas and Kapetanakis pigmented purpura is scaly and eczematous. The eczematous patches also demonstrate petechiae and hemosiderin staining. Pruritus is common, and the lesions are often more extensive than the other PPEs. It is distinguished histologically by the presence of spongiosis. Purpuric pityriasis rosea may resemble Ducas and Kapetanakis purpura.

Lichen aureus is characterized by the sudden appearance of one or several, golden or rust-colored, closely packed macules or lichenoid papules. The macules may be grouped into a patch and may occur on any part of the body, but the vast majority of lesions occur on the feet or lower leg. The patches are usually solitary and asymptomatic but may occasionally be painful. Adults predominate, but children may also be affected.

Rare variants of the pigmented purpuric dermatoses are the linear or zosteriform type and the transitory type. These tend to be more transient than the other variants. A single case of evolution to linear morphea has been reported. Granulomatous pigmented purpuric dermatosis has been reported with increasing frequency, often in the setting of coexistent hyperlipidemia. Notably, one case describes PPD-like sarcoidosis, and multisystem disease should be excluded in these rare presentations.

Histologically, all forms of PPE demonstrate superficial perivascular lymphocytic (and at times granulomatous) infiltrate associated with extravasation of RBCs and, in later lesions, hemosiderin deposition. The degree of hemosiderin deposition may be variable and is insufficient to confirm the diagnosis histologically. The infiltrating cells are primarily CD4+ lymphocytes. There may be a lichenoid band of lymphoid inflammatory cells (Gougerot-Blum type) or spongiosis (Ducas and Kapetanakis type). An iron stain (Perl, Prussian blue, ferricyanide) is sometimes used to demonstrate the hemosiderin deposition. Granulomatous variants tend to show superficial loosely organized granulomatous inflammation.

Cutaneous T-cell lymphoma (CTCL) may begin with clinical lesions that resemble pigmented purpura. In addition, lesions of pigmented purpuric dermatosis may demonstrate clonality. Patients with more widespread lesions, or involvement above the knee/buttocks, are much more likely to have clonal infiltrates and eventually meet histologic criteria for the diagnosis of CTCL.

In most cases of pigmented purpuric dermatosis, the etiology is unknown. Patients with stasis dermatitis and venous insufficiency may develop lesions that bear a superficial clinical resemblance to Schamberg disease. Their lesions are more diffuse and do not form well-circumscribed macules. Oral medications can induce PPEs that closely resemble Ducas and Kapetanakis purpura, including acetaminophen, aspirin, glipizide, IFN-α, and medroxyprogesterone injections. Dietary supplements have induced PPD, including one with selenium, vitamin E, and a parsley concentrate. Stopping the medication will lead to resolution of the eruption. Pigmented purpuric contact dermatitis may simulate a PPE. Inciting allergens include nickel sulfate, fragrance mix, and Disperse Blue dyes. Patch testing on the back may be negative, but a positive response may be seen when the causative allergen is applied to a lesion. As with pigmenting drug eruptions, pigmented purpuric contact dermatitis should be suspected when the lesions are more widespread (sites other than the legs) and especially if they have an eczematous character.

Anecdotal reports of benefit from topical corticosteroids make a therapeutic trial for 4–6 weeks reasonable. Oral rutoside, 50 mg twice daily, and ascorbic acid, 500 mg twice daily, may be beneficial. One study with 35 patients demonstrated 71% complete clearance and 20% improvement of more than 50%. Psoralen plus ultraviolet A (PUVA) and narrow-band UVB have demonstrated efficacy and should be considered when the other modalities fail. Immunosuppressive therapy with cyclosporine and methotrexate has also been effective but is usually not warranted given the lack of significant symptoms. If immunosuppression is considered, CTCL must be excluded, and patch testing and drug withdrawal should be undertaken.

Battle LR, et al: Granulomatous pigmented purpuric dermatosis. Clin Exp Dermatol 2015; 40: 387.

Engin B, et al: Patch test results in patients with progressive pigmented purpuric dermatosis. J Eur Acad Dermatol Venereol 2009; 23: 209.

Georgala S, et al: Persistent pigmented purpuric eruption associated with mycosis fungoides. J Eur Acad Dermatol Venereol 2001; 15: 62.

Hanson C, et al: Granulomatous pigmented purpuric dermatosis. Dermatol Online J 2014; 21.

Hoesly FJ, et al: Purpura annularis telangiectodes of Majocchi. Int J Dermatol 2009; 48: 1129.

Kaplan R, et al: A case of isotretinoin-induced purpura annularis telangiectodes of Majocchi and review of substance-induced pigmented purpuric dermatosis. JAMA Dermatol 2014; 150: 182.

Komericki P, et al: Pigmented purpuric contact dermatitis from Disperse Blue 106 and 124 dyes. J Am Acad Dermatol 2001; 45: 456.

Morrissey K, et al: Granulomatous changes associated with pigmented purpuric dermatosis. Cutis 2014; 94: 197.

Ozkaya DB, et al: Dermatoscopic findings of pigmented purpuric dermatosis. An Bras Dermatol 2016; 91: 584.

Schober SM, et al: Early treatment with rutoside and ascorbic acid is highly effective for progressive pigmented purpuric dermatosis. J Dtsch Dermatol Ges 2014; 12: 1112.

Sezer E, et al: Pigmented purpuric dermatosis-like sarcoidosis. J Dermatol 2015; 42: 629.

Unal E, Ergul G: Pigmented purpuric dermatosis after taking a dietary supplement. Cutan Ocul Toxicol 2016; 35: 260.

■ VASCULITIS

Vasculitis is a clinicopathologically defined process characterized by inflammation and necrosis of blood vessels. Because the clinical morphology correlates with the size of the affected blood vessel(s), these disorders are classified by the vessel(s) affected. Diseases may involve vessels of overlapping size. In general, small-vessel disease (affecting postcapillary venules) causes urticarial lesions and palpable purpura; small-artery disease manifests with subcutaneous nodules; medium-sized arteries with necrosis of major organs, livedo, purpura, and mononeuritis multiplex; and large-vessel disease with symptoms of claudication and necrosis.

Classification

Numerous vasculitis classification schemes have been proposed, most recently the 2012 Revised International Chapel Hill Consensus Conference Nomenclature of Vasculitides; all have limitations. It is important to remember that infectious and thrombotic conditions, which "classically" show thrombosis of vessels histologically, at times may also show true leukocytoclastic vasculitis. Therefore infectious, embolic, and thrombotic causes of vessel damage must

---

BOX 35.1 Classification of Vasculitis

I. Cutaneous small-vessel (postcapillary venule) vasculitis
   A. Idiopathic cutaneous small-vessel vasculitis
   B. Henoch-Schönlein purpura
   C. Acute hemorrhagic edema of infancy
   D. Urticarial vasculitis
   E. Cryoglobulinemic vasculitis
   F. Erythema elevatum diutinum
   G. Granuloma faciale
   H. Other diseases with leukocytoclastic vasculitis: drug-induced vasculitis, malignancy (lymphoreticular more common than solid tumor), connective tissue diseases, hyperglobulinemic purpura, inflammatory bowel disease, bowel-associated dermatitis–arthritis syndrome (bowel bypass), HIV infection, and neutrophilic dermatoses (Behçet; Sweet; erythema nodosum leprosum; septic vasculitis; autoinflammatory conditions–familial Mediterranean fever, and serum sickness)

II. Medium-vessel vasculitis
   A. Polyarteritis nodosa
      1. Benign cutaneous forms
      2. Systemic form

III. Mixed size (medium and small)–vessel disease
   A. Connective tissue disease associated (usually rheumatoid vasculitis)
   B. Septic vasculitis
   C. Antineutrophil cytoplasmic antibody associated
      1. Microscopic polyangiitis
      2. Granulomatosis with polyangiitis(Wegener)
      3. Eosinophilic granulomatosis with polyangiitis (Churg-Strauss)
      4. Occasional drug induced (most are postcapillary venule only)

IV. Large-vessel vasculitis
   A. Giant cell arteritis
   B. Takayasu arteritis

---

always be considered before unequivocally diagnosing a case as an "inflammatory" vasculitis. Leukocytoclastic vasculitis is also frequently seen adjacent to suppurative folliculitis and at the base of chronic ulcers. The discovery of the association of some forms of small-vessel and medium-vessel vasculitides with positive ANCAs has made their diagnosis and classification much easier (Box 35.1).

Grzeszkiewicz TM, Fiorentino DF: Update on cutaneous vasculitis. Semin Cutan Med Surg 2006; 25: 221.

Jennette JC, et al: 2012 Revised International Chapel Hill Consensus Conference Nomenclature of Vasculitides. Arthritis Rheum 2013; 65: 1.

Sunderkotter C, Sindrilaru A: Clinical classification of vasculitis. Eur J Dermatol 2006; 16: 114.

SMALL-VESSEL VASCULITIS

Cutaneous Small-Vessel Vasculitis (Cutaneous Leukocytoclastic Vasculitis)

The vast majority of cases of cutaneous LeukoCytoclastic Vasculitis (LCV) follow an acute infection or exposure to a new medication. Palpable purpura is the hallmark of this disease, with lesions ranging from pinpoint to several centimeters in diameter (Fig. 35.18). Annular, vesicular, bullous, or pustular lesions may develop. Small ulcerations may develop, but when ulceration is prominent, one must suspect either a vasculitis of larger vessels (small to medium arterioles) or the presence of both a vasculitis and a hypercoagulable

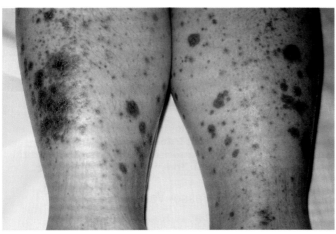

Fig. 35.18 Leukocytoclastic vasculitis. (Courtesy Steven Binnick, MD.)

state. Lesions of LCV predominate on the ankles and lower legs, affecting mainly dependent areas or areas under local pressure. Edema, especially of the ankles, is usually noted. In the hospitalized or bedridden patient, the buttocks and posterior thighs are dependent areas and may be the initial or primary site of involvement. Mild pruritus, fever, and malaise may occur. Arthralgias or less often frank arthritis may be seen. Other systemic involvement is rare and should lead to consideration of another diagnosis. Although in general, systemic involvement is not found or is minimal, serious systemic disease can accompany cutaneous LCV and should be sought in every patient.

The lesions usually resolve in 3–4 weeks, with residual postinflammatory hyperpigmentation. Ten percent of cutaneous LCV patients may have recurrences. A persistent underlying cause must be sought in chronic or recurrent cases.

Histology

There is angiocentric segmental inflammation of the postcapillary venule, with expansion of the vessel wall, fibrin deposition, and infiltration by neutrophils that show fragmentation of their nuclei (karyorrhexis or leukocytoclasia). Endothelial cell swelling is common, and fibrinoid necrosis of the vessel walls is seen. Vascular thrombosis may be present. The presence of tissue eosinophilia favors a medication as the cause. Immunofluorescence and ultrastructural studies have shown the presence of immunoglobulins, complement components, and fibrin deposits within postcapillary venule walls, if the biopsy is taken within the first 24 hours. Later, fibrin is prominent, but immunoglobulin deposits may have been destroyed. An important exception is Henoch-Schönlein purpura, which usually demonstrates prominent IgA deposits even in more advanced lesions.

Pathogenesis

Cutaneous small-vessel vasculitis is thought to be caused by circulating immune complexes. These complexes lodge in vessel walls and activate complement. Various inflammatory mediators are produced, contributing to endothelial injury.

Etiology

In most series, the majority of cutaneous LCV cases are idiopathic. Of the remaining 50% of cases, most are either drug induced or postinfectious. Drugs in virtually every class have been reported as causing LCV, and the time from start of the medication to onset of the eruption may be hours to years, making any ingested

agent a possible cause, including illicit substances such as cocaine. A host of infectious agents, such as β-hemolytic *Streptococcus* group A, *Mycoplasma*, and rarely *Mycobacterium tuberculosis*, may cause palpable purpura. Cutaneous LCV can occur in association with a connective tissue disease or as its presenting sign. Patients with lymphoproliferative neoplasms, as well as solid tumors (lung, colon, genitourinary, and breast cancer), may experience cutaneous small-vessel vasculitis at some time during the course of their disease. A recurrence of the LCV may mark the return of a treated malignancy. Cutaneous LCV may also be the initial manifestation of mixed small-vessel and medium-vessel vasculitis.

Clinical Evaluation

The clinical evaluation is critical in separating cases of benign cutaneous vasculitis (usually after an infection or induced by a medication) from those cases associated with more serious underlying disease or that have significant systemic involvement. One study of 112 patients with LCV demonstrated that 51% had associated systemic involvement. It may not be possible on initial physical examination to make this distinction. The history should focus on possible infectious disorders, prior associated diseases, drugs ingested, and a thorough review of systems. Screening laboratory tests may help to elucidate the underlying cause or extent of organ involvement. When the history suggests a recent drug and the patient is clinically well, nothing more than a urinalysis may be required. A CBC, basic metabolic panel, urinalysis, strep throat culture or ASO titer, hepatitis B and C serologies, and ANA and RF are a reasonable initial screen for patients with no obvious cause for their vasculitis. Serum protein electrophoresis, serum complements, ANCAs, and cryoglobulins may be required in some cases. Paraneoplastic LCV is relatively uncommon, but may be seen with both solid tumors and hematologic disorders. A skin biopsy should be performed to confirm the diagnosis of LCV. DIF should be performed to identify IgA vasculitis (Henoch-Schönlein purpura). Delayed organ involvement may occur, and patients should report any concerning symptoms.

Treatment

The initial treatment of most cases of LCV in patients who are clinically well and have a normal urinalysis should focus on symptom management and should not be aggressive, because the majority of cases are acute and self-limited, affect only the skin, and do not threaten progressive deterioration of internal organs. Rest and elevation of the legs will likely be helpful. Analgesics and avoidance of trauma and cold are prudent general measures. An identified antigen or drug should be eliminated and any identified infectious, connective tissue, or neoplastic disease treated.

A variety of systemic treatments may be required for severe, intractable, or recurrent disease, especially if significant organ involvement is present. For disease limited to the skin, NSAIDs can be considered for arthralgias. Colchicine, 0.6 mg two or three times daily, or dapsone, 50–200 mg/day, may be useful for chronic vasculitis. Low doses of colchicine and dapsone may be combined if either medication alone is unsuccessful or effective doses of either drug cannot be tolerated. Although one controlled trial (the only such trial for cutaneous small-vessel vasculitis) suggested that colchicine was ineffective for LCV, some of the patients did respond and flared when the drug was stopped. Oral antihistamines, by blocking the vasodilation induced by histamine, may reduce immune complex trapping and improve LCV. Systemic corticosteroids, in doses ranging from 60–80 mg/day, are recommended for patients with serious systemic manifestations or necrotic lesions. Usually, a brief course leads to resolution, and chronic treatment is rarely required. Unfortunately, systemic corticosteroids are not good long-term options for patients with chronic LCV. For those with chronic or refractory disease in whom colchicine or dapsone is ineffective, immunosuppressive agents, such as MMF, 2–3 g/day; methotrexate, 5–25 mg/week; or azathioprine, 50–200 mg/day (2–3.5 mg/kg/day), may be considered. Azathioprine dosing is based on thiopurine methyltransferase (TPMT) levels. In more difficult cases, cyclophosphamide, monthly IV pulses of steroids or cyclophosphamide, or cyclosporine, 3–5 mg/kg/day, may be effective. The tumor necrosis factor (TNF) blockers, especially infliximab and to a lesser degree etanercept, may be effective in cutaneous small-vessel vasculitis. However, these agents may also cause vasculitis. Rituximab has been effective in refractory cases. Patients with skin-only disease appear less likely to relapse and develop chronic involvement.

Arora A, et al: Incidence of leukocytoclastic vasculitis, 1996 to 2010. Mayo Clin Proc 2014; 89: 1515.

Bahrami S, et al: Tissue eosinophilia as an indicator of drug-induced cutaneous small-vessel vasculitis. Arch Dermatol 2006; 142: 155.

Barile-Fabris L, et al: Vasculitis in systemic lupus erythematosus. Curr Rheumatol Rep 2014; 16: 440.

Bouiller K, et al: Etiologies and prognostic factors of leukocytoclastic vasculitis with skin involvement. Medicine (Baltimore) 2016; 95: e4238.

Carlson JA, et al: Cutaneous vasculitis. Clin Dermatol 2006; 24: 414.

Fain O, et al: Vasculitides associated with malignancies. Arthritis Rheum 2007; 57: 1473.

Goeser MR, et al: A practical approach to the diagnosis, evaluation, and management of cutaneous small-vessel vasculitis. Am J Clin Dermatol 2014; 15: 299.

Haeberle MT, et al: Treatment of severe cutaneous small-vessel vasculitis with mycophenolate mofetil. Arch Dermatol 2012; 148: 887.

Khetan P, et al: An aetiological and clinicopathological study on cutaneous vasculitis. Indian J Med Res 2012; 135: 107.

Loricera J, et al: The spectrum of paraneoplastic cutaneous vasculitis in a defined population. Medicine (Baltimore) 2013; 92: 331.

Loricera J, et al: Single-organ cutaneous small-vessel vasculitis according to the 2012 Revised International Chapel Hill Consensus Conference Nomenclature of Vasculitides. Rheumatology (Oxford) 2015; 54: 77.

Mang R, et al: Therapy for severe necrotizing vasculitis with infliximab. J Am Acad Dermatol 2004; 51: 321.

Marzano AV, et al: Skin involvement in cutaneous and systemic vasculitis. Autoimmun Rev 2013; 12: 467.

Podjasek JO, et al: Cutaneous small-vessel vasculitis associated with solid organ malignancies. J Am Acad Dermatol 2012; 66: e55.

Podjasek JO, et al: Histopathological findings in cutaneous small-vessel vasculitis associated with solid-organ malignancy. Br J Dermatol 2014; 171: 1397.

Sais G, et al: Colchicine in the treatment of cutaneous leukocytoclastic vasculitis. Arch Dermatol 1995; 131: 1399.

Salehi M, et al: Levamisole-induced leukocytoclastic vasculitis with negative serology in a cocaine user. Am J Case Rep 2017; 18: 641.

Sokumbi O, et al: Vasculitis associated with tumor necrosis factor-α inhibitors. Mayo Clin Proc 2012; 87: 739.

Cutaneous Vasculitis and Connective Tissue Disease

Patients with various connective tissue diseases (SLE, Sjögren syndrome, rheumatoid arthritis [RA], dermatomyositis) may develop cutaneous vasculitic lesions. Vasculitis in the patient with connective tissue disease may be associated with significant internal organ involvement, especially of the peripheral and central nervous systems and the kidneys (glomerulonephritis). Ischemic digital infarcts are seen in addition to palpable purpura. Ulceration of vasculitic lesions can occur and may be particularly difficult to manage in patients with RA. The prevalence of vasculitis in patients with RA has decreased with improved treatment of RA, but this complication remains a significant source of morbidity and mortality for affected patients. Treatment is the same as for cutaneous LCV, along with management of the underlying connective tissue disease.

Barile-Fabris L, et al: Vasculitis in systemic lupus erythematosus. Curr Rheumatol Rep 2014; 16: 440.

Makol A, et al: Vasculitis associated with rheumatoid arthritis. Rheumatology (Oxford) 2014; 53: 890.

Subtypes of Small-Vessel Vasculitis

IgA Vasculitis (Henoch-Schönlein Purpura)

The term *IgA vasculitis* (IgAV) replaces the Henoch-Schönlein purpura eponym in the most recent vasculitis consensus criteria. IgAV is characterized by purpura, arthralgias, and abdominal and renal disease. Typically, mottled purpura appears on the extensor extremities, becomes hemorrhagic within 1 day, and starts to fade in about 5 days (Fig. 35.19). New crops may appear over a few weeks. Urticarial lesions, vesicles, necrotic purpura, and hemangioma-like lesions may also be present at some stages. There is a male predominance of cases, at least in adults. The disease occurs primarily in children (≈75% of cases), with a peak age between 2 and 8 years; however, adults may also be affected, with a broad age range and average age of 50. A viral infection or streptococcal pharyngitis is the usual triggering event. *Helicobacter pylori* infection has been implicated in some childhood and adult cases. Medication exposure can also trigger IgAV.

In about 40% of cases, the cutaneous manifestations are preceded by mild fever, headache, joint symptoms, and abdominal pain for up to 2 weeks. Once the vasculitis is fully established, skin lesions occur in all patients. GI symptoms are also common, occurring in about 65% of patients. Abdominal pain and GI bleeding may occur at any time during the disease; severe abdominal pain may even suggest—or portend—an acute surgical abdomen. Paralytic ileus may occur. Vomiting, rebound tenderness, and distention are other manifestations. GI radiographs may show "spiking" or a marbled "cobblestone" appearance. Arthralgia progressing to arthritis produces periarticular swelling around the knees and ankles; about 63% of patients have joint symptoms. Renal involvement manifests as microscopic or even gross hematuria and may occur in 40% or more of patients, with higher rates in adults (up

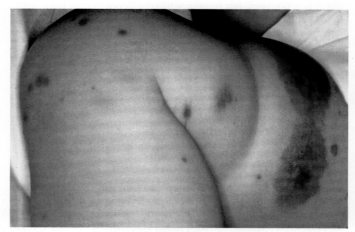

Fig. 35.19 Henoch-Schönlein purpura.

to 70% or more); usually it is mild. Pulmonary hemorrhage may occur and can be fatal. The long-term prognosis is generally favorable but is largely dictated by the severity of renal involvement. Children with gross hematuria usually do well; however, progressive glomerular disease and renal failure may develop in a small percentage, so careful follow-up is necessary for those with hematuria. Renal insufficiency is more common in adults, so the rate of long-term sequelae is higher in this population. Purpura above the waist may be a marker of renal involvement. Overall, persistent, usually mild nephropathy occurs in only 8% of patients. Relapses in disease activity, however, are common for months after initial diagnosis. IgA, C3, and fibrin depositions have been demonstrated in biopsies of both involved and uninvolved skin by immunofluorescence techniques. Abnormal IgA deposits in vessel walls are the defining pathophysiologic feature of IgAV (thus the name change) and may result from abnormal IgA1 glycosylation, leading to IgG-IgA1 immune complex deposition and resulting inflammation. In patients with abdominal pain suggestive of IgAV but with no skin lesions, histamine (as used as a control by allergists) can be injected into the skin and the area biopsied 4 hours later. This "histamine trap test" may identify IgA in vessels and confirm the diagnosis. The presence of IgM in lesional skin may be an indication of renal involvement. Patients with baseline renal impairment, proteinuria greater than 1 g/day, and certain renal biopsy findings are at higher risk of long-term severe renal disease.

In adult patients with IgAV and upper GI symptoms (gastritis), a search for *H. pylori* infection should be undertaken. If an association with *H. pylori* can be confirmed, treatment of the GI infection may lead to resolution. IgAV in adults can be associated with an underlying malignancy. Males represent 90% or more of malignancy-associated IgAV cases. Solid tumors are seen in more than half of patients, especially non–small cell lung cancer, prostate cancer, and renal cancer. About 40% have a hematologic malignancy. About half of patients present within 1 month of diagnosis of the malignancy.

Treatment is primarily supportive. The usual duration of illness is 6–16 weeks, and no therapy appears to shorten that duration significantly. Between 5% and 30% of patients will have persistent or recurrent disease. Close follow-up, including urinalysis and blood pressure monitoring, should be continued for at least 6 months. Dapsone, 50–200 mg/day, or colchicine, 0.6 mg/day to 1.2 mg twice daily, can be used initially if treatment is required and skin lesions are the primary concern. For abdominal pain, an H2 blocker and corticosteroids (prednisone at 1 mg/kg/day) can be effective. Corticosteroids are more effective for abdominal pain than analgesia. The value of systemic corticosteroids in the treatment of renal disease is controversial, but steroids may be used preventively or to treat active nephritis. Data from randomized trials unfortunately have not shown significant benefit to this or other therapies in decreasing the risk of long-term renal sequelae. IVIG can be used in refractory skin disease and persistent abdominal pain and to arrest rapidly progressive glomerulonephritis. Cyclophosphamide is also used and may be effective for renal disease. NSAIDs are best avoided because they may cause renal or GI complications.

Anil M, et al: Henoch-Schönlein purpura in children from western Turkey. Turk J Pediatr 51; 2009: 429.

Audemard-Verger A, et al: IgA vasculitis (Henoch-Schönlein) in adults. Autoimmun Rev 2015; 14: 579.

Audemard-Verger A, et al: Characteristics and management of IgA vasculitis in adults. Arthritis Rheumatol 2017; 69: 1862.

Bogdanovic R: Henoch-Schönlein purpura nephritis in children. Acta Paediatr 2009; 98: 1882.

Calvo-Río V, et al: Henoch-Schönlein purpura in northern Spain. Medicine (Baltimore) 2014; 93: 106.

Chartapisak W, et al: Prevention and treatment of renal disease in Henoch-Schönlein purpura. Arch Dis Child 2009; 94: 132.

Gonzalez-Gay MA, et al: Henoch-Schönlein purpura (IgA vasculitis). Clin Exp Rheumatol 2017; 35: 3.

Hoshino C: Adult-onset Schönlein-Henoch purpura associated with *Helicobacter pylori* infection. Intern Med 2009; 48: 847.

Jauhola O, et al: Renal manifestations of Henoch-Schönlein purpura in a 6-month prospective study of 223 children. Arch Dis Child 2010; 95: 877.

Jauhola O, et al: Cyclosporine A vs. methylprednisolone for Henoch-Schönlein nephritis. Pediatr Nephrol 2011; 26: 2159.

Okubo Y, et al: Nationwide epidemiological survey of childhood IgA vasculitis associated hospitalization in the USA. Clin Rheumatol 2016; 35: 2749.

Podjasek JO, et al: Henoch-Schönlein purpura associated with solid-organ malignancies. Acta Derm Venereol 2012; 92: 388.

Poterucha TJ, et al: A retrospective comparison of skin and renal direct immunofluorescence findings in patients with glomerulonephritis in adult Henoch-Schönlein purpura. J Cutan Pathol 2014; 41: 582.

Rigante D, et al: Is there a crossroad between infections, genetics, and Henoch-Schönlein purpura? Autoimmun Rev 2013; 12: 1016.

Takeuchi S, et al: IgM in lesional skin of adults with Henoch-Schönlein purpura is an indication of renal involvement. J Am Acad Dermatol 2010; 63: 1026.

Xiong LJ, et al: Is *Helicobacter pylori* infection associated with Henoch-Schönlein purpura in Chinese children? World J Pediatr 2012; 8: 301.

Acute Hemorrhagic Edema of Infancy

Also known as Finkelstein disease, Seidlmayer syndrome, medallion-like purpura, infantile postinfectious irislike purpura and edema, and purpura en cocarde avec oedème, acute hemorrhagic edema (AHE) of infancy affects children younger than 2 years with a recent history of upper respiratory illness (75%) or febrile prodrome, a course of antibiotics, or both. The children are often nontoxic in appearance. There is abrupt onset of large purpuric lesions involving the face, ears, and extremities (Fig. 35.20). Cockade, annular, or targetoid morphologies may be present. Scrotal purpura may also occur. Early in the course, there may first be acral edema, with subsequent proximal spread. The edema is nontender and may be asymmetric. A low-grade fever or prodrome is common, and involvement of internal organ systems (joint pains, GI symptoms, renal involvement) is rare. Routine laboratory tests are unremarkable. Spontaneous recovery without sequelae occurs within 12–20 days. The differential diagnosis includes IgAV (Henoch-Schönlein purpura), meningococcemia,

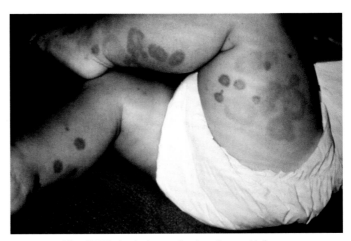

Fig. 35.20 Acute hemorrhagic edema of infancy.

erythema multiforme, urticaria, and Kawasaki disease. Some similarities exist between IgAV and AHE (postinfectious, seasonal, male predilection), but AHE is different in that it favors younger children (<2 years), resolves more quickly, lacks IgA on DIF in most cases, and is rarely associated with systemic symptoms. In one family, a child younger than 4 years developed AHE while the sibling age 16 developed IgAV after the same pharyngitis. From a clinical point of view, the most urgent need is to exclude septicemia, especially meningococcemia. Topical and systemic corticosteroids, as well as antihistamines and dapsone, have been reported as beneficial for relief of symptoms and rare complications of AHE of infancy.

Ferrarini A, et al: Acute hemorrhagic edema of young children. Eur J Pediatr 2016; 175: 557.

Fiore E, et al: Acute hemorrhagic edema of young children (cockade purpura and edema). J Am Acad Dermatol 2008; 59: 684.

Savino F, et al: Acute hemorrhagic edema of infancy. Pediatr Dermatol 2013; 30: e149.

Urticarial Vasculitis

A significant percentage of patients (reportedly as high as 5%–10%, but probably less) with fixed urticarial lesions will have vasculitis histologically. This is termed *urticarial vasculitis* (Fig. 35.21). This urticarial morphology is maintained throughout the course of the illness. Microscopic hemorrhage into the urticarial plaques may occur, resulting in a bruiselike appearance as the lesions fade. Determination of the serum complement levels (CH50, C3, C4, and anti-C1q precipitins) is critical in the evaluation of urticarial vasculitis. Patients with normal complement levels usually have an LCV, which is idiopathic, limited to the skin, self-resolving, and best considered a subset of cutaneous small-vessel vasculitis. Hypocomplementemic urticarial vasculitis is a distinctive syndrome seen virtually always in women. Clinical features include arthritis (50%–82%), arthralgias, angioedema, eye symptoms (up to 56%), asthma and obstructive pulmonary disease (20%), and GI symptoms (20%). Glomerulonephritis may be present. A rare subset of patients with hypocomplementemic urticarial vasculitis has Jaccoud arthropathy and serious valvular heart disease.

Underlying diseases associated with all forms of urticarial vasculitis include gammopathies (IgG and IgM gammopathy), SLE, Sjögren syndrome, serum sickness, and viral infections, especially hepatitis C. Medications can induce urticarial vasculitis, including penicillin, cimetidine, cocaine, saturated solution of potassium iodide (SSKI), NSAIDs, SSRIs, and multiple recent reports of TNF inhibitors. Patients with hypocomplementemic urticarial vasculitis can have anti-C1q antibodies directed against the collagen-like region of that molecule, a feature used to define the disease, and have low C1q levels and normal C1 inhibitor levels. Patients with SLE may also have these autoantibodies. Many patients with hypocomplementemic urticarial vasculitis will have positive ANAs, and up to one quarter will have positive anti-dsDNA antibodies. The vast majority (96%) will have a positive "lupus band test." Over time, more than 50% will meet the criteria for the diagnosis of SLE. For this reason, some consider hypocomplementemic urticarial vasculitis a form of SLE. Patients with HCV infection may develop hypocomplementemic or normocomplementic urticarial vasculitis without a detectable cryoglobulin.

The following three clinical features distinguish the skin lesions of urticarial vasculitis from true urticaria:

1. The lesions are often burning or painful, rather than pruritic.
2. The lesions last longer than 24 hours and are fixed, rather than transient and migrating.
3. On resolution, there is postinflammatory purpura or hyperpigmentation.

True urticaria is also more responsive to antihistamine therapy. More difficult is the distinction of urticarial vasculitis from neutrophilic urticaria, because patients with the latter condition can have painful, more persistent lesions. Histologic evaluation is critical.

Histologically, patients with hypocomplementemic urticarial vasculitis will show both LCV and diffuse interstitial neutrophils. Eosinophils are more likely to be seen in patients with neutrophilic urticaria or normocomplementemic urticarial vasculitis. Sweet syndrome shows a more intense dermal infiltrate with marked upper dermal edema. Sweet syndrome and vasculitis share the presence of karyorrhexis. Whereas virtually all biopsies of idiopathic urticaria demonstrate neutrophils, karyorrhexis is usually distinctly absent. In neutrophilic urticaria, neutrophils will be found in the dermis and in the vessel walls (moving from the vascular compartment into the skin). Finding neutrophils in the vessel walls alone without fibrinoid necrosis of vessel walls and leukocytoclasia is insufficient to make the diagnosis of urticarial vasculitis. Most patients with urticarial lesions with neutrophilic infiltrates and normal complements have neutrophilic urticaria rather than urticarial vasculitis.

Other neutrophilic disorders in the differential diagnosis of urticarial vasculitis include mixed cryoglobulinemia, Schnitzler syndrome, the autoinflammatory syndromes (*CIAS1/NALP3* mutations), and neutrophilic dermatosis associated with connective tissue disease. Mixed cryoglobulinemia will be seen most frequently in the context of HCV infection and may present with urticarial, purpuric, or even necrotic/ulcerative lesions. Vasculitis should be seen on biopsy. The other three conditions all can have cutaneous lesions that are urticarial and clinically similar. They tend to have less dermal edema than is typical of either urticaria or Sweet syndrome. Histologically, these conditions lack vasculitis but show tissue neutrophilia with leukocytoclasia. Schnitzler syndrome is diagnosed by the finding of an IgM monoclonal gammopathy. The autoinflammatory syndromes are diagnosed by their characteristic features and genetic testing. In some patients with adult-onset Still disease or SLE, transient macules and papules coalescing into plaques may be seen. This condition has been termed *neutrophilic urticarial dermatosis*, but its pathogenesis remains unknown. In patients with such neutrophilic urticarial lesions, ferritin measurement and a workup for SLE are appropriate.

The treatment of hypocomplementemic urticarial vasculitis is directed at the symptomatology and severity of the disease. Antihistamines may be used but are often ineffective. Indomethacin has been particularly effective. Dapsone, antimalarials, and

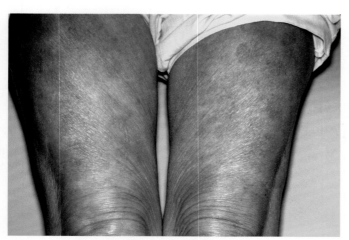

Fig. 35.21 Urticarial vasculitis.

colchicine may be tried. The addition of pentoxifylline to dapsone may be effective. Immunosuppressive therapy with prednisone and steroid-sparing agents such as MMF, azathioprine, rituximab, and canakinumab can be considered in refractory and severe cases. Omalizumab has used in one case with mixed results.

Breda L, et al: Hypocomplementemic urticarial vasculitis (HUVS) with precocious emphysema responsive to azathioprine. J Clin Immunol 2013; 33: 891.

Buck A, et al: Hypocomplementemic urticarial vasculitis syndrome. J Clin Aesthet Dermatol 2012; 5: 36.

Fadahunsi AW, et al: Hypocomplementemic urticarial vasculitis syndrome possibly secondary to etanercept. J Clin Rheumatol 2015; 21: 274.

Hamad A, et al: Urticarial vasculitis and associated disorders. Ann Allergy Asthma Immunol 2017; 118: 394.

Jachiet M, et al: The clinical spectrum and therapeutic management of hypocomplementemic urticarial vasculitis. Arthritis Rheumatol 2015; 67: 527.

Jara LJ, et al: Hypocomplementemic urticarial vasculitis syndrome. Curr Rheumatol Rep 2009; 11: 410.

Kai AC, et al: Improvement in quality of life impairment followed by relapse with 6-monthly periodic administration of omalizumab for severe treatment-refractory chronic urticaria and urticarial vasculitis. Clin Exp Dermatol 2014; 39: 651.

Kallenberg CG: Anti-C1q autoantibodies. Autoimmun Rev 2008; 7: 612.

Kieffer C, et al: Neutrophilic urticarial dermatosis. Medicine 2009; 88: 23.

Krause K, et al: Efficacy and safety of canakinumab in urticarial vasculitis. J Allergy Clin Immunol 2013; 132: 751.

Loricera J, et al: Urticarial vasculitis in northern Spain. Medicine (Baltimore) 2014; 93: 53.

Marzano AV, et al: Urticarial vasculitis and urticarial autoinflammatory syndromes. G Ital Dermatol Venereol 2015; 150: 41.

Pasini A, et al: Renal involvement in hypocomplementaemic urticarial vasculitis syndrome. Rheumatology (Oxford) 2014; 53: 1409.

Pinto-Almeida T, et al: Cutaneous lesions and finger clubbing uncovering hypocomplementemic urticarial vasculitis and hepatitis C with mixed cryoglobulinemia. An Bras Dermatol 2013; 88: 973.

Saeb-Lima M, et al: Autoimmunity-related neutrophilic dermatosis. Am J Dermatopathol 2013; 35: 655.

Swaminath A, et al: Refractory urticarial vasculitis as a complication of ulcerative colitis successfully treated with rituximab. J Clin Rheumatol 2011; 17: 281.

Cryoglobulinemic Vasculitis

About 15% of patients with a circulating cryoprecipitable protein are symptomatic and have cryoglobulinemic vasculitis. They typically have mixed (type II or III) cryoglobulinemia. Mixed cryoglobulinemia follows a benign course in half the cases, but in about one third, hepatic or renal failure occurs. About 15% of patients develop malignancy, usually B-cell lymphoma, and less frequently, hepatocellular or thyroid cancer. By far the most common cause of cryoglobulinemic vasculitis is HCV infection, but other chronic infections, lymphoproliferative disorders, and autoimmune diseases can also be associated. Cryoglobulinemic vasculitis usually presents with macular or palpable purpura, typically confined to the lower extremities. Lesions may be limited or severe. Two thirds of patients show confluent areas of hemosiderosis of the feet and lower legs, characteristic of prior episodes of purpura. Although only 30% of patients report an exacerbation with cold exposure, up to 50% will have Raynaud phenomenon and cold-induced acrocyanosis of the ears. Other morphologies include ecchymoses, livedo reticularis, urticaria, and ulcerations.

Neuropathy and other neurologic complications occur in 40% of patients. Arthralgias, xerostomia, and xerophthalmia are frequent complaints. Renal disease occurs in about 25% of patients; widespread systemic vasculitis occurs in about 10%. These complications can be significant and life threatening, as can therapy-related infections. Laboratory evaluation will reveal a cryoglobulin, hypocomplementemia (90%), and a positive RF (70%). ANCAs are rarely positive. A skin biopsy will show LCV.

The treatment of cryoglobulinemic vasculitis is the treatment of the underlying disease, if possible. With HCV infection, this may be IFN-α plus ribavirin, or newer direct antiviral agents. Cryoglobulinemic vasculitis associated with HCV may also flare with IFN treatment. Rituximab is being used with increasing frequency for severe cases, including to control the disease in cases of infection-induced cryoglobulinemia. Colchicine, dapsone, IVIG, and infliximab can be attempted. In severe cases, plasmapheresis may be beneficial.

Bryce AH, et al: Natural history and therapy of 66 patients with mixed cryoglobulinemia. Am J Hematol 2006; 81: 511.

Chandesris MO, et al: Infliximab in the treatment of refractory vasculitis secondary to hepatitis C–associated mixed cryoglobulinaemia. Rheumatology 2004; 43: 532.

Dammacco F, Sansonno D: Therapy for hepatitis C virus–related cryoglobulinemic vasculitis. N Engl J Med 2013; 369: 1035.

Dammacco F, et al: The expanding spectrum of HCV-related cryoglobulinemic vasculitis. Clin Exp Med 2016; 16: 233.

Damoiseaux J: The diagnosis and classification of the cryoglobulinemic syndrome. Autoimmun Rev 2014; 13: 359.

De Blasi T, et al: Cryoglobulinemia-related vasculitis during effective anti-HCV treatment with PEG-interferon alfa-2b. Infection 2008; 36: 285.

Farri C, et al: Mixed cryoglobulinemia. Semin Arthritis Rheum 2004; 33: 355.

Giuggioli D, et al: Cryoglobulinemic vasculitis and skin ulcers. Semin Arthritis Rheum 2015; 44: 518.

Mazzaro C, et al: Efficacy and safety of peginterferon alfa-2b plus ribavirin for HCV-positive mixed cryoglobulinemia. Clin Exp Rheumatol 2011; 29: 933.

Quartuccio L, et al: Retreatment regimen of rituximab monotherapy given at the relapse of severe HCV-related cryoglobulinemic vasculitis. J Autoimmune 2015; 63: 88.

Ramos-Casals M, et al: The cryoglobulinaemias. Lancet 2012; 379: 348.

Retamozo S, et al: Life-threatening cryoglobulinemic patients with hepatitis C. Medicine (Baltimore) 2015; 144: 410.

Viganò M, et al: HBV-associated cryoglobulinemic vasculitis. Kidney Blood Press Res 2014; 39: 65.

Zaja F, et al: Efficacy and safety of rituximab in type II mixed cryoglobulinemia. Blood 2003; 101: 3827.

Erythema Elevatum Diutinum

A rare condition, erythema elevatum diutinum (EED) is considered to be a chronic fibrosing leukocytoclastic vasculitis. Classically, multiple orange to yellow papules and plaques develop over the joints, particularly the elbows, knees, hands, and feet. Lesions may also involve the buttocks and areas over the Achilles tendon. Petechiae and purpura can be associated with early lesions. More rarely, large plaques with nodules at the periphery may affect the trunk and extremities. Scattered nodules on the trunk with no acral lesions constitute another rare variant. With time, the papules take on a doughy to firm consistency and develop a red or purple color (Fig. 35.22). In HIV infection, skin-colored or red nodules affect the soles, producing lesions resembling keloids, Kaposi sarcoma, or bacillary angiomatosis. Pruritus, arthralgias, and pain have been reported; however, most patients are asymptomatic. Some patients with EED will develop Sweet syndrome or pyoderma

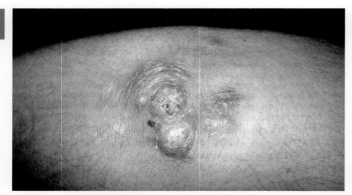

Fig. 35.22 Erythema elevatum diutinum.

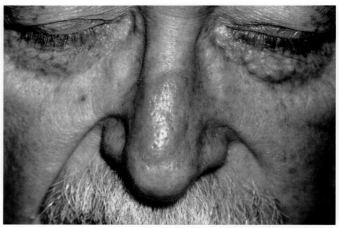

Fig. 35.23 Granuloma faciale. (Courtesy Steven Binnick, MD.)

gangrenosum–like ulcerations, which in one patient presented as a phagedenic penile ulceration. Systemic complications are rare, but an unusual and potentially rapidly destructive keratitis can lead to blindness. EED has been associated with HIV infection, SLE, Sjögren syndrome, lymphoma, breast cancer, lymphoepithelioma-like carcinoma, dermatitis herpetiformis, thyroid disease, hepatitis, and celiac disease. IgA monoclonal gammopathy may be detected. Chronic and recurrent streptococcal infections cause exacerbations of the disease in some patients. These may all represent conditions with persistent circulating immune complexes that might trigger a chronic vasculitis. Pathogenically, ANCAs (60% IgA and 33% IgG) are found in EED. ANCA-positive vasculitides, such as granulomatosis with polyangiitis and microscopic polyangiitis, have rarely been reported to have EED-like lesions.

Histologically, early lesions are an LCV, but with prominent interstitial neutrophils. Well-formed lesions are composed of nodular and diffuse mixed infiltrates of neutrophils and nuclear dust, eosinophils, histiocytes, and plasma cells that often extend into the subcutaneous fat. The prominence of eosinophils; the chronicity of the process, which results in an onion skin–like perivascular fibrosis; and the admixture of plasma cells and many lymphocytes are the hallmarks of EED. Erythrocyte extravasation may lead to extracellular cholesterol crystals in long-standing cases.

Dapsone is the treatment of choice for EED. Patients with celiac disease may respond to a gluten-free diet. Tetracycline and nicotinamide, sulfapyridine, colchicine, antimalarials, intralesional or systemic corticosteroids, topical dapsone, and surgical excision have all been reported as effective in a limited number of cases. Intermittent plasma exchange has been used successfully in patients with IgA paraproteinemia. The interstitial keratitis also responds to dapsone. Unfortunately, the late nodular lesions may not resolve with dapsone treatment.

Caucanas M, et al: Associated pyoderma gangrenosum, erythema elevatum diutinum, and Sweet's syndrome. Int J Dermatol 2013; 52: 1185.

Chan Y, et al: Erythema elevatum diutinum in systemic lupus erythematosus. Rheumatol Int 2011; 31: 259.

Chandrasekaran SS, et al: Erythema elevatum diutinum in association with dermatitis herpetiformis. Indian Dermatol Online J 2014; 5: 48.

Cirvidiu DC, et al: Erythema elevatum diutinum and hypothyroidism. An Bras Dermatol 2015; 90: 561.

Crichlow SM, et al: Is IgA antineutrophil cytoplasmic antibody a marker for patients with erythema elevatum diutinum? Br J Dermatol 2011; 164: 675.

Frieling GW, et al: Novel use of topical dapsone 5% gel for erythema elevatum diutinum. J Drugs Dermatol 2013; 12: 481.

Kawakami T, et al: Acceleration of pulmonary interstitial fibrosis in a patient with myeloperoxidase-antineutrophil cytoplasmic antibody–positive erythema elevatum diutinum. J Am Acad Dermatol 2011; 65: 674.

Kwon JL, et al: Erythema elevatum diutinum in association with celiac disease. Int J Dermatol 2009; 48: 787.

Liu TC, et al: Erythema elevatum diutinum as a paraneoplastic syndrome in a patient with pulmonary lymphoepithelioma-like carcinoma. Lung Cancer 2009; 63: 151.

Marie I, et al: Erythema elevatum diutinum associated with dermatomyositis. J Am Acad Dermatol 2011; 64: 1000.

Momen SE, et al: Erythema elevatum diutinum. J Eur Acad Dermatol Venereol 2014; 28: 1594.

Shimizu S, et al: Erythema elevatum diutinum with primary Sjögren syndrome associated with IgA antineutrophil cytoplasmic antibody. Br J Dermatol 2008; 159: 733.

Smitha P, et al: A case of extensive erosive and bullous erythema elevatum diutinum in a patient diagnosed with human immunodeficiency virus (HIV). Int J Dermatol 2011; 50: 989.

Zacaron LH, et al: Clinical and surgical therapeutic approach in erithema elevatum diutinum. An Bras Dermatol 2013; 88: 15.

Granuloma Faciale

Characterized by brownish red, infiltrated papules, plaques (Fig. 35.23), and nodules, granuloma faciale involves the facial areas, particularly the nose. Healthy, middle-aged (mean 53 years) white men (male/female ratio 5 : 1) are most often affected. Childhood cases have been reported. Extrafacial disease occurs in up to 20% of patients, usually affecting the upper trunk and extremities. The pathology of granuloma faciale is similar to that of EED, with focal LCV, diffuse dermal neutrophilia with leukocytoclasia, tissue eosinophilia, and perivascular fibrosis. Some histologic features, including an abnormal content of IgG4 plasma cells, may be similar to those of IgG4-related sclerosing diseases. A variety of treatment options are available. Intralesional corticosteroids are the recommended first approach. Cryotherapy in combination with intralesional corticosteroids has been shown to be very effective. Topical corticosteroids or tacrolimus may also be useful. Although controlled clinical trials are lacking, dapsone, colchicine, or antimalarials could be considered if the patient remains unresponsive. Topical dapsone and topical ingenol mebutate have been used in case reports. Pulsed dye or carbon dioxide (CO_2) laser therapy has been effective in multiple cases, making it a reasonable consideration as first-line treatment.

Bobyr I, et al: Granulomafaciale successfully treated with ingenol mebutate. Dermatol Ther 2016; 29: 325.

Cesinaro AM, et al: Granuloma faciale. Am J Surg Pathol 2013; 37: 66.

Dowlati B, et al: Granuloma faciale. Int J Dermatol 1997; 36: 548.

Erceg A, et al: The efficacy of pulsed dye laser treatment for inflammatory skin diseases. J Am Acad Dermatol 2013; 69: 609.

Lima RS, et al: Granuloma faciale. An Bras Dermatol 2015; 90: 735.

Oliveira CC, et al: Granuloma faciale. An Bras Dermatol 2016; 91: 803.

Paradisi A, et al: Drug-resistant granuloma faciale. Dermatol Ther 2016; 29: 317.

POLYARTERITIS NODOSA

Polyarteritis nodosa (PAN) is characterized by necrotizing vasculitis affecting primarily the small to medium-sized arteries. There are two major forms, the benign cutaneous and the systemic, although even long-standing benign cutaneous PAN can evolve into systemic disease. In 1990 the American College of Rheumatology selected the following 10 features of systemic PAN, at least three of which should be present for diagnosis:

1. Livedo racemosa
2. Polymorphonuclear arteritis
3. Leg pain/myopathy/weakness
4. Mononeuropathy/polyneuropathy
5. Positive hepatitis B virus (HBV) serology
6. Weight loss greater than 4 kg
7. Testicular pain/tenderness
8. Diastolic blood pressure greater than 90 mm Hg
9. Elevated blood urea nitrogen/creatinine
10. Arteriographic abnormality

Systemic PAN shares some clinical features with microscopic polyangiitis (MPA), but the strong association of MPA with ANCA positivity, the involvement of renal glomeruli and pulmonary capillaries, and the presence of vasculitis in arterioles, venules, and capillaries help distinguish MPA from PAN.

The mean age of presentation is 45–50 years, and PAN is two to four times more common in men than women. A cutaneous vasculitis identical to PAN has been seen in IV drug abusers (see later) and in association with SLE, inflammatory bowel disease, hairy cell leukemia, familial Mediterranean fever, and Cogan syndrome (nonsyphilitic interstitial keratitis and vestibuloauditory symptoms). Reported infectious associations include hepatitis B, hepatitis C, antecedent streptococcal infection, and many others. Vascular-based tuberculids (erythema induratum, nodular tuberculid) may have histology identical to PAN. The proportion of PAN cases associated with HBV was previously higher but is currently about 5%–7% of cases overall and decreasing with HBV immunization. The identification of associated hepatitis virus infection has therapeutic and prognostic implications. Patients with early-onset PAN and stroke should be evaluated for *CECR1* mutations and adenosine deaminase 2 deficiency (DADA2), because early recognition and treatment with anti-TNF agents is critical in this syndrome.

The skin is involved in up to 50% of patients with the systemic form of PAN, with wide-ranging findings. The most striking and diagnostic lesions (15% of patients) are 5–10 mm subcutaneous nodules occurring singly or in groups, distributed along the course of the blood vessels, above which the skin is normal or slightly erythematous (macular arteritis). These nodules are often painful and may pulsate and over time ulcerate. Common sites are the lower extremities, especially below the knee. Ecchymoses and peripheral gangrene of the fingers and toes may also be present (Fig. 35.24). Livedo reticularis in combination with subcutaneous

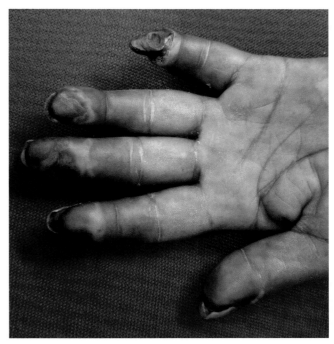

Fig. 35.24 Gangrene secondary to polyarteritis nodosa. (Courtesy Debabrata Bandopadhyay, MD.)

nodules strongly suggests the diagnosis of PAN. Palpable purpura with histologic features of cutaneous LCV may be seen in 20% of PAN patients. Urticaria is present in 6%. HBV-associated PAN is associated with cutaneous findings in only 30% of patients.

Classic systemic PAN may involve the vessels throughout the entire body. It has a particular predilection for the skin, peripheral nerves, GI tract, and kidneys. Hypertension (from renal involvement in 80%), tachycardia, fever, edema, and weight loss (>70%) are cardinal signs of the disease. Arthralgia/arthritis (up to 75%), myocardial and intestinal infarctions, and peripheral neuritis (75%) are also seen. Mononeuritis multiplex, most often manifested as footdrop, is a hallmark of PAN. Involvement of the meningeal, vertebral, and carotid arteries may lead to hemiplegia and convulsions. The lungs and spleen are rarely involved. Aneurysms develop, which may result in multiorgan infarcts. A five factor score (FFS) has been validated, with 1 point each for proteinuria (>1 g/day), renal insufficiency (serum creatinine >1.58 mg/dL), GI tract involvement, CNS involvement, and cardiomyopathy. The 5-year survival rates for patients with FFS of 0, 1, and more than 2 are 88%, 75%, and 54%, respectively. Among survivors, relapses remain common. Before the use of systemic immunosuppressives, the mortality rate for systemic PAN exceeded 90%.

A leukocytosis of as high as 40,000/mm³ may occur, with neutrophilia up to 80%; thrombocytosis, progressive normocytic anemia, and elevated ESR and C-reactive protein (CRP) may also be found. Hepatitis B and C studies should be performed. Urinary abnormalities, such as proteinuria, hematuria, and RBC casts, are present in 70% of patients. ANCA positivity in PAN is rare (if present, most often p-ANCA), whereas the more specific proteinase-3 and myeloperoxidase antibodies are negative.

The histology is that of an inflammatory necrotizing and obliterative panarteritis that affects the small and medium-sized arteries. Focal vasculitis forms nodular swellings that become necrotic, producing aneurysms and rupture of the vessels. Hemorrhage, hematoma, and ecchymosis may result. Obliteration of the lumen may occur, with ischemic necrosis of surrounding tissue. Characteristically, the arteries are affected at their branching points.

Biopsy samples of skin nodules or ulcers must be sufficiently deep to include affected vessels in the deep dermis or subcutis.

The mainstay of diagnosis is the presence of these histologic features and the constellation of clinical findings. The preferable site for biopsy is an accessible area such as skin, muscle, or testis. If these are not involved, angiography may detect aneurysmal dilations as small as 1 cm wide in the renal, hepatic, or other visceral vessels; the angiographic appearance of these aneurysms is characteristic, if not pathognomonic.

Treatment

Untreated classic PAN can be fatal, usually from renal failure or cardiovascular or GI complications. Death generally occurs early in the course of the disease, within weeks to months, highlighting the importance of early diagnosis and treatment. Patients with HBV- or HCV-associated PAN should receive appropriate antiviral treatments as part of their initial therapy. For PAN not associated with HBV or HCV, treatment with corticosteroids and cytotoxic agents has increased 5-year survival to more than 75%. Corticosteroids, in the range of 1 mg/kg/day of oral prednisone, are given initially. Once the disease remits, the dose should be reduced. After an average of 3–6 months, if the patient remains in remission, the corticosteroids are slowly tapered to discontinuation. The addition of azathioprine to corticosteroids for inducing remission was not associated with added benefit.

Cyclophosphamide is recommended for those with serious systemic involvement or steroid-refractory disease. It is given with corticosteroids or sometimes alone. Initially, 2 mg/kg/day as a single dose is recommended. Twice this amount may be required for severely ill patients. The oral cyclophosphamide dose is then adjusted to maintain the white blood cell (WBC) count between 3000 and 3500 cells/mm^3 and neutrophil count above 1500 cells/mm^3. When the disease has been quiescent for at least 1 year, the cyclophosphamide may be tapered and stopped. On average, 18–24 months of therapy are required. Pulsed IV cyclophosphamide is associated with a lower incidence of toxicity, especially the long-term risk of malignancy. Plasma exchange may be used for acute crises or treatment failures with corticosteroids and cyclophosphamide. Infliximab has been used in refractory cases. Ulcerations in PAN can be very painful because of the associated neuropathy and should be managed as nonhealing leg ulcers.

Cutaneous Polyarteritis Nodosa

About 10% of patients present with PAN localized to the skin and have limited systemic involvement. Neuropathy occurs in 20%. Subcutaneous nodules (80%), livedo (70%), and ulceration (44%) are the characteristic cutaneous features that should lead to suspicion of cutaneous PAN. Atrophie blanche–like lesions on the ankles may be the sole manifestation. Plaques on the trunk and proximal extremities, expanding slowly and centrifugally, are another manifestation. At the periphery of the plaques is a ring of 1–2 cm subcutaneous nodules. Cutaneous PAN has a better prognosis and requires less aggressive therapy. Patients rarely develop the systemic renal, GI, and cardiovascular complications of systemic PAN. Patients with cutaneous PAN and early-onset vasculopathy or strokes should be evaluated for deficiency in the ADA2 protein (DADA2, as discussed earlier). Whether there are two clear subsets of patients with cutaneous or systemic PAN, or whether they exist on a spectrum, is controversial. Patients with "cutaneous" PAN must be followed carefully and regularly evaluated to exclude the development of systemic involvement, which may appear as long as two decades after the initial diagnosis.

The diagnosis of cutaneous PAN is made by biopsy of a subcutaneous nodule. An excisional biopsy is recommended because the vasculitis is focal. The affected arteriole is at the junction of the dermis and subcutaneous tissue or in the subcutaneous fat.

Adjacent to the affected vessel, there is an inflammatory panniculitis, and inadequate evaluation of the biopsy or too small a sample may lead to the erroneous diagnosis of a panniculitis. Also distal to the affected arteriole, thrombosis usually occurs. If the biopsy is inadequate in depth or size, this bland thrombosis without inflammation is seen, and the erroneous diagnosis of a "vasculopathy" will be made. Cutaneous PAN has been associated with HBV surface antigenemia, HCV infection, Crohn disease, Takayasu arteritis, relapsing polychondritis, streptococcal infections, tuberculosis, and medications (minocycline). Typically, the only laboratory abnormality is an elevated ESR or CRP. In some cases, a p-ANCA may be present. Most patients respond well to aspirin, NSAIDs, prednisone, pentoxifylline, sulfapyridine, colchicine, dapsone, methotrexate, or MMF alone or in some combination. In childhood cutaneous PAN, because streptococcal infection is common, penicillin treatment may be used. In refractory cases, IVIG may be given.

Macular Lymphocytic Arteritis (Lymphocytic Thrombophilic Arteritis)

Macular lymphocytic arteritis is a rarely reported condition that affects predominantly non-Caucasian females. It presents with multiple, poorly defined brown macules on the lower legs resembling postinflammatory hyperpigmentation. Histologically, a vessel in the subcutaneous fat is infiltrated with lymphocytes, but usually without destruction of the vessel. Neutrophils are absent. Recent reports suggest this condition may actually represent an indolent form of cutaneous PAN with potential for ulceration. Two studies reviewing histopathology of cutaneous PAN versus macular arteritis failed to demonstrate significant differences.

Asano Y, et al: High-dose intravenous immunoglobulin infusion in polyarteritis nodosa. Clin Rheumatol 2006; 25: 396.

Beckum KM, et al: Polyarteritis nodosa in childhood. Pediatr Dermatol 2014; 31: e6.

Breda L, et al: Intravenous immunoglobulins for cutaneous polyarteritis nodosa resistant to conventional treatment. Scand J Rheumatol 2016; 45: 169.

Buffiere-Morgado A, et al: Relationship between cutaneous polyarteritis nodosa and macular lymphocytic arteritis. J Am Acad Dermatol 2015; 73: 1013.

Caorsi R, et al: ADA2 deficiency (DADA2) as an unrecognized cause of early onset polyarteritis nodosa and stroke. Ann Rheum Dis 2017; 76: 1648.

De Virgilio A, et al: Polyarteritis nodosa. Autoimmun Rev 2016; 15: 564.

Falcini F, et al: Clinical overview and outcome in a cohort of children with polyarteritis nodosa. Clin Exp Rheumatol 2014; 32: S134.

Fernanda F, et al: Mycophenolate mofetil treatment in two children with severe polyarteritis nodosa refractory to immunosuppressant drugs. Rheumatol Int 2012; 32: 2215.

Fortin PR, et al: Prognostic factors in systemic necrotizing vasculitis of the polyarteritis nodosa group. J Rheumatol 1995; 22: 78.

Garcia C, et al: Macular lymphocytic arteritis. Dermatology 2014; 228: 103.

Gonzalez Santiago TM, et al: Dermatologic features of ADA2 deficiency in cutaneous polyarteritis nodosa. JAMA Dermatol 2015; 151: 1230.

Guillevin L, et al: Prognostic factors in polyarteritis nodosa and Churg-Strauss syndrome. Medicine (Baltimore) 1996; 75: 17.

Hernández-Rodríguez J, et al: Diagnosis and classification of polyarteritis nodosa. J Autoimmun 2014; 48-49: 84.

Kermani TA, et al: Polyarteritis nodosa–like vasculitis in association with minocycline use. Semin Arthritis Rheum 2012; 42: 213.

Llamas-Velasco M, et al: Macular lymphocytic arteritis. J Cutan Pathol 2013; 40: 424.

Matsuo S, et al: The successful treatment of refractory polyarteritis nodosa using infliximab. Intern Med 2017; 56: 1435.

Matteoda Ma, et al: Cutaneous polyarteritis nodosa. An Bras Dermatol 2015; 90: 188.

Morimoto A, Chen KR: Reappraisal of histopathology of cutaneous polyarteritis nodosa. J Cutan Pathol 2016; 43: 1131.

Ozen S: The changing face of polyarteritis nodosa and necrotizing vasculitis. Nat Rev Rheumatol 2017; 13: 381.

Pichard DC, et al: Early-onset stroke, polyarteritis nodosa, and livedo racemose. J Am Acad Dermatol 2016; 75: 449.

Puechal X, et al: Adding azathioprine to remission-induction glucocorticoids. Arthritis Rheumatol 2017; 69: 2175.

Saadoun D, et al: Hepatitis C virus–associated polyarteritis nodosa. Arthritis Care Res (Hoboken) 2011; 63: 427.

Samson M, et al: Long-term follow-up of a randomized trial on 118 patients with polyarteritis nodosa or microscopic polyangiitis without poor-prognosis factors. Autoimmun Rev 2014; 13: 197.

Wee E, Kelly RI: The histopathology of cutaneous polyarteritis nodosa and its relationship with lymphocytic thrombophilic arteritis. J Cutan Pathol 2017; 44: 411.

ANCA-POSITIVE VASCULITIDES

Antineutrophil cytoplasmic antibodies (ANCAs) are an important laboratory finding used in the diagnosis and prognosis of systemic vasculitis. ANCAs occur in three patterns: cytoplasmic (c-ANCA), perinuclear (p-ANCA), and atypical ANCA. The initial screening is performed using indirect immunofluorescence, then confirmed using ELISA for characterization of target antigens. c-ANCA is associated with antibodies directed against proteinase 3 (PR3). Antibodies against myeloperoxidase (MPO) result in the p-ANCA pattern, but antibodies against other antigens may also give this pattern. Only ANCAs against PR3 or MPO are associated with primary vasculitic syndromes; atypical ANCAs are directed against neither. Most laboratories now perform specific tests to determine whether positive ANCAs are reactive against MPO or PR3. Anti-PR3 antibodies are relatively specific for granulomatosis with polyangiitis (Wegener granulomatosis) and microscopic polyangiitis. Antibodies against MPO are less specific and can be found in microscopic polyangiitis, eosinophilic granulomatosis with polyangiitis (Churg-Strauss syndrome), and drug-induced vasculitis. Usually, either anti-MPO or anti-PR3 antibodies are found, but not both. If both patterns are found, drug-induced vasculitis should be suspected, including levamisole-tainted cocaine exposure. A 2017 consensus statement proposed that high-quality immunoassays be used for PR3 and MPO without the need for initial IIF screening. There appear to be global ethnic and/or geographic differences in the patterns of ANCA-associated vasculitides, with MO-ANCA markedly more common in Japanese patients and somewhat more common in Chinese patients than in Europeans.

The ANCA-associated vasculitides—microscopic polyangiitis (MPA), granulomatosis with polyangiitis (GPA), and eosinophilic granulomatosis with polyangiitis (EGPA)—have overlapping features, characteristically demonstrating pulmonary hemorrhage and/or necrotizing glomerulonephritis (pulmonary-renal syndrome). Conversely, 60% of patients with the pulmonary-renal syndrome will have ANCA-associated vasculitis. Patients with ANCA-associated vasculitis have an increased risk of venous thromboembolism. With ANCA testing, these diseases can be diagnosed with 85% sensitivity and 98% specificity. However, although ANCAs are usually negative in Takayasu arteritis, giant cell arteritis, Kawasaki disease, and Behçet disease, positive ANCAs can be found in cryoglobulinemia and other forms of skin-limited vasculitis, SLE, RA, inflammatory bowel disease, and certain infectious diseases. ANCAs are most useful therefore when confirmed by ELISA testing in the setting of vasculitis with systemic features or in situations where the clinical findings suggest ANCA-associated vasculitis. ANCA testing, when used appropriately, is highly sensitive and specific, but it does not replace these clinical features, other relevant laboratory tests, or histologic confirmation of the presence of vasculitis.

Microscopic Polyangiitis

With the advent of ANCA serologies and clarification of the features of MPA, this diagnosis is becoming increasingly more common. There is a north-south gradient in incidence, with southern European countries having three to four times as many cases. Most patients with MPA have systemic symptoms, such as fever, weight loss, myalgias, and arthralgias, which can present with an acute flulike illness or evolve for months to years before a more explosive phase of the disease. These cases have been termed *slowly progressive MPA*. Most patients with MPA will have or develop segmental necrotizing and crescentic glomerulonephritis (80%–90%), with pulmonary involvement in 25%–65%. Pulmonary capillaritis, which can be complicated by hemorrhage, occurs in 12%–29% of MPA patients. Interstitial lung disease appears to be associated with worse outcome. Ear, nose, or throat involvement is found in significant numbers. The skin is involved in 44%. Purpuric papules and macules are most common, and livedo reticularis, retiform purpura, cutaneous ulcers, and digital ischemia are also seen. Urticarial lesions occur in 1% of cases. Patients with MPA may present with skin lesions as their initial clinical findings. Livedo is seen in two thirds of such patients. Biopsies of macules, papules, petechiae, or sites adjacent to ecchymoses may reveal a necrotizing LCV in the reticular dermis.

Vasculitic neuropathy is common (58%), and eye disease may occur. Eosinophilia and asthma are not seen. ANCAs are positive in 70% of cases, p-ANCA (from antibodies against MPO) more frequently than c-ANCA. MPA is differentiated from PAN by the presence of glomerulonephritis, pulmonary symptoms, and the absence of hypertension and microaneurysms. ANCAs are rarely positive in PAN.

MPA is managed similar to other forms of ANCA-associated vasculitis, with systemic corticosteroids and often cytotoxic agents from disease onset. Glucocorticoid monotherapy is associated with lower remission rates. In generalized but non–organ-threatening disease, methotrexate may be added to prednisone, 1 mg/kg/day or equivalent, as initial therapy. For more severe disease, cyclophosphamide is usually given instead with glucocorticoids in the early induction phase of treatment as monthly pulses (vs. daily treatment) for 6–12 months. This regimen has a lower relapse rate compared with the combination of methotrexate and corticosteroids. Rituximab in combination with glucocorticoids is another option for induction of remission shown not to be inferior to combination cyclophosphamide and prednisone for MPA and GPA. Other, less toxic immunosuppressives, such as methotrexate or azathioprine, may be used in milder cases or as maintenance therapy. MMF has also been used in milder cases. Low-dose rituximab may be superior for maintenance of remission. IVIG and anti-TNF agents (infliximab) may be considered in refractory cases. Tocilizumab has been used in one series of six patients as monotherapy. Relapses are frequent, in close to 70%. The 5-year survival is about 75%, and 7-year survival is 62%.

Bossuyt X, et al: Position paper: revised 2017 international consensus on testing of ANCAs in granulomatosis with polyangiitis and microscopic polyangiitis. Nat Rev Rheumatol 2017; 13: 683.

Cohen Tervaert JW, Damoiseaux J: Antineutrophil cytoplasmic autoantibodies. Clin Rev Allergy Immunol 2012; 43: 211.

Greco A, et al: Microscopic polyangiitis. Autoimmun Rev 2015; 14: 837.

Guilleven L, et al: Microscopic polyangiitis. Arthritis Rheum 1999; 42: 421.

Iatrou C, et al: Mycophenolate mofetil as maintenance therapy in patients with vasculitis and renal involvement. Clin Nephrol 2009; 72: 31.

Kallenberg CG: The diagnosis and classification of microscopic polyangiitis. J Autoimmun 2014; 48-49: 90.

Kluger N, et al: Comparison of cutaneous manifestations in systemic polyarteritis nodosa and microscopic polyangiitis. Br J Dermatol 2008; 159: 615.

Puechal X, et al: Long-term outcomes among participants in the WEGENT trial of remission-maintenance therapy for granulomatosis with polyangiitis (Wegener's) or microscopic polyangiitis. Arthritis Rheumatol 2016; 68: 690.

Sakai R, et al: Corticosteroid-free treatment of tocilizumab monotherapy for microscopic polyangiitis. Mod Rheumatol 2016; 26: 900.

Schirmer JH, et al: Clinical presentation and long-term outcome of 144 patients with microscopic polyangiitis in a monocentric German cohort. Rheumatology (Oxford) 2016; 55: 71.

Singer O, McCune WJ: Update on maintenance therapy for granulomatosis with polyangiitis and microscopic polyangiitis. Curr Opin Rheumatol 2017; 29: 248.

Sinico RA, Radice A: Antineutrophil cytoplasmic antibodies (ANCA) testing. Clin Exp Rheumatol 2014; 32: S112.

Stone JH, et al: Rituximab versus cyclophosphamide for ANCA-associated vasculitis. N Engl J Med 2010; 363: 221.

Wilke L, et al: Microscopic polyangiitis. J Clin Rheumatol 2014; 20: 179.

Granulomatosis With Polyangiitis (Wegener Granulomatosis)

Granulomatosis with polyangiitis (GPA) is a syndrome consisting of necrotizing granulomas of the upper and lower respiratory tract, generalized necrotizing angiitis affecting small and medium-sized blood vessels, and focal necrotizing glomerulitis. GPA is a rare disease, with a U.K. study finding 11.8/million person-years, more common in males, with peak incidence in ages 55–69. Approximately 90% of patients display ANCAs, with neutrophils acting as both the target and effector cells in this disease. Neutrophil extracellular traps (NETs) and NETosis are being increasingly evaluated as key mediators in the pathogenesis of vasculitis. Genetic risk factors identified include *CTLA4, PTPN22, COL11A2,* and *SERPINA1.*

By far the most common initial manifestation, present in 90% of patients, is the occurrence of rhinorrhea, severe sinusitis, and nasal mucosal ulcerations, with one or several nodules in the nose, larynx, trachea, or bronchi. Failure to respond to conventional treatment for sinusitis may prompt suspicion of the diagnosis. Fever, weight loss, and malaise occur in these patients, who are usually 40–50 years of age and more often male than female (1.3 : 1). Obstruction in the nose may also block the sinuses. The nodules in the nose frequently ulcerate and bleed. The parenchymal involvement of the lungs produces cough, dyspnea, and chest pain; 71% of patients have pulmonary infiltrates radiographically. Granulomas may occur in the ear and mouth, where the alveolar ridge becomes necrotic, and ulceration of the tongue and perforated ulcers of the palate develop. The combination of nasal and palatal involvement may lead to saddle-nose deformity. The "strawberry gums" appearance of hypertrophic gingivitis is characteristic, and biopsy of these lesions may be diagnostic (Fig. 35.25).

Cutaneous findings occur in 45% of GPA patients. Nodules may appear in crops, especially along the extensor surfaces of the extremities. The firm, slightly tender, flesh-colored or violaceous nodules may later ulcerate. These may be mistaken for ulcerating rheumatoid nodules. The necrotizing angiitis of the skin may present as a palpable purpura, petechial or hemorrhagic pustular

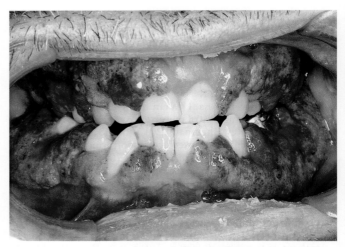

Fig. 35.25 Granulomatosis with polyangiitis (Wegener's), strawberry gingiva.

eruption, subcutaneous nodules, or ulcers. Livedo reticularis is rare in GPA. Patients may present with pyoderma gangrenosum–like lesions, and several patients have been reported presenting with features of temporal arteritis. The condition previously described as "malignant pyoderma" is now thought to represent GPA. Rarely patients may truly have both PG and GPA.

Limited forms of GPA involving the upper respiratory tract without renal involvement may also occur and have a better prognosis. Cutaneous findings can be associated with limited disease. Focal crescentic necrotizing glomerulonephritis occurs in 85% of GPA patients. It may be fulminant from the outset or may become more severe as the disease progresses. Renal failure was the most frequent cause of death before cyclophosphamide treatment. Other organs frequently involved include the joints (arthralgia in two thirds); eyes (conjunctivitis, episcleritis, and proptosis) in 58%; and the CNS and heart in 22% and 12% of patients, respectively.

Histologically, the cutaneous lesions may demonstrate an LCV, with or without granulomatous inflammation. Granulomatous vasculitis may be seen. Palisaded granulomas with multinucleated giant cells and a central core of neutrophils and debris are a characteristic finding. Often, if the lesions are ulcerated, they are nonspecific histologically. Biopsy of another affected organ, such as the kidney, lung, or upper respiratory tract, may be required to confirm the diagnosis. The early detection of GPA has improved with the availability of ANCA testing, because almost 100% of patients with active generalized GPA are ANCA positive by either indirect immunofluorescence or ELISA. Almost 90% are c-ANCA (anti-PR3) positive, with the remainder p-ANCA (anti-MPO) positive and very few ANCA negative. MPO-positive GPA patients should be distinguished from patients with MPA.

Untreated GPA has a mean survival time of 5 months and a 90% mortality over 2 years. Cyclophosphamide therapy has dramatically changed the prognosis; however, therapy-related adverse events now account for more deaths in the first year after diagnosis than the vasculitis itself. Treatment recommendations are cyclophosphamide, 2 mg/kg/day, and prednisone, 1 mg/kg/day, followed by slow tapering of the prednisone to not less than 15 mg/day during the first 3 months of therapy. Complete remission is achieved in up to 93% of patients and lasts an average of 4 years. Rituximab combined with high-dose glucocorticoids is an alternative to cyclophosphamide for induction therapy and was approved by the FDA in 2011. One study suggested that patients with PR3-ANCA–associated vasculitis respond better to rituximab than to cyclophosphamide/azathioprine regimens, and it may evolve where treatments differ based on ANCA pattern. In more limited disease, patients may respond to methotrexate alone or in combination with prednisone. After initial induction therapy and remission, methotrexate, azathioprine, leflunomide, MMF, or rituximab may be used instead of cyclophosphamide. Treatment should be continued for at least 1 year. Trimethoprim-sulfamethoxazole (TMP-SMX) may decrease the relapse rate and can be considered for long-term treatment of patients with limited upper respiratory tract involvement in remission, in combination with conventional immunosuppressive protocols. The benefit of long-term TMP-SMX results from its reduction of nasal carriage of *Staphylococcus aureus*, a possible trigger of GPA. In refractory cases, plasma exchange, IVIG, and anti-TNF therapy (infliximab) may be used. Tacrolimus, 0.1 mg/kg/day, was successful in treating a pyoderma gangrenosum–like ulceration in a patient with GPA.

Falk RJ, et al: Granulomatosis with polyangiitis (Wegener's). Arthritis Rheum 2011; 63: 863.

Guidelli GM, et al: Granulomatosis with polyangiitis and intravenous immunoglobulin. Autoimmun Rev 2015; 14: 659.

Hiemstra TF, et al: Mycophenolate mofetil vs azathioprine for remission maintenance in antineutrophil cytoplasmic antibody–associated vasculitis. JAMA 2010; 304: 2381.

Kallenberg CG: Key advances in the clinical approach to ANCA-associated vasculitis. Nat Rev Rheumatol 2014; 10: 484.

Lange C, et al: Immune stimulatory effects of neutrophil extracellular traps in granulomatosis with polyangiitis. Clin Exp Rheumatol 2017; 103: 33.

Miloslavsky EM, et al: Myeloperoxidase-antineutrophil cytoplasmic antibody (ANCA)-positive and ANCA-negative patients with granulomatosis with polyangiitis (Wegener's). Arthritis Rheumatol 2016; 68: 2945.

Pagnoux C, Guillevin L: Treatment of granulomatosis with polyangiitis. Expert Rev Clin Immunol 2015; 11: 339.

Pearce FA, et al: Global ethnic and geographic differences in the clinical presentations of anti-neutrophil cytoplasmic antibody-associated vasculitis. Rheumatology (Oxford) 2017; 56: 1962.

Pearce FA, et al: The incidence, prevalence and mortality of granulomatosis with polyangiitis in the UK Clinical Practice Research Datalink. Rheumatology (Oxford) 2017; 56: 589.

Relle M, et al: Genetics and pathophysiology of granulomatosis with polyangiitis and its main autoantigen proteinase 3. Mol Cell Probes 2016; 30: 366.

Specks U, et al: Efficacy of remission-induction regimens for ANCA-associated vasculitis. N Engl J Med 2013; 369: 417.

Takeuchi H, et al: Neutrophil extracellular traps in neuropathy with anti-neutrophil cytoplasmic antibody-associated microscopic polyangiitis. Clin Rheumatol 2017; 36: 913.

Tashtoush B, et al: Large pyoderma gangrenosum–like ulcers. Case Rep Rheumatol 2014; 2014: 2014: 850364.

Unizony S, et al: Clinical outcomes of treatment of anti-neutrophil cytoplasmic antibody (ANCA)-associated vasculitis based on ANCA type. Ann Rheum Dis 2016; 75: 1166.

Eosinophilic Granulomatosis With Polyangiitis (Churg-Strauss Syndrome)

Eosinophilic granulomatosis with polyangiitis (EGPA) occurs in three phases. The initial phase, often lasting many years, consists of allergic rhinitis, nasal polyps, and asthma. The average age of onset of the asthma is 35 years in EGPA (unlike allergic asthma, which often presents in childhood). After 2–12 years, a debilitated asthmatic patient begins to experience attacks of fever and eosinophilia (20%–90%), with pneumonia and gastroenteritis caused by eosinophilic infiltration (second phase). After a few more months or years, but on average 3 years after the initial symptoms, a diffuse small-vessel and medium-vessel vasculitis with granulomatous inflammation involves the lungs, heart, liver, spleen,

kidneys, intestines, and pancreas. Mononeuritis multiplex is common. Triggers of this third phase have included vaccination, desensitization, leukotriene inhibitors, azithromycin, inhaled fluticasone, and rapid discontinuation of corticosteroids. Renal involvement is less common than in GPA or MPA. A fatal outcome is likely in most untreated patients; congestive heart failure resulting from granulomatous inflammation of the myocardium is the most frequent cause of death. Increased rates of arterial and venous thrombosis are seen in EGPA, perhaps related to the dense infiltrates of eosinophils.

Cutaneous lesions are present in two thirds of EGPA patients. Palpable purpura is seen in almost 50%. Subcutaneous nodules on the extensor surfaces of the extremities and on the scalp are seen in 30%. Firm, nontender papules may be present on the fingertips; these may resemble the lesions seen with septic emboli or atrial myxoma but show vasculitis on biopsy. Urticaria, solar urticaria, and livedo reticularis can occur in EGPA. Plaques with the histologic features of eosinophilic cellulitis (Wells syndrome) can be seen.

Laboratory studies are significant for a peripheral eosinophilia, which correlates with disease severity. ANCAs are frequently positive (55%–70%), most often p-ANCA (anti-MPO) and less frequently c-ANCA (anti-PR3), and tend to correlate with disease severity.

Histologically, a small-vessel vasculitis is present that involves not only superficial venules, but also larger and deeper vessels. The tissue is often diffusely infiltrated with eosinophils, and granulomas may be present. Palisaded granulomas differ from those in Wegener granulomatosis in that they generally lack multinucleated giant cells, and the core contains eosinophils. In some patients, flame figures, similar to those in Wells syndrome, are noted in the dermis.

Corticosteroids alone may be used in patients with EPGA and FFS of 0 (see Polyarteritis Nodosa, earlier in this chapter) and are recommended to achieve remission, at a dose of approximately 1 mg/kg/day. Cyclophosphamide alone or in combination with corticosteroids should be used in patients with neuropathy, refractory glomerulonephritis, myocardial disease, severe GI disease, and CNS involvement. When treatment is stratified in this way, survival is good, about 90% at 7 years. However, 40% of patients experience one or more relapses, usually with steroid taper. Rituximab has been effective for other ANCA-associated vasculitides in clinical trials, but EGPA was excluded in most; emerging reports suggest this agent may be effective and well tolerated in patients with EGPA. Azathioprine, as well as methotrexate and leflunomide, is used as a steroid-sparing agent, especially to maintain a remission. IFN-α, MMF, IVIG, leukotriene-receptor antagonists, and the anti-TNF agents infliximab and etanercept have also been used successfully in patients with EPGA (Churg-Strauss syndrome). A 2017 randomized clinical trial of 136 patients with EGPA evaluating mepolizumab (an anti-interleukin [IL]-5 monoclonal antibody) demonstrated increased remission and reduced steroid use with good safety, though only 54% of patients in the treatment arm achieved remission. Rituximab followed by omalizumab was used in one patient with severe refractory EGPA. Notably omalizumab has been reported to induce EGPA in at least eight case reports to date.

Aguirre-Valencia D, et al: Sequential rituximab and omalizumab for the treatment of eosinophilic granulomatosis with polyangiitis (Churg-Strauss syndrome). Clin Rheumatol 2017; 36: 2159.

Black JG, et al: Montelukast-associated Churg-Strauss vasculitis. Ann Allergy Asthma Immunol 2009; 102: 351.

Comarmond C, et al: Eosinophilic granulomatosis with polyangiitis (Churg-Strauss). Arthritis Rheum 2013; 65: 270.

Davis MDP, et al: Cutaneous manifestations of Churg-Strauss syndrome. J Am Acad Dermatol 1997; 37: 199.

Djukanovic R, O'Byrne PM: Targeting eosinophils in eosinophilic granulomatosis with polyangiitis. N Engl J Med 2017; 376: 1985.

Gioffredi A, et al: Eosinophilic granulomatosis with polyangiitis. Front Immunol 2014; 5: 549.

Groh M, et al: Eosinophilic granulomatosis with polyangiitis consensus task force recommendations for evaluation and management. Eur J Intern Med 2015; 26: 545.

Ishibashi M, et al: Spectrum of cutaneous vasculitis in eosinophilic granulomatosis with polyangiitis (Churg-Strauss). Am J Dermatopathol 2015; 37: 214.

Jaworsky C: Leukotriene receptor antagonists and Churg-Strauss syndrome. J Cutan Pathol 2008; 35: 611.

Kim MY, et al: Clinical features and prognostic factors of Churg-Strauss syndrome. Korean J Intern Med 2014; 29: 85.

Mohammad AJ, et al: Rituximab for the treatment of eosinophilic granulomatosis with polyangiitis. Ann Rheum Dis 2016; 75: 396.

Mouthon L, et al: Diagnosis and classification of eosinophilic granulomatosis with polyangiitis (formerly named Churg-Strauss syndrome). J Autoimmun 2014; 48-49: 99.

Muñoz SA, et al: Rituximab in the treatment of eosinophilic granulomatosis with polyangiitis. Reumatol Clin 2015; 11: 165.

Nazir S, et al: Omalizumab-associated eosinophilic granulomatosis with polyangiitis. Ann Allergy Asthma Immunol 2017; 118: 372.

Nepal M, Padma H: Fluticasone-associated cutaneous allergic granulomatous vasculitis. South Med J 2008; 101: 761.

Samson M, et al: Long-term outcomes of 118 patients with eosinophilic granulomatosis with polyangiitis (Churg-Strauss syndrome) enrolled in two prospective trials. J Autoimmun 2013; 43: 60.

Sokolowska BM, et al: ANCA-positive and ANCA-negative phenotypes of eosinophilic granulomatosis with polyangiitis (EGPA). Clin Exp Rheumatol 2014; 32: S41.

Thiel J, et al: Rituximab in the treatment of refractory or relapsing eosinophilic granulomatosis with polyangiitis (Churg-Strauss syndrome). Arthritis Res Ther 2013; 15: R133.

Wechsler ME, et al: Mepolizumab or placebo for eosinophilic granulomatosis with polyangiitis. N Engl J Med 2017; 376: 1921.

COCAINE-ASSOCIATED VASCULITIS AND LEVAMISOLE-INDUCED VASCULOPATHY/VASCULITIS

There are numerous reports of various forms of cutaneous vasculitis associated with the IV or intranasal use of cocaine. Skin lesions have included typical LCV, as well as larger-vessel vasculitis resembling PAN. Localized nasal lesions with vasculitis resembling GPA (Wegener granulomatosis) have been observed in patients using inhaled cocaine. This has been termed *cocaine-induced pseudovasculitis* or *cocaine-induced midline destructive lesions* to try to distinguish it from true GPA. In addition, patients using cocaine may develop more widespread cutaneous and systemic vasculitis affecting the kidneys, lungs, and testes. The cutaneous lesions resemble LCV, but ecchymotic lesions (Fig. 35.26) and skin necrosis are more prominent in these patients than in the typical LCV patient. Purpura and necrosis of the earlobe and nose are especially common and characteristic; retiform purpura on the thighs, buttocks, cheeks, and other areas is frequently seen. Levamisole-tainted cocaine has also been reported to induce pyoderma gangrenosum-like cutaneous ulcerations. Agranulocytosis, not a typical feature of ANCA-positive vasculitis, also occurs. These patients have an elevated c-ANCA, similar to those with true GPA, but may display elevated p-ANCA as well. Notably the c-ANCA in patients with cocaine-induced vasculitis reacts with human neutrophil elastase (HNE-ANCA). Patients with GPA and MPA are negative for HNE-ANCA.

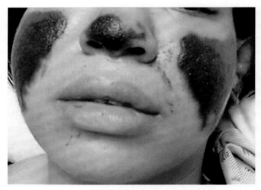

Fig. 35.26 Levamisole-induced vasculopathy. (Courtesy Antoine Sreih, MD.)

Street cocaine is often contaminated with pharmaceutical agents. Levamisole has been found in the cocaine seized by law enforcement in up to 70% of U.S. cases and 100% in Italy. Levamisole is associated with ecchymotic purpura and necrosis, with a predilection for the ears. It also causes agranulocytosis and c-ANCA positivity. It is therefore unclear whether the vasculitic lesions seen in recreational cocaine users are caused by the cocaine or by the levamisole excipient (levamisole-induced vasculopathy/vasculitis), or both. In every patient presenting with a cutaneous or systemic vasculitis, a detailed history of recreational drug use must be obtained, and toxicology screening should be considered in any patient with vasculitis having the features just outlined, especially agranulocytosis or cutaneous necrosis, or failing to respond to appropriate therapy. Because its half-life is only 5.6 hours, confirming the presence of levamisole in the urine can be difficult. In affected patients, stopping of the drug may lead to a gradual improvement of the vasculitis, although initial immunosuppressive therapy may be required. Treatment to eradicate nasal *S. aureus* should be considered if there are prominent nasal findings.

Buchanan JA, et al: Prevalence of levamisole in urine toxicology screens positive for cocaine in an inner-city hospital. JAMA 2011; 305: 1657.

Chung C, et al: Characteristic purpura of the ears, vasculitis, and neutropenia. J Am Acad Dermatol 2011; 65: 722.

Crowe DR, et al: Clinical, histopathologic, and immunofluorescence findings in levamisole/cocaine-induced thrombotic vasculitis. Int J Dermatol 2014; 53: 635.

Gaertner EM, Switlyk SA: Dermatologic complications from levamisole-contaminated cocaine. Cutis 2014; 93: 102.

Jeong HS, et al: Pyoderma gangrenosum associated with levamisole-adulterated cocaine. J Am Acad Dermatol 2016; 74: 892.

Jiménez-Gallo D, et al: Pyoderma gangrenosum and Wegener granulomatosis–like syndrome induced by cocaine. Clin Exp Dermatol 2013; 38: 878.

Keith PJ, et al: Pyoderma gangrenosum. Int J Dermatol 2015; 54: 1075.

Menni S, et al: Ear lobe bilateral necrosis by levamisole-induced occlusive vasculitis in a pediatric patient. Pediatr Dermatol 1997; 14: 477.

Neynaber S, et al: PR3-ANCA-positive necrotizing multi-organ vasculitis following cocaine abuse. Acta Derm Venereol 2008; 88: 594.

Pendergraft WF 3rd, Niles JL: Trojan horses: drug culprits associated with antineutrophil cytoplasmic autoantibody (ANCA) vasculitis. Curr Opin Rheumatol 2014; 26: 42.

Rachapalli SM, Kiely PD: Cocaine-induced midline destructive lesions mimicking ENT-limited Wegener's granulomatosis. Scand J Rheumatol 2008; 37: 477.

Sánchez-Cruz A, et al: Cocaine induced vasculitis. Case Rep Rheumatol 2012; 2012: 982361.

Strazzula L, et al: Levamisole toxicity mimicking autoimmune disease. J Am Acad Dermatol 2013; 69: 954.

Waller JM, et al: Cocaine-associated retiform purpura and neutropenia. J Am Acad Dermatol 2010; 63: 530.

GIANT CELL ARTERITIS/TEMPORAL ARTERITIS

Giant cell arteritis (GCA) is a systemic disease of people over age 50 (mean age >70), favoring women (2:1). It is uncommon in African Americans and favors whites. Its best-known location is the temporal artery, and it is also known as temporal arteritis, cranial arteritis, and Horton disease. GCA is characterized by a necrotizing arteritis with granulomas and giant cells, which produce unilateral headache and exquisite tenderness in the scalp over the temporal or occipital arteries in 50%–75% of patients. Temporal headaches are characteristically constant, severe, and boring. Ear and parotid pain and mastication-induced jaw claudication may occur. Fever, anemia, and a high ESR (>50) are usually present. Proximal, symmetric, and severe morning and even day-long limb girdle stiffness, soreness, and pain occur in 50% of patients (associated polymyalgia rheumatica). GCA is rarely fatal. Blindness may develop and is the most feared complication of the disease. Many patients who develop visual loss have premonitory symptoms, allowing for diagnosis and intervention, which may prevent permanent visual loss. However, failure to begin treatment within the first 48 hours of the onset of visual symptoms still may lead to permanent damage.

The cutaneous manifestations of GCA may be only inflammatory. The affected artery becomes evident as a hard, pulsating, tender, tortuous bulge under red or cyanotic skin. Another manifestation is necrosis of the scalp (Fig. 35.27). Lesions may begin as ecchymoses. Later, they may become vesicular or bullous and are followed by gangrene. Urticaria, purpura, alopecia, tender nodules, prurigo-like nodules, and livedo reticularis may be seen. Lingual artery involvement may cause an accompanying red, sore, or gangrenous tongue. Nasal septal perforation may develop. Actinic granuloma may be associated. Actinic damage of the arterial elastic tissue of the temporal artery may occur because of its superficial location. The elderly Caucasian is at greatest risk, and when lesions are biopsied, at times only the external half of the artery that received solar radiation is involved. Some posit that temporal arteritis may be an actinically induced disease.

Polymyalgia rheumatica (PMR) has a significant clinical association with GCA. Prompt treatment may forestall serious disease. About 10% of central retinal artery occlusions are caused by GCA. ESR is elevated in more than 90% of patients. Temporal artery biopsy is generally diagnostic and remains the gold standard, provided at least a 2-cm segment is provided. Even arteries that are normal on palpation may show diagnostic findings. Magnetic resonance angiography and color Doppler and duplex ultrasonography are noninvasive diagnostic methods that may aid in confirming the clinical suspicion and identifying the best site to biopsy, or may even obviate the need for biopsy, with a specificity of 78%–100% for ultrasound and 73%–97% for magnetic resonance imaging (MRI). Importantly, therapy should never be postponed waiting for a biopsy. Not all patients with arteritis of the temporal artery have GCA, because temporal arteritis may be a manifestation of a systemic vasculitis such as PAN, GPA, or microscopic polyarteritis. Conversely, GCA patients may have involvement of the aorta and its proximal branches, similar to Takayasu arteritis, and are at risk of aneurysm and dissection; it is not clear whether such patients with extracranial large-vessel vasculitis require more aggressive treatment or monitoring. Pathogenically, the presence of TNF polymorphisms in patients with PMR and temporal arteritis suggests a genetic predisposition. It is likely that a genetic predisposition plus an unknown environmental trigger leads to activated dendritic cell production of chemokines recruiting T cells, with both Th1 and Th17 inflammatory pathways likely involved, with IFN-γ in particular a key mediator of macrophage and giant cell inflammation. A genome-wide association study demonstrated HLA class II as the strongest risk-associated region, and specific gentes PLG and P4HA2. Varicella-zoster virus (VZV) is one suggested, albeit controversial, environmental trigger, with some studies demonstrating increased VZV antigen in GCA arteries.

Treatment begins with prednisone, 40–60 mg/day, and continues for 1 month or until all reversible clinical and laboratory parameters (e.g., ESR) return to normal. GCA is quite steroid responsive, and tapering to a prednisone dose of 7.5–10 mg/day is usually possible. Daily therapy seems to be important and is usually necessary for a minimum of 1–2 years. Most patients achieve complete remission, which is often maintained after therapy is withdrawn. Methotrexate may reduce total glucocorticoid requirement and decrease relapse rates. Cyclophosphamide, azathioprine, and anti-TNF agents may be used in refractory cases, but the data are mixed, and relapses occur when treatment is stopped. Tocilizumab (monoclonal antibody against IL-6 receptor) has been used in conjunction with steroids with increased efficacy in a 30-patient randomized trial. Abatacept (CTLA-4Ig) in conjunction with prednisone also demonstrated better relapse-free survival and longer remission.

Buttgereit F, et al: Polymyalgia rheumatica and giant cell arteritis. JAMA 2016; 315: 2442.

Carmona FD, et al: A genome-wide association study identifies risk alleles in plasminogen and *P4HA2* associated with giant cell arteritis. Am J Hum Genet 2017; 100: 64.

Ciccia F, et al: New insights into the pathogenesis of giant cell arteritis. Autoimmun Rev 2017; 16: 675.

Hoffman GS, et al: Infliximab for maintenance of glucocorticosteroid-induced remission of giant cell arteritis. Ann Intern Med 2007; 146: 621.

Langford CA, et al: A randomized, double-blind trial of abatacept for the treatment of giant cell arteritis. Arthritis Rheumatol 2017; 69: 837.

Martínez-Taboada VM, et al: A double-blind placebo-controlled trial of etanercept in patients with giant cell arteritis and corticosteroid side effects. Ann Rheum Dis 2008; 67: 625.

Rhee RL, et al: Infections and the risk of incident giant cell arteritis. Ann Rheum Dis 2017; 76: 1031.

Samson M, et al: Recent advances in our understanding of giant cell arteritis pathogenesis. Autoimmun Rev 2017; 16: 833.

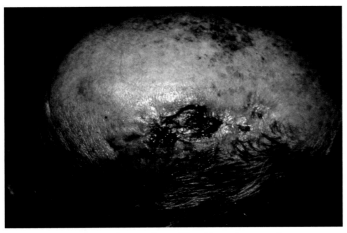
Fig. 35.27 Giant cell arteritis with scalp necrosis.

Tomasson G, et al: Risk for cardiovascular disease early and late after a diagnosis of giant-cell arteritis. Ann Intern Med 2014; 160: 73.

Tsianakas A, et al: Scalp necrosis in giant cell arteritis. J Am Acad Dermatol 2009; 61: 701.

Takayasu Arteritis

Known also as aortic arch syndrome and pulseless disease, Takayasu arteritis (TA) is a thrombo-obliterative process of the great vessels stemming from the aortic arch, occurring generally in young women (female/male ratio 9:1) in the second or third decade of life. It is more common in Japan, Southeast Asia, India, and South America. Radial and carotid pulses are typically obliterated. Most skin changes are caused by the disturbed circulation. There may be loss of hair and atrophy of the skin and its appendages, with underlying muscle atrophy. Occasional patients with cutaneous necrotizing or granulomatous vasculitis of small vessels have been reported. Erythematous nodules with or without livedo, simulating erythema nodosum or erythema induratum, may rarely occur. Sweet syndrome has also been reported in association with TA. Pyoderma gangrenosum–like ulcerations are well described in Japan; the lesions precede the diagnosis of TA by an average of 3 years. These lesions are more often generalized and in three quarters of cases occur on the upper extremities.

Treatment of TA with prednisone is recommended, 1 mg/kg/day tapered over 8–12 weeks to 20 mg/day or less. Methotrexate may be used for its steroid-sparing effects. The possible effectiveness of biologic therapies, such as the IL-6 receptor antagonist tocilizumab, is being actively investigated. With active medical and surgical intervention, the aggressive course of TA can be modified. The pyoderma gangrenosum–like lesions are also treated with systemic corticosteroids, but azathioprine, cyclophosphamide, MMF, cyclosporine, and tacrolimus have also been effective. TNF inhibitors, rituximab, and tocilizumab have been used increasingly in refractory cases. Abatacept and ustekinumab have also been suggested as potential options.

Koster MJ, et al: Recent advances in the clinical management of giant cell arteritis and Takayasu arteritis. Curr Opin Rheumatol 2016; 28: 211.

Loricera J, et al: Tocilizumab in patients with Takayasu arteritis. Clin Exp Rheumatol 2016; 34: s44.

Ma EH, et al: Sweet's syndrome with postinflammatory elastolysis and Takayasu arteritis in a child. Pediatr Dermatol 2012; 29: 645.

Minagawa A, et al: Takayasu's arteritis with pyoderma gangrenosum and necrotizing vasculitis. Clin Exp Dermatol 2010; 35: 329.

Rocha LK, et al: Cutaneous manifestations and comorbidities in 60 cases of Takayasu arteritis. J Rheumatol 2013; 40: 734.

Serra R, et al: Updates in pathophysiology, diagnosis, and management of Takayasu arteritis. Ann Vasc Surg 2016; 35: 210.

Seyahi E: Takayasu arteritis. Curr Opin Rheumatol 2017; 29: 51.

MALIGNANT ATROPHIC PAPULOSIS

Papulosis atrophicans maligna, also known as Degos disease, is a potentially fatal obliterative arteritis syndrome. Some affected patients, perhaps as many as 70%, have a long benign course with skin lesions only, whereas in others, death occurs within a few years. Degos disease occurs two to three times more frequently in men than in women, often presenting between ages 20 and 40. Familial kindreds are well reported. In patients with the more aggressive variant, survival averages 2–3 years after the disease has developed.

Skin lesions are usually the first sign of the disease. Clinically, Degos disease is characterized by the presence of pale-rose, round, edematous papules occurring mostly on the trunk. Similar lesions may occur on the bulbar conjunctiva and oral mucosa. Palms, soles, and face are spared, but the penis may be involved. Over days to weeks, the lesions become umbilicated, with an enlarging central depression. The center becomes distinctively porcelain white, while the periphery becomes livid red and telangiectatic. Central atrophy occurs eventually. The eruption proceeds by crops in which only a few new lesions appear at any one time. One patient was reported to develop panniculitis. Lesions characteristic of Degos disease may be seen in patients with LE, dermatomyositis, scleroderma, and GPA, as well as with "skin popping" of illicit drugs.

Systemically, ischemic infarcts involve the intestines, producing acute abdominal symptoms, which include epigastric pain, fever, and hematemesis. Death usually results from fulminant peritonitis caused by multiple perforations of the intestine. Imaging studies to evaluate for GI involvement are important, but laparoscopy may be the best means of detecting GI involvement. Less frequently, death occurs from cerebral infarctions.

Wedge-shaped necroses initiated by the occlusion of arterioles and small arteries account for the clinical lesions. Proliferation of the intima and thrombosis constitute the typical histologic picture. The thrombosing process is usually pauci-inflammatory, although neutrophils or lymphocytes may be found associated with the thrombosis. The overlying dermis, which is infarcted, contains abundant mucin, especially early in the lesion's evolution. Adnexae are typically necrotic, and the depressed central portion may be noted histologically.

The etiology of malignant atrophic papulosis is unknown, but based on the infarctive nature of the lesions and the universal presence of arteriolar thrombosis, a hyperthrombotic state or endothelial abnormality is suggested. Although most patients have not had abnormalities identified, abnormal platelet aggregation and abnormal coagulation have been identified in some cases. Antiphospholipid antibodies and anticardiolipin antibodies have been discovered in some patients, as has factor V Leiden mutation in one. Parvovirus B19 infection was associated with a fatal case in an adult. Prominent C5b-9 deposits and elevated IFN-α expression have also been described in vessels of the skin, GI tract, and brain, suggesting that complement-mediated vascular injury may play a role.

There is no proven therapy for Degos disease. Administration of immunosuppressives has been mostly unsuccessful and may even worsen the disease. IVIG has been of therapeutic benefit in one patient, but failed in another. Terminal complement inhibition using the C5 protein inhibitor eculizumab has been attempted. Although under investigation, eculizumab apparently has not consistently succeeded in preventing or forestalling systemic manifestations of the disease. Ingestion of low-dose acetylsalicylic acid alone or in combination with dipyridamole (Persantine) has been effective in some patients. Heparin, as described by Degos, has been helpful, and should be considered if antiplatelet therapy is ineffective. Nicotine patches, were effective in one patient. Subcutaneous treprostinil was used successfully in a case of eculizumab-resistant Degos disease. In severe crises, fibrinolytic therapy should be considered. The prognosis is guarded in patients with systemic involvement.

De Breucker S, et al: Inefficacy of intravenous immunoglobulins and infliximab in Degos' disease. Acta Clin Belg 2008; 63: 99.

Feci L, et al: Degos disease. G Ital Dermatol Venereol 2015; 150: 123.

Kanekura T, et al: A case of malignant atrophic papulosis successfully treated with nicotine patches. Br J Dermatol 2003; 149: 660.

Magro CM, et al: Degos disease. Am J Clin Pathol 2011; 135: 599.

Magro CM, et al: The effects of eculizumab on the pathology of malignant atrophic papulosis. Orphanet J Rare Dis 2013; 8:185.

Magro CM, et al: Opioid associated intravenous and cutaneous microvascular drug abuse (skin-popping) masquerading as Degos disease. Dermatol Online J 2015; 21.

Meephansan J, et al: Possible involvement of SDF-1/CXCL12 in the pathogenesis of Degos disease. J Am Acad Dermatol 2013; 68: 138.

Passarini B, et al: Lack of recurrence of malignant atrophic papulosis of Degos in multivisceral transplant. J Am Acad Dermatol 2011; 65: e49.

Scheinfeld N: Pairing and comparing nine diseases with Degos disease (malignant atrophic papulosis). Dermatol Online J 2009; 15: 10.

Shapiro LS, et al: Effective treatment of malignant atrophic papulosis (Köhlmeier-Degos disease) with treprostinil. Orphanet J Rare Dis 2013; 8: 52.

Theodoridis A, et al: Malignant atrophic papulosis (Köhlmeier-Degos disease). Orphanet J Rare Dis 2013; 8: 10.

Theodoridis A, et al: Malignant and benign forms of atrophic papulosis (Köhlmeier-Degos disease). Br J Dermatol 2014; 170: 110.

Toledo AE, et al: Laparoscopy shows superiority over endoscopy for early detection of malignant atrophic papulosis gastrointestinal complications. BMC Gastroenterol 2015; 15: 156.

Umemura M, et al: A case of Degos disease. Mod Rheumatol 2015; 25: 480.

Zhu KJ, et al: The use of intravenous immunoglobulin in cutaneous and recurrent perforating intestinal Degos disease (malignant atrophic papulosis). Br J Dermatol 2007; 157: 206.

THROMBOANGIITIS OBLITERANS (BUERGER DISEASE)

Thromboangiitis obliterans (TAO) is a nonatherosclerotic segmental occlusive disease affecting the arteries of multiple extremities. It is most often seen in men between ages 20 and 40 who smoke heavily. Smoking and rarely the use of smokeless tobacco are intimately tied to Buerger disease; the potential impact of cannabis remains uncertain—one group suggested the separate term *cannabis-associated arteritis*, though the disease appears similar in limited reports. The various diagnostic criteria proposed usually include age under 45 (or 50); history of tobacco use; distal extremity involvement (infrapopliteal segmental arterial occlusion with sparing of proximal vasculature); frequent distal upper extremity involvement (Raynaud or digital ulcers); consistent angiographic findings; superficial thrombophlebitis; and exclusion of autoimmune disease, diabetes mellitus, and hypercoagulable or embolic states.

The vasomotor changes in early cases may be transient or persistent; they produce blanching, cyanosis, burning, and tingling. Superficial thrombophlebitis in the leg and foot occurs in 38% of patients, and 44% may have Raynaud phenomenon. The color of the affected area may change when it is raised or lowered below heart level—red when dependent and white when elevated. Pain is a constant symptom, coming at first only after exercise and subsiding with rest. Instep and foot claudication is the classic complaint. Ultimately, the dorsalis pedis and posterior tibial pulses disappear, followed by others. In TAO, skin supplied by affected arterioles tends to break down, with central necrosis and ulceration and eventual gangrene (Fig. 35.28). GI involvement has been reported. Exposure to cold may cause exacerbations, and more cases are identified in the winter than in any other season.

Arteriography should be done to investigate for central atherosclerotic disease, which may be operable, rather than the inoperable distal damage of Buerger disease. A characteristic tapering and occlusion of the major arteries with "corkscrew" collateral arteries is found in Buerger disease on angiography. A vasculo-occlusive syndrome similar to Buerger disease has been reported in cannabis smokers, but venous thrombophlebitis does not occur. The pathogenic mechanism of the vascular occlusion

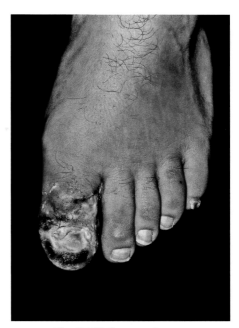

Fig. 35.28 Buerger disease.

in Buerger disease is unknown. In one report, G20210A prothrombin mutations, the majority homozygotic, were found, but these findings have not been reproduced.

The most important therapeutic step is the complete cessation of smoking. Even one or two cigarettes/day, smokeless tobacco, or nicotine replacement may keep the disease active. Vasodilatory therapy is often necessary, including iloprost, bosentan, sildenafil, or alprostadil. Limited data exist for most therapies, though IV iloprost (prostaglandin analog) has been effective in randomized trials and may help the patient with critical limb ischemia get through an acute episode. Oral iloprost is ineffective. Phosphodiesterase type 5 inhibitors have been used successfully. Sympathectomy can provide temporary relief. Implantation of a spinal cord stimulator may be tried. Autologous transplantation of bone marrow mononuclear cells into the calf muscle has benefited patients with TAO and other forms of limb ischemia. G-CSF–mobilized peripheral blood mononuclear cells have had similar efficacy. Endovascular recanalization may be useful in preventing the need for amputation. In patients who stop smoking and do not have gangrene, major amputation is rare. In continued smokers, at least 43% will require amputation.

Abeles AM, et al: Thromboangiitis obliterans successfully treated with phosphodiesterase type 5 inhibitors. Vascular 2013; 22: 313.

Bozkurt AK, et al: A stable prostacyclin analogue (iloprost) in the treatment of Buerger's disease. Ann Thorac Cardiovasc Surg 2013; 19: 120.

De Vriese AS, et al: Autologous transplantation of bone marrow mononuclear cells for limb ischemia in a Caucasian population with atherosclerosis obliterans. J Intern Med 2008; 263: 395.

Fazeli B, Ravari H: Mechanisms of thrombosis, available treatments, and management challenges presented by thromboangiitis obliterans. Curr Med Chem 2015; 22: 1992.

Galyfos G, et al: Conservative treatment of patients with thromboangiitis obliterans or cannabis-associated arteritis presenting with critical lower limb ischemia. Vasa 2017; 46: 471.

Graziani L, et al: Clinical outcome after extended endovascular recanalization in Buerger's disease in 20 consecutive cases. Ann Vasc Surg 2012; 26: 387.

Jimenez-Gallo D, et al: Treatment of thromboangitis obliterans (Buerger's disease) with high-potency vasodilators. Dermatol Ther 2015; 28: 135.

Jouanjus E, et al: Cannabis use: signal of increasing risk of serious cardiovascular disorders. J Am Heart Assoc 2014; 3: e000638.

Kothari R, et al: Thoracoscopic dorsal sympathectomy for upper limb Buerger's disease. JSLS 2014; 18: 273.

Malecki R, et al: The pathogenesis and diagnosis of thromboangitis obliterans. Adv Clin Exp Med 2015; 24: 1085.

Manfredini R, et al: Thromboangitis obliterans (Buerger's disease) in a female mild smoker treated with spinal cord stimulation. Am J Med Sci 2004; 327: 365.

Narvaez J, et al: Efficacy of bosentan in patients with refractory thromboangitis obliterans. Medicine (Baltimore) 2016; 95: e5511.

Vijayakumar A, et al: Thromboangitis obliterans (Buerger's disease). Int J Inflamm 2013; 2013: 156905.

Yuan L, et al: Clinical results of percutaneous transluminal angioplasty for thromboangitis obliterans in arteries above the knee. Atherosclerosis 2014; 235: 110.

ARTERIOSCLEROSIS OBLITERANS

Arteriosclerosis obliterans is an occlusive arterial disease most prominently affecting the abdominal aorta, as well as the small and medium-sized arteries of the lower extremities. The symptoms are caused by ischemia of the tissues. Intermittent claudication is manifested by pain, cramping, numbness, and fatigue in the muscles on exercise. These symptoms are relieved by rest. There may be "rest pain" at night when in bed. Also, sensitivity to cold, muscular weakness, stiffness of the joints, and paresthesia may be present. Sexual impotence is common, and there is increased frequency of coronary artery disease.

Reduced or absent pulses (dorsalis pedis, posterior tibial, or popliteal arteries) may be found on physical examination, confirming the diagnosis. The feet, especially the toes, may be red and cold. Striking pallor of the feet with elevation and redness with dependency are compatible findings. Decreased to absent hair growth may be observed on the legs. Ulceration and gangrene may supervene. If present, necrosis usually begins on the toes and is quite painful. Arteriography may be indicated as a preliminary to corrective surgery (arterial grafts). Occasionally, subclavian atherosclerosis may give rise to these signs in the distal upper extremity, producing painful nails and loss of digital skin. Diabetes mellitus, smoking, and hyperlipidemia are risk factors for the development of atherosclerosis.

Claudication and diminished blood pressure in the affected extremity are findings that may lead to earlier diagnosis and thus to curative surgical intervention. Usually, bypass of the affected artery or sympathectomy, or both, are the preferred treatment for arteriosclerosis obliterans. Balloon angioplasty or stent placement may also be effective. Oral beraprost, a prostaglandin I2 analog, appears to improve symptoms of intermittent claudication in these patients. When critical limb ischemia is present, injection of stem cells into the calf muscle may be beneficial.

Arai T: Long-term effects of beraprost sodium on arteriosclerosis obliterans. Adv Ther 2013; 30: 528.

Masaki H, et al: Collective therapy and therapeutic strategy for critical limb ischemia. Ann Vasc Dis 2013; 6: 27.

Matsumoto K, et al: Insulin resistance and arteriosclerosis obliterans in patients with NIDDM. Diabetes Care 1997; 20: 1738.

DIFFUSE DERMAL ANGIOMATOSIS

Diffuse dermal angiomatosis (DDA) is a disorder that preferentially affects women. The most common location is the breast, especially the dependent portion. Affected women tend to have large, pendulous breasts and are usually older than 45. Patients may have had a reduction mammoplasty (often decades earlier), and the disease tends to localize adjacent to the scar from that procedure. The clinical lesions may be reticulated groups of telangiectasias, ischemic (retiform) purpura, ulceration, or some combination. The erythematous/telangiectatic plaques are slightly palpable but not usually indurated. The nipple and areola are spared. The affected patients often have multiple risk factors for a hypercoagulable state or premature atherosclerosis, including a personal history of atherosclerotic cardiovascular disease, obesity, smoking, diabetes mellitus, hypertension, mutations in the thrombolytic pathway (analogous to those seen in livedoid vasculopathy), and a strong family history for premature atherosclerotic disease–related cardiovascular events. DDA can occur in association with calciphylaxis as well. It is likely that dermal vasculature proliferates in response to local tissue ischemia. The areas involved are similar to those affected by other prothrombotic disorders (e.g., warfarin necrosis, heparin necrosis)—skin with overly abundant adipose tissue. The breast is most often affected, but the abdomen and medial thighs are also sites of predilection. Usually, only one site is affected, but if the breast is involved, the process can be bilateral. Surgical procedures on the affected area may lead to ulceration that is painful and slow to heal. Because a surgical procedure triggered the ulceration, a mistaken diagnosis of pyoderma gangrenosum may be entertained.

Histologically, a diffuse dermal proliferation of endothelial cells and bland blood vessels occupies much of the dermis. Atypical cells and atypical vascular shapes (as seen in angiosarcoma and Kaposi sarcoma) are not seen. The dermal cells stain for markers of endothelial cells, CD31 and CD34. The pathogenesis is thought to be chronic local ischemia, which may lead to vascular proliferation (angiomatosis) or, if acute and severe, retiform purpura and ulceration. The fatty areas are poorly oxygenated (worse in obese patient), and the pendulous nature of the breasts may stretch or tether the vessels, further compromising the circulation. Inherited and acquired hypercoagulable risk factors (e.g., smoking, atherosclerosis) contribute to the pathogenesis.

The treatment of DDA involves reversing the contributing factors. This includes smoking cessation, weight reduction, and antithrombotic medications such as low-dose aspirin, 81 mg/day, and pentoxifylline, 400 mg twice daily. Reduction mammoplasty may lead to resolution. Atherosclerosis of the arteries serving the affected area may be found, and vascular surgery to enhance circulation may lead to improvement. More than one patient has been successfully treated with isotretinoin. Isotretinoin has fibrinolytic and antiangiogenic effects, which may explain its efficacy.

Crickx E, et al: Diffuse dermal angiomatosis associated with severe atherosclerosis. Clin Exp Dermatol 2015; 40: 521.

Ferreli C, et al: Diffuse dermal angiomatosis. G Ital Dermatol Venereol 2015; 150: 115.

Sanz-Motilva V, et al: Diffuse dermal angiomatosis of the breast. Int J Dermatol 2014; 53: 445.

Steele KT, et al: Diffuse dermal angiomatosis associated with calciphylaxis in a patient with end-stage renal disease. J Cutan Pathol 2013; 40: 829.

MUCOCUTANEOUS LYMPH NODE SYNDROME (KAWASAKI DISEASE)

The typical presentation is an irritable, ill-appearing, febrile infant or child younger than 5 years old. Clinical findings in mucocutaneous lymph node syndrome include a skin eruption; stomatitis (injected pharynx, strawberry tongue) and fissuring cheilitis; edema of the hands and feet; nonexudative conjunctival injection; and cervical lymphadenitis. The presence of four of these five cardinal features, plus fever for 5 days or longer, represent diagnostic criteria

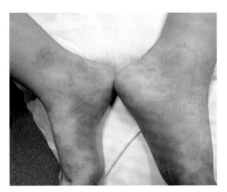

Fig. 35.29 Kawasaki disease.

established by the American Heart Association. The skin eruption is polymorphous and may be macular, morbilliform, urticarial, scarlatiniform, erythema multiforme–like, pustular, or erythema marginatum–like (Fig. 35.29). An early finding (within first week) is the appearance of an erythematous, desquamating perianal eruption in about two thirds of patients. Periorbital edema has been reported. From 15%–20% of children with Kawasaki disease (KD) and fever will not have one or more of the other cardinal features. These cases are termed *incomplete KD*. These patients are still at risk for cardiac disease. Adult KD is very rare, with fewer than 100 cases in the literature; a significant subset of those were in the setting of HIV infection.

Numerous cutaneous and systemic complications have been reported as accompanying or following KD. Pincer nail deformities may appear and resolve spontaneously. Intestinal pseudoobstruction may occur. Facial nerve paralysis has been described, and a severe peripheral vasculitis with vasospasm, digital ischemia, and gangrene can occur. Numerous children have developed guttate or plaque psoriasis 10–20 days after KD onset. The presumed mechanism is the triggering of psoriasis by the superantigens associated with the acute illness.

The acute illness evolves over 10–20 days. One or 2 weeks after the acute illness, the fingers and toes desquamate, starting around the nails. Coronary artery aneurysms occur in 20%–25% of untreated children and 3%–5% of treated children. This is the most common cause of acquired cardiac disease in young children. The cardiac involvement can also include decreased left ventricular function, arrhythmias, mitral regurgitation, and pericardial effusion. These complications can be immediate and are the major cause of morbidity and mortality. Over time, those with aneurysms can develop coronary artery stenosis, and as a result, acute cardiac events can occur in young adulthood.

Pathogenesis

A viral or infectious pathogenesis for KD is appealing for the following reasons:

1. Cases were rare before 1950.
2. KD affects children older than 3 months but younger than 8 years.
3. Seasonal peaks occur in the winter and spring.
4. Focal epidemics have been reported.
5. Oligoclonal IgA immune responses are found, suggesting a respiratory portal of entry of an infectious agent.

There are increased superantigens in the stool of children with KD, and a KD-like illness has been described with group A meningococcal septicemia. An infectious pathogenesis therefore remains the most plausible etiologic hypothesis; it is less clear whether this is caused by a single unknown agent or whether it represents an immunologic response to a variety of infectious triggers. There is some evidence suggesting a temporal relationship between KD and immunization; the benefits of vaccination greatly outweigh this potential risk.

It has long been suspected that there is a genetic basis for KD. The disease is 10–20 times more common in persons from Northeast Asia (Japan and Korea), where rates of up to 1 per 150 children are reported. When these Asians move to the United States, they still have this high rate of increased susceptibility. The risk of a sibling developing KD is increased tenfold. Children of parents who had KD in childhood have a twofold increased risk of developing KD. A genome-wide search of almost 1000 KD cases and family members found strong linkage to five genes, three of which form a single functional network. The central gene of this network is *CAMK2D*, which encodes a serine/threonine kinase expressed in cardiomyocytes and vascular endothelial cells. These genes are known to be involved in cardiac and inflammatory pathways. Their transcripts are also greatly suppressed during KD. Other genetic polymorphisms are associated with increased KD susceptibility, including the genes encoding inositol 1,4,5-trisphosphate 3-kinase C *(ITPKC)* and the immunoglobulin G receptor gene *(FCGR2A)*. The innate immune "inflammasome" is believed to play a major role in the vascular inflammation seen in KD.

KD is a systemic vasculitis of medium-sized arteries, of which the coronary arteries are most profoundly and characteristically affected. Coronary artery disease occurs after day 10 of the illness (subacute phase), in combination with thrombocythemia (up to 1 million cells). This combination of an altered endovascular surface and too many platelets, plus abnormal blood flow in the coronary aneurysms, leads to thrombosis and occlusion of the vessels and subsequent cardiac events.

Treatment

The cornerstone of therapy for KD patients is IVIG, given in a single dose of 2 g/kg infused over 10–12 hours. Response to treatment is best if given during the first 5–6 days of the illness; however, children with persistent fever beyond this period may benefit from later treatment. Aspirin is used to reduce inflammation and platelet aggregation. The dose is 80–100 mg/kg/day in four divided doses. Once the child has been afebrile for 3–7 days, the aspirin dose is decreased to a single daily dose of 3–5 mg/kg. If the child remains febrile 36 hours after initial treatment (which may occur in 10%–20% of patients), a second 2 g/kg dose of IVIG should be given. Such patients are at significantly higher risk of coronary artery aneurysms. A single dose of infliximab, 5 mg/kg, has been reported to be effective in refractory cases, but response, as with other treatments, is not universal. If there is no response to the second IVIG dose, systemic corticosteroid therapy is usually given. Cyclosporine, cyclophosphoamide, corticosteroids, and other immunosuppressive agents have been used in refractory cases. Angioplasty, thrombolytic therapy, or coronary artery bypass surgery may be required for patients with coronary disease. Overall, the rate of long-term adverse cardiovascular events appears to be low, although adult patients with a history of KD may be at increased risk of early atherosclerotic disease.

Agarwal S, Agarwal DK: Kawasaki disease. Expert Rev Clin Immunol 2017; 13: 247.

Bayers S, et al: Kawasaki disease. Part I. J Am Acad Dermatol 2013; 69: 501.e1.

Bayers S, et al: Kawasaki disease. Part II. J Am Acad Dermatol 2013; 69: 513.e1.

Burns JC, Newburger JW: Genetics insights into the pathogenesis of Kawasaki disease. Circ Cardiovasc Genet 2012; 5: 277.

Cohen E, Sundel R: Kawasaki disease at 50 years. JAMA Pediatr 2016; 170: 1093.

Falcini F, et al: Discrimination between incomplete and atypical Kawasaki syndrome versus other febrile diseases in childhood. Clin Exp Rheumatol 2012; 30: 799.

Galeotti C, et al: Kawasaki disease. Autoimmun Rev 2010; 9: 441.

Hara T, et al: Kawasaki disease. Clin Exp Immunol 2016; 186: 134.

Kobayashi T, et al: Efficacy of intravenous immunoglobulin combined with prednisolone following resistance to initial intravenous immunoglobulin treatment of acute Kawasaki disease. J Pediatr 2013; 163: 521.

McCrindle BW, et al: Diagnosis, treatment, and long-term management of Kawasaki disease. Circulation 2017; 135: e927.

Newburger JW: Kawasaki disease. Congenit Heart Dis 2017; 12: 641.

Onouchi Y, et al: ITPKC functional polymorphism associated with Kawasaki disease susceptibility and formation of coronary artery aneurysms. Nat Genet 2008; 40: 35.

Phuong LK, et al: Kawasaki disease and immunization. Vaccine 2017; 35: 1770.

Salguero JS, et al: Refractory Kawasaki disease with coronary aneurysms treated with infliximab. An Pediatr (Barc) 2010; 73: 268.

Seve P, et al: Adult Kawasaki disease. Semin Arthritis Rheum 2005; 34: 785.

Son MB, et al: Treatment of Kawasaki disease. Pediatrics 2009; 124: 1.

Uehara R, Belay ED: Epidemiology of Kawasaki disease in Asia, Europe, and the United States. J Epidemiol 2012; 22: 79.

TELANGIECTASIA

Telangiectasias are fine, linear vessels coursing on the surface of the skin. They may occur in normal skin at any age, in both genders, and anywhere on the skin and mucous membranes. Fine telangiectasias may be seen on the alae nasi of most adults. They are prominent in areas of chronic actinic damage. In addition, persons long exposed to wind, cold, or heat are subject to telangiectasias. Calcium channel blockers may lead to generalized or photodistributed telangiectatic lesions and contribute to the appearance of photoaging. Telangiectasias may also be found on the legs as a result of heredity, varicosities, pregnancy, and OC use.

Telangiectasias can be found in conditions such as radiodermatitis, xeroderma pigmentosum, lupus erythematosus, scleroderma and the CREST syndrome, rosacea, pregnancy, cirrhosis of the liver, AIDS, poikiloderma, basal cell carcinoma, necrobiosis lipoidica diabeticorum, lichen sclerosus et atrophicus, sarcoid, lupus vulgaris, keloid, adenoma sebaceum, kaposiform hemangioendothelioma, angioma serpiginosum, angiokeratoma corporis diffusum, hereditary benign telangiectasia, Cockayne syndrome, ataxia-telangiectasia, and Bloom syndrome.

Altered capillary patterns on the finger nailfolds (cuticular telangiectasias) are indicative of collagen vascular disease, such as LE, scleroderma, or dermatomyositis. These may infrequently be present in RA. These disorders are reviewed in Chapter 8.

Bakkour W, et al: Photodistributed telangiectasia induced by calcium channel blockers. Photodermatol Photoimmunol Photomed 2013; 29: 272.

Beaubien ER, et al: Kaposiform hemangioendothelioma. J Am Acad Dermatol 1998; 38: 799.

Cooper SM, Wojnaraowska F: Photo-damage in Northern European renal transplant recipients is associated with the use of calcium channel blockers. Clin Exp Dermatol 2003; 28: 588.

Huh J, et al: Localized facial telangiectasias following frostbite injury. Cutis 1996; 57: 97.

Kanekura T, et al: Lichen sclerosus et atrophicus with prominent telangiectasia. J Dermatol 1994; 21: 447.

Generalized Essential Telangiectasia

Generalized essential telangiectasia (GET) is characterized by the appearance of telangiectasias over a large segment of the body without preceding or coexisting skin lesions. Lesions tend to appear first on the legs and progress caudad. Women are more often affected, with the condition starting between age 20 and 50. Characteristic features include the following:

1. Widespread cutaneous distribution
2. Progression or permanence of the lesions
3. Accentuation in dependent areas and by dependent positioning
4. Absence of coexisting epidermal or dermal changes, such as atrophy, purpura, depigmentation, or follicular involvement

The telangiectasias may be distributed over the entire body or localized to some large area, such as the legs, arms, and trunk. They may be discrete or confluent. Distribution along the course of the cutaneous nerves may occur. Systemic symptoms are absent, although conjunctival telangiectasias can also be seen. GET is generally not believed to be associated with an increased risk of epistaxis, but GI bleeding has been reported. Families with this disorder, inherited as an autosomal dominant trait, have been reported. The cause of essential telangiectasia is unknown. Treatment is with vascular lasers, if required.

Cutaneous Collagenous Vasculopathy

Cutaneous collagenous vasculopathy, a condition initially reported in middle-aged men but now described in both genders, is clinically similar to GET (Fig. 35.30) but histologically distinct. Histologically, both disorders exhibit greatly dilated subepidermal vessels. However, in cutaneous collagenous vasculopathy, these blood vessels have thickened vascular walls and eosinophilic hyaline material within and around the vessels, whereas in GET, they do not. This material stains positive for collagen type IV.

Unilateral Nevoid Telangiectasia

In unilateral nevoid telangiectasia (UNT), fine, threadlike telangiectases develop in a unilateral, sometimes dermatomal distribution (or following lines of Blaschko). Spider angiomas may also be

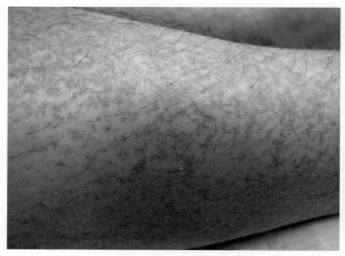

Fig. 35.30 Cutaneous collagenous vasculopathy.

present. The most common distribution is unilateral or bilateral involvement of the third and fourth cervical dermatomes. The condition is rare in men; in affected women, it starts in adulthood. The familial form (very rare) favors males, is autosomal dominant, and appears postnatally. UNT is associated with conditions that have increased levels of estrogen or VEGF: puberty, pregnancy, OC use, HCV infection, and cirrhosis, as well as with neurologic disorders such as hypoesthesia of the affected area. Treatment with pulse dye laser can be effective.

Akman-Karakaş A, et al: Unilateral nevoid telangiectasia accompanied by neurological disorders. J Eur Acad Dermatol Venereol 2011; 25: 1356.

Brady BG, et al: Cutaneous collagenous vasculopathy. J Clin Aesthet Dermatol 2015; 8: 49.

Gambichler T, et al: Generalized essential telangiectasia successfully treated with high-energy, long-pulse, frequency-doubled Nd:YAG laser. Dermatol Surg 2001; 27: 355.

Gordon Spratt EA, et al: Generalized essential telangiectasia. Dermatol Online J 2012; 18: 13.

Oliveira A, et al: Unilateral nevoid telangiectasia. Int J Dermatol 2014; 53: e32.

Perez A, et al: Cutaneous collagenous vasculopathy with generalized telangiectasia in two female patients. J Am Acad Dermatol 2010; 63: 882.

Smith J, et al: Unilateral nevoid telangiectasia syndrome (UNTS) associated with chronic hepatitis C virus and positive immunoreactivity for VEGF. Dermatol Online J 2014; 20.

Tanglertsampan C, et al: Unilateral nevoid telangiectasia. Int J Dermatol 2013; 52: 608.

Toda-Brito H, et al: Cutaneous collagenous vasculopathy. BMJ Case Rep 2015 Jul 8; 2015.

HEREDITARY HEMORRHAGIC TELANGIECTASIA (OSLER DISEASE)

Also known as Osler-Weber-Rendu disease, hereditary hemorrhagic telangiectasia (HHT) is characterized by small tufts of dilated capillaries scattered over the mucous membranes and the skin. These slightly elevated lesions develop mostly on the lips, tongue, palate, nasal mucosa, ears, palms, fingertips, nailbeds, and soles. They may closely simulate the mat telangiectases of the CREST variant of scleroderma, without the other features of CREST syndrome. Diagnostic criteria have been proposed and include the following:

1. Epistaxis—spontaneous, recurrent nosebleeds
2. Telangiectases—multiple at characteristic sites (lips, oral cavity, fingers, nose) (Fig. 35.31)

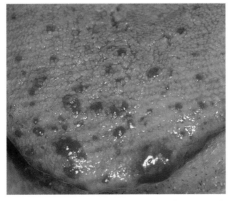

Fig. 35.31 Hereditary hemorrhagic telangiectasia.

3. Visceral lesions—GI bleeding; pulmonary, hepatic, cerebral, or spinal arteriovenous malformation (AVM)
4. Family history—one affected first-degree relative

The presence of three of the four criteria indicates a definite diagnosis, and two of four indicates a possible diagnosis. There are at least three variants: HHT1 and HHT2, and a third associated with juvenile polyposis.

Frequent nosebleeds and melena are experienced because of the telangiectasias in the nose and GI tract. Epistaxis is the most frequent and persistent sign. Worsening epistaxis may herald high-output cardiac failure from AVMs. Pregnancy can also exacerbate HHT. GI bleeding is the presenting sign in up to 25% of patients; however, 40%–50% develop GI bleeding sometime during the course of their disease. Chronic persistent anemia requiring iron and blood transfusions is characteristic of severe cases. The spleen may be enlarged. Pulmonary and CNS AVMs may appear later in life. Liver failure can result from diffuse intrahepatic shunting—hepatic artery to vein, bypassing the liver parenchyma. Retinal arteriovenous aneurysms occur only rarely. Other sites of bleeding may be the kidney, spleen, bladder, liver, meninges, and brain. The risk of cerebral hemorrhage from cerebral AVMs, cerebral abscesses, and pulmonary hemorrhage from pulmonary AVMs is probably high enough that asymptomatic patients should be screened for the presence of cerebral and pulmonary AVMs. Because of the risk of cerebral abscess, some have advocated antibiotic prophylaxis for dental and contaminated skin procedures.

The telangiectasias tend to increase in number in middle age; however, the first appearance on the undersurface of the tongue and floor of the mouth is at puberty. Pulmonary or intracranial arteriovenous fistulas and bleeding in these areas may be a cause of death.

Osler disease (HHT) is inherited as an autosomal dominant trait. The vascular abnormalities found in HHT consist of direct arteriovenous connections without an intervening capillary bed. Affected patients have mutations that affect transforming growth factor (TGF)–β signaling. Multiple gene mutations are known; mutations in endoglin *(ENG)* and ALK-1 *(ACVRL1)* together make up 85% of cases. These encode a homodimeric integral membrane glycoprotein, which is a TGF-β receptor. HHT1 is associated with *ENG* mutations, and HHT2 with *ACVRL1* mutations. HHT1 patients have a higher prevalence of pulmonary AVMs, whereas HHT2 patients tend to have a milder phenotype and later age of onset, but increased liver manifestations. Patients with HHT and juvenile polyposis have mutations in the *MADH4* gene, a downstream effector of TGF-β signaling. TGF-β is a potent stimulator of VEGF production. VEGF leads to disorganized and tortuous vessels, as seen in HHT. VEGF levels are increased in patients with HHT.

Treatment is directed at controlling the specific complications and identifying and treating AVMs before they become symptomatic. The tendency to epistaxis has been reduced by estrogen therapy, and some recommend estrogen preparations or tamoxifen. Thalidomide has also been used in a small study. Dermoplasty of the bleeding nasal septum may be performed by replacing the mucous membrane with skin from the thigh or buttock. Repeated laser treatments of the nasal and GI mucosa are often required. Topical tranexamic acid has been used to control epistaxis. Laser treatments, including Nd:YAG, may help the cutaneous telangiectasias. Topical timolol was ineffective. Bleeding episodes are treated supportively with iron and RBC transfusions. Interventional radiology with selective embolization can treat pulmonary and CNS AVMs, avoiding invasive surgeries. In patients with liver failure or high-output heart failure due to liver AVMs, liver transplantation may be required. Blocking VEGF with thalidomide (or more effectively with lenalidomide) can reduce GI bleeding and transfusion dependence. Bevacizumab, a monoclonal inhibitor of VEGF delivered intravenously, has dramatically improved some severely ill HHT patients, reducing the size and flow of their hepatic AVMs, reversing heart and liver failure, and reducing transfusion requirements. It has also been used successfully as a submucosal injection and topical spray for epistaxis.

Bose P, et al: Bevacizumab in hereditary hemorrhagic telangiectasia. N Engl J Med 2009; 360: 2143.

Fang J, et al: Thalidomide for epistaxis in patients with hereditary hemorrhagic telangiectasia. Otolaryngol Head Neck Surg 2017; 157: 217.

Faughnan ME, et al: International guidelines for the diagnosis and management of hereditary haemorrhagic telangiectasia. J Med Genet 2011; 48: 73.

Franchini M, et al: Novel treatments for epistaxis in hereditary hemorrhagic telangiectasia. J Thromb Thrombolysis 2013; 36: 355.

Fuchizaki U, et al: Hereditary haemorrhagic telangiectasia (Rendu-Osler-Weber disease). Lancet 2003; 362: 1490.

Guilhem A, et al: Intravenous bevacizumab in hereditary hemorrhagic telangiectasia. PLoS One 2017; 12: e0188943.

Jeon H, Cohen B: Lack of efficacy of topical timolol for cutaneous telangiectasias in patients with hereditary hemorrhagic telangiectasia. J Am Acad Dermatol 2017; 76: 997.

Karnezis TT, Davidson TM: Efficacy of intranasal bevacizumab (Avastin) treatment in patients with hereditary hemorrhagic telangiectasia-associated epistaxis. Laryngoscope 2011; 121: 636.

McDonald J, et al: Hereditary hemorrhagic telangiectasia. Genet Med 2011; 13: 607.

Papaspyrou G, et al: Nd:YAG laser treatment for extranasal telangiectasias. ORL J Otorhinolaryngol Relat Spec 2016; 78: 245.

Shovlin CL, et al: Ischaemic strokes in patients with pulmonary arteriovenous malformations and hereditary hemorrhagic telangiectasia: associations with iron deficiency and platelets. PLoS One 2014; 9: e88812.

Yaniv E, et al: Anti-estrogen therapy for hereditary hemorrhagic telangiectasia. Rhinology 2011; 49: 214.

LEG ULCERS

Leg ulcers are a common medical condition, affecting 3%–5% of the population over age 65. The cause of chronic leg ulceration is venous insufficiency alone in 45%–60% of cases, arterial insufficiency in 10%–20%, diabetes mellitus in 15%–25%, or combinations thereof in 10%–15%. Smoking and obesity increase the risk for ulcer development and persistence, independent of the underlying cause. Defining the cause of the leg ulceration is important for treatment.

The wound-healing response is complex, involving intricate interactions between different cell types, structural proteins, growth factors, and proteinases. Normal wound repair consists of three phases—inflammation, proliferation, and remodeling—which occur in a predictable sequence.

VENOUS DISEASES OF THE EXTREMITIES

Stasis Dermatitis

Stasis dermatitis presents as erythema and a yellowish or light-brown pigmentation of the lower third of the lower legs, especially in the area just superior to the medial malleolus. An associated eczematous dermatitis may occur. The dermatitis may be weepy or dry, scaling or lichenified; it is almost invariably hyperpigmented by melanin and hemosiderin. Varicose veins are usually present, although they need not be numerous or conspicuous. Stasis dermatitis is a cutaneous marker for venous insufficiency. The

approach to management should be twofold: relief of symptoms and treatment of the underlying venous insufficiency. Patients with pruritus and an eczematous component should be treated with emollients and topical corticosteroids. The daily use of elevation and support stockings is strongly recommended.

Venous Insufficiency and Obesity-Associated Mucinosis

Localized areas of mucin deposition can be observed directly over the perforators on the lower extremity. These present as blushed, red-blue, partially compressible, agminated papules. On biopsy, deposits of dermal mucin against a background of the changes of venous insufficiency are seen. In the setting of morbid obesity and lower extremity edema, pretibial translucent papules can appear and merge into plaques. The plaques are composed of dermal mucin (hyaluronic acid). The diagnosis of "pretibial myxedema" is usually made, but thyroid functions are normal. With weight loss, the lesions improve, suggesting that they were caused by the lower extremity edema and venous insufficiency of obesity.

Venous Insufficiency Ulceration

Stasis dermatitis and venous ulceration result from increased pressure in the venous system of the lower leg. The most common cause is insufficiency of the valves in the deep venous system and lower perforating veins of the lower leg. With each contraction of the calf, blood should be pumped to the heart via this "muscle pump." Intact valves in the lower leg are required to prevent this "pumped" blood from refluxing out through the perforators into the superficial system. Increased flow through the superficial system results in enlargement of the superficial venous plexus and the appearance of "varicose veins." Increased pressure on the iliac veins from pregnancy or obesity, or simple inactivity may also result in the appearance of "venous insufficiency." The valvular insufficiency results in disorder in the venous and capillary circulation of the leg. Valve insufficiency may occur from prior thrombophlebitis or congenital "weakness." Prolonged standing without walking or contracting the calf muscles, sitting for long periods, anemia, zinc deficiency, and a defective fibrinolytic system may accelerate the process. If a history of thrombophlebitis is present, an evaluation for a hypercoagulable state, such as a deficiency of factor V Leiden, should be considered.

Edema and fibrosis develop in the skin over the medial aspect of the ankle and lower third of the shin (Fig. 35.32). After minor trauma, a macular hemorrhage appears. This is the premonitory sign of an impending ulceration. Venous ulcers usually occur on the lower medial aspect of the leg. They may appear on the background of stasis dermatitis with lipodermatosclerosis (Fig. 35.33). Venous ulcerations can be painful, but not as painful as pyoderma gangrenosum or arterial or embolic ulcerations. The ulcer tends to be round or oblong and has a characteristic yellow, fibrinous base. Multiple lesions may occur.

In most cases, the diagnosis of a venous ulceration can be made on clinical grounds. If there is no clear history or physical findings of venous insufficiency, venous rheography can be performed. An ankle:brachial index (ABI; the ratio of blood pressure in the leg to the arm) should be performed, especially in cases where peripheral pulses are diminished and hair on the lower legs is lost. This will identify coexistent arterial disease. More extensive vascular studies may be necessary to identify the presence and extent of arterial disease or focal venous valvular incompetence or congenital absence. In leg ulcers of the lower medial leg, even if cutaneous findings of venous insufficiency are absent, venous insufficiency will still be the most common cause of the ulcer. Lesions in atypical locations, those that do not respond appropriately to therapy, and those in which venous rheography is normal may require a biopsy to exclude other causes, including a cutaneous neoplasm. Additional

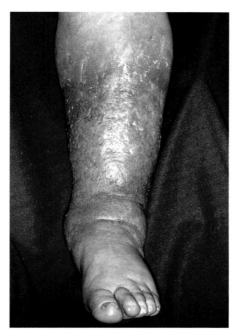

Fig. 35.32 Stasis dermatitis, venous insufficiency.

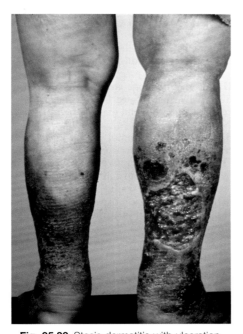

Fig. 35.33 Stasis dermatitis with ulceration.

workup may also be required to identify other, less common causes of leg ulcers, such as cholesterol emboli, atherosclerotic disease, diabetes mellitus, sickle cell disease, vasculitis, infection, and pyoderma gangrenosum.

Despite extensive research and the marketing of many new products and devices for the treatment of leg ulcers, little has changed in their management over the last decades. Treatment is primarily to improve venous return and reduce edema. Compression therapy is the mainstay of treatment. This involves, preferably, the use of inelastic/short-stretch bandages or multilayer compression dressings such as Unna boots, versus elastic/long-stretch bandages such as Coban or ACE wraps, which are significantly less effective at reducing venous hypertension and edema. Elevation

of the leg above the heart, for as much of the time as possible (at least 2 hours twice daily), is also beneficial. Elastic support of the legs must be continued after the ulcer heals. Other causes of edema, such as cardiac failure, must be addressed. The avoidance of long, cramped sitting (in airplanes or vehicles) or prolonged standing is advisable. Diuretics are overused and not proven to be of benefit. If there is a central cause of fluid retention (cirrhosis, heart failure, renal failure), diuretics may be beneficial, but otherwise they should be avoided. Avoidance of trauma is important. Pentoxifylline, 400–800 mg three times daily, in addition to compression, is beneficial in healing refractory venous ulcerations. Aspirin (300 mg/day) may have some benefit as well. A cooperative patient and a patient physician are necessary in the long-term management of venous disease. Topical antiinfectives are usually not necessary (except metronidazole gel to prevent or treat anaerobic overgrowth in cases of malodourous biofilm). There is a high risk of allergic contact dermatitis from other topical antibiotics. Oral antibiotics should only be used to treat associated invasive infection. A rim of erythema usually surrounds an ulcer. Expanding erythema, an enlarging ulcer, or increasing pain or tenderness may be signs of infection. Surface cultures and Gram stains may demonstrate colonizing, but not pathogenic, bacteria. Biopsy for histology and tissue homogenate culture is the most effective way to demonstrate a true invasive pathogen.

Many treatment options have been developed for chronic ulcers. Unfortunately, conclusive comparative studies between the various treatment alternatives are lacking. All are to be used in combination with compression treatment, which by itself leads to healing in 73% of cases without other interventions. Occlusive and semipermeable biosynthetic wound dressings can be very effective when combined with compression. They can speed healing, reduce pain, make dressing changes infrequent, and help debridement. If a hard eschar is present over the ulcer when first seen, a dressing will assist in its removal. Early in the treatment of an ulcer, a highly inflammatory and exudative phase occurs. This will often wash off the semipermeable dressing and may require the use of fenestrated dressings and even the application of absorbent padding over the dressing for the first few weeks. The patient might interpret this increased wound exudate, which is normal and indicates the conversion of a nonhealing to a healing wound, as an infection, and should be appropriately educated before such dressings are applied. Dressings containing dilute acetic acid or silver may help reduce bacterial overgrowth in the wound but fail to decrease the time to healing. However, metronidazole gel 0.75% instilled into the wound will help to reduce the amount of wound exudate and remove unpleasant odor by eliminating anaerobic bacteria. The smell of a chronic leg ulcer may reduce the patient's quality of life. Topical cadexomer iodine may be used for contaminated ulcers without clear-cut infection, or in addition to systemic antibiotics if there is documented infection. Topical growth factors applied to the wound bed, such as platelet-derived growth factor and epidermal growth factor, can promote wound healing but are limited by high cost. Topical timolol has been reported to help heal chronic leg ulcers in limited reports. Granulation tissue formation is enhanced, so they may be useful in wounds that are unable to develop a granulation tissue base despite local care and conservative debridement. Weekly debridement of the anesthetic, dead fibrinous tissue can be useful in stimulating granulation tissue at the base of slow-to-heal venous ulcerations. Sharp debridement down to visible bleeding tissue is most often employed, though enzymatic agents (collagenase) may be considered as less painful albeit slower options. Injection of granulocyte-macrophage colony-stimulating factor (GM-CSF) into the ulcer base may also stimulate refractory ulcers to heal, but is very expensive. Grafts and skin substitutes can be considered for refractory ulcers that have failed conservative therapy. Bilayer artificial skin grafts, in conjunction with compression, increases venous ulcer healing compared with compression plus dressing alone.

In more than 90% of patients, only simple but persistently applied measures are required. Enhanced compliance, longer elevation, and removal of leg edema are the first steps in attempting to heal refractory leg ulcers. If these are not optimized, expensive dressing and medications will not lead to healing. The role of vascular surgery or venous ablation in the healing of leg ulcers is controversial. Vascular surgery does not affect wound healing significantly compared with compression alone, but it appears to diminish rates of recurrence.

Risk factors that predict failure to heal within 24 weeks of limb compression therapy include a large wound area, history of venous ligation or stripping, history of hip or knee replacement, ABI less than 0.80, fibrin on 50% or more of the wound surface, and presence of the ulcer for an extended time. For every 6 months of duration, the ulcer healing time doubles.

ARTERIAL INSUFFICIENCY (ISCHEMIC) ULCER

Ischemic ulcers are mostly located on the lateral surface of the ankle or the distal digits. The initial red, painful plaque breaks down into a painful superficial ulcer with a surrounding zone of purpuric erythema. Granulation tissue is minimal, little or no infection is present, and a membranous inactive eschar forms over the ulcer. Patients at risk are those with long-standing hypertension, smokers, diabetic patients, and those with hyperlipidemia. The presence of an arterial ulceration identifies patients at increased risk for limb loss.

Signs and symptoms indicating that arterial disease is the cause of the ulceration include thinning of the skin, absence of hair, decreased or absent pulses, pallor on elevation, coolness of the extremity, dependent rubor, claudication on exercise, and pain on elevation (especially at night) relieved with dependency. In progressive disease, the diagnosis of TAO, or Buerger disease, should be considered. Patients with arterial insufficiency are also at risk for cholesterol emboli, another arterial cause of lower leg ulceration. Eosinophilia, palpable peripheral pulses, sudden onset, and associated renal insufficiency are clues to the diagnosis of cholesterol emboli.

The diagnosis of arterial insufficiency can usually be confirmed by physical examination and careful palpation of the leg pulses. For more accurate evaluation, the blood pressure in the arm and leg is taken, which should be almost identical. The ratio of the popliteal to brachial pressure is called the ABI; if less than 0.75, arterial insufficiency exists, and if less than 0.5, the insufficiency is substantial.

Surgical intervention may be required to heal the ulceration. If the blood supply cannot be improved, little can be done, except to prevent infection by the measures described for venous ulcers. The area should be protected from injury and cold, and smoking and tight socks should be avoided. Hyperbaric oxygen may be of some use but is limited by availability and cost. A recent Cochrane review highlighted the dearth of high-quality studies but suggested that hyperbaric oxygen improves ulcer healing in the short term but not the long term.

NEUROPATHIC ULCERS

Foot ulcers in diabetic patients are usually related to sensory neuropathy. Offloading the ulcer is the primary principle of management. Necrotic tissue should be debrided back to bleeding, viable tissue. Because the foot is typically insensate, this can be done in the office without the need for anesthetic. Associated osteomyelitis is best treated by removal of the infected bone. Consultation with or referral to a podiatrist or orthopedic surgeon may be indicated. Various shoes and padded boots can be used to offload different areas of the foot. An orthotics consultation is usually indicated. Clinical infection should be treated, but simple colonization typically does not require treatment. After the ulcer

heals, a shoe of appropriate depth and width will help to prevent recurrence. Frequent foot inspections for the presence of "hot spots," as well as debridement of dystrophic nails, are important facets of prevention of leg ulcers in diabetic patients.

Alavi A, et al: Diabetic foot ulcers: part I. J Am Acad Dermatol 2014; 70: 1.e1.

Alavi A, et al: Diabetic foot ulcers: part II. Am Acad Dermatol 2014; 70: 21.e1.

Cianfarani F, et al: Granulocyte/macrophage colony-stimulating factor treatment of human chronic ulcers promotes angiogenesis associated with de novo vascular endothelial growth factor transcription in the ulcer bed. Br J Dermatol 2006; 154: 34.

Gohel MS, et al: Long-term results of compression therapy alone versus compression plus surgery in chronic venous ulceration (ESCHAR). BMJ 2007; 335: 7610.

Jones JE, et al: Skin grafting for venous leg ulcers. Cochrane Database Syst Rev 2013; 1: CD001737.

Kranke P, et al: Hyperbaric oxygen therapy for chronic wounds. Cochrane Database Syst Rev 2012; 4: CD004123.

Lev-Tov H, et al: Successful treatment of a chronic venous leg ulcer using a topical beta-blocker. J Am Acad Dermatol 2013; 69: e204.

Margolis DJ, et al: Risk factors associated with failure of a venous leg ulcer to heal. Arch Dermatol 1999; 135: 920.

Meissner MH: Venous ulcer care. Phlebology 2014; 29: 174.

Michaels JA, et al: Randomized controlled trial and cost-effectiveness analysis of silver-donating antimicrobial dressings for venous leg ulcers (VULCAN) trial. Br J Surg 2009; 96: 1147.

Rico T, et al: Vascular endothelial growth factor delivery via gene therapy for diabetic wounds. J Invest Dermatol 2009; 129: 2084.

Samson RH, et al: Stockings and the prevention of recurrent venous ulcers. Dermatol Surg 1996; 22: 373.

Singer AJ, et al: Evaluation and management of lower-extremity ulcers. N Engl J Med 2017; 377: 1559.

Thomas B, et al: Topical timolol promotes healing of chronic leg ulcer. J Vasc Surg Venous Lymphat Disord 2017; 5: 844.

Van Gent WB, et al: Conservative versus surgical treatment of venous leg ulcers. J Vasc Surg 2006; 44: 563.

Wong IK, et al: Randomized controlled trial comparing treatment outcome of two compression bandaging systems and standard care without compression in patients with venous leg ulcers. J Vasc Surg 2012; 55: 1376.

◼ LYMPHEDEMA

Lymphedema is the swelling of soft tissues in which an excess amount of lymph has accumulated. Chronic lymphedema is characterized by long-standing, nonpitting edema. Box 35.2 provides a working classification of lymphedema.

The most prevalent worldwide cause of lymphedema is filariasis. In the United States the most common cause is postsurgical. If lymphedema is long standing, a verrucous appearance to the affected extremity develops (elephantiasis verrucosa nostra).

Lymphedema of the lower extremity must be distinguished from "lipedema." This syndrome is characterized by bilateral, symmetric lower extremity enlargement caused by subcutaneous fat deposition. The buttocks to the ankles are affected in women, starting at puberty with gradual progression. The feet are spared in lipedema but usually involved in lower extremity lymphedema. Lipedema does not respond to compression therapy. The skinfold at the base of the second toe is too thick to pinch in lymphedema but normal in lipedema (Stemmer sign). Verrucous changes do not occur in lipedema but do occur in lymphedema. Women with lipedema will have tenderness to pressure on the affected area. There is frequently a family history of lipedema. MRI will separate

BOX 35.2 Classification of Lymphedema

PRIMARY LYMPHEDEMA

- Congenital lymphedema (Milroy disease)
- Lymphedema praecox
- Lymphedema tarda

SYNDROMES ASSOCIATED WITH PRIMARY LYMPHEDEMA

- Yellow nail syndrome
- Turner syndrome
- Noonan syndrome
- Pes cavus
- Phakomatosis pigmentovascularis
- Distichiasis-lymphedema
- Emberger syndrome
- WILD (warts, immunodeficiency, lymphedema, anogenital dysplasia) syndrome
- Hypotrichosis-telangiectasia-lymphedema syndrome

CUTANEOUS DISORDERS SOMETIMES ASSOCIATED WITH PRIMARY LYMPHEDEMA

- Yellow nails
- Hemangiomas
- Xanthomatosis and chylous lymphedema
- Congenital absence of nails

SECONDARY LYMPHEDEMA

- Postmastectomy lymphedema
- Melphalan isolated limb perfusion
- Malignant occlusion with obstruction
- Extrinsic pressure
- Factitial lymphedema
- Post–radiation therapy
- Following recurrent lymphangitis/cellulitis
- Lymphedema of upper limb in recurrent eczema
- Granulomatous disease
- Rosaceous lymphedema
- Primary amyloidosis

COMPLICATIONS OF LYMPHEDEMA

- Cellulitis of lymphedema
- Elephantiasis nostra verrucosa
- Ulceration
- Lymphangiosarcoma

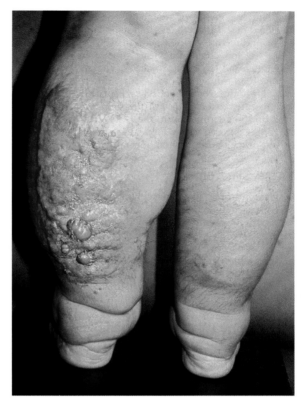

Fig. 35.34 Milroy disease. (Courtesy Dr. Lawrence Lieblich.)

the two entities if the diagnosis cannot be confirmed on a clinical basis.

TYPES

Lymphedema is classified by clinical type (see Box 35.2). Primary types include congenital and early-onset and late-onset lymphedema. Other primary types of lymphedema are associated with characteristic features or syndromes. Some cutaneous disorders are associated with, or a complication of, primary lymphedema. Secondary lymphedema can occur from numerous causes, including neoplasia and its treatment, infections, and physical factors.

Lymphedema Praecox

Lymphedema praecox accounts for the majority of primary lymphedema cases; it usually develops in females between ages 9 and 25. Swelling appears around the ankle and then extends upward to involve the entire leg; the condition is unilateral in 70% and affects the left leg more often than the right. With the passage of time, the leg becomes painful, with a dull, heavy sensation. Once this stage has been reached, the swollen limb remains swollen,

because fibrosis has occurred. These changes are caused by a defect in the lymphatic system. Lymphangiography demonstrates hypoplastic lymphatics in 87% of patients, aplasia in approximately 5%, and hyperplasia with varicose dilation of the lymphatic vessels in 8%. Because the condition typically occurs in women around menarche, estrogen may play a pathogenic role.

Nonne-Milroy-Meige Syndrome (Hereditary Lymphedema)

Milroy hereditary edema of the lower legs is characterized by a unilateral or bilateral lymphedema present at, or soon after, birth and is inherited as an autosomal dominant trait. The edema is painless, pits on pressure, is not associated with any other disorder, and persists throughout life (Fig. 35.34). It may involve the genitalia and produce lymphangiectasias superficially. Chylous discharge can occur. The face and arm may also be involved. Most frequently, the lymphedema is bilateral, and females are predominantly affected.

Treatment of this particular type of edema is extremely difficult, because the disease is an anomaly of the lymph-draining vessels. Decongestive physiotherapy can be considered. In some cases, surgical procedures to remove affected tissue can be performed. This condition may be linked to a mutation in *FLT4*, the gene for VEGFR3, which is expressed in lymphatic endothelial cells and is necessary for normal lymphatic function.

Lymphedema-Distichiasis Syndrome

The association of distichiasis (double row of eyelashes) and late-onset lymphedema is a form of hereditary lymphedema called lymphedema-distichiasis syndrome, or Meige syndrome. It is an autosomal dominant syndrome with the appearance of bilateral lymphedema, beginning between ages 8 and 10 in affected boys, and between 13 and 30 in affected girls. Lymphatic vessels are increased (not hypoplastic or absent, as in other forms of congenital lymphedema) in the affected legs, but lymphatic valves are aplastic. Associated findings are varicose veins in 50% by age 64; congenital ptosis (31%); and congenital heart disease (6.8%), cleft palate (4%), scoliosis, and renal abnormalities. There may be phenotypic heterogeneity in this syndrome, because different mutations may lead to slightly different phenotypes, especially in regard to the ancillary features associated with the syndrome. This syndrome is caused by a gene mutation in the FOXC2 transcription factor. This factor is expressed in developing eyelids, lymphatics, lymphatic valves, and other tissues with abnormalities in this syndrome.

Emberger Syndrome

Emberger syndrome is primary lymphedema associated with myelodysplasia. This genetic syndrome presents with lymphedema of one or both lower limbs and often the genitalia between infancy and puberty. Myelodysplastic syndrome and acute myeloid leukemia developing in adolescence or childhood are preceded by pancytopenia with a high incidence of monosomy 7 in the bone marrow. Associated features include mild skeletal abnormalities, deafness, and multiple warts. This syndrome is associated with gene mutations in GATA2, a hematopoietic transcription factor.

Wild Syndrome (Warts, Immunodeficiency, Lymphedema, Anogenital Dysplasia)

Lymphedema appears in early childhood and may progress to involve all four extremities and the genitalia. Widespread flat warts appear during childhood, resembling the numerous flat warts seen in epidermodysplasia verruciformis. The anogenital region develops numerous warts and anogenital dysplasia. Helper T cells are reduced.

Hypotrichosis-Telangiectasia-Lymphedema Syndrome

Lymphedema appears in childhood. Vascular dilations and telangiectasias appear on the palms and soles. Both autosomal recessive and autosomal dominant patterns of inheritance occur, but both forms are caused by mutations in the gene for SOX18.

Primary Lymphedema Associated With Yellow Nails and Pleural Effusion (Yellow Nail Syndrome)

Lymphedema is confined mostly to the ankles and occurs in about 60% of patients with yellow nail syndrome. The nails show a distinct yellowish discoloration and thickening. Recurrent pleural effusion or bronchiectasis may be a feature.

Secondary Lymphedema

In some malignant diseases, involvement of the axillary or pelvic lymph nodes will produce blockage and lymphedema. Malignant disease of the breast, uterus, prostate, skin, bones, or other tissues may cause such changes. Hodgkin disease and especially Kaposi sarcoma may be accompanied by significant lymphedema well beyond the amount expected from the degree of skin involvement. Such patients require chemotherapy; lymphedema is the hallmark of lymphatic involvement. Chronic lymphedema is seen in more than one in five women after mastectomy and removal of the axillary nodes; it may occur after varying time periods.

Postmastectomy Lymphangiosarcoma (Stewart-Treves Syndrome)

This type of vascular malignancy usually arises in chronic postmastectomy lymphedema. The lesions are bluish or reddish nodules arising on the arm. Similarly, primary or secondary lymphedema of the lower extremity may be complicated by angiosarcoma. Angiosarcoma arising in a lymphedematous extremity often presents with multiple lesions. Metastasis and death frequently result. Early, aggressive surgical treatment with amputation may be lifesaving. The treatment of breast cancer with lumpectomy and local radiation therapy may be complicated by angiosarcoma of the breast with minimal or no associated lymphedema. This is called "cutaneous postradiation angiosarcoma of the breast." This form of angiosarcoma also frequently results in metastasis and death. Benign lymphangiomatous papules may occur on the chest or axilla in breast cancer patients after radiotherapy as red or translucent grouped papules resembling lymphangioma circumscriptum.

Obesity-Related Lymphedema

Morbid obesity may impair lymphatic return, resulting in lymphedema. It is also an independent risk factor for developing lymphedema after surgery or cancer therapy. A recently described entity called "massive localized lymphedema" occurs in morbidly obese patients, presenting with a painless mass, usually on the medial thigh, characterized by typical cutaneous clinical and histologic changes of chronic lymphedema.

Postinflammatory Lymphedema

The lymphedematous extremity may be caused and worsened by repeated bacterial cellulitis or lymphangitis. These recurrent infectious episodes, when they complicate filariasis, cause the elephantiasis. Streptococcal cellulitis after venectomy in patients who have undergone coronary bypass surgery is a well-documented cause. However, almost any chronic or recurrent infection can cause lymphatic damage. Chronic antibiotic therapy can halt the progression by preventing the attacks of bacterial cellulitis.

Bullous Lymphedema

Frequently misdiagnosed as an immunobullous disease, bullous lymphedema usually occurs with poorly controlled edema related to heart failure and fluid overload. Compression results in healing.

Factitial Lymphedema

Also known as hysterical edema, lymphedema can be produced by wrapping an elastic bandage, cord, or shirt around an extremity, and/or holding the extremity in a dependent and immobile state. Self-inflicted causes of lymphedema are usually difficult to prove and may occur in settings of known causes of lymphedema, such as postphlebitic syndrome or surgical injury to the brachial plexus. Factitial lymphedema caused by blunt trauma localized to the dorsum of the hand or forearm is referred to as Secretan syndrome or l'oedème bleu, respectively. It often is unilateral, and significant purpura may occur. Effective care of such patients requires psychiatric intervention. Occupational causes must be excluded.

Podoconiosis

Podoconiosis, or mossy foot, is a noninfectious form of lymphedema. It is restricted to tropical regions in Central Africa, Central America, and North India. It occurs in persons walking barefoot in soil of volcanic origin. This soil has high concentrations of aluminum, silicon, beryllium, zirconium, magnesium, and iron. Colloid-sized particles of the dust penetrate the sole, are ingested by macrophages, and migrate to lymph nodes. Lymphatic drainage is impaired by fibrosis of lymphatic channels induced by microscopic deposits of the substances. Males and females are equally affected, and in endemic areas, up to 5% of the population can develop the disease. Moving into an endemic area from a nonendemic area can lead to the condition appearing over the next 5 years. Podoconiosis begins in childhood or adolescence with mild swelling of the feet. Burning of the feet occurs at night. The dorsal surface of the foot itches, is rubbed, and becomes lichenified. Increased skin markings result and, finally, marked hyperkeratosis caused by repeated infections. This closely resembles elephantiasis verrucosa cutis. The condition is usually asymmetric. Podoconiosis is prevented by wearing shoes. Elevation, compression, and local wound care all aid in treating this condition. Extensive surgery, as done for filariasis, has had disappointing results.

Occupational Hand Edema

Occupational persistent hand edema in divers can occur, related to the constrictive action of the divers' suits and pricks from sea urchin spines.

EVALUATION

The diagnosis of lymphedema is usually based on a classic presentation; in the early stages, however, the disease may require further investigation. Considerations include isotopic lymphoscintigraphy, fluorescence microlymphography, MRI, computed tomography, and ultrasonography. These imaging modalities have replaced lymphangiography, a more invasive technique that can cause further damage to remaining lymphatics.

TREATMENT

Most patients with lymphedema are treated conservatively by means of various forms of compression therapy, complex physical therapy, pneumatic pumps, and compressive garments. Chronic antibiotic treatment may be beneficial in patients with repeated episodes of erysipelas or cellulitis. In diabetic patients with insensate feet, the frequency of infection can be reduced by wearing properly fitting shoes. Volume-reducing surgery and lymphatic microsurgery are rarely performed, although a few centers consistently report favorable results. It is best to refer these patients to a center versed in the treatment of these complicated conditions, to optimize patient compliance and customize therapy to the patient's lifestyle.

Ameen M, et al: Clinicopathological case 2: lymphoedema-distichiasis syndrome. Clin Exp Dermatol 2003; 28: 463.

Angelini G, et al: Occupational traumatic lymphedema of the hands. Dermatol Clin 1990; 8: 205.

Asch S, et al: Massive localized lymphedema. J Am Acad Dermatol 2008; 59: S109.

Badger C, et al: Physical therapies for reducing and controlling lymphoedema of the limbs. Cochrane Database Syst Rev 2004; 4: CD003141.

Campisi C, Boccardo F: Microsurgical techniques for lymphedema treatment. World J Surg 2004; 28: 609.

Cerri A, et al: Lymphangiosarcoma of the pubic region. Eur J Dermatol 1998; 8: 511.

Connell F, et al: A new classification system for primary lymphatic dysplasias based on phenotype. Clin Genet 2010; 77: 438.

DiSipio T, et al: Incidence of unilateral arm lymphoedema after breast cancer. Lancet Oncol 2013; 14: 500.

Downes M, et al: Vascular defects in a mouse model of hypotrichosis-lymphedema-telangiectasia syndrome indicate a role for *SOX18* in blood vessel maturation. Hum Mol Genet 2009; 18: 2839.

Durr HR, et al: Stewart-Treves syndrome as a rare complication of hereditary lymphedema. Vasa 2004; 33: 42.

Fonder MA, et al: Lipedema, a frequently unrecognized problem. J Am Acad Dermatol 2007; 57: S1.

Grada AA, Phillips TJ: Lymphedema: diagnostic workup and management. J Am Acad Dermatol 2017; 77: 995.

Grada AA, Phillips TJ: Lymphedema: pathophysiology and clinical manifestations. J Am Acad Dermatol 2017; 77: 1009.

Karkkainen MJ, et al: Missense mutations interfere with VEGFR-3 signalling in primary lymphoedema. Nat Genet 2000; 25: 153.

Kreuter A, et al: A human papillomavirus–associated disease with disseminated warts, depressed cell-mediated immunity, primary lymphedema, and anogenital dysplasia. Arch Dermatol 2008; 144: 366.

Madke B: Benign lymphangiomatous papules or plaques after radiotherapy is the correct terminology. Indian J Dermatol 2015; 60: 199.

McEnery-Stonelake M, et al: Asymptomatic vesicular eruption on the chest in a breast cancer survivor. Arch Dermatol 2011; 147: 1443.

Mellor RH, et al: Lymphatic dysfunction, not aplasia, underlies Milroy disease. Microcirculation 2010; 17: 281.

Mendola A, et al: Mutations in the VEGFR3 signaling pathway explain 36% of familial lymphedema. Mol Syndromol 2013; 4: 257.

Miller TA, et al: Staged skin and subcutaneous excision for lymphedema. Plast Reconstr Surg 1998; 102: 1486.

Nenoff P, et al: Podoconiosis–non-filarial geochemical elephantiasis. J Dtsch Dermatol Ges 2010; 8: 7.

Nikitenko LL, et al: Adrenomedullin haploinsufficiency predisposes to secondary lymphedema. J Invest Dermatol 2013; 133: 1768.

Ostergaard P, et al: Mutations in *GATA2* cause primary lymphedema associated with a predisposition to acute myeloid leukemia (Emberger syndrome). Nat Genet 2011; 43: 929.

Ruocco V, et al: Lymphedema. J Am Acad Dermatol 2002; 47: 124.

Sharma A, Schwartz RA: Stewart-Treves syndrome. J Am Acad Dermatol 2012; 67: 1342.

Wagamon K, et al: Benign lymphangiomatous papules of the skin. J Am Acad Dermatol 2005; 52: 912.

36 Disturbances of Pigmentation

The visible pigmentation of the skin or hair is a combination of the amount of melanin, type of melanin (eumelanin vs. pheomelanin), degree of vascularity, presence of carotene, and thickness of the stratum corneum. Other materials can be deposited abnormally in the skin, leading to exogenous pigmentation. Eumelanin is the primary pigment producing brown coloration of the skin. Pheomelanin is yellow or red and is also produced solely in melanocytes. Melanin is formed from tyrosine, through the action of tyrosinase, in the melanosomes of melanocytes. A multitude of genes are expressed only in melanosomes and are important in melanin production and delivery. Melanosomes are lysosome-related organelles (LROs). Melanosome formation and the end result, pigmentation, require both the adequate manufacture of melanin and the appropriate transport of melanosomes within the melanocyte. The melanosomes are transferred from a melanocyte to a group of 36 keratinocytes called the epidermal melanin unit, to which they provide melanin. The variations in skin color between people are related to the degree of melanization of melanosomes, their number, and their distribution in the epidermal melanin unit. Disorders of loss or reduction of pigmentation may be related to loss of melanocytes or the inability of melanocytes to produce melanin or transport melanosomes correctly. Wood's light examination is often performed to evaluate lesions of hyperpigmentation or hypopigmentation. Hyperpigmented lesions that enhance with Wood's light usually have increased epidermal melanocyte number or activity. If the lesions do not enhance, the melanin is located in the dermis. Wood's light will greatly enhance depigmented lesions (complete loss of pigment) but does not enhance lesions with partial pigment loss (hypopigmentation).

PIGMENTARY DEMARCATION LINES

Pigmentary demarcation boundaries of the skin can be classified into groups based on their anatomic location, orientation, and degree of pigmentation (hyperpigmentation or hypopigmentation):

1. Group A: lines along the outer upper arms with variable extension across the chest
2. Group B: lines along the posteromedial aspect of the lower limb
3. Group C: paired median or paramedian lines on the chest, with midline abdominal extension
4. Group D: medial, over the spine
5. Group E: bilaterally symmetric, obliquely oriented, hypopigmented macules on the chest
6. Groups F, G, and H: facial pigmentary demarcation lines

The lines are more easily seen in patients with darker skin. Group B lines often appear for the first time during pregnancy.

The term *acquired, idiopathic, patterned facial pigmentation* (AIPFP) has been used to encompass pigmentary demarcation lines of the face, as well as idiopathic periorbital and perioral pigmentation. These are patterned, bilateral, and homogeneous and have various shades of brown with a variable gray undertone. Periorbital and perioral hyperpigmentation occur in the late teens and early twenties. Other forms of facial hyperpigmentation occur later (average age >30). Periorbital pigmentation usually is demarcated by a band of normal skin beneath the upper eyebrow superiorly and the orbital rim inferiorly. It may extend outward onto the lateral cheek or over the root of the nose. One third of patients with perioral pigmentation have a family history. These patterns of facial pigmentation may represent variations of embryologic pigmentation.

Pigmentary demarcation lines must be distinguished from the much rarer condition, acquired dermal melanocytosis (ADM). This primarily affects Asian and Hispanic women (male/female ratio 1:17). The face is the most common location, and it includes the entities bilateral and unilateral nevus of Ota–like macules (Hori and Sun nevus, respectively). ADM can first appear during pregnancy or therapeutic use of estrogen/progesterone. Lesions present as blue-gray patches, with superimposed brown macules. Infrequently, the trunk or extremities may be affected. Lesions do not enhance with Wood's light. They may be localized (after trauma) or may be more diffuse. Ultraviolet (UV) light and psoralen plus UVA (PUVA) therapy are possible precipitants. Biopsy shows melanocytes in the dermis, similar to the findings in mongolian spot, nevus of Ota, and nevus of Ito. The lesions appear to represent activation of melanin production by residual dermal melanocytes because biopsies in "normal" skin adjacent to the pigmented lesions show dermal melanocytosis.

Cho E, et al: Type B pigmentary demarcation lines of pregnancy involving the anterior thighs and knees. Ann Dermatol 2012; 24: 348.

Chuah SY, et al: Acquired dermal melanocytosis of the nose. J Eur Acad Dermatol Venereol 2015; 29: 827.

Fauconneau A, et al: Acquired dermal melanocytosis of the back in a Caucasian woman. Am J Dermatopathol 2012; 34: 562.

Mintz S, Velez I: Pigmentary demarcation lines (Futcher lines). Quintessence Int 2010; 41: 873.

Nagase K, et al: Acquired dermal melanocytosis induced by psoralen plus ultraviolet A therapy. Acta Derm Venereol 2012; 92: 691.

Peck JW, Cusack CA: Futcher lines. Cutis 2013; 92: 100.

Permatasari F, et al: Late-onset acquired dermal melanocytosis on the hand of a Chinese woman. Indian J Dermatol Venereol Leprol 2013; 79: 269.

Purnak S, et al: Pigmentary demarcation lines of pregnancy in two Caucasian women. J Eur Acad Dermatol Venereol 2015; 29: 2058.

Sarma N, et al: Acquired, idiopathic, patterned facial pigmentation (AIPFP) including periorbital pigmentation and pigmentary demarcation lines on face follows the lines of Blaschko on face. Indian J Dermatol 2014; 59: 41.

Xu C, et al: Types E and C of pigmentary demarcation lines in two Chinese sisters. Eur J Pediatr Dermatol 2014; 24: 71.

ABNORMAL PIGMENTATION

Hemosiderin Hyperpigmentation

Pigmentation resulting from deposits of hemosiderin occurs in purpura, hemochromatosis (see section later in chapter), hemorrhagic diseases, and stasis dermatitis. Clinically, hemosiderin hyperpigmentation is distinguished from postinflammatory dermal melanosis by a golden-brown hue, unlike the brown or gray-blue

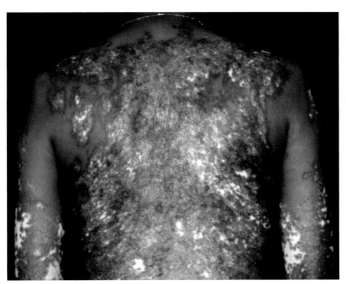

Fig. 36.1 Postinflammatory dyspigmentation resulting from lupus erythematosus.

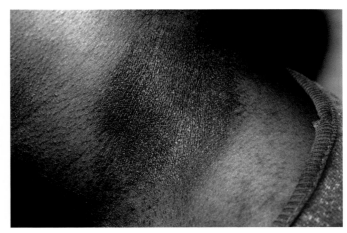

Fig. 36.2 Postinflammatory hyperpigmentation. (Courtesy Steven Binnick, MD.)

pigmentation of epidermal or dermal melanin, respectively. At times, a biopsy is required to distinguish melanin-induced from hemosiderin-induced hyperpigmentation. Extravasation of iron into the soft tissue from a poorly functioning venous catheter can cause local hemosiderosis of a limb. Multiple transfusions (>20) can result in cutaneous iron deposits in about 20% of patients. Drinking tea while ingesting an iron-containing solution can result in iron staining of the tongue and teeth, simulating black hairy tongue.

Medication Pigment

Some medications, including minocycline, deposit in the skin and complex with both iron and melanin, making uniquely colored (usually blue-gray) deposits.

Postinflammatory Hyperpigmentation (Postinflammatory Pigmentary Alteration)

Any natural or iatrogenic inflammatory condition can result in hyperpigmentation or hypopigmentation (Fig. 36.1). Postinflammatory dyspigmentation is more common in persons with Fitzpatrick skin types IV, V, and VI, especially types IV and V. It is more likely to occur after laser treatment when performed in premenstrual women. It affects both genders equally.

Hyperpigmentation may result from the following two mechanisms:

1. Increased epidermal pigmentation via increased melanocyte activity
2. Dermal melanosis from melanin dropout from the epidermis into the dermis

Wood's light examination will distinguish these two patterns of postinflammatory hyperpigmentation. Lesions of hyperpigmentation tend to be tan to brown and may have a gray hue, caused by dermal melanin (Fig. 36.2).

Hypopigmented lesions are prominently lighter than the surrounding area. Histologically, there is melanin in the upper dermis and around upper dermal vessels, located primarily in macrophages (melanophages). The pattern of the dermal melanosis does not predict whether the lesion will be lighter or darker as a result of the prior inflammatory process—thus the tendency of pathologists to provide a diagnosis of "postinflammatory pigmentary alteration" (PIPA) in such cases.

Postinflammatory dyspigmentation will often resolve on its own as long as the process that lead to the dyspigmentation (such as acne) does not continue and replace those areas that have normalized. Postinflammatory hypopigmentation (such as pityriasis alba) should be treated by treating the underlying disease. For hyperpigmented lesions, hydroquinone may be used in cases that enhance with Wood's light. Tretinoin application may enhance the effect of hydroquinone. Laser treatments and chemical peels must be done with extreme caution, because results are unpredictable and increased pigmentation may result. In darker patients, especially with lichenoid diseases such as lichen planus, the dyspigmentation can last for years.

Abad-Casintahan F, et al: Frequency and characteristics of acne-related post-inflammatory hyperpigmentation. J Dermatol 2016; 43: 826.

Al Mohizea S: The effect of menstrual cycle on laser-induced hyperpigmentation. J Drugs Dermatol 2013; 12: 1335.

Grimes PE: Management of hyperpigmentation in darker racial ethnic groups. Semin Cutan Med Surg 2009; 28: 77.

Kasuya Y, et al: Glossal pigmentation caused by the simultaneous uptake of iron and tea. Eur J Dermatol 2014; 24: 493.

Lobo C, et al: Retrospective epidemiological study of Latin American patients with transfusional hemosiderosis. Hematology 2011; 16: 265.

Oram Y, Akkaya AD: Refractory postinflammatory hyperpigmentation treated with fractional CO_2 laser. J Clin Aesthet Dermatol 2014; 7: 42.

Payette MJ, et al: Lichen planus and other lichenoid dermatoses. Clin Dermatol 2015; 33: 631.

Thompson J, et al: Severe haemosiderin pigmentation after intravenous iron infusion. Intern Med J 2014; 44: 706.

MELASMA (CHLOASMA)

Melasma is a common disorder, with two predisposing factors: sun exposure and sex hormones. It tends to affect darker-complexioned individuals, especially East, West, and Southeast Asians, Hispanics, and black persons who live in areas of intense sun exposure and who have Fitzpatrick skin types IV and V. Subtle melasma, as identified by UV light examination, may be seen in up to 30% of middle-aged Asian females. Men are also affected, especially those from Central America.

The pathogenesis of melasma is not known. However, many observations strongly suggest that sun exposure is the primary trigger. Melasma affects the face, a sun-exposed area, and worsens in the summer. Melasma patients have a lower minimal erythema dose (MED) to UV light, and pigment more easily with UV exposure. An association exists between the number of melanocytic nevi and the development of melasma. The prevalence of melasma increases with age in both men and women. Solar elastosis is more marked in areas of melasma than unaffected facial skin. Melasma-affected skin has reduced WIF-1 (Wnt antagonist) expression and resultant increased Wnt expression; Wnt stimulates melanogenesis.

After sun exposure, the second most important trigger for melasma is female hormones. Melasma is more common and severe in women than men. It occurs frequently during pregnancy, with oral contraceptive (OC) use, or with hormone replacement therapy (HRT) at menopause. Discontinuing OC use or HRT rarely clears the pigmentation, which still may last for many years. In contrast, melasma of pregnancy usually clears within a few months of delivery. Melasma may be seen in other endocrinologic disorders, as well as with phenytoin and finasteride therapy.

Melasma is characterized by brown patches, typically on the malar prominences and forehead. The forearms may also be affected. There are three clinical patterns of facial melasma: centrofacial, malar, and mandibular. The centrofacial and malar patterns constitute the majority (Fig. 36.3), but most patients have multiple types, so this classification is not very useful therapeutically. The pigmented patches are usually sharply demarcated. Although melasma has classically been classified as epidermal or dermal, based on the presence or absence of Wood's light enhancement, respectively, most cases show both epidermal and dermal melanin. There are nuclear changes within keratinocytes that indicate that epidermal melanin units are altered. Dermal melanophages are a normal finding in sun-exposed Asian skin. Independent of Wood's light findings, a therapeutic trial of some form of hypopigmenting agent should be offered.

Therapeutically, a sunblock with broad-spectrum UVA (even visible light) coverage should be used daily; it will modestly improve the melasma, but more important, will enhance the efficacy of bleaching creams and help prevent new lesions. Bleaching creams with hydroquinone are the gold standard and are moderately efficacious, containing 2% (available over the counter) to 4% hydroquinone. Tretinoin cream may be added to increase efficacy. Tretinoin alone may reduce melasma, but it is not as effective as hydroquinone. The combination of hydroquinone and tretinoin, administered with a topical corticosteroid, has been called "Kligman's formula" and is the most effective topical regimen available to treat melasma. Twice-weekly application of the triple combination can be effective for maintenance. Overuse can lead to fixed erythema and telangiectasias, acneiform eruptions, and hypertrichosis. Overuse of hydroquinone can lead to exogenous ochronosis. When 4% hydroquinone is ineffective, higher concentrations may be recommended. Satellite pigmentation and local ochronosis are potential complications from use of these higher-concentration preparations. Methimazole, azelaic acid, kojic acid, vitamin C, and arbutin are other therapies with minimal to moderate efficacy. Many of these agents are added to cosmetic products for skin lightening and may be combined, because they act on different steps of melanogenesis. All these topical agents are generally less effective than 4% hydroquinone but may be used in the patient intolerant of hydroquinone. Oral tranexamic acid may play a role as a systemic agent in treating refractory melasma.

Various surgical procedures, such as peels and light-based treatments, have been proposed as effective for melasma, but results are mixed. Peels with glycolic acid, salicylic acid, trichloroacetic acid (TCA), and tretinoin 1% have not reproducibly enhanced the efficacy of 4% hydroquinone and can cause hyperpigmentation if irritation ensues. The use of light-based modalities for the treatment of melasma should be approached with caution. These therapies may be complicated by hyperpigmentation, irritation, hypopigmentation, and even scarring, if not used appropriately. Intense pulse light (IPL) can improve melasma, but there is a high relapse rate. Pulsed dye laser may enhance combination topical treatment, and improvement may continue after therapy is discontinued. Q-switched neodymium:yttrium-aluminum-garnet (Nd:YAG) laser therapy can lead to increased pigmentation.

Adalatkhah H, et al: Melasma and its association with different types of nevi in women. BMC Dermatol 2008; 8: 3.

Brianezi G, et al: Changes in nuclear morphology and chromatin texture of basal keratinocytes in melasma. J Eur Acad Dermatol Venereol 2015; 29: 809.

Castanedo-Cazares JP, et al: Near-visible light and UV photoprotection in the treatment of melasma. Photodermatol Photoimmunol Photomed 2014; 30: 35.

Córdova ME, et al: Exogenous ochronosis in facial melasma. Actas Dermosifiliogr 2017; 108: 381.

Famenini S, et al: Finasteride-associated melasma in a Caucasian male. J Drugs Dermatol 2014; 13: 484.

Fisk WA, et al: The use of botanically derived agents for hyperpigmentation. J Am Acad Dermatol 2014; 70: 352.

Handel AC, et al: Melasma. An Bras Dermatol 2014; 89: 771.

Handel AC, et al: Risk factors for facial melasma in women. Br J Dermatol 2014; 171: 588.

Hernandez-Barrera R, et al: Solar elastosis and presence of mast cells as key features in the pathogenesis of melasma. Clin Exp Dermatol 2008; 33: 305.

Hexsel D, et al: Epidemiology of melasma in Brazilian patients. Int J Dermatol 2014; 53: 440.

Hexsel D, et al: Objective assessment of erythema and pigmentation of melasma lesions and surrounding areas on long-term management regimens with triple combination. J Drugs Dermatol 2014; 13: 444.

Jutley GS, et al: Systematic review of randomized controlled trials on interventions for melasma. J Am Acad Dermatol 2014; 70: 369.

Kandhari R, Khunger N: Skin lightening agents. Indian J Dermatol Venereol Leprol 2013; 79: 701.

Kim MJ, et al: Punctate leucoderma after melasma treatment using 1064-nm Q-switched Nd:YAG laser with low pulse energy. J Eur Acad Dermatol Venereol 2009; 23: 960.

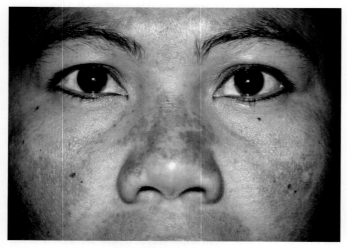

Fig. 36.3 Melasma.

Kim NH, et al: Cadherin 11, a miR-675 target, induces N-cadherin expression and epithelial-mesenchymal transition in melasma. J Invest Dermatol 2014; 134: 2967.

Li Y, et al: Treatment of melasma with oral administration of compound tranexamic acid. J Eur Acad Dermatol Venereol 2014; 28: 388.

Malek J, et al: Successful treatment of hydroquinone-resistant melasma using topical methimazole. Dermatol Ther 2013; 26: 69.

Passeron T: Long-lasting effect of vascular targeted therapy of melasma. J Am Acad Dermatol 2013; 69: e141.

Rivas S, Pandya AG: Treatment of melasma with topical agents, peels and lasers. Am J Clin Dermatol 2013; 14: 359.

Sardana K, Garg VK: Lasers are not effective for melasma in darkly pigmented skin. J Cutan Aesthet Surg 2014; 7: 57.

Sardana K, et al: Which therapy works for melasma in pigmented skin. Indian J Dermatol Venereol Leprol 2013; 79: 420.

Trivedi MK, et al: A review of laser and light therapy in melasma. Int J Womens Dermatol 2017; 3: 11.

Tse TW, et al: Tranexamic acid. J Cosmet Dermatol 2012; 12: 57.

RETICULATE PIGMENT DISORDERS OF THE SKIN

This group of disorders is linked by similar clinical features: reticulate pigmentation of various skin sites and characteristic histology—adenoid pigmented proliferations of the rete ridges of the interfollicular and infundibular follicular epidermis, at times with focal acantholysis. Patients may have overlapping features of several different syndromes, but now that the genetic basis for disease is being discovered, correct categorization should be easier.

Dyschromatosis Symmetrica Hereditaria (Reticulate Acropigmentation of Dohi)

Originally described and still reported primarily in the Japanese, acropigmentation of Dohi has been found to affect individuals from Europe, India, and the Caribbean region. It is also referred to as dyschromatosis symmetrica hereditaria (DSH) or symmetric dyschromatosis of the extremities. It is inherited most often as an autosomal dominant trait, although autosomal recessive kindreds have been reported. Patients develop progressive hyperpigmented and hypopigmented macules, often mixed in a reticulate pattern, concentrated on the dorsal extremities, especially the dorsal hands and feet. The lesions vary in size from pinpoint to pea sized. Freckle-like macules can present on the face. Long hair on the forearms, hypopigmented or hyperpigmented hair, acral hypertrophy, and dental abnormalities also have been reported. Lesions appear in infancy or early childhood and usually stop spreading before adolescence. The pigmentary lesions last for life although there is a report of spontaneous resolution. The autosomal dominant form of DSH is caused by a mutation in the *DSRAD (ADAR1)* gene.

Kantaputra PN, et al: Dyschromatosis symmetrica hereditaria with long hair on the forearms, hypo/hyperpigmented hair, and dental anomalies. Am J Med Genet A 2012; 158: 2258.

Mohana D, et al: Reticulate acropigmentation of Dohi. Indian J Dermatol 2012; 57: 42.

Murata T, et al: Dyschromatosis symmetrica hereditaria with acra hypertrophy. Eur J Dermatol 2011; 21: 649.

Shi BJ, et al: First report of the coexistence of dyschromatosis symmetrica hereditaria and psoriasis. J Eur Acad Dermatol Venereol 2012; 26: 657.

Zhang SD, et al: Pathogenicity of *ADAR1* mutation in a Chinese family with dyschromatosis symmetrica hereditaria. J Eur Acad Dermatol Venereol 2017; 31: e483.

Dyschromatosis Universalis Hereditaria, Familial Progressive Hyperpigmentation and Hypopigmentation

Dyschromatosis universalis hereditaria (DUH) is a rare autosomal dominant genodermatosis characterized by asymptomatic hyperpigmented and hypopigmented macules (Fig. 36.4) in a generalized distribution on the trunk and limbs, or sometimes the face. Lesions are irregular in size and shape and appear in infancy or childhood, often in the first few months of life. The palms, soles, and mucous membranes are usually spared. Most DUH patients do not show other symptoms and are otherwise well. Infrequently reported associations include ocular and auditory abnormalities, photosensitivity, developmental delay, and short stature. Histologically, there are normal numbers of melanocytes in both the lighter and the darker skin, but more melanized, mature melanosomes in the darker areas and empty, immature melanosomes in the hypopigmented areas. A mutation in the *ABCB6* gene (mitochondrial porphyrin transporter localized to outer membrane of mitochondria) has been identified in numerous cases of autosomal dominant DUH (DUH-1). The wild-type protein localizes to the dendrites of melanocytes and is probably involved in melanosome transport. The mutant protein remains in the Golgi complex, which could disrupt melanosome transport.

A much rarer variant of DUH is DUH-2. It is inherited as an autosomal recessive genodermatosis, with a putative gene location on chromosome 12.

Familial progressive hyperpigmentation (FPH) is an autosomal dominant genodermatosis characterized by hyperpigmented patches presenting in early infancy and progressing with age. Hypopigmented lesions are absent, distinguishing it from DUH-2, which FPH otherwise closely resembles. Familial progressive hyperpigmentation and hypopigmentation (FPHH) is an autosomal dominant disorder characterized by diffuse, partly blotchy hyperpigmentation, hyperpigmented macules, café au lait macules, and larger hypopigmented ash-leaf macules on the face, neck, trunk, and limbs present at birth or early in infancy (Fig. 36.5). Lesions increase in size and number with age. FPHH and FPH have also been associated with mutations in the same region of chromosome 12 as DUH-2, mapping to the gene *KITLG* (also known as steel factor or mast cell growth factor/stem cell factor), which codes for the ligand of c-KIT. The mutations in FPHH

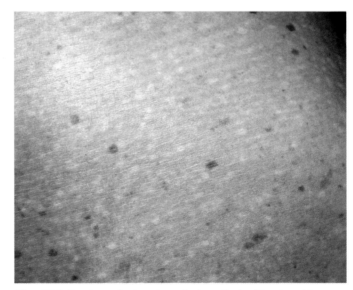

Fig. 36.4 Dyschromatosis universalis hereditaria. (Courtesy Vasanop Vachiramon, MD.)

and FPH are gain-of-function mutations. c-KIT mutations are also implicated in mastocytomas and there is a report of a patient with both FPH and mastocytomas.

Amyere M, et al: *KITLG* mutations cause familial progressive hyper- and hypopigmentation. J Invest Dermatol 2011; 1331: 1234.

Cui YX, et al: Novel mutations of *ABCB6* associated with autosomal dominant dyschromatosis universalis hereditaria. PLoS One 2013; 8: e79808.

Nogita T, et al: Removal of facial and labial lentigines in dyschromatosis universalis hereditaria with a Q-switched alexandrite laser. J Am Acad Dermatol 2011; 65: e61.

Piqueres-Zubiaurre T, et al: Familial progressive hyperpigmentation, cutaneous mastocytosis, and gastrointestinal stromal tumor as clinical manifestations of mutations in the c-KIT receptor gene. Pediatr Dermatol 2017; 34: 84.

Sorensen RH, et al: Dyschromatosis universalis hereditaria with oral leukokeratosis. Pediatr Dermatol 2015; 32: e283.

Zhang C, et al: Mutations in *ABCB6* cause dyschromatosis universalis hereditaria. J Invest Dermatol 2013; 133: 2221.

Dowlin-Degos Disease (Reticular Pigmented Anomaly of Flexures)

Reticular pigmented anomaly of the flexures is a rare autosomal dominant pigmentary disorder; it is now more often called Dowling-Degos disease (DDD). Pigmentation usually appears at puberty or in early adolescence but may present later in adulthood. The skin lesions primarily affect the intertriginous areas, such as the axillae, neck, genitalia, and inframammary/sternal areas. In some cases, the dorsal hands are involved. The pigmentation is reticular; at the periphery, discrete, brownish black macules surround the partly confluent, central pigmented area and progresses very slowly. In more mildly affected patients, the pigmentation is dappled. A follicular variant of DDD has been reported. There are frequently acneiform, pitted scars, sometimes pigmented, around the mouth. Comedonal and cystic lesions have been described on the flexures and in the axillae. Hidradenitis suppurativa–like lesions in the groin and axilla may occur. Patients may complain that the condition is worse during hot weather. Squamous cell carcinoma of the buttocks or perianal area has been described.

Histologically, in addition to the typical lentiginous adenoid proliferations of the rete ridges, small horn cysts may be present, so that the pattern resembles that of a reticulated seborrheic keratosis. Comedones may be present. Classic autosomal dominant DDD is caused by mutations in the keratin 5 gene (*KRT5*). Similar mutations occur in Galli-Galli disease, suggesting that the two conditions represent variants of the same disorder rather than separate diseases. In DDD patients who lack mutation in *KRT5*, mutations have been found in *POGLUT1* and *POFUT1*, both of which are essential regulators of Notch activity.

Galli-Galli Disease

Galli-Galli disease is now recognized as an acantholytic variant of DDD, also caused by mutations in the *KRT5* gene. The skin lesions are 1–2 mm, slightly keratotic, red to dark-brown papules, which are focally confluent in a reticulate pattern (Fig. 36.6). The skin lesions favor skinfolds, although other skin sites may also be involved. The neck, axillae, upper extremities, dorsal hands, trunk, groin, and even the scrotum and lower extremities may be affected. Histologically, there is prominent digitate downgrowth of the rete ridges, identical to that seen in DDD. The characteristic histologic feature is a suprabasilar cleft and suprapapillary thinning of the epidermis. There is no dyskeratosis, as seen in Grover disease. Ablative laser treatment led to axillary symptom resolution in one patient.

Basmanav FB, et al: Mutations on *POGLUT1*, encoding protein O-glucosyltransferase 1, cause autosomal-dominant Dowling-Degos disease. Am J Hum Genet 2014; 94: 135.

Gomes J, et al: Galli-Galli disease. Case Rep Med 2011; 2011: 703257.

Hanneken S, et al: Systematic mutation screening of *KRTS* supports the hypothesis that Galli-Galli disease is a variant of Dowling-Degos disease. Br J Dermatol 2010; 163: 197.

Horner ME, et al: Dowling-Degos disease involving the vulva and back. Dermatol Online J 2011; 17: 1.

Muller CS, et al: The spectrum of reticulate pigment disorders of the skin revisited. Eur J Dermatol 2012; 22: 596.

Schmieder A, et al: Galli-Galli disease is an acantholytic variant of Dowling-Degos disease. J Am Acad Dermatol 2012; 66: e250.

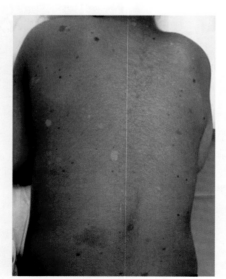

Fig. 36.5 Familial progressive hypopigmentation and hyperpigmentation (*KITLG* mutation). (Courtesy Lara Wine-Lee, MD, PhD.)

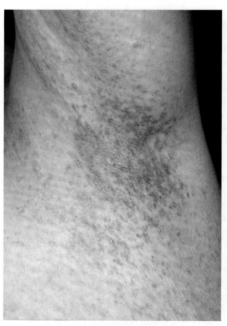

Fig. 36.6 Galli-Galli disease.

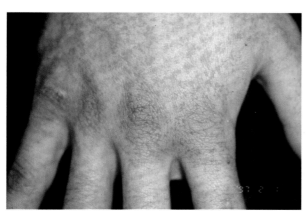

Fig. 36.7 Reticulate acropigmentation of Kitamura. (Courtesy Department of Dermatology, Keio University, School of Medicine, Tokyo, Japan.)

Singh S, et al: Follicular Dowling-Degos disease. Indian J Dermatol Venereol Leprol 2013; 79: 802.
Taskapan O, et al: Dowling-Degos disease with diffuse penile pigmentation. J Eur Acad Dermatol Venereol 2014; 28: 1405.
Voth H, et al: Efficacy of ablative laser treatment in Galli-Galli disease. Arch Dermatol 2011; 147: 317.

Reticulate Acropigmentation of Kitamura

Reticulate acropigmentation of Kitamura (RPK) is a rare autosomal dominant disease that initially was recognized in Japan but now has been seen in many countries. The characteristic presentation is pigmented, angulated, irregular, freckle-like lesions with atrophy (Fig. 36.7), arranged in a reticulate pattern on the dorsal feet and hands. Lesions start in the first to second decade of life, gradually progress, and slowly darken over time. The axillae and groin may be affected, as can the skin of the trunk and more proximal extremities. Linear irregular breaks in the dermatoglyphics of the palms are characteristic and help to distinguish this disorder from the other "reticulate flexural anomalies." Patients with mixed features of DDD and RPK have been reported. RPK is caused by a loss-of-function mutation in *ADAM10*, which also affects the NOTCH pathway explaining the similarities with DDD.

Koguchi H, et al: Characteristic findings of handprint and dermoscopy in reticulate acropigmentation of Kitamura. Clin Exp Dermatol 2014; 39: 58.
Ralser DJ, et al: Functional implications of novel *ADAM10* mutations in reticulate acropigmentation of Kitamura. Br J Dermatol 2017; 177: e340.

DERMATOPATHIA PIGMENTOSA RETICULARIS

Dermatopathia pigmentosa reticularis (DPR) is an extremely rare dominant ectodermal dysplasia characterized by the triad of generalized reticulate hyperpigmentation, noncicatricial alopecia, and onychodystrophy. Additional associations include loss of dermatoglyphics, hypohidrosis or hyperhidrosis, pigmented lesions of the oral mucosa, palmoplantar hyperkeratosis, and nonscarring blisters on the dorsa of the hands and feet. Wiry scalp hair and digital fibromatosis have also been reported. Both Naegeli-Franceschetti-Jadassohn syndrome (NFJS) and DPR are caused by mutations in the keratin 14 gene. Patients with NFJS can be differentiated from DPR because NFJS patients have dental anomalies their pigmentation may fade.

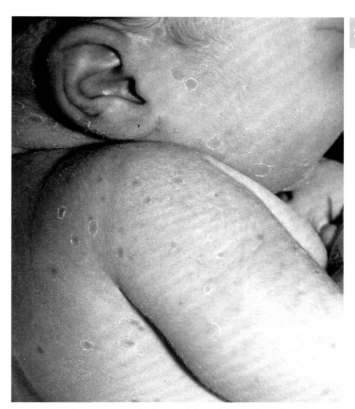

Fig. 36.8 Transient neonatal pustular melanosis.

Al Saif F: Dermatopathia pigmentosa reticularis. Indian J Dermatol 2016; 61: 468.
Goh BK, et al: A case of dermatopathia pigmentosa reticularis with wiry scalp hair and digital fibromatosis resulting from a recurrent *KRT14* mutation. Clin Exp Dermatol 2009; 34: 340.

TRANSIENT NEONATAL PUSTULAR MELANOSIS

Also called transient pustular melanosis (TPM) is present at birth. Newborns present with 1–3 mm, flaccid, superficial fragile pustules. Some of the pustules may have already resolved in utero, leaving pigmented macules (Fig. 36.8). Lesions can occur anywhere. Numerous lesions and lesions up to 1 cm in diameter have been reported, but any new pustules forming after birth should raise suspicion for another benign pustulosis such as erythema toxicum neonatorum or, more important, infections such as *Staphylococcus aureus* or herpes simplex. In dark-skinned infants, pigmented macules may persist for weeks or months after the pustules have healed. Transient neonatal pustular melanosis is observed more frequently in infants with skin types III-VI (approximately 5% vs less than 1% of infants with skin types I-II) and may be more common after vaginal than cesarean delivery.

Histologically, there are intracorneal or subcorneal aggregates, predominantly of neutrophils, although eosinophils may also be found. Dermal inflammation is composed of a mix of neutrophils and eosinophils.

Brazzelli V, et al: An unusual case of transient neonatal pustular melanosis. Eur J Pediatr 2014; 173: 1655.
Ekiz O, et al: Skin findings in newborns and their relationship with maternal factors. Ann Dermatol 2013; 25: 1.
Paloni G, Cutrone M: Giant transient pustular melanosis in an infant. Arch Dis Child Fetal Neonatal Ed 2013; 98: F492.

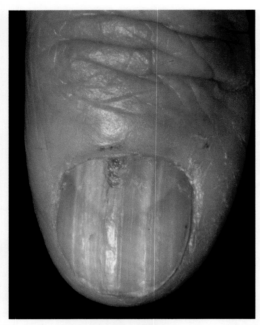

Fig. 36.9 Peutz-Jeghers syndrome. (Courtesy Steven Binnick, MD.)

PEUTZ-JEGHERS SYNDROME

Peutz-Jeghers syndrome (PJS) is characterized by hyperpigmented macules on the lips and oral mucosa, polyposis of the gastrointestinal (GI) tract, and greatly increased cancer risk. The dark-brown or black macules appear typically on the lips, especially the lower lip, in infancy or early childhood (Fig. 36.9). Similar lesions may appear on the buccal mucosa, tongue, gingiva, and the perianal mucosa; macules may also occur around the mouth, on the central face, perianally, and on the backs of the hands, especially the fingers, toes, and tops of the feet. More than two thirds of patients have lesions on the hands and feet, and 95% have perioral lesions. Skin lesions grow in size and number until puberty, after which they begin to regress. Buccal pigmented macules tend to persist. Similar pigmentation may be seen in the bowel.

The diagnosis of PJS is made with any of four major criteria: (1) two or more histologically confirmed PJS polyps; (2) any number of PJS polyps and a family history of PJS; (3) characteristic mucocutaneous pigmentation and a family history of PJS; or (4) any number of PJS polyps and characteristic mucocutaneous pigmentation. In 94% of patients who fulfill these criteria, a mutation in the *STK11* gene will be found. Almost half of patients are de novo mutations.

The associated polyps, which are histologically characteristic, are most common in the small intestine, but may also occur in the stomach, colon, and least commonly the rectum. The polyposis of the small intestine may cause repeated bouts of abdominal pain and vomiting. Bleeding and intussusception are common; intussusception is frequent (47%). Boys with PJS often have evidence of estrogen excess with gynecomastia and advanced bone age.

Patients with PJS have a 10-fold to 18-fold greater lifetime cancer risk (81%–94%) than the general population. The greatest risk is for GI malignancy, which is increased 130-fold in PJS patients. These cancers occur in the colon (39% of patients), stomach (29%), and small intestine (13%). Cancers begin to appear about age 30 years. Cancers also occur in extraintestinal sites, especially the breast, genitourinary (GU) tract, and pancreas (100-fold increase in PJS patients). The prevalence of cancers by anatomic site is pancreas (26%), breast (54%, can be bilateral),

and ovary (21%). Sertoli-Leydig cell stromal tumors occur in 9% of PJS males, and sex cord tumors with annular tubules can occur in female PJS patients. Given the high risk of cancer in PJS patients, standard screening protocols have been recommended. Because 40% of patients develop significant GI and potentially GU complications by age 6 years, GI screening may need to begin as early as age 4 or 5, with testicular examination in males with PJS. The syndrome is caused by a germline mutation of the *STK11/LKB1* tumor suppressor gene. Patients with truncation of the gene rather than a missense mutation are more severely affected, suggesting a phenotype/genotype correlation. In Chinese PJS patients, mutations in *OR4C45*, *ZAN*, pre–micro-RNAs, and other genes have been identified, suggesting that multiple different genes can cause this syndrome.

Laugier-Hunziker syndrome, Carney syndrome, and Cronkhite-Canada syndrome should be considered in the differential diagnosis of PJS. Laugier-Hunziker syndrome presents with mucosal pigmentation and pigmented nail streaks. Cronkhite-Canada syndrome consists of melanotic macules on the fingers and GI polyposis, as well as generalized, uniform darkening of the skin, extensive alopecia, and onychodystrophy. The polyps that occur are usually benign adenomas and may involve the entire GI tract. A protein-losing enteropathy may develop and is associated with the degree of intestinal polyposis. Onset is typically after age 30 in this sporadically occurring, generally benign condition. Hypogeusia (reduced taste) is the dominant initial symptom in Cronkhite-Canada, followed by diarrhea and ectodermal changes. The majority of all cases have been reported from Japan. Zinc therapy may improve the hypogeusia and other symptoms. Carney syndrome patients may also develop Sertoli cell tumors and gynecomastia, which, in combination with their mucocutaneous pigmentation, may lead to an erroneous diagnosis of PJS.

Banno K, et al: Hereditary gynecological tumors associated with Peutz-Jeghers syndrome (review). Oncol Lett 2013; 6: 1184.

Campos-Munoz L, et al: Dermoscopy of Peutz-Jeghers syndrome. J Eur Acad Dermatol Venereol 2009; 23: 730.

Goldstein SA, Hoffenberg EJ: Peutz-Jegher syndrome in childhood. J Pediatr Gastroenterol Nutr 2013; 56: 191.

Ham S, et al: Overexpression of aromatase associated with loss of heterozygosity of the *STK11* gene accounts for prepubertal gynecomastia in boys with Peutz-Jeghers syndrome. J Clin Endocrinol Metab 2013; 98: E1979.

Jelsig AM, et al: Hamartomatous polyposis syndromes. Orphanet J Rare Dis 2014; 9: 101.

Korsse SE, et al: Pancreatic cancer risk in Peutz-Jeghers syndrome patients. J Med Genet 2013; 50: 59.

Resta N, et al: Cancer risk associated with *STK11/LKB1* germline mutations in Peutz-Jeghers syndrome patients. Dig Liv Dis 2013; 45: 606.

Richey JD, et al: Carney syndrome in a patient previously considered to have Peutz-Jeghers syndrome. J Am Acad Dermatol 2014; 70: e44.

Shah KR, et al: Cutaneous manifestations of gastrointestinal disease. Part I. J Am Acad Dermatol 2013; 68: 189.e1.

Tsai HL, et al: Rectal carcinoma in a young female patient with Peutz-Jeghers syndrome. Med Princ Pract 2014; 23: 89.

Wang HH, et al: Exome sequencing revealed novel germline mutations in Chinese Peutz-Jeghers syndrome patients. Dig Dis Sci 2014; 59: 64.

Wangler MF, et al: Unusually early presentation of small-bowel adenocarcinoma in a patient with Peutz-Jeghers syndrome. J Pediatr Hematol Oncol 2013; 35: 323.

METALLIC DISCOLORATIONS

Pigmentation may develop from the deposit of fine metallic particles in the skin. The metal may be carried to the skin hematogenously or directly inoculated into the skin. Discolorations from medications containing silver and gold are discussed in Chapter 6.

Arsenic

Acute arsenic poisoning is associated with flushing on day 1 of exposure and facial edema on days 2–5. A morbilliform eruption appears on days 4–6. Hepatic dysfunction occurs simultaneously with the appearance of an eruption of discrete red-brown, erythematous papules in the intertriginous areas (areas of friction) of the lower abdomen, buttocks, and lateral upper chest. It regresses after 2–3 weeks, at times accompanied by acral desquamation. Three months after exposure, Mees' lines, total leukonychia, Beau's lines, and onychodystrophy may be seen. Periungual pigmentation occurs in up to half of acutely poisoned patients at 3 months.

Arsenic is an elemental metal that is ubiquitous, existing in nature as metalloids, alloys, and a variety of chemical compounds. These various forms of arsenic may be deposited into water, soil, and vegetation, producing serious health risks. Certain regions of Pakistan, India (West Bengal and Eastern India), Mongolia, China, Cambodia, and Vietnam have high levels of arsenic in their drinking water, exposing millions of people to levels of arsenic that result in health consequences. Evidence indicates that polymorphisms in arsenic-metabolizing (methylation) pathways, specifically converting monomethylarsonic acid to dimethylarsinic acid, may portend higher risk. Arsenic exposure is also associated with a significant reduction in circulating helper T cells, perhaps contributing to increased cancer risk. One study identified polymorphisms in the *XPD* gene as a risk factor for arsenic-induced skin lesions. Numerous cases of arsenic-induced skin lesions have occurred. Skin lesions usually occur only when arsenic concentrations in drinking water are 50 µg/L or more.

Two characteristic forms of skin disease occur. Cutaneous hyperpigmentation is the most common and earliest side effect. The hyperpigmentation is usually diffuse, most prominent on the trunk. Patchy hyperpigmentation may be accentuated in the inguinal folds, on the areolae, and on palmar creases. This can simulate Addison disease. Areas of hypopigmentation may be scattered in the hyperpigmented areas, giving a "raindrop" appearance. Focal melanotic macules may also be present. The pigmentation may resolve or persist indefinitely. Punctate keratoses on the palms and soles are characteristic. Diffuse palmoplantar keratoderma may rarely occur. Blackfoot disease—arsenic-induced peripheral vascular disease that can lead to vasospasm and peripheral gangrene—and a severe peripheral neuropathy can also occur with chronic arsenic ingestion.

Histologically, the arsenical keratosis on the palms and soles shows hyperkeratosis, parakeratosis, acanthosis, and papillomatosis. Approximately 6%–7% of hyperkeratotic skin lesions will demonstrate basilar atypia, and about 1% will show cancer. Arsenic exposure leads to the development of nonmelanoma skin cancers. Bowen disease represents the majority of arsenic-induced skin cancers and may appear on sun-exposed or sun-protected skin. Basal cell carcinomas are frequent, are usually multiple, are most common on the trunk, and can be in sun-protected sites. Squamous cell carcinoma may also occur. Acitretin may improve "arsenical" keratoses. Arsenic exposure results in increased risk for lung, liver, and renal carcinoma.

Lead

Chronic lead poisoning can produce a "lead hue," with lividity and pallor, and a deposit of lead in the gums may occur: the "lead line."

Iron

In the past, soluble iron compounds were used in the treatment of allergic contact and other dermatitides. In eroded areas, iron

was sometimes deposited in the skin, like a tattoo. The use of Monsel solution can produce similar tattooing, so aluminum chloride is now preferred, especially if biopsying melanocytic lesions, because the monsels can be mistaken for recurrent disease. If Monsel solution is used, to minimize tattooing, it is best applied with a cotton-tipped applicator barely moistened with the solution, then rolled across a wound that has just been blotted dry.

Hemochromatosis

Hemochromatosis is a disorder caused by mutations in at least five different genes involved in iron absorption. It is very common in the white European population, in whom most mutations are at two genetic loci, C282Y and H63D in the *HFE* gene. Two autosomal recessive forms of juvenile hereditary hemochromatosis are described, caused by mutations in the Hemojuvelin and the Hepcidin gene. Mutations in the transferrin receptor 2 gene lead to a form of autosomal recessive adult-onset hemochromatosis. Ferroportin mutation leads to an adult-onset form of autosomal dominant hemochromatosis.

Only a minority of persons with the most common genetic defects causing hemochromatosis will develop disease. Men are affected more frequently and at an earlier age, usually 30–50. With widespread genetic testing, the age of diagnosis has been decreased, and the number of asymptomatic affected females has dramatically increased. The characteristic cutaneous manifestation is gray to brown generalized mucocutaneous hyperpigmentation. This is enhanced in sun-exposed areas of the forearms, dorsal hands (Fig. 36.10), and face, as well as in the inguinal area. The mucous

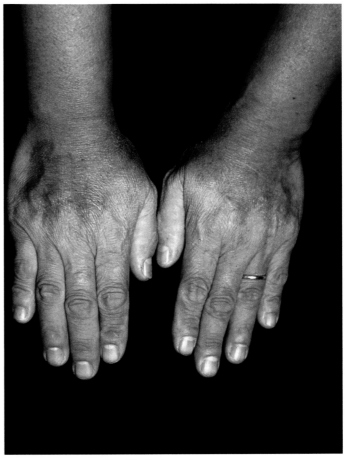

Fig. 36.10 Hemochromatosis.

membranes are pigmented in up to 20% of patients. The percentage of affected males with pigmentation is about 30%, and in women, fewer than 10% of diagnosed patients have skin changes. Biopsy of affected hyperpigmented skin shows dermal iron deposition, but the visible pigmentation is actually increased epidermal melanin in the basal cell layer. Other skin changes can include koilonychia and localized ichthyosis. Alopecia is common, and pruritus can occur. Porphyria cutanea tarda occurs more commonly in patients with hemochromatosis due to inhibition of uroporphyrinogen decarboxylase in the liver by iron overload. In patients with chronic venous insufficiency, the risk of lower leg ulceration is increased sixfold in those also carrying the C282Y mutation, leading some to suggest that this test should be ordered in at-risk patients at the initial stages of venous insufficiency.

The most seriously affected organ is the liver. Hepatomegaly and elevated liver function tests (LFTs) are signs of hepatic iron overload. Cirrhosis and hepatocellular carcinoma may develop. The endocrine system is also affected, with hypogonadism the primary complaint. Arthropathy is seen in about 50% of women and 40% of men. Cardiac abnormalities include heart failure and arrhythmias. Consuming alcohol and smoking, as well as coexistent hepatitis C virus infection, make it more likely that persons with genetic predisposition will develop clinical disease.

Levels of plasma iron and the serum iron-binding protein are elevated. The transferrin saturation (TS = serum iron/total iron-binding capacity) is a useful screening measure. A score of 45 or less is normal, except in premenopausal women, in whom greater than 35 may be considered abnormal. High serum ferritin levels are also present. Genotyping is now performed in persons with TS greater than 45 and elevated ferritin level, and confirms the diagnosis. Liver biopsy is reserved for persons with elevated LFTs, ferritin greater than 1000 µg/L, or age over 40.

All forms of hemochromatosis are treated with phlebotomy until satisfactory iron levels are attained. Vitamin C supplementation must be avoided, because it can worsen the disease. Raw seafood should be avoided because *Vibrio vulnificus* infection may occur. Phlebotomy can prevent cirrhosis. Once cirrhosis is present, phlebotomy does not prevent development of hepatocellular carcinoma, which occurs in 30% of patients.

Bardou-Jacquet E, Brissot P: Diagnostic evaluation of hereditary hemochromatosis (HFE and non-HFE). Hematol Oncol Clin North Am 2014; 28: 625.

Barton JC: Hemochromatosis and iron overload. Am J Med Sci 2013; 346: 403.

Elmariah SB, et al: Invasive squamous-cell carcinoma and arsenical keratoses. Dermatol Online J 2008; 14: 24.

Fatmi Z, et al: Burden of skin lesions of arsenicosis at higher exposure through groundwater of Taluka Gambat district Khairpur, Pakistan. Environ Geochem Health 2013; 35: 341.

Liao WT, et al: Differential effects of arsenic on cutaneous and systemic immunity. Carcinogenesis 2009; 30: 1064.

Lin GF, et al: Association of *XPD/ERCC2* $G_{23591}A$ and $A_{35931}C$ polymorphisms with skin lesion prevalence in a multiethnic, arseniasis-hyperendemic village exposed to indoor combustion of high arsenic coal. Arch Toxicol 2010; 84: 17.

Loh TY, et al: An unusual presentation of seborrheic keratoses in a man with hereditary hemochromatosis. Dermatol Online J 2016; 23.

Maiti S, et al: Antioxidant and metabolic impairment result in DNA damage in arsenic-exposed individuals with severe dermatological manifestations in Eastern India. Environ Toxicol 2012; 27: 342.

Majumdar KK, Guha Mazumder DN: Effect of drinking arsenic-contaminated water in children. Indian J Public Health 2012; 56: 223.

Park JY, et al: Metallic discoloration on the right shin caused by titanium alloy prostheses in a patient with right total knee replacement. Ann Dermatol 2013; 25: 356.

Pinto B, et al: Chronic arsenic poisoning following Ayurvedic medication. J Med Toxicol 2014; 10: 395.

Schuhmacher-Wolz U, et al: Oral exposure to inorganic arsenic. Crit Rev Toxicol 2009; 39: 271.

Sengupta SR, et al: Pathogenesis, clinical features and pathology of chronic arsenicosis. Indian J Dermatol Venereol Leprol 2008; 74: 559.

Xia Y, et al: Well water arsenic exposure, arsenic-induced skin lesions and self-reported morbidity in Inner Mongolia. Int J Environ Res Public Health 2009; 6: 1010.

Zamboni P, et al: Hemochromatosis C282Y gene mutation increases the risk of venous leg ulceration. J Vasc Surg 2005; 42:3 09.

Titanium

A titanium-containing ointment caused yellowish papules on the penis in a patient. Titanium screws used for orthopedic procedures, if close to the skin, can cause cutaneous blue-black hyperpigmentation. In cases of degeneration of artificial knee joints, periprosthetic black pigment can be seen, resulting from titanium deposition. Rarely, this pigment may migrate to the skin, resulting in dermal blue-gray patches over the shin. Titanium pigment was recently reported due to intralesional and topical application of triamcinolone in a patient with alopecia areata. Melanin stains are positive, but polarizing foreign material can be seen, and x-ray spectrophotometry reveals titanium in the tissue.

Akimoto M, et al: Metallosis of the skin mimicking malignant skin tumor. Br J Dermatol 2003; 149: 653.

Cohen BE, et al: Dermal titanium dioxide deposition associated with intralesional triamcinolone injection. Am J Dermatopathol 2016; 38: e163.

Dupre A, et al: Titanium pigmentation. Arch Dermatol 1985; 121: 656.

IDIOPATHIC GUTTATE HYPOMELANOSIS (LEUKOPATHIA SYMMETRICA PROGRESSIVA)

Idiopathic guttate hypomelanosis is a common acquired disorder that affects women more frequently than men. It usually occurs after age 40, and its prevalence increases with age, exceeding 90% in Koreans over age 60. The lesions occur chiefly on the shins (Fig. 36.11) and forearms, suggesting that sun exposure plays a role. Widespread lesions have occurred in patients receiving UV

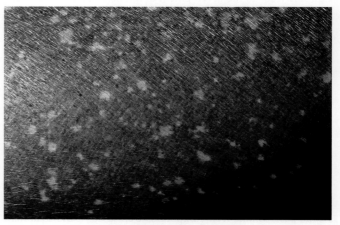

Fig. 36.11 Idiopathic guttate hypomelanosis.

36

phototherapy. Individual lesions are small (average 2–5 mm), hypopigmented macules. They usually number 10–30, but numerous lesions may occur. A few lesions can occur on the face. The lesions are irregularly shaped and sharply defined, similar to depigmented ephelides. Histologically, there is epidermal atrophy and reduced numbers of hypoactive melanocytes. Skin injury with cryotherapy, phenol, and carbon dioxide (CO_2) laser can improve the appearance of the lesions. Topical calcineurin inhibitors, by their stimulation of melanocyte migration and activity, can be therapeutic. Recent reports have investigated the use of tattoo needles to deliver 5-fluorouracil, which may help melanocyte migration by decreasing fibrosis.

Arbache S, et al: Activation of melanocytes in idiopathic guttate hypomelanosis after 5-fluorouracil infusion using a tattoo machine. J Am Acad Dermatol 2018; 78: 212.

Friedland R, et al: Idiopathic guttate hypomelanosis–like lesions in patients with mycosis fungoides. J Eur Acad Dermatol Venereol 2010; 24: 1026.

Kakepis M, et al: Idiopathic guttate hypomelanosis. J Eur Acad Dermatol Venereol 2015; 29: 1435.

Kim SK, et al: Comprehensive understanding of idiopathic guttate hypomelanosis. Int J Dermatol 2010; 49: 162.

Rerknimitr P, et al: Topical tacrolimus significantly promotes repigmentation in idiopathic guttate hypomelanosis. J Eur Acad Dermatol Venereol 2013; 27: 460.

Shilpashree P, et al: Therapeutic wounding: 88% phenol in idiopathic guttate hypomelanosis. Indian Dermatol Online J 2014; 5: 14.

Shin J, et al: The effect of fractional carbon dioxide lasers on idiopathic guttate hypomelanosis. J Eur Acad Dermatol Venereol 2013; 27: e243.

Shin MK, et al: Clinical features of idiopathic guttate hypomelanosis in 646 subjects and association with other aspects of photoaging. Int J Dermatol 2011; 50: 798.

Wambier CG, et al: Therapeutic pearl: 5-fluorouracil tattoo for idiopathic guttate hypomelanosis. J Am Acad Dermatol 2017 Nov 1; ePub ahead of print.

VITILIGO

Vitiligo usually begins in childhood or young adulthood, with a peak onset between ages 10 and 30, but it can occur much earlier in life. About half of cases begin before age 20. The prevalence ranges from 0.5%–1% in most countries, but more than 8% in some regions of India. Although females are disproportionately represented among patients seeking care, it is not known whether they are actually more frequently affected or simply more likely to seek medical care. Vitiligo has developed in recipients of bone marrow transplant or lymphocyte infusions from patients with vitiligo.

Clinical Features

Vitiligo is an acquired pigmentary anomaly of the skin manifested by depigmented white patches surrounded by a normal or a hyperpigmented border. There may be intermediate tan zones or lesions halfway between the normal skin color and depigmentation, so-called trichrome vitiligo, especially in early disease. Blue-gray hyperpigmented macules representing melanin incontinence may be present focally. The hairs in the vitiliginous areas usually become white as well. Rarely, the patches may have a red, inflammatory border. The patches are of various sizes and configurations, but the margins are usually smooth and convex.

Six types of vitiligo have been described, according to the extent and distribution of the involved areas: localized or focal (single or a few macules in one anatomic area, often the trigeminal area, especially in children); segmental (Fig. 36.12); generalized

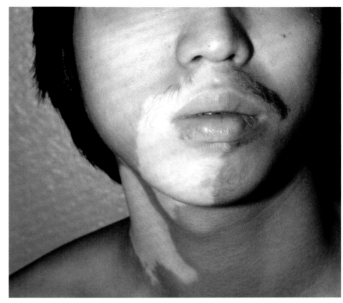

Fig. 36.12 Segmental vitiligo.

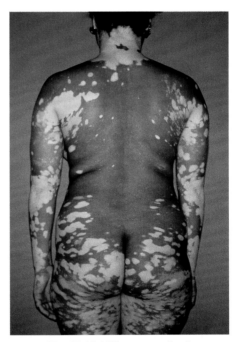

Fig. 36.13 Vitiligo, generalized.

(common symmetric); universal; acrofacial; and mucosal. The generalized pattern is most common (Fig. 36.13). Involvement is symmetric. The most commonly affected sites are the face, upper part of the chest, dorsal aspects of the hands, axillae, and groin. The skin around orifices tends to be affected: the eyes (Fig. 36.14), nose, mouth, ears, nipples, umbilicus, penis, vulva, and anus. Lesions appear at areas of trauma, so vitiligo favors the elbows and knees. Universal vitiligo applies to cases where the entire body surface is depigmented. The acrofacial type affects the distal fingers and facial orifices (lips and tips). Focal vitiligo may affect one nondermatomal site, such as the glans penis, or asymmetrically affect a single region. Focal vitiligo is distinguished from segmental vitiligo which tends to present in a unilateral bklaschkoid pattern

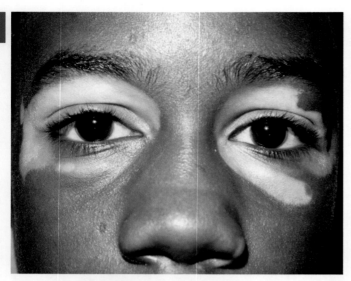

Fig. 36.14 Vitiligo. (Courtesy Steven Binnick, MD.)

Up to 30% of patients with vitiligo have an affected relative; however, it is not inherited as an autosomal dominant or recessive trait, but rather seems to have a multifactorial genetic basis. In addition to the autoimmune pathogenic hypothesis, which is most likely, oxidant/antioxidant and neural theories have been proposed.

The psychological effect of vitiligo should not be underestimated. Patients are frequently anxious or depressed because of the appearance of their skin and the way it affects their social interactions. This is true for both children and adults. Determining how the vitiligo psychosocially affects the patient (if it does) should be documented in the record and could be used as a metric to guide therapy. It is important to treat children who may not be having a psychological complication, because when they become young adults they frequently develop quality-of-life impairment as a result of their vitiligo. Referring the patient to a mental health professional or the National Vitiligo Foundation (www.nvfi.org) may be helpful in this situation.

Histopathology

Biopsies demonstrate an absence of melanocytes. Usually, there is no inflammatory infiltrate, but lichenoid or spongiotic inflammation may be detected at the edge of vitiligo lesions. This explains the scaling or hyperpigmentation sometimes observed around lesions of vitiligo.

Differential Diagnosis

Wood's light is key to evaluation because the lesions of vitiligo are depigmented. Vitiligo must be differentiated from morphea and lichen sclerosus, both of which are hypopigmented and associated with a change in the skin *texture*. Pityriasis alba has a fine scale, is slightly papular, and is poorly defined. Tinea versicolor favors the center back and chest and has a fine scale; yeast and hyphal forms are demonstrable with potassium hydroxide (KOH) examination. The tertiary stage of pinta might easily lead to diagnostic confusion, but a travel history and serologic testing will help elucidate the diagnosis. Patients with severe chronic actinic dermatitis may develop vitiligo-like depigmentation. Chemical leukoderma may closely resemble vitiligo (see later section).

Treatment

Vitiligo can be a frustrating condition to treat. Spontaneous repigmentation occurs in no more than a quarter of cases. Response is typically slow, taking weeks to months of therapy. Segmental vitiligo is reported to be the least responsive form. But, because pigmentary mosaicism can be confused for segmental vitiligo and because pigmentary mosaicism will not respond to therapy, the lack of response of segmental vitiligo to therapy may be overstated.

Treatment of vitiligo can be approached in two steps: (1) stopping progression and (2) repigmenting the depigmented areas. Many treatments may stop the progression, but fewer lead to durable repigmentation. For rapidly progressive, generalized vitiligo, a short course of systemic corticosteroids can be considered. Because early treatment may result in better response, the duration and stability of the vitiligo should be factored into any treatment decision. Specifically, if one hopes to recruit melanocytes from hair follicles in the affected area, if the hair is still pigmented in the vitiligo-affected skin, the likelihood of response may be higher. Some forms of treatment, such as phototherapy, may actually worsen the appearance of the vitiligo initially by pigmenting surrounding normal skin, accentuating the depigmented areas. This is particularly true in persons of lower Fitzpatrick phototypes (I and II). The anatomic location of the lesion predicts the likelihood

earlier in life and be less associated with autoimmune phenomena. Segmental vitiligo must in turn be differentiated from pigmentary mosaicism which is non-inflammatory and will not respond to therapy.

In patients with vitiligo, the initial local loss of pigment may occur around melanocytic nevi and melanomas, the so-called halo phenomenon, but not all patients with halo nevi or melanoma will develop vitiligo. Vitiligo-like leukoderma occurs in about 1% of melanoma patients. In those with previously diagnosed melanoma, this suggests metastatic disease. Paradoxically, however, because the reaction indicates an autoimmune response against melanocytes, patients who develop it have a better prognosis than patients without leukoderma. Lesions of vitiligo burn readily when exposed to the sun due to the lack of pigmentation. However, with repeated sun exposure lesions of vitiligo can tolerate additional UV exposure (photoadaptation), allowing for increasing doses of therapeutic UV phototherapy. Interestingly, the risk of nonmelanoma skin cancer in lesions of vitiligo appears to be lower than in nonaffected skin, likely due to the overactivity of the immune system in vitiligo lesions.

Ocular abnormalities are increased in patients with vitiligo, including iritis and retinal pigmentary abnormalities. Patients have no visual complaints. Idiopathic uveitis is also associated with vitiligo or poliosis.

Vitiligo is an autoimmune disease and affected patients who are at risk for other autoimmune diseases. Autoimmune thyroid disease is the most common autoimmune association and should be screened for at least clinically in every vitiligo patient, although some advocate for baseline blood tests in all patients. In children, it is reasonable not to do regular blood work because this can be very stressful. Other autoimmune conditions include type 1 diabetes mellitus, pernicious anemia, Addison disease, and alopecia areata. Additional screening should be directed by signs and symptoms. Cochlear dysfunction was found in 60% of vitiligo patients in one study. Vitiligo occurs in 13% of patients with the autoimmune polyendocrinopathy–candidiasis–ectodermal dystrophy (APECED) syndrome, caused by mutations in the autoimmune regulator gene (*AIRE*). Polymorphisms in *AIRE* are found more often in vitiligo patients than controls. Patients should be screened with a proper history, review of systems, and physical examination to help evaluate for the associated conditions. In patients with new symptoms or rapidly worsening vitiligo, screening blood work should be done, although some will advocate for blood work at regular intervals even in the absence of symptom change.

of response and the rate of response, independent of the modality used for therapy. Areas with higher density of hair follicles tend to repigment more easily, likely due to melanocyte migration out of the hair follicle. Therefore facial vitiligo has an excellent prognosis, with many patients achieving cosmetically significant improvement. The dorsal hands and feet, by contrast, respond to most forms of treatment only about 10%–20% of the time. Truncal vitiligo demonstrates an intermediate response. Mucosal vitiligo (of the lips) and periungual and dorsal hand vitiligo currently have essentially no reproducibly effective form of medical therapy.

The major problems for the vitiligo patient is appearance. For vitiligo patients who are not concerned about the appearance, non treatment is an option. These patients are treated with sun protection, supplemented with cosmetic camouflage as required. Phototherapy may more dramatically increase the risk of skin cancer in those with lower Fitzpatrick phototypes, suggesting that alternative approaches should be considered. Camouflage is therefore an important therapeutic modality for the vitiligo patient. Self-tanning creams often contain dihydroxyacetone, which is a brown dye that stains the skin. In lower concentrations, it can be used in persons with lower phototype, because it is a golden or tan color (self-tanning products). In high concentrations, it is dark brown and can be used in patients with type V and VI phototypes to camouflage their lesions. Dihydroxyacetone is a stain, so it does not rub off, but rather needs to be reapplied because it is sloughed off from the epidermis (every 5–10 days). Numerous cosmetic products are available and can be effective in making the vitiliginous skin blend completely into the normal surrounding skin. However, it is technically difficult for patients to match their skin color so patients will benefit by consulting an esthetician trained in medical camouflage. Once applied, the products tend to rub off. Application of Cavilon "No Sting Barrier Film" as a spray over the camouflage cosmetic may prevent the product from rubbing off during daily activities.

Topical treatment is appropriate for limited skin areas (<10%–20% body surface area [BSA]). Occlusion of all forms of topical therapy may enhance efficacy. Topical potent to superpotent corticosteroids are used for a 2-month trial. In children, the potency is often lowered and/or the medicine is onbly applied 5 days per week. Up to 80% of patients with facial vitiligo will achieve more than 90% repigmentation. This usually occurs diffusely, not perifollicularly, as occurs on the trunk. On the trunk, only 40% of patients achieve greater than 90% repigmentation. The total length of treatment should be limited to 4–6 months, and the patient must be monitored for acne, atrophy, and telangiectasias. Low dose intralesional triamcinolone has rarely been reported to be effective but caution is advised due to risk of atrophy. The response is reported to be durable and remains after the injections are stopped.

Topical pimecrolimus cream and tacrolimus ointment have been particularly efficacious in treating facial vitiligo. In some series, these have been as effective as superpotent topical corticosteroids and avoid the steroid-induced complications of atrophy and acne. Patients who initiate treatment in the summer have a higher rate of response. Continual application may be required; patients who discontinue treatment may develop new lesions. With topical therapies, new areas of vitiligo appear in untreated areas, suggesting there is no systemic effect. Topical pimecrolimus may enhance the efficacy of narrow-band (NB) UVB in repigmenting facial, but not other, vitiligo. Topical calcipotriene and other vitamin D analogs have had variable results. Alone, these agents lack efficacy. When they are used in combination with other treatments, some studies have demonstrated additive benefit and others no benefit.

Use of NB-UVB two to three times weekly has become the preferred form of phototherapy to treat vitiligo. It avoids the need for prolonged eye protection and the occasional psoralen-induced nausea associated with PUVA. About half of patients will achieve more than 75% repigmentation of the face, trunk, proximal arms, and legs. Hand and foot lesions repigment in less than 25% of patients. Children may have slightly higher response rates than adults. In patients with greater than 20% BSA involvement, only about 5% will show complete repigmentation with phototherapy. Long courses of treatment may be required. Repigmentation from phototherapy may begin after 15–25 treatments; however, significant improvement may take as many as 100–200 treatments (6–24 months). On average, maximum improvement is seen after about 9 months of therapy. If follicular repigmentation has not appeared after 3 months, phototherapy should be discontinued. Home phototherapy is a good option in UV-responsive vitiligo patients. Known photosensitivity, porphyria, and systemic lupus erythematosus are contraindications to phototherapy. Excimer laser phototherapy can be as effective as or more effective than NB-UVB, and the response is more rapid. It can be used on limited areas, avoiding whole-body UV exposure. Whereas 25% of treated patches repigment completely, treatment-resistant areas (elbows, knees, wrists, dorsal hands and feet) have only a 2% rate of at least 75% repigmentation. The addition of topical corticosteroid to excimer laser treatment will enhance efficacy. Topical tacrolimus used in combination with NB-UVB light therapy increases the efficacy, although the combined benefit may wane after 6 months. Afamelanotide, a synthetic melanocyte-stimulating hormone analog delivered by monthly implant, may enhance the efficacy of NB-UVB treatment. Oral khellin or L-phenylalanine and antioxidants have shown variable and not always reproducible benefit.

Topical application of 8-methoxypsoralen at a concentration of 0.01%–0.1%, followed by UVA exposure, may lead to repigmentation. Topical PUVA is used for focal or limited lesions. Inadvertent burns with blistering are frequent complications during treatment in the United States, even when the patient is treated by professionals. For this reason, topical PUVA therapy has been difficult for patients to perform at home. Topical PUVA, however, is widely used in India with success.

In certain situations, use of systemic immunosuppressives may be appropriate in the treatment of vitiligo. This is usually in the setting of rapidly progressive disease, with the goal of reducing the total amount of pigment loss. Systemic corticosteroids are usually used and are tapered over several months. Once the disease is arrested, the patient can be converted to phototherapy. The long-term use of systemic immunosuppressives is not recommended. These initially may control the disease, but with chronic use, unacceptable toxicity often develops.

Surgical treatments can be applied to limited lesions if the previous methods do not prove beneficial, but these are time consuming. Surgery is recommended primarily in patients with treatment-resistant vitiligo, specifically segmental vitiligo, which does not reactivate with injury. Patients must have stable disease (no new lesions or expansion of lesions for 1 year). Surgical procedures are not effective in patients who exhibit Koebner phenomenon or have active vitiligo. Given its expense, surgical treatment should be reserved for exposed skin sites covering less than 2%–3% of BSA. Minigrafting, transplantation of autologous epidermal cell suspension, and ultrathin epidermal grafts have all been used. UV phototherapy is often given after the surgical procedure. In some patients with refractory head and neck lesions of vitiligo, skin injury with various lasers combined with sunlight may lead to repigmentation.

Total Depigmentation

If more than 50%–80% of BSA is affected by vitiligo, the patient can consider depigmentation. This form of treatment should be considered permanent, and the goal is total depigmentation. Limited areas, such as those exposed daily, may be treated, but satellite and distant depigmentation may occur, so the action of the medication cannot be limited to the applied area. Monobenzone (monobenzyl ether of hydroquinone) 20% is applied twice daily for 3–6 months to residual pigmented areas. Up to 10 months may be required to complete the treatment. About one in six patients treated experiences acute dermatitis, usually confined to the still-pigmented areas, but this rarely limits treatment. Consultation with a psychiatrist before the depigmentation is recommended so that the patient understands the implications of the permanent change. Topical 4-methoxyphenol 20% cream (mequinol, monomethylether of hydroquinone) can also be used for depigmentation. The Q-switched laser selectively destroys melanocytes and can also achieve depigmentation. Laser can be combined with a topical depigmenting agent for added efficacy.

CHEMICAL LEUKODERMA (OCCUPATIONAL VITILIGO)

Chemical leukoderma is an acquired, depigmented dermatosis caused by repeated exposure to chemicals. It is frequently misdiagnosed as vitiligo. Patients with vitiligo or a family history of vitiligo are at much greater risk of developing chemical leukoderma. The diagnostic criteria follow:

1. Acquired, vitiligo-like depigmented lesions
2. History of repeated exposure to a specific chemical compound
3. Patterned, vitiligo-like macules conforming to site of exposure
4. Confetti macules

The majority of cases are caused by exposure to aromatic or aliphatic derivatives of phenols and catechols, including paratertiary butylphenol (adhesive in shoes), amylphenol, butylcatechol, and alkyl phenols. However, sulfhydryls, mercurials, arsenics, cinnamic aldehyde, p-phenylenediamine, chloroquine, and azelaic acid have also been implicated. Some of these compounds have a structure similar to tyrosine and may be converted by tyrosine-related protein-1 to compounds toxic to the melanocyte. This process is considered to be different from depigmentation after allergic contact dermatitis. The clinical pattern may be similar to idiopathic vitiligo, but lesions tend to be concentrated in areas of repeated contact with the substance. The first recognized cases of occupational vitiligo occurred in individuals who worked in rubber garments or wore gloves that contained monobenzyl ether of hydroquinone. Phenolic antiseptic detergents used in hospitals and in industrial cleaners have caused chemical leukoderma in janitorial and housekeeping employees (Fig. 36.15). Adhesives and glues containing incriminated chemicals may be found in shoes, wristbands, adhesive tape, and rubber products used in brassieres, girdles, panties, or condoms. Self-sticking bindis (cosmetic used by many Indian women on forehead) have been reported to induce leukoderma from the adhesive material. Also, electrocardiograph electrodes may cause similar round, hypopigmented spots at the site of contact. Radiation therapy and imiquimod application for genital wart treatment can also cause cutaneous depigmentation resembling vitiligo.

The most common location for chemical leukoderma is the face (40% of cases), followed by the hands and feet. The scalp is rarely affected. Hair dye (at rim of scalp but not on scalp), deodorant (axilla), detergent, adhesives (face, bindis), rubber sandals (feet), black socks and shoes (feet), and rubber condoms (penis) are the exposures associated with lesions in various anatomic regions. Pruritus occurs in more than 20% of patients (rare complaint in vitiligo patients). The clinical lesions are sharply marginated macules and patches, often with "confetti" or pea-sized macules seen at the periphery. This clinical pattern is atypical for idiopathic vitiligo and should suggest the diagnosis of chemical leukoderma. More than 25% of patients have lesions outside the area of contact with

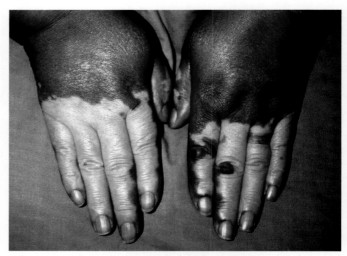

Fig. 36.15 Phenolic depigmentation.

the implicated chemical. In about 10% of patients, new vitiliginous lesions will continue to develop, even after exposure to the chemical is stopped. Treatment is avoidance and measures used for idiopathic vitiligo. Chemical leukoderma in a person without vitiligo has a good prognosis, with repigmentation in up to 75% of cases. If a person with vitiligo develops a chemical leukoderma, repigmentation occurs in only 20% of patients. Histologically, the vitiliginous areas of a chemical leukoderma show an absence of melanocytes identical to lesions of true vitiligo.

Alajlan A, et al: Transfer of vitiligo after allogeneic bone marrow transplantation. J Am Acad Dermatol 2002; 46: 606.

Alikhan A, et al: Vitiligo. J Am Acad Dermatol 2011; 65: 473.

Anbar TS, et al: Beyond vitiligo guidelines. Exp Dermatol 2014; 23: 219.

Anbar TS, et al: Most individuals with either segmental or non-segmental vitiligo display evidence of bilateral cochlear dysfunction. Br J Dermatol 2015; 172: 406.

Ashique KT, Srinivas CR: Resizing blister roof grafts for vitiligo surgery. J Am Acad Dermatol 2014; 71: e39.

Attili VR, Attili SK: Lichenoid inflammation in vitiligo. Int J Dermatol 2008; 47: 663.

Au WY, et al: Generalized vitiligo after lymphocyte infusion for relapsed leukaemia. Br J Dermatol 2001; 145: 1015.

Austin M: Fighting and living with vitiligo. J Am Acad Dermatol 2004; 51: S7.

Aziz Jalali M, et al: Treatment of segmental vitiligo with normal-hair follicle autograft. Med J Islam Repub Iran 2013; 27: 210.

Basak PY, et al: The role of helper and regulatory T cells in the pathogenesis of vitiligo. J Am Acad Dermatol 2009; 60: 256.

Bisen N, et al: Target-like pigmentation after minipunch grafting in stable vitiligo. Indian J Dermatol 2014; 59: 355.

Colucci R, et al: High prevalence of circulation autoantibodies against thyroid hormones in vitiligo and correlation with clinical and historical parameters of patients. Br J Dermatol 2014; 171: 786.

Dayal S, et al: Treatment of childhood vitiligo using tacrolimus ointment with narrowband ultraviolet B phototherapy. Pediatr Dermatol 2016; 33: 646.

Felsten LM, et al: Vitiligo. J Am Acad Dermatol 2011; 65: 493.

Ghosh S, Mukhopadhyay S: Chemical leucoderma. Br J Dermatol 2009; 160: 40.

Grimes PE, et al: The efficacy of afamelanotide and narrowband UV-B phototherapy for repigmentation of vitiligo. JAMA Dermatol 2013; 149: 68.

Hélou J, et al: Fractional laser for vitiligo treated by 10,600 nm ablative fractional carbon dioxide laser followed by sun exposure. Lasers Surg Med 2014; 46: 443.

Hsu S: Camouflaging vitiligo with dihydroxyacetone. Dermatol Online J 2008; 14: 23.

Krüger C, Schallreuter KU: A review of the worldwide prevalence of vitiligo in children/adolescents and adults. Int J Dermatol 2012; 51: 1206.

Li W, et al: Indication of vitiligo after imiquimod treatment of condylomata acuminata. BMC Infect Dis 2014; 14: 329.

Linthorst Homan MW, et al: Impact of childhood vitiligo on adult life. Br J Dermatol 2008; 159: 915.

Martin-Garcia RF, et al: Chloroquine-induced, vitiligo-like depigmentation. J Am Acad Dermatol 2003; 48: 981

Morrison B, et al: Quality of life in people with vitiligo. Br J Dermatol 2017; 177: e338.

Pacific A, Leone G: Photo(chemo)therapy for vitiligo. Photodermatol Photoimmunol Photomed 2011; 27: 261.

Paradisi A et al: Markedly reduced incidence of melanoma and nonmelanoma skin cancer in a nonconcurrent cohort of 10,040 patients with vitiligo. J Am Acad Dermatol 2014; 71: 1110.

Park JH, et al: Clinical course of segmental vitiligo. Ann Dermatol 2014; 26: 61.

Park KK, et al: A review of monochromatic excimer light in vitiligo. Br J Dermatol 2012; 167: 468.

Park OJ, et al: A combination of excimer laser treatment and topical tacrolimus is more effective in treating vitiligo than either therapy alone for the initial 6 months, but not thereafter. Clin Exp Dermatol 2016; 41: 236.

Patel NS, et al: Advanced treatment modalities for vitiligo. Dermatol Surg 2012; 38: 381.

Pavithran K, et al: Report of a case of radiation-induced new-onset vitiligo with collective review of cases in the literature of radiation-related vitiligo. Case Rep Med 2013; 2013: 345473.

Sassi F, et al: Randomized controlled trial comparing the effectiveness of 308-nm excimer laser alone or in combination with topical hydrocortisone 17-butyrate cream in the treatment of vitiligo of the face and neck. Br J Dermatol 2008; 159: 1186.

Sawicki J, et al: Vitiligo and associated autoimmune disease. J Cutan Med Surg 2012; 16: 261.

Shan X, et al: Narrow-band ultraviolet B home phototherapy in vitiligo. Indian J Dermatol Venereol Leprol 2014; 80: 336.

Silverberg NB: Recent advances in childhood vitiligo. Clin Dermatol 2014; 32: 524.

Spritz RA: Six decades of vitiligo genetics. J Invest Dermatol 2012; 132: 268.

Suga Y, et al: Medical pearl: DHA application for camouflaging segmental vitiligo and piebald lesions. J Am Acad Dermatol 2002; 47: 436.

Wang E, et al: Intralesional corticosteroid injections for vitiligo. J Am Acad Dermatol 2014; 71: 391.

Yang Y, et al: Clinical analysis of thyroglobulin antibody and thyroid peroxidase antibody and their association with vitiligo. Indian J Dermatol 2014; 59: 357.

Yazdani Abyaneh M, et al: Narrowband ultraviolet B phototherapy in combination with other therapies for vitiligo. J Eur Acad Dermatol Venereol 2014; 28: 1610.

VOGT-KOYANAGI-HARADA SYNDROME

Vogt-Koyanagi-Harada syndrome (VKHS) is a rare multisystem disease that affects the eyes, skin, auditory system, and central nervous system (CNS). It is less common in patients with type I and II skin. It is twice as common in females and affects all ages. The disease occurs in four phases. First is the prodromal phase or meningoencephalitic phase, with fever, malaise, headache, nausea, and vomiting. The CNS involvement can include meningismus, headaches, mental status changes, cerebrospinal fluid pleocytosis, tinnitus, and dysacusis. Recovery is usually complete. The second, uveitic phase is characterized by anterior and/or posterior uveitis and inflammation of many other parts of the eye. The third, convalescent phase begins 3 weeks to 3 months after the uveitis appears, usually as it begins to improve. This stage is characterized by noncicatricial alopecia, vitiligo-like depigmentation, and poliosis of scalp, eyebrows, eyelashes, and hairs of the axillae. The vitiligo-like lesions occur in only 20%–60% of patients with VKHS. The skin of the back or buttocks may be the initial or only anatomic area involved. The skin lesions must begin after the ocular symptoms to be considered diagnostic. The fourth phase is one of recurrent attacks of uveitis. Most ocular complications result from this stage of the disease, including permanent decreased visual acuity, cataracts, and glaucoma.

VKHS is a cell-mediated autoimmune disease, with the autoantigen(s) thought to be expressed solely in melanin-containing cells. The target antigens may be the tyrosinase family proteins. Supporting this hypothesis are the rare observations that vitiligo, interferon therapy for hepatitis C, and melanoma can all be associated with the appearance of VKHS. Aggressive immunosuppressive therapy with systemic corticosteroids and immunomodulatory medications (cyclosporine, azathioprine, mycophenolate, tacrolimus, infliximab) may preserve ocular function and prevent ocular complications. Th17 CD4+ cells stimulated by high levels of interleukin (IL)–23 and secreting IL-17 are present in VKHS patients with active uveitis. At least 10 patients with psoriasis and VKHS have been reported. They present at an older age than VKHS patients without psoriasis, and they often have HLA genotypes that have been associated with both VKHS and psoriasis (DR4, Cw6).

Abu El-Asrar AM, et al: Prognostic factors for clinical outcomes in patients with Vogt-Koyanagi-Harada disease treated with high-dose corticosteroids. Acta Ophthalmol 2013; 91: e486.

Abu El-Asrar AM, et al: The outcomes of mycophenolate mofetil therapy combined with systemic corticosteroids in acute uveitis associated with Vogt-Koyanagi-Harada disease. Acta Ophthalmol 2012; 90: e603.

Aisenbrey S, et al: Vogt-Koyanagi-Harada syndrome associated with cutaneous malignant melanoma. Graefe's Arch Clin Exp Ophthalmol 2003; 241: 996.

Chuang CT, et al: Reversible alopecia in Vogt-Koyanagi-Harada disease and sympathetic ophthalmia. J Ophthalmic Inflamm Infect 2013; 3: 41.

Liu X, et al: Inhibitory effect of cyclosporin A and corticosteroids on the production of IFN-gamma and IL-17 by T cells in Vogt-Koyanagi-Harada syndrome. Clin Immunol 2009; 131: 333.

O'Keefe GA et al: Vogt-Koyanagi-Harada disease. Surv Ophthalmol 2017; 62: 1.

Takahashi H, et al: Psoriasis vulgaris associated with Vogt-Koyanagi-Harada syndrome. J Dermatol 2013; 40: 933.

Tsuruta D, et al: Inflammatory vitiligo in Vogt-Koyanagi-Harada disease. J Am Acad Dermatol 2001; 44: 129.

Xiang Q, et al: TRAF5 and TRAF3IP2 gene polymorphisms are associated with Behçet's disease and Vogt-Koyanagi-Harada syndrome. PLoS One 2014; 9: e84214.

ALEZZANDRINI SYNDROME

Alezzandrini syndrome is an extremely rare condition (<10 reported cases) characterized by a unilateral degenerative retinal pigment epithelia degeneration, ipsilateral vitiligo on the face, ipsilateral poliosis, and ipsilateral sensorineural deafness. Interestingly, patients with multiple pigmentary anomalies such as Alezzandrini,

Vogt-Kayanagi-Harada, Waardenburg, and vitiligo can all have hearing problems.

Andrade A, Pithon M: Alezzandrini syndrome. Dermatology 2011; 222: 8.

de Jong MA, et al: Hearing loss in vitiligo. Eur Arch Otorhinolaryngol 2017; 274: 2367.

Gupta M, et al: Alezzandrini syndrome. BMJ Case Rep 2011 Aug 17; 2011.

LEUKODERMA

Postinflammatory leukoderma may result from many inflammatory dermatoses, such as pityriasis rosea, psoriasis, herpes zoster, secondary syphilis, and morphea. Sarcoidosis, tinea versicolor, mycosis fungoides, leprosy, scleroderma, and pityriasis lichenoides chronica may all present with hypopigmented lesions (only rarely are these actually depigmented). Burns, scars, postdermabrasion, and intralesional steroid injections with depigmentation are other examples of leukoderma. IL-17 and tumor necrosis factor (TNF)–α synergistically suppress pigmentation-related signaling and melanin production, partly through induction of β-defensin 3, an antagonist for melanocortin 1 (MC1R), and may represent the mechanism by which psoriasis and other inflammatory dermatoses are complicated by hypopigmentation.

Wang CQ, et al: IL-17 and TNF synergistically modulate cytokine expression while suppressing melanogenesis: potential relevance to psoriasis. J Invest Dermatol 2013; 133: 2741.

Yamaguchi Y, Hearing VJ: Melanocytes and their diseases. Cold Spring Harb Perspect Med 2014; 4: a017046.

CONGENITAL DISORDERS OF HYPOPIGMENTATION

Melanosomes are members of the LRO family. Congenital disorders of hypopigmentation can be caused by four groups of genetic defects: (1) mutations in genes controlling melanoblast migration (Waardenburg syndrome); (2) mutations in genes controlling enzymes involved in melanin synthesis (oculocutaneous albinism); (3) mutations in genes of melanosome structural proteins (genes controlling melanosome cell membrane or scaffolding on which melanins are deposited within melanosome—Chédiak-Higashi and Hermansky-Pudlak syndromes); or (4) mutations in genes controlling melanosome-trafficking proteins (surface proteins on melanosome that direct melanosome movement from Golgi complex to melanocyte periphery—Griscelli syndrome). Clinically, this group of disorders can be characterized as generalized (systemic) or localized. Within each of these subgroups are those conditions with associated comorbidities and those without comorbidities (Box 36.1).

Disorders of Melanin Synthesis

The seven genetic forms of nonsyndromal OCA are all caused by disruption of various parts of the melanin synthesis pathway and are all autosomal recessive disorders. Their prevalence varies widely around the world but is estimated at about 1 in 17,000. About 1 in 70 persons carries an OCA mutation. Given the phenotypic overlap of the various forms of OCA, genetic testing is recommended to differentiate the forms. Because both parents are obligate carriers and two thirds of healthy siblings are at risk for being carriers, genetic counseling is recommended. Carriers are asymptomatic.

Disorders of Melanosome Formation and Trafficking

These multisystem syndromes are associated with albinism and are caused by genes that function in intracellular organelle

---

BOX 36.1 Classification of Hypopigmentation Disorders

I. SYSTEMIC HYPOPIGMENTATION (GENERALIZED HYPOPIGMENTATION)

A. Without comorbidities
   i. Oculocutaneous albinism types 1–4
   ii. Griscelli syndrome type 3
B. With comorbidities
   i. Bleeding: Hermansky-Pudlak syndrome
   ii. Infection: Chédiak-Higashi syndrome, Griscelli syndrome, Hermansky-Pudlak syndrome type 2

II. LOCALIZED HYPOPIGMENTATION

A. Without comorbidities
   i. Nevus depigmentosus
   ii. Piebaldism
B. With comorbidities
   i. Deafness: Waardenburg syndrome
   ii. Megacolon and neural disorders: Hirschsprung disease type 2
   iii. Neural disorders: hypomelanosis of Ito

---

formation and movement in a variety of specialized cell types, such as melanocytes, neurons, immune cells, monocytes, platelets, and type II epithelial cells in lungs; therefore there are may extracutaneous signs and symptoms. The silver hair associated with some of these syndromes may demonstrate pigment clumping, allowing the diagnosis to be suspected.

Chédiak-Higashi Syndrome

Chédiak-Higashi syndrome (CHS) is a progressively degenerative, fatal disease characterized by partial oculocutaneous albinism (decreased skin, eye, and hair pigment), giant intracellular granules, pigment clumping in hair shafts, and a bleeding diathesis caused by absent or reduced platelet-dense bodies. There is irregular melanin clumping within hair follicles and on light microscopy and on transmission electron microscopy after the hair is cut longitudinally, large, irregular melanosomes can be seen. This finding can be used to support early diagnosis, although Griscelli can have similar clumping on light microscopy.

CHS presents in childhood, usually with infections of the skin, gut, and lungs due to decreased natural killer (NK)– and T-cell cytotoxicity. Common pathogens are *S. aureus*, streptococcus, gram-negative organisms, *Candida*, and *Aspergillus*. Immunoglobulins, antibody production, and phagocytosis are normal, but neutropenia is common and leukocytes display impaired migration. NK cells are decreased in function, and cytotoxic T-lymphocyte (CTL) cytotoxicity is impaired. The hair of these patients is blond and sparse. The ocular albinism is accompanied by nystagmus and photophobia. In darker-skinned races, affected patients are lighter-skinned than their parents and siblings and may have speckled hyperpigmentation and hypopigmentation.

CHS results from mutations in the *LYST or CHS1* gene, the exact biologic function of which is unknown. The gene must be important in lysosome and LRO trafficking or size regulation. Melanosomes are giant, and platelets, eosinophils, basophils, and monocytes have giant intracellular granules that are azurophilic.

About 85% of patients with CHS develop hemophagocytic lymphohistiocytosis (HLH), referred to as the "accelerated phase." This occurs during infancy or childhood and can be fatal. It is caused by the unfettered proliferation of lymphocytes creating a lymphoma-like condition with fever, anemia, neutropenia, hepatosplenomegaly, and lymphadenopathy. The likelihood of developing HLH is related to the degree of deficiency of CTL cytotoxicity,

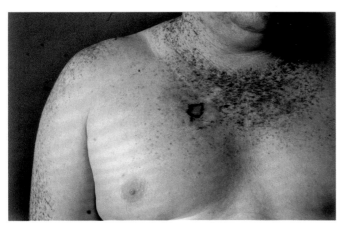

Fig. 36.16 Hermansky-Pudlak syndrome; freckling of V of neck and basal cell carcinoma in Puerto Rican man.

independent of genotype. Hematopoietic stem cell transplantation (HSCT) before the onset of this phase may be lifesaving, and it also prevents the infections. Unfortunately, even with HSCT, if patients with CHS survive into adulthood, they develop progressive neurologic involvement, including dementia, spinocerebellar impairment, parkinsonism, and spastic paraparesis.

Hermansky-Pudlak Syndrome

Hermansky-Pudlak syndrome (HPS) is an autosomal recessive disorder consisting of oculocutaneous albinism, a hemorrhagic diathesis secondary to the absence of dense bodies in platelets. There is progressive accumulation of a ceroid-like material in the reticuloendothelial system and visceral organs. It is hypothesized that this ceroid material can lead to interstitial lung disease (HPS-ILD) and inflammatory bowel disease (HPS-IBD). The hypopigmentation is caused by impaired melanosome trafficking. Patients with this disorder have a history of easy bruisability, epistaxis, gingival bleeding, hemoptysis, and bleeding after various surgical procedures and childbirth. Major bleeding occurs in 40% of patients with HPS.

Currently, nine human genes (for HPS1, *AP3B1* gene, and for HPS subtypes 3–9) have been identified, which, when independently mutated, lead to a clinical picture consistent with HPS. All these genes form protein complexes that regulate vesicle trafficking in the endolysosomal system (LROs). These proteins complex together to form various lysosomal-trafficking protein complexes: AP-3, BLOC-1, BLOC-2, and BLOC-3. Although many of the HPS subtypes share the clinical signs and symptoms previously noted, a few subtypes either lack some of these or have additional unique features that serve to distinguish them from the other HPS subtypes. Mutations in any gene that produces a protein that contributes to a specific BLOC tend to create a similar clinical phenotype. For example, in mice and men, HPS1 and HPS4 (BLOC-3 proteins) and HPS subtypes 3, 5, and 6 (BLOC-2 proteins) have relatively similar phenotypes. The most common subtype is HPS1, which, together with HPS4, accounts for 50% of the known worldwide cases of HPS. One in 21 Puerto Ricans has a mutation (usually 16–base pair [bp] duplication) in the HPS1 gene. HPS accounts for 80% of albinos in Puerto Rico, and 1 in 1800 Puerto Ricans in the northwest region of the country has HPS. HPS1 and HPS4 are clinically similar because together they form the BLOC-3 complex. These are the two most severe forms of HPS. Skin pigmentation can vary from total lack of pigment to lighter hair and skin coloring than in other members of the family. Ocular changes similar to those of OCA can occur, including iris transillumination, hypopigmented retina, visual impairment, horizontal nystagmus, and strabismus. Atypical nevi, acanthosis nigricans–like lesions in the axillae and neck, and trichomegaly also occur. Solar damage, as evidenced by solar lentigines, actinic keratoses, and nonmelanoma skin cancers, occurs in 80% of patients with the 16-bp duplication in HPS1 (Fig. 36.16). Interstitial pulmonary fibrosis, IBD, renal failure, and cardiomyopathy are late complications and can cause premature mortality between ages 20 and 50. About 60% of patients with HPS have pulmonary symptoms, starting at a mean age of 35 years. Pirfenidone, an antifibrotic agent, can slow the progression of pulmonary fibrosis in HPS1 patients with significant residual lung function (initial forced ventilatory capacity >50%). Lung transplantation can be considered.

Hermansky-Pudlak syndrome type 2 is caused by a mutation in the gene (*AP3B1*) coding for the 3βA subunit of AP3, a molecule necessary for normal protein trafficking to the lysosome. HPS2 is notable for immunodeficiency and persistent neutropenia, with recurrent bacterial infections of the upper respiratory system and middle ear, possibly caused by the lack of antigen presentation by the CD1b molecule, because CD1b fails to gain access to the lysosome. Initially, patients may be misdiagnosed as having CHS resulting from pigment dilution and recurrent infections. However, the large intracellular granules of CHS are absent. Mild pulmonary fibrosis and a mild hearing defect can be associated with HPS2.

Patients with HPS3, HPS5, and HPS6 have mild clinical findings, without reported pulmonary or GI involvement. These types are caused by mutations in three proteins that make up BLOC2. HPS7 and HPS8 are very rare and present with a phenotype of oculocutaneous albinism and a bleeding tendency caused by platelet dysfunction. The HPS7 gene (*DTNBP1*) encodes dysbindin; the HPS8 gene is *BLOC1S3*, both BLOC-1 subunits.

Disorders of Melanocyte Transport

Griscelli Syndrome

The myosin-5a/RAB27A/melanophilin tripartite protein complex is required to capture mature melanosomes in the peripheral actin network for subsequent transfer to keratinocytes. Mutation in each of these genes causes one type of Griscelli syndrome (GS), with a distinct clinical phenotype with features unique to each type. All types of GS are rare, autosomal recessive inherited, and characterized by mild skin and hair hypopigmentation (silver hair). Light microscopy of the hair shows irregular pigment clumping. The silvery hair and lack of a bleeding tendency distinguishes Griscelli from HPS, and the lack of immunodeficiency helps differentiate Griscelli from CHS. GS1 is caused by mutations in the *MYO5A* gene encoding the actin-associated myosin Va motor protein. Patients have primary neurologic dysfunction but no immunologic disease. GS1 and Elejalde syndrome are thought to be the same disease. GS2 is caused by mutation in the *RAB27A* gene. Patients have silver hair, infections, and hemophagocytic lymphohistiocytosis (HLH), usually triggered by viruses. Leukocytes infiltrating the brain can cause secondary neurologic disease, but patients have no primary neural defects. GS3 is caused by mutations in melanophilin (*MLPH*) and results only in cutaneous hypopigmentation and silver hair.

Vici Syndrome

Vici is an extremely rare syndrome characterized by hypopigmentation, immunodeficiency, and agenesis of the corpus collosum caused by mutations in the EPG5 gene involved in autophagy.

Çağdaş D, et al: Griscelli syndrome types 1 and 3. Eur J Pediatr 2012; 171: 1527.

Chiang SC, et al: Differences in granule morphology yet equally impaired exocytosis among cytotoxic T cells and NK cells from Chediak-Higashi syndrome patients. Front Immunol 2017; 8: 426.

Cullinane AR, et al: The BEACH is hot: a LYST of emerging roles for BEACH-domain containing proteins in human disease. Traffic 2013; 14: 749.

Cullup T, et al: Recessive mutations in *EPG5* cause Vici syndrome, a multisystem disorder with defective autophagy. Nature Genet 2013; 45: 83.

de Almeida HL, et al: Ultrastructural aspects of hairs of Chediak-Higashi syndrome. J Eur Acad Dermatol Venereol 2017 Dec 10; ePub ahead of print.

Dotta L, et al: Clinical, laboratory and molecular signs of immunodeficiency in patients with partial oculo-cutaneous albinism. Orphanet J Rare Dis 2013; 8: 168.

Durmaz A, et al: Molecular analysis and clinical findings of Griscelli syndrome patients. J Pediatr Hematol Oncol 2012; 34: 541.

Elevli M, et al: Chediak-Higashi syndrome. Turk J Haematol 2014; 31: 426.

Jessen B, et al: The risk of hemophagocytic lymphohistiocytosis in Hermansky-Pudlak syndrome type 2. Blood 2013; 121: 2943.

Kamaraj B, Purohit R: Mutational analysis of oculocutaneous albinism. Biomed Res Int 2014; 2014: 905472.

Kaur S, et al: A rare pigmentary disorder in two non-identical siblings. Dermatol Online J 2014; 20.

Lipsker D: Haemophagocytic lymphohistiocytosis and silvery hair in Griscelli syndrome. Br J Haematol 2016; 175: 11.

Lolli V, et al: Chédiak-Higashi syndrome. Pediatr Radiol 2015; 45: 1253.

Montoliu L, et al: Increasing the complexity. Pigment Cell Melanoma Res 2013; 27: 11.

Nagai K, et al: Clinical characteristics and outcomes of Chédiak-Higashi syndrome. Pediatr Blood Cancer 2013; 60: 1582.

Nouriel A, et al: Griscelli syndrome type 3. Pediatr Dermatol 2015; 32.

Peralta R, et al: Proposal for management and dermoscopy follow-up of nevi in patients affected by oculocutaneous albinism type Ia. Dermatol Pract Concept 2017; 7: 39.

Sánchez-Guiu, et al: Hermansky-Pudlak syndrome. Hamostaseologie 2014; 34: 301.

Seward SL Jr, Gahl WA: Hermansky-Pudlak syndrome. Pediatrics 2013; 132: 153.

Shahzad M, et al: Molecular outcomes, clinical consequences, and genetic diagnosis of oculocutaneous albinism in Pakistani population. Sci Rep 2017; 7: 44185.

Singh A, et al: An Indian boy with Griscelli syndrome type 2. Indian J Dermatol 2014; 59: 394.

Westbroek W, et al: Cellular and clinical report of new Griscelli syndrome type III cases. Pigment Cell Melanoma Res 2011; 25: 47.

Disorders of Melanoblast Migration and Survival

These disorders cause "spotting," with patches of white hair and depigmented skin.

Waardenburg Syndrome

Patients with WS have features of piebaldism, with a white forelock, hypopigmentation, and premature graying, caused by absence of melanocytes in affected areas. Other characteristic findings include synophrys (eyebrows growing together), lateral displacement of the medial canthus (dystopia canthorum), congenital deafness, and ocular changes, including heterochromia iridis (Fig. 36.17). Types I and III are both characterized by dystopia canthorum; in WS type I, white forelock and depigmented skin patches are more frequent; in WS type III, musculoskeletal anomalies (flexion contractures, muscle

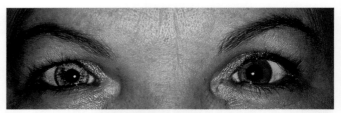

Fig. 36.17 Waardenburg syndrome with heterochromia iridis.

hypoplasia of the upper limbs, and camptodactyly) occur. In WS type II, no dystopia canthorum is observed, but hearing loss and heterochromia iridis are more frequently found. WS type IV is identical to type I, except for its association with Hirschsprung disease (congenital megacolon), because the migration of neural crest cells into the Auerbach plexus requires *EDN3/EDNRB* and *SOX10*. *SOX10* mutations are associated with neurologic defects, and there is a poor phenotype/genotype correlation in *SOX10*-associated WS. Developmental delay occurs in many of these patients, suggesting that other genes required for neural development may influence *SOX10* mutation–associated phenotype. This association between WS type IV caused by *SOX10* and neurologic disease has been termed *PCWH* (peripheral demyelinating neuropathy, central demyelinating leukodystrophy, Waardenburg syndrome, Hirschsprung disease).

Six genes are associated with WS. Types I and III are caused by mutations in the *PAX3* gene, encoding a transcription factor. Most cases of WS type II are caused by mutations in the *MITF* gene; however, some, more mildly affected patients with mutations in *SOX10*, *EDN3*, *EDNRB*, and *SNA12* may present as WS type II. WS type IV is caused either by a heterozygous mutation in the *SOX10* gene or by homozygous mutations in the endothelin-3 (*EDN3*) or the endothelin B receptor (*EDNR3*) gene. These mutations impair the ability of melanoblasts to reach their final target sites (inner ear, eye, skin) during embryogenesis.

Piebaldism

Piebaldism is a rare, autosomal dominant syndrome with variable phenotype, presenting at birth. The characteristic clinical features are a white forelock and patchy absence of skin pigment. The depigmented lesions are congenital and static (thus differentiating from vitiligo) and characteristically occur on the anterior and posterior trunk, mid–upper arm to wrist, midthigh to midcalf, and shins (Fig. 36.18). A characteristic feature of piebaldism is the presence of hyperpigmented macules within the areas lacking pigmentation and also on normally pigmented skin. The depigmented lesions may repigment spontaneously, or especially after injury. The white forelock is a triangular or diamond-shaped midline white macule on the frontal scalp or forehead, and it is the only manifestation in 80%–90% of patients. The medial portions of the eyebrows and eyelashes may be white. Histologically, melanocytes are completely absent in the white macules.

Piebaldism is caused by mutations in the *KIT* gene. The phenotypic differences between families are caused by different locations of mutations in the gene. A mild phenotype occurs in cases associated with haploinsufficiency or a truncated mutation in the TK domain. Severe phenotypes are associated with dominant-negative inhibition caused by a missense mutation in the TK domain. The white lesions may respond to camouflage cosmetics or surgical corrections (see Vitiligo). Rarely, neurofibromatosis type I has been associated with piebaldism.

Agarwal S, Ojha A: Piebaldism. Indian Dermatol Online J 2012; 3: 144.

Horner ME, et al: The spectrum of oculocutaneous disease. J Am Acad Dermatol 2014; 70: 795.e1.

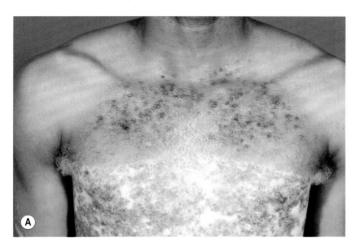

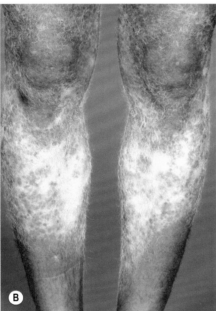

Fig. 36.18 (A and B) Piebaldism.

Jelena B, et al: Phenotypic variability in Waardenburg syndrome resulting from a 22q12.23-q13.1 microdeletion involving *SOX10*. Am J Med Genet 2014; 164: 1512.
Oiso N, et al: Piebaldism. J Dermatol 2013; 40: 330.
Park SY, et al: Piebaldism with neurofibromatosis type I. Ann Dermatol 2014; 26: 264.
Pingault V, et al: Review and update of mutations causing Waardenburg syndrome. Hum Mutat 2010; 31: 391.
Sleiman R, et al: Poliosis circumscripta. J Am Acad Dermatol 2013; 69: 625.
Yaar M, et al: Cutaneous pigmentation in health and disease: novel and well-established players. J Invest Dermatol 2013; 133:11.

OCULOCUTANEOUS ALBINISM

Oculocutaneous albinism (OCA) is an autosomal recessively inherited trait with reduction or absence of melanin in skin, hair, and eyes. Eye problems are frequently present, including moderate to severe impairment of visual acuity, nystagmus, strabismus, and photophobia. The cutaneous phenotype of the various forms of albinism is broad, but the ocular phenotype is reasonably specific in most forms.

The most serious sequelae of albinism are gross visual disturbances and increased risk for development of skin cancer. All persons with OCA and their parents should be educated regarding aggressive sun protection with sunscreens, appropriate clothing, and sun avoidance. Vitamin D supplementation may be required due to sun avoidance. Patients should be examined for skin lesions suspicious for melanoma and nonmelanoma skin cancer. Dermoscopy may be challenging in OCA patients given the lack of pigment, but a recent report proposes biopsying any nevus with a different pattern and any changing nevus and to consider reflectance confocal microscopy. A number of syndromes associated with albinism can also cause premature mortality from impaired functioning of other involved organs and systems.

Oculocutaneous Albinism 1. OCA1 results from mutations in the tyrosinase gene and accounts for approximately 40% of OCA worldwide. It is the most severe form of albinism and is the most common type of albinism in Japanese, non-Hispanic Caucasians and Europeans with a prevalence of about 1 in 40,000. Affected patients are homozygous for the mutant gene or are compound heterozygotes for different mutations in the tyrosinase gene *(TYR)*. OCA1 is divided into two forms: OCA1A and OCA1B. At birth, these are indistinguishable. OCA1A is the most severe form, with complete absence of tyrosinase activity and of melanin in the skin and eyes. Visual acuity is decreased to 20/400. The hair, eyelashes, and eyebrows are white, and the skin is white and does not tan (Fig. 36.19). Irises are light blue to pink and fully translucent. Amelanotic nevi may be present. In OCA1B, tyrosinase activity is greatly reduced but not absent. Affected patients may show an increase in skin, hair, and eye color beginning at age 1–3 years, and they can tan. Iris color may also darken over time. OCA1B was originally called "yellow mutant" albinism. Temperature-sensitive OCA (OCA1-TS) is considered a variant of OCA1B; it results from mutations in *TYR* that produce an enzyme with limited activity below 37°C (98°F) and no activity above this temperature. Affected patients have white hair, skin, and eyes at birth. At puberty, dark hair develops in cooler acral areas: legs, arms, and chest. Visual acuity is not as severely affected in OCA1B.

Oculocutaneous Albinism 2. *OCA2* has a prevalence of 1 in 36,000 in white Europeans, but as much as 1 in 4000 in some parts of Africa. It is the most common form of OCA, accounting for approximately 50% of OCA worldwide. *OCA2* was formerly called "tyrosinase-positive" albinism or "brown OCA." Inheritance is autosomal recessive and results from mutations in the *OCA2* gene, formerly known as the P-gene. The *OCA2* gene encodes an integral melanosomal protein that is important for normal biogenesis of melanosomes and normal processing and transport of melanosomal proteins such as tyrosinase and tyrosinase-related protein 1 (TYRP1). The cutaneous phenotype of *OCA2* patients is broad, ranging from near-normal pigmentation to virtually no pigment. Newborns have pigmented hair. Nevi and ephelides are common. Pink irises are usually not seen. Visual defects are not as severe as in OCA1. Pigmentation increases with age, and visual acuity improves from infancy to adolescence. Prader-Willi and Angelman syndromes are caused by deletions in the chromosomal region contiguous to and sometimes including the *OCA2* gene. About 1% of patients with these syndromes also have *OCA2*.

Oculocutaneous Albinism 3. OCA3 is caused by mutations in the *TYRP1* gene. TYRP1 is involved in the maintenance of melanosome structure and affects melanocyte proliferation and cell death. It also is an essential cofactor for tyrosinase activity. This form of OCA has been most frequently found in African patients and was called "rufous" or red OCA. Patients have red hair and reddish brown skin. Visual abnormalities may not be detectable.

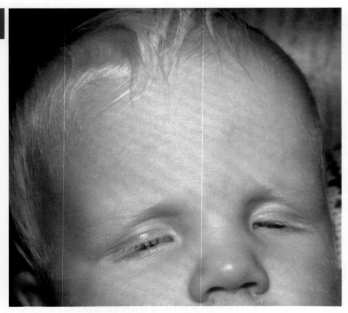

Fig. 36.19 Oculocutaneous Albinism.

Oculocutaneous Albinism 4.   OCA4 is caused by mutations in the *MATP* (also known as *SLC45A2*) gene encoding a membrane-associated protein, predicted to span the membrane 12 times and to function as a transporter. Patients are hypopigmented to a variable degree and are phenotypically identical to patients with OCA2. Visual acuity is decreased, and nystagmus is found in many but not all patients.

Oculocutaneous Albinism 5.   OCA5 has been mapped to the 4q24. It has been described in a Pakistani family with golden hair, white skin, nystagmus, photophobia, and impaired visual acuity.

Oculocutaneous Albinism 6.   OCA6 is caused by mutations in *SLC24A5*, the gene product of which is a solute carrier protein important in melanosomal architecture, linking closely the structure of the melanosome to melanin synthesis. This form of OCA is found in diverse ethnicities, and the phenotype is heterogeneous with hair color from white to blond to dark brown. Most mutations occur in position 111 of the gene, with a Thr111 mutation in European or American OCA and Ala111 in African or Asian OCA6.

Oculocutaneous Albinism 7.   OCA7 is caused by mutation in the C10 or Fll gene, the gene product of which is a member of the leucine-rich repeat proteins.

37 Dermatologic Surgery

Dermatology has always been a surgically oriented specialty. Although procedures such as curettage, biopsy, destruction, and excision have been key components of the field, the practice has evolved to include a greater number and extent of surgical procedures. This progression can be attributed to a variety of factors. Dermatologists have a greater understanding of cutaneous pathology, which places them in a unique role to manage complex surgical procedures that arise in the skin. In addition, outpatient dermatologic surgery has been shown to be cost-effective, safe, and efficacious, delivering a greater degree of patient convenience, particularly compared with other fields. The American Board of Dermatology therefore mandates surgical exposure and experience for all residents in dermatology residency programs. Furthermore, with the Accreditation Council for Graduate Medical Education (ACGME) accreditation of Micrographic Surgery and Dermatologic Oncology fellowships, dermatologic surgery has become recognized as a mainstream medical option for patients. This chapter and Chapters 38 and 39 provide a survey of procedures, indications, and appropriate management within the spectrum of the dermatologic surgery field.

Hanke CW, et al: Current status of surgery in dermatology. J Am Acad Dermatol 2013; 69: 972.
Hansen TJ, et al: Patient safety in dermatologic surgery. J Am Acad Dermatol 2015; 73: 1.

PREPARATION FOR SURGERY

A thorough and complete preoperative evaluation is required before performing any surgical procedure. A detailed medical history must be obtained, including information on drug allergies, current medications (including herbal or natural supplements), smoking/tobacco status, presence of a pacemaker or implantable cardioverter/defibrillator, recently implanted prosthetic devices, history of prior wound infection or perioperative bleeding, and history of endocarditis or cardiac valvular or congenital malformation.

Anticoagulants

Much has been written regarding the role of antithrombotic agents (including both antiplatelet and anticoagulant medications) and surgical bleeding. Dermatologists are frequently presented with the dilemma of whether to discontinue blood thinners in the setting of surgery. Data and multiple reviews have shown that continuous treatment with blood thinners perioperatively in patients undergoing Mohs and cutaneous surgery is not associated with an increase in surgical complications leading to significant morbidity. In contrast, discontinuation of these medications may increase the risk of catastrophic cerebral and cardiovascular complications. Multiple authors believe that the potential adverse effects of discontinuing essential medical blood thinners far outweigh the potential side effects of surgical bleeding (e.g., managing a postoperative hematoma). In fact, despite some surgeons' claims to the contrary, studies have demonstrated that blinded surgeons are unable to identify intraoperatively which patients are taking anticoagulation medication based on the subjective amount of surgical oozing. As such, it is recommended that patients be maintained on all medically necessary blood thinners during cutaneous surgery. In contrast, patients taking aspirin for primary prevention may discontinue use 2 weeks before any surgical procedure.

Herbal supplements are becoming increasingly popular with patients who are looking for a "natural" option to traditional medication. Patients may not readily volunteer that they are taking these supplements, either because they do not characterize supplements as medication or because they are concerned that physicians will not be accepting of alternative treatments. Therefore physicians should ask patients specifically if they are taking any supplements. Ginkgo, garlic, ginseng, ginger, and vitamin E may increase the risk of perioperative bleeding. These herbal supplements are not medically necessary, so patients should discontinue them for several weeks before undergoing dermatologic surgery.

Brown DG, et al: A review of traditional and novel oral anticoagulant and antiplatelet therapy for dermatologists and dermatologic surgeons. J Am Acad Dermatol 2015; 72: 524.
Callahan S, et al: The management of antithrombotic medication in skin surgery. Dermatol Surg 2012; 38: 1417.
Chang TW, et al: Complications with new oral anticoagulants dabigatran and rivaroxaban in cutaneous surgery. Dermatol Surg 2015; 41: 784.
Dinehart SM, Henry L: Dietary supplements: altered coagulation and effects on bruising. Dermatol Surg 2005; 31: 819.
Gill JF, et al: Tobacco smoking and dermatologic surgery. J Am Acad Dermatol 2013; 68: 167.
O'Neill JL, et al: Postoperative hemorrhage risk after outpatient dermatologic surgery procedures. Dermatol Surg 2014; 40: 74.
Otley CC: Perioperative evaluation and management in dermatologic surgery (review). J Am Acad Dermatol 2006; 54: 119.
Palamaras I, Semkova K: Perioperative management of and recommendations for antithrombotic medications in dermatological surgery. Br J Dermatol 2015; 172: 597.
Plovanich M, Mostaghimi A: Novel oral anticoagulants: what dermatologists need to know. J Am Acad Dermatol 2015; 72: 535.
West SW, et al: Cutaneous surgeons cannot predict blood-thinner status by intraoperative visual inspection. Plast Reconstr Surg 2002; 110: 98.
Zwiebel SJ, et al: The incidence of vitamin, mineral, herbal, and other supplement use in facial cosmetic patients. Plast Reconstr Surg 2013; 132: 78.

Surgical Site Infection

As a general rule, wound infections associated with skin surgery procedures occur at an extremely low rate. There is an extensive literature documenting the safety and overall low infection rate of skin procedures (ranging from surgical excisions, to laser, to liposuction). Postoperative wound infections, when they do occur, most commonly appear in the first 4–10 days after the procedure. In some cases, making a proper diagnosis of infection can be challenging, with other conditions being mimickers (e.g., allergic contact dermatitis or fibrin deposition over the granulation wound).

The Centers for Disease Control and Prevention defines a surgical site infection as occurring within 30 days of the procedure and involving only skin and subcutaneous tissue of the incision. In addition, at least one of the following criteria should also be present: (1) purulent drainage from the incision site, (2) organism isolation from culture of the fluid drainage or tissue, (3) pain/

Treatment of Wound Infection

Postoperative surgical site infection is uncommon in dermatologic surgery procedures, with an incidence of 1%–3%. Infections typically present 4–7 days after surgery with increased erythema, tenderness, warmth, and purulent drainage. Sutures can be removed to allow for drainage of exudate. In cases where infection leads to dehiscence, the wound can be packed or allowed to heal by second intention. Scar revision can be performed at a later date should that be necessary. A culture should be performed before initiating empiric antibiotics to determine sensitivities.

Staphylococcus aureus is the most common pathogen, and cephalexin or dicloxacillin is an appropriate first-line treatment. Patients with a penicillin allergy can be treated with clindamycin. Although this antibiotic has been associated with colitis, the short courses of clindamycin typically used with surgical site infection generally do not present a problem. In communities or institutions with a high incidence of methicillin-resistant *S. aureus* (MRSA), antibiotic choice can be modified based on community sensitivities (e.g., doxycycline, trimethoprim-sulfamethoxazole [TMP-SMX]). Ciprofloxacin can be used for infections with a higher likelihood of gram-negative or *Pseudomonas* organisms (e.g., ear). Antibiotic choice should be modified based on culture results.

The use of topical antibiotics after routine skin surgery has not been shown to reduce the incidence of surgical site infection. Several studies have demonstrated that petrolatum was as effective as topical antibiotics in terms of incidence of infection. In addition, many patients on topical antibiotics had a higher incidence of allergic contact dermatitis. Finally, studies have shown the overall cost saving of switching from postoperative bacitracin to petrolatum. As such, routine use of topical antibiotics ought to be avoided in the postoperative period.

Antibiotic Prophylaxis

Dermatologists performing cutaneous surgery are often faced with the decision of whether to prescribe prophylactic antibiotics. The main issues surrounding antibiotic prophylaxis are prevention of surgical site infections and reduction of the risk of endocarditis or contamination of prosthetic devices in high-risk patients. As a general rule, wound infections associated with skin surgery procedures occur at an extremely low rate. Although reducing infection is one objective in the use of antibiotics, dermatologists must consider the risks of such treatment, including adverse drug reactions, serious drug reactions, drug interactions, development of resistant strains of bacteria, and increased cost.

Determining the indications for antibiotic prophylaxis for surgical site infections requires an understanding of the various types of wound that the dermatologist may encounter. Wounds can be categorized into the following four groups:

1. Clean wounds (class I) are created on normal skin using clean or sterile technique. Examples include excision of neoplasms, noninflamed cysts, biopsies, and most cases of Mohs surgery. The majority of dermatologic surgery falls into this category. The infection rate of these wounds is less than 5%. Of note, this incidence is based on general surgery cases, which are often of longer duration and a greater extent than most dermatologic procedures. This explains the lower actual infection rate in dermatologic surgery, which is in the 1%–3% range.
2. Clean-contaminated wounds (class II) are created on contaminated skin or any mucosal or moist intertriginous surface, such as the oral cavity, upper respiratory tract, axilla, or perineum. The infection rate of these wounds is 10%.

3. Contaminated wounds (class III) involve visibly inflamed skin with or without nonpurulent discharge and have an infection rate of 20%–30%. Examples included inflamed cysts or traumatic wounds.
4. Infected wounds (class IV) have contaminated foreign bodies, purulent discharge, or devitalized tissue. Examples included necrotic tumors, ruptured cysts, or active hidradenitis suppurativa. These wounds have an infection rate of 40%.

Clean (class I) wounds, which constitute the vast majority of dermatologic surgery procedures, do not require antibiotic prophylaxis.

Although antibiotic prophylaxis in clean-contaminated (class II) wounds is not a clear issue, most cases do not require routine antibiotics. It is preferable to treat infections should they arise (because these are not a common occurrence, even in class II wounds), rather than expose all patients to antibiotics and the increased rate of drug-related adverse events. Some exceptions to this that have been advocated include surgical cases that violate mucosal membranes (oral, nasal, anogenital) and patients with heavily colonized skin (atopic dermatitis, infected skin), as well as those in whom a wound infection would result in significant morbidity. However, dermatologic surgeons do not universally agree on these exceptions, and the role for antibiotic prophylaxis is still debated.

In contaminated (class III) and infected (class IV) wounds, antibiotics serve a therapeutic, rather than a prophylactic, role and should be used routinely in these cases.

Antibiotic Selection and Timing

To achieve optimal prophylaxis, antibiotics should be in the bloodstream, and thus at the surgical site, at the time of incision. Antibiotics given at the conclusion of the procedure are not as effective in preventing infection, because they are not incorporated into the coagulum of the wound. Once the surgical wound is closed, the risk of infection decreases significantly. Most dermatologic procedures are of short duration, so a single preoperative dose of antibiotics 1 hour before the start of the case is sufficient. In rare cases with an extended dermatologic procedure, a second dose of antibiotics can be administered 6 hours postoperatively.

The choice of antibiotic is based on the most likely causative organism at the surgical site (Table 37.1). *S. aureus* is the most common wound infection in cutaneous surgery. Other pathogens to consider in some situations include *Streptococcus viridans* (oral mucosa) and *Escherichia coli* (perineal and genital location).

First-generation cephalosporins are an ideal initial choice for the treatment of wound infection because of their coverage of

TABLE 37.1 Antibiotic Prophylaxis for Heavily Colonized or High-Risk Patients

Surgical Site	Antibiotic	Regimen (Single Dose 1 Hour Preoperatively)
Skin	Cephalexin	1 g orally
	Dicloxacillin	1 g orally
	Clindamycin	300 mg orally
	Vancomycin	500 mg intravenously
Oral and respiratory mucosa	Cephalexin	1 g orally
	Amoxicillin	1 g orally
	Clindamycin	300 mg orally
Gastrointestinal and genitourinary mucosa	Cephalexin	1 g orally
	Trimethoprim-sulfamethoxazole	1 double-strength tablet orally
	Ciprofloxacin	500 mg orally

TABLE 37.2 Endocarditis Prophylaxis Regimen (Single Dose 1 Hour Preoperatively)

Situation	Agent	Adults	Children
Able to take oral medication	Amoxicillin	2 g	50 mg/kg
Unable to take oral medication	Ampicillin	2 g IM/IV	50 mg/kg IM/IV
	or		
	Cefazolin or ceftriaxone	1 g IM/IV	50 mg/kg IM/IV
Allergic to penicillins or ampicillin and able to take oral medication	Cephalexin*	2 g	50 mg/kg
	or		
	Clindamycin	600 mg	20 mg/kg
	or		
	Azithromycin or clarithromycin	500 mg	15 mg/kg
Allergic to penicillins or ampicillin and unable to take oral medication	Cefazolin or ceftriaxone*	1 g IM/IV	50 mg/mg IM/IV
	or		
	Clindamycin	600 mg IM/IV	20 mg IM/IV

Modified from Wilson W, et al: Prevention of infective endocarditis. Circulation 2007; 116: 1736–1754.
*Cephalosporins should not be used in patients with a history of anaphylaxis, angioedema, or urticaria with penicillins or ampicillin.
IM, Intramuscularly; IV, intravenously.

staphylococcal organisms, common gram-negative organisms such as *E. coli*, and certain *Proteus* species. Cephalosporins are rapidly absorbed when taken orally and have good tissue penetration. Their estimated cross-reactivity in penicillin-allergic patients is 5%–10%.

Isoxazolyl penicillins, such as dicloxacillin and nafcillin, can also be used because they provide coverage for most strains of streptococci and β-lactamase–producing bacterial strains, such as *S. aureus*. Aminopenicillins, such as ampicillin and amoxicillin, have better gram-negative, enterococcal, and group A streptococcal coverage. However, aminopenicillins are not effective against β-lactamase–producing bacteria and thus are used more often in procedures involving oral mucosa.

Clindamycin, macrolides (e.g., erythromycin, azithromycin), TMP-SMX, and ciprofloxacin can all be considered in patients with a penicillin or cephalosporin allergy, with the specific choice based on the site of surgery and thus the presumed causative organism. Vancomycin is generally limited to those cases where MRSA is suspected, because it requires intravenous administration and adjustment in patients with impaired renal function.

Endocarditis Prophylaxis

The American Heart Association (AHA) updated its recommendations on infective endocarditis (IE) prophylaxis in 2007. The overall conclusions were that bacteremia from daily activities is much more likely to cause IE than bacteremia associated with dental procedures, and that far fewer patients are now recommended to have antibiotic prophylaxis. Antibiotic prophylaxis has been limited to patients with the conditions listed in Box 37.1. All other cardiac conditions, including mitral valve prolapse and other forms of congenital heart disease, no longer require prophylaxis for any procedure.

Antibiotic prophylaxis is reasonable when procedures involve manipulation of gingival tissue, perforation of oral mucosa, or incision or biopsy of the respiratory mucosa, or when performed on infected skin, but only in patients with underlying cardiac conditions associated with the highest risk of adverse outcome, as outlined in Box 37.1. Antibiotic prophylaxis solely to prevent IE is not recommended for gastrointestinal or genitourinary procedures. The AHA reaffirmed its 1997 statement regarding medical procedures, including incision or biopsy of surgically scrubbed skin, that do not require antibiotic prophylaxis. Antibiotic prophylactic regimens for those select high-risk patients should be a single dose of antibiotic administered 1 hour before the procedure (Table 37.2).

BOX 37.1 Cardiac Conditions Associated With Highest Endocarditis Risk

Prosthetic cardiac valve or prosthetic material used for cardiac valve repair
Previous infectious endocarditis
Congenital heart disease (CHD)*
- Unrepaired cyanotic CHD, including palliative shunts and conduits
- Completely repaired congenital heart defect with prosthetic material or device, during the first 6 months after the procedure
- Repaired CHD with residual defects at the site or adjacent to the site of a prosthetic patch or prosthetic device (which inhibit endothelialization)

Cardiac transplantation recipients who develop cardiac valvulopathy

*Except for conditions listed above, antibiotic prophylaxis is not recommended for any other form of CHD.
Modified from Wilson W, et al: Prevention of infective endocarditis. Circulation 2007; 116: 1736–1754.

There are no formal guidelines regarding the use of antibiotics in patients with orthopedic prosthetic devices undergoing dermatologic surgery. However, guidelines for dental procedures in patients with joint replacement can be extrapolated to certain procedures. Patients with joint replacement probably do not need prophylactic antibiotics for clean wounds. If mucosa is invaded, prophylaxis may be appropriate and reasonable in the small number of patients who might be at high risk of joint infection. Consultation with orthopedic surgery is appropriate in determining whether antibiotic prophylaxis is necessary.

American Dental Association, American Academy of Orthopedic Surgeons: Antibiotic prophylaxis for dental patients with total joint replacements. J Am Dent Assoc 2003; 134: 895.

Bae-Harboe YS, Liang CA: Perioperative antibiotic use of dermatologic surgeons in 2012. Dermatol Surg 2013; 39: 1592.

Levender MM, et al: Use of topical antibiotics as prophylaxis in clean dermatologic procedures. J Am Acad Dermatol 2012; 66: 445.

Lilly E, Schmults CD: A comparison of high- and low-cost infection-control practices in dermatologic surgery. Arch Dermatol 2012; 148: 859.

Maragh SL, et al: Antibiotic prophylaxis in dermatologic surgery. Dermatol Surg 2005; 31: 83.

Maragh SL, Brown MD: Prospective evaluation of surgical site infection rate among patients with Mohs micrographic surgery without the use of prophylactic antibiotics. J Am Acad Dermatol 2008; 59: 275.

Rogers HD: Prospective study of wound infections in Mohs micrographic surgery using clean surgical technique in the absence of prophylactic antibiotics. J Am Acad Dermatol 2010; 63: 842.

Rossi AM, Mariwalla K: Prophylactic and empiric use of antibiotics in dermatologic surgery. Dermatol Surg 2012; 38: 1898.

Saco M, et al: Topical antibiotic prophylaxis for prevention of surgical wound infections from dermatologic procedures: a systematic review and meta-analysis. J Dermatolog Treat 2015; 26: 151.

Wilson W, et al: Prevention of infective endocarditis. Circulation 2007; 116: 1736.

Wright TI, et al: Antibiotic prophylaxis in dermatologic surgery. J Am Acad Dermatol 2008; 59: 464.

Preoperative Antisepsis

Many surgical preparations are available for preoperative antisepsis. Alcohol is frequently used for minor clean procedures, such as biopsies. However, because it has only weak antimicrobial activity, alcohol is not recommended for more extensive procedures.

Chlorhexidine has a broad spectrum against gram-positive and gram-negative organisms, a rapid onset of activity, and sustained residual activity even after being wiped off, and it is nonstaining. Chlorhexidine has been reported to cause both ototoxicity and keratitis from direct tympanic or ocular contact. However, this is mainly in patients under general anesthesia who cannot respond to immediate irritation associated with ocular contact, a problem that is avoided in most dermatologic procedures performed under local anesthesia.

Betadine (povidone-iodine) and all iodine-containing preparations have an excellent bactericidal activity within several minutes of application. However, these agents are often irritating to the skin, leave a residual color, can be absorbed in premature infants, and must dry before the procedure if they are to act as an effective antimicrobial agent.

Hexachlorophene is not bactericidal against many gram-negative organisms. It has the potential for neurotoxicity in children and teratogenicity in pregnancy. Hydrogen peroxide has no significant antiseptic properties, and thus it is not suitable for sterile skin preparation.

If hair must be removed before surgery, this should be done in a manner that does not leave open skin (cuts or scratches), which can serve as a conduit for infection. Preoperative shaving has been associated with a higher rate of bacterial infection secondary to cutting of the skin surface.

Dumville JC, et al: Preoperative skin antiseptics for preventing surgical wound infections after clean surgery. Cochrane Database Syst Rev 2015; 4: CD003949.

Echols K, et al: Role of antiseptics in the prevention of surgical site infections. Dermatol Surg 2015; 41: 667.

Kamel C, et al: Preoperative skin antiseptic preparations for preventing surgical site infections. Infect Control Hosp Epidemiol 2012; 33: 608.

Anesthesia

Anesthetics work by blocking sodium influx into neurons and preventing depolarization and blockage of action potential. Small, unmyelinated C fibers, which carry pain and temperature sensation, are more easily blocked than larger, myelinated A fibers, which carry pressure sensation and motor function. This difference translates clinically, with patients under local anesthesia not experiencing pain from the sharp incision, but still maintaining the sensation of pressure during the procedure.

All local anesthetics have a similar structure, consisting of three parts: an aromatic hydrophobic ring, intermediate chain, and amine end. The aromatic hydrophobic portion is lipophilic and facilitates diffusion through nerve cell membranes, correlating to the potency of the anesthesia. The hydrophilic amine end contributes to the aqueous solubility of the anesthetic and is involved in binding of the molecule to the sodium channel. The intermediate chain consists of either an amide or an ester. Amides are metabolized by hepatic microsomal enzymes, and esters are metabolized in plasma by pseudocholinesterase and excreted by the kidney.

The choice of anesthetic is based on a variety of factors, including patient allergy, renal or hepatic impairment, and type of procedure being performed. The "workhorse" anesthetic of dermatologic surgery is lidocaine, because of its rapid onset of action and intermediate duration of action. Longer-acting anesthetics, such as bupivacaine, have a delayed onset of action, but can be used in special procedures or in combination with lidocaine to maximize duration of anesthesia.

All local anesthetics, with the exception of cocaine and prilocaine, cause vasodilation from relaxation of smooth muscle. As a result, patients experience increased surgical bleeding and shorter duration of action as the anesthesia is cleared from the surgical site because of vasodilation. Epinephrine, which causes vasoconstriction, is often added to local anesthetics to decrease bleeding, increase duration of anesthesia, and reduce systemic side effects caused by systemic absorption. Concentrations of 1:100,000 to 1:400,000 are typically used, with lower concentrations having fewer side effects while still maintaining clinical efficacy. The vasoconstrictive effect of epinephrine takes 15 minutes for onset, so the surgeon must allow adequate time before starting the procedure. Epinephrine is a strong α- and β-adrenergic receptor agonist and has an absolute contraindication in hyperthyroidism and pheochromocytoma. Large amounts of epinephrine must be used cautiously in patients with severe hypertension or narrow-angle glaucoma, as well as in pregnancy. Patients taking β-blockers, monoamine oxidase inhibitors, tricyclic antidepressants, and phenothiazines are more sensitive to epinephrine. Although the subject of much controversy, epinephrine is safe to use in well-vascularized areas, such as the ear, nose, and genitals. Reports of necrosis are likely the result of excessive volume being placed, which can cause a physical tamponade of vessels, rather than being a direct result of epinephrine.

Sodium bicarbonate (8.4%) can be added (1:10 ratio) to reduce the pain and burning associated with the lower pH of lidocaine with epinephrine. However, sodium bicarbonate can reduce epinephrine activity with time, thus requiring freshly mixed preparations on a regular basis.

Side Effects

The most common side effect of local anesthetic is injection site pain. Buffering with sodium bicarbonate, using a small-gauge needle (e.g., 30 gauge), using ice or vibratory distraction at the injection site, injecting slowly into the subcutaneous tissue (rather than the dermis), warming the anesthesia, minimizing the number of injections, and placing subsequent injections in an already-anesthetized location can minimize the pain associated with local anesthesia. Vasovagal reactions are common during anesthesia administration. Patients should lie flat during the injection to reduce this occurrence. Cold compresses and placing the patient in a Trendelenburg position can help if symptoms occur.

Maximum dosage of anesthesia has traditionally been accepted as 5 mg/kg of 1% plain lidocaine and 7 mg/kg of 1% lidocaine with epinephrine. These numbers have been based on traditional industry-based studies, not found in the medical literature. Experience with tumescent liposuction has taught that dosages up to 55 mg/kg are well tolerated and safe in certain clinical situations. Bupivacaine has a greater risk of cardiac toxicity than lidocaine because of its longer duration of action.

Most true allergic reactions to local anesthetics have been reported with esters. The metabolite *p*-aminobenzoic acid (PABA) is responsible for ester allergies. There is no cross-reactivity between ester and amide classes of anesthetics, so allergy to one type does not preclude the use of the other. True systemic amide allergy is extremely rare. Thorough questioning of patients who report allergy often reveals a vasovagal reaction or epinephrine sensitivity. If local anesthetic use is precluded, intradermal injection with diphenhydramine can be used. Drowsiness can be a side effect when large doses of this agent are used. Bacteriostatic saline, with the benzyl alcohol preservative acting as the anesthetic agent, is often sufficient to provide the brief anesthesia needed to perform small procedures.

Topical anesthetics can be effectively used for many laser procedures, as well as decreasing pain associated with pinpricks of local anesthesia. These products require an extended time of application and/or occlusion to penetrate the stratum corneum and work effectively. The level of anesthesia obtained with these agents is often inconsistent. Topical anesthetics are more effective on mucosa because of the absence of the corneal barrier. There are numerous lidocaine-containing products in a variety of preparations. Eutectic mixture of 2.5% lidocaine and 2.5% prilocaine has also been used extensively. Prilocaine-induced methemoglobinemia has been reported in children from the increased systemic absorption of prilocaine from certain topical products.

Direct application of ice can reduce injection site pain. Ethyl chloride spray rapidly chills the skin and can be used for minor curettage procedures or needle insertion. Refrigerated forced air or water-chilled sapphire crystals can help reduce pain associated with laser procedures. Ophthalmic solutions of proparacaine 0.5% or tetracaine 0.5% can provide rapid anesthesia and are useful when placing corneal shields.

Alam M, et al: Safety of peak serum lidocaine concentration after Mohs micrographic surgery. J Am Acad Dermatol 2010; 63: 87.

Kouba DJ, et al: Guidelines for the use of local anesthesia in office-based dermatologic surgery. J Am Acad Dermatol 2016; 74: 1201.

Park KK, Sharon VR: A review of local anesthetics. Dermatol Surg 2017; 43: 173.

Sobanko JF, et al: Topical anesthetics for dermatologic procedures. Dermatol Surg 2012; 38: 709.

Anatomy

A thorough understanding of anatomy is critical when performing dermatologic surgery. The vascular supply, sensory and motor innervation, and muscles of facial expression all play a role in the successful surgical outcome (Figs. 37.1–37.3 and Box 37.2).

Although a full description of the entire anatomy that is relevant to dermatology is beyond the scope of this text, several key danger zones are worthy of mention. The temporal branch of the facial nerve is at greatest risk for injury when it runs superficial to the deep temporalis fascia as it crosses the zygomatic arch. Care must be taken to undermine bluntly in a plane above the superficial muscular aponeurotic system (SMAS). Injury to the temporal nerve results in brow ptosis and inability to raise the eyebrow. The danger zone for the marginal mandibular nerve lies where it crosses over the body of mandible, just anterior to the masseter muscle. Injury to the marginal mandibular nerve causes asymmetric ipsilateral lip elevation and inability to show the lower teeth. The spinal accessory nerve is at risk in a region of the neck delineated by the clavicle inferiorly, sternocleidomastoid muscle anteriorly, and trapezius muscle laterally and posteriorly. Damage to the nerve causes a winged scapula, inability to shrug the shoulder,

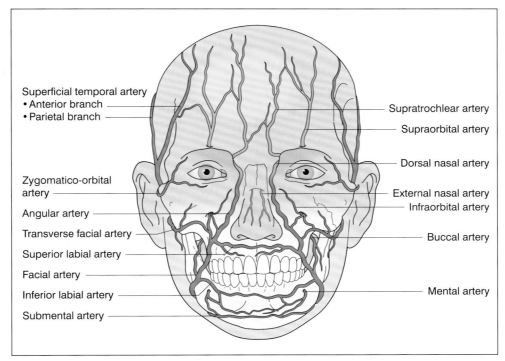

Fig. 37.1 Arterial supply of the face. Light pink designates arteries derived from the internal carotid artery; dark pink, from the external carotid artery.

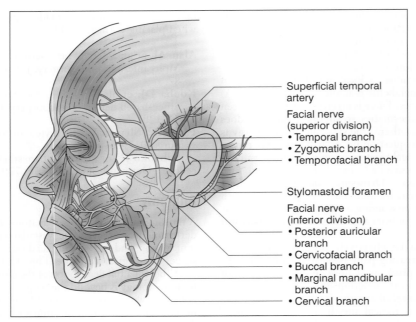

Fig. 37.2 Facial (motor) nerve.

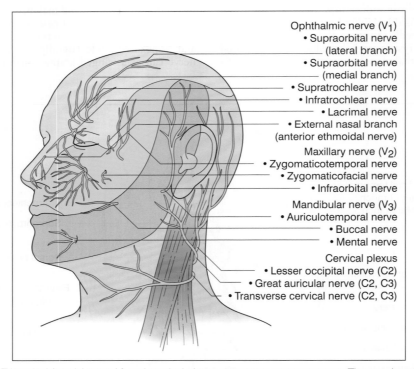

Fig. 37.3 Trigeminal (cranial nerve V) and cervical plexus cutaneous sensory nerves. The concha and external auditory canal are variably innervated by branches of the vagus, glossopharyngeal, and facial nerves.

BOX 37.2 Innervation of Muscles of Facial Expression via Cranial Nerve Vii (Facial Nerve)

TEMPORAL BRANCH

Frontalis muscle (m.)
Corrugator supercilii m.
Orbicularis oculi m. (upper portion)
Auricular m. (anterior and superior; also known as temporoparietalis m.)

POSTERIOR AURICULAR BRANCH

Occipitalis m.
Auricular m. (posterior)

ZYGOMATIC BRANCH

Orbicularis oculi m. (lower portion)
Nasalis m. (alar portion)
Procerus m.
Upper lip muscles
- Levator anguli oris m.
- Zygomaticus major m.

BUCCAL BRANCH

Buccinator m. (muscle of mastication)
Depressor septi nasi m.
Nasalis m. (transverse portion)
Upper lip muscles
- Zygomaticus major and minor muscles
- Levator labii superioris m.
- Orbicularis oris m.
- Levator anguli oris m.
Lower lip muscles (orbicularis oris m.)

MARGINAL MANDIBULAR BRANCH

Lower lip muscles
- Orbicularis oris m.
- Depressor anguli oris m.
- Depressor labii inferioris m.
- Mentalis m.
Risorius m.
Platysma m. (upper portion)

CERVICAL BRANCH

Platysma m.

BOX 37.3 Cutaneous Surgical Instruments and Supplies

- Scalpel handle (flat No. 3)
- Blade (No. 15)
- Needle holder (appropriate size)
- Sharp curved iris scissors, tissue-cutting scissors
- Blunt undermining scissors
- Skin hook (dull-tipped, two to four prongs)
- Hemostats
- Forceps (1 × 2 teeth, with suture platform)
- Skin preparatory scrub in sterile basin
- Sterile towels
- Sterile gauze and cotton-tipped swabs
- Hyfrecator cover
- Suture
- Suture scissors
- Blade remover

TABLE 37.3 Examples of Common Skin Suture Material

Material	Type
Absorbable	
Gut (chromic, plain)	Twisted
Polyglycolic acid (Dexon)	Braided
Polyglactin 910 (Vicryl)	Braided
Polydioxanone (PDS)	Monofilament
Polytrimethylene carbonate (Maxon)	Monofilament
Poliglecaprone 25 (Monocryl)	Monofilament
Glycomer 631 (Biosyn)	Monofilament
Nonabsorbable	
Silk	Braided
Nylon (Ethilon, Dermalon)	Monofilament
Nylon (Surgilon, Nurolon)	Braided
Polypropylene (Prolene, Surgipro)	Monofilament
Polyester (Ethibond, Mersilene, Dacron)	Braided
Polybutester (Novafil)	Monofilament

---

difficulty abducting the shoulder, shoulder drop, and chronic shoulder pain.

Chow S, Bennett RG: Superficial head and neck anatomy for dermatologic surgery. Dermatol Surg 2015; 41: S169.

Equipment

The choice of instruments and suture depends on the procedure being performed. Most simple, in-office biopsies are performed in a "clean" rather than sterile manner and require minimal instrumentation. More complex excisional and reconstructive surgery is generally performed with sterile technique and employs a surgical tray with a wider range of instruments (Box 37.3).

For procedures requiring sutures, absorbable material is used for deeper, layered closures, whereas surface sutures are generally nonabsorbable or fast-absorbing (Table 37.3). The large number of suture choices relates to both the type of procedure performed and the anatomic location treated. Choices include absorbable and nonabsorbable, synthetic and nonsynthetic, monofilament and braided. The surgeon must consider a variety of other characteristics when choosing which suture to use. Memory is the ability of the

suture to return to its original shape after deformation, which results in poor handling and decreased knot security. Plasticity is the ability of the suture to retain its new shape after it has been stretched. Elasticity is the ability of a suture to return to its original length and shape after stretching, an important factor to consider in relation to the resulting edema associated with surgery. The coefficient of friction is the ease with which the suture slides through tissue and is directly related to knot security. Capillarity is the ability of the suture to wick away fluid, with braided sutures having an increased tendency to trap fluid and bacteria. All have appropriate applications.

In general, for procedures requiring buried suture, a synthetic braided suture is a common choice. The 50% tensile strength for this class of suture is about 3 months, and this suture is less palpable under the skin. For these reasons, synthetic braided sutures are often used across all anatomic locations. For procedures on the trunk and extremities (i.e., areas under tension), a monofilament absorbable suture may be considered, because the tensile strength may last longer than with synthetic braided suture, and reports indicate decreased incidence of "spitting" suture. The thicker skin in the trunk and extremities may hide the palpability of monofilament absorbable suture, making it more acceptable to patients. Epidermal approximation in more delicate areas is more appropriately closed with smaller, 5-0 or 6-0 sutures, whereas 4-0 or 3-0 sutures are used in more high-tension areas (e.g., trunk, extremities). Absorbable sutures (e.g., gut) may be considered in sensitive areas where suture removal may be painful or difficult (e.g., eyelids) or in children. Facial sutures are often taken out in 5–7 days to decrease the risk of forming track marks from epithelialization of the suture puncture site, whereas sutures on the scalp, neck, and body are often left in for about 2 weeks. Running subcuticular sutures can be left in for 3 weeks to add tensile strength to wounds without the risk of suture marks. In some instances an absorbable buried running subcuticular suture is an appropriate choice for patients that travel great distance and have difficulty returning for suture removal. Surgical staples can be used on locations such as the scalp to accommodate the higher tension and avoid pulling hair into the wound. Staples can be applied more quickly than traditional suturing and can provide good wound eversion to facilitate healing.

Cyanoacrylates are liquid tissue adhesives that rapidly polymerize when applied to the skin. These adhesives are easy to apply, avoid suture marks, minimize postoperative wound care, and eliminate the need to return to the clinic for suture removal. N-butyl-2-cyanoacrylate (Indermil; Connexicon Medical Ltd) and octylcyanoacrylate (Dermabond; Ethicon, Bridgewater, NJ) are the more frequently used adhesives. The longer length of the side chain of octylcyanoacrylate has been shown to be stronger and more flexible when applied. Studies report various results compared with traditional sutures. Sutures, when properly placed, have the ability to evert wound edges, which may result in a more desirable final esthetic result. In addition, there are numerous reports of contact dermatitis from the use of tissue adhesives. As such, care must be taken in choosing the right clinical situations to use these products.

Bowen C, et al: Allergic contact dermatitis to 2-octyl cyanoacrylate. Cutis 2014; 94: 183.

Dumville JC, et al: Tissue adhesives for closure of surgical incisions. Cochrane Database Syst Rev 2014; 11: CD004287.

Regan T, Lawrence N: Comparison of poliglecaprone-25 and polyglactin-910 in cutaneous surgery. Dermatol Surg 2013; 39: 1340.

Regula CG, Yag-Howard C: Suture products and techniques. Dermatol Surg 2015; 41: S187.

Sniezek PJ, et al: A randomized controlled trial of high-viscosity 2-octyl cyanoacrylate tissue adhesive versus sutures in repairing facial wounds following Mohs micrographic surgery. Dermatol Surg 2007; 33: 966.

Tajirian AL, Goldberg DJ: A review of sutures and other skin closure materials. J Cosmet Laser Ther 2010; 12: 296.

Tierney EP, et al: Rapid absorbing gut suture versus 2-octylethylcyanoacrylate tissue adhesive in the epidermal closure of linear repairs. J Cosmet Laser Ther 2010; 12: 296.

BIOPSIES

When performing a skin biopsy, the clinician should consider the lesion characteristics, reason for biopsy (diagnostic vs. cosmetic), and site. Shave biopsies can range from a superficial scissor snip of an epidermal growth to deep shave excisions of papillary dermal processes. Punch biopsies are most often used for dermal lesions, sampling deeper than shave biopsies, but requiring sutures. Excisional biopsies remove an entire clinical lesion and are the biopsy of choice for pigmented lesions suspicious for melanoma. Incisional biopsies remove a portion of a clinical lesion and are often performed on larger plaques or patches when an excisional biopsy is not cosmetically acceptable or feasible. A wedge biopsy is a deep incisional biopsy that can sample pathologic tissue and adjacent normal tissue; it is especially useful for pathologic diagnosis of certain inflammatory conditions (e.g., panniculitis, fasciitis).

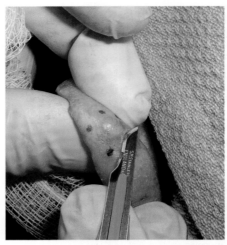

Fig. 37.4 Shave biopsy. Lesion is pinched up with thumb and finger and biopsy performed with sweeping strokes.

Shave biopsies are best suited for pedunculated, papular, or otherwise exophytic lesions. Using a deep or rolled shave, samples can also be obtained of macular or indurated lesions, provided the necessary histologic changes reside in the epidermis or papillary dermis. Infiltration of local anesthesia distends and elevates the lesion, increases skin turgor, affords greater resistance to the blade, and facilitates undercutting the lesion. Using either a No. 15 blade scalpel or a razor blade, which can be flexed to achieve the desired depth, a horizontal incision is made and the lesion removed with sweeping strokes (Fig. 37.4). Hemostasis is typically attained with topical application of 35% aluminum chloride solution.

Sharp scissor biopsy is best suited for pedunculated lesions. Iris or Gradle scissors are used to snip the base of the lesion. In many cases, this can be done without anesthesia. Chemical hemostasis, electrocautery, or simple pressure can be used to control bleeding.

The dermatologic punch is frequently used for both excisional and incisional biopsies (Fig. 37.5). When performing a punch biopsy, the skin should be stretched perpendicular to the relaxed skin tension lines. The elliptical wound resulting from the release of the tension can be suture-closed in a linear fashion, without redundancy or puckering associated with circular wounds. The punch is placed on the skin perpendicular to the surface. While the surgeon applies gentle pressure, it is rotated back and forth and advanced to the hub. The specimen is carefully grasped to avoid crush artifact, and the base is cut. Sutures are typically placed to achieve hemostasis, but punch sites that are allowed to heal by second intention have been shown to heal with a similar cosmetic outcome.

A variation of the punch biopsy can be used to remove larger subcutaneous nodules. Narrow-hole extrusion is a surgical technique that uses a punch biopsy to make a small cutaneous portal through which larger benign growths (e.g., lipoma) can be extruded (Fig. 37.6). This technique allows the evacuation of large subcutaneous growths with a relatively small surface incision.

Suture Technique

Proper suture placement is essential to obtain the desired final result. Sutures are used to close any dead space, reduce bleeding, provide tensile strength and minimize tension to facilitate wound healing, and achieve epidermal wound approximation to maximize cosmetic outcome. Instrument-tied knots are the most common

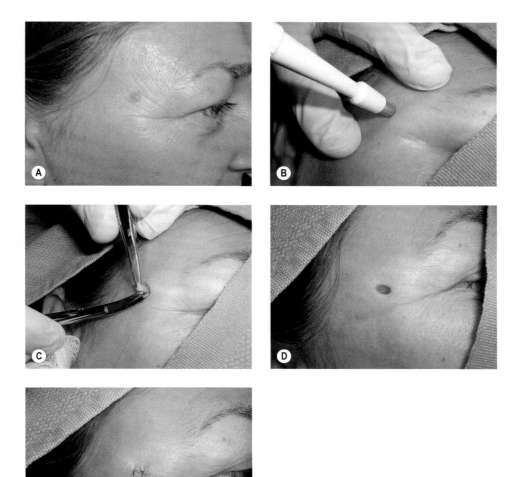

Fig. 37.5 Punch biopsy. (A) Lesion to be removed. (B) Skin stretched perpendicular to relaxed skin tension lines and punch inserted with twisting motion. (C) Specimen is carefully grasped and removed. (D) Resultant elliptical defect. (E) Sutures in place.

sutures used in dermatologic surgery. Various suturing techniques can be employed, based on factors such as size, anatomic location, and thickness of the surgical wound.

Buried subcutaneous sutures are used for larger or deeper wounds to reduce the risk of wound dehiscence. Proper placement is key to achieving eversion of the wound edges and decreasing tension (Fig. 37.7). The stitch is in the dermis and fat, with the knot cut short and buried to reduce tissue reaction and "spitting" sutures. A variation of this technique is the purse-string closure. The surgeon takes multiple horizontal bites every 5 mm or so around the circumference of a circular wound. After completing a complete circle, the suture is pulled tight and the wound is closed circumferentially. This technique can be used to partially or completely close a circular defect to help minimize the amount of time required for the remaining wound to close by second intention. The amount of closure achieved can vary based on the size and laxity of the defect.

Simple epidermal interrupted sutures are one of the most versatile stitches used in dermatology. These are best used for closure of small punch biopsies or for larger, layered excision or flap repairs. Interrupted sutures are especially useful in high-tension wounds; a single suture can be removed, and the surgeon can assess the wound for any dehiscence. For wound edges with a step-off from the opposing epidermal edges, the surgeon places

the suture more superficially at the higher side and deeper on the lower side to even the edges (Fig. 37.8).

The vertical mattress suture is useful for reducing tension, closing dead space, and achieving wound eversion (Fig. 37.9). It can function as both the buried and the superficial suture. Because it tends to leave track marks and strangulate the skin, the vertical mattress suture must be used strategically and removed sooner than traditional sutures.

The horizontal mattress suture reduces tension and can be used as a retention suture when attempting to close larger wounds (Fig. 37.10). It can cause strangulation and necrosis of poorly vascularized tissue and should be used with caution when closing flaps.

Running sutures can be used for epidermal closure in wounds under minimal tension and with closely approximated wound edges. Placement is much faster than with simple interrupted sutures because knots are only used at each end of the wound. The running locked suture is a variant of the simple running suture and involves passing the needle through the previous loop (Fig. 37.11). This technique creates pressure along the wound edge and can be used in highly vascularized regions for additional hemostasis.

Running subcuticular sutures typically use a nonabsorbable suture and are used for trunk and extremity closures where sutures are left for 2–3 weeks. Because the suture is buried, it can be left

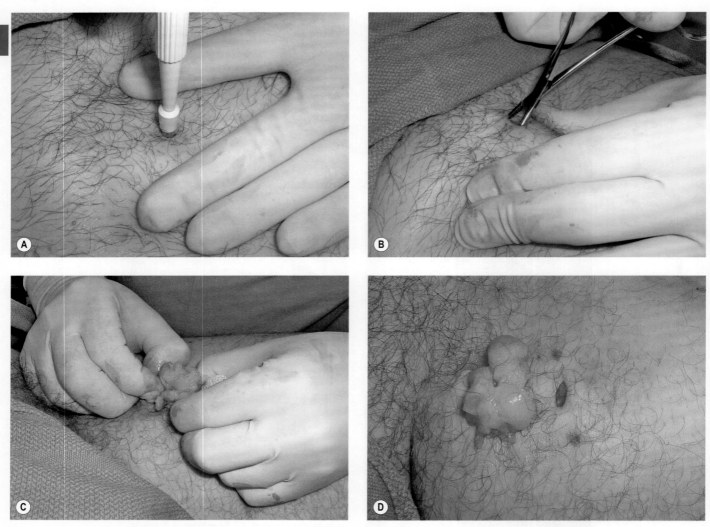

Fig. 37.6 Narrow-hole extrusion of lipoma. (A) The 4-mm punch is in center of lipoma. (B) Hemostat used to loosen lipoma. (C) Extrusion of lipoma through narrow hole. (D) Entire lipoma removed.

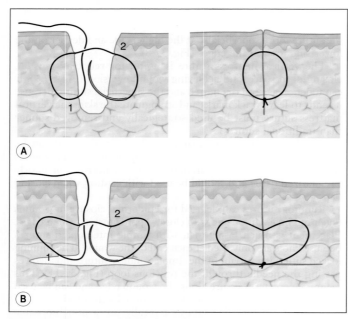

Fig. 37.7 Buried dermal sutures. Numbers indicate entry points of the needle. (A) Conventional buried suture placement results in mild wound eversion. (B) Buried vertical mattress suture placement results in moderate to significant wound eversion.

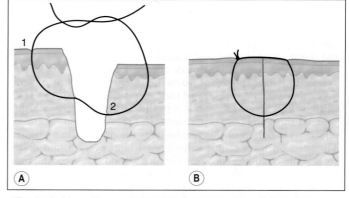

Fig. 37.8 Step-off correction. (A) To correct a step-off deformity, place a simple interrupted suture superficially on the higher wound edge (1) and deeply on the lower wound edge (2). Numbers indicate entry points of the needle. (B) Tying this suture results in even wound edges.

37

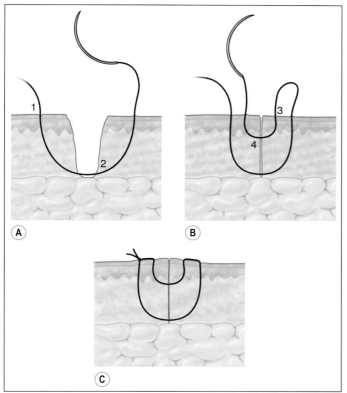

Fig. 37.9 Placement of vertical mattress stitch. (A) The needle is placed 5–10 mm from the wound edge, and a deeply seated simple interrupted suture is placed *(1) (2)*. Numbers indicate entry points of the needle. (B) The needle is redirected back across the wound more superficially, penetrating the skin edge 2–4 mm from the wound on both sides *(3)*. (C) Final appearance of this suture after tying.

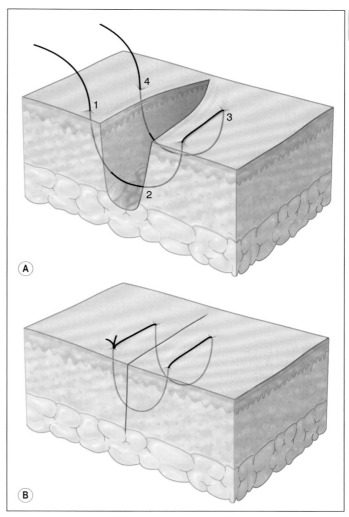

Fig. 37.10 Horizontal mattress suture. (A) To place this suture, begin with a widely spaced, simple interrupted suture *(1) (2)*. Numbers indicate entry points of the needle. Move laterally down the wound 3–5 mm, and place another interrupted suture in the opposite direction as the first *(3) (4)*. (B) Appearance of this suture when tied.

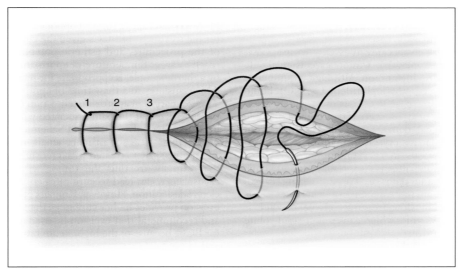

Fig. 37.11 Running block suture. A running simple suture is placed, passing the needle through the loop created by the last suture. This locking suture facilitates hemostasis. Numbers indicate entry points of the needle.

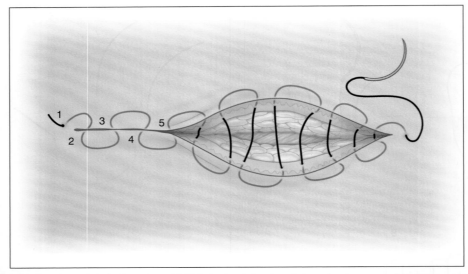

Fig. 37.12 Running subcuticular suture. Multiple horizontally placed dermal sutures are placed in succession on alternating wound edges. This results in epidermal and dermal closure without visible suture marks. Numbers indicate entry points of the needle.

in place for a longer period without developing cross-hatch marks (Fig. 37.12). A single loop coming out in the middle of larger wounds can help facilitate removal of the suture. Alternatively, absorbable suture can be used and can eliminate the need for removal. This option is ideal for patients who live a distance from the clinic or for patients who have difficulty returning for postoperative visits.

Christenson LJ, et al: Primary closure vs second-intention treatment of skin punch biopsy sites. Arch Dermatol 2005; 141: 1093.

Krunic AL, et al: Running combined simple and vertical mattress suture. Dermatol Surg 2005; 31: 1325.

Lam TK, et al: Secondary intention healing and purse-string closures. Dermatol Surg 2015; 41: S178.

Lee KK, et al: Surgical revision. Dermatol Clin 2005; 23: 141.

Moy RL, et al: A review of sutures and suturing techniques. J Dermatol Surg Oncol 1992; 18: 785.

CRYOSURGERY

Cryosurgery is used for the treatment of numerous benign, premalignant, and malignant skin lesions. Most dermatologists employ cryosurgery extensively because it is easy to use, cost-effective, and versatile. Postoperative wound care is relatively simple, and complications are uncommon. Although a number of cryogens have been used (e.g., ethyl chloride, CO_2, NO), liquid nitrogen, with a boiling point of $-195.6°C$, is most widely used.

The mechanism of injury in cryosurgery is the result of multiple factors, including mechanical damage to cells resulting from intracellular and extracellular ice crystal formation, exposure to high electrolyte concentrations in surrounding nonfrozen or thawing fluid, recrystallization patterns during thaw, and ischemia caused by vascular stasis and damage. Rapid freezing causes intracellular ice crystals that are more destructive than the extracellular crystals formed during slow freezing. Tissue damage is maximized with a slow thaw time, which causes increased solute gradients and greater cell destruction. Multiple freeze-thaw cycles can further increase damage to the target lesion.

There are several techniques for cryosurgery. The simplest is the use of a cotton-tipped applicator. Varying the amount of pressure applied and duration of contact of the applicator to the skin can control the depth of freeze. Additionally, the volume of liquid nitrogen can be increased or decreased by adding or removing cotton from the applicator tip. Viruses have been shown to survive in liquid nitrogen, so cotton-tipped applicators should never be reintroduced to the storage container. Rather, a small amount of liquid nitrogen should be transferred to an individual container and discarded after use.

Spray application is one of the most common methods of cryosurgery. This technique uses a handheld liquid nitrogen spray unit with an adjustable nozzle to vary the size of the stream delivered. An insulating cone or a disposable otoscope speculum can be used to focus the delivery of liquid nitrogen, resulting in a deeper freeze and finer control with less damage to uninvolved skin (Fig. 37.13).

Contact technique with a metal probe can also be used for treating skin lesions. This technique consists of applying a smooth metal tip in direct contact with the treated lesion. Typically it requires longer freeze time than the spray technique and is best used for small, round, flat lesions that can have an even contact with the probe.

Basal cell carcinomas (BCCs) can be treated with cryosurgery. However, alternative surgical options are more routinely performed for the treatment of BCCs given the cure rates obtained, tolerance of the procedure, and esthetic outcomes achieved. Freezing to reach a target temperature of approximately $-50°C$, as measured by a thermocouple, is appropriate for management of these tumors. This translates to a thaw time of approximately 60 seconds, with a freeze margin of approximately 5 mm (Fig. 37.14). It is important to recognize that the pain associated with such treatment requires local anesthesia. Kokoszka and Scheinfeld found a recurrence rate of less than 10% for primary small, noninfiltrating (superficial and nodular) BCC treated with cryosurgery. Some have suggested that initially treating the tumor with curettage, followed by cryosurgery, can lead to cure rates consistent with curettage and electrodesiccation. However, Kuijpers et al. suggested that standard excision provides higher cure rates than curettage and cryosurgery and recommend that excision be used as the preferred treatment for BCC, because of the higher cure rate, better cosmetic outcome, and faster healing.

Side effects of cryosurgery are similar to those of other ablative procedures (e.g., curettage and electrodesiccation) and include blistering, crusting, pain, a 3- to 4-week healing period, and scarring.

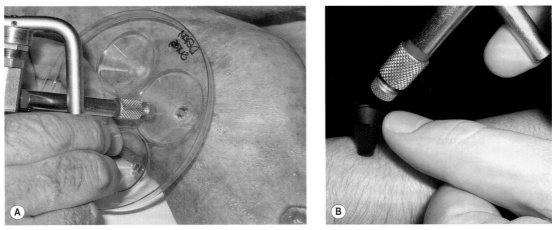

Fig. 37.13 (A) Cryoplate with multiple-sized openings. (B) Disposable otoscope speculum with tip cut off.

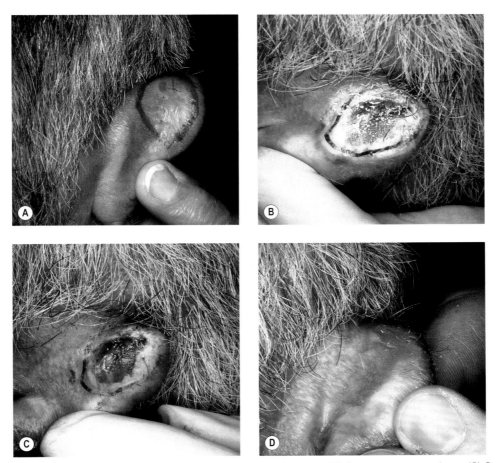

Fig. 37.14 Cryosurgery. (A) Basal cell carcinoma on the posterior helix. (B) Cryosurgery to neoplasm. (C) One week later, with necrosis and sloughing of treatment area. (D) Final result several months later.

Because melanocytes are more susceptible to thermal damage than keratinocytes, hypopigmentation can often be seen, especially in individuals with darker skin tones. Although more frequently seen with longer freeze-thaw times, pigment alterations can be observed even with very brief treatment cycles. A self-limited hyperplastic or pseudoepitheliomatous healing response may occur approximately 2–4 weeks after freezing. Nerve injury can occur during cryosurgery. Anatomic locations with superficial nerves

(e.g., lateral aspects of fingers, ulnar groove of elbow, preauricular and postauricular skin) are especially susceptible to this complication. Techniques to limit this risk include tenting the skin up and away from the nerve, ballooning the skin with lidocaine, or sliding the skin back and forth over the underlying fascia during treatment to limit exposure to the underlying nerve. Alopecia can occur when treating hair-bearing areas. Both atrophic and hypertrophic scars can be seen after cryosurgery.

Kokoszka A, Scheinfeld N: Evidence-based review of the use of cryosurgery in treatment of basal cell carcinoma. Dermatol Surg 2003; 29: 566.

Kuijpers DI, et al: Surgical excision versus curettage plus cryosurgery in the treatment of basal cell carcinoma. Dermatol Surg 2007; 33: 579.

Lindemalm-Lundstam B, Dalenbäck J: Prospective follow-up after curettage-cryosurgery for scalp and face skin cancers. Br J Dermatol 2009; 161: 568.

Nordin P: Curettage-cryosurgery for non-melanoma skin cancer of the external ear. Br J Dermatol 1999; 140: 291.

CURETTAGE

The curette has long been a standard tool in the dermatologist's surgical management of neoplasm. This round, semisharp knife is available in sizes from 0.5–10 mm, allowing for the removal of a variety of lesions. Because it is not as sharp as a scalpel, the curette does not easily cut through normal skin. Therefore it is best suited for use on soft or friable lesions, such as warts, seborrheic and actinic keratoses, the papules of molluscum contagiosum, and select BCCs and squamous cell carcinomas (SCCs). The proper selection of lesion, location, and size of the curette, combined with the surgeon's technique, all play a role in both the therapeutic and the cosmetic outcome.

The skin should be stabilized with the nondominant hand while the curette is held like a pencil. Curettage should be performed in a centripetal manner (from the outside in) to avoid stripping sun-damaged skin and creating a larger wound. To ensure complete destruction, curettage should be performed in multiple directions to produce symmetric wound margins. A large curette can be used for initial debulking, followed by a smaller curette to remove any residual foci or extensions. Curettage is complete when the "gritty," firm sensation of normal dermis is felt, and slight punctate dermal bleeding occurs.

Curettage combined with electrodesiccation (C&E) is widely used for the treatment of BCC and SCC (Fig. 37.15). Silverman et al. reviewed the cure rates of primary BCC treated with C&E over a 27-year period at New York University, stratifying low-, middle-, and high-risk anatomic locations and the risk of recurrence after C&E of primary BCC. Low-risk anatomic sites (neck, trunk, and four extremities) had a 5-year recurrence rate of 3.3%. Middle-risk sites (scalp, forehead, preauricular/postauricular, and malar areas) had an overall recurrence rate of 12.9%, but this was

reduced to 5% when limited to noninfiltrative carcinomas of less than 1 cm. High-risk sites (nose, paranasal, nasolabial groove, ear, chin, mandibular, perioral, and periocular areas) had an overall recurrence rate of 17.5%, but a more acceptable 5% recurrence rate was achieved when treatment was limited to lesions of less than 6 mm.

In addition to size and anatomic location, the histologic subtype is an important factor in the effectiveness of C&E. Infiltrative and micronodular BCCs are not appropriate for C&E, whereas it can be considered a therapeutic option in superficial and nodular subtypes. Blixt et al. demonstrated that tumors with high-risk histologic subtypes (e.g., infiltrating, micronodular, desmoplastic) had overall recurrence rates of 27% when treated with C&E alone. SCC in situ may be appropriately treated with C&E, although in most circumstances, invasive SCC would not typically be amenable to this modality.

There is little agreement regarding the requisite number of cycles of C&E. In fact, treating all lesions identically with a particular number of cycles may lead to overtreatment of some lesions and undertreatment of others. In general, accepted therapy employs three cycles to treat most malignant lesions. However, smaller superficial malignancies may be treated with fewer cycles; the rationale is to improve cosmetic outcome while still achieving acceptable cure rates. Nonetheless, the success of C&E relies on the surgeon's ability to identify by feel and appearance the tissue to be ablated. Finally, C&E should be replaced by excision if curettage extends into subcutaneous tissue. As such, lesions previously biopsied using a punch that has extended into the subcutaneous fat may be less amenable to C&E.

Barlow JO, et al: Treatment of basal cell carcinoma with curettage alone. J Am Acad Dermatol 2006; 54: 1039.

Blixt E, et al: Recurrence rates of aggressive histologic types of basal cell carcinoma after treatment with electrodesiccation and curettage alone. Dermatol Surg 2013; 39: 719.

Galles E, et al: Patient-reported outcomes of electrodessication and curettage for treatment of nonmelanoma skin cancer. J Am Acad Dermatol 2014; 71: 1026.

Goldman G: The current status of curettage and electrodesiccation. Dermatol Clin 2002; 20: 569.

Rodriguez-Vigil T, et al: Recurrence rates of primary basal cell carcinoma in facial risk areas treated with curettage and electrodesiccation. J Am Acad Dermatol 2007; 56: 91.

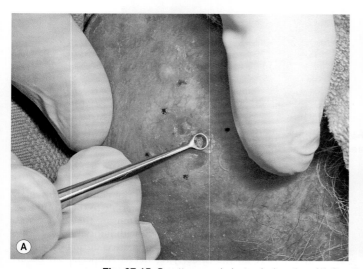
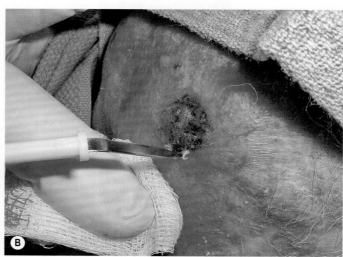

Fig. 37.15 Curettage and electrodesiccation. (A) Curettage of squamous cell carcinoma in situ. (B) Electrodesiccation immediately after curettage.

Silverman MK, et al: Recurrence rates of treated basal cell carcinomas. Part 2. Curettage-electrodesiccation. J Dermatol Surg Oncol 1991; 17: 720.

ELECTROSURGERY

Electrosurgery comprises a variety of surgical techniques, applications, and apparatuses. In general, the tissue effect is created by heat delivered to or generated in the tissue as a result of an electric current. Various forms of electrosurgery are routinely used by dermatologists for applications such as destruction, hemostasis, excisions, and cosmetic procedures. An understanding of the different modalities and their applications can improve surgical outcome (Fig. 37.16).

Data suggest that smoke produced by electrosurgery may pose some health risk to physicians and providers during the procedure. Surgical smoke contains high concentrations of known carcinogens, such as benzene, butadiene, and acetonitrile. Smoke evacuation and proper high-filtration masks may provide some protection during the procedures.

Electrocautery

Electrocautery is most often performed today with battery-powered, handheld, disposable units. Direct current is passed through a metal treatment tip. Resistance to the flow of current causes heat to be generated, which can be adjusted by the intensity of the current. Hemostasis is achieved by direct heating of the tissue; no electric current passes through the patient. Therefore this device is often considered in patients with implantable cardiac devices sensitive to electric current.

Electrodesiccation and Electrofulguration

Electrodesiccation (*desiccate*, "dry up") and electrofulguration (*fulgur*; "lightning") represent the most common uses of electrosurgery in dermatology. In electrodesiccation, the electrode tip is in contact with the tissue; with electrofulguration, a 1–2 mm separation between the tip and the tissue produces a spark. Electrodesiccation causes a deeper wound, whereas electrofulguration is more superficial.

A highly damped (decreasing amplitude) waveform of high voltage and low amperage is produced by a spark-gap generator. This is a monoterminal current, so a grounding electrode on the patient is not required. Electrodesiccation/fulguration produces superficial destruction, because the carbonization on the treated surface limits damage to deeper tissue.

This type of electrosurgery has numerous applications in the daily practice of dermatology. Superficial, small dermal tumors, such as syringomas or seborrheic keratoses, may be treated with electrodesiccation. Insertion of the fine, epilating needle into the tumor is followed by the application of low current until a surface bubbling occurs. The small amount of char is then removed with a curette, resulting in a smooth surface appearance. In addition, skin tags, warts, and fine telangiectases may all be effectively removed by this technique. Electrodesiccation or fulguration is typically employed in treatment of many BCCs and SCCs (see Curettage earlier in this chapter). It is also useful in excisional surgery to obtain hemostasis. The field must be dry, because the destruction by this current is superficial and will not be transmitted through blood.

Electrocoagulation

Electrocoagulation employs moderately damped current with a lower voltage and higher amperage. The patient is incorporated into a biterminal circuit. Electrocoagulation causes greater tissue damage and deeper penetration than electrodessication or electrofulguration.

Electrosection

Electrosection employs an undamped, low-voltage, high-amperage current in a biterminal manner. This technique has the advantage

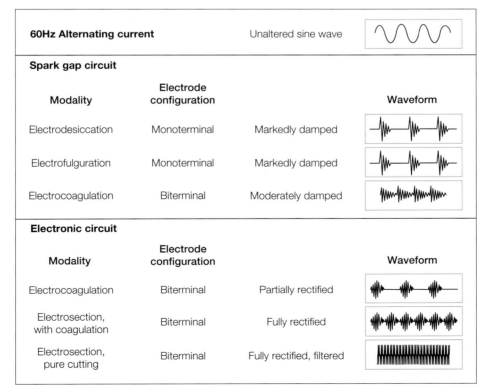

60Hz Alternating current		Unaltered sine wave	

Spark gap circuit			
Modality	**Electrode configuration**		**Waveform**
Electrodesiccation	Monoterminal	Markedly damped	
Electrofulguration	Monoterminal	Markedly damped	
Electrocoagulation	Biterminal	Moderately damped	

Electronic circuit			
Modality	**Electrode configuration**		**Waveform**
Electrocoagulation	Biterminal	Partially rectified	
Electrosection, with coagulation	Biterminal	Fully rectified	
Electrosection, pure cutting	Biterminal	Fully rectified, filtered	

Fig. 37.16 Electrosurgery waveforms.

of cutting with simultaneous hemostasis. As such, it is used for bloodless excisional surgery of protuberant masses and growths, such as rhinophyma. There is vaporization of tissue with minimal heat spread. Extra care must be taken with this technique; maintaining an appropriate depth can be difficult, given the ease with which the device can cut through skin. When the device is properly used, fine surgical excisions can be produced, with minimal trauma to surrounding tissue and excellent hemostasis. Various handpiece attachments, including scalpels, needles, wire loops, and balls, can further adapt the instrument to the specific procedure.

Special care must be taken when using electrosurgery in a patient with a pacemaker or implantable cardioverter-defibrillator, especially if the procedure is performed within a few centimeters of the device. Although modern devices are better shielded and less likely to respond to external electrical interference, it is always prudent to deliver current in short bursts. The physician should also consider the use of electrocautery (heat only, no electrical transmission) or a bipolar device (current transmitted between two tips) when treating these patients. Yu et al. reviewed the use of electrosurgery in patients with cardiac devices.

Howe N, Cherpelis B: Obtaining rapid and effective hemostasis. Part II. Electrosurgery in patients with implantable cardiac devices. J Am Acad Dermatol 2013; 69: 677.

Lewin JM, et al: Surgical smoke and the dermatologist. J Am Acad Dermatol 2011; 65: 636.

Matzke TJ, et al: Pacemakers and implantable cardiac defibrillators in dermatologic surgery. Dermatol Surg 2006; 32: 1155.

Oganesyan G, et al: Surgical smoke in dermatologic surgery. Dermatol Surg 2014; 40: 1373.

Rex J, et al: Surgical management of rhinophyma. Dermatol Surg 2002; 28: 347.

Taheri A, et al: Electrosurgery. Part 1. J Am Acad Dermatol 2014; 70: 591.

Taheri A, et al: Electrosurgery. Part 2. J Am Acad Dermatol 2014; 70: 607.

Voutsalath MA, et al: Electrosurgery and implantable electronic devices. Dermatol Surg 2011; 37: 889.

Yu SS, et al: Cardiac devices and electromagnetic interference revisited. Dermatol Surg 2005; 31: 932.

EXCISIONAL TECHNIQUE

The fusiform or elliptical excision is the workhorse procedure used to treat invasive skin cancers, as well as benign skin lesions needing extirpation (Fig. 37.17). The basic principle of the fusiform ellipse is excision of a specimen oriented with its longest axis along skin tension lines and its width not exceeding one third of its length. The ellipse can be curved in a crescentic or "lazy S" pattern to align the final scar better with skin tension lines. If the procedure is performed with the correct dimensions (usually a length/width ratio of 3:1) and a 30-degree angle at each pole, standing cutaneous cones at the two extremes of the excision are generally avoided. Standing cutaneous cones represent excess tissue bunching at the poles of a skin closure and should be "sewn out" or excised by triangulation or M-plasty, if needed. Undermining, using sharp or blunt dissection of the skin from underlying subcutaneous tissue, reduces wound tension and helps with wound edge eversion.

SKIN FLAPS AND GRAFTS

Choosing whether to close a wound by linear closure, local skin flap, or skin graft or to allow it to heal by second intention can be complex. Important considerations include patient concerns and ability to perform required wound care, local tissue movement, adjacent anatomic structural preservation and function, and cosmesis.

Healing by Second Intention

Wound healing by second intention yields excellent results in select clinical settings. Because contraction occurs in wound healing, wounds adjacent to a free margin may result in a pull and distortion. This may affect surrounding anatomic structures (e.g., pull on a nasal rim or eyelid). The wounds may heal with hypertrophic or pigmentary changes. In some areas and situations, however, allowing a wound to heal by second intention is appropriate. These include superficial wounds in concave areas (e.g., medial canthus, conchal bowl, junction between nose and cheek), partial-thickness wounds involving the mucosa of the lip, or certain clinical situations, such as elderly or frail patients with decreased cosmetic concerns (Fig. 37.18). Wound care is straightforward, and postoperative restrictions are minimal.

Flaps

Local skin flaps are geometric segments of tissue contiguous with a skin defect that are advanced, rotated, or transposed to close a wound. Advantages of flaps include better approximation of skin texture and color, hiding incision lines, redirecting tension vectors, and covering exposed cartilage and bone. Flap survival is based on the preservation of the random blood supply along the pedicle. Consideration of both the primary movement of the flap (actual movement of flap into defect) and secondary movement (movement of surrounding tissue in reaction to flap movement) is critical when designing the repair (Fig. 37.19).

Advancement Flap

An advancement flap moves almost entirely in one linear direction (Fig. 37.20). The classic advancement flap involves the creation of a rectangular pedicle, which slides into position over the primary surgical defect. The key suture advances the flap and closes the primary defect. Tissue redundancies at the base of the flap can be removed by triangulation. Survival of the distal tip of the flap depends on blood supply from the base, and thus a maximum length/width ratio of 3:1 should be designed.

If insufficient movement is obtained with a single advancement flap, a bilateral advancement (O-H) can be employed, such that each flap advances to cover half the defect. This repair can be used in eyebrow or helical rim repairs. Single advancement flaps (O-L) and bilateral single arm advancement flaps (O-T) are similar to classic advancement flaps, except that only a single incision is made and the standing cone is removed by triangulation. These flaps have the advantage of a larger pedicle providing blood supply and allow a linear portion of the flap to be hidden in an existing rhytid for better cosmetic outcome. Common sites for single arm advancement flaps include the nasal side wall, helical rim, upper lip, forehead, and eyebrow.

The island pedicle flap (or "V-Y flap") is a specific variant of an advancement flap (Fig. 37.21). This flap depends on a subcutaneous vascular pedicle for its blood supply and has all the epidermal connections severed by incisions. Care must be taken in designing island pedicle flaps because the incision lines surrounding the flap can result in a patchlike appearance in the final outcome. The best cosmetic results are achieved when at least one of the incision lines can be hidden in an existing rhytid or anatomic boundary.

Rotation Flap

The rotation flap can conceptually be considered a variation of the advancement flap, in that it slides into position in much the same way, although in an arcuate manner. Tension vectors from this pulling action are directed along the arc of rotation in reverse

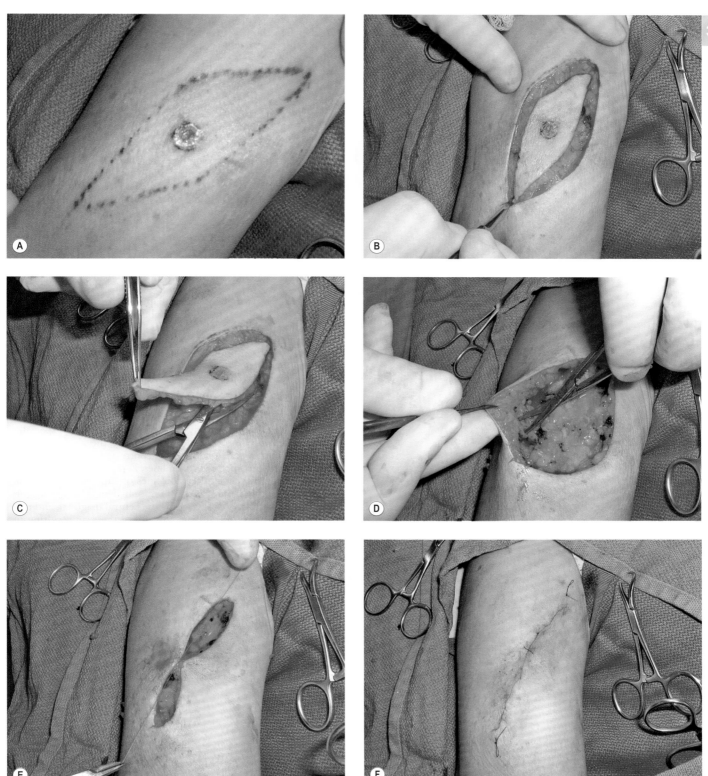

Fig. 37.17 Elliptical excision. (A) Ellipse is designed along relaxed skin tension lines with a 3:1 length-to-width ratio. (B) Incision made into subcutaneous tissue. (C) Removal using tissue scissors in even plane. (D) Blunt undermining of skin edges using skin hook. (E) Buried interrupted tension-bearing absorbable sutures placed. (F) Epidermal approximation using nonabsorbable running subcuticular sutures, with interruption in center of wound for easier removal.

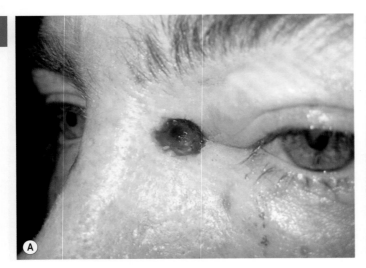

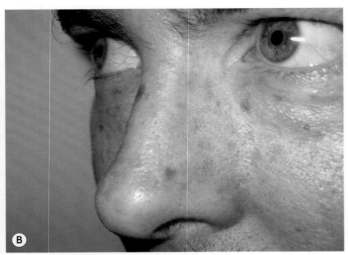

Fig. 37.18 Healing by second intention. (A) Mohs defect. (B) Final result, 1 year later.

fashion (Fig. 37.22). Rotation flaps are often used to close large defects when there is insufficient tissue laxity (Fig. 37.23). The flap has the advantage of good survival secondary to the large pedicle and the ability to recruit skin from a great distance. A back cut can be used to reduce pivotal restraint and provide greater tissue movement, but this may compromise the vascular pedicle. Variations include bilateral rotation flap (O-Z) (Fig. 37.24) or dorsal nasal rotation flap (Fig. 37.25).

Transposition Flaps

In the case of the transposition flap, the flap is elevated, transposed over intervening tissue, and sutured into the primary defect. The tension vector is redirected across the closure of the secondary defect (i.e., area originally occupied by flap). This is especially helpful for defects that are adjacent to anatomic free margins. The key suture closes the secondary defect, and the flap is then lifted and transposed into position over the primary defect. The prototype of this flap is the rhombic flap (Fig. 37.26). Other examples include bilobed flaps (Fig. 37.27), nasolabial/melolabial flaps, banner flap, Z-plasty, and Webster's 30-degree flap (Fig. 37.28).

Choice of a particular type of flap involves multiple factors, including location of defect, availability of tissue movement, surrounding structures, effects of tissue movement, and blood supply. Full discussion of flaps is beyond the scope of this chapter and is available in multiple referenced texts. The successful design and execution of flap repairs can be complex and requires appropriate and extensive training.

Z-plasty

The Z-plasty is useful for any reconstructive surgeon, especially as part of scar revision. When used properly, the Z-plasty alters the direction of the scar, lengthens the contracted scar, and changes a linear scar into geometric, broken lines. Z-plasty can thus redirect a scar into the relaxed skin tension lines or can reduce anatomic distortion resulting from scar contracture by lengthening the scar.

In the classic Z-plasty, the scar is the central diagonal, and two symmetric limbs are taken from the end of the scar, resulting in a "Z" appearance. The length and angle of these peripheral arms determine the degree of wound lengthening and redirection. In a classic 60-degree Z-plasty, the scar is redirected 90 degrees and the wound lengthened by 75% (Fig. 37.29). Smaller angles result in a less dramatic gain in length. Once the limbs are incised, the two triangular flaps are "flip-flopped" into position and sutured into place. One disadvantage of Z-plasty is the increase in incisions, which often are more difficult to camouflage.

Text continued on p. 903

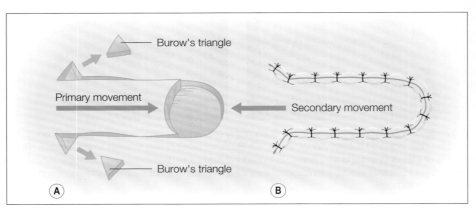

Fig. 37.19 Advancement flap movement.

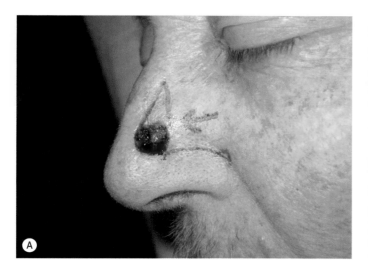
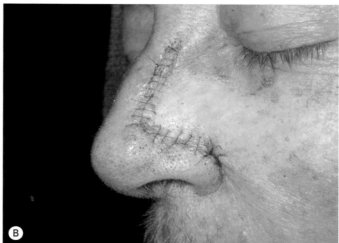
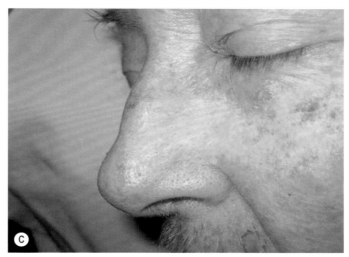

Fig. 37.20 Single arm advancement flap. (A) Advancement flap designed on nasal side wall. (B) Final wound closure. (C) Three months postoperatively.

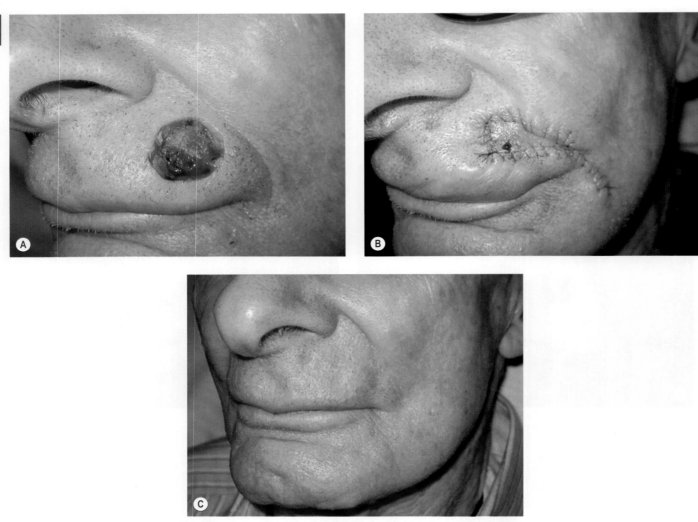

Fig. 37.21 Island pedicle flap. (A) Mohs defect. (B) Final wound closure. (C) One year postoperatively.

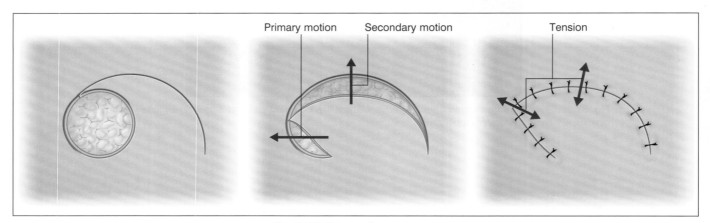

Fig. 37.22 Rotation flap movement.

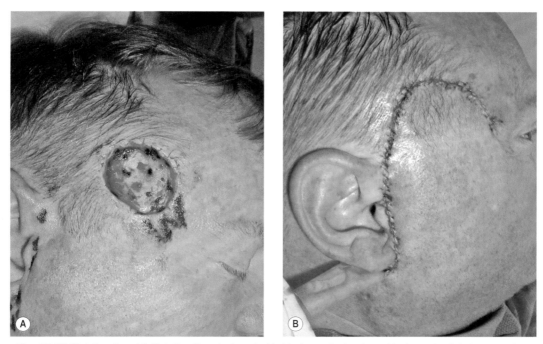

Fig. 37.23 Rotation flap. (A) Rotation flap designed with M-plasty. Redundant skin from cheek is borrowed to repair defect. (B) Final closure.

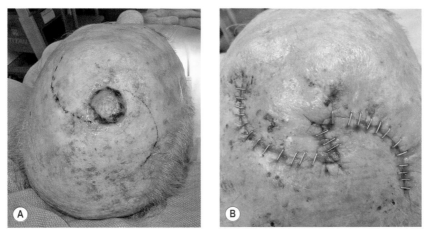

Fig. 37.24 O-Z rotation flap. (A) Flap designed. (B) Final wound closure.

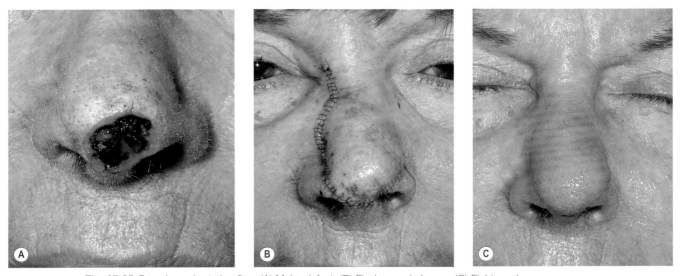

Fig. 37.25 Dorsal nasal rotation flap. (A) Mohs defect. (B) Final wound closure. (C) Eight weeks postoperatively.

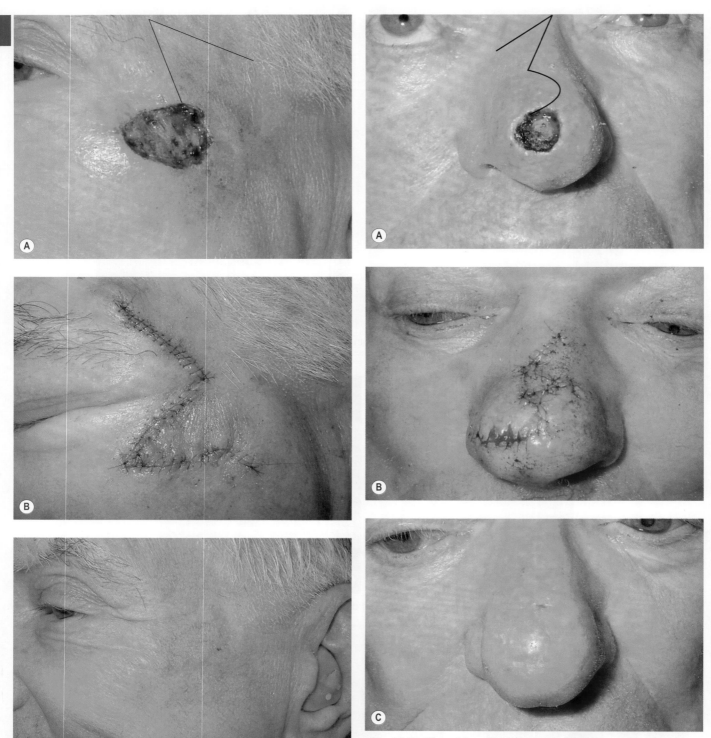

Fig. 37.26 Transposition flap. (A) Mohs defect. (B) Final wound closure. (C) Follow-up at 3 months.

Fig. 37.27 Bilobed flap. (A) Mohs defect. (B) Final wound closure. (C) Follow-up at 6 weeks.

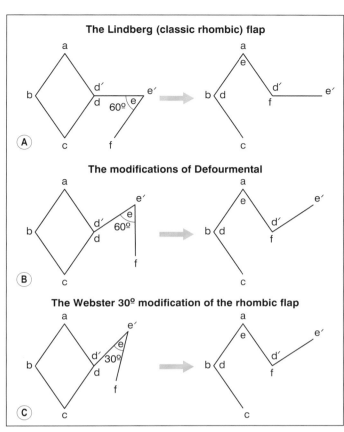

The Lindberg (classic rhombic) flap

The modifications of Defourmental

The Webster 30° modification of the rhombic flap

Fig. 37.28 Variations of transposition flap.

Skin Grafts

Skin grafts are employed when primary closure or flap closure is not an available option. By definition, a graft is completely excised from the donor site and is devitalized (i.e., no intrinsic blood supply). Success is predicated on the reattachment of vascular supply to the graft from the defect. Grafts offer the advantage of fewer incision lines compared with local flaps. However, the lack of color and texture match resulting from the remote donor location of grafts is a potential disadvantage.

Grafts can be categorized as full, split, or composite; when to use each depends on the depth of the defect, vascular supply, and concern about skin cancer recurrence. Full-thickness skin grafts have a full dermis and are the most common grafts used in dermatologic surgery. The graft is defatted, trimmed to fit the defect, anchored in place with peripheral and basting sutures, and secured with a tie-over dressing. Common donor sites include the preauricular cheek, postauricular crease, conchal bowl, upper eyelid, upper inner arm, and clavicle. Full-thickness grafts can produce an excellent cosmetic result if executed properly (Fig. 37.30). However, the increased skin thickness results in an increased metabolic demand and a higher rate of necrosis and failure.

Imbibition occurs during the first 24–48 hours after graft placement. The graft is sustained by passive diffusion of nutrients from the wound bed during this stage. The graft becomes edematous, and the fibrin network attaches the graft to the bed. Inosculation is the next stage of wound healing, with revascularization resulting from linkage of dermal vessels in the graft to the wound bed. Neovascularization occurs from capillary ingrowth to the graft from the recipient base and side walls. Full circulation can be restored in 7 days and depends on graft thickness and vascularity of the wound bed.

Split-thickness skin grafts have only a partial dermis and are useful for covering large areas or improving surveillance in tumors with a high risk of recurrence. Small grafts can be harvested freehand with No. 15 blade or with a handheld Weck blade, using various guards to determine graft thickness (Fig. 37.31). Larger grafts can be obtained using a power dermatome (Fig. 37.32). Grafts can be meshed, which results in an expanded size to provide coverage for larger defects. Compared with full-thickness skin grafts, split-thickness grafts have a higher rate of survival and shorter healing time, do not require repair of the donor site, and are a good choice for areas that are poorly vascularized because

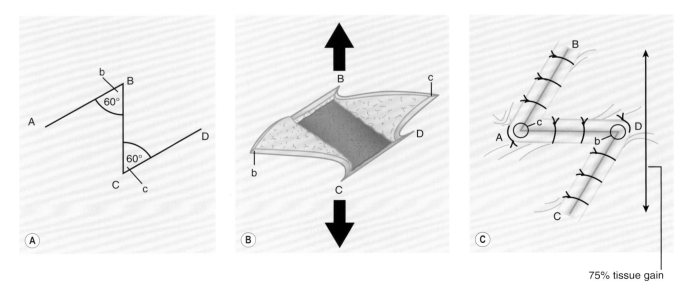

75% tissue gain

Fig. 37.29 Single Z-plasty, 60 degrees. (A) Central scar is the common diagonal. (B) Two triangular flaps are lifted and transposed. (C) Result is approximately 75% increased tissue length.

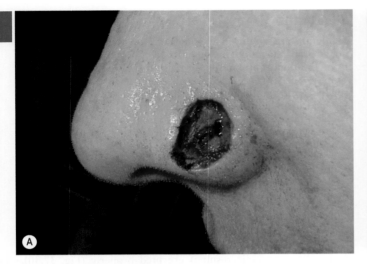

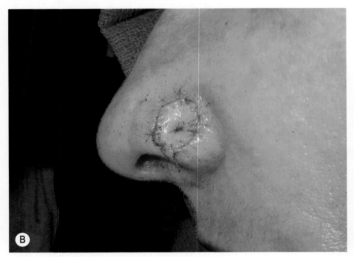

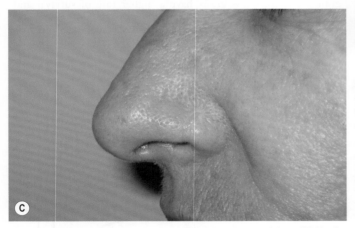

Fig. 37.30 Full-thickness skin graft. (A) Mohs surgery defect. (B) Final wound closure. (C) Follow-up at 3 years.

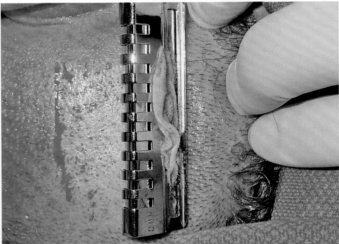

Fig. 37.31 Harvesting of split-thickness skin graft. Mastoid process is an excellent source. Hair will regrow at donor site and hide the wound. Hairs remaining in the graft are above the level of the bulb and will not persist once the graft takes.

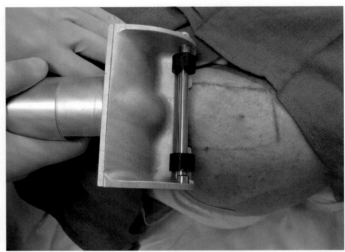

Fig. 37.32 Harvesting of split-thickness skin graft with powered dermatome.

of lower metabolic demand. However, split-thickness grafts have a higher degree of contraction, lack skin appendages, and provide a poorer cosmetic match than full-thickness grafts.

Composite grafts usually consist of skin and underlying structure (e.g., cartilage) and are predominantly used to repair such wounds as full-thickness alar rim defects. These grafts have an increased nutrient requirement and thus are more likely to fail. Free cartilage grafts can be used for reconstruction of the ear and nasal ala or tip.

Adams DC, Ramsey ML: Grafts in dermatologic surgery. Dermatol Surg 2005; 31: 1055.

Blake BP, et al: Transposition flaps. Dermatol Surg 2015; 41: S255.

Donaldson MR, Coldiron BM: Scars after second intention healing. Facial Plast Surg 2012; 28: 497.

Jacobs MA, et al: Clinical outcome of cutaneous flaps versus full-thickness skin grafts after Mohs surgery on the nose. Dermatol Surg 2010; 36: 23.

Kruter L, Rohrer T: Advancement flaps. Dermatol Surg 2015; 41: S239.

Lam TK, et al: Secondary intention healing and purse-string closures. Dermatol Surg 2015; 41: S178.

Leonard AL, Hanke CW: Second intention healing for intermediate and large postsurgical defects of the lip. J Am Acad Dermatol 2007; 57: 832.

LoPiccolo MC: Rotation flaps. Dermatol Surg 2015; 41: S247.
Neuhaus IM, Yu SS: Second-intention healing of nasal alar defects. Dermatol Surg 2012; 38: 697.
Sobanko JF: Optimizing design and execution of linear reconstructions on the face. Dermatol Surg 2015; 41: S216.

MOHS MICROGRAPHIC SURGERY

Frederic Mohs initially developed this technique at the University of Wisconsin in the 1930s as a means for margin control during surgical excision of skin cancer. The original technique used zinc chloride paste to fix tissue in vivo, followed by surgical excision. Drs. Ted Tromovitch and Sam Stegman in San Francisco modified Mohs technique in the 1970s to a fresh frozen tissue variant that continues to be used today. The basic surgical principles in Mohs micrographic surgery are similar to those used in standard excision, although unique challenges are encountered with Mohs surgery. A complete understanding of pathology, anatomy, cutaneous oncology, advanced surgical reconstruction, and management of surgical complications is critical to a successful patient outcome. Any dermatologist performing Mohs micrographic surgery should be well trained in this technique and all the accompanying challenges of surgical and postoperative care. In an effort to recognize the needed skills to be proficient in Mohs surgery, the ACGME has accredited postresidency fellowships in Micrographic Surgery and Cutaneous Oncology.

Mohs micrographic surgical excision is a tissue-sparing technique that employs frozen-section control of 100% of the surgical margin. This evaluation of the entire surgical margin using horizontal sections (not vertical, as used in standard sectioning) combined with precise mapping allows for the highest cure rate of cutaneous neoplasms (Fig. 37.33). In addition, the sparing of normal adjacent tissue can improve cosmesis and decrease the risk of functional defects in a sensitive anatomic location. Any tumor that has a contiguous growth pattern is a candidate for Mohs micrographic surgical excision. Immunohistochemical stains can be used in specific cases to help identify residual tumor.

Multiple indications exist for Mohs micrographic surgical excision (Fig. 37.34 and Box 37.4). In an effort to help identify which patients and tumors are appropriate for treatment with Mohs surgery, a joint task force has established guidelines for appropriate-use criteria. These guidelines should be followed to prevent overuse of Mohs surgery for inappropriate clinical situations. A smartphone "app" is available for easy reference when evaluating patients in the clinic. Mohs surgery provides cure rates of 99% for primary BCCs and 95% for recurrent BCCs. SCCs on the skin and lip treated with Mohs surgery have a 5-year recurrence rate of 3.1% (vs. 10.9% for other modalities). SCC on the ear treated with Mohs surgery has a 5-year recurrence rate of 5.3% (vs. 18.7% for other modalities). Locally recurrent SCC also has reduced recurrence when treated with Mohs surgery compared with other modalities (10% vs. 23.3%). Other tumors that can be successfully treated by Mohs surgery include dermatofibrosarcoma protuberans, atypical fibroxanthoma, and microcystic adnexal carcinoma. Mohs micrographic surgical excision of melanoma continues to be debated. Several studies have demonstrated comparable local recurrence, metastasis, and disease-specific survival rates in head and neck melanomas treated with Mohs micrographic surgery compared with standard excision. The use of MART-1 and other rapid immunohistochemistry stains has proven very beneficial in the frozen section Mohs analysis of melanoma.

> **BOX 37.4** Indications for Mohs Surgery
>
> - Recurrent or incompletely excised nonmelanoma skin cancer
> - Tumors with aggressive histologic subtypes (infiltrative, morpheaform, micronodular, perivascular, or perineural involvement)
> - Tumors with poorly defined clinical margins
> - High-risk location >0.4 cm (H-zone of the face, eyes, ears, nose)
> - Large tumors (>1.0 cm on face; >2.0 cm on trunk or extremities)
> - Cosmetically and functionally important areas, including genital, anal, perianal, hand, foot, and nail units
> - Tumors arising in immunosuppressed patients
> - Tumors arising in previously irradiated skin or scar
> - Genetic conditions with increased risk of neoplasms (basal cell nevus syndrome or xeroderma pigmentosa)

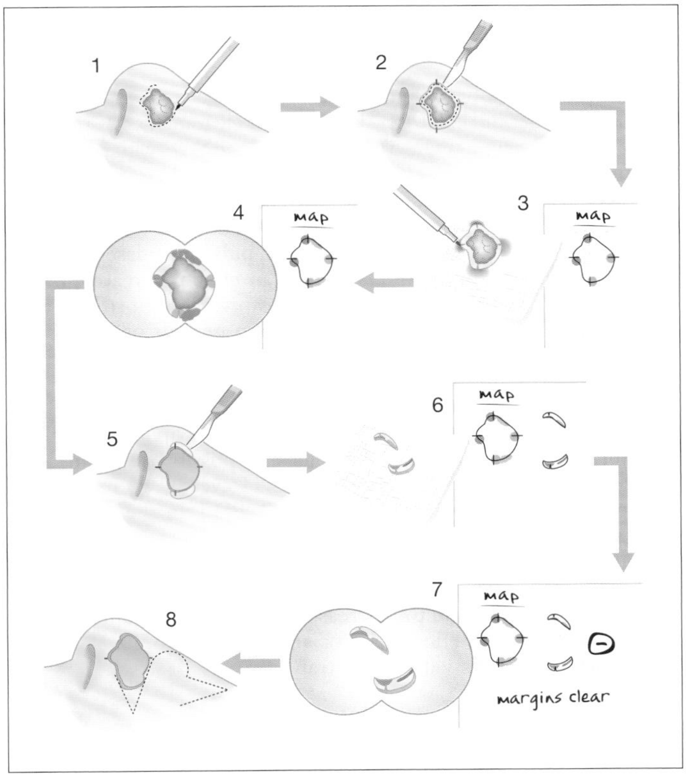

Fig. 37.33 Mohs micrographic surgery process.

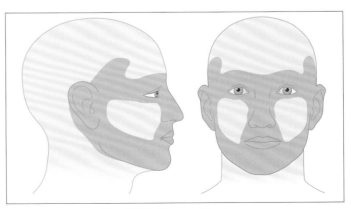

Fig. 37.34 H-zone of the face.

Alam M, et al: Adverse events associated with Mohs micrographic surgery. JAMA Dermatol 2013; 149: 1378.

Bae JM, et al: Mohs micrographic surgery for extramammary Paget disease. J Am Acad Dermatol 2013; 68: 632.

Chang KH, et al: The operative management of melanoma. Dermatol Surg 2011; 37: 1069.

Chin-Lenn L, et al: Comparison of outcomes for malignant melanoma of the face treated using Mohs micrographic surgery and wide local excision. Dermatol Surg 2013; 39: 1637.

Connolly SM, et al: Ad Hoc Task Force. AAD/ACMS/ASDSA/ASMS 2012 appropriate use criteria for Mohs micrographic surgery. J Am Acad Dermatol 2012; 67: 531.

El Tal AK, et al: Immunostaining in Mohs micrographic surgery. Dermatol Surg 2010; 36: 275.

Etzkorn JR, et al: Low recurrence rates for in situ and invasive melanomas using Mohs micrographic surgery with melanoma antigen recognized by T cells 1 (MART-1) immunostaining. J Am Acad Dermatol 2015; 72: 840.

Foroozan M, et al: Efficacy of Mohs micrographic surgery for the treatment of dermatofibrosarcoma protuberans. Arch Dermatol 2012; 148: 1055.

Leibovitch I, et al: Basal cell carcinoma treated with Mohs surgery in Australia. II. Outcome at 5-year follow-up. J Am Acad Dermatol 2005; 53: 452.

Leibovitch I, et al: Cutaneous squamous cell carcinoma treated with Mohs micrographic surgery in Australia. I. Experience over 10 years. J Am Acad Dermatol 2005; 53: 253.

Lowe GC, et al: A comparison of Mohs micrographic surgery and wide local excision for treatment of dermatofibrosarcoma protuberans with long-term follow-up. Dermatol Surg 2017; 43: 98.

Nosrati A, et al: Outcomes of melanoma in situ treated with Mohs micrographic surgery compared with wide local excision. JAMA Dermatol 2017; 153: 436.

Pugliano-Mauro M, Goldman G: Mohs surgery is effective for high-risk cutaneous squamous cell carcinoma. Dermatol Surg 2010; 36: 1544.

Rowe DE, et al: Long-term recurrence rates in previously untreated (primary) basal cell carcinoma. J Dermatol Surg Oncol 1989; 15: 315.

Rowe DE, et al: Mohs surgery is the treatment of choice for recurrent (previously treated) basal cell carcinoma. J Dermatol Surg Oncol 1989; 15: 424.

Rowe DE, et al: Prognostic factors for local recurrence, metastasis, and survival rates in squamous cell carcinoma of the skin, ear, and lip. J Am Acad Dermatol 1992; 26: 976.

Stigall LE, et al: The use of Mohs micrographic surgery (MMS) for melanoma in situ (MIS) of the trunk and proximal extremities. J Am Acad Dermatol 2016; 75: 1015.

Thomas CJ, et al: Mohs micrographic surgery in the treatment of rare aggressive cutaneous tumors. Dermatol Surg 2007; 33: 333.

Valentín-Nogueras SM, et al: Mohs micrographic surgery using MART-1 immunostain in the treatment of invasive melanoma and melanoma in situ. Dermatol Surg 2016; 42: 733.

PHOTODYNAMIC THERAPY

Photodynamic therapy (PDT) involves the activation of a photosensitizer by visible light in the presence of oxygen, resulting in the creation of reactive oxygen species, which selectively destroy the target tissue. The first requirement for PDT is delivery of either a systemic or a topical photosensitizing drug. Systemic photosensitizing molecules are large, lipophilic molecules that require intravenous administration to reach the target site. One of the major disadvantages of these systemic drugs is the prolonged period of phototoxicity. Examples include porfimer sodium and hematoporphyrin derivative. The benzoporphyrin derivative monoacid ring A (verteporfin) has a shorter period of photosensitivity (<72 hours) than other systemic agents.

Topical agents offer the advantage of limiting photosensitivity to the application site and have become widely used in dermatology. Delta-aminolevulinic acid (ALA) is the most common photosensitizing agent used in dermatology. It is applied and left on the skin for a sufficient period to allow for accumulation within the target cells. ALA is subsequently converted to the photosensitizer protoporphyrin IX (PpIX), which can then be stimulated through the controlled use of a light source. Tumor cells are thought to be selectively targeted by increased penetration of ALA through the abnormal epidermis overlying the tumor cells. In addition, the iron-deficient, rapidly proliferating tumor cells have an increased production of PpIX compared with normal epidermal cells, resulting in selective photosensitivity and damage to the target site. Methyl aminolevulinate (mALA) is also used as a topical photosensitizing agent. Gentle scraping or curettage before application is performed to increase penetration. Once absorbed, mALA is converted to ALA within the target tissue.

The second requirement of PDT is an appropriate light source to activate the photosensitizer. The light source must match the absorption peak of the photosensitizer. Lasers, intense pulsed-light devices, or an incoherent light source can be used. Red light uses the 630-nm peak of PpIX as its target and has deeper penetration, which is appropriate for dermal processes. Blue light targets the 417-nm peak and has a more superficial penetration, making it an appropriate choice for the treatment of epidermal lesions such as actinic keratoses.

Following absorption of light, the photosensitizer is converted from a stable ground state to an excited triplet state. The excited-triplet-state electrons interact with tissue oxygen, creating singlet oxygen. Singlet oxygen causes oxidative damage to cellular membranes (mitochondria and other cellular organelles) and direct cell death, the key mechanism of action in topical PDT. This entire process occurs over microseconds. In comparison, PDT using systemic photosensitizers predominantly causes destruction of target sites through vascular injury that leads to tissue ischemia.

Actinic Keratosis

Numerous studies have demonstrated the efficacy of PDT in the treatment of actinic keratoses, with overall clearance rates ranging from 50%–70% for a single treatment and up to 90% with additional treatment sessions. Facial lesions tend to respond better than acral or extremity lesions. Initial studies used an extended application of topical ALA for 14–18 hours, followed by activation with a variety of light sources (e.g., blue light, red light, pulsed dye laser, intense pulsed light). This protocol resulted in an effective treatment for actinic keratoses on the scalp and face. However, recent studies and clinical practice show that short incubation periods of 1–3 hours with ALA are an effective protocol for the treatment of actinic keratoses, vastly improving the convenience of this therapy.

Methyl ALA may offer several advantages over δ-ALA, including improved skin penetration from mALA's increased lipophilic quality, greater selectivity for neoplastic cells, and possibly less pain and discomfort associated with treatment. However, there are no comparative studies for ALA and mALA PDT in the treatment of actinic keratosis. Pariser et al. showed that mALA applied for 3 hours, followed by noncoherent red light, resulted in an almost 90% response rate in actinic keratosis. Given the absence of stratum corneum on the lips and the increased penetration of topical ALA, PDT has been used effectively for actinic cheilitis. This may be an option in patients with recalcitrant disease.

Basal Cell Carcinoma

Studies suggest that topical PDT for the treatment of BCC can have initial clearing and excellent cosmetic results, with cure rates ranging from 64%–97%. However, despite the initial success, BCCs treated with PDT often have a higher recurrence rate on long-term follow-up. In addition, comparative studies of PDT and traditional surgical treatments (e.g., excision or Mohs surgery) are limited or lacking.

Superficial BCC tends to have better response rates than nodular BCC, likely caused by the limited penetration of both the ALA and the activating light into the deeper portion of the dermis for nodular tumors. Pretreatment with curettage for thicker lesions may help to facilitate penetration of ALA and may result in improved cure rates. Infiltrative tumors have an even higher recurrence rate, suggesting that PDT should not be considered a first-line treatment for this histologic subset of BCC.

Arits et al. compared PDT, topical 5-fluorouracil (5-FU), and imiquimod for the treatment of superficial basal cells. Although all modalities were effective, imiquimod was demonstrated to have higher success rate. Both PDT and 5-FU had similar cure rates over 1-year follow-up. However, individual patient factors must be considered when choosing a treatment option.

Subsets of patients with numerous and extensive BCCs (e.g., basal cell nevus syndrome) may be unique cases in whom PDT can be considered for nodular or more extensive tumors, because of the tissue-sparing and chemopreventive advantages over traditional surgical treatments.

Squamous Cell Carcinoma in situ

In situ SCC is quite responsive to PDT. Multiple studies demonstrate an initial cure rate of 54%–100%, with variable long-term efficacy. Red light should be used instead of blue light because it penetrates more deeply and thus more effectively treats adnexal extensions. Truchuelo et al. demonstrated a 76% clearance of Bowen disease after two mALA PDT sessions. Calzavara-Pinton et al. used mALA PDT for SCC in situ and reported cure rates of 87.8% at 3 months and 70.7% at 24 months. These patients had good cosmetic outcomes and tolerated the procedure well. In contrast, patients with invasive SCC fared much more poorly with mALA PDT, with a 45.2% cure rate at 3 months falling to 25.8% at 24 months.

Few reports detail the use of PDT for invasive cutaneous SCC. Given the limited success in treating these tumors and the potential for metastatic spread, PDT is not recommended as standard therapy for invasive SCC.

Arits AH, et al: Photodynamic therapy versus topical imiquimod versus topical fluorouracil for treatment of superficial basal-cell carcinoma. Lancet Oncol 2013; 14: 647.

Babilas P, et al: Photodynamic therapy in dermatology. Photodermatol Photoimmunol Photomed 2010; 26: 118.

Basset-Seguin N, et al: Consensus recommendations for the treatment of basal cell carcinomas in Gorlin syndrome with topical methylaminolaevulinate-photodynamic therapy. J Eur Acad Dermatol Venereol 2014; 28: 626.

Braathen LR, et al: Guidelines on the use of photodynamic therapy for nonmelanoma skin cancer. J Am Acad Dermatol 2007; 56: 125.

Calzavara-Pinton PG, et al: Methylaminolaevulinate-based photodynamic therapy of Bowen's disease and squamous cell carcinoma. Br J Dermatol 2008; 159: 137.

Christensen E, et al: High and sustained efficacy after two sessions of topical 5-aminolaevulinic acid photodynamic therapy for basal cell carcinoma. Br J Dermatol 2012; 166: 1342.

Dirschka T, et al: Long-term (6 and 12 months) follow-up of two prospective, randomized, controlled phase III trials of photodynamic therapy with BF-200 ALA and methyl aminolaevulinate for the treatment of actinic keratosis. Br J Dermatol 2013; 168: 825.

Hadley J, et al: Results of an investigator-initiated single-blind split-face comparison of photodynamic therapy and 5% imiquimod cream for the treatment of actinic keratoses. Dermatol Surg 2012; 38: 722.

Morton CA, et al: European guidelines for topical photodynamic therapy. Part 1. J Eur Acad Dermatol Venereol 2013; 27: 536.

Mosterd K, et al: Fractionated 5-aminolaevulinic acid-photodynamic therapy vs. surgical excision in the treatment of nodular basal cell carcinoma. Br J Dermatol 2008; 159: 864.

Ozog DM, et al: Photodynamic therapy. Dermatol Surg 2016; 42: 804.

Pariser DM, et al: Photodynamic therapy with topical methyl aminolevulinate for actinic keratosis. J Am Acad Dermatol 2003; 48: 227.

Piacquadio DJ, et al: Photodynamic therapy with aminolevulinic acid topical solution and visible blue light in the treatment of multiple actinic keratoses of the face and scalp. Arch Dermatol 2004; 140: 41.

Rhodes LE, et al: Five-year follow-up of a randomized, prospective trial of topical methyl aminolevulinate photodynamic therapy vs surgery for nodular basal cell carcinoma. Arch Dermatol 2007; 143: 1131.

Roozeboom MH, et al: Overall treatment success after treatment of primary superficial basal cell carcinoma. Br J Dermatol 2012; 167: 733.

Scola N, et al: A randomized, half-side comparative study of aminolaevulinate photodynamic therapy vs. CO_2 laser ablation in immunocompetent patients with multiple actinic keratoses. Br J Dermatol 2012; 167: 1366.

Serra-Guillen C, et al: A randomized comparative study of tolerance and satisfaction in the treatment of actinic keratosis of the face and scalp between 5% imiquimod cream and photodynamic therapy with methyl aminolaevulinate. Br J Dermatol 2011; 164: 429.

Serra-Guillén C, et al: A randomized pilot comparative study of topical methyl aminolevulinate photodynamic therapy versus imiquimod 5% versus sequential application of both therapies in immunocompetent patients with actinic keratosis: clinical and histologic outcomes. J Am Acad Dermatol 2012; 66: e131.

Tierney E, et al: Photodynamic therapy for the treatment of cutaneous neoplasia, inflammatory disorders, and photoaging. Dermatol Surg 2009; 35: 725.

Truchuelo M, et al: Effectiveness of photodynamic therapy in Bowen's disease. J Eur Acad Dermatol Venereol 2012; 26: 868.

Zaiac M, Clement A: Treatment of actinic cheilitis by photodynamic therapy with 5-aminolevulinic acid and blue light activation. J Drugs Dermatol 2011; 10: 1240.

RADIATION THERAPY FOR SKIN CANCER

Radiation therapy (x-ray therapy [XRT]) has a long history of use for treatment of both benign and malignant skin conditions. The use of ionizing radiation in dermatologic therapy of benign conditions has all but disappeared, because of highly effective medical therapies and the potential genetic and somatic hazards of radiation. However, XRT for malignant skin conditions remains an important primary and adjuvant therapeutic modality. When used properly in the appropriate clinical situation, XRT can provide effective treatment while sparing normal tissue and eliminating the need for surgical reconstruction.

Radiation is an appropriate primary treatment for skin cancer in patients who refuse surgery or who are not optimal surgical candidates. However, patients who are relatively young are less ideal candidates for XRT because of the increased risk of developing additional primary tumors within the radiation field, as well as the long-term cosmetic complications associated with this therapy. Tumors located on the eyelids, nose, ears, and lips can be treated with excellent cosmetic outcomes with XRT, whereas lesions on the extremities are frequently treated by excision because of the larger surgical area that can be easily achieved. Treatment of small primary BCC with XRT can produce cure rates greater than 90%, although primary SCC may have slightly lower cure rates. It is important to stress that Mohs micrographic surgical excision of primary tumors can achieve cure rates of 97%–99%, often with excellent long-term cosmetic outcomes. Furthermore, Mohs surgery can generally be completed in a single day, whereas XRT is routinely delivered in many fractions over weeks.

Recently superficial XRT and electronic surface brachytherapy have been presented as alternative nonsurgical methods to treat superficial small skin cancers. These technologies differ from traditional XRT and classic forms of radionuclide-based brachytherapy. Superficial XRT is "low-energy" therapy. In contrast to other XRT types, where the goal is usually to treat tumors that extend deeply beneath the skin surface, superficial x-rays have very limited penetration and thus primarily target the skin. Electronic surface brachytherapy delivers radiation without using an isotope using a miniaturized x-ray tube. This form of treatment contains no actively radioactive isotope components, so it is subject to much less regulation and offers the advantage of less shielding requirements for patients and staff. Both superficial XRT and brachytherapy have been used for skin cancer increasingly over the past few years. In a retrospective analysis of 1715 BCCs and SCCs treated with superficial XRT, Cognetta et al. reported cumulative recurrence rates of all tumors at 2 and 5 years of 1.9% and 5.0%, respectively. Long-term outcomes for electronic brachytherapy are not yet available, but many centers have reported initial cohorts with good short-term cosmesis. At present, additional comparative research is needed for these modalities to determine their proper role in the treatment and management of cutaneous malignancies relative to surgery.

Radiation therapy may also be considered if surgical margins show microscopic evidence of residual tumor after excision. XRT can also be used for recurrent BCC and SCC not previously treated with radiation, although not with the same success as primary tumors. Cacialanza et al. demonstrated an 84% 5-year cure rate for recurrent BCC and SCC in a group of about 250 recurrent tumors, with almost all having an acceptable cosmetic result. Locke et al. showed that primary tumors treated with radiation had a response rate of 93%, versus 80% for recurrent neoplasms. Mohs micrographic surgical excision of recurrent nonmelanoma skin cancer (NMSC) produces higher cure rates (95%), but if cancers have recurred multiple times, consideration should be given to addition of adjuvant XRT based on concerning pathologic features.

Several studies indicate that recurrence of NMSC after primary XRT may be more aggressive and invasive than recurrence after primary surgical treatment. Smith et al. demonstrated that BCCs recurring after primary XRT had deeper subcutaneous tissue invasion and a larger percentage increase between clinical preoperative tumor area and final postoperative defect area than recurrent tumors that had initially been treated with other modalities. Therefore salvage surgeries for post-XRT recurrences generally should be undertaken with large clinical margins.

Radiation therapy offers a valuable adjunctive treatment option for particularly aggressive perineural SCC and BCC. Detection of single-cell tumor spread may be particularly difficult after excisional surgery. In addition, perineural carcinoma may spread more rapidly along nerve sheaths than by contiguous growth. With either primary surgery or primary radiation, overall control rates are lower for tumors with perineural invasion. Given the increased risk of metastasis and recurrence in this group of tumors, adjuvant XRT should be considered as prophylactic treatment after surgical excision for this aggressive feature.

Alam M, et al: The use of brachytherapy in the treatment of nonmelanoma skin cancer. J Am Acad Dermatol 2011; 65: 377.

Bhatnagar A: Nonmelanoma skin cancer treated with electronic brachytherapy. Brachytherapy 2013; 12: 134.

Caccialanza M, et al: Radiotherapy of recurrent basal and squamous cell skin carcinomas. Eur J Dermatol 2001; 11: 25.

Cognetta AB, et al: Superficial x-ray in the treatment of basal and squamous cell carcinomas. J Am Acad Dermatol 2012; 67: 1235.

Han A, Ratner D: What is the role of adjuvant radiotherapy in the treatment of cutaneous squamous cell carcinoma with perineural invasion? Cancer 2007; 109: 1053.

Hanke CW, et al: Current status of surgery in dermatology. J Am Acad Dermatol 2013; 69: 972.

Jambusaria-Pahlajani A, et al: Surgical monotherapy versus surgery plus adjuvant radiotherapy in high-risk cutaneous squamous cell carcinoma. Dermatol Surg 2009; 35: 574.

Linos E, et al: A sudden and concerning increase in the use of electronic brachytherapy for skin cancer. JAMA Dermatol 2015; 151: 699.

Locke J, et al: Radiotherapy for epithelial skin cancer. Int J Radiat Oncol Biol Phys 2001; 51: 748.

Silverman MK, et al: Recurrence rates of treated basal cell carcinomas. Part 4. X-ray therapy. J Dermatol Surg Oncol 1992; 18: 549.

Smith SP, et al: Use of Mohs micrographic surgery to establish quantitative proof of heightened tumor spread in basal cell carcinoma recurrent following radiotherapy. J Dermatol Surg Oncol 1990; 16: 1012.

Starling J 3rd, et al: Determining the safety of office-based surgery. Dermatol Surg 2012; 38: 171.

Veness MJ: The important role of radiotherapy in patients with non-melanoma skin cancer and other cutaneous entities. J Med Imaging Radiat Oncol 2008; 52: 278.

Wang Y, et al: Indications and outcomes of radiation therapy for skin cancer of the head and neck. Clin Plast Surg 2009; 36: 335.

38 Cutaneous Laser Surgery

Cutaneous laser surgery is a continually evolving area of dermatology. Development of new lasers, as well as improvements in existing lasers, continues to advance the field. As a result of this progress, laser surgery has become an extremely effective therapeutic modality for a multitude of dermatologic conditions.

LASER PRINCIPLES

Laser is an acronym for light amplification by stimulated emission of radiation. The first laser was a ruby laser operated in 1960 by Theodore Maiman. Medical applications were quickly recognized, and Leon Goldman pioneered their dermatologic use.

Although technology has advanced through the years, several distinctive characteristics have remained in all lasers. Compared with other light sources, laser light is defined as monochromatic (i.e., a single wavelength), collimated (i.e., nondivergent), coherent (i.e., in phase, with peaks and troughs of the light all aligned), and having high intensity that can travel over long distances (Fig. 38.1). Laser energy is measured in joules (J). *Fluence* is defined as the amount of energy delivered per unit area (J/cm²). *Power* is the rate at which energy is delivered and is measured in watts (1 watt is defined as 1 J/second).

The wavelength is determined by the active medium of each particular laser. Active medium can consist of a gas (e.g., argon, CO_2), liquid (e.g., dye), or solid (e.g., ruby, yttrium-aluminum-garnet crystal) (Table 38.1). The choice of wavelength is determined by the target tissue and depth of penetration required (Fig. 38.2).

Continuous-wave lasers emit a beam of light whose output power is constant over time, resulting in a long, continuous exposure. Quasi–continuous-wave lasers shutter the continuous beam into short segments, producing interrupted emissions of constant laser emission. Pulsed lasers produce short, high-energy pulses of light. Q-switched (quality-switched) lasers are able to generate extremely high-energy pulses over very short pulse durations (nanoseconds or picoseconds) and are used primarily for treating pigmented lesions.

Light can interact with incident targets in one of several ways: reflected, transmitted, scattered, or absorbed (Fig. 38.3). Approximately 5% of laser light is reflected from the epidermis and not absorbed. Transmitted light passes unaltered through the tissue. Light is scattered by the various skin structures, molecules, and cells, thus limiting its depth of penetration and effect on tissue. When reflected, transmitted, or scattered, the light has no effect on the target tissue. When absorbed, however, the light energy is transformed into heat. In most cases of laser therapy, it is the heat generated by absorption that produces the desired therapeutic effect.

The concept of selective photothermolysis, originally promoted by Parish and Anderson, is the basis for all laser-tissue interactions. Lasers in cutaneous surgery are selected by matching their particular wavelength with the absorption spectrum of a desired target. The target structures that absorb laser light are defined as chromophores, with the most common in the skin being water, hemoglobin, and melanin (Fig. 38.4). The goal is to deliver a wavelength that is specifically absorbed by the chromophore, inducing heat buildup and the resultant destruction of that target. In an ideal situation, this wavelength would have little or no absorption by surrounding structures. By controlling the laser's exposure times and energy delivered, the amount of heat buildup can be confined to the desired target with minimal or no collateral damage to surrounding

structures from heat dissipation. A target's thermal relaxation time (TRT) is defined as the time required for the heated target tissue to dissipate half the absorbed heat from the laser. TRT is related to the size and shape of the target structure. Selective photothermolysis is achieved by ensuring that the laser pulse duration is equal to or less than the TRT of the target tissue. Thus larger structures (e.g., hair follicles) have a longer TRT and are best treated with longer pulse widths. Smaller structures (e.g., melanosomes) have a shorter TRT and can be treated with much shorter pulse durations (Table 38.2).

The beam diameter of the laser, or spot size, is a factor in depth of laser penetration. Small spot sizes produce significantly more scatter of the laser outside the effective beam, thus resulting in smaller effective treatment areas. In contrast, larger spot sizes produce more photons that remain within the beam diameter, resulting in higher fluences at a given depth. Therefore with any given wavelength, a larger beam diameter results in a deeper level of penetration (Fig. 38.5).

Epidermal melanin and heat transfer from dermal structures can result in inadvertent epidermal heating and injury. By selectively cooling the overlying skin, while still maintaining sufficient dermal heat to damage the target, the laser surgeon can reduce the chances of epidermal injury. Precooling, parallel cooling, and postcooling have all been used to protect the skin. Dynamic cooling devices use a cryogen spray to cool the skin before and after laser exposure. Contact cooling with a chilled sapphire tip can be used throughout the treatment and is especially useful for parallel cooling. Contact cooling can also be achieved with a chilled metal plate to achieve precooling and postcooling. However, when using this kind of device, the operator must be especially careful to ensure adequate cooling is achieved, as it requires coordinated movement of the handpiece before and after firing the laser. Forced cooled air provides less effective cooling than other methods but can be useful in reducing pain associated with laser treatment. Direct application of ice can also be used for postcooling.

The laser is a technologically advanced instrument that has been used effectively and safely for a wide variety of dermatologic conditions. However, as with any surgery or therapeutic intervention, side effects and complications can occur. Short-term side effects include purpura, edema, and crusting. More concerning, long-term adverse events include scarring (both atrophic and hypertrophic), dyspigmentation, infection, and persistent erythema. Although not a complication, lasers sometimes show a lack of efficacy even when used properly in appropriate clinical settings. Detailed informed consent is critical before performing any laser treatment. Appropriate instruction and supervision in the use of lasers must be obtained by dermatologic surgeons to ensure optimum safety and surgical outcome. Adverse outcomes in laser-treated patients have a significant medicolegal impact, with nonphysician operators accounting for a significant proportion of these cases. Caution is required for any physician who is supervising these providers when performing laser treatment.

Anderson RR, Parrish JA: Selective photothermolysis. Science 1983; 220: 524.

Carroll L, Humphreys TR: Laser-tissue interactions. Clin Dermatol 2006; 24: 2.

Das A, et al: Cooling devices in laser therapy. J Cutan Aesthet Surg 2016; 9: 215.

Dawson E, et al: Adverse events associated with nonablative cutaneous laser, radiofrequency, and light-based devices. Semin Cutan Med Surg 2007; 26: 15.

Jalian HR, et al: Common causes of injury and legal action in laser surgery. JAMA Dermatol 2013; 149: 188.

Tanzi EL, et al: Lasers in dermatology. J Am Acad Dermatol 2003; 49: 1.

Vanaman M, et al: Complications in the cosmetic dermatology patient. Dermatol Surg 2016; 42: 12.

LASER TREATMENT OF VASCULAR LESIONS

A number of congenital and acquired vascular lesions can be effectively treated with laser. Given the variety of choices available, the laser surgeon must have a complete understanding of the inherent differences in wavelengths, pulse durations, and the vessel size of the particular lesion being targeted. Over the years, lasers have become more selective and the treatment of vascular lesions more effective.

Pulsed Dye Laser

The pulsed dye laser (PDL) was the first laser developed specifically to take advantage of selective photothermolysis. The laser medium is a rhodamine dye, which initially was developed to deliver a wavelength of 577 nm, coinciding with a specific hemoglobin absorption peak. Older lasers used a wavelength of 585 nm, but for various technical and clinical reasons, the wavelength has evolved in the current generation of PDL to be 595 nm. Initial pulse durations were about 500 microsecond (μs)/pulse. This was based on calculations that the target, hemoglobin, had a TRT of 1 ms or less. These parameters resulted in immediate postoperative purpura lasting up to 2 weeks.

Newer configurations of the laser allow for pulse durations from 0.45 to 40 ms, based on newer understandings of TRTs in the context of the size of the target (e.g., capillaries vs. larger vessels) and clinical effects (purpuric vs. nonpurpuric treatment). By using longer pulse durations, gentler and more uniform heating results in reduced or absent posttreatment purpura (more acceptable to patients) than the earlier PDL configurations, while still maintaining clinical efficacy.

The PDL is an extremely useful instrument for the treatment of vascular lesions. These lasers have traditionally been used for port wine stains, telangiectasias, erythematotelangiectatic rosacea, and hemangiomas. The risk of scarring and pigment change is

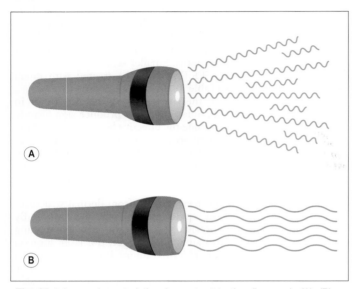

Fig. 38.1 Laser characteristics. In contrast to the diagram in (A), (B) demonstrates laser light that is both collimated and coherent.

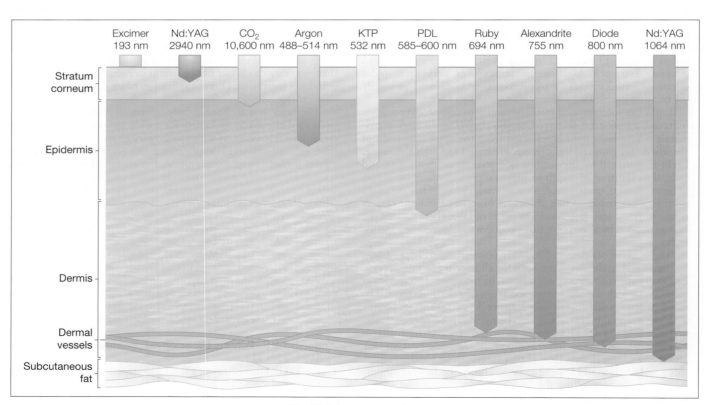

Fig. 38.2 Laser penetration.

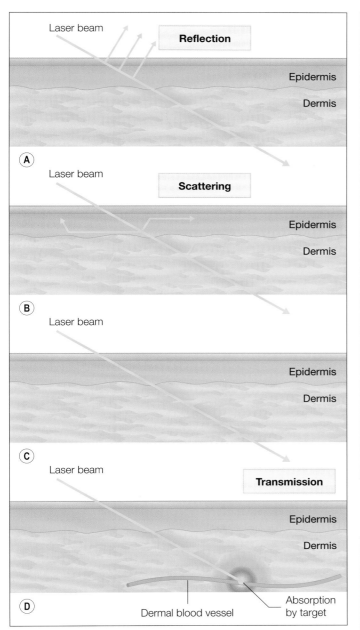

Fig. 38.3 Laser interaction with skin.

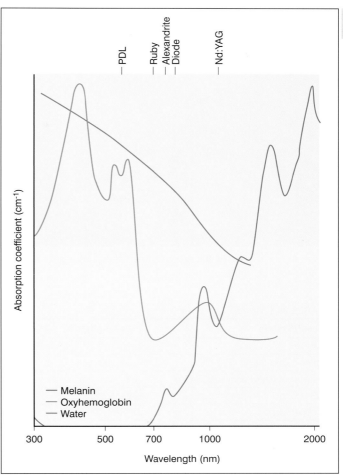

Fig. 38.4 Absorption spectra. The heterogeneous absorption spectra of chromophores allow selective photothermolysis to work.

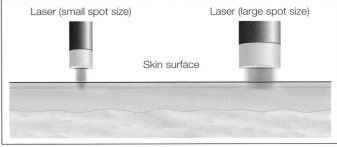

Fig. 38.5 Effects of spot size on scattering. The larger spot size allows more photons to remain within a beam's diameter, whereas with a smaller spot size, a greater fraction of photons scatters outside the beam and is ineffective. Thus a beam of a given wavelength penetrates to a deeper level with a larger spot size.

very low with this technology. PDL is used in a wide range of patients, including newborns. The newer, long-pulsed and longer-wavelength lasers allow for treatment of larger and deeper vessels. By combining these treatments with surface-cooling devices, the epidermis can be protected, which allows for the delivery of greater energy in a safer and less painful manner.

The PDL is the treatment of choice for port wine stains. A series of treatments every 4–6 weeks is required for maximum benefit, with gradual improvement after each session. Although most patients will show improvement, total clearance of lesions is extremely rare (Fig. 38.6). Rate of improvement is related to anatomic location, with lesions on the extremity having a less robust response than facial lesions. Size also plays a role in the response rate of port wine stains, with smaller lesions having a greater rate of improvement than larger lesions. Treatments are typically performed with short pulse durations (i.e., 0.45 or 1.5 ms),

with resulting purpura lasting for 10–14 days. When the treatment is performed with proper cooling and appropriate technique, the risk of atrophic scarring and pigmentary alterations is extremely low. Redarkening of treated port wine stains after treatment with PDL can occur over time and may necessitate repeat treatments years later.

Ulcerated hemangiomas have been successfully treated by PDL. In addition, after spontaneous resolution of infantile hemangiomas,

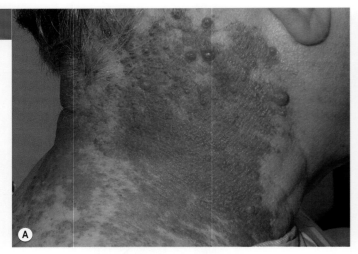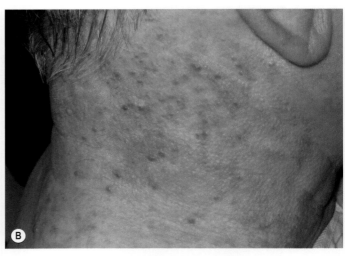

Fig. 38.6 Laser treatment of port wine stain. (A) Before treatment. (B) After eight treatments with pulsed dye laser.

TABLE 38.1 Dermatologic Lasers

Laser/System	Wavelength (nm)	Color	Applications
Argon	488–514	Blue-green	Vascular lesions
Intense pulsed light (IPL)	515–1200	Green-red and infrared	Vascular lesions, pigmented lesions, epilation, photodamage
Potassium titanyl phosphate (KTP)	532	Green	Vascular lesions, pigmented lesions
QS Nd:YAG (frequency doubled)	532	Green	Vascular lesions, pigmented lesions; tattoo—red
Copper vapor	578/511	Yellow-green	Vascular lesions, pigmented lesions
Flashlamp-pumped pulsed dye (PDL)	585–600	Yellow	Vascular lesions
QS ruby	694	Red	Deep and superficial pigmented lesions; tattoo—black, blue, green
Long-pulsed ruby	694	Red	Epilation
QS alexandrite	755	Infrared	Tattoo—blue, black, green
Long-pulsed alexandrite	755	Infrared	Epilation
Diode	810	Infrared	Epilation
QS Nd:YAG	1064	Infrared	Deep and superficial dermal pigment; tattoo—black, blue
Long-pulsed Nd:YAG	1064	Infrared	Epilation, vascular lesion
Er:YAG	2940	Infrared	Superficial skin resurfacing; destruction of superficial growths
Carbon dioxide	10,600	Infrared	Skin resurfacing; destruction of warts, keloids, superficial cancers, and benign growths

Nd:YAG, Neodymium-doped yttrium-aluminum-garnet; *QS,* Q-switched.

TABLE 38.2 Pulse Durations and Targets of Selective Photothermolysis

Chromophore	Diameter	TRT	Typical Laser Pulse Duration
Tattoo ink particle	0.1 μm	10 ns	10 ns
Melanosome	0.5 μm	250 ns	10–100 ns
Port wine stain vessels	30–100 μm	1–10 ms	0.4–20 ms
Terminal hair follicle	300 μm	100 ms	3–100 ms
Leg vein	1 mm	1 second	0.1 second

TRT, Thermal relaxation time.

PDL can be used for any persistent telangiectasias. PDL has a limited depth of penetration, however, and thus is not effective in the treatment of deeper components of hemangiomas, which are likely to continue to proliferate despite laser therapy. The use of PDL for superficial hemangiomas in the proliferative phase remains controversial. Some studies have demonstrated that early treatment with PDL results in improved clearing. However, other authors have advocated that the natural course of hemangiomas is of regression, and that potential risk of ulceration and atrophy from PDL treatment is not warranted for uncomplicated lesions.

Erythematotelangiectatic rosacea is a common condition characterized by persistent facial erythema, telangiectasias, and flushing. PDL has been shown to be an effective and safe treatment option (Fig. 38.7). The long-pulsed PDL has the advantage of purpura-free treatment, which is better tolerated by patients desiring cosmetic improvement.

Pulsed KTP lasers have pulse durations ranging from 1 to 100 ms. The advantage of these lasers is the strong absorption of their wavelength by hemoglobin. In addition, purpura is not present with the longer pulse widths. The 532-nm wavelength has a limited depth of penetration, making it an excellent choice for the treatment of fine facial vessels. However, it can be absorbed by epidermal pigment to a greater degree than other, longer-wavelength vascular lasers, which increases the risk of pigmentary complications. KTP lasers can be quite compact, allowing for easy transport between various locations. With few moving parts, they are also relatively maintenance free.

The KTP lasers are suited to treatment of individual telangiectasias of the face, cherry angiomas, and small spider angiomas. Because individual vessels must be traced out using a narrow beam diameter, the number of vessels treated in any given session is limited when using certain KTP lasers with smaller spot sizes. However, models with larger spot size and cooling can be effectively used for the treatment of erythematotelangiectatic rosacea and port wine stain.

Long-Pulsed Infrared Lasers

Lasers are now being used to take advantage of the broad oxyhemoglobin absorption band in the near-infrared range. Long-pulsed lasers include the alexandrite (755 nm), diode (800 nm, 940 nm), and neodymium:yttrium-aluminum-garnet (Nd:YAG; 1064 nm). These lasers are best used for larger and deeper vessels, such as large-vessel venous malformations, vascular blebs in port wine stains, blue reticular veins, venous lakes, and lower extremity spider veins (Fig. 38.8).

Intense Pulsed Light

The intense pulsed light (IPL) system, although technically not a laser, uses a flashlamp that emits a noncoherent broad spectrum of light (400–1200 nm) at various pulse durations and intervals. By employing filters to eliminate the lower wavelengths, light from 560 nm and above can be used to treat various cutaneous conditions. IPL technology has the advantage of treating more than one specific chromophore at a time and is especially useful in improving both vascular and pigmentary changes typically seen in photodamaged skin (see later discussion). In addition, IPL has a relatively large beam size and rapid pulse rate, allowing for the treatment of a large area in a relatively short amount of time. IPL has been used for the treatment of facial telangiectasia and rosacea. There is generally no purpura when appropriate settings are used, but care must be taken to avoid dyspigmentation and blistering in darker skin types. As with other light sources, a series of treatment sessions spaced out every 4–6 weeks is typically required for maximum improvement with IPL systems.

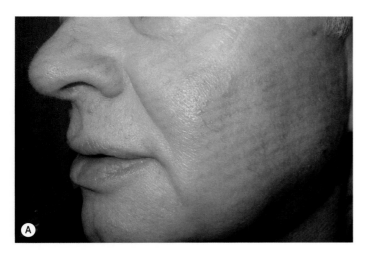

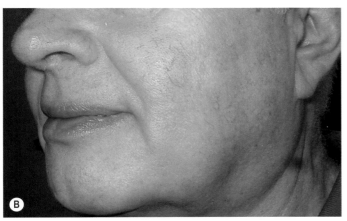

Fig. 38.7 Laser therapy for rosacea. (A) Before treatment. (B) After two treatments with subpurpuric pulsed dye laser.

The PDL has been effectively used for the treatment of warts, producing similar cure rates as traditional therapy. Several reports address the use of PDL for hypertrophic scars. Manuskiatti and Fitzpatrick demonstrated that PDL, intralesional corticosteroid, and 5-fluorouracil (5-FU) produced similar beneficial effects in the treatment of hypertrophic sternotomy scars. The mechanism of action in warts and hypertrophic scars is not clear but may be related to injury to vessels supporting the lesions or simply to heat-related injury. As with other treatment modalities for these two conditions, results are variable.

PDL has been demonstrated to reduce the immediate postprocedure purpura that may arise after various dermatologic procedures such as filler/toxin injections, or even bruising associated with PDL treatment itself. PDL using nonpurpuric settings can quicken the resolution of purpura and can be offered to all patients that undergo relevant procedures. Typically PDL is offered 1–2 days after the initial procedure

Potassium Titanyl Phosphate Laser

The potassium titanyl phosphate (KTP) laser produces a visible green beam of 532 nm. Because there is significant hemoglobin and melanin absorption of this wavelength, the KTP laser can be used to treat both vascular and superficial pigmented lesions. The KTP laser is actually an Nd:YAG laser that emits a wavelength of 1064 nm. The beam is passed through a crystal of KTP that reduces the wavelength by 50%, producing the 532-nm wavelength.

Becher GL, et al: Treatment of superficial vascular lesions with the KTP 532-nm laser. Lasers Med Sci 2014; 29: 267.

Chinnadurai S, et al: Laser treatment of infantile hemangioma. Lasers Surg Med 2016; 48: 221.

Civas E, et al: Clinical experience in the treatment of different vascular lesions using a neodymium-doped yttrium aluminum garnet laser. Dermatol Surg 2009; 35: 1933.

Clark C, et al: Treatment of superficial cutaneous vascular lesions. Lasers Med Sci 2004; 19: 1.

Faurschou A, et al: Pulsed dye laser vs. intense pulsed light for port-wine stains. Br J Dermatol 2009; 160: 359.

Galeckas KJ: Update on lasers and light devices for the treatment of vascular lesions. Semin Cutan Med Surg 2008; 27: 276.

Groot D, et al: Algorithm for using a long-pulsed Nd:YAG laser in the treatment of deep cutaneous vascular lesions. Dermatol Surg 2003; 29: 35.

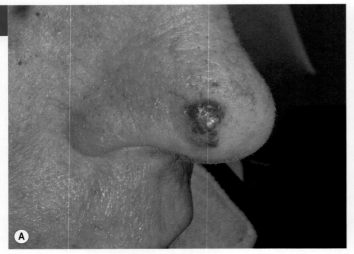

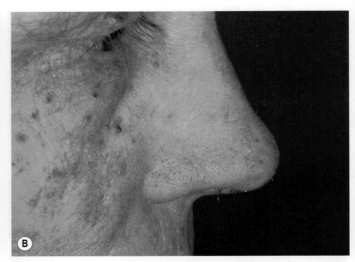

Fig. 38.8 Laser treatment of venous lake. (A) Before treatment. (B) After two treatments with long-pulsed Nd:YAG laser.

Huikeshoven M, et al: Redarkening of port-wine stains 10 years after pulsed-dye-laser treatment. N Engl J Med 2007; 356: 1235.

Kessels JP, et al: Superficial hemangioma: pulsed dye laser versus wait-and-see. Dermatol Surg 2013; 39: 414.

Manuskiatti W, Fitzpatrick RE: Treatment response of keloidal and hypertrophic sternotomy scars. Arch Dermatol 2002; 138: 1149.

Mayo TT, et al: Comparative study on bruise reduction treatments after bruise induction using the pulsed dye laser. Dermatol Surg 2013; 39: 1459.

Neuhaus IM, et al: Comparative efficacy of nonpurpuragenic pulsed dye laser and intense pulsed light for erythematotelangiectatic rosacea. Dermatol Surg 2009; 35: 920.

Nouri K, et al: Comparison of the effects of short- and long-pulse durations when using a 585-nm pulsed dye laser in the treatment of new surgical scars. Lasers Med Sci 2010; 25: 121.

Reddy KK, et al: Treatment of port-wine stains with a short pulse width 532-nm Nd:YAG laser. J Drugs Dermatol 2013; 12: 66.

Robson KJ, et al: Pulsed-dye laser versus conventional therapy in the treatment of warts. J Am Acad Dermatol 2000; 43: 275.

Savas JA, et al: Pulsed dye laser–resistant port-wine stains. Br J Dermatol 2013; 168: 941.

Schellhaas U, et al: Pulsed dye laser treatment is effective in the treatment of recalcitrant viral warts. Dermatol Surg 2008; 34: 67.

Schroeter CA, et al: Effective treatment of rosacea using intense pulsed light systems. Dermatol Surg 2005; 31: 1285.

Stier MF, et al: Laser treatment of pediatric vascular lesions. J Am Acad Dermatol 2008; 58: 261.

Tan SR, Tope WD: Pulsed dye laser treatment of rosacea improves erythema, symptomatology, and quality of life. J Am Acad Dermatol 2004; 51: 592.

Uebelhoer NS, et al: A split-face comparison study of pulsed 532-nm KTP laser and 595-nm pulsed dye laser in the treatment of facial telangiectasias and diffuse telangiectatic facial erythema. Dermatol Surg 2007; 33: 441.

Veitch D, et al: Pulsed dye laser therapy in the treatment of warts. Dermatol Surg 2017; 43: 485.

Witman PM, et al: Complications following pulsed dye laser treatment of superficial hemangiomas. Lasers Surg Med 2006; 38: 116.

TABLE 38.3 Q-Switched (QS) Lasers

Laser Type	Wavelength (nm)	Pulse Duration (ns)
QS Nd:YAG (frequency doubled)	532	5–7
QS ruby	694	25–40
QS alexandrite	755	50–100
QS Nd:YAG	1064	5–7

Nd:YAG, Neodymium-doped yttrium-aluminum-garnet.

LASER TREATMENT FOR PIGMENTED LESIONS

Highly pigment-selective Q-switched (QS) lasers are used extensively in the treatment of both epidermal and dermal pigmented lesions. In most cases, the target chromophore is the melanosome. These tiny structures have a very short TRT (250–1000 ns), and the development of Q-switching allows for production of extremely high energies and short, nanosecond (ns) pulse durations. Recent technologic advances have allowed the creation of laser in the picosecond range, which results in an even shorter pulse duration. As a result, these lasers can produce damage to the selected target while minimizing injury to surrounding tissue.

QS lasers are used to treat epidermal pigmented lesions and tattoos. The delivery of tremendous amounts of energy over a very short period (nanoseconds or picoseconds) produces pressure waves. This photoacoustic effect results in shock waves that shatter the larger ink particles into smaller fragments. The fragmented ink is then expelled via the scale/crust that is produced during the laser treatment, or removed via lymphatic drainage. Repeated treatments are necessary for complete response as a partial response is typically seen after each laser session. QS lasers include the ruby (694 nm), alexandrite (755 nm), and Nd:YAG, in both a frequency-doubled (532 nm) and standard (1064 nm) mode (Table 38.3). Because of the longer wavelength, the Nd:YAG laser penetrates much more deeply and therefore is more useful in treating more deeply seated or thicker lesions compared with shorter-wavelength QS lasers.

Less pigment-selective lasers can be used in some clinical settings. The variable-pulsed KTP laser can be used to treat

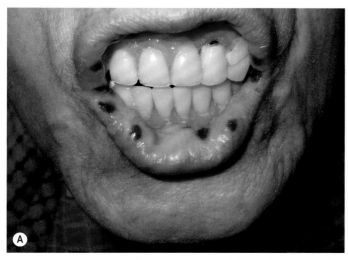
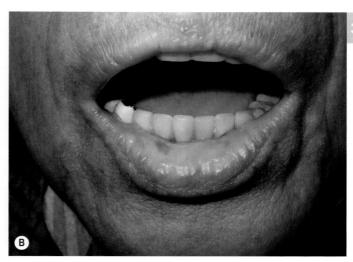

Fig. 38.9 Laser therapy for labial melanotic macules. (A) Before treatment. (B) After single treatment with Q-switched (QS) 532-nm laser.

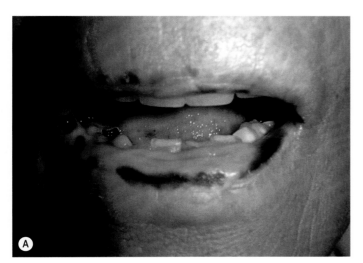
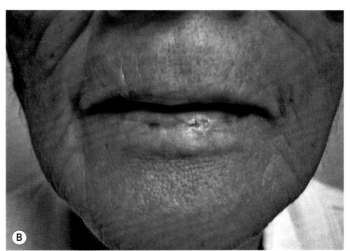

Fig. 38.10 Laser treatment of lip lentigines in patient with Peutz-Jeghers syndrome. (A) Before treatment. (B) After treatment with QS ruby laser.

epidermal pigmentation, such as lentigines, ephelides, thin seborrheic keratoses, and dermatosis papulosis nigra. Because the KTP laser has a limited depth of penetration, it is not effective in the treatment of deeper dermal lesions. Long-pulsed ruby, alexandrite, and Nd:YAG lasers can also be used to treat pigmented lesions, but are not as effective as their QS or picosecond counterparts.

Non–pigment-specific ablative lasers have been used in the treatment of pigmented lesions and tattoos. Carbon dioxide (10,600 nm) and erbium:YAG lasers (2940 nm) target water. They nonselectively remove the entire epidermis and a variable level of dermis tissue, as well as any associated pigment present.

Epidermal Pigmented Lesions

Lentigines are hyperpigmented macules composed of an increased number of basal melanocytes. These lesions can be effectively treated with a variety of laser and light sources because of their superficial position in the skin. QS lasers can be used to treat solar lentigines and those associated with certain syndromes (e.g.,

Peutz-Jeghers) (Figs. 38.9 and 38.10). Variable-pulsed KTP provides effective treatment. IPL is an excellent choice for patients with widespread photodamage consisting of both vascular and pigmentary changes.

Café au lait macules and Becker's nevus can be treated with QS lasers. Unfortunately, treatment often results in variable clinical efficacy. Short-term lightening or clearing with multiple treatments is frequently seen, but recurrence is common.

Dermal Pigmented Lesions

Nevus of Ota and nevus of Ito are dermal melanocytoses that can be effectively treated with QS lasers. A series of treatments can significantly improve or even clear the lesion (Fig. 38.11). These treatments are generally well tolerated and the results long-lasting.

Melasma is an acquired hypermelanosis that is often associated with sun exposure, pregnancy, and oral contraceptives and other hormone medications. First-line treatment includes strict sun protection, discontinuing any offending systemic medication, and

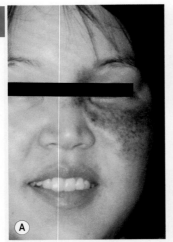 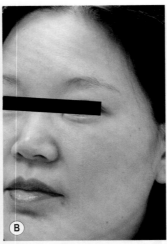

Fig. 38.11 Laser therapy for patient with nevus of Ota. (A) Before treatment. (B) After treatment with QS ruby laser.

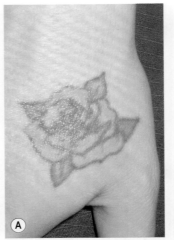 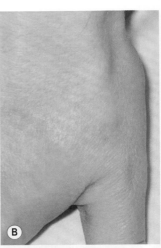

Fig. 38.12 Laser therapy for tattoo removal. (A) Before treatment. (B) After six treatments with QS ruby and QS Nd:YAG laser.

the use of topical agents such as hydroquinone and retinoids. Laser treatment is often ineffective, and recurrence is frequently seen in patients after initial improvement.

Postinflammatory hyperpigmentation does not generally respond to QS laser. Recurrence or worsening is typically seen because of additional epidermal injury associated with laser treatment perpetuates the deposition of pigment in the treated area.

Tattoos

Pigmentation to mark the skin for decorative purposes has been used by humans for thousands of years and remains a popular practice today. As a result of the increasing number of people with tattoos, it should come as no surprise that many patients desire removal. Regardless of the type of tattoo—cosmetic, medical, or traumatic—effective treatment can be frequently offered.

In the past, tattoos were removed by a variety of nonselective destructive techniques, including excision, dermabrasion, cryosurgery, and ablative laser. Although effective in eliminating the ink, these techniques produced significant scarring. With the advent of newer technology that is more specific and less traumatic, these destructive modalities are not generally employed today.

Currently, QS lasers are the first-line treatment for tattoo removal. The delivery of high energy in very short pulse durations causes fragmentation of the tattoo ink particle, which is then eliminated from the body by phagocytosis of macrophages and lymphatic drainage. Repeat treatments are required to achieve maximum benefit (Fig. 38.12).

Patients frequently inquire as to the number of treatment sessions needed for maximum improvement. Unfortunately, a precise answer is difficult to provide and depends on the amount of ink in the tattoo, size of tattoo, location, and color being treated. Traumatic tattoos typically respond extremely well with a short course of treatments. Amateur tattoos typically have less ink and generally have a good response to laser treatment. Traumatic tattoos from an injury typically respond very well with a limited number of treatments (Fig. 38.13). In contrast, multicolored professional tattoos have a more unpredictable response and require more treatments, sometimes 10–15 or more, to achieve maximum benefit. The choice of which laser to use depends on the specific tattoo color being targeted (Table 38.4).

Evidence of the superiority of picosecond lasers compared with nanosecond devices has been mixed. Although there have

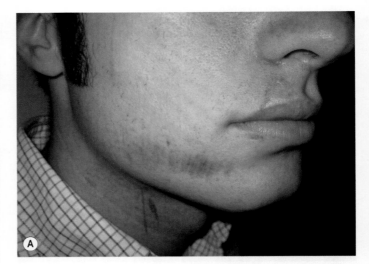

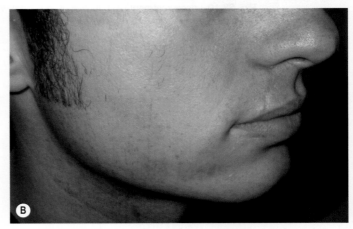

Fig. 38.13 Traumatic tattoo. (A) Before laser treatment. (B) After two treatments with QS Nd:YAG laser.

TABLE 38.4 Tattoo Colors and Pigments, With Lasers Used for Treatment

Color/Etiology	Pigment	Laser
Traumatic	Lead, asphalt, carbon, gunpowder	QS ruby; QS alexandrite; QS Nd:YAG (1064 nm)
Amateur black	India ink, carbon	QS ruby; QS alexandrite; QS Nd:YAG (1064 nm)
Professional black	Carbon, iron oxide, logwood extract	QS ruby; QS alexandrite; QS Nd:YAG (1064 nm)
Blue	Cobalt aluminate (azure blue)	QS ruby; QS alexandrite; QS Nd:YAG (1064 nm)
Green	Chromium oxide (casalis green), hydrated chromium sesquioxide (guignet green), malachite green, lead chromate, ferroferric cyanide, curcumin green, phthalocyanine dyes (copper salts with yellow coal tar dyes)	QS ruby; QS alexandrite
Red	Mercury sulfide (cinnabar), cadmium selenide (cadmium red), sienna (red ochre; ferric hydrate and ferric sulfate), azo dyes	QS Nd:YAG (532 nm)
Yellow	Cadmium sulfide (cadmium yellow), ochre, curcumin yellow	QS Nd:YAG (532 nm)
Brown	Ochre	Tan/light brown: QS Nd:YAG (532 nm) Dark brown: QS ruby; QS alexandrite; QS Nd:YAG (1064 nm)
Violet	Manganese violet	QS Nd:YAG (532 nm)
White	Titanium dioxide, zinc oxide	QS Nd:YAG (532 nm)
Flesh	Iron oxides	QS Nd:YAG (532 nm)

Nd:YAG, Neodymium-doped yttrium-aluminum-garnet; *QS,* Q-switched.

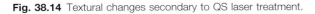

Fig. 38.14 Textural changes secondary to QS laser treatment.

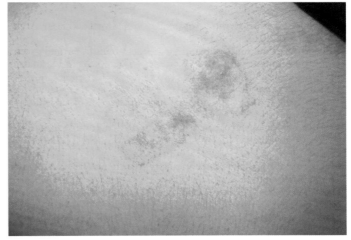

Fig. 38.15 Hypopigmentation secondary to QS laser treatment.

been many anecdotal reports of improved outcome, fewer treatment sessions, and overall outcomes with picosecond lasers, there have been limited comparative data. Pinto et al. did not demonstrate any difference between the picosecond and nanosecond QS laser devices in the treatment of black ink in a side by side study. Further studies and time will be needed to determine the efficacy of picosecond versus nanosecond technology.

Tattoo Complications

Textural changes can occur as a result of the repetitive injury associated with laser treatment (Fig. 38.14). Epidermal injury can be seen with excessive fluences and with short treatment intervals. By spacing out treatment sessions, lowering fluences, and using longer wavelengths to protect the epidermis, this can often be avoided.

Hypopigmentation is sometimes seen in patients with darker skin types (Fig. 38.15). Similar to textural changes, pigmentary changes are more common with shorter wavelengths (ruby and

alexandrite), which can cause more epidermal damage. Similar precautions can be used to minimize these changes.

Paradoxic darkening of flesh, brown, or white tattoos (with red and yellow ink less frequently) can occur immediately after treatment with QS lasers. The reduction of rust-colored ferric oxide to black-colored ferrous oxide or the white-colored titanium^{4+} dioxide to blue titanium^{3+} dioxide is thought to be responsible for the color change. This reaction is typically seen is cosmetic tattoos used for lip liners and eyebrows. However, many brightly colored tattoos have some white mixed in with them, so caution must be taken in these circumstances (Fig. 38.16). A test treatment in a limited area should be done if paradoxic darkening is possible. The darkened tattoo can be treated with the appropriate QS wavelength, but response is unpredictable and requires numerous treatments.

Despite appropriate treatment, tattoos may not respond completely. This may result from the color, ink density, anatomic location, or age of the tattoo. Appropriate preoperative counseling is required before embarking on any treatment course.

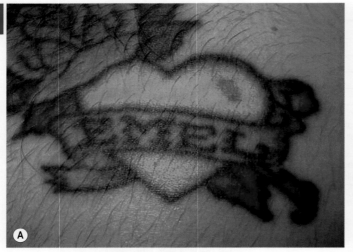
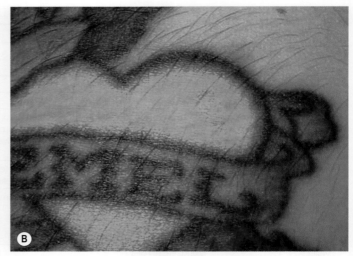

Fig. 38.16 Paradoxic darkening of red tattoo after single test pulse with QS 532-nm laser. (A) Single pulse with resulting darkening. (B) After treatment of darkening with QS Nd:YAG laser.

Treatment of gunpowder traumatic tattoos can result in microexplosions and scars. Care must be taken when treating these patients.

Bencini PL, et al: Removal of tattoos by Q-switched laser. Arch Dermatol 2012; 148: 1364.

Brauer JA, et al: Successful and rapid treatment of blue and green tattoo pigment with a novel picosecond laser. Arch Dermatol 2012; 148: 820.

Felton SJ, et al: Our perspective of the treatment of naevus of Ota with 1,064-, 755- and 532-nm wavelength lasers. Lasers Med Sci 2014; 29: 1745.

Fusade T, et al: Treatment of gunpowder traumatic tattoo by Q-switched Nd:YAG laser. Dermatol Surg 2000; 26: 1057.

Halachmi S, et al: Melasma and laser treatment. Lasers Med Sci 2014; 29: 589.

Holzer AM, et al: Adverse effects of Q-switched laser treatment of tattoos. Dermatol Surg 2008; 34: 118.

Hsu VM, et al: The picosecond laser for tattoo removal. Lasers Med Sci 2016; 31: 1733.

Kent KM, Graber EM: Laser tattoo removal. Dermatol Surg 2012; 38: 1.

Levin MK, et al: Treatment of pigmentary disorders in patients with skin of color with a novel 755 nm picosecond, Q-switched ruby, and Q-switched Nd:YAG nanosecond lasers. Lasers Surg Med 2016; 48: 181.

Liu J, et al: A retrospective study of Q-switched alexandrite laser in treating nevus of Ota. Dermatol Surg 2011; 37: 1480.

Park JM, et al: Combined use of intense pulsed light and Q-switched ruby laser for complex dyspigmentation among Asian patients. Lasers Surg Med 2008; 40: 128.

Pinto F, et al: Neodymium-doped yttrium aluminium garnet (Nd:YAG) 1064-nm picosecond laser vs. Nd:YAG 1064-nm nanosecond laser in tattoo removal. Br J Dermatol 2017; 176: 457.

Sadighha A, et al: Efficacy and adverse effects of Q-switched ruby laser on solar lentigines. Dermatol Surg 2008; 34: 1465.

Vachiramon V, et al: Comparison of Q-switched Nd:YAG laser and fractional carbon dioxide laser for the treatment of solar lentigines in Asians. Lasers Surg Med 2016; 48: 354.

Xi Z, et al: Q-switched alexandrite laser treatment of oral labial lentigines in Chinese subjects with Peutz-Jeghers syndrome. Dermatol Surg 2009; 35: 1084.

Yu P, et al: Comparison of clinical efficacy and complications between Q-switched alexandrite laser and Q-switched Nd:YAG laser on nevus of Ota. Lasers Med Sci 2016; 31: 581.

Zhou X, et al: Efficacy and safety of Q-switched 1,064-nm neodymium-doped yttrium aluminum garnet laser treatment of melasma. Dermatol Surg 2011; 37: 962.

LASER HAIR REMOVAL

Laser hair removal is widely used for the permanent reduction of hair and is one of the most popular laser procedures performed. Hair removal lasers target the melanin within the follicle, and given the size of the target chromophore, longer pulse durations are required to generate enough heat to damage the bulbar stem cells. Patients with dark hair and lightly pigmented skin are the best candidates for treatment. In contrast, white, blond, and gray hairs generally respond poorly given their absence of a sufficient pigment target.

Patients must avoid waxing, electrolysis, or plucking of hairs before laser treatment, because hair is required to be present as a target. Shaving before laser treatment is acceptable and will not interfere with efficacy. In fact, shaving is mandatory immediately before treatment to avoid epidermal injury from absorption of the laser by hairs on the surface of the skin. Only hairs in the anagen growth phase are permanently injured. Therefore sufficient time must elapse between treatments for hair to regrow and provide an appropriate chromophore for subsequent laser treatment, generally 6–8 weeks.

Devices currently used for hair removal include the long-pulsed ruby, alexandrite, diode, and Nd:YAG lasers and IPL. Multiple treatments are required for maximum benefit. In addition, these longer-pulsed lasers can produce a significant reduction in both hair and papules/pustules in patients with pseudofolliculitis barbae, acne keloidalis nuchae, pilonidal sinus, or folliculitis decalvans.

Complications are rare with proper patient selection and treatment parameters. Excessive fluences or insufficient cooling can result in epidermal injury (Fig. 38.17). Caution must be employed in treating patients with increased skin pigmentation caused by sun tanning, because pigmentary changes and cutaneous burns can occur. Because melanin is the target for these lasers, care must be taken in treating more darkly pigmented patients to avoid epidermal damage. In this patient population, the longer-pulsed Nd:YAG laser has allowed safe treatment with fewer

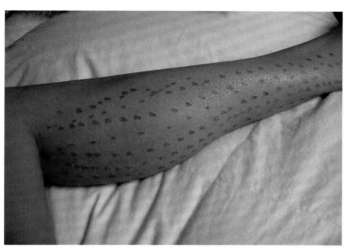

Fig. 38.17 Epidermal burns secondary to laser hair removal performed by an unlicensed provider at a "medi-spa."

complications, because of the deeper penetration and reduced melanin absorption of this wavelength. Paradoxic hypertrichosis as a result of laser hair treatment has been reported. The etiology is unclear, but the condition seems to occur more frequently in darker skin types. Rarely, atypical cutaneous infections have been reported. Interestingly, studies have shown that laser hair removal is the most common litigated laser procedure, with nonphysician providers accounting for a significant proportion of these cases.

Davoudi SM, et al: Comparison of long-pulsed alexandrite and Nd:YAG lasers, individually and in combination, for leg hair reduction. Arch Dermatol 2008; 144: 1323.

De Benito V, et al: *Mycobacterium chelonae* infection after laser hair removal. J Am Acad Dermatol 2013; 69: e255.

Desai S, et al: Paradoxical hypertrichosis after laser therapy. Dermatol Surg 2010; 36: 291.

Esmat SM, et al: The efficacy of laser-assisted hair removal in the treatment of acne keloidalis nuchae. Eur J Dermatol 2012; 22: 645.

Gan SD, Graber EM: Laser hair removal. Dermatol Surg 2013; 39: 823.

Haak CS, et al: Hair removal in hirsute women with normal testosterone levels. Br J Dermatol 2010; 163: 1007.

Ismail SA: Long-pulsed Nd:YAG laser vs. intense pulsed light for hair removal in dark skin. Br J Dermatol 2012; 166: 317.

Jalian HR, et al: Increased risk of litigation associated with laser surgery by nonphysician operators. JAMA Dermatol 2014; 150: 407.

Khan MA, et al: Control of hair growth using long-pulsed alexandrite laser is an efficient and cost effective therapy for patients suffering from recurrent pilonidal disease. Lasers Med Sci 2016; 31: 857.

Klein A, et al: Photoepilation with a diode laser vs. intense pulsed light. Br J Dermatol 2013; 168: 1287.

Rao K, Sankar TK: Long-pulsed Nd:YAG laser-assisted hair removal in Fitzpatrick skin types IV–VI. Lasers Med Sci 2011; 26: 623.

Schulze R, et al: Low-fluence 1,064-nm laser hair reduction for pseudofolliculitis barbae in skin types IV, V, and VI. Dermatol Surg 2009; 35: 98.

ABLATIVE LASER RESURFACING

Both carbon dioxide (CO_2) and erbium:YAG (Er:YAG) lasers are absorbed by water. Because water makes up 72% of the skin, these lasers effectively ablate the skin to varying depths depending on the energy delivered. Ablative lasers can be used therapeutically to treat conditions such as warts, adnexal tumors, and actinic damage. In addition to these medical indications, ablative lasers can also be employed to remove very superficial external layers and resurface the skin for cosmetic enhancement (e.g., acne scarring, photorejuvenation). Despite all the efforts to produce nonablative resurfacing technology, ablative lasers remain unparalleled in producing meaningful and dramatic rejuvenation.

Early systems employed a continuous-wave mode of emission, which led to a greater degree of thermal damage and risk of scarring. Newer, high-energy, ultrapulsed and computerized scanning systems have allowed a greater degree of control with laser ablation, resulting in more predictable outcomes.

Carbon Dioxide Lasers

The CO_2 laser emits an invisible infrared beam of 10,600 nm and can be used in continuous-wave or superpulsed mode. Water nonselectively absorbs laser energy, turning it instantly into steam, and producing ablative and thermal damage. Used in the superpulsed mode, the laser beam can be delivered in short bursts, allowing thermal destruction of the epidermis and papillary dermis while limiting deeper thermal damage. Delivery in this mode is more uniform and much faster when the optomechanical scanner is employed. Superpulsed CO_2 lasers are extremely effective for the treatment of actinic damage and photoaging. The thermal injury causes conformational changes within the collagen, leading to clinical tightening. As such, ablative laser resurfacing produces significant improvement in wrinkling, scarring, and skin tone.

Ablative laser surgery can be performed safely and comfortably under local anesthesia in the outpatient setting. Oral anxiolytics are routinely employed before starting the procedure. Regional blocks and local infiltration of anesthesia can provide effective pain control. Metal eye shields and anesthetic eye drops (e.g., proparacaine) should be used to provide eye protection. Wet towels are placed around the treatment site to prevent fire or heat injury.

Side effects include postinflammatory pigmentary changes, especially in patients with Fitzpatrick skin types III–VI. Treatment with hydroquinone at the first sign of hyperpigmentation can effectively reduce the skin darkening. Hypopigmentation is frequently seen after resurfacing and is often caused by the contrast between treated and untreated skin. To minimize the esthetic impact, the entire face should be treated. If this is not possible, regional subunits can be addressed to avoid a clear line of demarcation between treated and untreated skin. Scarring and textural changes can rarely be seen. Prolonged erythema can last 3–10 months, but patients can generally use make up to cover the redness. Bacterial, viral, and fungal infections have all been reported with resurfacing but have a relatively low incidence. Prophylactic antiviral agents are typically started on the day of the procedure, even in patients with no history of orolabial herpes simplex virus infection. There is no role for universal antibiotic or antifungal prophylactic treatment in patients undergoing resurfacing. Rather, treatment can be started empirically if patients develop infection, then tailored based on culture results. Given the morbidity of the postoperative course and prolonged recovery associated with ablative resurfacing, patients must be properly counseled during the preoperative visit.

Used in the quasi–continuous-wave mode, the CO_2 laser is an excellent therapeutic choice for very large plantar and periungual warts that have failed to respond to routine office modalities. Both a cutting mode and a defocused ablative mode can be used with these systems to excise the visible verrucae effectively and to treat any residual human papillomavirus in surrounding skin.

The CO_2 laser is also a treatment option for refractory keloids. Other benign lesions amenable to CO_2 laser ablation include xanthelasma, rhinophyma, and syringomas. Various malignant and premalignant lesions are also effectively treated by laser ablation, including actinic cheilitis and superficial basal and squamous cell carcinomas.

Erbium:Yttrium-Aluminum-Garnet Laser

The Er:YAG laser emits an invisible near-infrared beam of 2940 nm, resulting in significantly more efficient absorption by water (16 times) and a more explosive ablative effect than with the CO_2 laser. As such, the Er:YAG laser results in tissue ablation with less surrounding thermal damage. In addition, this wavelength is close to a collagen absorption peak, thus allowing for greater collagen ablation than the CO_2 laser. The decreased thermal injury and collagen ablation is an advantage for treatment of scars, photodamaged skin, rhytids, and rhinophyma (Figs. 38.18 and 38.19). Some maintain that healing may be slightly faster, with less risk of prolonged erythema and scarring. Nonetheless, the depth of injury produced (regardless of technology used) is the primary determinant for the healing process and incidence of side effects, not the laser used.

Compared with the photocoagulation effects of the CO_2 laser, the decreased thermal damage produced by the Er:YAG laser can result in poor hemostasis. To address this limitation, certain Er:YAG systems have a programmable coagulation mode to limit the amount of intraoperative bleeding. In addition, the collagen-tightening effect may not be as pronounced as with the CO_2 laser. However, when similar clinical injuries and depth are achieved, studies have shown that the Er:YAG and CO_2 lasers have comparable

photorejuvenating effects, as well as similar postoperative healing times and complication profiles.

Fractional Resurfacing

In fractional photothermolysis, an ablative laser is administered in a pixilated pattern over a grid. These lasers created small columns of thermal injury, or microthermal zones (MTZ), which are separated by areas of untreated skin. Only 15%–25% of the skin surface is typically ablated during a treatment session, so this technique allows for more rapid reepithelialization, compared with the confluent patch of laser-induced injury typically created with traditional ablative resurfacing. The injury created by MTZ results in the stimulation of collagen synthesis and cutaneous remodeling, much in the same manner as traditional resurfacing, but to a proportionately lesser degree.

Fractional resurfacing has been used for the treatment of photoaging, with the advantage of more rapid healing, reduced erythema and swelling, and fewer side effects. Fractional resurfacing has also been used for such indications as acne scars, residual hemangioma residuum, and pigmentary disorders. An additional advantage of this technology is the ability to treat any anatomic location, including hands, chest, neck, and arms. However, patients often need multiple treatment sessions to achieve maximum benefit, and the final result is not nearly as impressive as with traditional ablative resurfacing. In addition, the cumulative downtime required with multiple treatments may exceed that of a single ablative resurfacing treatment, thus negating the perceived benefit of fractional resurfacing.

Fractional ablative resurfacing has been used for the treatment of acne scarring. It has also been used for residual hemangioma and pigmentary disorders such as melasma.

Brightman LA, et al: Ablative fractional resurfacing for involuted hemangioma residuum. Arch Dermatol 2012; 148: 1294.

El-Domyati M, et al: Fractional versus ablative erbium:yttrium-aluminum-garnet laser resurfacing for facial rejuvenation. J Am Acad Dermatol 2013; 68: 103.

Farshidi D, et al: Erbium:yttrium aluminum garnet ablative laser resurfacing for skin tightening. Dermatol Surg 2014; 40: S152.

Graber EM, et al: Side effects and complications of fractional laser photothermolysis. Dermatol Surg 2008; 34: 301.

Hedelund L, et al: Fractional CO_2 laser resurfacing for atrophic acne scars. Lasers Surg Med 2012; 44: 447.

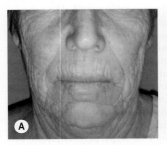 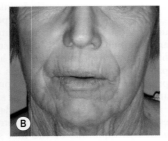

Fig. 38.18 Ablative resurfacing using Er:YAG laser. (A) Before treatment. (B) Six months after full-face resurfacing. (Courtesy Roy Grekin, MD.)

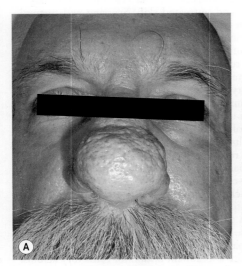 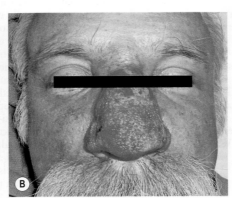 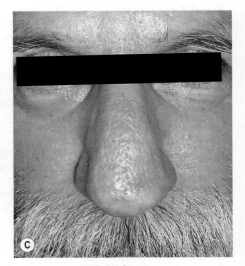

Fig. 38.19 Laser therapy for rhinophyma. (A) Before treatment. (B) Immediately after treatment with Er:YAG laser. (C) Final result 3 months later, with marked improvement in shape and appearance.

Madan V, et al: Carbon dioxide laser treatment of rhinophyma. Br J Dermatol 2009; 161: 814.

Metelitsa AI, Alster TS: Fractionated laser skin resurfacing treatment complications. Dermatol Surg 2010; 36: 299.

Orringer JS, et al: Direct quantitative comparison of molecular responses in photodamaged human skin to fractionated and fully ablative carbon dioxide laser resurfacing. Dermatol Surg 2012; 38: 1668.

Ortiz AE, et al: Ablative CO_2 lasers for skin tightening: traditional versus fractional. Dermatol Surg 2014; 40: S147.

Riggs K, et al: Ablative laser resurfacing. Clin Dermatol 2007; 25: 462.

Tierney EP, Hanke CW: Fractionated carbon dioxide laser treatment of photoaging. Dermatol Surg 2011; 37: 1279.

Tierney EP, et al: Review of fractional photothermolysis. Dermatol Surg 2009; 35: 1445.

Cosmetic Dermatology

Dermatologists have been leaders in the field of cosmetic surgery. Many procedures, products, and technologies in esthetic dermatologic surgery have been developed and researched by dermatologists. In addition, patients are increasingly turning to dermatologists for the management of concerns related to appearance. As a result, the specialty must continue to be at the forefront of cosmetic procedures and remain committed to advancing the field through innovation and scientific progress.

SOFT TISSUE AUGMENTATION

Soft tissue augmentation continues to remain popular as patients seek cosmetic improvement without undergoing invasive procedures. Numerous fillers are available to correct soft tissue contour abnormalities and provide cosmetic enhancement. Although they provide numerous advantages over surgical techniques, the temporary nature of most fillers requires repeated treatment to maintain a desired outcome. Some patients find that the temporary nature of these agents is less than ideal, but one must also consider that any undesired outcomes that may potentially occur due to treatment are also temporary. In the last few years the number of available agents has increased. In Europe there are as many as 30 different filler choices. The U.S. Food and Drug Administration (FDA) has approved fewer fillers, although several new products have recently become available.

Bovine Collagen

Bovine-derived collagen has been used for decades and is the gold standard against which all filler substances are compared. However, due to advances in newer products, as well as some of the limitations of collagen (discussed later), the use of collagen for soft tissue augmentation has fallen out of popularity. However, for historical perspective and completeness as a comparison with the newer products used today, a full discussion of collagen is included here.

There are currently three FDA-approved brand-name products for use in soft tissue augmentation: Zyderm I, Zyderm II, and Zyplast (Allergan, Irvine, CA). The source for all three bovine types is a closed herd in the United States, and there have been no cases of bovine spongiform encephalopathy associated with these products. All are composed of 95% type I collagen and the remainder of type III collagen, suspended in buffered saline and 0.3% lidocaine. Zyderm I consists of 35 mg/mL of collagen, and Zyderm II has a higher concentration of 65 mg/mL. Zyplast is cross-linked with glutaraldehyde, making it more resistant to proteolytic degradation, which provides longer duration. All three products come preloaded into syringes and are stored at 4°C.

Bovine collagen hypersensitivity occurs in about 3% of the population, making skin testing a requirement before using these products. Additionally, 1%–2% of patients with a negative skin test will subsequently develop an allergic reaction after treatment. Therefore many dermatologists recommend a second skin test after an initial negative test. Patients may also develop allergy after multiple treatments. Therefore in patients with a span between treatments of more than 2 years, repeated skin testing is indicated.

Zyderm I and Zyderm II are injected into the superficial dermis, whereas Zyplast is placed deeper. A combination of threading, fanning, and serial puncture injection techniques with a 30-gauge needle can be used. Anesthesia may not be required because the product already contains lidocaine; however, regional nerve blocks may be helpful in sensitive patients or when injecting the lips. Slight overcorrection is recommended when using bovine collagen because a reduction of volume is noted due to the amount of water in the product that is absorbed.

Patients can expect 2–5 months of improvement, depending on the location of placement. Dynamic rhytids (e.g., caused by muscular activity) have a shorter duration of correction, unlike more static conditions (e.g., acne scars). Zyplast may have a longer duration because of its relative protection from enzymatic degradation. However, it must be placed deeper in the dermis to avoid a beaded surface appearance and is therefore less useful for correction of superficial rhytids.

Complications with bovine collagen include delayed hypersensitivity reactions. Although rare, allergic reactions can occur in 1% of patients who have had two negative skin tests. This presents as swollen granulomas or sterile abscesses at the treatment site. Although self-limiting, these reactions can take up to 1 year to resolve. Intralesional steroid injections, antibiotics, and systemic antiinflammatory drugs can be considered for treatment. Zyplast placed in the glabellar complex has resulted in vascular occlusion and necrosis. This may be caused by the deeper placement required with this product and the associated adverse pressure-related effects on cutaneous vasculature.

Human Collagen

One of the main shortcomings of bovine collagen is the risk of hypersensitivity reaction. Synthetic human collagen has been developed as an alternative that does not require multiple skin testing and can be administered immediately. There has been no documented cross-reaction between bovine and bioengineered human collagen, allowing patients with a documented allergy to bovine collagen to be treated safely with human collagen.

Cosmoderm 1 and 2 and Cosmoplast (Allergan) are FDA-approved bioengineered human collagen derived from neonatal foreskin. Synthetic human collagen has a very similar formulation to its bovine counterpart and is packaged in similar concentrations. Cosmoderm 1 has a concentration of 35 mg/mL and is in phosphate-buffered saline with 0.3% lidocaine. Cosmoderm 2 has a concentration of 65 mg/mL. Cosmoplast has 35 mg/mL of human-derived collagen and is cross-linked with glutaraldehyde. All products have the same indications, are injected in a similar manner to their bovine counterparts, and have similar cosmetic results and longevity.

The clinical use of collagen continues to decline as manufacturers have decreased production and transitioned to the manufacturing and promotion of hyaluronic acid fillers.

Hyaluronic Acid

Hyaluronic acid, a polysaccharide, is a natural component of human connective tissue. A member of the family of glycosaminoglycans, hyaluronic acid is composed of repeating disaccharide units. This molecule has the advantage of being identical across all species. As such, hypersensitivity reactions should not occur, and skin testing is not required before treatment. However, early formulations of hyaluronic acid did produce rare hypersensitivity reaction, although the incidence has declined with the introduction of a more purified product. Granulomatous foreign body reactions have been described in case reports.

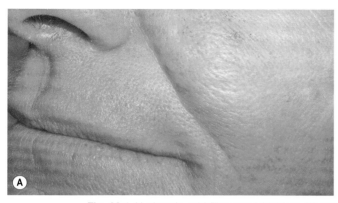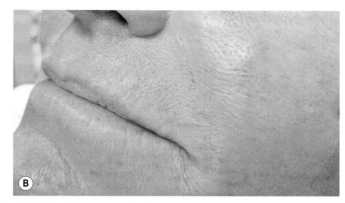

Fig. 39.1 Hyaluronic acid filler, nasolabial fold. (A) Before treatment. (B) Immediately after placement of hyaluronic acid, with marked improvement and reduction of rhytids.

Hyaluronic acid avidly binds water, and patients may experience redness, swelling, and bruising in the first few days after treatment. Most of the volume is maintained after placement, making overcorrection unnecessary when injecting. Hyaluronic acid products consist of a clear gel in a prepackaged syringe. Early products did not contain lidocaine, often necessitating the use of local anesthesia and regional blocks for patient comfort. However, many current preparations of hyaluronic acid now include lidocaine premixed in the syringe, thus eliminating the need for adjuvant anesthesia and making them significantly more comfortable for patients. Hyaluronic acid fillers can produce a more durable esthetic improvement than collagen, often lasting from 5 to 8 months (Fig. 39.1).

The two types of hyaluronic acid filler substances are streptococcal derived and animal (i.e., rooster comb) derived. Streptococcal-derived filler is by far the most common as manufacturers and consumers have moved away from animal-derived products due to lack of longevity. There are numerous evolving proprietary formulations, including Restylane and its various formulations (Silk, Lyft, Refyne, and Defyne) (Galderma, Fort Worth, TX), with the "L" designation for the lidocaine-containing formulation; Juvederm and its various formulations (Voluma, Ultra, Vollure, and Volbella) (Allergan, Irvine, CA), with the "XC" designation for the lidocaine-containing formulation; and Belotero Balance (Merz; Greensboro, NC). All these fillers come in prepackaged syringes and do not require refrigeration.

The characteristics and viscosity of the different products are largely determined by the size and concentration of the molecule within each preparation. Restylane contains 20 mg/mL of hyaluronic acid, with a particle size of 100,000/mL, and is injected with a 30-gauge needle. Restylane Silk also has a concentration of 20 mg/mL, but a much larger particle size of 8000/mL, and is appropriate for deeper contour abnormalities. In contrast, Restylane Silk has a similar concentration of 20 mg/mL, but a much smaller particle size, about one fifth the size of Restylane. This make it much more appropriate for fine perioral lines. Juvederm is available in two formulations, Ultra and Ultra Plus ("XC" indicates lidocaine-containing product). Both have a concentration of 24 mg/mL, with Ultra Plus being about 20% thicker, making it more appropriate for deeper folds. Voluma, Vollure, and Volbella all are manufactured with a propriety cross-linking technology that results in longer duration of action. They have varying concentrations of HA and as a result have different consistencies and indications for use. Voluma has a concentration of 20 mg/mL and is indicated for cheek augmentation of age-related volume loss to the middle of the face. Vollure has a concentration of 17.5 mg/mL and is indicated for moderate to severe facial wrinkles and folds. Volbella has a concentration of 15 mg/mL and is the indicated for lip augmentation or perioral rhytids. Belotero Balance has a concentration of 22.5 mg/mL and has an FDA indication for moderate facial wrinkles and folds. However, due to the "thin" nature of the product, it can be used for fine superficial lines, such as perioral rhytids.

Hyaluronic acids tend to produce more swelling and bruising than collagen. Proper preoperative consultation is necessary to ensure that the patient understands this and does not have upcoming social engagements. Some have advocated the use of cannulas instead of needles to minimize the risk of bruising. Injection site necrosis is an extremely uncommon but concerning complication that has been reported with fillers. This is typically due to occlusion of arterial vessels. Application of nitroglycerin paste may help to reduce the size of the resultant ischemia. Knowledge on the impending signs of ischemia and appropriate urgent management is required for all physicians who use fillers. Improper placement of hyaluronic acid too superficially can result in a blue discoloration or nodule on the skin surface, known as the Tyndall effect. An incision with a large-gauge needle or No. 11 blade and expression of the product can be performed. Hyaluronidase injections can dissolve the product if either a reaction or unevenness results, a considerable advantage over other filler substances.

Poly-L-Lactic Acid

Microparticles of poly-L-lactic acid (Sculptra; Galderma, Fort Worth, TX) are used as an injectable implant to replace diffuse volume loss, rather than the small-volume injections of other fillers. This product is currently FDA approved for correcting facial lipoatrophy in patients with human immunodeficiency virus (HIV) infection and for esthetic treatment of lines and contour deficiencies.

Poly-L-lactic acid (PLLA) is a biodegradable, biocompatible, and immunologically inert product that does not require skin testing. PLLA has been used as absorbable suture material (e.g., Vicryl). The material is absorbed gradually in the skin, inducing a fibroblastic response and de novo collagen synthesis. Multiple treatment sessions at intervals of 4–6 weeks are often required to achieve the final result (Fig. 39.2). Because correction depends on the formation of new collagen, patients must be counseled that an immediate effect does not occur with this product and they should be patient to await final improvement. Results can last for up to 2 years.

PLLA comes packaged as a freeze-dried powder and must be reconstituted for a minimum of 4 hours before injection to ensure adequate hydration of the particles. Lidocaine can be added to the vial to reduce injection pain. The product is injected using a 25-gauge needle at the level of the deep dermis and subcutaneous junction in a fanning or cross-hatch fashion. Postinjection massage for several days can help reduce nodule formation.

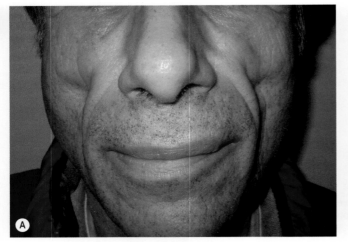 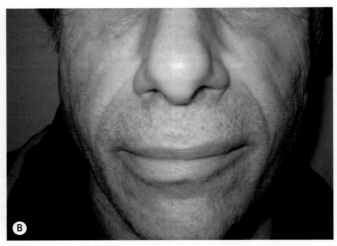

Fig. 39.2 Poly-L-lactic acid for HIV lipoatrophy. (A) Before treatment. (B) After five treatments.

Side effects include bruising, swelling, redness, and delayed foreign body granulomas at injection sites. Intralesional 5-fluorouracil (5-FU) or triamcinolone may be used for the treatment of these papules.

Calcium Hydroxylapatite

Calcium hydroxylapatite (Radiesse; Merz, Greensboro, NC) consists of fine particles (25–45 μm) of material traditionally used to reconstruct bone. Once injected into the dermal–subcutaneous junction, the particles act as scaffolding for autologous collagen synthesis. The ensuing fibrotic reaction results in soft tissue correction that can last for 9–12 months. It is FDA approved for correction of moderate to severe folds and wrinkles, such as nasolabial folds, and for HIV facial lipoatrophy.

Injections can be quite painful, and local anesthesia is generally used. Calcium hydroxylapatite is injected into the deep dermis and subcutaneous junction with a threading technique using a 27-gauge needle. It comes prepackaged in syringes and can be stored at room temperature.

Nodules are more often seen when calcium hydroxylapatite is injected into the lips, thus discouraging its use in the treatment of hypolabium. Caution must be exercised; any product that requires a fibrotic reaction to be effective can result in a granulomatous reaction and an untoward result. Because calcium is radiopaque, the product may be detected and may interfere with radiologic imaging.

Silicone

Silicone has been used in the past for soft tissue augmentation by dermatologists. This product was never FDA approved, and issues of purity and safety limited its widespread use. In 1994 the FDA removed silicone from the market. Recently, however, the FDA approved 1000-centistoke liquid silicone (Silikon 1000; Alcon Labs, Fort Worth, TX) for the treatment of retinal detachment. It is currently being used off-label as permanent filler for HIV-associated facial lipoatrophy, scars, and rhytids.

The potential for delayed and severe complications with this permanent filler, as well as legal concerns and restrictions, has limited use of silicone. Adverse reactions associated with silicone injections include granuloma formation and migration of implant, which are compounded by the permanent nature of the product. Many of the past reported complications of silicone injection were the result of using either an impure, non–medical-grade substance or an improper technique with large-volume injections. A multisession, microdroplet technique, placing multiple depot injections

of 0.01 mL of product into the deep dermis in 1–3 mm intervals, significantly reduces the complication rate. An additional consideration is that the current FDA-approved product is more concentrated than the previous silicone products. Further study is needed to evaluate the long-term safety and efficacy of silicone oil injections for correction of soft tissue contour deficiencies.

Polymethylmethacrylate

Bellafill (Suneva Medical, San Diego, CA), formerly ArteFill, is an FDA-approved suspension containing 20% polymethylmethacrylate (PMMA, commonly known as Lucite) microspheres of 30–40 μm in diameter, suspended in 80% bovine collagen, for soft tissue augmentation. The carrier collagen provides initial correction and is degraded over several months, leaving the PMMA microspheres. PMMA is nondegradable and serves as a permanent framework for connective tissue deposition and can produce long-term correction.

Technique is critical to successful outcomes. If injected too deeply, the implant is ineffective; superficial placement can cause prolonged erythema. Granuloma formation and hypertrophic scarring can occur and have been reported as a delayed reaction. Intralesional triamcinolone can be used for treatment of these reactions. One patient who developed a delayed foreign body granuloma 6 years after injection with PMMA was successfully treated with a 24-week course of 600 mg/day of allopurinol. Intralesional triamcinolone has also been used as a treatment for granulomas. Because the product contains bovine collagen, skin testing is required before use. Early indications suggest efficacy of triamcinolone treatment for acne scarring.

Expanded Polytetrafluoroethylene

Expanded polytetrafluoroethylene (ePTFE) is a synthetic solid material that is soft and pliable, is not degraded, and has the advantage of being permanent. The material is placed through a small skin incision and positioned in the desired location. Areas typically treated include lip margins or the muscular portion of the vermillion for enhancement, nasolabial folds, and soft tissue depressions. Complications associated with ePTFE include extrusion, migration, shrinkage, and hardening.

Autologous Fat Transplantation

Autologous lipotransfer allows for soft tissue augmentation without the risk of allergy, rejection, or infectious transmission. Unlike other filler techniques, fat transfer is truly a grafting procedure.

As such, its success is predicated on the survival of the transferred adipocytes. Fat is harvested from a choice of donor sites, typically the abdomen, buttock, thigh, or knee. There is no consensus as to the advantages of harvesting with a liposuction cannula, syringe extraction with a large-bore needle, or open surgical method. The fat is then separated from anesthetic fluid and blood and injected through a large-bore needle (16–18 gauge) into the desired location. Any remaining fat can be frozen at −70°C for use later, with varying claims regarding loss of efficacy.

The variable rate of graft survival, the recipient site reaction (bruising, swelling), and the added morbidity of a donor site are limiting factors in patient satisfaction with this technique. In some cases, partial survival results in uneven correction that may require additional treatments. Some argue that multiple smaller-volume injections spaced over two or three treatments are more effective than single, large-volume lipotransfer. If the fat survives, it can provide a very natural correction. However, local factors such as motor activity and gravitational effects will mitigate against permanent correction. This technique is not useful for the correction of superficial rhytids and mainly corrects deeper defects such as nasolabial folds, hypolabium, buccal depression, and deep scars.

Bachmann F, et al: The spectrum of adverse reactions after treatment with injectable fillers in the glabellar region. Dermatol Surg 2009; 35: 1629.

Benedetto AV, Lewis AT: Injecting 1000 centistoke liquid silicone with ease and precision. Dermatol Surg 2003; 29: 211.

Chen F, et al: HIV-associated facial lipoatrophy treated with injectable silicone oil. J Am Acad Dermatol 2013; 69: 431.

França Wanick FB, et al: Skin remodeling using hyaluronic acid filler injections in photo-aged faces. Dermatol Surg 2016; 42: 352.

Glogau RG: Fillers. Semin Cutan Med Surg 2012; 31: 78.

Goldman MP: Cosmetic use of poly-L-lactic acid. Dermatol Surg 2011; 37: 688.

Hexsel D, de Morais MR: Management of complications of injectable silicone. Facial Plast Surg 2014; 30: 623.

Jagdeo J, et al: A systematic review of filler agents for aesthetic treatment of HIV facial lipoatrophy (FLA). J Am Acad Dermatol 2015; 73: 1040.

Joseph JH, et al: Current concepts in the use of Bellafill. Plast Reconstr Surg 2015; 136: 171S.

Kadouch JA, et al: Delayed-onset complications of facial soft tissue augmentation with permanent fillers in 85 patients. Dermatol Surg 2013; 39: 1474.

Landau M: Hyaluronidase caveats in treating filler complications. Dermatol Surg 2015; 41: S347.

Ledon JA, et al: Inflammatory nodules following soft tissue filler use. Am J Clin Dermatol. 2013; 14: 401.

Levy RM, et al: Treatment of HIV lipoatrophy and lipoatrophy of aging with poly-L-lactic acid. J Am Acad Dermatol 2008; 59: 923.

Lorenc ZP, et al: Review of key Belotero Balance safety and efficacy trials. Plast Reconstr Surg 2013; 132: 33S.

Matarasso SL: Injectable collagens. Plast Reconstr Surg 2007; 120: 17S.

Moulonguet I, et al: Foreign body reaction to Radiesse. Am J Dermatopathol 2013; 35: e37.

Rayess HM, et al: A cross-sectional analysis of adverse events and litigation for injectable fillers. JAMA Facial Plast Surg 2017 Dec 21; ePub ahead of print.

Requena L, et al: Adverse reactions to injectable soft tissue fillers. J Am Acad Dermatol 2011; 64: 1.

Tzikas TL: A 52-month summary of results using calcium hydroxylapatite for facial soft tissue augmentation. Dermatol Surg 2008; 34: S9.

BOTULINUM TOXIN

The use of botulinum toxin (BTX) in dermatology has increased rapidly over the years, and at present it is one of the most common cosmetic procedure performed in the United States. In 2002 the FDA approved onabotulinumtoxinA for the treatment of dynamic glabellar frown lines. Although BTX is most frequently used for relaxation of dynamic rhytids in the upper third of the face, advanced esthetic treatment techniques for additional anatomic sites have been developed and are currently used off-label.

Produced by *Clostridium botulinum*, there are seven different serotypes of BTX: A, B, C1, D, E, F, and G. These serotypes inhibit the release of acetylcholine from the presynaptic motor neuron, resulting in chemodenervation and paralysis of the treated muscle. Over time, new nerve terminals form and create new neuromuscular junctions with the muscle fibers, which gradually restore motor function.

BTX type A (Botox Cosmetic [onabotulinumtoxinA], Allergan; Dysport [abobotulinumtoxinA], Medicis); Xeomin (incobotulinumtoxinA; Merz) is the most common serotype. Its mechanism of action is through the cleavage of SNAP-25, a presynaptic membrane protein required for fusion of neurotransmitter-containing vesicles. Effect is generally noted 2–5 days after treatment with BTX-A, but the delay can be as long as 2 weeks in some cases. Results can last 2–5 months. In addition to esthetic indications, onabotulinumtoxinA is FDA approved for the treatment of blepharospasm, strabismus, cervical dystonia, upper limb spasticity, chromic migraine, urinary incontinence, and axillary hyperhidrosis.

Each of these BTX-A products has a similar mechanism of action, but each formulation also has unique characteristics. For dosing purposes, onabotulinumtoxinA and incobotulinumtoxinA have a similar potency (clinical equivalency ratio of 1 unit = 1 unit). AbobotulinumtoxinA has equivalency of 3 : 1 compared with the other formulations. Therefore it is critical that physicians perform appropriate dosage conversions when switching among different products. AbobotulinumtoxinA appears to have greater spread once injected into the skin. IncobotulinumtoxinA is unique in that it is formulated with no complex proteins and thus, in theory, may have a lower risk of neutralizing antibody formation (although the risks of this occurring in esthetic use is exceedingly low with all current formulations of BTX-A). In addition, incobotulinumtoxinA has the advantage of being able to be stored refrigerated or at room temperature, whereas the other products require refrigeration. Newer formulations of BTX-A are currently under investigation and may result in even more options for the patient and physician in the future.

The only other serotype that is currently available commercially is BTX type B (Myobloc [rimabotulinumtoxinB]; Solstice Neurosciences, Malvern, PA). Its mechanism of action is through the cleavage of a vesicle-associated membrane protein (VAMP), also known as synaptobrevin. This serotype has more rapid onset of effect than BTX-A. In addition, differences in potency suggest that approximately 100 units of Myobloc are equivalent to 1 unit of Botox. It currently has FDA approval for the treatment of cervical dystonia.

BTX-A is distributed in vials as a vacuum-dried powder, which is reconstituted with 1.0–5.0 mL of saline. Many physicians think that the dilution of BTX does not a make a significant difference in patient outcome, and studies appear to confirm this. Others argue that higher concentrations with smaller injection volumes reduce the amount of unintended diffusion. It is more important to use the same dilution every time to ensure that the physician does not need to do "mental math," and to reduce confusion with each new vial of BTX.

Despite package insert recommendations, experience suggests that there is little loss of potency over several weeks after reconstitution with preserved saline. The American Society for Dermatologic

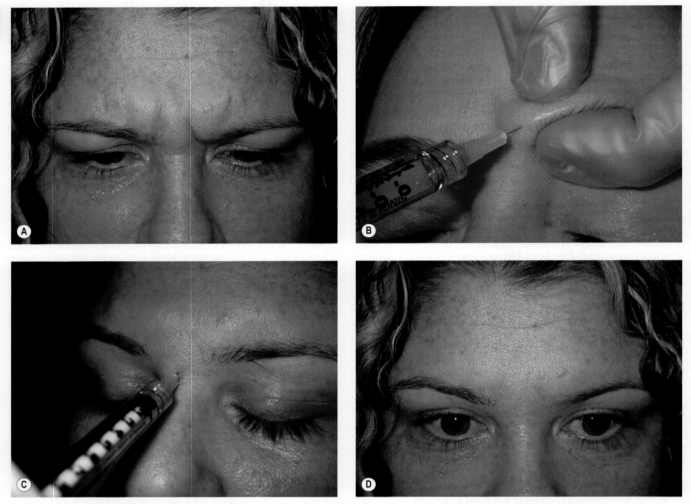

Fig. 39.3 Botulinum toxin injection technique for glabellar frown furrow. (A) Glabellar lines with frowning. (B) As patient frowns, the muscle is grasped between thumb and index finger; the injection is placed directly into the belly of the corrugator supercilii muscle. (C) Injection into the procerus muscle. (D) Patient attempting to frown after botulinum toxin injection.

Surgery has put out a consensus statement regarding the storage and reuse of previously reconstituted botulinum toxin. The use of preserved saline for reconstitution reduces the burning and pain associated with injection from the anesthetic properties of the benzyl alcohol in preserved saline.

BTX-A is predominantly used in dermatology for treatment of dynamic rhytids on the upper third of the face. The key to successful treatment is understanding the anatomy involved in facial expression, rather than performing the procedure by rote. Having the patient frown, squint, and raise the brows before treatment helps identify the active target muscles and serves as a guide for proper placement.

Glabellar Frown Lines

Currently, treatment of glabellar frown lines is the only FDA-approved cosmetic indication for BTX-A. These lines result from contraction of the corrugator supercilii muscle, which pulls the brows medially, and the procerus muscle, which pulls the brow inferiorly. In addition, by inactivating the brow depressors, unopposed action of the brow elevators (e.g., frontalis muscle) can result in a slight but noticeable brow lift.

Approximately 20–35 units of onabotulinumtoxinA (or equivalent if using different product) are typically injected into the corrugators and procerus in a five-point injection method (Fig. 39.3). Male patients and those with larger muscle mass may require a higher number of units (30–50). By having the patient furrow the brow, one can identify the origin and insertion of the corrugator supercilii. By grasping with the thumb and index finger, the physician can isolate the muscle and ensure accurate toxin placement.

If toxin diffuses through the orbital septum into the orbit, weakening of the levator palpebrae muscle can result in upper lid ptosis. Care should be taken to inject 1 cm above the superior bony orbital rim to reduce risk of diffusion of toxin and the resulting complication. The use of α-adrenergic agonist eye drops, such as apraclonidine 0.5% or phenylephrine 2.5%, can stimulate Müller muscles in the lid, providing some relief until the effects of the BTX-A dissipate.

Horizontal Forehead Lines

Horizontal forehead lines are caused by contraction of the frontalis muscle, which produces elevation and movement of the eyebrows.

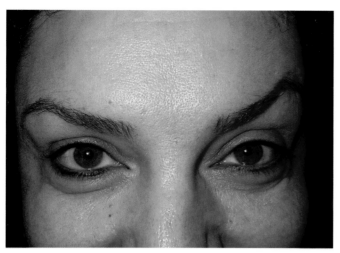

Fig. 39.4 Botulinum toxin complication: "quizzical" brow look.

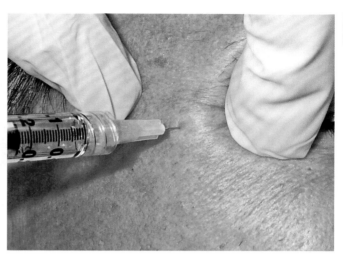

Fig. 39.5 Botulinum toxin injection technique for crow's feet. Superficial injection is approximately 1 cm from the orbital rim.

Care must be taken when treating this area with BTX-A to avoid ptosis or "heaviness" of the brow. Extra caution should be used in men with low-set brows or older patients who use their frontalis to raise their eyebrows to assist with vision.

Because the lower portion of the frontalis is primarily responsible for brow elevation, injections are often limited to the upper half or two thirds of the muscle. Between 10 and 25 units of onabotulinumtoxinA (or equivalent if using different product), delivered in multiple superficial injections across the forehead, is typically used for this area.

If upper lateral fibers of the frontalis remain totally untreated, the increased resting muscle tone will raise the lateral edge of the eyebrow, creating a quizzical look (Fig. 39.4). Injecting a small amount of BTX-A in the upper lateral brow can help correct this.

Crow's Feet

Crow's feet are rhytids that extend radially from the lateral canthus and are produced by contraction of the lateral orbicularis oculi. Even with successful treatment with BTX-A, rhytids may still persist because of the upward motion of the cheek when the patient smiles. Proper preoperative counseling is required to prevent frustrated patients.

Superficial blebs are raised approximately 1 cm lateral to the lateral canthus (Fig. 39.5). Between 8 and 12 units of onabotulinumtoxinA (or equivalent if using different product) are placed around each orbit. Care should be taken to orient the needle away from the globe as a safety precaution, in case the patient moves unexpectedly.

Bruising is common in this location because of the thinness of the skin and the presence of numerous periocular superficial veins. Purpura can be minimized by injecting superficially, ensuring proper illumination and stretching of the skin to help identify the veins, and limiting the total number of injections. Diffusion into the zygomaticus major and minor muscles, leading to ipsilateral lip ptosis and asymmetric smile, can occur with overzealous treatment of the inferior portion of the orbicularis oculi muscle.

Other Locations

Other sites that can be treated with BTX-A include platysmal bands, diagonal creases along the nasal side wall ("sniff lines" or "bunny lines"), mental crease, and depressor anguli oris muscle (for frowning of lateral corners of mouth). Care must be taken when treating the lower third of the face to avoid complications with mouth and lip control. Excessive or misplaced BTX-A in

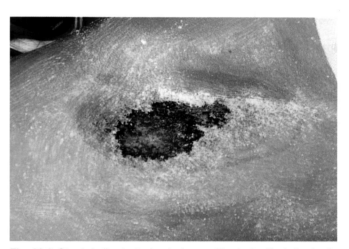

Fig. 39.6 Starch-iodine test; developing positive test with darkening in areas of hyperhidrosis.

the platysmal bands can cause dysphagia, dysphonia, and neck weakness.

Hyperhidrosis

In addition to cosmetic uses, onabotulinumtoxinA is FDA approved for the treatment of axillary hyperhidrosis. Before treatment, a Minor's starch-iodine test is used to document both the severity and the location of excessive sweating (Fig. 39.6). Effective treatment can be achieved with doses of 50 units/axilla, although some patients require higher doses. Intradermal injections are spaced in a grid 1 cm apart over the entire area. Anhidrosis is achieved within 1 week and typically lasts for 4–12 months. Side effects are generally limited to injection site bruising.

Treatment of palmar hyperhidrosis with BTX-A is more complicated than treating the axilla. Higher doses, typically 100–150 units/palm, are required because of the greater surface area involved and the limited diffusion of the toxin in acral skin. Pain is more significant when treating the palm and typically requires the use of wrist nerve blocks or ice applied to the skin. A slight muscle weakness of the hands, manifested by the loss of

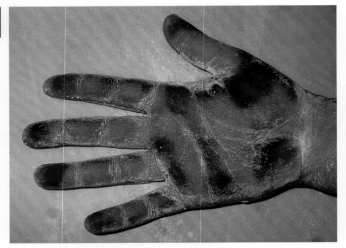

Fig. 39.7 Starch-iodine test; partial response to botulinum toxin.

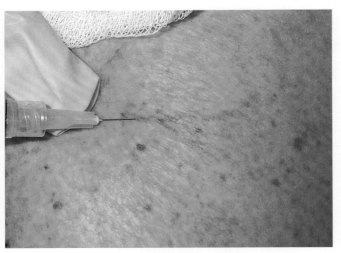

Fig. 39.8 Sclerotherapy; injection technique using fine needle to cannulate vein.

fine motor movement, is typically seen for several weeks after treatment.

Frequently, there are focal areas of activity after treatment for hyperhydrosis. However, because the sweat diffuses over the entire surface, patients often describe a false sensation of severe sweating and complain that the treatment "didn't work." By repeating the starch-iodine test, the focal areas of activity can be identified and directed touch-up performed (Fig. 39.7). Repeated treatments over time appear to increase the duration of efficacy for resulting injections.

Alam M, et al: Consensus statement regarding storage and reuse of previously reconstituted neuromodulators. Dermatol Surg 2015; 41: 321.

Allen SB, Goldenberg NA: Pain difference associated with injection of abobotulinumtoxinA reconstituted with preserved saline and preservative-free saline. Dermatol Surg 2012; 38: 867.

An JS, et al: Comparison of onabotulinumtoxinA and rimabotulinumtoxinB for the treatment of axillary hyperhidrosis. Dermatol Surg 2015; 41: 960.

Carruthers A, et al: The convergence of medicine and neurotoxins. Part I: botulinum toxin in clinical and cosmetic practice. Dermatol Surg 2013; 39: 493.

Carruthers A, et al: The convergence of medicine and neurotoxins. Part II: incorporating botulinum toxin into aesthetic clinical practice. Dermatol Surg 2013; 39: 510.

Carruthers A, et al: Evolution of facial aesthetic treatment over five or more years. Dermatol Surg 2015; 41: 693.

Carruthers A, et al: Multicenter, randomized, Phase III study of a single dose of incobotulinumtoxinA, free from complexing proteins, in the treatment of glabellar frown lines. Dermatol Surg 2013; 39: 551.

Carruthers A, et al: Repeated onabotulinumtoxinA treatment of glabellar lines at rest over three treatment cycles. Dermatol Surg 2016; 42: 1094.

Glaser DA, et al: A prospective, nonrandomized, open-label study of the efficacy and safety of onabotulinumtoxinA in adolescents with primary axillary hyperhidrosis. Pediatr Dermatol 2015; 32: 609.

Hanke CW, et al: A randomized, placebo-controlled, double-blind Phase III trial investigating the efficacy and safety of incobotulinumtoxinA in the treatment of glabellar frown lines using a stringent composite endpoint. Dermatol Surg 2013; 39: 891.

Kiripolsky MG, et al: A two-phase, retrospective analysis evaluating efficacy of and patient satisfaction with abobotulinumtoxinA

used to treat dynamic facial rhytides. Dermatol Surg 2011; 37: 1443.

Lecouflet M, et al: Duration of efficacy increases with the repetition of botulinum toxin A injections in primary axillary hyperhidrosis. J Am Acad Dermatol 2013; 69: 960.

Liu A, et al: Recommendations and current practices for the reconstitution and storage of botulinum toxin type A. J Am Acad Dermatol 2012; 67: 373.

Solish N, et al: Efficacy and safety of onabotulinumtoxinA treatment of forehead lines. Dermatol Surg 2016; 42: 410.

VARICOSE AND TELANGIECTATIC VEINS

Sclerotherapy

Patients frequently seek treatment of telangiectasias and reticular veins in the lower extremities. Historically, the treatment of choice for telangiectatic and reticular veins has been sclerotherapy (Fig. 39.8). However, some studies suggest that laser treatment for lower extremity telangiectasia can be as effective as sclerotherapy. In addition, laser therapy can be considered in patients who failed to respond to sclerotherapy or had significant complications from sclerotherapy. However, many believe that sclerotherapy should be first-line treatment for vessels that can be cannulated with a needle.

Sclerosing Solutions

There are three broad classes of sclerosing agent available to dermatologists: hyperosmotic agents, detergents, and chemical irritants (Table 39.1). Hyperosmotic agents cause endothelial cell damage through dehydration; detergents disrupt the cellular membrane; and chemical irritants act as a corrosive and lead to endothelial injury.

Hypertonic saline is an FDA-approved agent frequently used in sclerotherapy. At concentrations of 10%–30%, this agent has the advantage of a complete lack of allergenicity when used alone. The disadvantage of hypertonic saline is pain associated with injections and ulcerogenic potential. Often, anesthetic agents such as lidocaine are added to the mixture to minimize the discomfort involved, by decreasing the concentration of the saline and through the direct anesthetic effect.

Hypertonic saline (10%) mixed with dextrose (25%) is another hyperosmolar agent that has been used in vein sclerosing. This

TABLE 39.1 Sclerotherapy Agents

Agent	Class	FDA Approved	Comments
Hypertonic saline	Hyperosmotic	Yes	No allergenicity; painful
Hypertonic saline (10%) plus dextrose (25%)	Hyperosmotic	No	Lower allergenicity; painful
Sodium tetradecyl sulfate	Detergent	Yes	Can be used as foam; painless except with extravascular injection
Polidocanol	Detergent	Yes	Painless; can be used as foam
Sodium morrhuate	Detergent	Yes	High risk of allergic reaction
Chromated glycerin	Chemical irritant	No	Weak agent
Polyiodinated iodine	Chemical irritant	No	Highly caustic

FDA, Food and Drug Administration.

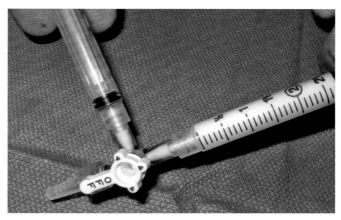

Fig. 39.9 Sclerosing foam. Sodium tetradecyl sulfate (STS) foam is made by mixing air with liquid using a three-way stopcock and two syringes.

agent has the advantages of low allergenicity and decreased pain compared with higher concentrations of plain hypertonic saline. However, this mixture is currently not FDA approved and is a relatively weak sclerosant compared with other options available.

Sodium tetradecyl sulfate (STS) or Sotradecol (AngioDynamics, Latham, NY) is a detergent sclerosant that has been FDA approved for 55 years. Typical concentrations used for superficial telangiectasias are 0.1%–0.2%, and reticular veins can be treated with 0.2%–0.5%. One advantage of STS is the lack of pain with injections; however, extravascular injection can be painful.

Polidocanol (Asclera; Merz Aesthetics, San Mateo, CA), a detergent, is FDA approved for use in sclerotherapy and comes in 0.5% (for vessels <1 mm in diameter) and 1% (for reticular veins <3 mm) concentrations. It possesses many of the same advantages as STS, including lack of pain with injection and the ability to be used as foam. Goldman demonstrated comparable efficacy and a similar adverse event profile between polidocanol and STS.

As detergents both STS and polidoconol can be made into foam. This is typically done with a three-way stopcock and a syringe filled with air (Fig. 39.9). Foam can increase contact between the agent and the vessel wall, can result in more effective sclerosis at a lower concentration, and allows treatment of larger-caliber vessels. Foam tends to degrade fairly quickly (1–2 minutes), so it should be mixed immediately before injection. The bubble size created correlates to the stability of the foam created, with microfoam (<50 μm) being more stable than larger foam (>100 μm). Foam technique has historically been an off-label use of polidocanol or STS but has been used widely with successful results and a high degree of safety. However, Varithena (BTG, London) is a polidocanol injectable nitrogen foam product approved by the FDA in 2013 and is indicated for the treatment of incompetent great saphenous veins, accessory saphenous veins, and visible varicosities of the great saphenous vein system above and below the knee. In addition to leg veins, foam sclerotherapy has been reported in the treatment of reticular veins of the chest and dorsal hands.

Sodium morrhuate is a detergent approved by the FDA for treatment of varicose veins. However, this sclerosing agent is not generally used for the treatment of cutaneous telangiectasias because of its highly caustic nature and higher anaphylaxis potential.

Glycerin and polyiodide iodine are chemical irritants used as sclerosing agents. Although not FDA approved for sclerotherapy, these act as corrosive agents and cause a direct injury to the vessel endothelium. Leach and Goldman report a significant decrease in bruising, swelling, and postprocedural hyperpigmentation with glycerin compared with STS.

Complications

Side effects and complications of sclerotherapy can be associated with all types of sclerosing agents. Ulceration can occur despite the meticulous technique of the dermatologist and regardless of the sclerosing agent used. Extravasation of sclerosing solution from the vein may occur, or injection into a dermal arteriole or arteriovenous anastomosis may result in cutaneous necrosis. If extravasation is suspected, injection of normal saline to dilute the sclerosing agent may prevent ulceration. Alternatively, application of 2% nitroglycerin ointment may prove beneficial. If ulceration does occur, conservative wound management should be undertaken until healed.

Hyperpigmentation along the course of treated veins has been reported to occur in 10%–30% of patients. This pigmentation is caused by hemosiderin deposition and has been reported with a variety of sclerosing agents, including hypertonic saline, polidocanol, and STS. Pigmentation often improves with time, with approximately 70% improvement over a 6-month period. Treatment options include trichloroacetic acid, hydroquinone, retinoic acid cream, intense pulsed light, and laser treatments.

Telangiectatic matting is the appearance of fine telangiectatic blush at the site of previously treated veins. This has been reported in 10%–15% of patients treated with sclerotherapy. Risk factors associated with this include estrogen therapy, obesity, and a family history of telangiectasia. Low injection pressures and limiting the amount of sclerosant per injection site may help reduce the incidence of telangiectatic matting. Spontaneous resolution often occurs in 3–12 months. Treatment options include intense pulsed light, pulsed dye laser, and injection of sclerosant into the matted vessels.

Arterial injection of sclerosant is the most serious complication of vein sclerosing. Although rare, it has considerable associated morbidity and necessitates timely action. Classically, the patient reports significant pain immediately after injection, accompanied by pallor and cyanosis. If arterial injection occurs, the physician should immediately apply ice and attempt to dilute the vessel

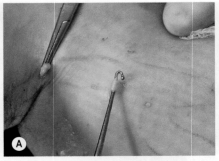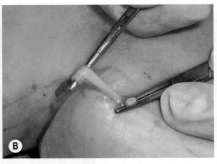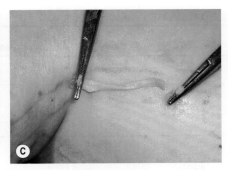

Fig. 39.10 Ambulatory phlebectomy. (A) Hook used to secure the vein. (B) Vein is clamped on either side and severed. Clamp is then used to remove the vein using a rolling and pulling technique. (C) Removed vein segment. The distal end can be tied off using absorbable suture, or additional segments can be removed using the same technique.

with injections of normal saline. Procaine can be used to inactivate STS. Intravenous heparin and thrombolysis should be considered.

Ambulatory Phlebectomy

Ambulatory phlebectomy is an outpatient procedure used to remove varicose veins, employing skin hooks through a series of stab incisions along the course of the varicosity. Tumescent anesthesia is often used during this technique and has the added benefit of compression of the vein and reduction of blood loss. Various hooks and clamps are used to remove the vein (Fig. 39.10). Incision sites heal with minimal scarring. Adverse effects are generally limited and consist of minor pain and bruising. Infection and nerve damage are extremely rare.

Endovenous Ablation

Endovenous ablation should be considered in patients with greater saphenous incompetence and is rapidly replacing traditional vein stripping. In patients with lower extremity telangiectasia and reticular veins, prior assessment of underlying saphenous reflux is necessary to prevent recurrence after treatment of the visible varicosities.

Radiofrequency or laser (using 810 nm or 1320 nm) can be used to heat and damage veins. Either method results in vein wall shrinkage and subsequent vessel thrombosis and occlusion. Tumescent anesthesia allows the procedure to be performed painlessly, surrounds and compresses the vein for greater contact between the catheter and vessel wall, and distends the skin away from the heat source, preventing cutaneous damage. A catheter is placed under ultrasound guidance and guided to the saphenofemoral junction. The catheter is slowly withdrawn along the length of the vein, and the thermal injury leads to vessel occlusion.

The most common complications include ecchymosis and pain. Thermal burns of the skin are infrequently seen when tumescent anesthesia is properly used. Nerve injury is uncommon, and paresthesias are often temporary. Deep vein thrombosis has been documented, but pulmonary embolism is extremely rare when the technique is performed properly.

Bertanha M, et al: Sclerotherapy for reticular veins in the lower limbs. JAMA Dermatol 2017; 153: 1249.

Friedmann DP, et al: Foam sclerotherapy for reticular veins of the chest. Dermatol Surg 2015; 41: 126.

Goldman MP: Treatment of varicose and telangiectatic leg veins. Dermatol Surg 2002; 28: 52.

Kern P, et al: A double-blind, randomized study comparing pure chromated glycerin with chromated glycerin with 1% lidocaine and epinephrine for sclerotherapy of telangiectasias and reticular veins. Dermatol Surg 2011; 37: 1590.

Leach BC, Goldman MP: Comparative trial between sodium tetradecyl sulfate and glycerin in the treatment of telangiectatic leg veins. Dermatol Surg 2003; 29: 612.

Lupton JR, et al: Clinical comparison of sclerotherapy versus long-pulsed Nd:YAG laser treatment for lower extremity telangiectases. Dermatol Surg 2002; 28: 694.

Malskat WS, et al: Endovenous laser ablation (EVLA). Lasers Med Sci 2014; 29: 393.

Moul DK, et al: Endovenous laser ablation of the great and short saphenous veins with a 1320-nm neodymium:yttrium-aluminum-garnet laser. J Am Acad Dermatol 2014; 70: 326.

Munia MA, et al: Comparison of laser versus sclerotherapy in the treatment of lower extremity telangiectases. Dermatol Surg 2012; 38: 635.

Palm MD, et al: Foam sclerotherapy for reticular veins and nontruncal varicose veins of the legs. Dermatol Surg 2010; 36: 1026.

Peterson JD, et al: Treatment of reticular and telangiectatic leg veins. Dermatol Surg 2012; 38: 1322.

Rao J, et al: Double-blind prospective comparative trial between foamed and liquid polidocanol and sodium tetradecyl sulfate in the treatment of varicose and telangiectatic leg veins. Dermatol Surg 2005; 31: 631.

Sadick NS: Choosing the appropriate sclerosing concentration for vessel diameter. Dermatol Surg 2010; 36: 976.

Stücker M, et al: Review of published information on foam sclerotherapy. Dermatol Surg 2010; 36: 983.

Tremaine AM, et al: Foam sclerotherapy for reticular veins of the dorsal hands. Dermatol Surg 2014; 40: 892.

Uurto I, et al: Single-center experience with foam sclerotherapy without ultrasound guidance for treatment of varicose veins. Dermatol Surg 2007; 33: 1334.

Van Den Bos RR, et al: Endovenous laser ablation-induced complications. Dermatol Surg 2009; 35: 1206.

Weiss MA, et al: Consensus for sclerotherapy. Dermatol Surg 2014; 40: 1309.

Wysong A, et al: Successful treatment of chronic venous ulcers with a 1,320-nm endovenous laser combined with other minimally invasive venous procedures. Dermatol Surg 2016; 42: 961.

FAT REMOVAL

Liposuction

Liposuction is used for the removal of local areas of adipose and to improve body contour. It is not a treatment for obesity and

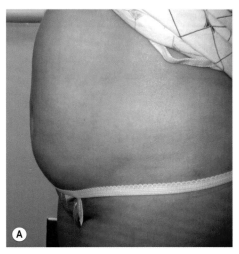 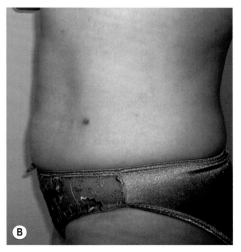

Fig. 39.11 Tumescent liposuction. (A) Before treatment of abdomen. (B) After treatment.

should not be used as a weight loss mechanism. The most common areas treated are the abdomen and thighs, neck, jowls, knees, ankles, and breasts (Fig. 39.11). Additional conditions, such as gynecomastia, buffalo hump, lipoma, lipodystrophy, and axillary hyperhidrosis, can be treated by liposuction.

The most common technique employed by dermatologists involves infiltrating the treated area with dilute anesthesia and aspirating the fat through cannulas attached to a vacuum. The choice of cannula can determine the amount of fat aspirated, with more aggressive cannulas having a larger bore, being pointier, and having multiple, larger holes placed near the tip. Tumescent anesthesia typically consists of 0.05%–0.1% lidocaine with 1:1 million epinephrine and sodium bicarbonate. The total safe concentration of lidocaine that can be used is 55 mg/kg. The benefits of tumescent anesthesia are the ability to perform the procedure comfortably under local anesthesia, hemostasis, and hydrodissection of adipocytes, which facilitates aspiration. Laser-assisted lipolysis has not been shown to be superior to traditional tumescent liposuction.

Much discussion surrounds the safety of office-based liposuction. It is important to stress that the serious complications seen in liposuction are associated with general anesthesia, not with procedures performed with local tumescent anesthesia. Although deaths have been reported during liposuction, none has occurred when patients were treated with tumescent anesthesia alone. Office-based tumescent liposuction performed by dermatologic surgeons is safe and has a lower complication rate than hospital-based procedures.

Cryolipolysis

In an effort to reduce the downtime and risks associated with traditional liposuction, the technique of cryolipolysis has been FDA approved for the reduction of unwanted fat in a variety of body locations (CoolSculpting, Allergan, Irvine, CA).

The technique is based on the principle that adipocytes are more sensitive to temperature changes than other skin cells. Therefore by using a controlled cooling system, the device can preferentially reduce the amount of unwanted fat, while minimizing any potential injury to surrounding tissue. Following treatment, the adipocytes undergo apoptosis, with resulting permanent reduction in the amount of fat in the treated location. Following apoptosis, an induced inflammatory response clears the cells over the proceeding 3 months.

The procedure is performed in an office setting with no anesthesia or sedation required. A vacuum suction–powered handpiece

(in various shapes and sizes, based on the desired location treated) is applied to skin and pulls the tissue up into contact with the cooling mechanism. After a preset amount of time, the machine turns off and the treatment is complete. The process is then repeated across the entire surface of the desired treatment area. The patient has no downtime and can immediately return to work, exercise, or other desired activity. In many instances, a repeat treatment 3 months later is required to achieve optimal results.

Cryolipolysis is generally well tolerated, but there have been some reported side effects. Short-term adverse events included erythema, edema, and bruising at the treatment site, all of which tend to resolve on their own with no long-term sequelae. Abnormal cutaneous sensation can occur over the treatment site, lasting up to 2 months in some cases. More severe delayed postprocedure pain has been reported as well. This persistent pain has been successfully managed with compression garments, lidocaine transdermal patches, or gabapentin. A rare (about 1 in 20,000) and potentially more serious long-term adverse event is the development of paradoxic adipose hyperplasia at the treated site. The pathoetiology of this fat deposition is unclear. Treatment with liposuction to remove the excess adipose can be curative.

Sodium Deoxycholate

Deoxycholate acid injection (Kybella, Allergan, Irvine, CA) is FDA approved as a "first in class" treatment for undesired fullness of submental fat. Endogenous deoxycholate acid is a secondary bile acid that is used in the emulsification of dietary fats, which facilitates absorption in the intestine. When used for fat reduction, deoxycholate acid initially causes direct damage to adipocytes via lysis of the cells. Following this direct effect, a local neutrophil-mediated inflammatory process ensues over the following days that helps further potentiate the desired response. As the inflammatory process resolves, fibroblasts are recruited to the area with fibrous septae thickening noted at 1 month after treatment.

Patients are treated with a series of injections over the submental region. Typically 2–4 sessions spaced about 4–6 weeks apart are required for maximum improvement. A grid is applied to the skin and a small aliquot is injected into each site. These minimally invasive treatments are very well tolerated, with typical side effects of discomfort, swelling, bruising, and numbness. Care must be taken when injecting to avoid underlying structures, such as the marginal mandibular nerve.

Coldiron BM, et al: Office surgery incidents: what seven years of Florida data show us. Dermatol Surg 2008; 34: 285.

Coleman WP 3rd, et al: Guidelines of care for liposuction. J Am Acad Dermatol 2001; 45: 438.

Dover JS, et al: Management of patient experience with ATX-101 (deoxycholic acid injection) for reduction of submental fat. Dermatol Surg 2016; 42: S288.

Fakhouri TM, et al: Laser-assisted lipolysis. Dermatol Surg 2012; 38: 155.

Habbema L: Safety of liposuction using exclusively tumescent local anesthesia in 3,240 consecutive cases. Dermatol Surg 2009; 35: 1728.

Housman TS, et al: The safety of liposuction. Dermatol Surg 2002; 28: 971.

Humphrey S, et al: ATX-101 for reduction of submental fat. J Am Acad Dermatol 2016; 75: 788.

Ibrahim O, et al: The comparative effectiveness of suction-curettage and onabotulinumtoxin-A injections for the treatment of primary focal axillary hyperhidrosis. J Am Acad Dermatol 2013; 69: 88.

Ingargiola MJ, et al: Cryolipolysis for fat reduction and body contouring. Plast Reconstr Surg 2015; 135: 1581.

Jalian HR, et al: Paradoxical adipose hyperplasia after cryolipolysis. JAMA Dermatol 2014; 150: 317.

Karcher C, et al: Paradoxical hyperplasia post cryolipolysis and management. Dermatol Surg 2017; 43: 467.

Shridharani SM: Early experience in 100 consecutive patients with injection adipocytolysis for neck contouring with ATX-101 (deoxycholic acid). Dermatol Surg 2017; 43: 950.

CHEMICAL PEELS

Superficial Peel

Peels are categorized by the level of injury they cause. Superficial peels cause wounding to the epidermis and may reach the papillary dermis. These peels are well tolerated by patients who require limited "downtime" after treatment. Superficial peels are used in the treatment of photoaging, acne, actinic keratoses, solar lentigines, and pigmentary dyschromias. Given the limited nature of the injury induced by these peels, patients often need multiple treatments on a weekly or monthly basis to reach a desired result. However, patients need to be properly counseled regarding the limited benefit of superficial peels, which cannot provide the improvement in wrinkles and deep furrows that may be possible with deeper injury peels. Repeated superficial peels cannot produce the same results as a single, deeper peel.

Alpha-hydroxy acids (AHAs) are naturally occurring agents that are typically derived from foods, include glycolic acid (sugarcane), lactic acid (sour milk), malic acid (apples), and citric acid (citrus fruits). Glycolic acid has the smallest molecular size and thus the greatest bioavailability, making it one of the most frequently used AHAs. The depth of injury is determined by the pH, concentration of the acid, amount applied, and length of treatment time. Glycolic acid, in concentrations up to 70%, is often used for melasma, acne, and photoaging. Following rapid application to the entire face, it must be neutralized with sodium bicarbonate or plain water. Glycolic acid has been used in combination with 5-FU for the treatment of actinic keratoses.

Salicylic acid, a β-hydroxy acid, can be used in concentrations of 20%–30% for the treatment of acne and mild photoaging. It is especially useful as an adjunctive treatment for acne because of both the keratolytic and the comedolytic properties of salicylic acid. It is also used in combination with other agents as part of Jessner solution. Salicylic acid tends to be less inflammatory than other superficial chemical peels. After application, patients experience some mild stinging and discomfort. A whitening of the skin, termed *frosting*, from the precipitation of salicylic acid crystals is noted within several minutes of application. Salicylic acid does not require neutralization, although cool compresses after application can soothe the skin.

TABLE 39.2 Jessner Solution	
Agent	**Amount**
Resorcinol	14 g
Salicylic acid	14 g
85% lactic acid	14 g
95% ethanol qs ad	100 mL

Trichloroacetic acid (TCA) in concentrations of 10%–25% is used extensively as a superficial peel. The depth of injury is related to the concentration and the number of applications, with repeated coats of a low-concentration TCA leading to greater penetration. The agent is applied, and erythema and a white frost are noted within 1 minute. Patients experience a burning sensation. Handheld fans and postprocedural cool compresses can reduce discomfort. TCA does not require neutralization after application.

Jessner solution combines resorcinol, salicylic acid, and lactic acid in ethanol (Table 39.2). This superficial peel has keratolytic activity and is typically used for acne or hyperkeratotic lesions. It is self-neutralizing, and multiple applications can be performed to obtain a deeper injury.

Solid CO_2 (dry ice) has been used alone and in combination with TCA to obtain a deeper peel. It has been proposed as an effective treatment for acne scars and as a way to potentiate the effect of TCA to achieve a deeper peel.

Medium-Depth Peel

Medium-depth chemical peeling is defined as a controlled wound through the epidermis and down to the deep papillary dermis. In contrast to the multiple treatments that are often performed with superficial peels, medium-depth peels are generally done as a single procedure because of the more significant injury produced and more robust clinical response. These peels cause epidermal necrosis and dermal injury, which result in increased collagen production during the wound-healing process over the next several months. Medium-depth peels are indicated for the treatment of mild to moderate photodamage, rhytids, pigmentary dyschromias, actinic keratoses, solar lentigines, and other epidermal growths.

The classic medium-depth peel is 50% TCA. However, it is generally not used currently as a single-agent peel because of its unpredictable results and increased incidence of scarring and dyspigmentation. Rather, combining 35% TCA with an initial application of another agent, such as Jessner solution or glycolic acid, can produce a medium-depth injury without the complications associated with higher concentrations of TCA alone. As a result of the damage to the epidermis produced with the initial peel, the lower-strength TCA is able to penetrate deeper and produce a more significant and even result.

Antiviral prophylaxis should be used in any full-face medium-depth peel because of the potential risk of herpes simplex virus activation. Acyclovir, 400 mg three times daily, or valacyclovir, 500 mg twice daily, can be started at the time of peel and continued until complete reepithelialization has occurred, typically 7–10 days. Prophylactic antibiotic therapy has no role in these full-face peels.

Deep Peel

Deep chemical peels are defined as those that cause an injury down to the midreticular dermis. These peels are indicated for patients with moderate to severe photodamage and advanced rhytids. Deep peels produce significant injury, and patients have an extended period of postoperative healing.

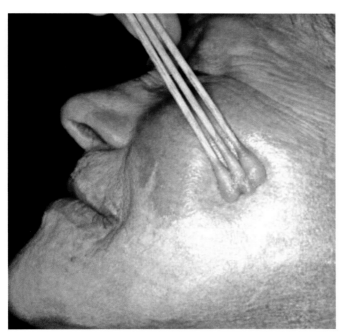

Fig. 39.12 Baker-Gordon phenol peel; white frosting after application. (Courtesy Richard G. Glogau, MD.).

TABLE 39.3 Baker-Gordon Formula

Agent	Amount
88% liquid phenol, USP	3 mL
Tap water	2 mL
Septisol liquid soap	8 drops
Croton oil	3 drops

are treated individually. A 15-minute wait is required between treating each subunit, spreading the entire procedure over 1–2 hours, thus further limiting the systemic concentration of phenol. After application, occlusive tape can be applied if a deeper wound is desired. The patients are managed conservatively in the postoperative period with petrolatum and wound care until the skin heals. In addition to the cardiac and systemic concerns associated with deep peels, other risks include hypopigmentation, textural abnormalities, and scarring. If any of the phenol solution accidentally contacts the eyes, mineral oil should be used to flush, because water can potentiate the effect of the phenol. Antiviral prophylaxis should be administered.

Baker-Gordon formula phenol peel is the traditional deep peel (Fig. 39.12). Undiluted 88% phenol does not produce a deep or consistent injury because it causes complete coagulation of epidermal keratin proteins, thus blocking further penetration. The Baker-Gordon formula reduces the concentration of phenol to 55%; the croton oil acts as a keratolytic and potentiates the depth of penetration of the phenol (Table 39.3). Cardiac monitoring is required because phenol can produce arrhythmias. Intravenous fluids are given before and during the peel to limit the serum concentrations of phenol and any potential renal complications. In addition, the face is divided into smaller cosmetic units, which

Bae BG, et al: Salicylic acid peels versus Jessner's solution for acne vulgaris. Dermatol Surg 2013; 39: 248.
Jackson A: Chemical peels. Facial Plast Surg 2014; 30: 26.
Kaminaka C, et al: Clinical evaluation of glycolic acid chemical peeling in patients with acne vulgaris. Dermatol Surg 2014; 40: 314.
Kubiak M, et al: Evaluation of 70% glycolic peels versus 15% trichloroacetic peels for the treatment of photodamaged facial skin in aging women. Dermatol Surg 2014; 40: 883.
Landau M: Cardiac complications in deep chemical peels. Dermatol Surg 2007; 33: 190.
Reserva J, et al: Chemical peels. Dermatol Surg 2017; 43: S163.
Salam A, et al: Chemical peeling in ethnic skin. Br J Dermatol 2013; 169: 82.
Sarkar R, et al: Comparative evaluation of efficacy and tolerability of glycolic acid, salicylic mandelic acid, and phytic acid combination peels in melasma. Dermatol Surg 2016; 42: 384.

Index

Page numbers followed by "*f*" indicate figures, "*t*" indicate tables, "*b*" indicate boxes, and "*e*" indicate online content.

A

AA amyloidosis, 516
Abacavir, adverse reactions, 119–120
"ABCD" criteria, for melanoma, 695
Abdomen, allergic contact dermatitis in, 97
Aberrant basal cell carcinoma, 650
ABI (ankle:brachial index), 856–857
Ablative laser resurfacing, 919–921
Abrasions, 13
Abscess
    metastatic tuberculous, 328, 328*f*
    staphylococcal, 255, 255*f*, 290.*e1f*
Absorbable sutures, 887–888
Acanthamoeba, 421
Acantholysis
    pityriasis rubra pilaris and, 207
    suprabasilar, 455
Acantholytic acanthoma, 640
Acantholytic dyskeratotic acanthoma, 640
Acanthoma
    acantholytic, 640
    clear cell, 639–640, 639*f*
    epidermolytic, 640
    granular parakeratotic, 641
    pilar sheath, 677
    reticulated, with sebaceous differentiation, 664
Acanthosis, 76
Acanthosis nigricans, 502–504, 502*f*–504*f*, 504.*e1f*, 635.*e7f*
    associated with insulin-resistant states and syndromes, 503–504
    associated with malignancy, 503
    diagnosis and treatment, 504
    drug-induced, 504
    familial, *Fgfr* gene mutation syndromes and, 503
    miscellaneous associations, 504
Acanthosis palmaris, 503, 503*f*
Acarina, order of, 446–450
Acatalasemia, 808
Acatalasia, 808
ACE inhibitors. *see* Angiotensin-converting enzyme (ACE) inhibitors
Acetic acid
    stings, 429
    venous leg ulcers, 857
Acetylsalicylic acid, Degos disease, 850–851
Achenbach syndrome, 834
Acid maltose lozenges, for Sjögren syndrome, 179–180
Acid-fast bacilli (AFB)
    Buruli ulcer, 333
    tuberculosis verrucosa cutis, 326
Acids, 92, 93*f*
Acitretin
    for palmoplantar pustulosis, 203
    for pityriasis rubra pilaris, 208
    for pustular psoriasis, 194–195
Acne, 231–251
    pyoderma faciale and, 249
    severe truncal, 233*f*

Acne *(Continued)*
    tropical, 240, 240*f*
    upper chest involvement with, 251.*e1f*
Acne, steroid, 138
Acne conglobata, 239, 239*f*, 251.*e1f*
Acne corne, 94
Acne estivalis, 240
Acne excoriée des jeunes filles, 240–241
Acne fulminans, 240
Acne keloidalis, 242, 242*f*
Acne keloidalis nuchae, 759
Acne miliaris necrotica, 245
Acne necrotica, 760
Acne neonatorum, 233
Acne scars, 231, 233*f*
Acne varioliformis, 245
Acne venenata, 241
Acne vermoulanti, 761
Acne vulgaris, 231–239, 232*f*
    clinical features of, 231, 232*f*
    complications of, 238–239, 238*f*
    pathogenesis of, 231–233
    pathology of, 233
    treatment of, 233–238, 234*b*
Acneiform eruptions, 241
Acquired aquagenic syringeal acrokeratoderma, 213, 213*f*
Acquired arteriovenous fistula, 600*f*
Acquired C1 esterase inhibitor deficiency, 155–156
Acquired clubbing, 780
Acquired dermal melanocytosis (ADM), 862
Acquired digital fibrokeratoma, 635.*e4f*
Acquired dyskeratotic leukoplakia, 805, 805*f*
Acquired generalized lipodystrophy, 495
Acquired hyperostosis syndrome (AHYS), 240
Acquired hypertrichosis lanuginosa, 769, 770*f*
Acquired ichthyosis, 565
Acquired immunodeficiency syndrome (AIDS)
    "advanced", 416
    cryptococcosis and, 312
    cytomegalovirus in, 381
    ecthymatous zoster in, 420.*e3f*
    hair disorders and, 763
    herpes zoster and, 377, 378*f*
    Kaposi sarcoma and, 418–420, 418*f*
    molluscum contagiosum, 392–393
    Mycobacterium avium intracellulare complex, 334
    oral hairy leukoplakia, 802, 803*f*
    pruritus, 47
    pyoderma gangrenosum and, 148
Acquired lipodystrophy, 494–495
Acquired localized trichorrhexis nodosa, 764
Acquired partial lipodystrophy, 494–495, 494*f*, 495.*e2f*
Acquired perforating collagenosis, 772
Acquired perforating dermatosis, 773, 773*f*
Acquired progressive lymphangioma, 602–603
Acral erythema, chemotherapy-induced, 129–134, 130*f*
Acral fibrokeratoma, 616
Acral mycosis fungoides, 737–738
Acral neuromatosis, 674–675
Acral nevi, 689

Acral persistent papular mucinosis, 186, 186*f*
Acral-lentiginous melanoma, 696–697, 696*f*
Acrocephalosyndactyly, 583
Acrochordons, 502
Acrocyanosis, 21–22, 21*f*
Acrodermatitis chronica atrophicans, 288, 513
    scleroderma *vs.*, 175
Acrodermatitis continua (of Hallopeau), 195, 204.*e2f*
Acrodermatitis enteropathica, 16
    zinc deficiency and, 481, 481*f*–482*f*, 484.*e2f*
Acrodynia, 136
Acrofacial vitiligo, 871–872
Acrokeratoelastoidosis, 210
Acrokeratosis verruciformis, 573
Acrokeratotic poikiloderma, 561
Acromegaly, 496, 497*f*, 504.*e1f*
Acromelalgia, 815, 815*f*
"Acropetechial syndrome", 399
Acrosclerosis, 174
Acrospiromas, 666–667, 667*f*
    malignant, 667
Acrosteolysis, 194
Acrosyringeal lichen planus, 222–223
Acrosyringeal nevus of Weedon and Lewis, 670
Acrosyringium, 4
Acrylic bone cement, 106
Acrylic monomers, dermatitis, 106
ACTH. *see* Adrenocorticotropic hormone (ACTH)
Actinic cheilitis, 794–795, 795*f*
Actinic dermatitis, chronic, 34–35, 34*f*, 45.*e2f*
Actinic elastotic plaque, 26
Actinic granuloma, 708–709, 708*f*
Actinic injury, 24–28
Actinic keratosis, 644–645, 644*f*
    photodynamic therapy for, 906
Actinic lichen nitidus, 225
Actinic prurigo, 32, 32*f*
Actinomyces, 268
Actinomyces actinomycetemcomitans, 212
Actinomycetomas, 318
Actinomycosis, 268, 268*f*
Action spectrum, 28
Acute febrile neutrophilic dermatosis, 145–147, 145*f*
    diagnostic criteria for, 146*b*
Acute generalized exanthematous pustulosis (AGEP), 120–121, 121*f*
    T-cells in, 113
Acute hemorrhagic edema of infancy, 839–840, 839*f*, 813.*e3f*
Acute infectious mononucleosis, urticaria and, 151
Acute intermittent porphyria, 525
Acute meningococcemia, 275
Acute myelogenous leukemia (AML), 746
Acute necrotizing ulcerative gingivitis (ANUG), 807–808, 807*f*
Acute seroconversion syndrome, 416
Acute-onset painful acral granuloma annulare, 705–706
Acyclovir
    for erythema multiforme, 141
    for genital herpes, 365

Acyclovir *(Continued)*
  for herpes simplex, 369
  for herpes zoster, 375–376
  for herpetic gingivostomatitis, 363–364
  for neonatal herpes simplex, 367
  for varicella, 371
Adalimumab, for sarcoidosis, 717
Adams-Oliver syndrome, 578
ADAMTS13, 825
Adapalene
  for acne vulgaris, 234
  for photoaging, 28
Addison disease, 497–498, 497*f*
Adenitis, neutrophilic sebaceous, 708–709
Adenomas
  adrenal, 496–497
  sebaceous, 664, 664*f*
Adenopathy, sarcoidosis and, 714
Adhesive dermatitis, 105
Adhesive tape reactions, 105
Adhesives, occupational vitiligo and, 874
Adiposis dolorosa, 628
Adnexa, 1–4
Adolescents
  acne vulgaris and, 231
  atopic dermatitis in, 66–67, 67*f*
Adrenal adenomas, 496–497
Adrenal hyperplasia, 498–499
Adrenal insufficiency, 497–498
Adrenergic urticaria, 152
Adrenocorticotropic hormone (ACTH),
      496–497
  acne vulgaris and, 232
  stimulation test, 770
Adrenogenital syndrome, 498, 498*f*, 770
Adrenoleukodystrophy, 545
Adriamycin, adverse reactions, 130
Adult, atopic dermatitis, 63–64, 66–67, 67*f*
Adult Langerhans cell histiocytosis, 727–728
Adult progeria, 579
Adult T-cell leukemia-lymphoma (ATL),
      414–415, 415*f*, 742–743
Advancement flap, 896, 899*f*–900*f*
Adverse drug reactions (ADRs), 112–113
AEC syndrome, 575, 576*f*
Aedes mosquitoes, 400
AEIOU, in Merkel cell carcinoma, 661
Aeromonas hydrophilia, 276
Aeromonas infections, 276
Afibrinogenemia, 831
African histoplasmosis, 310
African trypanosomiasis, 426, 426*f*
Agave americana, 100, 829
Agglutination test, latex
  for coccidioidomycosis, 309
  for cryptococcosis, 312
Aggressive angiomyxoma, 621
Aggressive digital papillary adenocarcinoma,
      671–672
Aggressive infantile fibromatosis, 613
Agminated Spitz nevi, 692, 692*f*
Aicardi-Goutieres syndrome, 150
AIDS. *see* Acquired immunodeficiency
      syndrome (AIDS)
Ainhum, 614
Airbag dermatitis, 93
AL amyloidosis, 515–516
Alagille syndrome, 533
  pruritus and, 48
Albendazole
  for creeping eruption, 433
  for cysticercosis cutis, 431
  for pinworm, 432
  for trichinosis, 437
Albinism, 3, 879, 880*f*

Albopapuloid lesions, dominant dystrophic
      epidermolysis bullosa, 560
Albright disease, 583
Albright sign, 501–502, 502*f*
Albright's hereditary osteodystrophy (AHO),
      529
Alcohol
  flushing and, 140
  irritant contact dermatitis and, 95
  nutritional disease, 475
Alcyonidium hirsutum, 100
Alefacept, 199
Aleppo boil, 422
"Aleukemic leukemia cutis", 746
Alexandrite laser, for nevus spilus, 686
Alezzandrini syndrome, 875–876
Algae, 100
  disease caused by, 322–323
Alitretinoin, oral, for hand eczema, 76
Alkaline phosphatase, zinc deficiency and,
      481–482
Alkaline sulfide, 92
Alkalis, contact dermatitis, 92, 93*f*
Alkaptonuria, 541–543, 542*f*
Allergic contact cheilitis, 794, 795*f*
Allergic contact dermatitis, 95–109
  adhesive dermatitis, 105
  from clothing, 101–102, 101*f*
  contact stomatitis, 104
  cosmetic dermatitis, 106–108
  juvenile plantar dermatosis, 77–78
  keratinocytes in, 3
  from metals and metal salts, 102–104
  from plants, 97–101
  preservatives, 108–109
  pruritus ani and, 50
  regional predilection, 96–97
  sensitivity, testing for, 96
  from shoes, 102, 102*f*, 139.*e1f*
  synthetic resin dermatitis, 105–106
  from topical drugs, 109–111, 110*f*
  vehicles, 109
Allergic granulomas, 716
Allergy, bovine collagen and, 922
Allodynia, zoster-associated pain, 376
Allopurinol
  for hairy cell leukemia, 747
  hypersensitivity syndrome, 116, 116*f*
  Stevens-Johnson syndrome, 117
All-*trans*-retinoic acid, Sweet syndrome and, 146
Allylamines, 291
Alopecia, 16, 585
  biopsy, 751
  causes of, 750
  cicatricial, 757–758, 757*f*–758*f*
  diagnosis of, 750
  frontal fibrosing, 220
  noncicatricial, 750–756
  pattern, 754–755
  in sarcoidosis, 713–714
  secondary syphilis, 361.*e2f*
Alopecia areata, 16, 57–58, 750–752, 793.*e1f*
  clinical features of, 750, 751*f*
  differential diagnosis of, 751
  etiologic factors of, 750–751
  histology of, 751
  prognosis of, 752
  tinea capitis and, 293–294
  treatment of, 751–752
Alopecia cicatrisata, 760
Alopecia mucinosa, 756
  in mycosis fungoides, 734–735, 734*f*–735*f*
  see also Follicular mucinosis
Alopecia neoplastica, 632, 633*f*, 761, 762*f*
Alopecia syphilitica, 756, 756*f*

Alopecia totalis, 750
Alopecia universalis, 750
Alphavirus, 401–402
Alport syndrome, 834
Alternaria, 318
Alternariosis, 318
Aluminum chlorhydroxide, for hyperhidrosis,
      774
Aluminum chloride
  for bromhidrosis, 776
  for hyperhidrosis, 774
Aluminum salts, dermatitis, 108
Amalgam tattoo, 806, 806*f*
Amantadine (Symmetrel), and livedo, 818
Amblyomma americanum, 446
Ambulatory phlebectomy, 930, 930*f*
Amebas, 421, 422*f*
Amebiasis cutis, 421
Amelanotic blue nevus, 703
Amelanotic melanoma, 697, 697*f*
  malignant, 703.*e4f*
Ameloblastoma, peripheral, 806
American Joint Committee on Cancer
      (AJCC), in melanoma, 699, 699*b*
American trypanosomiasis, 427
Amides, 884
  allergic contact dermatitis, 110
Amikacin
  for *Mycobacterium fortuitum*, 334
  for nocardiosis, 269
p-Aminobenzoic acid esters, 110
5-Aminolevulinic acid, for hidradenitis
      suppurativa, 243
Aminopenicillins
  adverse reactions, 112–113
  for wound infection, 883
Amiodarone
  photosensitivity, 124, 124*f*
  pigmentation, 127–128
Amitriptyline
  for erythromelalgia, 816
  for zoster-associated pain, 376–377
Amlexanox, aphthous stomatitis, 810
Amlodipine, for Raynaud disease, 814
Amoxicillin
  for acne vulgaris, 235
  for infectious mononucleosis, 380
  for wound infection, 883
Amoxicillin-clavulanate, HIV and, 119
Amphotericin B
  for aspergillosis, 322
  for chromoblastomycosis, 316–317
  for cryptococcosis, 312
  for fusariosis, 321–322
  for histoplasmosis, 311
  for hyalohyphomycosis, 321
  for leishmaniasis, 424
  for mucormycosis, 321
  for North American blastomycosis, 313
  for prototheosis, 323
  for sporotrichosis, 316
  for systemic candidiasis, 305
Ampicillin
  for infectious mononucleosis, 380
  for wound infection, 883
Ampicillin-amoxicillin, adverse reactions, 114
Amyloid, 515
Amyloidosis, 511, 515, 516*f*, 546.*e1f*
  classification, 515
  cutaneous, 517–519
    primary localized, 517–518
    secondary, 518
  familial syndromes associated with,
      519–520
  macular, 59

Amyloidosis (Continued)
nodular, 518, 518f
pharmaceutical, 519
systemic, 511, 515–517
dialysis-associated, 516–517
primary, AL amyloidosis, 515–516
secondary, AA amyloidosis, 516
Amyloidosis cutis dyschromica, 518
Anagen effluvium, 753–754, 754f
Anagen hairs, 750, 752f
Anagen phase, hair follicles, 5f–7f, 6, 10.e1f
Anal neurodermatitis, 49
Anamnestic (recalled) eruption, 110
Anaphylaxis, 156
Ancylostomiasis, 432
Androgen
acne vulgaris and, 231
hirsutism and, 770
Androgen-dependent syndromes, 498–499
Androgenetic alopecia
female-pattern, 755
male-pattern, 754–755, 793.e1f
Anergic leishmaniasis, 452.e1f
Anesthesia, 884–885
side effects of, 884–885
Anetoderma, 512, 512f, 744–745
Angelman syndromes, 879
"Angel's kiss", 595
Angina bullosa hemorrhagica, 807
Angioblastoma, 593
Angiocentric lymphoma, 742
Angioedema, 122, 123f, 154–156, 155f
acquired C1 esterase inhibitor deficiency
in, 155–156
episodic, with eosinophilia, 156
hereditary, 155
urticaria and, 151
vibratory, 153
Angioendotheliomatosis, malignant, 744
Angiofibromas, 502, 555f, 615, 586.e1f
Angioid streak, 507
Angioimmunoblastic lymphadenopathy, with
dysproteinemia, 741–743
Angioimmunoblastic T-cell lymphoma,
741–743
Angiokeratoma, 605
of Mibelli, 605
of scrotum, 605, 605f
Angiokeratoma circumscriptum, 605, 635.e2f
Angiokeratoma corporis diffusum, 537–538
Angioleiomyoma (vascular leiomyoma), 631
Angiolipoleiomyoma, 631
Angiolymphoid hyperplasia with eosinophilia
(ALHE), 605–606, 606f
Angioma
spider, 603, 635.e2f
tufted, 593, 593f, 635.e1f
Angioma serpiginosum, 606–607
Angiomatosis
bacillary, 280–281, 280f
diffuse dermal, 852
Angiosarcoma, 36–37, 609, 45.e2f, 635.e3f
Angiotensin receptor antagonist, for Raynaud
disease, 814
Angiotensin-converting enzyme (ACE) inhibitors
adverse reactions, 123
sarcoidosis and, 715
for scleroderma, 176
Angiotropic large cell lymphoma, 744
Angular cheilitis, 303, 795–796
Anhidrosis, 776
Anhidrotic ectodermal dysplasia, 81, 575
Anise-scented mokihana berry, 29
Ankle:brachial index (ABI), 856–857
Annular atrophic lichen planus, 217

Annular elastolytic giant cell granuloma
(AEGCG), 708–709, 708f, 730.e1f
Annular elastolytic granuloma, 708–709, 708f
Annular erythema, eosinophilic, 144
Annular lesions, 15
Annular lichen planus, 217, 217f,
230.e1f–230.e3f
Annular sarcoidosis, 711–712, 712f
Annular syphilid, 351
Annulus migrans, 799, 799f
Anogenital dysplasia, 860
Anonychia, 782
Anoplura, order of, 441–442
Anorexia nervosa
acrocyanosis and, 21
pruritus and, 47
ANOTHER syndrome, 499
Anthralin
for alopecia areata, 751–752
for flat warts, 406
for psoriasis, 198
Anthrax, 264–265, 389
with severe edema, 265f
Anthrenus scrophulariae, 444
Antibiotic (iatrogenic) candidiasis, 304
Antibiotics
for acne vulgaris, 235
for frostbite, 23
for Gram-negative folliculitis, 241
for granuloma annulare, 707
for hidradenitis suppurativa, 243
oral, for breast eczema, 73
prophylaxis, 882–884, 882t
for rosacea, 247–248
selection and timing, 882–883
for venous leg ulcers, 857
Anticentromere antibodies, in CREST
syndrome, 173
Anticholinergic agents, for hyperhidrosis, 775
Anticoagulants, 881–888
for frostbite, 23
for skin necrosis, 123–125, 125f
Anticonvulsants, 46–47, 116
hypersensitivity syndrome, 115–117
Antidepressants
for burning mouth syndrome, 59
for prurigo nodularis, 54
Antifibrinolytic agents, for acquired C1
esterase inhibitor deficiency, 155–156
Antifungal therapy, 291–292
for allergic contact dermatitis, 110
for breast eczema, 73
Antigen-presenting cells, in graft-versus-host
disease, 89
Antihistamines, 31–32
for acute urticaria, 154
for allergic contact dermatitis, 109–110
for aquagenic urticaria, 153
for atopic dermatitis, 69
for cholinergic urticaria, 151–152
for chronic urticaria, 154
for cold urticaria, 152
for dermatographism, 151
for eosinophilic folliculitis, 417
for exercise-induced urticaria, 153
oral, for prurigo simplex, 52
for polycythemia vera, 749
for prurigo nodularis, 54
for pruritus, 46
for small-vessel vasculitis, 837–838
for solar urticaria, 33–34, 152
for vibratory angioedema, 153
Antimalarials
for dermatomyositis, 170
for porphyria cutanea tarda, 522

Antimalarials (Continued)
for sarcoidosis, 717
for systemic lupus erythematosus, 165–166
for urticarial vasculitis, 840–841
Antimicrobial therapy
for allergic contact dermatitis, 110
for atopic dermatitis, 70
flushing and, 140
Antimony n-methyl glutamine, leishmaniasis,
424
Antineutrophil cytoplasmic antibody (ANCA)
polyarteritis nodosa, 844
positive vasculitides, 845–848
Sweet syndrome and, 146
Antinuclear antibodies (ANAs), 135
in mixed connective tissue disease, 178
in progressive systemic sclerosis, 174–175
in Raynaud disease, 813
subacute cutaneous lupus erythematosus
and, 160–161
systemic lupus erythematosus and, 164–165
Antinuclear ribonucleic acid protein
(anti-nRNP), systemic lupus
erythematosus and, 165
Antioxidants
in rubber, 105
for scleroderma, 176
Anti-p105 pemphigoid, 461
Antiphospholipid antibodies
anetoderma, 512
systemic lupus erythematosus and, 163, 165
Antiphospholipid antibody syndrome, 818
Antiproliferative therapy, for common warts,
406
Antipruritics, for atopic dermatitis, 70
Antipsychotic agents
for delusions of parasitosis, 56
for factitious dermatitis, 57
Antiretroviral-associated lipoatrophy, 494
α₁-Antitrypsin deficiency panniculitis, 492
Antivirals, for erythema multiforme, 143
Ants, 444–445, 444f
Anxiety, excoriated acne and, 241
Anxiolytics, for prurigo nodularis, 54
Aortic arch syndrome, 850
Apert syndrome, 583, 637
Aphthosis, 809–810
Aphthous ulcer, major, 810–811, 810f
Aplasia cutis congenita, 577–578, 662–663
Apocrine chromhidrosis, 5
Apocrine gland carcinoma, 672
Apocrine sweat units, 1, 5, 5f
Aponeurotic fibroma, 612
Apoptosis, 1
Apremilast, for sarcoidosis, 717
Aquadynia, 51–52
Aquagenic pruritus, 51–52
Aquagenic urticaria, 153
Aquagenic wrinkling, of palms, 213, 213f
Aquaporin family, of water channels, 179
Arachnida, order of, 446–450
Arachnidae, 450–451
Arachnidism, 450
Arbovirus group, 399–402
Arcanobacterium haemolyticum infection, 266
Arcuate dermal erythema, 86
Arcuate lesions, 15
Areolas, 9
hyperkeratosis of, 639
Argininosuccinic acid synthetase (ASS1 gene),
540
Argyria, pigmentation and, 128
Armadillos, Hansen disease, 336
Arms, allergic contact dermatitis in, 97
Aromatherapy, 100

Arrectores pilorum, 9
Arsenic, 869
Arsenical keratoses, 209, 643, 643*f*, 685.*e2f*
Arsenical melanosis, 128
Arterial insufficiency (ischemic) ulcer, 858
Arteriography, Buerger disease, 851
Arteriosclerosis obliterans, 852
Arteriovenous fistula, 635.*e1f*
Arthralgias
    erythema multiforme major and, 141–142
    subacute cutaneous lupus erythematosus
        and, 160–161
    Sweet syndrome and, 145–146
Arthritis
    in pancreatic panniculitis, 491–492
    pyoderma gangrenosum and, 148
    subacute cutaneous lupus erythematosus
        and, 160–161
    Sweet syndrome and, 145–146
Arthropod-related disease, prevention of,
    437–438
Asboe-Hansen sign, 13, 453
Ascher syndrome, 511–512, 512*f*, 797
Ascorbic acid
    pigmented purpura, 836
    for scurvy, 479
Ash-leaf macules, 555*f*
"Ashy dermatosis", 224
Aspergillosis, 322
Aspergillus, 322, 323.*e5f*
    colonization of, 291
    infection, chronic granulomatous disease,
        86
Aspergillus flavus, 322
Aspergillus fumigatus, 322
Aspergillus niger, 322
Asphyxia, traumatic, 39–40
Aspirin
    adverse reactions, 122
    diffuse dermal angiomatosis, 852
    for erythema nodosum, 486–487
    for erythromelalgia, 815–816
    for frostbite, 23
    Kawasaki disease, 853–854
    pruritus in polycythemia vera, 49
    for sunburn, 24–25
    varicella and, 371
Assassin bug, 427, 440–441
Asteatotic eczema, 77
Asthma
    adult-onset, with periocular
        xanthogranuloma, 709–711
    Churg-Strauss syndrome, 847
Asymmetric periflexural exanthem of
    childhood (APEC), 397
Ataxia telangiectasia, 84–85, 84*f*, 557, 586.*e2f*
Athlete's foot, 297
ATM gene, 557
ATM protein, 83
Atopic dermatitis, 20, 63–91
    in adolescents and adults, 66–67, 67*f*
    antimicrobial therapy for, 70
    antipruritics in, 70
    associated features and complications of,
        67–69
    barrier repair in, 69
    childhood, 66, 66*f*
    clinical manifestations of, 65–67
    criteria for, 65*b*
        modified, for children with, 65*b*
    cyclosporine, 71
    differential diagnosis for, 69
    education and support in, 69
    environmental factors in, 70
    epidemiology of, 63–64

Atopic dermatitis (*Continued*)
    food allergy and, 64–65
    general management of, 69–70
    genetic basis of, 64–65
    herpesvirus infection in, 367–368
    histopathology of, 69
    immunosuppressive agents for, 71–72
    infantile, 66, 66*f*
    management of acute flare, 72–73
    pathogenesis of, 64–65
    phototherapy for, 71
    prevention of, 64
    severe, 66, 66*f*
    systemic corticosteroids for, 71
    systemic therapy for, 71
    tar for, 71
    tinea capitis and, 294
    topical calcineurin inhibitors for, 70–71
    topical corticosteroid therapy for, 70
    treatment modalities for, 70–73
    warts in, 420.*e8f*
ATP7A gene, 763
ATP7B gene, 543
Atrichia
    with papular lesions, 762
    with papules, 584
Atrophic glossitis, 800, 800*f*
Atrophie blanche, 819, 819*f*
Atrophoderma, disorders with, 586
Atrophoderma of Pasini and Pierini, 172,
    173*f*
Atrophoderma reticulatum, 761
Atrophoderma vermiculatum, 586, 761
Atrophodermia reticulata symmetrica faciei,
    761
Atropine ointment, for hidrocystomas, 666
Atypical decubital fibroplasia, 618
Atypical fibroxanthoma, 619, 620*f*
Atypical lipomatous tumor, 629
Atypical mycobacteriosis, tuberculosis
    verrucosa cutis and, 326
Atypical nevus, 693–695
Atypical vascular lesion, 609
Auricular endochondral pseudocyst, 683, 683*f*
Australian sea wasp, 428
Autoantibodies
    cicatricial pemphigoid, 467
    dermatitis herpetiformis and, 470
    lichen sclerosus and, 227
    in urticaria, 153
Autoeczematization, 76
Autoerythrocyte sensitization, 834–835, 834*f*
Autoimmune bullous diseases, erythema
    multiforme major and, 142
Autoimmune diseases
    drug-induced, 136–137
    in vitiligo, 872
Autoimmune estrogen dermatitis, 78
Autoimmune progesterone dermatitis, 78
Autoinflammatory syndromes, 149–150
    and urticarial vasculitis, 840
Autologous fat transplantation, 924–925
Automeris io, 439
Autosensitization, 77
Autosomal recessive congenital ichthyosis,
    564–565
Autosomal recessive neonatal progeroid
    syndrome, 494
Avidin, 480
Axilla
    allergic contact dermatitis, 97
    extramammary Paget's disease of, 659–660
Axillary antiperspirants, 108
Axillary deodorants, 108
"Axillary web syndrome", 832–833

Azathioprine, 35
    adverse reactions, 134
    for atopic dermatitis, 71
    for dermatomyositis, 170
    for erythema multiforme, 143
    for pemphigus foliaceus, 458
    for pemphigus vulgaris, 455
    for pyoderma gangrenosum, 149
    for sarcoidosis, 717
    for scleroderma, 176
    for small-vessel vasculitis, 837–838
    for systemic lupus erythematosus, 166
Azelaic acid, for acne vulgaris, 235
Azithromycin
    for cat-scratch disease, 279–280
    for chancroid, 273
    for granuloma inguinale, 274
    for leishmaniasis, 424
    for pityriasis lichenoides et varioliformis
        acuta, 740
Azure lunulae, 543

B
Baboon syndrome, 95, 136, 399
Bacillary angiomatosis, 280–281, 280*f*
Bacille Calmette-Guérin (BCG) vaccination,
    325
Bacillus anthracis, 264
Bacitracin
    allergy to, 110, 112*f*
    contact urticaria, 112
Bacterial cellulitis, 261
Bacterial infections, 252–290
Bacterial resistance, for acne vulgaris, 235–236
Baghdad boil, 422
Baker-Gordon formula phenol peel, 933,
    933*f*, 933*t*
Bakers, hand eczema and, 74
Balamuthia, 421, 422*f*
Balanitis
    micaceous, 659
    Zoon. *see* Zoon balanitis
Balanitis plasmacellularis, 658, 658*f*
Balanoposthitis chronica circumscripta
    plasmacellularis, 658
Baldness, male-pattern, 754–755, 793.*e1f*
Balloon cell nevus, 690
Balloon cells, 378
Balneol, pruritus ani, 50
Balsam of Peru, 74
"Bamboo hair", 764
Banal nevi, 689
Banker type, of childhood dermatomyositis,
    169
Bannayan-Riley-Ruvalcaba syndrome (BRRS),
    599, 629, 675
Bannwarth syndrome, 287
BAP1-mutated nevi, 693
Barber's itch, 254, 294
"Bare underbelly" sign, 735
Barraquer-Simons syndrome, 494–495
Barrier repair
    in atopic dermatitis, 69
    for hand eczema, 76
Bart syndrome, 558
Bartonella, infections caused by, 279–281
Bartonella henselae, 279
Bartonella quintana, 279–280
Basal cell carcinoma (BCC), 4, 648–651, 651*f*,
    685.*e3f*
    association with internal malignancies, 650
    basaloid follicular hamartoma *vs.*, 678
    cryosurgery for, 892, 893*f*
    curettage combined with electrodesiccation
        for, 894

Basal cell carcinoma (BCC) *(Continued)*
  differential diagnosis of, 651
  etiology and pathogenesis of, 650
  histopathology of, 650–651
  immunosuppression in, 650
  large, 650*f*
  metastasis of, 650
  Mohs micrographic surgery for, 905–906
  natural history of, 650
  photodynamic therapy for, 906–907
  squamous cell carcinoma *vs.*, 653–655, 654*f*
  superficial, 649*f*
  treatment of, 651
Basaloid follicular hamartoma (BFH),
    677–678, 678*f*
Basaloid follicular hamartoma syndrome,
    Gorlin syndrome *vs.*, 653
Basement membrane zone (BMZ), 4
Basidiobolus ranarum, 320
Bathing suit ichthyosis, 564
Bathing trunk nevus, 691
Bazex syndrome, Gorlin syndrome *vs.*, 653
Bazin disease, 330
B-cell, cutaneous lymphoid hyperplasia and,
    731
BCNU, topical, for mycosis fungoides, 736
"Beaded hairs", 765, 765*f*
Beam diameter, of laser, 909
Beau lines, 783, 783*f*
Beaver lodges, in North American
    blastomycosis, 313
Becker nevus, 688, 688*f*, 915, 703.*e1f*
Beckwith-Wiedemann syndrome, 598
Bedbug, 452.*e2f*
  bites, 440, 440*f*, 452.*e2f*
Bedsore, 38
Bees, 444
Behçet syndrome, 486, 811–812, 811*f*, 812.*e2f*
Bejel, 360
Belimumab, for systemic lupus erythematosus,
    166
Benadryl, aphthous stomatitis, 810
Benign cephalic histiocytosis (BCH), 721,
    721*f*
Benign compound nevi, 689
Benign familial pemphigus, 586.*e3f*
Benign lichenoid keratoses, 642–643, 642*f*,
    685.*e2f*
Benign lipoblastoma, 630
Benign lymphangioendothelioma, 602–603
Benign melanocytic nevi, 689–695, 689*f*
Benign mucosal pemphigoid. *see* Cicatricial
    pemphigoid
Benign nevi, 703.*e1f*
Benign recurrent Spitz nevi, 690
Benign solitary fibrous papule, 615
Benign tumors, 587–590
Benzalkonium chloride, 109
Benznidazole, for trypanosomiasis, 427
Benzocaine, 110
  pruritus and, 46
Benzoyl peroxide
  for acne vulgaris, 231, 234
  for acneiform eruptions, 241
  with dapsone, 235
  for dermatitis, 106
  for hidradenitis suppurativa, 243
  for pseudofolliculitis barbae, 767
  for rosacea, 247
Benzyl benzoate, for scabies, 448
Berardinelli-Seip syndrome, 493
Bergapten, 29
Beriberi, 477
Berloque dermatitis, 29, 45.*e2f*
Bermuda fire sponge, 100

Bernard-Soulier syndrome, 834
Beryllium granuloma, 42
Besnier, prurigo gestationis, 466
Beta carotene, erythropoietic protoporphyria,
    524
Betadine (povidone-iodine), for preoperative
    antisepsis, 884
Betaine supplementation, homocystinuria, 511
Bevacizumab
  adverse reactions to, 132, 133*f*
  Osler disease, 855–856
Bexarotene, 132
  for lymphomatoid papulosis, 739
  for mycosis fungoides, 737
Bichloracetic acid, for genital warts, 409
Bier spots, 822
Bilharziasis, 430–431
Biliary cirrhosis, xanthomatous, 533
Biliary pruritus, 48–49
Bilobed flap, 902*f*
Biologic agents
  adverse reactions to, 134
  alopecia areata, 751–752
  psoriasis, 199–200
"Biologic false-positive" (BFP) test, for
    syphilis, 348
Biologic response modifiers, for mycosis
    fungoides, 736
Biopsies, 14, 888–892
  for alopecia, 750
  for bacillary angiomatosis, 280
  for calciphylaxis, 821
  for cicatricial alopecia, 756
  of dysplastic nevi, 694–695
  for erythema migrans, 287
  for erythroplasia of Queyrat, 657–658
  for granuloma annulare, 706
  for herpes simplex, 362
  for Kaposi sarcoma, 418
  for livedoid vasculopathy, 819
  for melanomas, 698
  for telogen effluvium, 753
  for thrombotic thrombocytopenic purpura,
    825
Biotin
  deficiency in, 480–481
  for onychoschizia, 783
Birth defects, in Gorlin syndrome, 652–653
Birt-Hogg-Dubé syndrome, 676–677, 676*f*,
    685.*e6f*
BIS-GMA, 106
Biskra button, 422
Bisphenol A, 106
Bisphosphonate therapy
  for mixed connective tissue disease, 178
  systemic lupus erythematosus and, 165
Bites, 421–452
  configuration of lesions, 15
Björnstad syndrome, 763
B-K mole syndrome, 693
Black dermatographism, 102
Black dot ringworm, 292, 292*f*
Black dot sign, 98*f*
Black fly, 442
Black hairy tongue, 799–800, 800*f*
Black heel, 39, 39*f*
"Black measles", 396
Black piedra, 306
Black widow spider, 450, 450*f*
Blackfoot disease, 869
Blackhead, 231, 232*f*
Blaschkitis, adult, 227
Blastic NK-cell lymphoma, 747
Blastic plasmacytoid dendritic cell neoplasm,
    747

Blastomyces dermatitidis, 312
Blastomycosis
  coccidioidomycosis and, 309
  keloidal, 319, 319*f*
  North American, 312–313, 313*f*, 323.*e3f*
  South American, 313–314
Blastomycosis-like pyoderma, 257, 270
Blau syndrome, 150, 715
Bleaching creams
  for dermatitis, 107
  for melasma, 864
  for Mongolian spot, 702
Bleomycin
  adverse reactions, 130–131, 131*f*
  for common warts, 406
  for keratoacanthoma, 647
Blepharochalasis, 511–512
Blindness, giant cell arteritis, 849
Blister beetle dermatitis, 443–444, 443*f*
Blistering dermatoses, chronic, 453–474
Blistering distal dactylitis, 262, 262*f*
Blisters, 11–12, 12*f*
Bloch-Sulzberger disease, 547–548
Blood eosinophilia, erythema gyratum repens
    and, 144
Bloom syndrome, 581, 581*f*
Bloom-Torre-Machacek syndrome, 581,
    581*f*
Blue light, photodynamic therapy and, 906
Blue nails, 790
Blue nevi, 15, 698, 702–703, 702*f*, 17.*e2f*
  Spitz nevi and, 690
Blue nevus of Jadassohn-Tieche, 702
Blue nevus-like melanoma, 703
Blue rubber bleb nevus syndrome, 599, 599*f*
Blue sclerae, 513–514, 514.*e2f*
Blueberry muffin baby, 381, 831
Blushing, 140
Bockhart impetigo, 254
Body cavity-based B-cell lymphoma, 383
Body dysmorphic disorder, 54–55, 58
Body louse, 441–442
Body mass index (BMI), calciphylaxis,
    820–821
Bone beetles, 444
Bone marrow
  myelofibrosis, 747–748
  transplantation
    for chronic granulomatous disease, 86
    for thromboangiitis obliterans, 851–
    852
    for Wiskott-Aldrich syndrome, 83
Bony lesions, in Langerhans cell histiocytosis,
    728–729, 729*f*
Borderline borderline (BB) leprosy, 338
Borderline lepromatous (BL) leprosy, 338,
    339*f*, 342
Borderline leprosy, 342, 346.*e1f*
Borderline tuberculoid (BT) leprosy, 338,
    338*f*, 342, 346.*e1f*
Borrelia, Lyme disease from, 286
Borrelia afzelii, 731
Borrelia burgdorferi, 286
Borrelia infections
  cutaneous lymphoid hyperplasia and, 731
  granuloma annulare and, 706
Borreliosis, 286–288
Bosentan
  for Raynaud disease, 814
  for scleroderma, 176
Botfly, 443
Botryomycosis, 256–257, 256*f*
Botulinum toxin, 925–928, 926*f*
  other locations, 927
  for Raynaud disease, 814–815

Botulinum toxin (*Continued*)
  for scleroderma, 176
  type A
    for hand eczema, 76
    for hyperhidrosis, 775
    for lichen simplex chronicus, 53–54
    for notalgia paresthetica, 59
  type B, 925
  for zoster-associated pain, 376–377
Bouba. *see* Yaws
Boutonneuse fever, 285, 285*f*, 290.*e4f*
Bovine collagen, 922
Bovine farcy, 278
Bovine papular stomatitis (BPSV), 389
Bovine-associated parapoxvirus infections,
  389
Bowel bypass syndrome, Sweet syndrome and,
  146–147
Bowen disease, 20–21, 656–657, 790, 791*f*,
  685.*e4f*
  clinical features of, 656, 656*f*
  differential diagnosis of, 657
  histopathology of, 656–657
  photodynamic therapy for, 907
  treatment of, 657
  trichilemmal carcinoma *vs.*, 676
Bowenoid papulosis, 408, 408*f*
Brachioradial pruritus, 32–33, 33*f*, 60
Braided suture, 887–888
Branchial cleft cysts, 684
Breakfast-lunch-and-dinner sign, 15
Breast
  eczema, 73–74, 74*f*
  see also Nipples
Brill-Zinsser disease, 284
Bristleworms, 429
Brittle nails, 784
Bromhidrosis, 776–777
  delusions of, 58
Bromidrosiphobia, 58
Bromocriptine
  acromegaly and, 496
  flushing and, 140
Bromoderma, 136–137
Bronchogenic cysts, 683–684
Brooke-Spiegler syndrome (BSS), 668,
  673–674, 673*f*
Brown hairy tongue, 799–800, 800*f*
Brown oculocutaneous albinism, 879
Brown recluse spider, 451, 451*f*
Brown-tail moth caterpillar, 439
Brucellosis, 283
Brunsting type, of childhood dermatomyositis,
  169
Brunsting-Perry pemphigoid, 467, 467*f*,
  474.*e3f*
Bruton syndrome, 80
Bubble hair deformity, 766
Bubo, in lymphogranuloma venereum, 289
Buck disease, 136
"Buckshot" scatter, of nevi, 689
Budesonide, 110–111
Buerger disease, 851–852, 851*f*
Buffalo hump, 496
Buffalopoxvirus, 389
Bulimia, 55
Bullae, 12–13, 17.*e1f*
Bullous amyloidosis, 516
Bullous drug reactions, 117–118, 118*f*
Bullous impetigo, 253, 253*f*
Bullous lichen planus, 218–219
Bullous lupus erythematosus, 162, 162*f*,
  183.*e3f*
Bullous lymphedema, 860
Bullous mastocytosis, 622, 622*f*

Bullous pemphigoid, 461–464,
  474.*e2f*–474.*e3f*
  antigen, 4
  clinical features of, 461, 461*f*–462*f*
  course and prognosis of, 463–464
  etiologic factors of, 462
  histopathology of, 462
  treatment of, 462–463
  urticarial, 474.*e2f*
Bullous pyoderma gangrenosum, 134, 147
Bullous scabies, 462
Bullous tinea, 298*f*
Bupivacaine, 884
Bupropion, adverse reactions, 123
Buried subcutaneous sutures, 889, 890*f*
Burning lips syndrome, 59
Burning mouth syndrome, 59
Burns, electrical, 18–19
Buruli ulcer, 333, 333*f*
Buschke-Lowenstein tumor, 408, 408*f*,
  655–656
Buschke-Ollendorff syndrome, 614
Busulfan, adverse reactions, 130
Butchers, warts in, 403
B virus, 383

C
C1 complement deficiency, 88
C1 esterase deficiency, 154
C2 complement deficiency, 88
C3 complement deficiency, 88
"C3 nephritic factor", 494–495
C4 complement deficiency, 88
C9 complement deficiency, 88
CADASIL syndrome, 544
Café au lait macules, 687, 915, 586.*e1f*
Café noir spots, 687
Calabar swelling, 435, 435*f*
Calamine lotion, for toxicodendron sensitivity,
  99
Calcifying epithelioma of Malherbe, 672, 672*f*
Calcineurin inhibitors
  for eczema herpeticum, 367–368
  flushing and, 140
  for granuloma annulare, 706
  lichen planus and, 219
  for pruritus, 46
  topical
    for atopic dermatitis, 70–71
    for necrobiosis lipoidica, 539
    for pemphigus foliaceus, 458
Calcinosis, in dermatomyositis, 168
Calcinosis cutis, 502, 527–530
  in dermatomyositis, 168, 183.*e5f*
  dystrophic, 527
  iatrogenic and traumatic, 528
  idiopathic, 528–529
  metastatic, 527–528
  systemic lupus erythematosus and, 162
Calciphylaxis, 820–822, 821*f*
  and livedo, 818
Calcipotriene
  ointment, for prurigo nodularis, 54
  for psoriasis, 198
  for scleroderma, 176
  topical, for ichthyosis, 565–566
Calcipotriol
  for inflammatory linear verrucous
    epidermal nevus, 639
  for psoriatic nails, 779
Calcitriol
  for inflammatory linear verrucous
    epidermal nevus, 639
  for scleroderma, 176
Calcium carbonate crystals, 429

Calcium channel blockers
  for erythromelalgia, 816
  flushing and, 140
  photosensitivity, 124–125
  pruritic dermatitis in the elderly, 77
  for Raynaud disease, 814
  for scleroderma, 176
  and telangiectasia, 854
Calcium deposits, in dermatomyositis, 168
Calcium hydroxylapatite, 924
Calcium oxide, 92
Calliphoridae flies, 443
Callus, 37–41, 38*f*, 45.*e3f*
Calomel disease, 136
Camphor
  for pruritus, 46
  topical, for chronic urticaria, 154
Cancer, lichen sclerosus and, 229
Candida albicans, 301
  diaper dermatitis and, 76
  onycholysis and, 786
Candida glabrata vaginitis, 303
Candida onychomycosis, 299–300
Candidal intertrigo, 302, 302*f*
Candidal paronychia, 303
Candidal vulvovaginitis, 303
Candidiasis, 301–305
  antibiotic (iatrogenic), 304
  breast eczema, 73
  candidal intertrigo and, 302, 302*f*
  candidid, 304
  chronic mucocutaneous, 304–305, 304*f*
  congenital cutaneous, 303
  diaper, 302
  erosio interdigitalis blastomycetica, 303–304
  oral, 302–303, 302*f*
  paronychia, 303
  perianal, 303
  perlèche and, 303
  pruritus ani, 50
  systemic, 305
  tongue, 800
  topical anticandidal agents for, 301–302
  vaginal, 51
  vulvovaginitis, 303
Candidid, 304
Canities segmentata sideropenica, 763
Canker sores, 809–810
Cannabinoids, for dermatomyositis, 170
Cantharidin, 68
  molluscum contagiosum, 392
Cantharone
  for common wart, 405
  for molluscum contagiosum, 392
Capillarity, of suture, 887
Capillary aneurysms, 603
Capillary loops, 162, 174
Capillary malformation-arteriovenous
    malformation 2 (CM-AVM2), 598
Capillary malformation-arteriovenous
    malformation (CM-AVM), 597–598
Capillary malformations, 594–595
Capnocytophaga canimorsus, 278
Capsaicin
  flushing and, 140
  for irritant contact dermatitis, 93
  for lichen simplex chronicus, 53
  for notalgia paresthetica, 59
  for pruritus, 46
  for zoster-associated pain, 376–377
Captopril, adverse reactions, 123
Carabidae, 444
Carbamazepine
  bullous drug reactions and, 117
  drug-induced hypersensitivity syndrome, 115

Carbamoyl phosphate synthetase deficiency, 540
Carbaryl, for pediculosis capitis, 441
Carbon dioxide (CO_2) laser, 919–920
  for genital warts, 410
  for hidrocystoma, 666
  for nevus of Ota, 702
  resurfacing, 41–42
  for trichilemmomas, 675–676
Carbon stain, 43, 44f
  fireworks and, 43
Carcinoid, 633–635
Carcinoid syndrome, flushing and, 140
Carcinoma
  metastatic, 632
  sebaceous, 664, 664f
  see also specific carcinoma
Carcinoma cuniculatum, 655–656, 655f
Carcinoma erysipeloides, 632, 632f, 635.e6f
Cardiofaciocutaneous syndrome, 554
Cardiolipin-cholesterol-lecithin antigen, 348
Cardol, 99
Carmustine, for mycosis fungoides, 736
Carney complex, 688, 703
Carney syndrome, 621f
Carotenemia, 484, 484f
Carotenosis, 539, 540f
Carpenter syndrome, 583
Carpet beetle, 444
Cartilage-hair hypoplasia, 584, 584f
Carvajal syndrome, 766
Carybdea marsupialis, 428
Casal necklace, 479
Cashew nutshell oil, 99
Caspofungin, 292
  for aspergillosis, 322
  in systemic candidiasis, 305
Cassia oil, allergic contact dermatitis, 100
Castor bean, 99
Cat flea, 445, 445f
Catagen hairs, 6f, 750, 10.e1f
Cataracts, atopic dermatitis, 67–68
Catastrophic antiphospholipid antibody
  syndrome (CAPS), 830, 830f
Caterpillar dermatitis, 439, 439f
Cat-scratch disease, 279–280, 279f
Cattle grub, 443
Caviar tongue, 801
CD4/CD56+ hematodermic neoplasm, 747
CD30, 739
CD30+ cutaneous T-cell lymphoma, 740–741,
  740f
CD34+ dermal dendrocyte, 8
CD40, 176
CD56, 740
CD154, 176
CD163, 176
Cedar poisoning, 99–100
Cefaclor, adverse reactions, 129
Cefotaxime, photosensitivity, 124–125
Cefoxitin, for Mycobacterium fortuitum
  infection, 334
Ceftazidime, for glanders, 278
Ceftriaxone
  for chancroid, 273
  for gonococcemia, 275
  for Lyme disease, 288
  for meningococcemia, 275
  for Vibrio vulnificus infection, 276
Celery
  allergic contact dermatitis, 99
  phytophotodermatitis, 29
Cellular blue nevus, 702–703
Cellulitis, 261, 261f
  dissecting, of scalp, 244–245, 245f
  eosinophilic, 144–145, 144f

Cellulitis (Continued)
  Haemophilus influenzae, 272
  Helicobacter, 277
  metastatic tuberculous, 328, 328f
  pneumococcal, 264
Cement workers, hand eczema and, 74
Centipede bites, 438, 438f
Central America, onchocerciasis, 435–436
Central centrifugal cicatricial alopecia, 759, 760f
Central dell sign, 674
Central nervous system (CNS)
  cryptococcosis on, 311
  epidermal nevi, 636
  herpes simplex, 367
  herpes zoster, 375
  sarcoidosis in, 715
  syphilis, 354
  systemic lupus erythematosus and, 163
  thrombotic thrombocytopenic purpura, 825
  trypanosomiasis and, 427
  Vogt-Koyanagi-Harada syndrome in, 875
Central nevus, 690–691
Centrifugal abdominal lipodystrophy, 495
Centroblasts, 743–744
Centrocytes, 743–744
Centrofacial lentiginosis, 687
Centruroides scorpion, 450f
Cephalexin, for wound infection, 882
Cephalosporins
  adverse reactions, 112–113
  for wound infection, 882–883
Ceratophyllus gallinae, 445
Cerebral cavernous malformations, 599
Cerebrospinal fluid (CSF)
  herpes simplex, 367
  syphilis, 354
Cerebrotendinous xanthomatosis, 533–534
Ceruloplasmin, 543
Ceruminoma, 669
Ceruminous glands, 669
Cestodes, 430
Cetirizine
  for chronic urticaria, 154
  for erythema gyratum repens, 144
Cevimeline, for Sjögren syndrome, 179–180
Chagas disease, 427
Chancre, 348–350, 349f, 361.e1f
  genital herpes and, 369
  tuberculous, 325–326
Chancre redux, 349
Chancroid, 272–273, 272f, 290.e3f
  genital herpes and, 369
Chancroidal genital ulcer disease, 273
Chapping, 13
Chédiak-Higashi syndrome (CHS), 876–877
Cheilitis, 794–796
  in actinic prurigo, 32
  causes of, 96–97
Cheilitis exfoliativa, 794
Cheilitis glandularis, 795, 795f
Cheilitis granulomatosa, 797–798
Chemical leukoderma, 874–875
Chemical peels, 863, 932–933, 932t, 933f
Chemically induced photosensitivity, 28–30
Chemotherapy
  acral erythema, 129–134, 130f
  for actinic keratosis, 644–645
  agents of, adverse reactions to, 129
  anagen effluvium and, 753
  for cutaneous B-cell lymphoma, 743
  dyspigmentation, 130
  flushing and, 140
  hair growth and, 6
  -induced dyspigmentation, 131f
  for Merkel cell carcinoma, 662

  for mycosis fungoides, 737
  neutrophilic eccrine hidradenitis and, 778
  onycholysis and, 786
  for plasmacytoma, 745
  for primary cutaneous anaplastic large cell
    lymphoma, 741
  for primary cutaneous follicle center cell
    lymphoma, 744
  toxicity of, 129–134, 139.e2f
Cherry angiomas, 593–594, 635.e2f
Cherubism, 806
Cheveux incoiffables, 766, 766f
Chevron nail, 785
Cheyletiella blakei, 449, 449f
Cheyletiella dermatitis, 449
Cheyletiella parasitovorax, 449
Cheyletiella yasguri, 449
Chiclero ulcer, 423
Chiggers
  bite, 449, 449f
  prevention of disease from, 438
Chigoe, 445
Chikungunya virus, 401, 420.e6f
Chilblain lupus erythematosus, 22, 159
Chilblains, 22, 22f, 45.e1f
  treatment for, 22
CHILD syndrome, 534, 568–569, 569f
  epidermal nevi and, 636
Children
  abused, 833, 833f
  acne in, 231, 233f
  atopic dermatitis in, 66, 66f
  bullous pemphigoid in, 462f, 463–464
  DEET and, 437
  dermatomyositis, 169, 169f, 183.e5f
  discoid lupus erythematosus, 157
  genital warts in, 410, 410f
  granulomatous perioral dermatitis in,
    250–251, 250f
  immune thrombocytopenic purpura (ITP)
    in, 823
  keratosis lichenoides chronica in, 225
  Langerhans cell histiocytosis in, 727
  lichen striatus in, 227
  linear IgA disease, 472–473, 472f–473f
  melanoma in, 695
  progressive systemic sclerosis, 174
  sarcoidosis in, 715
  solitary basal cell carcinoma in, 650
  systemic lupus erythematosus, 164
  varicella in, 370
  waxy keratoses of, 640
Chilopoda, 438
CHIME syndrome, 570
Chimney sweep's cancer, 94–95
Chinese herbs, for atopic dermatitis, 71
Chironex fleckeri, 428
Chlamydial infections, 289
Chloasma, 863–865, 864f
Chloracne, 94
Chlorambucil, bullous pemphigoid, 463
Chlorhexidine, for preoperative antisepsis, 884
Chlorhexidine gluconate, for hidradenitis
  suppurativa, 243
Chloroacetophenone, 93
2-Chlorodeoxyadenosine
  for hairy cell leukemia, 747
  for xanthoma disseminatum, 722
Chloroma, 747
Chloroquine, 127
  hair color and, 763
  for polymorphous light eruption, 31–32
  pruritus and, 52
  for sarcoidosis, 717
  for systemic lupus erythematosus, 165

Chlorpromazine, hyperpigmentation, 128, 128*f*
Cholesterol, 533
Cholesterol emboli, 818–819, 818*f*
Cholinergic urticaria, 151–152, 152*f*, 156.*e3f*
Chondrodermatitis nodularis chronica helicis, 616
Chondrodysplasia punctata, 566, 566*f*
Chondroid syringoma, 669
   malignant, 669
Chordomas, 628
Christ-Siemens-Touraine syndrome, 575
Chromates, allergic contact dermatitis, 102
Chromhidrosis, 5, 777
Chromium, 103
Chromobacteriosis, 276
Chromobacterium, 276
Chromobacterium violaceum, 276
Chromoblastomycosis, 316–317, 316*f*, 323.*e4f*
Chronic actinic dermatitis, 34–35, 34*f*, 45.*e2f*
Chronic atypical neutrophilic dermatosis with lipodystrophy and elevated temperature (CANDLE), 150
Chronic bullous disease of childhood (CBDC), 472–473, 472*f*–473*f*, 474.*e4f*
Chronic erythema nodosum, 485–487, 486*f*, 495.*e1f*
Chronic granulomatous disease, 86–87
Chronic kidney disease (CKD), 47–48, 48*f*
Chronic lymphangitis, 261
Chronic lymphocytic leukemia (CLL), 746–747
Chronic meningococcemia, 275
Chronic mucocutaneous candidiasis, 304–305, 304*f*, 323.*e2f*
Chronic myelogenous leukemia (CML), 746
Chronic pruritic dermatoses of unknown cause, 52–54
Chronic recurrent erysipelas, 261
Chronic spontaneous urticaria, 154
Chronic undermining burrowing ulcers, 268
Chrysanthemums, 99
Chrysiasis, 128
Chrysops dimidia, 435
Chrysops silacea, 435
Churg-Strauss syndrome, 847–848
   leukotriene receptor antagonist associated, 137
   solar urticaria and, 152
Cicatricial alopecia, 757–758, 757*f*–758*f*
   lichen planopilaris and, 222–223, 222*f*
Cicatricial basal cell carcinoma, 648–649
Cicatricial pemphigoid, 466–468, 474.*e3f*
   antilaminin, 467*f*, 474.*e3f*
   clinical features of, 466–467, 466*f*
   etiologic factors of, 467
   histopathology of, 467
   treatment of, 467–468
Cidofovir
   for common warts, 406
   for molluscum contagiosum, 392–393
Ciliata, 421
Cimetidine
   for chronic mucocutaneous candidiasis, 305
   for warts, 406
Cimicosis, 440
Cinnamic aldehyde, topical, flushing and, 140
Cinnamon oil, allergic contact dermatitis, 100
Ciprofloxacin
   for tularemia, 283
   for wound infection, 882
Circle of Hebra, 447
Circumostomy eczema, 77
Circumscribed neurodermatitis, 53, 53*f*
Citric acid, 100

Citronella, 437
Citrullinemia, 540
Civatte, poikiloderma of, 26, 27*f*
"Civatte bodies", 220
Clarithromycin
   for bacillary angiomatosis, 280–281
   for fish tank granuloma, 332
   for *Mycobacterium haemophilum* infection, 333
Clark nevus, 693–695
Clark's level, in melanoma, 698
Classic basal cell carcinoma, 648, 648*f*
Class-switch recombination defects, 82
Clavus, 37–38
Claw hand, of Hansen disease, 341*f*
Clean wounds, 882
Clear cell acanthoma, 639–640, 639*f*
Clear cell hidradenoma, 666–667
Clear cell papulosis, 661
Clear cell sarcoma, 697
"Clear cell syringoma", 666
Clefts, 13
Cleridae, 444
Clindamycin
   for acne vulgaris, 235
   for folliculitis decalvans, 759
   for hidradenitis suppurativa, 243
   for pseudofolliculitis barbae, 767
   for rosacea, 245
   for wound infection, 882
Clip test, in telogen effluvium, 752
Clobetasol
   for lichen planus, 229
   ointment, aphthous stomatitis, 810
Clofazimine treatment, pigmentation and, 128
Clomiphene citrate, flushing and, 140
Clomipramine, 128
   for trichotillomania, 58
Clonal seborrheic keratoses, 667
Clonidine, allergic contact dermatitis, 109–110
Clostridial infections, 267–269
Clostridial myonecrosis, 267–268, 267*f*
Clothing, dermatitis from, 101–102, 101*f*
Clotrimazole
   for oral candidiasis, 302–303
   for pitted keratolysis, 267
Clotting disorders, 828–829
Clouston syndrome, 670
CLOVES syndrome, 597
   epidermal nevi and, 636
Clubbing, 780–781, 781*f*, 793.*e5f*
Coal briquette makers, 94
Coal tar, 94–95
   for atopic dermatitis, 70
Cobalt, allergic contact dermatitis, 103–104
Cobb syndrome, 628
Cocaine
   chronic use of, 22
   injections of, 40
   local anesthetic and, 884
Cocaine-associated vasculitis, 848–849, 848*f*
Cocaine-induced midline destructive lesions, 848
Cocaine-induced pseudovasculitis, 848
Coccidioidal granuloma, 308
Coccidioides immitis, 308
Coccidioidomycosis, 14, 308, 323.*e3f*
Cochliomyia hominivorax, 443
Cockayne syndrome, 580
Coefficient of friction, of suture, 887
Colchicine
   for α₁-antitrypsin deficiency panniculitis, 492
   for aphthous stomatitis, 810
   for Behçet syndrome, 811

Colchicine (*Continued*)
   for chronic urticaria, 154
   for familial Mediterranean fever, 149
   for Henoch-Schönlein purpura, 839
   for small-vessel vasculitis, 837–838
Cold exposure, Raynaud disease, 813
Cold injuries, 21–24
Cold panniculitis, 490, 490*f*, 495.*e1f*
"Cold sore", 363
Cold urticaria, 152, 156.*e2f*–156.*e3f*
Coleoptera, order of, 443–444
Collagen, 1, 8
   in BMZ, 8
   in dermis, 8, 9*f*
   in subcutaneous tissue, 9–10
   synthesis and degradation of, 505
   types of, 505, 506*t*
Collagenosis, reactive perforating, 505–507
Collagenous fibroma, 612
Collagenous vasculopathy, 854, 854*f*
Collodion baby, 564*f*, 566
Colloid milium, 27–28, 45.*e1f*
   prevention and treatment of, 28
Color of lesions, 15
Colored sweat, 777
Combination therapy
   for psoriasis, 200
   topical, for acne vulgaris, 235
Combined melanocytic nevi, 690
Comedones, 231, 232*f*
Common baldness, 754
Common blue nevus, 702
Common carpet beetle, 444
Common variable immunodeficiency, 81, 81*f*
Common warts, treatment of, 405–410
Complement deficiency, 88–89, 88*f*
   syndromes, 161
Complement factor H (CFH), 825
Complement fixation tests, 314
Complex regional pain syndrome, 60–61, 60*f*, 62.*e2f*
Composite grafts, 904–905
Compound nevi, 689, 692
Compression therapy, venous leg ulcers, 857
Conditioned irritability, 77
Condylomata, of scrotum, 361.*e3f*
Condylomata acuminata, 352, 407–408, 407*f*–408*f*, 420.*e8f*
   giant, 408
   molluscum contagiosum and, 420.*e5f*
Condylomata lata, 352, 352*f*, 361.*e2f*
Conenose bug, 440–441
Confluent and reticulated papillomatosis, 209, 209*f*, 214.*e1f*
Congenital alopecia, 756, 757*f*
Congenital anetoderma, 512
Congenital cutaneous candidiasis, 303
Congenital erythropoietic porphyria, 524–525, 524*f*
Congenital fibrinogen disorders, 831
Congenital generalized lipodystrophy, 493, 493*f*
Congenital hypertrichosis lanuginosa, 769, 769*f*
Congenital ichthyosiform erythroderma, 564, 565*f*
Congenital inclusion dermoid cysts, 680, 680*f*
Congenital leukemia, 747
Congenital leukemia cutis, 747
Congenital lipodystrophies, 493–494
Congenital melanocytic nevus, 691–692
Congenital onychodysplasia of index fingers, 781, 793.*e5f*
Congenital preauricular fistula, 684–685
Congenital rubella syndrome, 397

Congenital self-healing reticulohistiocytosis (CSHR), 727f, 730.e2f
Congenital smooth muscle hamartoma, 631
Congenital syphilis, 355–357
  diagnosis of, 356–357
  early, 355–356, 355f
  late, 356, 356f
Congenital varicella syndrome, 372
Conidiobolus coronatus, 320
Conjunctival nevi, 690
Conjunctivitis
  actinic prurigo and, 32
  allergic, 73
Connective tissue diseases, 157–183
  definition of, 8
  mixed, 178, 178f, 183.e7f
Connective tissue nevi, 614, 615f, 635.e4f
Conradi-Hünermann syndrome, 566
Conradi-Hünermann-Happle syndrome, 566
Consistency of lesions, 16
Contact Allergen Management Program (CAMP), 96
Contact allergy
  atopic dermatitis and, 66
  to corticosteroids, 69
Contact dermatitis, 92–139, 254
  allergic, 95–109
  irritant, 92–95
  occupational, 110–111, 139.e1f
    management of, 111–112
  onychomycosis and, 300
  pruritus vulvae and, 51
  systemic, 95
Contact stomatitis, 104
Contact urticaria, 111
  immunologic mechanism in, 111
  management of, 112
  nonimmunologic mechanism in, 111–112
  substances causing, 112
  syndrome, 74
  testing, 112
  uncertain mechanism in, 112
Contaminated wounds, 882
Continuous-wave lasers, 909
Contraceptives. *see* Oral contraceptives
Cooling, laser treatment, 909
Copper, 543
  deficiency, 763
Coproporphyrins, 520
"Coral bead" appearance, in multicentric reticulohistiocytosis, 724
Coral cuts, 38, 38f
Coral dermatitis, 428–429
"Corkscrew hairs", 478–479, 479f
Cornification, disorders of, 563–566
Corns, 37–38
Cornu cutaneum, 645–646, 646f
Corps ronds, 1
Corticosteroids, 110
  adverse reactions to, 137
  for alternariosis, 318
  for Churg-Strauss syndrome, 847–848
  for Cushing syndrome, 496–497
  for ear eczema, 75
  for Henoch-Schönlein purpura, 839
  for immune thrombocytopenic purpura (ITP), 824
  injected/intralesional
    for acne vulgaris, 237–238
    adverse reactions to, 137–138, 139.e3f
    for alopecia areata, 751
    aphthous stomatitis, 810
    granuloma faciale, 842–843
    for lichen planus of nails, 778
    Melkersson-Rosenthal syndrome, 798

Corticosteroids (*Continued*)
  for lichen planopilaris, 758
  for meralgia paresthetica, 60
  for microscopic polyangiitis, 845–846
  for mixed connective tissue disease, 178
  for oral erythema multiforme, 143
  for polyarteritis nodosa, 844
  for psoriasis, 197–199
  for rhinoscleroma, 277
  systemic
    for acute urticaria, 154
    adverse reactions to, 138
    for α_1-antitrypsin deficiency panniculitis, 492
    for atopic dermatitis, 71
    for common variable immunodeficiency, 81
    complications of, 138
    for granuloma annulare, 707
    for hand eczema, 76
    for herpes zoster, 375
    for multicentric reticulohistiocytosis, 725
    for polymorphous light eruption, 31–32
    for pressure urticaria, 152–153
    for pyoderma gangrenosum, 148–149
    for relapsing polychondritis, 182–183
    for sarcoidosis, 716–718
    for small-vessel vasculitis, 837–838
    Stevens-Johnson syndrome and, 118, 118f
    for Sweet syndrome, 146–147
    for vitiligo, 873
  for systemic lupus erythematosus, 166
  topical
    adverse reactions to, 137–139, 138f
    for alopecia areata, 751
    for atopic dermatitis, 70
    for breast eczema, 73
    for circumostomy eczema, 76
    for common variable immunodeficiency, 81
    for cutaneous lymphoid hyperplasia, 731
    for dermatomyositis, 170
    for eosinophilic folliculitis, 417
    for erythema gyratum repens, 144
    for folliculitis decalvans, 759
    for granuloma annulare, 706
    for granuloma faciale, 842–843
    for hand eczema, 76
    for inflammatory linear verrucous epidermal nevus, 639
    for juvenile plantar dermatosis, 77
    for lichen planus, 220–221
    for lichen planus of nails, 778
    for mycosis fungoides, 736
    for necrobiosis lipoidica, 539
    from nickel dermatitis, 103
    for occupational contact dermatitis, 111
    for prurigo simplex, 52
    for pruritus ani, 50
    for pruritus scroti, 50–51
    for radiodermatitis, 37
    rosacea and, 247
    for toxicodendron sensitivity, 99, 111
Cortisol, screening test for Cushing syndrome and, 497
Corymbose syphilid, 351
Corynebacterium jeikeium sepsis, 266
Cosmetic camouflage, for vitiligo, 873
Cosmetic dermatitis, 106–108
  preservatives, 108–109
  vehicles, 109
Cosmetic dermatology, 922–933
Cosmetic intolerance syndrome, 108
Cosmoderm 1, 922

Cosmoderm 2, 922
Cosmoplast (Allergan), 922
Costello syndrome, 511, 553–554
Cosyntropin, diagnosis of Addison disease and, 498
Cotton, dermatitis from, 101
Cotton gloves, 75
Cotton-tipped applicator, for cryosurgery, 892
Counseling, genital herpes, 366
Cowden syndrome, 674–676, 675f, 685.e6f
Cowpox, 389
Coxiella burnetii, 283
Coxsackievirus A6, 394, 394f
Coxsackievirus A10, 394
Crab louse, 441f, 442
Cracks, 13
Cranial arteritis, 849
C-reactive protein (CRP), in systemic lupus erythematosus, 164
Creeping eruption, 432–433
Creosote, 94
CREST syndrome, 173, 173f, 527, 183.e6f
  and Osler disease, 855
Cretinism, 499
Crohn disease, 796–797
  pyoderma gangrenosum and, 148
Cromolyn sodium ophthalmic drops, for eyelid eczema, 73
Cronkhite-Canada syndrome, 583, 868
Crotamiton, scabies and, 441
Crotch itch, 297
Crouzon syndrome, 583
Crowe sign, 550
Crow-Fukase (POEMS) syndrome, 583
Crow's feet, 927, 927f
Crusted scabies, 448, 448f
Crusts, 13
Cryofibrinogenemia, 826–827
Cryofiltration apheresis, cryoglobulinemia, 827
Cryoglobulinemia, 152, 826–827, 826f
  and urticarial vasculitis, 840
Cryoglobulinemic vasculitis, 826, 826f, 841
Cryolipolysis, 931
Cryopyrin-associated periodic syndromes, 150
Cryospray cooling, nevus flammeus, 604
Cryosurgery, 892–894, 893f
  side effects of, 892–894
Cryotherapy
  for Bowen disease, 657
  for chromoblastomycosis, 316–317
  for common warts, 405
  for genital warts, 409
  granuloma faciale, 842–843
  for Kaposi sarcoma, 419–420
  for lichen sclerosus, 229–230
  for molluscum contagiosum, 392
  prurigo nodularis, 54
Cryptococcosis, 311–312, 311f, 323.e3f
Cryptococcus neoformans, 312
Cryptogenic organizing pneumonia, erythema gyratum repens and, 144
Ctenocephalides felis, 284
Culiseta mosquito, 401
Culture
  in coccidioidomycosis, 308–309
  for herpes simplex, 362
  in onychomycosis, 300
Curettage, 894–895, 894f
  for Bowen disease, 657
  for molluscum contagiosum, 392
  for seborrheic keratosis, 641
Curry-Jones syndrome, 674
Cushing disease, 496–497
Cushing syndrome, 9–10, 496–497, 497f

Cushingoid changes, corticosteroids adverse reactions, 138
Cutaneous B-cell lymphoma, 732, 743–745, 743*f*
Cutaneous blastomycosis, 312
Cutaneous ciliated cysts, 684
Cutaneous collagenous vasculopathy, 854, 854*f*
Cutaneous columnar cysts, 683–684
Cutaneous Crohn disease, 796–797
Cutaneous diphtheria, 265–266
Cutaneous dysesthesia syndromes, 58–62
Cutaneous endometriosis, 632–635
Cutaneous focal mucinosis, 189
Cutaneous horn, 645–646, 646*f*, 685.*e3f*
Cutaneous immunosuppression, 25
Cutaneous laser surgery, 909–921, 912*t*
    principles of, 909–910, 910*f*–911*f*
Cutaneous leishmaniasis, 422–423
Cutaneous lesions, syphilis, 350–352
Cutaneous leukocytoclastic vasculitis, 836–838, 837*f*, 813.*e3f*
Cutaneous listeriosis, 265
Cutaneous lymphadenoma, 674
Cutaneous lymphocyte antigen (CLA), 735
Cutaneous lymphoid hyperplasia, 731–749
    bandlike T-cell pattern of, 731–732
    nodular B-cell pattern of, 731, 732*f*
Cutaneous lymphomas, 732–741
Cutaneous mastocytosis, 622
Cutaneous melanoacanthoma, 688
Cutaneous meningioma, 627
Cutaneous meningospinal angiomatosis, 597–598
Cutaneous mixed tumor, 669
Cutaneous myelofibrosis, 747–748
Cutaneous myxofibrosarcoma, 620
Cutaneous necrotizing vasculitis, 384
Cutaneous North American blastomycosis, 312
Cutaneous plasmacytosis, 745
Cutaneous polyarteritis nodosa, 844–845
Cutaneous pseudosarcomatous polyps, 617
Cutaneous signs and diagnosis, 11–17
Cutaneous sinus of dental origin (dental sinus), 802, 802*f*
Cutaneous small-vessel vasculitis, 836–838
Cutaneous stigmata, atopic dermatitis, 67–68
Cutaneous T-cell lymphoma (CTCL), 122, 731–749
    milia in, 683
    and pigmented purpura, 835
    primary, 732–741
    sarcoidosis and, 716
Cutaneous vascular anomalies, 587
Cutaneous vascular diseases, 813–861
Cutaneous vasculitis, in Sjögren syndrome, 179
Cuterebra cuniculi, 443
Cutis laxa, 511, 514.*e1f*
Cutis marmorata, 817
Cutis marmorata telangiectatica congenita, 596, 596*f*
Cutis rhomboidalis nuchae, 26, 27*f*
Cutis verticis gyrata, 577, 586.*e5f*
CXCR4 mutation, in WHIM syndrome, 84
Cyanoacrylates, 106
Cyanocobalamin, deficiency in, 478
CYBB gene, 86
Cyclic neutropenia, 808
Cyclin D1 gene, 695
Cyclin-dependent kinase 4 (CDK4), in atypical nevus, 693
Cyclophosphamide
    adverse reactions, 130
    anagen effluvium and, 753
    for bullous pemphigoid, 463
    for Churg-Strauss syndrome, 847–848

Cyclophosphamide *(Continued)*
    for cicatricial pemphigoid, 467–468
    for dermatomyositis, 170
    for microscopic polyangiitis, 845–846
    for pemphigus vulgaris, 455
    for polyarteritis nodosa, 844
    for relapsing polychondritis, 182–183
    for sarcoidosis, 717
    for scleroderma, 176
    for small-vessel vasculitis, 837–838
    for systemic lupus erythematosus, 166
    for Wegener granulomatosis, 846–847
Cyclosporin A
    actinic dermatitis, 35
    actinic prurigo, 32
    solar urticaria, 33–34
Cyclosporine
    for acute generalized exanthematous pustulosis, 122
    for atopic dermatitis, 71
    for bullous pemphigoid, 463
    for chronic urticaria, 154
    for erythema multiforme, 143
    for erythromelalgia, 816
    flushing and, 140
    milia and, 683
    and pigmented purpura, 836
    for prurigo nodularis, 54
    for psoriasis, 199
    for psoriatic nails, 779
    for pyoderma gangrenosum, 148–149
    for small-vessel vasculitis, 837–838
    for Stevens-Johnson syndrome, 118
    for thrombotic thrombocytopenic purpura, 825
Cyclosporine ophthalmic emulsion (Restasis), for eyelid eczema, 73
CYLD gene, 673–674
Cylindroma, 668–669, 668*f*, 685.*e5f*
Cyproterone acetate, for hirsutism, 771
Cystathionine β-synthase, 511
Cystic acne, 239
Cystic basal cell carcinoma, 648
Cystic fibrosis
    basaloid follicular hamartoma in, 677–678
    essential fatty acid deficiency and, 482
"Cystic fibrosis nutrient deficiency dermatitis" (CFNDD), 482
Cystic hygroma, 602*f*
Cystic papillomas, 683
Cysticercosis cutis, 431
Cytoid bodies, 758, 759*f*
"Cytokine storm", 705–706
Cytokines, adverse reactions to, 134
Cytomegalic inclusion disease, 381–382
Cytomegalovirus (CMV), 381–382
    adverse drug reactions in, 113
Cytophagic histiocytic panniculitis (CHP), 492–493

D
DAB389IL-2 fusion toxin, for mycosis fungoides, 737
Dabska tumor, 592–593
Dactylitis, blistering distal, 262, 262*f*
Dactylolysis spontanea, 614
Danazol
    for cholinergic urticaria, 151–152
    flushing and, 140
    for immune thrombocytopenic purpura (ITP), 824
Dapsone
    for acne vulgaris, 235
    for α₁-antitrypsin deficiency panniculitis, 492

Dapsone *(Continued)*
    for aphthous stomatitis, 810
    for Behçet syndrome, 811
    for bullous pemphigoid, 463
    for chronic urticaria, 154
    for cicatricial pemphigoid, 467–468
    for erythema elevatum diutinum, 842
    for erythema multiforme, 143
    for Henoch-Schönlein purpura, 839
    for hypersensitivity syndrome, 116–117
    for pemphigus foliaceus, 458
    for pemphigus vulgaris, 456
    for prurigo pigmentosa, 52–53
    for psoriasis, 199
    for pyoderma gangrenosum, 148
    for relapsing polychondritis, 182–183
    for small-vessel vasculitis, 837–838
    for systemic lupus erythematosus, 165
    topical, benzoyl peroxide with, 235
Darier disease, 572–573, 572*f*, 780, 780*f*, 586.*e4f*
    tumors of the follicular infundibulum *vs.*, 678
Darier sign, 14
Darier-Roussy sarcoid, 713
Darier-White disease, 572–573
Darkfield examinations, chancre, 349–350
Dasatinib, adverse reactions to, 132
de Morgan spots, 593–594
Debridement, pressure ulcers, 39
Deck-chair sign, 53, 828
Decubitus, 38
Deep granuloma annulare, 704–705
Deep mycoses, 291–292, 308–309
Deep peel, 932–933, 933*f*, 933*t*
Deep penetrating nevus, 703
Deep venous thrombosis (DVT), 831–832
Deer fly fever, 282
Deerfly, 442
DEET, 437
β-Defensins, 3
Degos acanthoma, 639, 639*f*
Degos disease, 850
Dehydroepiandrosterone sulfate (DHEAS)
    acne vulgaris and, 232
    androgen-dependent syndromes and, 498–499
Delayed pressure urticaria, 152–153, 153*f*
Delta-aminolevulinic acid (ALA), 906
Delusions of parasitosis, 55–56, 62.*e2f*
Demodex mites, 449
    eosinophilic folliculitis, 417
    rosacea and, 247
Dengue, 400–401, 400*f*
Dengue hemorrhagic fever, 400
Dengue shock syndrome, 400
Dennie-Morgan fold, 66–67, 91.*e1f*
Dental defects, in incontinentia pigmenti, 548
Dental sinus, 802, 802*f*
Dentifrices, dermatitis, 108
Deodorant dermatitis, 97
Depigmentation, total, 873–874
Depression
    hand eczema and, 73
    isotretinoin and, 237
Dercum disease, 628
Dermabrasion
    actinic cheilitis, 794–795
    in trichilemmomas, 675–676
Dermacentor andersoni, 446
Dermacentor variabilis, 446, 446*f*
DermaGard film, polymorphous light eruption, 31
Dermal dendrocyte hamartoma, 618, 618*f*
Dermal duct tumor, 666–667
Dermal fibrosis, 175, 505

Dermal fibrous tissue, abnormalities of, 505–514
Dermal melanocytic lesions, 701–703
Dermal melanocytosis, 543, 701–702, 701f
Dermal pigmented lesions, 915–916, 916f
Dermal tumors, 587–635
Dermanyssus, 449
"Dermatitic" epidermal nevus, 638–639
Dermatitis
  actinic, 34–35, 34f, 45.e2f
  atopic, 63–91
  contact, 254
  factitious, 57, 57f, 62.e2f
  gonococcal, 274–275
  perianal, 262, 262f
  perioral, 249–250, 249f
    granulomatous, 250–251, 250f
  periorbital, 250
  phototoxic tar, 29
  plant-associated, 100
  from plants, 97–101
  rhus, 30
Dermatitis artefacta, 57
Dermatitis bullosa striata pratensis, 30
Dermatitis herpetiformis, 469–471, 474.e4f
  associated disease of, 470
  clinical features of, 469–470, 470f
Dermatitis repens, 202
Dermatobia hominis, 443
Dermatofibroma, 617, 617f, 635.e5f
  systemic lupus erythematosus and, 162
Dermatofibrosarcoma protuberans, 619f, 635.e5f
  black, 102
  white, 67
Dermatoheliosis, 26–28, 26f
Dermatologic surgery, 881–908
  anatomy and, 885–887, 886f, 887b
  equipment for, 887–888, 887b, 887t
  preparation for, 881–888
Dermatomal zoster, 377
Dermatomes, 14, 15f
  herpes zoster, 374–375
Dermatomyositis, 8, 167–171, 183.e4f
  amyopathic, 168
  associated diseases to, 169
  childhood, 169, 169f, 183.e5f
  diagnostic criteria for, 168–169
  differential diagnosis of, 170
  etiology of, 169–170
  histopathology of, 170
  hypomyopathic, 168
  incidence of, 170
  laboratory findings of, 170
  muscle changes in, 168
  prognosis for, 171
  sine myositis, 168
  skin findings in, 167–168, 167f–168f
  treatment for, 170–171
Dermatopathia pigmentosa reticularis (DPR), 867, 880.e1f
Dermatophagia, 55
Dermatophytids, 294
Dermatophytosis, 270, 297
  erythema annulare centrifugum and, 143
Dermatoses
  blistering, chronic, 453–474
  hormone-induced, 79–80
  nail-associated, 779–780
  neurocutaneous, 46–62
  neutrophilic, of dorsal hand, 147, 147f, 156.e2f
  from physical factors, 18–45
  reactive neutrophilic, 145–149
  rheumatoid neutrophilic, 180, 181f
Dermatosis papulosa nigra, 641–642, 642f

Dermatothlasia, 58
Dermestidae, 444
Dermis, 8–9, 9f
Dermoepidermal junction, 4
Dermoid cyst, 680–681, 680f, 807
Dermoplasty, nasal septum, 855–856
Dermoscopy, 14
  for seborrheic keratoses, 641
Desmoid tumors, 612
Desmoplakin mutations, 559
Desmoplastic fibroblastoma, 612
Desmoplastic melanoma, 697, 697f
Desmoplastic Spitz nevi, 693
Desmoplastic squamous cell carcinoma, 654
Desmoplastic trichoepithelioma, 674, 674f
Desmosine, 8
Desmosomes, 1
Desquamation, of palms and soles, 258, 258f
Dexamethasone
  for acne vulgaris, 236
  Cushing syndrome, 496–497
  for pemphigus vulgaris, 456
  suppression tests, for hirsutism, 770
Diabetes mellitus
  bullae, 539, 539f
  carotenosis, 539, 540f
  dermopathy, 539
  limited joint mobility, 539–540
  necrobiosis lipoidica, 538–540
  pruritus, 47
  skin disorders in, 538–540
  waxy skin, 539–540
Diabetic dermopathy, 539
Diabetic foot ulcer, 62.e2f
Diabetic scleredema, 175
Diagnosis, 14–17
Dialysis, hypervitaminosis A, 476
Dialysis-associated amyloidosis, 516–517
Diamanus montanus, 445
Diane 35, hirsutism and, 771
Diaper candidiasis, 302
Diaper dermatitis, 76–77
Diazoxide, hair color and, 763
Diclofenac, for actinic keratosis, 644–645
Dicloxacillin, for wound infection, 882
Didymosis aplasticosebacea, 662–663
Diet
  acne vulgaris and, 232
  for psoriasis, 199
  telogen effluvium and, 752–753, 753f
Diethylcarbamazine
  for filariasis, 434
  for loiasis, 435
  for onchocerciasis, 436
Dietzia papillomatosis, 209
Diffuse cutaneous mastocytosis, 622
Diffuse dermal angiomatosis (DDA), 852
Diffuse infantile fibromatosis, 612
Diffuse large B-cell lymphoma, 744, 744f
Diffuse palmoplantar keratodermas, 211
  with transgrediens, 211
  without transgrediens, 211
DiGeorge syndrome, 82, 501
Digital fibromyxoma, 616
Digital papillary adenocarcinoma, 671–672
Dihydroxyacetone
  hair color and, 763
  for vitiligo, 873
Diisocyanates, 102
Dilated pore, 677, 685.e6f
Diltiazem, hyperpigmentation, 128
Dimethyl sulfoxide (DMSO), 293
Dimple sign, 617
Dinitrochlorobenzene, for melanoma, 700–701

Diphenhydramine
  for acute urticaria, 154
  for atopic dermatitis, 69
Diphtheria, cutaneous, 265–266
Diplopoda, 439
Diptera, order of, 442–443
Dipyridamole (Persantine), Degos disease, 850–851
Direct fluorescent antibody (DFA) test, 350, 362
  for herpes zoster, 377–378
Direct immunofluorescence (DIF)
  for pemphigus foliaceus, 458
  for pemphigus vulgaris, 453–454
  for Senear-Usher syndrome, 459
  systemic lupus erythematosus and, 165
  for Waldenström macroglobulinemia, 828
Discoid eczema, 78–79, 79f, 91.e2f
Discoid lupus erythematosus, 13–15, 16f, 157–159, 158f, 183.e1f, 17.e2f
  alopecia in, 756, 758f
  childhood, 157
  differential diagnosis of, 157–159
  dyspigmentation and scarring of, 183.e1f
  generalized, 157, 158f
  histology of, 157
  localized, 157, 158f
  and tattoo, 41
Discrete papular lichen myxedematosus, 185–186
Dissecting cellulitis, 760, 760f, 793.e2f
  of scalp, 244–245, 245f
Dissecting terminal folliculitis, 242
Disseminate infundibulofolliculitis, 774, 793.e4f
Disseminated coccidioidomycosis, 308, 308f, 323.e3f
Disseminated cryptococcosis, 311
Disseminated granuloma annulare, 704, 705f
Disseminated herpes zoster, 374–375
Disseminated intravascular coagulation, 830–831
Disseminated juvenile xanthogranuloma, 720
Disseminated sporotrichosis, 314
Disseminated superficial actinic porokeratosis (DSAP), 571, 571f
Disseminated xanthosiderohistiocytosis, 722
Distal onycholysis, in psoriasis, 193f
Distal subungual onychomycosis, 299, 299f
Distal trichorrhexis nodosa, 764
Distichiasis, 859–860, 813.e5f
Distribution of lesions, 14, 15f
Disulfiram, flushing and, 140
"Ditz", 694
Diuretics, venous leg ulcers, 857
DNA virus, 362
Docetaxel, chemotherapy-induced acral erythema and, 130
DOCK8 deficiency, 85, 86f
Dog bite pathogens, 278
Dog tick, 446
Dogger Bank itch, 429–430
Dominant dystrophic epidermolysis bullosa, 560–561, 561f
Donovanosis, 273–274
"Dory flop", 349
Double-filtration plasmapheresis (DFPP), for bullous pemphigoid, 463
Double-stranded DNA, systemic lupus erythematosus and, 164–165
Doucas and Kapetanakis pigmented purpura, 835
Douglas fir tussock moth caterpillar, 439
Dowling-Degos disease, 866
Down syndrome, 499
  and elastosis perforans serpiginosa, 505

Doxepin, 46
  for allergic contact dermatitis, 109–110
  for chronic urticaria, 154
  cream, pruritus and, 46
  for excoriation disorder, 56–57
  for lichen simplex chronicus, 53
  for pruritus scroti, 50–51
Doxorubicin
  anagen effluvium and, 753
  chemotherapy-induced acral erythema and, 130
Doxycycline
  for acne vulgaris, 235
  for α₁-antitrypsin deficiency panniculitis, 492
  for bacillary angiomatosis, 280–281
  for ehrlichiosis, 286
  for epidemic typhus, 284
  for filariasis, 434–435
  for fish tank granuloma, 332
  for glanders, 278
  for leptospirosis, 286
  for Lyme disease, 288
  for lymphogranuloma venereum, 290
  for Marfan syndrome, 510
  for *Mycobacterium fortuitum* infection, 334
  for onchocerciasis, 436
  for rickettsialpox, 285
  for rosacea, 247–248
  for tularemia, 283
  for *Vibrio vulnificus* infection, 276
Dracontiasis, 433–434
Dracunculiasis, 433–434, 434*f*
Drug reaction with eosinophilia and systemic symptoms (DRESS), 113
Drug reactions, 112
  acute generalized exanthematous pustulosis, 120–121, 121*f*
  anticoagulant-induced skin necrosis, 123–125, 125*f*
  autoimmune diseases, 136–137
  biologic agents, 134
  bromoderma, 136–137
  bullous, 117–118, 118*f*
  chemotherapeutic agents, 129
  clinical morphology of, 113–114
  corticosteroids, 137, 138*f*
  cytokines, 134
  drug-induced hypersensitivity syndrome (DIHS), 114–115, 115*f*
  with eosinophilia and systemic symptoms (DRESS), 113
  epidemiology of, 112–139
  evaluation of, 112–113
  exanthems, 114, 114*f*
  fixed, 119–120, 120*f*, 139.*e2f*
  fluoroderma, 136–137
  HIV disease and, 119
  interstitial granulomatous, 709
  iododerma, 136, 136*f*
  leukemia and, 747
  lichenoid reactions, 129
  melanonychia and, 788
  mercury, 135–136
  pathogenesis of, 113
  photosensitive, 123
  pigmentation, 127, 127*f*–128*f*
  pseudolymphoma, 121–122
  radiation-induced epidermal necrolysis, 117–119, 119*f*
  red man syndrome, 122–123
  serum-sickness-like reactions, 127–129
  toxic epidermal necrolysis, 117
  urticaria/angioedema, 122, 123*f*
  vasculitis, 127–129

Drug reactions (*Continued*)
  vitamin K reactions, 125–126, 126*f*
  Wells syndrome and, 144–145
Drug-induced autoimmune diseases, 136–137
Drug-induced hypersensitivity syndrome (DIHS), 114–115, 115*f*
Drug-induced lupus erythematosus, 137, 164
Drug-induced pruritus, 52
Drug-induced pseudolymphoma, 121–122
Drug-induced psoriasis, 197
Drug-induced purpura, 829
Drug-induced thrombocytopenia, 824
Drug-induced ulcer, of lip, 796
Drugs
  anhidrosis from, 776
  history, 14
  livedo, 818
  topical, contact dermatitis from, 109–111, 110*f*
Drummer's digits, 39
Dry ice, for chemical peels, 932
"Dry riverbed sign," of eosinophilic fasciitis, 177
Dsg1 antigen, in pemphigus foliaceus, 458
Dsg3 antigen, in pemphigus vulgaris, 453–454
DSRAD (ADAR1) gene, 865
Dull-pink globules, 692
Dumdum fever, 425–426
Dunnigan type, in familial partial lipodystrophy, 493
Dupuytren contracture, 610–611
Dusts, irritant contact dermatitis, 93
Dutasteride, for male-pattern alopecia, 754
Dutcher bodies, 743
Dyclonine hydrochloride (Dyclone), aphthous stomatitis, 810
Dyes, allergic contact dermatitis, 101
Dynamic rhytids, 922
Dyschromatosis symmetrica hereditaria (DSH), 865
Dyschromatosis universalis hereditaria (DUH), 865–866, 866*f*, 880.*e1f*
Dysesthesia, scalp, 58–59
Dysfibrinogenemia, 831
Dyshidrosiform pemphigoid, 461
Dyshidrosis, 75
Dyskeratosis congenita, 574, 574*f*
Dysmorphic syndrome, 58
Dysmorphophobia, 58
Dysplastic gangliocytoma, of cerebellum, 675
Dysplastic nevus, 689, 693–695, 694*f*
  fried-egg appearance of, 703.*e3f*
Dysplastic nevus syndrome (DNS), 693
Dysproteinemia, angioimmunoblastic lymphadenopathy with, 741–743
Dysproteinemic purpura, 826–828
Dystrophia unguis mediana canaliformis, 786, 786*f*
Dystrophic calcinosis cutis, 527, 527*f*

E
Earlobe
  dermatitis, 96–97
  nickel dermatitis, 103
Early neurosyphilis, 354
Ear(s)
  eczema, 73, 73*f*, 91.*e1f*
  seborrheic dermatitis in, 191
Easy bruising syndromes, 834
Ebola virus (EBOV), 395
EBV nuclear antigen 1 (EBNA-1), 379–380
Ecchymosis, 823
  corticosteroids adverse reactions, 138
  painful bruising syndrome, 834, 834*f*
Eccrine angiomatous hamartoma, 594

Eccrine carcinoma, 671, 671*f*
Eccrine chromhidrosis, 777
Eccrine sweat units, 1, 4–5
  occlusion of, 19
Echidnophaga gallinacea, 445
Echinocandins, 292
Echinococcosis, 431
Echovirus 9, 393
Ecthyma, 259, 290.*e1f*
Ecthyma contagiosum, 389–390
Ecthyma gangrenosum, 269–270, 269*f*
Ectodermal dysplasias, 575–577
Ectopia lentis, Marfan syndrome, 510
Eczema, 11, 13, 63–91
  autosensitization and conditioned irritability, 77
  breast (nipple), 73–74, 74*f*
  circumostomy, 77
  diaper (napkin) dermatitis, 76–77, 77*f*
  ear, 73, 73*f*, 91.*e1f*
  eyelid dermatitis, 73
  hand, 74–76, 74*f*, 91.*e1f*
  in hepatitis C, 384–385
  id reactions, 77
  juvenile plantar dermatosis, 77–78
  mycosis fungoides *vs.*, 736
  nummular (discoid), 78–79, 79*f*, 91.*e2f*
  onychomycosis and, 300
  pruritic, dermatitis in elderly persons, 78
  regional, 73–78
  xerotic, 78, 78*f*
Eczema craquelé, 77, 62.*e1f*
Eczema herpeticum, 68, 69*f*, 367–368, 367*f*–368*f*
Eczema vaccinatum, 388
Edema
  dermatomyositis and, 167
  solid facial, acne vulgaris and, 238–239
Edema indurativum, 349
EEC syndrome, 575–576, 576*f*
Eflornithine, trypanosomiasis and, 427
EGR. *see* Erythema gyratum repens (EGR)
Ehlers-Danlos syndromes (EDSs), 8, 508–510, 508*f*, 509*t*, 514.*e1f*
Ehrlichiosis, 285–286
Elastic fibers, 8
Elasticity, of suture, 887
Elastin, 8
Elastofibroma dorsi, 614–615
Elastolysis, generalized, 511
Elastosis perforans serpiginosa (EPS), 505, 506*f*
Elastotic marginal plaques, of hands, 212
Elastotic nodules of the ear, 26
Elastotic striae, 513
Elbows
  hairy, 769
  spring and summer eruptions of, 31
Elderly
  bullous pemphigoid, 461
  immune thrombocytopenic purpura (ITP) in, 824
  Merkel cell carcinoma in, 661
  pruritic dermatitis in, 78
  varicella in, 373
  vitamin D deficiency and, 476–477
Electrical burns, 18–19
Electrocauterization, 895
  for genital warts, 409–410
Electrocoagulation, 895
Electrodesiccation, 895
  for actinic cheilitis, 794–795
  curettage and, 894, 894*f*
  for dermatosis papulosa nigra, 642
Electrofulguration, 895
  for genital warts, 409–410

Electrosection, 895–896
Electrosurgery, 895–896, 895f
Elejalde syndrome, 877
Elephantiasis arabum, 434–435
Elephantiasis tropica, 434–435
Elephantiasis verrucosa nostra, 813.e4f
Elephantoid fever, 434
Elliptical excision, 896, 897f
Emberger syndrome, 860
Embolia cutis medicamentosa, 126
EMLA cream
    for drug-induced and food-induced
        purpura, 829
    pruritus and, 46
Emodepside, for onchocerciasis, 436
Emollients
    for CKD-associated pruritus, 48
    for erythema ab igne, 21
    for friction blisters, 39
    for photoaging, 28
    for winter itch, 49
Emotional flushing, 140
Emperipolesis, 749
Emphysema, subcutaneous, 39, 40f, 57
En coup de sabre, 172
Enalapril, adverse reactions, 123
Enanthem, viral, 420.e6f
Encephalitis, granulomatous amebic, 421
Encephalocele, 627–628
Enchondroma, of the distal phalanx, 791
Endemic pemphigus, 458–459, 458f
Endemic syphilis, 360
Endemic typhus, 284
Endocarditis prophylaxis, 883–884, 883b, 883t
Endocrine diseases, 496–504
Endocrine system, hemochromatosis and, 870
Endogenous vasoactive substances, flushing
    and, 140
Endometrial cancer, trichilemmomas and, 675
Endothrix hair mount, 323.e1f
Endovascular papillary angioendothelioma,
    592–593
Endovenous ablation, 930
English ivy, 99
Engraftment syndrome, 89
Enoxaparin
    for lichen planus, 220–221
    skin necrosis and, 126
Entamoeba histolytica, 421
Enterobiasis, 431–432
Enteropathy, dermatitis herpetiformis and,
    470
Enterovirus 71, 393–394
Enterovirus infections, 393–395
Entomophthoromycosis, 320
Enzyme immunoassay (EIA), syphilis, 348
Enzyme replacement therapy, Fabry disease,
    537–538
Enzyme-linked immunosorbent assay
    (ELISA), for pemphigus foliaceus, 458
Enzyme-related panniculitis, 491–493
Eosinophilia, episodic angioedema with, 156
Eosinophilic annular erythema, 144
Eosinophilic cellulitis, 144–145, 144f, 261
Eosinophilic eruption, radiotherapy, 35–36
Eosinophilic fasciitis, 177–178, 177f, 183.e7f
Eosinophilic folliculitis, 417, 417f
Eosinophilic granulomatosis with polyangiitis
    (EGPA), 847–848
Eosinophilic pustular folliculitis (EPF), 202
Eosinophilic ulcer, of oral mucosa, 801
Ephelides, 805
Ephelis, 26, 686
Epidemic typhus, 283–284, 283f
Epidermal appendages, 4–8

Epidermal cyst, 678–679
Epidermal growth factor receptor (EGFR)
    inhibitors, cutaneous side-effects of, 132,
    132f, 139.e2f
Epidermal inclusion cyst, 678–679, 679f,
    685.e7f
Epidermal melanin unit, 862
Epidermal melanocytic lesions, 686–688
Epidermal necrolysis, radiation-induced,
    117–119, 119f
Epidermal nevi, 636–639
Epidermal nevus syndrome, 554–555,
    637–638
Epidermal pigmented lesions, 915, 915f
Epidermis, 1–4
Epidermization, of lip, 803
Epidermodysplasia verruciformis, 411–412,
    411f, 420.e8f
    squamous cell carcinoma and, 653
Epidermolysis bullosa, 558–561, 558b
    dermolytic or dystrophic form, 560–561
    junctional, 560, 560f
        with pyloric atresia, 560
        recessive, 561, 561f
Epidermolysis bullosa acquisita (EBA), 162,
    462, 468–469, 468f, 474.e4f
    criteria for, 468
    inflammatory, 468, 469f
    noninflammatory, 468
    treatment of, 469
Epidermolysis bullosa simplex, 558–560, 559f,
    586.e2f
    basalar, 559
    generalized
        intermediate, 559, 559f
        severe, 559
    localized, 559
    migratory circinate, 559
    with mottled pigmentation, 559
    with muscular dystrophy, 560
    Ogna, 560
    with pyloric atresia, 560
    suprabasal, 558
Epidermolysis bullosa-associated nevus, 695
Epidermolytic acanthoma, 640
Epidermolytic hyperkeratosis, 565f
Epidermolytic ichthyosis (EI), 565
Epinephrine, 154, 884
Epiphysitis, 356
Episodic angioedema with eosinophilia, 156
Epistaxis, Osler disease, 855
Epithelial cysts and sinuses, 678–684
Epithelioid blue nevus, 703
Epithelioid cell histiocytoma, 617–625
Epithelioid cell nevus, 692–693
Epithelioid hemangioendothelioma, 592, 592f
Epithelioid sarcoma, 620, 620f
Epithelioid sarcoma-like (pseudomyogenic)
    hemangioendothelioma, 592
Epithelioma, sebaceous, 664
Epithelioma adenoides cysticum, 673–674,
    673f
Epoprostenol, for scleroderma, 176
Epoxy resins, 105–106
Epstein-Barr virus (EBV), 379–381
    adverse drug reactions in, 113
Epulis, 806–807
Equestrian panniculitis, 490
Erbium:yttrium-aluminum-garnet laser
    (Erbium:YAG)
    ablative laser resurfacing, 920, 920f
    pigmented lesions, 915
Erdheim-Chester disease (ECD), 718–719, 723
Ergot derivatives, for erythromelalgia, 816
Erosio interdigitalis blastomycetica, 303–304

Erosions, 13, 17.e1f
Erosive lichen planus, 217–218
Erosive pustular dermatitis, of scalp, 760
Eruptive keratoacanthomas, of lower leg, 647
Eruptive lingual papillitis, 800–801, 801f
Eruptive nevi, 689
Eruptive pseudoangiomatosis, 395
Eruptive syringomas, 665–666
Eruptive vellus hair cysts (EVHCs), 682
Eruptive xanthoma, 532, 532f, 546.e2f
Erysipelas, 260–261, 260f, 290.e1f–290.e2f
    chronic recurrent, 261
Erysipeloid of Rosenbach, 264, 264f
Erythema, 140–144
    chemotherapy-induced acral, 129–134, 130f
    color, 15
    dermatomyositis and, 167
    venous leg ulcers, 857
Erythema ab igne, 20–21, 21f, 45.e1f
Erythema annulare centrifugum, 143–144,
    143f, 156.e2f
Erythema contusiforme, 485
Erythema dyschromicum perstans, 224
Erythema elevatum diutinum (EED),
    841–842, 842f, 813.e3f
Erythema gyratum, 635.e3f
Erythema gyratum repens (EGR), 144, 144f,
    156.e1f
Erythema induratum, 330, 330f, 487–488
Erythema infectiosum, 398, 398f
Erythema marginatum, 263, 263f
Erythema migrans, 286, 287f
Erythema multiforme, 141–143, 141f–142f
    grouping of lesions, 15
    major, 141–142
    minor, 141
    oral, 143, 156.e1f
Erythema necroticans, 339
Erythema nodosum (EN), 145, 485–487, 486f,
    495.e1f
    chronic, 485–487, 486f, 495.e1f
    in sarcoidosis, 711
Erythema nodosum leprosum, 343, 343f, 346.e1f
Erythema nodosum migrans, 486
Erythema palmare, 140
"Erythema punctatum Higuchi", 395
Erythema toxicum neonatorum, 140–141,
    141f, 156.e1f
Erythematotelangiectatic rosacea, 912, 913f
Erythermalgia, 815, 815f
Erythrasma, 50, 266, 266f, 290.e2f
    tinea cruris and, 297
Erythremia. see Polycythemia vera
Erythroderma, 213–214, 214f
    in mycosis fungoides, 732, 749.e2f
    primary immunodeficiency diseases, 80
    in Sézary syndrome, 738
Erythrodermic mastocytosis, 623, 623f
Erythrodermic pemphigoid, 461
Erythrodermic polyneuropathy, 136
Erythrodermic psoriasis, 195, 195f, 204.e2f
Erythrodermic sarcoidosis, 713
Erythrodontia, congenital erythropoietic
    porphyria, 524–525
Erythrokeratodermia variabilis (EKV), 569,
    569f
Erythrokeratodermia variabilis et progressiva
    (EKVP), 569–570
Erythrokeratodermias, 569–570
Erythromelalgia, 815–817, 815f
Erythromelanosis follicularis faciei et colli,
    585, 774
Erythromycin
    for acne vulgaris, 231
    for bacillary angiomatosis, 280–281

Erythromycin (*Continued*)
   for chancroid, 273
   for cutaneous diphtheria, 265–266
   for granuloma inguinale, 274
   for lymphogranuloma venereum, 290
   for pityriasis lichenoides et varioliformis
     acuta, 740
Erythroplakia, 803, 803*f*
Erythroplasia of Queyrat, 657–658, 657*f*, 685.*e4f*
   Zoon balanitis *vs.*, 658
Erythropoietic porphyria, congenital,
   524–525, 524*f*
Erythropoietic protoporphyria (EPP), 33,
   523–524, 523*f*
Erythropoietin, porphyria cutanea tarda, 522
Erythrotelangiectatic rosacea, 245, 245*f*
Esophageal carcinoma, leukoplakia with, 803
Esophagus
   lichen planus in, 216
   progressive systemic sclerosis in, 174
Espundia, 424–425
Essential fatty acid deficiency, 482
Essential hyperhidrosis, 774
Essential oils, 100
Esters, 884
Estrogens
   cancer risk and, 140
   in erythema nodosum, 485
Etanercept
   for acute generalized exanthematous
     pustulosis, 122
   adverse reactions, 137
   for common variable immunodeficiency, 81
   for dermatomyositis, 170
   injection sites, 135
   for pityriasis lichenoides et varioliformis
     acuta, 740
   for small-vessel vasculitis, 837–838
   for Stevens-Johnson syndrome, 118
Ethambutol, for *Mycobacterium kansasii*
   infection, 334–335
Ethyl chloride spray, 885
Ethyl-butyl-acetyl aminopropionate, 437
Ethylene urea melamine formaldehyde resin,
   101
Ethylenediamine, 109
Etretinate, for mycosis fungoides, 737
Eumelanin, 3, 762, 862
Eumycetomas, 318–319
European processionary caterpillar, 439
Euxyl K 400, 108–109
Evolution of lesions, 14–15
Examination, 14
Exanthem subitum, 382
Exanthems
   adverse drug reactions, 114, 114*f*
   mercury and, 136
Excisional biopsies, 888
Excisional technique, 896, 897*f*
Excited skin syndrome, 96
Excoriated acne, 241
Excoriations, 13
Exercise-induced anaphylaxis, 156
Exercise-induced urticaria, 153
Exercise-related "vasculitis", 829
Exfoliation, 13
Exfoliative dermatitis, 213–214, 214*f*
Exogenous ochronosis, 542–543, 542*f*
Expanded polytetrafluoroethylene (ePTFE),
   924
External genital warts, 406–407
External otitis, 271, 271*f*
Extracorporeal photochemotherapy
   for mycosis fungoides, 737
   for pemphigus vulgaris, 456

Extracutaneous juvenile xanthogranuloma,
   719–720
Extracutaneous mastocytoma, 623
Extramammary Paget disease, 659–661, 660*f*,
   685.*e7f*
Extramedullary hematopoiesis, 747–748
Extremities, venous diseases of, 856–858
Exudative hyponychial dermatitis, 132
Eye makeup, 107
Eyelash trichomegaly, 769
Eyelids
   allergic contact dermatitis, 96–97, 97*f*
   atopic dermatitis, 66, 67*f*
   dermatitis, 73
   dermatomyositis and, 167
   lipoid proteinosis in, 536*f*
   seborrheic dermatitis in, 191
Eye(s)
   granuloma annulare and, 706
   herpes simplex infection of, 365
   herpes zoster in, 375, 375*f*
   in incontinentia pigmenti, 548
   juvenile xanthogranuloma in, 719–720
   sarcoidosis in, 715
   vitamin A deficiency and, 476
   vitiligo in, 871–872
   Vogt-Koyanagi-Harada syndrome in, 875

F
Fabric finishers, allergic contact dermatitis,
   101
Fabry disease, 537–538, 537*f*, 546.*e3f*
Face
   arterial supply of, 885*f*
   redness, 140
Facial (motor) nerve, 886*f*
   temporal branch of, 885–887
Factitial lymphedema, 860
Factitial panniculitis, 491
Factitious dermatitis, 57, 57*f*, 62.*e2f*
Factor XIIIa-positive dermal dendrocytes, 8
Famciclovir
   for erythema multiforme, 143
   genital herpes, 365
   herpes simplex, 369
   herpes zoster, 375–376
   herpetic gingivostomatitis, 363–364
   varicella, 373–374
Familial acanthosis nigricans, 503
Familial α-lipoprotein deficiency, 534–535
Familial apoprotein CII deficiency, 533
"Familial atypical multiple mole-melanoma"
   (FAMM) syndrome, 693
Familial benign chronic pemphigus, 562–563,
   562*f*
Familial cold autoinflammatory syndrome,
   150, 152
Familial hypercholesterolemia, 532–533, 533*f*
Familial Mediterranean fever (FMF), 149
Familial medullary thyroid carcinoma
   (FMTC), 518–519
Familial myxovascular fibromas, 616–617
Familial partial lipodystrophy, 493–494
Familial presenile sebaceous hyperplasia, 663
Familial primary localized cutaneous
   amyloidosis, 518
Familial progressive hyperpigmentation and
   hypopigmentation (FPHH), 865–866,
   867*f*
Familial rectal pain syndrome, 816
Famotidine, for dermatographism, 151
Fanconi syndrome, 575
Farber disease, 545
Farber lipogranulomatosis, 545
"Farcy buds", 278

Farmer's neck, 26
Farmyard pox, 389–390
Fascial hernia, 616–617
Fasciotomy, purpura fulminans, 830
Fat microcysts, 488
Fat removal, 930–932
Fatal shock, cold urticaria and, 152
Favre-Racouchot syndrome, 26, 27*f*
Favus, 293
Febrile ulceronecrotic Mucha-Habermann
   disease, 740
Fechtner syndrome, 834
Feet, tinea of, 297–299, 298*f*
   KOH examination, 298*f*
Felted hair, 767
Female hormones, systemic lupus
   erythematosus and, 164
Female-pattern alopecia, 755
Feminine hygiene sprays, dermatitis, 108
Ferguson Smith type keratoacanthoma, 647
FERMT3 gene, mutation in, leukocyte
   adhesion deficiency and, 87
Ferreira-Marques syndrome, 495
Ferritin, 870
Ferrochelatase (FECH), 523
Fetal alcohol syndrome, 769
Fetal hydantoin syndrome, 769
Fetal valproate syndrome, 769
"Fever blister", 363
Fexofenadine, for chronic urticaria, 154
Fiberglass dermatitis, 93
Fibrinogen, congenital disorders, 831
Fibrinolysis syndrome, 830
Fibrinolytic therapy, Degos disease, 850–851
Fibroblast, 8
Fibroblastic rheumatism, 182
Fibroepithelioma of Pinkus, 649
Fibrofolliculoma, 676–677
Fibroma
   aponeurotic, 612
   collagenous, 612
   familial myxovascular, 616–617
   gingival, 556
   perifollicular, 676–677
   periungual, 586.*e2f*
   of tendon sheath, 635.*e4f*
Fibromatosis colli, 613
Fibrous hamartoma of infancy, 613
Fibrous histiocytoma, 617
Fibrous papule, of nose/face, 615, 615*f*
Fibrous tissue abnormalities, 609–610
Fifth disease, 398
Figurate erythemas, 143–144
FIGURE (facial idiopathic granulomas with
   regressive evolution), 250
Filaggrin, 2
   atopic dermatitis and, 64
Filarial elephantiasis, 434*f*, 452.*e2f*
Filariasis, 434–435, 452.*e2f*
Filovirus, 395
Finasteride
   for female-pattern alopecia, 755
   for hirsutism, 771
   for male-pattern alopecia, 754
Finkelstein disease, 839–840
Fipronil, 438
Fire ants, 444–445
Fish odor syndrome, 776
Fish tank granuloma, 332, 332*f*
Fissured tongue, 799, 799*f*
Fissures, 13
Fixed cutaneous sporotrichosis, 314, 315*f*
Fixed drug reactions, 119–120, 120*f*, 139.*e2f*
   erythema multiforme and, 142
   lip ulcers, 796, 796*f*

FLAER (fluorescent aerolysin) flow cytometry test, paroxysmal nocturnal hemoglobinuria, 833–834
Flannel moth caterpillar, 439
Flaps, 896–898, 898f
Flash burns, 18–19
Flat warts, 403–404, 404f
Flatworms, 430
FLCN gene, 676–677
Flea bites, 445, 445f
Flea-borne illness, prevention of, 438
Flegel disease, 642
Flegel hyperkeratosis, 1–2
FLG gene, mutations in, 64
Flowers, allergic contact dermatitis from, 99
Fluconazole, 291–292
  for candidal vulvovaginitis, 303
  for candidiasis, 302
  for coccidioidomycosis, 309
  for cryptococcosis, 312
  for leishmaniasis, 424
  for onychomycosis, 300
  for *Pityrosporum* folliculitis, 307
  for protothecosis, 323
  for systemic candidiasis, 305
  for tinea capitis, 294
  for tinea corporis, 296
  for tinea of hands and feet, 299
  for tinea versicolor, 307
Fluence, 909
Fluocinonide ointment, aphthous stomatitis, 810
Fluorescent treponemal antibody absorption (FTA-ABS) test, 348
Fluoroderma, 136–137
Fluoroquinolones
  photosensitivity reactions and, 124
  for rhinoscleroma, 277
5-Fluorouracil (5-FU)
  actinic cheilitis, 794–795
  for Bowen disease, 657
  chemotherapy-induced acral erythema and, 130
  for epidermal nevi, 636–637
  for erythema ab igne, 20–21
  for extramammary Paget disease, 660–661
  for genital warts, 410
  for milia, 683
  for molluscum contagiosum, 392–393
  for psoriatic nails, 779
  for serpentine hyperpigmentation, 131, 131f
Flushing, 140, 247
Flutamide, flushing and, 140
Fluticasone, adverse reactions, 137
Focal acral hyperkeratosis, 211
Focal dermal hypoplasia, 578–579
Focal palmoplantar keratodermas, 209–211
Focal preauricular dermal dysplasia, 578
Focal vitiligo, 871–872
Fogo selvagem, 458–459, 458f
Folded skin with scarring, 630
Folic acid deficiency, 478
Follicular atrophoderma, 585
Follicular infundibulum, tumors of, 678
Follicular lichen planus, 222–223, 230.e3f
Follicular mucinosis, 188–189, 188f–189f, 756, 190.e2f
"Follicular occlusion triad", 239
Follicular ostia, loss of, 756, 757f
Follicular spicules, 745
Folliculitis, 255
  dissecting terminal, 242
  eosinophilic, 417, 417f
  fungal, 296

Folliculitis (Continued)
  Gram-negative, 241–242, 242f, 271–272
  Pityrosporum, 307
  pruritic, of pregnancy, 466
  Pseudomonas aeruginosa, 270–271, 290.e3f
  staphylococcal, 254, 254f
  superficial pustular, 254
  suppurative, pyoderma gangrenosum and, 148
Folliculitis decalvans, 760, 760f
Folliculitis nares perforans, 773
Folliculitis ulerythematosa reticulata, 761
Folliculosebaceous cystic hamartoma, 678
Fong syndrome, 785, 785f
Fonsecaea pedrosoi, 316
Food additives
  flushing and, 140
  urticaria and, 151
Food allergy, atopic dermatitis and, 64–65
Food-induced purpura, 829
Foot, neuropathic ulcers, 858
"Footprints in the snow," alopecia cicatrisata, 760
Forchheimer spots, 380
Fordyce's disease (spots), 7, 798f
Forehead lines, 926–927, 927f
Foreign body reactions, 40–41
Foresters, allergic contact dermatitis, 99–100
Formaldehyde, allergic contact dermatitis, 109
Formaldehyde-releasing agents, allergic contact dermatitis, 109
Fournier gangrene, of penis/scrotum, 268
FOXC2 transcription factor, 859–860
Fox-Fordyce disease, 777, 777f, 793.e4f
FOXP3 gene, IPEX syndrome and, 82
Fractional resurfacing, 920–921
Fracture blisters, 39
Fragrances, allergic contact dermatitis, 106, 106f
Frambesia. *see* Yaws
Franceschetti-Klein syndrome, 582
Francisella tularensis, 282
Freckles, 3, 26, 686
Free cartilage grafts, 904–905
Frey syndrome, 774
Friction blisters, 38–39
Frictional acne, 231–232
Fried-egg appearance, of dysplastic nevus, 703.e3f
Frontal fibrosing alopecia, 220, 759, 759f
Frontalis, 927
Frontalis-associated lipoma of the forehead, 635.e6f
Frostbite, 22–23, 23f, 45.e1f
  treatment for, 23
Fruit, allergic contact dermatitis from, 99
Fucosidosis, 538
Fugitive swelling, 435, 435f
Full-thickness grafts, 903, 904f
Fumaric acid esters, for granuloma annulare, 707
Fungal folliculitis, 296
Fungal infections, 291–323
  primary immunodeficiency diseases and, 80
  pruritus ani, 50
  pruritus scroti, 50
Funnel web spiders, 451
Furocoumarins, 29
Furrowed tongue, 799, 799f
Furuncles, hidradenitis suppurativa and, 243
Furuncular myiasis, 443
Furunculosis, 255–256
Fusariosis, 321–322
Fusarium, 321

Fusiform excision, 896
Fusion toxin, for mycosis fungoides, 737

G
Gabapentin
  for CKD-associated pruritus, 48
  for meralgia paresthetica, 60
  for zoster-associated pain, 376–377
Gadfly, 442
Gadolinium-associated plaques, 178
Gain-of-function mutations, erythromelalgia, 816
Galli-Galli disease, 865f, 866–867
Galvanic urticaria, 153
Gamasoidosis, 449
Gambian trypanosomiasis, 427
Ganglioneuroma, 627
Gangrene
  Fournier, of penis or scrotum, 268
  gas, 267–268, 267f
  Meleney, 268
  of skin, 267–269
  symmetric peripheral, 830
  in trench foot, 23
GAPO syndrome, 584
Gardner syndrome, 629
Gardner-Diamond syndrome, 834–835, 834f
Gas gangrene, 267–268, 267f
Gastrointestinal (GI) tract, bleeding, in Osler disease, 855
Gastrointestinal polyps, Peutz-Jeghers syndrome and, 688
GATA2 deficiency, 85–86
Gaucher disease, 535–536, 536f
Gene therapy
  for osteogenesis imperfecta, 514
  for recessive dystrophic epidermolysis bullosa, 561
Generalized acquired hypertrichosis, 769–770
Generalized congenital hypertrichosis, 769, 769f
Generalized eruption
  adult type, 622–623
  childhood type, 622
Generalized eruptive histiocytoma, 721–722
Generalized eruptive histiocytosis, 721–722
Generalized eruptive keratoacanthomas, 647
Generalized erythema, 140
Generalized essential telangiectasia (GET), 604, 854, 813.e4f
Generalized granuloma annulare, 704
Generalized hair follicle hamartoma, 677–678
Generalized hyperhidrosis, 774–776
Generalized lentiginosis, 687
Generalized morphea, 172, 172f
Generalized pustular psoriasis, 194–195, 195f
Generalized vitiligo, 871–872, 871f
Genetic testing, porphyrias, 520
Genetics, Hansen disease, 336
Genital herpes, 365–366, 366f
Genital leiomyomas, 630–631
Genital nevi, 689
Genital syringomas, 665–666
Genital warts, 406–407
  in children, 410, 410f
  diagnosis of, 408–409
  treatment of, 409–410
Genitalia, lichen planus in, 229
Genodermatoses, 547–586
Gentamicin
  for granuloma inguinale, 274
  for plague, 281
  for tinea of hands and feet, 298–299
  for tularemia, 283
Gentian violet, breast eczema, 73

Geographic tongue, 799, 799f
Geometric port wine stain, 596
Geotrichosis, 305–306
Geotrichum candidum, 305
Geraniol candles, 437
German measles, 397
"Ghost cells"
    in lipodermatosclerosis, 488
    in pancreatic panniculitis, 492
Gianotti-Crosti syndrome (GCS), 380, 385–386, 385f–386f, 420.e4f
Giant cell arteritis/temporal arteritis, 849–850, 849f
Giant cell tumor, 613, 614f
Giant condyloma acuminatum, 408
Giant hairy nevus, 691, 691f
Giant pigmented nevus, 691
Giant solitary trichoepithelioma, 674
Gigantism, 496
Gila monster, 452
Gingiva
    lichen planus on, 218, 218f
    ulceration, in Langerhans cell histiocytosis, 728, 729f
Gingival fibromas, 556
Gingivitis, vitamin C deficiency and, 478–479, 479f
Gingivostomatitis, herpetic, 363, 363f, 369–370
Ginkgo biloba, for scleroderma, 176
Ginkgo tree dermatitis, 99
Glabellar frown lines, 926, 926f
Glanders, 278
Glandular rosacea, 245, 246f
Glandular tularemia, 282–283
Glanzmann thrombasthenia, 834
Gleich syndrome, 156
Gliadins, dermatitis herpetiformis, 470
Glomangioma, 790
Glomeruloid hemangioma, 594
Glomus bodies, 9
Glomus tumor, 599–600
Glossitis, 515
Glossodynia, 59
Glove powder, 112
Gloves-and-socks syndrome, papular-purpuric, 398–399, 399f, 420.e6f
Glucocorticoids
    excess of, 496
    for hypereosinophilic syndrome, 748
Glues, occupational vitiligo and, 874
Gluten free, dermatitis herpetiformis, 471
Glycerin, for sclerotherapy, 929
Glycolic acid
    for chemical peels, 932
    for melasma, 864–865
Glycolipids, 1–2
Glycopyrrolate, oral, for hidrocystomas, 666
Gnathostomiasis, 433
Goat moth, 439–440
Goeckerman technique, for psoriasis, 198
Gold
    allergic contact dermatitis, 104, 104f
    pemphigus vulgaris, 456
    pigmentation, 128
    reactions, 95
Golfer's vasculitis, 829
Golimumab, for sarcoidosis, 717
Goltz syndrome, 578–579, 578f, 586.e5f
Gonadal dysgenesis, 550
Gonadal mosaicism, 547
Gonococcal dermatitis, 274–275
Gonococcemia, 274–275, 275f, 290.e3f
Good syndrome, 81
Gorham-Stout syndrome, 602

Gorlin sign, 510
Gorlin syndrome, 652–653, 652f
Gottron papules, 167–168, 168f, 183.e5f
Gottron sign, 167, 169f, 183.e4f
Gougerot and Carteaud papillomatosis, 209, 209f
Gougerot-Blum syndrome, 835
Gout, 545, 545f
    juvenile, 545–546
    nodules or tophi of, 180
Gouty panniculitis, 493
Graft-*versus*-host disease (GVHD), 89–91, 89f
    chronic, 90f
    erythema multiforme and, 142
    in solid-organ transplantation, 90–91
Graham-Little-Piccardi-Lasseur syndrome, 220, 222–223, 758
Grain itch, 449
Grains, 1
Gram-negative folliculitis, 241–242, 242f
Gram-negative infections, 269–283
    folliculitis, 271–272
    toe web, 270, 270f, 290.e2f
Gram-positive infections, 252–269
Gram-positive toxic shock syndromes, 257–259
Granular cell tumor, 625, 625f
Granular layer, 1
Granular parakeratotic acanthoma, 641
Granulocyte colony-stimulating factor (G-CSF)
    adverse reactions, 134
    cyclic neutropenia, 808
    thromboangiitis obliterans, 851–852
Granulocytic sarcoma, 747
Granuloma annulare, 704–707, 705f, 17.e1f, 730.e1f–730.e2f
Granuloma faciale, 842–843, 842f
Granuloma fissuratum, 807
Granuloma gluteal infantum, 76
Granuloma inguinale, 273–274, 274f, 290.e3f
Granuloma multiforme (GM), 709
Granuloma venereum, 273–274
Granulomas, 42
    allergic, 716
    beryllium, 42
    cutaneous noninfectious, ataxia telangiectasia, 83
    mercury, 42, 42f
    noninfectious, in common variable immunodeficiency, 81
    primary immunodeficiency diseases, 80
    pyogenic, 806–807
    related palisading, 181
    silica, 42–43, 43f
    silicone, 42–43, 42f
    zirconium, 42, 43f
Granulomatosis with polyangiitis (GPA), 846–847, 846f
Granulomatous amebic encephalitis, 421
Granulomatous lesions, rosacea and, 247
Granulomatous perioral dermatitis, in children, 250–251, 250f
Granulomatous slack skin, 738, 738f
Granulosis rubra nasi, 778
Graves disease, 500
Gray hair, 762
Gray nevus, 703
Green blowfly, 443
Green foot syndrome, 270
Green hair, 763
Green nail syndrome, 270, 270f, 790
Green tea extract, for genital warts, 409
Grenz ray radiotherapy, for hand eczema, 76

Grenz zone, in multicentric reticulohistiocytosis, 725
Griffith's classification, of pityriasis rubra pilaris, 207
Griscelli syndrome, 877
Griseofulvin, 291
    for tinea capitis, 294
    for tinea corporis, 296
    for tinea imbricata, 296
    for tinea of hands and feet, 299
Grocer's itch, 449
Groin, allergic contact dermatitis in, 97
"Groove sign," of eosinophilic fasciitis, 177, 177f
"Grosshans-Marot disease", 227
Ground itch, 432
Ground substance, 184
Group B streptococcal infection, 263
Grouping of lesions, 15
Grover disease, 453, 473–474, 473f
Growth hormone, 496
    deficiency in, 498
Grzybowski variant keratoacanthoma, 647
Guinea worm disease, 433–434
Gummas, 354
Gustatory hyperhidrosis, 774
Guttate lesions, 15
Guttate morphea, 172
    lichen sclerosus and, 229
Guttate psoriasis, 193f, 194, 204.e2f
Gypsy moth, 439–440
Gyrate erythemas, 143–144
Gyrate lesions, 15

H
H syndrome, 586
Haber syndrome, 247
Haemophilus ducreyi
    chancre (primary stage), 349
    chancroid and, 272
Haemophilus influenzae
    cellulitis, 272
    X-linked agammaglobulinemia, 80
Hailey-Hailey disease, 562–563, 562f
Haim-Munk syndrome, 212
Hair, 16–17, 16f
    anagen, 5f–7f, 6–7, 10.e1f
    bulb, 5, 6f
    casts, 763
    color of, 7, 762–763
    corticosteroids adverse reaction, 138
    diseases of, 750–756
    dyes, 107, 107f
    growth, 6, 7f
    ingestion of, 57
    structure defects of, 763–769
    telogen, 6–7, 7f, 10.e1f
    transplantation
        for female-pattern alopecia, 755
        for male-pattern alopecia, 754
    tuft, sacral, 793.e3f
Hair follicles, 5–7
    associated diseases, 772–774
Hair straighteners, 107
HAIR-AN syndrome, 503–504
Hairdressers, hand eczema and, 74
Hairy cell leukemia, 747
Hairy elbows, 769
Half and half nails, 783, 783f
Hallermann-Streiff syndrome, 583
Hallopeau type, of pemphigus vegetans, 456
Halo nevus, 690–691, 690f, 703.e2f
Halo phenomenon, 872
Halofuginone, for scleroderma, 176
Halogenoderma, 136

Hamartoma
  basaloid follicular, 677–678, 678f
  congenital smooth muscle, 631
  folliculosebaceous cystic, 678
  generalized hair follicle, 677–678
Hand eczema, 74–76, 74f, 91.e1f
  protection for, 76
  pulpitis, 75
  treatment for, 76
    barrier repair in, 76
    botulinum toxin A in, 76
Hand swelling, 436–437
Hand-arm vibration syndrome, 813
Hand-foot syndrome, 129–134, 130f
Hand-foot-and-mouth disease, 394–395, 394f
Hands
  allergic contact dermatitis in, 97, 99f–100f
  atopic dermatitis, 66, 67f
  chronic mucocutaneous candidiasis on, 304f
  dorsal, neutrophilic dermatosis of, 147, 147f, 156.e2f
  tinea of, 297–299, 297f
    KOH examination, 298f
Hanging curtain sign, 205
"Hanging groin", 436
Hangnail, 787
Hansen disease, 9, 14, 16, 336–346
  adjunctive treatments, 345
  borderline borderline (BB) leprosy, 338
  borderline lepromatous (BL) leprosy, 338, 339f, 342
  borderline leprosy, 342, 346.e1f
  borderline tuberculoid (BT) leprosy, 338, 338f, 342, 346.e1f
  classification of, 337–339, 337t
  diagnosis of, 336–337
  early, 337–338
  epidemiology of, 336
  grouping of lesions, 15
  histoid leprosy, 339
  histopathology of, 342
  human immunodeficiency virus and, 341
  immunopathogenesis of, 342
  indeterminate, 337–338
  infectious agent of, 336
  lepromatous leprosy, 339, 339f–340f, 342, 346.e1f
  management of reactions, 345
  mucous membrane involvement, 341, 341f
  nerve involvement, 339–341, 341f
  ocular involvement, 341
  organ transplantation and, 341–342
  pregnancy and, 341
  prevention of, 345–346
  reactional states, 342–343
    type 1, 342–343, 343f, 346.e1f
    type 2, 343, 343f
  special clinical considerations and, 341–342
  treatment of, 343–345, 344t
  tuberculoid leprosy, 338, 338f, 342
  visceral involvement, 341
Hapalonychia, 785
Happle syndrome, 566
Happle-Tinschert syndrome, 677–678
Hapten, 113–114
Hard corns, 38
Hard nevus of Unna, 636
Harlequin ichthyosis (HI), 564–565
Hartnup disease, 540–541
Hashimoto thyroiditis, 499
Hay-Wells syndrome, 575
Head, allergic contact dermatitis in, 96–97, 97f
Head louse, 441
Headlight sign, 66–67
Healing, by second intention, 896, 898f

Heat injuries, 18–21
Heat treatment, for common warts, 405
Heat urticaria, 152
Heating, laser, 909
Heavy-metal poisoning, melanosis, 806
Heberden nodes, 180
Heck disease, 411
Hedgehog signaling, 4
Heerfordt syndrome, 715
Helicobacter cellulitis, 277
Helicobacter pylori
  Henoch-Schönlein purpura, 838
  urticaria and, 151
Heliotrope, in dermatomyositis, 167, 167f
Heloderma suspectum, 452
Hemangioendotheliomas, 590
  spindle cell, 592, 592f
Hemangioma
  glomeruloid, 594
  infantile, 587–590, 588f, 635.e1f
  microvenular, 607
  noninvoluting congenital, 590
  pulse dye laser for, 911–912
Hemangiopericytoma, 593
  lesions formerly classified as, 593
Hematologic malignancy
  reactive neutrophilic dermatoses and, 145
  Sweet syndrome, 146
Hematoma, 823, 813.e2f
Hematopoietic diseases, pruritus, 47
Hematopoietic stem cell transplantation (HSCT)
  for Hurler syndrome, 543
  for paroxysmal nocturnal hemoglobinuria, 833–834
  sarcoidosis and, 716
Hemenocampa pseudotsugata, 439–440
Hemidesmosomes, 4
Hemileuca maia, 439
Hemiptera, order of, 440–441
Hemochromatosis, 521, 521f, 869–870, 869f
Hemoglobin, skin color, 15
Hemolytic uremic syndrome (HUS), 825–826
Hemorrhagic bullae, 13
Hemorrhagic gingivitis, 478–479, 479f
Hemosiderin hyperpigmentation, 862–863
Henderson-paterson bodies, 392
Henoch-Schönlein purpura, 838–839, 838f, 813.e3f
Heparin
  Degos disease, 850–851
  for disseminated intravascular coagulation, 830–831
  for livedoid vasculopathy, 820
  skin necrosis, 125
Heparin-induced thrombocytopenia (HIT), 125, 824
Hepatitis B virus (HBV), 383–384
  lichen planus and, 219
  polyarteritis nodosa, 844
  urticaria and, 151, 151f
Hepatitis C virus (HCV), 384–385, 384f
  cryoglobulinemic vasculitis, 841
  lichen planus and, 219
  polyarteritis nodosa, 844
  porphyria cutanea tarda, 520–521
  pruritus, 47
  pyoderma gangrenosum and, 148
  urticarial vasculitis, 840
Hepatitis-associated lichen planus, 219
Hepatoerythropoietic porphyria, 523
Hepatolenticular degeneration, 543
Herald patch, 353
Herbal supplements, surgery and, 881
Hereditary angioedema, 155

Hereditary coproporphyria, 523
Hereditary cutaneous amyloidosis syndromes, 518–519
Hereditary hemorrhagic telangiectasia, 604
Hereditary hemorrhagic telangiectasia (HHT), 855–856, 855f, 813.e4f
Hereditary lymphedema, 859, 859f
Hereditary nonpolyposis colorectal cancer syndrome (HNCCS), 665
Hereditary osteo-onychodysplasia, 785, 785f
Hereditary sclerosing poikiloderma, 582
Hereditary sensory and autonomic neuropathies, 62
Heredofamilial amyloidosis, 519–520
Hermansky-Pudlak syndrome, 877, 877f
Heroin, narcotic dermopathy, 40, 40f
Herpangina, 394, 394f
  and herpes simplex, 809
Herpes gestationis, 464–465
Herpes gladiatorum, 364, 364f, 420.e1f
Herpes labialis, 369
Herpes simplex, 362–370, 420.e1f
  atopic dermatitis and, 68, 69f
  differential diagnosis, 369–370
  erythema multiforme, 141
  genital, 420.e1f
  histopathology, 369
  HSV-1 infection, 362, 420.e2f
  HSV-2 infection, 362, 420.e2f
  in immunocompromised patients, 368–369, 368f–369f
  intrauterine, 366–367
  neonatal, 366–367, 367f
  recurrent intraoral infection, 809, 809f
Herpes zoster, 374–379, 374f, 420.e2f–420.e3f
  acquired immunodeficiency syndrome, 377, 378f
  complications of, 375
  dermatomal distribution, 420.e2f
  diagnosis of, 377–378
  differential diagnosis of, 378
  disseminated, 374–375
  distribution of lesions, 14
  herpes simplex and, 369
  histopathology of, 378
  in immunosuppressed patients, 377, 378f
  inflammatory skin lesions after, 378–379, 379f
  necrotic, 420.e2f
  ophthalmic, 375, 375f
  oral, 374, 374f
  pain, 376–377
  prevention of, 378
  treatment of, 375–376
Herpes zoster ophthalmicus, 375
Herpesvirus group, 362–383
Herpesvirus simiae, 383
Herpetic gingivostomatitis, 363, 363f, 369–370
Herpetic keratoconjunctivitis, 365
Herpetic sycosis, 364, 364f
Herpetic whitlow, 364–365, 365f
Herpetiform aphthae, 809
Herpetiform pemphigus, 457–458
Herringbone nail, 785
Hertoghe sign, 67
Herxheimer reaction. *see* Jarisch-Herxheimer reaction
Hexachlorophene, for preoperative antisepsis, 884
Hidradenitis, 130, 778
Hidradenitis suppurativa, 242–244
  of axilla, 242f
  of groin, 243f
Hidradenoma papilliferum, 669
Hidroacanthoma simplex, 666–667

Hidrocystomas, 666, 666f
Hidrotic ectodermal dysplasia, 575, 575f
Highly active antiretroviral therapy (HAART)
    for HIV infection, 416
    for Kaposi sarcoma, 419
    for lipodystrophy, 493
Hirsutism, 770–772, 770f, 793.e3f
Histamine
    flushing and, 140
    itching and, 46
Histiocytic medullary reticulosis, 745–746
Histiocytoses, 718–729
    malignant, 745–746, 749.e4f
Histoid leprosy, 339
Histones, 1
Histopathology, 14
Histoplasmosis, 14, 309–311
    African, 310
    epidemiology of, 310–311
    etiology and pathology of, 310
    immunology of, 311
    primary cutaneous, 310
    primary pulmonary, 309
    progressive disseminated, 309–310, 310f
    treatment of, 311
History, 14
HIV infection, 415–420
    adverse drug reactions in, 113
    atopic dermatitis and, 66
    cryptococcosis and, 311
    cytomegalovirus, 381
    drug reactions and, 119
    erythema elevatum diutinum, 841–842
    erythroderma and, 214
    granuloma annulare in, 706
    Hansen disease and, 341
    in lipodystrophy, 493
    Merkel cell carcinoma and, 661
    molluscum contagiosum, 390–391
    neoplasia, 417–418
    photosensitivity, 35
    in porphyria cutanea tarda, 521
    primary, 416, 416f
    pruritus, 416–417
    pyoderma gangrenosum and, 148
    Sjögren syndrome and, 179
    syphilis and, 358–359
    tuberculosis and, 324
    varicella, 373–374
Hives, 11, 12f, 150–156
HMB-45, in Spitz nevus, 692–693
Hobnail hemangioma, 594
Hodgkin disease, 745
    cutaneous, 732
    exfoliative dermatitis and, 214
    pruritus, 47
Holmes-Adie syndrome, 776
"Holster sign," of dermatomyositis, 167
Home tanning solutions, 29
Homme orange, 622
Homocysteine, 511
Homocystinuria, 511
Honeycomb atrophy, 761
Hookworm disease, 432
Horizontal forehead lines, 926–927, 927f
Horizontal mattress suture, 889, 891f
Horizontal plexus, 8
Hormone replacement therapy (HRT)
    for acne vulgaris, 236, 236f
    for erythema nodosum, 485
    flushing and, 140
    for melasma, 864
Hormone-induced dermatoses, 79–80
Hortaea werneckii, 299
Horton disease, 849

"Hot comb alopecia", 759
Hot foot syndrome, 271
Hot tar burns, 19
Hot tub folliculitis, 270–271, 271f
Housefly, 442
Houseplants, allergic contact dermatitis from, 99
HRAS-duplicated Spitz nevi, 693
HTLV-1-associated myelopathy, 414–415
Human bite pathogens, 278
Human botfly, 443
Human collagen, for soft tissue augmentation, 922
Human flea, 452.e3f
Human herpesvirus
    type 3, 374–379
    type 4, 379–381
    type 5, 381–382
    type 6, 382
        adverse drug reactions in, 113
        Rosai-Dorfman disease and, 749
    type 7, 382
        adverse drug reactions in, 113
    type 8, 382–383, 382f
Human immunodeficiency virus (HIV)
    infection. see HIV infection
Human leukocyte antigen (HLA), 113
    dermatitis herpetiformis, 470
    pemphigoid gestationis, 464
    pemphigus vulgaris and, 455
    Stevens-Johnson syndrome, 119–120
Human monkeypox, 389
Human monocytic ehrlichiosis (HME), 285
Human papillomavirus (HPV)
    epidermodysplasia verruciformis and, 411–412
    genital, 407, 407f
    -induced genital dysplasia, 408
    lichen sclerosus and, 229
    vaccination, 410
    warts, 402
Human tanapox, 390
Human T-lymphotropic virus 1 (HTLV-1), 414–415, 415f, 742–743
Human trypanosomiasis, 426–427
Hunter syndrome, 543–544, 544f
Hunterian chancre, 348–349
Huriez syndrome, 582
Hurler syndrome, 543
Hutchinson sign, 356, 356f, 375, 690, 696
Hutchinson-Gilford syndrome, 579–580
Hyaline fibromatosis syndrome, 613–616
Hyalinosis cutis et mucosae, 536
Hyalohyphomycosis, 321, 321f
Hyaluronan (hyaluronic acid), 3–4, 8
    for actinic keratosis, 644–645
    for scar sarcoid, 714
    for soft tissue augmentation, 922–923, 923f
Hydatid disease, 431
Hydroa vacciniforme, 34
    differential diagnosis of, 34
Hydroactive adhesive (Biore) pads, for trichostasis spinulosa, 768
Hydrocarbons, 29, 94–95
Hydrochloric acid burns, 92, 93f
Hydrocortisone, for atopic dermatitis, 69
Hydroid, 428–429
Hydroquinone
    antioxidants, 105
    dermatitis, 107
    in exogenous ochronosis, 542–543
    for melasma, 864–865
    for nevus of Ota, 702
    occupational vitiligo and, 874
    for solar lentigo, 687

α-Hydroxy acids, ichthyosis, 565
4-Hydroxyanisole (4-HA), for solar lentigo, 687
Hydroxychloroquine, 127
    for chronic urticaria, 154
    for granuloma annulare, 707
    for lichen planus, 220–221
    for livedoid vasculopathy, 820
    for pemphigus foliaceus, 458
    for sarcoidosis, 717
    for Sjögren syndrome, 179–180
    for systemic lupus erythematosus, 165
    Waldenström hyperglobulinemic purpura, 828
Hydroxychloroquine sulfate, polymorphous light eruption, 31–32
Hydroxyethyl starch (HES), pruritus, 52
21-Hydroxylase deficiency, 498–499
17-Hydroxyprogesterone (17-HP), 498–499
    stimulation test, 770
Hydroxyurea
    for atopic dermatitis, 71
    for chronic actinic dermatitis, 35
    dermopathy, 137
Hydroxyzine, 109
    for acute urticaria, 154
    for atopic dermatitis, 69
    for polycythemia vera, 749
Hymenoptera, 444–445
Hyperalgesia, zoster-associated pain, 376
Hyperbaric oxygen, for necrobiosis lipoidica, 539
Hypercalcemia, 489
Hypercholesterolemia, familial, 532–533
Hyperesthesia of lesions, 16
Hyperhidrosis, 20, 774–776
    axillary, 793.e4f
    botulinum toxin injection for, 927–928, 927f–928f
    tinea infections and, 298
Hyper-IgD syndrome (HIDS), 150
Hyperimmunoglobulinemia E syndrome, 87–88
Hyperkeratosis, of nipple and areola, 639, 685.e1f
Hyperkeratosis lenticularis perstans, 642
Hyperkeratotic hand dermatitis, 75, 75f, 91.e1f
Hyperkeratotic scabies, 300, 448
Hyperlipoproteinemia
    primary, 532–533
    secondary, 533–535
Hyperosmotic agents, for sclerotherapy, 928
Hyperparathyroidism, 502
Hyperphosphatemic familial tumoral calcinosis, 528–529
Hyperpigmentation, 15–16, 17.e2f
    in Addison's disease, 497–498, 497f, 504.e1f
    chemotherapy-induced, 130
    drug induced, 127
    familial progressive, 865–866, 867f
    fixed drug reactions and, 120
    hemosiderin, 862–863
    laser resurfacing for, 919
    of nails, 788, 789f
    postinflammatory, 863, 863f
    as sclerotherapy complications, 929
Hyperplasias, 605–607
Hypersensitivity syndromes, 113
Hyperthyroidism, 500–501
    pruritus, 47
Hypertonic saline, for sclerotherapy, 928
Hypertrichosis, 769–770
Hypertrichosis cubiti, 769

Hypertriglyceridemia
  in familial partial lipodystrophy, 493
  isotretinoin and, 237
Hypertrophic actinic keratoses, 644, 685.e2f
  of arms and hands, 685.e2f
Hypertrophic lichen planus, 217, 217f
Hypertrophic lupus erythematosus, 159, 159f,
  183.e2f
Hypertrophic osteoarthropathy, 780
Hypertrophic scars, 13–14
Hypervitaminosis A, 476
Hypoalphalipoproteinemia, 534–535
Hypoderma lineatum, 443
Hypofibrinogenemia, 831
Hypohidrosis, 776
  postmiliarial, 20
Hypohidrotic ectodermal dysplasia, 575, 586.e5f
Hypomelanosis of Ito, 549
Hypomelanotic blue nevus, 703
Hypoparathyroidism, 501–502
Hypophosphatemic rickets, 663
Hypopigmentation
  congenital disorders of, 876–879, 876b
  familial progressive, 865–866, 867f
  laser resurfacing for, 919
  mycosis fungoides, 733, 734f
  tattoo laser removal, 917
Hypopigmented sarcoidosis, 712
Hypopigmented tinea versicolor, 306–307
Hypothyroidism, 499–500
  alopecia in, 756
  congenital, 499
  mild, 499
  pruritus, 47
Hypotrichosis-telangiectasia-lymphedema
  syndrome, 860
Hypovitaminosis A, 475–476
Hysterical edema, 860

I

Iatrogenic calcinosis cutis, 528
Iatrogenic candidiasis, 304
Ibuprofen, for frostbite, 23
Ice, anesthesia and, 885
Ichthyosiform sarcoidosis, 713, 713f
Ichthyosis, 13, 565
  congenital syndromes with, 566–570
Ichthyosis follicularis, 585, 762
Ichthyosis hystrix, 636
Ichthyosis vulgaris, 2–3, 64, 563
Id reactions, eczema, 77
Idiopathic arthritis, juvenile, 181–182
Idiopathic calcinosis cutis, 528–529, 528f
Idiopathic chronic telogen effluvium, 752–753
Idiopathic clubbing, 780
Idiopathic eruptive macular pigmentation
  (IEMP), 224
Idiopathic guttate hypomelanosis, 870–871,
  870f, 880.e2f
Idiopathic hypereosinophilic syndrome, 748
Idiopathic hypertrophic osteoarthropathy, 577
Idiopathic nodular vasculitis, 330
Idiopathic photosensitivity disorders, 30–35
Idiopathic scrotal calcinosis, 528
"Idiopathic" thrombocytopenic purpura,
  823–824
Idiopathic thrombocytopenic purpura,
  systemic lupus erythematosus and,
  163–164
α-Iduronidase, 543
IgA vasculitis, 838–839, 838f
IgG autoantibodies, in urticaria, 153
IgG4-related skin disease, 745
Igneous rock sign, 217
IGRAs, in tuberculosis, 325

IKBKG gene, mutations in, 81
IL-1 receptor antagonist, deficiency, 149–150
IL-36 receptor antagonist, deficiency,
  149–150
Iloprost
  for Raynaud disease, 814
  for thromboangiitis obliterans, 851–852
Imatinib, depigmentation, 131
Imatinib mesylate
  for hypereosinophilic syndrome, 748
  for polycythemia vera, 749
Imidazoles, 110, 291
Imipenem
  for glanders, 278
  for nocardiosis, 269
Imipramine, 128
Imiquimod
  actinic cheilitis, 794–795
  for actinic keratosis, 644–645
  for Bowen disease, 657
  for erythema ab igne, 20–21
  for erythroplasia of Queyrat, 658
  for extramammary Paget disease, 660–661
  for flat warts, 406
  for genital warts, 409
  for Gorlin syndrome, 651
  for granuloma annulare, 706
Immediate pigment darkening, 24
Immersion foot syndromes, 23–24
Immune reconstitution inflammatory
  syndrome (IRIS), 416
Immune thrombocytopenia, 823–824, 823f
Immune thrombocytopenic purpura (ITP),
  823–824, 823f
Immunoadsorption, for pemphigus vulgaris,
  456
Immunocompromised patients, herpes
  simplex in, 368–369, 368f–369f
Immunocytoma, primary cutaneous, 743
Immunodeficiency, 860
Immunodeficiency syndromes, 80–91
Immunodiffusion tests, for South American
  blastomycosis, 314
Immunofluorescence antibody test, 437
Immunoglobulin
  for immune thrombocytopenic purpura
    (ITP), 824
  for Kawasaki disease, 853
Immunoglobulin A (IgA), linear bullous
  dermatosis, 137
Immunoglobulin G (IgG), syphilis, 348
Immunoglobulin M (IgM)
  syphilis, 348
  Waldenström macroglobulinemia, 828
Immunologic urticaria, 122
Immunology
  in coccidioidomycosis, 309
  in cryptococcosis, 312
  in histoplasmosis, 311
  in South American blastomycosis, 314
Immunomodulatory therapy, multimodality,
  for mycosis fungoides, 736
Immunoprecipitation, in paraneoplastic
  pemphigus, 458
Immunosuppressed patients
  herpes zoster in, 377, 378f
  Merkel cell polyomavirus in, 661
  oral hairy leukoplakia in, 380
  warts in, 412–414
Immunosuppression
  adverse reactions to, 133–134
  in Merkel cell carcinoma, 661
  and pigmented purpura, 836
  in squamous cell carcinoma, 653
  in Stevens-Johnson syndrome, 119

Immunosuppressive therapy
  for lichen planus, 221
  for systemic lupus erythematosus, 166
  for Wiskott-Aldrich syndrome, 83
Immunotherapy
  for genital warts, 410
  for warts, 406
Impetigo, 252–254, 253f, 290.e1f
  of Bockhart, 254
  bullous, 253, 253f
  circinata, 253
  contagiosa, 253
  herpes simplex, 369
Impetigo herpetiformis, 195, 466
Incisional biopsies, 888
Incontinentia pigmenti, 1, 547–548, 548f,
  586.e1f
Incontinentia pigmenti achromians, 548–549,
  549f
Indeterminate cell histiocytosis (ICH),
  725–726
Indirect immunofluorescence (IIF)
  for bullous pemphigoid, 462
  for epidermolysis bullosa acquisita,
    468–469
  for paraneoplastic pemphigus, 459
  for pemphigus foliaceus, 458
Indomethacin
  for urticarial vasculitis, 840–841
  Waldenström hyperglobulinemic purpura,
    828
Infantile acne, 231, 233f
Infantile acropustulosis, 203–204
Infantile atopic dermatitis, 66, 66f
Infantile digital fibromatosis, 613
Infantile digital myofibroblastoma, 613
Infantile hemangioma, 587–590, 588f, 635.e1f
Infantile neuroblastoma, 626–627
Infantile perianal pyramidal protrusion, 617
Infantile postinfectious irislike purpura and
  edema, 839–840, 839f
Infantile systemic hyalinosis, 613–616
Infants
  postnatal telogen effluvium of, 752–753
  zinc deficiency and, 481
Infections
  in erythema nodosum, 486–487
  Gram-negative, 269–283
  Gram-positive, 252–269
  surgical site, 881–882
  wounds, 882
Infectious hepatitis, 383–386
Infectious mononucleosis, 380
Infective dermatitis, 86, 415
Infective endocarditis (IE) prophylaxis, 883b,
  883t
Infiltrative basal cell carcinoma, 649
Inflammatory bowel disease (IBD)
  isotretinoin and, 237
  reactive neutrophilic dermatoses and, 145
Inflammatory carcinoma, 632, 632f, 635.e6f
Inflammatory lesions, syphilis, 356
Inflammatory linear verrucous epidermal
  nevus, 638–639, 638f
Inflammatory oncotaxis, 744
Inflammatory skin lesions
  after herpes zoster, 378–379, 379f
  in autoinflammatory syndromes, 149
Infliximab
  for acne conglobata, 243
  for acute generalized exanthematous
    pustulosis, 122
  adverse reactions of, 135
  atopic dermatitis and, 71
  for common variable immunodeficiency, 81

Infliximab (*Continued*)
  for dermatomyositis, 170
  for Kawasaki disease, 853–854
  for multicentric reticulohistiocytosis, 725
  for pyoderma gangrenosum, 148–149
  for sarcoidosis, 717
  for small-vessel vasculitis, 837–838
  for Stevens-Johnson syndrome, 118
Infundibular cyst, 678–679
Infundibular segment, hair follicles, 5
Ingram technique, for psoriasis, 198
Ingrown nail, 787–788
Inhalants, urticaria and, 151
Inherited patterned lentiginosis, 688, 688*f*,
  703.*e1f*
Injected filler substances, 43–44, 44*f*
Injection site reactions, 126, 134
  corticosteroids, 137–138
Ink spot lentigo, 687
Inoculation cutaneous tuberculosis from an
  exogenous source, 325–327
Insecta, class of, 439–445
Insecticides, 93
Insulin-induced lipohypertrophy, 495.*e2f*
Insulin-resistant states, acanthosis nigricans
  associated with, 503–504
Intense pulsed light (IPL), 913–914
  nevus flammeus, 593
  for rosacea, 248
  for solar lentigo, 687
Interface dermatitis, 120
Interface reactions, 15
Interferon (IFN) alpha
  for cutaneous lymphoid hyperplasia, 731
  hepatitis C infection, 384–385
  herpes simplex, 369
  for primary cutaneous follicle center cell
    lymphoma, 744
  sarcoidosis and, 716
Interferon (IFN) alpha-2, for polycythemia
  vera, 49
Interferon (IFN) alpha-2b
  for cutaneous lymphoid hyperplasia, 731
  for melanoma, 701
Interferon (IFN)-β, 126
Interferon (IFN)-γ, for atopic dermatitis, 71
Interferon therapy, hair color and, 763
Interferon-mediated diseases, 150
Interferonopathies, 159
Interleukin-2 (IL-2), adverse reactions to, 134
Intermittent hair follicle dystrophy, 766
Internal organ cancer, pruritus and, 47
Internal solid-tissue malignancies, pruritus, 47
Interstitial granulomatous dermatitis (IGD),
  181
Interstitial granulomatous drug reaction
  (IGDR), 709
Interstitial lung disease (ILD),
  dermatomyositis and, 169
Intertrigo, 266–267
  streptococcal, 262
Intestinal parasites, pruritus, 47
Intradermal Spitz nevi, 693
Intraepidermal neutrophilic IgA dermatosis,
  460, 460*f*, 474.*e2f*
Intraepidermal spiral duct, 4
Intrahepatic cholestasis of pregnancy, 465
  pruritus, 48
Intralesional injections
  corticosteroids
    for acne vulgaris, 237–238
    for alopecia areata, 751
    for aphthous stomatitis, 810
    for granuloma faciale, 842–843
    for herpes zoster lesions, 378–379

Intralesional injections (*Continued*)
    for lichen planus of nails, 778
    for Melkersson-Rosenthal syndrome, 798
  steroids
    for cutaneous lymphoid hyperplasia, 731
    for lichen planus, 221–222
    for pyoderma gangrenosum, 148
  triamcinolone
    for alopecia areata, 751
    for granuloma annulare, 706
    for necrobiosis lipoidica, 539
    for prurigo, 52
Intraoral leukoplakia, 802
Intrauterine herpes simplex, 366–367
Intravascular large B-cell lymphoma, 744
Intravascular lymphoma, 635.*e3f*
Intravascular papillary endothelial hyperplasia,
  606
Intravenous contrast material, flushing and,
  140
Intravenous immunoglobulin (IVIG)
  for atopic dermatitis, 71
  for bullous pemphigoid, 463
  chemotherapy-induced acral erythema and,
    130
  for dermatomyositis, 170
  for pemphigus vulgaris, 455
  for Stevens-Johnson syndrome, 118
Invasive staphylococcal infections, 257
Inverse psoriasis, 194, 194*f*
"Invisible" mycosis fungoides, 733
Io moth caterpillar, 439
Iodine, for preoperative antisepsis, 884
Iododerma, 136, 136*f*
Iontophoresis, 76
  for hyperhidrosis, 774
Ipilimumab, for melanoma, 700
IR3535, 437
Iris pearls, 341
Iron
  deposition, dermal, 15–16
  metallic discoloration and, 869–870
  overload, porphyria cutanea tarda, 521
Iron deficiency, 483
  hair color and, 763
  in polycythemia vera, 749
  smooth tongue, 800
  in telogen effluvium, 753
Irritant contact dermatitis, 92–95
  pruritus ani and, 50
Irritant dermatitis, of hands, 55, 55*f*
Irritants, 93
Isavuconazole
  for aspergillosis, 322
  for mucormycosis, 321
Ischemic ulcer, 858
Island pedicle flap, 896, 900*f*
Isodesmosine, 8
Isolated IgA deficiency, 81
Isopropyl alcohol, erythromelalgia, 816
Isotopic response, herpes zoster, 378–379,
  379*f*
Isotretinoin
  for acne conglobata, 243
  for acne vulgaris, 231, 236–237, 237*f*
  for dissecting cellulitis of scalp, 245
  for Gram-negative folliculitis, 241–242
  for mycosis fungoides, 737
  for nevus comedonicus, 637
  for pityriasis rubra pilaris, 208
  for prurigo nodularis, 54
  for staphylococcal infection, 251.*e1f*
  for systemic lupus erythematosus, 166
Isoxazolyl penicillins, for wound infections,
  883

Isthmus, 5
Isthmus-catagen cyst, 679, 679*f*
Itch-scratch cycle, 66
Itchy points, 51
ITGB2 gene, mutation in, leukocyte adhesion
  deficiency and, 86–87
Itraconazole, 291
  for alternariosis, 318
  for candidiasis, 302
  for chromoblastomycosis, 316–317
  for coccidioidomycosis, 309
  for cryptococcosis, 312
  for eosinophilic folliculitis, 417
  for histoplasmosis, 311
  for hyalohyphomycosis, 321
  for North American blastomycosis, 313
  for onychomycosis, 300
  for phaeohyphomycosis, 317
  for prototheosis, 323
  for South American blastomycosis, 314
  for sporotrichosis, 315
  for tinea capitis, 294
  for tinea corporis, 296
  for tinea imbricata, 296
  for tinea of hands and feet, 299
  for tinea versicolor, 307
Ivermectin, for creeping eruption, 433
Ixodes scapularis, 438

J

Jacobi ulcer, 649
Jacquet erosive diaper dermatitis, 76
Janeway spot, 252, 253*f*
Janus kinase (JAK) inhibitors, 200
Jarisch-Herxheimer reaction, 357
Jaw cysts, in Gorlin syndrome, 652
Jellyfish dermatitis, 428, 428*f*
Jessner lymphocytic infiltrate of the skin, 732,
  749.*e1f*
Jessner solution, 932, 932*t*
Jigger, 445
Job syndrome, 87
Jock itch, 297
Jogger's nipples, 73
Joint mobility, limited, in diabetes mellitus,
  539–540
Joules (J), 909
Junctional acral nevus, 689*f*
Junctional epidermolysis bullosa, 560, 560*f*,
  586.*e3f*
  with pyloric atresia, 560
Junctional nevi, 689
Junctional Spitz nevi, 693
Juvederm, 923
Juvenile gout, 545–546
Juvenile hyaline fibromatosis, 613–616, 613*f*
Juvenile idiopathic arthritis, 181–182
Juvenile myelomonocytic leukemia (JMML),
  720
Juvenile plantar dermatosis, 77–78
Juvenile rheumatoid arthritis (JRA), 181–182
Juvenile xanthogranuloma (JXG), 718–721,
  719*f*

K

Kaempferol, for candidiasis, 302
Kala-azar, 425–426
Kamino bodies, 692
Kandahar sore, 422
Kaolin, aphthous stomatitis, 810
Kaposi sarcoma, 36–37, 607–609, 608*f*, 420.*e3f*
  acquired immunodeficiency syndrome and,
    418–420, 418*f*
  bacillary angiomatosis and, 280
  clinical features of, 607–609

Kaposi sarcoma *(Continued)*
  course, 608–609
  epidemiology of, 608
  etiopathogenesis of, 608
  histology of, 608
  human herpesvirus 8 in, 382f, 383
  internal involvement of, 608
  lymphedema in, 860
  treatment of, 608
Kaposi varicelliform eruption, 367–368,
    367f–368f
Kaposiform hemangioendothelioma, 590–591,
    591f
Kaposiform lymphangiomatosis, 602–605
Karyorrhexis
  Sweet syndrome and, 146–147
  urticarial vasculitis, 840
Kasabach-Merritt syndrome (KMS), 591, 591f
Kathon CG, 108–109
Kawasaki disease, 852–854, 853f, 813.e4f
Kayser-Fleischer rings, 543
Ked itch, 443
Keloidal blastomycosis, 319, 319f
Keloids, 13–14, 610–625, 610f, 919–920,
    635.e4f
  acne vulgaris and, 238
Keratin, 1
  laminated, 13
  in nail, 8
  types of, 1
Keratinization, 1
  abnormal, 1
Keratinocytes, 1–3
Keratinocytic epidermal nevi, 636–637
Keratitis-ichthyosis-deafness syndrome, 568,
    568f
Keratoacanthoma, 646–648, 685.e3f
  clinical features of, 646
  histopathology of, 646–647
  in Muir-Torre syndrome, 664–665
  squamous cell carcinoma *vs.*, 654
  treatment of, 647
Keratoacanthoma centrifugum marginatum,
    647–648, 648f
Keratoacanthoma-visceral carcinoma
    syndrome (KAVCS), 646
Keratoconjunctivitis, herpetic, 365
Keratoconus, atopic dermatitis and, 67–68
Keratoderma, palmoplantar, 209
Keratoderma blennorrhagicum, 195, 201f
Keratoderma climactericum, 212
Keratohyalin granules, 2–3
Keratolysis, pitted, 267, 267f, 290.e2f
Keratolysis exfoliativa, 212, 213f, 214.e1f
Keratolytics
  for calluses, 37–38
  for trichostasis spinulosa, 768
Keratosis
  arsenical, 643, 643f, 685.e2f
  benign lichenoid (lichen planus-like),
    642–643, 642f
  lichen planus-like, 642–643, 642f
  seborrheic, 640–641, 641f, 685.e1f–685.e2f
  solar, 644–645
  stucco, 642, 685.e2f
Keratosis follicularis, 572–573
Keratosis follicularis spinulosa decalvans,
    585–586, 761–762
Keratosis lichenoides chronica, 224–225, 224f
Keratosis pilaris, 67, 538, 585
Keratosis pilaris atrophicans, 585–586, 762
Keratosis pilaris rubra faceii, 67
Keratosis punctata, 38
  atopic dermatitis and, 66
  of palmar creases, 209–210, 210f

Keratosis spinulosa, 774
Kerinokeratosis papulosa, 640
Kerion celsii, 292, 292f
Ketamine, for erythromelalgia, 816
Ketoconazole, 291
  for leishmaniasis, 424
  for South American blastomycosis, 314
  for tinea capitis, 294
  for tinea versicolor, 307
KID syndrome, 679–680
Kikuchi disease, 380–381
Kimura disease, 606, 606f
Kindler syndrome, 561
Kinking hair, 766–767
Kissing bugs, 427, 440–441
"Kissing lesions", 443–444
Klebsiella granulomatis, granuloma inguinale
    and, 274
Klebsiella pneumoniae, rhinoscleroma and, 277
"Kligman's formula," for melasma, 864
Klinefelter syndrome, 550
Klippel-Feil syndrome, 584
Klippel-Trenaunay syndrome (KTS), 597,
    597f
Knee, papular sarcoidosis of, 711
Knockdown resistance (KDR), pediculosis
    capitis, 441–442
Knuckle pads, 611, 612f
Koebner phenomenon
  erythema multiforme, 141
  lichen nitidus and, 225
  in psoriasis, 195–196, 196f
  in tattoos, 41
Koenen tumors, 556, 556f
Koilonychia, 781, 781f
Koplik spots, 396, 396f
Korean yellow moth dermatitis, 440–441
KTS-Parkes-Weber, 597
Kwashiorkor, 483–484, 483f–484f
  hair color and, 763
Kyrle disease, 772
Kytococcus sedentarius, 267

L
Labial artery, prominent inferior, 601
Labial melanosis, 687
Laboratory examination, for tinea capitis, 293
Lacaziosis, 319, 319f
Lacquer dermatitis, 99
Lacrimal gland, sarcoidosis in, 715
Lacrimators, 93–94
Lactic acid
  for nevus of Ota, 702
  for winter itch, 49
Lafora disease, 544, 544f
Lagoa crispata, 439
Lahore sore, 422
LAMB syndrome, 688
Lamellar bodies, 1–2
Lamellar dyshidrosis, 212
Lamellar granules, 1–2
Lamellar ichthyosis, 1–2, 564, 564f
Lamina densa, 4
Lamina lucida, 4
Lamins, 493
Lamotrigine, drug-induced hypersensitivity
    syndrome, 115
Langerhans cell histiocytosis (LCH), 726–728
  adult, 727–728
  bony lesions in, 728–729, 729f
  childhood, 727
  oral mucosa lesions in, 728, 729f
  skin lesions in, 727–728, 728f
  treatment and prognosis of, 729–730
  visceral involvement in, 729

Langerhans cells, 3–4, 114
Lanolin, dermatitis, 108
Lanreotide, for acromegaly, 496
Lanugo hair, 750
Large-spore endothrix, 292–293
Large-vessel vasculitis, 836b
Laron syndrome, 763
Larva currens, 433
Larva migrans, 432–433
  cutaneous, 433f, 452.e2f
Larva migrans profundus, 433
Laryngeal papillomatosis, 410–411
Laser hair removal, 918–919, 919f
  hidradenitis suppurativa and, 243
  for pseudofolliculitis barbae, 767
Laser therapy, 18
  for alopecia areata, 751–752
  for common warts, 405
  for hidrocystomas, 666
  for nevus flammeus, 597
  for Osler disease, 855–856
  for pigmented lesions, 914–918
  for solar lentigo, 687
  of vascular lesions, 910–914
  for vitiligo, 873
  see also specific lasers
Latanoprost, hair color and, 763
Latex, anaphylaxis, 112
Latex agglutination test
  for coccidioidomycosis, 309
  for cryptococcosis, 312
Latex gloves, 76
Latrodectism, 450–451, 450f
Laugier-Hunziker syndrome, 868
Lead, 869, 880.e2f
Leeches, 431
Leflunomide
  for dermatomyositis, 170
  for sarcoidosis, 717
Leg ulcers, 856
  arterial, 858
  venous, 856–858, 857f
Legius syndrome, 553
Leiker granuloma multiforme, 709
Leiomyoma, 630–632
Leiomyosarcoma, 631
Leishman-Donovan bodies, 426
Leishmania, 422
Leishmaniasis, 14, 422–426
Leishmaniasis americana, 424–425
Leishmaniasis recidivans, 423, 452.e1f
Leishmanioma, 425
Lelis syndrome, 576
Lemon oil, 100
Lenalidomide
  for prurigo nodularis, 54
  for systemic lupus erythematosus, 166
Lennert lymphoma, 741
Lentigines, 3
  laser treatment for, 914–915
  multiple, 553
Lentiginosis profusa syndrome, 553
Lentiginous melanoma, on sun-damaged skin,
    695
Lentigo, 26, 26f, 686–688
Lentigo maligna, 687, 689, 695, 696f
Lentigo senilis, 686–687
Lentigo simplex, 686
Lenz-Majewski syndrome, 576
LEOPARD syndrome, 553, 553f, 687
Lepidoptera, order, 439–440
Lepromatous leprosy, 339, 339f–340f, 342,
    346.e1f
Lepromin test, 337t
Leptin, 9–10

Leptomeningeal angiomatosis, 596

Leptospirosis, 286

Lesch-Nyhan syndrome, 545–546, 546f

Leser-Trélat sign, 641

"Lester iris", 785

Leukemia

nonspecific conditions associated with, 747

pruritus of, 47

pyoderma gangrenosum and, 148

Sweet syndrome and, 145, 145f, 156.e2f

varicella vaccine and, 372

Leukemia cutis, 22, 746–747, 749.e4f

clinical features of, 746–747

specific eruptions of, 746–747, 746f–747f

Leukemids, 747

Leukocyte adhesion deficiency, 87

Leukocyte adhesion glycoproteins (LAD), deficiency of, 148

Leukocytoclastic vasculitis, 828, 836–838, 837f, 813.e3f

neutrophilic dermatosis of the dorsal hands and, 147

Sweet syndrome and, 146

Leukocytosis, Sweet syndrome and, 146

Leukoderma, 3, 876

chemical, 874–875

vitiligo and, 872

Leukoderma acquisitum centrifugum, 690–691

Leukonychia, 788, 788f

Leukonychia trichophytica, 299

Leukopathia symmetrica progressiva, 870–871, 870f

Leukopenia, subacute cutaneous lupus erythematosus and, 160–161

Leukoplakia, 802–803, 812.e1f

with tylosis and esophageal carcinoma, 803

Leukotriene receptor antagonists, Churg-Strauss syndrome, 137

Leuprolide acetate, flushing and, 140

Levamisole, 848–849

Levamisole-induced vasculopathy/vasculitis, 848–849, 848f

Lhermitte-Duclos disease, 675

Lichen, allergic contact dermatitis from, 99–100

Lichen amyloidosis, 517, 518f, 546.e1f

Lichen aureus, 835

Lichen myxedematosus, 184–187

generalized, 184–185, 185f

localized, 185–186

Lichen nitidus, 11, 225–226, 225f, 230.e3f

Lichen planopilaris, 222–223, 222f

alopecia in, 759, 759f, 793.e2f

Lichen planus, 13, 209, 215–224, 216f, 230.e1f

annular and annular atrophic, 217, 217f, 230.e1f–230.e3f

bullous, 218–219

cancer risk and, 219

differential diagnosis of, 220

erosive/ulcerative/mucosal, 217–218, 218f

follicular, 222–223, 230.e3f

generalized, 220f

hepatitis C and, 384

hepatitis-associated, 219

hypertrophic, 217, 217f

koebnerized, 216f, 230.e2f

linear, 217, 639

of nails, 779, 779f

onychomycosis and, 300

pathogenesis and histology of, 219–220

pruritus vulvae and, 51

and related conditions, 215–230

and tattoos, 41

treatment of, 220–224

Lichen planus follicularis tumidus, 222–223

Lichen planus pemphigoides, 461

Lichen planus pigmentosus, 223–224, 223f

Lichen sclerosus, 227–230, 230.e4f

pruritus vulvae and, 51

vitiligo and, 872

Lichen sclerosus et atrophicus, 227–230, 228f

Lichen scrofulosorum, 330

Lichen simplex chronicus, 53–54, 53f, 62.e1f

tinea capitis and, 294

treatment for, 53–54

Lichen spinulosus, 774

Lichen striatus, 226–227, 226f, 639, 230.e3f–230.e4f

Lichenification, 50, 53

in atopic dermatitis, 66

Lichenoid drug reaction, 129, 135

from gold, 139.e2f

lichen planus and, 220

TNF and, 135

Lichenoid syphilids, 350–351

Liddle sign, 496, 497f

Lidocaine

for anesthesia, 884

for aphthous stomatitis, 810

dosage of, 884–885

for notalgia paresthetica, 59

for pruritus, 46

topical, for pruritus, 51

for zoster-associated pain, 376–377

Light

laser, 909

photodynamic therapy and, 906

Lightning, burns from, 45.e1f

Lime oil, 100

Linalool, 437

Lindane, for scabies, 448

Linear epidermal nevus, 636, 637f

verrucous, 638–639, 638f, 685.e1f

Linear focal elastosis, 513, 513f

Linear IgA bullous dermatosis, 137, 471–473

adult linear IgA disease, 471–472, 472f

childhood linear IgA disease and, 472–473, 472f–473f

Linear IgM dermatosis of pregnancy, 466

Linear lesions, 15

Linear lichen planus, 217, 639

Linear porokeratosis, 571, 572f

"Linear" psoriasis, 639

Linear unilateral basal cell carcinoma syndrome, 653

Linezolid, for nocardiosis, 269

Lingua plicata, 799, 799f

Lingual artery, giant cell arteritis, 849

γ-linolenic acid cream, for CKD-associated pruritus, 48

Linuche unguiculata, 428

Lip licking, 55, 794, 62.e1f

Lip plumper, contact urticaria, 107

Lipedema, lymphedema, 858–859

Lipedematous alopecia, 756

Lipid disturbances, 530–538

Lipids, 7

intravenous therapy, essential fatty acid deficiency and, 482

Lipoatrophia annularis, 495

Lipoatrophy, 493–495

acquired, 494–495

centrifugal abdominal, 495

congenital, 493–494

localized, 495

Lipodermatosclerosis, 488–489, 488f

"Lipodystrophia centrifugalis abdominalis infantilis", 495

Lipodystrophy, 493–495

acquired, 494–495

centrifugal abdominal, 495

congenital generalized, 493, 493f

localized, 495

Lipofibromatosis, 611

Lipohypertrophy, insulin-induced, 495.e2f

Lipoid proteinosis, 536–537, 536f

Lipomas, 628–630

HIV-associated, 417

multiple, 628, 628f

Lipomembranous fat necrosis, 488

α-Lipoprotein deficiency, familial, 534–535

Lipoprotein lipase deficiency, 532, 533f

Liposarcoma, 630

Liposomal amphotericin B, 424

Liposuction, 930–931, 931f

Lipsticks, 107

Liquid nitrogen, 892

for seborrheic keratosis, 641

for solar lentigo, 687

Lisch nodules, 551–552

Lisinopril, adverse reactions, 123

Listeria monocytogenes, 265

Listeriosis, 265

Livedo racemosa, 817–819, 817f, 821, 813.e1f

Livedo reticularis, 817–819

photoinduced, 813.e1f

purpura, 817

with summer/winter ulceration, 819

Livedoid dermatitis, 126

Livedoid vasculopathy, 819–820

Liver

disease

erythropoietic protoporphyria, 524

obstructive, 533

porphyria cutanea tarda, 520–521

pruritus and, 47

hemochromatosis in, 870

transplantation, for α₁-antitrypsin deficiency panniculitis, 492

Liver spots, 686

Liverwort, 99–100

Lizard bite, 452

Loa loa, 435

Lobomycosis, 319, 319f, 323.e5f

Lobstein syndrome, 513

Lobular panniculitis, 487–491

Local anesthetics, 884

for allergic contact dermatitis, 110–111

for zoster-associated pain, 376–377

Localized acquired cutaneous PXE, 508

Localized acquired hypertrichosis, 769

Localized congenital hypertrichosis, 769

Localized granuloma annulare, 704

Localized lipodystrophy, 495

Localized morphea, in scleroderma, 171–172, 171f

Localized vitiligo, 871–872, 880.e1f

L'oedème bleu, 860

Loeffler syndrome, 433

Loeys Dietz syndrome, 510–511

Lofgren syndrome, 485, 711

Loiasis, 435, 435f

Lone star tick, 446, 446f

Longitudinal erythronychia, 788–789

Longitudinal melanonychia, 789

Long-pulsed infrared lasers, 913, 914f

Lonomia achelous, 439

Loose anagen syndrome, 753, 754f, 793.e1f

Loss of heterozygosity (LOH), 547

Louse-borne epidemic typhus, 283

Low-dose rechallenge, HIV and, 119

Lower extremities, allergic contact dermatitis in, 97

Loxoscelism, 451, 451*f*
  treatment of, 451
Lubricants, Sjögren syndrome and, 179–180
Lucio phenomenon, 343, 344*f*
Lues maligna, 351
Lufenuron, 438
LUMBAR syndrome, 589
Lumber workers, allergic contact dermatitis,
  99–100
Lumbosacral radiculopathy, pruritus ani and,
  50
Lung cancer, erythema gyratum repens and,
  144
Lunulae, 8
  red, 790
  spotted, 790
Lupus erythematosus, 8, 137, 157–167
  alopecia in, 758
  annular lesions of, 183.*e2f*
  bullous, 162, 162*f*, 183.*e3f*
  chilblain, 22, 159
  chronic cutaneous, 157–160
  classification of, 158*b*
  complement deficiency syndromes and,
    161
  discoid. *see* Discoid lupus erythematosus
  drug-induced, 164
  erythema multiforme and, 142
  hypertrophic, 159, 159*f*, 183.*e2f*
  Jessner lymphocytic infiltrate of the skin
    vs., 732
  of lip, 183.*e2f*
  neonatal, 161, 161*f*, 183.*e3f*
  polymorphous light eruption and, 31
  subacute cutaneous, 160–161, 160*f*, 183.*e2f*
  systemic. *see* Systemic lupus erythematosus
  tumid, 159–160, 159*f*
Lupus erythematosus panniculitis, 160, 160*f*
Lupus erythematosus-lichen planus overlap
  syndrome, 159, 183.*e2f*
Lupus hair, 183.*e3f*
Lupus miliaris disseminatus faciei, 250, 250*f*
Lupus pernio, 712, 712*f*
Lupus vulgaris, 326–327, 327*f*
"Lupus vulgaris postexanthematicus",
  326–327
Lycopenemia, 484
Lycosidae, 451
Lymantria dispar, 439–440
Lyme disease, 286–288
  granuloma annulare and, 706
  prevention of, 438
Lymph nodes
  mycosis fungoides in, 733, 736
  in secondary syphilis, 352
Lymphadenoma, cutaneous, 674
Lymphadenopathy, 350
  cat-scratch disease and, 279, 279*f*
Lymphadenosis benigna cutis. *see* Cutaneous
  lymphoid hyperplasia
Lymphangioma circumscriptum, 601–602
Lymphangiomatosis, 602
Lymphangiosarcoma, 633
Lymphangitis, 261, 261*f*
  chronic, 261
  tularemia and, 282
Lymphatic system, in secondary syphilis, 352
Lymphedema, 858–860
  classification of, 859*b*
  evaluation of, 861
  treatment of, 861
  types of, 859–861
Lymphedema praecox, 859
Lymphedema-distichiasis syndrome, 859–860
Lymphocyte transformation test (LTT), 113

Lymphocytic hypereosinophilic syndrome,
  748
Lymphocytic thrombophilic arteritis, 844–845
Lymphocytoma cutis. *see* Cutaneous lymphoid
  hyperplasia
Lymphoepithelioid lymphoma, 741
Lymphogranuloma venereum (LGV),
  289–290, 289*f*
  primary lesion of, 290.*e4f*
  scrofuloderma and, 328
Lymphoid-mediated disorders, alopecia in,
  758–759
Lymphomas
  B-cell, 749.*e3f*
  cutaneous, 732–741
  cutaneous T-cell, 122
  intravascular, 749.*e4f*
  lymphomatoid papulosis and, 739
  primary effusion, 383
  Sweet syndrome and, 146
Lymphomatoid papulosis, 738–739, 739*f*, 745,
  749.*e3f*
  type C, 739
Lymphopenia, 83
Lynch syndrome, 665
Lyngbya majuscula Gomont, 100, 429
Lysophosphatidic acid, 48
Lysophosphatidylcholine, 48

M
Maalox, aphthous stomatitis, 810
Macaques, 383
Mace, 94, 94*f*
Macrocomedones, 231
Macrocystic lymphatic malformations, 602
Macrolactams (calcineurin inhibitors), for
  psoriasis, 198
Macrophage activation syndrome (MAS), 123
Macrophage receptor protein, 176
Macrophage/monocyte disorders, 704–730
Maculae ceruleae, 442
Macular amyloidosis, 59, 517, 517*f*, 546.*e1f*
"Macular angiomas", 537
Macular atrophy, 512
Macular depigmentation, 17.*e1f*
Macular eruptions, syphilis, 350
Macular granuloma annulare, 704
Macular lymphocytic arteritis, 844–845
Macular syphilid, tinea versicolor and, 307
Macules, 11
"Maculopapular" cutaneous mastocytosis, 621
Maculopapular reactions, 114, 114*f*
MADH4 gene, 855
Madura foot, 318
Maduromycosis, 318
Mafenide acetate, allergic contact dermatitis,
  110
Maffucci syndrome, 599
MAGIC syndrome, 182
Magnetic resonance angiography, giant cell
  arteritis, 849
Magnification, 14
Majocchi disease. *see* Purpura annularis
  telangiectodes
Majocchi granuloma, 296, 297*f*, 323.*e1f*
Major aphthous ulcer, 810–811, 810*f*
Major histocompatibility complex (MHC), 3
Mal de Meleda, 211
Mal perforans pedis, 61, 61*f*
Malacoplakia, 272
Malaria prophylaxis, 437–438
Malassezia
  fungus, 307
  in tinea versicolor, 306
Malathion gel, 441

Male-pattern baldness, 754–755, 793.*e1f*
Malherbe calcifying epithelioma, 672
Malignancy
  flushing and, 140
  in Henoch-Schönlein purpura, 839
  in multicentric reticulohistiocytosis,
    724–725
  palmoplantar keratoderma and, 211
  Peutz-Jeghers syndrome and, 868
  radiation therapy and, 907–908
  in sarcoidosis, 716
Malignant "angioendotheliomatosis", 744
Malignant atrophic papulosis, 850–851
Malignant blue nevus, 703
Malignant degeneration, 689–690
Malignant fibrous histiocytoma, 36–37,
  619–620
Malignant histiocytosis, 745–746, 749.*e4f*
Malignant melanoma, 703.*e4f*
  see also Melanomas
Malignant mixed tumor, 669
Malignant pilomatricoma, 672–673
Malignant trichilemmal cyst, 679–680, 680*f*
Malingering, 57
Mallorca acne, 240
Malnutrition, 479
  protein-energy, 483–484
Malpighian layer, 1
MALT-type lymphoma, 743
Mandibuloacral dysplasia, 494
Mandibulofacial dysostosis, 582
Mango dermatitis, 99
β-Mannosidase deficiency, 538
Mantleomas, 676–677
Mantoux test, tuberculosis, 325
Marasmus, 483
Marburg virus (MARV), 395
Marfan syndrome, 8, 510, 510*f*
Marginal mandibular nerve, 885–887
Marginal plaques, collagenous and elastotic,
  of hands, 212
Marine plants, allergic contact dermatitis
  from, 100
Marinesco-Sjögren syndrome, 583
Marshall syndrome, 147
Marshall-White syndrome, 822
Marsupialization, for dissecting cellulitis of
  scalp, 245
MASP2 deficiency, 88
Mast cells, 9
  sarcoma, 623
  staining of, 9
Masters disease, 286
Mastigophora, class of, 421–427
Mastocytosis, 9, 621, 635.*e5f*
  biochemical studies, 623
  clinical classification of, 621, 622*b*
  cutaneous, 622
  diagnosis of, 624
  differential diagnosis of, 624
  flushing and, 140
  histopathology of, 623–624
  prognosis of, 624
  systemic, 622
  treatment of, 624
Matchbox sign, 55
Maternal allergen avoidance, 64
MATP gene, oculocutaneous albinism in, 880
Matrix keratinization, 8
Maxacalcitol, for ichthyosis, 565–566
May-Hegglin anomaly, 834
Mayo Muir-Torre Syndrome (MTS), 665*t*
McKusick syndrome, 584
Mckusick-type metaphyseal chondrodysplasia,
  584

Measles, 395–397, 396f
Mebendazole
for hookworm, 432
for pinworm, 432
Mechanical injuries, 37
"Mechanic's hands," in dermatomyositis, 167, 168f
Mechlorethamine hydrochloride, for mycosis fungoides, 736
Medallion-like purpura, 839–840, 839f
Median nail dystrophy, 786, 786f
Median raphe cysts, 684, 684f
Median rhomboid glossitis, 801, 801f
Medication pigment, 863
Medication-induced hyperlipoproteinemia, 533
Medina worm, 433–434
Mediterranean spotted fever, 285
Mediterranean visceral leishmaniasis, 423
Medium-depth peel, 932
Medium-sized congenital nevocytic nevus, 691–692, 703.e2f
Medium-vessel vasculitis, 836b
Medullary thyroid carcinoma, flushing and, 140
Mees lines, 783–784, 784f
Meffert sign, 798
MEFV gene, 149
Megalencephaly capillary malformation, 597
Megalopyge crispata, 439
Meglumine antimoniate, 424
Meibomian glands, 7
Meige syndrome, 859f
Meirowsky phenomenon, 24
Meissner corpuscles, 9
Melaleuca oil, 99
Melanin, 3, 686, 862
hair color and, 762
in phaeohyphomycosis, 317
pigmentation, abnormalities in, 14
skin color, 15
Melanoacanthoma, 641, 688–689, 689f
Melanoblast, migration and survival disorders of, 878–879
Melanocortin 1 receptor (MC1R), 3
Melanocytes, 3
in hair, 7, 762
transport disorders, 877–878
"Melanocytic matricoma", 672
Melanocytic nevi, 686–703
benign, 689–695, 689f
congenital, 691–692
Melanocytic oral lesions, 805–806, 805f
Melanocytosis, acquired dermal, 862
Melanoderma, 94
Melanogenesis, delayed, 24
Melanomas, 3, 11, 695–701, 703.e3f
biopsy for, 698
differential diagnosis of, 697–698
dysplastic nevus and, 693
etiologic factors of, 695
giant pigmented nevus and, 691
histopathology of, 698
metastasis in, 698–699, 698f
Mohs micrographic surgery and, 905–906
nevus spilus and, 686
in preexisting nevi, 689–690
prognosis of, 699–700
regressing, 691
in situ, 687
skin type risk for, 26
in Spitz nevus, 692–693
staging of, 699, 699b
subungual, 790, 792f
treatment of, 700–701

Melanomas (Continued)
types of, 695–697
in vitiligo, 872
workup and follow-up for, 700
Melanonychia, 789–790, 789f
Melanosis, 806, 806f
arsenical, 128
labial, penile, and vulvar, 687, 687f
neurocutaneous, 691
oral, 805–806, 805f
transient neonatal pustular, 867, 867f
Melanosomes, 3, 762, 862
in hair, 7
Melanotic macules, 687
Melarsoprol, trypanosomiasis and, 427
MELAS syndrome, 586
Melasma, 863–865, 864f
Melasma, laser treatment for, 915–916
Melatonin, for female-pattern alopecia, 755
Meleney gangrene, 268
Melioidosis, 279
Melkersson-Rosenthal syndrome, 798, 798f, 812.e1f
Meloidae, 443
Melophagus ovinus, 443
Meningitis, cryptococcosis and, 311
Meningocele, 627–628
Meningococcemia, 275, 275f, 290.e3f
Meningovascular neurosyphilis, 354
Menkes steely (kinky) hair syndrome, 764, 793.e2f
Menopausal flushing, 140
Menthol
pruritus, 46
topical, for chronic urticaria, 154
Mequinol, for solar lentigo, 687
Meralgia paresthetica, 60
Mercaptobenzothiazole, 105
Mercury
adverse reactions, 135–136
allergic contact dermatitis, 103
Mercury granuloma, 42, 42f
Merkel cell carcinoma, 661–662, 661f, 685.e4f
Merkel cell polyomavirus (MCPyV), 661
Merlin, 553
Metabolism, errors in, 515–546
Metal salts, allergic contact dermatitis, 102–104
Metallic discolorations, 868–870
Metals
allergic contact dermatitis, 102–104
hyperpigmentation, 128
Metastases
of basal cell carcinoma, 655
of melanomas, 698–699, 698f
of Merkel cell carcinoma, 661
of squamous cell carcinoma, 655
Metastatic calcinosis cutis, 527–528
Metastatic carcinoma, 632
Metastatic malignant melanoma, 703.e5f
Metformin
for acquired lipodystrophy, 494
for androgen-dependent syndromes, 499
for hirsutism, 771
Methicillin-resistant Staphylococcus aureus (MRSA), 252, 882
Methionine, homocystinuria, 511
Methotrexate
adverse reactions to, 134
for alopecia areata, 751–752
for atopic dermatitis, 71
for Behçet syndrome, 811–812
for bullous pemphigoid, 463
for Churg-Strauss syndrome, 847–848

Methotrexate (Continued)
for dermatomyositis, 170
for keratoacanthoma, 647
for Langerhans cell histiocytosis, 729
for lymphomatoid papulosis, 739
for multicentric reticulohistiocytosis, 725
for mycosis fungoides, 737
and pigmented purpura, 836
for pityriasis lichenoides et varioliformis acuta, 740
for pityriasis rubra pilaris, 208
for psoriasis, 199
for pyoderma gangrenosum, 149
for rheumatoid arthritis, 180
for sarcoidosis, 717
for scleroderma, 176
for Sézary syndrome, 738
for small-vessel vasculitis, 837–838
for systemic lupus erythematosus, 165
for Takayasu arteritis, 850
Methoxsalen, for alopecia areata, 751–752
8-Methoxypsoralen, for vitiligo, 873
Methyl aminolevulinate (mALA), 906
Methyl bromide, 93
Methylchloroisothiazolinone/ methylisothiazolinone (MCI/MI), 108–109
Methyldibromoglutaronitrile, 108–109
Methylnicotinate-induced flushing, 140
Methylparaben, allergic contact dermatitis, 110
Methylprednisolone
for alopecia areata, 751
for dermatomyositis, 170
for pemphigus vulgaris, 455
for pyoderma gangrenosum, 148–149
Metronidazole
for creeping eruption, 433
flushing and, 140
for Guinea worm disease, 434
for trichomoniasis, 422
for venous leg ulcers, 857
Mevalonate kinase (MVK) gene, mutations in, 150
Meyerson's nevus, 691
MIB-1 (Ki-67), in Spitz nevus, 692–693
Micaceous balanitis, 659
Micafungin, 292
for aspergillosis, 322
"Michelin tire baby" syndrome, 630, 630f
Miconazole
for diaper dermatitis, 76
for pitted keratolysis, 267
Microcephaly capillary malformation syndrome, 598
Microcystic adnexal carcinoma, 670–671, 671f
Microcystic lymphatic malformation, 601–602, 601f
β$_2$-Microglobulin amyloidosis, 516–517
Microhemagglutination assay for T. pallidum (MHA-TP), 348
Micronodular basal cell carcinoma, 649
Microsatellite instability, in Muir-Torre syndrome, 665
Microscopic polyangiitis, 845–846
Microsporum audouinii, 292
Microsporum canis, 292
Microsporum nanum, 295
Microvenular hemangioma, 607
MIDAS syndrome, 579
Miescher granuloma, 708–709, 708f, 730.e1f
Mikulicz syndrome, 715
Milia, 682–683, 682f
Milia-like idiopathic calcinosis cutis, 528
Milian citrine skin, 26

Miliaria, 19–20
  treatment for, 20
Miliaria crystallina, 19–20, 19f
Miliaria profunda, 20
Miliaria pustulosa, 20
Miliaria rubra, 20, 20f
Miliary (disseminated) tuberculosis, 328
Miliary sarcoid, 711
Milker's nodules, 389, 389f
Millipede burns, 439, 439f
Milroy disease, 859f
Miltefosine, leishmaniasis, 424, 426
Mineral oils, 94
Minocycline
  for acne vulgaris, 235, 235f
  for acneiform eruptions, 241
  for confluent and reticulated papillomatosis, 209
  for hyperpigmentation, 127, 127f–128f
  for hypersensitivity syndrome, 116
  for livedo, 818
  for milia en plaque, 683
  for nocardiosis, 269
  for prurigo pigmentosa, 52–53
  for pyoderma gangrenosum, 149
Minor's starch-iodine test, 927, 927f–928f
Minoxidil
  for alopecia areata, 751–752
  for female-pattern alopecia, 755
  hair color and, 763
  for male-pattern alopecia, 754
Mismatch repair (MMR) genes, 665
Mites, 447–450
Mixed connective tissue disease, 178, 178f, 183.e7f
Mixed porphyria, 523
Mixed size vasculitis, 836b
MMP-1, 27
MMP-3, 27
MMP-9, 27
Modified varicella-like syndrome, 372
Mohs micrographic surgery, 905–906, 905f
  indications for, 905–906, 905b, 905f
  for melanoma, 700
  for verrucous carcinoma, 659
Moisturizers
  for atopic dermatitis, 68
  for hand eczema, 75
  for photoaging, 28
Mokihana burn, 29
Moles, 689
Molluscoid pseudotumors, 510
Molluscum bodies, 392
Molluscum contagiosum, 390–393, 391f, 420.e5f–420.e6f
  in atopic dermatitis, 68
Molluscum contagiosum-like lesions, cryptococcosis and, 311
Molluscum-like lesions, of cryptococcosis, 323.e3f
Mometasone, 110–111
Mondor disease, 39, 832–833, 832f
Mongolian spots, 15, 702
Monilethrix, 765–766, 765f
Monobenzone, for total depigmentation, 873–874
Monobenzyl, occupational vitiligo and, 874
Monoclonal gammopathy, pyoderma gangrenosum and, 148
Monocyte disorders, 704–730
Monofilament absorbable suture, 887–888
Monosymptomatic hypochondriacal disorder, 55
Montelukast
  for cholinergic urticaria, 151–152
  for pressure urticaria, 152–153

Montgomery syndrome, 722
Montgomery tubercles, 7
Morbilliform reactions, 114, 114f
Morgellons disease, 56
Morphea, 8, 183.e5f
  alopecia in, 757
  generalized, 172, 172f
  guttate, 172
  linear, 172, 172f
  localized, in scleroderma, 171–172, 171f
  pansclerotic, 172
  vitiligo and, 872
Morphea profunda, 172
Morpheaform basal cell carcinoma, 648–649
Morpheaform sarcoidosis, 714
Morphea-lichen sclerosus et atrophicus overlap, 172
Morpheic basal cell carcinoma, 648–649
Mosaicism, 547–555
Mosquito bites, 442–443
Mosquito Magnet, 437–438
Mosquito traps, 437–438
Mosquitoes
  Chikungunya virus and, 401
  dengue and, 400
  filariasis and, 434
  Sindbis virus and, 401
Mossy foot, 860–861
Moth dermatitis, 439–440
Motor nerve neuropathy, 375
Mottled pigmentation, epidermolysis bullosa simple with, 559
Mouth, pemphigus vulgaris in, 453
Mouthwashes, dermatitis, 108
Moxidectin, for onchocerciasis, 436
Moyamoya disease, 818
Moynahan syndrome, 687
MQX-503, for Raynaud disease, 814
MRSA. *see* Methicillin-resistant *Staphylococcus aureus* (MRSA)
Mucha-Habermann disease, 739–740, 739f, 749.e3f
Mucin, extramammary Paget disease, 659–660
Mucinoses, 184–190
  cutaneous focal mucinosis, 189
  follicular mucinosis, 188–189, 188f–189f, 190.e2f
  lichen myxedematosus, 184–187
    generalized, 184–185, 185f
    localized, 185–186
  myxoid cysts, 189–190, 189f, 190.e2f
  reticular erythematous mucinosis, 188, 188f, 190.e2f
  scleredema, 187–188, 187f, 190.e2f
  venous insufficiency and obesity-associated, 856
Mucinous carcinoma, 671
Muckle-Wells syndrome, 150
Mucocele, 807, 807f
Mucocutaneous leishmaniasis, 424–425, 425f, 452.e1f
Mucocutaneous lymph node syndrome, 852–854, 853f
Mucolipidosis type I, 538
Mucopolysaccharides, deposits of, 499, 500f
Mucopolysaccharidoses, 184
Mucopolysaccharidosis I, 543
Mucopolysaccharidosis II, 543–544
Mucormycosis, 320–321
Mucosal lentigines, 687
Mucosal lesions, filovirus, 395
Mucosal lichen planus, 217–218, 218f
Mucosal melanoma, 697
Mucosal sarcoidosis, 714
Mucosal vitiligo, 872–873

Mucous extravasation phenomenon, 807
Mucous membrane
  disorders of, 794–812
  Hansen disease and, 341, 341f
Mucous membrane lesions
  in Epstein-Barr virus, 380
  in secondary syphilis, 352, 352f
  in systemic lupus erythematosus, 162
Mucous retention cysts, 807
Muehrcke lines, 783, 784f
Muir-Torre syndrome, 664–665
Multicentric reticulohistiocytosis (MRH), 724–725, 724f
Multifocal lymphangioendotheliomatosis, 602–603
Multikinase inhibitors, cutaneous side effects of, 132, 133f
Multimodality immunomodulatory therapy, for mycosis fungoides, 736
Multiple carboxylase deficiency, 480, 481f
Multiple cutaneous leiomyomas, 630, 631f
Multiple endocrine neoplasia type I (MEN-1), 502, 502f
Multiple endocrine neoplasia type IIA (MEN-2A) syndrome, 518–519
Multiple familial trichoepithelioma, 673–674
Multiple hamartoma syndrome, 674–676
Multiple keratoacanthomas, 647
Multiple leiomyomas, 635.e6f
Multiple lentigines, 553
  syndrome, 687
Multiple lipomas, 628, 628f
Multiple minute digitate hyperkeratosis (MMDH), 640
Multiple mucosal neuromas, 625, 626f
Multiple myeloma, 744–745, 745f
Multiple sclerosis, pruritus, 47
Multiple spindle cell nevi, 703.e3f
Multiple sulfatase deficiency, 569
Multisystem Langerhans cell histiocytosis, 729
MUM1, 744
Munchausen syndrome, 57
Murine typhus, 284
Muscidae, 442
Muscles
  biopsy, for trichinosis, 437
  changes, in dermatomyositis, 168
  skin, 9
Muscular dystrophy, epidermolysis bullosa simple with, 560
Mushroom poisoning, erythromelalgia, 816
"Music box spines", 210, 210f
Myalgias, Sweet syndrome and, 145–146
Mycetoma, 318–319, 318f, 323.e4f
Mycobacteria, classification of, 332
Mycobacterial diseases, 324–335
  nontuberculous mycobacteriosis, 332–335
  tuberculosis, 324–332
Mycobacterium avium intracellulare complex, 334, 334f, 335.e2f
Mycobacterium bovis, 325
Mycobacterium chelonae/abscessus, 333–334, 334f
Mycobacterium fortuitum, 333–334, 334f
Mycobacterium haemophilum, 333
Mycobacterium kansasii, 334–335
Mycobacterium marinum, 38, 332, 332f, 335.e1f–335.e2f
Mycobacterium tuberculosis, 324
Mycobacterium ulcerans, 333
Mycolactone, 333
Mycophenolate, for chronic urticaria, 154
Mycophenolate mofetil (MMF)
  for atopic dermatitis, 71
  for dermatomyositis, 170
  for pemphigus vulgaris, 455

Mycophenolate mofetil (MMF) *(Continued)*
  pyoderma gangrenosum and, 149
  for sarcoidosis, 717
  for scleroderma, 176
  for small-vessel vasculitis, 837–838
  for systemic lupus erythematosus, 166
  for urticarial vasculitis, 840–841
Mycoplasma, 288–289
Mycoplasma infection, erythema multiforme
    and, 141
Mycoplasma pneumoniae, 288–289
Mycoses, superficial and deep, 291–292
Mycosis fungoides, 214, 732–737,
    749.e1f–749.e2f
  clinical features of, 733–735, 733f–734f
  differential diagnosis of, 736
  erythroderma and, 214
  evaluation and staging of, 733
  histopathology of, 735–736
  HIV-associated, 418
  natural history of, 732–733
  pathogenesis of, 735
  syringotropic, 749.e2f
  systemic manifestations of, 735
  treatment of, 736–737
Mycosis fungoides palmaris et plantaris,
    737–738
Mycotic pruritus ani, 50
Myelodysplastic syndromes, 746
  Sweet syndrome and, 146
Myelofibrosis, 747–748
Myeloid leukemia, 746
Myeloid metaplasia, pyoderma gangrenosum
    and, 148
Myeloma
  multiple, 744–745, 745f
  pyoderma gangrenosum and, 148
Myeloperoxidase (MPO), 845
Myeloproliferative hypereosinophilic
    syndrome, 748
Myiasis, 443, 443f
Myocarditis, systemic lupus erythematosus
    and, 163
Myoepithelioma, cutaneous, 669
Myoepitheliomas, 628
Myopericytoma, 593
Myospherulosis, 490
Myriapoda, class of, 438–439
Myrmecia, 404, 404f
Myroxylon pereirae, 95, 106
Myxedema, 499, 500f
  pretibial, 500–501, 504.e1f
Myxedema, scleroderma *vs.*, 175
Myxoid cysts, 189–190, 189f, 190.e2f
Myxomas, 620–621, 621f

N
Naegeli-Franceschetti-Jadassohn syndrome
    (NFJS), 548–549, 867
Nafcillin, for wound infection, 883
Nagashima-type PPK, 211
Nail bed
  neoplasms of, 791–793
  purpura of, 790
Nail en raquette, 785, 785f
Nail isthmus keratinization, 8
Nail matrix nevi, 690
Nail plate, 8
  staining of, 790
Nail products, 107
Nail-patella syndrome, 785, 785f
Nails, 7–8, 16–17
  avulsion
    onychocryptosis and, 787
    onychomycosis and, 300

Nails *(Continued)*
  biting, 785
  discolorations of, 788–793
  diseases of, 778–788
  epidermal growth factor receptors (EGFR)
      and, 132, 132f
  keratosis lichenoides chronica and, 224–225
  Langerhans cell histiocytosis in, 728
  lichen planus and, 215, 216f, 230.e2f
  lichen striatus and, 226
  pitting, in psoriasis, 193f, 204.e1f
  sarcoidosis, 714
  toxicity of, 132
  Zinsser-Cole-Engman syndrome in, 574
Nakajo-Nishimura syndrome, 22
"Naked tubercle", 715
Nalfurafine
  for CKD-associated pruritus, 48
  for pruritus, 46–47
Naloxone
  for biliary pruritus, 48
  for pruritus, 46–47
Naltrexone, for pruritus, 46–47
NAME syndrome, 688
Naphthalene oils, 94
Napkin dermatitis, 76–77
Napkin psoriasis, 76, 77f, 194, 91.e2f
Naproxen, photosensitivity, 125
Narcotic dermopathy, 40
Narrow-band (NB) UVB phototherapy
  for CKD-associated pruritus, 48
  for pigmented purpura, 836
  for vitiligo, 873
Narrow-hole extrusion, 888, 890f
Nasal bridge collapse, 341, 341f
Nasal crease, 66–67, 91.e1f
Nasal glioma, 627, 627f
Nasal/nasal-type NK/T-cell lymphoma, 742,
    742f
National Alopecia Areata Foundation, 752
Nattrassia mangiferae, 299–300
NDDH. *see* Neutrophilic dermatoses, of
    dorsal hands
Necatoriasis, 432
Neck, allergic contact dermatitis in, 96–97, 97f
"Neck sign," of progressive systemic sclerosis,
    174
Necrobiosis lipoidica, 538–540, 539f
Necrobiosis lipoidica diabeticorum, 538–540,
    546.e3f
Necrobiotic xanthogranuloma (NXG),
    709–711, 710f
Necrolytic acral erythema, 384, 384f, 420.e3f
Necrotizing fasciitis, 261–262, 262f, 290.e2f
Necrotizing glomerulitis, 846
Necrotizing livedo, 817
Nectinopathies, 576–577
Neem oil, 437
Neisseria gonorrhoeae, 274–275
Neisseria meningitidis, 275
Nemathelminthes, 431–437
Nematoda, class, 431–432
Nematode dermatitis, 432
NEMO gene, 548
  mutations in, 81
Neodymium:yttrium-aluminum-garnet
    (Nd:YAG) laser therapy, 914
  for Mongolian spot, 702
  for onychomycosis, 300
Neomycin, 95, 110
Neonatal acne, 231
Neonatal lupus erythematosus, 161, 161f,
    183.e3f
Neonatal-onset multisystem inflammatory
    disease, 150

Neonates
  herpes simplex in, 366–367, 367f
  varicella in, 372
Neoplasms
  with dermatomyositis, 169
  oral, 802–806
Nephrogenic systemic fibrosis, 178–179,
    190.e1f
Nerve blocks
  for lichen planus of nails, 778
  for meralgia paresthetica, 60
  for psoriatic nails, 779
  for zoster-associated pain, 376–377
Nerve sheath myxoma, 625–626
Nerves
  dermis and, 9
  Hansen disease and, 339–341, 341f
Netherton syndrome, 567, 567f
Neumann type, of pemphigus vegetans, 456
Neural tissue, 624–625
Neurilemmoma, 635.e6f
Neurocutaneous dermatoses, 46–62
Neurocutaneous melanocytosis, 691
Neurofibromas, 550–551, 551f
Neurofibromatosis, type 1, 550–553, 551f
  juvenile xanthogranuloma and, 720
Neurofibromin, 552
Neuroleptics, for vulvodynia, 59
Neurologic alopecia, 756
Neurologic disorders, and livedo, 818
Neuroma cutis, 625
Neuromediators, itching and, 46
Neuropathic pain, Fabry disease, 537
Neuropathic ulcers, 61, 858
Neuropeptides, itching and, 46
Neurosarcoidosis, 715
Neurosyphilis, 354–355
  early, 354
  late (parenchymatous), 354–355
  meningovascular, 354
Neurothekeoma, 625–626
Neurotic excoriations, 56, 56f
Neurotrophins, 3
Neutral lipid storage disease, 567
Neutropenia
  cyclic or periodic, 808
  in fusariosis, 321–322
Neutrophilia, Sweet syndrome and, 146
Neutrophilic dermatoses
  acute febrile, 145–147, 145f
    diagnostic criteria for, 146b
  of dorsal hands (NDDH), 147, 147f,
    156.e2f
  reactive, 145–149
  rheumatoid, 180, 181f, 183.e8f
Neutrophilic eccrine hidradenitis, 778
Neutrophilic figurate erythema of infancy,
    144
Neutrophilic sebaceous adenitis, 708–709
Neutrophilic urticaria, 153
  with systemic inflammation, 150
  urticarial vasculitis and, 840
Neutrophil-mediated disorders, alopecia in,
    760–761
Nevi, 3
  blue, 15, 17.e2f
  distribution of lesions, 14
  epidermal, 636–639
  sebaceous, 662–665, 685.e5f
Nevirapine, hypersensitivity syndrome, in
    HIV patients, 119–120
Nevocytic nevi, 689
Nevoid basal cell carcinoma syndrome
    (NBCCS), 652–653, 652f
"Nevoid" psoriasis, 639

Nevus anemicus, 600, 601f, 635.e2f
Nevus araneus, 603
Nevus ceruleus, 702
Nevus comedonicus, 637, 637f, 685.e1f
"Nevus comedonicus syndrome", 637
Nevus flammeus, 11, 603
Nevus fuscoceruleus ophthalmomaxillaris, 702
Nevus lipomatosus superficialis, 629
Nevus of Ito, 702
    laser treatment for, 915
Nevus of Ota, 702, 702f, 703.e5f
    laser treatment for, 915, 916f
Nevus oligemicus, 600
Nevus sebaceus, 662–663, 663f
Nevus sebaceus syndrome, with lipodermoid of conjunctiva, 685.e1f
Nevus simplex, 595, 595f
Nevus spilus, 687f, 703.e1f
Nevus verrucosus, 636
New World leishmaniasis, 423f, 452.e1f
Newborn, subcutaneous fat necrosis of, 489, 489f
Niacin
    deficiency in, 479–480, 480f
    flushing and, 140
Nickel
    allergic contact dermatitis and, 102–103, 103f
    hand eczema and, 74
Nicolau syndrome, 126
Nicotinamide
    for pellagra, 480
    for pemphigus vulgaris, 456
Nicotine patches, Degos disease, 850–851
Niemann-Pick disease, 535
Nifedipine
    for chilblains, 22
    for Raynaud disease, 814
    for Raynaud of the nipple, 813
    for scleroderma, 176
Nifurtimox, trypanosomiasis and, 427
Nigua, 445
Nikolsky sign, 13
Nipples
    eczema, 73–74, 74f
    hyperkeratosis of, 639, 685.e1f
    Paget disease of, 659, 659f
Nit, 441
Nitric acid, 92
Nitrile gloves, for hand eczema, 76
Nitrites, flushing and, 140
Nitrogen mustard, topical, for mycosis fungoides, 736
Nitroglycerin
    for chondrodermatitis nodularis chronica helicis, 616
    for Raynaud disease, 814
Nitrosoureas, anagen effluvium and, 753
Nits, 763
NK/T-cell lymphoma, 742, 742f
NLRP3 gene, mutations in, 150
Nocardia, 269, 269f
Nocardia asteroides, 269
Nocardia brasiliensis, 269
Nocardiosis, 269, 269f, 290.e2f
NOD2 gene, mutations in, 150
Nodal nevi, 690
Nodular basal cell carcinoma, 648, 648f
Nodular fasciitis, 618
Nodular granulomatous phlebitis, 330
Nodular hidradenoma, 666–667
Nodular lichen myxedematosus, 186
Nodular lymphoid, 8
Nodular melanoma, 697

Nodular primary localized cutaneous amyloidosis, 518
Nodular pseudosarcomatous fasciitis, 618
Nodular syphilid, 353
Nodular tuberculid, 330
Nodular vasculitis, 487–488, 487f
Nodules, 11
Noma, 808
Nonabsorbable sutures, 889–892
Noncicatricial alopecia, 750–756
Nonepidermolytic epidermal nevi, 636
Non-Hodgkin lymphoma, 732
Noninfectious immunodeficiency disorders, 63–91
Noninvoluting congenital hemangioma, 590
Nonmelanoma skin cancer (NMSC), 643–644, 643f
    HIV-associated, 417–418
    radiation therapy for, 908
Non-mycosis fungoides CD30-cutaneous large T-cell lymphoma, 741
Non-mycosis fungoides CD30-pleomorphic small/medium-sized cutaneous T-cell lymphoma, 741
Nonne-Milroy-Meige syndrome, 859, 859f
Nonsteroidal antiinflammatory drugs (NSAIDs)
    adverse drug reactions of, 112–113
    for erythema nodosum, 486–487
    fixed drug reactions and, 120
    for meralgia paresthetica, 60
    photosensitivity and, 124, 124f
    for pseudoporphyria, 522
    for small-vessel vasculitis, 837–838
    for sunburn, 24–25
    for TRAPS, 149
    urticaria and, 122
Nonsynthetic sutures, 887
Nonthrombocytopenic purpura, 826–828
Nontreponemal tests, 348
Nontuberculous mycobacteriosis, 332–335
Nonvenereal treponematoses, 359–361
Non-X histiocytoses, 718–726
Noonan syndrome, 553
Noonan syndrome-like disorder with loose anagen hair (NSLAH), 553
Norape cretata, 439
Norepinephrine, adrenergic urticaria and, 152
Normolipemic papuloeruptive xanthomatosis, 532
Normolipemic xanthoma, 532
North American blastomycosis, 312–313, 313f, 323.e3f
Norwegian scabies, 448
Nose
    pellagra and, 480
    perforating folliculitis of, 772
Nosebleeds, in Osler disease, 855
Notalgia paresthetica, 16, 59
NOTCH3 gene, 544
NSAIDs. see Nonsteroidal antiinflammatory drugs (NSAIDs)
NSDHL gene, 534
N-serrated pattern, of immunoglobulins, 453
Nummular lesion, 15
Nutritional deficiency, diagnosis of, 475
Nutritional disease, 475–484
Nutritional status, telogen effluvium and, 752–753
Nystatin, 291

O

Obesity
    lymphedema and, 860
    mucinosis and venous insufficiency, 856

Obestatin, 9–10
O'Brien actinic granuloma, 708–709, 708f
Obstructive liver disease, 533
Obstructive purpura, 833, 833f
Occipital horn syndrome, 508, 763
Occlusive dressings
    for pressure ulcers, 39
    for pyoderma gangrenosum, 148
    for venous leg ulcers, 857
Occlusive therapy, for common warts, 405
Occupational contact dermatitis, 110–111, 139.e1f
    management of, 111–112
Occupational hand edema, 861
Occupational vitiligo, 874–875
Ochronosis, 15–16, 541–543, 542f
    exogenous, 542–543, 542f
Ochronotic arthropathy, 542
Octreotide
    for acromegaly, 496
    for nevus sebaceus, 663
Ocular rosacea, 246–247, 246f
Oculodermal melanocytosis, 702
Oculoglandular syndrome of Parinaud, 279
Oculoglandular tularemia, 282–283
Oculo-oral-genital syndrome, 811–812, 811f
Odontogenic sinus, 812.e1f
Odontogenous sinus, 802, 802f
Odonto-tricho-ungual-digital-palmar syndrome, 576
Oedemeridae, 443
Ogna, epidermolysis bullosa simplex, 560
Ohara disease, 282
Ointments
    for atopic dermatitis, 69
    for nummular eczema, 78
Oklahoma puss caterpillar, 439
Olanzapine, for delusions of parasitosis, 56
Old World leishmaniasis, 422, 422f
Ollendorf (Buschke-Ollendorff) sign, 350–351
Ollier disease, 599
Olmsted syndrome, 212, 212f
Omalizumab, for chronic urticaria, 154
Omenn syndrome, 82
Onchocerca volvulus, 436
Onchocerciasis, 435–436, 435f–436f
Ondansetron, pruritus, 48
Onion, allergic contact dermatitis, 99
"Onion skin," alopecia cicatrisata, 760
Onychauxis, 782
Onychoatrophy, 782
Onychocryptosis, 787–788
Onychogryphosis, 782
Onycholemmal carcinoma, 791
Onycholysis, 786
    in lichen planus, 215
Onychomadesis, 782–783, 783f
Onychomatricoma, 790, 791f
Onychomycosis, 299–301, 299f
    diagnosis of, 300
    differential diagnosis of, 300
    treatment for, 300–301
    types of, 299
Onychopapillomas, 790
Onychophagia, 55, 55f, 785–786, 793.e5f
Onychophosis, 782
Onychorrhexis, 784
Onychoschizia, 784–785, 784f
Onychotillomania, 786
Ophiasis, 750, 751f, 793.e1f
Ophthalmia nodosa, 439
Ophthalmic zoster, 375, 375f
Ophthalmologic abnormalities, in atopic dermatitis, 68
Opiate analgesia, zoster-associated pain, 377

Opioids, for pruritus, 46–47, 52
Orabase, aphthous stomatitis, 810
Oral antimicrobial therapy, for psoriasis, 199
Oral candidiasis, 302–303
Oral commissure burns, 18, 19*f*
Oral contraceptives
    for acne vulgaris, 236
    for androgen excess, 499
    erythema nodosum, 485
    for hirsutism, 771
    lichen sclerosus and, 228
    for melasma, 864
Oral Crohn disease, 796–797
Oral erythema multiforme, 143, 156.*e1f*
Oral florid papillomatosis, 803
Oral hairy leukoplakia, 380, 380*f*, 802, 803*f*,
    420.*e3f*
Oral immunomodulatory therapy, for
    necrobiosis lipoidica, 539
Oral lichenoid lesion (OLL), 218
Oral melanoacanthoma, 688–689, 805
Oral melanotic macules, 805
Oral mucosa, 16–17, 16*f*
    lesions, in Langerhans cell histiocytosis,
        728, 729*f*
Oral papillomas, in Cowden syndrome, 675*f*,
    685.*e6f*
Oral papillomatosis, 555
Oral submucous fibrosis, 616, 617*f*
Orf, 389–390, 390*f*, 420.*e5f*
Organoid nevus, 662–663, 663*f*
Orgyia pseudotsugata, 439
Oriental sore, 422
Ornithonyssus, 449
Orolabial herpes, 363–364, 363*f*
Oropharyngeal actinomycosis, 268
Oropharyngeal form, of tularemia, 282–283
Oroya fever, 281
Orthostatic purpura, 833
Osler disease, 855–856, 855*f*
Osler node, 252
Osler sign, 542*f*
Osler-Weber-Rendu disease, 855–856, 855*f*
Osseous choristoma, of tongue, 806
Osseous sarcoidosis, 715*f*
Osseous syphilis, late, 354
Osteoarticular changes, in multicentric
    reticulohistiocytosis, 724
Osteogenesis imperfecta, 8, 513–514, 514*f*
Osteoma cutis, 529–530, 529*f*, 546.*e2f*
Osteoporosis
    atopic dermatitis and, 70
    in complex regional pain syndrome, 61
    steroid induced, 138
Otitis externa, 72, 73*f*, 271, 271*f*
Otomycosis, 322
Ovarian tumors
    acne vulgaris and, 232
    hirsutism and, 770
Oxalic acid, 92
Oxalosis, 818
Oxandrolone, for lipodermatosclerosis,
    488–489
Oxyhemoglobin, skin color, 15
Oxyuriasis, 431–432

P
p16 tumor-suppressor gene, 693
P16m alleles, 693
p53 gene mutations, 643–644
PABA (*p*-Aminobenzoic acid), 107
Pachydermodactyly, 611–612
Pachydermoperiostosis, 577, 577*f*
Pachyonychia congenita, 573–574, 573*f*,
    586.*e4f*

Paclitaxel, for angiosarcoma, 609
Paecilomyces, 321, 321*f*, 323.*e5f*
Paederus dermatitis, 444*f*, 452.*e2f*
Paget cells, 659
Paget disease
    of breast, 659, 659*f*, 685.*e4f*
    extramammary, 659–661, 660*f*, 685.*e7f*
Pagetoid reticulosis, 737–738, 749.*e3f*
Pain
    in angioleiomyoma, 631
    in Fabry disease, 537
    local anesthetic and, 884
    zoster-associated, 376–377
Painful bruising syndrome, 834–835, 834*f*
Painful fat herniation, 40, 40*f*
Painful piezogenic pedal papules, 40*f*
Palatal melanoma, 703.*e4f*
Pale cell acanthoma, 639–640, 639*f*
Palifermin-associated papular eruption,
    130–131
Palisaded granulomatous dermatoses,
    704–709
Palisaded neutrophilic granulomatous
    dermatitis, 162, 163*f*, 183.*e4f*, 183.*e8f*
Palmar granuloma annulare, 705–706
Palmar keratoderma, erythropoietic
    protoporphyria, 524
Palmar peeling, recurrent, 212
Palmar xanthomas, 531, 531*f*
Palmoplantar erythrodysesthesia syndrome,
    129–134
Palmoplantar hyperhidrosis, 774
Palmoplantar keratoderma, 209, 499
    diffuse, 211
    and malignancy, 211
Palmoplantar pustulosis, 203, 203*f*–204*f*,
    204.*e3f*
Palms
    aquagenic wrinkling of, 213, 213*f*
    desquamation of, 258, 258*f*
    diffuse hyperkeratosis of, 211*f*
    keratosis lichenoides chronica and, 224–225
    pits of, in Gorlin syndrome, 652
    pityriasis rubra pilaris on, 206–207
    punctate keratoses of, 210
Palpation, 16
Pamidronate
    for complex regional pain syndrome, 61
    for Menkes disease, 763–764
    for osteogenesis imperfecta, 514
Pancreatic panniculitis, 491–492, 491*f*
Pancreatitis, 533
Panhypopituitarism, 498
Panniculitides, 10, 488
Panniculitis, lupus erythematosus, alopecia in,
    757–758
Panniculitis-like T-cell lymphoma, 741–742,
    742*f*
Panniculus, 1, 2*f*, 9–10
Pansclerotic morphea, 172
PAPA syndrome, 149, 240
    pyoderma gangrenosum and, 148
Papillary eccrine adenoma, 670
Papillomas, cystic, 683
Papillomatosis
    confluent and reticulated, 209, 209*f*, 214.*e1f*
    oral, 555
    oral florid, 803
Papillon-Lefèvre syndrome, 212, 584
Papovavirus group, 402–414
Pappataci fever, 400
Papular acrodermatitis, of childhood, 385–386
Papular dermatitis, of pregnancy, 465–466
Papular eruptions, syphilis, 350–352
Papular mucinosis of infancy, 186

"Papular pruritic eruption", 416–417
Papular sarcoid, 711, 712*f*
"Papular sarcoidosis of the knee", 711
Papular syphilid, 353
Papular urticaria, 11
Papular xanthoma (PX), 723
Papular-purpuric gloves-and-socks syndrome
    (PPGSS), 398–399, 399*f*, 420.*e6f*
Papules, 11, 12*f*, 17.*e1f*
Papuloerythroderma of Ofuji, 53, 736
Papulonecrotic tuberculid, 329–330, 330*f*
Papulonodular mucinosis, systemic lupus
    erythematosus and, 162, 162*f*
Papulopustular rosacea, 246*f*
Papulosis, clear cell, 661
Papulosis atrophicans maligna, 850
Papulosquamous syphilids, 350–351
Papulovesicular acrolocated syndrome,
    385–386
Papulovesicular dermatitis, 444
Parabens, dermatitis, 109
Parachordomas, 628
Paracoccidioides brasiliensis, 314
Paracoccidioidomycosis, 314*f*, 323.*e3f*–323.*e4f*
Paraffin oils, 94
Paraffinoma, 41–42
Parakeratosis, 1
Paralytic footdrop, 61–62
Paramyxovirus group, 395–397
Paraneoplastic pemphigus, 142, 459–460, 459*f*
Paraneoplastic rheumatism, 182
Paraneoplastic syndrome, 632–633
Paraphimosis, lichen sclerosus and, 228
Parapoxvirus infections, bovine-associated, 389
Parasitic infections, 421–452
Parasitosis, delusions of, 55–56, 62.*e2f*
Parathyroid hormone
    deficiency in, 501
    excess of, 502
Parenchymatous neurosyphilis, 354–355
Paronychia, 256, 256*f*
    candidal, 303
Parotid duct cyst, 807
Parotid gland, sarcoidosis in, 715
Paroxetine
    flushing and, 140
    for polycythemia vera, 749
    pruritus in polycythemia vera, 49
Paroxysmal extreme pain disorder, 816
Paroxysmal hand hematoma, 834
Paroxysmal nocturnal hemoglobinuria
    (PNH), 833–834
Parrot pseudoparalysis, 356
Parry-Romberg syndrome, 172
Parthenium hysterophorus, 99
Partial unilateral lentiginosis, 688
Parvovirus B19
    immune thrombocytopenic purpura (ITP),
        823
    skin findings attributed to, 399
Parvovirus group, 397–399
Pasteurella multocida, 277–278, 278*f*
Pasteurellosis, 277–278
Patch testing, 35, 51
    for acute generalized exanthematous
        pustulosis, 122
    for allergic contact dermatitis, 96, 96*f*
    for contact urticaria, 112
    for cosmetics-associated, 107
    for eyelid eczema, 73
    for fiberglass dermatitis, 93
    fixed drug reactions and, 120
    for hand eczema, 73
Patches, 11
Patch-type granuloma annulare, 704

Pathergy
  Behçet syndrome, 811
  pyoderma gangrenosum and, 147
Patient evaluation, cutaneous vascular
    disorders, 819
Pattern alopecia, 754–755
Patterned acquired hypertrichosis, 769–770
Paucibacillary cutaneous tuberculosis,
    326–327
Pearly penile papules, 615–616
Pediatric sarcoidosis, 715
Pediculosis, 441–442
Pediculosis capitis, 441–442
Pediculosis corporis, 442, 442f
Pediculosis pubis, 442
  pruritus ani and, 50
Pediculosis vestimenti, 442
Pegvisomant, for acromegaly, 496
Pelea anisata, 29
Pellagra, 479–480, 480f, 484.e1f
  atrophic glossitis, 800
Pelodera, 433
Pelvic computed tomography, in melanoma,
    700
Pemphigoid gestationis, 464–465, 464f,
    474.e3f
Pemphigoid nodularis, 461
Pemphigus
  familial benign chronic, 562f
  paraneoplastic, 142
  syphilitic, 355–356
Pemphigus erythematosus, 459, 474.e2f
Pemphigus foliaceus, 457–458, 457f,
    474.e1f–474.e2f
  treatment of, 458
Pemphigus vegetans, 12, 456–457
  tinea cruris and, 297
Pemphigus vulgaris, 453–456, 454f, 474.e1f
  clinical features of, 453, 454f
  epidemiology of, 453
  etiologic factors of, 453–455
  histopathology of, 455
  oral, 474.e1f
  treatment of, 455–456
Penicillamine
  for pemphigus vulgaris, 454–455
  systemic lupus erythematosus and, 164
D-Penicillamine, Wilson disease, 543
Penicillamine-associated disease, 505
Penicillin
  for actinomycetomas, 319
  adverse reactions of, 113
  in erythema nodosum, 485
  for infectious mononucleosis, 380
  for leptospirosis, 286
  for Lyme disease, 288
  for rat-bite fever, 282
Penicillin G
  for actinomycosis, 268
  for cutaneous diphtheria, 265
  for meningococcemia, 275
Penicillium marneffei, 321
Penile melanosis, 687
Penile papules, 635.e4f
Penile venereal edema, 349
Penis
  calciphylaxis, 821
  erythroplasia of Queyrat in, 658
  Fournier gangrene of, 268
  median raphe cysts of, 684
  sclerosing lymphangiitis, 39, 39f
  vitiligo in, 871–872, 880.e2f
Pentamidine, 424
Pentamidine isethionate, trypanosomiasis and,
    427

Pentoxifylline
  chilblains, 22
  diffuse dermal angiomatosis, 852
  frostbite, 23
  for sarcoidosis, 717
  venous leg ulcers, 857
Perforating calcific elastosis, 508
Perforating folliculitis of the nose, 772
Perforating granuloma annulare, 705, 706f
Perforating ulcer, 61
Perfume dermatitis, 96–97
Periadnexal dermis, 8
Perianal candidiasis, 303
Perianal dermatitis, 262, 262f
Perianal tuberculosis, 327
Pericarditis, systemic lupus erythematosus
    and, 163
Periderm, 1, 2f
Perifollicular fibromas, 676–677
Perifolliculitis capitis abscedens et suffodiens,
    244–245
Perifolliculitis capitis abscedens et suffodiens
    of Hoffman, 760, 760f
Perineal erythema, recurrent toxin-mediated,
    260
Perineal skin tag, 617
Perineurioma, 625
Perinevoid vitiligo, 690–691
Periocular hyperpigmentation, 129
Periodic acid-Schiff (PAS)-positive basement
    membrane, 4
Periodic fever, aphthous stomatitis,
    pharyngitis, and adenitis (PFAPA)
    syndrome, 808
Periodic neutropenia, 808
Perioral dermatitis, 96–97, 100, 249–250, 249f
  rosacea and, 247
Periorbital dermatitis, 250
Periorbital hyperpigmentation, 862
Periorificial tuberculosis, 327–328
Peripheral ameloblastoma, 806
Peripheral T-cell lymphoma, 740
Perisynovitis (Clutton joints), 356
Periumbilical perforating PXE, 508
Periungual fibromas, 586.e2f
Periungual squamous cell carcinoma, 654
Periungual warts, 403
Perlèche, 303
Permanent wave preparations, dermatitis, 107
Permethrin
  for eosinophilic folliculitis, 417
  for pediculosis capitis, 442
  for scabies, 448
Pernio, 22, 22f, 45.e1f
Perniosis, 22
Persistent palmar erythema, 140
Perspiration, menopausal flushing and, 140
Petechiae, 823
Petrolatum dermatitis, 94
Petroleum jelly, 42
  for aquagenic urticaria, 153
  for atopic dermatitis, 68
  irritant properties of, 94
Peutz-Jeghers syndrome (PJS), 688, 868, 868f,
    880.e1f
PEX7 gene, 567–568
Peyronie disease, 611
PFAPA syndrome. *see* Periodic fever, aphthous
    stomatitis, pharyngitis, and adenitis
    (PFAPA) syndrome
Pfeiffer syndrome, 583
PG factor, 465
PHACE syndrome, 589
Phaeohyphomycosis, 291, 317, 317f, 321
Phaeomycotic cysts, 317

Phagedena, 273
Phagedenic chancre, 349
Phagocyte defects, 86–87
Phakomatoses, 555–586
Phakomatosis pigmentovascularis, 603, 603f,
    686, 702
Pharmaceutical amyloidosis, 519
Pheidole ants, 751
Phenol, 92
Phenolic antiseptic detergents, occupational
    vitiligo and, 874
Phenolic depigmentation, 874f
Phenolic glycolipid 1 (PGL-1), 336
Phenylalanine, 541
p-Phenylenediamine (PPDA), 107
Phenylketonuria (PKU), 541, 541f
Phenytoin, radiation-induced epidermal
    necrolysis, 119
Pheochromocytoma, flushing and, 140
Pheomelanin, 3, 762, 862
Philodendron, 99
Phimosis, 273
  lichen sclerosus and, 228, 228f
Phlebectomy, ambulatory, 930, 930f
Phlebitis, nodular granulomatous, 330
Phlebotomus fever, 400
Phlebotomus papatasii, 400
Phlebotomy
  for polycythemia vera, 749
  for porphyria cutanea tarda, 522
Phosphodiesterase inhibitors, for psoriasis, 200
Photoaccentuation, 141
Photoaging, 26–28, 26f
Photoallergy, 28, 123–124
Photochemotherapy, for scleroderma, 176
Photocontact dermatitis, 96–97
Photodistributed telangiectasia, 124–125
Photodynamic therapy (PDT), 906–907
  for acne vulgaris, 238
  for actinic cheilitis, 794–795
  for flat warts, 406
  for granuloma annulare, 706
  for hidradenitis suppurativa, 243
  for lichen planus, 220–221
  for lichen sclerosus, 229–230
  for mycosis fungoides, 737
  for onychomycosis, 301
Photo-onycholysis, 28–29, 29f, 786
Photopatch test, 96
Photophobia syndrome, 585
Photosensitivity, 28–35
  atopic dermatitis and, 66
  chemically induced, 28–30
  dermatomyositis and, 170
  HIV infection, 35
  idiopathic, 30–35
  reactions, 124, 124f
  severe, 25
  systemic lupus erythematosus and, 165
Photosensitizers, 28
Phototherapy
  for atopic dermatitis, 71
  for chronic urticaria, 154
  for eosinophilic folliculitis, 417
  for granuloma annulare, 707
  for hand eczema, 76
  for hydroa vacciniforme, 34
  for lichen planus, 220–221
  for necrobiosis lipoidica, 539
  for pityriasis lichenoides et varioliformis
      acuta, 740
  for pruritic dermatitis in elderly persons, 77
  for pruritus, 46–47
  for scleroderma, 176
  for vitiligo, 872–873

Photothermolysis, selective, 909
Phototoxic reactions, 28–30
Phototoxic tar dermatitis, 29
Phototoxicity, 28
Phrynoderma, 475–476, 476f
Phycomycosis, 320–321
Phylum Annelida, 431
Phylum Arthropoda, 437–451, 437f
Phylum Chordata, 451–452
Phylum Cnidaria, 428–430
Phylum Nemathelminthes, 431–437
Phylum Platyhelminthes, 430–431
Phylum Protozoa, 421–428
Physical (inducible) urticaria, 151–153
Physical panniculitis, 489–491
Phytophotodermatitis, 28, 29f–30f, 45.e2f
Phytosterolemia, 534
Pian. see Yaws
Picaridin, 437
Picker's acne, 240–241
Picornavirus group, 393–395
Picosecond lasers, for Mongolian spot, 702
Piebaldism, 878–879, 879f, 880.e2f
Piedra, 306, 306f
Piezogenic pedal papules, 40
Pigment granules, 3
Pigmentary demarcation lines, 862, 880.e1f
Pigmentary mosaicism, 548–549
    with hyperpigmentation, 549
    with hypopigmentation, 549
Pigmentary purpuric eruptions (PPEs),
        835–836
Pigmentation
    abnormal, 862–863
    disturbances of, 862–880
    drug-induced, 127, 127f–128f
    Gaucher disease, 535–536
    metallic discolorations and, 868–869
    minocycline-induced, 251.e1f
    mottled, epidermolysis bullosa simplex
        with, 559
    as sclerotherapy complications, 929
Pigmented basal cell carcinoma, 649, 649f
Pigmented epithelioid melanocytoma, 703
Pigmented lesions, 14
    laser treatment for, 914–918
Pigmented purpuric dermatosis, 813.e2f
Pigmented purpuric lichenoid dermatitis, 835
Pigmented spindle cell nevus, 693
Pigmented villonodular tenosynovitis, 613
Pigmented warts, 403
PiK3CA-related overgrowth syndromes
    (PROS), 597
Pilar cyst, 679, 679f
Pilar sheath acanthoma, 677
Pilar tumors, 4
Pili annulati, 765
Pili bifurcati, 768
Pili multigemini, 768, 768f
Pili pseudoannulati, 765
Pili torti, 763–764, 764f
Pilocarpine, for Sjögren syndrome, 179–180
Pilomatrical carcinoma, 672–673
Pilomatricoma, 672, 672f
Pilomatrix carcinoma, 672–673
Pilonidal sinus, 681, 685.e7f
Pimecrolimus cream
    for atopic dermatitis, 70
    for lichen simplex chronicus, 53
    for rosacea, 249–250
    topical, for acneiform eruptions, 241
    for vitiligo, 873
Pimozide, for delusions of parasitosis, 56
Pincer nails, 787, 787f
Pinch purpura, 515

Pine caterpillars, 439
Pink disease, 136
Pink rot fungus, 29
Pinpoint, papular polymorphous light
        eruption (PMLE), 225
Pinta, 360–361
    histopathology of, 360–361
    late dyschromic stage, 360, 361.e3f
    primary stage, 360
    secondary stage, 360
    treatment of, 361
    vitiligo and, 872
Pinworm
    infection, 431–432
    pruritus ani and, 50
Pirfenidone, for Hermansky-Pudlak
        syndrome, 877
Piroxicam, photosensitivity, 124, 124f
Pitch warts, 94–95
Pitted keratolysis, 267, 267f, 290.e2f
Pituitary hormone, deficiency in, 498
Pityriasis alba, 67, 91.e1f
    vitiligo and, 872
Pityriasis amiantacea, 772
Pityriasis lichenoides, 739–740
    erythema multiforme and, 142
Pityriasis lichenoides chronica, 740
Pityriasis lichenoides et varioliformis acuta,
        739–740, 739f
Pityriasis rosea, 205–206
    clinical features of, 205, 206f
    differential diagnosis of, 205
    distribution of lesions, 14
    etiology of, 205
    histology of, 205
    treatment of, 205–206
Pityriasis rotunda, 570, 570f
Pityriasis rubra pilaris, 15, 206–208, 214.e1f
    clinical features of, 206–207, 207f
    diagnosis of, 208
    etiology of, 207
    histology of, 207
    treatment of, 208
Pityriasis versicolor, 306–307
Pityrosporum folliculitis, 307
Plague, 281
Plakoglobin mutation, 558–559
Plakophilin mutation, 559
Plane xanthoma, 531–532, 531f
Plant sterols, 534
Plantar bromhidrosis, 776
Plantar fibromatosis, 611
Plantar verrucous cysts, 404
Plantar warts, 404, 404f
Plant-associated dermatitis, 100
Plants
    derivatives, allergic contact dermatitis from,
        100–101
    dermatitis from, 97–101
Plaques, 11, 12f, 17.e1f
    in sarcoidosis, 713, 713f
Plaque-type porokeratosis (mibelli), 571
"Plaque-type" syringoma, 665–666
Plasma cell cheilitis, 796
Plasma cell gingivitis, 796
Plasma cell orificial mucositis, 796
Plasmacytoma, 744–745, 745f
    in myeloma, 749.e4f
Plasmacytosis, cutaneous and systemic, 745
Plasmacytosis circumorificialis, 658
Plasmapheresis
    for cryoglobulinemia, 827
    for pemphigus vulgaris, 456
    for purpura fulminans, 830
    for Waldenström macroglobulinemia, 828

Plasmoacanthoma, 796
Plasticity, of suture, 887
Platelet
    accelerated destruction, 823
    deficient production, 823
    transfusions, 824
        in disseminated intravascular coagulation,
            830–831
Platelike osteoma cutis, 529
Platinum dermatitis, 104
Platonychia, 785
Platysma muscle, 9
Pleomorphic T-cell lymphoma, 741
Pleural effusion, 860
Plexiform fibrohistiocytic tumor, 619
Plica neuropathica, 767
Plummer nails, 500
Plummer-Vinson syndrome, 483
Pneumococcal cellulitis, 264
Pneumocystis jiroveci, 321
Pneumocystosis, 321
Pneumonia
    cryptogenic organizing, erythema gyratum
        repens and, 144
    varicella and, 371
Pneumonic tularemia, 282–283
Pneumothorax, Birt-Hogg-Dubé syndrome
    and, 677
Podo, 443–444
Podoconiosis, 860–861
Podophyllin
    for genital warts, 409
    for oral hairy leukoplakia, 380
POEMS syndrome, 21, 594, 744–745
Pohl-Pinkus constrictions, 753
Poikiloderma, with neutropenia, 582
Poikiloderma congenitale, 581–582, 582f
Poikiloderma of Civatte, 26, 27f
Poikiloderma vasculare atrophicans, 733
Polidocanol, for sclerotherapy, 929
Pollens, allergic contact dermatitis from, 100
Polyangiitis, granulomatosis with, pyoderma
    gangrenosum and, 148
Polyarteritis nodosa (PAN), 843–845, 843f
    cutaneous, 844–845
    treatment of, 844
Polyarthralgias, sarcoidosis and, 714–715
Polyarthritis, in progressive systemic sclerosis,
    174
Polychondritis, relapsing, 182–183, 182f
Polycyclic lesions, 15
Polycystic ovarian syndrome (PCOS), 498
    acne vulgaris and, 232–233
    hirsutism and, 770
Polycythemia vera, 49, 749
    pyoderma gangrenosum and, 148
Polyester resins, 106
Polyiodide iodine, for sclerotherapy, 929
Poly-L-lactic acid, 923–924, 924f
Polymerase chain reaction (PCR), 422
    for erythema multiforme, 142
    herpes simplex, 362
    Mycobacterium leprae, 336
    for nodular vasculitis, 487–488
Polymethylmethacrylate (PMMA), for soft
    tissue augmentation, 924
Polymorphic eruption
    associated with radiotherapy, 35–36
    of pregnancy, 465–466
Polymorphous light eruption (PMLE), 30–32,
        30f–31f
    action spectrum of, 31
    differential diagnosis of, 31
    Jessner lymphocytic infiltrate of the skin
        vs., 732

Polymyalgia rheumatica (PMR), giant cell arteritis, 849
Polyostotic fibrous dysplasia, 583
Polyoxyethylene sorbitan, 19
Polypoid basal cell carcinoma, 649
Polypoid melanoma, 697
Polyposis, Peutz-Jeghers syndrome (PJS) and, 868
Polytetrafluoroethylene, expanded, 924
Polyurethane varathane 91, 103
Polyvinyl resins, allergic contact dermatitis, 101
Pompholyx, 75, 75f
Popliteal pterygium syndrome, 582–583
Popsicle panniculitis, 490
Porelike basal cell carcinoma, 649
Pork tapeworm, 431
Porocarcinoma, 667
Porokeratosis, 570–572, 570f, 586.e3f
Porokeratosis et disseminata, 571–572
Porokeratosis palmaris, 571–572
Porokeratosis plantaris, 571–572
Porokeratosis plantaris discreta, 38, 211
Porokeratotic eccrine ostial and dermal duct nevus (PEODDN), 568, 568f
Poroma, 666–667, 667f
    malignant, 667
Porphyria cutanea tarda, 33, 384, 520–522, 521f–522f, 546.e1f
Porphyrias, 520–527
    hypertrichosis in, 769
Porphyrinogens, 520
Port wine stains, 595, 595f, 635.e1f
    pulse dye laser for, 911, 912f
Portuguese man-of-war dermatitis, 428
Posaconazole, 292
    for aspergillosis, 322
    for chromoblastomycosis, 316–317
    for coccidioidomycosis, 309
    for eumycetoma, 319
    for fusariosis, 321–322
    for hyalohyphomycosis, 321
    for mucormycosis, 321
    for phaeohyphomycosis, 317
    for prototheosis, 323
    for systemic candidiasis, 305
Postcardiotomy syndrome, 833
Postganglionic adrenergic fibers, 9
Postherpetic neuralgia, 376–377
Postinflammatory hyperpigmentation, 15–16, 863, 863f
Postinflammatory leukoderma, 876
Postinflammatory lymphedema, 860
Postinflammatory pigmentary alteration (PIPA), 863, 863f
Post-kala-azar dermal leishmaniasis, 426
Postmastectomy lymphangiosarcoma, 860
Postmenopausal women, lichen sclerosus and, 228
Postmiliarial hypohidrosis, 20
Postnatal telogen effluvium of infants, 752–753
Poststeroid panniculitis, 490
Postvaccination follicular eruption, 388
Potassium dichromate, 102
Potassium iodide
    for entomophthoromycosis, 320
    for erythema nodosum, 486–487
    for sporotrichosis, 315
    Sweet syndrome and, 146–147
Potassium titanyl phosphate (KTP) laser, 913
Power, laser energy, 909
Poxvirus group, 386–393
Prairie crocus, allergic contact dermatitis from, 99

Pramoxine
    for pruritus, 46–47
    for pruritus ani, 50
    for pruritus scroti, 50–51
Prayer calluses, 37
Praziquantel, for cysticercosis cutis, 431
Prednisolone, for pyoderma gangrenosum, 148–149
Prednisone
    for acne fulminans, 240
    for acne vulgaris, 236
    for bullous pemphigoid, 462–463
    for chronic urticaria, 154
    for cicatricial pemphigoid, 467–468
    for dermatomyositis, 170
    for giant cell arteritis, 849–850
    for lichen planus of nails, 778
    for mixed connective tissue disease, 178
    for pemphigus vulgaris, 455–456
    for PFAPA syndrome, 809
    for Sweet syndrome, 146–147
    for systemic lupus erythematosus, 165
    for Takayasu arteritis, 850
    for TRAPS, 149
    for urticarial vasculitis, 840–841
    for Wegener granulomatosis, 846–847
Pregabalin
    for prurigo nodularis, 54
    for pruritus, 46–47
    for zoster-associated pain, 377
Pregnancy
    dermatoses and, 465–466
    hair growth and, 6
    Hansen disease and, 341
    herpes simplex, 367
    intrahepatic cholestasis of, 465
    lichen sclerosus and, 228
    linear IgM dermatosis of, 466
    nevi during, 689
    papular dermatitis of, 465–466
    pemphigoid gestationis, 464
    pigmented nevi during, 695
    polymorphic eruption of, 465–466
    pruritic folliculitis of, 466
    pruritic urticarial papules and plaques of, 465, 465f, 474.e2f
    pyoderma gangrenosum and, 148
    Sweet syndrome and, 146
    syphilis, 357
    systemic lupus erythematosus in, 164
    telogen, 752
    varicella during, 372
Premature sebaceous hyperplasia, 663
Prematurity, anetoderma of, 512
Prenatal syphilis, 355
Preoperative antisepsis, 884
Preservatives, cosmetics, 108–109
Pressure alopecia, 761, 761f
Pressure ulcers, 38
    prevention of, 39
Pressure urticaria, 152–153, 153f
Pretibial fever, 286
Pretibial myxedema, 500–501, 504.e1f
Prickly heat, 20
Prilocaine, local anesthetic and, 884
Primary biliary cirrhosis, 48–49, 49f
    lichen planus and, 219
Primary cutaneous adenoid cystic carcinoma, 672
Primary cutaneous anaplastic large cell lymphoma, 740–741, 740f, 749.e2f
Primary cutaneous aspergillosis, 322, 322f
Primary cutaneous blastomycosis, 313
Primary cutaneous coccidioidomycosis, 308

Primary cutaneous follicle center cell lymphoma, 743–744
Primary cutaneous histoplasmosis, 310
Primary cutaneous immunocytoma, 743
Primary cutaneous large B-cell lymphoma, 744, 744f
Primary cutaneous marginal-zone lymphoma (PCMZL), 743
Primary cutaneous staphylococcal infections, 252–257
Primary effusion lymphoma, 383
Primary gonococcal dermatitis, 274
Primary immunodeficiency diseases, 80
Primary inoculation cryptococcosis, 311–312
Primary inoculation tuberculosis, 325–326, 326f, 335.e1f
Primary lesions, 11–13, 12f
Primary localized cutaneous amyloidosis, 517–518
Primary lymphedema, associated with yellow nails and pleural effusion, 860
Primary pulmonary coccidioidomycosis, 308
Primary pulmonary cryptococcosis, 311
Primary pulmonary histoplasmosis, 309
Primary sclerosing cholangitis, pruritus, 48
Primary systemic amyloidosis, 515–516
Primrose dermatitis, 99
Prodrome, erythema multiforme major and, 141–142
Profilaggrin, 2
Progeria, 579–580, 579f, 586.e5f
Progesterone, acute intermittent porphyria, 525
Progressive disseminated histoplasmosis, 309–310, 310f
Progressive mucinous histiocytosis, in women, 723–724
Progressive nodular histiocytosis (PNH), 722–723
Progressive osseous heteroplasia, 529
Progressive pigmentary dermatosis, 835–836
Progressive pigmenting purpura, 835–836
Progressive systemic sclerosis, 173–175
    internal involvement of, 174
    laboratory findings in, 174–175
    prognosis of, 174
    radiographic findings in, 175
    skeletal manifestations, 174
    skin findings in, 174, 174f
Prolactin, hirsutism and, 770
Prolidase deficiency, 541
Proliferating angioendotheliomatosis, 607, 607f
Proliferating epidermoid cyst, 679
Proliferating trichilemmal cyst, 679–680, 680f
Proliferative verrucous leukoplakia, 804, 804f
Prominent inferior labial artery, 601
Properdin, 88
Propionibacterium acnes, 231
Propranolol
    for adrenergic urticaria, 152
    for cholinergic urticaria, 151–152
    for Marfan syndrome, 510
    for rosacea, 248
Propylene glycol
    for dermatitis, 109
    for ichthyosis, 565–566
Prostaglandin analogs, 129
Prostaglandins
    itching and, 46
    sunburn, 24–25
Prostate cancer, finasteride for, 754
Protein C concentrate, disseminated intravascular coagulation, 830–831
Protein C deficiency, 125–126

Protein deprivation, in telogen effluvium, 752–753
Protein highly expressed in testis (PHET), 175–176
Proteinase 3 (PR3), 845
Protein-energy malnutrition, 483–484
Proteus syndrome, 555, 557f, 598, 586.e2f
    epidermal nevi and, 636
Proton pump inhibitors, 291
Prototheca, 322–323
Protothecosis, 322–323
Provocative use test, 96
    for adrenergic urticaria, 152
    fixed drug reactions and, 121
Proximal subungual onychomycosis, 299, 299f
Proximal trichorrhexis nodosa, 764
"Prozone" phenomenon, 348
Prurigo gestationis, 466
Prurigo gravidarum, 465
Prurigo nodularis, 54, 54f, 62.e1f
    treatment for, 54
Prurigo papule, 52
Prurigo pigmentosa, 52–53, 52f, 62.e1f
Prurigo simplex, 52
    treatment for, 52
Pruritic dermatitis, elderly, 78
Pruritic dermatoses, 49–58
Pruritic eruption, radiotherapy, 35–36
Pruritic folliculitis of pregnancy, 466
Pruritic urticarial papules and plaques of pregnancy (PUPP), 465f, 474.e2f
Pruritogenic stimuli, 46
Pruritus, 46–62
    anhidrosis with, 776
    aquagenic, 51–52
    biliary, 48–49
    brachioradial, 32–33, 33f, 60
    categories of, 46
    dermatoses, 49–58
    drug-induced, 52
    in erythema gyratum repens, 144
    with excoriations, 47f
    HIV-associated, 416–417
    internal causes of, 47–49
    in lichen planus, 215
    patterns of, 46
    in polycythemia vera, 749
    scalp, 52
    treatment of, 46–47
Pruritus ani, 49–50
    treatment for, 50
Pruritus scroti, 50–51, 50f
Pruritus vulvae, 51, 51f
Pseudoacromegaly, 496
Pseudoainhum, 614
Pseudoangiomatosis, eruptive, 395
Pseudo-atrophoderma colli, 209
Pseudocowpox (PCPV), 389
Pseudocyst of the auricle, 683, 683f
Pseudoephedrine, nonpigmenting fixed dry eruption from, 139.e2f
Pseudoephedrine hydrochloride, fixed drug reactions, 121
Pseudoepitheliomatous hyperplasia, 4
    squamous cell carcinoma *vs.*, 654–655
Pseudoepitheliomatous keratotic and micaceous balanitis, 659
Pseudofolliculitis barbae, 759, 767–768, 767f
Pseudohypoparathyroidism (PH), 501–502, 502f
Pseudolymphoma, 122
Pseudomelanoma, 690
Pseudomonas aeruginosa, 322
    ear eczema, 72
    folliculitis, 270–271, 290.e3f

Pseudomonas hot foot syndrome, 271
Pseudomonas infections, 269–272
    onycholysis and, 786
    X-linked agammaglobulinemia, 80
Pseudomonas septicemia, 270
Pseudonits, 763
Pseudopelade of Brocq, 761
Pseudoporphyria, 124, 125f, 524
Pseudorheumatoid nodule, 704–705, 705f
Pseudosarcomatous ischemic fasciitis, 618
Pseudoverrucous papules and nodules, 38
Pseudoxanthoma elasticum (PXE), 8, 507–508, 507f, 514.e1f
Psittacosis, urticaria and, 151
Psoriasis, 13, 16, 192–201, 204.e1f, 204.e3f
    acute generalized exanthematous pustulosis and, 121–122
    clinical differential diagnosis, 197
    clinical features, 192–193, 193f
    course, 195–196, 196f
    eczema herpeticum, 368
    epidemiology, 196
    evolving therapies, 200–201
    hand, 73
    HIV-associated, 416
    inheritance, 196
    napkin, 76, 77f, 91.e2f
    "nevoid" or "linear", 639
    onychomycosis and, 300
    at ostomy sites, 76
    pathogenesis, 196–197
    pathology, 197
    and pityriasis rubra pilaris, 207
    and tattoos, 41
    tinea capitis and, 294
    TNF and, 134, 135f
    treatment, 197–200
        biologic agents, 199–200
        combination therapy, 200
        hyperthermia, 198–199
        Janus kinase (JAK) inhibitors, 200
        occlusive, 199
        phosphodiesterase inhibitors, 200
        surgical, 198
        systemic, 199
        topical, 197–198
    types, 193–195
Psoriatic arthritis, 194, 194f
Psoriatic nails, 779–780, 780f, 793.e5f
Psychiatric illness, signs of, 55
Psychodermatology, 54–55
Psychodidae sandflies, 442
Psychogenic (neurotic) excoriations, 56, 56f
Psychogenic pruritus, 50
Psychogenic purpura, 834–835, 834f
Psychosis, 55
Psychotherapy, for factitious dermatitis, 57
PTCH gene, 652
PTEN gene mutations, 555
PTEN hamartoma tumor syndrome, 675
Pterygium, lichen planus of the nails and, 778, 779f
Pterygium inversum unguis, 174, 787, 787f, 183.e6f–183.e7f
Pterygium unguis, 787
Puffy hand syndrome, 21
Pulex irritans, 445
Pulicosis, 445
Pull test, in telogen effluvium, 752
Pulmonary capillaritis, 845
Pulmonary embolism, deep venous thrombosis, 831
Pulmonary fibrosis, in progressive systemic sclerosis, 174
Pulmonary Langerhans cell histiocytosis, 729

Pulmonary sarcoidosis, 714
Pulmonary tuberculosis, erythema gyratum repens and, 144
Pulsed dye laser (PDL), 910–913, 912f
    for hidrocystomas, 666
    for lupus erythematosus, 165
    for nevus flammeus, 597
    for rosacea, 248
    for striae, 513
Pulseless disease, 850
Punch biopsies, 888, 889f
Puncta pruritica, 51
Punctate keratoses, of palms and soles, 210, 210f
Punctate palmoplantar keratoderma, 210, 214.e2f
Punctate superficial necrosis, of fingertips, 813
Purified protein derivative (PPD), in tuberculosis, 324
Purine nucleoside phosphorylase deficiency, 81
PURPLE, 819
Purpura, 822–823
    amyloidosis, 515
    corticosteroids adverse reactions, 138
    evaluation of, 823
    of nail beds, 790
    pathogenesis of, 823
    secondary to clotting disorders, 828–829
    secondary to vomiting, 813.e2f
    thrombocytopenic. *see* Thrombocytopenic purpura
Purpura annularis telangiectodes, 835
Purpura en cocarde avec oedème, 839–840, 839f
Purpura fulminans, 829–830, 829f–830f
    in varicella, 371
Purpura gangrenosa, 829–830, 829f–830f
Purpura hyperglobulinemica, 827–828
Purpura pigmentosa chronica, 835–836
Purpuric agave dermatitis, 829
Purpuric phototherapy-induced eruption, 525–527
Puss caterpillar, 439, 439f
Puss moth, 439–440
Pustular bacterid, 203
Pustular psoriasis
    of extremities, 203
    of hand, 193f
Pustular syphilids, 351
Pustules, 13, 13f
    in miliaria pustulosa, 20
Pustulosis, transient neonatal, 867, 867f
PUVA therapy
    for acquired perforating dermatosis, 773
    for actinic dermatitis, 35
    for alopecia areata, 751–752
    for atopic dermatitis, 70
    for graft-*versus*-host disease, 89
    for hand eczema, 75
    for lentigines, 687
    for lichen planus, 220–221
    for lymphomatoid papulosis, 739
    for mycosis fungoides, 736–737
    for necrobiosis lipoidica, 539
    for onychomycosis, 301
    for pigmented purpura, 836
    for prurigo, 52
    for pruritus, 46–47
    for psoriasis, 198
    for solar urticaria, 33–34
    for vitiligo, 873
PV antigen, 454
PXE-like papillary dermal elastolysis, 508

Pyloric atresia
  epidermolysis bullosa simplex with, 560
  junctional epidermolysis bullosa with, 560
Pyoderma, blastomycosis-like, 270
Pyoderma faciale, 249, 249f
Pyoderma gangrenosum, 147–149, 148f
  bullous, 147
  classic, 147
  clinical picture of, 148
  granulomatosis with polyangiitis, 148
  local treatment for, 148
  management of, 148
  pustular, 147
  systemic treatment for, 148–149
  vegetative, 147
Pyogenic arthritis, PG, acne, and suppurative
    hidradenitis (PA-PASH) syndrome, 149
Pyogenic granuloma, 590, 590f, 806–807,
    635.e1f
  acne vulgaris and, 238–239
Pyogenic lymphoma, 741
Pyogenic paronychia, 256
Pyomyositis, 257
Pyostomatitis vegetans, 797, 797f
  pyoderma gangrenosum and, 147
Pyrantel pamoate, pinworm, 432
Pyrexia, tick bite, 446
Pyridoxine
  chemotherapy-induced acral erythema and,
    130
  deficiency of, 478
  excess of, 478
  pemphigoid gestationis, 465
Pyrin, 149

Q
Q fever, 283
Q-switched (QS) lasers, 909
  for blue nevi, 703
  and carbon stains, 43–44
  for epidermal melanocytic lesions, 686
  for Mongolian spot, 702
  for nevus spilus, 686
  for pigmented lesions, 914, 914t, 915f–
    918f
  tattoo-associated dermopathies, 41–42
Quasi-continuous-wave lasers, 909
Quicklime, 92
Quinacrine, 127
  for lichen planus, 220–221
  for systemic lupus erythematosus, 165
Quincke edema, 155
Quinidine, 127
  and livedo, 818
Quinine, and livedo, 818

R
Rabbit botfly, 443
Raccoon eyes, 627
Racquet nails, 785, 785f
Radiation cancer, 36, 37f
Radiation dermatitis, 133
  malignant fibrous histiocytosis, 635.e5f
Radiation enhancement, 133
Radiation recall, 133, 133f
Radiation therapy, 907–908
  for acneiform eruptions, 241
  for cutaneous B-cell lymphoma, 743
  for cutaneous lymphoid hyperplasia, 731
  for extramammary Paget disease, 660–661
  for Merkel cell carcinoma, 662
  for mycosis fungoides, 737
  for plasmacytoma, 745
  for primary cutaneous follicle center cell
    lymphoma, 744

Radiation-induced epidermal necrolysis,
    117–119, 119f
Radioallergosorbent test (RAST), 112, 154
  food allergy, 64
Radiodermatitis, 35–37
  acute, 35–36, 36f
  chronic, 36, 36f–37f, 45.e2f
  treatment for, 36–37
Ragweed oil dermatitis, 100
Ramsay Hunt syndrome, 375, 420.e3f
Randox, 100
Ranitidine
  for chronic urticaria, 154
  for flat warts, 406
Ranula, 807
Rapamycin, for trichilemmoma, 675–676
Rapid plasma reagin (RPR) test, 348
Rapidly growing mycobacteria, 332–335
Rapidly involuting congenital hemangioma, 590
Rapp-Hodgkin ectodermal dysplasia
    syndrome, 576, 576f
Rapunzel syndrome, 57
Rasopathies, 550–554
Rat flea, 445
Rat flea-borne endemic typhus, 283
Rat-bite fever, 281–282
Raynaud disease, 813–815, 814f
  treatment of, 814–815
Raynaud of the nipple, 813
Raynaud phenomenon, 813–815, 813.e1f
  in progressive systemic sclerosis, 174
Raynaud syndrome, 21
Reactive arthritis, with conjunctivitis/
    urethritis/diarrhea, 201–202
  clinical features, 201–202, 201f
"Reactive eccrine syringofibroadenoma", 670
Reactive granulomatous dermatitis, 709
Reactive lymphoid hyperplasia, 749.e1f
Reactive neutrophilic dermatoses, 145–149
Reactive perforating collagenosis, 505–507,
    506f, 773, 773f
Recalcitrant palmoplantar eruptions, 202–204
Recall reactions, 133, 133f
Recreational activity-associated purpura, 829
Recurrent aphthous stomatitis, 809–810, 809f
Recurrent infundibulofolliculitis, 774
Recurrent intraoral herpes simplex infection,
    808–809, 809f
Recurrent nevus, 690
Recurrent palmar peeling, 212
Recurrent palmoplantar hidradenitis, 778
Recurrent respiratory papillomatosis, 410–411
Recurrent Spitz nevus, 690
Recurrent toxin-mediated perineal erythema,
    260
Red baby syndrome, 399
Red ear syndrome, 816–817
Red edematous plaques, Sweet syndrome and,
    146–147
Red light, photodynamic therapy and, 906
Red lunulae, 790
Red man syndrome, 122–123
Red oculocutaneous albinism, 879
5α-Reductase deficiency, 754
Reduviid bites, 440–441, 441f
Refsum syndrome, 567–568
Regional lymphangitic sporotrichosis, 314
Regressing melanoma, 691
Reiter syndrome, 195, 201–202
  clinical features, 201–202, 201f
Relapsing polychondritis, 182–183, 182f
Related palisading granulomas, 181
Renal disease
  Henoch-Schönlein purpura and, 839
  sarcoidosis and, 715

Renal failure
  chronic, 517
  in metastatic calcinosis cutis, 527
  pruritus, 47
Renal transplantation, in chronic kidney
    disease, 48
Renal tumors, in Birt-Hogg-Dubé syndrome,
    677
Repetitive phototherapy, for solar urticaria, 152
Residual dyspigmentation, 15
Resorcin, for acne vulgaris, 235
Restrictive dermopathy, 579
Restylane, 923
Rete ridges, 8
Reticular erythematous mucinosis (REM),
    188, 188f, 190.e2f
Reticular pigmented anomaly, of flexures, 866
Reticulate acropigmentation of Dohi, 865
Reticulate acropigmentation of Kitamura
    (RPK), 866f, 867
Reticulate pigment disorders, of skin,
    865–867
Reticulated acanthoma with sebaceous
    differentiation, 664
Reticulated port wine stain, 595
Reticulohistiocytoma, 724
Reticulohistiocytosis, 724–725
Retiform hemangioendothelioma, 592
"Retiform" purpura, 817, 823
Retinoid embryopathy, 237
Retinoids, 67
  for confluent and reticulated papillomatosis,
    209
  for Gorlin syndrome, 653
  for granuloma annulare, 707
  for hypertrophic lupus erythematosus, 165
  for inflammatory linear verrucous
    epidermal nevus, 639
  for lichen planopilaris, 758
  for lichen planus, 220–221
  for lichen planus of nails, 778
  for mycosis fungoides, 737
  onycholysis and, 786
  oral
    for acne vulgaris, 236–237
    for hand eczema, 76
    for pityriasis rubra pilaris, 208
    for psoriasis, 199
    for rosacea, 247
    for sarcoidosis, 717
    for squamous cell carcinoma, 655
  topical
    for acne vulgaris, 234
    for keratosis pilaris, 585
Retinyl palmitate, for measles, 396
Retronychia, 788
Retroviruses, 414–420
Reye syndrome, 371
Rheumatism
  fibroblastic, 182
  paraneoplastic, 182
Rheumatoid arthritis, 180–182
  erythema gyratum repens and, 144
  juvenile, 181–182
Rheumatoid neutrophilic dermatosis, 180,
    181f, 183.e8f
Rheumatoid nodules, 180, 180f
Rheumatoid vasculitis, 180, 183.e8f
Rhinitis sicca, in Sjögren syndrome, 179
Rhinophyma, 246, 246f, 920f
Rhinoscleroma, 277, 277f
Rhinosporidiosis, 319–320, 320f
Rhinosporidium seeberi, 319–320
Rhipicephalus tick, 452.e3f
Rhodesian trypanosomiasis, 427

Rhopilema nomadica, 428
Rhus dermatitis, 30
Rhytids, dynamic, 922
Ribavirin
for hepatitis C infection, 384–385
in sarcoidosis, 716
Riboflavin deficiency, 477–478, 477*f*
perlèche in, 484.*e1f*
Richner-Hanhart syndrome, 209, 543, 570
Richter syndrome, 380–381
Ricin, 99
Rickets, hypophosphatemic, 663
Rickettsia felis, 445
Rickettsia prowazekii, 283
Rickettsia tsutsugamushi, 283
Rickettsia typhi, 283
Rickettsial diseases, 283–290
Rickettsialpox, 285, 285*f*
Ridged wart, 404
Ridley and Jopling scale, 337, 337*t*
Rifampin
for biliary pruritus, 48
for Buruli ulcer, 333
flushing and, 140
for furunculosis, 256
for lichen planopilaris, 759
for meningococcemia, 275
Ringed hair, 765
Risperidone, for delusions of parasitosis, 56
Rituximab
for bullous pemphigoid, 463
for dermatomyositis, 170
for pemphigus vulgaris, 456
for primary cutaneous follicle center cell
lymphoma, 744
for sarcoidosis, 717
for scleroderma, 176
for small-vessel vasculitis, 837–838
for systemic lupus erythematosus, 166
for thrombotic thrombocytopenic purpura,
825
for Waldenström macroglobulinemia, 828
River blindness, 436
RNA viruses, 362
Roberts-SC syndrome, 598
Rocky Mountain spotted fever, 284, 284*f*
Rodent ulcer, 649
Romana sign, 427, 440–441
Rombo syndrome, 586
Romiplostim, for erythromelalgia, 815–816
Rosacea, 245–249, 251.*e1f*
clinical considerations with, 246–247
clinical features of, 245–246, 245*f*–246*f*
differential diagnosis of, 247
erythrotelangiectatic, 245, 245*f*
etiology of, 246
extrafacial lesions on, 247
flushing and, 140
glandular, 245, 246*f*
granulomatous lesions and, 247
ocular findings on, 246–247
papulopustular, 246*f*
perioral dermatitis and, 247
steroid, 137–138
topical corticosteroid use and, 247
treatment of, 247–248
Rosacea fulminans, 249
Rosai-Dorfman disease, 748–749
see also Sinus histiocytosis with massive
lymphadenopathy
Rosenbach, erysipeloid of, 264, 264*f*
Roseola infantum, 382
Ross syndrome, 776
Rotation flap, 896–898, 900*f*–901*f*
Roth-Bernhardt disease, 60

Rothmund-Thomson syndrome, 581–582,
582*f*, 586.*e5f*
"Round finger-pad sign," of progressive
systemic sclerosis, 174
Rubber accelerators, dermatitis, 105
Rubber dermatitis, 97, 104–105, 105*f*
Rubber gloves, 75, 104–105
testing, 112
Rubella, 397, 420.*e6f*
Ruby laser
for blue nevi, 703
for Mongolian spot, 702
for nevus of Ota, 702
for nevus spilus, 686
Rud syndrome, 568
"Rufous" oculocutaneous albinism, 879
Running locked suture, 889, 891*f*
Running subcuticular sutures, 889–892, 892*f*
Running sutures, 889
Russell sign, 55
Rutoside, for pigmented purpura, 836

S
S-100A6, in Spitz nevus, 692–693
Sabra dermatitis, 100
Saddleback caterpillar, 439, 440*f*
Sailor's neck, 26
Salicylates, varicella and, 371
Salicylazosulfapyridine, for pyoderma
gangrenosum, 149
Salicylic acid, 68
for acne vulgaris, 235
for chemical peels, 932
for common warts, 405
for corns, 38
for ichthyosis, 565–566
for psoriasis, 198
Salmon patch, 594
Salmonella, 276
Salmonellosis, 276
Salt-split-skin preparations, 453
Samitz sign, of dermatomyositis, 167*f*
San Joaquin Valley fever, 14
see also Coccidioidomycosis
Sandflies, leishmaniasis, 424
Sandfly fever, 400
Sandworm, 433
SAPHO syndrome, 240
Sarcodina, class of, 421
Sarcoidal plaque, 713*f*
Sarcoidosis, 711–718, 730.*e2f*
alopecia in, 761
annular, 711–712, 712*f*
differential diagnosis of, 716
erythema nodosum in, 485, 711
erythrodermic, 713
histopathology of, 715–716
hypopigmented, 712
ichthyosiform, 713, 713*f*
morpheaform, 714
mucosal, 714
nail, 714
papular, 711, 712*f*
pediatric, 715
in scars (scar sarcoid) and tattoos, 714, 714*f*
in the setting of immunologic
abnormalities, 716
silica granuloma and, 43
subcutaneous, 713
systemic, 714–715, 715*f*
treatment of, 716–718
ulcerative, 712–713
Sarcoma
clear cell, 697
epithelioid, 620, 620*f*

Sarcoma (*Continued*)
granulocytic, 747
mast cell, 623
undifferentiated pleomorphic, 619–620
Sarcoptes scabiei, 447
Sarna lotion, topical, for chronic urticaria,
154
Scab mites, 448
Scabies, 447–448, 447*f*–448*f*, 452.*e3f*
Scabs, 13
Scales, 13, 72
Scalp
allergic contact dermatitis and, 96–97
dissecting cellulitis of, 244–245, 245*f*
dysesthesia, 58–59
erosive pustular dermatitis of, 760
giant cell arteritis, 849, 849*f*
pruritus, 52
ringworm, 292
Scalp electrodes, neonatal herpes simplex, 367
SCALP syndrome, 578, 662–663
Scarlet fever, 259, 260*f*
Scarring alopecia, 757, 757*f*–758*f*
Scars, 13–14
lichen planus, 13–14
sarcoidosis, 714, 714*f*
Schamberg disease, 835*f*
Schamroth sign, 780
Schilder disease, 545
Schimmelpenning syndrome, 637, 638*f*,
662–663
Schistocytes, thrombotic thrombocytopenic
purpura, 825
Schistosoma mansoni, ova of, 430*f*
Schistosome cercarial dermatitis, 430
Schistosomiasis, visceral, 430–431
Schizophrenia, 55–56
Schnitzler syndrome, 150–151
urticarial vasculitis and, 840
Schopf-Schulz-Passarge syndrome (SSPS),
666
Schwannoma, 626, 626*f*
Schwannomin, 553
Sciatic nerve injury, 61–62
Scleredema, 187–188, 187*f*, 190.*e2f*
Sclerema neonatorum, 489
Scleroatrophic syndrome of Huriez, 582
Sclerodactyly, 173*f*
Scleroderma, 8, 171–177, 183.*e6f*
cutaneous types of, 171–172
differential diagnosis of, 175
histology of, 175
linear, 172, 172*f*, 183.*e6f*
nodular, 174
pathogenesis of, 175–176
Raynaud phenomenon, 813
systemic types of, 173–175
treatment for, 176–177
Scleroderma-like reactions to taxanes, 132
Sclerodermatomyositis, 169
Scleromyxedema, 184, 185*f*, 190.*e1f*
Sclerosing lipogranuloma, 41–42, 491
Sclerosing lymphangiitis, 39, 39*f*
Sclerosing panniculitis, 488
Sclerosing sweat duct carcinoma, 670–671,
671*f*
Sclerosis, in graft-*versus*-host disease, 89
Sclerotherapy, 928–930, 928*f*
complications of, 929–930
for pyogenic granuloma, 590
solutions, 928–929, 929*f*, 929*t*
for venous malformation, 598
Sclerotinia sclerotiorum, 29
Scolopendra, 438
Scombroid fish poisoning, flushing and, 140

Scopolamine cream, for hidrocystomas, 666
Scopulariopsis brevicaulis, 299–300
Scorpion sting, 450
Scorpionidae, order of, 450
SCORTEN, 118
Scratch marks, 13
Scrofuloderma, 324, 327–328, 328*f*, 335.*e1f*
Scrotal tongue, 799, 799*f*
Scrotum
  angiokeratoma of, 605, 605*f*
  condylomata of, 361.*e3f*
  elephantiasis tropica, 434
  extramammary Paget disease of, 659–660
  fat necrosis of, 490
  Fournier gangrene of, 268
  pruritus ani, 50, 50*f*
  in riboflavin deficiency, 477–478
Scrub typhus, 283–284
Scurvy, 478–479, 478*f*, 484.*e1f*
Scytalidium hyalinum, 299–300
Sea anemone, 428–429, 429*f*
Sea chervil, 429–430
Sea urchin injuries, 429, 429*f*
Sea wasp, 428
Seabather's eruption, 428, 428*f*
Sea-blue histiocytosis, 726
Seatworm infection, 431–432
Seaweed dermatitis, 100, 429
Sebaceoma, 664, 685.*e5f*
Sebaceous adenoma, 664, 664*f*
Sebaceous carcinoma, 664, 664*f*
Sebaceous duct, 7
Sebaceous epithelioma, 664
Sebaceous glands, 5, 7
Sebaceous hyperplasia, 663
Sebaceous nevi, 662–665
Sebaceous trichofolliculoma, 673
Sebaceous tumors, 664–665
Sebastian syndrome, 834
Sebocytes, 7
Seborrheic dermatitis, 191–192, 192*f*, 204.*e1f*
  in anal area, 50
  clinical features of, 191
  differential diagnosis of, 191–192
  discoid lupus erythematosus *vs.*, 157–159
  etiology and pathogenesis of, 191
  histology of, 191
  in HIV-infected patient, 417*f*
  Langerhans cell histiocytosis and, 727
  pityriasis rosea and, 205
  psoriasis *vs.*, 197
  tinea capitis and, 294
  tinea cruris and, 297
  treatment of, 192
Seborrheic keratosis, 640–641, 641*f*,
  685.*e1f*–685.*e2f*
Seborrheic-like psoriasis, 193
Second intention, healing by, 896, 898*f*
Secondary clubbing, 780
Secondary cutaneous plasmacytoma, 744
Secondary hyperlipoproteinemia, 533–535
Secondary lesions, 13–14
Secondary lymphedema, 860
Secondary Raynaud phenomenon, 813
Secondary systemic amyloidosis, 516
Secretagogues, for Sjögren syndrome,
  179–180
Secretan syndrome, 860
Seeds, allergic contact dermatitis from, 100
Segmental anhidrosis, 776
Segmental hyalinizing vasculitis, 819
Segmental neurofibromatosis, 552*f*
Segmental vitiligo, 871–872, 871*f*
Seidlmayer syndrome, 839–840, 839*f*
Selective photothermolysis, 909

Selective serotonin reuptake inhibitors
  (SSRIs), 57
  for Raynaud disease, 814
Selenium deficiency, 483
Selenium sulfide
  for folliculitis decalvans, 759
  hair color and, 763
  for pityriasis amiantacea, 772
  for tinea capitis, 294
  for tinea versicolor, 307
Self-biting, 55, 55*f*
Self-examination, 16–17
Self-healing papular mucinosis, 186, 186*f*
Self-induced panniculitis, 491
Self-tanning creams, for vitiligo, 873
Semipermeable biosynthetic wound dressings,
  for venous leg ulcers, 857
Senear-Usher syndrome, 459
Senile angiomas, 593–594
Senile systemic amyloidosis, 517
Sensitivity, testing for, 96
Sensitization, 109
Sentinel node biopsy
  for melanoma, 700
  for Merkel cell carcinoma, 661–662
Sepsis, *Corynebacterium jeikeium*, 266
Septal panniculitis, 485–487
Septicemia, 282
Serologic tests
  for epidemic typhus, 284
  for Hansen disease, 337
  for syphilis, 348
Serotonin agonists, flushing and, 140
Serotonin toxicity, flushing and, 140
Serpiginous lesions, 15
Serratia species, 86
Sertraline, in biliary pruritus, 48
Serum complement, systemic lupus
  erythematosus and, 165
Serum sickness-like reactions, 127–129
Severe combined immunodeficiency, 82–83
Severe pruritus, 46, 47*f*
Severe serotonin toxicity, flushing and, 140
Sex partners, treatment of, 357
Sézary syndrome, 214, 735, 738, 738*f*,
  749.*e3f*
Shagreen plaque, 555, 555*f*
Sharp scissor biopsy, 888
Shave biopsies, 888, 888*f*
"Shawl sign," of dermatomyositis, 167, 167*f*
Shell nail syndrome, 781
Shelley "shoreline" nails, 782
Sherpas, 781
Shigellosis, 276–277
Shiitake flagellate dermatitis, 130–131, 131*f*
Shin spots, 539
Shingles, 374–379
Shoe dermatitis, 102, 102*f*, 139.*e1f*
Shoulder pad sign, 516
Sialidosis, 538
Sicca syndrome, 179–180
Sicca-like syndrome, 119
Siemens-1 syndrome, 585–586
Sildenafil
  for chilblains, 22
  flushing and, 140
  for Raynaud disease, 814
  for scleroderma, 176
Silica granuloma, 42–43, 43*f*
Silicone, for soft tissue augmentation, 924
Silicone granuloma, 42–43, 42*f*
Silk, dermatitis from, 101
Silver
  pigmentation, 128
  venous leg ulcers, 857

Silver nitrate
  for pemphigus vulgaris, 455
  for pyogenic granuloma, 590
Silver sulfadiazine, for pemphigus vulgaris,
  455
Simple epidermal interrupted sutures, 889,
  890*f*
Sindbis virus, 401
Sinequan, for atopic dermatitis, 69
Single-system Langerhans cell histiocytosis,
  729
Sinus histiocytosis with massive
  lymphadenopathy (SHML), 718,
  748–749, 748*f*, 749.*e4f*
Sinusoidal hemangioma, 600–601
Siphonaptera, order of, 445
Sirukumab, for systemic lupus erythematosus,
  166
Sisaipho, 750
Sister Mary Joseph nodule, 632, 633*f*
Sitosterolemia, 534
Sixth disease, 382
Sjögren syndrome, 179–180, 518
Sjögren-Larsson syndrome, 567
Skeletal abnormalities, in incontinentia
  pigmenti, 548
Skeletal defects, in Gorlin syndrome, 652–653
Skin
  appendages, diseases of, 750–793
  color, 3, 15–16
  gangrene of, 267–269
  structure and function of, 1–10, 2*f*
  types (phototypes), 25, 25*t*
Skin beetles, 444
Skin biopsy, 56
  for bullous drug reactions, 118
Skin flaps, 896–905, 898*f*–903*f*
Skin fragility, 558–559
  woolly hair syndrome, 559
Skin fragility-ectodermal dysplasia syndrome,
  559
Skin grafts, 896–905, 904*f*
  for necrobiosis lipoidica, 539
  for venous leg ulcers, 857
Skin infections
  with cryptococcosis, 311
  Gram-negative, 269–283
  Gram-positive, 252–269
  miscellaneous, 264–267
  streptococcal, 259–264
Skin lesions
  in Langerhans cell histiocytosis, 727–728, 728*f*
  at vaccination scars, 388
Skin popping, 40, 40*f*, 45.*e3f*
Skin prick test, for food allergy, 64
Skin puncture, Behçet syndrome, 811
Skin shavings, 436
Skin testing, for adverse drug reactions, 113
Skin toxicity, from cytokines, 134
Skin tumors, in Gorlin syndrome, 652
"Sky-blue moons," of nails, 543
SLC24A5 gene, oculocutaneous albinism in,
  880
Sleep, loss of, atopic dermatitis and, 68
Small plaque parapsoriasis (SPP), 208–209, 208*f*
Smallpox, 386–387, 386*f*
  in atopic dermatitis and, 68
  scars, 420.*e4f*
Small-sized congenital nevocytic nevus,
  691–692
Small-spore ectothrix, 292
Small-vessel vasculitis, 836–843, 836*b*
Smears
  for chancroid, 273
  for Hansen disease, 337

Smoker's keratosis, 798
Smoker's patches, 798
Smoking
    livedoid vasculopathy and, 820
    thromboangiitis obliterans and, 851–852
Smooth atrophy, 354
Smooth tongue, 800, 800*f*
"Snail-track" ulcers, 797
Snakebite, 452, 452.*e3f*
Sneddon syndrome, 818
    systemic lupus erythematosus and, 163
Sneddon-Wilkinson disease, 202, 457–458
Snuffles, 355
Soak and smear technique
    for atopic dermatitis, 68
    for prurigo simplex, 52
    for winter itch, 49
Sodium antimony gluconate, leishmaniasis,
        424
Sodium bicarbonate, local anesthetic and, 884
Sodium channel, erythromelalgia and, 816
Sodium deoxycholate, 931–932
Sodium morrhuate, for sclerotherapy, 929
Sodium silicate, 92
Sodium sulfacetamide, for acne vulgaris, 235
Sodium tetradecyl sulfate (STS), for
        sclerotherapy, 929
"Sodoku", 282
Soft corns, 38
Soft epidermal nevus, 636
Soft tissue
    augmentation, 922–925
    melanoma, 697
Solar elastosis, 26
Solar erythema, 24–25
Solar keratosis, 644–645, 644*f*
Solar lentigo, 642, 686–687, 703.*e1f*
Solar urticaria, 33–34, 33*f*, 152
Solenonychia, 786, 786*f*
Soles
    desquamation of, 258, 258*f*
    keratosis lichenoides chronica and, 224–225
    lichen planus of, 230.*e2f*
    pits of, in Gorlin syndrome, 652
    pityriasis rubra pilaris on, 206–207
    psoriasis in, 192–193
    punctate keratoses of, 210, 210*f*
Solid CO₂, for chemical peels, 932
Solid tumors, Sweet syndrome and, 146
Solid-organ transplantation, graft-*versus*-host
        disease in, 90–91
Solitary basal cell carcinoma, in young
        person, 650
Solitary cutaneous leiomyoma, 630–631
Solitary fibrous tumor, 618–619
Solitary keratoacanthoma, 646–647, 646*f*
Solitary mastocytoma, 622
Solitary neurofibroma, 625–628
Solitary trichoepitheliomas, 674
Solvents, irritant contact dermatitis, 95
Sorafenib
    chemotherapy-induced acral erythema and,
        130
    cutaneous side effects of, 132
    palmoplantar keratoderma and, 209
Sorbic acid, 109
Sore throat, syphilitic, 352
South American blastomycosis, 313–314
Southern tick-associated rash illness (STARI),
        286
Spandex, 101–102
Spangled hair, 765
Spanish pine caterpillar, 439
Spare collagenases, 8
Sparfloxacin, 124

Sparganosis, 431, 431*f*
"Spark" nevus, 694
"Spastic" nevus, 694
Speckled lentiginous nevus, 686
Spherulocytosis, 490
Spicules, follicular, 745
Spider angioma, 603, 635.*e2f*
Spider bites, pyoderma gangrenosum *vs.*, 148
Spider nevus, 603
Spinal accessory nerve, 885–887
Spindle cell hemangioendothelioma, 592, 592*f*
Spindle cell nevus, 692–693
Spiny keratoderma, 210, 210*f*
Spiradenoma, 667–668, 668*f*
Spirillum minor, 281–282
Spironolactone
    for acne vulgaris, 236
    for androgen-dependent syndromes, 499
    for hirsutism, 771
Spitz nevi, 689, 692–693, 692*f*, 703.*e2f*
    recurrent, 690
Splenectomy
    for immune thrombocytopenic purpura
        (ITP), 823
    for thrombotic thrombocytopenic purpura,
        825
    for Wiskott-Aldrich syndrome, 83
Splinter hemorrhages, 8
"Split ends", 764
Split-thickness skin grafts, 903–904, 904*f*
Sponges, 429
Spongiosis, in eczema, 73
Spoon nails, 781, 781*f*
Sporothrix schenckii, 314–315
Sporotrichoid staphylococcal abscesses,
        290.*e1f*
Sporotrichoid tuberculosis, 328–329, 329*f*
Sporotrichosis, 314–316, 315*f*, 323.*e4f*
Sporozoa, class of, 427–428
Spots, 11
    size, laser, 909
Spotted fever group, 284–285
Spotted lunulae, 790
Spray application, for cryosurgery, 892, 893*f*
SPRED1 gene, 553
Squalene, 7
Squamous cell carcinoma in situ, 656–657
    see also Bowen disease
Squamous cell carcinoma (SCC), 653–655,
        654*f*, 685.*e3f*
    basal cell carcinoma *vs.*, 653–655
    bowenoid papulosis and, 408
    clinical features of, 653–654, 654*f*
    curettage combined with electrodesiccation
        for, 894
    differential diagnosis of, 654–655
    epidermodysplasia verruciformis and, 411,
        411*f*
    erythroplasia of Queyrat and, 657
    genital, 418
    histopathology of, 654
    HIV-associated, 418
    keratoacanthoma *vs.*, 654
    lichen planus and, 216
    metastases of, 655
    Mohs micrographic surgery for, 905–906
    of nail bed, 790, 792*f*
    oral, 804, 804*f*, 812.*e1f*
    prevention/treatment of, 655
    radiation cancer and, 36–37
    in situ, 907
    of skin, aggressive, 124
Squirrel flea, 445
Stable heel ulcers, 39
Stablefly, 443

Stanozolol, for lipodermatosclerosis, 488–489
Staphylinidae, 443
Staphylococcal infections, 252–259
    abscess, 255, 255*f*, 290.*e1f*
    folliculitis, 254, 254*f*
    folliculitis decalvans and, 759
    furunculosis, 255–256, 255*f*
    invasive, 257
    paronychia, 256
    primary cutaneous, 252–257
    systemic, 257
Staphylococcal scalded skin syndrome (SSSS),
        257, 257*f*, 290.*e1f*
Staphylococcal superinfection, breast eczema,
        73
Staphylococcus aureus
    chronic granulomatous disease, 86
    diaper dermatitis, 76
    impetigo, 253
    staphylococcal scalded skin syndrome, 257
    X-linked agammaglobulinemia, 80
Staphylococcus epidermidis, 19
Starch-iodine test, 927, 927*f*–928*f*
Starfish, 429
Stasis dermatitis, 856, 813.*e4f*
Stasis purpura, 833
Statins, for Raynaud disease, 814
Steatocystoma multiplex, 15, 681–682, 681*f*
Steatocystoma simplex, 681
Steely hair disease, 764
Stellate pseudoscars, 26–27, 45.*e1f*
Stem cells, 1
    chronic granulomatous disease, 86
    transplantation
        for herpes zoster, 377
        for severe combined immunodeficiency,
            82
Steroid acne, 138, 241, 241*f*
Steroid phobia, 69
Steroidal agents, intralesional, for cutaneous
        lymphoid hyperplasia, 731
Steroid-modified tinea, 296*f*
Steroids
    cream, for lichen simplex chronicus, 53
    for giant cell arteritis, 849–850
    intralesional, for pyoderma gangrenosum,
        148
    for lichen planus, 220–221
    for prurigo nodularis, 54
    for pruritus scroti, 50–51
    rosacea, 251.*e1f*
    systemic
        for actinic dermatitis, 35
        for papuloerythroderma of Ofuji, 53
        for sunburns, 24–25
        for *Toxicodendron* dermatitis, 99
    for tattoo-associated dermopathies, 41–42
    topical
        for acne keloidalis, 242
        for acneiform eruptions, 241
        for actinic dermatitis, 35
        for pruritus, 46
        for psychogenic pruritus, 51
        for sunburns, 24–25
Stevens-Johnson syndrome (SJS), 117, 118*f*,
        142*f*
    erythema multiforme and, 141
Stewart-Treves syndrome, 609, 609*f*, 633, 860,
        635.*e3f*
"Stiff skin syndrome", 175
Stigmata, syphilis, 356, 356*f*
Still disease, 181–182, 181*f*
STING-associated vasculopathy with onset in
        infancy (SAVI), 150
Stingray injury, 451–452

Stings, 421–452
  treatment of, 429
Stippled nails, 785
Stomatitis
  contact, 104
  eczema herpeticum, 368
Stomatitis nicotina, 798
"Stork bite", 595
Stratum corneum, 1, 24
Stratum germinativum, 1
Stratum spinosum, 1
"Strawberry gums", 714
Streptobacillus moniliformis, 281–282
Streptococcal infections
  erythema elevatum diutinum, 841–842
  erythema nodosum, 485
  group B, 263
  intertrigo, 262
  psoriasis, 196–197
  skin, 259–264
Streptococcus iniae infections, 263–264
Streptococcus pneumoniae, X-linked
    agammaglobulinemia, 80
Streptococcus pyogenes, impetigo, 253
Streptomycin
  for Buruli ulcer, 333
  for plague, 281
  for tularemia, 283
Stress
  psoriasis and, 197
  Raynaud phenomenon/disease and, 813
Stretch marks, 512–513
Striae, corticosteroid adverse reaction, 138,
    139.e3f
Striae distensae, 512–513, 513f
Striae gravidarum, 512–513
Striate keratodermas, 210, 210f
Striated beaded lines, 26
Strongyloidiasis, 433
Stucco keratosis, 642, 685.e2f
Sturge-Weber syndrome, 596–597, 596f
Subacute cutaneous lupus erythematosus
    (SCLE), 137, 160–161, 160f
Subacute prurigo, 77
Subacute spongiotic dermatitis, 78
Subcorneal pustular dermatosis, 202
  pyoderma gangrenosum and, 147
Subcutaneous emphysema, 39, 40f
  factitial, 57
Subcutaneous fat, diseases of, 485–495
Subcutaneous fat necrosis
  of newborn, 489, 489f, 495.e1f
  pancreatic, 491–492, 495.e2f
  of scrotum, 490
Subcutaneous granuloma annulare, 704–705,
    705f
Subcutaneous panniculitis-like T-cell
    lymphoma (SPTCL), 160
Subcutaneous plexiform neurofibromas, 551
Subcutaneous sarcoidosis, 713
Subcutaneous T-cell lymphoma, 741–742, 742f
Subcutaneous tissue, 9–10, 10f
Subcutaneous tumors, 587–635
Subepidermal calcified nodule, 528, 528f
Subpapillary plexus, 8
Subungual exostosis, 616
Subungual glomus tumor, 635.e3f
Subungual keratoacanthomas, 646
Subungual melanoma, 790, 792f
Sucralfate
  aphthous stomatitis, 810
  Behçet syndrome, 811
SUFU gene, 652
Sulfapyridine
  for bullous pemphigoid, 463
  for pyoderma gangrenosum, 149

Sulfasalazine
  for alopecia areata, 751–752
  for chronic urticaria, 154
  for pyoderma gangrenosum, 149
Sulfated acid mucopolysaccharide, 8
Sulfites, flushing and, 140
Sulfonamides
  for acne vulgaris, 235
  erythema nodosum and, 485
  hypersensitivity syndrome, 116
  long-acting, 115
  photosensitivity reactions and, 124
Sulfur, for acne vulgaris, 235
Sulfur mustard gas, 93
Sulfuric acid, 92
Summer actinic lichenoid eruption, 225
Sun nevus, 702
Sun protection factor, 25
Sunburn, 24–25, 24f
  clinical signs and symptoms of, 24
  lentigo, 687
  prophylaxis for, 25
  treatment for, 24–25
Sun-damaged skin, lentiginous melanoma on,
    695
Sunflower oil, 19
Sunitinib
  chemotherapy-induced acral erythema,
    130
  hair depigmentation and, 131
Sunscreens, 25
  for allergic contact dermatitis, 107
  broad-spectrum, 25
  for chronic actinic dermatitis, 35
  for dermatomyositis, 170
  for erythema multiforme, 143
  for rosacea, 247
  for solar urticaria, 33–34, 152
  for systemic lupus erythematosus, 165
Superantigens, staphylococcal, 68
Superficial acral fibromyxoma, 616
Superficial basal cell carcinoma, 649, 649f
Superficial lymphatic malformation, 635.e2f
Superficial migratory thrombophlebitis, 634f,
    635.e7f
Superficial muscular aponeurotic system
    (SMAS), 9
Superficial mycoses, 291–307
Superficial peel, 932
Superficial pustular folliculitis, 254
Superficial spreading malignant melanoma,
    703.e4f
Superficial spreading melanoma, 696, 696f
Superficial thrombophlebitis, 832, 832f
Superficial white onychomycosis, 323.e2f
Superior vena cava syndrome, flushing and,
    140
Superpotent topical corticosteroids, for
    granuloma annulare, 706
Support stocking, Waldenström
    hyperglobulinemic purpura, 828
Suppurative dermatitis, 86
Suppurative folliculitis, pyoderma
    gangrenosum and, 148
Surgery
  for cicatricial alopecia, 757
  for eumycetoma, 319
  for giant pigmented nevus, 691
  for hyperhidrosis, 775–776
  for melanoma, 700
  for plasmacytoma, 745
  for prototheccosis, 323
  for psoriasis, 198
  for trichilemmoma, 675–676
  for vitiligo, 873
Surgical ablation, for common warts, 405

Surgical excision
  for Buruli ulcer, 333
  for desmoplastic trichoepithelioma, 674
  for epidermal cyst, 679
  for keloid, 610
Surgical intervention, for rosacea, 248
Surgical site infection, 881–882
Sutton disease, 810
Sutton nevus, 690–691
Sutures, 887, 887t
  technique, 888–892
Sweat
  formation of, 5
  secretion of, 5
Sweat glands
  disorders of, 774–778
  tumors of, 665–672
Sweet syndrome, 134, 145–147, 145f, 156.e2f
  diagnostic criteria for, 146b
  erythema nodosum and, 486
  urticarial vasculitis, 840
Swimmer's itch, 429, 430f
Sycosis barbae, 254, 254f
Sycosis vulgaris, 254, 295
Symmetric drug-related intertriginous and
    flexural exanthema (SDRIFE), 95, 121
Symmetric peripheral gangrene, 830
Symmetric synovitis, 182
Sympathectomy
  for hyperhidrosis, 775
  for Raynaud disease, 814–815
  for thromboangiitis obliterans, 851–852
Syndrome of inappropriate antidiuretic
    hormone secretion (SIADH), 377
Synovitis, symmetric, 182
Synthetic resin dermatitis, 105–106
Synthetic sutures, 887
Syphilids, 350–351
Syphilis, 347–359
  alopecia in, 352, 756, 756f
  cardiovascular, late, 355
  chancre (primary stage), 348–350, 349f,
    361.e1f
  congenital, 355–357
    diagnosis of, 356–357
    early, 355–356, 355f
    late, 356, 356f
  cutaneous, 348–353
    diagnosis of, 353
    differential diagnosis of, 353
  endemic, 360
  histopathology of, 352–353
  HIV disease and, 358–359
  late, 353–355
  osseous, 354
  latent, 353
  North American blastomycosis and, 313
  secondary, 350–352, 351f, 361.e1f–361.e2f
  serologic tests, 348
  tertiary cutaneous, 353–354, 353f,
    361.e2f–361.e3f
  treatment of, 357–358
Syringadenoma papilliferum, 669–670
Syringocystadenoma papilliferum, 669–670, 670f
Syringofibroadenoma, 670
Syringoid carcinoma, 671, 671f
Syringoma, 665–666, 665f, 685.e5f
Syringomyelia, 62
Syringotropic cutaneous T-cell lymphoma,
    734–735, 735f
Systemic agents
  for bullous drug reactions, 118
  for hand eczema, 76
  for systemic lupus erythematosus, 165–166
Systemic candidiasis, 305
Systemic contact dermatitis, 95, 110

Systemic corticosteroids
  for α₁-antitrypsin deficiency panniculitis, 492
  for granuloma annulare, 707
  for multicentric reticulohistiocytosis, 725
  for sarcoidosis, 717–718
Systemic juvenile xanthogranuloma, 720
Systemic lupus erythematosus (SLE), 161–167
  childhood, 164
  complement deficiency and, 88
  cutaneous manifestations of, 162
  differential diagnosis of, 165
  drug-induced, 137
  epidermolysis bullosa acquisita and, 469
  etiology of, 164
  female hormones in, 164
  immunologic findings in, 164–165
  laboratory findings in, 164
  oral lesions of, 162, 162f, 183.e3f
  palmar erythema in, 183.e3f
  photosensitive, 30
  in pregnancy, 164
  pyoderma gangrenosum and, 148
  systemic manifestations of, 163–164, 163f
  TNF inhibitors and, 135
  treatment for, 165–167
  urticarial vasculitis, 840
Systemic mastocytosis, 622–623
Systemic plasmacytosis, 745
Systemic sarcoidosis, 714–715
Systemic sclerosis sine scleroderma, 174
Systemic staphylococcal infections, 257

T
Tabes dorsalis, 354–355
Tacrolimus, 31–32
  for pityriasis lichenoides et varioliformis acuta, 740
  for pyoderma gangrenosum, 148
  for rosacea, 247
  topical
    for acneiform eruptions, 241
    for atopic dermatitis, 70
    for chronic actinic dermatitis, 35
    for lichen planus, 220–221
    for lichen sclerosus, 229–230
    for pruritus ani, 50–51
    for vitiligo, 873
  for Wegener granulomatosis, 846–847
Taenia solium, 431
Takahara disease, 808
Takayasu arteritis, 850
Talc granuloma, 43
Talcum powder, 93
  tinea cruris and, 297
Talon noir, 39
Tamoxifen, flushing and, 140
Tangier disease, 534–535
Tanning, 24
TAP1/TAP2 gene deficiencies, 82
Tape-stripping, fixed drug reactions and, 120
Tapioca granule, 395
Tar dermatitis, phototoxic, 29
TAR syndrome, 598
Tarantula, 451
Target lesions, of erythema multiforme, 141, 141f, 156.e1f
Targetoid hemosiderotic hemangioma, 594, 594f
Tars
  for atopic dermatitis, 71
  for psoriasis, 198
Tattoos, 41–45, 41f, 45.e3f
  complications of, 917–918, 917f–918f
  laser treatment of, 916, 916f, 917t
  sarcoidosis in, 714

Taxanes, scleroderma-like reactions to, 132
Tazarotene
  for acne vulgaris, 234
  for eruptive vellus hair cysts, 682
  for Gorlin syndrome, 653
  photoaging and, 28
  for pityriasis rubra pilaris, 208
  for psoriasis, 198
  for psoriatic nails, 779
  for trachyonychia, 781
T-cells
  in adverse drug reactions, 113
  cutaneous lymphoid hyperplasia and, 731–732
  deficiency, 82
  in fixed drug reactions, 118
  reactions of, 113
Tea tree oil, 109, 441
Tear gas dermatitis, 93–94, 94f
Telangiectasia, 604, 854–855
  corticosteroids adverse reaction, 137
  photoaging, 26–27
  pulse dye laser for, 910–911
Telangiectasia macularis eruptiva perstans, 9, 623
Telangiectatic mats, 173
Telangiectatic matting, 929
Telangiectatic veins, 928–930
Telangiectatic vessels, dermatomyositis and, 167
Telaprevir, for hepatitis C infection, 385
Telogen effluvium, 7f, 752–753, 753f
  biopsy, 753
Telogen hairs, 750, 752f
Telogen phase, hair follicles, 6, 7f, 10.e1f
Temperature-sensitive oculocutaneous albinism (OCA1-TS), 879
Temporal arteritis, 849–850, 849f
Temporal nerve, 885–887
Tendinous xanthomas, 546.e2f
Tendon sheath, fibroma of, 635.e4f
Tennis toe, 37, 38f
"Tent sign", 672
Teratoma, 632
Terbinafine, 291
  for candidiasis, 301
  for chromoblastomycosis, 316–317
  for onychomycosis, 300
  for tinea capitis, 294
  for tinea corporis, 296
  for tinea imbricata, 296
  for tinea of hands and feet, 299
Terminal deoxynucleotidyl transferase-mediated deoxyuridine triphosphate-biotin nick end labeling (TUNEL) method, 9
Terminal hairs, 750
Ternatin, 9–10
Terry nails, 784, 784f
Tertiary cutaneous syphilis, 353–354, 353f, 361.e2f–361.e3f
Testosterone
  acne vulgaris and, 232
  androgen-dependent syndrome and, 498
  for hirsutism, 770
2,3,7,8-Tetrachlorodibenzo-p-dioxin, 94
Tetracycline
  for acne keloidalis, 243
  for acne vulgaris, 235
  for aphthous stomatitis, 810
  for bullous pemphigoid, 463
  for folliculitis decalvans, 759
  for hidradenitis suppurativa, 243
  for leptospirosis, 286
  for pemphigus foliaceus, 458
  for pemphigus vulgaris, 456
  for pityriasis lichenoides et varioliformis acuta, 740

Tetramethylthiuram disulfide, 105
Texture of lesions, 16
Th17 cells, 114
Thalidomide, 46–47
  for actinic dermatitis, 35
  for actinic prurigo, 32
  for aphthous stomatitis, 810
  for Behçet syndrome, 811
  for CKD-associated pruritus, 48
  for cryoglobulinemia, 827
  for cutaneous lymphoid hyperplasia, 731
  for erythema multiforme, 143
  for lichen planus, 220–221
  for necrobiosis lipoidica, 539
  for prurigo nodularis, 46–47
  for sarcoidosis, 717
  for systemic lupus erythematosus, 165
Thaumetopoea pityocampa, 439
Thaumetopoea processionea, 439
Theraphosidae, 451
Thermal burns, 18, 19f
  electrical burns, 18–19
  hot tar burns, 19
  treatment for, 18
Thermal relaxation, 909
Thermoregulation, 5
Thiabendazole, creeping eruption and, 433
Thiamine deficiency, 477
Thimble jellyfish, 428
Thimerosal, allergic contact dermatitis, 95, 103
Thin-layer rapid-use epicutaneous (TRUE) test, 96
Thioglycolates, dermatitis, 107
Thiopurine methyltransferase (TPMT) level, pemphigus vulgaris and, 456
Thioridazine, 128
Thromboangiitis obliterans (TAO), 851–852, 851f
Thrombocytopenia
  drug-induced, 824
  immune, 823–824, 823f
  Sweet syndrome and, 146–147
  in varicella, 371
Thrombocytopenic purpura, 823–824
Thrombophlebitis
  in Klinefelter syndrome, 550
  superficial, 832, 832f
Thrombosis, systemic lupus erythematosus and, 163, 163f
Thrombotic microangiopathy, 824–826
Thrombotic thrombocytopenic purpura, 825
Thrush, 302–303, 302f
Thymoma with immunodeficiency, 82
Thyroglossal duct cysts, 684
Thyroid acropachy, 500, 501f
Thyroid autoantibodies, 153
Thyroid carcinoma, 36–37
Thyroid disease, flushing and, 140
Thyroid hormone, deficiency in, 499
Thyroid-stimulating hormone (TSH) receptor, congenital hypothyroidism and, 499
Ticks
  bite, 446, 446f
  Lyme disease from, 286
  paralysis, 446–447
  prevention of disease from, 438
  Rocky Mountain spotted fever from, 284
Tinea amiantacea, 772, 793.e4f
Tinea barbae, 294–295, 295f
Tinea capitis, 292, 292f
  diagnosis of, 293
  differential diagnosis of, 293–294
  pathogenesis and natural history in, 293
  prognosis of, 294
  treatment of, 294

Tinea circinata, 295–297
Tinea corporis, 295–297, 295*f*, 323.*e1f*
  diagnosis of, 296
  other forms of, 296–297
  and pityriasis rosea, 205
  treatment for, 296
Tinea cruris, 297, 323.*e1f*
Tinea faciei, 295, 295*f*, 323.*e1f*
Tinea gladiatorum, 296
Tinea imbricata, 323.*e1f*
Tinea incognita, 296
Tinea nigra, 299–301, 323.*e2f*
Tinea of hands and feet, 297–299, 297*f*–298*f*
  KOH examination for, 298*f*
Tinea pedis, 297–298
Tinea sycosis, 294
Tinea unguium, 299–301
Tinea versicolor, 13, 306–307, 306*f*, 323.*e2f*
  pityriasis rosea and, 205
  vitiligo and, 872
Tissue plasminogen activator, frostbite, 23
Tissue transglutaminase (TTG), dermatitis
  herpetiformis, 470
Titanium, 870
Titanium hydrochloride, 92
Tixocortol pivalate, 110–111
T lymphocytes, activated, in erythema
  multiforme, 142
TNF-receptor-associated periodic syndrome
  (TRAPS), 149
TNFRSF1A gene, 149
TNMB system, for mycosis fungoides, 733
"Toadskin", 475
Toe web infection, Gram-negative, 270, 270*f*,
  290.*e2f*
Togaviridae, 399–402
Tokelau, 296
Toker cell, 659
Tolnaftate powder, for tinea of hands and feet,
  298
Tomatoes, erythema annulare centrifugum
  and, 143
Tongue
  black hairy, 799–800, 800*f*
  caviar, 801
  fissured, 799, 799*f*
  geographic, 799, 799*f*
  lichen planus of, 230.*e2f*
  osseous choristoma of, 806
  smooth, 800, 800*f*
Tonic pupils, 776
Tonofilaments, 1
Tophi, gout, 545, 546.*e3f*
Topical agents, for hand eczema, 76
Topical anesthetics, 885
Topical anticandidal agents, for candidiasis,
  301–302
Topical calcineurin inhibitors, for granuloma
  annulare, 706
Topical cinnamic aldehyde, flushing and,
  140
Topical drug contact dermatitis, 109–111,
  110*f*
Topical therapy
  for basal cell carcinoma, 651
  for rosacea, 247
TORCH syndrome, 427
Torus palatinus, 798–799, 812.*e2f*
Total depigmentation, 873–874
Touraine-Solente-Gole syndrome, 577
Touton giant cells, 720
Toxic epidermal necrolysis (TEN), 117
  erythema multiforme and, 141
Toxic pustuloderma, 121
Toxic shock syndromes (TSS), 257–258

Toxicodendron (poison ivy), dermatitis from,
  98–99, 98*f*, 139.*e1f*
  impetigo and, 254
Toxicoderma, 130–131
Toxin-mediated perineal erythema, recurrent,
  260
Toxoplasma gondii, 427
Toxoplasmosis, 427–428
Trabecular carcinoma, 661–662, 661*f*
Trachyonychia, 782
Traction alopecia, 761, 761*f*
Tramadol, for zoster-associated pain, 377
Tranexamic acid, for Osler disease, 855–856
Transepidermal water loss (TEWL), 64
Transferrin, 870
Transient acantholytic dermatosis, 453,
  473–474, 473*f*
Transient erythroporphyria of infancy,
  525–527
Transient neonatal pustular melanosis, 867, 867*f*
Transposition flaps, 898, 902*f*–903*f*
Trastuzumab, for extramammary Paget
  disease, 660–661
Traumatic anserine folliculosis, 773–774
Traumatic asphyxia, 39–40
Traumatic calcinosis cutis, 528
Traumatic neuroma, 635.*e5f*
Traumatic panniculitis, 490
Traumatic purpura, 833, 833*f*
Treacher Collins syndrome, 582
Tree-associated plants, allergic contact
  dermatitis, 99–100
Trees, allergic contact dermatitis from, 99
Treg, in adverse drug reactions, 114
Trematoda, class of, 430–431
Trench fever, 280
Trench foot, 23
Trench mouth, 807–808
Treponema pallidum, 347
Treponema pallidum particle assay (TPPA), 348
Treponemal tests, 348
Tretinoin
for acne vulgaris, 234
  for acneiform eruptions, 241
  for actinic keratosis, 644–645
  for epidermal nevi, 636–637
  for eruptive vellus hair cysts, 682
  for flat warts, 406
  for melasma, 864
  for milia, 683
  for nevus of Ota, 702
  for oral hairy leukoplakia, 380
  photoaging, 28
  for solar lentigo, 687
  for striae, 513
Triamcinolone
  for acquired perforating dermatosis, 773
  for atopic dermatitis, 69
  injection of
    for alopecia areata, 751
    for granuloma annulare, 706
    for keloid, 610
    for necrobiosis lipoidica, 539
  for lichen simplex chronicus, 53–54
  for lipodermatosclerosis, 488–489
  for pretibial myxedema, 501
  for prurigo, 52
  for winter itch, 49
Triamcinolone acetonide
  for acne keloidalis, 242
  for acne vulgaris, 237–238
  for lichen planus of nails, 778
  for lupus erythematosus, 165
  for psoriatic nails, 779
  for sarcoidosis, 716

Triangular alopecia, 756, 757*f*
Triatome reduviid bug, 427*f*, 441*f*
Triazoles, 291
Trichilemmal carcinoma, 676
Trichilemmal cyst, 679, 679*f*
Trichilemmoma, 674–676
Trichinosis, 436–437
Trichloroacetic acid (TCA)
  for chemical peels, 932
  for genital warts, 409
  for molluscum contagiosum, 392
Trichloroethylene
  eosinophilic fasciitis and, 177
  inhalation, 95
Trichoadenoma, 677
Trichoblastoma, 674, 685.*e6f*
Trichodiscoma, 676–677
Trichodynia, 753
Trichodysplasia spinulosa, 414, 414*f*, 769
Trichoepithelioma, 674, 685.*e6f*
  desmoplastic, 674, 674*f*
  giant solitary, 674
  multiple familial, 673–674, 673*f*
  solitary, 674
Trichofolliculoma, 673, 673*f*
Trichogram evaluation, in telogen effluvium, 752
Trichomalacia, 57–58
Trichomonas vaginalis, 422
  infection, 51
Trichomoniasis, 421–422
Trichomycosis axillaris, 772, 772*f*, 793.*e3f*
Trichophagia, 755, 793.*e2f*
Trichophyton, 291
Trichophyton mentagrophytes, 294
  onychomycosis from, 299
Trichophyton rubrum, 291
  onychomycosis from, 299
Trichophyton tonsurans, 292
Trichophyton verrucosum, 294
Trichophyton violaceum, 292
Trichoptilosis, 767
Trichorhinophalangeal syndrome, 584
Trichorrhexis invaginata, 765, 765*f*
Trichorrhexis nodosa, 764–765, 764*f*
Trichoschisis, 764
Trichoscopy, 57–58
Trichostasis spinulosa, 768–769, 768*f*, 793.*e2f*
Trichothiodystrophy, 580–581
Trichotillomania, 57–58, 58*f*, 755, 755*f*
  biopsy, 755
  tinea capitis and, 294
Trichotillosis, 755–756, 755*f*
  see also Trichotillomania
Trichrome vitiligo, 871
Tricyclic antidepressants (TCA), for
  zoster-associated pain, 377
Trientine, Wilson disease, 543
Trifluorothymidine (Viroptic), herpes simplex,
  369
Trigeminal nerve (cranial nerve V), 886*f*
Trigeminal trophic syndrome, 61
Trimethoprim, for acne vulgaris, 231
Trimethoprim-sulfamethoxazole (TMP-SMX)
  for acne vulgaris, 235
  adverse reactions, in HIV patients, 119
  for glanders, 278
  for granuloma inguinale, 274
  for nocardiosis, 269
  for pneumocystosis, 321
  for South American blastomycosis, 314
  for Stevens-Johnson syndrome, 117
  for Wegener granulomatosis, 846–847
Trimethylamine, 776
Tripe palms, 503, 503*f*
Tropical acne, 239*f*, 240

Tropical anhidrotic asthenia, 20
Tropical immersion foot, 23, 24f
Tropical spastic paraparesis, 414–415
Tropical swelling, 435, 435f
True depigmentation, 15
Trumpeter's wart, 806
Trunk, allergic contact dermatitis in, 97
Tryptase, itching and, 46
L-Tryptophan, eosinophilic fasciitis and, 177
TSEB radiation
    for mycosis fungoides, 737
    for Sézary syndrome, 738
Tsetse fly, 442
Tsutsugamushi fever, 284
Tuberculids, 329–330
    granuloma annulare and, 706
Tuberculin testing, 325
Tuberculoid leprosy, 338, 338f, 342, 346.e1f
Tuberculosis cutis orificialis, 328
Tuberculosis (TB), 324–332
    categories of, 324
    cutaneous, inoculation of, from an
        exogenous source, 325–327
    diagnosis of, 330–331
    from endogenous source by direct
        extension, 327–328
    epidemiology of, 324
    erythema induratum by, 330
    erythema nodosum and, 485
    from hematogenous spread, 328–329
    treatment of, 331–332
    tuberculids, 329–330
    tuberculin testing, 325
    vascular reactions by, 330
Tuberculosis verrucosa cutis, 324, 326, 326f,
        335.e1f
Tuberculous abscess, metastatic, 328, 328f
Tuberculous cellulitis, 328, 328f
Tuberculous chancre, 325–326
Tuberculous mastitis, 329
Tuberculous ulceration, 328, 328f
Tuberous sclerosis, 502, 555–557, 555f, 586.e1f
Tuberous xanthomas, 546.e2f
Tubular apocrine adenoma, 670
Tufted angioma, 593, 593f, 635.e1f
Tufted folliculitis, 760–761, 761f
Tularemia, 282–283, 282f, 290.e4f
Tumescent liposuction, 930–931, 931f
Tumid lupus erythematosus, 159–160, 159f
    Jessner lymphocytic infiltrate of the skin
        vs., 732
Tumor alopecia, 761–762
    see also Alopecia neoplastica
Tumor necrosis factor (TNF) blockers
    for giant cell arteritis, 849
    for microscopic polyangiitis, 845–846
    for small-vessel vasculitis, 837–838
Tumor necrosis factor (TNF) inhibitors
    for acne vulgaris, 237
    adverse reactions, 134–135
    interstitial granulomatous drug reaction
        and, 709
    for multicentric reticulohistiocytosis, 725
    for sarcoidosis, 717
Tumor necrosis factor (TNF)-α, 3
Tumor suppressor gene, 547
Tumoral calcinosis, 528–529
Tumor-infiltrating lymphocytes (TILs), 735
Tumors, 11
    dermal, 587–635
    of hair follicle, 672–678
    oral cavity, 802
    sebaceous, 664–665
    subcutaneous, 587–635
    of sweat glands, 665–672

TUNEL (terminal deoxynucleotidyl
        transferase-mediated deoxyuridine
        triphosphate-biotin nick end labeling)
        method, 9
Tunga penetrans, 445
Tungiasis, 445, 445f
Tunica dartos, 7
Turner syndrome, 499, 550
Turpentine, 100–101
Twenty-nail dystrophy, 778
"Twisted hairs", 763, 764f
Tylosis, 803
Tyndall effect, 15
Type C lymphomatoid papulosis, 739
Typhoidal type, of tularemia, 282–283
Typhus group, 283–284
Tyrosinase gene (TYR), oculocutaneous
        albinism in, 879
"Tyrosinase-positive" albinism, 879
Tyrosinemia II, 543
TYRP1 gene, in oculocutaneous albinism, 879
Tyson glands, 7
Tzanck smear
    for herpes simplex, 362
    for herpes zoster, 377–378

U
"Ugly duckling" sign, 689–690, 694f
Ulceration
    in dermatomyositis, 168
    of fingertip, 183.e7f
    tuberculous, 328, 328f
Ulcerative colitis, pyoderma gangrenosum
        and, 148
Ulcerative lichen planus, 217–218
Ulcerative sarcoidosis, 712–713
Ulceroglandular type, of tularemia, 282
Ulcers, 13, 14f, 17.e1f
Ulerythema acneiforme, 761
Ulerythema ophryogenes, 585f, 761
Ultraviolet (UV) light
    blockers of, 31
    chronic actinic dermatitis, 35
    on onychomycosis, 301
    psoriasis, 198
    solar urticaria, 33–34
    sunburn, 24
Ultraviolet (UV) therapy
    for acquired perforating dermatosis, 773
    for mycosis fungoides, 736–737
    for polycythemia vera, 749
Ultraviolet B (UVB) light
    for biliary pruritus, 48
    for pityriasis rosea, 205–206
Ultraviolet radiation (UVR)
    nonmelanoma skin cancer from, 643–644
    squamous cell carcinoma from, 653
Umbilical pseudosarcomatous polyps, 617
Uncinariasis, 432
Uncombable hair syndrome, 766, 766f
Undifferentiated pleomorphic sarcoma,
        619–620
Undulant fever, 283
Unguis incarnatus, 787–788
Unilateral laterothoracic exanthem, 397
Unilateral nevoid telangiectasia (UNT),
        604–605, 604f, 854–855
Universal vitiligo, 871–872
Unna boots
    lipodermatosclerosis, 488–489
    venous leg ulcers, 857
Unna-Thost keratoderma, 211, 211f, 214.e2f
Upper thoracic sympathectomy, for
        hyperhidrosis, 775
Upshaw-Schulman syndrome, 825

Urbach-Wiethe disease, 536
Urea, for winter itch, 49
Uremia, acquired perforating disease in,
        793.e4f
Uric acid crystals, 493
Uroporphyrinogen decarboxylase (UROD),
        521
Uroporphyrins, 522–523
Ursodeoxycholic acid, for biliary pruritus, 48
Urticaria, 150–156, 150f–151f
    adrenergic, 152
    annular and polycyclic, 156.e3f
    aquagenic, 153
    atopic dermatitis and, 67
    cholinergic, 151–152, 152f, 156.e3f
    chronic spontaneous, 154
    classification of, 151
    clinical evaluation of, 153–154
    cold, 152, 156.e2f–156.e3f
    diagnosis of, 153
    drug-induced, 122, 123f
    etiologic factors of, 151–153
    exercise-induced, 153
    galvanic, 153
    heat, 152
    hypothyroidism and, 499
    neutrophilic, 153
    papular, 11
    pathogenesis/histopathology of, 153
    physical (inducible), 151–153
    pigmentosa, 14
    pressure, 152–153, 153f
    solar, 33–34, 33f, 152
    treatment of, 154
    urticarial vasculitis and, 840
"Urticaria multiforme", 141–142
Urticaria pigmentosa, 622, 623f, 635.e5f
Urticarial dermatitis, 444
Urticarial fever, 430
Urticarial vasculitis, 840–841, 840f
Urushiol, 98
U-serrated pattern, of immunoglobulins, 453
Ustekinumab, atopic dermatitis and, 71
Uta, 423
UV protection factor, 25
UV recall-like phenomenon, 114
Uveitis, granuloma annulare and, 706
Uveoparotid fever, 715

V
Vaccination
    for herpes zoster, 378
    human papillomavirus, 410
    measles, 396–397
    scars, skin lesions at, 388
    for vaccinia, 387
    for varicella, 372
Vaccinia, 387–388
    atopic dermatitis, 68
    benign hypersensitivity reactions to, 388
    cutaneous immunologic complications,
        388
    eczema vaccinatum, 388
    generalized, 387–388
    inadvertent inoculation and
        autoinoculation, 387, 387f, 420.e4f
    progressive, 388
    roseola, 420.e4f
    vaccination for, 387
Vaccinia gangrenosum, 388
Vaccinia necrosum, 388, 388f
Vacuolar interface dermatitis, 161
"Vagabond's disease", 442
Vagina, with lichen planus, 218
Vaginal candidiasis, 51

Valacyclovir
    for erythema multiforme, 143
    for genital herpes, 365
    for herpes simplex, 369
    for herpes zoster, 375–376
    for herpetic gingivostomatitis, 363–364
    for varicella, 373–374
    for zoster-associated pain, 376–377
Valley fever. *see* Coccidioidomycosis
Valproate, 116
van der Woude syndrome, 583
Vancomycin
    adverse reactions, 123
    drug-induced hypersensitivity syndrome, 115
    flushing and, 140
    for wound infections, 883
Vanillin, 100
Variable livedo, 817
Varicella, 14–15, 370–374, 371f, 420.*e2f*
    atopic dermatitis, 68
    in immunocompromised patients, 372–374,
        373f
    in pregnant women and neonates, 372
    treatment of, 371
    vaccine for, 372
Varicella-zoster immune globulin (VZIG), 372
Varicella-zoster virus, 374–379
Varicose veins, 928–930
Variegate porphyria, 523
variola major, 386–387
Vascular alopecia, 756
Vascular anomalies, cutaneous, 587
Vascular diseases, cutaneous, 813–861
Vascular lesions, laser treatment of, 910–914
Vascular malformations, 594
Vascular reactions, to tuberculosis, 330
Vascular stigmata, atopic dermatitis, 68
Vascular tumors, 587–596
Vasculature, dermis, 8
Vasculitis, 836
    adverse drug reactions and, 127–129
    classification of, 836, 836b
    cocaine-associated, 40, 848–849
    connective tissue disease, 838
    in hairy cell leukemia, 747
    large-vessel, 836b
    leukocytoclastic, 826
    livedoid, 819–820
    medium-vessel, 836b
    mixed size, 836b
    nodular, 487–488, 487f
    rheumatoid, 180, 183.*e8f*
    in Sjögren syndrome, 179
    small-vessel, 836–843, 836b
    TNF inhibitors and, 135
Vasculopathy, herpes zoster, 375
Vasodilators
    for chilblains, 22
    flushing and, 140
    for scleroderma, 176
Vasovagal reactions, during anesthesia, 884
Vater-Pacini corpuscles, 9
Vectors, of disease, 445
Vegetable gums, dermatitis, 105
Vegetables, allergic contact dermatitis from,
    99
Vegetative pyoderma gangrenosum, 147
Vellus hairs, 750
Vemurafenib
    for melanoma, 700–701
    side effect of, 124
Venereal Disease Research Laboratories
    (VDRL) tests, 348
Venlafaxine, for zoster-associated pain, 377
Venous diseases, of extremities, 856–858

Venous insufficiency
    lipodermatosclerosis, 488–489
    livedoid vasculopathy, 819–820
    obesity-associated mucinosis, 856
    ulceration, 856–858, 857f
Venous lakes, 603, 604f, 635.*e2f*
Venous malformation, 598–600
Venous thromboembolism (VTE), 831
Verruca, 402–411, 420.*e8f*
Verruca plana, 403–404, 404f, 420.*e7f*
Verruca plantaris, 404, 404f
Verruca vulgaris, 403, 403f, 420.*e6f*–420.*e7f*
Verruciform xanthoma, 534–535, 534f, 546.*e3f*
    epidermal nevi and, 636
Verrucous carcinoma, 655–656, 655f
Verrucous cysts, 683
Verrucous nevus, 636
Verruga peruana, 281, 281f
Vertical mattress suture, 889, 891f
Vesicles, 11–12, 12f, 17.*e1f*
Vesicopustules, 13
Vesiculobullous hand eczema, 74f, 75
    chronic, 75
Vessel-based lobular panniculitis, 487
Vibices, 823
Vibration white finger, 813
Vibratory angioedema, 153
Vibrio vulnificus infection, 275–276, 276f
Vici syndrome, 877–878
Vinblastine
    for Kaposi sarcoma, 419–420
    for Langerhans cell histiocytosis, 729
Vincent disease, 807–808
Vinyl gloves, for hand eczema, 75
Violaceous lesions, 15
Viral diseases, 362–420
Viral infections, primary immunodeficiency
    diseases, 80
Viral-associated trichodysplasia, 769
Visceral involvement, in Langerhans cell
    histiocytosis, 729
Visceral leishmaniasis, 423, 425–426
    clinical features of, 425–426
    diagnosis of, 426
    epidemiology of, 426
    etiologic factors of, 426
    treatment of, 426
Visceral manifestations, of progressive
    systemic sclerosis, 174
Visceral schistosomiasis, 430–431
Viscerotropic leishmaniasis, 426
Vitamin A, 475–476
    for measles, 396
Vitamin B$_1$, deficiency in, 477
Vitamin B$_2$, deficiency in, 477–478
Vitamin B$_3$, deficiency in, 479
Vitamin B$_6$, 478
Vitamin B$_{12}$ deficiency, 478
    hair color and, 763
Vitamin C deficiency, 478–479
Vitamin D, 476–477
Vitamin D$_3$, supplementation of, 476–477
Vitamin K
    deficiency, 477
    reactions, 125–126, 126f
Vitiligo, 3, 11, 871–874, 880.*e1f*–880.*e2f*,
    17.*e1f*
    clinical features of, 871–872, 871f–872f
    differential diagnosis of, 872
    Graves disease and, 501
    histopathology of, 872
    occupational, 874–875
    scleroderma *vs.*, 175
    total depigmentation and, 873–874
    treatment of, 872–874

Vitiligo-like leukoderma, 872
Vogt-Koyanagi-Harada syndrome (VKHS),
    875
Vohwinkel keratoderma, 211, 214.*e2f*
    mutilating, 211–212, 212f
von Hippel-Lindau syndrome, 557
von Recklinghausen disease, 550
von Willebrand factor (vWF), 825
von Zumbusch psoriasis, 194–195, 195f
Voriconazole, 292
    for aspergillosis, 322
    for coccidioidomycosis, 309
    for fusariosis, 321–322
    for hyalohyphomycosis, 321
    for phaeohyphomycosis, 317
    photosensitivity and, 124
    for prototheccosis, 323
    for systemic candidiasis, 305
Vulva
    amyloidosis, 546.*e1f*
    bullous pemphigoid, 461
    ciliated cysts, 684
    extramammary Paget disease of, 659–660
    leukoplakia, 802–803
    lichen planus, 215, 218
    lichen sclerosus, 228, 230.*e4f*
    melanosis, 687, 687f
    pruritus vulvae, 51, 51f
    vulvodynia, 59
Vulvitis chronica plasmacellularis, 658
Vulvodynia, 59
Vulvovaginal-gingival (VVG) syndrome, 218
Vulvovaginitis
    candidal, 303
    herpetic, 365
    Trichomonas, 421–422

W
Waardenburg syndrome, 878, 878f
Waldenström hyperglobulinemic purpura,
    827–828, 827f
Waldenström macroglobulinemia (WM), 828
"Walking dandruff", 449
Warfarin
    -induced skin necrosis, 125, 125f
    for livedoid vasculopathy, 820
Warm water immersion foot, 23–24, 23f
Warts, 402–411, 403f, 860
    in atopic dermatitis, 68
    flat, 403–404, 404f
    histologic features of, 404
    immunodeficiencies associated with, 412
    in immunosuppressed patients, 412–414
    laser treatment for, 919
    pigmented, 403
    plantar, 404, 404f
    primary immunodeficiency diseases
        associated with, 85–86
    pulse dye laser for, 913
    treatment of, 405–410
Warty dyskeratoma, 640
WASP gene, mutations in, 83
Wasps, 444
    parasitic, 438
Water glass, 92
Watts, 909
Wavelength, laser, 909
Wax esters, 7
Waxy keratoses of childhood, 640
Waxy skin, diabetes mellitus, 539–540
Weary-Kindler syndrome, 561
Wedge biopsy, 888
Wegener granulomatosis, 82, 846–847, 846f
Wells syndrome, 144–145, 144f, 444
Wen, 679, 679f

Werlhof disease, 823, 823*f*
Werner syndrome, 579
West African trypanosomiasis, 427
West Nile fever, 399–400
Wet pellagra, 479
Wheals (hives), 11, 12*f*
WHIM syndrome, 85, 85*f*, 402–403
Whistling face syndrome, 583
White Addison disease, 497–498
White clot syndrome, 126
White dermatographism, 67
White nails, 788, 788*f*
White piedra, 306, 306*f*, 323.*e2f*
White sponge nevus, 805
White superficial onychomycosis, 299, 323.*e2f*
Whitmore disease, 279
Whorled nevoid hypermelanosis, 549
Wiesner nevi, 693
WILD syndrome, 85–86, 860
Wilson disease, 543, 790
Winer, dilated pore of, 677, 685.*e6f*
Winter itch, 49, 49*f*, 77
Winterbottom sign, 426
Wiskott-Aldrich syndrome, 84, 84*f*, 91.*e2f*
Wood tick, 446
Wood's light, 862
    examination under, 14
    hyperpigmentation, 15–16
    tinea capitis, 293
Wool, dermatitis from, 101
Woolly hair, 767, 767*f*
Woolly hair nevus, 766
Woringer-Kolopp disease, 737–738
Workplace modifications, for hand eczema,
    76
Wounds
    categories of, 882
    infection, treatment of, 882

X
Xanthelasma, 532, 532*f*, 546.*e2f*
Xanthelasma palpebrarum, 532
Xanthogranuloma
    juvenile, 718–721, 719*f*
    necrobiotic, 709–711, 710*f*
Xanthoma disseminatum, 722, 722*f*
Xanthoma planum, 531–532
Xanthoma tendinosum, 531, 531*f*
Xanthoma tuberosum, 530–531, 531*f*
Xanthomas, 11, 15, 16*f*, 530–532, 546.*e3f*
    normolipemic, 532
    primary biliary cirrhosis, 48, 49*f*
Xanthomatous biliary cirrhosis, 533
Xanthotrichia, 763
Xenopsylla braziliensis, 445
Xenopsylla cheopis, 281, 284, 445, 445*f*
Xeroderma pigmentosum, 580, 580*f*, 586.*e5f*
Xerosis, 48
    atopic dermatitis and, 68
    corticosteroid adverse reaction, 138
    in diabetes mellitus, 538
Xerostomia, in Sjögren syndrome, 179
Xerotic eczema, 78, 78*f*
X-linked agammaglobulinemia, 80–81
X-linked disorders, 547–555
X-linked dominant chondrodysplasia
    punctata, 566
X-linked dominant protoporphyria, 524
X-linked ichthyosis, 563–564, 563*f*, 586.*e3f*
X-linked neutropenia, 83
X-linked recessive chondrodysplasia punctata
    (CDPX1), 566
X-linked thrombocytopenia, 83
X-type histiocytoses, 726–728
    see also Langerhans cell histiocytosis
XXYY genotype, 550
XYY genotype, 550

Y
Yaws, 359–360, 359*f*, 361.*e3f*
Yeasts, diseases resulting from, 291–323
Yellow nail syndrome, 790–791, 791*f*, 860
Yellowjackets, 444
Yersinia pestis, 281
Yperite, 93

Z
Zanolimumab, for Sézary syndrome, 738
ZAP-70 deficiency, 82
Zebra fish, 763–764
Zidovudine, pigmentation and, 128
Zika virus, 401–402
Zinc
    deficiency, 481–482, 481*f*
    supplementation, Wilson's disease, 543
Zinc chromate paint, dermatitis, 103
Zinc sulfate, 481–482
Zinsser-Cole-Engman syndrome, 574
Zirconium granuloma, 42, 43*f*
Zirconium salt preparations, 108
Zoon balanitis, 658, 685.*e4f*
    erythroplasia of Queyrat *vs.*, 657–658
Zoonotic poxvirus infections, 389–390
Zoonotic scabies, 448
Zostavax, 378
Zoster, 374–379
    see also Herpes zoster
Zoster sine herpete, 374
"Zosteriform" lentigo, 686
Z-plasty, 898, 903*f*
Zyderm I, 922
Zyderm II, 922
Zygomycosis, 320–321
Zyplast (Allergan, Irvine, CA), 922